P9-CER-730

WORLD HEALTH ORGANIZATION

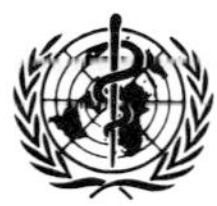

INTERNATIONAL AGENCY FOR RESEARCH ON CANCER

TOBACCO: A MAJOR INTERNATIONAL HEALTH HAZARD

Proceedings of an International Meeting organized by the IARC
and co-sponsored by the All-Union Cancer Research Centre
of the Academy of Medical Sciences of the USSR, Moscow, USSR
held in Moscow,
4–6 June 1985

EDITORS

D. G. ZARIDZE R. PETO

IARC Scientific Publications No. 74

INTERNATIONAL AGENCY FOR RESEARCH ON CANCER
LYON
1986

The International Agency for Research on Cancer (IARC) was established in 1965 by the World Health Assembly, as an independently financed organization within the framework of the World Health Organization. The headquarters of the Agency are at Lyon, France.

The Agency conducts a programme of research concentrating particularly on the epidemiology of cancer and the study of potential carcinogens in the human environment. Its field studies are supplemented by biological and chemical research carried out in the Agency's laboratories in Lyon and, through collaborative research agreements, in national research institutions in many countries. The Agency also conducts a programme for the education and training of personnel for cancer research.

The publications of the Agency are intended to contribute to the dissemination of authoritative information on different aspects of cancer research.

Distributed for the International Agency for Research on Cancer
by Oxford University Press, Walton Street, Oxford OX2 6DP, UK

London New York Toronto
Delhi Bombay Calcutta Madras Karachi
Kuala Lumpur Singapore Hong Kong Tokyo
Nairobi Dar es Salaam Cape Town
Melbourne Auckland

Oxford is a trade mark of Oxford University Press

Distributed in the USA
by Oxford University Press, New York

ISBN 92 832 1174 X
ISSN 0300-5085

PRINTED IN SWITZERLAND

CONTENTS

I. IMPLICATIONS AND RECOMMENDATIONS

II. TOBACCO – A MAJOR HEALTH HAZARD

III. DISEASE PATTERNS AND SMOKING

IV. TOBACCO – SPREAD OF THE HABIT AND TRENDS

V. SMOKING – CURRENT RESEARCH ISSUES

VI. HEALTH EFFECTS OF LOW-TAR, LOW-NICOTINE CIGARETTES

VII. SMOKING CONTROL IMPLEMENTATION

FOREWORD

Tobacco smoking is one of the major causes of disease and death today: it causes cancer, pulmonary obstructive disease and cardiovascular disease. The list of target sites for tobacco-related cancers is impressive: lung, urinary bladder, renal pelvis, oral cavity, pharynx, larynx, oesophagus, pancreas and possibly kidney and liver.

The evidence, therefore, of the severe consequence for health of smoking is so compelling and so overwhelming that it is difficult to understand why it has been, and still is, so difficult to initiate successful preventive measures. The answer is probably two-sided.

The first is the difficulty that individuals have in renouncing a habit that has become solidly rooted in their culture and in their daily life. Most people believe that making the choice to smoke is their privilege and is made freely. They derive satisfaction from it and, at the same time, they are unable to perceive or to accept the evidence of chronic accumulation of risk. The second part of the answer is the interest of governments around the world in tobacco-derived income. Many governments, although genuinely concerned about the good health of their citizens, still continue to allow the sale of tobacco and to make money out of it; and, of course, in many countries powerful private interests are involved. When these private interests coincide with those of the governments, the resulting alliance is probably the strongest possible. Governments should perhaps be convinced that not only is the sale of tobacco inconsistent with public health, but also that there are other ways of supporting the national economy.

Recently, evidence has become available that smokers of cigarettes yielding high levels of tar and nicotine have a greater risk of developing lung cancer than smokers of cigarettes that yield less tar. Tobacco is a mixture containing a large number of chemicals, many of which are recognized carcinogens and/or mutagens. Tar, which results from the pyrolysis of tobacco, certainly contains carcinogenic chemicals, and one can therefore assume that, by decreasing the delivery of at least one of the carcinogenic fractions of smoke, a less intense carcinogenic activity of the total mixture may result. Tobacco smoke will, however, clearly continue to be a carcinogen even if it contains less tar.

The abolition of cigarettes with high levels of tar will potentially reduce the risk of lung cancer, but there is absolutely no doubt that any measure that still involves the production and use of cigarettes is only provisional and represents only a preliminary step towards the truly adequate measure of preventing damage to health from smoking, i.e., avoidance of smoking, and replacement of tobacco as a widespread crop. It must also be clearly stressed that there is no evidence whatsoever that the consumption of so-called 'low-tar' cigarettes has any effect on decreasing the incidence of and mortality from cardiovascular diseases.

The achievement of complete avoïdance of smoking and replacement of tobacco by another crop will necessitate, inevitably, a phase of intense and widespread education of the public, which should begin early in life. It is important that everybody becomes aware that the introduction of tobacco into our culture is a very recent event and that the consumption of cigarettes is a habit that became widely disseminated only within the last century. There is therefore no reason that humanity cannot continue its course without tobacco.

It is also important to stress that tobacco is carcinogenic not only when it is burned and smoked, but also when it is chewed. Recent advertising in which it is claimed that tobacco chewing is harmless contradicts very clear, definite evidence that tobacco is carcinogenic when it is chewed.

The diffusion of the habit of smoking all over the world makes the problem a truly international one of public health, and the All-Union Cancer Research Center of the Academy of Medical Sciences of the USSR is to be commended on its initiative in calling this meeting jointly with the IARC. Professor Blokhin and Professor Trapeznikov, in particular, are to be congratulated on their foresight and for the excellent organization of this international forum.

L. Tomatis, MD
Director,
IARC

LIST OF PARTICIPANTS

F. Adelkofer	Forschungsgesellschaft Rauchen und Gesundheit, Mittelweg 17, 2000 Hamburg 13, Federal Republic of Germany
K. Aoki	Department of Preventive Medicine, Nagoya University School of Medicine, 65 Tsurumai-cho, Showa-ku, Nagoya 466, Japan
F. Berrino	Istituto Nazionale per lo Studio e la Cura dei Tumori, via Venezian 1, 20133 Milan, Italy
K. Bjartveit	Norwegian Council on Smoking and Health, PO Box 8155, DEP 0033, Oslo 1, Norway
N.N. Blokhin	Director, All-Union Cancer Research Center of the Academy of Medical Sciences of the USSR, ul. Solianka 14, Moscow 109801, USSR
P.A. Bogovski	Director, Institute of Experimental and Clinical Medicine, Ministry of Public Health of the Estonian SSR, Ilmarise 25-6, Tallinn 200015, Estonia, USSR
J. Cullen	Deputy Director, Division of Cancer Prevention and Control, National Cancer Institute, Building 31, Room 4A-32, Bethesda, MD 20205, USA
I.I. Djachkin	Tobacco Production and Research Institute, Krasnodar, USSR
R. Doll	Cancer Epidemiology and Clinical Trials Unit, Radcliffe Infirmary, Oxford OX2 6HG, United Kingdom
V.V. Dvoirin	Head of Department, All-Union Cancer Research Center of the Academy of Medical Sciences of the USSR, Kashirskoye shosse 24, Moscow 115478, USSR
S. Eckhardt	Director, National Oncological Institute, Rath Gyorgy Str. 7, 1525 Budapest, 114 Pf21, Hungary

Y.T. Gao	Departement of Epidemiology, Shanghai Cancer Institute, 270 Dong An Road, Shanghai, China
V.N. Gerasimenko	Director, Institute of Clinical Oncology, All-Union Cancer Research Center of the Academy of Medical Sciences of the USSR, Kashirskoye shosse 24, Moscow 115478, USSR
I.S. Glasunov	Head, Division of Cooperative Preventive Programmes, Institute of Preventive Cardiology, All-Union Cardiology Research Center, 10 Petroverigsky Lane, Moscow, USSR
L.A. Griciute	Director, Lithuanian Cancer Research Institute, 341 Dzerzhinskio str., 232021 Vilnius, USSR
P.C. Gupta	WHO Collaborating Center for Oral Cancer Prevention, Tata Institute of Fundamental Research, Homi Bhabha Road, Bombay 40005, India
E. Heseltine	International Agency for Research on Cancer, 150 cours Albert-Thomas, 69372 Lyon Cedex 08, France
D. Hoffmann	Naylor Dana Institute for Disease Prevention, American Health Foundation, Dana Road, Valhalla, NY 10595, USA
V.V. Khudoley	N.N. Petrov Research Institute of Oncology, USSR Ministry of Public Health, Leningradskaya st. 66, Pesochny-2, 188646 Leningrad, USSR
H. Klus	Department of Research and Development, Austria Tabakwerke AG, Hasnerstrasse 124, 1160 Vienna, Austria
V.A. Kobljakov	All-Union Cancer Research Center of the Academy of Medical Sciences of the USSR, Kashirskoye shosse 24, Moscow 115478, USSR
I.P. Komjakov	N.N. Petrov Research Institute of Oncology, USSR Ministry of Public Health, Leningradskaya st. 66, Pesochny-2, 188646 Leningrad, USSR
M. Kunze	Institute of Social Medicine, University of Vienna, Kinderspitalgasse 15, 1095 Vienna, Austria
E. Leparski	World Health Organization, Regional Office for Europe, 8 Scherfigsvej, 2100 Copenhagen Ø, Denmark

C.S. Muir	International Agency for Research on Cancer, 150 cours Albert-Thomas, 69372 Lyon Cedex 08, France
R.S. Paffenbarger, Jr	Department of Family, Community and Preventive Medicine, Medical Center, School of Medicine, Stanford University, Stanford, CA 94308, USA
H. Peach	Department of Community Medicine, United Medical and Dental Schools, St Thomas' Campus, London SE1 7EH, United Kingdom
R. Peto	Nuffield Department of Clinical Medicine, Radcliffe Infirmary, Oxford OX2 6HE, United Kingdom
V.P. Pisklov	Head of Department, All-Union Research Institute of Tobacco, 350072 Krasnodar, USSR
L.M. Ramström	Director, NTS, National Smoking and Health Association, Sveavägen 166, 113 45 Stockholm, Sweden
R. Saracci	International Agency for Research on Cancer, 150 cours Albert-Thomas, 69372 Lyon Cedex 08, France
M. Sorsa	Department of Industrial Hygiene and Toxicology, Institute of Occupational Health, Haartmaninkatu 1, 00290 Helsinki 29, Finland
S.D. Stellman	American Cancer Society Inc., 4 West 35th Street, New York, NY 10001, USA
S. Tanneberger	Director, Zentralinstitut für Krebsforschung, Akademie der Wissenschaften der DDR, Lindenberger Weg 80, 1115 Berlin-Buch, German Democratic Republic
L. Tomatis	Director, International Agency for Research on Cancer, 150 cours Albert-Thomas, 69372 Lyon Cedex 08, France
S. Tominaga	Chief, Division of Epidemiology, Aichi Cancer Center Research Institute, Tashiro-cho, Chikusa-ku, Nagoya, Japan
N.N. Trapeznikov	Deputy Director, All-Union Cancer Research Center of the Academy of Medical Sciences of the USSR, Kashirskoye shosse 24, Moscow 115478, USSR
V.G. Veitsler	Head of Department, Scientific Research Institute of Food Industry, USSR Food Industry Ministry, Krasnodar, USSR

U. Veronesi — Director, Istituto Nazionale dei Tumori, via Venezian 1, 20133 Milan, Italy

D.G. Zaridze — International Agency for Research on Cancer, 150 cours Albert-Thomas, 69372 Lyon Cedex 08, France

I. IMPLICATIONS AND RECOMMENDATIONS

IMPLICATIONS

These pages highlight the scientific deliberations, but do not represent a full summary of the proceedings.

Despite the fact that the main adverse health effects of smoking have been well known for many years, smoking remains one of the most important public health problems both in developed and in developing countries. Between one-quarter and three-quarters of the men smoke in virtually all countries from which survey data are available. Women generally smoke less than men, but the proportion of adult women smokers in many parts of Europe and North America is about 30%, and increasing numbers of women are taking up the habit. Smoking continues to increase in many (though not all) developed and almost all developing countries.

Tobacco smoking, particularly of cigarettes, is an important cause of chronic disability and death from a wide range of neoplastic, vascular and respiratory diseases. The neoplastic diseases caused by smoking include cancers of the lung, oral cavity, pharynx, larynx, oesophagus, urinary bladder, renal pelvis and pancreas. The most important of these neoplastic diseases is lung cancer. In most developed countries for which data are available, the proportion of lung cancer attributable to smoking is 80–90% in men and the attributable proportion in women is approaching this level in many of these countries. Even if a smaller fraction of lung cancers in other countries is induced by tobacco, a substantial proportion of the global total must be attributable to this single cause.

Tobacco is probably the most important known carcinogen for human society today. It accounts for more cancer deaths than all other reliably known effects put together, and the annual number of lung cancer deaths due to tobacco is still rising rapidly. By the end of the century, this number is expected to exceed one million, to which must be added an even greater number of tobacco-induced deaths from diseases other than lung cancer.

In countries where the oral consumption of smokeless tobacco in various forms is popular, it is also a cause of cancer, chiefly of the oral cavity. Oral use of smokeless tobacco is spreading to other countries and this can only be considered deleterious.

In addition, smoking causes even more deaths from non-neoplastic diseases than from cancer. Coronary heart disease (CHD) is the leading cause of death in most developed countries and in those where prolonged smoking is widespread about one-third of all CHD deaths in middle-aged people may be attributed to cigarette smoking. Smoking also contributes to the development of various other arterial diseases, and is the predominant cause of chronic obstructive lung disease (a term that includes chronic bronchitis and emphysema).

On the basis of knowledge of the chemical composition of sidestream smoke, experimental data and human exposure measurements, 'passive' exposure to other people's tobacco smoke must be presumed to cause some risk of developing lung cancer. However, the exact extent to which it does so requires additional research. Although less firm, evidence has emerged that involuntary smoking may also increase the incidence of CHD.

Those who stop smoking before they have cancer or serious heart or lung disease can avoid much of the excess risk of death from smoking that they would have suffered if they had continued. The longer the period of cessation, the greater the diminution of risk.

Cessation of smoking results in a rapid and substantial reduction in death rates from CHD. Approximately 10 years after cessation, the primary onset rate of coronary heart disease for exsmokers approaches that of lifelong nonsmokers. An important part of the treatment of atherosclerotic diseases – coronary, cerebral, aortic and peripheral vascular and obstructive lung disease – is persuading patients who are smokers to give up the habit.

The rise in cigarette consumption observed in many countries in the past few decades suggests that, in future decades, important increases will be observed in the rates of lung cancer and other smoking-related diseases in those countries, unless some measures are taken to prevent at least part of these long-term adverse effects.

The excess risks of death produced by smoking in middle and old age depend strongly not only on what is currently smoked but also, perhaps surprisingly, on what was smoked in early adult life, even if this was several decades earlier. Hence, there is a potentially misleading delay of several decades between the widespread adoption of cigarette smoking by the young adults in a particular country and the eventual emergence of its full effects. Indeed, during the period while large increases in cigarette smoking are taking place among young adults, there may (temporarily) be little increase in mortality for decades after the main increases in cigarette usage cease. Thus, large increases in conditions such as lung cancer may be observed as a delayed result of long-past increases in cigarette usage by young adults.

Because of the long delay that may occur between the adoption of a particular smoking habit and the emergence of its full effects on cancer risks, there has been uncertainty about the effects on health of changes in design of cigarettes. Evidence on this subject has, however, emerged (IARC, 1986) and the present meeting endorsed the conclusion of the IARC Working Group that: '. . . the risk of lung cancer associated with the types of cigarettes commonly smoked before the middle 1950s is greater than that for modified cigarettes with low tar levels now generally available in some countries.

'The health benefits from the cessation of smoking, however, greatly exceed those to be expected from changes in cigarette composition.' But, it was considered by no means certain that current changes in cigarette composition would have any comparable effect on the risk of other tobacco-related diseases. Particularly, it was uncertain whether such changes would have any effect on the risk of developing CHD.

Worldwide, the number of tobacco-induced deaths is still increasing rapidly, so the elimination of smoking would ultimately result in the avoidance of several million tobacco-induced deaths each year, and even moderate decreases in smoking would prevent substantial numbers of such deaths.

RECOMMENDATIONS

The ultimate response to the disastrous facts outlined above must be the eradication of virtually all tobacco use. All responsible bodies should declare their commitment to such a programme in all countries, which would probably be the most effective means of protecting present and future public health.

A series of measures is therefore urgently needed, as intermediate steps towards this final goal. As a first step, reduction in the consumption of tobacco would be the most important means. Each country should therefore formulate a specific strategy for reduction of smoking rates within a defined period.

Measures to discourage the use of cigarettes are of substantial public health importance in areas such as the USSR, Europe, North America and Australia, where cigarettes have been used widely for many decades, and where they may already account for 20–35% of all cancer deaths. They are also important in areas such as China, other parts of Asia, and Africa, where widespread use of cigarettes is so recent that even though at present the habit may account for only a small percentage of all cancer deaths, causation of a much higher proportion in future decades can already be foreseen.

The meeting consequently RECOMMENDS that in all countries specific measures should be taken to discourage continuation of the habit among smokers and adoption of the habit among nonsmokers.

The measures that are most appropriate to achieve this will, of course, differ widely from country to country. Expert committees of the World Health Organization (1979) and International Union Against Cancer (1977) have already formulated extensive lists of recommendations that deserve detailed consideration, as they contain much carefully thought out advice. These recommendations emphasize the need to give national smoking control programmes a multicomponent nature.

Most of the measures recommended, however, are concerned not with restriction but with education. Partly as a result of these, the majority of smokers in most industrialized countries may by now be aware that smoking is hazardous, but probably most remain unaware of the relative magnitude of the hazards involved.

The meeting consequently RECOMMENDS that responsibility be taken for ensuring that the majority of cigarette smokers be led to understand the approximate size of the excess risk of disability and death associated with the habit, and of the benefits of cessation of the smoking habit.

One method that might be particularly appropriate in all countries, since it gains access to all cigarette smokers at negligible cost, is to have on each pack of cigarettes a quantitatively informative health warning (or a set of health warnings that are cyclically altered, some of which are quantitatively informative). The warning should be large enough to be prominent, and its wording should be reviewed (and perhaps revised) at regular intervals to help it communicate the *size* of the hazard to ordinary smokers.

Appropriate health education programmes could be given a prominent position in the school curriculum. Health education could be made a routine part of many clinic visits, for some patients in ill health are influenced by doctors and nurses to cease smoking. In order to achieve implementation on a really broad basis, special efforts must be made to give specific training to key professionals such as teachers and health workers. Health education programmes could be offered through various mass media. Finally, a systematic effort could be made to discourage smoking by various particularly influential individuals such as teachers, health professionals and media personalities – indeed, schools, clinics and television studios might exert a useful influence by becoming completely nonsmoking areas.

One programme component that is consistently recommended, and for which there is particularly clear evidence that it is helpful, is substantial increases in the real price of cigarettes, maintaining those increases against inflation. Increases in price should make any very hazardous cigarettes (e.g., nonfilter, high-tar) at least as expensive as hazardous cigarettes.

Other widely recommended components include a ban on all forms of tobacco sales promotion, and various measures to give nonsmokers freedom from the annoyance and hazards of breathing other people's smoke. Such measures may also help to change smokers' perception of their habit.

A complementary approach to the elimination of tobacco consumption could be changes in cigarette design. It would be necessary to analyse cigarette composition, especially for nicotine and tar delivery. If tar deliveries are relatively high, they should be lowered, since there is evidence that the risk of lung cancer associated with high-tar cigarettes is greater than that for low-tar cigarettes.

The meeting therefore RECOMMENDS that, although elimination of tobacco consumption should be the final goal, an upper limit, such as, perhaps, 15 mg, on cigarette tar deliveries be introduced as quickly as possible.

It should be noted, however, that there is no evidence that this step will reduce the incidence of other smoking-related diseases, such as heart disease. An initiative to reduce tar levels should not provide an excuse to avoid introducing other, much more important aspects of a smoking and health programme, and great care should be taken to ensure that efforts to reduce tar levels do not give the impression that smoking of low-tar cigarettes is without substantial hazard.

In view of the global extent of the smoking problem, international collaboration should be sought in controlling smoking. Several of the agencies of the United Nations family are ready to act, and it is recommended that member states stimulate these organizations to give priority to such activities and to seek their active assistance in national work, e.g., the World Health Organization could be asked to assist in planning and implementing various actions. Further, the Food and Agriculture Organization and the World Bank could be asked for assistance in finding alternative crops to replace tobacco in national agriculture.

Substantial assistance could be supplied by various nongovernmental organizations, e.g., the UICC.

To be fully effective, measures may have to be maintained for many years. The achievement and maintenance of a strong, consistent and effective strategy over such a long period poses obvious difficulties.

The meeting consequently RECOMMENDS that some permanent mechanism be established in each country where there are appreciable numbers of tobacco smokers to ensure that the control of tobacco-related diseases continues, over a long period, to receive an appropriate degree of attention.

REFERENCES

IARC (1986) *IARC Monographs on the Evaluation of the Carcinogenic Risk of Chemicals to Humans,* Vol. 38, *Tobacco Smoking,* Lyon

International Union Against Cancer (1977) *Lung Cancer Prevention: Guidelines for Smoking Control (UICC Tech. Rep. Ser., Vol. 28),* Geneva

World Health Organization (1979) *Controlling the Smoking Epidemic. Report of the WHO Expert Committee (WHO Tech. Rep. Ser., No. 636),* Geneva

II. TOBACCO – A MAJOR HEALTH HAZARD

TOBACCO: AN OVERVIEW OF HEALTH EFFECTS

R. DOLL

Emeritus Professor of Medicine, University of Oxford,
Honorary Member Imperial Cancer Research Fund,
Cancer Epidemiology and Clinical Trials Unit,
Radcliffe Infirmary, Oxford, UK

INTRODUCTION

When tobacco was first introduced into Europe at the end of the sixteenth century, smoking was recommended for medicinal purposes; but its use soon became controversial and it was condemned as a noxious vice as often as it was praised for its prophylactic value. Little scientific evidence was, however, obtained about its effects until the late 1940s, at which period medical textbooks either ignored the subject altogether or referred briefly to tobacco amblyopia, a form of blindness associated with heavy pipe smoking and poor nutritional status, to tobacco angina, a rare form of angina in which chest pain was precipitated by smoking, and to cancers of the lip and tongue, which experienced surgeons had for long suspected were associated with the smoking of pipes. Then, in 1950, five papers appeared in the UK and the USA describing studies in which the smoking habits of large numbers of patients with cancer of the lung or, in some studies, with cancers of the mouth, pharynx, or larynx, were compared with the smoking habits of control patients (Doll & Hill, 1950; Levin *et al.*, 1950; Mills & Porter, 1950; Schrek *et al.*, 1950; Wynder & Graham, 1950). In one of these it was concluded that 'smoking is a factor, and an important factor, in the production of carcinoma of the lung' (Doll & Hill, 1950), and the modern era of the study of the health effects of smoking had begun.

The results of these studies are summarized in Table 1, together with those of three smaller and less detailed studies that had been published in Germany and the Netherlands in the preceding 11 years. In six, comparisons could be made between heavy smokers and nonsmokers, the results of which suggested that the risk of lung cancer among the former might be some 3–30 times greater than that among the latter, the differences being due partly to the different methods of smoking in different countries, but more importantly to the different definitions employed in the categorization of nonsmokers, who in at least one study included exsmokers.

The obvious way to check the conclusions drawn from these studies was to record the smoking habits of large numbers of men and women who smoked different amounts, to

Table 1. Smoking and lung cancer: results of early case-control studies

Reference	No. of men		Percentage of 'nonsmokers'		Percentage of 'heavy smokers'	
	With lung cancer	Without lung cancer	With lung cancer	Without lung cancer	With lung cancer	Without lung cancer
Müller, 1939[a]	86	86	3.5	16.3	65	36
Schairer & Schöniger, 1943[a]	93	270	3.2	15.9	52	27
Wassink, 1948[b]	134	100	4.5	19.0	55	19
Doll & Hill, 1950[c]	649	649	0.3	4.2	26	13
Levin *et al.*, 1950[d]	236	481	15.3	21.7	–	–
Mills & Porter, 1950[d]	444	430	7	31	–	–
Schrek *et al.*, 1950[d]	82	522	14.6	23.9	18	9
Wynder & Graham, 1950[d]	605	780	1.3	14.6	51	19

[a] Germany
[b] The Netherlands
[c] UK
[d] USA

follow them up over a period of years, and to see whether the recorded habits would serve to predict the risk of developing disease. By this method, it was, moreover, possible to study not only the relationship between smoking and lung cancer, but also that between smoking and all other diseases that were common enough for a substantial number of cases to be observed within the period of observation.

Many such studies have now been carried out, eight of which cover a large enough number of individuals for a long enough period for useful information to be obtained about a wide range of diseases (Hammond & Horn, 1958; Dunn *et al.*, 1960; Best *et al.*, 1961; Hammond, 1966; Kahn, 1966; Cederlöf *et al.*, 1975; Doll & Peto, 1976; Hirayama, 1977; Doll *et al.*, 1980). All have been limited to the study of mortality and all give qualitatively similar results, despite the fact that four were carried out in the USA, and one each in Canada, the UK, Japan and Sweden. All agree in showing that cigarette smoking is, in general, associated with a higher mortality than the smoking of pipes and cigars and most agree that pipe and cigar smoking are only weakly associated with any disease other than cancers of the upper respiratory and digestive tracts (lip, tongue, mouth, pharynx other than nasopharynx, larynx and oesophagus).[1] The rest of this paper will, therefore, be largely confined to the effects of cigarette smoking, which is, outstandingly, the principal way in which tobacco is now smoked throughout the world, apart from some parts of Asia and Africa where tobacco continues to be smoked in local forms that resemble small cigars more closely than cigarettes. When smoked, some of these local preparations deliver very large amounts of nicotine and tobacco tar, and the health effects of each need to be studied separately.

All these cohort studies show large differences in risk of the order of ten- to 40-fold between men smoking 20 or more cigarettes a day and lifelong nonsmokers for death due to cancer of the lung, some other cancers of the upper respiratory and digestive tracts, chronic bronchitis and emphysema (now preferably called chronic obstructive lung dis-

[1] Exceptionally, in Sweden the relative risk of lung cancers is equally high in pipe and cigarette smokers.

ease), respiratory heart disease, and aortic aneurysm, and smaller differences for the risk of death from several other cancers and a wide variety of other diseases ranging from ischaemic heart disease through pulmonary tuberculosis and peptic ulcer to cirrhosis of the liver and suicide. For many of these diseases, however, it has not been easy to decide how far these differences in mortality rates reflect the role of cigarette smoking in the production of disease and how far they are due to confounding, that is, to an association between smoking and other aspects of the individual's way of life, or aspects of his character, which are the direct cause of the condition.

PROOF OF CAUSATION

Intervention studies to produce disease are unacceptable in a civilized society, while intervention studies with random allocation of a measure to prevent disease are possible in theory but are seldom practicable for they cannot be carried out until people are already convinced that the proposed measure is likely to be beneficial, and if they are, it may be unethical to conduct the study. In these circumstances, we have to make up our minds on the basis of epidemiological observations combined with the results of animal experiments. The latter are, however, less helpful in relation to cigarette smoking than they are in relation to many other putative agents of human disease, partly because it is difficult to make animals smoke in the way that humans do, partly because of different anatomical features which modify the distribution of inhaled smoke droplets, and partly because cigarette smoke interacts with other aspects of human disease, such as diet-induced atheroma, that are not easily reproducible in laboratory experiments. The epidemiological evidence alone is, however, sometimes so clear that there is no difficulty in concluding that the factor being studied is a cause of the disease, just as Snow was able to conclude that water polluted with human faeces was a cause of cholera, before the cholera vibrio was discovered. Proof of causation, in the strict logical sense, is not, in these circumstances, obtainable, although the range of evidence that has accumulated about the relationship between smoking and some of the diseases with which it is associated – lung cancer, for example – is now sufficient to provide proof of causation, in the legal sense (i.e., proof beyond reasonable doubt).

Before reaching a conclusion that cigarette smoking actually causes many of the diseases with which the habit is associated, however, we have to consider not merely the fact of the association, but many other features as well. These include the strength of the association (a ten-fold increase in risk being, for example, much less easily explained on other grounds than an increase of, say, only 50%), the existence of a graduated risk proportional to the amount smoked, a reduction in risk following the cessation of smoking, the correspondence between the incidence of the disease in the two sexes, in different populations, and at different times with group figures for the consumption of cigarettes, and the results of laboratory investigations. In some cases, too, it has been possible to obtain biological evidence that is almost impossible to explain on any grounds other than that cigarette smoking causes the disease.

We have noted, for example, two such observations relating to lung cancer in the cohort study of British doctors whose smoking habits were recorded in 1951 and subsequently again at intervals of five to seven years. One showed that the mortality from lung cancer in the British doctors fell relative to that in the country as a whole, corresponding to the relative reduction in the amount smoked, while the relative mortality from other cancers remained the same (Doll & Peto, 1976). The other showed that, among those who stopped smoking, the incidence of the disease hardly changed with the passage of time, something that has never been observed to occur under any other circumstances (Doll, 1978). Another example was recorded by Fletcher *et al.* (1976) and Fletcher and Peto (1977) when they followed 800 men for eight years, taking detailed smoking histories and making measurements of their respiratory function every six or 12 months. Their results showed that the deterioration in respiratory function progressed with time more rapidly in cigarette smokers than in non-smokers, but that when cigarette smokers stopped smoking, the rate of deterioration slowed down and approximated to that in men who had never smoked and whose deterioration was dependent on age alone.

These three observations, together with all the other human evidence, leave no room for doubt that cigarette smoking is one of the principal causes of both cancer of the lung and chronic obstructive lung disease and, in view of its relation to the latter, it must also be regarded as a cause of respiratory heart disease. Nor can there be any doubt that cigarette smoking contributes to the causation of several other diseases, including myocardial infarction, which because of its importance as a cause of death has been subject to intensive investigation in many countries, peripheral vascular disease (the clinical progress of which is clearly dependent on the continuation of smoking), aneurysm of the descending aorta, and half a dozen types of cancer, the relations of which to tobacco have recently been reviewed by the IARC (1986). These include cancers of the upper respiratory and digestive tracts and cancers of the bladder and pancreas.

For many of the other diseases that are associated with smoking, the conclusion that it contributes to their causation or lethality is more fairly described as presumptive than proved. This is unimportant for public health policy, as several of those diseases for which smoking is sufficiently well established as a cause to justify its avoidance are so common, and the death rate attributed to them so high, that it is immaterial whether another one or two dozen less common diseases are added to them. A proper understanding of the role of tobacco is, however, important medically, as, for some diseases, we need to know whether the cessation of smoking improves the results of treatment (as in the case of gastric ulcer) and, for all diseases, it helps our attempts to unravel the mechanism by which they are produced – or hinders them if we have judged incorrectly.

QUANTITATIVE ASSESSMENT OF EFFECTS OF SMOKING

For some of the diseases which, it is agreed, smoking helps to cause, it is not possible to say that the whole of the difference in incidence between smokers and nonsmokers is due to the effect of tobacco, as smoking is confounded with other factors that contribute independently to the aetiology of disease. This is certainly so for those cancers of the upper respiratory and digestive tracts that are also due to the consumption of alcohol, and this makes it very difficult to assess what proportion of the total incidence of these diseases can properly be ascribed to the effects of either.

Associations reflecting causation

For the other diseases that we can now confidently assert are caused by smoking, most or all of the difference in mortality between smokers and nonsmokers can be attributed directly to the habit. These are listed in Table 2. Three are among the most common causes of death in developed countries, as is shown in Table 2 by the proportion of deaths attributed to them in three of the countries for which detailed enumeration of deaths by cause are regularly published (that is, Denmark, England and Wales, and the USA). Reasonable proportions to attribute to smoking, taking into account that smaller proportions are attributable to smoking in women than in men, would be about 85% for the combined group of deaths due to cancer of the lung, chronic obstructive lung disease and aortic aneurysm, and 25% for the combined group of deaths due to cancers of the pancreas and bladder and ischaemic heart disease. This leads to the conclusion that 14–17% of all deaths in the three countries referred to in Table 2 would be caused prematurely by smoking, as a result of the contribution of smoking to these nine causes of death alone.

Positive associations of mixed or uncertain character

Table 3 lists 18 other diseases (or groups of diseases) that have nearly always been associated with smoking, whenever they have been examined separately. Five are specific types of cancer, one is a group of cancers of the upper respiratory and digestive tracts, and one consists of cancers of unspecified types, composed of a variety of cancers that are associated with smoking in different ways. Smoking and alcohol are both causes of cancers of the tongue, mouth, pharynx and larynx and of cancer of the oesophagus, and both act independently and synergistically. The attribution of risk is, moreover, complicated by the fact that smoking and the consumption of alcohol tend to be associated in the same individual so that very large numbers of people would have to be studied before it was possible to make any accurate estimate of the proportion of these cancers that would be avoided in the absence of smoking. In many countries it would certainly be large. In others,

Table 2. Proportion of deaths due to diseases the excess of which in smokers is attributable to smoking (three countries)

Cause of death	No. of deaths as % of total		
	Denmark 1982	England & Wales 1983	USA 1979
Cancer of lip	<0.1	<0.1	<0.1
Cancer of lung	5.2	6.1	5.1
Cancer of pancreas	1.4	1.0	1.1
Cancer of bladder	0.9	0.8	0.5
Ischaemic heart disease	29.9	27.0	28.8
Respiratory heart disease	<0.1	<0.1	<0.1
Aortic aneurysm	0.5	1.2	0.7
Peripheral vascular disease	0.1	0.2	0.1
Chronic obstructive lung disease	3.1	4.0	2.4
Total	41.1	40.3	38.9

Table 3. Proportion of deaths due to diseases the excess of which in smokers may be attributable to smoking in whole or in part (three countries)

Cause of death	No. of deaths as % of total		
	Denmark 1982	England & Wales 1983	USA 1979
Cancer of oesophagus	0.4	0.7	0.4
Cancer of tongue, mouth, pharynx and larynx	0.5	0.4	0.6
Cancer of stomach	1.4	1.8	0.7
Cancer of liver	0.3	0.2	0.3
Cancer of kidney	0.6	0.4	0.4
Cancer of cervix uteri	0.5	0.3	0.3
Cancer of unspecified site	0.9	1.4	1.3
Respiratory tuberculosis	<0.1	<0.1	<0.1
Hypertension	0.7	1.0	1.7
Myocardial degeneration	0.2	1.0	3.7
Arteriosclerosis	1.7	1.1	1.5
Cerebral thrombosis	1.5	1.7	2.0
Other cerebrovascular disease	8.1	10.0	6.8
Pneumonia	2.9	9.6	2.3
Other respiratory disease	1.0	1.3	1.1
Gastric ulcer	0.4	0.3	0.2
Duodenal ulcer	0.2	0.4	0.2
Hernia	0.1	0.1	<0.1
Total	21.4	31.5	23.6

where other and as yet unknown factors cause extremely high risks of cancer of the oesophagus (as in parts of the USSR, China and South and East Africa) and where chewing various mixtures of tobacco, betel and lime are responsible for high risks of cancers of the buccal cavity, the proportion of deaths from these causes that are attributable to smoking may be relatively low.

Whether any cancers of the stomach, liver, kidney and cervix uteri are attributable to smoking is still uncertain. Cohort studies have regularly shown higher rates in smokers than in nonsmokers, but the possibility of confounding with other factors exists – specially for cancers of the liver and cervix uteri – and the IARC (1986) was unable to come to a conclusion about them. It seems likely, however, that some cancers of the renal pelvis can be attributed to smoking, along with cancer of the bladder, even if adenocarcinomas of the body of the kidney cannot.

The relationship between smoking and the other 11 causes of death has not yet been studied in great detail. The excess mortality in smokers is generally relatively small (though sometimes absolutely large) and may, perhaps, be attributed to smoking on the grounds of analogy with, or misdiagnosis of, a disease that smoking is known to cause. On these grounds, for instance, some deaths from cerebral thrombosis may be attributed to smoking because of the known effect of smoking on the development of atheroma, and some deaths attributed to myocardial degeneration or nonspecifically to arteriosclerosis may also be due to smoking because they were really due to undiagnosed ischaemic heart disease.

For others the evidence is confused. Gastric ulcer, for example, has become less common as smoking has increased, yet controlled trials have shown that gastric ulcers heal more quickly when smoking is stopped and it seems very unlikely that the grossly increased mortality in smokers that has been found consistently in cohort studies does not reflect, at least in part, the inhibitory effect of smoking on an ulcer's healing. In part, too, it may reflect the greater liability of smokers to die of postoperative complications following haemorrhage or perforation.

Other diseases, such as pulmonary tuberculosis and inguinal hernia, can hardly be said to be caused by tobacco in the ordinary sense; but they may be aggravated by the cough that accompanies chronic productive bronchitis (which is certainly due to smoking) and they may, consequently, have a higher fatality in those who smoke than in those who do not. Some of the excess mortality from respiratory tuberculosis in smokers could, however, be due to confounding with alcoholism.

Associations reflecting confounding

For a few other causes of death that are more common in smokers than in nonsmokers, the difference in mortality can be attributed wholly to confounding. These are listed in Table 4. In people who die from these causes, smoking is presumably confounded with the consumption of alcohol, personality features, psychological stress, or even with all three.

For these causes of death, cultural differences that affect the nature and prevalence of the factors that are truly responsible for them may well also affect their confounding with tobacco, and it need not be assumed that similar relationships would be observed in studies in other countries. In any case, none of the deaths due to these causes need be attributed to tobacco — unless perhaps it proves that toxic chemicals in cigarette smoke make a small contribution to the grossly increased mortality from cirrhosis of the liver that is regularly observed in heavy cigarette smokers.

Associations possibly reflecting protection

Against the large number of diseases caused, or aggravated, by smoking there are some that smoking may help to prevent or ameliorate. That this should be so is hardly surprising, since tobacco smoke contains some 3000 chemicals with many different pharmacological

Table 4. Proportion of deaths due to diseases the excess of which in smokers is attributable to confounding (three countries)

Cause of death	No. of deaths as % of total		
	Denmark 1982	England & Wales 1983	USA 1979
Alcoholism	0.1	<0.1	0.3
Cirrhosis of liver	1.0	0.4	1.6
Poisoning	0.3	0.2	0.2
Suicide	2.7	0.7	1.4
Total	4.1	1.3	3.4

Table 5. Proportion of deaths due to diseases that smoking may help to prevent or ameliorate (three countries)

Cause of death	No. of deaths as % of total		
	Denmark 1982	England & Wales 1983	USA 1979
Cancer of endometrium	0.4	0.2	0.1
Parkinsonism	0.3	0.4	0.2
Ulcerative colitis	<0.1	<0.1	<0.1
Pre-eclampsia	<0.1	<0.1	<0.1
Total	0.7	0.6	0.4

effects. Four diseases that may fall into this category are listed in Table 5. Only parkinsonism has been studied intensively (Godwin-Austen *et al.*, 1982). The evidence that has been obtained from both case-control and cohort studies is strong, and suggests that the mortality attributable to it may be reduced by at least a half. Less data are available for ulcerative colitis, but those that have been obtained certainly suggest that smoking may help to prevent relapse (Jick & Walker, 1983). It is probable, too, that it reduces the risk of some hormone-dependent diseases, particularly cancer of the endometrium, as it reduces the level of oestrogens in the blood and lowers slightly the age of menopause (Baron, 1984), and it may (perhaps because of the hypotensive effect of thiocyanate) reduce the risk of pre-eclampsia (Palmgren *et al.*, 1973; US Surgeon General 1979a). It may also protect against post-operative venous thrombosis (Emerson & Marks, 1977), but this has not been included in Table 5, as the evidence is too incomplete.

Diseases generally unrelated to smoking

There remain, of course, many diseases that are unrelated to smoking. Few, however, are common in the three countries represented in Tables 2–5 and, in these countries, they account, in total, only for between a quarter and a third of all deaths.

Involuntary (or passive) smoking

In addition to the many effects on the smoker, smoking may also affect others, either by releasing smoke into the ambient atmosphere, where it is inspired involuntarily by non-smokers or by causing the absorption of toxic products into the circulation which, in pregnant women, may cross the placenta and affect the fetus.

The sidestream smoke that is not directly inspired by smokers differs in composition from the mainstream smoke that is directly inspired and from the remains of the mainstream smoke that is eventually exhaled. The differences are, however, differences in quantity rather than quality, so that involuntary smoking may have similar effects on non-smokers as voluntary smoking has on smokers, although the chance of the effects occurring will be very much less. Whether it represents a hazard or not will depend on whether the effect is one that occurs in proportion to the dose received down to the lowest levels, as is believed to be the case with the production of cancer, or whether there is a threshold dose for the effect, below which none is produced. How great the risk is for individual nonsmokers will be discussed later in this Symposium, but it is generally too small to have any measurable effect nationally in comparison with that produced by smoking voluntarily. An exception is the effect on young children, who have been found to have more respiratory symptoms and twice as many attacks of bronchitis and pneumonia when their parents smoke as when they refrain (Colley *et al.,* 1974; Leeder *et al.,* 1976).

The fetus, as would be expected, responds differently from the child and adult, the principal effect of the mother's smoking being a reduction in weight at each stage of gestation with, in consequence, a small increase in perinatal mortality (US Surgeon General, 1979b). Whether any of the chemicals in smoke are absorbed in sufficient amounts to be teratogenic is still in dispute; but if any malformations are produced, the increase in incidence over the background rate in children born to nonsmoking mothers is certainly small (see Landesman-Dwyer & Emmanuel, 1979 and Johnston, 1981, for reviews). The fetus might also be affected if smoking had damaged the germ cells in either parent. No such effect has, however, yet been observed.

CONCLUSION

The smoking of tobacco, it is now clear, has many gross effects on health which, in some countries, lead to premature death in a substantial proportion of the whole population. For the three countries for which data are given in Tables 3–5, the proportion must be at least one in seven and may be materially greater, depending on the proportion of the excess mortality from the diseases listed in Table 3 which occurs in smokers that is attributed to smoking, and the proportion that is attributed to the confounding of smoking with other etiological agents.

In many other countries the proportion must be much the same, while in others it is likely to be less, depending on the amount of illness due to other causes, the prevalence of etiological agents that interact with smoking in the production of disease, and the smoking habits of the population, both now and in the past.

In countries where infectious diseases are common, particularly tropical countries where a great deal of illness is due to parasitic infections, the proportion of illness attributable to smoking is small; and, as the consumption of tobacco in these countries tends also to have been small in the past, the proportion of all illness that is now attributable to smoking is, in some of these countries, very small indeed at present, although in those where large increases in the habit have emerged recently, large increases in smoking-related disease are likely to follow eventually.

In other countries smoking may be common and may have been so for many years, yet the effects may be different, because of variation in the prevalence of other agents with which it interacts. It interacts, for example, with alcohol in the production of cancer of the oesophagus and with asbestos in the production of cancer of the lung. The former interaction results in a grossly increased risk of cancer of the oesophagus in north-west France, where the consumption of alcohol is both common and heavy, and the latter grossly increases the amount of lung cancer attributable to smoking in some occupational groups. It is, however, relatively unimportant everywhere at the national level, as the proportion of the population exposed to material amounts of asbestos is generally small.

Smoking interacts, too, with the level of blood cholesterol, approximately multiplying the effect of high levels (Mann *et al.*, 1976) and, in countries where these levels are low, the amount of myocardial infarction it produces, though still absolutely large, can be relatively small. This is so, for example, in Japan and some other parts of Eastern Asia, where low levels of blood cholesterol are due to a diet that includes relatively little fat, much of which is polyunsaturated. How far smoking interacts with other factors to increase the risk of many other smoking-related diseases is still unclear. It is, for example, uncertain how far the effect of smoke in producing chronic obstructive lung disease is modified by background levels of atmospheric pollution and by social conditions that lead to respiratory infection in childhood.

The third factor – the variation in smoking habits – is obviously important as the amount of disease produced by smoking cannot be large when smoking is uncommon. The effect is, however, much more complex than may appear at first sight, not only because of the importance of the method of smoking and the type of cigarettes (particularly the amount of tar that they deliver) but also because heavy consumption is associated with little disease until smoking has been common for many years. The relationship between the risk of disease and the duration of smoking has been worked out most clearly for cancer of the lung and chronic obstructive lung disease, but a similar relationship probably holds for the other smoking-induced cancers and may hold for many other smoking-induced diseases as well. The importance of the relationship between risk and duration of smoking has been shown most clearly in the trends in mortality from lung cancer in the UK, Finland and the USA, which will be discussed later in this Symposium. Because duration of smoking is so important, it not infrequently happens that the amount of tobacco consumed may be much greater in one country than in another while the lung cancer mortality rate may be temporarily much lower, as is the case in Japan in comparison with the UK.

All these factors combined make it very difficult to estimate the contribution of smoking to morbidity and mortality in different countries. It certainly cannot be estimated solely from knowledge of current smoking habits, and the figures for each country can be determined only after detailed study of the local conditions.

REFERENCES

Baron, J.A. (1984) Smoking and estrogen-related disease. *Am. J. Epidemiol.*, ***119,*** 9–22

Best, E.W.R., Josie, G.H. & Walker, C.B. (1961) A Canadian study of mortality in relation to smoking habits: A preliminary report. *Can. J. public Health,* **52,** 99–106

Cederlöf, R., Friberg, L., Hrubec, Z. & Lorich, U. (1975) *The Relationship of Smoking and Some Social Covariables to Mortality and Cancer Morbidity,* Stockholm, Department of Environmental Hygiene, Karolinska Institute

Colley, J.R.T., Holland, W.W. & Corkhill, R.T. (1974) Influence of passive smoking and parental phlegm on pneumonia and bronchitis in early childhood. *Lancet,* ***ii,*** 1031–1034

Doll, R. (1978) An epidemiological perspective of the biology of cancer. *Cancer Res.,* ***38,*** 3573–3583

Doll, R. & Hill, A.B. (1950) Smoking and carcinoma of the lung. *Br. med. J.,* ***ii,*** 739

Doll, R. & Peto, R. (1976) Mortality in relation to smoking: 20 years' observations on male British doctors. *Br.med. J.,* ***ii,*** 1525–1536

Doll, R., Gray, R., Hafner, B. & Peto, R. (1980) Mortality in relation to smoking: 22 years' observations on female British doctors. *Br. med. J.*, ***i,*** 967–971

Dunn, J.E., Linden, G. & Brelow, L. (1960) Lung cancer mortality experience of men in certain occupations in California. *Am. J. public Health*, ***50,*** 1475–1487

Emerson, P.A. & Marks, P. (1977) Preventing thromboembolism after myocardial infarction: Effect of low dose heparin on smoking. *Br. med. J.*, ***i,*** 18–20

Fletcher, C. & Peto, R. (1977) The natural history of chronic airflow obstruction. *Br. med. J.*, ***i,*** 1645–1648

Fletcher, C., Peto, R., Tinker, C. & Speizer, F.E. (1976) *The Natural History of Chronic Bronchitis and Emphysema,* Oxford, Oxford University Press

Godwin-Austen, R.B., Lee, P.N., Marmot, M.G. & Stern, G.M. (1982) Smoking and Parkinson's disease. *J. neurol. neurosurg. Psychiatry*, ***45,*** 577–581

Hammond, E.C. (1966) *Smoking in relation to the death rates of one million men and women.* In: Haenszel, W., ed., *Epidemiological Approaches to the Study of Cancer and Other Chronic Diseases (National Cancer Institute Monograph No. 19),* Bethesda, MD, National Cancer Institute, pp. 127–204

Hammond, E.C. & Horn, D. (1958) Smoking and death rates: Report on forty-four months of follow-up of 187,783 men. *J. Am. med. Assoc.*, ***166,*** 1159–1172 and 1294–1308

Hirayama, T. (1977) *Smoking and cancer: A prospective study on cancer epidemiology based on census population in Japan.* In: *Health Consequences, Education, Cessation Activities, and Governental Action. Smoking and Health II (Proceedings of the Third World Conference on Smoking and Health, DHEW Publication No. (NIH) 77-1413),* Washington DC, US Government Printing Office, pp. 65–72

IARC (1986) *IARC Monographs on the Evaluation of the Carcinogenic Risk of Chemicals to Humans,* Vol. 38, *Tobacco Smoking,* Lyon

Jick, H. & Walker, A.M. (1983) Cigarette smoking in ulcerative colitis. *New Engl. J. Med.*, ***308,*** 261–263

Johnston, O. (1981) Cigarette smoking and the outcome of human pregnancies: A status report on the consequences. *Clin. Toxicol.*, ***18,*** 189–209

Kahn, H.A. (1966) *The Dorn study of smoking and mortality among US veterans: Report on eight and one half years of observation.* In: Haenszel, W., ed., *Epidemiological Approaches to the Study of Cancer and Other Chronic Diseases (National Cancer Institute Monograph No. 19),* Bethesda, MD, National Cancer Institute, pp. 1–125

Landesman-Dwyer, S. & Emmanuel, I. (1979) Smoking during pregnancy, *Teratology*, ***19,*** 119–126

Leeder, S.R., Corkhill, R.T., Irwig, L.M., Holland, W.W. & Colley, J.T.R. (1976) Influence of family factors on the incidence of lower respiratory illness during the first year. *Br. J. prev. soc. Med.*, ***30,*** 203–213

Levin, M.L., Goldstein, H. & Gerhardt, P.R. (1950) Cancer and tobacco smoking. *J. Am. med. Assoc.*, ***143,*** 336–338

Mann, J.I., Doll, R., Thorogood, M., Vessey, M.P. & Waters, W.E. (1976) Risk factors for myocardial infarction in young women. *Br. J. prev. soc. Med.*, ***30,*** 94–100

Mills, C.A. & Porter, M.M. (1950) Tobacco-smoking habits and cancer of the mouth and respiratory system. *Cancer Res.*, ***10,*** 539–542

Müller, F.H. (1939) Tobacco abuse and carcinoma of the lung (Ger.). *Z. Krebsforsch.*, ***49,*** 57–85

Palmgren, B., Wahlen, T. & Wallander, B. (1973) Toxaemia and cigarette smoking during pregnancy: Prospective consecutive investigation of 3,927 pregnancies. *Acta obstet. gynecol. scand.*, ***52,*** 183–185

Schairer, E. & Schöniger, E. (1943) Lung cancer and tobacco use (Ger.). *Z. Krebsforsch.*, ***54,*** 261–269

Schrek, R., Baker, L.A., Ballard, G.P. & Dolgoff, S. (1950) Tobacco smoking as an etiologic factor in disease: Cancer. *Cancer Res.*, ***10,*** 49–58

US Surgeon General (1979a) *Smoking and Health,* Washington DC, US Government Printing Office, pp. 8/41–8/42

US Surgeon General (1979b) *Smoking and Health,* Washington DC, US Government Printing Office, pp. 8/11–8/30

Wassink, W.F. (1948) Etiology of lung cancer (Dutch). *Med. Tijdschr. Geneesk,* ***92,*** 3732–3747

Wynder, E.L. & Graham, E.A. (1950) Tobacco smoking as a possible etiologic factor in bronchogenic carcinoma. *J. Am. med. Assoc.*, ***143,*** 329–336

INFLUENCE OF DOSE AND DURATION OF SMOKING ON LUNG CANCER RATES

R. PETO

Imperial Cancer Research Fund,
Reader in Cancer Studies,
Nuffield Department of Clinical Medicine,
Radcliffe Infirmary, Oxford, UK

SUMMARY

Lung cancer risks depend far more strongly on the duration than on the daily dose-rate of cigarette smoking. For example, a three-fold increase in the daily dose-rate may produce only about a three-fold increase in effect, while a three-fold increase in duration might produce about a 100-fold increase in effect. Hence, a few decades after cigarette smoking becomes widespread, national lung cancer rates may remain very misleadingly low, even though they will eventually become extremely high.

INTRODUCTION

Worldwide, lung cancer already kills more people than any other neoplastic disease does, and the annual number of deaths it causes is still rising rapidly in many countries. For example, in the USSR, the number of men diagnosed each year as having lung cancer was about 40000 in 1970, but it will be about 80 000 in the mid-1980s and well over 100 000 by the early 1990s, and still rising rapidly (Zaridze & Gurevicius, this volume, p. 87). These increases are due partly to increases in the numbers of older men and partly to increases in the thoroughness of detection of the disease, but chiefly they are due to the *delayed* effects of past increases in cigarette usage. This delay between cause and full effect may mean that the main increase in cigarette usage in a country takes place over a decade or two during which no large absolute increase in lung cancer incidence occurs, and that later on a vast increase in lung cancer incidence then takes place over the course of a few decades during which no large further increase in smoking is occurring. Obviously, without a quantitative understanding of the relevance of *dose* and of *time* in tobacco carcinogenesis, there would be plenty of scope for misunderstandings to become established during the decades while tobacco smoke exposure is approximately constant but lung cancer rates are increasing rapidly. Hence, the present chapter is on dose and time relationships for tobacco-induced lung cancer, although some other aspects of the epidemiology of lung cancer will also be drawn in. The first section discusses the time relationships, and then other aspects of the effects of smoking are reviewed.

THE NEED FOR PROLONGED EXPOSURE

There are a few key features of the effects of tobacco on lung cancer incidence that are slightly counter-intuitive. Chief among them, and the key to any proper understanding of tobacco carcinogenesis, is the extraordinary relevance of the *duration* of smoking to lung cancer onset rates. For example, after 45, 30 and 15 years of cigarette smoking, the excess annual incidence rates of lung cancer might be about 0.5%, 0.1% and under 0.01% (Table 1). The annual lung cancer incidence rates to be expected among smokers may be estimated by adding up a *background* (i.e., nonsmoker) rate, which, like the onset rates of many other types of cancer, depends strongly on age (but not, by definition, on tobacco exposure), plus an *excess* rate, which depends strongly on duration of regular tobacco exposure (but not otherwise, at least to a first approximation, on age). Typical background and excess rates for males are depicted in Figure 1 (from Doll, 1971), and those for females might be about two-thirds as great.

Thus, a three-fold increase in the duration of regular tobacco use can increase the annual incidence of lung cancer about 100-fold. This particular relationship, which has been derived from detailed epidemiological studies on defined populations, may apply quite widely, even though in other populations the absolute risks may differ slightly. For example, in the entire adult male population of England and Wales in the 1970s, the

Table 1. Approximate[a] effects of various durations of cigarette smoking on annual incidence of lung cancer

Years of cigarette smoking	Annual[b] excess incidence	
	Moderate smokers	Heavy smokers
15	0.005%	0.01%
30	0.1%	0.2%
45	0.5%	1%
(60)	(1.5%?)	(3%?)

[a] Estimated from data reported by Doll and Peto (1978) for male British doctors. The cumulative risks would be far greater than these annual risks, of course, so an eventual total of over 10% of regular cigarette smokers may die of tobacco-induced cancer, depending on the number and type of cigarettes smoked.

[b] The *cumulative* incidence will, of course, be far greater than the annual incidence. For example, at the above lung cancer rates (and in the absence of other causes of death), men who smoked cigarettes regularly from early adult life onwards would have about a 10% (if moderate) or 20% (if heavy) probability of developing lung cancer at or before their mid-seventies. Since, in addition, smoking kills more people by diseases other than lung cancer than it kills by lung cancer, a minimal statement of the total risks associated with the habit would be that *about a quarter of all young adults who smoke cigarettes regularly will be killed before their time by the habit.* (Some of those killed would have died soon anyway, but others would have lived on for another 5, 10, 20, 30 or more years, the average amount of life lost being 10–15 years.)

Fig. 1. Background and excess risks. Lung cancer death rates among nonsmokers (lower line) in relation to age, and among regular cigarette smokers (upper line) in relation to approximate years of smoking (from Doll, 1971).

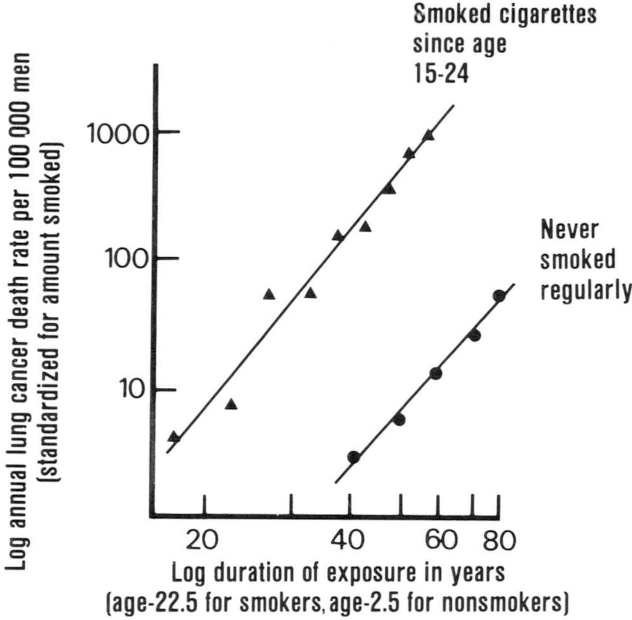

These two lines can be used directly to indicate the approximate background and excess risks, for in middle and old age the lung cancer incidence rates among people who have smoked cigarettes throughout adult life greatly exceed the rates among nonsmokers of similar age. (This might not, however, be true for people who did not begin to smoke substantial numbers of cigarettes until middle age, for the background and the excess risks indicated by these lines are, respectively, approximately 10^{-9} of the fourth power in years of age and 10^{-11} of the fourth power of years of regular cigarette smoking.)

proportions of smokers at various different ages were not very different, but the male lung cancer death rate at 80 years of age was about 100 times that at 40 years of age. This is probably because the 80-year-old smokers had been smoking cigarettes for about three times as long as the 40-year-old smokers (and not chiefly because of the frailty of the old; Peto, 1985).

The most surprising consequence of the overwhelming effects of the *duration* of smoking is illustrated, using real data[1], in Figure 2, which shows how strongly the annual excess risk of death from lung cancer at 60 years of age depends on whether men started smoking at 15 or at 25 years of age (i.e., on whether by the age of 60 they had smoked for 45, or for only 35, years). Failure to appreciate the relationship illustrated in Figure 2 has led to a variety of unjustifiable conclusions, e.g., that cigarettes do not cause lung cancer or, less perversely, that low-tar cigarettes have at least as great an effect as high-tar ones (National Academy of Sciences/National Research Council, 1982), that air pollution is of com-

[1] The data utilized are from the third largest prospective survey yet reported, and are similar to the findings of the larger two surveys; the corresponding results from all three of these surveys are presented in the US Surgeon-General's 1982 report (US Department of Health and Human Services, 1982).

Fig. 2. The relevance of smoking in early adult life

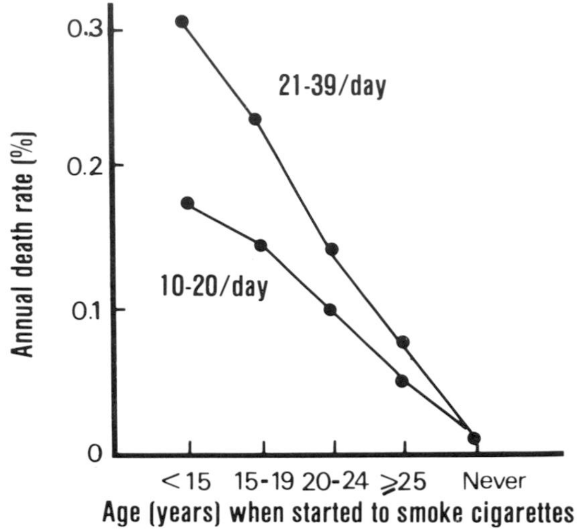

Relationship, in prospective survey data of regular smokers, between the age when regular cigarette smoking began in early adult life and lung cancer death rates at age 55–64 (mean, age 60) for US males (from Doll & Peto, 1981, Appendix E). Data are presented separately for heavy and for moderate smokers.

Fig. 3. Trends in US cigarette consumption

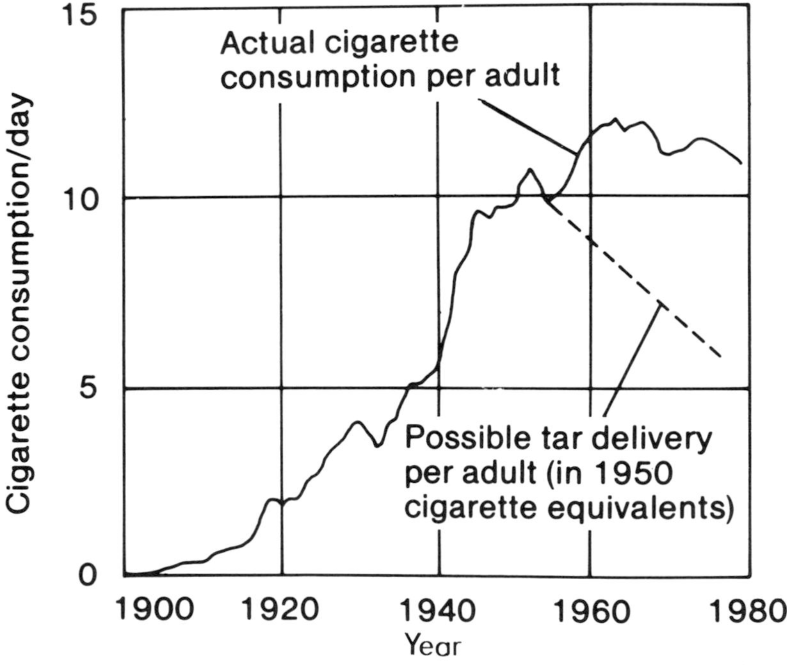

Mean daily sales of manufactured cigarettes per US adult aged over 18 years, with a crude estimate of tar yield per adult (from Doll & Peto, 1981). The estimate of tar yield allows approximately for decreases since the 1950s in tar yield per cigarette smoked in a standard manner, but not for any systematic changes in the manner in which cigarettes are smoked.

parable importance to tobacco (but see, however, Cederlöf *et al.*, 1978), or that new causes of lung cancer (rather than the delayed effects of past changes in tobacco usage) are chiefly responsible for the rapid increase in lung cancer in recent years. In each case, the point that is often overlooked is that current patterns of lung cancer mortality in late middle age or in old age depend strongly not only on current patterns of tobacco usage, but also on the patterns of cigarette usage among young adults as much as half a century ago.

Thus, current trends, current urban/rural differences and current international differences in lung cancer reflect, among other things, past trends, past urban/rural differences

Fig. 4. Recent trends in US cancer mortality

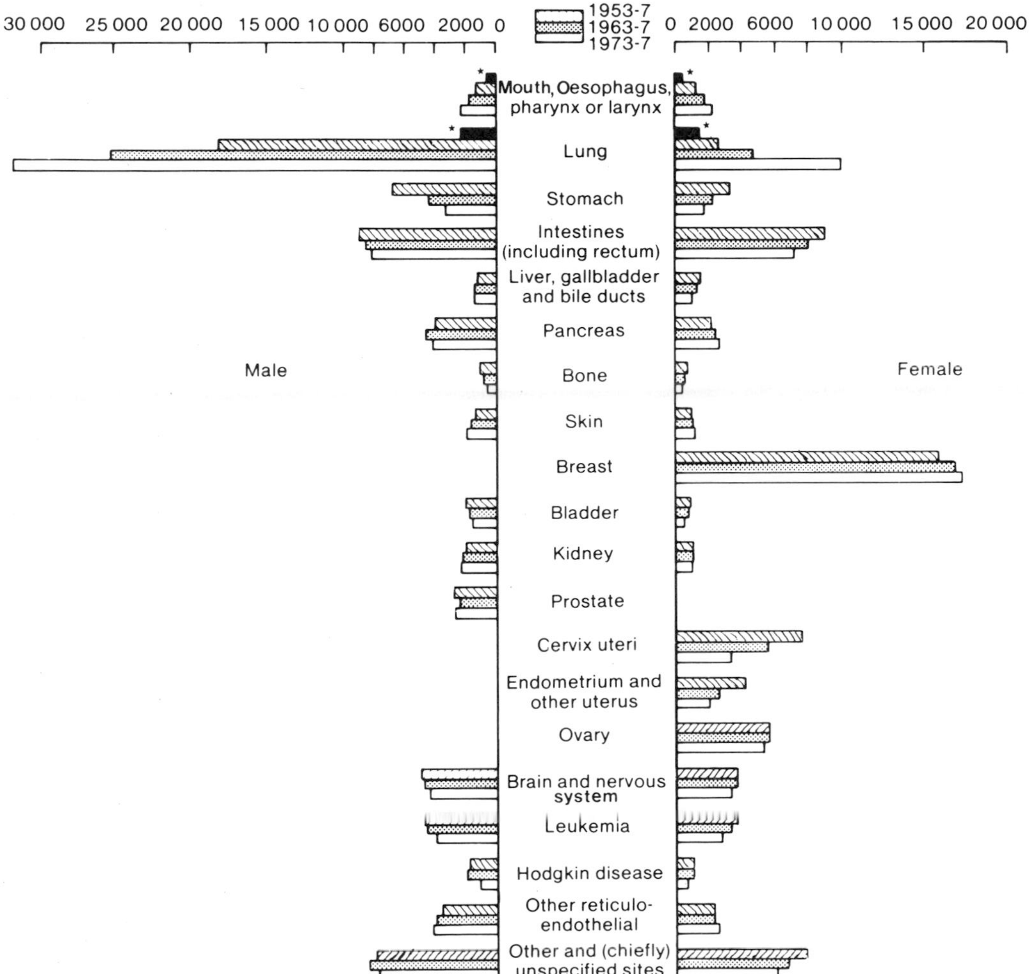

Age-standardized death certification rates (per 100 million people aged under 65) in the 1950s (top bar), the 1960s (middle bar) and the 1970s (bottom bar) for various types of cancer in the USA (from Doll & Peto, 1981). For cancers of the lung and upper respiratory and digestive tracts, estimated rates for lifelong nonsmokers are also given (bar*, above the rates for the 1950s).

and past international differences in cigarette usage by young adults. Consider, for example, the extent to which current trends in US lung cancer mortality rates among men now aged 70 might be affected by the large trends in cigarette consumption 50 years ago among people then aged 20. (For details, see Appendix E of Doll & Peto, 1981.) In 1930, US cigarette consumption was increasing rapidly among young men, and national sales rose from 1 cigarette/adult per day in 1915 to about 10/adult per day in 1945. The effects of those increases are only now becoming fully apparent, and largely or wholly as a delayed result of them US lung cancer rates in men in late middle and old age are still rising steeply, despite the fact that cigarette sales per adult have remained at a fairly steady 10–12/day ever since 1945, and that tar levels per cigarette have fallen substantially (Fig. 3). Contrary to various suggestions, the 'discrepancy' that has been seen for the past 25 years in the USA between rising lung cancer rates (see Fig. 4) and falling tar levels does *not* imply, or even suggest, that Americans are exposed to increasing levels of carcinogenic pollutants other than tobacco, nor, as a recent report (National Academy of Sciences/National Research Council, 1982) suggested, that tar-level reductions in cigarettes have been ineffective. (Indeed, but for tar-level reductions, the current increases in US lung cancer mortality rates would probably be appreciably more rapid.)

Likewise, in many countries, the smoking of manufactured cigarettes by young adults may have tended to become widely established in towns before it became so in the

Fig. 5. Lung cancer and smoking in the same generation

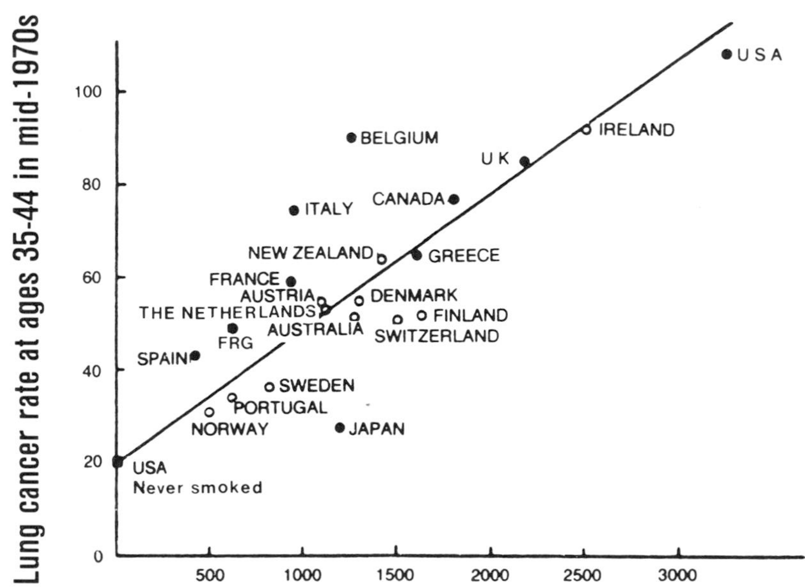

Relationship between lung cancer mortality rates (mean of male and female rates) for one generation in early middle age with manufactured (excluding hand-rolled cigarettes in Belgium and smuggled cigarettes in Italy) cigarette consumption when that generation of people were in early adult life: data for various countries, and for US nonsmokers estimated by fitting a power-law relationship to the prospective survey data reported by Garfinkel (1981). From Doll & Peto (1981)

surrounding countryside. If so, then half a century ago cigarette smoking was probably more prevalent among young men in towns than among young men in the country. Disparities in recent years between urban and rural lung cancer rates among today's old smokers may therefore be chiefly due not to air pollution, but rather to a delayed effect of past urban/rural differences in cigarette usage among the people who were then young but who are now old.

Finally, it is wholly wrong to suggest that the poor international correlation between *current* smoking habits and *current* lung cancer rates indicates that smoking is not the chief determinant of worldwide lung cancer mortality. For, such a correlation effectively relates the lung cancer rates of the grandparents to the smoking habits of their grandchildren. If instead the national lung cancer rates *for one generation* are related to national cigarette consumption rates when *that* generation consisted of young adults, a moderately close relationship does emerge (Fig. 5).

OTHER FEATURES OF THE EPIDEMIOLOGY OF SMOKING AND LUNG CANCER

Dose-response relationships

In Table 1, it may be seen that doubling the dose may *approximately* double the excess risk at each age. Partly because of difficulties of dosimetry[2], it is not really known whether, as Doll and Peto (1978) tentatively suggested, a doubling of the true dose-rate produces an approximately four-fold increase in the age-specific effect, or whether, as is suggested by much other data, it produces merely a two-fold increase. (Whatever the exact truth, however, it is clear that smoking two packs/day for 20 years is far less hazardous than smoking one pack/day for 40 years, so any analyses based on inappropriate concepts such as 'pack-years' should be treated warily.)

Time course of the effects of stopping smoking

If smoking ceases, the annual excess risk remains roughly (perhaps to within a factor of two?) constant thereafter. Referring to Table 1, it may be seen that the annual excess risk after 30 years of smoking is about 0.1%, so if a smoker stops after 30 years then approximately this annual excess risk may persist indefinitely. Thus, for example, 15 years later the annual excess risk might still be about 0.1% instead of the 0.5% that it would have been had smoking continued, so about 80% of the excess risk is being avoided. (It is not, however, true that the annual *absolute* excess risk decreases substantially, and still less is it true that it decreases to zero after 10 years; only one prospective study has suggested that,

---

[2] The effective dose may not be simply proportional to the number of cigarettes smoked per day, for the carbon monoxide uptake per cigarette appears to be less for heavy than for moderate smokers. Also, since the chief target area is the main airways, rapid inhalation may deposit less on them than slow inhalation does (a suggestion reinforced by reports, e.g., Doll & Peto, 1976, that in some, although not all, studies heavy smokers who describe themselves as 'not inhaling' get *more* lung cancer than do comparably heavy smokers who 'do inhale'!).

and the others clearly refute it.) Because the large increases in annual risk that would otherwise develop are avoided by stopping smoking, from a practical public health viewpoint this means that cessation works, since *people who stop smoking before they have cancer thereby avoid most of the risk of getting cancer from the habit.* The time course of the effects of changes in smoking that fall short of complete cessation will be discussed in the chapter on the effects on national mortality rates of changes in cigarette manufacture that reduce the amount of 'tar' delivered per cigarette (see p. 211).

The importance of cigarettes as opposed to pipes

In the UK and the USA, cigarettes appear to have a far greater effect than pipe or cigar tobacco did, and so the switch earlier this century from pipes to cigarettes has produced vast increases in lung cancer rates. The reasons for this difference are not adequately known, especially as the smoke from pipes and cigars is about as carcinogenic for laboratory animals as that from cigarettes. One suggestion is that the difference depends chiefly on the greater alkalinity of the smoke from pipes and cigars, which might make inhalation less pleasant and facilitate the transport of nicotine across the oral mucosa, thereby obviating the need to inhale (see Wald *et al.*, 1981). This suggestion might not be difficult to test, and, if confirmed, might point to an important way of diminishing the hazards of cigarettes, although at present this remains speculative.[3] A related suggestion is that the 'air-cured' tobacco of, for example, certain French cigarettes somewhat resembles pipe tobacco and is therefore substantially less carcinogenic than the 'flue-cured' tobacco typical of British and American cigarettes; but the international differences in lung cancer rates on which this suggestion rested were not reliable, because they owed so much to differences in *duration* of cigarette smoking. (During the 1930s and 1940s, for example, British cigarette consumption was four times that in France.) Recently, evidence has emerged from a large case-control study (Benhamou *et al.*, 1985) that, if anything, the converse is likely to be true – that is, that regular use of cigarettes made of dark French tobacco may be early twice as hazardous as similar use of cigarettes made of 'light' tobacco.

'Interaction' with other causative factors

A variety of other causative factors for lung cancer are known, of which the best studied are asbestos, ionizing radiations and urban air pollution. All these have a far greater absolute extra effect on smokers than on nonsmokers (illustrated, for asbestos, in Table 2), as may various other causative factors. Some of the benefits of control of certain other causes of lung cancer may therefore be attainable indirectly by reducing exposure to tobacco. Since, however, effective exposures to tobacco are currently increasing in many countries (and, even where they are decreasing, the immediate decreases are unlikely to be

[3] In the study of Cederlöf *et al.* (1975), in Sweden, pipe smokers had the same ten-fold excess risk of lung cancer that cigarette smokers had, which rather suggests that the smallness of the effects in the UK or the USA might be due more to traditions of pipe smoking than to the pharmacology of the smoke – and, it is unlikely that such traditions are themselves *wholly* determined by pharmacological factors.

Table 2. Multiplicative effects of heavy exposure to asbestos and of smoking on lung cancer risks[a]

	Relative risk of lung cancer for	
	Nonsmokers	Smokers
No known asbestos exposure	1 (reference category)	11
Heavy asbestos exposure (prolonged employment as a lagger before 1968 US dust controls were introduced)	5	53

[a] Data from Selikoff (1981). Note that although such heavy exposure to asbestos is no longer permitted in many countries, places where heavy occupational exposures do still occur may offer excellent opportunities for limited disease prevention, since even if the workers do not smoke (so the excess risk of bronchial carcinoma is low) the risk of mesothelioma, which does not depend on synergy with tobacco, will still be high.

enormous), the theoretical possibility of avoiding exposure to tobacco clearly does not justify inaction when other substantial causes of lung cancer can be materially reduced.[4]

Miscertification of lung cancer deaths

People, and especially old people, dying of lung cancer may never have their disease recognized, and may be miscertified as dying of some other condition. Progressive rectification of such errors produces large, purely artefactual, increases in lung cancer death certification rates. In middle-aged people, such effects were substantial during the first half of the century, even in developed countries – for example, when diagnostic radiology was introduced during the 1920s it produced about a three-fold increase in British lung cancer death *certification* rates. Now, for middle-aged people, such effects are chiefly limited to the developing countries. In people in old age, however, large (e.g., two-fold) artefactual increases have continued to emerge since 1950, even in various developed countries, while among old people in many developing countries lung cancer death certification rates are still grossly unreliable [as are 'age-standardized' lung cancer death certification rates, unless standardization is to the truncated age-range 35–64 recommended by the IARC (Waterhouse *et al.,* 1976) to circumvent such difficulties].

Effects of age

The effects of the duration of smoking are so strong, and so closely correlated with age, that it is virtually impossible to determine exactly whether ageing *per se* has any independent effect on excess lung cancer rates among people of different ages who have all smoked similarly for a similar number of years, or whether it has no material effect. If age has any

[4] Apart from smoking, asbestos, ionizing radiations and combustion products, the other reliably established causes of lung cancer are bis(chloromethyl) ether, mustard gas, and certain compounds or oxidation states of arsenic, chromium and nickel (Doll & Peto, 1981).

independent effect, however, this is small compared with the effect of duration of smoking (e.g., Peto, 1985). For practical purposes, of course, the reason smoking in the teenage years produces high risks (see Fig. 2) is immaterial: it does not matter whether it acts merely through increasing the total duration of smoking by a few extra years, or whether in addition the teenage lung is slightly more, or slightly less, vulnerable than the adult lung. What chiefly matters from a public health viewpoint is that damage to the body accumulates so *those who start to smoke in their teens will be at much greater risk of being killed by tobacco in middle or old age than those who start later in life.*

CONCLUSION

Among regular cigarette smokers, the excess lung cancer risk depends strongly not only on smoking habits during the past few years, but also on smoking habits during early adult life. Hence, current lung cancer rates in countries where smoking among young adults became widespread less than half a century ago may be serious underestimates of the eventual magnitude of the tobacco-induced lung cancer hazard.

REFERENCES

Benhamou, S., Benhamou, E., Tirmarche, M. & Flamant, R. (1985) Lung cancer and use of cigarettes: a French case-control study. *J. natl Cancer Inst.*, ***74,*** 1169–1175

Cederlöf, R., Friberg, L., Hrubec, Z. & Lorich, U. (1975) *The Relationship of Smoking and Some Covariables to Mortality and Cancer Morbidity,* Stockholm, Department of Environmental Hygiene, Karolinska Institute

Cederlöf, R., Doll, R., Fowler, B., Friberg, L., Nelson, N. & Vouk, V. (1978) Air pollution and cancer: risk assessment methodology and epidemiological evidence. *Environ. Health Perspect.*, ***22,*** 1–12

Doll, R. (1971) The age distribution of cancer: implications for models of carcinogenesis (with discussion). *J. R. Statist. Soc. A*, ***134,*** 133–136

Doll, R. & Peto, R. (1976) Mortality in relation to smoking: 20 years' observations on male British doctors. *Br. med. J.*, ***ii,*** 1525–1536

Doll, R. & Peto, R. (1978) Cigarette smoking and bronchial carcinoma: dose and time relationships among regular smokers and lifelong non-smokers. *J. Epidemiol. Commun. Health*, ***32,*** 303–313

Doll, R. & Peto, R. (1981) Quantitative estimates of avoidable risks of cancer in the United States today. *J. natl Cancer Inst.*, ***66,*** 1191–1308

Garfinkel, L. (1981) Time trends in lung cancer mortality among non-smokers and a note on passive smoking. *J. natl Cancer Inst.*, ***66,*** 1061–1066

National Academy of Sciences/National Research Council (1982) *Reduced Tar and Nicotine Cigarettes: Smoking Behavior and Health,* Washington DC, National Academy Press

Peto, R. (1985) *There is no such thing as ageing, and cancer is not related to it.* In: Likhachev, A., Anisimov, V. & Montesano, R., eds, *Age-related Factors in Car-*

cinogenesis (IARC Scientific Publications No. 58), Lyon, International Agency for Research on Cancer, pp. 43–53

Selikoff, I.J. (1981) *Constraints in estimating occupational cancer mortality.* In: Peto, R. & Schneiderman, M.A., eds, *Quantification of Occupational Cancer,* Cold Spring Harbor, NY, Cold Spring Harbor Laboratory, pp. 3–17

US Department of Health and Human Services (1982) *The Health Consequences of Smoking: Cancer. A Report of the Surgeon General,* Washington DC, US Public Health Service

Wald, N., Idle, M., Boreham, J., Bailey, V. & Van Vunakis, H. (1981) Serum cotinine levels in pipe smokers: evidence against nicotine as a cause of coronary heart disease. *Lancet,* ***ii,*** 775–777

Waterhouse, J., Muir, C., Correa, P. & Powell, J., eds (1976) *Cancer Incidence in Five Continents Vol. III (IARC Scientific Publications No. 15),* Lyon, International Agency for Research on Cancer

SMOKELESS TOBACCO AND CANCER: AN OVERVIEW

C.S. MUIR & D.G. ZARIDZE[1]

*International Agency for Research on Cancer,
Lyon, France*

Tobacco is used in many ways other than smoking. This communication describes briefly those habits associated with the use of smokeless tobacco and reviews the key evidence linking most of them to an increased risk of cancer of the mouth and pharynx.

SNUFF: INHALED

In 1761, Hill described two patients with nasal cancer which was ascribed to heavy snuff inhalation (Redmond, 1970). However Harrison (1967), describing antral lesions in a series of confirmed snuff users, remarked that the use of commercial snuffs available in the UK did not appear to be associated with an increased risk of sinus cancer. Brinton *et al.* (1984) in a case-control study in North Carolina and Virginia (1970–1980) found an increased relative risk of 3.1 for adenocarcinoma of the nasal cavity and sinuses and of 1.9 for squamous-cell carcinoma in snuff users in the USA, but the snuff was 'dipped' (see below) rather than inhaled.

The snuffs currently used for inhalation in Europe and North America, denoted as dry (Scotch) snuff, comprise powdered tobacco and a variety of additives which blenders guard secret. In South Africa, the snuffs used by the Bantu peoples comprise tobacco leaves admixed with the ash of aloes *(Liliaceae* family), oil, lemon juice and a variety of herbs. Keen *et al.* (1955) obtained a history of prolonged and heavy use of these snuffs in 80% of patients with cancer of the maxillary sinus compared to 34% in persons with cancer at other sites. It has been suggested that the relatively high nickel and chromium content of these snuffs, as well as their benzo[*a*]pyrene content may explain part of their carcinogenic action (Baumslag *et al.*, 1971).

SNUFF: 'DIPPED'

Snuff 'dipping' is the name given in the southern USA to the habit of placing snuff between cheek and gum. The highly alkaline snuff used for this purpose is termed wet. The

[1] Present address: All-Union Cancer Research Center of the Academy of Medical Sciences of the USSR, Kashirskoye shosse 24, Moscow 115478, USSR.

Table 1. Relative risk (RR) for cancers of oral cavity and pharynx associated with snuff use and smoking by 196 white women in North Carolina[a]

Habit	RR	Numbers	
		Cases	Controls
Snuff only	4.2	79	80
Smoking only	2.9	70	101
Snuff and smoking	3.3	11	14
None	1.0	36	153

[a] Adapted from Winn *et al.*, (1981)

snuff so deposited, usually many times a day, is chewed or sucked, a proportion being eventually expectorated. As early as 1915, Abbe had reported on a case of tongue cancer in a woman who habitually rubbed powdered tobacco along the lingual edge. In 1957, Wilkins and Vogler reported on persons with gingival cancer in Georgia in the USA: 23 of 44 women patients dipped snuff and 12 of 37 men either snuffed or chewed tobacco, frequencies considered much higher than expected.

The *US Cancer Mortality Atlas* (Mason *et al.*, 1975) revealed an unexpectedly high level of oral cancer in females in several southern and eastern states (Blot & Fraumeni, 1977). Investigations showed that many women employed in the textile industry, unable to smoke at work for safety reasons, had recourse to snuff.

A case-control study (Winn *et al.*, 1981) of females in North Carolina with cancers of the tongue, gum, floor of mouth, other mouth, oropharynx, hypopharynx and pharynx unspecified (*International Classification of Diseases,* 8th revision, codes 141, 143–146 and 148–149; WHO, 1967) showed considerable excess of risk for snuff dippers (Table 1). For snuff dippers only, use for 1–24 years, 25–42 years and 50 years and more carried relative risks of 14, 13 and 48 respectively for the gum and buccal mucosa. One third of snuff dippers had developed the habit by the age of 10 years; the average duration of use was 45 years.

The results for a large prospective study of about 250 000 US veterans holding Government insurance policies followed up from 1954 to 1982, whose use of chewing tobacco and snuff is known, are expected in 1986 (Winn, personal communication).

CHEWING TOBACCO

Tobacco, whether cut from a roll or plug, twist, or in the commoner loose-leaf form, is still chewed in parts of the USA and elsewhere. Few of the published studies have taken smoking into account and many of the chewers probably had both habits. Williams and Horm (1977) conducted a population-based case-control study based on the interview of a random sample of patients from the Third National Cancer Survey of the USA. Controls were persons with other cancers – lung, larynx and bladder excluded. Among men, use of chewing tobacco and snuff was strongly associated with cancer of the gum and mouth, but not with cancer of the lip or tongue. Controlling for age, race and smoking, a highly significant relative risk of 3.9 was observed for moderate use; for heavy use, the relative risk was 6.7 (not significant). Brinton *et al.* (1984) found, however, a relative risk of 0.7 for tobacco chewing in a case-control study using hospital and death certificate controls.

In recent years, tobacco chewing and snuff-dipping habits have increased among US college students, especially athletes. For example, in a survey of 1119 high-school students, Greer and Poulsen (1983) found that 117 (11%) used 'smokeless tobacco'; among these, 43% had oral mucosal lesions in the labial groove in the form of hyperkeratotic or erythroplakic areas. The tobacco was kept in the mouth for from one to three hours daily.

NASS

The word *nass* means a state of oblivion. The use of *nass* is widespread in Soviet Central Asia, northern Iran, and parts of Pakistan and Afghanistan *(nasswar)*. *Nass* is a mixture of variable composition and usually contains tobacco (50%), wood ash (20–30%), lime (9–10%) and oil (10–15%) (Table 2). In some areas, lime is not added to *nass* (Paches & Milievskaya, 1980). In Afghanistan, cardamom oil and menthol are added to the mixture.

Akin in many ways to Bantu snuff, *nass* is placed in the oral cavity. In Chimkent (Kazakh SSR), 60% of users place the *nass* under the tongue and 40% between the lower lip and the gums (Nugmanov & Baimakanov, 1970). In Djambul in the same republic, 96% are said to place the *nass* between the lower lip and the gums (Alexandrova, 1970), whereas in Samarkand (Uzbek SSR), most place the mixture under the tongue (Zaridze *et al.*, 1985). Depending on the republic, sex and age, some 5–50% of the population are *nass* users.

The habitual use of *nass* is associated with oral leukoplakia (Table 2).

Table 2. Frequency of oral leukoplakia in *nass* users and smokers, Djambul, Kazakh SSR

Habit	No.	% with leukoplakia
Nass[a]	289	7.3
Smoking[a]	243	2.1
Neither habit[a]	1480	0.5
Nass[b]	1510	6.5
Neither habit[b]	4674	0.3

[a] Data from Alexandrova (1970)
[b] Data from Chasanov & Fasiev (1970)

Zaridze *et al.* (1985) presented data in which the relative risk for oral leukoplakia in smokers, *nass* users, and *nass* users who also smoked was examined (Table 3). Relative risks were significantly elevated in *nass* users and in smokers; the combined habits were accompanied by an additive increase in risk.

Leukoplakia usually occurs more frequently at the sites within the oral cavity that are in direct contact with *nass* (Zaridze *et al.*, 1985). There seems little doubt that this habit not only increases the risk of leukoplakia, as does betel-quid chewing (see below), but is also associated with oral cancer. In a study of 93 oral cancer cases and 247 controls, Nugmanov and Baimakanov (1970) found that 30% of cancer patients were *nass* users, compared to only 8% of controls. Chasanov (1965), in a series of 248 oral cancers in Bukhara (Uzbek

Table 3. Relative risks (95 % confidence intervals) for oral leukoplakia associated with use of *nass* with and without smoking in 1569 men aged 55–69 years in Samarkand, Uzbek SRR [a]

Habit	Relative risk	
	Nonsmoker	Smoker
Non-user of *nass*	1.0	7.8 (4.4–14.2)
Nass user	5.6 (3.4–9.5)	11.5 (5.4–24.3)

[a] Data from Zaridze *et al.* (1985)

SSR), noted that their distribution followed that of the use of *nass*, namely: floor of mouth, 25%; tongue, 49%; palate, 17%; cheek, 17%; and alveolar ridge, 1%.

BETEL QUID

The chewing of the betel quid, with or without tobacco, is a very widespread habit in the Indian sub-continent, South-East Asia and parts of Oceania. The habit is of great antiquity, tobacco being added from the sixteenth century onwards. The basic quid comprises the leaf of the betel vine *(Piper betle),* sliced or shaved areca nut from the so-called betel palm *(Areca catechu),* and powdered slaked lime, to which are added one or more of a wide variety of additives (gambier, catechu, cardamom, cloves, aniseed, etc.) which frequently depend on locality (for an exhaustive review see Peeters, 1970). The method of preparation of ingredients varies and this may entail differences in chemical composition. For example, the uncured areca nuts used in Assam have a much higher content of tannin and arecoline than those used elsewhere.

The leaf contains the essential oil eugenol (a weak animal carcinogen), terpenes and potassium nitrate, but the main pharmacological effect comes from the alkaloids in the areca nut, mainly the arecoline present at a level of 0.1%. It is this alkaloid which induces a sensation of well-being as well as sweating and a considerable increase in saliva output.

There is still debate as to whether the habit as outlined above is carcinogenic. However when tobacco (usually of the sun-dried variety) is added to the chew, the risk of oral and,

Table 4. Relative risks of oral cancer in chewers and nonchewers in the case-control studies of Orr (1933) and Hirayama (1966)

Frequency of chewing	Relative risk	
	Orr study	Hirayama study
Never	1 [a]	1
Occasional	5	8
3–5 times per day	18	15
>5 times per day	34	18
Sleeps with quid in mouth	200 [a]	63

[a] Risk estimate based on two cases

probably, oropharyngeal, hypopharyngeal and oesophageal cancer is substantially increased.

One of the first case-control studies ever conducted, that by Orr (1933) in Travancore, South India, showed not only very large increases in the relative risk for oral cancer but also a strong dose-response. It is of interest to compare the results of Orr, who contrasted the habits of 100 cases of oral cancer with those of 100 controls (how these were chosen is not stated) without cancer, with those obtained by Hirayama (1966), who interviewed 545 cases and 440 controls, over 30 years later – the similarity is quite remarkable (Table 4), suggesting that Orr's controls were properly chosen.

Unfortunately Orr (1933) did not distinguish between chewers who included tobacco in the quid and those who did not, nor did he mention whether smoking was prevalent at the time, let alone by those in his study. Hirayama (1966) addressed this question and the salient findings are presented in Table 5.

Table 5. Relative risk and attributable risk % due to betel-quid chewing, with or without tobacco, in smokers and nonsmokers [a]

Habit	Relative risk	Attributable risk %
No habit	1	–
Smoking only (S)	4	67
Betel-quid chewing only (B)	3	22
B+S	4	50
Betel quid chewed with tobacco (T)	15	89
B+T+S	22	92

[a] Data from Hirayama (1966)

From Table 5 it is clear that smoking and chewing of the tobacco-less betel quid are associated with modest increases in risk of about the same order. Addition of tobacco to the quid increases risk very substantially and if this category of chewers also smoke there is a small incremental risk.

The data of Sanghvi *et al.* (1955) can be interpreted as showing that the combined habit of chewing and smoking is somewhat more carcinogenic for the oropharynx and hypopharynx than for the mouth. In this pioneering paper, however, betel-quid chewers who included tobacco in the quid were not separated from those who did not.

The findings are thus consistent: oral use of smokeless tobacco, whether prepared industrially or by artisanal means, increases the risk of oral cancer (IARC, 1985).

OTHER HABITS

There are numerous other ways in which tobacco is used – several are mentioned below. In general, their carcinogenicity has not been formally studied.

Mishri

Mishri is prepared by heating sun-dried Indian tobacco on a heated metal plate until it turns black. The powder prepared thereafter is used for cleaning the teeth. The habit is usually practised by women and may give rise to habituation, users applying and retaining *mishri* in the mouth several times a day.

Khaini

Powdered sun-dried Indian tobacco and lime are the main ingredients of *khaini*. The powder, like snuff, is placed between cheek and gum and allowed to dissolve away rather than being chewed. This habit has been linked with oral cancer (Khanolkar & Suryabai, 1945).

Zarda, kiwan

During *zarda* manufacture tobacco leaf is first broken into small pieces and boiled in water with lime and spices. The residue is dried and coloured with vegetable dyes. To prepare *kiwan,* the leaves are soaked and boiled in rose-water and spices. The mixture is allowed to macerate and pills or granules prepared.

Gudakhu

This is a paste consisting of sun-dried tobacco, molasses and other ingredients used mainly for cleaning teeth in Orissa and southern Bihar, India.

Shammah

This mixture of powdered tobacco leaf, carbonate of lime and ash is used in parts of southern Saudi Arabia. Some 68% of *shammah* users have leukoplakic lesions at the point of contact and in a series of 29 biopsies of such lesions squamous-cell carcinoma was diagnosed in seven (Salem *et al.,* 1984).

DISCUSSION

The foregoing brief review[2] outlines the evidence linking most of the habits involving the use of smokeless tobacco to cancer, cancer which usually arises at the point of contact. Unfortunately, many of the epidemiological studies do not separate such tobacco habits from smoking and a proportion do not define the sites of cancer studied precisely. Thus it is not always easy to decide what is meant by 'oral cancer'.

These habits are far from being esoteric curiosities in that they are very widely practised by large numbers of people, possibly as many as 400 million, and give rise to an estimated 100 000 and 50 000 cancers each year in males and females respectively (Parkin *et al.,* 1985).

[2] For further details, including manufacture, consumption statistics, particulars of other epidemiological studies, the chemistry of the substances mentioned, the results of animal testing for carcinogenicity and of mutagenicity assays, etc., see Volume 37 of the *IARC Monographs* (IARC, 1985).

The preparation of snuff and chewing tobacco in the USA is on an industrial scale, some 40 million lb of snuff being produced in 1980. Estimates of the number of current users of smokeless tobacco range from 7–22 million (Squier, 1984). In the Orient, however, much of the preparation of the betel quid and its components is at the artisan level and production figures are difficult to obtain. Nonetheless, the sums spent on the habit must be relatively very large.

Perusal of a series of records of the Bombay Cancer Registry, which collects information on selected habits from all cancer patients, indicates that the average daily expenditure on the betel quid is stated to be 50 paise or 15 rupees a month. This represents a very high proportion of income as the monthly family cash income is frequently given as 150 rupees. The poor man's luxury is expensive. (Permission to examine these records was kindly given by Dr D. Jussawalla, Director of the Bombay Cancer Registry.)

For control measures to have a chance of success the motives underlying adoption of a habit should be understood. Much work has been done in this area for smoking but very little for the oral use of tobacco.

Schonland and Bradshaw (1969) examined these questions in Indian betel-quid chewers in Natal Province, South Africa. The effects as perceived by habitués (tobacco is not a common ingredient in the chew) are listed in Table 6. The results are of the greatest interest in that over one-third were chewing by force of habit. More females considered the habit good for health than considered it pleasurable. Paradoxically, health reasons were often advanced to explain diminution or cessation of habit.

Burton-Bradley (1979) writing from Papua New Guinea, where tobacco is rarely added to the chew, although concomitant smoking is common, refers to arecadainism or addiction to the areca nut alkaloids, and is of the opinion that to give this habit up may lead to others which are more harmful.

However, arecoline may not be without its dangers, as in-vitro nitrosation yields 3-methylnitrosaminopropionitrile which is highly carcinogenic for the experimental animal (Wenke & Hoffmann, 1983).

Mehta *et al.* (1982) have shown that, in the setting of the Indian village, it is possible to influence behaviour and reduce the frequency of betel-quid chewing, and Warnakulasuriya *et al.* (1984) have shown in Sri Lanka that paramedical personnel can be trained to reliably identify leukoplakia and other oral lesions with a view to referral for

Table 6. Effects of betel-quid chewing as perceived by chewers, by sex, in Natal Province, South Africa [a]

Effect	% observing effect	
	Men	Women
Soothing	40	30
Stimulating	9	12
Both above effects	12	15
No effect	39	32

[a] Data from Schonland & Bradshaw (1969). Numbers in sample: 77 men, 479 women

treatment. It remains to be seen whether these pioneering efforts are applicable on a wider scale and at what cost.

Improvement of diet is likely to reduce risk as Notani and Sanghvi (1976) and Jafarey *et al.* (1977) suggest. However, in many parts of the world it is the poorest who are most likely to have an oral tobacco habit and least likely to have an adequate diet. Winn *et al.* (1984) noted that fruit and vegetable consumption reduced risk in cigarette smokers and those without tobacco habits, but not, apparently, in snuff dippers.

The tobacco companies, faced with lower sales of cigarettes in the developed countries are now, despite clear evidence of the carcinogenicity of the habit, promoting the use of chewing snuff, the product being sold in the form of sachets for oral use (Cameron, 1985). If the sale of these products, which do not carry any health warning, is allowed to continue, the toll of periodontal disease and oral cancer will be high.

REFERENCES

Abbe, R. (1915) Cancer of the mouth: The case against tobacco. *N.Y. med. J.*, ***102,*** 1–2

Alexandrova, H.M. (1970) *Role of nass in the development of pathological changes in the mouth.* In: *Epidemiology of Malignant Tumours,* Alma-Ata, Nauka, pp. 243–246

Baumslag, N., Keen, P. & Petering, H.G. (1971) Carcinoma of the maxillary antrum and its relationship to trace metal content of snuff. *Arch. environ. Health,* ***23,*** 1–5

Blot, W.J. & Fraumeni, J.F. (1977) Geographic patterns of oral cancer in the United States: etiologic implications. *J. chron. Dis.,* ***30,*** 745–757

Brinton, L.A., Blot, W.J., Becker, J.A., Winn, D.M., Browder J.P., Farmer, J.C. & Fraumeni, J.F. (1984) A case-control study of cancers of the nasal sinuses and paranasal sinuses. *Am. J. Epidemiol.,* ***119,*** 896–906

Burton-Bradley, B.G. (1979) Arecaidinism. Betel chewing in transcultural perspective. *Can. J. Psychiatry,* ***24,*** 481–488

Cameron, D. (1985) Warning against US tobacco sachets. *The Scotsman,* July 26 1985, Edinburgh

Chasanov, T.K. (1965) *Cancer of the oral mucosa in relation to use of nass.* In: *Problems of Geographic Pathology of Oropharyngeal Tumours,* Alma-Ata, Nauka, pp. 84–87

Chasanov, T.K. & Fasiev, K.T. (1970) *Epidemiological study of oral precancer in the Bukhara region of Uzbekistan.* In: *Epidemiology of Malignant Tumours,* Alma-Ata, Nauka, pp. 236–238

Greer, R.O. & Poulsen, T.C. (1983) Oral tissue alteration associated with the use of smokeless tobacco by teen-agers. Part 2, Clinical findings. *Oral Surg.,* ***56,*** 275–284

Harrison, D.F.N. (1967) *Snuff – its use and abuse: An essay on nasal physiology.* In: Muir, C.S. & Shanmugaratnam, K., eds, *Cancer of the Nasopharynx,* Copenhagen, Munksgaard, pp. 119–123

Hirayama, T. (1966) An epidemiological study of oral and pharyngeal cancer in central and South-East Asia. *Bull. World Health Organ.,* ***34,*** 41–69

IARC (1985) *IARC Monographs on the Evaluation of the Carcinogenic Risk of Chemicals to Humans,* Vol. 37, *Tobacco Habits Other than Smoking; Betel-Quid and Areca-Nut Chewing; and Some Related Nitrosamines,* Lyon

Jafarey, N.A., Mahmoud, Z. & Zaidi, S.H.M. (1977) Habits and dietary pattern of cases of carcinoma of the oral cavity and pharynx. *J. Pak. Med. Assoc.*, ***27,*** 340–343

Keen, P., de Moor, N.G., Shapiro, M.P. & Cohen, L. (1955) The aetiology of respiratory tract cancer in the South African Bantu. *Br. J. Cancer,* ***9,*** 528–538

Khanolkar, V.R. & Suryabai, B. (1945) Cancer in relation to usages. Three new types in India. *Arch. Pathol.,* ***40,*** 351–361

Mason, T.J., McKay, F.W., Hoover, R., Blot, W.J. & Fraumeni, J. (1975) *Atlas of Cancer Mortality for US Counties: 1950–1969 (DHEW Publication No. [NIH] 75–780),* Washington DC, Department of Health, Education, and Welfare

Mehta, F.J., Gupta, P.C., Pindborg, J.J., Bhonsk, R.B., Jalnawalla, P.N. & Sinar, P.N. (1982) An intervention study of oral cancer and precancer in rural Indian populations: A preliminary report. *Bull. World Health Organ.,* ***60,*** 441–446

Nugmanov, S.W. & Baimakanov, S.Sh. (1970) *The results of an epidemiological study of oropharyngeal tumours in Kazakhstan following the WHO projects.* In: *Epidemiology of Malignant Tumours.* Alma-Ata, Nauka, pp. 227–231

Notani, P.N. & Sanghvi, L.D. (1976) Role of diet in cancers of the oral cavity. *Ind. J. Cancer,* ***13,*** 156–160

Orr, I.M. (1933) Oral cancer in betel nut chewers in Travancore. Its aetiology, pathology and treatment. *Lancet,* ***ii,*** 575–580

Paches, A.I. & Milievskaya, I.L. (1980) *Epidemiological study of cancer of the mucous membrane of the oral cavity in the USSR.* In: Levin, D.L., ed., *Cancer Epidemiology in the USSR and USA (NIH Publication No. 80-2044),* Bethesda, MD, US Department of Health and Human Services, pp. 177–184

Parkin, D.M., Stjernswärd, J. & Muir, C. (1984) Estimates of the worldwide frequency of twelve major cancers. *Bull. World Health Organ.,* ***62,*** 163–182

Peeters, A. (1970) *La Chique de Betel. Etude Ethnologique [Betel quid. Ethnological study],* Volume I, Thesis, University of Paris

Redmond, D.E. (1970) Tobacco and cancer: The first clinical report, 1761. *New Engl. J. Med.,* ***282,*** 18–23

Salem, G., Juhl, R. & Schiodl, T. (1984) Oral malignant and premalignant changes in 'Shammah' – users from the Gizam Region, Saudi Arabia. *Acta odont. Scand.,* ***42,*** 41–45

Sanghvi, L.D., Rao, K.C.M. & Khanolkar, V.R. (1955) Smoking and chewing of tobacco and relation to cancer of the upper alimentary tract. *Br. med. J.,* ***i,*** 1111–1114

Schonland, M. & Bradshaw, E. (1969) Upper alimentary tract cancer in Natal Indians with special reference to the betel-chewing habit. *Br. J. Cancer,* ***23,*** 670–682

Squier, C.A. (1984) Smokeless tobacco and oral cancer: A cause for concern? *Ca Cancer J. Clin.,* ***34,*** 242–247 (and following Editor's Note)

Warnakulasuriya, K.A.A.S., Ekanayeke, A.W.I., Sivayoham, S., Stjernsward, J.J., Pindborg, J., Sobin, L.H. & Perera, K.S.G.P. (1984) Utilisation of primary health care workers for early detection of oral cancer and pre-cancer cases in Sri Lanka. *Bull. World Health Organ.,* ***62,*** 243–250

Wenke, G. & Hoffmann, D. (1983) A study of betel quid carcinogenesis. I. On the in-vitro *N*-nitrosation of arecoline. *Carcinogenesis,* ***4,*** 169–172

Wilkins, S.A. & Vogler, W.R. (1957) Cancer of the gingiva. *Surg. Gynecol. Obstet.,* ***105,*** 145–152

Williams R.R. & Horm, H.W. (1977) Association of cancer sites with tobacco and alcohol consumption and socio-economic status of patients: Interview study from the Third National Cancer Survey. *J. natl Cancer Inst.*, ***58,*** 525–547

Winn, D.M., Blot, W.J., Shy, C.N., Pickle, L.W., Tolodo, A. & Fraumeni, J.F. (1981) Snuff dipping and oral cancer among women in the Southern United States. *New Engl. J. Med.*, ***304,*** 745–749

Winn D.M., Ziegler, R.G., Pickle, L.W., Gridley, J., Blot, W.J. & Hoover, R.W. (1984) Diet in the aetiology of oral and pharyngeal cancer among women from the Southern United States. *Cancer Res.*, ***44,*** 1216–1222

WHO (1967) *International Classification of Diseases. 1965 Revision. Manual of the International Statistical Classification of Diseases, Injuries and Causes of Death,* Vol. I, Geneva

Zaridze, D.G., Kuvshinov, J.P., Matiakin, E., Polakov, B.I., Boyle, P. & Blettner, M. (1985) Chemoprevention of precancerous lesions of the mouth and oesophagus in Uzbekistan, USSR. Proceedings of the Fourth Symposium on Epidemiology and Cancer Registries in the Pacific Basin, Hawaii, January 16–20. *Natl Cancer Inst. Monograph* (in press)

CIGARETTE SMOKING AND CARDIOVASCULAR DISEASES[1]

R.S. PAFFENBARGER, Jr[2] & R.T. HYDE

Stanford University School of Medicine,
Stanford, CA 94305, USA

A.L. WING & C. HSIEH

Havard University School of Public Health,
Boston, MA 02115, USA

SUMMARY

That cigarette smoking is causally associated with development of cardiovascular disease is recognized unequivocally. Epidemiological studies worldwide have documented the many pathways of influence and synergism by which this ubiquitous but artificial habit exerts its ill effects on cardiorespiratory and other body systems, leading not only to cardiovascular disease but to cancer and other ailments. Current investigations among college alumni, women, elderly, and other subgroups provide data on how various independent influences combine with smoking to establish risk and promote pathogenesis of cardiovascular disease. Their findings also confirm that cigarette smoking is one of the strongest instigators. All of this knowledge has implications for the design and implementation of effective intervention programmes.

INTRODUCTION

Cigarette smoking is a major cause of cardiovascular disease among both men and women. Numerous investigations since the mid-1950s have documented higher rates of disease and earlier mortality in cigarette smokers than in nonsmokers. Reports of the US

[1] This is Report No. XXXII in a series on chronic diseases in former college students.

[2] To whom requests for reprints should be sent.

Surgeon General (US Department of Health, Education and Welfare, 1964; US Department of Health and Human Services, 1983) have strongly urged that concerted actions be taken to reduce the causes and incidence of cardiovascular disease throughout all levels of society. Cigarette smoking contributes to development of atherosclerotic lesions, the predominant underlying cause of cardiovascular disease, and to the clinical manifestations of atherosclerotic vascular disease – coronary, cerebral, aortic and peripheral vascular disease, and sudden unexpected death. Although understanding of the precise pathophysiological basis of these clinical manifestions is incomplete, it may relate to several deleterious effects of cigarette smoking on cardiovascular health, accelerating the atherosclerotic process, promoting myocardial oxygen insufficiency, inducing an abnormal plasma lipoprotein-cholesterol profile, disrupting the haemostatic system, and lowering the threshold for ventricular fibrillation. While nicotine and carbon monoxide are the constituents of tobacco smoke most prominent as agents, hydrogen cyanide, oxides of nitrogen, and carbon disulphide also are highly suspect in the pathogenesis of coronary heart disease.

Recognition of the seriousness of the cigarette smoking problem leads to questions as to what to do about it. Strategies of intervention are becoming prominent topics of research and debate. Epidemiological studies may be of value to the establishment of realistic directions and goals for action. The present report seeks to explore some of these contributions.

So much has been published on smoking and cardiovascular disease in the past two decades that a brief initial review of several representative reports from various nations seems appropriate. Consideration will be directed to the effects of cigarette smoking, in combination with other influences, on the risks of cardiovascular disease, as revealed in current studies. These and other recent investigations have implications for intervention strategies. A few comments on trends and perceptions will complete the discussion.

REPRESENTATIVE WORLD STUDIES

Cigarette smoking and incidence of specific clinical manifestations of coronary heart disease were studied among men in the Framingham Heart Study in 1950–1968 (Kannel & Gordon, 1974). Age-adjusted rates for total coronary heart disease increased in a gradient from nonsmokers, to exsmokers, to light smokers, to more than double for smokers of a pack or more of cigarettes per day. About one-fifth of the events recorded were sudden deaths, which displayed a similar gradient. Heavy smokers had higher rates of coronary insufficiency, angina pectoris and myocardial infarction than nonsmokers. The parallel trends corroborate a real association between the level of cigarette smoking and development of coronary heart disease. Similar parallels noted in other populations lend further credence to that causal hypothesis (Friedman *et al.*, 1979; Keys, 1980; US Department of Health and Human Services, 1983; Kuller *et al.*, 1985).

Table 1 shows that studies throughout the world have implicated cigarette smoking in exacerbating the risk of coronary heart disease everywhere. The study of 290 000 US military veterans (Dorn, 1959; Kahn, 1966; Rogot & Murray, 1980) spans a time, 1917–1940, when cigarette smoking and coronary heart disease were rising. Coronary

Table 1. Relative risks[a] of death from coronary heart disease among selected populations, by cigarette smoking habit

Population studied	Composition of study (age in years)	Years of follow-up	No. of deaths	Relative risk of death	
				Nonsmoker	Smoker
USA veterans (Rogot & Murray, 1980)	290 000 men (35–84)	16	34 874	1.00	1.58
American Cancer Society (9 states) (Hammond & Horn, 1958)	188 000 men (50–70)	4	5 297	1.00	1.70
Japanese (29 health districts) (Hirayama & Hamano, 1981)	122 000 men (40+)	13	3 351	1.00	1.71
	143 000 women (40+)	13	2 653	1.00	1.78
American Cancer Society (25 states) (Hammond, 1966; Hammond & Garfinkel, 1969)	358 000 men (35–84)	4	10 771	1.00	1.24–2.81
	483 000 women (35–84)	4	4 048	1.00	1.19–2.00
Canadian veterans (Best, 1966)	78 000 men (30–90)	6	3 405	1.00	1.60
British physicians (Doll & Peto, 1976; Doll *et al.*, 1980)	34 000 men	20	3 191	1.00	1.62
	6 194 women	22	179	1.00	2.00
Swedish random sample (Cederlöf *et al.*, 1975)	27 000 men (18–69)	10	916	1.00	1.70
	28 000 women (18–69)	10	457	1.00	1.30
California (9 occupations) (Weir & Dunn, 1970)	68 000 men (35–64)	8	1 718	1.00	1.60
Swiss physicians (Gsell *et al.*, 1979)	3 749 men	18	280	1.00	1.33–2.18

[a] Age-adjusted

heart disease mortality data on these men for the 16-year follow-up, 1953–1969, showed that the risk was 58% higher for smokers than for nonsmokers.

The American Cancer Society studies of huge populations of volunteer study subjects followed for four years yielded detailed information on types of tobacco used, number of cigarettes smoked daily, age at which smoking began, inhalation practices, and other variables that might influence mortality (Hammond & Horn, 1958; Hammond, 1966). Compared with death rates among nonsmokers, more than 11 500 excess deaths were attributable to smoking, amounting to 46% in men and 41% in women.

Canadian veterans (Best, 1966) and Californians in a wide selection of occupations (Weir & Dunn, 1970) experienced similar hazards of smoking.

Among 122 000 men and 143 000 women followed in Japan for 13 years (over 3 million person-years of risk), coronary heart disease mortality ratios for smokers were 1.7 for men and 1.8 for women (Hirayama & Hamano, 1981). After adjustment for predisposing influences of social class and consumption of meat, milk and alcohol, the risk of death from coronary heart disease remained higher for smokers than for nonsmokers. The proportion of smokers was 76% in men and 10.5% in women, and their proportions of coronary heart disease mortality attributed to cigarette smoking were 34.3% and 9.5%, respectively.

When 34 400 male British physicians were followed for 20 years, 1951–1971, coronary heart disease accounted for 3191 of 10 072 deaths (Doll & Peto, 1976; Doll *et al.*, 1980). Risk of coronary heart disease mortality was 62% higher for the cigarette smokers. Risk was doubled over nonsmokers for British women physicians who smoked 15 or more cigarettes daily.

Among 55 000 Swedish men and women followed for ten years through 1972 (Cederlöf *et al.*, 1975), overall coronary heart disease mortality was 70% higher for male cigarette smokers, and 30% higher for women smokers, than for nonsmokers. A sub-sample queried in 1969 revealed that smoking habits were unchanged since 1963.

Data on 1212 deaths among 3749 Swiss physicians during an 18-year follow-up, 1955–1973, showed that coronary heart disease mortality rates increased with dosage in cigarettes smoked per day, being up 33% for use of ten or fewer, and up 118% for 35 or more smoked per day, over the rate for nonsmokers (Gsell *et al.*, 1979). This pattern is corroborated in each of the studies listed in Table 1.

MECHANISMS OF RISK

Dosage effects are consistent as indicated not only by cigarettes smoked per day but by data on inhalation, use of filters, age at beginning to smoke, years of smoking, cessation of smoking, and risks to nonsmokers in the vicinity of cigarette smokers (passive or secondary exposure). The dose-dependent influence of cigarette smoking on coronary heart disease risk is considered strong evidence that the relationship between the cigarette habit and coronary heart disease is causal.

Cigarette smoking and atherosclerosis

The epidemiological evidence linking cigarette smoking and cardiovascular diseases is reinforced by pathological findings that smoking aggravates and accelerates development of the underlying lesions and occlusive events in coronary, cerebral, aortic and peripheral arteries (Auerbach *et al.*, 1965, 1976; Strong & Richards, 1976; McMillan, 1978; McGill, 1979). A variety of studies have shown more severe atherosclerotic change in smokers than in nonsmokers, and a concomitant increase in the degree of both macroscopic and microscopic pathological change with the amount of cigarette smoking. In addition, some evidence exists to incriminate smoking in altering the serum lipoprotein profile in ways that increase the development of atherosclerosis, e.g., reduction of the high-density lipoprotein cholesterol. Smoking affects the haemostatic system by decreasing platelet survival time and increasing platelet stickiness and tendency to aggregate. The manifold gaseous constituents in cigarette smoke have complex pharmacological and toxic effects that alter metabolism, reduce oxygen transport, lower the threshold of ventricular fibrillation, and promote the atherosclerotic process (Astrup & Kjeldsen, 1979).

COMBINED INFLUENCES ON RISK

College alumni health study

A study of cigarette smoking habits, other ways of living, and health status among male college alumni (former college students) in the USA has shown how past and present characteristics relate to risk of cardiovascular disease in middle and later life (Paffenbarger *et al.*, 1978, 1984). Data on 16 936 former students aged 35–74 years and initially free of coronary heart disease, who had entered Harvard University in the period 1916–1950, were reviewed for personal characteristics, including the cigarette habit. These had been recorded in college student health archives and in post-college, mailed questionnaires returned by alumni in 1962 or 1966. Follow-up data were obtained from repeat questionnaires in 1972 for nonfatal coronary heart disease and from official death certificates through 1978 for fatal cardiovascular disease. The overall experience represented by this study population spans the twentieth century from 1900 to the present, as in 1978 the ages of surviving study subjects ranged from 45-85 years.

During the follow-up interval of six or ten years (1966 or 1962 to 1972), there were 572 first attacks of coronary heart disease, 357 nonfatal and 215 fatal. Incidence rates for coronary heart disease were computed per 10 000 man-years. Overall, the risk for smokers was 68% higher than that for nonsmokers. Mortality rates for fatal cardiovascular diseases were computed similarly for the 12–16-year follow-up from 1966 or 1962 to 1978, in which there were 640 deaths from some form of cardiovascular disease. Excess mortality risks for smokers over nonsmokers were 77% for total cardiovascular disease, 78% for coronary heart disease, 52% for stroke, and 100% (double) for other cardiovascular diseases.

Table 2 shows age-adjusted rates and relative risks of total coronary heart disease and fatal cardiovascular disease, for their respective follow-up intervals, by level of cigarette smoking habit. Prevalence for smoking categories, given as the percentage of man-years, shows a distribution of about one-quarter heavy smokers, one-third nonsmokers, and one-quarter exsmokers. For coronary heart disease, as the number of cigarettes smoked per

Table 2. Age-adjusted rates and relative risks of coronary heart disease and cardiovascular death among Harvard College alumni, by cigarette smoking habit

No. of cigarettes smoked per day	Prevalence in man-years (%)	No. of cases	Cases per 10 000 man-years	Relative risk of disease	*p* for trend
Coronary heart disease (nonfatal and fatal), 1962–1972					
20+	28	179	70.9	1.82	
10–19	6	40	67.2	1.72	
1–9	5	26	48.4	1.24	<0.0001
0	37	178	39.0	1.00	
Former	25	90	42.9	1.10	
All cardiovascular disease (fatal), 1962–1978					
20+	27	214	49.2	1.91	
10–19	6	38	35.9	1.39	
1–9	5	29	30.7	1.19	<0.0001
0	38	208	25.8	1.00	
Former	24	84	22.1	0.86	

day increases from none to a pack or more, a gradient increase in risk to smokers over nonsmokers is seen ranging steadily upward to nearly double (82%) in an evidently dose-dependent trend. Exsmokers have a slightly higher risk (10%) than nonsmokers. The pattern is similar for fatal cardiovascular disease. If the difference for exsmokers is meaningful, it may imply that some may have improved their lifestyle in other respects also.

Figure 1 presents a series of graphic cross-tabulations of cigarette smoking habit with other alumnus characteristics (blood pressure status, physical activity, body weight-for-height, and history of parental coronary heart disease) for which cardiovascular mortality rates were computed (shown as numbers on tops of bars). Numbers of deaths are given in a corresponding key beneath each cross-tabulation. Breakpoints were chosen to provide three levels of each characteristic for comparison. Relative risks were established by assigning 1.00 to the death rate for the presumed highest-risk combination, represented by the back corner bar in each cross-tabulation. Mortality trends are sought as the influence of each characteristic is assessed, holding constant the influences of age and the paired characteristic. This permits identification of any confounding of influences, or any gradient effect of contemporary cigarette habit with these other alumnus characteristics.

Three categories of cigarette smoking level were set: nonsmoker (61% of man-years of observation), smoking less than one pack a day (11%), and smoking one or more packs a day (28%). Blood pressure categories consisted of normotensive alumni with student systolic blood pressure below 130 mm Hg (70%), normotensive alumni with student systolic blood pressure of 130 mm Hg or higher (21%), and alumni with physician-diagnosed hypertension (9%). Physical activity was expressed in kilocalories per week, calculated as an estimate of leisure-time energy expended in walking, stair climbing, and sports play; then groups were established as alumni expending 2000 or more kilocalories per week (40% of man-years), 500–1999 kilocalories per week (45%), and less than 500 kilocalories per week (15%). Weight-for-height groups were determined by body mass index (Quetelet's index; 1000 × weight in pounds divided by height in inches squared) and classified as men with an index below 34 units (38% of man-years), 34–35 units (25%), and 36 units or more (37%). The three categories for parental history of coronary heart disease identified alumni having neither parent with such a history (64% of man-years), those having one parent with coronary heart disease (33%), and those having both parents afflicted (3%).

Figure 1A gives rates and relative risks of fatal cardiovascular disease by alumnus cigarette habit cross-tabulated with student and alumnus blood pressure status. For normotensive alumni, risk was 10–20% lower with decreasing amounts smoked, irrespective of whether student systolic blood pressure was below 130 mm Hg or higher. Among alumni with physician-diagnosed hypertension, however, the relative risk of fatal cardiovascular disease was reduced by nearly one half (relative risk, 0.55) when smoking level was decreased from heavy (a pack or more per day) to none. The effect of the cigarette habit on risk of fatal cardiovascular disease is strong and independent of the influence of hypertension, which is even stronger.

At each level of cigarette smoking in Figure 1B there was a decline in cardiovascular disease mortality as leisure-time exercise increased and when the data were adjusted for the influence of smoking, exercise continued to be inversely related to death. Cigarette habit is directly related to cardiovascular disease mortality when exercise is held constant.

Fig. 1. Death rates and relative risks of cardiovascular disease per 10 000 man-years of observation among Harvard University alumni, by cross-tabulations of cigarette smoking habit and (A) blood pressure status, (B) physical activity index (kilocalories per week), (C) body mass index (1000 × weight in pounds divided by height in inches squared), and (D) history of parental coronary heart disease. Death rates are given on top of bars, and corresponding numbers of deaths in the diamond keys. A relative risk of 1.00 is assigned to the paired combination with presumed highest risk (each back-corner bar)

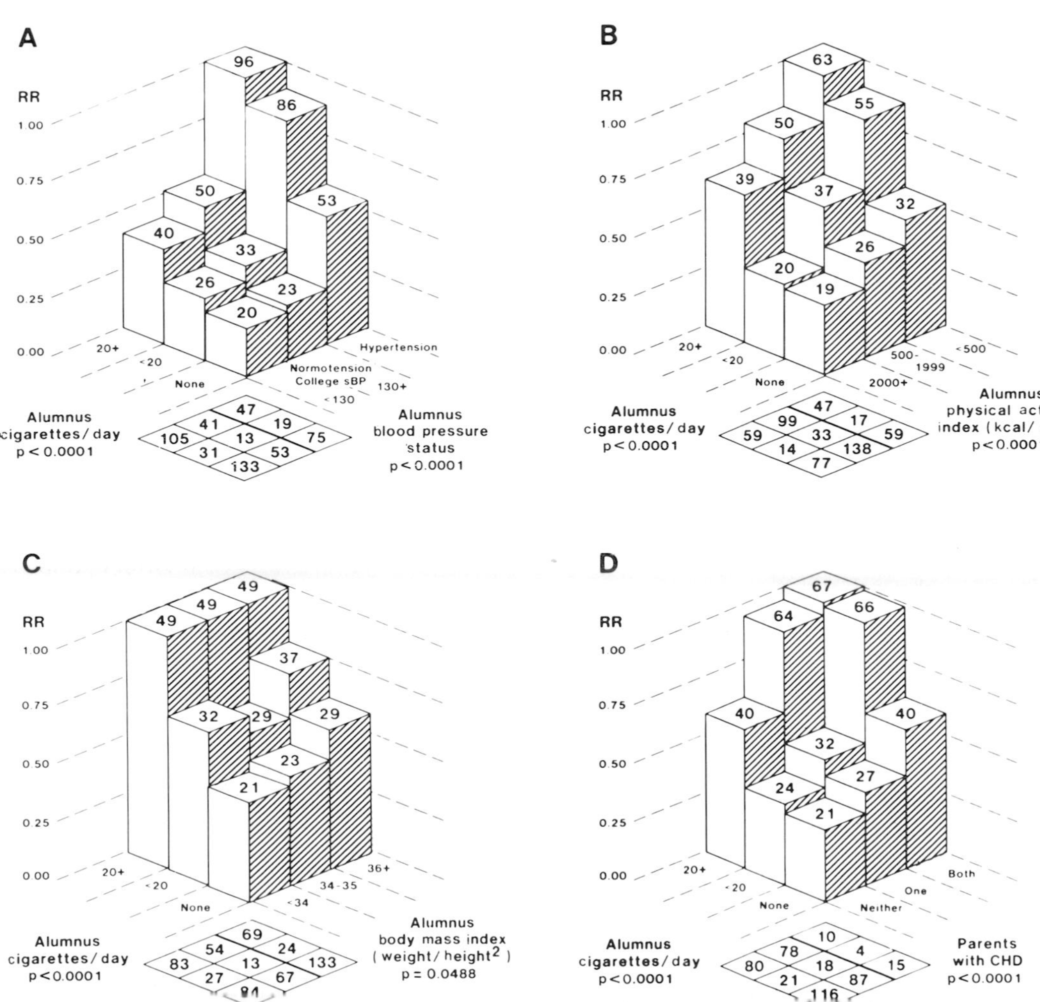

The most physically active nonsmokers had only 30% as much fatal cardiovascular disease as the sedentary heavy smokers, and the least physically active nonsmokers 52%.

Figure 1 C shows that cardiovascular disease mortality is related directly to the cigarette habit when body mass index is held constant. If smoking is held constant, risk of fatal cardiovascular disease is related directly also to weight-for-height, but less strongly than to smoking. The most lean nonsmokers (men no more than 10% over 'ideal' weight, having a body mass index below 34) had only 43% the risk of their heavy-smoking, more obese classmates, 20% or more overweight (smoking a pack or more of cigarettes per day and having a body mass index of 36 or higher). The figure shows substantial benefit from reduced smoking patterns in each weight-for-height group, but among heavy smokers there was no benefit for reduced weight-for-height.

Cross-tabulation of cardiovascular disease mortality risks by cigarette smoking and history of parental coronary heart disease is shown in Figure 1 D. To the extent that such parental history reflects a familial or hereditary tendency toward fatal cardiovascular disease in alumni, the risk implied by that tendency is cut nearly in half (0.60) even among nonsmoking alumni with a double parental history of coronary heart disease. The trend of lower cardiovascular disease mortality with reduced cigarette smoking is substantial, and the influence of parental coronary heart disease status is similarly strong. Throughout this cross-tabulation, as in each of the others, there is a consistent lowering of cardiovascular disease mortality rates as alumnus cigarette smoking declines from heavy to light to none.

Table 3 gives relative and attributable risks of total coronary heart disease in ten years of follow-up and of fatal cardiovascular disease in 16 years of follow-up, by selected characteristics known to predispose to these outcomes. The risks are derived from a multivariate analysis (Cox, 1972) and computed for the presence *versus* the absence of each adverse characteristic, with adjustments for age and each of the other characteristics listed. After allowance for each other variable, it is evident that cigarette smokers were at a 67% greater risk of coronary heart disease, nonfatal or fatal, than nonsmokers; hypertensive men had twice the risk of normotensives; sedentary alumni were at a 38% higher risk than men more physically active; heavier men were at a 23% greater risk than men more lean; and alumni with an adverse parental history of coronary heart disease had a 20% greater risk of

Table 3. Relative and attributable risks [a] of coronray heart disease and cardiovascular death among Harvard College alumni, by selected adverse characteristics

Alumnus characteristic	Prevelance in man-years (%)	Relative risk of disease (95% CL) [b]		P	Attributable risk (%)
Coronary heart disease (nonfatal and fatal), 1962–1972					
Cigarette smoking [c]	40	1.67	(1.43–1.91)	<0.0001	21
Hypertension [d]	9	1.99	(1.71–2.27)	<0.0001	8
Sedentary lifestyle [e]	61	1.38	(1.12–1.64)	0.0015	19
Overweight for height [f]	37	1.23	(0.99–1.47)	0.0755	8
History of parental CHD [g]	37	1.20	(0.96–1.44)	0.1185	7
All cardiovascular disease (fatal), 1962–1978					
Cigarette smoking [c]	39	1.84	(1.64–2.04)	<0.0001	25
Hypertension [d]	9	2.18	(1.94–2.42)	<0.0001	9
Sedentary lifestyle [e]	62	1.31	(1.09–1.53)	0.0172	16
Overweight for height [f]	37	1.18	(0.98–1.38)	0.1081	6
History of parental CHD [g]	37	1.33	(1.13–1.53)	0.0062	11

[a] Adjusted for differences in age and each of the other characteristics listed
[b] CL, confidence limits
[c] Any amount
[d] Physician-diagnosed
[e] Energy expenditure of <2000 kilocalories/week in walking, stair-climbing, and sports play
[f] 20% or more over ideal weight for height (1959 Metropolitan Life Insurance Company standards), i.e., body mass index 36+
[g] CHD, coronary heart disease, in either or both parents

developing coronary heart disease themselves than classmates whose parents were free from such affliction. Attributable risk estimates for the corresponding characteristics suggest that cigarette smoking might account for 21% of the coronary heart disease among alumni; hypertension, 8%; sedentary living, 19%; overweight, 8%; and the genetic or familial tendencies implied by parental coronary heart disease, a further 7%. If all of these adversities for alumni could have been avoided there might have been half as many attacks of coronary heart disease.

Relative and attributable risks of cardiovascular disease mortality for these same alumnus characteristics are of the same general order of magnitude as for coronary heart disease (Table 3). They indicate that there might have been 65% fewer cardiovascular disease deaths during the study interval 1962–1978 in the absence of all five characteristics, or a loss of only 224 alumni instead of the observed 640 decedents from underlying cardiovascular disease causes.

Women smokers

Current study of the relation of cigarette smoking and nonfatal myocardial infarction in women aged 25–49 years living in the north-eastern USA provides new evidence on dose-response and interaction with other personal characteristics known or suspected to predispose to infarction (Rosenberg *et al.*, 1985). This case-control study contrasted 555 women who survived first attacks with 1864 women of similar age hospitalized for a variety of conditions judged to be unrelated to cigarette smoking. The proportion of current smokers among myocardial infarction patients was 80%, as contrasted with 50% among control patients. Relative risk estimates of myocardial infarction increased steadily from 1.4 for smokers of 1–14 cigarettes per day to 2.4 for those using 15–24 cigarettes, to 5.0 for use of 25–34, to 7.0 for smokers of 35 or more cigarettes daily. Among former smokers who had abstained for at least one year, relative risks were the same as for women who had never smoked.

As shown in Table 4, risk of myocardial infarction among current oral contraceptive users was increased 23-fold for heavy smokers over nonsmokers. Women heavy smokers with a serum cholesterol level below 200 mg/dl had a five-fold increased risk of myocardial infarction over comparable nonsmokers; with higher levels the risk for smokers over nonsmokers was ten-fold greater. Furthermore, the risk of myocardial infarction was higher for smokers than nonsmokers among these women with and without such predisposing characteristics as hypertension, angina pectoris, diabetes, obesity, a tendency to time-urgency and competitiveness (so-called type A behaviour), and an adverse history of cardiovascular disease in a parent or sibling.

Elderly smokers

Among elderly (65-74 years) white males from an impoverished urban setting, current cigarette smokers were at 52% higher risk of fatal coronary heart attack in five years of follow-up over nonsmokers, exsmokers, and pipe or cigar smokers (Jajich *et al.*, 1984). The excess risk of mortality in this population of 2674 persons declined within one to five years of cessation of smoking. Smokers of all ages should be encouraged to quit (see Table 5).

Table 4. Relative risks estimates[a] of nonfatal myocardial infarction among women aged <50 years in north-eastern USA, by cigarette habit and selected characteristics [b]

Characteristic	Level	Relative risk of nonfatal myocardial infarction		
		Nonsmokers	Smokers (95% CL) [c]	
Oral contraceptive use	Current	1.00	23	(6.6–82)
	Past	1.00	6.8	(4.5–10)
	Never	1.00	4.8	(3.5–6.6)
Serum cholesterol (mg/dl)	<200	1.00	4.6	(2.5–8.7)
	200–249	1.00	12	(6.4–21)
	250+	1.00	10	(4.0–25)
HDL-cholesterol (mg/dl) [d]	<40	1.00	4.7	(2.7–8.2)
	40+	1.00	14	(8.3–25)
Type A personality	Present	1.00	6.8	(3.3–14)
	Absent	1.00	11	(6.7–17)
Family history CVD [e]	Present	1.00	7.1	(3.9–13)
	Absent	1.00	11	(6.5–18)
Hypertension	Yes	1.00	4.0	(2.4–6.7)
	No	1.00	8.0	(6.0–11)
Angina pectoris	Yes	1.00	5.1	(1.5–17)
	No	1.00	6.2	(4.8–8.0)
Diabetes mellitus	Yes	1.00	3.2	(1.2–8.7)
	No	1.00	6.7	(5.2–8.7)
Pre-menopausal		1.00	8.3	(6.1–11)
Post-menopausal		1.00	3.9	(2.5–6.0)
Body mass index	40+	1.00	5.5	(3.6–8.6)
	<40	1.00	7.1	(5.3–9.7)

[a] Age-adjusted
[b] From Rosenberg *et al.* (1985)
[c] Smokers of 25+ cigarettes per day; CL, confidence limits
[d] HDL-cholesterol, high-density lipoprotein-cholesterol
[e] CVD, cardiovascular disease

Filter cigarette risks

In the Framingham study (Castelli *et al.*, 1981) men were classified as to whether they smoked filter or nonfilter cigarettes. The 58% of men who used filtered brands had been smoking for a shorter period than the comparison group, but despite this more favourable cigarette-smoking history, their incidence rates of coronary heart disease (myocardial infarction, coronary heart disease death, or total coronary heart disease) in 14 years of follow-up showed no differences from those of nonfilter cigarette users. Findings were unchanged when rates were adjusted for differences in levels of blood pressure and serum cholesterol. Thus there was no evidence that filter cigarettes of the 1960s and 1970s conferred any protection against coronary heart disease for Framingham men. Perhaps this is not unexpected, since smokers may alter their smoking behaviour when they switch to low-yield brands to compensate for nicotine. This altered behaviour may induce accelerated atherogenesis through increased uptake of carbon monoxide, hydrogen cyanide and nitrous oxides (Astrup & Kjeldsen, 1979).

Passive smoking

The effects of passive (involuntary) smoking on nonsmokers are receiving increased attention. Aronow (1978) demonstrated that nonsmoking patients with angina pectoris exposed in a confined space to the cigarette smoke of others experienced an increase in serum carboxyhaemoglobin levels, coronary symptomatology, and electrographic changes indicative of myocardial ischaemia at lower levels of exercise testing than when not so exposed. Garland *et al.* (1985) studied 695 nonsmoking women from a retirement community in California who were classified according to their husbands' cigarette-smoking status as wives of those who had never smoked, and former and current smokers. In ten years of follow-up, nonsmoking wives of current or former smokers experienced an elevated death rate of coronary heart disease compared with nonsmoking wives of those who had never smoked. A dose-response relationship was shown for the quantity of cigarettes smoked by the husband. These findings held when adjustments were made for multiple characteristics predisposing to coronary heart disease. Although the added risk of disease among exposed wives was 14.9, the experience was small and not statistically significant ($p < 0.10$).

The issues relative to coronary heart disease are unsettled, but when passive smokers protest, their complaints against heavy smoking at close quarters often are based on more immediate irritations than remote fears of heart attack. Difficulties of determining atmospheric concentrations of toxic substances are likely to complicate the epidemiological problem of studying the patterns and intensities of involuntary exposure to cigarette smoke and of assessing any influences of subtle exposures of long duration.

TRENDS

Cessation of smoking

Table 5 summarizes several studies in which influence of cessation of cigarette smoking on risk of total coronary heart disease among men is examined in terms of interval since quitting the habit, age at time of cessation, intensity of cigarette use, and duration of use (Hammond, 1966; Hammond & Garfinkel, 1969; Cederlof *et al.*, 1975; Doll & Peto, 1976). There is a consistent gradient of reduction in risk as the interval since cessation increases, so that men who have abandoned cigarettes for a decade or more have little if any excess risk over men who have never smoked. The risk-reduction benefit is seen in all age groups and for both light and heavy smokers who have dropped the habit. Among men aged 65 years or older, percentage reduction appears less impressive than for younger men aged 30–54 but, in view of age-related rates of coronary heart disease mortality, the numbers spared would be substantial. In general, the greater the relative risk attached to cigarette smoking, the greater the benefit or reduction in risk achieved by quitting the habit.

Table 5. Relative risks of death from coronary heart disease among selected populations, by years since cigarette smoking cessation

Population studied	Years since cessation	Relative risk of death		
		Attained age (years)		
		30–54	55–64	65+
British physicians	None	3.5	1.7	1.3
(Men who smoked cigarettes	1–4	1.9	1.9	1.0
only for 5+ years;	5–9	1.3	1.4	1.3
20-year follow-up)	10–14	1.4	1.7	1.2
(Doll & Peto, 1976)	15+	1.3	1.3	1.1
	Nonsmoker	1.0	1.0	1.0
		No. of cigarettes smoked per day		
		1–19	20+	
American Cancer Society (25 states)	None	1.90	2.55	
(Men who smoked cigarettes only;	<1	1.62	1.61	
6-year follow-up)	1–4	1.22	1.51	
(Hammond, 1966; Hammond &	5–9	1.26	1.16	
Garfinkel, 1969)	10–19	0.96	1.25	
	20+	1.08	1.05	
	Nonsmoker	1.00	1.00	
		Years of smoking cigarettes		
		<20	20+	Total
Swedish random sample	None	–	–	1.7
(Men; 10-year follow-up)	1–9	0.9	1.6	1.5
(Cederlöf *et al.*, 1975)	10+	0.9	1.1	1.0
	Nonsmoker	1.0	1.0	1.0

In five worldwide intervention trials (Puska *et al.*, 1979; Hjermann *et al.*, 1981; Multiple Risk Factor Intervention Trial, 1982; Rose *et al.*, 1982; World Health Organization European Collaborative Group, 1982), cigarette smoking was reduced 10–15% more in the intervention group than in the control group. The intervention group had some 10% fewer coronary heart disease deaths than the comparable control group, but the differences within the individual trials were not significant. When the results of four of these trials were combined, however, coronary heart disease deaths were significantly less common in the intervention group than in the control group.

Chapman (1985) reports that small stop-smoking encounter groups and clinics are inept, expensive and hopeless approaches to the problem of effective intervention. He recommends massive education programmes and dedicated medical collaboration to reach the millions of smokers who must be persuaded to kick the cigarette habit. In the meantime recidivism and prevarication by subjects tend to limit the credibility of data on cessation and weaken results of many studies based on them. Nevertheless, the findings on benefits of smoking-behaviour modification are meaningful because they do echo strong evidence from other nonexperimental studies of cardiovascular disease and may forecast eventual success for broad, long-range intervention programmes.

Mortality and other patterns

Cardiovascular disease mortality has declined in the USA by 38% since 1950, while deaths from all other causes were declining by about 21% (Epstein, 1984; Feinleib, 1984). Since 1968, coronary heart disease mortality has fallen 27%, as mirrored by 280 000 fewer deaths in the following decade than would have been expected on the basis of 1968 mortality rates. The decline in cigarette smoking since the first Surgeon General's Report (US Department of Health, Education, and Welfare, 1964), 25% among men and 14% among women aged 20 years and over, together with improvement in other lifestyle habits and better blood pressure control, may explain a large segment of the decline in cardiovascular disease mortality. Feinleib (1984) has translated trends in cigarette smoking, blood cholesterol patterns and blood pressure levels into equations and related them to risk of cardiovascular death. From these he made the following predictions: (1) a 20% reduction in numbers of smokers would have induced a 10% decline in mortality; (2) a 5 mg/dl average reduction in serum cholesterol would have induced a 4% drop in mortality; and (3) a 2 mm Hg decrease in diastolic blood pressure would have induced a 9% decline in cardiovascular mortality. Together, such trends might account for a 22% reduction in cardiovascular disease death rates, very similar to the observed decline over the period concerned.

DISCUSSION

The existence of a strong adverse relationship between cigarette smoking and cardiovascular disease is no longer a topic for debate. This report has presented new data and summarized findings that may offer important contributions to the planning of effective large-scale programmes of intervention designed to minimize the cigarette habit as an element of lifestyle. Knowledge of how cigarette smoking promotes disease can be used to educate against it, and no other intervention strategy is likely to be as successful. These aspects have been considered directly or by implication throughout the report. In summary, they reveal that the potential benefits from solving the problem are as manifold as the array of hazards associated with it. Whenever cigarette smoking is abandoned to reduce risk of cardiovascular disease, cancer will be reduced, and other chronic diseases as well. After all, cigarette smoking is an artificial enemy that was created by man himself, and he has the power to destroy it.

ACKNOWLEDGEMENTS

This work was supported by Grant HL37174 from the National Heart, Lung and Blood Institute of the US Public Health Service; and by the G. Unger Vetlesen Foundation; the E.I. du Pont de Nemours Company; the Marathon Oil Foundation, Inc.; and the Mobil Foundation.

REFERENCES

Aronow, W.S. (1978) Effect of passive smoking on angina pectoris. *New Engl. J. Med.*, ***299***, 21–24

Astrup, P. & Kjeldsen, K. (1979) Model studies linking carbon monoxide and/or nicotine to arteriosclerosis and cardiovascular disease. *Prev. Med.*, ***8***, 295–302

Auerbach, O., Hammond, E.C. & Garfinkel, L. (1965) Smoking in relation to atherosclerosis of the coronary arteries. *New Engl. J. Med.*, ***273***, 775–779

Auerbach, O., Carter, H.W., Garfinkel, L. & Hammond, E.C. (1976) Cigarette smoking and coronary artery disease: A macroscopic and microscopic study. *Chest*, ***70***, 697–705

Best, E.W.R. (1966) *A Canadian Study of Smoking and Health*, Ottawa, Epidemiology Division, Health Services Branch, Biostatistics Division, Research and Statistics Directorate

Castelli, W.P., Garrison, R.J., Dawber, T.R., McNamara, P.M., Feinleib, M. & Kannel, W.B. (1981). The filter cigarette and coronary heart disease: the Framingham study. *Lancet*, ***ii***, 109–113

Cederlöf, R., Friberg, L., Hrubec, Z. & Lorich, U. (1975) *The Relationship of Smoking and Some Social Covariables to Mortality and Cancer Morbidity. A Ten-year Follow-up in a Probability Sample of 55 000 Swedish Subjects, Age 18–69*, Part 1 and Part 2, Stockholm, Department of Environmental Hygiene, The Karolinska Institute

Chapman, S. (1985) Stop-smoking clinics: A case for their abandonment. *Lancet*, ***i***, 918–920

Cox, D.R. (1972) Regression models and life tables (with discussion). *J. R. Soc. Biostat.*, ***34***, 187–200

Doll, R. & Peto, R. (1976) Mortality in relation to smoking: 20 years' observations on male British doctors. *Br. med. J.*, ***274***, 1525–1536

Doll, R., Gray, R., Hafner, B. & Peto, R. (1980) Mortality in relation to smoking: 22 years' observations on female British doctors. *Br. med. J.*, ***280***, 967–971

Dorn, H.F. (1959) Tobacco consumption and mortality from cancer and other diseases. *Public Health Rep.*, ***74***, 581–593

Epstein, F.H. (1984) Lessons from falling coronary heart disease mortality in the United States. *Postgrad. Med. J.*, ***60***, 15–19

Feinleib, M. (1984) Changes in cardiovascular epidemiology since 1950. *Bull. N. Y. Acad. Med.*, ***60***, 449–464

Friedman, G.D., Dales, L.G. & Ury, H.K. (1979) Mortality in middle-aged smokers and nonsmokers. *New Engl. J. Med.*, ***300***, 213–217

Garland, C., Barrett-Connor, E., Suarez, L., Criqui, M.H. & Wingard, D.L. (1985) Effects of passive smoking on ischemic heart disease mortality of nonsmokers: a prospective study. *Am. J. Epidemiol.*, ***121***, 645–650

Gsell, O., Abelin, T. & Wieltchnig, E. (1979) Smoking and mortality of Swiss physicians: Results after 18 years of observation (Ger.). *Bull. schweiz. Akad. med. Wiss.*, ***35***, 71–82

Hammond, E.C. (1966) Smoking in relation to the death rates of one million men and women. In: Haenszel, W., ed., *Epidemiological Approaches to the Study of Cancer and Other Chronic Diseases (Natl Cancer Inst. Monograph No. 19)*, Bethesda, MD, National Cancer Institute, pp. 127–204

Hammond, E.C. & Garfinkel, L. (1969) Coronary heart disease, stroke, and aortic aneurysm. Factors in the etiology. *Arch. Environ. Health*, ***19***, 167–182

Hammond, E.C. & Horn, D. (1958) Smoking and death rates – Report on forty-four months of follow-up of 187 783 men: II Death rates by cause. *J. Am. med. Assoc.*, ***166***, 1294–1308

Hirayama, T. & Hamano, Y. (1981) Smoking and mortality from major causes of death (Jpn.) *Eisei No Shibyo*, ***28***, 3–18

Hjermann, I., Velve Byre, K., Holme, I. & Leren, P. (1981) Effect of diet and smoking intervention on the incidence of coronary heart disease. Report from the Oslo study group of a randomized trial in healthy men. *Lancet*, ***ii***, 1303–1310

Jajich, C.L., Ostfeld, A.M. & Freeman, D. H., Jr (1984) Smoking and coronary heart disease mortality in the elderly. *J. Am. med. Assoc.*, ***252***, 2831–3834

Kahn, H.A. (1966) The Dorn study of smoking and mortality among U.S. veterans: Report on eight and one-half years of observation. In: Haenszel, W., ed., *Epidemiological Approaches to the Study of Cancer and Other Chronic Diseases (National Cancer Institute Monograph No. 19)*, Bethesda, MD, National Cancer Institute, pp. 1–125

Kannel, W.B. & Gordon, T. (1974) *The Framingham Study, Section 30. Some Characteristics Related to the Incidence of Cardiovascular Disease and Death: 18-year Follow-up (Department of Health, Education, and Welfare Publication No. NIH 74–599)*, Washington DC

Keys, A. (1980) *Seven Countries: A Multivariate Analysis of Death and Coronary Heart Disease*, Cambridge, MA, Harvard University Press

Kuller, L., Meilahn, E. & Ockene, J. (1985) Smoking and coronary heart disease. In: Connor, W.E. & Bristow, J.D., eds, *Coronary Heart Disease: Prevention, Complications, and Treatment*, Philadelphia, PA, J.B. Lippincott

McGill, H.C., Jr (1979) Potential mechanisms for the augmentation of atherosclerosis and atherosclerotic disease by cigarette smoking. *Prev. Med.*, ***8***, 390–403

McMillan, G.C. (1978) Atherogenesis: The process from normal to lesion. In: Chandler, A.B., Eurenius, K., McMillan, G.C., Nelson, C.B., Schwartz, C.J., Wessler, S., eds, *The Thrombotic Process in Atherogenesis*, New York, Plenum Press, pp. 3–10

Multiple Risk Factor Intervention Trial (1982) Risk factor changes and mortality results. *J. Am. med. Assoc.*, ***248***, 1465–1477

Paffenbarger, R.S., Jr, Wing, A.L. & Hyde, R.T. (1978) Physical activity as an index of heart attack risk in college alumni. *Am. J. Epidemiol.*, ***108***, 161–175

Paffenbarger, R.S., Jr, Hyde, R.T., Wing, A.L. & Steinmetz, C.H. (1984) A natural history of athleticism and cardiovascular health. *J. Am. med. Assoc.*, ***252***, 491–495

Puska, P., Tuomilehto, J., Salonen, J., Neittaanmaki, L., Maki, J., Virtamo, J., Nissinen, A., Koskela, K. & Takalo, T. (1979) Changes in coronary risk factors during a comprehensive five-year community programme to control cardiovascular diseases (North Karelia project). *Br. med. J.*, ***ii***, 1173–1178

Rogot, E. & Murray, A.J. (1980) Smoking and causes of death among U.S. veterans: 16 years of observation. *Public Health Rep.*, ***95***, 213–222

Rose, G., Hamilton, P.J.S., Colwell, L. & Shipley, M.J. (1982) A randomised controlled trial of anti-smoking advice: 10-year results. *J. Epidemiol. Commun. Health*, ***36***, 102–108

Rosenberg, L., Kaufman, D.W., Helmrich, S.P., Miller, D.R., Stolley, P.D. & Shapiro,

S. (1985) Myocardial infarction and cigarette smoking in women younger than 50 years of age. *J. Am. med. Assoc.*, ***253,*** 2965–2969

Strong, J.P. & Richards, M.L. (1976) Cigarette smoking and atherogenesis in autopsied men. *Atherosclerosis,* ***23,*** 451–476

US Department of Health and Human Services (1983) *The Health Consequences of Smoking: Cardiovascular Disease. A Report of the Surgeon General,* Washington DC, Public Health Service, Office on Smoking and Health

US Department of Health, Education, and Welfare (1964) *Smoking and Health Report of the Advisory Committee to the Surgeon General of the Public Health Service (PHS Publication* No. 1103), Washington DC, US Department of Health, Education, and Welfare, Public Health Service, Center for Disease Control

Weir, J.M. & Dunn, J.E., Jr (1970) Smoking and mortality: a prospective study. *Cancer,* ***25,*** 105–112

World Health Organization European Collaborative Group (1982) Multifactorial trial in the prevention of coronary heart disease: 2. Risk factor changes at two and four years. *Eur. Heart J.*, ***3,*** 184–190

SMOKING AND RESPIRATORY DISEASE EXCLUDING LUNG CANCER

H. PEACH

*Department of Community Medicine,
United Medical and Dental Schools, St Thomas' Campus
London SE1 7EH, UK*

INTRODUCTION

This paper is concerned with a group of diseases which, in the 1950s, would have been called 'chronic non-specific respiratory disease' (Ciba Foundation Guest Symposium, 1959) namely, chronic obstructive lung disease, chronic mucus hypersecretion and asthma. Specific airway diseases such as tuberculosis, sarcoidosis, pneumoconiosis and diseases of the pulmonary interstitium are excluded. Chronic obstructive lung disease, often referred to as chronic obstructive airways disease or chronic obstructive pulmonary disease, is an important burden in terms of morbidity and mortality in many economically developed countries. Chronic mucus hypersecretion, which describes a chronic productive cough independent of airflow limitation and was previously called simple and mucopurulent bronchitis (Thurlbeck, 1977), may not itself lead to mortality (Peto *et al.*, 1983) but is important in terms of morbidity.

Table 1 shows the deaths and admissions to hospital in the UK due to 'chronic bronchitis and emphysema', a term which embraces both chronic mucus hypersecretion and chronic obstructive lung disease. There is little doubt that death rates from bronchitis and emphysema are related to the number of cigarettes smoked. However, the increase in cigarette smoking over the decades before 1956 did not result in correspondingly more deaths from bronchitis, as happened with lung cancer. In the 25 years before 1956, death rates from bronchitis in men remained fairly constant, while in women there was a steady decline. Since then, the death rates in men have shown an accelerating decline. Since 1978, the decline in death rates among men and women have appeared to accelerate even more (Fig. 1), but this may be a recent certification artefact. Generally, diagnosis and methods of certification for respiratory disease have probably been more stable in the UK than in most countries, and the marked drop in mortality rates over time probably reflects a real fall in disease incidence. This fall is probably due to improvements in living standards, improvements in the control of air pollution, and possibly decreasing tar delivery from cigarettes.

Table 1. Mortality and hospital discharges for chronic bronchitis and emphysema in England and Wales, 1981[a]

	Rates per 10 000 population				
	All ages	25–44 years	45–64 years	65–74 years	75+ years
Mortality					
Men	53.03	0.73	31.29	198.32	647.00
Women	18.60	0.28	10.92	43.46	141.74
Hospital discharges					
Men	97.27	3.94	83.44	371.82	729.91
Women	40.59	4.01	46.14	96.18	167.81

[a] From Office of Population Censuses and Surveys (1981a, b)

MUCUS HYPERSECRETION

Surveys from many countries show that cigarette smokers cough more often and produce more phlegm than do nonsmokers. Even teenagers who smoke more than five cigarettes a day cough almost as much as adult cigarette smokers (Addington *et al.*, 1970; Seely *et al.*, 1971). The risk increases with number of cigarettes smoked, earlier age of starting to smoke, and depth of inhalation. That cough and phlegm usually disappear or diminish when cigarette smoking is given up shows that smoking is the main cause of these symptoms. At all ages, cigarette smokers have more chest illnesses than nonsmokers (Finklea *et al.*, 1971; Colley *et al.*, 1973). Cough, expectoration, and recurrent respiratory infections lead to much absence from work and are often treated with expensive antibiotics. Airways obstruction is often more severe during an infective episode but recovery is usual, and these episodes do not seem to accelerate the progression of chronic obstructive lung disease (Fletcher & Peto, 1977). Pipe and cigar smokers are much less affected than are cigarette smokers by cough, phlegm and recurrent chest infection (Boudik *et al.*, 1970; Comstock *et al.*, 1970; Mueller *et al.*, 1971). Morning phlegm has been found to be commoner in smokers of nonfilter cigarettes than in smokers of filter-tipped cigarettes (Rimington, 1972).

OBSTRUCTIVE LUNG DISEASE

Obstructive lung disease is as specifically related to smoking as is lung cancer. Forced expiratory volume in one second (FEV_1) falls gradually and irreversibly over several decades among both nonsmokers and smokers. The range of rates of loss of FEV_1 is much wider among smokers than nonsmokers. Some smokers suffer such unusually rapid rates of loss of FEV_1 that, if they continue to smoke, they will first become disabled, once their FEV_1 falls to about one litre, and then killed by their obstructive lung disease. If such people stop smoking their FEV_1 will not recover but their subsequent rate of loss of FEV_1 will usually revert to about that seen in nonsmokers. Thus, if susceptible smokers stop well before they are disabled, they will not die from chronic obstructive lung disease.

That there was no rise in death rates from chronic bronchitis and emphysema following the rise in tobacco consumption indicated that extrinsic factors must exist that alone or in

Fig. 1. Age and age-specific mortality rates for chronic bronchitis and emphysema in England and Wales, 1953–1983 (from Holland, 1984)

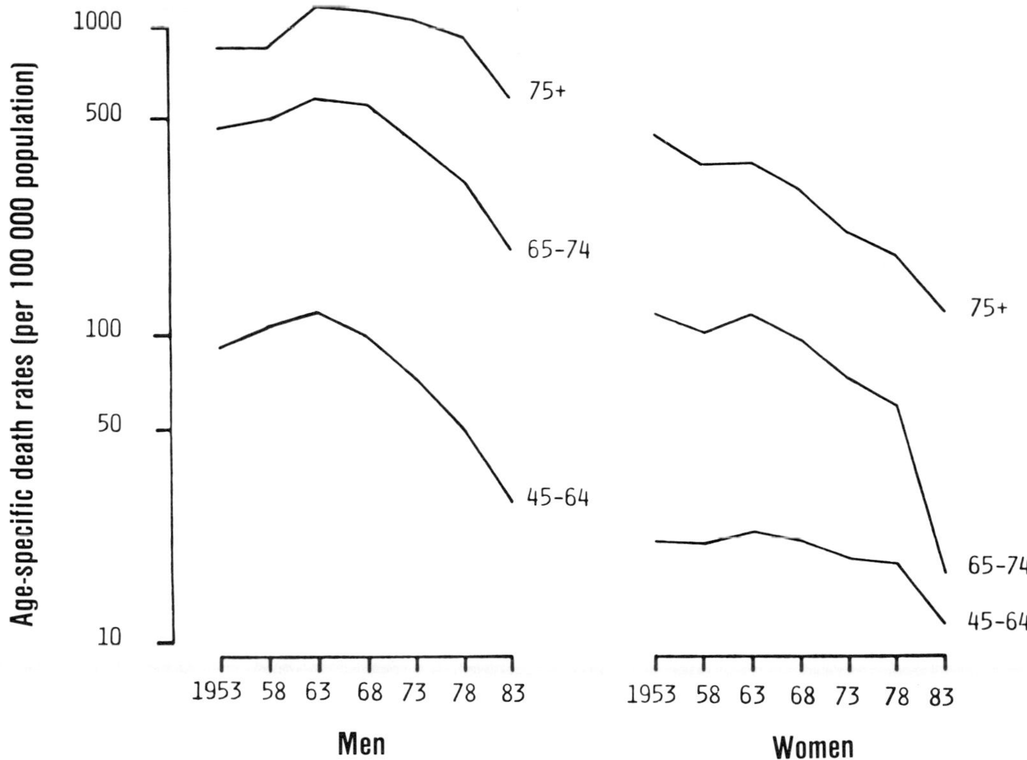

conjunction with smoking are responsible for some of the mortality from chronic bronchitis and emphysema. Studies in the UK and elsewhere have shown that chronic obstructive lung disease is more common among poorer groups in a population than among the economically better off (Reid, 1963). This appears to reflect general environmental exposures rather than specific occupational factors, since married women classified by their husband's socioeconomic status also have an excess of chronic bronchitis and emphysema (Fig. 2). Such factors might include poor housing conditions, domestic overcrowding, or indoor and outdoor air pollution, but they have never been precisely identified. Acute episodes of high-level particulate air pollution can exacerbate symptoms in susceptible groups in a population such as the elderly, the chronically ill, and, possibly also, young children. Similarly, the long-term chronic effects of exposure to high levels of air pollution have been well documented. Both these aspects of air pollution were thoroughly reviewed by Holland *et al.* (1979). In many countries, the introduction of measures to control particulate air pollution has meant that this is now a less important factor than it was in the past, except in particular populations occupationally or otherwise exposed to high levels of local pollution. It must be emphasized that, at present, only the effects of tobacco are reliably known to be of substantial importance and amenable to change.

Fig. 2. Mortality among men (□) and women (■) aged 15–64 years from chronic bronchitis and emphysema by social class in England and Wales, 1970–1972 (from Holland, 1984); N, nonmanual; M, manual

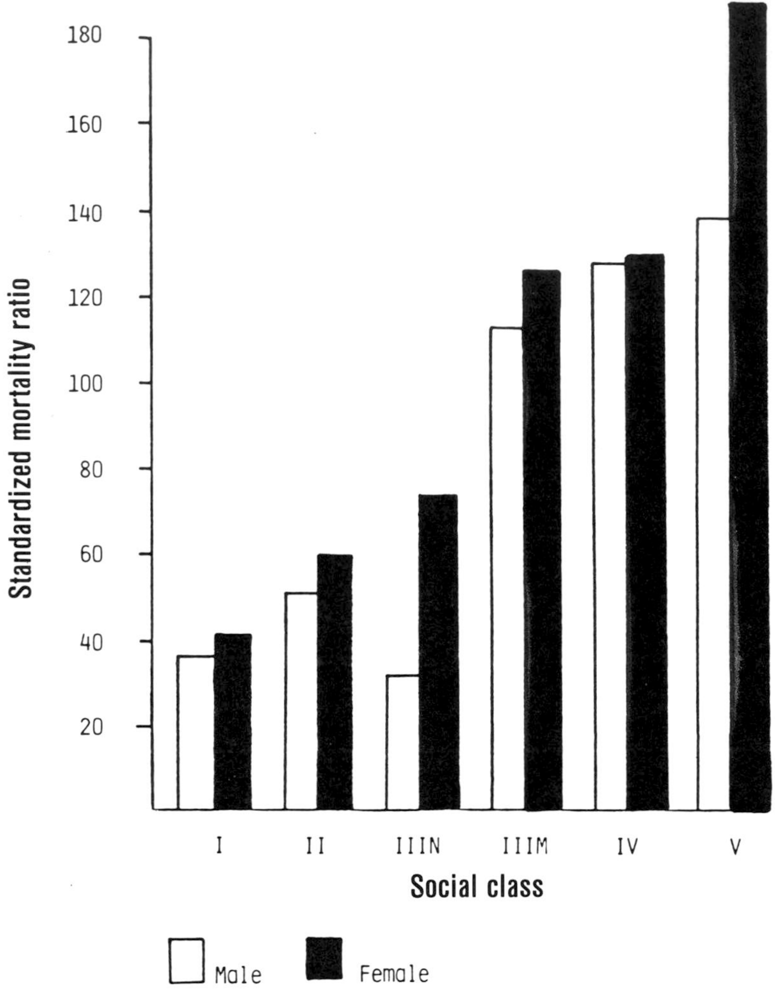

CHILDREN, RESPIRATORY DISEASE AND SMOKING

Although cough and phlegm usually disappear or diminish when cigarette smoking is given up, and the rate of loss of FEV_1 will usually revert to about that seen in nonsmokers, priority in prevention should not be given to persuading adults with chronic mucus hypersecretion or chronic obstructive lung disease to stop smoking. It is better to dissuade children from ever taking up the habit or at least from becoming regular smokers. Traditionally, smoking has been the habit of adults, but, since the late 1950s, it has been established that a measurable proportion of school children smoke regularly. Estimates of

Table 2. Annual incidence (per 100 infants) of 'bronchitis' or pneumonia in the first year of life[a]

Parental asthma or wheeze	Parental smoking habit			
	Neither	One	Both	Habit changed
Neither	6.7	9.6	13.7	8.7
One	8.9	18.0	22.3	7.4
Both	14.3	13.6	39.3	30.0

[a] From Leeder *et al.* (1976)

the prevalence of smoking one or more cigarettes per week among school children, vary from 7% of boys aged 10–11 years to over 16% in two populations of boys aged 11–14 years and up to 20–40% in youths of 14–17 years (Bewley *et al.*, 1973). The role of cigarette smoking in the development of respiratory disease in childhood has more relevance to attempts to persuade children from ever taking up the habit than has rates of decline of FEV_1 in middle age.

Holland *et al.* (1969a) followed a cohort of 2000 children born between 1963 and 1965 in Harrow, a suburb in north-west London. A one in three random sample had 'crying' ventilatory function tests performed using a pneumotachograph. Of the original 623 who had these initial tests, ventilatory function measured each year was available for 487 at the age of five. No events before, during or immediately after pregnancy had an effect on incidence of respiratory illness or on ventilatory function up to six weeks of age, and ventilatory function was not affected by any other environmental or familial factors. No large or consistent differences in 'crying' ventilatory function were found between children who subsequently suffered from pneumonia or bronchitis and those who did not (Colley *et al.*, 1976), which suggests that children who suffer from pneumonia or bronchitis in early life do not start life with a defective respiratory system.

The factors which appeared to be most closely associated with 'bronchitis' or pneumonia in the first year of life were a history of asthma or wheeze in the parents and parental smoking habits. If both these factors were present, the annual incidence of 'bronchitis' and pneumonia per 100 infants was 39.3, compared to 6.7 where neither existed (Table 2). A higher incidence of 'bronchitis' and pneumonia was also associated with parental cough or phlegm. This association may have resulted from shared genetic susceptibility to respiratory disease, parents and children living in the same home environment, or to cross-infection within the family. Work in France (Liard *et al.*, 1982) showed that wheezy bronchitis was strongly related to mother's cigarette consumption but simple bronchitis was not. This supports the hypothesis that passive inhalation of cigarette smoke irritates the child's lung and facilitates the spread of infection to the lower respiratory tract.

In the Harrow study, the main factors influencing the incidence of 'bronchitis' and pneumonia and other respiratory symptoms during the first five years of life were similar to those which affected disease incidence in the first year of life. However, ventilatory function, measured as peak expiratory flow rate (PEFR) using the Wright Peak Flow Meter, at the age of five was related to past history of bronchitis and pneumonia (the earlier the onset of disease, the greater the effect of past history) and also to the history of asthma, but not to parental smoking habits (Leeder *et al.*, 1976).

The normal practice of school medical examinations at the ages of five, 11 and 15 years was utilized in the Kent studies, which began in 1964 (Holland *et al.*, 1969a,b). The parents of 4707 children were interviewed. Examination of the children included PEFR measurements. Older children answered questions about respiratory symptoms and smoking habits. Re-examinations, when parents were asked about their child's respiratory illnesses over the preceding 12 months, took place at the age of 11 years for those aged five at the start of the study, and at 14 for those aged 11 at the start of the study. Prevalence of respiratory tract symptoms was found to be influenced by area of residence, parent's social class, age and sex, and particularly smoking habits; even exsmokers had more symptoms of cough and phlegm production than those who had never smoked. In contrast, PEFR was significantly influenced by area of residence, parent's social class, number of siblings and past history of bronchitis, pneumonia and asthma but not smoking.

Only 1978 children could be traced at the time of the first re-examination, and because the percentage loss varied between area and social class groups it was not possible to use the data to draw conclusions about the relationship between respiratory disease and social and environmental factors. However, it was possible to establish that children with a history of 'bronchitis', pneumonia or asthma before the age of five years (partly caused by parental smoking) were more likely to have 'bronchitis', wheezy chest and phlegm production at the age of 11. Children with reported symptoms at 11 also had on average a lower PEFR at 11 and at five. Those who had had low ventilatory function at the age of five were more likely to have respiratory symptoms and low ventilatory function at 11.

The most recent follow-up of the children in the Kent cohort was in 1974–1975. The relative risks of reporting respiratory symptoms in children with an early history of 'bronchitis', asthma or pneumonia was unchanged for those at ages five, 11 and 15. Thus, once a child's respiratory system has been compromised by early disease, there appears to be a lasting increased risk of having persistent symptoms.

Further evidence is needed to link factors experienced in early life with the development of chronic disease in much later life. It is unlikely that a single birth cohort could be satisfactorily followed from birth to old age. For example, a 1946 cohort was difficult to follow because the numbers remaining in 1966 had dwindled so that the reliability of conclusions was reduced (Douglas & Waller, 1966). Nonetheless, the study showed that a relationship between lower respiratory tract infection and air pollution levels exists until at least the age of 15. In 1966 it was only possible to collect data from 3899 of the original sample, then aged 20 (Colley *et al.*, 1973). The major finding of the 20-year follow-up was that prevalence of cough during the day or night was most closely related to current smoking habits and to a history of lower respiratory tract illnesses before the age of two. In the most recent follow-up, it was possible to collect data from 2088 men and women aged 25 (Kiernan *et al.*, 1976). At this age certain changes in the factors affecting respiratory symptom prevalence appeared to have taken place, namely that the association of cough prevalence with past history of respiratory illness and current smoking was even stronger.

Studies of respiratory disease in childhood have thus demonstrated that the environmental factors which are associated with respiratory disease in adults, for example air pollution, past respiratory illness and smoking, are also present amongst children. The relationship of respiratory disease in childhood to that developed in adults is more tenuous. No good prospective studies have yet been completed or undertaken to demonstrate the link, and merely showing that the same factors are responsible for disease at both ages is insufficient to prove that there is any real association. From a prevention viewpoint, it is not necessary to wait until such a link is demonstrated, because respiratory disease in children is more relevant than respiratory disease in adults to persuading children not to take up smoking. Smoking habits are associated with bronchitis and pneumonia in teenagers, and young adults and antismoking campaigns could emphasize this. However, respiratory disease in childhood is also related to infection in earlier years. It is quite possible that we may be able to treat respiratory infection in the early years better and thus perhaps avoid some of the troubles of later childhood. But also, if it could be shown that those children with respiratory infections were susceptible to chronic bronchitis and emphysema in later life, campaigns directed toward preventing those children from taking up cigarette smoking may be even more effective.

The Medical Research Council Derbyshire smoking study was the first longitudinal study of children's smoking to be performed in the UK (Banks *et al.*, 1978). At the start of the study in 1974, questionnaires were administered to children aged 11–12 years. These children were followed up until 1978. Factors which induce children to take up smoking are many and varied, but considerable importance seems to be attached to parental and sibling smoking, especially for the same sex. The fact that parental smoking is also associated with bronchitis and pneumonia among children under five years of age and that children's smoking habits are associated with bronchitis and pneumonia in teenagers and young adults suggest that antismoking efforts could be directed at the family rather than at adults or children separately.

LESS HAZARDOUS SMOKING

If children cannot be dissuaded from taking up smoking, the next best thing is to persuade adults to stop smoking. Various surveys of British men carried out in the 1950s and early 1960s have recently yielded sufficient data on deaths from chronic obstructive lung disease to show that the single original forced expiratory volume in one second (FEV_1) measured when these men were in their fifties can be used to predict reliably which men would have a high risk of death from chronic obstructive lung disease during the subsequent 20 years (Peto *et al.*, 1983). Antismoking campaigns directed toward these men could be very effective. However, the age-standardized chronic obstructive lung disease death rates per 100 000 British doctors who smoked 1–14, 15–24 and 25+ cigarettes a day were 51, 78 and 114 respectively, suggesting that if people cannot cease smoking, diminution of the dose might produce diminution of the effect (Doll & Peto, 1976).

Because of this dose-response relationship, it has also been suggested that the smoking of cigarettes in a lower tar group would be less deleterious to the lungs. Several studies have suggested that there might be a direct relationship between reduction in the tar yield of cigarettes and a reduced prevalence of cough (Comstock *et al.*, 1970; Freedman & Fletcher, 1976; Fletcher *et al.*, 1976; Dean *et al.*, 1978; Schenker *et al.*, 1982), and phlegm production (Rimington, 1972; Hawthorne & Fry, 1978; Higenbottam *et al.*, 1980). Fewer studies have examined the potential importance of tar yield for change in pulmonary function. One prospective study (Comstock *et al.*, 1970) found that smokers of nonfilter cigarettes, compared to those smoking filter-tipped cigarettes, had a lower FEV_1 at entry into the study but a smaller reduction of FEV_1 after five years. However, in another longitudinal survey, multiple regression analysis did not show any significant association between tar yield and lung function (Sparrow *et al.*, 1983). Cross-sectional surveys also indicate no relationship between pulmonary function and the use of filter-tipped *versus* nonfilter cigarettes (Beck *et al.*, 1981) or cigarette tar yield (Higenbottam *et al.*, 1980).

It has been suggested that mucus hypersecretion and chronic airflow obstruction are essentially distinct lung diseases (Fletcher *et al.*, 1976; Peto *et al.*, 1983), and it is possible that they might differ in their susceptibility to tar intakes. However, it would be premature to conclude that tar intake might not be an important factor in chronic airflow obstruction. Firstly, cross-sectional studies cannot define the natural history of a disease. Secondly, Fletcher *et al.* (1976) suggested that approximately eight years are necessary to establish rates of change of FEV_1 with sufficient confidence even to distinguish between smokers and nonsmokers. Thirdly, there is usually no information on the lung function of smokers at the time they change from high- to low-tar cigarettes. It is possible that similar function differences may exist in subjects who choose between high- and low-tar cigarettes as have been observed in adults choosing to smoke or not (Tashkin *et al.*, 1983).

Government tables of the tar yields of cigarettes in the UK advise committed smokers to choose a cigarette in a lower tar group. In 1971–1973, data on smoking habits including cigarette brand smoked, phlegm production and lung function were recorded on factory workers as part of the Heart Disease Prevention Project (HDPP) (Rose *et al.*, 1980). Assessment of their 1984 smoking habits, phlegm production and lung function permitted

Table 3. Characteristics of cigarette smokers at the start of the Heart Disease Prevention Project[a]

Variable	Type of cigarette smoked 1971–1984: mean (SE)		
	Same tar group	Dropped one tar group	Dropped two tar groups
Age (years)	47.5 (0.44)	48.0 (0.27)	48.3
Social class[b] I-III NM (%)	28.2	21.8	27.3
IIIM-V (%)	71.7	78.3	72.8
Cigarettes/day	17.4 (0.73)	17.7 (0.56)	18.5 (0.79)
Tar yield (mg/cigarette)	19.7 (0.20)	22.5 (0.23)	23.0 (0.39)
Nicotine yield (mg/cigarette)	1.28 (0.02)	1.44 (0.02)	1.47 (0.03)
Inhale (%)	87	86	94
Morning phlegm usually (%)	28	32	37
FEV_1 % FVC[c]	77.5 (0.59)	77.2 (0.40)	78.0 (0.66)
FEV_1[c] (litres)	3.1 (0.05)	3.0 (0.03)	3.1 (0.05)
FVC[c] (litres)	4.0 (0.05)	3.9 (0.04)	4:0 (0.03)
Number	145	322	132

[a] From Peach *et al.* (1986)

[b] Social class in the UK is divided into six categories: I, II, III nonmanual (NM), III manual (M), IV and V, on the basis of present occupation

[c] FEV_1, forced expiratory volume in one second; FVC, forced vital capacity; FEV_1 % FVC, the ratio of FEV_1 to FVC expressed as a percentage

Fig. 3. Mean prevalence of bronchial reactivity according to age, atopic status and smoking history; (–·–·) current smokers, 3-mm mean skin-weal diameter; (------) nonsmokers, 3-mm mean skin-weal diameter; (——) current smoker, 0-mm mean skin-weal diameter; (·······) non-smoker, 0-mm mean skin-weal diameter

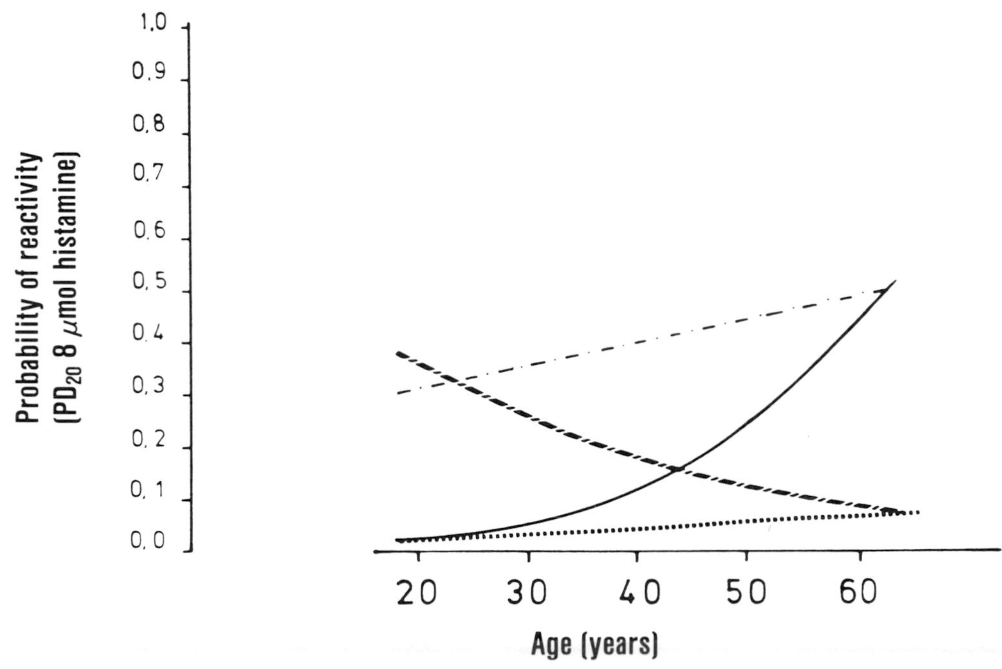

a comparison between cigarette smokers who had changed tar groups with those who had not.

Table 3 shows the age, social class, smoking habits, phlegm production and mean pulmonary function levels of men at the start of the HDPP. Smokers who subsequently changed to a lower tar group smoked cigarettes with higher tar and nicotine yields in 1971. If high-tar cigarettes were particularly deleterious, men who smoked them might have had more phlegm and poorer lung function before they changed tar groups. A comparison between men changing and not changing to a cigarette in a lower tar group would then be biased. However, there was no difference in mean pulmonary function levels (forced expiratory volume in one second [FEV_1], forced vital capacity [FVC] and the ratio of FEV_1 to FVC expressed as a percentage) between these types of smoker in the HDPP. There was a tendency for the prevalence of phlegm at the start of the study to increase from 28% among men who always smoked a cigarette in the same tar group to 37% among those who subsequently dropped two or more tar groups, but this trend was not significant. Although smokers who changed tar groups did not differ in phlegm production and pulmonary function before they changed, a comparison with non-changers could still be biased if the effects of smoking the higher-tar cigarettes were long-term. Only a controlled trial in which 'middle'-tar cigarette smokers, who are unwilling to stop smoking, are allocated at random to smoke a cigarette of the same or a lower tar group will provide definitive evidence of the potential benefit of changing tar groups on respiratory disease.

ASTHMA

Bronchial reactivity is beginning to appear as an important cause of continuing deterioration in patients with chronic obstructive lung disease. Barter *et al.* (1974) and Barter and Campbell (1976) showed that the deterioration in FEV_1 over a four-year period was related to the degree of bronchial reactivity. Mann (1976) related the improvement in FEV_1 of patients who stopped smoking to the bronchial reactivity measured by a bronchial challenge with 0.15 mg methacholine. Patients with the most bronchial reactivity had the best response, suggesting that increased bronchial reactivity is an important factor in lowering FEV_1. This bronchial reactivity is not in the asthmatic range and does not appear to be related to atopic status. However, the role of tobacco products as allergens is only just beginning to be assessed. Burney and his colleagues (personal communication) carried out tests of bronchial reactivity to histamine in 511 subjects randomly selected from a population who had returned questionnaires on respiratory symptoms. Bronchial reactivity was associated with positive skin tests to common allergens and with smoking history (Fig. 3). Both of these effects were in turn affected by the age of the subjects, the skin sensitivity being the more important determinant of reactivity in the young, and smoking the more important in older subjects. If bronchial reactivity is to be taken as the defining characteristic of asthma, it must follow that cigarette smoking is commonly associated with this condition.

REFERENCES

Addington, W.W., Carpenter, R.L., McCoy, J.E., Duncan, K.A. & Mogg, K. (1970) The association of cigarette smoking with respiratory symptoms and pulmonary function in a group of a high school students. *Oklahoma State med. Assoc.*, ***63,*** 525–529

Banks, M.H., Bewley, B.R., Bland, J.M., Dean, J.R. & Pollard, V. (1978) Longterm study of smoking by secondary schoolchildren. *Arch. Dis. Child.*, ***53,*** 12–19

Barter, C.E. & Campbell, A.H. (1976) Relationship of constitutional factors in cigarette smoking to decrease in the one second forced expiratory volume. *Am. Rev. resp. Dis.*, ***113,*** 305–314

Barter, C.E., Campbell, A.H. & Tandon, M.K. (1974) Factors affecting the decline of FEV_1 in chronic bronchitis. *Aust. N. Z. J. Med.*, ***4,*** 339

Beck, G.J., Doyle, C.A. & Schachter, E.N. (1981) Smoking and lung function. *Am. Rev. resp. Dis.*, ***123,*** 149–155

Bewley, B.R., Day, I. & Idle, L. (1973) *Smoking by Children in Great Britain: A Review of the Literature.* London, Social Science Research Council, Medical Research Council

Boudik, F., Goldsmith, J.R., Teichman, V. & Kaufmann, P.C. (1970) Epidemiology of chronic bronchitis in Prague. *Bull. World Health Organ.*, ***42,*** 711

Ciba Foundation Guest Symposium (1959) Terminology, definitions and classification of chronic pulmonary emphysema and related conditions. *Thorax*, ***14,*** 286–299

Colley, J.R.T., Douglas, J.W.B. & Reid, D.D. (1973). Respiratory disease in young adults: influence of early childhood lower respiratory tract illness, social class, air pollution and smoking. *Br. med. J.*, ***3,*** 195–198

Colley, J.R.T., Holland, W.W., Leeder, S.R. & Corkhill, R.T. (1976) Respiratory function of infants in relation to subsequent respiratory disease: an epidemiological study. *Bull. Eur. Physio-Pathol.*, ***12***, 651–657

Comstock, G.W., Brownlow, W.J., Stone, R.W. & Startwell, P.E. (1970) Cigarette smoking and changes in respiratory findings. *Arch. Environ. Health*, ***20***, 50–57

Dean, G., Lee, P.N., Todd, G.F., Wicken, A.J. & Sparks, D.N. (1978) Factors related to respiratory and cardiovascular symptoms in the United Kingdom. *J. Epidemiol. Community Health*, ***32***, 86–96

Doll, R. & Peto, R. (1976) Mortality in relation to smoking: 20 years' observations on male British doctors. *Br. med. J.*, ***ii***, 1525–1536

Douglas, J.W.B. & Waller, R.E. (1966) Air pollution and respiratory infection in children. *Br. J. prev. soc. Med.*, ***20***, 1–8

Finklea, J.F., Hasselbad, V., Sadifer, S.H., Hammer, D.I. & Lowrimore, G.R. (1971) Cigarette smoking and acute non-influenzal respiratory disease in military cadets. *Am. J. Epidemiol.*, ***93***, 457–462

Fletcher, C.M. & Peto, R. (1977) The natural history of chronic airflow obstruction. *Br. med. J.*, ***i***, 1645–1648

Fletcher, C., Peto, R., Tinker, C. & Speizer, F.E. (1976) *The Natural History of Chronic Bronchitis and Emphysema. An Eight-year Study of Early Chronic Obstructive Lung Disease in Working Men in London*, New York, Oxford University Press

Freedman, S. & Fletcher, C.M. (1976) Changes of smoking habits and cough in men smoking cigarettes with 30% NSM tobacco substitute. *Br. med. J.*, ***i***, 1427–1430

Hawthorne, V.M. & Fry, J.S. (1978) Smoking and health: the association between smoking behaviour, total mortality and cardio-respiratory disease in west central Scotland. *J. Epidemiol. Community Health*, ***32***, 260–266

Higenbottam, T., Shipley, M.J., Clark, T.J.H. & Rose, G. (1980) Lung function and symptoms of cigarette smokers related to tar yield and number of cigarettes smoked. *Lancet*, ***i***, 409–412

Holland W.W. (1984) 'Chronic bronchitis – what has to be done. What should we do next? An epidemiologist's dreams', Ninth Annual Theodore L. Badger Lecture delivered at Harvard Medical School 26 November, 1984

Holland, W.W., Halil, T., Bennett, A.E. & Elliott, A. (1969a) Factors influencing the onset of chronic respiratory disease. *Br. med. J.*, ***ii***, 205–208

Holland W.W., Halil, T., Bennett, A.E. & Elliott, A. (1969b) Indications for measures to be taken in childhood to prevent chronic respiratory disease. *Milbank Mem. Fund Q.*, ***48***, 215–227

Holland, W.W., Bennett, A.E., Cameron, I.R., Florey, C.V., Leeder, S.R., Schilling, R.S., Swan, A.V. & Waller, R.E. (1979) Health effects of particulate pollution: reappraising the evidence. *Am. J. Epidemiol.*, ***110***, 525–659

Kiernan, K.E., Colley, J.R.T., Douglas, J.W.B. & Reid, D.D. (1976) Chronic cough in young adults in relation to smoking habits, childhood environment and chest illness. *Respiration*, ***33***, 236

Leeder, S.R., Corkhill, R.T., Wysocki, M.J., Holland, W.W. & Colley, J.R.T. (1976) Influence of personal and family factors on ventilatory function of children. *Br. J. prev. soc. Med.*, ***30***, 219–224

Liard, R., Perdrizet, S. & Reinert, P. (1982) Wheezy bronchitis in infants and parents' smoking habits. *Lancet*, ***i***, 334–335

Mann, J.S. (1976) *Cigarette Smoking and Lung Function,* MD thesis, University of Sydney

Mueller, R.E., Keble, D.L., Plummer, J. & Walker, S.H. (1971) The prevalence of chronic bronchitis, chronic airway obstruction and respiratory symptoms in a Colorado city. *Am. Rev. resp. Dis.,* ***103,*** 209–228

Office of Population Censuses and Surveys (1981a) *Mortality Statistics in England and Wales,* London, Her Majesty's Stationery Office

Office of Population Censuses and Surveys (1981b) *Hospital Inpatient Statistics in England and Wales,* London, Her Majesty's Stationery Office

Peach, H., Hayward, D.M., Ellard, D.R., Morris, R.W. & Shak, D. (1986) Phlegm productions and lung function among cigarette smokers changing tar groups during the 1970s. *Epidemiol. Commun. Health* (in press)

Peto, R., Speizer, F.E., Cochrane, A.L., Moore, F., Fletcher, C.M., Tinker, C.M., Higgins, I.T.T., Gray, R.G., Richards, S.M., Gillilard, J. & Norman-Smith, B. (1983) The relevance in adults of airflow obstruction but not of mucus hypersecretion to mortality from chronic lung disease: 20-year results from prospective surveys. *Am. Rev. resp. Dis.,* ***128,*** 491–500

Reid, D.D. (1963) *The Epidemiology of Chronic Bronchitis,* Edinburgh, Royal College of Physicians of Edinburgh

Rimington, J. (1972) Phlegm and filters. *Br. med. J.,* ***ii,*** 262–264

Rose, G., Heller, R.F., Pedoe, H.T. & Christie, D.G.S. (1980) Heart disease prevention project: a randomised controlled trial in industry. *Br. med. J.,* ***i,*** 747–751

Schenker, M.B., Samet, J.M. & Speizer, F.E. (1982) Effect of cigarette tar content and smoking habits on respiratory symptoms in women. *Am. Rev. resp. Dis.,* ***125,*** 684–690

Seely, J.E., Zuskin, E. & Bouhuys, A. (1971) Cigarette smoking: objective evidence for lung damage in teenagers. *Science,* ***172,*** 741–743

Sparrow, D., Stafos, T., Bosse, R. & Weiss, S. (1983) The relationship of tar content to decline in pulmonary function in cigarette smokers. *Am. Rev. resp. Dis.,* ***127,*** 56–58

Tashkin, D.P., Clark, V.A., Coulson, A.H., Bourque, L.B., Simmons, M., Reems, C., Detels, R. & Rokaw, S. (1983) Comparison of lung function in young non-smokers and smokers before and after initiation of the smoking habit: a prospective study. *Am. Rev. resp. Dis.,* ***128,*** 12–16

Thurlbeck, W.M. (1977) Aspects of chronic airflow obstruction. *Chest,* ***72,*** 3

III. DISEASE PATTERNS AND SMOKING

SMOKING PATTERNS IN THE USSR

D.G. ZARIDZE[1]

International Agency for Research on Cancer,
Lyon, France

V.V. DVOIRIN & V.A. KOBLJAKOV

All-Union Cancer Research Center of the
Academy of Medical Sciences of the USSR,
Moscow, USSR

V.P. PISKLOV

All-Union Research Institute of Tobacco,
Krasnodar, USSR

SUMMARY

Smoking is widespread in the USSR. The prevalence of smoking among males ranges from 35–80%, although some of the very high rates may be the result of surveying selected population groups. Smoking appears to be more frequent among young people, and the proportion of adolescent smokers is high. There are reported to be fewer women smokers (about 10%) than in most countries of Europe and North America. The *per capita* production of smoking materials (cigarettes and *papyrossi)* increased substantially during the post-war period, reached its maximum in the year 1971, and decreased thereafter. The highest *per capita* sales of smoking materials were reported in the years 1976–1980, and they have declined slightly since. Presently, 70% of the smoking materials produced in the USSR are cigarettes. The proportion of filter cigarettes has increased from 1.1% in 1963 to 30% in 1982. However, about 90% of cigarettes produced in the USSR still fall within the category of high-tar cigarettes (20 mg/cigarette and over). To avoid a continuation of the

[1] Present address: All-Union Cancer Research Center of the Academy of Medical Sciences of the USSR, Kashirskoye shosse 24, Moscow 115478, USSR.

increase in the frequency of smoking and, consequently, an increase in mortality from lung cancer and other diseases caused by smoking, serious consideration should be given to a wide range of smoking control measures.

INTRODUCTION

It has been established that smoking is carcinogenic to humans. The malignant tumours caused by smoking include lung, oral, oropharyngeal, hypopharyngeal, laryngeal, oesophageal, urinary bladder, renal pelvic, pancreatic and, possibly, renal and cervical cancer (IARC, 1986).

Smoking also contributes to the development of coronary heart disease, which is the leading cause of death in many developed countries, and to diseases of other arteries. One-third of all deaths from coronary heart disease in middle age are attributable to cigarette smoking, as is a smaller proportion of cerebrovascular disease. Finally, smoking is a cause of most cases of chronic obstructive lung disease (US Department of Health and Human Services, 1983; Royal College of Physicians, 1983).

Despite the fact that the main adverse health effects of smoking are well known, tobacco consumption remains high in many areas. Consequently, smoking remains one of the most important public health problems in developed countries and is becoming increasingly important in developing countries. A substantial proportion of men (20–85%) smoke in virtually all countries from which smoking survey data are available. Women generally smoke less than men but, even so, the proportion of women who smoke in most countries of Europe and North America is of the order of 30% (IARC, 1986), with generally higher proportions among younger women.

As judged by trends in cigarette sales, smoking continues to increase in most developed and developing countries although, in a few countries such as the UK, the USA, Belgium and Finland, sales of cigarettes have been declining since the mid-1970s (IARC, 1986).

The introduction of filter cigarettes and several other changes in cigarette manufacture have resulted in a decrease in the yield of certain noxious products in tobacco smoke, such as tar and nicotine, when the cigarettes are smoked under standard conditions (though people who smoke such cigarettes tend to compensate for these decreases by inhaling more smoke per cigarette; Lee, 1980). The proportion of filter cigarettes has increased steadily and, in many countries, filter cigarettes now dominate the market (IARC, 1986).

Information has recently been accumulating that the use of 'high-tar' cigarettes is associated with greater lung cancer risks than the use of 'low-tar' cigarettes (Peto & Doll, 1984). However, there is no evidence that the use of 'low-tar' cigarettes will affect the risk of cardiovascular and respiratory diseases or smoking-related cancers at any other sites.

PRODUCTION AND SALES OF SMOKING MATERIALS IN THE USSR

The statistics available on the production of smoking materials (cigarettes/*papyrossi*[2] in the USSR go back to 1913. In that year, 117 900 million pieces of smoking materials were

[2] Type of cigarettes characterized by a long, hollow mouthpiece.

Table 1. Trends in production of smoking materials in the USSR

Year	All smoking materials (*papyrossi* + cigarettes)		*Papyrossi*			Cigarettes		
	Total no. in million pieces	No. *per capita*	Total no. in million pieces	% [a]	No. *per capita*	Total no. in million pieces	% [a]	No. *per capita*
1963	257 800	1152	196 000	76	876	61 800	24	276
1964	280 300	1235	209 700	73	898	76 600	27	337
1965	304 400	1325	212 700	70	926	91 700	30	399
1966	303 500	1307	203 900	67	878	99 600	33	429
1967	286 600	1220	174 100	61	741	112 500	39	479
1968	288 500	1215	160 000	55	674	128 500	45	541
1969	307 600	1283	166 300	54	694	141 300	46	589
1970	322 700	1334	174 700	54	722	148 000	46	612
1971	334 400	1369	178 600	53	732	155 400	47	637
1972	347 800	1411	180 000	52	730	167 800	48	681
1973	362 700	1458	179 400	49	721	183 300	51	737
1974	369 300	1471	173 700	47	692	195 600	53	779
1975	364 300	1438	162 400	45	641	201 900	55	797
1976	375 200	1467	157 100	42	614	218 100	58	853
1977	378 500	1467	149 600	40	580	228 900	60	887
1978	377 400	1450	137 400	36	528	240 000	64	922
1979	360 200	1371	119 100	33	453	241 100	67	918
1980	364 000	1375	116 200	32	439	247 800	68	936
1981	365 400	1372	113 900	31	426	251 500	69	946
1982	359 400	1336	106 200	30	395	253 200	70	941

[a] Percentage of total amount of smoking materials (*papyrossi* + cigarettes)

Table 2. Trends in annual *per capita* sales of smoking materials (*papyrossi* and cigarettes) in the USSR

Years	Annual *per capita* sales of smoking materials
1961–1965	1200.0
1966–1970	1392.0
1971–1975	1583.0
1976–1980	1641.7
1981–1983	1595.7

produced. By 1940 this number had increased to 318 600 million. Production of tobacco products declined drastically during the Second World War but production again reached pre-war levels in the 1960s, and has increased thereafter (Table 1). Although the *per capita* production of smoking materials has decreased somewhat during the last few years, the same period has seen a marked increase in cigarette imports. The number of imported cigarettes is now about 70 000 million annually.

The *per capita* consumption of smoking materials, as judged by the *per capita* sales of smoking materials, reached its maximum in the years 1976–1980 and has not increased since then (Table 2).

Cigarette production has drastically increased since 1960 while, during the same period, we observe a decline in *papyrossi* production (Table 1). There are considerable differences in types of smoking materials produced and probably consumed in different areas of the Soviet Union. In 1982, cigarettes represented 54% of the smoking materials produced in the Kazakh SSR, 57% in the Russian Soviet Federated Socialist Republic (RSFSR), 78% in the Armenian SSR, 91% in the Georgian SSR, 99% in Azerbaidjan, and 100% in the Tadjik, Estonian and Lithuanian republics. In the year 1982, for the whole of the Soviet Union the proportion of cigarettes in all smoking materials was 70%.

TRENDS IN THE PRODUCTION OF FILTER CIGARETTES AND CONSTITUENTS OF TOBACCO SMOKE OF CIGARETTES AND *PAPYROSSI* IN FREQUENT USE IN THE USSR

The proportion of filter cigarettes has increased from 0.3% of all smoking materials in 1963 to 21.3% in 1982. The proportion of filter cigarettes represented 1% of all cigarettes in 1963, and has increased since to 30% and 60% for the USSR and Moscow, respectively (Tables 3 and 4). The proportion of cigarettes with a paper filter, which were introduced in the early 1960s, has been declining since 1975, and is presently 1.7% and 5% for the USSR and Moscow, respectively. By 1985 the proportion of cigarettes with a cellulose acetate filter had reached 28% and 55% for the USSR and Moscow, respectively (Table 4).

Table 3. Trends in production of filter cigarettes in the USSR

Year	Total no. (million pieces)	No. *per capita*	Percentage of all smoking materials (*papyrossi* + cigarettes)	Percentage of all cigarettes
1963	700	3	0.3	1.1
1964	900	4	0.3	1.2
1965	4 100	17	1.3	4.5
1966	6 900	29	2.3	6.9
1967	10 700	45	3.7	9.5
1968	21 700	91	7.5	16.9
1969	29 400	122	9.6	20.8
1970	32 600	134	10.1	22.0
1971	36 300	148	10.9	23.4
1972	40 100	162	11.5	23.9
1973	43 030	173	11.9	23.5
1974	51 100	203	13.9	26.1
1975	58 600	231	16.1	29.0
1976	62 000	240	16.5	28.4
1977	62 600	242	16.5	27.3
1978	69 800	268	18.5	29.1
1979	74 200	282	20.6	30.8
1980	75 900	287	20.9	30.6
1981	76 800	288	21.0	30.5
1982	76 700	285	21.3	30.3

Table 4. Trends in production of different types of filter cigarettes in the USSR and in Moscow

		USSR				Moscow			
		All cigarettes	Filter cigarettes	With paper filter	With cellulose acetate filter	All cigarettes	Filter cigarettes	With paper filter	With cellulose acetate filter
1960	No. (million pieces)	54 200	500	500	0	–	–	–	–
	% of all cigarettes		0.9	0.9	0		–	–	–
1965	No. (million pieces)	91 700	4 100	4 100	0	–	–	–	–
	% of all cigarettes		4.5	4.5	0		–	–	–
1970	No. (million pieces)	147 900	32 600	16 100	16 500	12 600	5 900	1 800	4 100
	% of all cigarettes		22.0	10.9	11.1		46.7	14.0	32.7
1975	No. (million pieces)	202 000	58 600	25 100	33 500	16 300	8 900	2 000	6 900
	% of all cigarettes		29.0	12.4	16.6		54.5	12.5	41.9
1980	No. (million pieces)	247 800	75 900	11 300	64 600	20 600	12 700	1 500	11 200
	% of all cigarettes		30.6	4.6	26.0		61.3	7.0	54.3
1985	No. (million pieces)	302 700	89 700	5 100	89 600	22 600	13 600	1 200	12 500
	% of all cigarettes		29.6	1.7	27.9		60.2	5.3	54.9

Fig. 1. Tar and nicotine yields in 45 popular brands of cigarettes in the USSR and Bulgaria

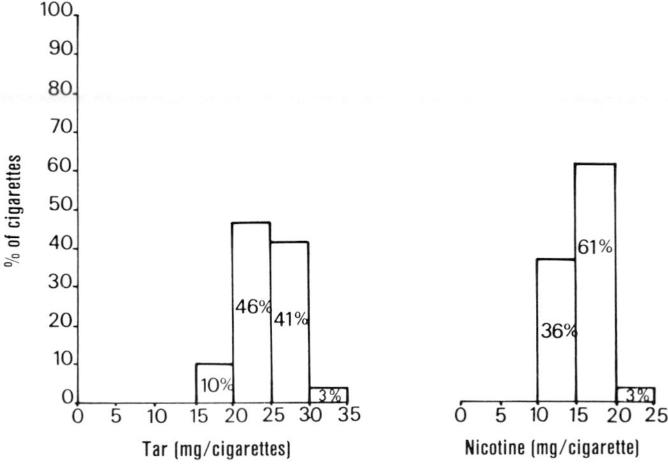

An analysis of tobacco smoke of a sample of 41 brands of cigarettes and *papyrossi* produced in Moscow, Leningrad, Tbilisi, Tallin and Kaunas and four brands of Bulgarian cigarettes was carried out[3]. The sample included two brands of *papyrossi,* and 11 brands of nonfilter and 32 brands of filter cigarettes. Following the classification of tar yields adopted in Volume 38 of the *IARC Monographs* series (IARC, 1986), tar yields in the above sample

[3] Chemical analysis of smoke was undertaken by Dr Kobljakov at the Laboratory of the Austrian Tobacco Industry, Vienna, Austria, at the Laboratory of the Government Chemist, Department of Industry, London, UK, and at the Naylor Dana Institute, American Health Foundation, Valhalla, N.Y., USA.

Table 5. Tar and nicotine levels (mg/cigarette) of different types of Soviet cigarettes

'Class' [a]	Type	No. of brands analysed	Tar	Nicotine
1	Filter	4	23	1.0
2	Filter	4	27	1.3
3	Filter	5	23	1.2
3	Nonfilter	5	28	1.6
4	Filter	4	24	1.2
5	Filter	4	19	1.1
5	Nonfilter	5	28	1.5
6	Nonfilter	4	29	1.8
7	Nonfilter	4	27	1.8

[a] Cigarettes are classified by 'class' according to their quality (from 1 'high' to 7 'low').

were found to be very high (20 mg/cigarette and over) in 90% of cigarettes; in 10%, tar yields were found to be high, i.e., 19 mg/cigarette (Fig. 1).

Nicotine levels were found to be above 1.5 mg/cigarette in 64% of cigarettes analysed. In 36%, nicotine yield was 1.0–1.5 mg/cigarette (Fig. 1). The tar yield in the cigarettes ranged from 19–31 mg/cigarette, and the range in nicotine yield was 1.0–2.1 mg/cigarette.

Table 5 shows results of tobacco smoke analysis[4] of 39 brands of cigarettes produced by seven different factories in the USSR according to their type, i.e., 'class'. (In the USSR cigarettes are classified by class, i.e., quality from 1'high' to 7 'low'.) All but four brands analysed contained 19 mg/cigarette tar or more.

PREVALENCE OF SMOKING

According to Chazov *et al.* (1984) there are about 70 million smokers in the Soviet Union, i.e:, 26% of the population. The existing literature on the prevalence of the smoking habit in the USSR covers the period between the early 1960s and the early 1980s (Table 6).

According to surveys carried out in the early 1960s in Armenia, Azerbaidjan and Georgia, about 69–79% of men and 5–7% of women were cigarette smokers (Orlovski, 1977). According to Oleynikov *et al.* (1981), in the middle 1970s, 44–48% of men living in Moscow and Kaunas and about 10% of women living in Moscow reported smoking. Comparable results have been obtained in other areas. A survey of 1687 men and women in eight towns of the USSR in 1981 showed that 64.5% of men and 11% of women smoke, the proportion of smokers in this survey varied from 51% to 78% for men and 2% to 24% for women (Loransky *et al.,* 1983). A survey of 1529 men and women aged 14–60 years,

[4] Chemical analysis of tobacco smoke was undertaken at the All-Union Research Institute of Tobacco, Krasnodar, USSR.

Table 6. Prevelance of smoking in the USSR

Area	Reference	Year of survey	Total no. surveyed	Men	Women	% of smokers	
						Men	Women
Armenia	Orlovski (1977)	1960	1685	792	893	77.9	6.9
Azerbaidjan	Orlovski (1977)	1963	2079	695	1384	68.6	4.8
Georgia	Orlovski (1977)	1960	1238	544	694	78.5	7.5
Moscow	Oleynikov *et al.* (1983)	1975	966	–	–	44.2	10.1
Moscow	Oleynikov *et al.* (1981)	1978	3966	3966 [a]	–	48.1	10.1
Kaunas	Oleynikov *et al.* (1981)	1978	5482	5482 [a]	–	43.1	–
Zelinograd	Loransky *et al.* (1983)	1981	204	66	138	53.0	6.5
Lipetsk	Loransky *et al.* (1983)	1981	280	183	97	66.1	8.2
Ufa	Loransky *et al.* (1983)	1981	165	76	89	77.6	2.2
Tula	Loransky *et al.* (1983)	1981	206	72	134	51.4	8.9
Stavropol	Loransky *et al.* (1983)	1981	284	42	242	64.3	6.2
Kiev	Loransky *et al.* (1983)	1981	87	53	34	62.3	23.5
Daugavpils	Loransky *et al.* (1983)	1981	203	139	64	66.9	12.5
Erevan	Loransky *et al.* (1983)	1981	258	57	201	68.4	20.4
Lipetsk	Shevtshuk & Tarasova (1983)	1981	1529	813	716	54.2	5.9
Burjat ASSR	Orlovski (1977)	1957	1444		Ethnic Burjats		
				–	541	–	80.8
					Others		
				–	903	–	9.6

[a] All were males between 40 and 59 years of age

Table 7. Prevalence of smoking in the USSR by age

Area	Reference	Total no. surveyed	Age (years)	% of smokers	
				Men	Women
Moscow	Oleynikov *et al.* (1981)	966	16–70+ [a]	44.2	10.1
			16–19	24.7	7.3
			20–29	60.4	16.8
			30–39	62.6	19.0
			40–49	46.3	8.3
			50–59	38.6	6.4
			60–69	35.7	10.8
			70+	20.0	6.2
Moscow	Oleynikov *et al.* (1983)	619	40–44	51.3	–
		537	45–49	48.9	–
		515	50–54	48.3	–
		242	55–59	40.7	–
Kaunas	Oleynikov *et al.* (1983)	690	40–44	47.1	–
		698	44–49	42.7	–
		604	50–54	42.5	–
		660	55–59	38.4	–
8 towns	Loransky *et al.* (1983)	681	20–40	78.0	15.0
			50+	55.0	3.0

[a] The whole group

Table 8. Prevalence of smoking in the USSR in adolescents

Area	Reference	School or grade	Approx. age	Total no. surveyed	M	F	% of smokers	
							M	F
11 towns[a]	Loransky *et al.* (1983)	4–10	11–17	2819	1424	1395	25.9	11.5
		7	14				10.8	2.5
		10	17				46.2	8.1
Lipetsk	Shevtshuk & Tarasova (1983)	10	17				69.2	16.7
Lipetsk	Shevtshuk & Tarasova (1983)	7	14				12.5	–
Lipetsk	Shevtshuk & Tarasova (1983)	8	15				37.5	4.3
Lipetsk	Shevtshuk & Tarasova (1983)	9	16				17.6	3.8
Lipetsk	Shevtshuk & Tarasova (1983)	Primary technical school	10–14				56.4	5.2
Lipetsk	Shevtshuk & Tarasova (1983)	Secondary technical school	14–17				55.9	5.9
Lipetsk	Shevtshuk & Tarasova (1983)	University	17–22				50.5	5.0

[a] Moscow, Zelinograd, Dmitrov, Lipetsk, Ufa, Daugavpils, Essentuki, Chabarovsk, Sukhumi, Vilnius, Kaunas

Table 9. Prevelance of smoking in males in the USSR according to level of education

Area	Reference	Education (no. surveyed)	Age (years)	% of smokers
Moscow	Oleynikov *et al.* (1983)	1. Primary (298)	40–59	64.8
		2. Unfinished secondary (1059)	40–59	59.7
		3. Secondary (459)	40–59	50.1
		4. University (1693)	40–59	37.2
Kaunas	Oleynikov *et al.* (1983)	1. Primary (950)	40–59	51.2
		2. Unfinished secondary (1284)	40–59	50.5
		3. Secondary (967)	40–59	41.9
		4. University (919)	40–59	33.0
6 towns	Chazov *et al.* (1984)	1. Primary	40–59	64.8
		2. Secondary	40–59	59.7
		3. University	40–59	37.2

carried out in Lipetsk revealed that 54.2% of men and 5,9% of women were smokers (Shevtshuk & Tarasova, 1983).

It is of interest to mention certain ethnic differences in smoking. Orlovski (1977) reported that, as part of a study carried out in the Burjat ASSR, he surveyed 541 Burjat women and 903 other women; of the Burjat women 81% were cigarette smokers compared to only 9.6% of the other women. Oleynikov *et al.* (1981, 1983) and Loransky *et al.* (1983) reported that the highest proportion of smokers is observed in the younger age groups (Table 7). The highest proportion of smokers was observed among men and women in the age group 20–29 years (Oleynikov *et al.*, 1981); more men smoked in the age group 40–44 years than in older age groups (Oleynikov *et al.*, 1983); 78% of men and 15% of women in the age group 24–40 years reported smoking, compared to only 55% of men and 3% of women over the age of 50 (Loransky *et al.*, 1983).

Surveys among adolescents revealed a high proportion of smokers in both sexes (Table 8). A survey carried out in 11 towns and cities of the USSR, which included about 2819 adolescents, revealed that 25.9% of boys and 11.5% of girls in the age group 11–17 years and attending secondary school smoke cigarettes. The proportion of smokers among those attending grade 7 (about 13–14 years of age) was 10.8% for boys and 2.5% for girls; the proportion of smokers increases to 46.2% for boys and 8.1% for girls attending grade 10 (aged about 16–17) (Loransky *et al.*, 1983). High proportions of smokers were observed in school, technical school and university students in Lipetsk (Shevtshuk & Tarasova, 1983).

Surveys in which the educational status of respondents was evaluated have shown that smoking is more frequent among less educated people (Table 9) (Oleynikov *et al.*, 1983; Chazov *et al.*, 1984).

DISCUSSION

Smoking is widespread in the USSR. The prevalence of smoking among males, which, according to population surveys, ranges from 35% to 80%, is comparable with the highest rates in the world, although no data are available from nationwide surveys, and some of the very high rates may be the results of surveying selected population groups. Smoking appears to be more frequent among young people, and the proportion of adolescent smokers is very high. There are reported to be fewer women smokers than in most countries of Europe and North America (IARC, 1986).

Unfortunately, no data are available on which to judge trends in the prevalence of the smoking habit. However, data from sales of smoking materials (cigarettes and *papyrossi)* indicate that the consumption of smoking materials in the USSR reached 1642 pieces per person per year in the years 1976–1980, placing the USSR among the 30 countries with the highest *per capita* cigarette consumption. *Per capita* cigarette consumption in 110 countries for which statistics are available ranges from 17 to 3000 (IARC, 1986).

Consumption of smoking materials in the USSR increased by about 32% from 1961 to 1980, suggesting that the vigorous antismoking campaign (which includes a ban on tobacco sales promotion, restriction of smoking in public places, the dissemination of information on the adverse health effects of smoking, health warnings on cigarette packets, etc.) carried out in this country (Chazov *et al.*, 1984) has not yet produced significant results although, in the last few years, a small decrease in cigarette consumption has been seen.

The rise in cigarette consumption up to the year 1980 in the USSR suggests that, in coming decades, important increases will be observed in the rates of lung and other cancers caused by smoking, as well as in the rates of cardiovascular and obstructive lung diseases.

About 90% of the cigarettes consumed in the USSR fall within the category of 'high-tar' cigarettes (20 mg and over), as defined by the IARC (1986). Data recently obtained from both descriptive and analytical epidemiological studies suggest that the risk of lung cancer is less for 'low-tar' than for 'high-tar' cigarettes. The substantial reduction (about 50–70 %) in the lung cancer mortality rates in young and middle-aged men in England and Wales and Finland could be attributed to decreases in tar deliveries in cigarettes consumed in these countries (Peto & Doll, 1984). In addition, the results obtained in several case-control and prospective studies suggest that those who smoke 'low-tar' cigarettes are at lower risk of lung cancer (Hammond *et al.*, 1977; Lee & Garfinkel, 1981; Lubin *et al.*, 1984). Thus, if the 'tar yields' of cigarette smoke are lowered in the USSR, this could result in a decrease in lung cancer risk, and would gradually produce a substantial decrease in lung cancer incidence and mortality compared to that expected if no changes in cigarette composition are made.

The health benefits of stopping smoking greatly exceed those obtained by changing cigarette composition. The prevention of cancer by the elimination of smoking would result in about a 20–25% decrease in the total cancer mortality in the USSR. It is estimated that about 30% of cancer deaths in the USA could be prevented by the elimination of smoking (Doll & Peto, 1981). No comparable result could be achieved by the treatment of cancer, even using the most advanced and expensive treatment. The impact of complete cessation of smoking on the mortality from cardiovascular diseases will be even greater.

To avoid a continuation of the increase in the frequency of smoking and, consequently, an increase in the mortality and incidence rate of lung cancer and other diseases caused by smoking, and to achieve decreases in the above rates, serious consideration should be given to a wide range of smoking control measures recommended by the World Health Organization (1979) and the International Union against Cancer (Gray & Daube, 1980), including modification of cigarette manufacture, with the aim of decreasing their carcinogenicity.

The majority of smokers are still unaware of the real dangers of smoking. To fill this important gap, serious efforts should be made to ensure that scientifically accurate and adequately presented information be delivered to the general population through the media. Schools and teachers should play an important role in antismoking campaigns. Health education programmes should be given a central position in the curriculum. Smoking in schools should be discouraged, not only for students but also for teachers.

The greatest responsibility for antismoking action lies with the medical profession. All opportunities of meeting patients should be used to explain to them the health hazards related to smoking. Nonsmoking should be considered to be the norm in all types of medical or health care premises, including hospitals, outpatient clinics, research institutions and medical faculties.

Now that it is widely accepted that tobacco products should carry a health warning, an effort should be made for health warning messages to contain explicit information about diseases caused by smoking, and estimates of the risk of acquiring these diseases or dying from them. Every cigarette packet should contain, along with the health warning, information about the level of the various tobacco smoke constituents such as tar, carbon monoxide and nicotine. Upper limits for the harmful substances contained in tobacco smoke should be established, and sales of tobacco exceeding these limits should be banned.

It has been accepted that increasing the price of tobacco products is a useful tool for the control of smoking. Increases in the price of the more hazardous brands (nonfilter, high-tar) would encourage cigarette smokers to switch to less hazardous brands (filter, 'lower tar'). The increase in price should make more hazardous cigarettes (nonfilter, high-tar) as expensive as less hazardous cigarettes.

It is known that the revenues from tobacco are higher than from any other crop. However, the short-term positive effect on the economy of the country produced by high revenues from tobacco growing is negligible in comparison with the long-term damage to the national economy which is produced by an increased use of tobacco products, in view of the increase in disability and death from diseases caused by smoking. It is essential, therefore, that tobacco be replaced by other, probably less profitable, crops which in the long run will not have an adverse effect on the national economy through damage to the health of a considerable proportion of the population.

REFERENCES

Chasov, E.I., Oganov, R.G. & Glasunov, I.S. (1984) Prevention of diseases by annual screening of the population (Russ.). *Sov. Sdravochranenie,* ***10,*** 3–6

Doll, R. & Peto, R. (1981) *The Causes of Cancer. Quantitative Estimates of Avoidable Risks of Cancer in the United States Today,* Oxford, Oxford University Press

Gray, N. & Daube, M., eds (1980) *Guidelines for Smoking Control (UICC Tech. Rep. Ser. Vol.* 52), Geneva, International Union Against Cancer

Hammond, E.C., Garfinkel, L., Seidman, H. & Lew, E.A. (1977) *Some recent findings concerning cigarette smoking.* In: Hiatt, N.H., Watson, J.D. & Winston, J.A., eds, *Origin of Human Cancer. Book A: Incidence of Cancer in Humans,* Cold Spring Harbor Conferences on Cell Proliferation, Vol. 4, New York, Cold Spring Harbor Laboratory, pp. 101–112

IARC (1986) *IARC Monographs on the Evaluation of the Carcinogenic Risk of Chemicals to Humans,* Vol. 38, *Tobacco Smoking,* Lyon

Lee, P.N. (1980) Low tar cigarette smoking. *Lancet,* ***i,*** 1365–1366

Lee, P.N. & Garfinkel, L. (1981) Mortality and types of cigarettes smoked. *J. Epidemiol. Community Health,* ***35,*** 16–22

Loransky, D.N., Popova, E.B., Chakimova, L.S. & Shevtshuk, A.G. (1983) State of the smoking problem (Russ.). *Sov. Sdravochranenie,* ***6,*** 33–38

Lubin, J.H., Blot, W.J., Berrino, F., Flamant, R., Gillis, C.R., Kunze, M., Schmal, D. & Wisco, G. (1984) Patterns of lung cancer risk according to type of cigarettes smoked. *Int. J. Cancer,* ***33,*** 569–576

Oleynikov, S.P., Glasunov, E.S. & Chazova, L.V. (1981) Smoking among men and women of various age groups (Russ.). *Ter. Arkh.,* ***2,*** 111–115

Oleynikov, S.P., Shazova, L.V., Glasunov, I.S., Deev, A.D., Baubine, A.V., Prochorkis, R.P. & Damarkene, S.B. (1983) Smoking and various sociodemographic patterns (results of collaborative studies in Moscow and Kaunas) (Russ.) *Ter. Arkh.,* ***1,*** 57–61

Orlovski, L.V. (1977) *Importance of education in the anti-smoking campaign* (Russ.). In: *Proceedings of the Meeting of the USSR Academy of Medical Sciences Commission on the Problem of Medical Education,* Archangelsk, pp. 122–130

Peto, R. & Doll, R. (1984) *Keynote address: The control of lung cancer.* In: Mizell, M. & Correa, P., eds, *Lung Cancer. Causes and Prevention, Proceedings of the International Lung Cancer Update Conference held in New Orleans, 3–5 March 1983,* Deerfield Beach, USA, Verlag Chemie International, pp. 1–19

Royal College of Physicians (1983) *Health or Smoking? Follow-up Report of the Royal College of Physicians,* London, Pitman Publishing Ltd

Shevtshuk, A.G. & Tarasova, R.N. (1983) Organization of an anti-smoking campaign (Russ.). *Sdravochranemie Ross. Fed.*, **5**, 27–28

US Department of Health and Human Services (1983) *The Health Consequences of Smoking. Cardiovascular Diseases. A Report of the Surgeon General,* Rockville, MD

World Health Organization (1979) *Controlling the Smoking Epidemic. Report of the WHO Expert Committee on Smoking Control (WHO Tech. Rep. Ser. No. 636),* Geneva

LUNG CANCER IN THE USSR: PATTERNS AND TRENDS

D.G. ZARIDZE[1] & R. GUREVICIUS

International Agency for Research on Cancer,
Lyon, France

SUMMARY

Lung cancer in the USSR has become the most frequent type of tumour in males. In females, however, lung cancer rates are far behind rates for cancer of the breast, stomach and cervix. In 1980, lung cancer accounted for about one-fourth of newly diagnosed cancer cases in males and about one-sixth of all cancer cases in both sexes. The incidence of lung cancer is increasing in the USSR. In the five Soviet republics for which time trends have been examined in this paper, increases in lung cancer incidence have been observed in men for all ages, with the exception of the age group 30–39 years. Modest increases in lung cancer are seen in women in the older age groups, while small decreases or stabilization of rates are observed in younger age groups. However, there are two exceptions: statistically significant increases in Georgia for women aged 40–49 years, and an upward trend in Lithuania in urban females born in the years 1932 and 1937, suggesting that these particular groups of women smoke more than other women in the areas for which lung cancer time trends have been analysed. The continued increase in cigarette consumption in this country explains the rising trends in lung cancer and, moreover, leads to the prediction that this increase will continue for another 30–40 years.

INTRODUCTION

Lung cancer is presently the most important cause of death from cancer in the world, with an estimated total number of deaths of about one million annually (IARC, 1986). In males in developed countries, the proportion of lung cancers attributable to smoking is of the order of 90% (IARC, 1986). Even if a smaller fraction of lung cancers in other countries are induced by tobacco, 60–75% of the global total must be attributable to this single cause (Muir & Parkin, 1985).

[1] Present address: All-Union Cancer Research Center of the Academy of Medical Sciences of the USSR, Kashiskoye shosse 24, Moscow 115478, USSR

Incidence of and mortality from lung cancer is increasing in most countries (Campbell, 1980; Pollack & Horm, 1980; Plesko *et al.*, 1981; Mastrandrea *et al.*, 1984; Muir & Parkin, 1985), and even larger increases can be predicted on the basis of the large increase in cigarette smoking in young adults since the Second World War (Royal College of Physicians, 1983). However, in a few countries, a decline in lung cancer mortality has been observed, particularly among young and middle-aged men (Doll & Peto, 1981; Wald *et al.*, 1981; Osmond *et al.*, 1982; Peto & Doll, 1984; IARC, 1986). This trend has been attributed to the lowering of the tar delivery per cigarette (Doll & Peto, 1981; Wald *et al.*, 1981; Peto & Doll, 1984).

MATERIALS AND METHODS

The incidence data on lung cancer for five Soviet republics – Byelorussia, Estonia, Georgia, Moldavia and Lithuania – i.e., numbers of cases of cancers of the trachea, bronchus and lung (ICD.8 – 162.0) for a 12-year period (1971–1982), were provided by the Department of Statistics of the Ministry of Public Health of the USSR. Data for six 10-year age groups (0–29, 30–39, 40–49, 50–59, 60–69, 75+) for males and females separately for each calendar year from 1971 to 1982 were abstracted from special data collection forms (Napalkov *et al.*, 1983). The rates are based on the population census (1980) and, for between-census years, on the mid-year population estimates provided by the same Department.

The annual rates per 100 000 of the population for all ages were standardized for age, using the world standard population (Waterhouse *et al.*, 1982). The age-specific rates were calculated for 10-year age groups using the direct method of standardization.

Incidence trends were calculated using exponential regression analysis following the formula, $\log \hat{y} = a + bx$, based on the logarithm of the observed incidence rates (Cancer Registry of Norway, 1982) where:

$\hat{y}$ is the estimated annual incidence rate,
x is the time point in the calendar year
$a = \overline{\log y} - b\bar{x}$, where

$$b \text{ (regression coefficient)} = \frac{\Sigma\,(x_i - \bar{x})\,(\log y_i - \overline{\log y})}{\Sigma\,(x_i - \bar{x})^2}$$

The average annual percentage change (AAPC) equals $(10^b - 1)100$, where the standard error of b is defined by the formula:

$$S_b = \sqrt{S^2 / \Sigma\,(x_i - \bar{x})^2} \text{ where } S^2 \text{ is the standard deviation from regression.}$$

The values for AAPC are given in Tables 1 and 2, together with the standard deviation and the *p* values. In addition, the coefficient of determination (r^2) has been calculated, showing formal goodness of fit for each time series. A level of r^2 close to one indicates an 'excellent' fit, or linear relationship with time, and a level close to zero shows large fluctuations and absence of linear relationship with time. Goodness of fit (r^2) was estimated using a Hewlett-Packard standard programme.

The graphs are drawn on a semilogarithmic scale. The male/female ratios are the quotients of male and female age-standardized rates for all ages.

RESULTS

The incidence of lung cancer in the USSR varies in the different Soviet republics (Fig. 1), the highest rates in males being observed in Estonia, the Russian Soviet Federated Socialist Republic (RSFSR) and Lithuania, and in females in the Ukraine, Kazakhstan, Moldavia and RSFSR. The age-standardized incidence rates of lung cancer per 100 000 population in the USSR increased from 37.7 in 1965 to 61.7 in 1984 in males, and from 5.6 in 1965 to 7.6 in 1984 in females.

The age-standardized incidence rates of lung cancer increased in all the four Soviet republics for which we have examined time trends. The increase in incidence is observed in both males and females (Fig. 2, Table 1), the increase in age-standardized rates in males being statistically significant in all four areas while, in females, statistically significant increases are seen only in Georgia and Estonia.

The increase in the incidence of lung cancer in Estonia has occurred in all age groups in males and in the age groups 50–59, 60–69 and 75+ in females (Fig. 3, Table 2).

In Lithuania an increase in lung cancer incidence is seen in males of all ages. A very important and statistically significant increase is observed in the age group 30–39 (Fig. 4, Table 2). In females an increase in incidence is seen only for the age group 50–59, while in all other age groups incidence rates have decreased, although these decreases are not statistically significant. Analysis of lung cancer incidence trends between 1957 and 1981 by birth cohort has revealed that, in males, the incidence of lung cancer increases with each successive cohort. The increases in the slopes for males start with cohorts born around the turn of the century. The curve becomes steeper for those who were born in 1912–1917 and continues to rise in male cohorts born in 1932 and 1937 (Fig. 5). The pattern observed in

Fig. 1. Lung cancer incidence in the USSR in 1980, age-standardized rates (world standard population) per 100 000 population; RSFSR, Russian Soviet Federated Socialist Repub ic

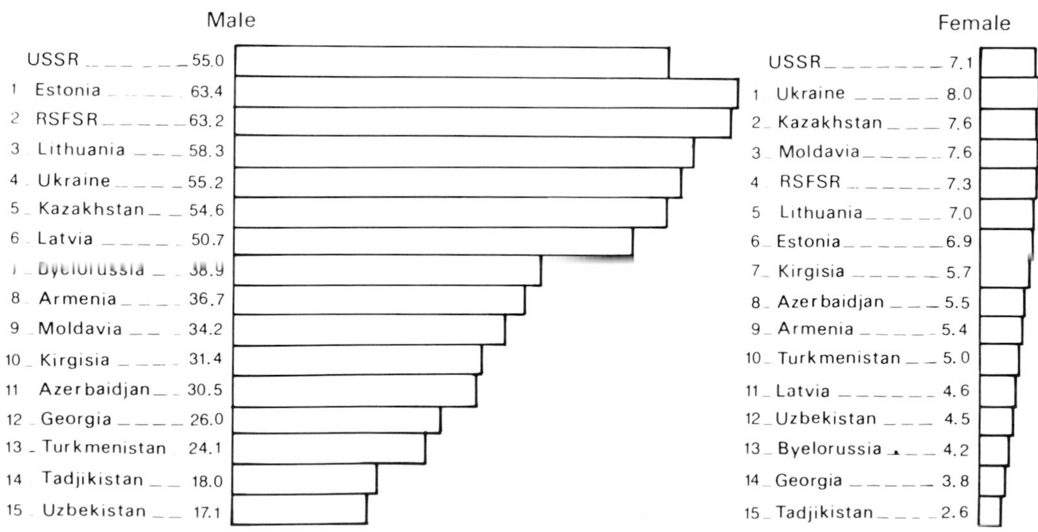

Fig. 2. Lung cancer in the USSR

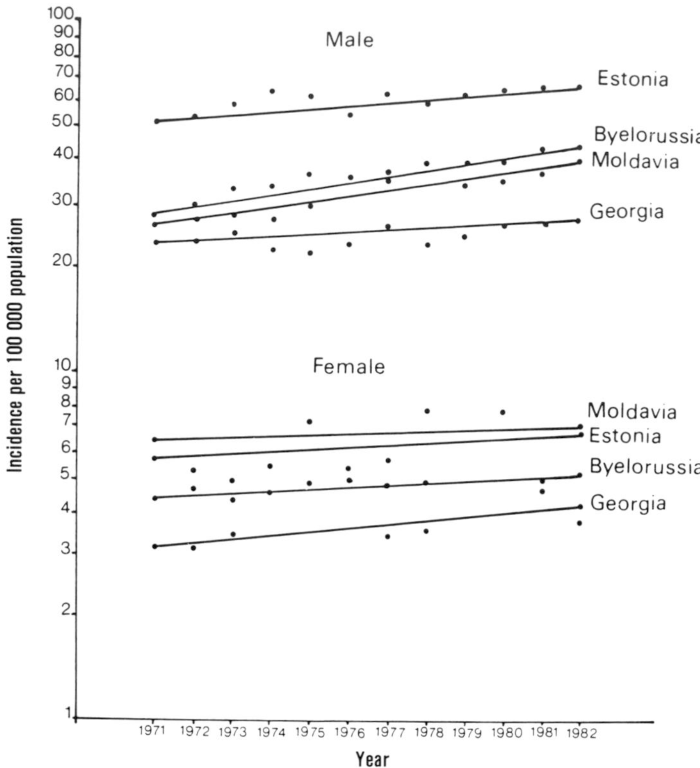

Table 1. Estimates from regression analysis of age-standardized[a] lung cancer incidence rates and male/female ratios in selected republics in the USSR during the period 1971–1982

Republic	Sex	Age-specific rate per 100 000 population		Goodness of fit (r^2)	Average annual percentage change (standard deviation)	Significance of trend (p)
		1971	1982			
Byelorussia	M	29.5	45.2	0.941	3.9 (0.3)	p <0.001
	F	4.4	4.9	0.258	0.9 (0.5)	NS[b]
	M/F	6.7	9.3	0.820	3.0 (0.4)	p <0.001
Estonia	M	55.0	67.0	0.621	1.8 (0.4)	p <0.001
	F	6.1	7.6	0.287	2.0 (1.0)	p <0.05
	M/F	9.1	8.8	0.006	–0.2 (1.0)	NS
Georgia	M	22.3	26.8	0.506	1.7 (0.5)	p <0.01
	F	3.1	4.1	0.668	2.5 (0.6)	p <0.01
	M/F	7.2	6.5	0.121	–0.9 (0.7)	NS
Moldavia	M	26.1	40.9	0.804	4.2 (0.6)	p <0.01
	F	5.7	7.2	0.260	2.2 (1.2)	NS
	M/F	4.6	5.6	0.167	1.9 (1.3)	NS

[a] Six age groups (0–29, 30–39, 40–49, 50–59, 60–69, 70+) standardized to the world standard population
[b] NS, not significant

Fig. 3. Lung cancer in Estonia

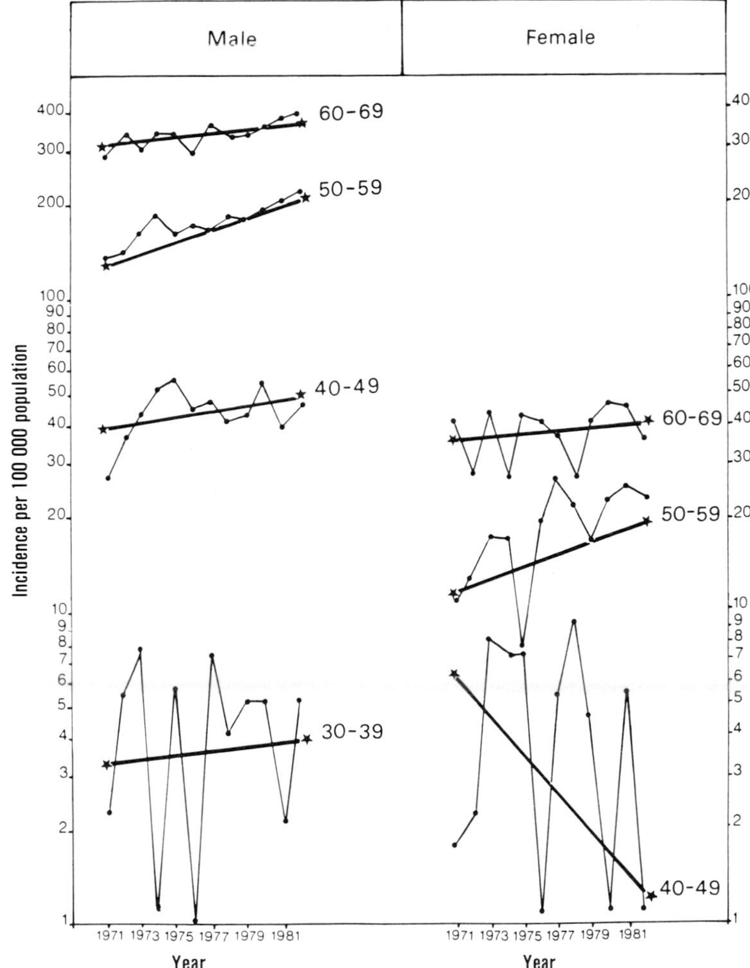

females is different, showing decreases or stabilization of lung cancer incidence in successive cohorts. However, small increases seem to occur for the cohorts born in 1932 and 1937 in the urban female population (Fig. 6) while, in rural females of the same birth cohorts, decreases in lung cancer are observed (Fig. 7).

In Byelorussia, a statistically significant increase in lung cancer incidence is observed in males of all ages except for the age group 30–39, in which a small, statistically non-significant decrease in lung cancer incidence is seen. In females, increases in incidence are seen for the age groups 40–49, 60–69 and 70+, while a decrease in incidence is observed for the age group 50–59 (Fig. 8, Table 2).

Table 2. Estimates from regression analysis of age-specific incidence rates of lung cancer in five Soviet republics during the period 1971–1982

Republic	Sex	Age group	Age-specific rate per 100 000 population 1971	1982	Goodness of fit (r^2)	Average annual percentage change	(standard deviation)	Significance of trend (p)
Byelorussia	Male	30–39	4.2	3.9	0.013	–0.6	(1.8)	NS [a]
		40–49	24.9	34.8	0.748	3.9	(0.7)	p <0.001
		50–59	87.3	139.7	0.926	4.4	(0.4)	p <0.0001
		60–69	180.3	254.0	0.875	3.2	(0.4)	p <0.0001
		70+	137.0	242.2	0.895	5.3	(0.6)	p <0.0001
	Female	30–39	0.7	0.7	0.000	–0.2	(12.9)	NS
		40–49	2.8	3.3	0.133	1.3	(1.1)	NS
		50–59	11.4	9.9	0.159	–1.3	(1.0)	NS
		60–69	24.8	28.1	0.101	1.1	(1.0)	NS
		70+	27.4	35.8	0.470	2.5	(0.8)	p <0.05
Estonia	Male	30–39	3.3	3.9	0.006	1.6	(6.5)	NS
		40–49	39.3	49.2	0.141	2.1	(1.6)	NS
		50–59	144.3	207.9	0.788	3.4	(0.5)	p <0.001
		60–69	305.7	372.4	0.506	1.8	(0.6)	p <0.05
		70+	377.8	392.5	0.026	0.3	(0.7)	NS
	Female	30–39	–	–	–	–		–
		40–49	6.1	1.3	0.148	–13.2	(11.4)	NS
		50–59	11.4	19.1	0.066	4.8	(5.7)	NS
		60–69	35.4	40.3	0.050	1.3	(1.8)	NS
		70+	38.5	47.7	0.144	1.0	(1.5)	NS
Georgia	Male	30–39	4.8	2.3	0.318	–6.3	(3.1)	p <0.05
		40–49	18.5	20.7	0.125	1.1	(0.9)	NS
		50–59	67.5	81.3	0.290	1.7	(0.8)	p <0.05
		60–69	133.0	160.6	0.253	1.7	(0.9)	NS
		70+	103.0	136.9	0.414	2.6	(1.0)	p <0.01
	Female	30–39	0.9	0.6	0.005	–2.9	(13.8)	NS
		40–49	2.2	5.2	0.508	7.9	(2.4)	p <0.01
		50–59	8.0	10.5	0.151	2.5	(1.9)	NS
		60–69	17.2	18.4	0.012	0.6	(1.7)	NS
		70+	15.2	24.2	0.509	4.3	(1.3)	p <0.05
Lithuania	Male	30–39	3.2	7.4	0.328	8.7	(4.1)	p <0.05
		40–49	35.7	44.0	0.159	2.1	(1.6)	NS
		50–59	122.5	170.5	0.388	3.4	(1.4)	p <0.05
		60–69	275.6	325.5	0.252	1.7	(1.0)	NS
		70+	–	–	–	–		
	Female	30–39	1.7	0.5	0.204	–11.5	(8.4)	NS
		40–49	5.1	4.6	0.016	–0.9	(2.2)	NS
		50–59	12.9	21.6	0.535	5.3	(1.6)	p <0.01
		60–69	34.6	30.4	0.098	–1.3	(1.3)	NS
		70+	–	–	–	–		
Moldavia	Male	30–39	5.5	5.0	0.007	–0.9	(3.6)	NS
		40–49	26.5	38.4	0.329	3.4	(1.6)	p <0.05
		50–59	81.1	132.0	0.789	4.5	(0.7)	p <0.001
		60–69	152.4	216.4	0.706	3.2	(0.7)	p <0.001
		70+	102.1	210.4	0.706	6.8	(1.4)	p <0.001

Republic	Sex	Age group	Age-specific rate per 100 000 population		Goodness of fit (r^2)	Average annual percentage change (standard deviation)		Significance of trend (p)
			1971	1982				
	Female	30–39	1.9	1.4	0.038	–2.8	(4.6)	NS
		40–49	5.7	6.9	0.155	1.7	(1.3)	NS
		50–59	16.8	21.8	0.132	2.4	(2.0)	NS
		60–69	29.1	37.8	0.408	2.4	(0.9)	p <0.05
		70+	22.8	38.7	0.246	4.9	(2.7)	NS

[a] NS, not significant

Fig. 4. Lung cancer in Lithuania

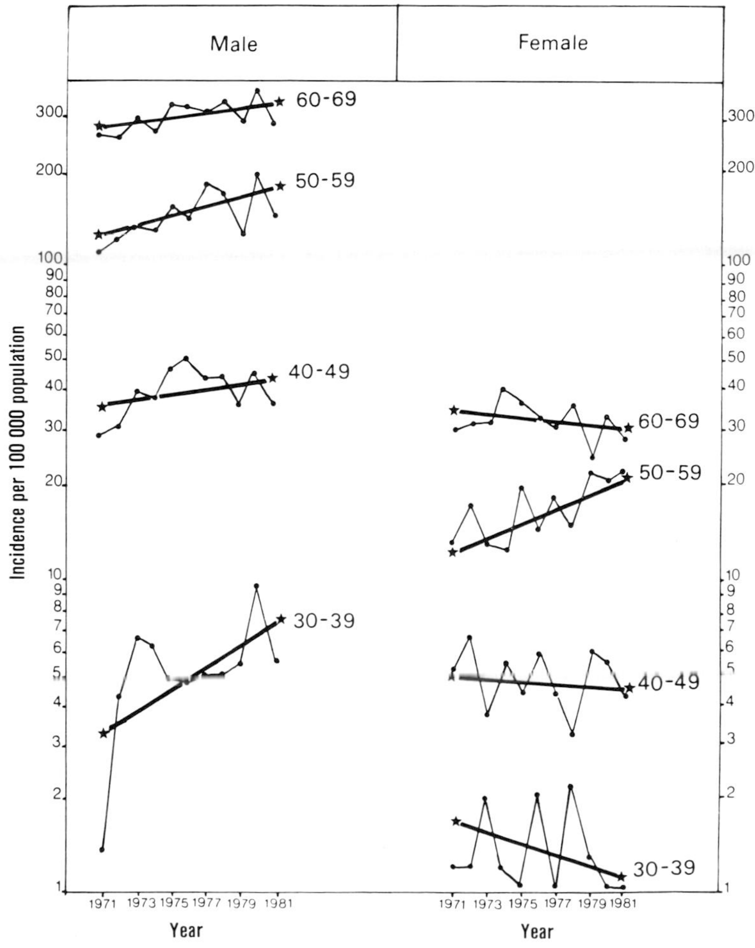

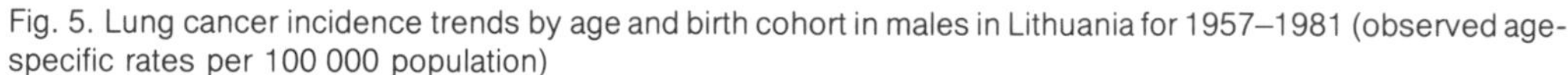

Fig. 5. Lung cancer incidence trends by age and birth cohort in males in Lithuania for 1957–1981 (observed age-specific rates per 100 000 population)

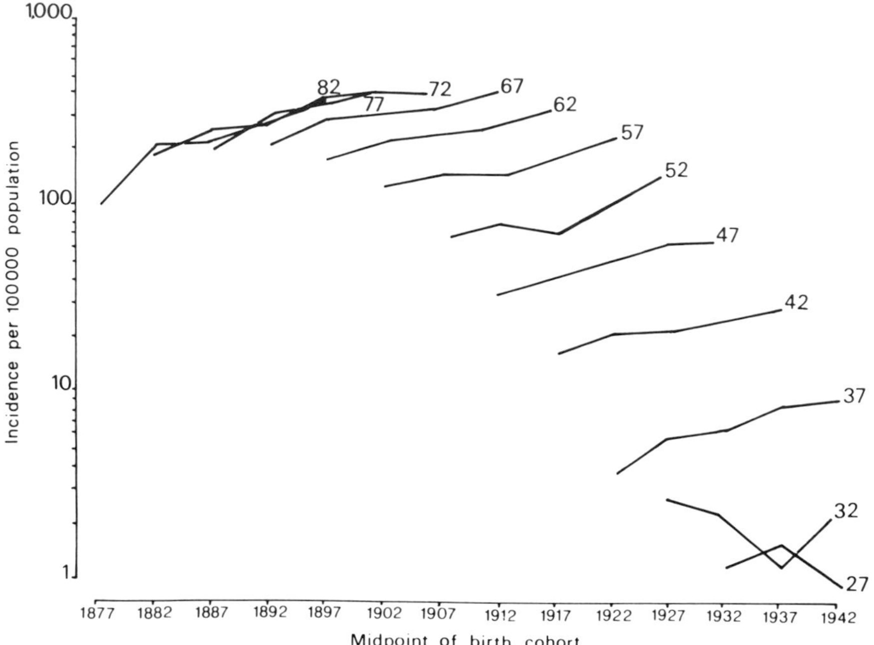

In Moldavia, lung cancer incidence is on the increase for all age groups (except 30–39) for both males and females (Fig. 9, Table 2).

Similar trends are observed in Georgia (Fig. 10, Table 2) but the data show two interesting features: (1) an increase observed in females of all ages, with the steepest increase in the age group 40–49, which is statistically significant; and (2) a statistically significant decrease in the rates in males aged 30–39.

DISCUSSION

Lung cancer in the Soviet Union has become since 1980 the most frequent type of tumour in males, with age-standardized rates reaching 55.0 per 100 000 population for the year 1980. The next most frequent site in males was the stomach (47.2 per 100 000). In females, however, lung cancer rates (7.1 per 100 000) were far behind rates for cancer of the breast (22.2 per 100 000), stomach (21.0 per 100 000) and cervix (16.2 per 100 000) (Napalkov *et al.*, 1983).

In 1980, lung cancer accounted for about one-fourth of all cancer cases in males and about one-sixth of all newly diagnosed cancer cases in both sexes. International comparisons show that the incidence of lung cancer in men in the USSR is approaching the world's highest rates (Waterhouse *et al.*, 1982).

Fig. 6. Lung cancer incidence trends by age and birth cohort in urban females in Lithuania for 1957–1981 (observed age-specific rates per 100 000 population)

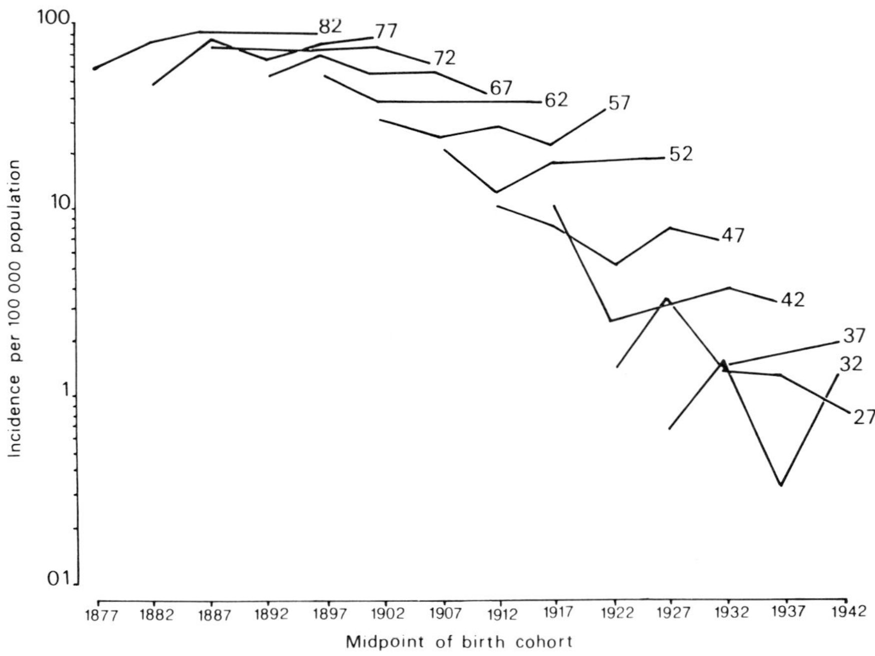

Lung cancer incidence in females in the USSR is lower, and the latter could be explained by the fact that women in the USSR seem to smoke considerably less than men. According to the various smoking surveys carried out in the USSR, about 40–80% of the men and only 6–10% of the women reported smoking cigarettes (Orlovski, 1977; Oleynikov *et al.*, 1981; Loransky *et al.*, 1983; Shevtshuk & Tarasova, 1983). However, recent surveys report that 23.5% of women in Kiev and 20.5% in Erevan are cigarette smokers (Loransky *et al.*, 1983).

A comparison of trends in lung cancer rates in the USSR with those in other countries shows that the various patterns of trends observed internationally are represented in the various Soviet populations. An increase in incidence of and mortality from lung cancer is observed in virtually all countries for which trends have been examined (Teppo *et al.*, 1975; Saracci, 1977; Benjamin, 1977; Devesa & Silverman, 1978; Campbell, 1980; Trichopoulos *et al.*, 1980; Clemmesen, 1981; Plesko *et al.*, 1981; Mastrandrea *et al.*, 1984), and a similar pattern of increases is seen in the USSR. In the five republics for which time trends have been examined in this paper, increases in lung cancer incidence have been observed in age-standardized incidence rates in both sexes and in men of all ages, with the exception of the age group 30–39. The increase in cigarette consumption in this country which has been seen until the late 1970s (Zaridze *et al.*, in this volume[2]) explains the increasing trends in lung cancer and, moreover, predicts that this increase will continue for another 30–40 years.

[2] See p. 75.

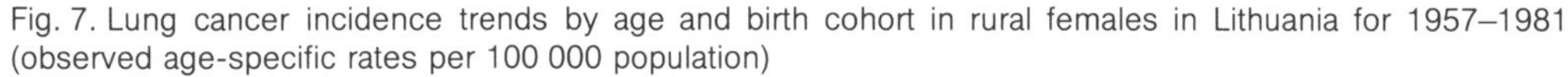

Fig. 7. Lung cancer incidence trends by age and birth cohort in rural females in Lithuania for 1957–1981 (observed age-specific rates per 100 000 population)

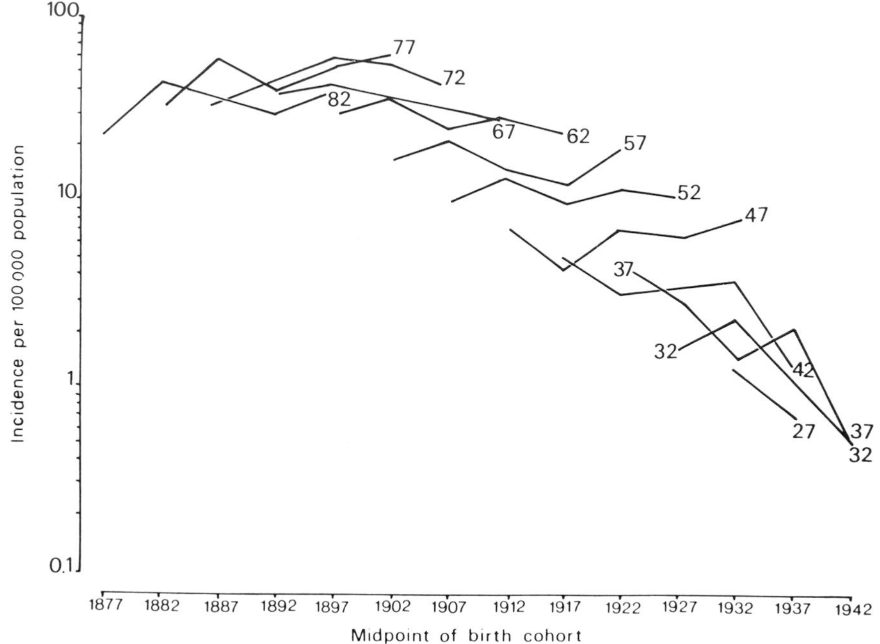

There are certain differences in lung cancer trends in females internationally. In most countries, lung cancer rates in females are increasing less rapidly than in males, resulting in an increase in the male/female ratio with time. Examples of such countries are Czechoslovakia, France, Finland, Greece, the Netherlands, Switzerland, the Federal Republic of Germany and Italy (Teppo *et al.*, 1975; Benjamin, 1977; Saracci, 1977; Foster, 1978; Trichopoulos *et al.*, 1980; Plesko *et al.*, 1981; Mastrandrea *et al.*, 1984). However, in countries such as the UK, the USA, Denmark, Australia and New Zealand, lung cancer rates are increasing more rapidly in females than in males, accompanied by a gradual decrease in the male/female ratio (Foster, 1978).

Modest increases in lung cancer incidence rates are seen in Soviet women in the older age groups, while small decreases or stabilization of rates are observed in the age group 30–39 and in some areas in the age group 40–49. However, there are two alarming exceptions: a statistically significant increase in lung cancer in Georgia in women aged 40–49 years, and an upward trend in Lithuania in urban females born in the years 1932 and 1937, suggesting either that these particular groups of women smoke more than other women in the areas analysed, or that they are exposed to some other factor related to lung cancer, the latter explanation being less probable. Judging by the change in the male/female ratio, the rate of increase in lung cancer incidence remains higher in men in Byelorussia and Moldavia. The increase is slightly more pronounced in Estonian women

Fig. 8. Lung cancer in Byelorussia

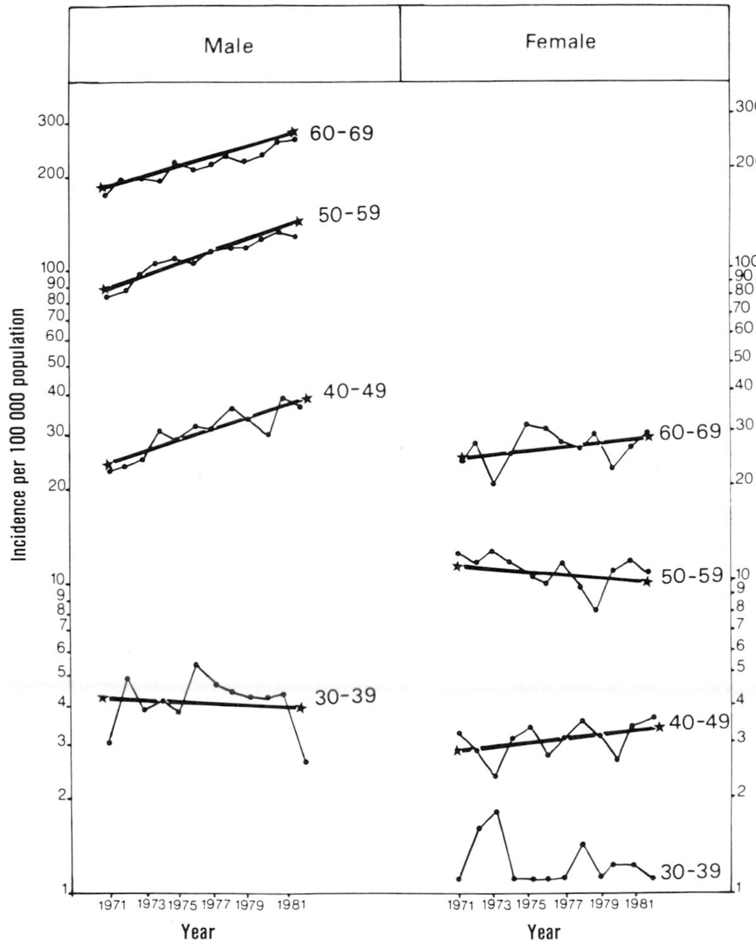

than in Estonian men and very much more so in Georgian women compared to Georgian men. In fact, the decrease in the male/female ratio in Georgia has occurred in the age groups 30–39 and 40–49, while no change has been observed in older age groups.

In a few countries (the UK and Finland), a decrease in lung cancer mortality is being observed in young and middle-aged men, these trends being attributed to a decrease in tar delivery per cigarette which has occurred in these countries during the last 30 years or so (Doll & Peto, 1981; Wald *et al.*, 1981; Peto & Doll, 1984; IARC, 1986).

In the USSR a statistically significant decrease in lung cancer incidence is observed in men in Georgia in the age group 30–39, slight decreases in rates or stabilization of trends are seen in this age group in Byelorussia, Moldavia and Estonia, while a statistically significant increase has been observed in the same age group in Lithuania. Stabilization of

Fig. 9. Lung cancer in Moldavia

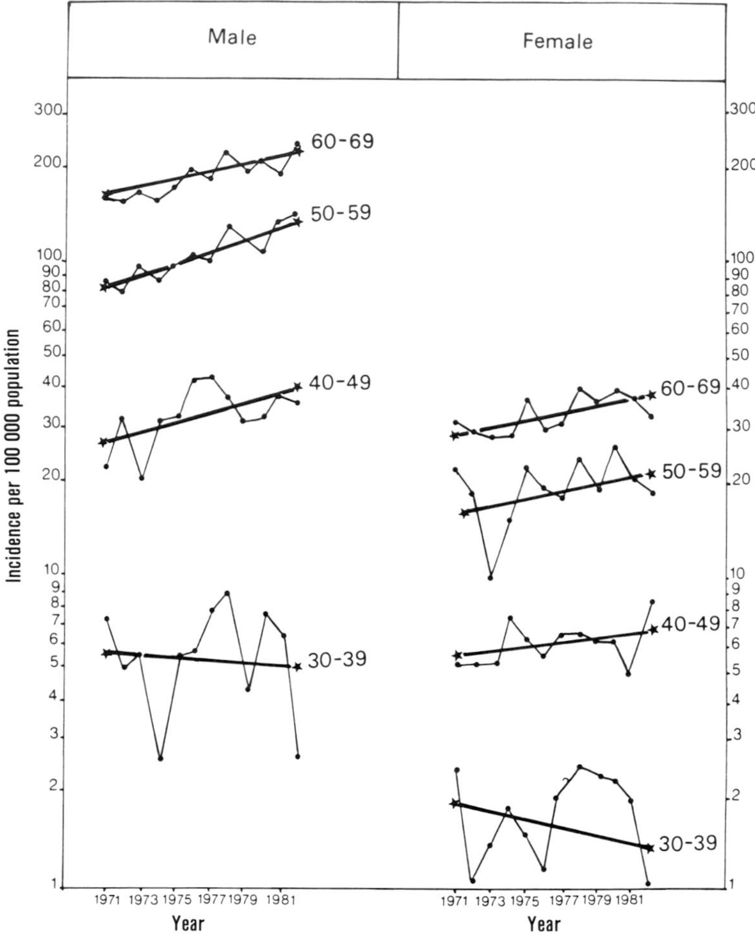

or decrease in incidence rates in young males suggests either that the younger generation of men smoke less or that the cigarettes they smoke are less carcinogenic. Unfortunately, no data are available either on trends in the smoking habit by age or on trends in the smoke composition of Soviet cigarettes. However, we know that filter cigarettes started to appear in the USSR only in the early 1970s and that by the mid-1970s they represented only 17% of all cigarettes sold; in addition, about 90% of cigarettes are still 'high-tar' (Zaridze *et al.*, in this volume[3]). Thus the decreasing trends in young males (if at all real) cannot be explained by changes in cigarette composition but rather by a change in the smoking habits of the younger generation.

[3] See p. 75.

Fig. 10. Lung cancer in Georgia

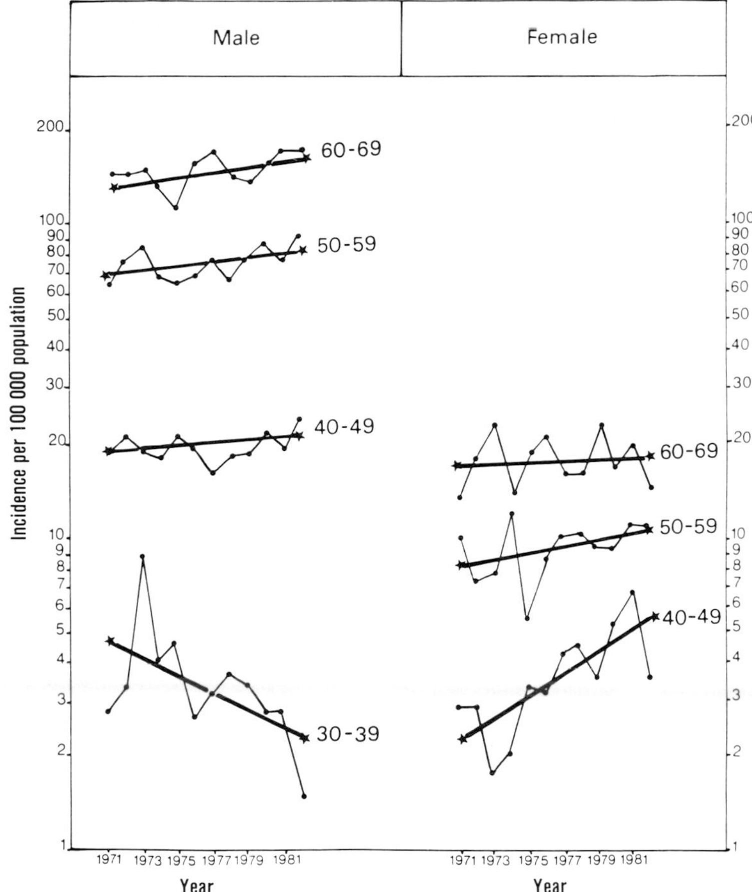

Lung cancer in the USSR has become the major public health problem. The number of newly diagnosed lung cancer cases has increased rapidly over the last 20 years: in 1965, lung cancer was diagnosed in 31 400 men and 8800 women, in 1970 in 39 800 men and 10 600 women, in 1975 in 50 700 men and 13 400 women, in 1980 in 63 200 men and 14 700 women and in 1984 in 75 000 men and 16 700 women. By the end of the century the number will be well above 100 000. By the most conservative estimates, about 70–80% of lung cancer in the USSR is attributable to smoking. Thus, about 80 000 lung cancer cases or 80 000 deaths from lung cancer, which would occur annually by the end of this century, are preventable.

Based on the experience of a few countries (the UK, Finland), where there have been 50–70% declines in lung cancer mortality rates in young and middle-aged men, attributed to a decrease in the 'tar yield' of cigarettes used in these countries over the last 20–30 years (Doll & Peto, 1981; Wald *et al.*, 1981; Peto & Doll, 1984; IARC, 1986), it can be predicted that similar declines could be produced by reducing the 'tar yield' of cigarettes in countries where such changes in cigarette composition have not yet been introduced.

REFERENCES

Benjamin, B. (1977) Trends and differentials in lung cancer mortality. *World Health Stat. Rep.*, ***30***, 118–145

Campbell, H. (1980) Cancer mortality in Europe. Site-specific patterns and trends 1955 to 1974. *World Health Stat. Q.*, ***33***, 241–280

Cancer Registry of Norway (1982) *Trends in Cancer Incidence in Norway*, Oslo

Clemmesen, J. (1981) Uses of cancer registration in the study of carcinogenesis. *J. natl Cancer Inst.*, ***67***, 5–13

Devesa, S.S. & Silverman, D.T. (1978) Cancer incidence and mortality trends in the United States: 1935–74. *J. natl Cancer Inst.*, ***60***, 545–571

Doll, R. & Peto, R. (1981) *The Causes of Cancer. Quantitative Estimates of Avoidable Risks of Cancer in the United States Today*, Oxford, Oxford University Press

Foster, F. (1978) Sex differentials in cancer mortality and morbidity. *World Health Stat. Q.*, ***31***, 360–383

IARC (1986) *IARC Monographs on the Evaluation of the Carcinogenic Risk of Chemicals to Humans*, Vol. 38, *Tobacco Smoking*, Lyon, International Agency for Research on Cancer

Loransky, D.N., Popova, E.B., Chakimova, L.S. & Shevtshuk, A.G. (1983) State of the smoking problem (Russ.). *Sov. Sdravochranenie*, ***6***, 33–38

Mastrandrea, V., La Rosa, F. & Cresci, A. (1984) Trends of lung cancer mortality in Italy in relation to consumption of tobacco products. *Am. J. Epidemiol.*, ***120***, 257–264

Muir, C.S. & Parkin, D.M. (1985) The world cancer burden: Prevent or perish. *Br. med. J.*, ***290***, 5–6

Napalkov, N.P., Tserkovny, G.F., Merabishvili, V.M., Parkin, D.M., Smans, M. & Muir, C.S., eds (1983) *Cancer Incidence in the USSR (IARC Scientific Publications No. 48)*, Lyon, International Agency for Research on Cancer

Oleynikov, S.P., Glasunov, E.S. & Chazova, L.V. (1981) Smoking among men and women of various age groups (Russ.). *Ter. Arkh.*, ***2***, 111–115

Orlovski, L.V. (1977) *Importance of education in the anti-smoking campaign*. In: *Proceedings of the Meeting of the USSR Academy of Medical Sciences Commission on the Problem of Medical Education* (Russ.), Archangelsk, pp. 122–130

Osmond, C., Gardner, M.J. & Acheson, E.D. (1982) Analysis of trends in cancer mortality in England and Wales during 1951–80 separating changes associated with period of birth and period of death. *Br. med. J.*, ***284***, 1005–1008

Peto, R. & Doll, R. (1984) *Keynote address: The control of lung cancer*. In: Mizell, M. & Correa, P., eds, *Lung Cancer. Causes and Prevention, Proceedings of the International Lung Cancer Update Conference held in New Orleans, 3–5 March 1983*, Deerfield Beach, USA, Verlag Chemie International, pp. 1–19

Plesko, I., Dimitrova, E., Hostynova, E. & Somogyi, J. (1981) Trends in cancer mortality in Czechoslovakia 1949–78. *Neoplasma*, ***28***, 233–243

Pollak, E.S. & Horm, J.W. (1980) Trends in cancer incidence and mortality in the United States, 1969–76. *J. natl Cancer Inst.*, ***64***, 1091–1103

Royal College of Physicians (1983) *Health or Smoking?* Follow-up Report of the Royal College of Physicians, London, Pitman Publishing Ltd.

Saracci, R. (1977) *Epidemiology of lung cancer in Italy*. In: Mohr, V., Schmael, D.,

Tomatis, L. & Davis, W., eds, *Air Pollution and Cancer in Man (IARC Scientific Publications No. 16),* Lyon, International Agency for Research on Cancer, 205–215

Shevtshuk, A.G. & Tarasova, R.N. (1983) Organization of an anti-smoking campaign [in Russian]. *Sdravochranenie Ross. Fed.,* **5,** 27–28

Teppo, L., Hakama, M., Hakulinen, T., Lehtonen, M. & Saxen, E. (1975) Cancer in Finland 1953–1970: Incidence, mortality, prevalence. *Acta pathol. microbiol. Scand.* (Suppl. 252)

Trichopoulos, D., Kalandidi, A. & Tzonou, A. (1980) *Incidence and distribution of lung cancer in Greece.* In: Pontifex, G., ed., *Lung Cancer: Aetiology, Epidemiology, Prevention, Early Diagnosis, Treatment,* 1st European Symposium of Lung Cancer, Chalkidiku, 1980. Amsterdam, Oxford and Princeton, Excerpta Medica, pp. 10–17

Wald, N.J., Doll, R. & Copeland, G. (1981) Trends in tar, nicotine and carbon monoxide yields of UK cigarettes manufactured since 1934. *Br. med. J.,* **282,** 763–765

Waterhouse, J.A.H., Muir, C.S., Shanmugaratnam, K. & Powell, J., eds (1982) *Cancer Incidence in Five Continents,* Vol. IV *(IARC Scientific Publications No. 42),* Lyon, International Agency for Research on Cancer

SMOKING AND CANCER PATTERNS AND TRENDS IN JAPAN

S. TOMINAGA

Aichi Cancer Center Research Institute,
Nagoya, Japan

SUMMARY

In Japan, cancer has become the leading cause of deaths since 1981. Of all sites of cancer, lung cancer, which is presently the second most common cancer in males and the fourth most common cancer in females, has increased markedly over the last 35 years. The reason for the marked increase of lung cancer in Japan is not clear, but it is likely that a marked increase in cigarette consumption has greatly contributed to it. In Japan, cigarette consumption has been decreasing slightly in recent years and the percentage of smokers among adult males has decreased from the highest, 83.7%, in 1966 to 65.5% in 1984. However, lung cancer mortality is still increasing, although the rate of increase has been getting smaller among middle to young age groups in recent years. To prevent further increase in lung cancer and to prevent other tobacco-related diseases, much stronger smoking control measures are necessary in Japan.

MATERIALS AND METHODS

Cancer mortality data were obtained from the Japan vital statistics series 1935–1983 (Ministry of Health and Welfare of Japan, 1984). The age-adjusted mortality rate for each site of cancer was calculated by using the Japanese population of 1935. Cigarette consumption data for 1920–1970 were obtained from a report for the Tobacco Research Council (Beese, 1972) and cigarette consumption data from 1971–1984 and data on smoking habits for 1958–1984 were obtained from the reports of the Japan Tobacco and Salt Public Corporation (unpublished data). A survey on smoking habits for adults of 20 years old and over has been conducted annually by the Japan Tobacco and Salt Public Corporation (now Japan Tobacco, Inc.) since 1958.

RESULTS

Trends in cancer mortality in Japan

Figure 1 shows trends in the crude death rate of major causes of deaths in Japan (1935–1983). Stroke was the leading cause of deaths from 1951 to 1980, but cancer has become the leading cause of deaths since 1981 and cancer deaths accounted for 23.8% of all deaths in 1983.

Figure 2 shows trends in the age-adjusted cancer death rate by site in Japan from 1935 to 1982. Stomach cancer is the most common cancer in both sexes, but the mortality rate has

Fig. 1. Trends in the crude death rate of major causes of deaths in Japan (1935–1983) (data from Ministry of Health and Welfare of Japan, 1984)

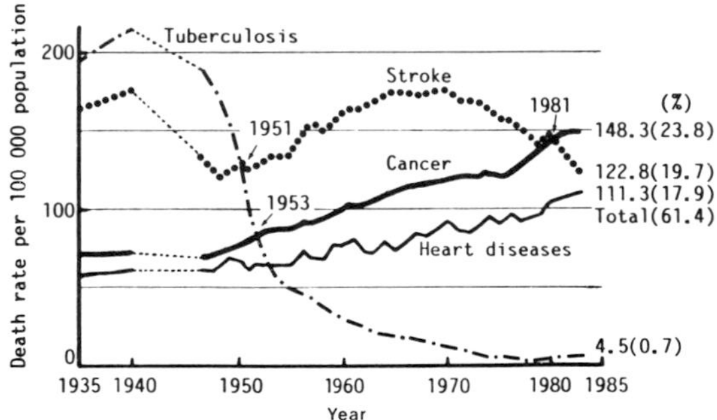

Fig. 2. Trends in the age-adjusted death rate (standardized on age distribution of Japanese in 1935) of cancer by site in Japan (1935–1982) (data from Ministry of Health and Welfare of Japan, 1984)

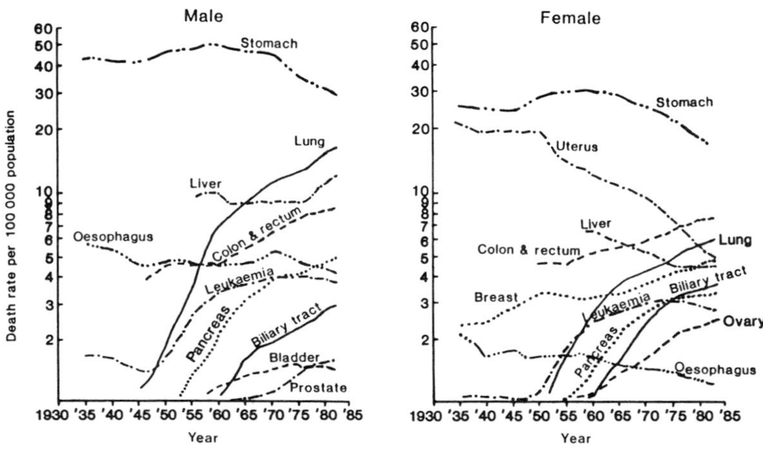

Fig. 3. Trends in the age-adjusted incidence rate (standardized on world population) of cancer by site in Osaka (1963–1980) (data from Hanai & Fujimoto, 1984)

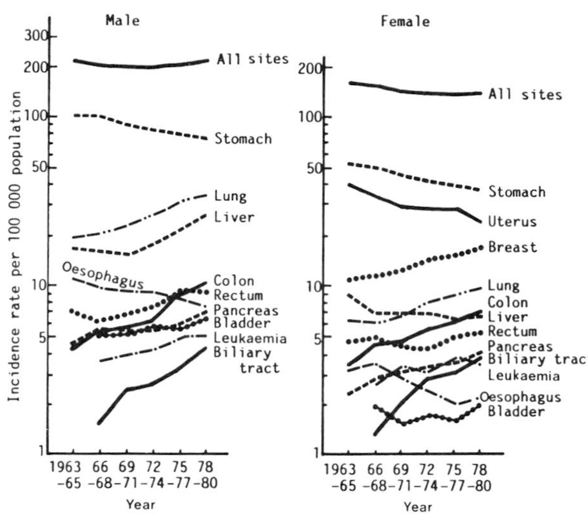

been decreasing in recent years. Cancer of the uterus, most of which is cervical cancer, has shown a marked decreasing trend since 1950. These decreasing trends in death rates of cancers of the stomach and uterus were also observed in the incidence rates of cancer as determined from the population-based cancer registry in Osaka (Hanai & Fujimoto, 1984) as shown in Figure 3.

Lung cancer was a rare cancer until around 1950, when tuberculosis was the leading cause of deaths. The number of deaths from lung cancer in Japan was only 768 (520 for males and 248 for females) in 1947, but it increased to 25 651 (18 644 for males and 7007 for females) in 1983. The crude death rate of lung cancer per 100 000 population was 1.4 for males and 0.6 for females in 1947, but it increased to 31.9 (22.8 times) for males and 11.6 (10.3 times) for females in 1983. The age-adjusted death rate of lung cancer per 100 000 population was 1.3 for males and 0.6 for females, but it also increased to 16.6 (12.8 times) for males and 6.0 (10.0 times) for females in 1983 (Table 1).

As seen in Figure 2 and Table 1, lung cancer mortality is still increasing. Figure 4 shows a prediction of future age-adjusted death rates of cancer by site in Japan, based on observed time trends from 1972 to 1981 (Tominaga, 1984). It was predicted that, in males, the lung cancer death rate would exceed the stomach cancer death rate in around 1992 and in females the former would exceed the latter in around 1997, assuming that the observed time trends from 1972 to 1981 continue until 2000.

Table 1. Mortality statistics on lung cancer in Japan (1935-1983)

	Total no. of deaths		Crude death rate per 100 000		Age-adjusted death rate per 100 000 [a]	
Year	Male	Female	Male	Female	Male	Female
1935	–	–	–	–	–	–
1940	–	–	–	–	–	–
1947	520	248	1.4	0.6	1.3	0.6
1948	553	266	1.4	0.7	1.4	0.6
1949	721	306	1.8	0.7	1.8	0.7
1950	789	330	1.9	0.8	1.9	0.8
1951	809	387	1.9	0.9	1.9	0.9
1952	1 084	496	2.6	1.1	2.5	1.1
1953	1 234	158	2.9	1.2	2.7	1.1
1954	1 599	685	3.7	1.5	3.4	1.5
1955	1 893	818	4.3	1.8	3.9	1.7
1956	2 318	999	5.2	2.2	4.7	2.0
1957	2 568	1 085	5.7	2.3	5.1	2.2
1958	2 919	1 352	6.5	2.9	5.6	2.6
1959	3 329	1 410	7.3	3.0	6.2	2.7
1960	3 638	1 533	7.9	3.2	6.6	2.8
1961	3 932	1 766	8.5	3.7	7.0	3.2
1962	4 336	1 891	9.3	3.9	7.5	3.3
1963	4 768	1 968	10.1	4.0	8.1	3.4
1964	5 067	2 105	10.6	4.3	8.4	3.5
1965	5 404	2 321	11.2	4.6	8.6	3.8
1966	5 857	2 508	12.0	5.0	9.1	4.0
1967	6 296	2 566	12.9	5.1	9.6	4.0
1968	6 666	2 699	13.5	5.3	9.8	4.0
1969	7 209	2 924	14.4	5.6	10.3	4.2
1970	7 502	2 987	14.8	5.7	10.5	4.2
1971	8 042	3 087	15.7	5.8	10.9	4.2
1972	8 837	3 453	17.0	6.4	11.5	4.5
1973	9 256	3 600	17.5	6.5	11.6	4.5
1974	9 986	3 730	18.6	6.7	12.1	4.5
1975	10 711	4 048	19.6	7.2	12.6	4.7
1976	11 440	4 429	20.7	7.8	13.1	5.0
1977	12 542	4 693	22.5	8.1	13.9	5.1
1978	13 417	5 113	23.8	8.8	14.2	5.3
1979	14 597	5 323	25.7	9.1	14.9	5.3
1980	15 438	5 856	27.0	9.9	15.3	5.6
1981	16 638	6 161	28.9	10.3	15.9	5.7
1982	17 555	6 661	30.2	11.1	16.2	5.9
1983	18 644	7 007	31.9	11.6	16.6	6.0

[a] Standardized on age distribution of population of Japan, 1935

Fig. 4. Prediction of the future age-adjusted death rate (standardized on age distribution of Japanese in 1935) of cancer by site in Japan based on observed trends from 1972–1981 (data from Tominaga, 1984)

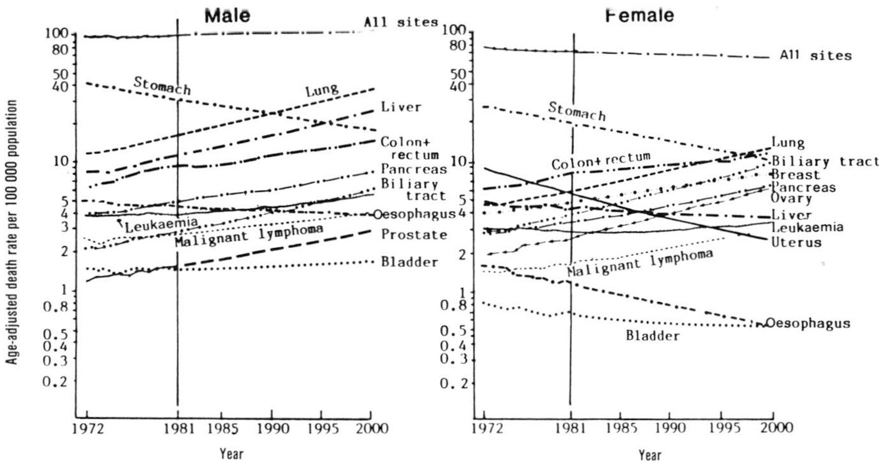

Table 2. Trends in cigarette consumption and percentage of smokers in Japan [a]

Year	No. of cigarettes consumed per adult of 15 years and over per year	Percentage of smokers aged 20 years and over		Average number of cigarettes smoked per day per smoker	
		Males	Females	Males	Females
1920	600	–	–	–	–
1925	730	–	–	–	–
1930	750	–	–	–	–
1935	880	–	–	–	–
1940	1 130	–	–	–	–
1943	1 140	–	–	–	–
1944	950	–	–	–	–
1945	310	–	–	–	–
1946	310	–	–	–	–
1947	360	–	–	–	–
1948	660	–	–	–	–
1949	1 000	–	–	–	–
1950	1 220	–	–	–	–
1955	1 650	–	–	–	–
1958	1 690	75.9	12.4	–	–
1960	1 880	80.5	13.2	–	–
1965	2 350	82.3	15.7	19.4	12.2
1966	2 440	83.7	18.0	19.8	13.6
1970	2 810	77.5	15.6	20.9	14.3
1975	3 422	76.2	15.1	23.8	16.6
1977	3 497	75.1	15.1	24.0	15.6
1980	3 393	70.2	14.4	24.6	15.7
1984	3 270	65.5	14.0	24.9	16.7

[a] Data from Beese (1972); Japan Tobacco and Salt Public Corporation (unpublished data)

Table 3. Sex- and age-specific percentage of smokers aged 20 years old and over in Japan (1967–1984) [a]

Sex	Age (years)	1967	1968	1969	1970	1971	1972	1973	1974	1975	1976	1977	1978	1979	1980	1981	1982	1983	1984
Male	20–29	83.2	78.0	78.5	79.9	79.2	80.0	80.1	82.9	81.5	80.8	79.9	78.2	80.3	77.1	76.4	76.2	70.9	71.3
	30–39	84.1	79.3	80.6	78.4	77.3	77.0	78.7	79.7	77.0	74.8	76.0	76.0	76.1	73.4	75.9	74.7	71.3	70.9
	40–49	85.8	82.5	83.7	81.0	79.7	81.0	82.2	80.6	76.3	75.4	74.5	75.3	71.2	69.1	68.6	67.5	65.2	64.1
	50–59	82.3	81.3	80.3	78.3	78.8	79.8	77.7	78.0	78.6	77.5	75.5	76.3	74.6	70.0	69.6	72.2	65.7	67.2
	60+	73.3	70.8	71.1	67.8	69.8	68.5	70.1	69.7	65.8	64.4	67.4	65.5	62.0	60.0	60.9	58.8	56.5	52.8
	All ages	82.3	78.5	79.1	77.5	77.4	77.6	78.3	78.8	76.2	75.1	75.1	74.7	73.1	70.2	70.8	70.1	66.1	65.5
Female	20–29	11.0	8.1	9.9	9.8	10.2	12.7	11.0	12.9	12.7	14.3	16.0	14.9	16.4	16.2	17.4	17.4	15.0	17.1
	30–39	16.4	13.6	13.1	13.7	13.4	13.4	12.4	14.1	13.5	14.4	13.2	15.7	14.0	14.2	14.9	16.2	14.8	15.0
	40–49	20.9	17.8	16.8	16.1	16.1	14.9	15.5	17.6	15.7	14.6	14.5	16.6	15.5	14.4	16.5	15.7	13.4	13.3
	50–59	23.1	21.1	20.7	23.3	17.9	20.6	18.0	21.1	17.9	17.4	16.0	16.8	16.3	12.8	13.5	14.1	11.8	11.3
	60+	20.3	20.4	19.8	20.0	19.4	18.5	21.2	20.5	16.8	17.5	17.0	17.3	15.4	14.6	14.1	13.3	12.4	13.3
	All ages	17.7	15.4	15.4	15.6	14.7	15.5	15.1	16.7	15.1	15.4	15.1	16.2	15.4	14.4	15.3	15.4	13.5	14.0

[a] Data from Japan Tabocco and Salt Public Corporation (unpublished)

Trends in cigarette consumption and smoking habit in Japan

Table 2 shows the average annual number of cigarettes consumed per person of 15 years old and over from 1920 to 1984, the percentage of smokers among adults of 20 years old and over from 1958 to 1984, and the average number of cigarettes smoked per day per smoker from 1965 to 1984 in Japan.

The average annual number of cigarettes consumed per person of 15 years old and over gradually increased from 600 in 1920 to 1140 in 1943, but sharply decreased to 310 immediately after the Second World War. However, it recovered quickly and exceeded the pre-war level in 1950. Thereafter, the average annual number of cigarettes consumed showed a marked increase and reached the world's highest level in around 1975. It peaked in 1977 and has shown a decreasing trend for the last several years, as the percentage of male smokers has decreased.

Since 1958, the Japan Tobacco and Salt Public Corporation has conducted an annual nationwide survey on smoking habits in randomly selected adults of 20 years old and over. The percentage of smokers was 75.9% in males and 12.4% in females in 1958. The percentage increased gradually and reached the highest level of 83.7% in males and 18.0% in females in 1966. Thereafter the percentage of smokers decreased gradually especially in males, and in 1984 was 65.5% in males and 14.0% in females. A marked decrease has been observed in the percentage of male smokers in recent years.

The sex- and age-specific percentages of smokers from 1967 to 1984 are shown in Table 3, and relative time trends of smokers by sex and by age group are shown in Figure 5. A decreasing trend is observed in all age groups in males, and in age groups of 40 years and over in females. But a marked increase is observed in young females of 20–29 years old. The percentage of smokers in girls is not available, but is estimated to show the same increasing trend as for women in the their twenties.

Fig. 5. Relative trends in the percentage of smokers by sex and by age group in Japan (1967–1984) (data from Japan Tobacco and Salt Public Corporation, unpublished)

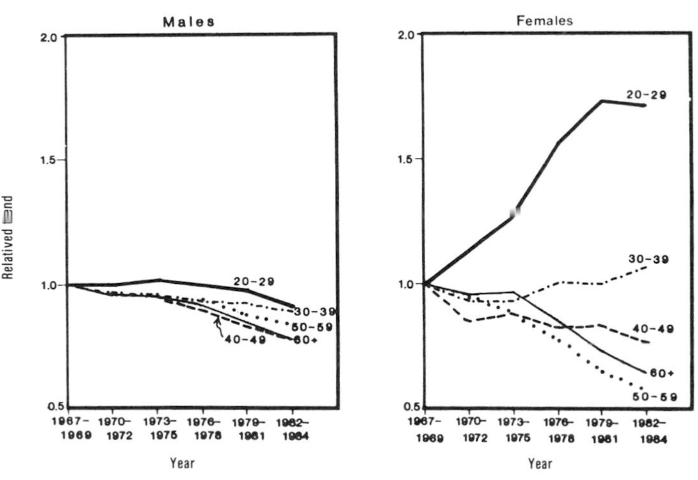

Table 4. Percentage of smokers aged 20 years old and over by sex and by occupation in Japan (1967–1984) [a]

Sex	Occupation	1967	1968	1969	1970	1971	1972	1973	1974	1975	1976	1977	1978	1979	1980	1981	1982	1983	1984
Males	Service workers and salesmen	88.4	83.7	84.2	84.6	83.2	83.1	83.7	87.3	84.7	85.3	83.2	81.0	80.8	78.8	80.7	78.3	75.4	83.6
	Manual workers	85.6	80.0	83.1	81.3	81.5	80.6	83.3	83.5	80.5	79.9	78.3	79.4	77.4	76.5	78.3	75.6	72.2	74.1
	Merchants and proprietors	83.8	79.2	80.0	76.4	80.4	79.2	80.2	79.4	78.1	75.4	76.0	74.7	76.1	70.7	72.4	70.9	69.2	66.3
	Clerical workers	83.2	79.6	81.2	78.5	76.6	77.8	77.5	78.0	75.1	75.1	76.1	73.9	72.1	70.1	68.7	69.2	64.0	63.5
	Farmers and fishermen	85.3	81.4	82.2	79.4	72.3	77.6	77.0	78.5	75.0	72.5	72.8	74.5	68.4	68.7	67.6	70.5	62.2	62.0
	Students	69.3	62.6	64.8	73.4	74.6	68.6	61.8	73.5	72.0	70.9	72.2	60.8	66.6	64.7	60.5	–	–	–
	Executives and liberal professionals	77.8	75.8	74.3	73.5	75.5	77.4	77.1	74.6	71.9	73.7	71.0	72.9	71.0	64.5	67.2	67.0	61.7	59.8
	Men without jobs	66.3	63.9	67.7	63.8	67.1	61.1	66.5	64.9	65.5	61.6	65.2	65.6	63.5	57.7	57.6	56.8	57.3	53.8
	Total	82.3	78.5	79.1	77.5	77.4	77.6	78.3	78.8	76.2	75.1	75.1	74.7	73.1	70.2	70.8	70.1	66.1	65.6
Females	Service workers and saleswomen	45.1	42.4	46.7	42.4	31.8	38.8	32.8	43.3	43.0	43.2	42.6	40.4	39.8	37.3	38.5	37.9	35.7	38.3
	Manual workers	24.2	21.3	19.3	19.1	16.3	19.1	17.8	19.8	20.5	21.4	18.7	20.0	17.7	17.0	19.3	20.8	16.3	15.1
	Merchants and proprietors	41.1	19.3	27.0	21.5	25.6	19.2	19.4	23.5	24.7	24.2	22.4	25.1	25.9	26.1	21.2	24.0	19.5	19.6
	Clerical workers	15.2	10.4	13.3	14.1	11.2	12.7	12.7	13.5	14.2	15.3	14.0	14.7	16.2	14.3	15.7	15.3	14.0	13.1
	Executives and liberal professionals	33.7	32.5	27.8	37.0	24.0	29.5	25.5	28.6	27.1	25.0	16.2	21.1	25.6	28.3	25.0	–	–	–
	Students	6.5	2.2	9.1	3.6	23.2	19.5	2.7	20.7	8.3	20.8	25.0	10.6	14.3	11.5	21.3	–	–	–
	Farmers and fisherwomen	8.5	8.5	9.9	7.0	7.9	7.7	8.6	8.9	6.2	8.4	6.2	6.8	4.7	5.4	4.9	8.7	4.4	3.9
	Women without jobs	19.4	19.4	17.4	19.0	17.1	17.4	20.7	19.6	17.2	16.2	16.9	19.3	16.2	15.7	15.7	14.3	13.8	13.1
	Housewives	14.6	13.2	11.8	11.9	12.9	12.9	12.7	14.4	12.6	12.3	13.2	14.0	13.3	12.0	13.1	12.6	11.2	12.6
	Total	17.7	15.4	15.4	15.6	14.7	15.5	15.1	16.7	15.1	15.4	15.1	16.2	15.4	14.4	15.3	15.4	13.5	14.0

[a] Data from Japan Tabocco and Salt Public Corporation (unpublished)

The percentages of smokers by occupation in adults aged 20 years and over from 1967 to 1984 are shown in Table 4. Service workers and salesmen showed the highest percentage of smokers, while female farmers showed the lowest percentage of smokers.

The average number of cigarettes smoked per day per smoker was 19.4 for males and 12.2 for females in 1965, but it increased gradually to 24.9 for males and 16.7 for females in 1984, probably reflecting the switch from high-tar, high-nicotine cigarettes to low-tar, low-nicotine cigarettes and a greater probability of relatively light smokers stopping smoking.

Comparisons of the time trends in lung cancer mortality, cigarette consumption and percentage of smokers in Japan

Figure 6 shows comparisons of the time trends in the lung cancer mortality, the average annual cigarette consumption per person of 15 years and over and the percentage of smokers in adults of 20 years and over in Japan. A close similarity in time trends is observed between cigarette consumption and lung cancer mortality in both males and females. However, a marked discrepancy is observed between the trends of percentage of smokers and lung cancer mortality. This discrepancy may be explained partly by the increasing number of cigarettes smoked per day per smoker and the delayed effect of stopping smoking on the incidence/mortality of lung cancer. From Figure 7, which shows trends in the lung cancer mortality by age group in Japan in 1950–1980, it can be observed that the increasing trend is more marked in older age groups and is getting smaller in middle to young age groups. It is interesting to note that persons in age groups of 45–59 years, who were young adults in 1940–1950, when the supply of cigarettes was least, have not shown a marked increasing trend in lung cancer mortality. Persons of younger age groups as well as middle to older age groups who do not show a marked increasing trend in the lung cancer

Fig. 6. Comparisons of trends of the age-adjusted lung cancer mortality; (——), cigarette consumption per adult (........) and the percentage of smokers in adults (– – – –) in Japan (data from Ministry of Health and Welfare of Japan, 1984; Japan Tobacco and Salt Public Corporation, unpublished)

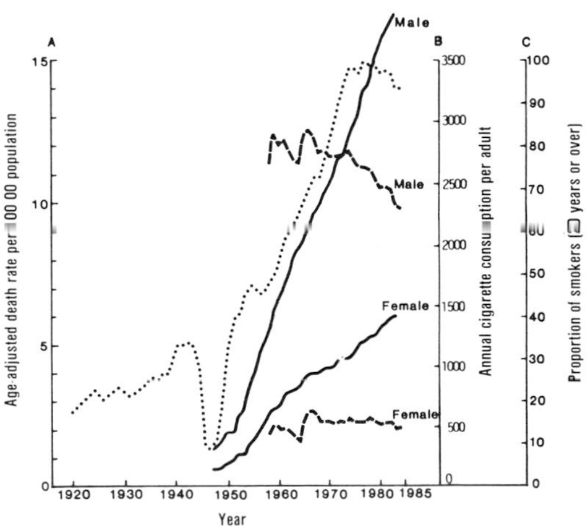

Fig. 7. Trends in the sex- and age-specific death rate of lung cancer in Japan (1950–1980) (data from Ministry of Health and Welfare of Japan, 1984)

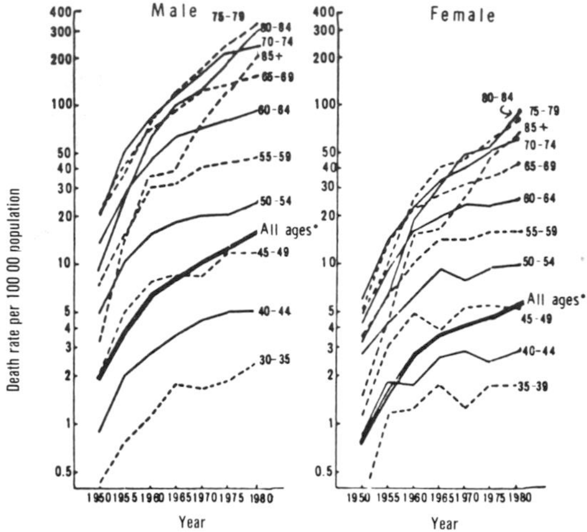

mortality. Persons of younger age groups as well as middle to older age groups who do not show a marked increasing trend in the lung cancer mortality may have benefited from the availability of filter-tip, low-tar cigarettes in recent years.

DISCUSSION

On the evidence from many epidemiological studies, cigarette smoking is considered a major risk factor for lung cancer as well as for cancers of the oral cavity, larynx and oesophagus. It is known that cigarette smoking is also related to cancers of the pharynx, stomach, pancreas, liver, bladder and cervix (US Department of Health, Education, and Welfare, 1979; Royal College of Physicians, 1983).

The chronological relationship between cancer pattern, especially lung cancer mortality and cigarette consumption and percentage of smokers in Japan revealed that there was a good similarity between the trends of cigarette consumption and lung cancer mortality. However, there was a discrepancy between the trends of lung cancer mortality and the percentage of smokers. This discrepancy could be due partly to increasing cigarette consumption among smokers, selection of smokers (light smokers tended to stop smoking more easily) and a delay in the effect of stopping smoking on the risk of lung cancer. The increasing trend of lung cancer mortality has been more marked in old age groups. Lung cancer mortality is reaching a plateau in middle to young age groups. It is predicted from the decreasing trends of cigarette consumption and percentage of smokers in males that the male lung cancer mortality rate will begin to decrease in the future in Japan as has been observed already in the USA and the UK (Doll & Peto, 1981).

To prevent future increases in lung cancer mortality and to prevent other tobacco-related diseases, much stronger smoking control measures are necessary in Japan.

ACKNOWLEDGEMENTS

The author is grateful to Ms K. Hirose and Ms M. Hanaki for their technical assistance and help in preparation of the manuscript.

REFERENCES

Beese, D.H., ed. (1972) *Tobacco Consumption in Various Countries (Tobacco Research Council Research Paper 6, third edition)*, London, Tobacco Research Council

Doll, R. & Peto, R. (1981) The causes of cancer: Quantitative estimates of avoidable risks of cancer in the United States today. *J. natl Cancer Inst.*, ***66***, 1192–1308

Hanai, A. & Fujimoto, I. (1984) Time trends in cancer incidence (Jpn.). *Gan-To-Kagakuryoho*, ***11***, 367–376

Ministry of Health and Welfare of Japan, ed. (1984) *Japan Vital Statistics Series 1935–1983*, Tokyo

Royal College of Physicians of London (1983) *Health or Smoking? Follow-up Report of the Royal College of Physicians of London*, London, Pitman

Tominaga, S. (1984) Epidemiology of cancer of the Japanese (Jpn.). *Diagn. Ther.*, ***72*** (9), 19–26

US Department of Health, Education, and Welfare (1979) *Smoking and Health: A Report of the Surgeon General (DHEW Publication No.* (PHS) 79-50066), Washington DC, US Public Health Service

SMOKING AND LUNG CANCER IN SHANGHAI

Y.T. GAO

Department of Epidemiology,
Shanghai Cancer Institute,
Shanghai, People's Republic of China

SUMMARY

The effect of smoking on lung cancer and other diseases in Shanghai is described. The tar yield of cigarettes consumed by the residents is still high. About half of the male adults in Shanghai are smokers. The prevalence of smoking varies with level of education and occupation. The new generation tends to start smoking earlier. Lung cancer ranks second after stomach cancer, but the incidence rate for lung cancer has increased considerably in recent years. It is estimated that the population attributable risk (PAR) of smoking for lung cancer is 80.5% for males and 19.3% for females. There is an urgent need to adopt effective measures against smoking in the general public.

GENERAL INFORMATION ON PRODUCTION OF MANUFACTURED CIGARETTES IN SHANGHAI

Smoking is a very popular habit among male adults in Shanghai. It is estimated that about half of the male adults in Shanghai are smokers. Manufactured cigarettes were introduced into China from western Europe. The first factory to produce manufactured cigarettes in Shanghai was established in 1925 by a British company. After 1950 this factory became the main monopolized enterprise producing cigarettes in Shanghai.

The production and sales of manufactured cigarettes increased year by year. Taking the production of cigarettes by this monopoly during 1955 as 1, the production levels in 1965, 1975 and 1984 were 1.74, 2.62 and 3.01, respectively. The tar yield and nicotine content of cigarettes produced by this monopoly have remained high in recent years. Based upon the measurements made in 1983 for some brands of cigarettes, which are commonly available on the market, the tar yield ranges from 19–32 mg per cigarette, and the nicotine content ranges from 0.8–1.6 mg per cigarette.

The monopoly started producing filter cigarettes in 1959. In 1967, filter cigarettes accounted for only 0.23% of total production of cigarettes but the proportion has since increased considerably, accounting for 2.0% and 25.8% of total production in 1975 and 1984, respectively.

Because the cigarettes produced in Shanghai are distributed to the whole of China, and because the cigarettes produced in other places also come onto the market in Shanghai, we cannot directly relate the production and sales of cigarettes in Shanghai to the health problems of local residents. However, several field studies have been completed in recent years and some studies are still on-going. The effect of smoking on the health of the residents may be evaluated to some extent by these studies.

PREVALENCE OF SMOKING AMONG ADULTS IN THE SHANGHAI URBAN AREA

In order to obtain basic information on prevalence of smoking among residents, and as the initial stage of a cohort study, a cross-sectional survey was completed in 1982 among about 220 000 adults residing in the urban area and rural counties of Shanghai (Deng & Gao, 1985). The method and results of the survey conducted in the urban area are briefly described below.

Three urban residential areas of Shanghai were selected for the study and 110 367 adults aged 20 years and over (94% of the total number of adults residing in these areas) were interviewed by trained interviewers and by use of a unified questionnaire including items such as smoking habit, occupation and residential history. The distribution of age and level of education of persons interviewed was similar to that of the total population of the Shanghai urban area as presented in the 1982 population census report (Office of Population Census of Shanghai, 1984).

Table 1 shows that, in these areas, 47.2% of male adults are current smokers; persons who have never smoked account for 41.5%; the proportion of exsmokers who have given up smoking for more than one year is small, only 2.6%; others (8.6%) smoke irregularly and infrequently. It is worth noting that a relatively high prevalence of smoking is observed among young people aged 20–29 years; smokers account for 45.7% of the total male population in this age group.

Table 1. Smoking habits of male adults in three urban residential areas of Shanghai (1982)

Age (years)	No. of persons interviewed	Nonsmoker		Current smoker		Infrequent smoker		Exsmoker	
		No.	%	No.	%	No.	%	No.	%
20–	18 878	7 885	41.8	8 623	45.7	2 319	12.3	51	0.3
30–	10 512	4 741	45.1	4 594	43.7	1 132	10.8	45	0.4
40–	7 388	3 205	43.4	3 520	47.6	531	7.2	132	1.8
50–	8 864	3 288	37.1	4 786	54.0	402	4.5	388	4.4
60–	6 002	2 185	36.4	3 119	52.0	210	3.5	488	8.1
70–	2 639	1 172	44.4	1 083	41.0	104	3.9	280	10.6
80+	369	223	60.4	88	23.8	14	3.8	44	11.9
Total	54 652	22 699	41.5	25 813	47.2	4 712	8.6	1 428	2.6

Table 2. Smoking habits of female adults in three urban residential areas of Shanghai (1982)

Age (years)	No. of persons interviewed	Nonsmoker		Current smoker		Infrequent smoker		Exsmoker	
		No.	%	No.	%	No.	%	No.	%
20–	17 763	17 748	99.9	6	0	9	0.1	0	0
30–	9 102	9 080	99.8	16	0.2	6	0.1	0	0
40–	8 311	7 944	95.6	287	3.5	71	0.9	9	0.1
50–	10 180	8 843	86.9	1 105	10.9	176	1.7	56	0.6
60–	6 516	5 070	77.8	1 104	16.9	180	2.8	162	2.5
70–	3 009	2 358	78.4	476	15.8	83	2.8	92	3.1
80+	834	703	84.3	98	11.8	20	2.4	13	1.6
Total	55 715	51 746	92.9	3 092	5.6	545	1.0	332	0.6

In contrast to the male population, the proportion of current smokers among female adults is very small, only 5.6%; 92.9% of female adults are nonsmokers (Table 2). In addition, in general, women smokers in Shanghai started to smoke after the age of 40 years.

The prevalence of smoking in Shanghai varies with level of education and occupation. A higher prevalence is observed among persons with a lower educational level. The proportions of current male smokers are 54.7%, 47.1% and 27.4% among persons with a primary, middle and university education, respectively. After adjusting for age (the age distribution of the total population interviewed being used as the standard) the corresponding figures are 52.3%, 47.1% and 25.5%, respectively. Among females the proportions of current smokers in the above-mentioned education groups are 10.5%, 1.1% and 0.7%. After adjusting for age, the corresponding figures are 5.9%, 4.3% and 1.7%, respectively. The highest prevalence is observed among labourers and tradespeople, the lowest prevalence is among teachers and medical workers, both in males and females.

Of the male adults interviewed, 12.3% started smoking before 20 years of age, 22.7% started between 20–24 years of age. But 18.1% of the young people aged 20–29 years started smoking before 20 years of age, which means that people are tending to start smoking earlier.

Based upon the data on proportions of nonsmokers and smokers, and distribution of daily consumption of cigarettes among smokers, we have estimated that, in recent years, the average consumption of manufactured cigarettes in the Shanghai urban area has risen to 2183 cigarettes per male adult per year and 213 cigarettes per female adult per year.

DESCRIPTIVE AND ANALYTICAL EPIDEMIOLOGIAL DATA ON LUNG CANCER IN SHANGHAI

Cancer is one of the most important problems of public concern in Shanghai. Since 1962, among all causes of deaths, cancer has ranked second after circulatory diseases (including cerebrovascular diseases) in the urban area.

Table 3. The ten leading sites of cancer incidence for males in the Shanghai urban area in 1978–1982

Site (ICD9)[a]	No. of cases	Crude rate (per 10^5)	Age-adjusted rate (per 10^5)	% among all cases
Stomach (151)	9501	64.3	58.3	23.7
Lung (162)	8880	60.1	54.7	22.1
Liver (155)	5872	39.7	34.4	14.6
Oesophagus (150)	3328	22.5	20.8	8.3
Rectum (154)	1521	10.3	9.4	3.8
Colon (153)	1412	9.6	8.5	3.5
Bladder (188)	1083	7.3	7.1	2.7
Pancreas (157)	878	5.9	5.5	2.2
Leukaemia (204-208)	814	5.5	5.4	2.0
Nasopharynx (147)	770	5.2	4.4	1.9

[a] ICD9, Code in the International Classification of Diseases, Ninth revision

Table 4. The ten leading sites of cancer incidence for females in the Shanghai urban area in 1978–1982

Site (ICD9)[a]	No. of cases	Crude rate (per 10^5)	Age-adjusted rate (per 10^5)	% among all cases
Stomach (151)	4593	31.9	24.6	16.0
Lung (162)	3492	24.2	18.5	12.2
Breast (174)	3401	23.6	19.1	11.9
Liver (155)	2190	15.2	11.6	7.6
Oesophagus (150)	1685	11.7	8.9	5.9
Cervix (180)	1628	11.3	8.5	5.7
Colon (153)	1432	9.9	7.6	5.0
Rectum (154)	1325	9.2	7.0	4.6
Ovary (183)	925	6.4	5.0	3.2
Pancreas (157)	723	5.0	3.8	2.5

[a] ICD9, Code in the International Classification of Diseases, Ninth revision

Based upon the cancer incidence data reported by the Shanghai Cancer Registry, lung cancer ranked second after stomach cancer, but it has become an increasingly striking problem in Shanghai in recent years. Considering that the incidence rate for stomach cancer was rather stable for many years, and the rate for lung cancer increased rapidly, we predicted in 1982 that the rate for lung cancer among males in Shanghai will exceed that for stomach cancer in the near future, probably in the 1990s (Shanghai Cancer Institute, Shanghai Sanitary-antiepidemic Center, 1982). The ten leading cancer sites for both sexes during 1978–1982 in the Shanghai urban area (with a total population of 6.3 million by the middle of 1982) are listed in Tables 3 and 4 (Shanghai Cancer Registry, 1985).

In comparison with the incidence rates for lung cancer listed in a 1982 compilation (Waterhouse *et al.*, 1982), the rate for males in Shanghai was somewhat higher than the typical middle level, but the rate for females was among the highest in the world.

Table 5. Time trend of the standardized mortality rates (per 10^5) for lung cancer in the Shanghai urban area

Period	Standardized mortality rate	
	Male	Female
1963–1965	28.4	11.1
1966–1968	35.2	13.7
1969–1971	36.8	12.8
1972–1974	43.1	16.2
1975–1977	49.7	18.5
1978–1980	51.8	18.4

Table 6. Survival rates and median survival time for lung cancer cases registered in the Shanghai urban area during the period 1972–1979

Sex	No. of cases followed up	Survival rate (%)			Median survival time (months)
		1 year	3 years	5 years	
Male	11 833	34	10	7	7.4
Female	4 960	33	11	7	7.0

The standardized mortality rates for lung cancer for six time periods are shown in Table 5 (Shanghai Cancer Registry, unpublished data). There has been a sizeable increase in lung cancer mortality over this time period.

The prognosis of lung cancer patients is still very poor. Based upon the data on new cases of lung cancer registered in the total population of the Shanghai urban area during the period 1972–1979, the five-year survival rate calculated by the life-table method was 7% for both males and females, the median survival time (the time period from diagnosis to death) was only 7.4 months for male cases and 7.0 months for female cases (Table 6) Shanghai Cancer Institute, Shanghai Sanitary-antiepidemic Center, 1982).

Based upon data on 1936 new cases of lung cancer with confirmed histological diagnoses registered by the Shanghai Cancer Registry during 1980–1982, the predominant histological type of lung cancer in males was squamous-cell carcinoma (55.0%); adenocarcinoma accounted for 29.3%, other types for 15.7%. The predominant type in females was adenocarcinoma (57.4%); squamous-cell carcinoma accounted for 27.8%, other types for 14.8% (Zheng & Gao, 1986).

A hospital-based, case-control study of lung cancer with different histological types matched by sex, age and residence conducted in the Shanghai urban area showed that the association of squamous-cell carcinoma of lung cancer for smoking was very strong, the relative risks for males and females were 12.00 and 7.00, respectively. The association of adenocarcinoma for smoking was weak, the relative risks for males and females were 1.77 and 1.10, respectively (Table 7) (Zheng & Gao, 1986).

Using the data on proportions of smokers among male and female populations aged 40 years and over (55.1% and 11.8%), and the relative risks of lung cancer for smoking in

Table 7. Association of lung cancer with smoking in the Shanghai urban area (1982–1984)

Sex	Histological type	No. of pairs	Odds ratio	95% confidence limits
Male	Squamous-cell carcinoma	160	12.00	5.40–26.66
	Adenocarcinoma	152	1.77	1.06–2.95
Female	Squamous-cell carcinoma	76	7.00	3.13–15.64
	Adenocarcinoma	152	1.10	0.61–1.98

both sexes (8.4 and 3.0), it was estimated that the population attributable risk (PAR) of lung cancer for smoking was 80.5% in males and 19.3% in females (Zheng & Gao, 1986). Thus the major part of male lung cancer cases in the Shanghai urban area can be explained by the popular habit of smoking among male adults, but the risk factors attributable to the majority of female lung cancer cases, especially adenocarcinoma, are still unknown and remain to be explored. There is an on-going large-scale, population-based, case-control study of lung cancer in Shanghai, which is aimed at generating hypotheses on the remaining unknown risk factors of lung cancer, with special attention to female nonsmoking cases.

The results of other studies on association of lung cancer with smoking carried out in Shanghai and other places in China were similar to those mentioned above, and also showed that smoking is a major cause of lung cancer. Li *et al.* (1984) reported the results of a cohort study in which 1636 male factory workers were followed up in Shanghai for nine years (1972–1981). Using age-adjusted mortality rates for lung cancer in smokers and non-smokers, the authors estimated the relative risk of lung cancer for smokers to be 8.3. In Beijing, Huang *et al.* (1981) conducted a hospital-based, case-control study of lung cancer, in which 284 male cases, 50 female cases and 1189 controls were involved. The relative risks of squamous-cell carcinoma, adenocarcinoma and undifferentiated carcinoma of lung cancer for smokers were 11.0, 2.2 and 3.6, respectively. In Tianjing, 99 male cases and 36 female cases of lung cancer were matched with the same number of controls by sex and age. The results showed that the relative risks of lung cancer for smokers were 6.0 (95% confidence intervals, 2.6–13.5) in males and 3.9 (95% confidence intervals, 1.4–10.7) in females (Xu *et al.*, 1983).

Associations of bladder cancer and heart diseases with smoking have also been reported in China. In Shanghai, You *et al.* (1981) matched 317 male cases of bladder cancer with the same number of controls by age and residential area. The relative risk of bladder cancer for smokers was 1.53. In Nanjing, 162 cases of coronary heart disease matched with 324 controls by a ratio of one to two were interviewed. The relative risk of coronary heart disease for smokers was found to be 1.57 (Yao *et al.*, 1984). In the above-mentioned cohort study, Li *et al.* (1984) also reported a relative risk of death due to cardiovascular disease for smokers of 1.51.

In conclusion, there is enough convincing evidence to show that smoking has a serious effect on the health of the population of Shanghai. Considering that half of the male adults are smokers, that the tar yield of cigarettes consumed by the residents is still high, and that people are tending to start smoking at an earlier age, it is evident that there is an urgent need to adopt measures against smoking in the general public.

REFERENCES

Deng, J. & Gao, Y.T. (1985) The prevalence of smoking habit among 110 000 adult residents in the Shanghai urban area. *Ch. J. prev. Med.*, ***5***, 271–274

Huang, G.J., Wang, L.D., Lin, H., Jiang, L.J., Zheng, D.H., Lu, J.S. & Li, J.Y. (1981) Association of lung cancer with smoking. *Ch. med. J.*, ***61***, 636–637

Li, W.X., Wang, H.Z., Jing, H.G., Qin, H.D. & Chen, X.B. (1984) Smoking and excess mortality. *Ch. J. Epidemiol.*, ***5***, 91–94

Office of Population Census of Shanghai (1984) *Data on 1982 Population Census*, Shanghai

Shanghai Cancer Institute, Shanghai Sanitary-antiepidemic Center (1982) Analysis of cancer incidence, mortality and survival rates in the Shanghai urban area during the period 1972–79. *Shanghai Tumor*, ***2***, 1–7

Shanghai Cancer Registry (1985) In: *Cancer Incidence in Five Continents*, Vol. V, Lyon, International Agency for Research on Cancer (in press)

Waterhouse, J., Muir, C., Shanmurgaratnam, K. & Powell, J., eds (1982) *Cancer Incidence in Five Continents*, Vol. IV *(IARC Scientific Publications No. 42)*, Lyon, International Agency for Research on Cancer

Xu, R.H. & Geng, G.Y. (1983) A case-control study on association of lung cancer with smoking in Tianjing. *Ch. J. Epidemiol.*, ***4***, 193–197

Yao, C.L., Du, F.C., Xu, Y.C. & Hong, L.J. (1984) Smoking and coronary heart disease. *Ch. J. Epidemiol.*, ***5***, 88–90

You, X.Y., Deng, J., Mou, D.J. & Yao, Y.F. (1981) Searching for the etiologic factors of bladder cancer. *Shanghai Tumor*, ***4***, 12–14

Zheng, W. & Gao, Y.T. (1986) Association of squamous-cell carcinoma and adenocarcinoma of lung cancer with smoking. *Shanghai Tumor*, ***1***, 17–20

IV. TOBACCO – SPREAD OF THE HABIT AND TRENDS

SPREAD OF SMOKING TO THE DEVELOPING COUNTRIES

S. TOMINAGA

Aichi Cancer Center Research Institute,
Nagoya, Japan

SUMMARY

In most developing countries, tobacco consumption was relatively low in the past. It has been increasing in recent years as developed countries have exported more cigarettes to developing countries, and as developing countries have cultivated more tobacco themselves to produce cheaper tobacco, at the sacrifice of food production. Tobacco sales are an important source of revenue for governments in the developing countries as in the developed countries. The spread of smoking to developing countries and the increase in tobacco consumption have had several adverse effects: (1) an increase in lung cancer and other smoking-related diseases; (2) an increase in economic burdens resulting from imports of cigarettes from developed countries and increased medical costs for smoking-related diseases; and (3) decreases in production and import of foods. There are many obstacles and constraints to smoking control in the developing countries, but smoking control is badly needed to prevent lung cancer and other smoking-related diseases, to alleviate economic burdens and to increase the production and import of foods.

INTRODUCTION

In 1971, an editorial in the *British Medical Journal* discussing the Second World Conference on Smoking and Health said, 'There is a real danger of this deadly habit [smoking] being exported to the younger countries of Africa and Asia. The Western World has a responsibility to see that this is not done.' (Anon., 1971). But this is unfortunately what has happened.

A meeting of the WHO Expert Committee on Smoking Control, held in Geneva, 23–28 October, 1978 (World Health Organization, 1979) reported that, 'The spread of the smoking habit has occurred like an epidemic. The habit has spread from country to country, from continent to continent, and even between different population groups within the same country . . . the burden of two health problems [has] moved in opposite directions during the past 25 years. While tuberculosis has been decreasing in most countries, there has been a rapid increase in smoking-related diseases, of which lung cancer is the most striking example. The trends vary from country to country, the cross-over of curves taking place at different times.

'The increasing trend in smoking-related diseases, as exemplified by lung cancer, parallels the trend in smoking . . ..

'In some developing countries there has been a similar increase in cigarette consumption but again the curves are many years behind those for the developed countries . . . Developing countries have not yet had time to experience the same grim increase in smoking-related mortality as has taken place in the industrialized countries, but they must expect it unless they halt and reverse the increase in cigarette consumption.' As the WHO Expert Committee on Smoking Control has warned, the spread of smoking and the increase of cigarette consumption will be accompanied by an epidemic of smoking-related diseases even in the developing countries where infectious diseases and malnutrition are still major public health problems.

There are at least three major reasons for the spread of smoking and the increase of tobacco consumption in the developing countries: (1) an increase in exports of cigarettes from the developed countries to the developing countries owing to a decline in smoking

Table 1. Annual tobacco consumption per adult (15 years old and over) in the developing countries and selected developed countries in 1973 [a]

Country/area	No. of manufactured cigarettes	All tobacco goods (kg)
India	170	0.6
Malawi	200	0.2
Indonesia	230	0.8
Sierra Leone	430	0.6
Kenya	470	0.4
Ghana	480	0.6
Morocco	690	0.8
Pakistan	760	1.7
El Salvador	1020	1.5
Chile	1320	1.4
Jamaica	1350	1.4
Mexico	1360	1.4
South Africa	1380	2.3
Brazil	1490	2.0
Nicaragua	1520	1.2
Malaysia	1600	1.5
Barbados	1620	1.7
Mauritius	1920	1.5
Costa Rica	2060	1.6
Venezuela	2210	–
Japan	3240	3.3
Canada	3450	4.5
UK	3230	2.8
USA	3850	4.2

[a] Data from World Health Organization, 1979

and a shrinking cigarette market in the developed countries; (2) an increase in cultivation of tobacco in the developing countries to decrease imports of expensive tobacco and tobacco products; and (3) the failure or negligence of smoking control by governments and public health professionals in the developing countries.

In this paper, the recent trends in cigarette consumption and the percentage of smokers in the developing countries are reviewed, and methods of estimating the percentage of smokers and effects of smoking or smoking-related diseases are presented. The impact of spread of smoking to developing countries is also discussed.

Fig. 1. Growth rates in cigarette markets in developed and developing countries 1975–1980 (data from Royal College of Physicians of London, 1983; Japan Tobacco and Salt Public Corp., unpublished data)

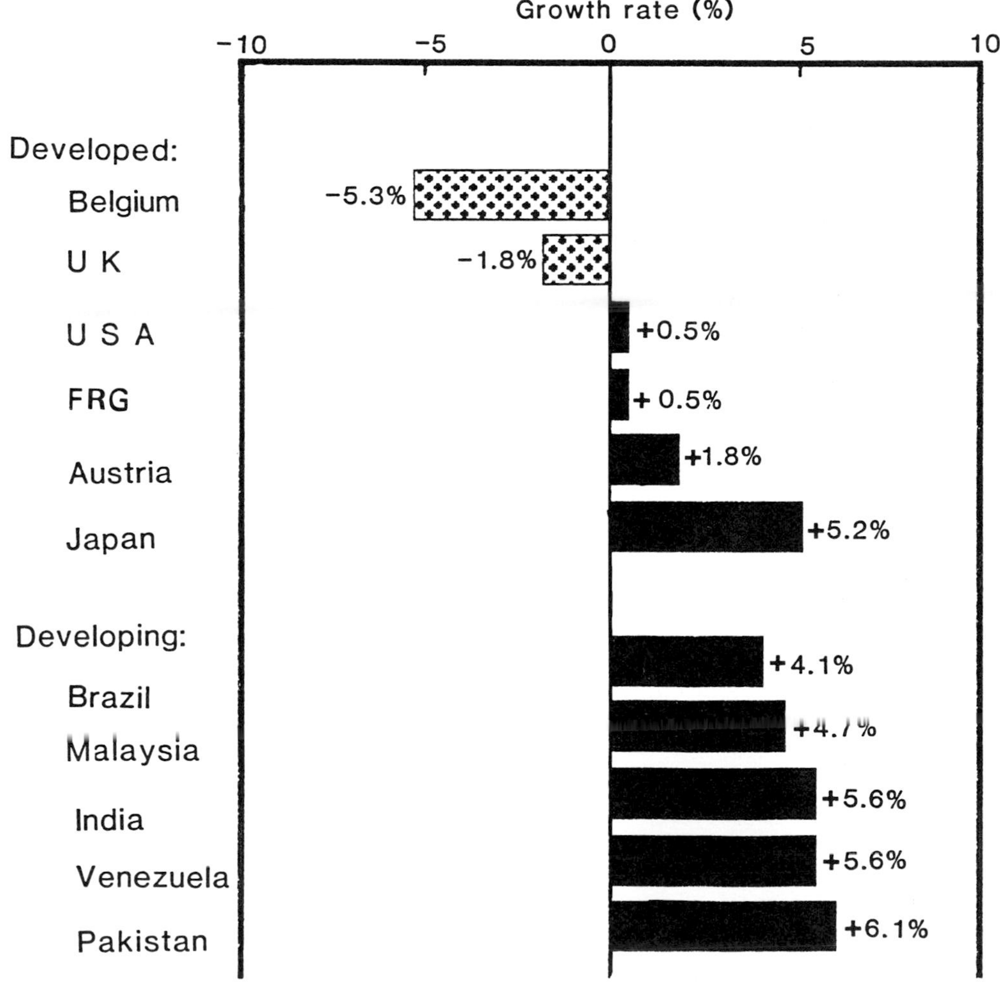

TOBACCO CONSUMPTION IN THE DEVELOPING COUNTRIES

In most developing countries, tobacco consumption, especially cigarette consumption, used to be low compared to that in developed countries (Table 1). But the growth rates of cigarette consumption in the developing countries have been greater than those of the developed countries (Fig. 1). Although the data shown in Table 1 and Figure 1 are not strictly comparable between countries, the consumption of tobacco per adult in each country/area is a good index of spread and growth of smoking. Thus, as the WHO Expert Committee on Smoking Control (World Health Organization, 1979) stressed, it is necessary to standardize the method of data collection of tobacco consumption in the future.

In several countries in southern Asia such as India, Bangladesh, Pakistan, Sri Lanka and Nepal, tobacco has been consumed in various forms; cigarettes, *bidis* (hand-rolled cigarettes), *hookah* and *chuttas*. It is desirable to estimate tobacco consumption for each form of tobacco because the effect may vary from one form to another.

PERCENTAGE OF SMOKERS IN THE DEVELOPING COUNTRIES

It is important to know the percentage of smokers for each population, and the amount of tobacco consumed per smoker when there is a large difference in smoking behaviour between males and females. However, in most developing countries the percentage of smokers has not been studied systematically. A variety of forms of traditional smoking materials in the developing countries make any survey of smoking more complicated. Estimates of percentage of smokers of any form of tobacco product in various parts of the developing world, especially in southern Asia and Africa, have been summarized (Royal College of Physicians of London, 1983) and are illustrated in Figure 2. Most of the original data were reported at the WHO Workshop on Smoking and Health Issues in Developing Countries held in Colombo, Sri Lanka, in 1981. Most surveys show a lower prevalence of smoking in females than in males and a higher consumption of manufactured cigarettes in professional and office workers (Jayant, 1983). Besides varying by sex and occupation, smoking habits in large countries such as India and China may vary widely by region, socioeconomic status, ethnicity and many other factors.

A desirable way of surveying smoking habits is a population-based survey or a survey on randomly selected samples. But a case-control study on lung cancer or other smoking-related diseases will also show us relatively good estimates of smoking habits. For example, a case-control study on lung cancer in Cuba (Joly *et al.*, 1984) showed that 80.3% of male controls and 31.0% of female controls had smoked cigarettes regularly. The percentages of smokers for hospital controls (80.5% for males, 30.5% for females) and neighbourhood controls (80.1% for males, 31.8% for females) were virtually the same. From these results it is suggested that the percentage of adults who had ever smoked regularly was about 80% in males and 30% in females in Cuba. This study also showed that the relative risk of lung cancer was 14.1 for male smokers and 7.3 for female smokers and that the attributable risk of smoking was 66% for male lung cancer cases and 91% for female lung cancer cases. Thus, a carefully conducted case-control study on lung cancer or other smoking-related diseases will give us useful information on various aspects of smoking.

Fig. 2. Estimates of percentage of adult smokers in various parts of the developing world (data from Jayant, 1983; Royal College of Physicians of London, 1983)

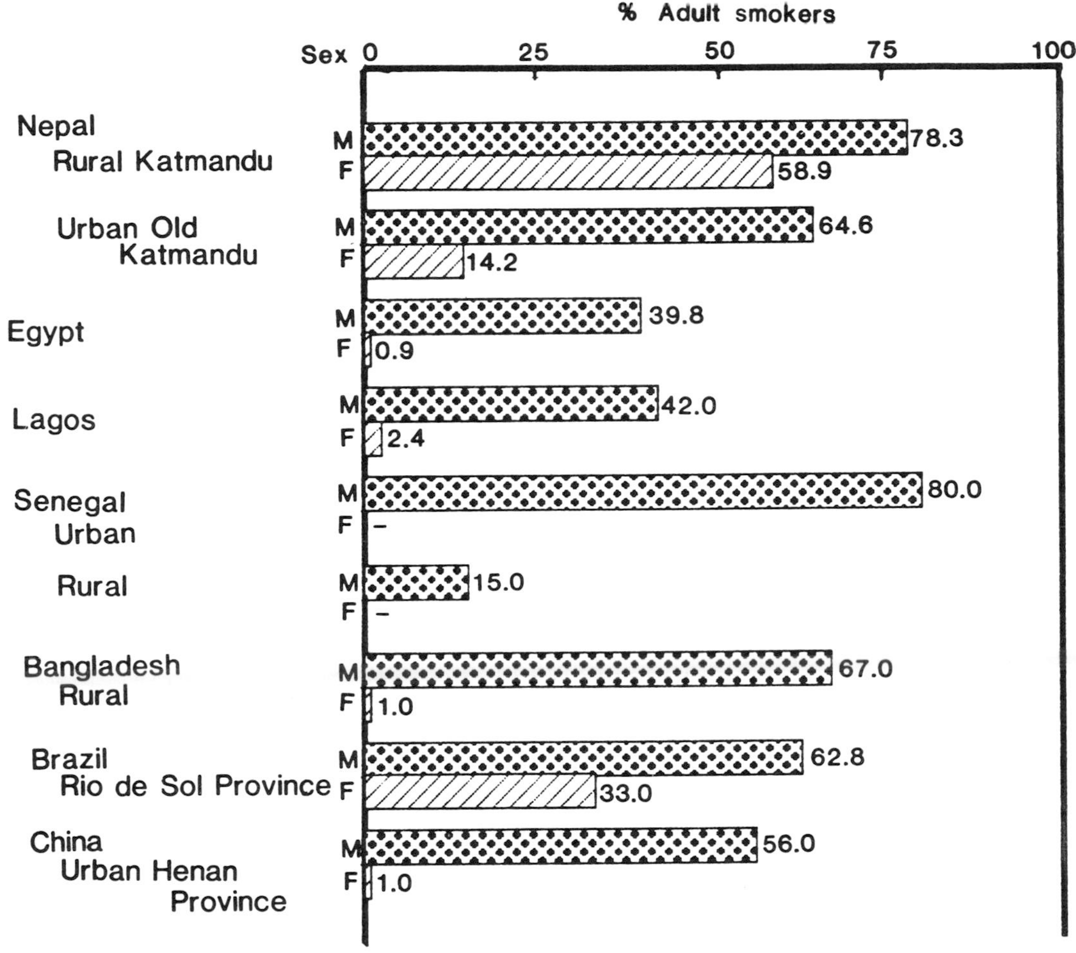

TRENDS IN LUNG CANCER IN THE DEVELOPING COUNTRIES

Lung cancer mortality is relatively low in most developing countries (Fig. 3). As the consumption of tobacco products, especially cigarettes has increased in the developing countries, it is likely that lung cancer incidence and mortality have increased or will increase many years later. But the trends in the incidence and mortality of lung cancer in most developing countries have not been studied systematically, largely due to inadequate vital statistics and/or cancer registries. Perhaps it is too late to begin smoking control after we see a significant increase in lung cancer and other smoking-related diseases. A good correlation between consumption of manufactured cigarettes per adult and lung cancer mortality, as well as decreasing trends in lung cancer mortality among relatively young age

Fig. 3. Age-adjusted death rates for lung cancer in 1978–1979 in 39 countries (rate per 100 000 population) (data from Kurihara *et al.*, 1984); *1978 only

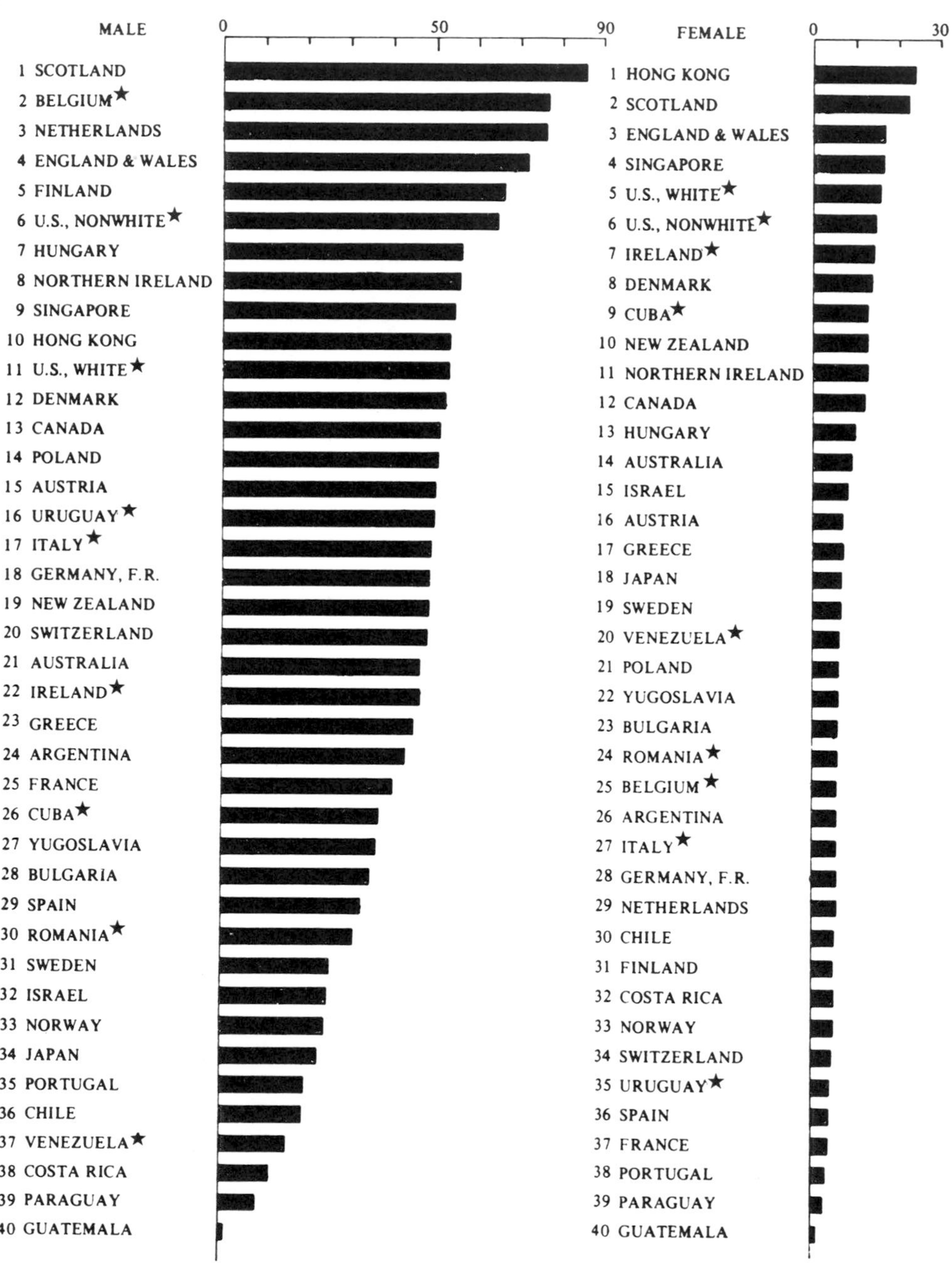

groups following decreases of possible tar intake per adult, as observed in the UK and the USA (Doll & Peto, 1981), will justify initiation of smoking control without seeing an actual increase of lung cancer and other smoking-related diseases in the developing countries.

ADVERSE EFFECTS OF SPREAD OF SMOKING IN THE DEVELOPING COUNTRIES

The spread of smoking to developing countries has adverse effects in several respects: (1) it inevitably leads to an increase in lung cancer and other smoking-related diseases; (2) it increases economic burdens owing to increasing imports of more expensive cigarettes from developed countries, to increasing medical costs for smoking-related diseases and to increasing time lost from work due to smoking-related diseases; and (3) food production and food imports are hampered by cultivation of tobacco and imports of tobacco products. In many developing countries malnutrition is still a major problem. Food should get a higher priority in the trade-off, 'food or tobacco'.

OBSTACLES AND CONSTRAINTS TO SMOKING CONTROL IN THE DEVELOPING COUNTRIES

In many developing countries smoking is still socially accepted. Health education is hampered by a shortage of trained manpower in smoking control and a high rate of illiteracy. Low priority is given to smoking control measures in the health care systems compared to the priority given to control measures for infectious diseases and malnutrition. This reluctant attitude of governments to smoking control derives mainly from the fact that the tobacco industry is an important source of revenue. For example, in Malaysia, cigarette sales in the single year 1982 totalled nearly US $ 460 million. The Health Ministry budget was only US $ 273 million for five years. The government received over US $ 210 million or 47% of the total sales in various forms of taxes, a factor which influenced government handling of the smoking issue (Teoh, 1984).

THE NEED FOR SMOKING CONTROL IN THE DEVELOPING COUNTRIES AND RECOMMENDATIONS

Smoking control is necessary in both developed and developing countries, but particularly in the developing countries, in order to prevent lung cancer and other smoking-related diseases (which are preventable by smoking control), to alleviate economic burdens, and to increase production and import of foods.

The 1978 WHO Expert Committee on Smoking Control (World Health Organization, 1979) has made specific recommendations addressed to developing countries, which are as follows:

'1. Countries that have a recognizable smoking problem should attempt to control it by the means elaborated in this report, and countries so far without such a problem should give high priority to policies directed at the prevention of smoking. This implies the development of data collection systems to delineate the problem, the adoption of the necessary legislation, and the use of educational techniques suitable to the socio-cultural situation, particularly those where communication is difficult.

'2. No country should allow a tobacco-growing or manufacturing industry to be developed. Where such an industry exists, priority should be given to the development of substitute crops, with international cooperation.'

The 1978 WHO Expert Committee on Smoking Control (World Health Organization, 1979) has also made recommendations addressed to developed countries. Those recommendations were considered useful in alleviating the adverse effects of smoking in the developing countries. The recommendations were as follows:

'1. Exports of tobacco containing higher levels of toxic substances than those marketed under the same brand designation in the country of origin should cease immediately.

'2. All packaged tobacco that is exported should carry the health warnings and emission levels required in the country of origin printed in such a way as to be intelligible to the recipients.'

The 1982 WHO Expert Committee on Smoking Control Strategies in Developing Countries (World Health Organization, 1983) has made more specific, elaborate recommendations, but the basic concept and strategies are virtually same as in the recommendations made by the earlier Expert Committee.

It is easy to produce and repeat recommendations, but it is difficult to have them adopted. The Royal College of Physicians of London (1983) said in their fourth report, entitled *'Health or Smoking?'*

'Each of the previous College reports has concluded with a list of recommendations for actions. Sadly, through apathy and vested interests, very few of these have been adopted. That is no reason for us to fail to make similar recommendations again. The health risks of smoking do not lessen with the passage of years, rather they increase. As more and more suffer the consequences of this unnecessary habit the urgency for action remains as strong as ever.

'Action to control and eventually abolish the distress caused by smoking-related diseases and the burden they place on the National Health Service has to be taken by smokers, by nonsmokers, by educators both in school and beyond, by health care professionals and, most importantly, by the Government.'

This is true for both developed and developing countries.

ACKNOWLEDGEMENTS

The author is grateful to Ms K. Hiorse and Ms M. Hanaki for their technical assistance and help in preparation of the manuscript.

REFERENCES

Anon. (1971) An editorial: World action on smoking. *Br. med. J.*, ***4,*** 65

Doll, R. & Peto, R. (1981) The causes of cancer: Quantitative estimates of avoidable risks of cancer in the United States today. *J. natl Cancer Inst.*, ***66,*** 1192–1308

Jayant, K. (1983) Tobacco habits in relation to coronary heart disease. *World Smok. Health,* ***8,*** 24–27

Joly, O.G., Lubin, J.H. & Caraballoso, M. (1984) Dark tobacco and lung cancer in Cuba. *World Smok. Health,* ***9,*** 21–26

Kurihara, M., Aoki, K. & Tominaga, S., eds (1984) *Cancer Mortality Statistics in the World,* Nagoya, University of Nagoya Press

Royal College of Physicians of London (1983) *Health or Smoking? Follow-up Report of the Royal College of Physicians of London,* London, Pitman

Teoh, S.K. (1984) Smoking in Malaysia: promotion and control. *World Smok. Health,* ***9,*** 27–30

World Health Organization (1979) *Controlling the Smoking Epidemic: Report of the WHO Expert Committee on Smoking Control (WHO Tech. Rep. Ser. No. 636),* Geneva

World Health Organization (1983) Smoking control strategies in developing countries: Report of a WHO Expert Committee *(WHO Tech. Rep. Ser. No. 695),* Geneva

WORLDWIDE CHANGES AND TRENDS IN CIGARETTE BRANDS AND CONSUMPTION

L.M. RAMSTRÖM

NTS, National Smoking and Health Association
(WHO Collaborating Centre for Reference on Smoking and Health)
S-113 46 Stockholm, Sweden

INTRODUCTION

The cigarette is probably more widely spread and used on a global scale than any other commercial consumer product – the only possible exception being the match, a product which incidentally goes very well with the cigarette. During recent decades, cigarette consumption has been influenced by a variety of both upward and downward pressures. Consequently there have been various changes in cigarette consumption all over the world. Many such changes refer to the types and brands of cigarettes that are consumed. The purpose of the current study is to analyse how this 'inner structure' of cigarette markets can change and how such changes interact with changes in overall market size. This is especially important when it comes to estimating the possible effects of various interventions by smoking control activities.

TRENDS IN TOTAL CIGARETTE SALES

While tobacco for pipe smoking and chewing has been used for some five hundred years in Europe, and for still longer in other parts of the world, the cigarette is a quite recent phenomenon, emerging from the invention of cigarette machines towards the end of the nineteenth century. Being just around one hundred years old, the cigarette has been an enormous success and world output is now close to five million millions of pieces annually as reported by the Food and Agriculture Organization of the United Nations in 1982[1]. While the overall picture of the century-long lifetime of the cigarette has been one of

[1] Food and Agriculture Organization of the United Nations (1982) *The Economic Significance of Tobacco* (FAO unpublished document ESC:MISC 82/1), Rome.

Table 1. Changes in cigarette sales; annual average for the latest available three-year period[a]

Developed country	% change	Developing country	% change
USA	−2.5	Brazil	−2.3
Canada	−2.8	Ecuador	0.0
UK	−3.8	Zaire	+6.8
Germany, Federal Republic	−6.8	Tanzania	−5.2
Hungary	+0.8	Pakistan	+1.1
Italy	+0.5	Bangladesh	+5.5
Japan	+0.8	Malaysia	−4.8

[a] Data from Maxwell (1981, 1984a)

continuous growth, recent decades have shown a definite slow-down in growth rate. For the time being, the world output of cigarettes shows an annual growth rate of just a small percentage. At the same time, the global picture is a rather heterogeneous one. This is further illustrated by Table 1, which is derived from sales data reported by Maxwell (1981, 1984a).

In Table 1, the figures for each country show the average annual change in cigarette sales over a recent three-year period, in most cases 1981–1983. The incompleteness of available data has made it impossible to refer to that same period for all countries, so in some cases the actual period lies up to three years earlier. The left-hand column of Table 1 shows some developed countries. The growth rate is negative or just slightly positive. The right hand column shows some developing countries. Here the picture is even more heterogeneous, and some countries demonstrate a very strong growth rate in cigarette consumption. It is important to point out that figures of this kind are not particularly stable. Especially in the very poor countries, they change quite a lot from one period to another. However, Table 1 illustrates the general pattern of rather wide variation between individual countries in a framework of moderate total growth which is occurring mainly in developing countries.

TRENDS FOR DIFFERENT TYPES OF CIGARETTES

One of the weaknesses of sales figures such as those from which Table 1 is derived is their lack of specificity. For example, they do not distinguish between different categories of cigarettes such as traditional name-brands, generic or no-name cigarettes and hand-rolled cigarettes, or they fail to cover all of these categories altogether. Neither do they distinguish between subcategories of branded cigarettes such as, for example, low-tar versus high-tar cigarettes. The following sections will look a little bit further into some of these distinctions.

Traditional brands versus cheaper cigarettes

When studying the development of cigarette consumption in a country, it might be insufficient to look at traditional brands only. This is clearly illustrated by the situation in

Table 2. Case study: the Federal Republic of Germany; changes in cigarette consumption after an increase of 39% in cigarette duties in June 1982[a]

Category	Cigarette consumption (10^{12})		
	1982	1983	% change
Name-brands	130	108	−17
Generics and hand-rolled	17	30	+76
Total	147	138	−6

[a] Data from *Tobacco Reporter* (Anon., 1983a)

Table 3. Cigarette sales in Canada: some recent trends[a]

Cigarette type	Sales[b]	
	1982	1983
Factory-made	66.3	65.5
Home-rolled	5.5	6.1
Total	71.8	71.6

[a] Data from *World Tobacco* (Anon. 1983b)
[b] Figures indicate sales as 10^{12} pieces (number of home-rolled ones estimated from sales of fine-cut tobacco)

Table 4. Loyalty level in the USA, i.e., percentage of buyers who would abstain from switching to a generic equivalent at half the price[a]

Favourite brand	Market share (%)	Loyalty level (%)
Marlboro	19	45
Kool	8	57
Vantage	4	63
Camel	5	68
Tareyton	1	74

[a] Data from *World Tobacco* (Anon., 1982a)

the Federal Republic of Germany in 1982 and following years, which has been described in *Tobacco Reporter* (Anon., 1983a). In June 1982, there was a remarkable increase in cigarette duties of 39%. Table 2 shows what happened. The year after the tax increase, the sales of name-brands of cigarettes went down by as much as 17%. But, at the same time, the sales of fine-cut tobacco for hand-rolling were increasing very strongly. Further, the market was quickly supplemented by cheaper cigarettes, both generics and certain new brands that were specifically introduced with a low-price image. These previously very small categories were now growing so much as to compensate for about two-thirds of the decline in sales of traditional brands. The net reduction in cigarette consumption was thereby just 6% instead of 17%. More recent reports in *World Tobacco* (Anon., 1984a) tell us that the continued development represents a further recovery in terms of market size but with a partly new structure, where some of the new, cheaper brands have stabilized with quite high market shares and the total market share of generics and fine-cut tobacco has stabilized at a higher level than before. Consequently, the long-term effect of the dramatic price increase has mainly been a restructuring of the market rather than a reduction of its size.

Table 3 gives a similar example from Canada. According to estimates published by *World Tobacco* (Anon., 1983b) the sales of factory-made cigarettes were down by 800 million pieces from 1982 to 1983. At the same time the number of home-rolled cigarettes was estimated to have increased by 600 million pieces, so as to leave the total number of cigarettes virtually unchanged.

Generics are strengthening their position not only in the Federal Republic of Germany but in many other countries as well, for example, the USA. Figures reported by Maxwell (1984a) indicate a quick development from 1981 (0.4% market share), through 1982 (0.9%) to 1983 (2.9%) and further reports in *World Tobacco* (Anon., 1984b) seem to confirm a continued growth.

The overall growth of generics brings up the question of brand loyalty. Which smokers are most or least likely to switch from their favourite brand to a cheaper generic cigarette? In the USA, a study was made where smokers of various brands were asked about their willingness to stick to their old brand even if a generic equivalent were available at half the price. The percentage of those abstaining from switching to the cheaper alternative was taken as the 'loyalty level' for that brand. Table 4 indicates some examples of such loyalty levels as reported in *World Tobacco* (Anon., 1982a). Table 4 also indicates the popularity of the brand as expressed by its market share. Quite contrary to what might have been expected, the brands with the strongest positions on the market have the lowest loyalty levels. Obviously, those who smoke small brands do so because, more strongly than other smokers, they appreciate some brand-specific characteristics – maybe taste, maybe general image of the brand. This distribution of loyalties also means that there are many more smokers with limited brand loyalty than with a very strong loyalty. Consequently, generics may probably enjoy a continued increase in market share and they will therefore deserve increased attention when it comes to analysing future trends in cigarette consumption.

Filter cigarettes versus nonfilter ones

The most easily visible distinction between types of cigarettes is undoubtedly the one between filter cigarettes and nonfilter ones. The proportions of these two categories differ a lot between countries and have changed substantially over time during the last few decades. Table 5 gives some examples of market shares for filter brands in various countries in 1977 and 1982 as reported by Maxwell (1980, 1984a). In each one of the countries the current trend is one of growing market share for filter brands, but there are still large differences between the countries at the extreme ends of the scale. It is notewor-

Table 5. Market shares for filter brands; examples of national trends[a]

Country	Market share (%)	
	1977	1982
India	27	31
Netherlands	56	69
Hungary	72	84
Germany, Federal Republic	87	89
USA	90	93
Malaysia	96	98
Argentina	99	100

[a] From Maxwell (1980, 1984a)

Table 6. Market position of filter brands in 55 countries in 1982[a]

	Market share (%)			
	0–49	50–79	80–95	96–100
Number of countries	7	4	18	26

[a] Data from Maxwell (1983/1984)

thy that here we find both developing and developed countries at all parts of the scale. Table 6 gives a more comprehensive overview of the data. It includes all the 55 countries for which data regarding market shares of filter brands were available for the year 1982, and indicates the number of countries where the market share of filter brands falls in the range indicated in the upper line. The distribution of countries is an extremely uneven one. It is strongly shifted towards the right end, with almost half of the countries falling in the narrow top interval 96–100%, while the median value is 94%. This pattern means that in very many countries the distinction between filter and nonfilter cigarettes is quite irrelevant as a subject for statistical analysis. It should further be kept in mind that this distinction is rather irrelevant even from a more general point of view since so many filter brands yield larger amounts of tar and nicotine – and, even more often, larger amounts of gaseous smoke components – as compared to some nonfilter brands.

The above-mentioned observations suggest that consumption trends should preferably be studied separately for individual brands or groups of brands with different delivery levels for tar, nicotine, carbon monoxide and other components that play major roles in relation to the health effects of smoking.

Low-tar versus high-tar cigarettes

Table 7 combines data reported by *World Tobacco* (Anon., 1980a) and Maxwell (1981, 1984a). It shows how sales have developed for four different brands on the Japanese

Table 7. Market shares in Japan for brands yielding different tar levels[a]

Brand	Tar yield (mg)	Market share (%)		
		1979	1981	1983
Mild Seven	14	30.9	37.6	42.1
Seven Stars	16	19.5	17.1	14.1
Hi-lite	19	14.2	10.9	8.2
Hope	20	7.1	5.3	4.7

[a] Data from *World Tobacco* (Anon., 1980a); Maxwell (1981, 1984a)

Table 8. Market shares in Brazil for brands yielding different tar levels[a]

Brand	Tar yield (mg)	Market share (%)		
		1980	1981	1982
Galaxy	9	1.6	1.9	2.1
Continental	21	14.6	13.7	12.3

[a] Data from Frecker & Pischkitl (unpublished data, see footnote on p. 141); Maxwell (1981, 1984a)

Table 9. Market shares in Pakistan for brands yielding different tar levels[a]

Brand	Tar yield (mg)	Market share (%)		
		1978	1980	1982
Wills	22	3.3	5.5	4.8
Morven Gold	29	2.4	3.1	4.4

[a] Data from Frecker & Pischkitl (unpublished data, see footnote on p. 141); Maxwell (1981, 1984a)

Table 10. Market shares in Canada for brands yielding different tar levels[a]

Tar yield (mg)	Market share (%)		
	1977	1978	1979
0–5	4.0	4.9	6.1
6–9	3.6	4.5	5.0
10–14	20.2	26.5	33.7
0–14	27.8	35.9	44.8
15+	72.2	64.1	55.2

[a] Data from *World Tobacco* (Anon. 1980b)

Table 11. Low-tar brands: market shares in the USA[a]

Tar yield (mg)	Market share (%)				
	1979	1980	1981	1982	1983
7–15	(37)	(42)	50.2	48.7	43.0
0–6	(5)	(7)	9.4	10.1	10.2
0–15	42.4	48.5	59.6	58.8	53.2

[a] Data from Maxwell (1983, 1984b)

market during the period 1979–1983. Only one brand, Mild Seven, has enjoyed an increase in market share. This brand is the one with the lowest tar yield. There is a very clear correlation between tar level and sales trend, which is quite surprising in view of the rather modest differences between the tar levels in question. Basically the same kinds of trends have been observed in Brazil, as demonstrated in Table 8, which combines data from Frecker and Pischkitl (1984)[2] and Maxwell (1981, 1984a). The low-tar brand, Galaxy, is a small brand but its market share is growing. The high-tar brand, Continental, is on the decrease. An example from Pakistan shows an entirely different picture. As seen in Table 9, which is based on data from the same sources as Table 8, the very high-yielding brand, Morven Gold, has enjoyed almost a doubling of its market share from 1978 to 1982, while the less high-yielding brand, Wills, goes up and down.

It should be pointed out that these data are just examples of individual brands and cannot be taken as descriptions of the total trend pattern in the countries concerned. However, *World Tobacco* (Anon., 1980b) has reported more comprehensive data from Canada, as shown in Table 10. Here we can see the market development for brands at various tar levels during the period 1977–1979. The two bottom lines give the basic breakdown in low-tar and high-tar brands (low-tar defined as 'less than 15 mg'). During this short period there has been a substantial shift in market shares whereby the low-tar half of the assortment has gained market shares. It should, however, be noted that almost all of this increase has been confined to the 10–14-mg segment while the two lowest segments have enjoyed very limited gains only.

While Canadian data for exactly the same categories have not been available for years after 1979, similar kinds of data are available from the USA for the period 1979–1983 as reported by Maxwell (1983, 1984b) (Table 11). For the 'overlap' year, 1979, the US data are very similar to the Canadian ones. After 1979, the market share for low-tar brands increased up to 1981 but then began to go down. The lowest segment remains at a level of about 10%. This is a rather modest level but this segment seems to be more stable than the 7–15-mg segment which has gone down in market share from 50% to 43% between 1981 and 1983.

[2] Frecker, R.C. & Pischkitl, H. (1984) Constituents of cigarettes from developing countries: nicotine, tar, and carbon monoxide values for 50 brands selected by the World Health Organization (WHO unpublished document WHO/SMO/84.4), Geneva.

The trends are very complex indeed. Some statements published in tobacco industry journals suggest that one rather small group of smokers stick to ultra-low-yield brands for the mere sake of the low figures as such, while another, larger group of smokers is paying increased attention to taste and therefore disapproves of low-tar cigarettes. US tobacco industry spokesmen use expressions like 'The full-flavored product appears to be making a comeback' (Maxwell, 1983) or 'Obviously a cigarette with some tar in it tastes better than those with none' (Maxwell, 1984b). While these statements primarily refer to the US market and the US smoker, tobacco industry spokesmen express themselves even more eloquently when explaining why smokers in developing countries prefer 'robust cigarettes to mild ones'. This is said to be 'understandable in poor countries where imported cigarettes are a special luxury, to be savoured rarely; each has to yield a full quota of sensory satisfaction' (Anon., 1982b).

SUMMARY CONCLUSIONS

When looking at the above review of changes and trends in cigarette consumption some summary conclusions can be drawn:

– a continued growth in cigarette consumption will mainly take place in developing countries;

– price increases may have complex and unexpected effects, such as changing the brand structure of the market rather than reducing its size on a long-term basis;

– future studies of cigarette consumption trends will have to give increased attention to generic and hand-rolled cigarettes;

– in the future it will be irrelevant to look at the distinction between filter cigarettes and nonfilter ones; the important distinction will be between different types of filter cigarettes;

– an increasing taste consciousness among large groups of smokers will most probably constitute an additional obstacle to low-tar cigarettes ever becoming a viable vehicle for the limitation of smoking-related health risks.

REFERENCES

Anon. (1980a) Japan – Consumption up. *World Tob.*, ***67***, 49

Anon. (1980b) Canada – The ladder game. *World Tob.*, ***67***, 51–54

Anon. (1982a) Future retail threat to tobacco branding? *World Tob.*, ***78***, 57–60

Anon. (1982b) Saudia Arabia – Formula regulation. *World Tob.*, ***76***, 54

Anon. (1983a) Rough road to recovery. *Tob. Rep.*, ***110*** (12), 50–52

Anon. (1983b) Canada – Glimmers of hope. *World Tob.*, ***81***, 49–50

non. (1984a) German Federal Republic – Sales recovery. *World Tob.*, ***84***, 59–60

Anon. (1984b) United States – Generically-priced. *World Tob.*, ***85***, 44–45

Maxwell, J.C. (1980) How the brands ranked. *World Tob.*, ***69, 70***

Maxwell, J.C. (1981) How the brands ranked. *World Tob.*, ***73, 74***

Maxwell, J.C. (1983) Inventories cloud cigarette survey. *Tob. Rep.*, ***110*** (2), 34–35

Maxwell, J.C. (1983/1984) How the brands ranked. *World Tob.*, ***81, 82, 83, 85, 86***

Maxwell, J.C. (1984a) How the brands ranked. *World Tob.*, ***85, 86, 87***

Maxwell, J.C. (1984b) Cigarette sales in downspin. *Tob. Rep.*, ***111*** (1), 50–51.

V. SMOKING – CURRENT RESEARCH ISSUES

CHEMICAL CONSTITUENTS AND BIOACTIVITY OF TOBACCO SMOKE

D. HOFFMANN & E.L. WYNDER

Naylor Dana Institute for Disease Prevention,
American Health Foundation,
Valhalla, NY 10595, USA

INTRODUCTION

The occurrence of cancer of the respiratory tract and of the upper digestive tract is causally related to smoking of cigarettes, cigars, pipes and *bidis,* while malignant tumours of the bladder, renal pelvis and pancreas are causally related to smoking of cigarettes (IARC, 1986). Epidemiological studies have demonstrated an association of tobacco chewing with cancer of the oral cavity (IARC, 1985). These conclusions have been supported by a large number of bioassays. The application of tobacco extracts, the inhalation of tobacco smoke and the application of tobacco smoke condensate induce cancer in laboratory animals (Wynder & Hoffmann, 1967; Hoffmann *et al.*, 1983; IARC, 1985, 1986). It has been the joint task of chemists and biologists to identify those components in tobacco and tobacco smoke that contribute to their carcinogenic effects. However, it would be an insurmountable task to evaluate each of the more than 2500 constituents in tobacco leaf and more than 3900 compounds in tobacco smoke for possible tumorigenic effects (Table 1). Therefore, the research programme has to be limited to the identification of those tumorigenic and carcinogenic agents that can account for most of the carcinogenic activity of tobacco products. Despite this limitation, remarkable progress has been made by the laboratory scientists. This progress is well reflected in the reduced carcinogenic potential of 'low-tar' cigarettes (IARC, 1986). In evaluating the carcinogenic risk of environmental tobacco smoke exposure (passive smoking), the knowledge of the physicochemical nature of sidestream and mainstream smoke and the principles of chemical carcinogenesis were the primary data bases which led the IARC (1986) to conclude that 'passive smoking gives rise to some risk of cancer.'

THE PHYSICOCHEMICAL NATURE OF TOBACCO SMOKE

The combustion of tobacco products leads to the formation of mainstream smoke (MS) and sidestream smoke (SS). MS is generated during puff-drawing in the burning cone and

Table 1. Estimates of constituents in tobacco smoke (≃3900 known compounds)

Major classes of compounds[a]	No.
Amides, imides, lactones	240
Carboxylic acids, anhydrides	240
Lactones	150
Esters	475
Aldehydes	110
Ketones	520
Alcohols	380
Phenols	285
Amines	200
N-Nitrosamines	22
N-Heterocyclics	920
Hydrocarbons	755
Nitriles	105
Carbohydrates	45
Ethers	310
Total	4865

[a] Some compounds contain multiple functional groups, thus this list exceeds 3900

hot zones of cigarettes and cigars; it travels through the tobacco column and out of the mouthpiece. SS is formed between puffing and is emitted from the smouldering coal into the ambient air.

The data presented throughout this review are derived from machine-smoking under standardized laboratory conditions (Brunnemann *et al.*, 1976a; International Committee for Cigar Smoke Study, 1974). However, it has to be realized that machine-smoking parameters can differ substantially from the puff-drawing parameters of smokers, especially in the case of cigarettes with low nicotine delivery (Herning *et al.*, 1981).

About 30% of the total effluents of MS originate from the tobacco, the remainder comes from the air drawn through the cigarette. When leaving the mouthpiece, undiluted smoke from a nonfilter cigarette contains about 5×10^9 particles per millilitre, with a median particle size of about 0.4 μm (Keith & Tesh, 1965; Carter & Hasegawa, 1975).

The pH of tobacco smoke is of major significance, since it influences the degree of protonation and, therefore, the proportion of nicotine and other basic components in the vapour phase. This determines the inhalability of MS (Armitage & Turner, 1970). At about pH 5.4, all nicotine in tobacco smoke is monoprotonated and resides in the particulate phase (Fig. 1). The pH of the MS of air-cured tobaccos and of cigars increases with ascending number of puffs. Consequently, the smoke of these products contains proportionately larger amounts of nicotine in the vapour phase. The smoke pH of cigarettes filled with flue-cured tobaccos or with tobacco blends, on the other hand, decreases slightly or remains rather constant (Fig. 2; Brunnemann & Hoffmann, 1974).

The total MS of a cigarette weighs about 400–500 mg. More than 92% of the total is made up of 400–500 individual gaseous components with nitrogen (≃58%), oxygen (≃12%),

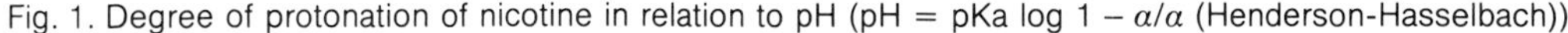

Fig. 1. Degree of protonation of nicotine in relation to pH (pH = pKa log 1 – α/α (Henderson-Hasselbach))

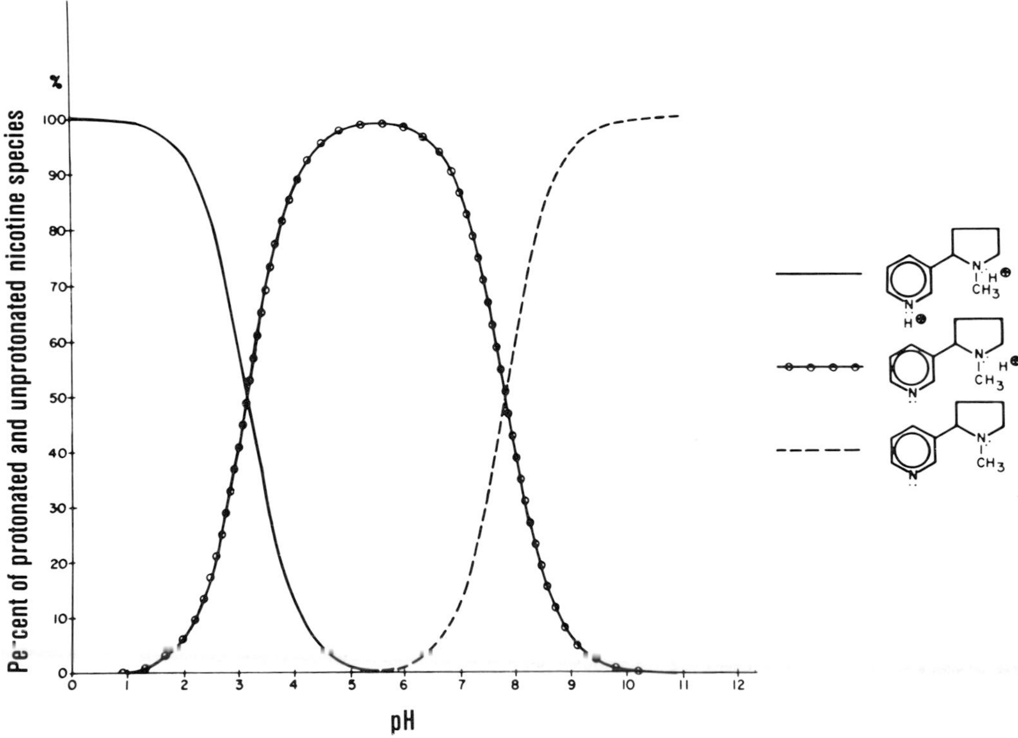

Fig. 2. pH of total mainstream smoke of various tobacco products: (1) little cigar I; (2) little cigar II; (3) cigar; (4) Kentucky reference cigarette (84 mm); (6) blended cigarette without filter (84 mm)

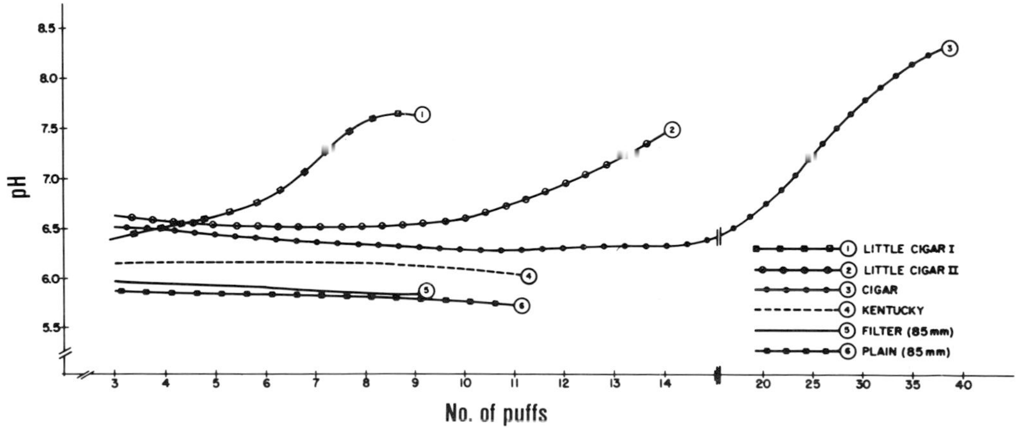

Fig. 3. Approximate chemical composition of mainstream smoke (from Norman, 1977)

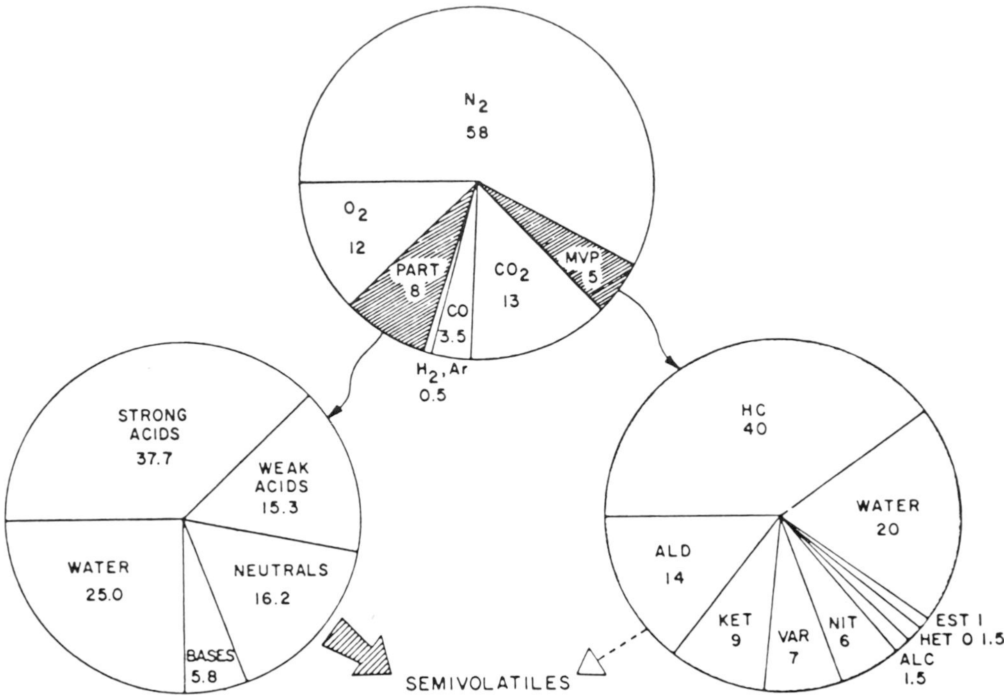

carbon dioxide (≃13%) and carbon monoxide (≃3.5%) as major constituents. The remainder is comprised of other vapour phase components and of compounds constituting the particulate phase (Fig. 3; Norman, 1977).

VAPOUR PHASE

Bioassays with total smoke have indicated that the majority of the genotoxic and cocarcinogenic agents reside in the particulate phase (Dontenwill *et al.*, 1973; Hoffmann *et al.*, 1979). Thus, specific methods have been developed for the quantitative determination of smoke particulates. The most widely applied technique is the Cambridge filter method, utilizing a glass fibre filter pad which retains 99.7% of all particles with diameters of >0.1 μm (Dube & Green, 1982). This manner of trapping does not effect a strict separation of the solid and gaseous components in the physicochemical sense, nevertheless, it permits reproducible, quantitative determination of the particulate matter in the smoke of cigarettes, cigars and pipes and analysis of the major vapour phase components by gas chromatography. In addition to nitrogen, oxygen, carbon dioxide and carbon monoxide, the vapour phase contains hydrogen, methane and other hydrocarbons, volatile aldehydes and ketones, nitrogen oxides, hydrogen cyanide and volatile nitriles and at least an additional 400–450 minor constituents (Keith & Tesh, 1965; Wynder & Hoffmann, 1967; Brunnemann & Hoffmann, 1982).

Table 2. Major toxic and tumorigenic agents in the vapour of freshly generated smoke of a nonfilter cigarette[a]

Agent	Conc./cigarette	Biol. effect[b]
Carbon monoxide	10–23 mg	T
Acetaldehyde	0.5–1.2 mg	CT
Nitrogen oxides (NO_x)	50–600 μg	T
Hydrogen cyanide	150–300 μg	CT, T
Ammonia	50–170 μg	T
Acrolein	50–100 μg	CT
Benzene	20–50 μg	HC
Formaldehyde	5–100 μg	C
2-Nitropropane	0.2–2.2 μg	C
Hydrazine	24–43 ng	C
Urethane	20–38 ng	C
Vinyl chloride	1.3–16 ng	HC

[a] Does not include volatile *N*-nitrosamines
[b] Abbreviations: T, toxic agent; CT, ciliatoxic agent; HC, human carcinogen; C, carcinogen

Fig. 4. Hamburg II smoke inhalation device for Syrian golden hamsters

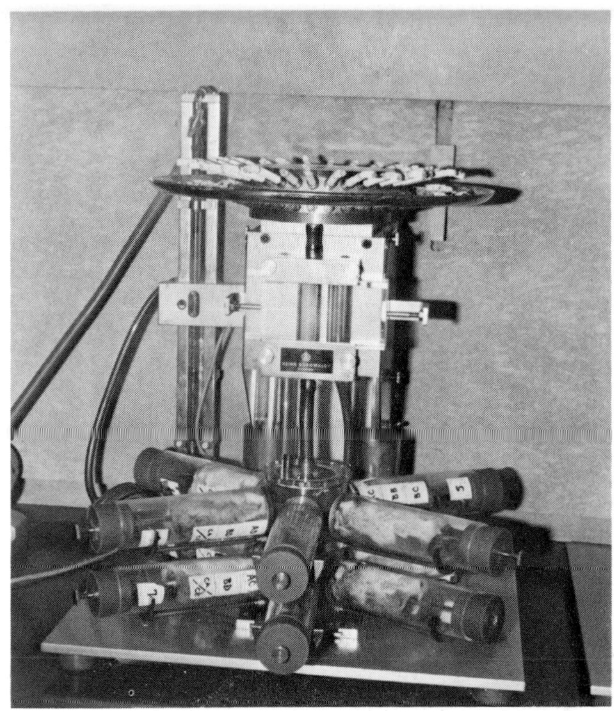

Table 2 presents a listing of the major known toxic and tumorigenic agents in the vapour phase of cigarette smoke. Each of the volatile smoke constituents was quantitatively assessed by analytical methods that had to be specifically developed for their determination in the smoke of cigarettes or cigars. Despite the presence of volatile carcinogens in the vapour phase of tobacco smoke, currently available bioassays – and here mainly inhalation experiments with hamsters (Fig. 4) – have not been sensitive enough to induce tumours by administering the vapour phase as such, aside from the induction of lung adenoma in mice (Mohr & Reznik, 1978).

PARTICULATE PHASE

While the vapour phase by itself is not tumorigenic in most of the inhalation assays, and the total smoke induces benign and malignant tumours in the upper respiratory tract of rats and hamsters (Dontenwill *et al.*, 1973; Hoffmann *et al.*, 1979), evidence from contact carcinogenesis studies indicates that the particulate phase contains most of the known tumorigenic and carcinogenic agents of tobacco smoke. Tobacco smoke particulates

Fig. 5. Fractionation of cigarette 'tar'; C, relative carcinogenic activity; P, relative tumour-promoting activity

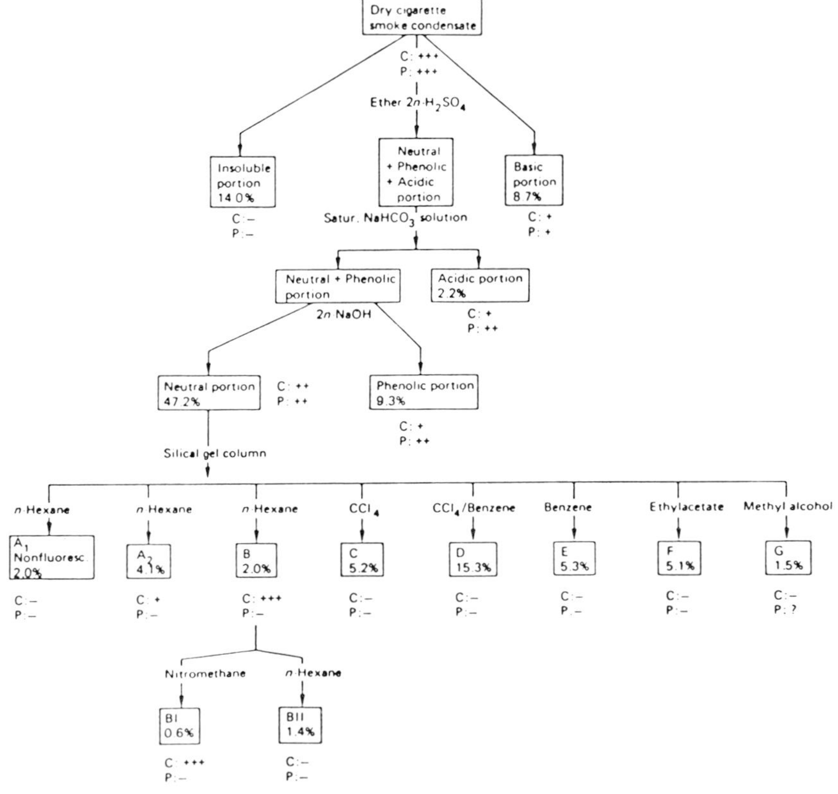

Fig. 6. Tumour-initiating activities of 80 end-fractions from BI subfractions. Each end-fraction was tested on 20 mice, negative control, no initiator: 1% croton oil as promoter; line a, fractions with activities significantly above those in negative control group ($p < 0.05$); line b, fractions with strong tumour-initiating activity ($p < 0.05$ above those in line a)

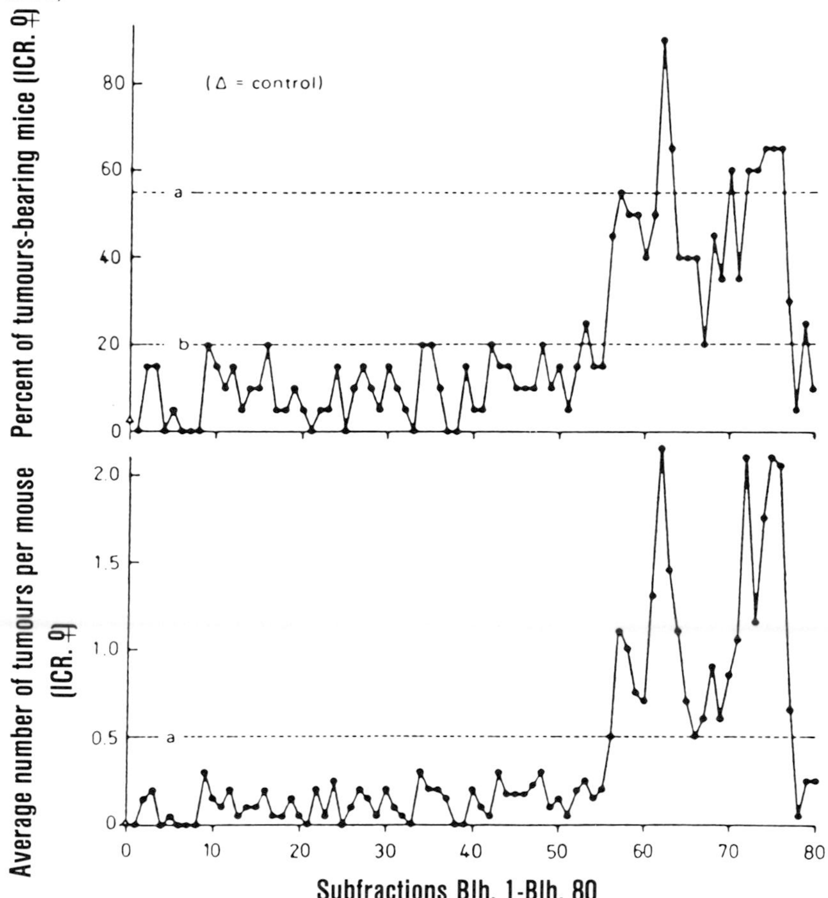

('tars') have consistently and in a dose-related response, induced benign and malignant tumours in the skin of mice and rabbits, and in the connective tissue and bronchial epithelium of rats (Wynder & Hoffmann, 1967; Mohr & Reznik, 1978; Hoffmann *et al.*, 1979; IARC, 1986).

Tumour initiators and cocarcinogens

The findings from bioassays with tobacco 'tars' have led to more detailed and systematic testing on mouse skin of the various fractions and subfractions of the particulate phase (Fig. 5; Hoffmann & Wynder, 1971). The only fractions found to have significant activity as complete carcinogens were the neutral fraction and its subfractions B and BI. A further breakdown of subfraction BI, which amounted to 0.6% of the total particulate phase, led

Table 3. Major compounds identified in neutral subfractions BIh 56–66 of the particulate phase of cigarette smoke

Chlorinated hydrocarbon insecticides	Benzofluorenes
DDD	11*H*-benzo[*a*]fluorene
o,p'-DDD	11*H*-benzo[*b*]fluorene
DDT	7*H*-benzo[*c*]fluorene
o,p'-DDT	17*H*-cyclopenta[*a*]phenanthrene
DDM (DDD-HCl)	17*H*-cyclopenta[*a*]phenanthrene
DDE (DDT-HCl)	x-Methyl-17*H*-cyclopenta[*a*]phenanthrene
Trans-4,4'-Dichlorostilbene	x-Ethyl-17*H*-cyclopenta[*a*]phenanthrene
N-Alkylcarbazoles	x-Phenylindene
9-Methylcarbazole	Pyrenes
9-Ethylcarbazole	Pyrene
1,9-, 2,9-, 3,9- and 4,9-Dimethylcarbazole	1-, 3- and 4-Methylpyrene
Fluoranthenes	x,x'-Dimethylpyrene(s)
Fluoranthene	
1-, 2-, 3-, 7- and 8-Methylfluoranthene	
X-Ethylfluoranthene(s)	
x,x'-Dimethylfluoranthenes	
Benzo[*mno*]fluoranthene	

Table 4. Major compounds identified in neutral subfractions BIh 71–78 of the particulate phase of cigarette smoke

Chrysenes	Benzofluoranthenes
Chrysene	Benzo[*b*]fluoranthene
1-, 2-, 3-, 4-, 5- and 6-Methylchrysene	Benzo[*j*]fluoranthene
x,x'-Dimethylchrysene(s)	Benzo[*k*]fluoranthene
x-Ethylchrysene(s)	Ideno[1, 2, 3,-*cd*]pyrene
Benz[*a*]anthracenes	Dibenzopyrenes
Benz[*a*]anthracene	Dibenzo[*a, h*]pyrene (?)
x-Methylbenz[*a*]anthracene	Anthanthrene
Benzo[*c*]phenanthrenes	Perylene
Benzo[*c*]phenanthrene	Benzo[*ghi*]perylene
x-Methylbenzo[*c*]phenanthrene	
Benzopyrenes	
Benzo[*a*]pyrene	
x-Methylbenzo[*a*]pyrenes	
Benzo[*e*]pyrene	

to a highly carcinogenic concentrate, BIh (representing 0.09% of the 'tar') and this, in turn, was chromatographically separated to yield 80 end fractions. Upon testing as tumour initiators on mouse skin (Fig. 6), end fractions BIh 56–66 and BIh 71–78 were found to be highly active. Their chemical analysis revealed that they consisted primarily of polynuclear aromatic hydrocarbons, many of which are known carcinogens in laboratory animals (Tables 3 and 4; Hoffmann & Wynder, 1971). Application to mouse skin of these highly active end fractions in doses proportionate to their occurrence in the total particulate

Table 5. Carcinogens and cocarcinogens in the smoke of a nonfilter cigarette

Agent	Relative carcinogenic activity	ng/cigarette
Carcinogens		
Benzo[*a*]pyrene	+++	10–50
5-Methylchrysene	+++	0.6
Dibenz[*a,h*]anthracene	++	40
Benzo[*b*]fluoranthene	++	30
Benzo[*j*]fluoranthene	++	60
Dibenzo[*a,i*]pyrene	++	present
Indeno[1, 2, 3-*cd*]pyrene	+	4
Benz[*a*]anthracene	+	40–70
Chrysene	+	40–60
Benzo[*e*]pyrene	?	5–40
Dibenz[*a,j*]acridine	++	3–10
Dibenz[*a,h*]acridine	+	0.1
Dibenzo[*c,g*]carbazole	+	0.7
Cocarcinogens		
Pyrene		50–200
Fluoranthene		100–260
Benzo[*g h i*]perylene		60
4,4'-Dichlorostilbene		1 500
Catechol		25 000–360 000
3-Methylcatechol		11 000–20 000
4-Methylcatechol		15 000–21 000
4-Ethylcatechol		10 000–24 000

matter did not lead to tumour induction. Yet, co-application of the active neutral subfractions with the inactive phenolic fraction of the particulate matter led to a tumour yield which accounted for approximately 65–75% of that induced with the total 'tar'. This indicated that the phenolic fraction had cocarcinogenic activity, and further studies showed that catechols were the major cocarcinogens in the phenolic portion (Hecht *et al.*, 1981). Catechol itself is the most abundant phenol in tobacco smoke, amounting to 26–360 μg per cigarette (Wynder & Hoffmann, 1967; Brunnemann *et al.*, 1976b). Table 5 lists the major epithelial carcinogens and cocarcinogens identified in the smoke of a non-filter cigarette.

Organ-specific carcinogens

Tobacco smoke contains, in addition to contact carcinogens and cocarcinogens, several organ-specific carcinogens. This supports the epidemiological observation that cigarette smoking is an important factor in the etiology of cancer of the oesophagus, pancreas, renal pelvis and urinary bladder (IARC, 1986). Table 6 lists the known organ-specific carcinogens in cigarette smoke. Polonium-210 (0.03–1.0 pCi/cigarette) has been incriminated as a possible contributing factor for the increased risk for cancer of the lung in cigarette smokers (Radford & Hunt, 1964; Harley *et al.*, 1980). The presence of aromatic amines in

Table 6. Organ-specific carcinogens in cigarette smoke

Carcinogen	ng/cigarette
N-Nitrosodimethylamine	1–180
N-Nitrosoethylmethylamine	1–40
N-Nitrosodiethylamine	0.1–28
N-Nitrosopyrrolidine	2–110
N-Nitrosopiperidine	0–9
N-Nitrosodiethanolamine	0–40
N'-Nitrosonornicotine	120–3700
4-(Methylnitrosamino)-1-(3-pyridyl)-1-butanone (NNK)	120–950
N'-Nitrosoanabasine	40–400
2-Toluidine	30–160
2-Naphthylamine	4.3–27
4-Aminobiphenyl	2.4–4.6
Nickel	20–3000
Polonium-210	0.03–1.0 pCi

Table 7. Estimated exposure of US residents to nitrosamines[a]

Source of exposure	Nitrosamines[b]	Primary exposure route	Daily intake (μg/person)	
Beer	NDMA	Ingestion	0.34	
Cosmetics	NDELA	Dermal absorption	0.41	
Cured meat; cooked bacon	NPYR	Ingestion	0.17	
Scotch whisky	NDMA	Ingestion	0.03	
Cigarette smoking	VNA[c]	Inhalation	0.3	
	NDELA	Inhalation	0.5	
	NNN	Inhalation	6.1	16.2[d]
	NNK	Inhalation	2.9	
	NAT+NAB	Inhalation	7.2	

[a] From National Research Council (1981)
[b] NDMA, *N*-nitrosodimethylamine; NDELA, *N*-nitrosodiethanolamine; NPYR, *N*-nitrosopyrrolidine; NNK, 4-(methylnitrosamino)-1-(3-pyridyl)-1-butanone; NAT, *N'*-nitrosoanatabine; NAB, *N'*-nitrosoanabasine
[c] VNA, volatile nitrosamines (NDMA+ *N*-nitrosomethylethylamine+ *N*-nitrosodiethylamine+NPYR)
[d] Tobacco-specific nitrosamines

smoke has been associated with the increased risk for bladder cancer in cigarette smokers (Doll, 1972).

The *N*-nitrosamines are the major group of organ-specific carcinogens in tobacco products. They are formed during the processing of tobacco and during smoking by *N*-nitrosation of secondary and tertiary amines. Tobacco smoke contains volatile, non-volatile and tobacco-specific *N*-nitrosamines (TSNA; Table 6). It has been estimated that US residents receive the highest degree of exposure to nitrosamines from cigarette smoking (Table 7). In fact, the concentration of these compounds in tobacco smoke exceeds by

Fig. 7. Tobacco alkaloids and nitrosamines which can be formed from them. With the exception of NNA, all of these compounds are present in tobacco and tobacco smoke

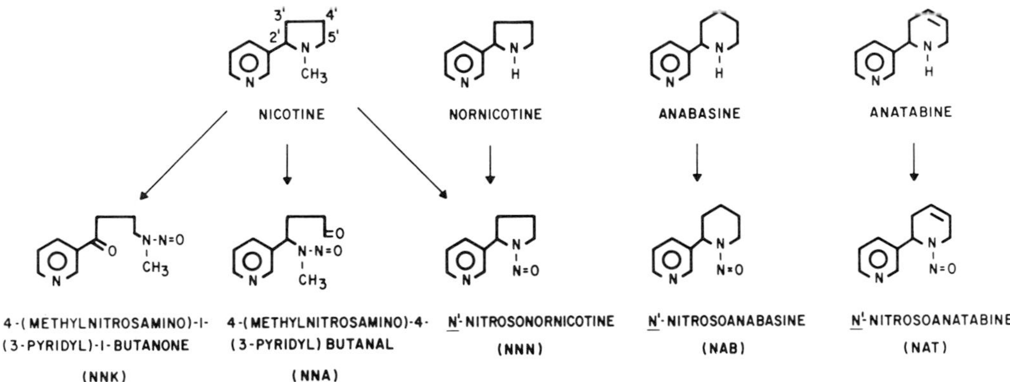

Table 8. *N*-Nitrosamines in cigarette smoke from different varieties of tobacco (ng/cigarette) [a]

N-Nitrosamine	Burley tobacco	Bright tobacco	French black tobacco
N-Nitrosodimethylamine	11–180	0.5–13.2	29–143
N-Nitrosomethylamine	9.1–13	>0.1	2.7–12
N-Nitrosodiethylamine	4–25	nd–1.8 [b]	0.6–6
N-Nitrosopyrrolidine	52–76	6.2	25–110
N'-Nitrosonornicotine	3700	620	590
4-(Methylnitrosamino)-1-(3-pyridyl)-1-butanone	320	420	220
N'-Nitrosoanatabine	4600	410	200
N'-Nitrosoanabasine	400	40	nd–150 [b]

[a] From Hoffmann *et al.*, 1984a
[b] nd, not detected

at least two orders of magnitude the levels of nitrosamines reported in any other consumer product or respiratory environment, except for a few, very limited occupational settings (National Research Council, 1981).

The most abundant nitrosamines in tobacco smoke are the TSNA. They are formed from nicotine and the minor tobacco alkaloids (Fig. 7). In the smoke, 25–45% of the TSNA originate by transfer from the tobacco, the remainder is formed by pyrosynthesis during smoking (Adams *et al.*, 1983; Hoffmann & Hecht, 1985). The single most important factor for the smoke yields of nitrosamines is the nitrate content of tobacco (Adams *et al.*, 1984), thus the smoke of air-cured tobacco is significantly richer in the nitrosamines (Table 8; Hoffmann *et al.*, 1984a). Utilization of cigarette blends with stems and ribs, which are the portions of the tobacco leaf with the greatest abundance of nitrate, can substantially elevate the nitrosamine content of the smoke (Brunnemann *et al.*, 1983).

The nicotine-derived *N*-nitrosamines, *N'*-nitrosonornicotine (NNN) and 4-(methylnitrosamino)-1-(3-pyridyl)-1-butanone (NNK), are by far the most powerful carcinogens in

Table 9. Carcinogenicity of tobacco-specific nitrosamines[a]

Nitrosamine[b]	Species and strain	Route of application	Principal target organs	Dose
NNN	A/J mouse	i.p.	Lung	0.12 mmol/mouse
	F344 rat	s.c.	Nasal cavity, oesophagus	0.2–3.4 mmol/rat
		oral	Oesophagus, nasal cavity	1.0–3.6 mmol/rat
	Sprague-Dawley rat	oral	Nasal cavity	8.8 mmol/rat
	Syrian golden hamster	s.c.	Trachea, nasal cavity	0.9–2.1 mmol/hamster
NNK	A/J mouse	i.p.	Lung	0.12 mmol/mouse
	F344 rat	s.c.	Nasal cavity, lung, liver	0.2–2.8 mmol/rat
	Syrian golden hamster	s.c.	Trachea, lung, nasal cavity	0.9 mmol/hamster 0.005 mmol/hamster
NAT	F344 rat	s.c.	None	0.2–2.8 mmol/rat
NAB	F344 rat	oral	Oesophagus	3-12 mmol/rat
	Syrian golden hamster	s.c.	None	2 mmol/hamster
NNA	A/J mouse	i.p.	None	0.12 mmol/mouse

[a] From Hoffmann and Wynder, 1985
[b] NNN, *N'*-nitrosonornicotine; NNK, 4-(methylnitrosamino)-1-(3-pyridyl)-1-butanone; NAT, *N'*-nitrosoanatabine; NAB, *N'*-nitrosoanabasine; NNA, 4-(methylnitrosamino)-4-(3-pyridyl)butanal

Fig. 8. Scheme linking nicotine, the major tobacco alkaloid and habituating factor in tobacco, to formation of the promutagenic DNA adduct O^6-methylguanine

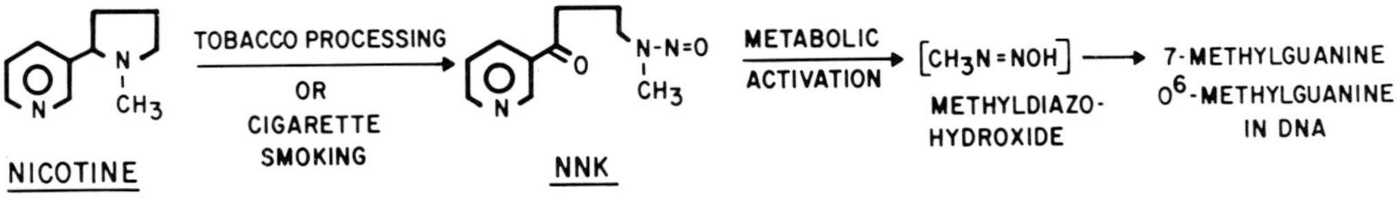

tobacco smoke, inducing carcinoma in mice, rats and Syrian golden hamsters (Table 9). Perhaps the most important observation is that NNK induces benign and malignant tumours in laboratory animals not only in the upper respiratory tract but also in the lung. In hamsters, a single application of 1 mg of NNK suffices to induce lung tumours. In rats, NNK induces also liver tumours, nasal cavity tumours, and a high incidence of squamous-cell carcinoma and adenocarcinoma in the lungs of males and, at a significantly lower rate, in females (Hoffmann *et al.*, 1984b; Hoffmann & Hecht, 1985). Although we are presently lacking definite evidence, it may be presumed that NNN and NNK are also formed endogenously when a smoker inhales the precursors, nitrogen oxides and nicotine, as smoke constituents. The inhalation of smoke from a single cigarette provides up to 600 μg of nitrogen oxides and up to 2 mg of nicotine. The known catalytic effects of thiocyanate for *N*-nitrosation (Boyland *et al.*, 1971) favour these reactions in smokers who have elevated levels of thiocyanate in the saliva and in blood (IARC, 1986), owing to the detoxification of hydrogen cyanide, inhaled as a smoke constituent in amounts of up to 500 μg per cigarette (Brunnemann *et al.*, 1977).

A most stimulating observation lies in the fact that NNK is metabolically activated by α-hydroxylation, yielding methyldiazohydroxide. This unstable compound is known to alkylate guanine in DNA to 7-methylguanine and O^6-methylguanine *in vitro* as well as *in vivo*. Thus, we know today, that nicotine is not only the major habituating agent in tobacco but that it is also a precursor for the powerful carcinogen NNK. Figure 8 depicts the pathway of NNK formation from nicotine. Metabolic activation leads to α-hydroxylation of NNK which gives rise to methyldiazohydroxide. The latter methylates DNA to the pro-mutagenic DNA adduct, O^6-methylguanine (Hoffmann & Hecht, 1985).

ENVIRONMENTAL TOBACCO SMOKE

Since 1981, a number of epidemiological studies have indicated a possible correlation between uptake of environmental tobacco smoke ('passive smoking') and an increased risk for cancer. The IARC concluded: 'The observations on nonsmokers that have been made so far are compatible with either an increased risk from "passive" smoking or an absence of risk. Knowledge of the nature of sidestream and mainstream smoke, of the materials absorbed during "passive" smoking, and of the quantitative relationships between dose and effect that are commonly observed from exposure to carcinogens leads to the conclusion that passive smoking gives rise to some risk of cancer.' (IARC, 1986).

A comparison of the constituents of mainstream (MS) and sidestream (SS) smoke reveals that these combustion effluents are similar but not the same (Table 10). The differences become particularly apparent when one compares the chemical composition of undiluted MS and SS. Considering that 35–40% of the tobacco is burned during puff-drawing and the remainder during smouldering, one would expect, in the case of a non-filter cigarette, that the release of smoke compounds in the SS would be 50–100% greater

Table 10. Comparisons of mainstream (MS) and sidestream (SS) smoke of cigarettes (physicochemical data)

Parameters	MS	SS
Peak temperature during formation (°C)	~900	~600
pH (total aerosol) [a]	6.0–6.2	6.4–6.6
Particle size (μm)	0.1–1.0	0.01–0.1
Median diameter	0.4	
Smoke dilution (vol. %) [b]		
Carbon monoxide	3–5	≃1
Carbon dioxide	8–11	≃2
Oxygen	12–16	16–20
Hydrogen	15–3	≃0.5

[a] 85-mm nonfilter cigarette
[b] At a distance of 10 mm from the burning coal

Table 11. Distribution of compounds in mainstream smoke (MS) and sidestream smoke (SS) of nonfilter cigarettes

Compound	MS	SS/MS
Vapour phase		
Carbon monoxide	10–23 mg	2.5–4.7
Carbon dioxide	20–40 mg	8–11
Benzene	20–50 μg	10
Formaldehyde	5–100 μg	0.1–~50
Acrolein	50–100 μg	8–15
Acetone	100–250 μg	2–5
Hydrogen cyanide	400–500 μg	0.1–0.25
Hydrazine	24–43 ng	3.0
Ammonia	50–170 μg	40–170
Methylamine	11.5–28.7 μg	4.2–6.4
Nitrogen oxides	50–600 μg	4–10
N-Nitrosodimethylamine	10–180 ng	20–100
N-Nitrosopyrrolidine	2–110 ng	6–30
Particulate phase		
Particulate matter	15–40 mg	1.3–1.9
Nicotine	1–2.5 mg	2.6–3.3
Phenol	60–140 μg	1.6–3.0
Catechol	100–350 μg	0.6–0.9
Hydroquinone	110–300 μg	0.7–0.9
Aniline	360 ng	30
2-Toluidine	30–160 ng	19
2-Naphthylamine	4.3–27 ng	30
4-Aminobiphenyl	2.4–4.6 ng	31
Benz[*a*]anthracene	40–70 ng	2–4
Benzo[*a*]pyrene	10–40 ng	2.5–3.5
N'-Nitrosonornicotine	120–3700 ng	0.5–3
4-(Methylnitrosamino)-1-(3-pyridyl)-1-butanone	120–950 ng	1–4
Cadmium	100 ng	7.2
Nickel	20–3000 ng	13–30
Polonium-210	0.03–1.0 pCi	?

than in the MS. However, this is not the case. As seen in Table 11, compounds generated by reduction reactions are formed in significantly higher yields and those formed by oxidation occur in lower yields during smouldering (SS formation) than during puff-drawing (MS formation). These differences are primarily due to the depletion of oxygen inside the burning cone during smouldering as opposed to only a partial oxygen deficiency during puff-drawing. Excessive formation of SS compounds is greatest for ammonia, amines including aromatic amines and, especially, for the volatile carcinogenic *N*-nitrosamines (VNA).

The high yields of VNA in SS explain the fact that they are detectable in smoke-polluted environments in spite of extensive dilution by air. The qualitative and quantitative differences of MS and SS composition and the effects of ageing of SS constituents in the environment make it clear that smoke polluted indoor-air cannot be regarded as 'diluted mainstream smoke'.

REDUCTION OF SMOKE CONSTITUENTS

One of the earliest and yet most important observations in the association of cancer risk and smoking was that of a dose-response relationship (Wynder & Graham, 1950; Doll & Hill, 1954; Hammond & Horn, 1958). Therefore, during the last two to three decades, a reduced exposure to tobacco smoke by modifying the smoke yields of cigarettes was

Fig. 9. US sales-weighted average tar and nicotine yields (adapted from Norman, 1982); RT, reconstituted tobacco; ET, expanded tobacco; F, cigarettes with filter tips; numbers, lengths of filter tips

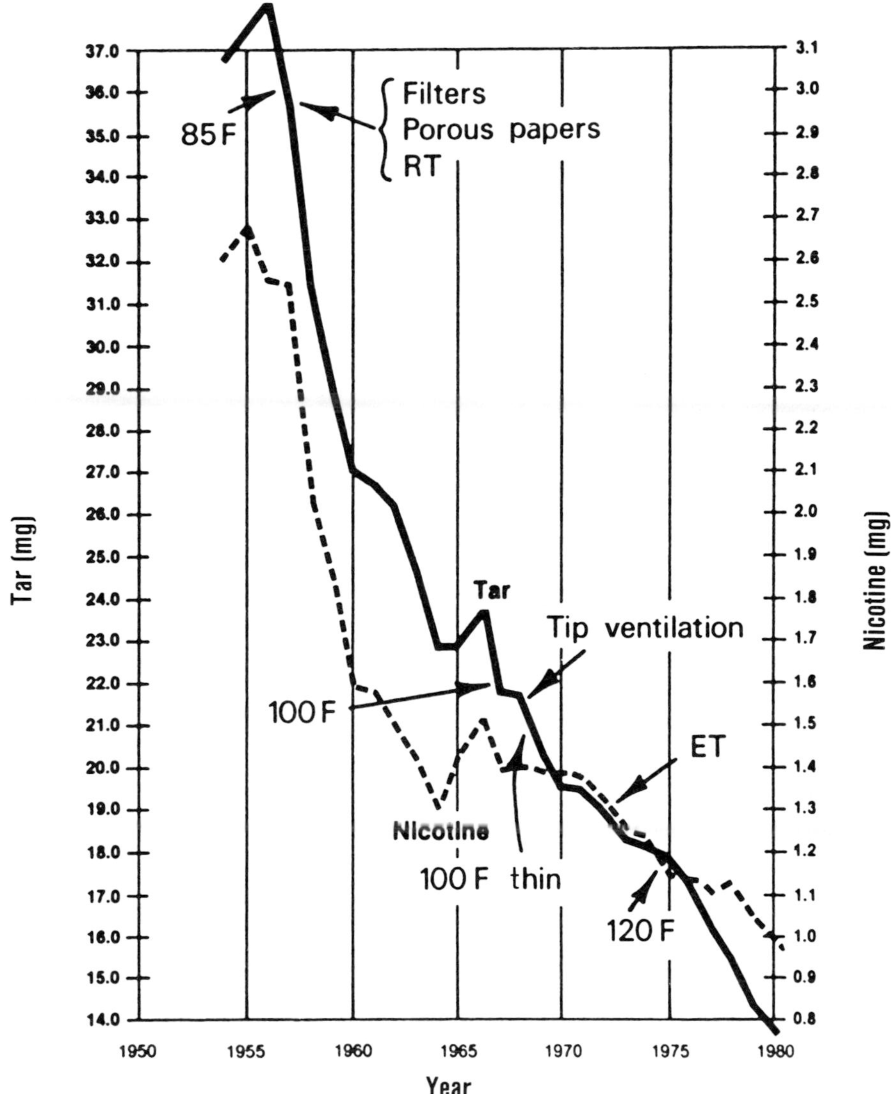

Table 12. Reductions of biological activity of smoke from experimental cigarettes[a]

Methods[b]	Smoke constituents			Selective reduction of biological activity[c]		Remarks
	'Tar'	Nicotine	Benzo[*a*]pyrene	Carcinogenicity	Tumour promotion	
Agricultural aspects						
Tobacco type (Bright-Burley)[d]	+	+	+	+	+	
New cultivars	+	+	+		?	
Fertilization (nitrate)	+	+	+	+	?	
Tobacco processing						
Cut	±	±	±	±?	?	
Use of tobacco midribs	+	+	+	++	++	
Reconstituted tobacco sheets (RTS)[e]	+	+	+	++	±	Some RTS give high CO
RTS-paper process	++	+	+	++	±	
Expanded tobacco laminae	+	++	+	±?	±	
Expanded tobacco midribs	+	++	+	++	?	
Cigarette production						
Paper porosity	+	+	+	±	?	
Cellulose acetate filters	+	+	+	±	±	
Charcoal filters[f]	+	+	+	±	±	
Perforated filters	++	++	++	±	±	Smoker's compensation

[a] From Wynder and Hoffmann (1982)
[b] Methdology known to be applied to commercial US cigarettes. Reductions: ++, >50%; +, significant; ±, insignificant; ±?, questionable; ?, unknown
[c] Comparison of gram-to-gram 'tar' on mouse skin tests and/or hamster smoke inhalations
[d] Replacing Bright with Burley tobaccos
[e] Data given for RTS relate to those not made by the paper process
[f] Reductions of 'tar', nicotine, benzo[*a*]pyrene (and other nonvolatiles) and volatile *N*-nitrosamines are, in general, greater with cellulose acetate filters than with charcoal filters.

regarded as one significant step towards diminishing the cancer risks associated with smoking. Measures to reduce the smoke yields included changes in the cultivation of tobacco, breeding and selection of new varieties, homogenized leaf curing, incorporation of stems and ribs into the tobacco blends, use of reconstituted and expanded tobaccos, and modification of wrappers and filter tips.

The most obvious results of these changes in the make-up of cigarettes have been reflected in a trend of declining sales-weighted average 'tar' and nicotine levels in the smoke of cigarettes since 1955. This trend has been observed in many countries.

In the USA, sales-weighted average 'tar' and nicotine values have dropped from 38 mg and 2.7 mg, respectively, in 1956 to 13 mg 'tar' and 1.0 mg of nicotine (Tobacco Institute, 1984). Figure 9 graphically documents the decline in 'tar' and nicotine while denoting the technical modifications that have contributed to the reduction of smoke yields of cigarettes (Norman, 1982).

For our own studies (Wynder & Hoffmann, 1967; Hoffmann & Wynder, 1976) and for studies by the US National Cancer Institute (1980), experimental cigarettes were made in which specific parameters were changed. The smoke of these cigarettes was analysed and the resulting 'tars' were assayed for carcinogenicity and tumour-promoting activity on mouse skin. The most encouraging results in respect to a selective reduction of tumorigenicity were observed for cigarettes made entirely of reconstituted tobacco, of stems and ribs, of expanded tobacco and of expanded stems and ribs (Table 12). In smoke inhalation studies with modified cigarettes, significant declines in activity were also observed in respect of tumours in the larynx of hamsters (Dontenwill, 1974).

We consider these changes in the make-up of cigarettes and a significant reduction of the tumorigenic potential of the resulting smoke as significant progress, although we need to acknowledge that the smoker of cigarettes with a low nicotine content tends to compensate by smoking more intensely (Herning *et al.*, 1981).

The IARC (1986) concluded that 'in a few countries, in which smoking has been established for many years, a substantial reduction in mortality from lung cancer has been observed in young and middle-aged men, which is greatest in the youngest age groups. This has occurred at a time when the number of cigarettes smoked by young men in these countries has remained approximately constant. No substantial cause (or cofactor) has so far been identified that offers a plausible explanation for the observed magnitude of the reduction of risk for lung cancer, other than changes in cigarette design which include reduction in tar content.'

SUMMARY

Tobacco smoke contains more than 3900 constituents. In this presentation we have summarized our present knowledge as to the physicochemical nature of tobacco smoke and specific agents therein. Emphasis has been placed on the discussion of formation and identification of toxic and, especially, of tumorigenic agents in tobacco smoke. In the concluding Table 13 we have listed those smoke constituents in the mainstream smoke of cigarettes that we regard as important contributors to the toxic and carcinogenic potential of tobacco smoke. This judgement is based on extensive laboratory studies. Finally, data

Table 13. Biologically active agents in mainstream smoke[a]

Smoke constituent	Conc./cigarette	Biological effect[b]
Total particulate matter	15–40 mg	T, HC
Carbon monoxide	10–23 mg	T
Nicotine	1.0–2.5 mg	T
Acetaldehyde	0.5–1.2 mg	CT
Acetone	100–250 μg	CT
NO_x	50–600 μg	T
Formic acid	80–600 μg	CT
Hydrogen cyanide	400–500 μg	CT, T
Catechol	140–500 μg	CoC
Ammonia	50–130 μg	T
Benzene	20–50 μg	HC
Acrolein	50–100 μg	CT
Acrylonitrile	3.2–15.0 μg	C
Phenol	60–140 μg	TP
Formaldehyde	5–100 μg	C
Carbazole	1 μg	C?
2-Nitropropane	0.2–2.2 μg	C
N'-Nitrosonornicotine	120–3700 ng	C
4-(Methylnitrosamino)-1-(3-pyridyl)-1-butanone	120–950 ng	C
N'-Nitrosoanabasine	120 ng	C?
N-Nitrosodiethanolamine	0–40 ng	C
N-Nitrosopyrrolidine	2–110 ng	C
N-Nitrosodimethylamine	2–180 ng	C
N-Nitrosomethylethylamine	0.1–40 ng	C
N-Nitrosodiethylamine	0.1–28 ng	C
N-Nitrosodi-*n*-propylamine	0–1 ng	C
N-Nitrosodi-*n*-butylamine	0–3 ng	C
N-Nitrosopiperidine	0–9 ng	C
N-Nitrosopyrrolidine	2–42 ng	C
Hydrazine	24–43 ng	C
Urethane	20–38 ng	C
Vinyl chloride	1.3–16 ng	HC
Benz[*a*]anthracene	40–60 ng	C
Benzo[*a*]pyrene	10–50 ng	C
5-Methylchrysene	0.6 ng	C
Dibenz[*a, j*]acridine	3–10 ng	C
2-Naphthylamine	4.3–27 ng	HC
4-Aminobiphenyl	2.4–4.6 ng	HC
2-Toluidine	30–160 ng	C
Polonium-210	0.03–1.0 pCi	

[a] Quantitative data refer to nonfilter cigarettes
[b] Abbreviations: T, toxic agent; HC, human carcinogen; CT, ciliatoxic agent; CoC, cocarcinogen; TP, tumour promoter; C, animal carcinogen

are presented in support of the concept that product modification can reduce the carcinogenic potential of cigarettes. However, it must be emphasized that the only safe way to avoid the cancer risks associated with smoking is to refrain from smoking.

ACKNOWLEDGEMENTS

We greatly appreciate the extensive contributions of our colleagues J.D. Adams, K.D. Brunnemann, S.S. Hecht, E.J. LaVoie and A.S. Rivenson. We thank B. Stadler, D. Conroy and I. Hoffmann for their editorial assistance.

Our studies in tobacco carcinogenesis are supported by Grants CA-17613, CA-29580, and CA-35667 from the National Cancer Institute, US Department of Health and Human Services. This is No. XXXIII of the series *'A Study of Tobacco Carcinogenesis'*.

REFERENCES

Adams, J.D., Lee, S.J., Vinchkoski, N., Castonguay, A. & Hoffmann, D. (1983) Chemical studies on tobacco smoke. 73. On the formation of the tobacco-specific carcinogen 4-(methylnitrosamino)-1-(3-pyridyl)-1-butanone during smoking. *Cancer Lett.*, ***17***, 339–346

Adams, J.D., Lee, S.J. & Hoffmann, D. (1984) Carcinogenic agents in cigarette smoke and the influence of nitrate on their formation. *Carcinogenesis*, ***5***, 221–223

Armitage, A.K. & Turner, D.M. (1970) Absorption of nicotine in cigarette and cigar smoke through the oral mucosa. *Nature*, ***226***, 1231–1232

Boyland, E., Nice, E. & Williams, K. (1971) The catalysis of nitrosation by thiocyanate in saliva. *Food Cosmet. Toxicol.*, ***9***, 639–643

Brunnemann, K.D. & Hoffmann, D. (1974) The pH of tobacco smoke. *J. Food Cosmet. Toxicol.*, ***12***, 115–124

Brunnemann, K.D. & Hoffmann, D. (1982) Pyrolytic origins of major gas phase constituents of cigarette smoke. *Recent Adv. Tob. Sci.*, ***8***, 103–140

Brunnemann, K.D., Hoffmann, D., Wynder, E.L. & Gori, G.B. (1976a) *Determination of tar, nicotine, and carbon monoxide in cigarette smoke. A comparison of international smoking conditions.* In: Wynder, E.L., Hoffmann, D. & Gori, G.B., eds, *Smoking and Health. I. Modifying the Risk for the Smoker (US Dept of Health, Education, and Welfare Publ. No. (NIH) 76–1221)*, Washington DC, pp. 441–449

Brunnemann, K.D., Lee, H.-C. & Hoffmann, D. (1976b) Chemical studies on tobacco smoke XLVII. On the quantitative analysis of catechols and their reduction. *Anal. Lett.*, ***9***, 939–955

Brunnemann, K.D., Yu, L. & Hoffmann, D. (1977) Gas chromatographic determination of cyanide and cyanogen in tobacco smoke. *J. anal. Toxicol.*, ***1***, 38–42

Brunnemann, K.D., Masaryk, J. & Hoffmann, D. (1983) Role of tobacco stems in the formation of *N*-nitrosamines in tobacco and cigarette mainstream and sidestream smoke. *J. Agric. Food Chem.*, ***31***, 1221–1224

Carter, W.L. & Hasegawa, I. (1975) Fixation of tobacco smoke aerosols for size distribution studies. *J. Colloid Interface Sci.*, ***53***, 134–141

Doll, R. (1972) *Cancers related to smoking.* In: *Proceedings of the 2nd World Conference on Smoking and Health*, London, Pitman Medical, pp. 10–23

Doll, R. & Hill, A.B. (1954) The mortality of doctors in relation to their smoking habits; a preliminary report. *Br. med. J.*, ***i***, 1451–1455

Dontenwill, D.P. (1974) *Tumorigenic smoke inhalation studies in inbred Syrian hamsters.* In: Karbe, E. & Park, J.F., eds, *Experimental Lung Cancer – Carcinogenesis and Bioassays,* New York, Springer, pp. 331–359

Dontenwill, W., Chevalier, H.J., Harke, H.P., Lafrenz, U., Reckzeh, G. & Schneider, B. (1973) Investigations on the effects of chronic cigarette smoke inhalation in Syrian golden hamsters. *J. natl Cancer Inst.* ***5,*** 1781–1832

Dube, M.F. & Green, C.R. (1982) Methods of collection of smoke for analytical purposes. *Recent Adv. Tob. Sci.,* ***8,*** 42–102

Hammond, E.C. & Horn, D. (1958) Smoking and death rates – report on forty-four months of follow-up in 187 783 men. II. Death rates by cause. *J. Am. med. Assoc.,* ***166,*** 1294–1308

Harley, N.H., Cohen, B.S. & Tso, T.C. (1980) *Polonium-210: A questionable risk factor in smoking-related carcinogenesis.* In: Gori, G.B. & Bock, F.G., eds, *A Safe Cigarette? (Banbury Report No. 3),* Cold Spring Harbor, NY, Cold Spring Harbor Laboratory, pp. 93–104

Hecht, S., Carmella, S., Mori, H. & Hoffmann, D. (1981) A study of tobacco carcinogenesis. XX. Role of catechol as a major cocarcinogen in the weakly acidic fraction of smoke condensate. *J. natl Cancer Inst.,* ***66,*** 163–169

Herning, R.I., Jones, R.T., Bachman, J. & Mines, A.H. (1981) Puff volume increases when low-nicotine cigarettes are smoked. *Br. med. J.,* ***283,*** 187–189

Hoffmann, D. & Hecht, S.S. (1985) Perspectives in cancer research. Nicotine-derived *N*-nitrosamines and tobacco-related cancer: Current status and future directions. *Cancer Res.,* ***45,*** 935–944

Hoffmann, D. & Wynder, E.L. (1971) A study of tobacco carcinogenesis. XI. Tumor initiators, tumor accelerators, and tumor promoting activity of condensate fractions. *Cancer,* ***27,*** 848–864

Hoffmann, D. & Wynder, E.L. (1976) *Selective reduction of tumorigenicity of tobacco smoke. III. The reduction of polynuclear aromatic hydrocarbons in cigarette smoke.* In: Wynder, E.L., Hoffmann, D. & Gori, G.B., eds, *Smoking and Health. I. Modifying the Risk for the Smoker, (US Department of Health, Education and Welfare Publ. No. (NIH) 76–1221),* Washington DC, pp. 495–504

Hoffmann, D., Rivenson, A., Hecht, S.S., Hilfrich, J., Kobayashi, N. & Wynder, E.L. (1979) Model studies in tobacco carcinogenesis with the Syrian golden hamster. *Prog. exp. Tumor Res.,* ***24,*** 370–390.

Hoffmann, D., Wynder, E.L., Rivenson, A., LaVoie, E.J. & Hecht, S.S. (1983) Skin bioassays in tobacco carcinogenesis. *Prog. exp. Tumor Res.,* ***26,*** 43–67

Hoffmann, D., Brunnemann, K.D., Adams, J.D. & Hecht, S.S. (1984a) *Formation and analysis of N-nitrosamines in tobacco products and their endogenous formation in tobacco consumers.* In: O'Neill, I.K., von Borstel, R.C., Miller, C.T., Long, J. & Bartsch, H., eds, N-*Nitroso Compounds: Occurrence, Biological Effects and Relevance to Human Cancer (IARC Scientific Publications No. 57),* Lyon, International Agency for Research on Cancer, pp. 743–762

Hoffmann, D., Rivenson, A., Amin, S. & Hecht, S.S. (1984b) Dose-response study of the carcinogenicity of tobacco-specific *N*-nitrosamines in F344 rats. *J. Cancer Res. clin. Oncol.,* ***108,*** 81–86

IARC (1985) *IARC Monographs on the Evaluation of the Carcinogenic Risk of Chemicals to Humans,* Vol. 37, *Tobacco Habits Other than Smoking; Betel-Quid and Areca-Nut Chewing; and Some Related Nitrosamines,* Lyon

IARC (1986) *IARC Monographs on the Evaluation of Carcinogenic Risk of Chemicals to Humans,* Vol. 38, *Tobacco Smoking,* Lyon

International Committee for Cigar Smoke Study (1974) Machine smoking of cigars. *Coresta Inf. Bull.,* ***1,*** 31–34

Keith, C.H. & Tesh, P.G. (1965) Measurement of the total smoke issueing from a burning cigarette. *Tob. Sci.,* ***9,*** 61–64

Mohr, U. & Reznik, G. (1978) Tobacco carcinogenesis. *Lung Biol. Health Dis.,* ***10,*** 263–367.

National Research Council (1981) *The Health Effects of Nitrate, Nitrite and N-Nitroso Compounds,* Washington DC, National Academy Press, p. 529

Norman, V. (1977) An overview of the vapor phase, semivolatile and nonvolatile components of cigarette smoke. *Recent Adv. Tob. Sci.,* ***3,*** 28–58

Norman, V. (1982) Changes in smoke chemistry of modern day cigarettes. *Recent Adv. Tob. Sci.,* ***8,*** 141–177

Radford, E.P. & Hunt, V.R. (1964) Polonium-210, a volatile radioelement in cigarettes. *Science,* ***143,*** 247–249

Tobacco Institute (1984) *US Sales-weighted Average Tar and Nicotine Yield,* Washington, DC, p. 2

US National Cancer Institute (1980) *Towards a Less Hazardous Cigarette (Report No. 5),* Bethesda, MD, p. 29

Wynder, E.L. & Graham, E.A. (1950) Tobacco smoking as a possible etiologic factor in bronchiogenic carcinoma. A study of six hundred and eighty-four proved cases. *J. Am. med. Assoc.,* ***143,*** 329–336

Wynder, E.L. & Hoffmann, D. (1967) *Tobacco and Tobacco Smoke. Studies in Experimental Carcinogenesis,* New York, Academic Press, p. 730

Wynder, E.L. & Hoffmann, D. (1982) *Tobacco.* In: Schottenfeld, D. & Fraumeni, J. F., Jr, eds, *Cancer Epidemiology and Prevention,* Philadelphia, W.B. Saunders Co., pp, 277–292

THE COMBINED EFFECTS OF SMOKING AND OTHER AGENTS

F. BERRINO

Epidemiology Unit,
National Institute for the Study and Treatment of Tumours,
Milan, Italy

Humans are exposed to many different carcinogenic and anticarcinogenic stimuli during their lifespan. Some of these factors modify the effect of the exposure to others, and the knowledge of the pattern of combined action may be of help in planning preventive strategies.

Tobacco smoking is the most extensively studied of all carcinogenic exposures. It is related to tumours at many sites, including the respiratory, the upper digestive and the urinary tract. A considerable amount of information has also been produced on the combined effect of smoking and other factors, mainly radiation, diet and occupational exposures.

In most cases, the available epidemiological evidence suggests that the combined agents act synergistically according to a multiplicative model (i.e., the relative risk associated with the combined exposure, with reference to the category of no exposure, is the product of the relative risks of subjects with a single exposure).

Tables 1 to 3 illustrate the results of five studies in which the interaction pattern was typically multiplicative. They refer to the interaction of smoking with alcohol in producing oesophageal cancer, of smoking with occupational exposure to asbestos in producing lung cancer among anthophyllite miners and insulation workers, and of smoking with occupational and, respectively, environmental exposure to radon daughters (Lundin *et al.*, 1969; Tuyns *et al.*, 1977; Hammond *et al.*, 1979; Meurman *et al.*, 1979; Edling *et al.*, 1984).

Table 4 shows the combined effect of cigarettes and occupational exposure on bladder cancer; subjects were classified as (possibly) exposed to bladder carcinogens if their occupational history included one or more of the following areas or activities: chemical industry, dye production, production of tyres and other rubber goods, petrol refining, gas plants, typography, furnaces, leather, shoe repair, textiles (Vineis *et al.*, 1981).

Table 5 shows a similar analysis from two population-based, case-control studies on lung cancer; in the study untertaken in Saronno (Italy) (Pastorino *et al.*, 1984), the judgement on exposure to lung carcinogens was derived from a blind analysis of the occupational histories by a panel of experts; in the Los Angeles (USA) study (Pike *et al.*, 1979), all blue collar workers were considered as possibly exposed. It is clear that, in this kind of study, some misclassification of exposure may occur. Random misclassifications, however, while

Table 1. Relative risks of oesophageal cancer as a function of alcohol and tobacco consumption[a]

Tobacco consumption (g/day)	Alcohol consumption (g/day)		
	0–40	41–80	81+
20+	5.1	12.3	44.4
10–19	3.4	8.4	19.9
0–9	1.0	7.3	18.0

[a] From Tuyns *et al.* (1977)

Table 2. Relative risks of lung cancer for tobacco and asbestos exposure[a] and tobacco and anthophyllite exposure[b] in two cohort studies

	Insulation workers	Unexposed controls	Anthophyllite miners	Unexposed controls
Nonsmokers	5.2	1.0	1.6	1.0
Smokers	53.2	10.8	12	19

[a] From Hammond *et al.* (1979)
[b] From Meurman *et al.* (1979)

Table 3. Relative risks of lung cancer for tobacco and radiation exposure: a cohort study on US uranium miners[a] and a case-control study on radon in homes in Sweden[b]

	Uranium miners	Unexposed population	Radon level in home	
			>50+ Bq/m³	<50 Bq/m³
Nonsmokers	4.0	1.0	2.8	1.0
Smokers	40.0	10.3	17.3	6.8

[a] Data from Lundin *et al.* (1969)
[b] Modified from Edling *et al.* (1984)

Table 4. Relative risks of bladder cancer for tobacco and occupational exposure to bladder carcinogens[a]

Average daily cigarette consumption	Nonoccupationally exposed	Occupationally exposed
Nonsmokers	1.0	1.2
1–9	2.4	2.8
10–19	5.4	11.1
20+	6.6	11.2

[a] From Vineis *et al.* (1981)

Table 5. Relative risks of lung cancer for tobacco and occupational exposure in two population-based case control studies

	Saronno[a]		Los Angeles[b]	
	Exposed	Unexposed	Exposed	Unexposed
Nonsmokers	2.5	1.0	2.8	1.0
Smokers	15.8	7.6	14.2	5.3

[a] From Pastorino *et al.* (1984)
[b] From Pike *et al.* (1979)

Table 6. Relative risks of lung cancer for tobacco and occupational exposure to asbestos and polynuclear aromatic hydrocarbons (PAH) [a]

Exposure	Cigarettes per day		
	0–9	10–19	20+
Not exposed	1.0	4.0	6.3
PAH only	1.3	7.0	9.9
Asbestos only	2.8	6.8	12.0
PAH and asbestos	2.8	34.5	16.4

[a] From Pastorino *et al.* (1984)

reducing relative risk estimates, do not necessarily affect the possibility of studying the pattern of interaction.

Table 6 shows that in the Saronno study the multiplicative model seems to hold also when the two major occupational factors, asbestos and polynuclear aromatic hydrocarbons, are considered separately (Pastorino *et al.*, 1984).

The studies on tobacco and alcohol usually provide some dose-effect estimates; most published studies on occupational factors, on the contrary, lack adequate quantitative assessment of exposure, and the knowledge of the interaction pattern at different dose levels is largely incomplete. At extreme dose levels, only very small sample sizes are usually available, so that it may prove impossible to detect a significant difference from what would be expected under a multiplicative model. A further limitation of these studies is that, with few exceptions, only two carcinogens have been studied at a time (e.g., tobacco and alcohol, tobacco and radiation, tobacco and asbestos). Moreover, the dose-response curves of each of the two carcinogens acting alone are frequently based on small samples. Noncarcinogenic exposures may interact in different ways (synergistically or antagonistically) with different (combinations of) carcinogenic exposures. For instance, chronic exposure to noncarcinogenic fumes or dusts may increase the susceptibility of the lung to the effect of carcinogenic chemicals (e.g., by impairing the clearance of the bronchial tree); the same noncarcinogenic factors, on the other hand, through the same mechanism – tending to increase the thickness of the mucous sheath – might protect against the short-ranging alpha radiation. This might explain why, in some underground mining conditions, the combined effect of smoking and radon daughter exposure was multiplicative (Lundin *et al.*, 1969, Whittermore & McMillan, 1983), while in other conditions, for example, in Scandinavian mines (Axelson & Sundell, 1978), it was more consistent with an additive model.

Times of exposure and induction-latency periods have been considered only rarely. The apparent synergism between tobacco and radiation in uranium miners and in domestic exposure might be due to the promotional effect of tobacco smoke on the initiating radiation (Reif, 1984). In other studies, however, the combined effect seems more consistent with an additive than with a multiplicative pattern. It is the case with lung and oesophageal cancer among atomic bomb survivors (Prentice *et al.*, 1983). This might indicate that the promotional effect of tobacco is time-dependent. The timing of different exposures may be relevant also for the potential preventive effect of some dietary factors. It has been consistently shown, for instance, that a diet rich in foods containing β-carotene is associated with a nearly two-fold lower incidence of lung cancer. The protective effect seems to be higher among heavy smokers and recent data from our laboratory suggest that the protection is confined to current smokers, while the protection among nonsmokers or exsmokers, if any, is much less (Pisani *et al.*, 1986). To clarify the mechanisms of interaction, the protection conferred by stopping smoking should be studied in relation to the times of exposure to other agents.

Irrespective of the biological mechanisms, however, the synergism usually observed for multiple exposures underlines the danger inherent in the exposure to all of them.

REFERENCES

Axelson, O. & Sundell, L. (1978) Mining, lung cancer and smoking. *Scand. J. Work environ. Health,* ***6,*** 227–231

Edling, C., Kling, H. & Axelson, O. (1984) Radon in homes – A possible cause of lung cancer. *Scand. J. Work environ. Health,* ***10,*** 25–34

Hammond, E.C., Selikoff, I.J. & Seidman, H. (1979) Asbestos exposure, cigarette smoking and death rates. *Ann. N.Y. Acad. Sci.,* ***330,*** 473–490

Lundin, F.E., Lloyd, W.J., Smith, E.M., Archer, V.E. & Holaday, D.A. (1969) Mortality of uranium miners in relation to radiation exposure, hard-rock mining and cigarette smoking – 1950 through September 1967. *Health Phys.,* ***16,*** 571–579

Meurman, L.O., Kiviluoto, R. & Hakama, M. (1979) Combined effect of asbestos exposure and tobacco smoking on Finnish anthophyllite miners and millers. *Ann. N.Y. Acad. Sci.,* ***330,*** 491–495

Pastorino, U., Berrino, F., Gervasio, A., Pesenti, V., Riboli, E. & Crosignani, P. (1984) Proportion of lung cancers due to occupational exposure. *Int. J. Cancer,* ***33,*** 231–237

Pike, M.C., Jing, J.S., Rosario, I.P., Henderson, B.E. & Menck, H.R. (1979) *Occupation: 'Explanation' of an apparent air pollution related localized excess of lung cancer in Los Angeles County.* In: Breslow, N.E. & Whittermore, A.S., eds, *Energy and Health,* Philadelphia, SIAM, pp. 3–16

Pisani, P., Berrino, F., Macaluso, M., Crosignani, P. & Baldasseroni, A. (1986) Carrots, green vegetables and lung cancer: a case-control study. *Int. J. Epidemiol.* (in press)

Prentice, R.L., Yoshimoto, Y. & Mason, M.W. (1983) Relationship of cigarette smoking and radiation exposure to cancer mortality in Hiroshima and Nagasaki. *J. natl Cancer Inst.*, ***70***, 611–622

Reif, A.E. (1984) Synergism in carcinogenesis. *J. natl Cancer Inst.*, ***73***, 25–39

Tuyns, A.J., Pequignot, G. & Jensen, O.M. (1977) Cancer of the oesophagus in Ille-et-Vilaine as a function of alcohol and tobacco consumption levels. Multiplicative risks (Fr.). *Bull. Cancer*, ***64***, 45–60

Vineis, P., Segnan, N., Costa, G. & Terracini, B. (1981) Evidence of a multiplicative effect between cigarette smoking and occupational exposure in the aetiology of bladder cancer. *Cancer Lett.*, ***14***, 285–290

Whittermore, A.S. & McMillan, A. (1983) Lung cancer mortality among U.S. uranium miners: A reappraisal. *J. natl Cancer Inst.*, ***71***, 489–499

PASSIVE SMOKING AND LUNG CANCER

R. SARACCI

International Agency for Research on Cancer
Lyon, France

INTRODUCTION

The health effects of involuntary, or passive, exposure to environmental tobacco smoke (ETS) have been the object, during the last ten years, of a relatively small number of studies (forerunners of a larger number now in progress or in the planning stage) which, however, have substantially changed the perception of both scientists and laymen of the relevance of this issue. No doubt this perceived relevance stems from the combination of three elements: (a) the possible existence of health risks for people passively exposed to ETS; (b) the extent of the exposure: as, for example, the data from the US population in Table 1 indicate (Friedman *et al.*, 1983), people's self-assessed exposure is neither rare nor unappreciable; (c) the involuntary nature of the exposure. Indeed, opinions may vary on how best to deal with the hazardous (to the smoker) habit of smoking, given the mixture of personal 'free' choice and social conditioning in its inception and maintenance; but there is little variation, throughout the history of public health theory and practice, in the opinion that involuntary hazards ought to be tackled mostly by regulatory and legislative restrictions.

The position on the health effects of ETS about a decade ago can be illustrated by a quotation from the US Surgeon General's 1975 report *Health Consequences of Smoking* (US Surgeon General, 1976):

'1. Tobacco smoke can be a significant source of atmospheric pollution in enclosed areas. Occasionally, with heavy smoking and poor ventilation, the maximum limit for an 8 hour work exposure to carbon monoxide may be exceeded.

'2. Carbon monoxide may produce some deterioration in psychomotor performance. These effects produced by CO may become important when added to factors such as fatigue and alcohol when operating a motor vehicle.

'3. Unrestricted smoking on buses and planes is annoying to a majority of nonsmoking passengers even under conditions of adequate ventilation. To some people even slight exposure to smoke brings on eye and throat irritations.

'4. Children of parents who smoke are more likely to have bronchitis and pneumonia during the first year of life.

Table 1. Distribution of total hours per week of any reported passive smoking

Total hours per week	% (N = 34 861)
0	36.7
1–9	28.8
10–39	18.6
40+	15.9
Total	100.0

[a] From Friedman *et al.* (1983)

'5. Levels of carbon monoxide commonly found in smoke-filled environments have been shown to decrease the exercise tolerance of patients with angina pectoris.'

Notice that all the listed effects are acute, the most prominent being bronchitic episodes in infants, as shown in the work of Colley *et al.* (1974). That the respiratory function could be adversely affected in older children as well was suggested by other investigations, such as that of Weiss *et al.* (1978) in children aged 6–9 years old. It should be noted that some reported associations with other adverse health outcomes, for example, that of maternal smoking with low birth weight (Sidle, 1982) derive from exposure circumstances different from the one considered here, i.e., passive exposure to *environmental* tobacco smoke.

A *British Medical Journal* editorial (Anon., 1978) concisely summarized the evidence, in a vein not dissimilar to the US Surgeon General's report of 1975, stating: 'For the moment most – but not all – of the pressure for people (including many smokers) to have the right to breathe smoke-free air must be based on aesthetic considerations rather than on known serious risks to health.' For those to whom aesthetics is not a sufficient motive the picture started to change in the 1980s, although only partially, with two studies (White & Froeb, 1980; Kauffmann *et al.*, 1983), criticized for their methodology (Adlkofer *et al.*, 1980; Lebowitz, 1984), suggesting chronic effects on some lung function tests in adults; more substantially with the study by Hirayama (1981; 1983) reporting an excess of lung cancer in nonsmoking wives of smokers. Evidence subsequently accruing on this issue has been the subject of commentaries and reviews cumulatively outnumbering the actual studies supplying the evidence (Lehnert, 1981; Lee, 1982; Shepherd, 1982; US Surgeon General, 1982; Rylander *et al.*, 1983; Wynder & Goodman, 1983; Lehnert & Wynder, 1984). A recent review, by an IARC Working Group evaluating the whole spectrum of neoplastic responses to active and passive exposure to tobacco smoke, has been carried out within the IARC programme on the evaluation of the carcinogenic risk of chemicals to humans (IARC, 1986). In the following pages I will borrow freely from this review.

THE EPIDEMIOLOGICAL STUDIES

At the time of writing this paper, there were six main studies, each involving at least 30 cases of lung cancer in non-smokers, directly bearing on the relationship of lung cancer to

Table 2. Cohort studies on passive smoking and lung cancer: standardized mortality ratios

Reference	Cigarettes/day smoked by husband				
	None	Exsmoker	1–14	15–19	20+
Hirayama (1981, 1983)	1.00	1.36	1.42	1.58	1.98
Garfinkel (1981)	1.00	–	1.27 (1–14 and 15–19 combined)		1.10
			1.37 [a] (1–14 and 15–19 combined)		1.04 [a]

[a] Adjusted for age, race, education, residence and husband's occupation

ETS exposure. Two studies have involved the observation of large cohorts while the other four are case-control studies, the total number of lung cancer cases in nonsmokers in the six investigations being 738.

Cohort studies

The key results of the two cohort studies are summarized in Table 2. In the Japanese study by Hirayama (1981; 1983) 91 540 nonsmoking women were followed up from 1966 to 1981 and 200 lung cancers were recorded in married women whose husband's smoking habits were known (for another 103 cases the smoking habits were unknown). In the study by the American Cancer Society (Garfinkel, 1981) 176 739 married women (out of 375 000 nonsmoking women) were followed up from 1960 to 1972: 153 cases of lung cancer were observed, 88 of which were in women married to smokers. The relative risks shown in the second line of Table 2 are adjusted by matching on the basis of the wife's five-year age-group, husband's occupational exposure, highest educational level of husband and wife, race, urban-rural residence and absence of serious disease at the start of the study. The mortality ratios, taking those in women married to nonsmoking husbands as equal to 1, show an increasing trend (statistically significant, $p<0.02$) with amount smoked by the husband in the Japanese study; they are not significantly elevated above 1, nor do they show a trend, in the US study. However, looking at the figures in a different way, the ratios in the US study are not significantly different from those in the Japanese one, both being compatible with a slightly elevated relative risk (say 1.2) or, alternatively, with a relative risk of 1.

Case-control studies

The first case-control study was conducted on nonsmoking female residents in Athens, Greece, from September 1978 to 1982 (Trichopoulos *et al.*, 1981; 1983). A total of 77 cases of lung cancer were interviewed in a cancer hospital, and 225 nonsmoking female controls interviewed at a different (orthopaedic) hospital. Cases were histologically confirmed and bronchial alveolar carcinomas excluded. The case and control series were reported as showing very close distribution on age, duration of marriage, occupation, years of school-

Table 3. Smoking habits of husbands of nonsmoking women with lung cancer and of nonsmoking control women[a]

Group	Nonsmokers	Exsmokers	Cigarettes/day (current smokers)				
			1–10	11–20	21–30	31+	Total
Lung cancer	24	15	2	22	7	7	77
Controls	109	35	16	40	8	17	225
RR[b]	1.0	1.9	2.4		3.4		

[a] From Trichopoulos *et al.* (1981, 1983)
[b] Relative risk, ratio of risk of lung cancer among women whose husbands belong to a particular smoking category to that among women whose husbands are nonsmokers. χ^2 (linear trend) = 6.7; p (two-tail) about 0.01

Table 4. Nonsmoking, ever-married lung cancer cases and controls and lifetime consumption of cigarettes by their spouses[a]

	Cigarettes smoked by spouse (pack-years)		
	None	1–40	≥41
Males			
Cases	6	2	0
Controls	154	20	6
Odds ratio	1.0	2.0	
Females			
Cases	8	5	9
Controls	72	38	23
Odds ratio	1.0	1.18	3.52[b]
		2.07	
Both sexes			
Odds ratio (adjusted for sex)	1.0	1.48	2.11[b]

[a] From Correa *et al.* (1983)
[b] $p < 0.05$

ing and recent residence. The results are shown in Table 3: a statistically significant trend of increasing relative risk with husband's intensity of smoking is present.

The second case-control study was reported by Correa *et al.* (1983) and included 30 ever-married nonsmoking lung cancer patients and 313 patients and 313 controls, matched for hospital, race, sex, age (plus or minus five years). Exposure to passive smoking was calculated as total lifetime number of cigarettes (in pack-years = average number of packs smoked per day × number of days/365) smoked by the spouses at the time of the interview. Histological confirmation of the cases was obtained and bronchoalveolar carcinomas were excluded. Table 4 shows the results, indicating an increase in relative risk for subjects with smoking spouses (the increase is statistically significant, $p<0.05$, for females and for both sexes when the spouse's lifetime consumption was >41 pack-years).

Table 5. Exposure to passive inhalation among a subset of cases and controls[a]

	Men		Women	
	Cases	Controls	Cases	Controls
At home[b]				
Yes	6	5	16	17
No	19	20	37	36
Total	25	25	53	53
At work[c]				
Yes	18	11	26	31
No	7	14	27	22
Total	25	25[d]	53	53
Spouse smoker[e]				
Ever	5	5	13	15
Never	7	7	11	10
Total	12	12	24	25

[a] From Kabat and Wynder (1984)
[b] Current exposure on a regular basis to family members who smoke
[c] Current exposure on a regular basis to tobacco smoke at work
[d] $p < 0.045$
[e] Spouse's current or past smoking habits

Table 6. Relative risk (RR) of lung cancer among never-smokers by levels of passive exposure[a]

Category	No. of patients	No. of controls	RR	*p* value
None	22	40	1.00	
Low[b]	57	81	1.28	<0.44
High[c]	9	16	1.02	<0.96
Total passive	66	97	1.24	<0.49

[a] From Koo *et al.* (1984)
[b] <35 000 hours
[c] >35 000 hours

The third study was carried out by Kabat and Wynder (1984) who interviewed 25 male and 53 female case-control pairs (matched on hospital, sex, age, within plus or minus two years, race). Their results are shown in Table 5 and indicate no differences between cases and controls for various passive exposure criteria to ETS, except for exposure of males to ETS at work (relative risk 3.27, $p < 0.045$).

Finally, Table 6 presents some key results from a study carried out by Koo *et al.* (1984) in Hong Kong on 200 female lung cancer patients and 200 healthy district controls, matched by district, age (plus or minus five years) and socioeconomic status. No association of lung cancer among never-smokers with level of passive smoking seems to emerge.

INTERPRETING THE STUDIES

The results briefly outlined may be interpreted in the light of a number of considerations. First, questionnaire information on passive exposure to ETS appears to reflect, at least qualitatively, as indicated by data such as those of Matsukura *et al.* (1984), the exposure as measured by the presence in the urine of the main metabolite of nicotine, i.e., cotinine. The quantitative aspect, particularly when intra-laboratory and inter-laboratory variation in cotinine assay and differences in questionnaire design come into play, are less well defined; we are, in fact, carrying out at IARC an international exercise on this very point. Second, passive exposure to ETS implies exposure to components of the sidestream smoke which are of the same nature as those of the mainstream smoke (Table 7) (IARC, 1986): indeed, some components from the combustion process escape mostly in the sidestream smoke, though of course they also become diluted in the air environment rather than in the much smaller respiratory air spaces of the smoker where the mainstream smoke flows. Some estimations of equivalent exposures of active and passive smoking have been attempted, involving several assumptions. According to one estimate (Table 8) (Hugod *et al.*, 1978), if the equivalence is based on total particulate matter (which includes tar), 11 hours of 'severe' exposure to ETS is equivalent to active smoking of one cigarette. This would imply that exposure to ETS would roughly amount, in most circumstances, to smoking one cigarette (or less) per day, up to perhaps a maximum of two. Third, no dose-response relating average number of cigarettes smoked per day in regular smokers to lung

Table 7. Concentrations of selected compounds in nonfilter cigarette mainstream smoke (MS) and the ratio of their relative distribution in sidestream smoke (SS): MS [a]

Compound	MS	SS:MS
Vapour phase		
Carbon monoxide	10–23 mg	2.5–4.7
Carbon dioxide	20–60 mg	8–11
Carbonyl sulphide	18–42 μg	0.03–0.13
Benzene	12–48 μg	10
Toluene	160 μg	6–8
Formaldehyde	70–100 μg	0.1~50
Acrolein	60–100 μg	8–15
Acetone	100–250 μg	2–5
Pyridine	16–40 μg	7–20
3-Vinylpyridine	15–30 μg	20–40
Hydrogen cyanide	400–500 μg	0.1–0.25
Hydrazine	32 ng	3.0
Ammonia	50–150 μg	40–170
Methylamine	17.5–28.7 μg	4.2–6.4
Dimethylamine	7.8–10 μg	3.7–5.1
Nitrogen oxides	100–600 μg	4–10
N-Nitrosodimethylamine	10–40 μg	20–100
N-Nitrosopyrrolidine	6–30 μg	6–30
Formic acid	210–478 μg	1.4–1.6
Acetic acid	330–810 μg	1.9–3.9

Compound	MS	SS/MS
Particulate phase		
Particulate matter	15–40 mg	1.3–1.9
Nicotine	1.7–3.3 mg	1.8–3.3
Anatabine	2.4–20.1 μg	0.1–0.5
Phenol	60–140 μg	1.6–3.0
Catechol	100–360 μg	0.6–0.9
Hydroquinone	110–300 μg	0.7–0.9
Aniline	360 ng	30
ortho-Toluidine	160 ng	19
2-Naphthylamine	1.7 ng	30
4-Aminobiphenyl	4.6 ng	31
Benz[*a*]anthracene	20–70 ng	2.2–4
Benzo[*a*]pyrene	20–40 ng	2.5–3.5
Cholesterol	14.2 μg	0.9
γ-Butyrolactone	10–22 μg	3.6–5.0
Quinoline	0.5–2 μg	8–11
Harman	1.7–3.1 μg	0.7–1.9
N'-Nitrosonornicotine	200–3000 ng	0.5–3
4-(Methylnitrosamino)-1-(3-pyridyl)-1-butanone	100–1000 ng	1–4
N-Nitrosodiethanolamine	20–70 ng	1.2
Cadmium	100 ng	3.6–7.2
Nickel	20–80 ng	0.2–30
Zinc	60 ng	0.2–6.7
Polonium-210	0.03–0.5 pCi	1.06–3.7
Benzoic acid	14–28 μg	0.67–0.95
Lactic acid	63–174 μg	0.5–0.7
Glycolic acid	37–126 μg	0.6–0.95
Succinic acid	112–163 μg	0.43–0.62

[a] From IARC, 1986

cancer mortality rates offers an indication of departure from linearity at low dose (whatever the shape at higher doses), implying that even small doses contribute some excess risk in lung cancer (Doll & Peto, 1978; US Surgeon General, 1982). Considerations of this kind led the IARC Working Group to the following conclusion (IARC, 1986):

'The observations on nonsmokers that have been made so far are compatible with either an increased risk from "passive" smoking or an absence of risk. Knowledge of the nature of sidestream and mainstream smoke, of the materials absorbed during "passive" smoking, and of the quantitative relationships between dose and effect that are commonly observed from exposure to carcinogens leads to the conclusion that passive smoking gives rise to some risk of cancer.'

One may attempt to give an approximate numerical expression to 'some risk', remembering that, for example, the data from the British doctors' study can be fitted by a line: incidence per 10^5 man-years $= 9 + 9 \times$ cigarettes per day. Using this as a general relation (it cannot be, if nothing else because it is dependent on the age structure of the investigated population), the relative risk due to passive exposure to ETS would range from 3 to 1.5 on

Table 8. Comparison of uptake of smoke constituents in smokers and passive smokers[a]

Smoke constituent	Mainstream yield inhaled by smoker (mg/cigarette)	Inhaled amount in passive smoking conditions (mg/hour)[b]	Cigarette equivalents/hour	Cigarette equivalent time (hours)
Nitrogen oxides	0.30	0.182	0.61	1.6
Carbon monoxide	18.40	9.160	0.50	2.0
Aldehyde	0.81	0.214	0.26	3.8
Acrolein	0.09	0.013	0.14	7.1
Total particulate matter	25.30	2.300	0.09	11.1
Nicotine	2.10	0.041	0.02	50.0
Cyanide	0.25	0.005	0.02	50.0

[a] Data from Hugod *et al.* (1978)

[b] Volunteers were exposed in a closed, unventilated room to quite severe passive smoke conditions in which the air carbon monoxide concentration was kept at 20 ppm over a 3-hour period

the already discussed assumption that passive exposure may be equivalent to active smoking of two to one or less (say 0.5) cigarettes per day. Relative risks at this low end of the range (1.5) may prove difficult to detect as statistically significant and cannot be validly estimated in their size unless: (a) large numbers of subjects are observed; *and* (b) major sources of bias do not operate. A critical bias in the specific context of passive smoking studies stems from the possibility that some self-reported nonsmokers are in fact smokers. If this rate of false reporting (whatever the reason) is negatively associated with the spouse's smoking habits, for example, if wives of smokers tend to report faithfully their own habits, while some wives of nonsmokers hide their smoking habit, an *under estimation* of the true relative risk associated with exposure to the husband's smoke will ensue, and may even make an increase in relative risk undetectable. On the other hand, if this rate of false reporting is positively associated with the spouse's smoking habits, i.e., wives of smokers, but not wives of nonsmokers, include a number of women who smoke but do not report it, an *over estimation* of any true relative risk would ensue.

No systematic attempt to control for this type of bias has been made in the studies hitherto published. To control for it or, failing this, to obtain some estimates of its actual direction and size within a given study, appears necessary, worth trying, but not easy.

Given these open problems, three points can be made by way of conclusion:

(a) the published studies, when considered by themselves, are compatible either with absence of excess risk of lung cancer due to passive exposure to ETS or with the presence of a 'small' excess risk;

(b) in the light of the other available evidence, external to the studies, the interpretation favourable to the presence of a risk becomes definitely more plausible than the alternative;

(c) under these circumstances further epidemiological studies aiming at a direct estimate of the risk may be justified provided steps are taken to overcome, in the study design and conduct, the play of biases, some of which have been alluded to. Unless this is done, the studies stand a good chance of contributing results of a confusing rather than of a clarifying nature.

REFERENCES

Adlkofer, F., Scherer, G. & Weissman, H. (1980) Small-airways dysfunction in passive smokers (letter). *New Engl. J. Med.*, ***302***, 392

Anon. (1978) Breathing other people's smoke (Editorial). *Br. med. J.*, ***ii***, 453

Colley, J.R.T., Holland, W.W. & Corkhill, R.T. (1974) Influence of passive smoking and parental phlegm on pneumonia and bronchitis in early childhood. *Lancet*, ***ii***, 1031–1034

Correa, P., Pickle, L.W., Fontham, E., Lin, Y. & Haenszel, W. (1983) Passive smoking and lung cancer. *Lancet*, ***ii***, 595–597

Doll, R. & Peto, R. (1978) Cigarette smoking and bronchial carcinoma: dose and time relationships among regular smokers and lifelong nonsmokers. *J. Epidemiol. Community Health*, ***32***, 303–313

Friedman, G.D., Petitti, D. & Bawol, R.D. (1983) Prevalence and correlates of passive smoking. *Am J. publ. Health*, ***73***, 401–405

Garfinkel, L. (1981) Time trends in lung cancer mortality among nonsmokers and a note on passive smoking. *J. natl Cancer Inst.*, ***66***, 1061–1066

Hirayama, T. (1981) Non-smoking wives of heavy smokers have a higher risk of lung cancer: a study in Japan. *Br. med. J.*, ***282***, 183–185

Hirayama, T. (1983) Passive smoking and lung cancer: consistency of association. *Lancet*, ***ii***, 1425–1426

Hugod, C., Hawkins, L.H. & Astrup, P. (1978) Exposure of passive smokers to tobacco smoke constituents. *Int. Arch. occup. environ. Health*, ***42***, 21

IARC (1986) *IARC Monographs on the Carcinogenic Risk of Chemicals to Humans*, Vol. 38, *Tobacco Smoking*, Lyon

Kabat, G.C. & Wynder, E.L. (1984) Lung cancer in nonsmokers. *Cancer*, ***53***, 1214–1221

Kauffmann, F., Tessier, J.F. & Oriol, W. (1983) Adult passive smoking in the home environment: a risk factor for chronic airflow limitation. *Am. J. Epidemiol.*, ***117***, 269–280

Koo, L.C., Ho, J.H.C. & Saw, D. (1984) Is passive smoking an added risk factor for lung cancer in Chinese women? *J. exp. clin. Cancer Res.*, ***3***, 277–284

Lebowitz, M.D. (1984) Influence of passive smoking on pulmonary function: a survey. *Prev. Med.*, ***13***, 645–655

Lee, P.N. (1982) Passive smoking. *Food Chem. Toxicol.*, ***20***, 223–229

Lehnert, G. (1981) Ill as a result of passive smoking? (Ger.). *Münchner med. Wochenschr.*, ***123***, 1485–1488

Lehnert, G. & Wynder, E.L., eds (1984) Symposium: Medical perspectives on passive smoking. *Prev. Med.*, ***13***, 557–746

Matsukura, S., Taminato, T., Kitano, N., Seino, Y., Hamada, H., Uchibashi, M., Nakajima, H. & Hirata, Y. (1984) Effect of environmental tobacco smoke on urinary cotinine excretion in nonsmokers – Evidence for passive smoking. *New Engl. J. Med.*, ***311***, 828–832

Rylander, R., Peterson, Y. & Snella, M.C. (1983) *ETS – Environmental Tobacco Smoke, Report from a Workshop on Effects and Exposure Levels*, University of Geneva

Shepherd, R.J. (1982) *The Risks of Passive Smoking*, London, Croom Helm, pp. 95–98

Sidle, N. (1982) *Smoking in Pregnancy – a Review*, London, Hero Unit, The Spastics Society

Trichopoulos, D., Kalandidi, A., Sparros, L. & MacMahon, B. (1981) Lung cancer and passive smoking. *Int. J. Cancer,* ***27,*** 1–4

Trichopoulos, D., Kalandidi, A. & Sparros, L. (1983) Lung cancer and passive smoking: conclusion of Greek study. *Lancet,* ***ii,*** 677–678

US Surgeon General (1976) *The Health Consequences of Smoking: A Reference Edition,* Washington DC, US Department of Health, Education and Welfare, US Government Printing Office

US Surgeon General (1982) *The Health Consequences of Smoking: Cancer,* Washington DC, US Department of Health and Human Services, US Government Printing Office, pp. 239–251

Weiss, S.T., Tager, I.B., Speizer, F.E. & Rosner, B. (1978) Persistent wheeze – Its relation to respiratory illness, cigarette smoking, and level of pulmonary function in a population sample in children. *Am. Rev. respir. Dis.,* ***18,*** 649–652

White, J.R. & Froeb, H.F. (1980) Small airways dysfunction in nonsmokers chronically exposed to tobacco smoke. *New Engl. J. Med.,* ***302,*** 720–723

Wynder, E.L. & Goodman, M.T. (1983) Smoking and lung cancer: some unresolved issues. *Epidemiol. Rev.,* ***5,*** 177–207

A SIMPLE, INEXPENSIVE URINE TEST OF SMOKING[1]

H. PEACH[2] & R.W. MORRIS

Department of Community Medicine,
United Medical and Dental Schools, St Thomas' Campus
London SE1 7EH, UK

G.A. ELLARD & P.J. JENNER

National Institute for Medical Research,
Mill Hill, London NW7 1AA, UK

SUMMARY

Three novel colorimetric methods of detecting urinary nicotine metabolites called the barbituric acid, diethylthiobarbituric acid (DETB) and DETB-extraction methods were evaluated for use as a simple cheap objective test of smoking. Urine samples were collected from 103 male smokers and 78 male nonsmokers working at two London factories. The smokers recorded the number of cigarettes smoked over the previous 36 hours. All three methods correctly classified the smokers. The DETB-extraction method had a lower false-positive rate (averaging 3% on morning and afternoon urine samples) than either the DETB or barbituric acid methods (12% and 6% respectively) and was the best procedure for classifying subjects as 'smokers' or 'non-smokers'. Using a quantitative variant of the barbituric acid method, there was a significant correlation (r = 0.85, $p<0.001$) between the urinary nicotine metabolites/creatinine ratios and number of cigarettes smoked. However, the ratios for smokers of 6–15, 16–25, and 26 or more cigarettes overlapped considerably. The methods can be performed very rapidly and reagent costs are equivalent to less than one penny per test.

---

[1] A version of this paper appeared in *Thorax, 40* (5) in May 1985; this version is included with the permission of the journal editor.

[2] To whom editorial correspondence should be addressed.

INTRODUCTION

Self-reports of smoking behaviour need to be supplemented by an objective test of smoking. Large discrepancies have been found between self-reported smoking status and objective tests of smoking (Ohlin *et al.*, 1976; Sillett *et al.*, 1978; Wilcox *et al.*, 1979; Gillies *et al.*, 1982). Although some nonsmokers may have detectable levels of urinary nicotine due to passive smoking (Feyerabend *et al.*, 1982), the discrepancy has been largely attributed to deception on the part of smokers (Ohlin *et al.*, 1976; Sillett *et al.*, 1978; Wilcox *et al.*, 1979).

Measurements of expired carbon monoxide, carboxyhaemoglobin or thiocyanate in the blood, or nicotine in urine or saliva have been used to validate self-reported smoking habits. However, none of these tests is really satisfactory for routine use by physicians, for example in antismoking clinics. Even the measurement of expired carbon monoxide, which is the most acceptable to subjects, still requires the training and supervision of fieldworkers in using expensive equipment. Measurement of urinary and salivary cotinine avoids the need for venepuncture but the present method of assay involving gas chromatography is expensive (about £4.00 per test), time consuming and subject to inter-technician variability. Analysis by radioimmunoassay does not confer any benefits in terms of the need for expensive equipment, cost (about £8.00 per test) and technician variability. A simpler, less expensive test of smoking would seem desirable.

In the past modifications of the König reaction have been used to measure urinary concentrations of isonicotinic acid and isonicotinylglycine, major metabolites of the anti-tuberculosis drug, isoniazid (Ellard *et al.*, 1972). Their sensitivity was such that they enabled a simple colorimetric urine test to be devised which was capable of detecting the ingestion of minute doses of isoniazid, thereby enabling it to be used as a marker to monitor patient compliance (Ellard & Greenfield, 1977; Ellard *et al.*, 1980; Stanley *et al.*, 1983). Urine samples from nonsmokers containing isonicotinic acid gave a characteristic blue colour when tested by the procedure. However, it was noticed that urine samples of smokers not taking isoniazid gave distinctive orange colours and it was thought that nicotine and its metabolites were being detected (Bowman *et al.*, 1959; Stanley *et al.*, 1983). Preliminary studies showed that if diethylthiobarbituric acid were used in place of barbituric acid as the condensing agent in the König reaction, a red product was obtained which was readily extractable into ethyl acetate. These observations formed the basis of three potential simple urine tests to monitor nicotine intake.

The main purpose of this study was to establish the false-positive and false-negative rates of the urine tests in identifying smokers and nonsmokers so that they could be compared with the rates which have been published for the other methods. The inter-observer variability as well as the variability of the test on duplicate urine samples was also determined.

METHOD

Subjects

Volunteers were recruited from men working in two London factories (Philips Electronics and Tate and Lyle Refineries Ltd) and included 78 nonsmokers and 103 regular smokers of manufactured and hand-rolled cigarettes. Pipe and cigar smokers were not enrolled.

Recording of smoking habits and collection of urine samples

At the start of a working day, the volunteers were each provided with two bottles for collecting urine and three randomly numbered tubes containing thymol, one also marked 'AM' and two 'PM'. The men were asked how many cigarettes they had already smoked that day, the brand of cigarette or tobacco used, and to keep a record of every cigarette smoked over the next 36 hours, since cotinine, a major metabolite of nicotine, has a half-life of about 20 hours (Benowitz *et al.*, 1983). As a check on the accuracy of recording, smokers of manufactured cigarettes were also asked to count the number of cigarettes in their packets at the start and end of each day, noting the number of new packets opened. All volunteers were asked whether they worked or lived with someone who smoked. The following day (24 hours after being given the bottles and tubes), the men were asked to provide one 5-ml specimen of urine first thing in the morning and two 5-ml specimens at a single voiding in the middle of the afternoon. The random numbering of the tubes and the removal of AM and PM labels before delivery to the laboratory ensured that the tests were carried out blind. The creatinine concentrations of the two afternoon samples should have been identical and distinct from that of the morning sample and this was checked to ensure that the subjects had not mixed up the tubes when collecting the morning and afternoon specimens. Samples were preserved with a crystal of thymol and frozen at –20° C prior to analysis. However, an investigation carried out on a random sample of the smokers' urines showed that they could be stored for at least a week at room temperature without significant decomposition of either nicotine metabolites or creatinine.

To provide additional evidence concerning the ability of the methods to detect low concentrations of nicotine metabolites, such as cotinine, 0.05-ml aliquots of aqueous cotinine with concentrations of 0, 1, 2, 4, 8 and 16 μg/ml respectively were added to 0.45-ml portions of each of the 24 afternoon urine samples from the nonexposed nonsmokers. The samples were coded and randomized before being tested by the three methods, and the results were read by the two observers.

Laboratory methods

The urine specimens were tested for the presence of nicotine metabolites by the three alternative qualitative procedures described below and classified by two observers (Ellard and Jenner) with the naked eye. Where it was very difficult to make a decision, the samples were classified as probably positive or probably negative, otherwise they were reported as definitely positive or definitely negative. No reference was made to any sort of comparison chart. The second observer had had no experience of using any of the methods before the study, while the first observer had only had some experience of the direct barbituric acid method prior to the investigation. Thorough mixing after each of the reagent or solvent additions was achieved by agitation on a vortex mixer for about three seconds.

Qualitative detection of nicotine metabolites: direct barbituric acid method. Aliquots (0.5 ml) of urine samples were pipetted into small test-tubes together with a 4 mol/l pH 4.7 acetate buffer (0.2 ml) and reacted by the sequential addition at 15-sec intervals of freshly prepared 10% aqueous potassium cyanide (0.1 ml), 10% aqueous chloramine-T (0.1 ml), and 1% barbituric acid in acetone/water (1:1 v/v) (0.5 ml). A positive result was indicated by the appearance of an orange colour within 20 minutes.

Qualitative detection of nicotine metabolites: direct diethylthiobarbituric acid (DETB) method. As above but employing 1,3-diethyl-2-thiobarbituric acid and noting the presence or absence of a pink/red colour at 20 minutes.

Qualitative detection of nicotine metabolites: diethylthiobarbituric acid-(DETB) extraction method. As above but extracting the reaction product into 0.5 ml ethyl acetate.

Quantitative determination of nicotine metabolites: barbituric acid method. After all the factory specimens had been read by both observers with the naked eye as positive or negative for the presence of nicotine metabolites and the results recorded, urinary concentrations of nicotine metabolites were determined quantitatively. The optical densities of the specimens tested by the barbituric acid method were measured at 506 nm 20 minutes after reaction and compared with the reading given by an aqueous solution of 10 μg/ml cotinine. Standard curves relating the optical density of the reaction product and cotinine concentration in aqueous solution and nonsmoker's urine were prepared. Statistical evaluations showed that both curves were linear and parallel to each other. From the errors, it was shown that the cotinine concentration could be predicted from the optical density with a residual standard deviation of only 0.08 μg/ml. A cotinine standard was used since, when the pH of the urine is uncontrolled, as in this study, urinary concentrations of cotinine exceed those of nicotine (Langone *et al.*, 1973).

Quantitative determination of nicotine metabolites: DETB-extraction method. The DETB-extraction method was carried out using double volumes and after 20 minutes the reaction product was extracted into 2 ml ethyl acetate. After centrifugation, 1.5 ml of the ethyl acetate extract was pipetted into a small test-tube, 0.2 ml ethanol was added and the mixture was shaken. The optical density was then measured at 532 nm and nicotine metabolite concentrations calculated by reference to the results obtained with an aqueous 10 μg/ml cotinine standard.

Determination of creatinine. In order to allow for the effects of diuresis (Langone *et al.*, 1973), nicotine metabolites/creatinine ratios (μg apparent cotinine/mg creatinine) were calculated after measuring creatinine concentrations by a modification of the alkaline picrate method (Ellard *et al.*, 1974).

Statistical methods

The recordings of the two observers on the morning and first afternoon samples were used to calculate inter-observer variability. The duplicate afternoon samples, read by each observer, were used to assess inter-test variability. The percentage agreement between two observers reading a series of nonidentical specimens or one observer reading a series of duplicate specimens as 'positive' or 'negative' can be high even when there is no real association between the readings. Therefore, it was necessary to calculate Kappa statistics, which allow for this phenomenon, where values of Kappa increasing from zero to one indicate how much greater the agreement was than could be attributed to chance (Fleiss, 1981). The false-positive and false-negative rates of the three qualitative methods read by each observer in identifying smokers and nonsmokers were calculated separately from the results obtained (a) on the morning samples, and (b) on the afternoon samples.

RESULTS

Qualitative results

Table 1 shows the inter-observer variability of the three colorimetric methods in identifying smokers and nonsmokers. The inter-test variability as read by one observer is also shown. The inter-test variability was similar for the second observer. Although inter-observer and inter-test variability was low for all three methods, the inter-test agreement was highest for the DETB-extraction method.

Table 2 shows the false-negative and false-positive rates of the three methods in identifying smokers and nonsmokers as read by one observer. For simplicity, probable negatives have been included with the definite negatives and probable positives with the definite positives. All the urine samples from the smokers were found to be definitely positive by each of the three methods by both observers. Significant false-positive rates were encountered but these were much lower for the DETB-extraction method (morning and afternoon rates averaging 3%) than for the direct barbituric acid and DETB procedures (morning and afternoon rates averaging 6% and 12%, respectively). Similar results were obtained by the second observer and the same specimens were nearly always misclassified by both observers. It was concluded that the DETB-extraction method was the most satisfactory procedure for classifying subjects as 'smokers' or 'nonsmokers'.

After the qualitative tests had been completed and the results recorded, the false-positive readings encountered among the nonsmokers by each of the three methods were analysed according to their estimated excretion of nicotine metabolites and reported

Table 1. Inter-observer and inter-test variability of the colorimetric methods in determining smoking status

Type of variability	Percentage reading in agreement (Kappa statistics ± s.e.) [a]			No.
	Barbituric acid method	DETB method	DETB-extraction method	
Inter-observer				
AM samples	98 (0.95±0.02)	97 (0.93±0.03)	98 (0.97±0.02)	181
PM samples	99 (0.99±0.01)	97 (0.94±0.03)	100 (1.00±0.00)	179 [b]
Inter-test				
PM samples	94 (0.87±0.04)	93 (0.85±0.04)	99 (0.98±0.02)	174 [c]

[a] See text for explanation of Kappa statistics
[b] Two specimens missing or broken
[c] Seven specimens missing or broken

Table 2. False-positive and false-negative rates of the three colorimetric methods for determining smoking status

Method	Morning sample		Afternoon sample	
	False-negatives	False-positives	False-negatives	False-positives
Barbituric acid	0%	4 (4%)	0%	10 (9%)
DETB	0%	11 (10%)	0%	16 (14%)
DETB extraction	0%	5 (5%)	0%	1 (1%)
True positives	103		102	
True negatives	78		77	
Total	181		179 [a]	

[a] Two specimens missing or broken

Table 3. Sensitivity study: number of positive observations

Method	Final cotinine concentration (μg/ml)						No. of subjects
	0	0.1	0.2	0.4	0.8	1.6	
Barbituric acid	1	0	1	9	18	24	24
DETB	3	3	6	14	24	24	24
DETB extraction	1	8	20	24	24	24	24

smoking exposures. The nicotine metabolites/creatinine ratios of all but one of the non-smokers were very similar and averaged (with standard deviations) 0.7 (0.2) and 0.9 (0.2) for morning and afternoon specimens respectively. The exception was a subject with ratios of 2.0 and 2.7 respectively who was exposed at home and at work. For this subject, definitely positive results were obtained by each of the three qualititative methods. For the remaining 77 subjects, about half of the false-positives by the direct barbituric acid and DETB methods were classified as definitely positive whereas all the false-positives by the DETB-extraction procedure were reported as only probably positive. Among these 77 nonsmoking subjects, there was no relationship between positivity and reported exposures to smoking at home and/or work. Most of the false-positives occurred among highly coloured urine samples with elevated creatinine concentrations.

The results obtained by one observer in the additional sensitivity study are summarized in Table 3. Similar results were obtained for the second observer. The findings suggest that a 50% positivity could be obtained with concentrations of about 0.45, 0.35 and 0.15 μg/ml cotinine for the barbituric acid, DETB, and DETB-extraction methods respectively. This indicates that the extraction procedure is considerably more sensitive than the direct barbituric acid method for detecting nicotine metabolites in the urine.

Quantitative results

Figure 1 shows that using the direct barbituric acid method there was a strong correlation ($r = 0.85$), significantly different from zero ($p<0.001$), between the nicotine metabolites/creatinine ratios of the morning samples of urine on the second day and the number of cigarettes smoked on the first day. The correlation remained significant ($r = 0.48$; $p<0.001$) after excluding the nonsmokers. Despite this, there was considerable overlap between the ranges of the nicotine metabolites/creatinine ratios of smokers of 6–15, 16–25 and 26 or more cigarettes. Figure 2 shows the range of the nicotine metabolites/creatinine ratios of the morning samples of urine for men grouped according to the number of cigarettes smoked on the previous day. Similar results were found using nicotine metabolites/creatinine ratios of the afternoon samples of urine on the second day and the number of cigarettes smoked on that day, as well as the total smoked over the first and second days. Investigations carried out on the afternoon samples showed that the quantitative variant of the DETB-extraction procedure did not give a significantly better discrimination between the nicotine metabolites/creatinine ratios of samples from smokers and nonsmokers than the simpler direct barbituric acid method.

Fig. 1. Relationship between nicotine metabolites/creatinine ratios of 181 morning urine samples on the second day and number of cigarettes smoked on the first day

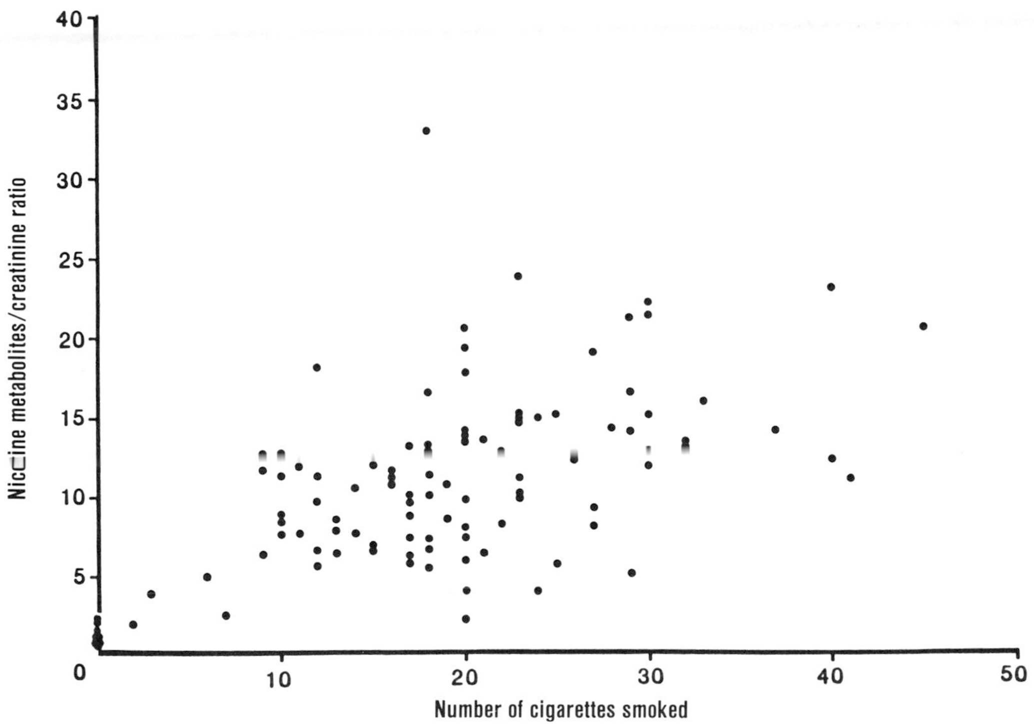

Fig. 2. Nicotine metabolites/creatinine ratios of 181 morning urine samples for men smoking different numbers of cigarettes over the previous day

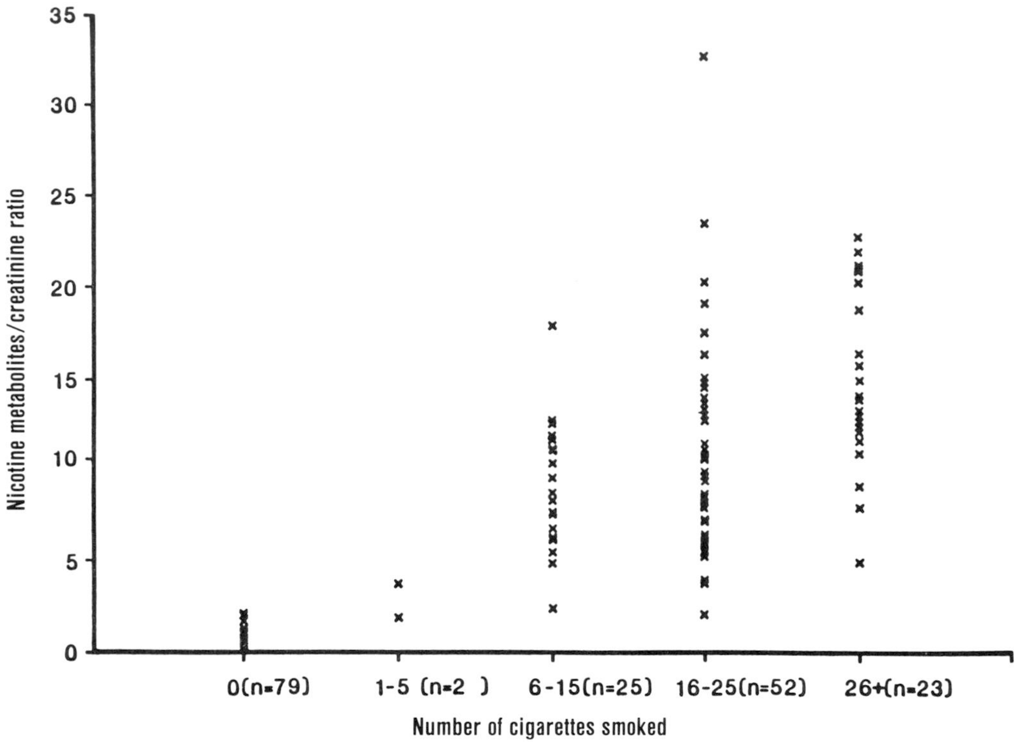

DISCUSSION

The reluctance of some people to admit to being smokers could create difficulties when trying to validate a new objective test of smoking. However, the greatest discrepancies between self-reported smoking status and objective tests of smoking have been reported among respondents from antismoking clinics (Ohlin *et al.*, 1976) and patients given anti-smoking advice (Sillett *et al.*, 1978; Wilcox *et al.*, 1979), where deception would be expected to be a problem. A factory rather than a hospital population was chosen to evaluate the colorimetric urine test in order to reduce deception on the part of respondents. Prior knowledge that a test of smoking is to be carried out sometimes increases self-reporting of smoking (Evans *et al.*, 1977; Bauman & Dent, 1982), and respondents in this study were sent a letter explaining fully the purpose of the work. The men also kept a record of cigarettes smoked over the two days of the study in order to eliminate recall errors.

Using the DETB-extraction method only four of the 78 nonsmokers in our study were misclassified. False-negative and false-positive rates for the DETB-extraction method in identifying smokers and nonsmokers of 0% and 3% respectively compared very favourably with the results of other tests published in the literature. Thus false-negative rates of 12–34% have been found using expired carbon monoxide, 5–17% with blood carboxyhaemoglobin, 7–36% with serum/plasma thiocyanate, 5% for plasma cotinine and 28% using a combination of serum thiocyanate and expired carbon monoxide (Ohlin *et al.*, 1976; Vogt *et al.*, 1977; Sillett *et al.*, 1978; Williams *et al.*, 1979; Cohen & Bartsch, 1980; Petitti *et al.*, 1981; Vesey *et al.*, 1982; Kornitzer *et al.*, 1983). The corresponding proportions of false-positives in these studies were 1–5%, 0–19%, 0–19%, 2% and 1% respectively.

It might be argued that considerable experience would be required to use this subjective qualitative procedure efficiently. However, the second observer, who was new to the procedures, performed as well as the other, more experienced, observer. Furthermore, the proportion of false-positives recorded among the first half of the samples analysed by the DETB-extraction method was no higher than among the remainder for either observer. It may therefore be concluded that the DETB-extraction test is robust and likely to perform as well in the hands of other observers reading small numbers of specimens for the first time.

It was hoped that a colorimetric estimation of the urinary concentration of nicotine metabolites might provide a useful measure of nicotine inhalation, and the possibility was envisaged that this might be directly related to the number of cigarettes smoked. Although there was a significant overall correlation between the urinary nicotine metabolites/creatinine ratios and number of cigarettes smoked (Fig. 1), the ratios for volunteers smoking 6–15, 16–25, and 26 or more cigarettes overlapped considerably. However, such estimates of nicotine intake correlated as closely with numbers of cigarettes smoked as other previously measured parameters. Thus correlations of 0.4–0.5 have been found between serum thiocyanate (Vogt *et al.*, 1977; Vesey *et al.*, 1982; Kornitzer *et al.*, 1983), carboxyhaemoglobin (Vesey *et al.*, 1982), expired carbon monoxide (Vogt *et al.*, 1977) and urinary nicotine (Feyerabend *et al.*, 1982) respectively and numbers of cigarettes smoked. In these studies, the levels in light smokers and nonsmokers also overlapped considerably, as did those in moderate and heavy smokers (Vogt *et al.*, 1977; Feyerabend *et al.*, 1982; Vesey *et al.*, 1982). It is now accepted that the intake of nicotine, cyanide or carbon monoxide depends not only on the number of cigarettes smoked but also on the puffing and inhaling patterns. As a consequence, the number of cigarettes smoked accounts for only about 25% of the variance in urinary nicotine, expired carbon monoxide and serum thiocyanate (Vogt *et al.*, 1979; Vesey *et al.*, 1982).

If self-reports of smoking need to be supplemented by an objective test of smoking it would be useful if such a test avoided venepuncture, did not require fieldworkers to be trained to use expensive equipment, could be applied to a large number of samples in a reasonable time, and was inexpensive. The DETB-extraction procedure meets these criteria. It requires only urine samples, is simple to perform, takes less than one minute per test on average to carry out, and reagent costs are less than one penny per specimen. Furthermore, the quantitative barbituric acid ratio method for estimating nicotine intake is also cheap and rapid to perform (about three minutes per sample) and both methods only require equipment which should be available in any biochemistry laboratory.

ACKNOWLEDGEMENTS

We would like to thank Professor Holland for encouraging us to do the study, Miss D. Shah for assistance with computing and Mr D.R. Ellard for help with the chemical analyses. We are indebted to Dr Terry and Sister Saku of Philips Electronics and Dr Biss and Sister Wilkinson of Tate and Lyle Thameside Refineries for their invaluable help in setting up the study. We thank Mrs L. Clarke for word processing the manuscript and Ms V. Norcott Martin, Department of Medical Illustration, Rayne Institute, St. Thomas's Hospital, for drawing the figures. The study was undertaken in connection with research being funded by the Tobacco Products Research Trust.

REFERENCES

Bauman, K.E. & Dent, C.W. (1982) Influence of an objective measure on self-reports of behaviour. *J. appl. Psychol.*, ***67***, 623–628

Benowitz, M.L., Kuyt, F., Jacob, P., Jones, R.T. & Osman, A. (1983) Cotinine disposition and effects. *Clin. Pharmacol. Therap.*, ***34***, 604–611

Bowman, E.R., Turnbull, L.B. & McKennis, H. (1959) Metabolism of nicotine in the human and excretion of pyridine compounds by smokers. *J. Pharmacol. exp. Therap.*, ***127***, 92–95

Cohen, J.D. & Bartsh, G.E. (1980) A comparison between carboxyhaemoglobin and serum thiocyanate determinations as indicators of cigarette smoking. *Am. J. Public Health*, ***70***, 284–286

Ellard, G.A. & Greenfield, C. (1977) A sensitive urine-test method for monitoring the ingestion of isoniazid. *J. clin. Pathol.*, ***30***, 84–87

Ellard, G.A., Gammon, P.T. & Wallace, S.M. (1972) The determination of isoniazid and its metabolites acetylisoniazid, monoacetyl hydrazine, diacetylhydrazine, isonicotinic acid and isonicotinylglycine in serum and urine. *Biochem. J.*, ***126***, 449–458

Ellard, G.A., Gammon, P.T., Helmy, H.B. & Rees, R.J.W. (1974) Urine test to monitor the self-administration of dapsone by leprosy patients. *Am. J. trop. Med. Hyg.*, ***23***, 404–407

Ellard, G.A., Jenner, P.J. & Downs, P.A. (1980) An evaluation of the potential use of isoniazid, acetylisoniazid and isonicotinic acid for monitoring the self-administration of drugs. *Br. J. clin. Pharmacol.*, ***10***, 369–381

Evans, R.I., Hansen, W.B. & Mittelmark, M.B. (1977) Increasing the validity of self reports of smoking behavior in children. *J. appl. Psychol.*, ***62***, 521–523

Feyerabend, C., Higenbottam, T. & Russell, M.A.H. (1982) Nicotine concentrations in urine and saliva of smokers and non-smokers. *Br. med. J.*, ***284***, 1002–1004

Fleiss, J.L. (1981) *Statistical Methods for Rates and Proportions*, 2nd ed., New York, Wiley, pp. 217–221

Gillies, P.A., Wilcox, B., Coates, C., Kristmundsdottir, F. & Reid, D.J. (1982) Use of objective measurement in the validation of self reported smoking in children aged 10–11 years: saliva thiocyanate. *J. Epidemiol. Community Health*, ***36***, 205–208

Kornitzer, M., Vanhemeldonck, A., Bourdoux, P. & Backer, G.D. (1983) Belgian heart disease prevention project: comparison of self-reported smoking behaviour with serum thiocyanate concentrations. *J. Epidemiol. Community Health,* ***37,*** 132–136

Langone, J.J., Gjika, H.B., van Vunakis, H. (1973) Nicotine and its metabolites. Radioimmunoassays for nicotine and cotinine. *Biochemistry,* ***12,*** 5025–5030

Ohlin, P., Lundh, B. & Westling, H. (1976) Carbon monoxide levels and reported cessation of smoking. *Psychopharmacology,* ***49,*** 263–265

Petitti, D.B., Friedman, G.D. & Kahn, W. (1981) Accuracy of information on smoking habits on self-administered research questionnaires. *Am. J. Public Health,* ***71,*** 308–311

Sillett, R.W., Wilson, M.B., Malcolm, R.E. & Ball, K.P. (1978) Deception among smokers. *Br. med. J.,* ***ii,*** 1185–1186

Stanley, J.N.A., Pearson, J.M.H. & Ellard, G.A. (1983) An investigation of dapsone compliance using an isoniazid-marked formulation. *Lepr. Rev.,* ***54,*** 317–325

Vesey, C.J., Saloojee, Y., Cole, P.V. & Russell, M.A.H. (1982) Blood carboxyhaemoglobin, plasma thiocyanate, and cigarette consumption implications for epidemiological studies in smokers. *Br. med. J.,* ***284,*** 1516–1518

Vogt, T.M., Selvin, S., Widdowson, S. & Hulley, S.B. (1977) Expired air carbon monoxide and serum thiocyanate and objective measures of cigarette exposure. *Am. J. Public Health,* ***67,*** 545–549

Vogt, T.M., Selvin, S. & Hulley, S.B. (1979) Comparison of biochemical and questionnaire estimates of tobacco exposure. *Prev. Med.,* ***8,*** 23–33

Wilcox, R.G., Hughes, J. & Roland, J. (1979) Verification of smoking history on patients after infarction using urinary nicotine and cotinine measurements. *Br. med. J.,* ***ii,*** 1026–1028

Williams, C.L., Eng, A., Botvin, G.J., Hill, P. & Wynder, E.L. (1979) Validation of students' self-reported cigarette smoking status with plasma cotinine levels. *Am. J. Public Health,* ***69,*** 1272-1274

VI. HEALTH EFFECTS OF LOW-TAR, LOW-NICOTINE CIGARETTES

CIGARETTE YIELD AND CANCER RISK: EVIDENCE FROM CASE-CONTROL AND PROSPECTIVE STUDIES

S.D. STELLMAN

American Cancer Society, Inc.
4 West 35th Street,
New York, NY 10001, USA

INTRODUCTION

The belief that cancer risk can be reduced by lowering the tar yield of cigarettes has been developed from three basic observations: (1) many cancers exhibit a dose-response with respect to the number of cigarettes smoked per day, as shown in Figure 1 (Wynder & Stellman, 1977); (2) cancer risk decreases with number of years of smoking cessation (Fig. 2); (3) tumours can be produced quantitatively in animals using cigarette combustion products (Wynder & Hoffmann, 1967).

Although quantitative relationships between cigarette smoking and cancer risk had been developed in both case-control and prospective studies in the 1950s and even earlier, epidemiological confirmation of a specific relationship with cigarette tar yield was not achieved consistently until the late 1960s. Since that time, differences in relative risk have been observed for at least four cancer sites: lung, larynx, oral cavity, and bladder.

In this paper we review the data which have led to these conclusions, and discuss some of the similarities and differences in the studies.

LUNG CANCER

Case-control studies

Three series of case-control studies have estimated the relative risk for developing lung cancer in relation to cigarette yield: Bross and Gibson (1968), the series begun by Wynder in the 1960s and continuing into the present (Wynder *et al.*, 1970; Wynder *et al.*, 1976; Wynder & Goldsmith, 1977; Wynder & Stellman, 1977; Mushinski & Stellman, 1978; Wynder & Stellman, 1979; Wynder *et al.*, 1984), and a cooperative European study begun in 1976 under the auspices of the US National Cancer Institute, covering five countries: Italy, France, Scotland, the Federal Republic of Germany and Austria. In the latter series, the results have been presented as a whole (Lubin *et al.*, 1984a,b) and the Austrian

Fig. 1. Relative risk for cancers of the lung (Kreyberg types I and II), oral cavity, larynx, oesophagus, and bladder for male current smokers, according to number of cigarettes smoked per day. N, number of cases in case-control study (from Wynder & Stellman, 1977)

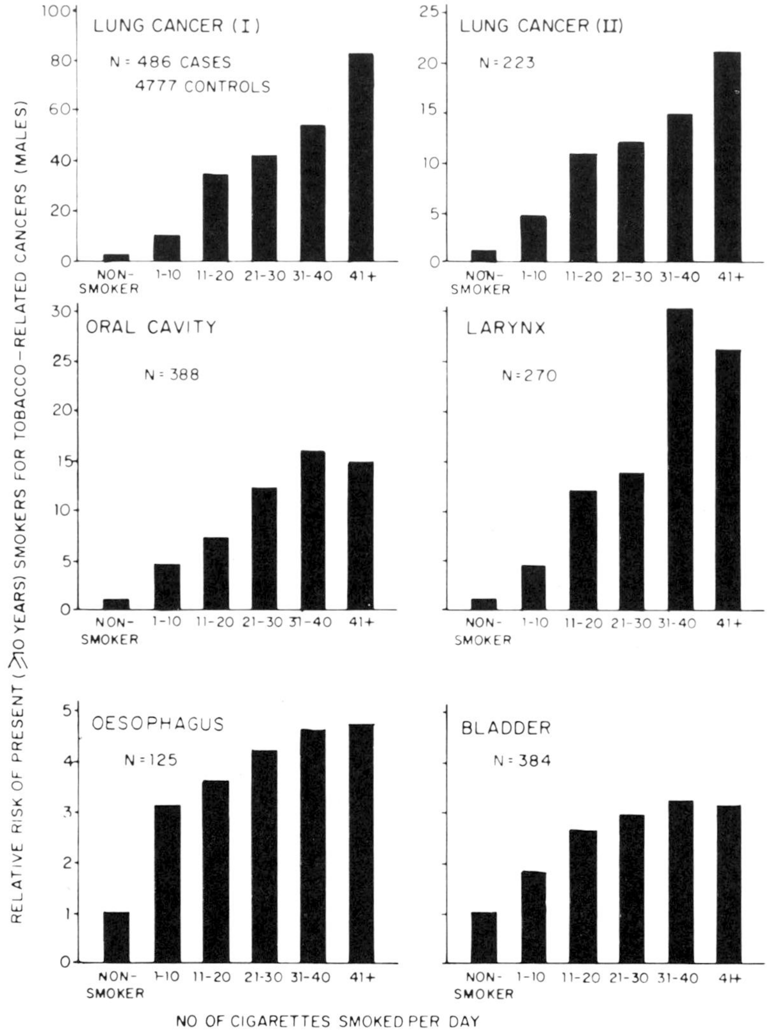

component has also been published separately (Kunze & Vutuc, 1980; Vutuc & Kunze, 1982a,b, 1983).

Results of these case-control studies are summarized in Table 1, in which comparisons are made between smokers of filter *versus* nonfilter cigarettes. The relative risk of lung cancer in nonfilter as compared to filter cigarette smokers as a referent ranges from 1.3 to 2.3. This must be understood in the context of an individual's lifetime exposure to cigarette tar. The average age of lung cancer diagnosis in the USA is now about 58 years. Most

Fig. 2. Relative risk for cancers of the lung (Kreyberg types I and II), oral cavity, larynx, oesophagus, and bladder for male former cigarette smokers, according to number of years since cessation of smoking. N, number of cases in case-control study (from Wynder & Stellman, 1977)

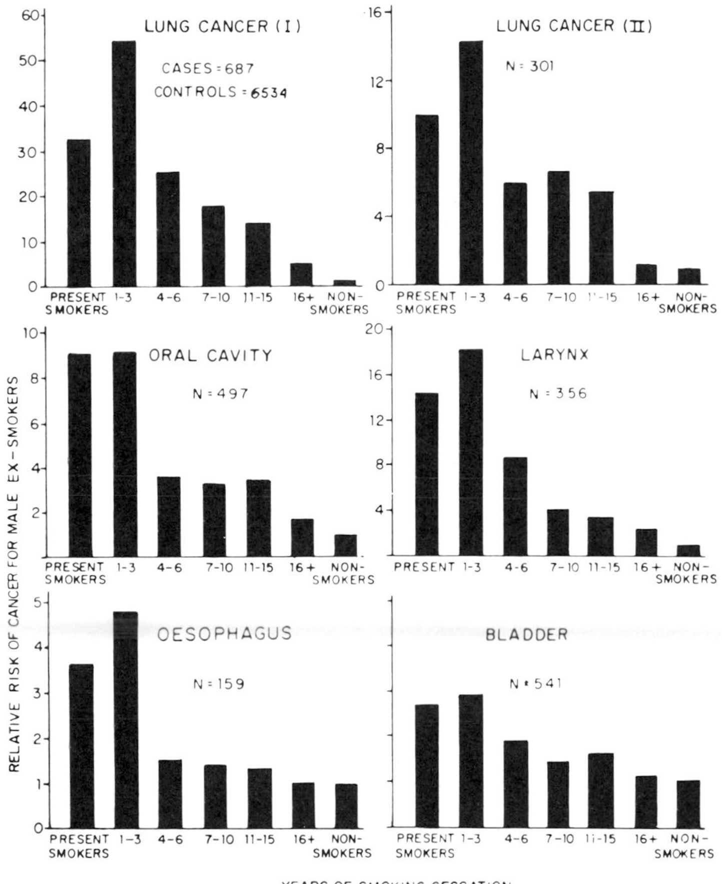

smokers in this cohort began smoking at a time when there were very few filter cigarettes on the market, and the tar yield of nonfilter cigarettes was over 30 mg. Data from the new American Cancer Society study (Stellman & Garfinkel, 1986) suggest that a wave of switching from nonfilter to filter cigarettes occurred in the mid-1960s immediately after the appearance of the Surgeon General's report in 1964, which received widespread publicity. Figure 3 shows the proportion of a smoker's lifetime which would have been spent with filter cigarettes, assuming smokers switched from nonfilter cigarettes at about that time, and assuming average ages of beginning to smoke characteristic of this population. It is obvious that recent lung cancer cases received a great deal of their tar exposure in their early smoking years from nonfilter, or from the early high-tar filter cigarettes, irrespective of the types of cigarette they smoke today.

Table 1. Relative risks for lung cancer reported from case-control studies, in relation to filter usage[a]

Study	Sex	Comparison	Relative risk
Bross & Gibson (1968)	Males	F to NSR	3.8
		NF to NSR	6.5
		NF to F	1.7
Wynder *et al.* (1970)[b]	Males	F to NSR	23.6
		NF to NSR	38.3
		NF to F	1.6
Wynder & Stellman (1979)	Males	NF to LTF	1.3
	Females	NF to LTF	1.4
Lubin *et al.* (1984 a, b)	Males	Mixed F and NF to F	2.1
		NF to F	2.1
	Females	Mixed F and NF to F	2.3
		NF to F	2.3

[a] Abbreviations: F, filter cigarette smokers; NSR, nonsmokers; NF, nonfilter cigarette smokers; LTF, long-term filter cigarette smokers

[b] Cases were Kreyberg type I only

In three of these case-control series, results have also been presented in terms of specific tar yields. These findings, shown in Table 2, demonstrate that, even allowing for substantial differences in schemes for estimating smokers' tar dosage, dose-response relationships are easily discernible.

Follow-up studies

There have been three important follow-up studies of lung cancer in relation to cigarette smoking in which cigarette yield has been studied in detail.

The American Cancer Society enrolled over one million men and women aged 40 years and over, in 25 states, in a prospective study in 1959. Follow-ups were conducted annually through 1966, and again in 1971 and 1972. Analyses of lung cancer death rates in relation to smoking habits were originally published by Hammond (1966).

Hammond *et al.* (1976, 1977) later presented evidence from this study showing that the lung cancer mortality rates for smokers of 'low tar-nicotine' cigarettes, compared to rates in smokers of 'high tar-nicotine' cigarettes, were reduced by about 20% in men and by about 40% in women. These estimates were made using a matched group analysis which permitted adjustment for many variables at once, including age, race, number of cigarettes smoked per day, age smoking began, urban/rural residence, education, job exposure to chemicals, X-rays, or other toxicants, history of prior illness, and calendar period (Hammond, 1985). Hammond's results are shown in Table 3.

For the present review we have re-calculated the standard mortality ratios (SMR) according to quantity smoked daily by current smokers, and by tar yield of cigarette at baseline, for lung cancer in men during 1960–1966, the six years when annual follow-up was done. Calculations were also restricted to this period to minimize effects of changes in

Fig. 3. Filter cigarette usage as a percentage of total smoking experience, by birth cohort (from Wynder & Stellman, 1979)

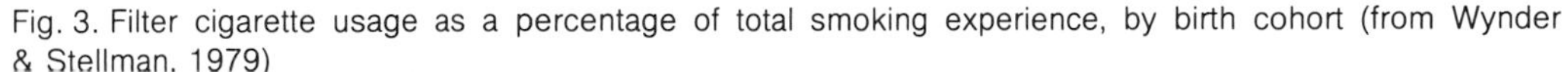

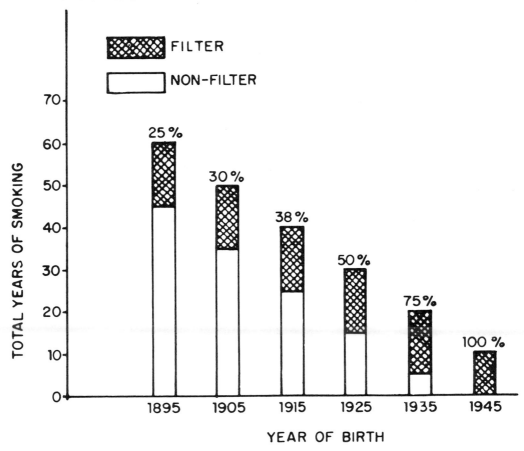

smoking habits. In addition, during the first six years of the study, additional confirmation was sought whenever cancer was mentioned on the death certificate, so that the cause of death was based upon 'best evidence'.

Results of this new calculation are shown in Figure 4. There were 967 deaths from lung cancer during this period. For statistical convenience, the reference population is the largest subgroup, namely, smokers of 'medium tar-nicotine' cigarettes, who smoked 20 cigarettes per day. For all other tar-nicotine and quantity categories of smokers, as well as for exsmokers and nonsmokers, expected numbers of deaths were computed by multiplying age-calendar-year-specific lung cancer death rates in the reference population by the person-years of exposure to risk of dying in the target group, and summing over age-calendar-year strata. The SMR is the number of observed divided by expected deaths. Data were renormalized to give lifetime nonsmokers an SMR of 1.0.

Table 2. Relative risk for lung cancer according to tar exposure indices proposed by various authors[a]

Reference	Sex	Relative risk								
Mushinski & Stellman (1978)		Current tar level (mg/day)								
		0	1–199	200–399	400–599	600–799	800–999	1000–1199	1200–1399	1400+
		Kreyberg I								
	Males	1.0	5.1	7.4	12.2	20.1	24.8	34.2	30.6	29.9
	Females	1.0	7.9	9.6	18.9	28.5	14.8			
Kunze & Vutuc (1980); Vutuc & Kunze (1982b)		Lifetime tar score								
		Below 500	501–1000	1001–2000	2001–3000	3001+				
		Kreyberg I								
	Males	2.0	2.6	5.3	7.2	8.3				
	Females	1.5	4.2	4.8	4.9	6.8				
		Kreyberg II								
	Males	–	1.8	1.8	3.5	3.9				
	Females	–	1.1	3.1	–	2.3				
Lubin *et al.* (1984a)		Mean cigarette tar content (mg)[b]								
		(15.6)	(18.5)	(20.6)	(23.6)	(25.2)	(28.8)			
		Lung cancer								
	Males	1.0	1.2	1.7	1.3	1.3	1.4			
	Females	1.0	1.9	1.3	1.1	1.5	–			

[a] Nonsmokers and referent; see Table 5 for definitions of tar exposure indices

[b] Categories were combined from within-country 10, 25, 50, 75, and 90th percentiles. Mean tar values (given in brackets) are within each such category

Table 3. Standardized mortality ratio for lung cancer among one million men and women followed up for twelve years, relative to lifetime nonsmokers, according to tar-nicotine yield of usual cigarettes, adjusted for age, calendar year, and many other variables (see text)[a]

	Standardized mortality ratio		
	'Low T/N'	'Medium T/N'	'High T/N'
Males	0.81	0.95	1.00
Females	0.60	0.79	1.00
'Adjusted' deaths:	235.2	285.5	318.4

[a] From Hammond *et al.* (1976)

Fig. 4. Standardized mortality ratios for lung cancer in males, among nonsmokers, exsmokers, and current smokers of low-, medium-, and high-tar/nicotine (T/N) cigarettes (defined by Hammond *et al.*, 1976). The group was enrolled in 1959, and followed up through 1966.

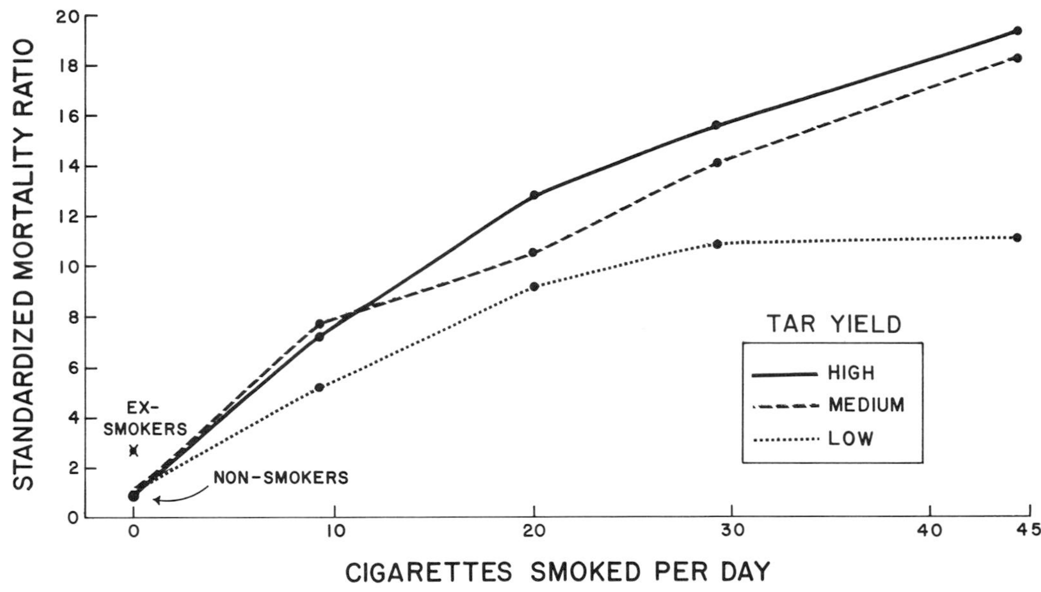

At each tar-nicotine level, the SMR increased with quantity smoked, in an approximately linear dose-response relationship. For current smokers of at least 20 cigarettes per day, at each value of daily quantity smoked, the SMR for the 'high tar-nicotine' cigarette smokers exceeded that for the 'medium' group, which in turn exceeded that for the 'low' group. Lifetime non-smokers had lung cancer death rates well below any of the current smokers, irrespective of cigarette yield for the latter.

Two other studies are worthy of mention. Rimington (1981) observed 104 lung cancer cases in a follow-up study of 10 414 male volunteers for a mass radiography screening in England. Subjects were enrolled in 1970–1971, and followed for 69 to 81 months. The relative risk for nonfilter *versus* filter cigarette smokers was reported as 1.54. The incidence was computed by dividing the numbers of cases by numbers enrolled, without considering person-years at risk. Adjustment was made for age and for quantity smoked.

In the Whitehall study (Higenbottam *et al.*, 1982), smoking data were available for 17 475 of 18 403 male civil servants aged 40–64 years who were enrolled during 1967–1969 and followed for at least ten years. Ten-year death rates, adjusted for age and employment grade, were computed for current smokers within categories of inhalation, quantity and tar-yield.

There were 108 deaths due to lung cancer among inhalers, and 35 among noninhalers, with tar- and quantity-specific rates for both groups shown in Table 4. Among inhalers, the data show a distinct dose-response at the two lowest consumption levels (1–9 and 10–19 cigarettes per day), although not at the highest, and among noninhalers there is a possible dose-response at the two highest levels (10–19 and 20 or more cigarettes per day).

Table 4. Ten-year lung cancer mortality rates (and number of deaths) among 17 475 male British civil servants in the Whitehall study, according to quantity smoked, tar yield, and inhalation[a]

No. cigarettes smoked per day	Tar yield (mg)		
	18–23	24–32	33+
Inhalers			
1–9	0.39 (2)	0.53 (1)	1.62 (7)
10–19	1.46 (19)	1.55 (8)	2.61 (20)
20+	2.23 (35)	2.00 (13)	1.79 (3)
Noninhalers			
1–9	1.08 (4)	0.00 (0)	0.93 (1)
10–19	1.25 (5)	1.28 (2)	4.18 (5)
20+	1.71 (7)	5.81 (9)	5.85 (2)

[a] From Higenbottam *et al.* (1982)

CANCERS OTHER THAN LUNG

Studies of cigarette yield and cancer have focused mainly on lung cancer, for the obvious reason that, having the greatest incidence and mortality rate of tobacco-related cancers, the numbers of cases available for study are greater than for other sites. Several studies, however, have examined the possible influence of cigarette yield on other cancers. In the American Health Foundation case-control studies, interviewers were instructed to see patients with cancers of the lung, mouth, oesophagus, larynx and bladder. Wynder and Stellman (1979) published relative risks for cancer of the larynx based on 286 male and 64 female cases. After adjusting for age, duration of smoking, number of cigarettes per day, and alcohol consumption, the risk of larynx cancer in nonfilter *versus* long-term filter cigarette smokers (at least ten years on filters) was 1.49 for men and 3.97 for women (both significant). The relative risk was greater for nonfilter than for filter cigarette smokers at every quantity level.

Lee and Garfinkel (1981) reported new analyses of data from the American Cancer Society follow-up study of 1959–1972, in which the relative mortality for smokers of low tar/nicotine cigarettes (as defined by Hammond *et al.*, 1976) was consistently lower in both men and women than for high tar/nicotine cigarettes for cancer of the buccal cavity and pharynx, oesophagus, larynx, bladder and pancreas. The adjustment procedure, based upon simultaneous matching for nine separate variables, rendered the numbers of effective ('adjusted') cases very small. The mortality ratios were statistically significant only for cancers of the oesophagus and bladder in women, and for none of the sites in men.

Wynder *et al.* (1976) gave relative risks for cancer of the oral cavity in a case-control study of 593 men and 280 women and matched controls: for nonfilter cigarette smokers *versus* nonsmokers, 7.8; for long-term filter cigarette smokers *versus* nonsmokers, 5.7; and for nonfilter *versus* long-term filter cigarette smokers, 1.4. Adjustment was made for age, but not for alcohol consumption. Significance levels were not given.

In a Canadian, population-based, case-control study of 480 male and 152 female case-control pairs, Howe *et al.* (1980) reported a reduced risk associated with the use of filter cigarettes compared to nonfilter cigarettes. A recent Italian study of 512 male bladder cancer cases and 596 controls gave a relative risk of 3.0 for nonfilter *versus* filter cigarette smokers (Vineis *et al.*, 1984). On the other hand, there was no difference for men between long-term filter and nonfilter cigarette smokers in the relative risk for bladder cancer in a case-control study by Wynder and Goldsmith (1977), which involved 574 cases and an equal number of matched controls.

DISCUSSION

There are many methodological issues which must be dealt with in the assessment of the relationship between cigarette yield and cancer outcomes. These fall roughly into four categories: questions of dosage, outcome, other etiological factors and confounding. The strengths and weaknesses of the studies described may be examined largely through attention to these four items.

Dosage

In any study of cigarette type and disease, dosage is the most important – and in some ways the most difficult – variable to estimate. There are many reasons for this.

In the first place, the average tar content of cigarettes has fallen considerably during the past 30 years, even within the same brand. Secondly, some smokers switch brands frequently, particularly in response to promotion of the new brands or in response to 'health' publicity. Thirdly, most smokers try to quit at some time in their lives; some are successful, others quit and begin again repeatedly. The actual lifetime dosage of persons in the latter category is quite difficult to determine. Finally, even in well-conducted interviews, subjects sometimes recall their smoking history imperfectly, especially regarding duration of smoking specific brands.

Many different ways of expressing cigarette dosage have been used, ranging from simple classification as filter *versus* nonfilter, to elaborate algorithms designed to account for 'complete' year-by-year smoking histories. Cumulative dosage measures have the advantage of taking into account the subject's entire history, including early smoking, which may have contributed disproportionately to lifetime tar exposure, since the cigarettes first smoked by persons now in the cancer age group had tar contents two to three times those of current cigarettes. It has the disadvantage of making cumulative scores 'pile up' at the beginning of a smoker's life, during the years when all cigarettes had high tar levels. Such scores may be insensitive to differences in tar levels between recent brands. Furthermore, cumulative dosage scores, particularly when expressed as 'pack-years', have the disadvantage of making two packs per day for 10 years equivalent to one pack per day for 20 years, necessitating further adjustment for duration or other parameters.

The wide range of tar exposure indices which have been used by various authors is shown in Table 5. These range from categorization of smokers as either filter or nonfilter cigarette smokers (Bross & Gibson, 1968; Wynder & Stellman, 1979), use of the tar rating of the

Table 5. Tar exposure indices used by various authors

Reference	Indices
Bross & Gibson (1968)	1. Quantity-duration combinations (low, medium, high) 2. Filter *versus* nonfilter
Hammond *et al.* (1976, 1977)	High, 25.8–35.7 mg; medium, 17.6–25.7 mg; low, below 17.6 mg
Mushinski & Stellman (1978)	Tar rating of current cigarette
Kunze & Vutuc (1980)	Σ (quantity $\times$ duration $\times$ k) where $k = 1$, below 15 mg; $k = 2$, 15–24 mg; $k = 3$, above 24 mg
Lubin *et al.* (1984a)	1. Lifetime filter *versus* mixed filter and nonfilter *versus* lifetime nonfilter 2. Within-country quintiles of: Σ (tar $\times$ quantity) / Σ (quantity) combined across five countries

current cigarette (Hammond *et al.*, 1976; Mushinski & Stellman, 1978), to fairly elaborate scoring systems presented by Lubin *et al.* (1984a), and Kunze and Vutuc (1980).

Finally, it has been repeatedly demonstrated and emphasized that people do not smoke identically to machines, and that the tar yields upon which machine analyses are based do not represent the true quantities of particulates or concentrations of vapour phase toxicants to which people were actually exposed (Kozlowski *et al.*, 1980; Benowitz *et al.*, 1983). At best, machine-determined yields give relative representations of degree of exposure to cigarette combustion products, such as tar.

Since, as has been seen in the preceding sections, the results of studies using different dosage measures are remarkably consistent, we may reasonably conclude that the basic principle that relative risk for lung cancer is in rough proportion to tar yield has been confirmed, despite these many difficulties and the disparities between studies, and that age-specific lung cancer rates may be expected eventually to reflect the falling average tar levels in many Western countries.

Outcome

In both case-control and follow-up studies, specification of the outcome under investigation is not trivial and may strongly influence interpretation of results. In the series of studies by Wynder and colleagues, and in those by Kunze and Vutuc, lung cancers were classified as Kreyberg Types I or II, the former invariably exhibiting a stronger dose-response to quantity of cigarettes smoked per day. If these observations are correct, it follows that any ameliorative effect of lower tar yield will be of lesser importance for adenocarcinoma of the lung than for squamous-cell carcinoma.

Other etiological factors

Smoking is the major cause of lung cancer in the populations studied, but it is not the only cause. Few of the studies mentioned have made adjustment for exposure to other factors related to occupation, environment, or nutrition. We have recently shown (Stellman, 1985) that smokers consume foods rich in vitamins A and C much less frequently than nonsmokers. Since vitamin A and similar compounds have been suggested as possible inhibitors of epidermoid cancers, it may in the future be desirable to examine dietary intake along with smoking history. None of the studies reviewed here have done so.

Other confounding factors

Most of the studies have adjusted for age and sex, but few have examined other potential biases in selection of subjects, differences in social class between cases and controls, etc. These are factors which, especially in hospitalized populations, can strongly affect smoking habits (Wynder *et al.*, 1984). Considering the consistency of results, despite the variety of study designs and populations summarized above, it is not likely that these confounding fachors have played a major role in the studies summarized here. However, it is important to keep them in mind when designing future studies.

CONCLUSIONS

In three series of case-control studies and three prospective studies conducted in the USA and Europe, the relative risk for lung cancer was found to be consistently lower in both male and female smokers of lower-yield cigarettes. This basic finding continued to hold irrespective of the many different ways in which dosage was expressed, whether qualitatively (filter *versus* nonfilter) or quantitatively (with explicit tar yields or ranges). Risks for other types of cancer, notably mouth, larynx and bladder, were also found to be lower in smokers of filter cigarettes in a number of North American and European studies.

This is all the more remarkable since the designs of studies differed considerably, and the designation of cigarette tar yields for specific cigarettes reflected only crudely true lifetime exposures for individuals. Smokers reaching lung cancer age during the past few years have almost invariably begun smoking nonfilter cigarettes, and many switched to filters during the 1960s, when health warnings gained prominence. It is very likely that as successive cohorts of smokers are exposed to cigarettes of much lower yield for much greater proportions of their lives, the associated risks will decline even further. However, it is to be emphasized that in all studies, risks of smokers of all types of cigarettes, no matter the yields, were significantly higher than those of lifetime nonsmokers.

REFERENCES

Benowitz, N.L., Hall, S.M., Herning, R.I., Jacob, P., Jones, R.T. & Osman, A.-L. (1983) Smokers of low-yield cigarettes do not consume less nicotine. *New Engl. J. Med.*, ***309***, 139–142

Bross, I.D.J. & Gibson, R. (1968) Risks of lung cancer in smokers who switch to filter cigarettes. *Am. J. Public Health*, ***58***, 1396–1403

Hammond, E.C. (1966) *Smoking in relation to the death rates of one million men and women.* In: Haenszel, W., ed., *Epidemiologic Approaches to the Study of Cancer and Other Chronic Diseases (National Cancer Institute Monograph No. 19),* Bethesda, MD, US Department of Health, Education, and Welfare, Public Health Service, National Institutes of Health, National Cancer Institute, pp. 127–204

Hammond, E.C. (1985) *Matched group analysis method.* In: Garfinkel, L., Ochs, O. & Mushinski, M. , eds, *Selection, Follow-up, and Analysis in Prospective Studies: A Workshop (National Cancer Institute Monograph, No.* 67; *NIH Publication No.* 85-2713), Bethesda, MD, US Department of Health and Human Services, Public Health Service, National Institutes of Health, National Cancer Institute, pp. 157–160

Hammond, E.C., Garfinkel, L., Seidman, H. & Lew E.A. (1976) "Tar" and nicotine content of cigarette smoke in relation to death rates. *Environ. Res., **12,*** 263–274

Hammond, E.C., Garfinkel, L., Seidman, H. & Lew E.A. (1977) *Some recent findings concerning cigarette smoking.* In: Hiatt, H.H., Watson, J.D. & Winsten, J.A., eds, *Origins of Human Cancer,* Book A, *Incidence of Cancer in Humans,* Cold Spring Harbor, NY, Cold Spring Harbor Laboratory, pp. 101–112

Higenbottam, T., Shipley, M.J. & Rose, G. (1982) Cigarettes, lung cancer, and coronary heart disease: the effects of inhalation and tar yield. *J. Epidemiol. Community Health, **36,*** 113–117

Howe, G.R., Burch, J.D., Miller, A.B., Cook, G.M., Esteve, J., Morrison, B., Gordon, P., Chambers, L.W., Fodor, G. & Winsor, G.M. (1980) Tobacco use, occupation, coffee, various nutrients, and bladder cancer. *J. natl Cancer Inst., **64,*** 701–713

Kozlowski, L.T., Frecker, R.C., Khouw, V. & Pope, M.A. (1980) The misuse of "less-hazardous" cigarettes and its detection: hole-blocking of ventilated filters. *Am. J. Public Health, **70,*** 1202–1203

Kunze, M. & Vutuc, C. (1980) *Threshold of tar exposure: analysis of smoking history of male lung cancer cases and controls.* In: Gori, G. & Bock, F.G., eds, *A Safe Cigarette? (Banbury Report No. 3),* Cold Spring Harbor, NY, Cold Spring Harbor Laboratory, pp. 29–34

Lee, P.N. & Garfinkel, L. (1981) Mortality and type of cigarette smoked. *J. Epidemiol. Commun. Health, **35,*** 16–22

Lubin, J.H., Blot, W.J., Berrino, F., Flamant, R., Gillis, C.R., Kunze, M., Schmahl, D. & Visco, G. (1984a) Patterns of lung cancer risk according to type of cigarette smoked. *Int. J. Cancer, **33,*** 569–576

Lubin, J.H., Blot, W.J., Berrino, F., Flamant, R., Gillis, C.R., Kunze, M., Schmahl, D. & Visco, G. (1984b) Modifying risk of developing lung cancer by changing habits of cigarette smoking. *Br. med. J., **288,*** 1953–1956

Mushinski, M.H. & Stellman, S.D. (1978) Impact of new smoking trends on women's occupational health. *Prev. Med., **7,*** 349–365

Rimington, J. (1981) The effect of filters on the incidence of lung cancer in cigarette smokers. *Environ. Res., **24,*** 162–166

Stellman, S.D. (1985) *Chairman's remarks on Session V: Data analysis in cohort studies.* In: Garfinkel, L., Ochs, O. & Mushinski, M., eds, *Selection, Follow-up, and Analysis in Prospective Studies: A Workshop (National Cancer Institute Monograph, No.* 67, *NIH Publication No.* 85-2713), Bethesda, MD, US Department of Health and Human Services, Public Health Service, National Institutes of Health, National Cancer Institute, pp. 145–147

Stellman, S.D. & Garfinkel, L. (1986) Smoking habits and tar levels in a new American Cancer Society prospective study of 1.2 million men and women. *J. natl Cancer Inst.* (in press)

Vineis, P., Estève, J. & Terracini, B. (1984) Bladder cancer and smoking in males: types of cigarettes, age at start, effect of stopping and interaction with occupation. *Int. J. Cancer,* ***34,*** 165–170

Vutuc, C. & Kunze, M. (1982a) Lung cancer risk in women in relation to tar yields of cigarettes. *Prev. Med.,* ***11,*** 713–716

Vutuc, C. & Kunze, M. (1982b) Cigarette tar exposure and occupation in female lung cancer patients. *Excerpta med. Int. Congr., Ser. 55B,* 41–48

Vutuc, C. & Kunze, M. (1983) Tar yields of cigarettes and male lung cancer risk. *J. natl Cancer Inst.,* ***71,*** 435–437

Wynder, E.L. & Goldsmith, R. (1977) The epidemiology of bladder cancer. A second look. *Cancer,* ***40,*** 1246–1268

Wynder, E.L. & Hoffmann, D. (1967) *Tobacco and Tobacco Smoke. Studies in Experimental Carcinogenesis,* New York, Academic Press

Wynder, E.L. & Stellman, S.D. (1977) Comparative epidemiology of tobacco-related cancers. *Cancer Res.,* ***37,*** 4608–4622

Wynder, E.L. & Stellman, S.D. (1979) Impact of long-term filter cigarette usage on lung and larynx cancer risk: a case-control study. *J. natl Cancer Inst.,* ***62,*** 471–477

Wynder, E.L., Mabuchi, K. & Beattie, E.J. (1970) The epidemiology of lung cancer. Recent trends. *J. Am. med. Assoc.,* ***213,*** 2221–2228

Wynder, E.L., Mushinski, M. & Stellman, S.D. (1976) *The epidemiology of the less harmful cigarette.* In: Wynder, E.L., Hoffmann, D. & Gori, G.B., eds, *Modifying the Risk for the Smoker.* Vol. I. *Proceedings of the Third World Conference on Smoking and Health, New York City, June 2–5, 1975, (DHEW Publication No. (NIH) 76-1221),* Bethesda, MD, US Department of Health, Education, and Welfare, Public Health Service, National Institutes of Health, National Cancer Institute, pp. 1–12

Wynder, E.L., Goodman, M.T. & Hoffmann, D. (1984) Demographic aspects of the low-yield cigarette: considerations in the evaluation of health risk. *J. natl Cancer Inst.,* ***72,*** 817–822

OVERVIEW OF CANCER TIME-TREND STUDIES IN RELATION TO CHANGES IN CIGARETTE MANUFACTURE

R. PETO

Imperial Cancer Research Fund
Reader in Cancer Studies,
Nuffield Department of Clinical Medicine,
Radcliffe Infirmary, Oxford, UK

SUMMARY

The chief purpose of the present chapter is not to review lung cancer trends in general, but merely to consider the extent to which trends in national lung cancer rates can help assess any differences between the carcinogenic effects of different types of cigarette. For this limited purpose, the British data are uniquely informative, for (1) British male lung cancer rates were already high but stable before the cigarette tar levels were halved, and (2) British male cigarette consumption remained stable for some years thereafter. Against this apparently stable background, an otherwise unexplained decrease of about one-half in British male lung cancer mortality in early middle age has followed the decrease in cigarette tar deliveries, which is consistent with Stellman's conclusion (this volume[1]), based on review of the case-control and prospective studies, that cigarette-induced lung cancer risks are approximately proportional to machine-measured tar deliveries. Lung cancer trends are also reviewed for males from the USA (where cigarette tar deliveries have been greatly reduced) and from the USSR (where they have not).

INTRODUCTION

Changes in machine-measured tar yield per cigarette

In many countries, cigarette manufacturing methods have undergone substantial changes over the past three decades. The most obvious alteration has been the progressive replacement of nonfilter cigarettes with filter-tipped cigarettes, but other changes have

[1] See p. 197.

Fig. 1. US sales-weighted average tar and nicotine yields per manufactured cigarette (from American Cancer Society, 1981)

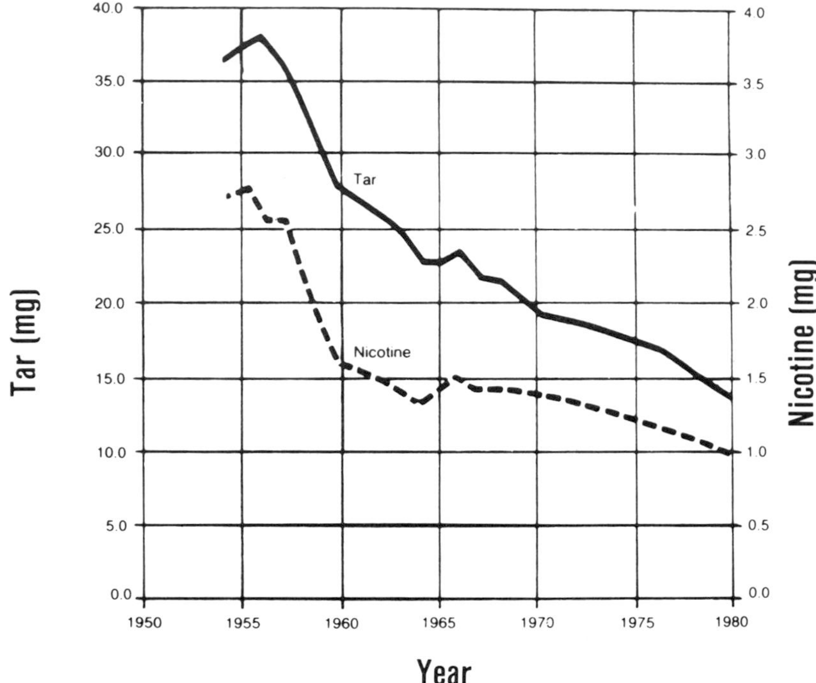

involved the use of different varieties of tobacco plant, different (and generally more porous) types of paper, different methods of shredding and processing the tobacco, and different additives.

The smoke from cigarettes yields a condensate that might typically contain several milligrams of 'tar'. This cigarette tar is a complex mixture of hundreds (or even thousands) of different chemicals, many of which can be used to cause cancer in laboratory animals. One of the chief purposes of changing the method of manufacture of cigarettes has been to reduce the amounts of 'tar' they deliver when smoked in a standard way by a machine (Fig. 1), in the hope that this would decrease the net adverse effects of smoking.

Before filter-tips began to be widely used, typical tar deliveries per cigarette might (depending on the country concerned) have been more than 30 mg. Even in countries where no systematic effort has yet been made to reduce tar deliveries, values in the range 20–30 mg might now be typical, whereas in countries where substantial reductions have been deliberately engendered the average tar delivery is likely now to be under 15 mg – indeed, in Finland an upper limit of 15 mg has recently been introduced.

Compensatory smoking

The extent to which such changes in cigarette tar deliveries will actually reduce risks is, however, not easy to predict, for smokers do not use cigarettes as predictably as machines do, and the composition of a cigarette can influence the manner in which it is smoked. Many studies (e.g., Peach, this volume[2]) have shown that if cigarettes with a medium nicotine delivery (as measured by a standard machine) are replaced by cigarettes with a lower one, then the amount of cigarette smoke that smokers choose to take into the periphery of their lungs will increase. At least for nicotine, this increase may suffice to compensate entirely, or almost entirely, for the change in the nature of the smoke, so there may be very little difference in the uptake per cigarette smoked of nicotine into the blood (except for cigarettes with yields so low that few smokers are currently prepared to use them). Moreover, many different components of smoke may vary approximately in parallel with any variations in nicotine, so this 'compensation' is likely to be of substantial relevance to the health hazards caused by the actual use of different types of cigarette by humans.

First, it suggests that there may be no great difference between one type of cigarette and another in the amount of pharmacological satisfaction that smokers get from each cigarette (and hence no great difference in the daily number of cigarettes they choose to smoke, or in the ease of adoption or cessation of the habit).

Second, it suggests that there may be no great difference between one type of cigarette and another in their production of those adverse health effects, such as heart disease or chronic obstructive lung disease, that are chiefly determined by the amounts of smoke products that reach the *periphery* of the lung.

Third, for adverse health effects, such as bronchial carcinoma, that generally involve not the periphery of the lung but instead anatomic subsites that are higher up in the bronchial tree, it emphasizes the potential unreliability of theoretical predictions about the magnitude (or even the direction) of any differences in lung cancer risk between actual use of one type of cigarette and actual use of another.

Difficulty in predicting carcinogenic effects on main airways

The type of lung cancer usually produced by cigarettes is bronchial carcinoma, arising from the walls and, particularly, the bifurcations of the *main* airways. For the chief carcinogenic factors in the smoke, however, it is difficult to predict what the effective dose to the bronchi will be as the smoke streams past these walls and bifurcations, especially since it is not reliably known which of the many chemicals in cigarette smoke are chiefly responsible for its carcinogenic (or cocarcinogenic) activity in the bronchus. Indeed, it is not even known with certainty whether these agents are only in the particulate phase or whether some in the gas phase are also importantly relevant. (Cigarette smoke is a mixture of particles, which may swell rapidly in a moist environment, and gases.) Moreover, it is already known that differences in the chemical composition of the smoke substantially alter inhalation practices. Differences in, for example, the speed of inhalation would affect the length of time that the tissues of the main airways are exposed to the gas phase, and these (or other) differences in inhalation might also substantially affect the proportion of particulate matter that is deposited on the walls of the airways.

[2] See p. 251.

The surprisingly substantial practical relevance of these speculations may be illustrated by two curious observations among men who are *heavy* smokers: (1) those who say they 'do not inhale' seem to get almost as much smoke into the periphery of their lungs as other equally heavy smokers who say they 'do inhale', but (2) these 'noninhalers' get it there in a manner that in several studies has been found to give them significantly *more* lung cancer in their main airways than otherwise similar 'inhalers' get! This apparent anomaly has been nicely reviewed and discussed by Wald *et al.* (1983) (see also Wald, 1985), who suggest that it could arise chiefly because *slow* inhalation may expose the walls of the main airways to more of the chief cancer-causing substances than *rapid* inhalation does. But, although reasonably plausible explanations for the data can certainly be developed from such ideas, there obviously still remains great uncertainty about the quantitative determinants of exposure of the main airways both to gas-phase and, especially, to particulate-phase smoke components.

Limitations of laboratory evidence

Thus, when comparing the lung cancer hazards that are likely to be conferred by different types of cigarette, evidence from laboratory studies is, for the present, of limited practical value. It is known that differences between different types of cigarette can engender large differences in the extent (and hence, presumably, also the manner) of inhalation; it is known that differences in the manner of inhalation can engender large differences in risk whose magnitude (and even direction!) are difficult to predict; it is not known which the chief cancer-causing agents in cigarette smoke are, and even if it were there would at present be no reliable way of measuring the average extent to which actual smoking patterns would deposit particular agents onto the key target areas in the main airways. (In particular, although the extent of deposition of smoke products into the periphery of the lung can be measured by analyses of blood samples, this is not likely to be proportional to the extent of action of cancer-causing factors on the main airways: Wald *et al.*, 1983.)

Restriction of attention to epidemiological evidence

From the foregoing, it appears that the only useful way to discover whether there are any important differences in the lung cancer risks caused by the habitual use of different types of cigarette is likely to be direct epidemiological observation. Two main types of epidemiological study may be considered: time-trend studies of an entire population (which will be dealt with below), and 'analytic' studies of individuals, i.e., studies that use standard case-control or prospective methods (Stellman, this volume[3]).

Both 'analytic' and time-trend studies have their strengths and weaknesses, but when (as is actually the case) the conclusions of each are concordant then their strengths reinforce each other, and together they may provide ample evidence to justify practical action.

---

[3] See p. 197.

Time-trend studies

Two of the main strengths of time-trend studies of an entire population are, first, that they may allow (at least in early middle age) direct comparison of *prolonged* high-tar usage with reasonably *prolonged* low-tar usage, and second, that they allow the study of extremely large numbers, so lung cancer rates can be studied meaningfully even for people as young as 30–34 or 35–39 years of age, among whom the disease is extremely rare but among whom the contrast in lifelong average tar delivery per cigarette may currently be greatest.

The main disadvantage of time-trend studies is, of course, that other causes of change of lung cancer incidence may also have been operating, so it may be difficult to be certain exactly how much of any trend that is observed can be ascribed to changes in cigarette composition. If, however, a time-trend study is undertaken in a population in which the big increase in lung cancer mortality in those of middle age due to the delayed effect of a previous increase in cigarette use was largely completed before the tar levels began to undergo their main decrease, and in which no large change in current cigarette consumption is in progress, then it may usefully complement the analytic studies.

Analytic studies

The great strength of analytic studies (i.e., of studies comparing different individuals within the same population) is that they should be less subject to certain systematic biases than a time-trend study might be. Their weaknesses, however, are that it is difficult to use them to study the crucially informative period in early middle age sufficiently accurately (because the disease is so rare at these ages), and that it is generally impossible to use them to compare the *prolonged* use of high-tar cigarettes with the *prolonged* use of low-tar cigarettes, simply because as low-tar cigarettes become widely available in a particular country high-tar ones tend to disappear, so that the two do not coexist widely for long. Hence, we may expect a systematic tendency for analytic studies to underestimate any true differences in risk between prolonged use of high-tar cigarettes and prolonged use of medium-tar cigarettes.

Despite this, the findings in analytic studies have actually been surprisingly substantial and consistent, and Stellman (this volume[1]), after reviewing them, concludes that 'relative risk for lung cancer is in rough proportion to tar yield' (i.e., to tar yield as measured by a standard smoking machine), adding that 'It is very likely that as successive cohorts of smokers are exposed to cigarettes of much lower yield for much greater proportions of their lives, the associated risks will decline even further.' (One further study – that of Alderson *et al.*, 1985 – has recently yielded unpromising results, but inclusion of it would merely dilute, rather than reverse, Stellman's conclusions.)

Review of some time-trend studies now follows, (1) to determine whether national trends, especially in people in early middle age, support Stellman's conclusion that substantial risk reductions have already been achieved, and (2) to determine how large the risk reductions in people in early middle age appear to be, especially in populations where the large increases in tobacco-induced lung cancer in people in early middle age had already been completed, or nearly completed, before substantial tar-level reductions emerged. Data will be presented from five developed populations, chosen to illustrate contrasting trends in patterns of cigarette usage and tar delivery.

Two (Finnish and, especially, UK males) involve countries where cigarette smoking by young men appears to have become widespread in the *first* quarter of the century (Lee, 1975) and where large changes in cigarettes, which lowered tar yields, were implemented in the third quarter (Lee, 1976; Wald *et al.*, 1981). Consequently, any moderate effects that these tar-level reductions may have on lung cancer can be assessed against a background rate of male lung cancer that had, at least in people in early middle age, already approximately stabilized, albeit at a very high level (Doll & Peto, 1981).

One (American males) involves a population where cigarette smoking by young adults increased substantially in the *second* quarter of the century (Lee, 1975) and where tar-level reductions were also implemented in the third quarter (Fig. 1; US Surgeon General, 1982). Consequently, any moderate effects of these tar-level reductions on lung cancer rates have to be assessed against a background of the rapid rises in lung cancer produced by the delayed effects of the earlier increase in cigarette usage (Doll & Peto, 1981).

The fourth example (French females) involves a population where smoking became common only in the *third* quarter of the century (Hill & Flamant, 1985), and because this increase in cigarette usage is so recent the large increase in lung cancer that it will eventually produce has not yet really begun to materialize.

The fifth and final example (males in the USSR) differs not so much in timing but in tar trends. The USSR is a country where cigarette smoking by young men appears (although reliable data are not available) to have become widespread during the first half of the century, but where tar levels still remain much higher than they currently are in the first three countries. Perhaps because of this, the lung cancer rates in early middle-aged men in the USSR appear for the present to be remaining as high as those in the UK before British tar levels were reduced (Napalkov *et al.*, 1983).

METHODS FOR TREND ASSESSMENT

Sources of data on history of cigarette usage

In developed countries, where cigarette sales are monitored quite closely, sales-weighted data on actual cigarette sales per head (Lee, 1975) are usually reasonably reliable, and trends in these can generally be accepted as real and meaningful. Trends in data from questionnaires on the proportion of smokers or on the total numbers of cigarettes smoked may in contrast be systematically misleading, as antismoking propaganda may have a much larger effect on people's self-reported smoking than on their actual smoking. [Recent divergences between the trends in self-reported smoking and actual sales in the USA (Warner, 1978), France (Hill & Flamant, 1985) and elsewhere illustrate this point.] If data from questionnaires are to be used at all, they should therefore perhaps be used merely to apportion total sales between various sex- and age-specific categories.

Another potentially misleading way of using questionnaires is to ask a sample of people what they used to smoke some decades previously, and then to extrapolate these answers back to well before 1950, when almost no direct information existed as to who smoked what. Such extrapolations may yield moderately useful (though not wholly reliable) estimates of the proportions of all cigarettes smoked previously by people of each sex, but may yield considerably less reliable estimates of age-specific, sex-specific past habits – as, perhaps, in the paper of Lee (1975) and in some of the US Surgeon-General's reports. For this reason, *excessively* detailed modelling of national lung cancer trends should generally be avoided (especially in old people, where the trends in lung cancer may depend particularly strongly on age-specific trends in smoking many decades previously).

Use of mortality data on people in middle age

Mortality data on people in *middle* age provide perhaps the most reliable source available for assessment of lung cancer trends, for reasons discussed in IARC (1986) and by Doll and Peto (1981).

REAL EFFECTS OF HISTORY OF TOBACCO USAGE ON LUNG CANCER TRENDS

The chief effects of tobacco on national lung cancer trends that need to be assessed are the long-delayed effects of nationwide adoption of cigarette usage, and the moderately delayed effects of nationwide decreases in the tar delivery per cigarette (Doll & Peto, 1981; Peto & Doll, 1984).

Effects of nationwide adoption of cigarette usage

Cigarettes cause a far greater risk of lung cancer than others forms of tobacco do (US Surgeon General, 1979, 1982). So, when a nation adopts widespread cigarette usage, large real increases in lung cancer will eventually follow, whether the switch is from nothing to cigarettes or whether it is from other forms of tobacco to cigarettes. These large increases in lung cancer may, however, appear many decades after the large increases in cigarette

Table 1. 40 years of evolution of British annual respiratory[a] cancer death certification rates per 100 000 men, emphasizing the high rates in men born about 1900

Age range (years)	1943 [b]	1953 [b]	1963 [b]	1973 [b]	1983 [c]
30–34	4	4	3	2	1
40–44	20	25	22	18	12
50–54	63	123	122	107	77
60–64	107	258	367	354	299
70–74	80	265	497	678	640
80–84	[d]	144	342	602	834
No. of cigarettes per man per day in preceding year	10.7	9.9	10.6	10.6	7.1

[a] All respiratory and intrathoracic in England and Wales, excluding nose, sinuses and larynx
[b] Mean for five years centred on index year
[c] Mean for 1982–1984 only (1985 not yet available, and 1981 subject to slight underestimation at older ages, due to temporary difficulties in central records office; Wald, 1985)
[d] Data for people aged 80 and above were not subdivided, and anyway were subject to gross under-certification
Data from Doll and Peto (1981; appendix E) and Office of Population Censuses and Surveys (1984a,b,c,d, 1985a,b)

usage, simply because it is those who start to smoke in early adult life who will be at greatest risk in middle and old age (Doll & Peto, 1981), and 30 years separate the late teenage years from the age-range 45–49, while 60 years separate the late teenage years from the age-range 75–79. Hence, if other things are equal, it will probably not be until about 20, 30, 40, 50 and 60 years after cigarette smoking in people in their late teens or early twenties approaches a maximum that lung cancer at ages 35–39, 45–49, 55–59, 65–69 and 75–79 can be expected to do so. Thus, for 30 years after cigarette smoking among teenagers finally becomes nearly maximal, lung cancer rates in people at ages 45–49 may continue to rise. Thereafter they may become stable, while lung cancer rates in people in the age-range 65–69 may continue to rise for another 20 years before they too stabilize. Thus, lung cancer rates in people at ages 35–39, 45–49, 55–59, 65–69 and 75–79 may approximately reach their maxima 20, 30, 40, 50 and 60 years after a common starting point. This possibility is exemplified by the British male lung cancer death certification rates (Table 1). The underlined rates are those for men born in about 1900, and are approximately maximal.

Modification of lung cancer hazard by changes in cigarette tar delivery

The general pattern in each age group is one of sharp increases preceding this maximum, followed by an approximate stability that is disturbed only by the recent decreases that have begun to take place in people in early middle age following substantial changes (Wald *et al.*, 1981) in tar delivery per British cigarette. Similar decreases are beginning to emerge in Finland (Fig. 2), where tar levels have also decreased substantially, due in part to progressive abandonment of the 'Russian-style' *papyrossi* cigarettes that used to be favoured in Finland (Lee, 1975).

It is interesting to contrast these figures from countries where tar levels have been reduced with the corresponding figures from a country such as the USSR, where they have not (Table 2). In the USSR, typical tar deliveries per cigarette are still running at about 20–30 mg (IARC, 1986; Zaridze *et al.*, this volume[4]), with a mean of perhaps 25 mg. This is nearly as high as the tar deliveries of US or UK cigarettes in the 1950s, before their tar deliveries were halved (Fig. 1, Fig. 3), and it may be noteworthy that the USSR lung cancer incidence rates in people in middle age (Table 2) appear to be converging towards the old high UK lung cancer rates of the 1950s and not towards the lower rates that now obtain in both the UK (Table 1) and Finland (Fig. 2).

If the hypothesis is true that tar-level decreases are important determinants of the recent decreases in lung cancer mortality in people in early middle age in the UK and Finland, then one may wonder why corresponding differences in risk are not seen in other countries. A possible answer might be that they are being seen but not recognized, simply because moderate (e.g., two-fold) differences such as these can easily be swamped by the vast increases in lung cancer that are being produced in many countries by the delayed effects of past changes in cigarette usage (Doll & Peto, 1981). On this view, the reason why men in the UK and Finland provide such a useful 'natural experiment' for observation of the effects of tar-level changes is that these are perhaps the only two countries in the world

[4] See p. 75.

Fig. 2. 20 years of evolution of Finnish lung cancer incidence (from IARC, 1986)

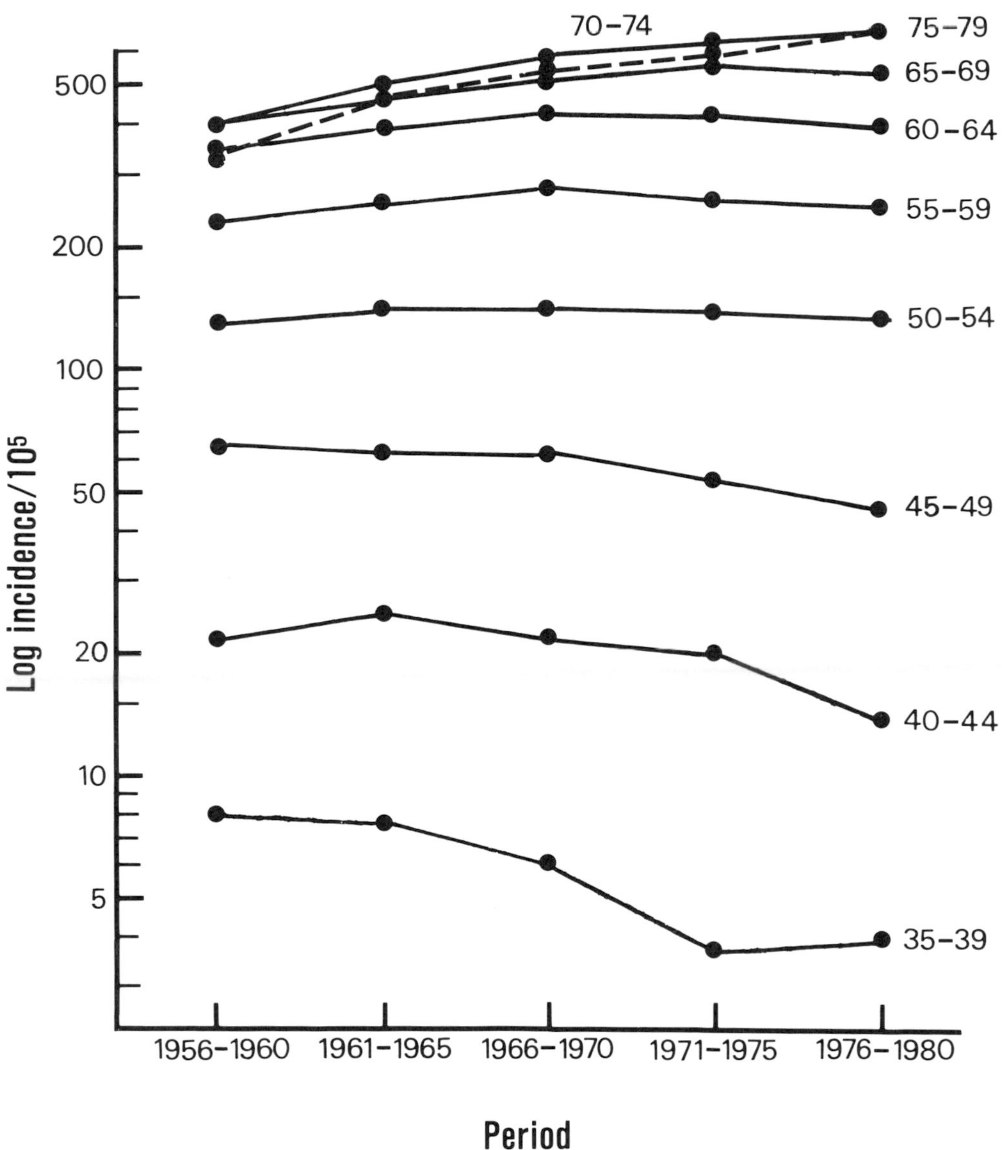

Owing to the use of a 'log' scale, the decreases over the past 15 years (i.e., 1963–1978) at ages 45–49, 40–44 and 35–39 may not look important, yet they would represent, respectively, avoidance of about 31%, 41% and 53% of the 1963 lung cancer deaths at these ages. As in the UK, changes in incidence are due chiefly to changes in the risk per cigarette rather than to changes in the number of cigarettes smoked. Indeed, except for a temporary decrease during the Second World War, cigarette consumption per Finnish adult has been fairly steady for more than 50 years, averaging about four/day and five/day in the second and third quarters of the present century, respectively (Lee, 1975).

Table 2. 20 years of evolution of USSR annual lung cancer incidence registration rates per 100 000 men, compared with the corresponding rates in the UK

Age range (years)	USSR incidence[a]					England & Wales mortality × 1.1 [b]	
	1960	1965	1970	1975	1980	1958	1983
30–39	3	5	6	7	6	7	3
40–49	24	29	35	46	47	47	24
50–59	85	127	142	153	176	197	136
c							

[a] From IARC (1986)
[b] By 1958, British mortality rates in people at ages 30–59 had reached their maxima and had stabilized. Rates for 10-year age groups are estimated as averages of the rates for the two corresponding five-year ages-groups in Table 4, and multiplication by 1.1 is intended to provide an approximate estimate of the ratio of incidence to mortality that might be expected in parts of the UK, such as Birmingham, where registration of all incident cases has been in progress for several years (Waterhouse *et al.*, 1976).
[c] USSR incidence data for 1960 are published for 60 years and over, without subdivision.

Fig. 3. Sales-weighted tar, nicotine and carbon monoxide yields of UK cigarettes (from Wald, 1985)

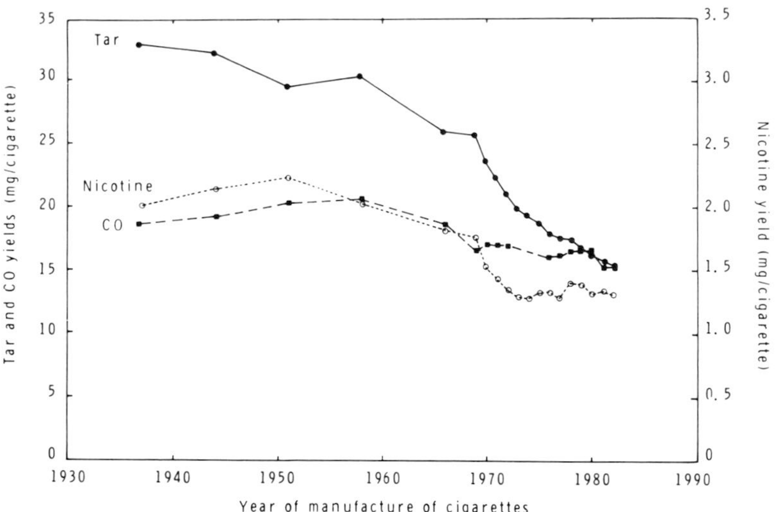

(Lee, 1975) where cigarette smoking by young men became established so long ago that the lung cancer rates in early middle-aged men had stabilized (or, in the case of Finland, nearly stabilized) by the late 1950s, i.e., before the large tar-level reductions began. Consequently, these were the only two populations in which the effects of tar-level changes on lung cancer were monitored against a background of roughly constant lung cancer rates instead of against a background of rapidly rising lung cancer rates, as, for example, in the USA (Table 3; Doll & Peto, 1981).

In the USA, cigarette sales increased between the two World Wars from one (in 1918) up to five (in 1939) cigarettes per adult per day and then during the Second World War they

Table 3. 40 years of US annual respiratory cancer death certification rates per 100 000 men, emphasizing the high rates in men born in the late 1920s[a]

Age range (years)	1940	1950	1960	1970	1980
30–34	1.5	1.7	2.4	2.1	1.3
40–44	7	11	15	22	19
50–54	24	47	67	87	102
60–64	41	97	166	225	261
70–74	38	103	211	355	444
80–84	30	77	152	291	467
Actual period studied	1938–1942	1948–1952	1958–1962	1968–1972	1978–1981
No. of cigarettes per adult per day in preceding year	5	10	11	11	11

[a] From IARC (1986)

quickly doubled, and have remained at about 10, 11 or 12 per adult per day ever since (Lee, 1976). As a delayed effect of this large increase before and, especially, during the Second World War in cigarette usage by young men, large increases in US male lung cancer death rates were taking place throughout the 1950s and 1960s, the maximal rate in any age group being seen among those who reached adulthood in the late 1940s (Doll & Peto, 1981). Thus, among US males aged 30–34, 35–39, 40–44 and 45–49 the maximum lung cancer rate has been reached, and in those at 50–54 it should recently have been reached (Table 3). Within each age group, the large increases before the maxima are clearly seen; in addition, however, there does appear to be a slight decrease after the maximum is attained (especially in those at ages 30–34). This *might* reflect the effects of tar-level changes. Even if it does, however, and even if these effects spread to older age groups over the remainder of this century, they cannot be expected to outweigh the large increase in US lung cancer death rates in old age that will presumably continue to emerge throughout this century as a delayed effect of the large increase in cigarette usage by young adults before and during the Second World War.

RECAPITULATION

Rationale for study of UK male trends

As already noted, large, but wholly artefactual, trends in lung cancer death certification rates can result merely from improvements in the accuracy of diagnosis and/or certification of the disease. Moreover, large real trends in lung cancer rates can result from changes in patterns of tobacco use. (In particular, large increases in rates of the disease can be expected a few decades after the widespread adoption of cigarette smoking by young adults.) The key question is whether, in addition to these *large* artefactual changes and *large* real changes in lung cancer, any *moderate* decreases in the disease during the 1970s or early 1980s can confidently be attributed to the approximate halving of cigarette tar

Table 4. Recent trends in England and Wales in lung[a] cancer death certification rates[b] per million men in middle age (Note *both* the approximate constancy before the large decreases in tar delivery per cigarette in about 1960, *and* the large – and accelerating – decrease thereafter)

Age range (years)	1953	1958	1978	1983	% Change from 1958 to 1978	% Change from 1958 to 1983
30–34	37	36	17	14	−54%	−62%
35–39	100	94	56	44	−41%	−53%
40–44	250	253	139	122	−45%	−52%
45–49	584	594	402	321	−33%	−46%
50–54	1232	1254	999	765	−20%	−39%
55–59	2018	2326	1897	1705	−18%	−27%

[a] Data include those for pleura, etc. (1953–1958: ICD6 and 7 162–164; 1976–1978: ICD8 162–163; 1979–1984: ICD9 162–165), and hence the downward trend in bronchial carcinoma rates is slightly diluted by the upward trend in rates of pleural mesothelioma.
[b] Each rate is for a five-year period centred on the index year (i.e., 1951–1955, 1956–1960, 1976–1980), except for the last one, which is for a three-year period (1982–1984).
[c] Sources of data: 1951–1955 and 1956–1960 numbers of deaths and populations are from Office of Population Censuses and Surveys (1975). 1976–1980 and 1982–1984 numbers of deaths are from the annual mortality returns of the Registrar-General (Office of Population Censuses and Surveys, 1978, 1979, 1980a,b, 1982, 1983, 1984a,b, 1985a). 1976-1984 population estimates are from the revisions published after the 1981 census (Office of Population Censuses and Surveys, 1984c,d, 1985b): these differ slightly from the original (unrevised) estimates in the annual mortality returns. Wald (1985) has suggested that there may have been some underascertainment of lung cancer in 1981 compared with adjacent years, but in fact inclusion of the 1981 data would not materially alter the above 1982–1984 rates.

deliveries that took place in some countries in the 1960s and late 1950s. The chief difficulty, of course, is that in general moderate decreases cannot *confidently* be identified against a background of large increases. Hence, very few national trends can yield really useful information about the effects of changes in cigarette tar deliveries. Obviously, populations in which the epidemic has not yet emerged (i.e., where lung cancer rates are not yet dominated by cigarette smoking) cannot do so, and nor can populations in which the epidemic was still emerging rapidly during the 1960s. Thus, the most informative populations would be those for which, at least in some age/sex categories, the cigarette-induced lung cancer rates were *high but stable* during the late 1950s and early 1960s.

The only two populations that really meet this criterion are UK and Finnish middle-aged males (Table 4, Fig. 2), and, in both countries, large changes in cigarette manufacture took place during the 1960s. In Finland, however, these changes involved, among other things, one rather unusual feature, viz., replacement of what were popularly called 'Russian-style' *papyrossi* cigarettes (i.e., cigarettes with a long hollow mouthpiece instead of a filter) by conventional manufactured cigarettes. In the UK, the change was merely from one conventional type of manufactured cigarette to another, and was accompanied by a decrease in sales-weighted tar delivery that has been reliably documented (see Fig. 3, from Wald, 1985). The fact that UK male lung cancer rates had already stabilized before the cigarette tar deliveries changed substantially, together with the nature of the change in the cigarettes that was involved, makes the UK lung cancer trends uniquely informative about differences between one type of conventional cigarette and another. Moreover, male cigarette consumption in the UK (Table 5) was remarkably steady throughout the period

Table 5. Daily consumption of manufactured cigarettes per UK male aged 15 or over, 1920–1982 [a]

Quinquennial 1920–1979			Annual, 1975–1982, as percentage of mean (10.4) during 1940–1974	
1920–1924	5.8			
1925–1929	6.6		1940–1974	100%
1930–1934	7.6		1975	98%
1935–1939	9.1		1976	93%
1940–1944	10.7		1977	87%
1945–1949	10.5		1978	88%
1950–1954	9.9	Mean 1940–1974=10.4	1979	87%
1955–1959	10.5	manufactured cigarettes	1980	85%
1960–1964	10.6	daily	1981	74%
1965–1969	10.3		1982	68%
1970–1974	10.6			
1975–1979	9.4			

[a] From Wald (1985)

Table 6. Approximate proportion of cigarette-induced[a] lung cancer likely[b] to have been avoided by the percentage reductions in daily cigarette consumption in Table 5 (last column)

Age range (years)	1978	1983
30–34	4.8% [a]	18.3% [a]
35–39	3.8%	15.6%
40–44	3.1%	13.5%
45–49	2.7%	11.9%
50–54	2.3%	10.6%
55–59	2.1%	9.6%

[a] Estimated on the assumption that the ratio of the cigarette-induced lung cancer mortality in the age range A to (A+4) years among regular smokers who have stopped for Y years is approximately proportional to the fourth power of (A-Y-15): Doll & Peto (1976, 1978)

[b] Since a small proportion of lung cancer is not ascribable to tobacco, the proportion of *all* lung cancer thus avoidable might be slightly less.

from 1940 to the mid-1970s, and the changes in it during the late 1970s were too small and too recent to have had any appreciable effect on UK lung cancer mortality in the late 1970s, which further simplifies matters. Indeed, the 13% decrease in cigarette consumption during the mid-1970s was, in 1978, still so recent that it would have been expected to produce a decrease of only 3 or 4% in male lung cancer mortality at ages 35–44 (Table 6).

The percentage of UK men who described themselves, in reply to survey questionnaires, as 'smokers' had decreased during the 1970s rather more than male cigarette consumption had done, indicating that the average daily consumption per smoker was slightly higher in 1978 than it had been a few years earlier. If this finding is accepted, it suggests either that as some smokers gave up others smoked slightly more, or (perhaps more plausibly) that light smokers were more likely to give up than heavy smokers were. In neither case, however, would this change have been expected to diminish the lung cancer rate, since the excess lung cancer incidence per cigarette among heavy smokers is at least as great as that among light smokers (Doll & Peto, 1978).

Results of study of UK male trends

Hence, changes in cigarette smoking alone can account for a decrease of only a few per cent in the 1978 UK lung cancer death rates (e.g., 3 or 4% or so), and no large change in the curability of the disease has taken place since the 1950s. The actual decrease between 1958 and 1978 in mortality among men aged 35–44 between 1958 and 1978 was 40–50%, suggesting about a 40% reduction over and above any changes due to differences in the numbers smoked or in cancer therapy. These decreases, moreover, continued if anything to accelerate over the next few years, so that by 1983 the UK lung cancer death rate among men aged 35–44 was less than half what it had been in 1958 and was approximately half what it would have been expected to be just on the basis of changes in the numbers of cigarettes actually smoked (Table 6).

It is too soon to know how great these decreases will ultimately become, but it certainly appears that the lung cancer incidence associated with a given history of cigarette usage will (at least in people in early middle age) be no more than half as great in the future as it was in the 1950s. This decrease by at least half in the lung cancer risks associated with a given habit has coincided with a halving of the tar delivery per cigarette, and although other factors may have influenced the lung cancer trends, none are known that, separately or together, would be expected to have had an effect even half as large as this.

As already noted, the conclusion from Stellman's review of the case-control and prospective studies (this volume[5]; see also, however, Alderson *et al.*, 1986) was that 'relative risk for lung cancer is in rough proportion to tar yield', and that 'It is very likely that as successive cohorts of smokers are exposed to cigarettes of much lower yield for much greater proportions of their lives, the associated risks will decline even further'. Now, in the one country where an analysis of national trends would be expected to be most informative, a halving of cigarette tar deliveries appears to have been followed by an otherwise unexplained halving of the lung cancer risk, with further rapid decreases in progress. The study of national trends is usually a rather crude epidemiological tool, since it is always possible that some unsuspected factor has been overlooked, but in this instance it does appear to offer substantial support for the conclusions suggested by the 'analytic' studies.

Eventual size of risk reduction suggested by UK male trends

If these national trends are indeed due in substantial part to changes in the carcinogenicity of cigarettes, then it would be of considerable interest to know how large the decrease

[5] See p. 197.

will eventually become. But, this cannot yet be answered for it is not possible to predict reliably whether the main effect of changing tar deliveries should be rapid or slow to emerge. If the timing of any effects of tar-level changes were analogous to the timing of the effects of cessation of smoking, then within only 10–15 years of tar-level decreases any changes in lung cancer would become apparent. In view, however, of the great importance of cigarette smoking in *early* adult life (Peto, this volume[6]), it is possible that tar levels experienced in early adult life might be importantly relevant to lung cancer risks many decades later, in which case the full effects of any changes in tar delivery might take several decades to emerge. If both effects applied, then one might expect to see (at least in a country such as the UK, where lung cancer rates had stabilized before tar-level reductions were introduced) decreases in lung cancer rates in adults of all ages as a result of the past 15 or 20 years of lowered tar levels, with the largest percentage decreases occurring, at least for the present, in people in the youngest age groups.

This does indeed appear to be more or less what is currently being seen among UK males (Tables 2 and 4), so it is possible that the percentage change in those in early middle age may provide the first clear indication of what can ultimately be expected for adults of all ages, even though only a small minority of cancer deaths take place in people in early middle age.

This would suggest that the introduction of cigarette tar-level reductions in countries where tar levels remain high might (unless it diverted attention from the much more important need to discourage smoking) ultimately avoid about half of all cigarette-induced lung cancer. In countries where lung cancer accounts for about one-third of all tobacco-related deaths, therefore, such changes might in turn avoid 10 or 20% of all tobacco-related deaths, if it is assumed that such changes have no comparable effect on other smoking-related diseases or on the extent to which people choose to smoke.

REFERENCES

Alderson, M.R., Lee, P.N. & Wang, R. (1985) Risk of lung cancer chronic bronchitis, ischaemic heart disease and stroke in relation to the type of cigarette smoked. *J. Epidemiol. Community Health*, ***39***, 286–293

American Cancer Society (1981) US tar/nicotine levels dropping. *World Smok. Health*, ***62***, 47

Doll, R. & Peto, R. (1976) Mortality in relation to smoking: 20 years' observations on male British doctors. *Br. med. J.*, ***ii***, 1524–1535

Doll, R. & Peto, R. (1978) Cigarette smoking and bronchial carcinoma: dose and time relationships among regular smokers and lifelong non-smokers. *J. Epidemiol. Community Health*, ***32***, 303–313

Doll, R. & Peto, R. (1981) The causes of cancer: quantitative estimates of avoidable risks of cancer in the United States today. *J. natl Cancer Inst.*, ***66***, 1191–1308

Hill, C. & Flamant, R. (1985) A major cause of epidemic: the tobacco consumption increase in France (Fr.) *Rev. Epidemiol. Santé publ.*, ***33***, 387–395

[6] See p. 23.

IARC (1986) *IARC Monographs on the Evaluation of the Carcinogenic Risk of Chemicals to Humans, Vol. 38, Tobacco Smoking,* Lyon

Lee, P.N. (1975) *Tobacco Consumption in Various Countries (Research Paper 6, Fourth Edition),* London, Tobacco Research Council

Lee, P.N. (1976) *Statistics of Smoking in the United Kingdom (Research Paper 1, Seventh Edition),* London, Tobacco Research Council

Napalkov, N.P., Tserkovny, G.F., Merabishvili, V.M., Parkin, D.M., Smans, M. & Muir, C., eds (1983) *Cancer Incidence in the USSR,* 2nd revised ed. *(IARC Scientific Publications No. 48),* Lyon, International Agency for Research on Cancer

Office of Population Censuses and Surveys (1975) *Cancer Mortality, England and Wales, 1911–1970 (Studies on Medical and Population Subjects No. 29),* London, Her Majesty's Stationery Office

Office of Population Censuses and Surveys (1978, 1979, 1980a,b, 1982, 1983, 1984a,b, 1985a) *Mortality Statistics, Cause, for the Years 1976, 1977, 1978, 1979, 1980, 1981, 1982, 1983, 1984 (Series DH2, Nos 3–11),* London, Her Majesty's Stationery Office

Office of Population Censuses and Surveys (1984c) *Final Mid-1981 and Revised Mid-1961 to Mid-1980 Population Estimates for England and Wales (OPCS Monitor PP1 84/1 (10 January 1984)),* London, Her Majesty's Stationery Office

Office of Population Censuses and Surveys (1984d) *Mid-1983, Final Mid-1981 and Mid-1982 Population Estimates for England and Wales (OPCS Monitor PP1 84/3 (8 May 1984)),* London, Her Majesty's Stationery Office

Office of Population Censuses and Surveys (1985b) *Mid-1984 Population Estimates for England and Wales (OPCS Monitor PP1 85/1 (14 May 1985)),* London, Her Majesty's Stationery Office

Peto, R. & Doll, R. (1984) *Keynote address: The control of lung cancer.* In: Mizell, M. & Correa, P., eds, *Lung Cancer Causes and Prevention,* Deerfield Beach, FL, Verlag Chemie International

US Surgeon-General (1979) *Smoking and Health – A Report of the Surgeon-General (Publication No. PHS 79–50066),* Washington DC, US Government Printing Office

US Surgeon-General (1982) *Smoking and Health: Cancer – A Report of the Surgeon-General (Publication No. DHHS PHS 82–50179),* Washington DC, US Government Printing Office

US Surgeon-General (1984) *The Health Consequences of Smoking: Chronic Obstructive Lung Disease – A Report of the Surgeon-General (Publication No. DHHS PHS 84–50205),* Washington DC, US Government Printing Office

Wald, N.J. (1985) *Smoking.* In: Vessey, M.P. & Gray, M., eds, *Cancer Risks and Prevention,* Oxford, Oxford University Press, pp. 44–67

Wald, N.J., Doll, R. & Copeland, G. (1981) Trends in tar, nicotine and carbon monoxide levels of UK cigarettes manufactured since 1934. *Br. med. J.,* ***282,*** 763–765

Wald, N.J., Idle, M., Boreham, J. & Bailey, A. (1983) Inhaling and lung cancer: an anomaly explained. *Br. med. J.,* ***287,*** 1273–1275

Warner, K.E. (1978) Possible increases in the under-reporting of cigarette consumption. *J. Am. stat. Assoc.,* ***73,*** 314–318

Waterhouse, J., Muir, C., Correa, P. & Powell, J., eds (1976) *Cancer Incidence in Five Continents Vol. III (IARC Scientific Publications No. 15),* Lyon, International Agency for Research on Cancer

EXPERIMENTAL STUDIES ON THE MUTAGENICITY AND RELATED EFFECTS OF LOW-TAR AND HIGH-TAR CIGARETTES IN RELATION TO SMOKER EXPOSURES

M. SORSA

Institute of Occupational Health,
Department of Industrial Hygiene and Toxicology,
Helsinki, Finland

INTRODUCTION

Tobacco smoke is a very complex mixture of particles and gases containing at least 3800 different compounds. An IARC Working Group recently evaluated 40 of the chemicals as having shown sufficient evidence of carcinogenicity in animals, and the number of chemical compounds having shown some carcinogenic effects is considerably higher (IARC, 1986). However, the toxicological properties of most of the chemicals are still unknown, and almost nothing is known about their interactions in the complex mixture.

During the last decade of research on the experimental mutagenicity/carcinogenicity of tobacco smoke, various compounds have been suggested as the candidate for the major carcinogenic determinant of smoking, including:

- polynuclear aromatic hydrocarbons in the tar fraction (e.g., Wynder & Hoffmann, 1967)
- protein and amino acid pyrolysates produced in the burning tip of the cigarette (e.g., Mizusaki *et al.*, 1977)
- tobacco-specific *N*-nitrosamines (e.g., Hoffmann *et al.*, 1974, 1984)
- active oxygen generated from cigarette smoke (Nakayama *et al.*, 1985).

The multistage character of the carcinogenic process together with the complexity of the exposing agent, the tobacco smoke, and the variables in exposure have as yet hindered firm conclusions about the identification and quantification of the significant carcinogens in tobacco smoke. The reasonable ease of short-term testing, as compared with long-term animal bioassays, provides crucial methods to determine which substances in cigarette smoke are those transforming human cells to malignant ones, and which would be the feasible ways to design less harmful cigarettes. The experimental data available on the mutagenicity of 'the less hazardous cigarette' is discussed below.

Reductions of the tar, nicotine and carbon monoxide components in cigarette smoke have mainly been achieved by filter technology, with few changes in the cigarettes themselves. The yields are analytically measured from smoke obtained in standardized machine smoking, while the levels of exposure of the smoker may vary considerably depending on his way of smoking. Reduction of the tar does not necessarily decrease other potentially hazardous compounds in smoke, e.g., nitrosamines (Hoffmann *et al.*, 1984). For this reason also, discussion on studies using biological and biochemical intake markers among smokers of low-tar and high-tar cigarettes have been included.

EXPERIMENTAL STUDIES ON MUTAGENICITY

Cigarette smoke condensate

Most of the studies related to tobacco mutagenesis have been performed on cigarette smoke condensates (CSCs) and using the *Salmonella*/microsome test system for detection of mutagenicity (see overview of *de Marini,* 1983). The results are almost boringly positive, showing variation in activity depending on the type of CSC, source and types of metabolic system, and the tester strains of *Salmonella* used. Since the first report of the mutagenicity of CSC appeared (Kier *et al.*, 1974), at least twenty reports have been published. These data have been summarized (IARC, 1986).

In most experiments CSC has been found to be mutagenic only in the presence of an exogenous metabolic system. Several characteristics of tobacco and cigarettes have been shown to affect the mutagenicity of CSC; amount of total nitrogen and amount of Burley tobacco were positively correlated with mutagenicity, while sugar content and age of tobacco leaves were negatively correlated with the mutagenicity of the CSC (Mizusaki *et al.*, 1977).

The findings on the mutagenicity of fractionated CSC reveal that in the *Salmonella* system, the basic fractions are the most potent, while the acidic and neutral fractions are usually only weakly mutagenic. This may be due to the specific sensitivity towards aromatic amines present in the basic fractions of the tester strain TA1538 used.

CSC has been shown to be mutagenic also in various eukaryotic organisms and with different genetic endpoints (Table 1).

Table 1. Positive responses obtained with cigarette smoke condensate in various eukaryotic tests[a]

Test organism	Endpoint studied	
	Point mutations	Chromosomal damage
Yeast	+	
Plant cells		+
Fruit fly	+	
Rodent cells *in vitro*	+	+
Human cells *in vitro*		+

[a] Data from de Marini (1983)

It is interesting to notice that in tests for chromosomal damage (sister chromatid exchanges, SCEs), CSC was found also to be active in the absence of an exogenous metabolic system (de Raat, 1979; Hopkin & Evans, 1979; Sorsa *et al.*, 1982; Salomaa *et al.*, 1985). These results show, contrary to findings in the *Salmonella* assay, that CSC also contains direct-acting mutagens that are usually not detected in the Ames test.

The role of benzo[*a*]pyrene, an indirect mutagen, was estimated to be of minor importance in the mutagen spectrum of CSC. In the human lymphocyte system, the amount of benzo[*a*]pyrene needed to produce a significant response of SCEs was equivalent to 50–250 cigarettes, while CSC produced from only one-eightieth of a cigarette induced a positive response in the test (Hopkin & Evans, 1979). In the Chinese hamster ovary (CHO) cell system, the potency difference of CSC and benzo[*a*]pyrene alone was even higher, while less than 10 mg (about one-hundreth) from the weight of a cigarette used to produce CSC was enough to induce SCEs (Salomaa *et al.*, 1985). The mutagenicity of CSC thus appears to be about 20 000 times higher than expected from the benzo[*a*]pyrene content of the cigarette.

CSC produced from low-tar and high-tar cigarettes

There are surprisingly few studies in which the efficiency of filter technology in relation to the mutagenicity of the CSC (or mainstream smoke) has been assessed. Sato *et al.* (1977) found that in the *Salmonella*/microsome test system, the number of revertants was nearly the same when calculated per weight of CSC from low-tar or high-tar cigarettes. Furthermore, on a weight-for-weight basis, CSCs produced from cigarettes of different tar categories induced a roughly similar response of SCEs in cultured human lymphocytes (Hopkin & Evans, 1984).

When very low-tar cigarettes (1 mg) were used to produce CSC, the SCE response in human lymphocytes was found to be even higher per weight basis than with the other low- or medium-tar CSCs (Sorsa *et al.*, 1982). In the CHO cell system, known to be especially sensitive for the direct-acting mutagens present in CSC, a negative correlation was observed between the tar content of seven brands of filter cigarettes and the ability of the condensate to induce SCEs; the CSC from cigarettes with the highest amount of tar had the lowest activity per weight basis in inducing SCEs, and vice versa (Salomaa *et al.*, 1985).

The experimental data on mutagenicity, both in prokaryotic as well as in eukaryotic test systems thus points to the insignificant role of the tar content in determining the genetic activity of the CSC, on a weight basis.

Cigarette smoke

Experimental studies on the mutagenicity of cigarette smoke are much fewer, even though their relevance considering human active or passive exposure would be much higher than studies on artificially produced smoke condensates.

Extracts of aged sidestream and exhaled smoke collected on filters were shown to be mutagenic in the *Salmonella*/microsome test (Bos *et al.*, 1983; Löfroth *et al.*, 1983). Ong *et al.* (1984) showed that sidestream smoke was mutagenic also when tested directly on the bacterial plates.

Table 2. Experimental evidence on mutagenicity and related effects of tobacco smoke in eukaryotic tests[a]

Test organism	Endpoint studied	
	Point mutations	Chromosomal damage
Yeast	+	
Plant cells		+[b]
Fruit fly	+	
Rodent cells *in vitro*		+
Human cells *in vitro*		+[b]
Rodents *in vivo*		+

[a] Data from de Marini (1983); see also text
[b] Gas phase of smoke only

In CHO cells, using SCE induction as the parameter of genetic activity, mainstream cigarette smoke collected on filters was highly active, so that a positive response was obtained already with smoke generated from $1/160$th of the cigarette, while $1/20$th of the same brand of medium-tar cigarette was needed to produce the amount of CSC causing a positive response (Salomaa *et al.*, unpublished data). Both the gas phase as well as the particulate phase of mainstream smoke were active both with and without an exogenous metabolic system.

In human lung carcinoma cells, smoke from one filter-tipped cigarette (tar amount not given) produced approximately 10 000 single-strand breaks in DNA (Nakayama *et al.*, 1985), thus demonstrating the high genotoxic potency of cigarette smoke. The available evidence on mutagenicity of tobacco smoke in eukaryotic assays is briefly summarized in Table 2.

STUDIES ON SMOKERS OF HIGH-TAR AND LOW-TAR CIGARETTES

Biochemical intake markers

Three constituents of tobacco smoke are routinely used to measure smoke exposure in human samples: carbon monoxide, nicotine and hydrogen cyanide; nicotine and its metabolite cotinine are the only tobacco-specific markers of intake.

A rough dose-response relationship is observed between the number of recently smoked cigarettes and levels of nicotine, its metabolite cotinine and carboxyhaemoglobin. Still, the nicotine and tar yields of cigarettes seem to be poor predictors of intake-marker levels in smokers.

Smokers of low-tar cigarettes have been shown to compensate for intake of nicotine, e.g., by inhaling more than smokers of high-tar yields (Herning *et al.*, 1981), or by behavioural misuse of ventilated filters (Kozlowski *et al.*, 1980). The modification of the smoking techniques is reflected by the finding that smokers of low-tar cigarettes had nicotine concentrations in blood, urine and saliva at the same range as middle-tar and high-tar cigarette smokers (Feyerabend *et al.*, 1980; Russell *et al.*, 1980). Furthermore, Benowitz *et al.* (1983) demonstrated that serum cotinine concentration is proportional to the number of cigarettes smoked and not to the certified nicotine content of the cigarette. In a study of 240 subjects with various smoking habits, no correlation was observed between brand yield of tar and the exposure markers carboxyhaemoglobin, breath carbon monoxide, plasma cotinine or salivary and plasma thiocyanate, when level of consumption was similar (Rickert & Robinson, 1981). In an experimental seven-week follow-up study, no differences were seen in carboxyhaemoglobin values of smokers of low-tar (5 mg) and medium-tar (16 mg) cigarettes (Sorsa *et al.*, 1984). In the same smoker groups, the urinary thioether excretion was similar in the low-tar and medium-tar cigarette smokers, although significantly higher than in nonsmokers (Heinonen *et al.*, 1983).

Even though the biochemical measures do not, in a simple way, quantitatively indicate the intake of carcinogenic compounds in cigarette smoke, the results of similar intake of these markers among low-tar and high-tar cigarette smokers show the importance of modifications of smoking for the actual exposure of the smoker.

Urine mutagenicity

Yamasaki and Ames (1977), employing XAD-2 resin to concentrate the urine and the *Salmonella*/microsome system as indicator, were the first to show that cigarette smokers have mutagenic urine. The mutagenicity of the urine of smokers has since been confirmed by several research groups. A trend for dose-response relationship seems to exist between the level of exposure to smoke and the extent of mutagenic activity in the urine (Jaffe *et al.*, 1983; Kriebel *et al.*, 1983). Concentrates of urine from cigarette smokers are usually mutagenic only after metabolic activation, suggesting that enzymatic splitting of conjugates may be necessary before activity can be detected.

Kobayashi and Hayatsu (1984) and Kado *et al.* (1985) have studied the kinetics of the excretion of mutagens in the urine of cigarette smokers. The peak mutagenic activity of urine collected from a smoker appeared in a few hours after the start of smoking and the activity decreased to pre-smoking levels in approximately 12 hours. The elimination of smoking-related mutagen from the body followed first-order kinetics (Kado *et al.*, 1985).

On the basis of the rapid excretion kinetics of urinary mutagenicity caused by smoking, the effects of high-tar or low-tar cigarette smoking can be rather easily evaluated. In groups of some 70 urine samples of low-tar and medium-tar cigarette smokers, no differences were observed in the urinary mutagenicity levels (Sorsa *et al.*, 1984). In a double-blind, cross-over study of volunteer smokers, a dose response in the number of cigarettes smoked and urinary mutagenicity was seen without differences among groups of low-tar and high-tar cigarette smokers (Tuomisto *et al.*, 1985).

Chromosomal effects

There is substantial evidence from a great number of studies that smoking is related to an increased prevalence of structural chromosome aberrations as well as sister chromatid exchanges (SCEs) in peripheral blood lymphocytes of cigarette smokers.

The increase of chromosome aberrations in smokers is usually not higher than three- or four-fold compared with otherwise unexposed nonsmokers, and very rarely is a clear dose response observed (Obe *et al.*, 1984). With regard to the intra-chromosomal exchange events seen as SCEs, the dose-response relationship has been reported in several studies (Lambert *et al.*, 1982, Vijayalaxmi & Evans, 1982). Such a dose-related effect is usually referred to groups of heavy, medium and light smokers, but also the duration of smoker years, measured as cumulative pack-years has been reported to be correlated to the level of SCEs observed (Livingstone & Fineman, 1983; Husgafvel-Pursiainen *et al.*, 1984).

Few studies have been designed to detect differences in the chromosomal parameters of low-tar and high-tar cigarette smokers. In a short-term follow-up study of smokers, no differences were observed in the levels of SCEs between groups of low-tar and medium-tar cigarette smokers (Sorsa *et al.*, 1984). In a larger study, where the smoking history of the subjects was determined only on the basis of the present status of smoking, no significant differences were found in the SCE frequencies of low-tar and high-tar cigarette smokers (Wulf *et al.*, 1983). Further studies should be designed on long-term, low-tar or high-tar cigarette smokers, since the response to smoking seen as increased SCEs in lymphocytes is known to persist a longer time and to be induced only gradually (Lambert *et al.*, 1982).

CONCLUSIONS

The chemical composition and the genetically active compartments of cigarette smoke are extremely complex, and the smoker exposure and intake of hazardous compounds from cigarette smoke greatly depend on the modifications of smoking habits.

Both cigarette smoke and cigarette smoke condensates have been shown to be mutagenic in various test organisms using different genetic endpoints. In smokers, the mutagenicity related to smoking can be detected in the urine of smokers. Tobacco smoking results in chromosomal damage observable as increased prevalence of structural chromosome aberrations and sister chromatid exchanges in blood cells of smokers. Positive evidence exists for a dose-response relationship between the number of cigarettes consumed and the prevalence of sister chromatid exchanges observed.

The experimental evidence on the mutagenic activity of cigarette smoke condensates produced from low-, medium- or high-tar cigarettes clearly shows, on the basis of both prokaryotic and eukaryotic test systems, that the activity measured on a weight-for-weight basis is similar or possibly even higher in some very low-tar CSCs. Naturally, a lot more low-tar than high-tar cigarettes will be needed to obtain the same amount of CSC.

The biochemical intake markers, e.g., carboxyhaemoglobin, nicotine, cotinine or thiocyanate in biological fluids, poorly differentiate smokers of low-tar and high-tar cigarettes. The few studies so far performed to investigate the relation of urinary mutagenicity or prevalence of sister chromatid exchanges and the tar yield of cigarettes smoked have not given evidence about differences in the response of these parameters in groups of smokers of low-tar or high-tar yield cigarettes.

On the basis of presently available experimental evidence and intake studies on smokers, the issue of smoking-induced cancer in relation to reductions of tar in cigarettes is still controversial.

REFERENCES

Benowitz, N.L., Hall, S.M., Herning, R.I., Jacob, P., III, Jones, R.T. & Osman, A.-L. (1983) Smokers of low-yield cigarettes do not consume less nicotine. *New Engl. J. Med.*, ***30,*** 139–142

Bos, R.P., Theuws, J.L.G. & Henderson, P.T. (1983) Excretion of mutagens in human urine after passive smoking. *Cancer Lett.*, ***19,*** 85–90

Feyerabend, C., Higenbottam, T. & Russell, M.A.H. (1980) Nicotine concentrations in urine and saliva of smokers and non-smokers. *Br. med. J.*, ***284,*** 1002–1004

Heinonen, T., Kytöniemi, V., Sorsa, M. & Vainio, H. (1983) Urinary excretion of thioethers among low-tar and medium-tar cigarette smokers. *Int. Arch. occup. environ. Health*, ***52,*** 11–16

Herning, R.I., Jones, R.T., Bachman, J. & Mines, A.H. (1981) Puff volume increases when low-nicotine cigarettes are smoked. *Br. med. J.*, ***283,*** 187–189

Hoffmann, D., Hecht, S.S., Orneff, R.M. & Wynder, E.L. (1974) *N*-Nitrosonor-nicotine in tobacco. *Science*, ***186,*** 265–267

Hoffmann, D., Brunnemann, K.D., Adams, J.D. & Hecht, S.S. (1984) *Formation and analysis of* N-*nitrosamines in tobacco products and their endogenous formation in consumers.* In: O'Neill, I.K., von Borstel, R.C., Miller, C.T., Long, J. & Bartsch, H., eds, N-*Nitroso Compounds: Occurrence, Biological Effects and Relevance to Human Cancer (IARC Scientific Publications No. 57)*, Lyon, International Agency for Research on Cancer, pp. 733–762

Hopkin, J.M. & Evans, H.J. (1979) Cigarette smoke condensates damage DNA in cultured human lymphocytes. *Nature*, ***279,*** 241–242

Hopkin, J.M. & Evans, H.J. (1984) Cellular effects of smoke from "safer" cigarettes. *Br. J. Cancer*, ***49,*** 333–336

Husgafvel-Pursiainen, K., Sorsa, M., Järventaus, H., & Norppa, H. (1984) Sister-chromatid exchanges in lymphocytes of smokers in an experimental study. *Mutat. Res.*, ***138,*** 197–203

IARC (1986) *IARC Monographs on the Evaluation of the Carcinogenic Risk of Chemicals to Humans*, Vol. 38, *Tobacco Smoking*, Lyon

Jaffe, R.L., Nicholson, W.J. & Garro, A.J. (1983) Urinary mutagen levels in smokers. *Cancer Lett.*, ***20,*** 37–42

Kado, N.Y., Eisenstadt, E. & Hsieh, D.P.H. (1985) The kinetics of mutagen excretion in the urine of cigarette smokers. *Mutat. Res.* (in press)

Kier, L.D., Yamasaki, E. & Ames, B.N. (1974) Detection of mutagenic activity in cigarette smoke condensates. *Proc. natl Acad. Sci. USA*, ***71,*** 1159–1163

Kobayashi, H. & Hayatsu, H. (1984) A time-course study on the mutagenicity of smoker's urine. *Gann*, ***75,*** 489–493

Kozlowski, L.T., Frecker, R.C., Khouw, V. & Pope, M.A. (1980) The misuse of "less-hazardous" cigarettes and its detection: hole blocking of ventilated filters. *Am. J. Public Health*, ***70,*** 1202–1203

Kriebel, D., Commoner, B., Bolinger, D., Bronsdon, A., Gold, J. & Henry, J. (1983) Detection of occupational exposure to genotoxic agents with a urinary mutagen assay. *Mutat. Res.*, ***108,*** 67–79

Lambert, B., Bredberg, A., McKenzie, W. & Sten, M. (1982) Sister chromatid exchange in human populations: the effect of smoking, drug treatment, and occupational exposure. *Cytogenet. Cell Genet.*, ***33***, 62–67

Livingstone, G.K. & Fineman, R.M. (1983) Correlation of human lymphocytes SCE frequency with smoking history. *Mutat. Res.*, ***119***, 59–64

Löfroth, G., Nilsson, L. & Alfheim, I. (1983) *Passive smoking and urban air pollution:* Salmonella*/microsome mutagenicity of simultaneously collected indoor and outdoor particulate matter.* In: Waters, M.D., Shandu, S.S., Lewtas, J., Claxton, L., Chernoff, N. & Nesnow, S., eds, *Short-term Bioassays in the Analysis of Complex Environmental Mixtures III,* New York and London, Plenum Press, pp. 515–525

de Marini, D.M. (1983) Genotoxicity of tobacco smoke and tobacco smoke condensate. *Mutat. Res.*, ***114***, 59–89

Mizusaki, S., Okamoto, H., Abiyama, A. & Fubukara, Y. (1977) Relation between chemical constituents of tobacco and mutagenic activity of cigarette smoke condensate. *Mutat. Res.*, ***48***, 319–326

Nakayama, T., Kanebo, M., Kodama, M. & Nagata, C. (1985) Cigarette smoke induces DNA single-strand breaks in human cells. *Nature*, ***314***, 462–464

Obe, G., Heller, W.-D. & Vogt, H.-J. (1984) *Mutagenic activity of cigarette smoke.* In: Obe, G., ed., *Mutation in Man,* Berlin, Springer-Verlag, pp. 223–246

Ong, T., Stewart, J. & Whong, W.-Z. (1984) A simple *in situ* mutagenicity test system for detection of mutagenic air pollutants. *Mutat. Res.*, ***139***, 177–181

de Raat, W.K. (1979) Comparison on the introduction by cigarette smoke condensates of sister-chromatid exchanges in Chinese hamster cells and of mutations in *Salmonella typhimurium. Mutat. Res.*, ***66***, 253–259

Rickert, W.S. & Robinson, J.C. (1981) Estimating the hazards of less hazardous cigarettes. II. Study of cigarette yields of nicotine, carbon monoxide, and hydrogen cyanide in relation to levels of cotinine, carboxyhemoglobin, and thiocyanate in smokers. *J. Toxicol. environ. Health*, ***7***, 391–403

Russell, M.A.H., Jarvis, M., Iyer, R. & Feyerabend, C. (1980) Relation of nicotine yield of cigarettes to blood nicotine concentrations in smokers. *Br. med. J.*, ***280***, 972–976

Salomaa, S., Sorsa, M., Alfheim, L. & Leppänen, A. (1985) Genotoxic effects of smoke emissions in mammalian cells. *Environ. Int.*, ***11*** (in press)

Sato, S., Seino, Y., Ohka, T., Yahagi, T., Nagao, M., Matsuhima, T. & Sugimura, T. (1977) Mutagenicity of smoke condensates from cigarettes, cigars and pipe tobacco. *Cancer Lett.*, ***3***, 1–8

Sorsa, M., Norppa, H., Leppänen, A. & Rimpelä, M. (1982) Induction of sister-chromatid exchange in human lymphocytes by smoke condensates from different brands of cigarette. *Mutat. Res.*, ***103***, 149–153

Sorsa, M., Falck, K., Heinonen, T., Vainio, H., Norppa, H. & Rimpelä, M. (1984) Detection of exposure to mutagenic compound in low-tar and medium-tar cigarette smokers. *Environ. Res.*, ***33***, 312–321

Tuomisto, J., Kolonen, S., Sorsa, M. & Einistö, P. (1985) No difference between urinary mutagenicity in smokers of low-tar and medium-tar cigarettes: A double-blind crossover study. *Arch. Toxicol.* (in press)

Vijayalaxmi & Evans, H.J. (1982) *In vivo* and *in vitro* effects of cigarette smoke on chromosomal damage and sister-chromatid exchange in human peripheral blood lymphocytes. *Mutat. Res.*, ***92***, 321–332

Wulf, H.C., Husum, B. & Niebuhr, E. (1983) Sister chromatid exchanges in smokers of high-tar cigarettes, low-tar cigarettes, cheroots and pipe tobacco. *Hereditas*, ***98***, 225–228

Wynder, E.L. & Hoffmann, D. (1967) *Tobacco and Tobacco Smoke. Studies in Experimental Carcinogenesis,* New York, Academic Press, 730 pp.

Yamasaki, E. & Ames, B.N. (1977) Concentration of mutagens from urine with the nonpolar resin XAD–2: cigarette smokers have mutagenic urine. *Proc. natl Acad. Sci. USA,* ***74***, 3555–3559

INFLUENCE OF CIGARETTE YIELD ON RISK OF CORONARY HEART DISEASE AND CHRONIC OBSTRUCTIVE PULMONARY DISEASE

S.D. STELLMAN

American Cancer Society, Inc.
4 West 35th Street,
New York, NY 10001, USA

INTRODUCTION

There is good reason to expect cigarette smoke to be toxic to the cardiovascular system. Nicotine produces numerous pharmacological effects, including increases in blood pressure and heart rate, increases in free fatty acids and catecholamines, and stimulation of the central nervous system. Carbon monoxide reduces the amount of oxygen available to heart muscle. The gas phase of cigarette smoke also contains numerous ciliatoxic chemicals, leading one to expect an effect on the respiratory system as well (US Department of Health and Human Services, 1984).

Therefore, there is some reason to expect that a lowering of the concentration of toxic agents in cigarette smoke inhaled by the smoker should lead to a reduction in the risk of diseases of the cardiovascular and respiratory systems. However, the situation is not so clearcut as for cancer risk in relation to tar yield (Stellman, this volume[1]). While lower nicotine yields (as determined with automatic smoking machines) are attributable in some measure to more efficient filtration, use of filter cigarettes may not necessarily lead to reduced risk of disease, especially if the role of carbon monoxide is comparable to that of nicotine. Whereas tar and nicotine yields are generally correlated with each other, carbon monoxide yield is correlated with neither, and in fact has been found to be higher in some filter cigarettes than in nonfilter cigarettes (Borland *et al.*, 1983).

In this paper we examine the epidemiological evidence relating to the risk of coronary heart disease (CHD) and chronic obstructive pulmonary disease (COPD) in smokers of cigarettes of varying yields. In spite of a fairly large number of published studies, the case for risk reduction is not a strong one. This is due to a number of design and methodological problems, as well as to problems in interpretation of results. For one thing, the literature

[1] See p. 197.

on CHD and COPD contains numerous cross-sectional studies, that is, studies of prevalence of specific symptoms among smokers of different types of cigarettes. While prevalence studies are useful in assessing the health status of different groups of individuals, they are notoriously difficult to interpret in etiological terms, because one can never be certain whether the disease has influenced the risk factor.

Estimation of dosage for the purpose of constructing dose-response relationships is difficult because of the uncertainty surrounding the choice of which smoke component to use. Some studies have used cigarette carbon monoxide yield, some have used serum carboxyhaemoglobin, some nicotine yield, and some have expressed exposure in terms of only filter *versus* nonfilter cigarette smoking.

Choice of endpoints to describe 'disease status' is also problematical. Some of the studies were designed to obtain incidence or death rates in large groups over a period of many years, while others examined only changes in lung function and various respiratory symptoms over a fairly short period. In many studies described below, health data were collected by questionnaire only, without clinical examination or other source of verification. Subjects in some of those studies have been classified as having 'possible angina' or 'possible claudication', but such rubrics lack the rigour attained in studies where uniform clinical examinations were conducted, and make it hard to compare different studies with each other.

Another difficulty which arises in attempting to reconcile the findings of the various studies with each other is the lack of uniformity with which rates are reported. Few of the follow-up studies were analysed according to the standard life-table type of procedures. In some, 'mortality' was calculated as nothing more than number dead over initial number alive, irrespective of when deaths occurred, or the length of the follow-up period. This makes it practically impossible to compare rates between studies.

A final methodological difficulty occurs particularly for CHD studies, where other major risk factors for CHD, such as blood pressure and serum lipids, have not always been measured, leading to the possibility of confounding or other biases.

CIGARETTE YIELD AND CORONARY HEART DISEASE

We have reviewed three cross-sectional studies which dealt with prevalence of atherosclerotic conditions, such as angina, four follow-up studies, and one case-control study of myocardial infarction.

Cross-sectional studies of CHD

In 1974, Heliovaara and colleagues examined 1068 Finnish men, aged 59–74 years, who had initially been enrolled in 1959 in a follow-up study of CHD. As shown in Table 1, the relative prevalence of three conditions, claudication, chest-pain attack, and definite CHD, was greater in men whose carboxyhaemoglobin (COHb) levels exceeded 0.5%, compared to men with COHb levels of 0.5% and below. A dose response was observed for claudication (Heliovaara *et al.,* 1978).

In 1969, Wald *et al.* (1973) examined 1085 male and female Danish workers, and found blood COHb levels significantly associated with the prevalence of ischaemic heart disease

Table 1. Prevalence odds ratios among 789 Finnish men for definite occurrence of three cardiovascular conditions relative to unaffected men[a]

Condition	Prevalence odds ratio			
	Carboxyhaemoglobin (%)			
	Below 0.5	0.6–2.0	2.1–4.0	4.1+
Claudication	1.00	1.42	2.54	5.75
Chest-pain attack	1.00	2.36	2.32	2.86
Definite CHD[b]	1.00	1.42	1.59	1.58

[a] From Heliovaara *et al.* (1978)
[b] CHD, coronary heart disease

and intermittent claudication. In the age group 30–69 years, a person with a COHb level of 5% or more was 21 times as likely to be affected as a person of the same age and sex, with similar smoking history, but with a level of less than 3%.

On the other hand, in home interviews conducted in 1972 in the UK with 12 736 men and women aged 37–67 years, Dean *et al.* (1978) observed no differences between smokers of filter and nonfilter cigarettes in the prevalence of angina, possible claudication and possible infarction.

Follow-up studies of CHD

Four studies of CHD incidence or mortality have been reported, and one very large study is now in progress in the USA.

The American Cancer Society enrolled over one million men and women aged 40 years and over, in 25 states, in a prospective study in 1959. Follow-ups were conducted annually through 1966, and again in 1971 and 1972. Analyses of CHD death rates in relation to smoking habits were previously published by Hammond (1966) and by Hammond and Garfinkel (1969).

Hammond *et al.* (1976, 1977) also presented evidence from this study showing that smokers of 'low tar-nicotine' cigarettes had CHD mortality rates 81–93% of those of smokers of 'high tar-nicotine' cigarettes, using a matched group analysis which permitted adjustment for many variables at once, including age, race, number of cigarettes smoked per day, age smoking began, urban/rural residence, education, job exposure to chemicals, X-rays, or other toxicants, history of prior illness, and calendar period.

For the present review we have re-calculated the standard mortality ratios (SMRs) according to quantity smoked daily by current smokers and by tar yield of cigarette at baseline, for CHD death in men during 1960–1966, the six years when annual follow-up was done. Calculations were also restricted to this period to minimize effects of changes in smoking habits.

Results are shown in Figure 1. There were 6050 deaths from CHD during this period. For statistical convenience, the reference population is the largest subgroup, namely, smokers of 'medium tar-nicotine' cigarettes, who smoked 20 cigarettes per day. For all other tar-nicotine and quantity categories of smokers, as well as for exsmokers and non-

Fig. 1. Standardized mortality ratios for coronary heart disease in males, among nonsmokers, exsmokers and current smokers of low-, medium- and high-tar/nicotine cigarettes (defined by Hammond *et al.*, 1976). The group was enrolled in 1959, and followed up through 1966.

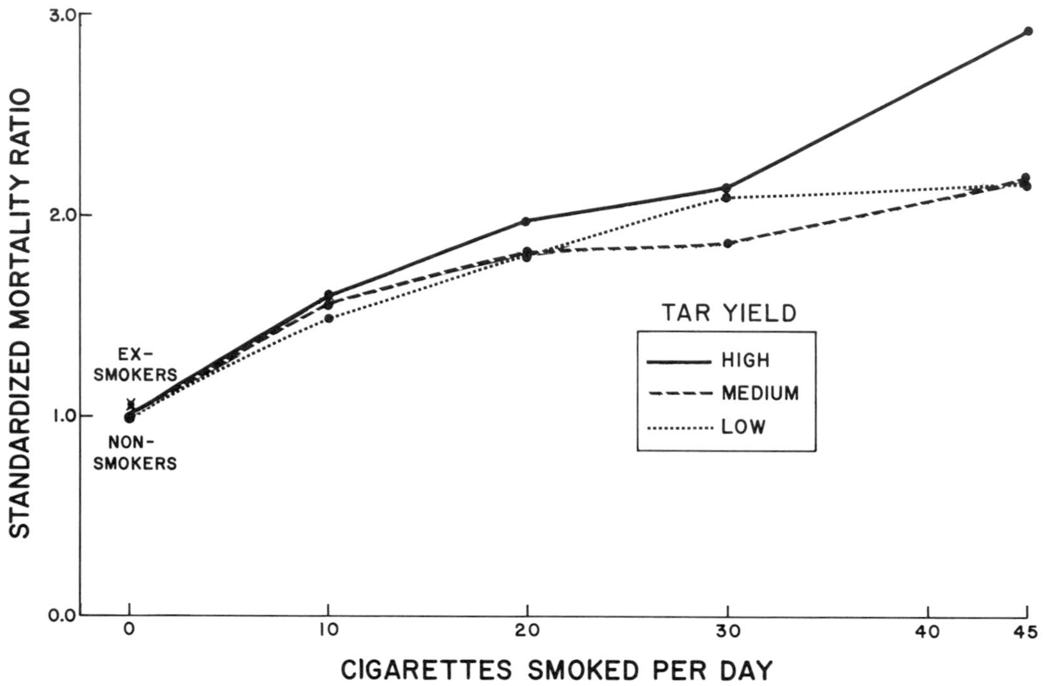

smokers, expected numbers of deaths were computed by multiplying age-calendar-year-specific rates of CHD death in the reference population by the person-years of exposure to risk of dying in the target group, and summing over age-calendar-year strata. The SMR is the number of observed divided by expected deaths. Data were renormalized to give lifetime nonsmokers an SMR of 1.0.

At each tar-nicotine level, the SMR increased with quantity smoked, in an approximately linear dose-response relationship. For current smokers, at each value of daily quantity smoked, the SMR for the 'high tar-nicotine' cigarette smokers exceeded that for the 'medium' group, which in turn exceeded that for the 'low' group, except at 30 cigarettes per day. Lifetime nonsmokers had death rates well below any of the current smokers, irrespective of cigarette yield for the latter.

We have recently begun a new prospective study of 1.2 million men and women in all 50 states, to examine, among other hypotheses, the effect on mortality from various causes of smoking the much lower-yield cigarettes now available in the USA (Stellman & Garfinkel, 1986). Follow-up is being conducted biennially through 1988.

Castelli *et al.* (1981) analysed the Framingham study data by classifying men according to their smoking habits at the seventh examination (1963–1964), and gave incidence rates as of the fourteenth examination (that is, follow-up through 1977). The 14-year CHD incidence was not lower in filter smokers than in nonfilter cigarette smokers, even after adjustment for age, blood pressure, and serum cholesterol. There were no differences between filter and nonfilter cigarette smokers in rates of new myocardial infarction or total dcaths.

Hawthorne and Fry (1978) followed up over 18 000 Scottish men and women aged 45–64 years between 1965 and 1977. There were 793 deaths reported among the 11 295 men, of which 360 were from ischaemic heart disease and 56 were from cerebrovascular disease. Comparing 'relative mortality' between smokers of filter *versus* nonfilter cigarettes, they reported no differences in men for deaths from all causes, ischaemic heart disease or cerebrovascular disease, or from all causes in women. (There were only 132 deaths among the 7491 women followed, which was apparently considered too few to analyse for specific causes of death by cigarette type.)

In the Whitehall study, ten-year CHD mortality rates were computed for 17 475 male civil servants aged 40–64 years, for whom smoking data (including tar yield, quantity, and inhalation) were available (Higenbottam *et al.*, 1982). There were 147 CHD deaths among male smokers who said they inhaled, and 26 among those who said they did not. Among inhalers, there was a marked increase in risk with increasing tar yield at 1–9 cigarettes per day but no clear trends with respect to tar yield at higher consumption levels (see Table 2). No relation to tar yield was seen in noninhalers. With a few minor exceptions, the CHD rates for both inhalers and noninhalers were higher than for nonsmokers.

A separate analysis of the same data with respect to cigarette carbon monoxide yields (Borland *et al.*, 1983) showed a ten-year mortality rate significantly *lower* in smokers of high-yield cigarettes: relative risk for CHD (adjusted for age, grade of employment, cigarettes per day and tar yield) was 0.68 among smokers of cigarettes yielding over 20 mg of carbon monoxide, compared with smokers of cigarettes yielding 18 mg or less. An inverse dose-response with respect to carbon monoxide yield was observed among men who inhaled (Table 2).

Table 2. Ten-year coronary heart disease mortality rates (per hundred) among smokers (inhalers only) according to cigarette tar and carbon monoxide yields in the Whitehall Study

	Mortality rate		
	No. of cigarettes smoked per day		
	1–9	10–19	20+
Tar yield [a]			
18–23 mg	2.68	5.63	6.60
24–32 mg	3.81	6.57	6.23
33 mg or more	7.42	6.47	7.84
Ratio: 33+ *versus* 18–23	2.77	1.15	1.19
Carbon monoxide yield [b]			
18 mg or less	6.12		
Above 18–20 mg	4.98		
Above 20 mg	3.01		

[a] From Higenbottam *et al.* (1982); no. of deaths, 147
[b] From Borland *et al.* (1983); no. of deaths, 200

Other studies of CHD

A case-control study of men aged 30–54 years with new cases of nonfatal myocardial infarction (MI) in US hospitals was reported by Kaufman *et al.* (1983). Between the 502 cases and 835 controls, there were no significant differences in mean yields of nicotine, tar, or carbon monoxide, and relative risks for MI did not vary with any of these yield parameters. It should be pointed out that the cigarette yields referred to the most recently smoked cigarette, relative to the time of the MI; historical data on smoking were not presented.

Finally, Wald *et al.* (1981) measured the serum cotinine in smokers of cigarettes, pipes and cigars, and found the highest levels by far in pipe smokers. Wald argued that as pipe smokers have little excess CHD risk, nicotine cannot be responsible for CHD in cigarette smokers. This paper led to considerable contention (McNicol & Turner, 1982; Wald *et al.*, 1982), but Wald has maintained his views.

Coronary heart disease: discussion

The evidence linking cigarette yield to increased risk of CHD and other cardiovascular diseases is not nearly as strong as the evidence for tar and lung cancer, and cannot at this time be said to be established beyond doubt. There are many possible reasons for this situation. One may be, of course, that we are looking at the wrong components of cigarette smoke, and that the factor (or factors) responsible for increasing the risk of CHD has not yet been identified. It may also be that carbon monoxide plays a more important role than we realize, and that the joint effect of carbon monoxide and nicotine (which are not correlated with each other and which in fact may go in opposite directions) may be crucial.

A second problem is how to interpret a smoker's level of serum carboxyhaemoglobin or other metabolite as measured today with respect to smoking exposures in the past, particularly since tar and nicotine yields of practically all cigarettes are now well below the levels of two or three decades ago.

A third problem is assignment of specific cigarette yield values to individuals. People, of course, do not smoke in the same fashion as the machines on which nicotine yields are measured, and smokers can inhale considerably different levels of toxicants than indicated on the cigarette package or in laboratory reports (Kozlowski, 1980).

Even if the nominal yield values are accepted, in most follow-up studies the mortality was related to yields of cigarettes at baseline, determined up to twelve years earlier, whereas average yields may have changed dramatically during the follow-up period. The usual excuse for this assignment is lack of new smoking data during the follow-up period, and the hope that the fall in yields occurred roughly in parallel in all brands, but this must surely lead to significant misclassification.

Figure 2 illustrates the difficulties encountered by the investigator who attempts to interpret data gathered from smokers followed over a long period of time. In the Figure, the calendar periods for a number of follow-up studies (and survey periods for some cross-sectional studies) have been superimposed upon a graph of the sales-weighted tar and nicotine levels in the USA. While British levels have fallen at a different rate than have American levels, the point is the same for both countries: tar and nicotine cigarette yields

Fig. 2. Observation or survey periods for studies of coronary heart disease, chronic obstructive pulmonary disease, and lung cancer, in relation to time trends in US sales-weighted average tar and nicotine levels; (●——●), tar; (●------●), nicotine

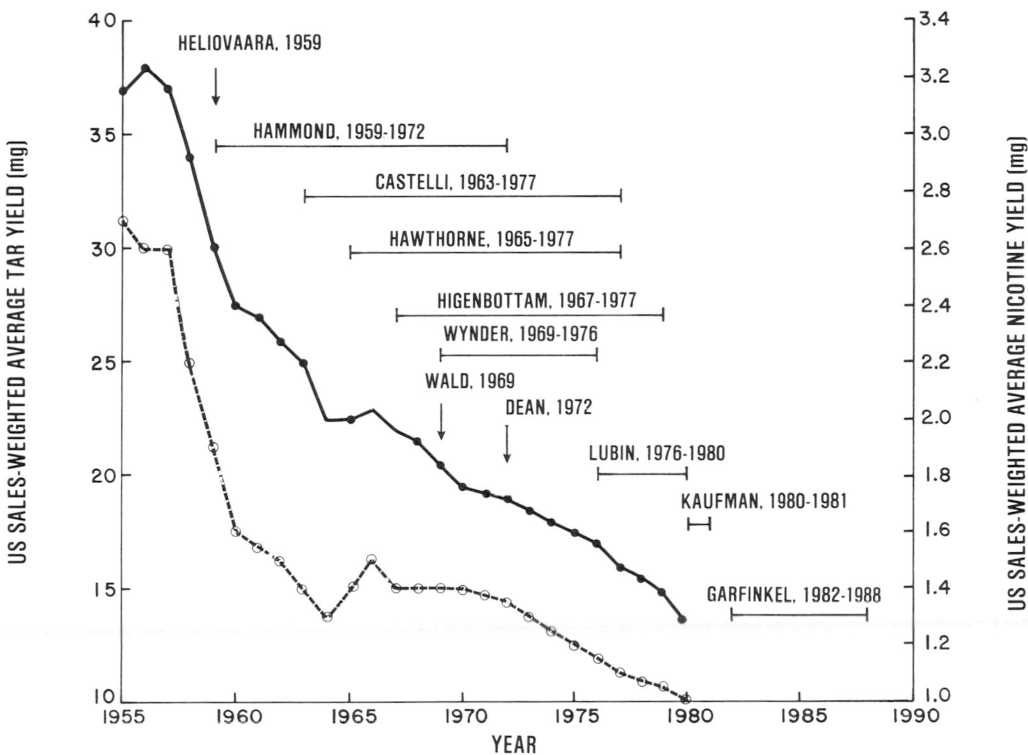

recorded at the start of a follow-up study almost invariably overstate the average exposure to the smoker throughout the observation period.

Other factors related to the design and analysis of specific studies must also colour our interpretation of these results. For one thing, the influence of other risk factors of the same level of importance as smoking (such as serum lipids and blood pressure) have not often been measured, and their importance is often ignored. Secondly, the weight to be attached to prevalence studies in general must be less than for either prospective or case-control studies. An association in a cross-sectional study cannot differentiate too well between cause and effect, and smokers who survive CHD often alter their smoking habits, sometimes in response to medical advice, and often out of plain fear. Thus, one does not know for certain whether a high prevalence of a particular symptom in a group of smokers is observed because smoking caused that symptom, or whether it would have been higher still except for large numbers of subjects who quit smoking because of it.

Finally, several of the follow-up studies presented mortality results in a very crude fashion, by dividing total deaths from a given cause by the number of men at the start of the study. Such analysis (or lack of it) fails to account for time periods of exposure to risk, and does not discriminate between deaths which may have occurred early in the follow-up period from those which occurred later, and can slight competing risks from other causes of death (and there are, of course, many for cigarette smoking).

Summary of findings for CHD

The prevalence rates of ischaemic heart disease or CHD and intermittent claudication were significantly associated with serum carboxyhaemoglobin in two studies, but not with filter *versus* nonfilter cigarette use in one study.

CHD death rate was associated with cigarette tar yield at all levels of daily quantity smoked in one prospective study, based on 6050 observed CHD deaths. CHD death rates increased with tar yield at low but not high daily consumption levels in another prospective study, based on 173 CHD deaths, and were *inversely* related to cigarette carbon monoxide yield in the same study. CHD death rates were not different in smokers of filter *versus* nonfilter cigarettes in two other prospective studies. The relative risk for new myocardial infarction in younger men was unrelated to cigarette tar, nicotine or carbon monoxide yield in one case-control study.

On the basis of tar-nicotine yield alone, and considering the magnitude of the American Cancer Society study, the evidence from prospective studies strongly favours a relationship between cigarette yield and risk of death from CHD. This conclusion seems at odds with the two prospective studies in which no relation was found with filter usage, as well as with the case-control study. It might be argued, however, that filter use is a less sensitive index of exposure to cardiotoxic components of cigarette smoke, especially given the wide range of tar and nicotine yields in filter cigarettes smoked by the cohorts in question. Lack of an association in the case-control study might possibly be due to its dealing with MI survivors only, who may have smoked lower yield cigarettes than those who succumbed immediately, and to use as an exposure index of cigarette yields at time of MI, rather than past exposures. This is only speculation, however. Fortunately, an American Cancer Society prospective study of 1.2 million men and women, now in progress, is designed to resolve many of these issues (Stellman & Garfinkel, 1986).

The totality of evidence, therefore, is weakly consistent with, but does not yet conclusively support, a relationship between cigarette yield and subsequent death from CHD.

CIGARETTE YIELD AND CHRONIC OBSTRUCTIVE PULMONARY DISEASE

Cross-sectional studies of COPD

Four studies were identified in which the prevalence rates of one or more respiratory symptoms were studied among smokers of various types of cigarettes. Three were conducted in the UK and one in the USA.

Rimington (1972) evaluated sputum production in 10 414 men aged 40 years and over who had volunteered for a mass radiographic screening programme, and found that 37.2% of those who smoked nonfilter cigarettes had persistent daily sputum, compared to 31.9% who smoked filter cigarettes.

Dean *et al.* (1978) reported on a representative cross-sectional sample of 6277 men and 6459 women interviewed at home in England, Scotland and Wales in 1972. Prevalence rates of four 'respiratory' symptoms (bronchitis, morning cough, shortness of breath, wheezing) increased with the number of cigarettes smoked per day, and with inhalation, and were higher in nonfilter than in filter cigarette smokers, but differences were significant only for morning cough (men and women) and shortness of breath (women only).

Higenbottam *et al.* (1980) reported an analysis of respiratory symptoms and lung function measurements in the Whitehall study of 18 403 male civil servants aged 40–64 years. Phlegm production increased with tar yield of current cigarette; forced expiratory volume in one second (FEV_1) did not decrease with tar yield according to the authors, but did according to a re-analysis by Lee (1980).

In an American study, 5686 women were selected at random from Western Pennsylvania telephone directories and interviewed by telephone (Schenker *et al.*, 1982). Tar was a significant risk factor for chronic cough (relative risk, 2.0) and chronic phlegm (relative risk, 1.6), but not for grade 3 dyspnoea or wheeze. The two former symptoms were more strongly affected by daily quantity smoked than by tar.

Follow-up studies of COPD

We have computed standardized mortality ratios (SMRs) for COPD deaths from the American Cancer Society study, in a fashion similar to that presented above for CHD, and in an earlier paper for lung cancer (Stellman, this volume[2]). A total of 322 deaths from COPD were observed during the first six years of follow-up (1960–1966). Results are shown in Figure 3. A dose-dependence of the SMR for COPD on quantity smoked per day was observed for smokers of high- and medium-tar cigarettes only. Among smokers of 20 cigarettes per day or less, the risk were not detectably different for high-tar compared to low-tar smokers, while for smokers of even greater numbers daily, COPD risks were actually highest among medium-tar smokers.

Comstock *et al.* (1970), who observed a group of 670 male telephone company employees for six years, found that smokers of nonfilter cigarettes had a higher initial prevalence of cough and phlegm than filter cigarette smokers, and experienced a greater increase in both symptoms. The mean FEV_1 was lower in nonfilter than in filter cigarette smokers at baseline, but decreased relatively less over time in the nonfilter group.

Hawthorne and Fry (1978) reported a follow-up study in Scotland of over 18 000 men and women aged 45–64 years. Both male and female nonfilter cigarette smokers had a higher prevalence at baseline than did filter cigarette smokers of bronchitis symptoms, shortness of breath, wheezing and phlegm. A similar finding was obtained with tar level. The mortality rate from chronic bronchitis in men appeared to be slightly higher in nonfilter than in filter cigarette smokers, but the numbers of deaths were small (28 in all), differences were not significant, and the information on mortality presented was very crude. Corresponding death rates for women were not given owing to the small numbers.

---

[2] See p. 197.

Fig. 3. Standardized mortality ratios for chronic obstructive pulmonary disease in males, among nonsmokers, exsmokers, and current smokers of low-, medium- and high-tar/nicotine cigarettes (defined by Hammond *et al.*, 1976). The group was enrolled in 1959, and followed up through 1966.

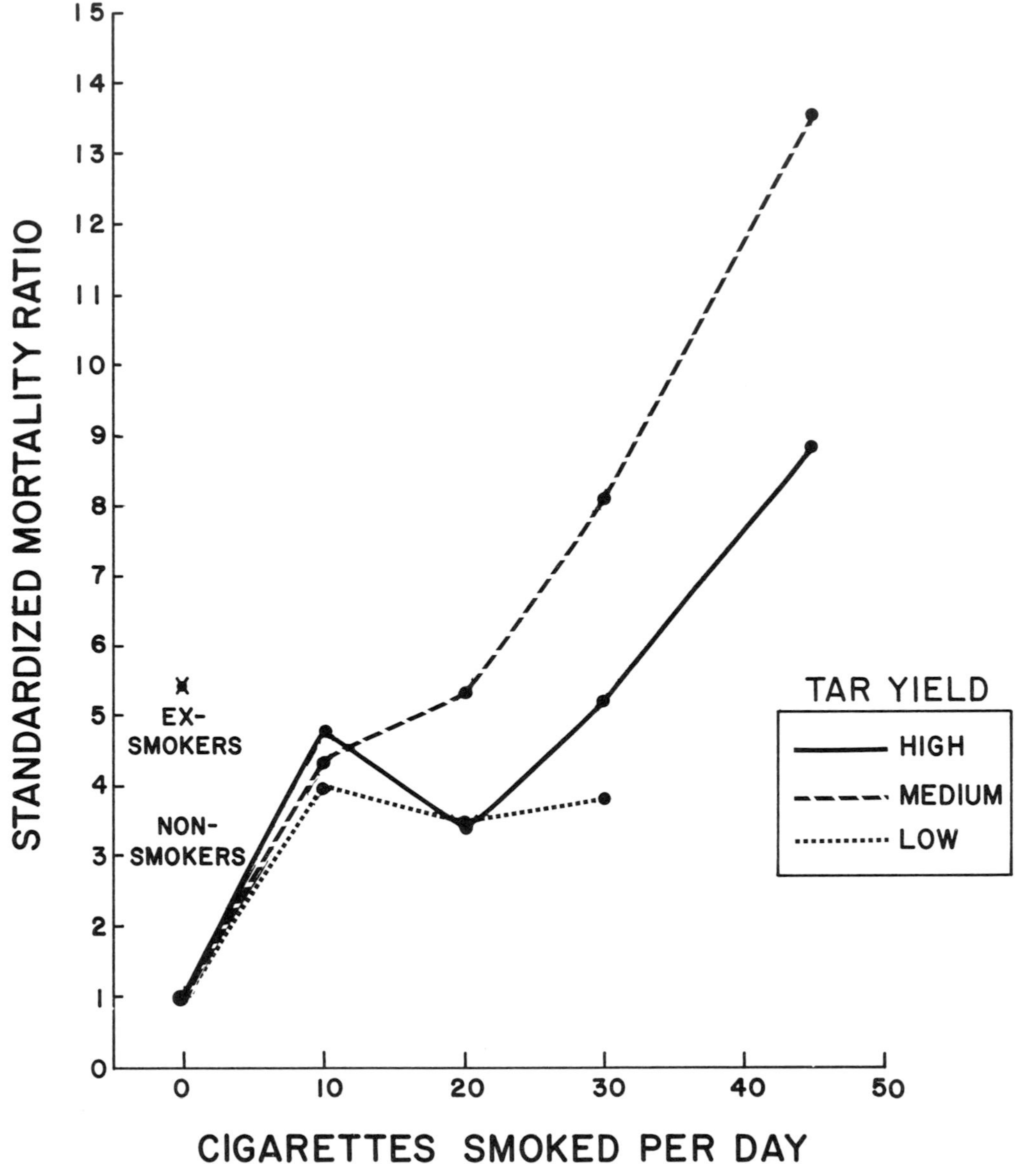

Peto *et al.* (1983) presented some interesting and useful data on COPD death rates in relation to smoking in a cohort of 2718 British men aged 25–64 years followed up for 20–25 years. While no specific data on tar or nicotine levels were presented, the COPD death rate was not related to mucous hypersecretion; the authors suggested that persons with severe airway obstruction may switch to lower-tar cigarettes, and that cross-sectional studies may be confounded by this phenomenon.

In a US study of 2144 men followed up from 1963 to 1968, Sparrow *et al.* (1983) found cigarette tar yield unrelated to pulmonary function (FVC or FEV_1), either at baseline or at follow-up five years later.

Summary of findings for COPD

Four cross-sectional and five prospective studies have been reviewed. Both filter use and low tar levels were consistently related to lower sputum or phlegm production in five studies, to reduced prevalence of cough in three studies, and to shortness of breath in two studies. Wheeze and dyspnoea were higher in nonfilter than in filter cigarette smokers in two cross-sectional analyses, but were unrelated to tar level in a third.

Lung function (as measured by FVC or FEV_1) was lower on average (that is, worse) in smokers of higher-tar or nonfilter cigarettes in two cross-sectional studies, but was unrelated to tar level in one prospective study either at baseline or after five years of follow-up.

Finally, mortality from chronic bronchitis was no different in filter than in nonfilter cigarette smokers in one follow-up study, and was about the same in high-tar/nicotine smokers compared to low-tar/nicotine smokers in another extremely large study.

In summary, there is good evidence that smoking low-yield cigarettes leads to lower phlegm production, reduced cough and less shortness of breath, but conflicting evidence for an effect on lung function, and none for an effect on mortality from COPD.

REFERENCES

Borland, C., Chamberlain, A., Higenbottam, T., Shipley, M. & Rose, G. (1983) Carbon monoxide yield of cigarettes and its relation to cardiorespiratory disease. *Br. med. J.*, ***287,*** 1583–1586

Castelli, W.P., Dawber, T.R., Feinleib, M., Garrison, R.J., McNamara, P.M. & Kannel, W.B. (1981) The filter cigarette and coronary heart disease: The Framingham Study. *Lancet, **ii,*** 109–113

Comstock, G.W., Brownlow, W.J., Stone, R.W. & Sartwell, P.E. (1970) Cigarette smoking and changes in respiratory findings. *Arch. environ. Health, **21,*** 50–57

Dean, G., Lee, P.N., Todd, G.F., Wicken, A.J. & Sparks, D.N. (1978) Factors related to respiratory and cardiovascular symptoms in the United Kingdom. *J. Epidemiol. Community Health, **32,*** 86–96

Hammond, E.C. (1966) *Smoking in relation to the death rates of one million men and women.* In: Haenszel, W., ed., *Epidemiologic Approaches to the Study of Cancer and Other Chronic Diseases (National Cancer Institute Monograph No. 19),* Bethesda, MD, US Department of Health, Education, and Welfare, Public Health Service, National Institutes of Health, National Cancer Institute, pp. 127–204

Hammond, E.C. & Garfinkel, L. (1969) Coronary heart disease, stroke, and aortic aneurysm. Factors in the etiology. *Arch. environ. Health,* ***19,*** 167–182

Hammond, E.C., Garfinkel, L., Seidman, H. & Lew, E.A. (1976) 'Tar' and nicotine content of cigarette smoke in relation to death rates. *Environ. Res.,* ***12,*** 263–274

Hammond, E.C., Garfinkel, L., Seidman, H. & Lew, E.A. (1977) *Some recent findings concerning cigarette smoking.* In: Hiatt, H.H., Watson, J.D. & Winsten, J.A., eds, *Origins of Human Cancer,* Book A, *Incidence of Cancer in Humans,* Cold Spring Harbor, NY, Cold Spring Harbor Laboratory, pp. 101–112

Hawthorne, V.M. & Fry, J.S. (1978) Smoking and health: the association between smoking behaviour, total mortality, and cardiorespiratory disease in west central Scotland. *J. Epidemiol. Community Health,* ***32,*** 260–266

Heliovaara, M., Karvonen, M.J., Vilhunen, R. & Punsar, S. (1978) Smoking, carbon monoxide, and atherosclerotic diseases. *Br. med. J., 1978,* ***i,*** 268–270;

Higenbottam, T., Shipley, M.J., Clark, T.H.J. & Rose, G. (1980) Lung function and symptoms of cigarette smokers related to tar yield and number of cigarettes smoked. *Lancet,* ***i,*** 409–412

Higenbottam, T., Shipley, M.J. & Rose, G. (1982) Cigarettes, lung cancer, and coronary heart disease: the effects of inhalation and tar yield. *J. Epidemiol. Community Health,* ***36,*** 113–117

Kaufman, D.W., Helmrich, S.P., Rosenberg, L., Miettinen, O.S. & Shapiro, S. (1983) Nicotine and carbon monoxide content of cigarette smoke and the risk of myocardial infarction in young men. *New Engl. J. Med.,* ***308,*** 409–413

Kozlowski, L.T., Frecker, R.C., Khouw, V. & Pope, M.A. (1980) The misuse of "less-hazardous" cigarettes and its detection: hole-blocking of ventilated filters. *Am. J. Public Health,* ***70,*** 1202–1203

Lee, P.N. (1980) Low tar cigarette smoking, *Lancet,* ***i,*** 1365–1366

McNicol, M.W. & Turner, J.A.McM. (1982) Nicotine, carbon monoxide, and heart disease. *Lancet,* ***i,*** 40

Peto, R., Speizer, F.E., Cochrane, A.L., Moore, F., Fletcher, C.M., Tinker, C.M., Higgins, I.T.T., Gray, R.G., Richards, S.M., Gilliland, J. & Norman-Smith, B. (1983) The relevance in adults of air-flow obstruction, but not of mucus hypersecretion, to mortality from chronic lung disease. *Am. Rev. resp. Dis.,* ***128,*** 491–500

Rimington, J. (1972) Phlegm and filters. *Br. med. J.,* ***ii,*** 262–264

Schenker, M.B., Samet, J.M. & Speizer, F.E. (1982) Effect of cigarette tar content and smoking habits on respiratory symptoms in women. *Am. Rev. resp. Dis.,* ***125,*** 684–690

Sparrow, D., Stefos, T., Bosse, R. & Weiss, S.T. (1983) The relationship of tar content to decline in pulmonary function in cigarette smokers. *Am. Rev. resp. Dis.,* ***127,*** 56–58

Stellman, S.D. & Garfinkel, L. (1986) Smoking habits and tar levels in a new American Cancer Society prospective study of 1.2 million men and women. *J. natl Cancer Inst.* (in press)

US Department of Health and Human Services (1984) *The Health Consequences of Smoking. Cardiovascular Disease. A Report of the Surgeon General,* Bethesda, MD, US Department of Health and Human Services, Public Health Service, Office of the Assistant Secretary for Health, Office on Smoking and Health (DHHS Publication No. (PHS) 84–50204)

Wald, N., Howard, S., Smith, P.G. & Kjeldsen, K. (1973) Association between atherosclerotic diseases and carboxyhaemoglobin levels in tobacco smokers. *Br. med. J.*, ***i***, 761–765

Wald, N., Idle, M., Borcham, J., Bailey, A. & Van Vunakis, H. (1981) Serum cotinine levels in pipe smokers: evidence against nicotine as cause of coronary heart disease. *Lancet*, ***ii***, 775–777

Wald, N., Idle, M., Boreham, J., Bailey, A. & Van Vunakis, H. (1982) Nicotine, carbon monoxide, and heart disease (Reply). *Lancet*, ***i***, 40–41

A DOUBLE-BLIND RANDOMIZED CONTROLLED TRIAL OF THE EFFECT OF A LOW- *VERSUS* A MIDDLE-TAR CIGARETTE ON RESPIRATORY SYMPTOMS – A FEASIBILITY STUDY

H. PEACH[1], D.M. HAYWARD & D. SHAH

Department of Community Medicine,
United Medical and Dental Schools, St Thomas' Campus,
London SE1 7EH, UK

G.A. ELLARD

National Institute for Medical Research,
Mill Hill,
London NW7 1AA, UK

SUMMARY

A feasibility study of a double-blind, randomized controlled trial of the effect of a low- *versus* a middle-tar cigarette on respiratory symptoms is described. A smoking questionnaire was sent to 19 366 households. Returned questionnaires (64%) yielded 604 middle-tar cigarette smokers aged 20–44 years; 342 replied to a health warning stating that they did not want to or had failed to stop smoking and of these 183 volunteered for the trial. Thus about every 100 households originally mailed yielded one volunteer. Of the volunteers, 95 men were randomly allocated to be sold a middle-tar cigarette and 88 to be sold a low-tar cigarette of identical appearance. The cigarettes were sold at three different reduced prices and the men were asked to smoke them for five weeks. There was a 22% drop-out and this was unrelated to type of cigarette smoked. A reduction in price of 20% was sufficient incentive for volunteers to participate. Cigarette butts were collected weekly or fortnightly

[1] To whom editorial correspondence should be addressed

and urine samples were collected initially and after three and five weeks. Compliance with the trial cigarettes was good. The excretion of nicotine metabolites, number of cigarettes smoked and average butt weight for men allocated the low-tar cigarette was not significantly different from that of those allocated the middle-tar cigarette. This suggested that the former compensated for the 37% reduction in the nicotine yield of their cigarette by taking more frequent or deeper puffs from their cigarette. The implications of these results for a large-scale, randomized controlled trial are discussed.

INTRODUCTION

As part of the Voluntary Agreement of 21 November 1980 between United Kingdom Health Ministers and the Tobacco Industry, the latter agreed to continue its long-standing policy of reducing the tar yield of cigarettes. In order to determine whether such a policy actually results in the smoking of less harmful cigarettes, the industry agreed to provide funds for supporting research as proposed by the Independent Scientific Committee on Smoking and Health, to monitor the effects on human health of such product modification. The Committee identified respiratory disease as an important area for such research.

There are three ways in which the potential effect of reducing tar yields of cigarettes on respiratory disease has been studied. Firstly, correlation studies of the relationship between the sales-weighted tar yields of cigarettes and long-term trends in mortality from tobacco-related diseases such as lung cancer (Royal College of Physicians, 1983). Secondly, cross-sectional (Higenbottam *et al.,* 1980; Schenker *et al.,* 1982) or prospective (Sparrow *et al.,* 1983) studies of respiratory disease in subjects who have chosen to smoke cigarettes of different tar yields. Thirdly, there are case-control studies in which the tar yields of cigarettes smoked by patients with lung cancer or chronic obstructive lung disease are compared with those of cigarettes smoked by controls (Kunze & Vutuc, 1980).

Because a smoker's choice of cigarette might be affected by his or her existing symptoms (Rimpela & Rimpela, 1985), the Independent Scientific Committee on Smoking and Health considered that it was essential to conduct 'intervention studies'. Such studies might compare the respiratory symptoms or function of committed smokers who had been randomly allocated to smoke cigarettes of differing tar yields.

Suitable populations for such studies would be male smokers aged 20–44 years, because men have a higher prevalence of respiratory symptoms and, in that age group, such symptoms are likely to be reversible. Subjects could be identified through a questionnaire mailed to households on the electoral register of a town. Committed smokers of middle-tar cigarettes (16–18 mg tar per cigarette) would be defined as middle-tar cigarette smokers who continue to smoke after being sent a health warning. Trial cigarettes would be selected from middle- and low-tar brands of cigarettes already on the market but, in order to prevent bias, they would need to be commercially manufactured for the study without their brand identifications.

It was envisaged that financial incentives would have to be given to encourage volunteers to participate in such investigations and that this could be conveniently done by selling the trial cigarettes at reduced prices. However, such a strategy could alter their smoking pattern as could changes in the nicotine and tar contents of the test cigarettes that they smoked (US Surgeon General, 1984). Changes in daily cigarette consumption could be monitored by counting regular collections of cigarette butts, while alterations in the way the cigarettes were smoked could be investigated by weighing the cigarette butts and estimating nicotine intake by urinary nicotine metabolite determinations (Peach *et al.*, 1985).

Intervention studies to assess the possible impact of smoking low-tar cigarettes on pulmonary function are impracticable since at least eight years of follow-up is necessary to distinguish between the one-second forced expiratory volumes of smokers and non-smokers (Fletcher *et al.*, 1976). Intervention studies can, however, be conducted within periods of about six months if the effect of smoking different types of cigarettes on respiratory symptoms is explored (Leeder *et al.*, 1977). A possible limitation to such an approach is that a change in mucus secretion may not be directly correlated with the progress of chronic obstructive airways disease (Peto *et al.*, 1983).

This paper describes a study to investigate the feasibility of conducting a double-blind randomized controlled trial of a low- *versus* a middle-tar cigarette. Specific aspects assessed were the response of households to the initial questionnaire and of middle-tar cigarette smokers to the health warnings they received; the influence of different financial incentives on the proportion of volunteers who dropped out from the trial; the acceptability of the low-tar cigarette to the middle-tar cigarette smokers; willingness of smokers to collect cigarette butts and compliance with the trial cigarettes; whether middle-tar cigarette smokers allocated the low-tar cigarettes compensated for the reduced nicotine yield of their cigarettes by altering their smoking patterns; and the proportions of middle-tar cigarette smokers who had respiratory symptoms. The investigation had the approval of the ethical committees of St Thomas's Hospital and the Medway District Health Authority.

METHODS

Recruitment of smokers to the study

The 14 electoral wards of a town, Gillingham, in Kent, England were ranked according to the numbers of men aged 16–44 years recorded in the previous census. The top eight wards with a total of 13 759 young men were selected for the study. A one-page questionnaire and a reply-paid envelope were then sent to the 19 366 households on the electoral registers of the eight wards. The questionnaire deliberately stated that the purpose of the enquiry was simply to collect information about men's smoking habits and no mention was made of the proposed trial. The questionnaire requested the names of all men in the households aged 18–50 years, their dates of birth, whether they smoked manufactured cigarettes or not, and if so, to enclose an empty packet or packets of the cigarettes usually smoked by each man, writing his name on the packet. Nonresponding households were sent a postcard reminder two weeks later and, if necessary, a second questionnaire in a third mailing after a further fortnight.

Men aged 20–44 years who were smoking a middle-tar cigarette were sent a letter informing them that smoking is dangerous and causes heart disease, bronchitis and lung cancer, and advising them to stop smoking. The letter also explained that help to give up smoking could be obtained by writing to the Health Education Council. They were asked to return a tear-off slip in the reply-paid envelope stating whether they did or did not wish to stop smoking. Nonresponders were sent a postcard reminder and then a second health warning two and four weeks later, respectively.

The responses yielded on average about 40 committed, male, middle-tar cigarette smokers from each ward. The wards were then divided up into two to four convenient districts containing about 15 suitable candidates for the study. The field workers (17 community nurses and two health visitors) generally chose to visit potential volunteers from districts in which they usually worked. Initial contacts were often made with the wives or parents of potential volunteers and an appointment then made to see the candidate within the next few days. The trial was carried out in two stages, and seven field workers helped in both stages.

Allocation of volunteers to middle- and low-tar cigarettes

The field workers had a fully structured questionnaire which began by checking the man's name, date of birth and whether he was still smoking a middle-tar cigarette. Information was also collected about the number of cigarettes usually smoked per day, age at which regular smoking had begun, occupation and respiratory symptoms, using the shorter Medical Research Council respiratory symptoms questionnaire (Holland *et al.*, 1976). Middle-tar cigarette smokers were then asked to take part in a study 'which involved smoking an experimental cigarette for five weeks'. Middle-tar cigarette smokers agreeing to take part in the trial were asked to continue smoking their usual cigarette for a further week, to collect as many of the butts as possible and to note the number of butts lost or cigarettes given away to friends. Meanwhile the men within each of the eight electoral wards were randomly allocated to be sold middle- or low-tar cigarettes at three alternative prices: £1.00, £0.76 or £0.43 per packet of 20. The tar yields of the middle- and low-tar cigarettes were 15.5 and 9.0 mg per cigarette, respectively, while their corresponding nicotine yields were 1.5 and 0.9 mg, respectively. Thus, on average, the smokers allocated to the low-tar cigarette smoked a cigarette with a nicotine yield about 40% lower than that of those continuing to smoke middle-tar cigarettes. Both were king-size filter cigarettes of virtually identical appearance. To enable any surreptitious smoking of nontrial cigarettes to be detected, the inside of the paper around their filters was dyed with a red non-toxic substance. The type of cigarettes and the price at which they were to be sold were distinguished by the number and positioning of asterisks within the frame of the health warning.

Conduct of the study

After collecting the butts of their usual cigarettes during the first week of the study, participants were visited by their field worker who collected a urine sample in a thymol-containing tube, noted the number of cigarettes smoked so far that day and on the previous day, and sold them a week's supply of the trial cigarette based on their normal weekly cigarette consumption. Participants were asked to collect the butts of the test cigarettes smoked over the subsequent week and to keep a record of the number of butts lost or cigarettes given away to friends. The men were requested to smoke only the trial cigarettes for the following five weeks. At the end of the first, third and fifth weeks on the trial cigarettes, participants were visited by their field worker who collected the previous week's or fortnight's cigarette butts, obtained a further urine sample and sold the men two weeks supply of the trial cigarettes. If the participants thought they were going to run out of cigarettes before the field worker was due to visit, they could telephone to arrange delivery of a further supply. At the end of the fifth week, any respiratory symptoms of the volunteers were once again elicited.

The cigarette butts were counted and weighed at St Thomas's Hospital before being opened and checked for the presence of the red dye. Nicotine intake was assessed by determining the ratios of the urinary concentrations of nicotine metabolites (as cotinine) to creatinine by the barbituric acid and alkaline picrate methods, respectively (Peach *et al.*, 1985).

RESULTS

Recruitment to the study

Table 1 summarizes the efficiencies of the three phases in the recruitment of potential volunteers for the study. Returned questionnaires were eventually received from two-thirds of the households that were originally mailed, and yielded 604 middle-tar cigarette smokers. The relative frequencies of the different cigarette brands that they smoked were typical of their current shares in the commercial market (Communication from the Laboratory of the Government Chemist to the Independent Scientific Committee on Smoking and Health). About a half of the 349 middle-tar cigarette smokers who returned their tear-off slips after receiving the health warning and admitted they were still smoking replied that they did not want to give up smoking.

In the third phase of recruitment to the trial, about a fifth of the men could not be contacted even after three visits, and a third of the remainder refused to participate. The proportions of noncontacts and refusals appeared not to vary greatly among the eight different wards (Table 2). When the performance of the seven field workers who helped in both the first and second part of the study was examined, it was apparent that with but a single exception they performed very similarly, and that they were no more successful in contacting potential volunteers and persuading them to participate in the second stage of the study than they had been in the first. A higher proportion of the men who refused to participate in the trial or could not be contacted initially stated that they did not want to give up smoking. 62% of 169 *versus* 32% of 173 ($\chi^2 = 30.4$, 1 df, $p < 0.001$).

Only 14 of the 93 men who refused to participate in the trial gave reasons; five were too busy, three were collecting coupons, two were unwilling to collect butts, two were unwilling to smoke king-size cigarettes, one was getting duty-free cigarettes and another felt himself to be too light a smoker.

Information about smoking habits, occupation and respiratory symptoms was collected from 40 of the 93 men who refused to take part in the trial. There was no significant difference between the findings for those refusing and the corresponding data from the 183 volunteers who agreed to participate in the study (Table 3).

Table 1. Recruitment into the study

Phase		Cumulative response		
1a	Initial questionnaires sent	Initial replies (2 weeks)	After postcard reminder (4 weeks)	After second questionnaire (6 weeks)
	19 366 (100%)	6388 (33%)	9178 (47%)	12 317 (64%)

Phase		Smokers of manufactured cigarettes				
1b	No. subjects aged 20–44 years	Middle-tar	Low-middle-tar	Low-tar	Other smokers/ brand unknown	Nonsmokers or exsmokers
	9044 (100%)	604 (7%)	565 (6%)	153 (2%)	457 (5%)	7265 (80%)

2	Candidates, middle-tar smokers	Returned tear-off slips	Claimed to have stopped smoking	Wanted to stop smoking	Unwilling to stop smoking
	604 (100%)	386 (64%)	37	180	169
3	Candidates, committed middle-tar smokers	No. contacted	Stopped smoking	Refused to participate	Entered into the study
	349 (100%)	66 (19%)	7 (2%)	93 (27%)	183 (52%)

Table 2. Non-contacts, refusals and drop-outs in the study in the eight Gillingham wards

Ward	Numbers (%) of smokers			
	Candidates[a]	Non-contacts and refusals	Drop-outs	Completed trial
Beechings	45	16 (36%)	3 (7%)	26 (58%)
Brampton	34	16 (47%)	2 (6%)	16 (47%)
Hempstead and Wigmore	47	14 (30%)	9 (19%)	24 (51%)
Parkwood	43	24 (56%)	2 (5%)	17 (40%)
Rainham	32	20 (63%)	2 (6%)	10 (32%)
Rainham Mark	35	17 (49%)	5 (14%)	13 (37%)
Riverside	51	25 (49%)	5 (10%)	21 (41%)
St Margarets	55	27 (49%)	12 (22%)	16 (29%)
All	342	159 (46%)	40 (12%)	143 (42%)

[a] Plus seven men who were found to have stopped smoking

Table 3. Characteristics of refusals and volunteers

Characteristic[a]	Refusals	Volunteers
Number of cigarettes per day		
1–4	3	3
5–14	7	23
15–24	22	96
25+	7	60
MD	1	1
Age began smoking regularly		
<10	1	3
11–20	36	173
21+	3	6
MD	0	1
Employment status		
Working	36	159
Not working	4	24
Social class		
I, II, III NM	18	84
IIIM, IV, V	22	97
MD	0	2
Respiratory symptoms		
Cough	6	59
No cough	27	120
MD	7	4
Phlegm	5	41
No phlegm	28	136
MD	7	6
Tar yield of cigarette		
16 mg	19	77
17 mg	13	60
18 mg	8	45
MD	0	1
Depth of inhalation		
Heavy	15	79
Moderate	21	98
Slight	4	5
Not at all	0	1

[a] MD, missing data; social class in the UK is divided into six categories: I, II, III nonmanual (NM), III manual (M), IV and V, on the basis of present occupation

Losses from the trial

Of those enrolled, 40 men dropped out of the trial. The proportions of drop-outs did not vary significantly from ward to ward (see Table 2) and overall were uninfluenced by either the price charged or the type of cigarette sold (Table 4). There was a suggestion that the drop-out rates among those allocated the low-tar cigarettes increased with decreasing price, but this was not statistically significant. In contrast a significantly lower drop-out rate

Table 4. Possible influence of type of cigarette and price per packet[a] charged in proportion of volunteers dropping out of study

Type of cigarette	Drop-out rate			
	Pack price			
	£ 1.00	£ 0.76	£ 0.43	All
Middle-tar	8/31 (26%)	9/32 (28%)	2/32 (6%)	19/95 (20%)
Low-tar	5/32 (16%)	6/27 (22%)	10/29 (34%)	21/88 (24%)
Both	13/63 (21%)	15/59 (25%)	12/61 (20%)	40/183 (22%)

[a] The average price paid by the smokers for their usual cigarettes was about £1.20 per pack

($p < 0.05$) was encountered among those sold the middle-tar cigarettes at the cheapest price (Table 4). Seven claimed to have dropped out because they had given up smoking, while four withdrew because they believed their cigarettes (all low-tar) gave them headaches or a sore throat. However, 21 gave no reason at all for opting out of the study.

Pattern of smoking during the study

The men were very willing to collect their cigarette butts and keep a record of the number lost. Thus during the six-week period of the study the men collected or recorded as lost about 75% of the butts of the cigarettes that they had been sold by the field workers (Table 5). Furthermore, less than 1% of the butts returned were not from the trial cigarettes. Moreover there was an excellent correlation ($r = 0.67$, $p < 0.001$) between the number of butts from their own brands of cigarettes smoked in the first week (butts returned plus butts recorded as lost) and the number of cigarettes which the men told the field workers that they usually smoked each week before the trial started.

The average daily purchases and consumption of cigarettes (based on butts returned or recorded as lost) together with the average weights of cigarette butts returned are summarized in Tables 5 and 6. It is clear that the pattern of cigarette consumption and the extent to which the cigarettes were smoked did not change significantly throughout the study, and that there was no apparent difference between those allocated to smoke either low-tar or middle-tar cigarettes. Urine samples were successfully collected from all the volunteers who completed the trial. The relative intake of nicotine by the two groups as estimated from the average ratios of the urinary excretion of nicotine metabolites to creatinine is illustrated in Figure 1. Nicotine intake did not change significantly throughout the study and was not affected by switching half of the volunteers to the low-tar cigarettes.

Respiratory symptoms

The prevalence of cough and phlegm among the volunteers at the start of the trial was 33% and 23%, respectively. As expected, after only five weeks these proportions did not change significantly (36% and 25%, respectively) whichever cigarette the men smoked.

Table 5. Average number of cigarettes bought from field workers and butts collected and lost per day during the trial

Week	Low-tar cigarette			Middle-tar cigarette		
	Cigarettes bought	Butts collected	Butts lost	Cigarettes bought	Butts collected	Butts lost
Pre-trial	–	9.9	3.7	–	10.3	5.7
1	20.0	11.4	3.6	21.4	11.4	5.0
2	20.4	12.1	3.0	20.7	11.5	4.6
3	20.0	11.8	3.5	20.3	11.1	4.3

Table 6. Number and weight of cigarette butts collected during trial

Week(s) ending	Low-tar cigarette			Middle-tar cigarette		
	No. of butts	Weight (g)	Weight per butt (g)	No. of butts	Weight (g)	Weight per butt (g)
Pre-trial	6 030	2045	0.34	6 815	2171	0.32
1st	5 550	1879	0.33	6 404	2095	0.33
3rd	11 357	3795	0.33	12 268	4163	0.34
5th	11 046	3666	0.33	11 791	3903	0.33

DISCUSSION

Recruitment of smokers to the study

It had been anticipated that as many as 80% of the households contacted might have responded to the initial questionnaire, that 75% of the responding middle-tar cigarette smokers might have returned their tear-off slips, and that the proportion of eligible, committed middle-tar smokers who could be contacted and would have agreed to participate in the study would have been about 50%. These proportions were in fact 64%, 64% and 52% giving a yield on entry into the study of only about two-thirds of that anticipated. Middle-tar cigarette smokers who failed to return the tear-off slip at the bottom of the health warning may have thought that the survey was a thinly disguised campaign aimed at persuading them to stop smoking. Some explanation of the true purpose of the study at this stage might have led to a higher response. However, the trial involved selling cigarettes at reduced prices to subjects, and the ethical committees were adamant that the health warning should not be undermined by any mention of details of the proposed study.

Judged by drop-out rates, selling the cigarettes at £1.00 for a pack of 20 (a price reduction of about 20%) was a sufficient financial incentive to join and participate fully in the five-week trial. Most of the 22% who dropped out of the study did so within the first couple of weeks. The great majority of the men who completed the trial said that they would have been willing to continue for several more months if asked. It would therefore seem reasonable to expect a drop-out rate of about 30% in the proposed large-scale, six-month study.

Fig. 1. Mean excretion of nicotine metabolites (μg/mg creatinine) during the trial; *, medium tar; +, low tar

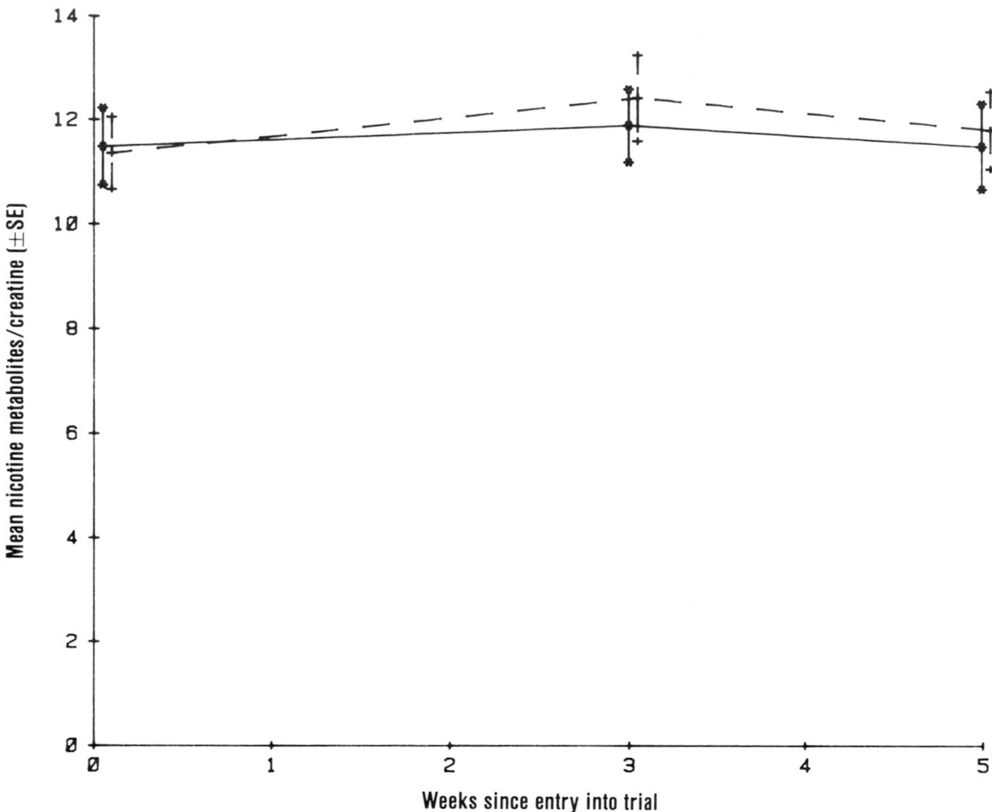

Apparent compensation by smokers who were allocated the low-tar/low-nicotine cigarette

The smoking patterns of the middle-tar cigarette smokers who were allocated to smoke the test middle-tar cigarette in the trial did not appear to change significantly; they purchased the same numbers of cigarettes each week, collected similar numbers of butts whose average weights did not differ from those of their own that they smoked during the first week of the trial. Furthermore, the extent of their nicotine inhalation, as indicated by the urinary excretion of nicotine metabolites, was unchanged. These findings suggest that the smoking patterns of the men were essentially uninfluenced by being sold cigarettes more cheaply or by participating in the trial itself.

The numbers of cigarettes smoked by the men who were changed from their normal middle-tar, middle-nicotine cigarettes to low-tar, low-nicotine cigarettes also did not change, nor did the apparent extent to which the cigarettes were smoked as indicated by their butt weights. Most importantly the amounts of nicotine that they continued to inhale remained constant despite the fact that the nicotine yield of their allocated cigarettes was some 40% less than those they normally smoked before entry into the trial. It must therefore be concluded that they had compensated for the reduced nicotine yield of the low-tar cigarettes by changing their smoking pattern in a subtle way. This might have been done by increasing the number or sizes of puffs taken.

Since the tar/nicotine ratios of the test low- and middle-tar cigarettes and of the great majority of all commercial brands of cigarettes are very similar (about 10:1), it follows that if complete compensation were a general phenomenon, changing from middle-tar to low-tar cigarettes would be unlikely to result in a significantly reduced amount of tar being inhaled each day.

It should however be emphasized that in view of the daily variations in the amount of nicotine inhaled each day by the individual smokers, as assessed by nicotine metabolite/creatinine ratios, and the relatively modest numbers of subjects taking part in the study, a 22% difference in the excretion of nicotine metabolites could have occurred between those allocated to smoke the middle-tar and low-tar cigarettes without it having being detected ($p = 0.05$). This therefore indicates that although some compensation undoubtedly occurred, it may well have been only partial.

Implications of the apparent compensation by those allocated to smoke low-tar cigarettes for the design of proposed large-scale trial

In view of the chronic nature of smoking, the prevalence of respiratory symptoms (25%) would not be expected to change significantly over the six-month observation period of the proposed large-scale trial, although a small proportion of those initially presenting with symptoms (perhaps 10% or 2.5% of the total smoking population) would probably lose them in this time, being replenished by a similar number developing symptoms from among those without symptoms at the start of the trial.

Since it is generally assumed that components in tar are responsible for the deleterious effects of smoking on respiratory symptoms, and it is possible that subjects who give up smoking lose their smoking-induced respiratory symptoms within the space of about six months (Leeder *et al.*, 1977), it is reasonable to hypothesize that if middle-tar cigarette smokers were switched to low-tar cigarettes and did not compensate for the 40% reduced nicotine yield of their cigarettes, about 30% might lose their symptoms over the proposed six-month observation period as compared with a 10% loss among those allocated to middle-tar cigarettes (a net loss of 20%).

The demonstration of compensation in this study when middle-tar cigarette smokers were switched to low-tar cigarettes confirms the findings of other recent studies (US Surgeon General, 1984), although the absolute extent of this compensation can only be established with greater precision by carrying out further studies involving considerably larger numbers of subjects. Nevertheless, it is apparent that an inevitable consequence of this phenomenon is that switching middle-tar cigarette smokers to low-tar cigarettes will result in substantially smaller reductions in tar intake than those suggested by differences in the tar yields of the cigarettes (40%), with the result that the net reduction in respiratory symptoms is likely to be considerably less than the 20% predicted if compensation did not occur. This emphasizes the importance of carrying out more extensive studies of nicotine intake in the proposed large-scale trial. It also suggests the value of having, in addition to a group of committed middle-tar cigarette smokers who either continue to smoke such a cigarette or are switched to low-tar cigarettes, the option of having a third group allocated to smoke a nicotine-enhanced, low-tar cigarette with a nicotine content similar to that of middle-tar cigarettes. An alternative approach would be to use a cigarette with a substantially lower tar/nicotine ratio than those currently on the UK market. The inclusion of such a group could therefore explore the hypothesis that, if there were no pharmacological incentive to compensate, the tar intake should be sufficiently reduced for the resultant decrease in respiratory symptoms to be detected with reasonable confidence.

Size of the proposed trial

In order to detect a net loss of symptoms by 20% of smokers with cough or phlegm at the start of the trial when allocated to one of the test cigarettes (30% loss *versus* 10% in those continuing to smoke standard middle-tar cigarettes) with reasonable confidence ($\alpha = \beta = 0.05$), it may be calculated that 140 men in the group would need to complete the trial. From the success rate of the recruitment into this feasibility study (one participant per 100 households originally mailed), an assumed likely drop-out rate of 30% and symptoms in 25% of the smokers, approximately 80 000 households would need to be mailed initially per group; 160 000 for a study of middle- *versus* low-tar cigarettes and 240 000 if a nicotine-enhanced, low-tar cigarette were also included.

Conclusion

Clearly, a double-blind, randomized controlled trial of this magnitude will be a very costly and demanding undertaking, and would only be justified if a suitable nicotine-enhanced, low-tar cigarette were available. Furthermore, it would be essential to establish early in such a trial the extent of compensation among smokers allocated to both the standard low-tar cigarette and the nicotine-enhanced, low-tar cigarette.

ACKNOWLEDGEMENTS

We would like to thank Professor Holland for his advice and help in carrying out the study; Ms C. Cousins and Ms C. Clarke for help with the mailing of questionnaires; Mrs Wales, Mrs Craddock, Mrs Baines, Mrs Chambers, Mrs Davis, Mrs Eaton, Mrs Ellis, Mr Gates, Mrs Holman, Mrs Hussain, Mrs Kitchingham, Mrs Liyanage, Mrs North, Ms Nuttar, Mrs Osborne, Mrs Parker-Smith, Mrs Pickett, Mrs Reiderman, Mrs Robson, Mrs Taylor and Mrs Wilson for the field work; and Miss P.L. Surgenor, Mrs Y.J. Smith and Mrs L. Clarke for word processing the manuscript. The study was funded by the Tobacco Products Research Trust.

REFERENCES

Fletcher, C.M., Peto, R., Tinker, C. & Speizer, F.E. (1976) *The Natural History of Chronic Bronchitis and Emphysema. An Eight Year Study of Early Chronic Obstructive Lung Disease in Working Men in London,* New York, Oxford University Press

Higenbottam, T. Shipley, M.J., Clark, T.J.H. & Rose, G. (1980) Lung function and symptoms of cigarette smokers related to tar yield and number of cigarettes smoked. *Lancet*, ***i***, 409–412

Holland, W.W., Ashford, J.B., Colley, J.R.T., Morgan, D.C. & Pearson, N.J. (1976) A comparison of two respiratory symptom questionnaires. *Br. J. prev. soc. Med.*, ***20***, 76–96

Kunze, M. & Vutuc, C. (1980) *Threshold of tar exposure. Analysis of smoking history of male lung cancer cases and controls.* In: Gori, G.B. & Bock, F.G., eds, *A Safe Cigarette? (Banbury Report No. 3)*, Cold Spring Harbour, NY, Cold Spring Harbour Laboratory, pp. 251–260

Leeder, S.R., Colley, J.R.T., Corkhill, R. & Holland, W.W. (1977) Change in respiratory symptom prevalence in adults who alter their smoking habits. *Am. J. Epidemiol.*, ***105***, 522–529

Peach, H., Ellard, G.A., Jenner, P.J. & Morris, R.W. (1985) A simple, inexpensive urine test of smoking. *Thorax*, ***40***, 351–357

Peto, R., Speizer, F.E., Cochrane, A.L., Moore, F., Fletcher, C.M., Tonker, C.M., Higgins, I.T.T., Gray, R.G., Richards, J.M., Gilliland, J. & Norman-Smith, B. (1983) The relevance in adults of airflow obstruction but not mucus hypersecretion, to mortality from chronic lung disease. *Am. Rev. resp. Dis.*, ***128***, 491–500

Rimpela, A.H. & Rimpela, M.K. (1985) Increased risk of respiratory symptoms in young smokers of low tar cigarettes. *Br. med. J.*, ***290***, 1461–1463

Royal College of Physicians (1983) *Health or Smoking? Follow-up Report of the Royal College of Physicians*, London, Pitman, pp. 21–25

Schenker, M.B., Samet, J.M. & Speizer, F.E. (1982) Effect of cigarette tar content and smoking habits on respiratory symptoms in women. *Am. Rev. resp. Dis.*, ***125***, 684–690

Sparrow, D., Stefos, T., Bosse, R. & Weiss, S.T. (1983) The relationship of tar content to decline in pulmonary function in cigarette smokers. *Am. Rev. resp. Dis.*, ***127***, 56–58

US Surgeon General (1984) *The Health Consequences of Smoking. Chronic Obstructive Lung Disease*, Rockville, MD, US Department of Health and Human Services, pp. 344–347

LOW-TAR CIGARETTES – POSSIBILITIES AND LIMITATIONS

H. KLUS

Research and Development,
Austria Tabakwerke AG,
A 1160 Vienna, Austria

INTRODUCTION

Tobacco is a remarkable product among modern luxuries. Possible health risks for tobacco consumers are described in numerous scientific papers and, owing to the mass media, are well known to the consumer (for a review see US Department of Health and Human Services, 1979). This is valid especially for inhalative cigarette smoking. However, the majority of smokers have not changed their habit (Statistisches Bundesamt, 1984). Therefore, product modifications should certainly have a place in the strategy to reduce health risks attributed to smoking.

This paper will be restricted primarily to the complex 'low-tar cigarette'. Possibilities and limitations of product modification of cigarettes will be discussed.

Hammond (1966), Doll and Peto (1976) and numerous other groups have shown in large prospective epidemiological studies that cancer, especially lung cancer, is found much more frequently in cigarette smokers than in nonsmokers. They were also able to establish a dose-response relationship between the incidence of cancer and the amount of cigarette smoke inhaled. As a consequence of these findings, the tobacco industry started to reduce the condensate and nicotine levels of cigarettes. Examples include the reductions in the USA (Anon., 1983), the Federal Republic of Germany (Verband der Cigarettenindustrie, unpublished data) and Austria (Klus, unpublished data) (Fig. 1, 2, 3).

Limited by the possibilities in the past, which only comprised the careful selection of raw tobaccos for the blend and the use of filters of different efficiency, the reduction of smoke nicotine and condensate was nearly parallel. Some authors, like Wynder and Stellman (1979), Lee and Garfinkel (1981), Lubin *et al.* (1984), and Peto and Doll (1985), attributed the declining lung cancer rate observed in younger cohorts in some countries at least partly to the reduction of tar of these cigarettes. Today, as a result of research worldwide, there are numerous additional possibilities for selectively influencing the composition of cigarette smoke. These possibilities, which might enable the tobacco industry to produce modified cigarettes that may be perhaps less harmful than the products in the past, are summarized below.

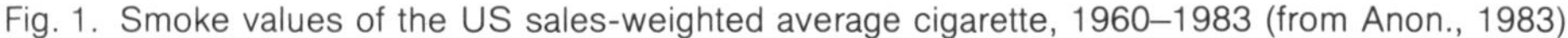
Fig. 1. Smoke values of the US sales-weighted average cigarette, 1960–1983 (from Anon., 1983)

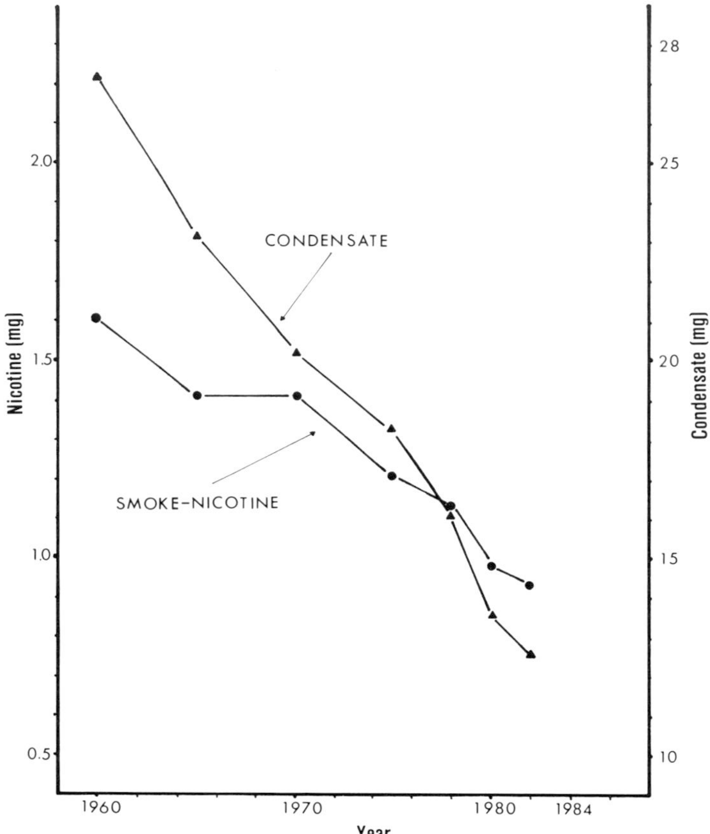

Breeding of tobacco plants is possible using classical (Matzinger *et al.*, 1984; Chaplin & Spurr, 1982) and recent biotechnical methods such as cell and tissue cultures, and haploid and protoplast cultures (Kumashiro, 1984). Genetic engineering is an additional possibility, which may lead to tailor-made tobacco plants in the future (Schell, 1984). Physical and chemical methods can be applied on leaf and cut tobacco during tobacco processing (e.g., homogenized leaf curing, expanding, reconstitution) to change the chemical composition of tobacco smoke (Gori, 1980). The chemical composition of the smoke can also be changed by varying the pyrolysis and burning conditions in the glowing cone of the cigarette (e.g., using filter technology, tip ventilation and paper technology) (Baker, 1984).

The cancer risk of cigarette smokers has been attributed to various compounds of tobacco smoke such as polynuclear aromatic hydrocarbons, volatile and tobacco-specific nitrosamines, heavy metals like nickel and cadmium, and radioactive elements like polonium-210 (US Department of Health and Human Services, 1982). It is possible to influence the amount of these substances in cigarette smoke but it is not yet known which

Fig. 2. Smoke values of the sales-weighted average cigarette from the Federal Republic of Germany, 1962–1982 (from Verband der Deutschen Cigarettenindustrie, unpublished data)

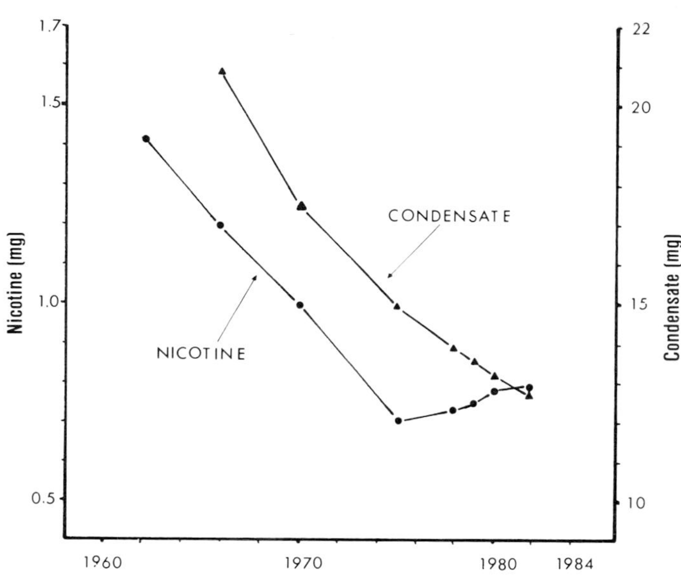

are the most important in the development of smoking-related cancer. This should be clarified in order to avoid a product modification in the wrong direction.

For example, some years ago, it was demonstrated that by increasing the nitrate content of cigarette tobacco the smoke yields of condensate and nicotine could be reduced significantly, and for catechol and polynuclear aromatic hydrocarbons an additional specific reduction could be achieved (Adams *et al.,* 1984) (Fig. 4). Animal experiments have also shown that addition of nitrate to the tobacco can significantly reduce the biological activity of the smoke condensate, e.g., on the mouse skin (Hoffmann & Wynder, 1972). On the basis of these findings some cigarette companies increased the amount of nitrate-rich tobaccos, especially the percentage of Burley stems used in their blends. However, this procedure results in an increase of nitrogen oxides and *N*-nitrosamines in the smoke, compounds which are of more and more interest with respect to their carcinogenic potential (Adams *et al.*, 1984; Hoffmann & Hecht, 1985) (Fig. 5).

A less harmful cigarette is worthless if nobody smokes it. That means that the acceptance of such a cigarette by the consumer is one of the most important points. In Figure 6 the complex interaction of various factors that influence smoking behaviour and also the acceptance of a cigarette is shown. According to the literature (Silvette *et al.,* 1962) the pharmacodynamic efficacy of nicotine is most important. There is evidence from the literature that the majority of cigarette smokers regulate their nicotine intake according to their individual requirements (for a review see McMorrow and Fox, 1983). The exact proof of this hypothesis is, however, still missing. But this assumption is supported by a lot of research obtained in many laboratories.

Fig. 3. Smoke values of the Austrian sales-weighted average cigarette, 1960–1984 (from Klus, unpublished data)

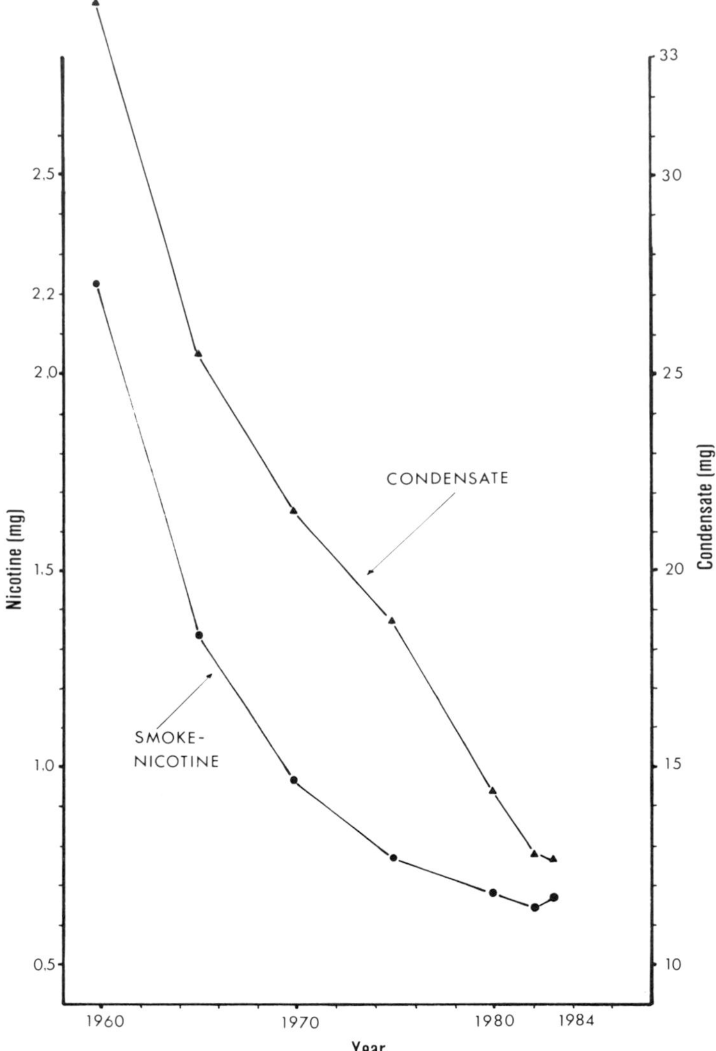

In a study of 200 cigarette smokers, Schievelbein *et al.* (unpublished data) found a high inter-individual variation in serum cotinine levels which ranged from almost 0 to more than 500 ng/ml serum. Cotinine is the main metabolite of nicotine. In contrast to nicotine, it shows a long half-life time and is, therefore, a good parameter by which to measure nicotine intake. There was only a weak correlation between nicotine intake and the number of cigarettes smoked per day and no correlation between the nicotine delivery of the brand determined by mechanical smoking under standard conditions (Coresta Stan-

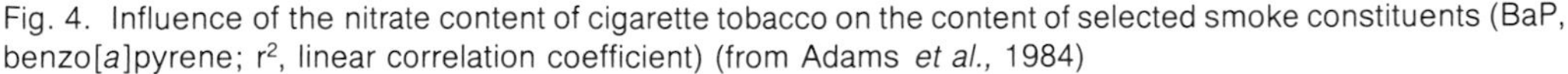

Fig. 4. Influence of the nitrate content of cigarette tobacco on the content of selected smoke constituents (BaP, benzo[*a*]pyrene; r^2, linear correlation coefficient) (from Adams *et al.*, 1984)

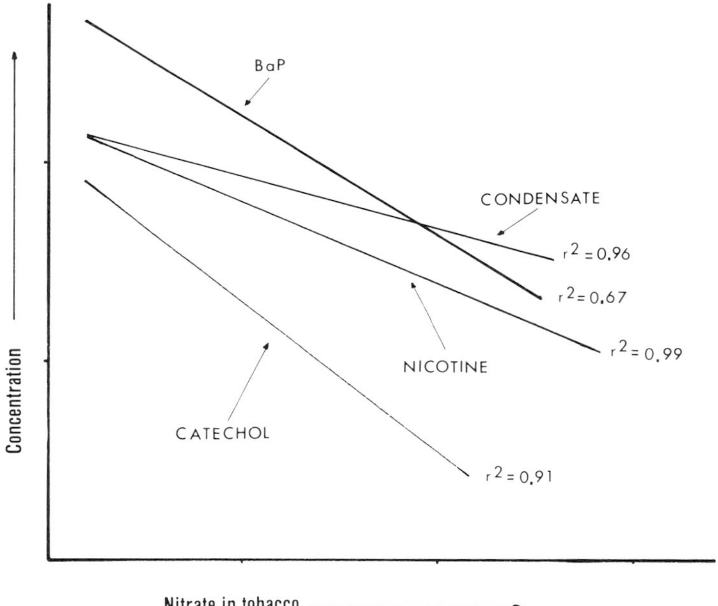

dard Method No.1; Cooperation Centre for Scientific Research Relative to Tobacco, 1966). Based on these investigations, all smokers were classified according to their serum cotinine levels as high, medium and low 'nicotine intakers'. The results of a second investigation four weeks later with the same subjects were similar. Except for an insignificant number of smokers, they showed nearly the same cotinine serum levels as in the first experiment, maintaining their 'nicotine-intaker' class. These results were confirmed by a third investigation, another four weeks later.

The authors concluded that, despite a rather high inter-individual variation, the intra-individual nicotine intake in cigarette smokers is relatively constant over time. It is this constancy which speaks in favour of nicotine-intake regulation. It seems that the individual smoker makes use of a certain stable amount of nicotine he is offered by his cigarette brand. It is not yet known what governs the constancy of cigarette smoke intake. There is substantial evidence that nicotine is the regulating factor at least for a number of cigarette smokers. If this is true, a change in nicotine delivery in the cigarette will be compensated by the consumer by changing his individual smoking habits as regards puff volume, mode of inhalation, puff number, and so on. This hypothesis is also substantiated by Benowitz *et al.* (1983), Russell *et al.* (1980) and Wald *et al.* (1981). Modification of cigarettes to reduce the condensate and nicotine delivery in the same degree may therefore, at least in part, be neutralized by compensating mechanisms and the positive effect for the consumer may be lost.

Fig. 5. Influence of the nitrate content of cigarette tobacco on the content of nitrogen oxides and *N*-nitrosamines in the smoke (NNN, *N'*-nitrosonornicotine; NPYR, *N*-nitrosopyrrolidine; NDMA, *N*-nitrosodimethylamine) NO, nitrogen oxides; r^2, linear correlation coefficient) (from Hoffmann *et al.,* 1984)

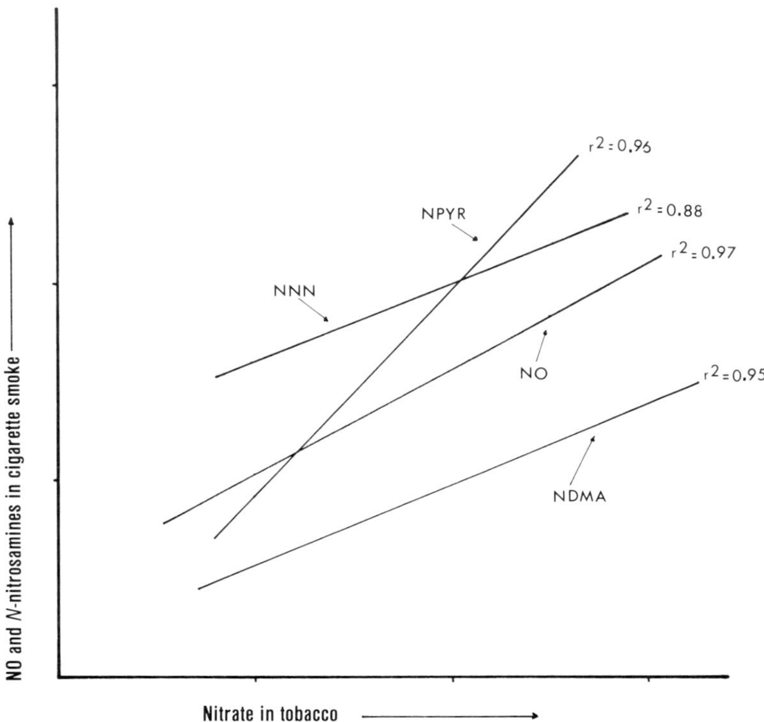

Therefore, product modification in the direction of a 'less harmful cigarette' has to consider possible compensating mechanisms. As a consequence of this, a modern cigarette should have a sufficient nicotine delivery, while the yields of condensate and gas-phase compounds should be as low as possible. Taste and smell experiences, which are essential for smoking pleasure are the natural limitations of such a product development (von Hees *et al.*, 1984). The technical possibilities for the realization of this concept are more or less available and are described below.

BREEDING AND AGRICULTURAL METHODS

Prerequisites for a 'less harmful cigarette' are tobacco varieties with sufficient amounts of nicotine which produce small amounts of condensate. Nicotine itself does not seem to be a factor in carcinogenesis. However, recently it was shown by Hoffmann and Hecht (1985) and also by our own working group (Klus & Kuhn, 1975) that the tobacco-specific *N*-nitrosamines are generated in part from nicotine. Tobacco-specific *N*-nitrosamines are

Fig. 6. The interaction of factors that influence smoking behaviour

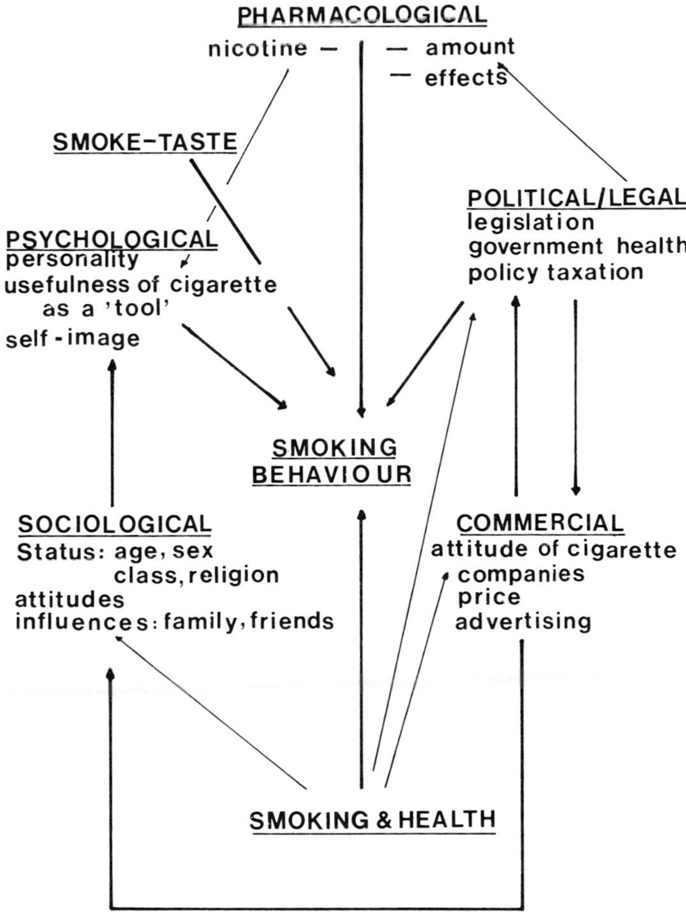

not found in freshly harvested tobaccos. They are formed during the curing and ageing processes.

The amount of nitrosamines in tobacco and tobacco smoke correlates with the nitrate content of tobacco (Adams *et al.*, 1984). As was shown recently, nitrate in tobacco is degraded to ammonia or nitrogen by bacteria and enzyme systems (Stangelberger, 1984). In both cases, nitrite is formed during the degradation pathway, and this is essential for nitrosamine formation in tobacco. Reduction of nitrate in tobacco, especially in Burley tobaccos, is possible by breeding varieties poor in nitrate. It may also be achieved by changing agricultural methods, such as reduction of fertilization with nitrate (Raper & McCants, 1967; Broaddus *et al.*, 1965; Merker, 1979). Additional offering of phosphate and molybdenum also leads to a reduction in nitrate (Schmid, 1966; Pal *et al.*, 1976; Sims & Atkinson, 1976; Eivazi *et al.*, 1982). Molybdenum is the cofactor of nitrate reductase, the enzyme which is responsible for nitrate degradation in tobacco.

Schell (1984) of the Max-Planck Institute for Breeding Research, Cologne, recently reported the first results obtained with genetic engineering in tobacco. According to Schell, tobacco is well suited for genetic engineering. Gene-vector systems for the cloning and re-introduction into tobacco of any type of foreign genetic information have been developed. Intervention in nitrate metabolism, and in the formation of proteins, aroma substances and alkaloids might be possible in the near future using this technique, achieving a reduction of nitrosamines in tobacco and tobacco smoke. It may also be possible to influence the cadmium uptake of the tobacco plant by genetic engineering.

TOBACCO PROCESSING

Homogenized leaf curing (HLC) was described by Tso *et al.* (1975). The process and goals of this tobacco treatment are shown schematically in Figure 7.

The composition of tobacco smoke can also be influenced by expansion of cut-tobacco as well as with the use of reconstituted tobacco sheets.

For expansion, the cut tobacco is soaked in a liquid with a low boiling point, like Freon-11, carbon dioxide or liquid nitrogen, at a pressure of 6–7 × 10^7 Pa the shock-like evaporation of the liquid leads to an expansion of the leaf structure to almost double its original volume. The percentage of nicotine in the cigarette smoke condensate has been shown to rise with increasing amounts of expanded tobacco in the blend (Klus & Kuhn, 1975).

The expansion of cut-rolled tobacco stem is also a widely used method of tobacco processing. The expansion medium is mostly steam. Dontenwill *et al.* (1977) showed, that, when tested on mouse skin, the smoke condensate of cigarettes containing 50% of expanded tobacco stem in the blend produces fewer tumour-bearing mice than the smoke condensate of cigarettes without expanded stem.

Fig. 7. Homogenized leaf curing of tobacco (schematic) (from Tso *et al.*, 1975)

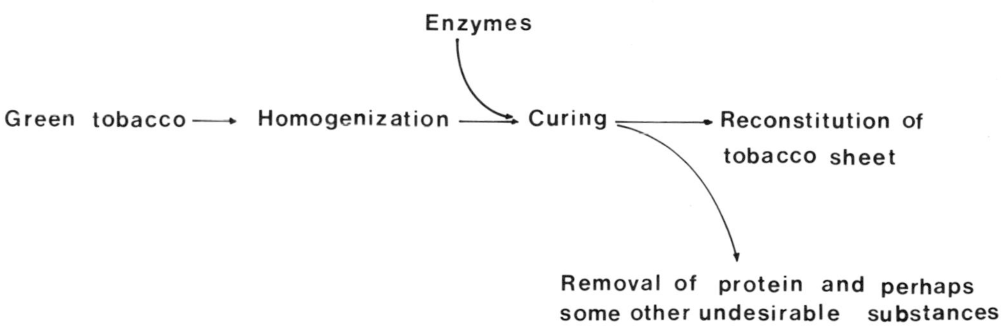

Reconstituted tobacco sheets have been used for more than three decades in the production of cigarettes. Originally, they were used primarily for economic reasons. Wynder and Hoffmann (1965) demonstrated that condensate from cigarettes made from reconstituted tobacco sheets produced a lower tumour rate in the skin of mice than condensate from cigarettes made from natural tobaccos. Dontenwill *et al.* (1972) confirmed these reports. Therefore, the use of reconstituted tobaccos is considered a step towards a 'less harmful cigarette'.

CIGARETTE PAPER

Spears (1974) stated that the paper used in the manufacturing of cigarettes can influence smoke composition in a number of ways:

– The combustion of the cigarettes may be modified leading to changes in aroma and smoke composition.

– Part of the gas phase of cigarette smoke, e.g., the carbon monoxide and nitrogen oxide, diffuses through the paper and air is drawn through the paper into the tobacco-rod of the cigarette, diluting the smoke.

– The quality of the paper influences the distribution of the air in and around the glowing cone and therefore the burning conditions. A change in smoke composition and burning rate is possible.

– The paper influences the amount of tobacco burned per puff and during the puffs.

The parameters that determine these effects of cigarette papers are porosity and the type and amount of burn additives.

FILTERS

The filter, an integral part of a modern cigarette, has evolved from being an implement purely for reducing the amount of smoke into a tool for influencing the quality and composition of the smoke. The parts of tobacco smoke that might be influenced by filters are shown in Figure 8 (Williamson, 1974).

The particulate phase or condensate can be filtered mechanically only. By contrast, many compounds of the gas phase and the semivolatile phase can be selectively reduced by filters. The aims of modern filters are shown in Figure 9.

They include selective and nonselective filtration by various mechanisms and also control of smoke formation by influencing combustion. An example of the possibilities for modifying smoke composition by selective filtration with the aid of a modern cellulose acetate filter is shown in Figure 10 (Williamson *et al.*, 1965; Hoffmann *et al.*, 1980). The filter contains triacetine, an additive widely used in acetate filters of modern cigarettes. In this connection it should be pointed out, that volatile *N*-nitrosamines, like *N*-nitrosodimethylamine, are selectively reduced in cigarette smoke by such a modern cellulose acetate filter (Hoffmann *et al.*, 1980).

Fig. 8. Possibilities for influencing the composition of tobacco smoke with the aid of filters (from Williamson, 1974)

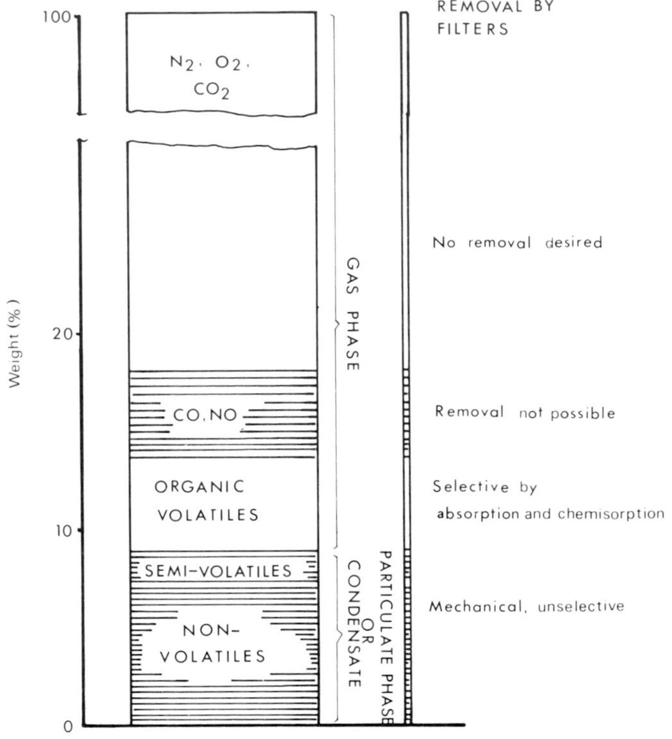

Fig. 9. The aims of a modern cigarette filter

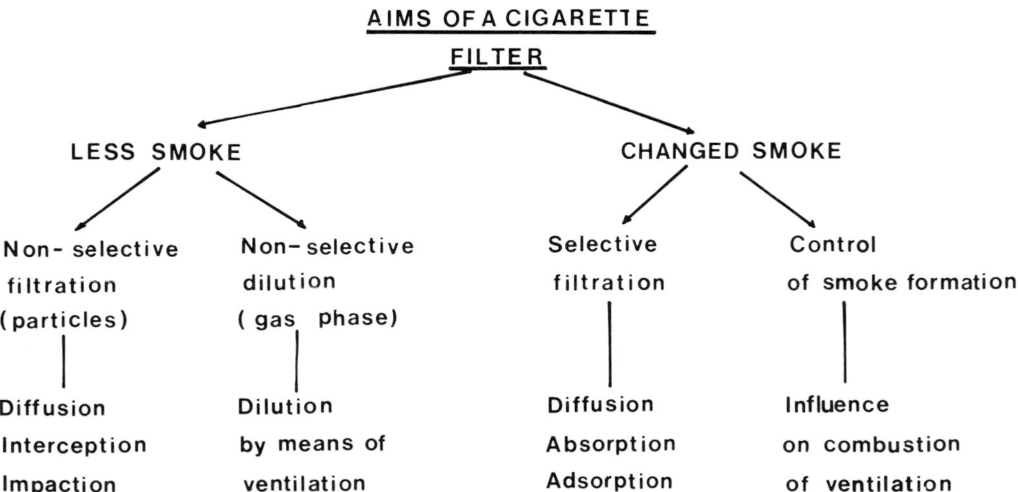

Fig. 10. Selective filtration of cigarette smoke with the aid of a modern cellulose acetate filter (+ 10 % triacetin) (NDMA, *N*-nitrosodimethylamine; NDEA, *N*-nitrosodiethylamine; NPYR, *N*-nitrosopyrrolidine) (from Williamson *et al.*, 1965; Hoffmann *et al.*, 1980)

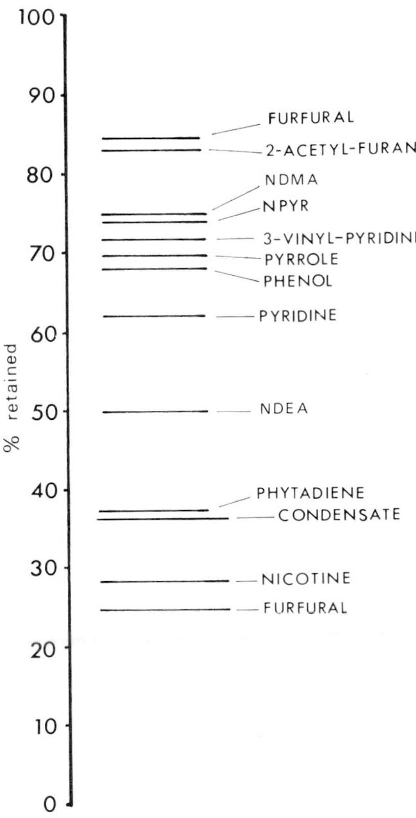

FILTER VENTILATION

In Figure 9, where the aims of a modern cigarette filter were shown, filter or tip ventilation is also shown. Filter ventilation primarily means the addition of an exactly determined amount of air to the mainstream smoke *via* a perforation zone in the tipping of the filter, thus reducing the amount of air flowing around and in the glow zone. This decreases the glow-temperature and changes the combustion characteristics (Baker, 1980), which leads to a change in the composition of the smoke. The influence of tip ventilation on cigarette smoke composition was first described by Norman (1974). This relationship is shown in Figure 11 (Klus *et al.*, 1984). Nicotine is selectively enriched, carbon monoxide selectively reduced. According to preliminary results, tobacco-specific and also volatile nitrosamines seem to be reduced selectively with filter ventilation (Klus *et al.*, unpublished data).

As reported recently, filter ventilation also affects the transfer of aroma compounds from tobacco into the smoke drastically (Klus *et al.*, 1984; Fig. 12).

Fig. 11. The influence of tip ventilation on selected cigarette smoke compounds; TPM, total particulate matter (from Klus *et al.*, 1984)

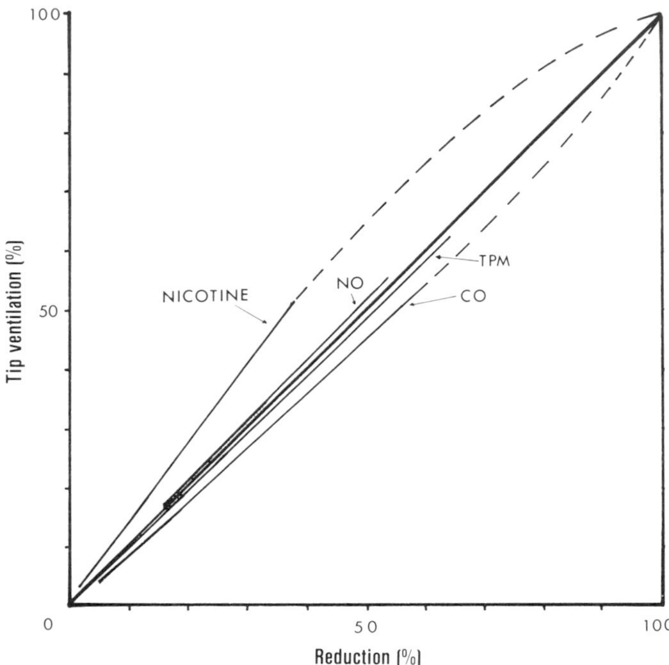

The pH of cigarette smoke is also changed by filter ventilation (Klus *et al.*, 1985) (Fig. 13). The pH increases with increasing filter ventilation, that is, the smoke becomes alkaline. The amount of free, unprotonated nicotine in the smoke is pH-dependent (Brunnemann & Hoffmann, 1974).

The quality factors in cigarette smoke, which have been variously described as 'bite' or 'strength', are connected to the acidic or basic nature of the smoke. The pharmacological effect of nicotine is, according to Armitage and Turner (1970), Schievelbein and Eberhardt (1972), and Russell *et al.* (1976), not only a function of the nicotine concentration per puff but also of the pH of the smoke.

Another factor connected with the pH of tobacco smoke is the so-called 'inhalability'. Cigar smoke showing an alkaline reaction is harder to inhale than, for example, the smoke of a cigarette made from bright tobaccos with a slightly acidic reaction of the smoke (Brunnemann & Hoffmann, 1974).

The use of filter ventilation is also limited by consumer acceptance. The change in the smoke taste due to the alteration of the smoke composition should be taken into consideration when making filter-ventilated cigarettes. If this is not done, there is a risk that consumers will not accept the new brand. In my opinion, the possible acceptance limit for filter ventilation is 40–50% at this stage.

Fig. 12. The influence of tip ventilation on selected aroma compounds in cigarette smoke (Klus *et al.*, 1984)

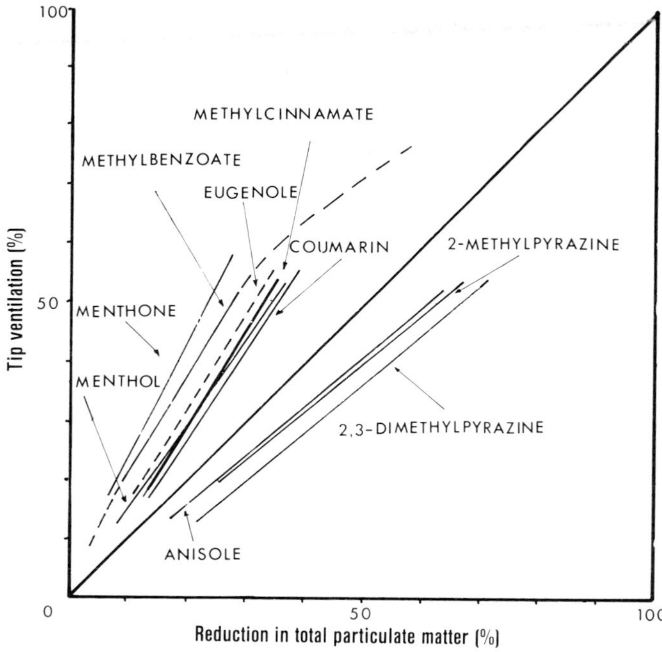

Fig. 13. The influence of tip ventilation on the pH of cigarette mainstream smoke (puff by puff analysis) (Klus *et al.*, 1985)

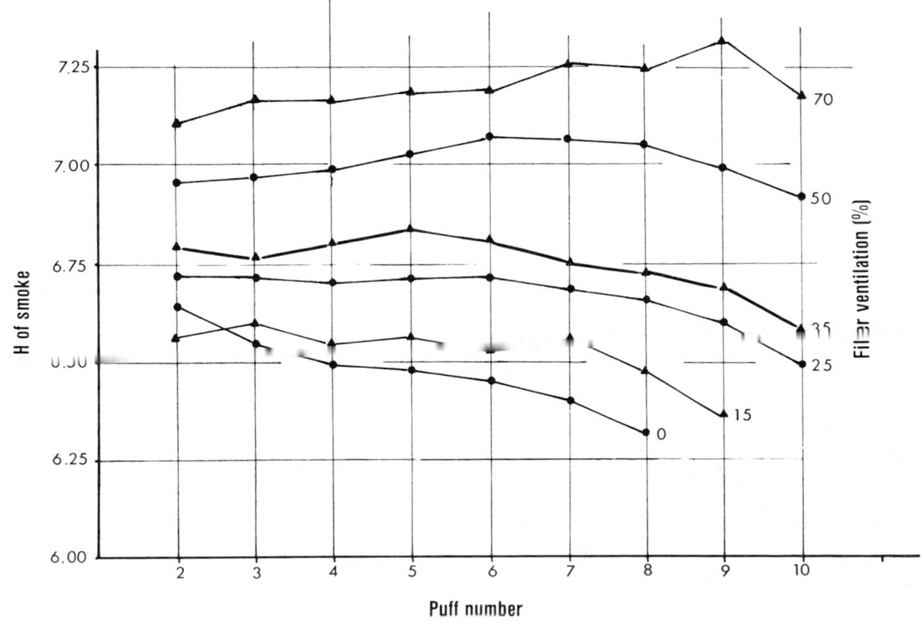

CONCLUSION

I have tried to show some methods already available which can be used to modify cigarettes. Other methods, similar or even more effective, must be developed. I would like to close with a statement by Russell at a conference in London (Richards, 1984). Russell replied to the question 'Can we have safer cigarettes?' as follows: 'The answer is yes, we have them already, but we can have them much more safe.' That is my strong belief too.

REFERENCES

Adams, J.D., Lee, S.J. & Hoffmann, D. (1984) Carcinogenic agents in cigarette smoke and the influence of nitrate on their formation. *Carcinogenesis,* ***5,*** 221–223

Anon. (1983) Cigarette report: Low tar in command. *Tob. Int.,* ***185,*** 68–69

Armitage, A.K. & Turner, D.M. (1970) Absorption of nicotine in cigarette and cigar smoke through the oral mucosa. *Nature,* ***226,*** 1231–1232

Baker, R.R. (1980) *Development of temperature distribution inside the reaction zone of a burning cigarette.* In: Wiedemann, H.G., ed., *Proceedings of the 6th International Conference on Thermal Analysis,* Vol. 1, Basle, Boston, Stuttgart, Birkhäuser Verlag, pp. 439–444

Baker, R.R. (1984) The effect of ventilation on cigarette combustion mechanisms. *Recent Adv. Tob. Sci.,* ***10,*** 88–150

Benowitz, N.L., Hall, S.M., Herning, R.I., Jacob, P., Jones, R.T. & Osman, A.L. (1983) Smokers of low-yield cigarettes do not consume less nicotine. *New Engl. J. Med.,* ***309,*** 139–142

Broaddus, G.M., York, J.E., Jr & Moseley, J.M. (1965) Factors affecting the levels of nitrate nitrogen in cured tobacco leaves. *Tob. Sci.,* ***9,*** 149–157

Brunnemann, K.D. & Hoffmann, D. (1974) The pH of tobacco smoke. *Food Cosmet. Toxicol.,* ***12,*** 115–124

Chaplin, J.F. & Spurr, M.W., Jr (1982) Altering condensate levels in tobacco smoke by genetic techniques. *Beitr. Tabakforsch. Int.,* ***11,*** 151–160

Cooperation Centre for Scientific Research Relative to Tobacco (CORESTA) (1966) *CORESTA Standard Method No. 1* Machine smoking of cigarettes and determination of moist and anhydrous smoke condensate, Paris

Doll, R. & Peto, R. (1976) Mortality in relation to smoking: 20 years observation on male British doctors. *Br. med. J.,* ***2,*** 1525–1536

Dontenwill, W., Chevalier, H.J., Harke, H.P., Klimisch, H.J., Lafrenz, U. & Reckzeh, G. (1972) Experimental investigations of the tumorigenic effect of cigarette smoke condensate on mouse skin. IV. Comparisons of condensates from different tobacco leaves, the influence of the addition of $NaNO_3$ to tobacco or tobacco leaves, the effect of volatile portions of the smoke, the influence of pretreatment with dimethylbezanthracene (Ger.). *Z. Krebsforsch.,* ***78,*** 236–264

Dontenwill, W., Chevalier, H.J., Harke, H.P., Klimisch, H.J., Reckzeh, G., Fleischmann, B. & Keller, W. (1977) Experimental investigations of the tumorigenic effect of cigarette smoke condensate on mouse skin. VII. Comparisons of condensates from various modified cigarettes (Ger.). *Z. Krebsforsch.,* ***89,*** 145–151

Eivazi, F., Sims, J.L. & Leggett, J.E. (1982) *Phosphorus and molybdenum interaction effects on uptake of molybdenum by Burley tobacco plants.* Paper presented at the *36th Tobacco Chemists Research Conference, NC, October 1982* (in press)

Gori, G.B. (1980) *Less hazardous cigarettes: Theory and practice.* In: Gori, G.B. & Bock, F.G., eds, *A safe cigarette? (Banbury Report No. 3),* Cold Spring Harbor, NY, Cold Spring Harbor Laboratory, pp. 261–279

Hammond, E.C. (1966) Smoking in relation to the death rates of one million men and women. *Cancer Monogr.,* ***19,*** 127–204

von Hees, U., Scherer, G. & Adlkofer, F. (1984) *Nicotine deliveries from various tobacco products.* Paper presented at the *8th CORESTA International Tobacco Scientific Congress, October 7–12, Vienna, Austria* (in press)

Hoffmann, D. & Hecht, S.S. (1985) Nicotine-derived *N*-nitrosamines and tobacco related cancer: Current status and future directions. *Cancer Res.,* ***45,*** 935–944

Hoffmann, D. & Wynder, E.L. (1972) Selective reduction of tumorigenicity of tobacco smoke. II. Experimental approaches. *J. natl Cancer Inst.,* ***48,*** 1855–1868

Hoffmann, D., Adams, J.D., Piade, J.J. & Hecht, S.S. (1980) *Chemical studies on tobacco smoke. LXVIII. Analysis of volatile and tobacco specific nitrosamines in tobacco products.* In: Walker, E.A., Griciute, L., Castegnaro, M., Borzsönyi, M. & Davis, W., eds, N-*Nitroso Compounds: Analysis, Formation and Occurrence (IARC Scientific Publications No. 31),* Lyon, International Agency for Research on Cancer, pp. 507–516

Hoffmann, D., Brunnemann, K.D., Adams, J.D. & Hecht, S.S. (1984) *Formation and analysis of* N-*nitrosamines in tobacco products and their endogenous formation in tobacco consumers.* In: O'Neill, I.K., von Borstel, R.C., Miller, C.T., Long, J. & Bartsch, H., eds, N-*Nitroso Compounds: Occurrence, Biological Effects and Relevance to Human Cancer (IARC Scientific Publications No. 57),* Lyon, International Agency for Research on Cancer, pp. 743–762

Klus, H. & Kuhn, H. (1975) Investigations of non-volatile *N*-nitrosamines of tobacco alkaloids (Ger.). *Fachl. Mitteil. Austria Tabakwerke,* ***16,*** 307–317

Klus, H., Novak, A. & Begutter, H. (1984) The influence of tip ventilation on the transfer of some selected flavouring compounds to cigarette mainstream smoke. Paper presented at the *8th CORESTA International Tobacco Scientific Congress, 7–12 October, Vienna, Austria* (in press)

Klus, H., Begutter, H. & Ultsch, I. (1985) The influence of filter ventilation on the pH of mainstream smoke (Ger.). *Beitr. Tabakforsch. Int.* (in press)

Kuhn, H. & Klus, H. (1975) *Possibilities for reduction of nicotine in cigarette smoke.* In: Wynder, E.L., Hoffmann, D. & Gori, G.B., eds, *Workshop II: Modifying the Risk for the Smoker. Proceedings of the 3rd World Conference on Smoking and Health, 2–5 June, Vol. 1, New York,* pp. 463–469

Kumashiro, T. (1984) *Statement to the presentation of J.S. Schell.* In: *8th CORESTA International Scientific Congress, 7–12 October, Vienna, Austria (CORESTA Inf. Bull. Special),* Paris, Cooperation Centre for Scientific Research Relative to Tobacco, pp. 30–32

Lee, P.N. & Garfinkel, L. (1981) Mortality and type of cigarette smoked. *J. Epidemiol. Community Health,* ***35,*** 16–22

Lubin, J.H., Blot, W.J., Berrino, F., Flamant, R., Gillis, C.R., Kunze, M., Schmähl, D.

& Visco, G. (1984) Patterns of lung cancer risk according to the type of cigarette smoked. *Int. J. Cancer,* ***33,*** 569–576

Matzinger, D.F., Weeks, W.W. & Wernsman, E.A. (1984) Genetic modification of total particulate matter. *Recent Adv. Tob. Sci.,* ***10,*** 15–51

Merker, J. (1979) Nitrate fertilization in tobacco cultivation (Ger.). *Ber. Inst. Tabakforsch. Dresden,* ***26,*** 5–27

McMorrow, M.J. & Fox, R.M. (1983) Nicotine role in smoking: An analysis of nicotine regulation. *Psychol. Bull.,* ***93,*** 302–327

Norman, V. (1974) The effect of perforated tipping paper in the yield of various smoke components. *Beitr. Tabakforsch.,* ***7,*** 282–287

Pal, U.R., Gosset, D.R., Sims, J.L. & Leggett, J.E. (1976) Molybdenum and sulfur nutrition effects on nitrate-reductase in Burley tobacco. *Can. J. Bot.,* ***54,*** 2014–2022

Peto, R. & Doll, R. (1985) The control of lung cancer. *New Sci.,* ***105,*** 26–30

Raper, C.D., Jr & McCants, C.B. (1967) Influence of nitrogen nutrition on growth of tobacco leaves. *Tob. Sci.,* ***11,*** 175–179

Richards, T. (1984) Can we have safer cigarettes? *Br. med. J.,* ***289,*** 1374

Russell, M.A.H., Feyerabend, C. & Cole, P.V. (1976) Plasma nicotine levels after cigarette smoking and chewing nicotine gum. *Br. med. J.,* ***i,*** 1043–1046

Russell, M.A.H., Jarvis, M., Iyer, R. & Feyerabend, C. (1980) Relation of nicotine yield of cigarettes in blood nicotine concentrations in smokers. *Br. med. J.,* ***280,*** 972–976

Schell, J.S. (1984) *Genetic engineering of tobacco: Possibilities and prospects.* Paper presented at the *8th CORESTA International Tobacco Scientific Congress, 7–12 October, Vienna, Austria (CORESTA Inf. Bull. Special),* Paris, Cooperation Centre for Scientific Research Relative to Tobacco, pp. 25–27

Schievelbein, H. & Eberhardt, R. (1972) Cardiovascular actions of nicotine and smoking. *J. natl Cancer Inst.,* ***48,*** 1785–1794

Schmid, K. (1966) *Investigations upon the effect of the trace-element molybdenum on the nitrate content of tobacco.* In: *Proceedings of the 4th International Tobacco Scientific Congress, Athens, Greece*

Silvette, H., Hoff, E.C., Larson, P.S. & Haag, H.B. (1962) The actions of nicotine on central nervous system functions. *Pharmacol. Rev.,* ***14,*** 137–173

Sims, J.L. & Atkinson, W.O. (1976) Lime, molybdenum and nitrogen source effects on yield and selected chemical components of Burley tobacco. *Tob. Sci.,* ***20,*** 174–177

Spears, A.W. (1974) *Effect of manufacturing variables on cigarette smoke composition.* Paper presented at the *CORESTA International Tobacco Scientific Symposium, 22–27 September, Montreux, Switzerland (CORESTA Inf. Bull. Special),* Paris, Cooperation Centre for Scientific Research Relative to Tobacco, pp. 65–78

Stangelberger, J. (1984) *Different possibilities for the reduction of the nitrate and nitrite content of tobacco* (Ger.). Thesis, Technical University of Vienna, Austria

Statistisches Bundesamt, ed. (1985) Statistical Yearbook 1961–1984 for the Federal Republic of Germany (Ger.), Stuttgart, Verlag W. Kohlhammer

Tso, T.C., Lowe, R. & DeJong, D.W. (1975) Homogenized leaf curing. I. Theoretical bases and some preliminary results. *Beitr. Tabakforsch.,* ***8,*** 44–51

US Department of Health and Human Services (1979) *The Health Consequences of Smoking. A Report of the Surgeon General (Publication No. PHS 79–50066),* Washington DC, US Government Printing Office

US Department of Health and Human Services (1982) *The Health Consequences of smoking: Cancer. A Report of the Surgeon General (Publication No. DHHS PHS 82–50179)*, Washington DC, US Government Printing Office

Wald, N.J., Idle, M., Boreham, J. & Bailey, A. (1981) The importance of tar and nicotine in determining cigarette smoking habits. *J. Epidemiol. Community Health*, ***35***, 23–24

Williamson, J.T. (1974) *The effect of filters on cigarette smoke compounds.* Paper presented at the *CORESTA International Tobacco Scientific Symposium, 22–27 September, Montreux, Switzerland (CORESTA Inf. Bull. Special)*, Paris, Cooperation Centre for Scientific Research Relative to Tobacco, pp. 79–95

Williamson, J.T., Graham, J.F. & Allman, D.R. (1965) The modification of cigarette smoke by filter tips. *Beitr. Tabakforsch.*, ***3***, 233–242

Wynder, E.L. & Hoffmann, D. (1965) Reduction of tumorogenicity of cigarette smoke. An experimental approach. *J. Am. med. Assoc.*, ***192***, 88–94

Wynder, E.L. & Stellman, S.D. (1979) The impact of long-term filter cigarette usage in lung and larynx cancer risk. A case-control study. *J. natl Cancer Inst.*, ***62***, 471–477

VII. SMOKING CONTROL IMPLEMENTATION

LEGISLATION AND POLITICAL ACTIVITY[1]

K. BJARTVEIT

Norwegian Council on Smoking and Health,
Oslo 1, Norway

Legislation is one of the cornerstones in a comprehensive national programme on smoking and health. This paper is intended to give a general introduction to this theme.

LEGISLATIVE MEASURES

What kinds of measures can be used in legislative action? Professor Ruth Roemer (1982) has given a brilliant and thorough presentation; and here I shall just try to summarize briefly the restrictive measures which have been implemented or proposed in an attempt to influence smoking behaviour (Bjartveit *et al.*, 1969; Bjartveit, 1971; World Health Organization, 1976; WHO Expert Committee on Smoking Control, 1979; Grey & Daube, 1980). They can be grouped as follows:

Restriction of influences encouraging smoking

(a) Reduction of explicit influence, for example, a ban on promotion.
(b) Reduction of implicit influence, for example, a ban on smoking on television.

Requirements for influences discouraging smoking

(a) Health warnings on tobacco packets, including packets for export.
(b) Health warnings in such tobacco advertisements as are permitted in the absence of a ban.
(c) Declaration on packets and in advertisements of emission levels of harmful substances.
(d) Mandated health education, included mandated funding.

---

[1] A version of this paper was presented at the 5th World Conference on Smoking and Health, Winnipeg, Canada, 10–15 July 1983; and this version is included with the permission of the organizers of that conference, the Canadian Council on Smoking and Health.

Sales restrictions

(a) Limitation of sales outlets, i.e., number of shops permitted to sell tobacco, and of vending machines.
(b) Limitation on hours of sale, for example, only during ordinary opening hours for shops.
(c) Age limitations, i.e., prohibition of sale to minors.
(d) End to sales in health premises.
(e) End to duty-free sales.

Product restrictions

(a) Upper limit of tobacco content per cigarette (concerns also goods for export).
(b) Upper limit for emissions of defined harmful substances (concerns also goods for export).

Taxation

(a) General tax increase on tobacco products. This is undoubtedly one of the most effective measures available. To achieve maximum impact and to prevent a waning of the effect over time, the exercise needs to be repeated at more or less regular intervals.
(b) Selective tax increase, i.e., a graded taxation according to emissions of defined harmful substances.

Restrictions on smoking

These establish nonsmoking as a norm, and limit smoking to defined zones and/or times.
(a) Restrictions on smoking in public places.
(b) Restrictions on smoking at places of work. This applies particularly to occupations where industrial pollution, e.g. asbestos, causes a synergistic risk increase for the smoker (probably also for the passive smoker).

A dilemma

This list, which is by no means complete and whose arrangement may be questioned, presents an arsenal of powerful weapons. A signal of their importance is the fact that, with few exceptions, these measures have been fought vigorously by the tobacco industry.

On the other hand, it is also clear from the list of restrictions that they may be met with irritation by the general population, and a feeling of being under the guardianship of the authorities. Boomerang effects may occur if restrictions are not introduced with caution. Therefore, it is important not to implement restrictions which will not be understood and respected.

This situation demonstrates our dilemma: if restrictions are not utilized, we may lose opportunities to influence a major health problem. If utilized too fast, and without intelligence, they may turn out to be useless and even counter-productive.

Table 1. Attitudes to restrictions on smoking in public places in a representative sample (2597) of the Norwegian population aged 16–74 years, in 1982, who were given the question: 'It has been discussed whether or not specific rules should be introduced for smoking in public places and work premises. Which of these arrangements would you prefer?'[a]

Area of restriction	Total prohibition	Separate rooms for smokers	Smoke-free zones	Total in favour of restrictions	Request to smokers not to smoke	Unlimited smoking
Waiting rooms for travellers	16	49	21	86	8	6
Waiting rooms in hospitals	53	36	6	95	3	2
Canteens at work	17	38	24	79	11	10
Offices and smaller work premises	37	23	9	69	22	9
Restaurant and cafés	8	13	28	49	11	40

[a] From Norwegian Central Bureau of Statistics, unpublished data. Don't-know answers were disregarded (20–29%)

To find a point of balance, it is necessary to observe public opinion in this field closely. Surprisingly, however, when public opinion is measured, it may reveal that people agree to restrictions more often than anticipated.

ATTITUDES TO LEGISLATION

In a 1982 survey (Norwegian Central Bureau of Statistics, unpublished data) of a representative sample of the entire Norwegian population aged 16–74 years, a substantial proportion wanted more or less strong restrictions on smoking in public places (Table 1): 86% in waiting rooms for travellers; 95% in waiting rooms in hospitals; 79% in canteens at work; 69% in offices and smaller work premises; and 49% in restaurants and cafés.

In a 1982 survey including a representative sample of the population across Canada, aged 15 years and above (no., 2340; don't-know answers disregarded, 1–2%): 90% wanted nonsmoking areas in restaurants which are large enough to have them; and 92% wanted nonsmoking areas on buses, trains and aircraft (Canadian Gallup Poll Ltd., 1982).

In a 1973 survey before the Norwegian Tobacco Act entered into force, 81% of the adult population aged 16–74 years (no., 2313; don't-know answers disregarded, 18%) were in favour of the advertising ban on tobacco and of the compulsory health labelling (Central Bureau of Statistics, 1974).

In 1982, 46% of Canadians wanted cigarette advertising to be eliminated altogether. Only 7% would have allowed it to increase (Table 2) (Canadian Gallup Poll Ltd., 1982)

In a 1979 Norwegian survey, 56% of the adult population aged 16–74 years (no., 1511; don't-know answers disregarded, 5.5%) supported an increase in cigarette prices as a measure to influence the damaging habit (Aaro & Brekke, 1984).

LEGISLATION: ONE PART OF A COMPREHENSIVE PROGRAMME

The positive attitude towards the restrictions referred to here probably reflects results of earlier information and education activities. Here we touch upon an indispensible prere-

Table 2. Attitudes toward cigarette advertising in a representative sample (2340) of the Canadian population aged 15+ in 1982 [a]

Option for cigarette advertising	Percentage response
Eliminated altogether	46
Reduced to lower level	19
Restricted to current level	28
Allowed to increase	7

[a] From Canadian Gallup Poll Ltd., 1982. Don't-know answers were disregarded (5%)

quisite for implementing legislative action: it must be integrated in a total, comprehensive, well-balanced smoking and health programme, which includes both information and education, as well as cessation activities. In such a programme, the restrictions will function as a catalyst to the other elements.

One advantage of legislation is that, in terms of money, it costs very little. However, some governments might think that legislation is a cheap alibi for not investing in more expensive education and cessation programmes – people will still have the impression that something is being done. To introduce legislation in a vacuum of other activities, however, would probably have no effect at all. The same applies to partial or inadequate legislation.

MEASURING THE EFFECT OF LEGISLATION

What effect has antismoking legislation? Let us take an advertising ban as an example. It is remarkable how the interest in this question has steadily increased, along with a demand for data. Enthusiasts ask obviously because they want proof that can convince their legislators about the necessity of an advertising ban. The tobacco industry asks obviously because they want proof that can convince their legislators that an advertising ban does not work. Bureaucrats ask because they want a solid basis for action, or a few of them may want excuses for postponing the trouble of preparing drafts for their legislators. Politicians ask because they want evidence that can convince their parliamentary colleagues in either direction.

I feel it is necessary to pour some cold water on the confidence in the measurements used for estimating an effect of an advertising ban (Bjartveit, 1980), and these are my reasons:

(1) I think that it is quite impossible, in the strict scientific sense, to quantify the effect of an advertising ban. I am somewhat afraid of making this statement, which I did at the 5th World Conference on Smoking and Health in Winnipeg. It has been misinterpreted and misused, giving the impression that my opinion is that an advertising ban has no effect. Nevertheless, my point was and is, that we are not dealing with a controlled trial, where we have two isolated communities, identical in demographic, social and cultural structure – and in smoking habits as well as in smoking and health programmes – one with and one without an advertising ban.

(2) Legislation is part of a comprehensive programme – and we want it to be so. It is impossible, however, to select one element from such a programme and estimate its isolated value.

(3) Legislation may have several phases of effectiveness: First a short-term effect due mainly to the publicity generated when an Act is announced, discussed and implemented. In this connection, we should also welcome resistance against legislation – so long as it fails – it may focus people's interest even more on the health consequences of smoking. Then we have the long-term effect, particularly on children and young people, who will grow up in an environment free of an advertising pressure which glorifies the smoking habit as a key to success, self-confidence and adulthood. This long-term effect is the important one, but this implies that it will take decades before new trends in smoking habits of young generations will substantially influence the total *per capita* consumption.

(4) We should never accept the challenge from the tobacco industry – and from politicians and bureaucrats – that we have to prove an effect of an advertising ban before this question can be decided upon. In my view, the burden of proof lies with the tobacco industry, it is up to them to prove that a worldwide investment of 1.8 billion US dollars a year[2] in tobacco advertising and promotion has no impact on consumption levels of and on youth.

In many countries today, politicians and bureaucrats sit on the fence, saying, 'Let us wait for results from countries which have already implemented legislation'. From what I have said, it is clear that they will have to wait for many years before so-called proof of effect can be given, and hence, an enormous amount of health benefits might be lost.

MOTIVES FOR LEGISLATION

Politicians must have the courage to go in for legislation without advance proof of its effect. Their decisions have to be motivated for other reasons, and I shall put forward two of them:

(1) If it is true that smoking is the cause of the greatest epidemic of modern times, then it is simply unethical to permit sales promotion of these deadly products. I think we should not make it more complicated than that. A child, a teenager, will argue along these lines, they will question the double set of morals of the government, and ask very logically, 'If you try to convince me that smoking is dangerous for my health, why don't you stop advertising?'.

(2) The industrialized countries should now become aware of the gigantic advertising campaign which the tobacco industry has launched in third world countries, in order to compensate the market they are losing in the rich countries. This campaign is the most cynical and reprehensible marketing activity I know of, because the tobacco industry knows very well what the health authorities have predicted as a result of an increasing tobacco consumption: these areas, where smoking-related diseases are as yet relatively seldom, will come to experience them in only a few years. It would be impossible for the

[2] The figure presented in 1979 (Wickström, 1980).

industry to introduce their products into third world countries at the same speed if they were unable to utilize their refined and skilled advertising techniques. The health authorities in these countries often look to the industrialized part of the world for signals to follow. If we don't ban advertising, it is not likely that they will do so. This forces us to review our attitude towards an advertising ban. We are dealing with a pandemic, and our responsibilities go beyond our own borders.

These two arguments touch upon one important working mechanism of legislation, namely, to underline how gravely governments look upon the smoking and health problem, thus reinforcing and increasing the effect of information work. The intention of legislation, together with all other antismoking activities, is to establish nonsmoking as the norm.

NORWEGIAN EXPERIENCES

Although difficulties are involved in presenting so-called proof, some indications of an early effect can be given from countries which have introduced legislation. In my own country, Norway, a Tobacco Act was enforced in 1975 (National Council on Smoking and Health, 1975; Bjartveit, 1977; Bjartveit *et al.*, 1981), including, *inter alia,* a total ban on advertising (also indirect advertising) and a health warning on packages[3]. In addition, from 1980 to 1982, we have had three price increases, due to taxation, of 29, 22 and 10%, respectively.

Because a government programme is expected primarily to have an effect upon young people, trends in their smoking rates are of particular interest. Since 1957, nationwide surveys of smoking rates among students in the basic school have been conducted four times (Fig. 1). Increasing rates were registered up to 1975, and smoking among girls in particular showed a dramatic and alarming increase, with rates in 1975 equal to or above those of the boys at all age-levels in the upper grades. In 1980, the rates were on the decline for both sexes, most pronounced for the girls, who at all age-levels were back again to lower smoking rates than the boys. Because these surveys have been carried out at long and irregular intervals, it is uncertain whether or not 1975 represents the peak year – the rates may have been even higher – but without doubt the top was reached during the 1970s. The decline in 1980 is most promising.

Sales figures also support a new trend after the Parliament decided to introduce a government programme (Fig. 2). There was an increase in *per capita* tobacco consumption

[3] It may be noted that the extent of tobacco promotion in Norway, measured by expenditures, was moderate compared for example with the UK and the USA. In 1974, the year before enforcement of the advertising ban, the equivalent of about US $ 2.75 million (1974 value) were spent in Norway on newspaper and magazine advertisements, films, trade papers and outdoor posters for tobacco promotion (Central Bureau of Statistics, 1974). The figures for roughly corresponding categories of promotion were US $ 55.89 million for the UK (Aarø & Brekke, 1984) and US $ 241.1 million for the USA (Bjartveit, 1980), the US figure referring to the 20 best selling brands with about 90% market share. Calculated expenditures per inhabitant: US $ 0.69 for Norway, 1.00 for the UK, and 1.14 for the USA (1974 values). It should also be remembered that large sums were, and are, used in the UK and the USA for other promotional expenditures which did not exist in Norway in 1974 (gift coupons, sports sponsorship, etc.).

Fig. 1. Percentage of daily smokers among school students, by age and sex, in Norway in 1957, 1963, 1975 and 1980

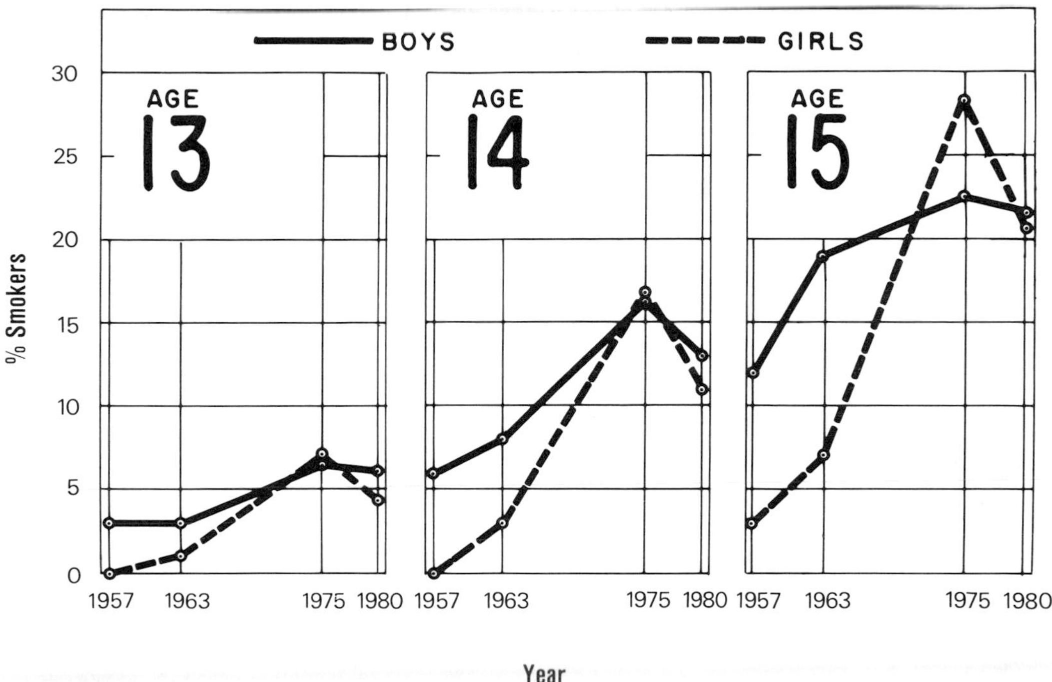

Surveys were carried out in 1957 and 1963 in Norwegian schools. Sample sizes within each age/sex-group ranged from 812–1245 in 1957 and from 440–605 in 1963 (Nilsen, 1959, 1963). On 4 November 1975 and 1980, all students in Norway in grades 7, 8 and 9 (aged 13, 14 and 15) were asked to fill out a questionnaire on smoking habits. Representative samples of these questionnaires were collected for analysis; sample sizes within each age/sex-group ranged from 790–957 (National Council on Smoking and Health, unpublished data).

until 1970, the year when the Parliament discussed the issue and endorsed a government programme on smoking and health, including legislation. Since then, the *per capita* consumption has levelled out, and during the last few years has shown a tendency to drop. Although some of this decline may be due to increased purchases abroad, there seems little doubt that a decrease in consumption has taken place.

The most important feature, however, is the extension of the regression line for consumption from 1950 to 1970. If the upward trend for the 1950s and 1960s had continued in the 1970s and 1980s, we would have had today a *per capita* consumption which would have been about 30% higher than it is. In my opinion, the shaded area of Figure 2 illustrates what has been gained in recent years.

Some may say that Norwegian consumption reached a mature level in the 1970s. However, the Norwegian consumption figures are far below the level for the UK (Fig. 3), and Norwegians do not differ that much from the British. *Per capita* consumption in Norway today corresponds with the figures the UK experienced more than 30 years ago. Our figures are also below those of the UK in other respects (Fig. 4): among males aged 60–69 years, the British lung cancer death rate is more than three times the Norwegian. Here again our figures are about 30 years behind the British.

Fig. 2. Consumption per adult (aged 15+) of manufactured cigarettes plus smoking tobacco, Norway, 1950/1951–1982/1983. The dotted line is an extension of the regression line for the years 1950/1951 to 1969/1970. The arrows indicate points of time for parliamentary endorsement of the governmental control programme, for enforcement of the Tobacco Act and for recent price increases due to taxation. (Data for sales figures from Reports from the Directorate of Customs and Excise, Oslo, and for population figures from Reports from the Central Bureau of Statistics, Oslo, unpublished data).

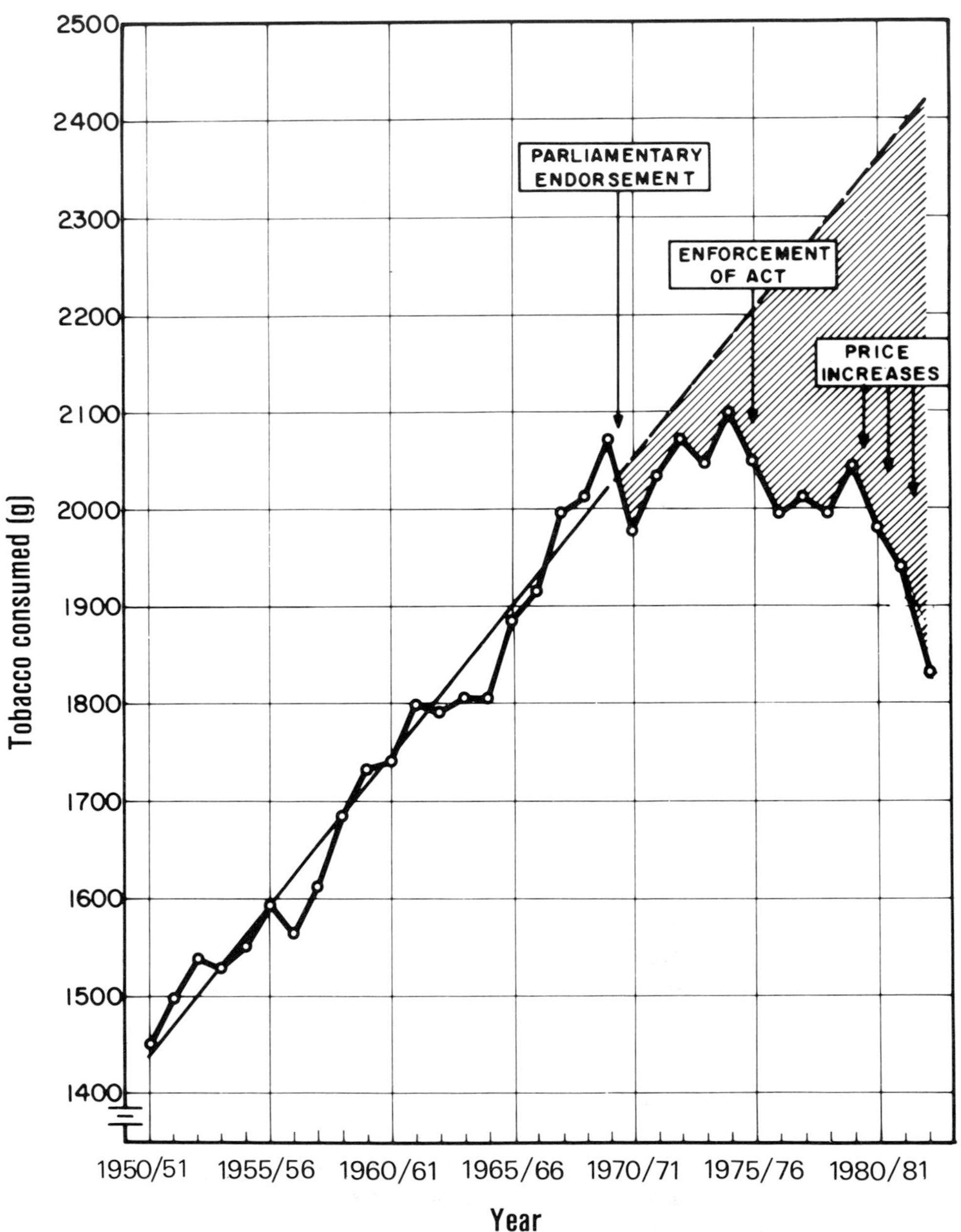

Fig. 3. Consumption per adult (aged 15+) of manufactured cigarettes plus smoking tobacco, UK and Norway, 1931 (1934/1935)–1978 (1979/1980) (Data for UK from Lee, 1969 and personal communications; and for Norway, as for Fig. 2).

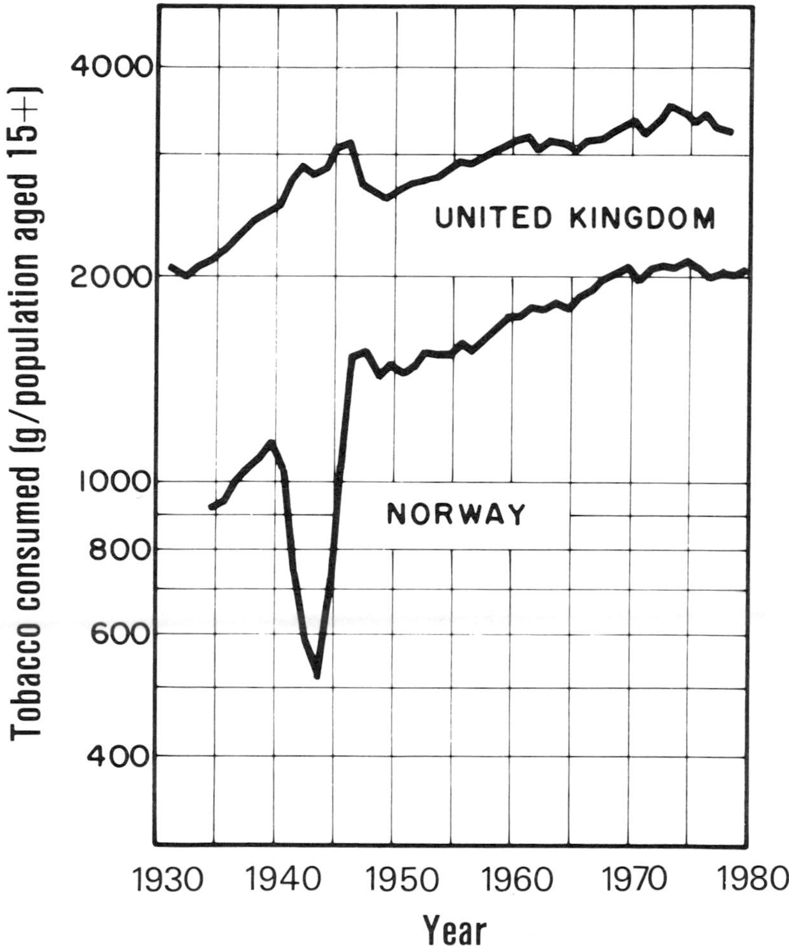

What does this imply? It implies that, since the increasing trend in tobacco consumption has now been stopped, thus avoiding a rise to the level experienced in other nations with a history of longer and heavier smoking, there is no doubt that a considerable amount of human suffering has been avoided.

THE FINAL GOAL

And now, are we satisfied with this new development in the smoking epidemic? No, we are not. I think it is time to call a spade a spade, and announce our final goal: the eradication of the problem.

Fig. 4. Lung cancer death rates in males aged 60–69 in England and Wales, and Norway, 1931 (mean 1931–1935)–1979 (ICD 8th revision: 162, and corresponding codes for previous revisions). (Data for England and Wales from General Register Office, 1974; Office of Population Censuses and Surveys, 1978; and for Norway, from annual reports from the Central Bureau of Statistics, Oslo, unpublished data)

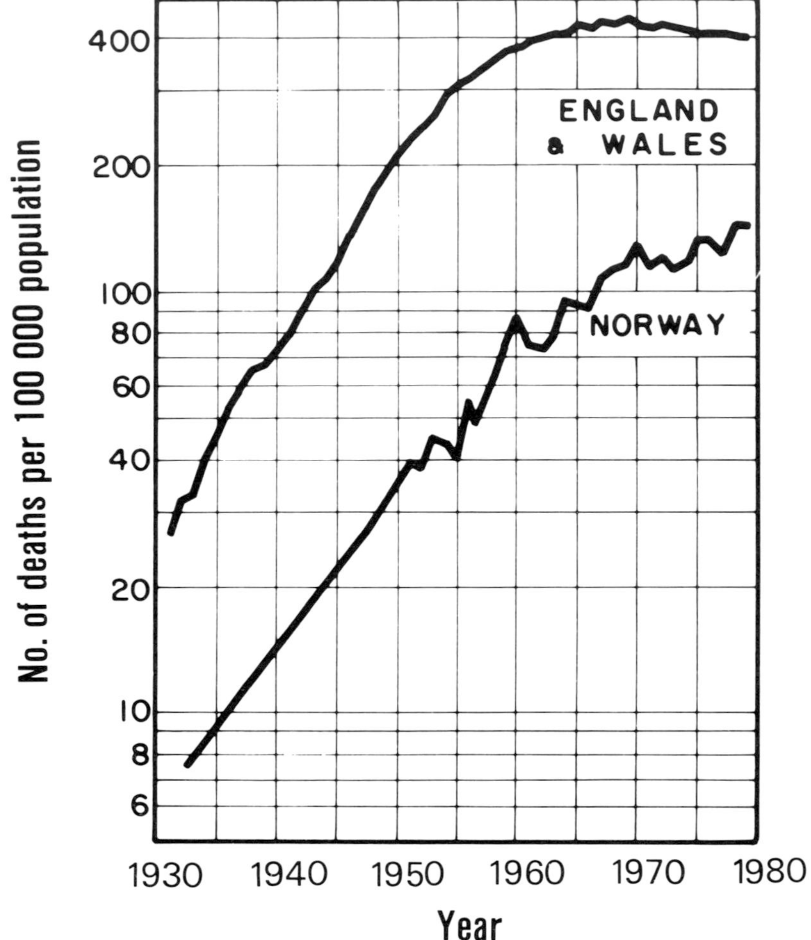

In 1981, the Norwegian Medical Association passed the following resolution:

'The Representative Body of the Norwegian Medical Association urges the Government to work towards making Norway a smoke-free society by the year 2000... Phasing out the consumption of tobacco is an important step towards improving the health of the nation.'

This resolution has received extensive publicity. The doctors ask the Government not only to turn its attention to this avoidable health problem, but to rid the country of it within a reasonable time.

Some will find this goal Utopian and unrealistic, and think that more time is needed. This may very well be so. The main point, however, is that eradication has been set up as an attainable goal, and that this goal should be reached within the foreseeable future. This ought to be possible. With few exceptions, cigarettes started to invade the industrialized countries at the beginning of this century. It should be possible to get them out before we have gone too far into the next.

POLITICAL VICTIMS

Now the question arises whether or not the politicians are willing to take the necessary steps to reach this goal. Such steps could cost them their political career. We have already seen a couple of victims. At the 4th World Conference on Smoking and Health in Stockholm, the US Secretary of Health, Education, and Welfare, Mr Joseph Califano, gave a plenary address, where he heavily attacked the tobacco industry (Califano, 1980):

'We can expect that the tobacco industry will do everything in its power to counteract our public-health efforts. We should, however, view such determined opposition not only as an obstacle, but also a challenge to our creativity and skill.'

One month later Secretary Califano was fired by President Carter. Politicians from tobacco-producing states cheered: '. . . that'll get a million votes alone', one of them said (Anon., 1979).

Another outstanding politician also spoke in Stockholm, Sir George Young, the UK Junior Minister of Health, who said (Young, 1980) that:

'. . . the solution to many of today's medical problems will not be found in the research laboratories of our hospitals, but in our Parliaments. For the prospective patient, the answer may not be cure by incision at the operating table, but prevention by decision at the Cabinet Table.'

In 1980 in Oslo, at a World Health Day Conference, Sir George was given the topic, 'Smoking or health – a choice for the politicians'. He then said, referring to what happened with Secretary Califano:

'The words might, I think, bear more than one meaning . . . Smoking is in every sense a political issue, and those politicians who concern themselves with it find themselves unexpectedly promoted or demoted.'

Did Sir George have a presentiment? One year later, Prime Minister Thatcher transferred him to another Ministry, where he would be less dangerous to the tobacco industry. Press comments underlined the connection between this event and Sir George's commitment to antismoking legislation: 'Representations by the tobacco industry against the Government's antismoking campaign are believed at Westminster to have played a part in persuading the Prime Minister to shift Ministers . . .' 'I never knew the tobacco industry was so powerful', said a top civil servant (Anon., 1981).

STATEMENTS BY NORWEGIAN POLITICIANS

In January 1983, the Norwegian Minister of Health, Dr Leif Arne Heløe, stated in the Parliament:

'The systematic work of the Government to influence public opinion has the same long term objective as requested by the Norwegian Medical Association. A smoke-free society is also the aim of the proposals in a planned White Paper.'

I also have the honour to draw your attention to a special message which the Norwegian Prime Minister, Mr Kåre Willoch (1983), sent to the 5th World Conference on Smoking and Health. Mr Willoch said, among other things:

'The Norwegian Government will continue its efforts to reduce the use of tobacco in Norway.

'Two main conditions are indispensable for a successful result: firstly, a ban on tobacco advertising and promotion and, secondly, an active, informed opinion and attitude against smoking, emphasizing nonsmoking as the normal social behaviour.'

MOBILIZING INTERNATIONAL ORGANIZATIONS

Some people may think, and rightly so, that such a statement is easy to make in a country which is economically independent of tobacco production. In many third world countries, tobacco production, manufacturing and trade count for a substantial fraction of the gross national product, and provide the daily living for people who have no other alternative than starvation and hardship. The tobacco industry has indeed very cleverly utilized this situation. With this background it seems at first glance hopeless to stem the epidemic. What we need, therefore, is a wordwide political strategy for reaching the final goal.

This means an active involvement by international organizations, in particular, members of the United Nations family, such as the Food and Agriculture Organization (FAO). This Organization has previously provided technical assistance for tobacco cultivation and marketing. In 1978, the following statement was made (WHO Expert Committee on Smoking Control, 1979):

'However, since the resolution on smoking and health passed by the Twenty-ninth World Health Assembly in May 1976, FAO has not promoted any activities leading to project execution.'

Although this is a good start, are we satisfied with this policy? No, certainly not. We want the international organizations to give priority to a comprehensive, global plan for development of substitute crops and industries, and to render all possible assistance to achieve this goal.

We cannot expect the tobacco industry to support such a plan. They have had their chance, and have failed to show genuine concern about the serious health consequences of their products.

MOBILIZING POLITICIANS

What, then, are the prospects? The simple answer is that our goal will not be obtained unless politicians and the general public all over the world are mobilized on our side.

If we are to talk at all about reasons for failure of a government programme, the main one is that the programme has not been comprehensive enough, not radical enough, not global enough. The first to blame is the medical profession, which has been too passive and too soft. We have to realize that if we want to do something about the smoking and health problem, we are in politics. Our task is to confront the politicians with the enormous magnitude of the problem, to get them to see what it is all about: the greatest epidemic of modern times. We have to get them out of a stage of only pretending serious concern, into a stage of active involvement and determination. Let us ask them the impertinent question 'Do you really want to do something about the problem? Or is your involvement only a question of lip-service?'.

Some of us may think that our job is merely to account for the scientific evidence, and that the medical journals are the only media acceptable as a communication channel. Involvement in political pressure is below one's dignity for many professional people. In my opinion, such an attitude is out of touch with real life. We should be aware that our opponents, the tobacco industry, are experts in lobby activities and creation of political pressure. Who is going to create a counter-pressure, and tell the decision-makers the other side of the story, if not us? This does not mean that we have to become politicians. But we should realize that we all are political human beings, and utilize all possible channels to make the politicians stand up and take responsibility.

One thing is for sure, without active political involvement, we shall never reach the final goal. Therefore, let us *act,* and let us act now.

REFERENCES

Aarø, L.E. & Brekke, T. (1984) *Health Education in Norway 1979/80. Description of Projects and Methods* (in press)

Anon. (1979) *International Herald Tribune,* 20 July

Anon. (1981) Tobacco barons and health reshuffle. *The Observer,* 16 Nov.

Bjartveit, K. (1971) Pavirkning av roykevaner ved restriktive tiltak (Nor.), *Social-medicinsk tidsskrift,* ***48,*** 123–127

Bjartveit, K. (1977) The Norwegian Tobacco Act. *Health Educ. J.,* ***36,*** 2–9

Bjartveit, K. (1980) *How to measure effects of a governmental programme.* In: Ramström, L.M., ed., *The Smoking Epidemic, a Matter of Worldwide Concern. Proceedings of the Fourth World Conference on Smoking and Health,* Stockholm, Almqvist & Wiksell International, pp. 155–157

Bjartveit, K., Christie, N., Holbaek-Hanssen, L., Mork, T., Nilsen, E., Vormeland, O. & Ås, B. (1969) *Influencing Smoking Behaviour (UICC Tech. Rep. Ser., Vol. 3),* Geneva, International Union Against Cancer

Bjartveit, K., Löchsen, P.M., Aarö, L.E. (1981) Controlling the epidemic: Legislation and restrictive measures. *Can. J. Public Health,* ***72,*** 406–412

Califano, J.A. (1980) *Remarks to the Fourth World Conference on Smoking and Health.* In: Ramström, L.M., ed., *The Smoking Epidemic, a Matter of Worldwide Concern. Proceedings of the Fourth World Conference on Smoking and Health,* Stockholm, Almqvist & Wiksell International, pp. 118–122

Central Bureau of Statistics (1974) *Survey on Smoking Habits, 4th Quarter 1973,* Report from the Division for Interview Surveys, Oslo

General Register Office (1974) *The Registrar-General's Statistical Review of England and Wales, 1921–1973,* London, Her Majesty's Stationery Office

Gray, N. & Daube, M., eds (1980) *Guidelines for Smoking Control,* 2nd ed. *(UICC Tech. Rep. Ser. Vol. 52),* Geneva, International Union Against Cancer

Lee, P.N., ed. (1969) *Statistics of Smoking in the United Kingdom,* London, Tobacco Research Council

National Council on Smoking and Health (1975) *The Act Relating to Restrictive Measures for the Marketing of Tobacco Products (Norway), No. 14 of March 9, 1973,* Oslo

Nilsen, E. (1959) Smoking habits among children in Norway. *Br. J. prev. soc. Med.,* ***13,*** 5–13

Nilsen, E. (1963) *Roykevaner og opplysningsarbeid* (Nor.), Oslo, Norwegian Cancer Society

Office of Population Censuses and Surveys (1978) *Mortality Statistics, Cause. Registrar-general on Deaths by Cause, Sex and Age in England and Wales, 1974–1977,* London, Her Majesty's Stationery Office

Roemer, R. (1982) *Legislative Action to Combat the World Smoking Epidemic,* Geneva, World Health Organization

WHO Expert Committee on Smoking Control (1979) *Controlling the Smoking Epidemic (WHO Tech. Rep. Ser., No. 636),* Geneva, World Health Organization

Wickström, B. (1980) *Cigarette marketing in the third world:* In: Ramström, L.M., ed., *The Smoking Epidemic, a Matter of Worldwide Concern. Proceedings of the Fourth World Conference on Smoking and Health,* Stockholm, Almqvist & Wiksell International, pp. 98–105

Willoch, K. (1983) Greeting to the 5th World Conference on Smoking and Health. The Smoking Epidemic Can Be Conquered. *Tobakken Vi Oslo, No. 2,* 1–2

World Health Organization (1976) *Legislative Action to Combat Smoking Around the World, a Survey of Existing Legislation,* Geneva

Young, G. (1980) *The politics of smoking.* In: Ramström, L.M., ed., *The Smoking Epidemic, a Matter of Worldwide Concern. Proceedings of the Fourth World Conference on Smoking and Health,* Stockholm, Almqvist & Wiksell International, pp. 123–127

EDUCATIONAL PROGRAMMES AND INFORMATION IN DEVELOPED COUNTRIES

M. KUNZE

Institute of Social Medicine,
University of Vienna, Austria

SUMMARY

Smoking control should be achieved by implementing comprehensive programmes including public information, health education, cessation 'treatment', and legislation. Health education for children will have only modest impact as long as smoking is still a symbol of being grown-up, of social status and prestige. Separate programmes should be designed for public information, school health education and hospitals and health professionals. Health education and public information are the prerequisites for comprehensive smoking control programmes because they create and maintain problem awareness. On the other hand, a ban on advertising for tobacco is a prerequisite for successful health education.

The ultimate goal of health education and information is promotion of the positive social image of nonsmoking behaviour.

INTRODUCTION

Educational programmes and information are an essential part of a comprehensive approach to smoking control. This paper has the following objectives:

– to demonstrate the importance of health education and information within the overall concept of smoking control;

– to mention principles of planning and performing health education and information;

– to report on international coordinating activities; and

– to issue recommendations for future health education and information activities.

COMPREHENSIVE APPROACH TO SMOKING CONTROL

Smoking control should be achieved by implementing comprehensive programmes including public information, health education, cessation campaigns and legislation. This approach needs careful planning and continuous evaluation.

Countries such as Norway and Finland have incorporated much of their progressive legislation within the framework of a comprehensive Tobacco Act. It would clearly be helpful if this were possible in all countries, both for purposes of administrative convenience and to demonstrate the determination of governments to recognize the magnitude of smoking problems by adopting a wide-ranging and forceful approach. The only caveat here is that it would be unfortunate if difficulties in producing comprehensive legislation prevented speedy action on any specific component.

Smoking: acquiring and maintaining a behavioural pattern

People usually start smoking in their youth. Before youngsters have their first experience of smoking they are concerned with this behaviour in various ways:

– one or both of their parents smoke or there are other models, such as friends, brothers and sisters or teachers, who are smoking;

– they recognize that smoking is often followed by positive consequences (it reduces stress, it looks very smart);

– an extensive propaganda for cigarettes suggests many advantages of cigarette-consumption;

– there is also the fact of curiosity young people want to experience the effects of smoking.

Although first attempts at smoking cause negative consequences – for example dizziness, nausea – many youngsters continue smoking because of positive reinforcements such as:

– smoking is a symbol of being grown-up;

– it increases prestige; and

– it is a sign of courage.

It will be difficult to resist smoking if the behaviour is maintained. There are three main reasons:

(1) the combination of certain situations and smoking produces a habit; the situation acts as conditioned stimulus, smoking is the conditioned response (respondential learning);

(2) the consumption of cigarettes is often reinforced by positive consequences; many smokers report a certain feeling of stimulation or a calming effect (instrumental learning);

(3) smokers also get used to the pharmacological effect; nicotine, activating the blood circulation, could be an important reinforcement for some smokers.

Health education: not a simple recipe

The psychosocial background of smoking outlined shows how health education and public information are to be designed; and that health education, especially for children and youngsters, is not a simple solution for the tobacco problem. One of the commonly used statements heard in discussions about smoking control refers to the fact that health education (in schools) is the most important strategy. Yet, knowing about the motivational factors which make young people try smoking, one would state that health education for children will have only modest impact as long as smoking is still a symbol of being grown-up, of social status and prestige.

Health education is important but will only work properly if it is accompanied by a process of 'social discrimination' against smoking. This can be achieved by various approaches within the context of a long-term comprehensive programme, which, among other strategies, bans advertising for tobacco which is targeted on young people by 'glamourizing' smoking.

It might not be important to stress the health consequences of smoking too much when dealing with children and youngsters, however, one has to mention why smoking is detrimental to health. When dealing with older (grown-up) target groups, the health aspects are increasingly important, because smokers start to experience the negative consequences and to look for solutions to their problems.

In industrialized countries, 60–70% of all smokers are 'dissonant smokers' who feel at least uneasy about their habit and want to change their behaviour (including smoking cessation).

Health education programmes: key elements

Wide experience of health education programmes on smoking (and other problems) has been gained over a period of years in many countries. One would propose development of separate programmes, as follows:

Public information programmes. Using mass media (television and radio programmes, films, advertisements, posters, etc.) and including special-focus programmes targeted at groups such as: pregnant women, businessmen, health professionals, etc.

School health education programmes. A wide variety of projects have been implemented around the world with varying degrees of success.

Other educational institutions. It is important to recognize that health education need not be limited to the classroom, nor, indeed, is the need for education on smoking. Therefore, education programmes should be prepared for colleges, other educational establishments, and youth organizations.

Hospitals and health professionals. It is crucial that doctors and health professionals set an example through: their own smoking habits (particularly in front of patients), restriction on smoking in health premises, advice to patients about smoking, and inclusion of appropriate information on smoking in training courses.

Health education and public information: prerequisites for comprehensive smoking control programmes

When a country starts to deal with its tobacco problem, public information measures are the first step, to create problem awareness. Then the need for health education programmes will be recognized by the public and by decision makers. All the other control measures can only be developed and implemented if the basis for political decision is provided by information. Price policy and taxation may serve as an example for the relationship between smoking control measures and health education and public information.

Price policy and taxation have lots of advantages (they are easily executed and very effective, and well accepted by governments, especially nowadays), but they cannot be applied properly if the population is not convinced that smoking is harmful. We now have quite good recipes for success: increase the price continuously, well above inflation rates, and implement also the concept of differential tax. The need for public information to explain these concepts to the public is obvious.

Advertising and marketing against health

When discussing the problems of health education and public information, the phenomenon of advertising and marketing of tobacco products should be mentioned as the main obstacle. This is the case in both developed and in developing countries. It is a relatively new phenomenon for a public health system to have an active opponent backed by tremendous financial resources which allow aggressive penetration into almost every sector of modern society. Sports events and cultural performances are the best examples of promotion campaigns by the tobacco multinationals. The public health system and its leaders sometimes seem to be a little helpless against marketing and advertising measures and the reaction very often is resignation, but we have to fight the opposition and to understand the psychological, social and political strategies and tactics used by the tobacco industry.

Ban on advertising for tobacco: a prerequisite for successful health education

A total ban on all activities promoting the consumption of tobacco products is necessary because:

– advertising for cigarettes creates a positive environment for tobacco, which is an obstacle to smoking control activities; and

– advertising not only influences children to start smoking but also prevents those who want to stop smoking from doing so.

Recommendations by international organizations

According to repeated official WHO statements the tobacco problem is the most important public health issue in industrialized countries and a matter of growing concern in developing countries. These statements were endorsed by other international governmental and nongovernmental bodies, among these, the International Union Against Cancer (UICC) being the most active, with a special programme on smoking and cancer which comprises a number of regional projects worldwide.

Three major workshops were held in Europe (WHO Regional Office for Europe, 1986) recently to improve cooperation between neighbouring countries as far as smoking control is concerned. One workshop focused on the situation in German-speaking countries, another on countries in the Eastern part of Europe, and the third dealt with smoking control activities in the Southern European Countries.

The Workshop on Smoking and Health held in Suzdal, USSR, 13–17 September 1983, issued among other results the following recommendations concerning health education and information:

– Effective programmes must be as broadly based as possible, involving education, legislation, fiscal and curative measures. Of these, education was seen as the first priority since legislation and fiscal measures were unlikely to be enacted until high levels of public awareness had been attained. (This statement is extremely important and has already been discussed in more detail in this paper.)

– Groups, e.g., health professionals, teachers, youth leaders, are of prime importance in drawing up an effective smoking control programme. At the same time, attention must be paid to educating decision-makers – especially those in government and other high authorities.

At the Symposium on Smoking and Health in Southern European Countries, held in Barcelona, 22–24 March, 1984, three major areas of concern were characterized: (1) the disturbingly high levels of cigarette smoking among children and young people; (2) the dramatic and still rising increase in smoking prevalence among women in many of the Southern European countries; and (3) the high prevalence of smoking among vital example groups, such as doctors, health professionals in general and teachers.

In this respect, the Symposium urged governments to implement WHO's recommendations on smoking, such as:

– establishment of a comprehensive governmental programme;
– a ban on all advertising and promotion of tobacco products;
– visible and clear health warnings on all cigarette packets;
– substantial financing for health and education programmes;
– use of taxation to discourage smoking; and
– measures to protect the rights of nonsmokers.

A UICC workshop on the tobacco problem in German-speaking countries stressed the need for better cooperation especially in the areas of restrictions on tobacco advertising and promotion activities, price policy and taxation and comprehensive legislative measures.

WHO's smoking control programme

As an example of WHO's commitment to the case, the smoking control programme developed by the WHO Regional Office for Europe is outlined, showing the emphasis on health education. It has the following objectives:

– to develop and support a European policy in which the reduction of smoking is seen as a continuing, top priority health-promotion issue and a long-term commitment;

– to stimulate and support the establishment and further development of effective national smoking control programmes in Member States;

– to stimulate the development and use of health promotion programmes which promote nonsmoking for specific target groups, with special reference to vulnerable and high-risk groups;

– to promote a positive social image of nonsmoking behaviour in Member States;

– to stimulate the search for better methods to help smokers stop smoking and to promote the wide accessibility of assistance to smokers;

The tobacco problem is now recognized to a much greater extent under the aspects of a newly designed policy of health education which is moving:

– from individual behaviour modification to a systematic public health-approach;
– from medical orientation to a recognition of lay competence;
– from health prescription to health promotion;
– from authoritarian health education to supportive health education.

Collaborative Survey of Smoking and other Health-related Behaviours: Finland, Norway, the UK, Austria

This Survey (WHO Regional Office for Europe, 1986) is an important step to coordinate health education in Europe and to provide scientific information for the planning and evaluation of programmes directed at children and youngsters.

The questionnaire covers:

- beliefs, attitudes and behaviour with respect to smoking
- use of other drugs
- behaviours detrimental to health such as use of alcohol and other drugs, tea, coffee and irregular sleeping and eating habits
- self-image
- general image of smoking and nonsmokers
- sense of alienation and degree of social support
- psychosomatic and respiratory symptoms.

The aims of the Survey are to map the development of smoking attitudes and behaviour in the countries involved and to examine how these are linked to other health-related behaviours. It is hoped to be able to locate smoking within the context of other health concerns and habits and to examine the ways in which these are similar and different between the countries. Any differences can then be linked to known differences between the countries in social and political climate.

Health warnings: are they any good?

This question is raised very often and is mainly used to discredit this piece of public information. If one is to judge from the impact of health warnings on packages for tobacco products it must not be seen as an isolated measure against smoking but as one activity within the overall framework of a long-term behaviour-modification programme.

There is good evidence that a system of rotating warnings serves to maintain public interest and attention, and to increase knowledge on the health hazards of smoking. The warnings should be amended to take account of local circumstances and changing knowledge, and amendments can themselves be the subject of mass media publicity.

Following the positive experiences in Sweden, Norway and Iceland, we propose that a system of 10 or more different health warnings be introduced, focusing on the health and social consequences of smoking. These warnings should be pre-tested and replaced annually by a new set of warnings. They should be the subject of legislation which mandates a minimum size and specific location (e.g., front of pack) for warnings on packs and any remaining advertisements. The warnings would be complementary to but separate from information on harmful components of cigarettes. A medical commission could be established to maintain constant review of the warnings and – in conjunction with publicity experts – produce new warnings.

Health education: does it work?

It already works when performed within the framework of a comprehensive smoking control programme which is a long-term commitment of society.

It works if it is based on the psychosocial factors creating the smoking behaviour and on the appropriate counteractions, including social discrimination against tobacco consumption.

It works if public health systems really acknowledge the magnitude of the tobacco problem.

REFERENCE

WHO Regional Office for Europe (1986) *Fourth European Survey on Smoking and Health*, Copenhagen (in press)

AN INTERVENTION STUDY OF TOBACCO CHEWING AND SMOKING HABITS FOR PRIMARY PREVENTION OF ORAL CANCER AMONG 12 212 INDIAN VILLAGERS

P.C. GUPTA[1], M.B. AGHI, R.B. BHONSLE, P.R. MURTI & F.S. MEHTA

WHO Collaborating Center for Oral Cancer Prevention
Tata Institute of Fundamental Research,
Bombay 40005, India

C.R. MEHTA

Department of Biostatistics,
WHO Collaborating Center for Biostatistics,
Harvard School of Public Health,
Boston, MA, USA

J.J. PINDBORG

Department of Oral Pathology,
Royal Dental College and Dental Department,
Rigshospitelet,
Copenhagen, Denmark

SUMMARY

In a house-to-house screening survey, 12 212 tobacco chewers and smokers were selected from the rural population in the Ernakulam district, Kerala state, India. These individuals were interviewed for their tobacco habits and examined for the presence of oral cancer and precancerous lesions, first in a baseline survey, and then annually, over a five-year period. They were educated using personal and mass media communication to give up their tobacco habits. The control group was provided from the results of the first five years of a 10-year follow-up study conducted earlier by the authors in the same area with the same methodology but on different individuals without any educational intervention. The

[1] Present address: Takemi Program in International Health, Harvard School of Public Health, 665 Huntington Avenue, I–1102, Boston, MA 02115, USA, to which requests for reprints should be directed.

stoppage of the tobacco habit was substantially higher in the intervention group (9.4%) compared to the control group (3.2%). A logistic regression analysis showed that the behavioural intervention was helpful to all categories of individuals, however, the effect was different for different categories: intervention was more helpful to men, chewers, and those with a long duration of the habit. These individuals rarely quit their habit without intervention.

INTRODUCTION

A high incidence of oral cancer in India and, indeed, in several other South-East Asian countries is directly attributable to the usage of tobacco in the form of chewing and smoking. Thus, oral cancer appears to be amenable to primary prevention. From the cost-benefit point of view, putting resources into the primary prevention of oral cancer would provide maximum returns (World Health Organization, 1985). Little is known, however, about the feasibility and the effectiveness of undertaking a primary prevention programme of oral cancer in the general population.

A prospective behavioural intervention study was, therefore, undertaken to study the feasibility and the effectiveness of the primary prevention of oral cancer as phase III of an on-going study of oral cancer and precancer in rural Indian populations. Phase I of the study, which began in 1966–1967, consisted of house-to-house cross-sectional surveys of over 150 000 individuals in six districts of India (Mehta *et al.*, 1969, 1972), and Phase II was a 10-year follow-up study (1967–1977) of 30 000 individuals in three districts of India (Gupta *et al.*, 1980).

The results so far have shown that the habits of tobacco chewing and smoking are strongly associated with oral cancer and precancer. All prevalent and incident cases of oral cancer, and almost all prevalent and incident cases of oral precancer were found only among tobacco chewers and smokers, although large proportions of baseline samples and followed-up cohorts consisted of individuals without any tobacco habit. In a preliminary report from the intervention study, it was shown that the spontaneous regression rate of oral precancerous lesions increased significantly within one year of stoppage or significant reduction of the tobacco habit (Mehta *et al.*, 1982).

The intervention study of tobacco habits was therefore undertaken with a view to educating the population to give up their tobacco habits and measuring the resultant change in the incidence rate of oral precancerous lesions. The aim of the present paper is to assess the effect of the behavioural intervention programme on the tobacco habits of the individuals after a five-year follow-up period. The analysis is confined to the Ernakulam district in Kerala state, one of the three areas where the intervention study was carried out.

MATERIALS AND METHODS

A complete screening of the population of some selected villages in the Ernakulam district was carried out and all available tobacco users aged 15 years and over were chosen (12 212 individuals) as the study sample. Only the temporary residents, very old, sick or infirm, psychologically disturbed, and treated oral cancer cases were excluded.

The baseline survey for the intervention study was conducted in 1977–1978. The selected individuals were questioned in detail about their tobacco habits by trained clerks and examined for the presence of oral cancer and leukoplakia by two of the authors (Bhonsle and Murti) and other dentists who were especially trained and standardized for the diagnosis of oral precancerous lesions. The clinical examination immediately followed the interview, and was done separately and independently.

All the individuals were re-interviewed and re-examined annually, using the house-to-house approach with the same methodology and criteria as in the baseline survey.

In this paper, oral lesions are divided into four categories: severe, comprising of oral cancer and submucous fibrosis; moderate, consisting of leukoplakia; mild, comprising all other lesions such as preleukoplakia, leukoedema, leukokeratosis nicotina palati, localized atrophy of the tongue papillae, lichen planus, etc.; and no oral lesion.

Tobacco habits

Tobacco was smoked as well as chewed in the Ernakulam district. The most common smoking habit was *bidi* smoking, practised almost solely by men. *Bidi* is a cheap smoking stick of 4–8 cm in length, consisting of a rolled piece of dried *temburni* leaf *(Diospyros melanoxylon)* with 0.15–0.25 g of coarsely ground tobacco. Tobacco was chewed, mostly in the form of a betel quid consisting of betel leaf, lime (calcium hydroxide), areca nut and tobacco. Further details regarding the tobacco habits are given elsewhere (Mehta *et al.*, 1971).

Intervention methods

Little is known about the psychology of tobacco addiction in India. Special in-depth studies in the three areas revealed that tobacco usage is a learned behaviour, generally from parents and other elders, or from peers. The rationale for initiating tobacco usage, and very often for its continuation, was its perceived medicinal value for various health-related problems, such as toothache. There was no awareness either regarding the oral mucosal health status or any possible ill-effect of tobacco usage.

Based on these findings, a sequential programme of intervention was devised. The individuals were made aware of the structures within the oral cavity and the concept of oral health. The link between tobacco habits and oral cancer was explained through the oral precancerous lesions. When the relationship seemed to be convincing, they were urged to think about their own tobacco habit. Various possible ways of giving up the tobacco habit were discussed. Withdrawal symptoms were explained as real, but emphasized as a temporary phenomenon. General benefits of giving up tobacco habits, e.g., financial, were pointed out. Further support and encouragement was given to those who attempted and failed to give up their tobacco habit. Reinforcement was provided to those who succeeded, and a model and leadership role was suggested to them. It ought to be pointed out that for different individuals, and even for the same individual at different times, there was an interplay and exchange between various stages of intervention.

This educational intervention programme utilized two approaches: personal communication and mass media. Personal communication was given by the dentist after oral examination in the form of oral diagnosis and then by a specially-trained social scientist in a one-to-one situation once a year. Most individuals also received personal communication in a group situation annually from the team.

The mass media used for intervention included films, posters, radio broadcasts and newspaper articles. A documentary film was specially made for the study sample, which detailed the relationship between tobacco habits and oral cancer. Posters were placed in villages primarily as reminders of intervention efforts. The radio in India is a Government-operated medium and periodic radio broadcasts helped in further increasing the credibility of the intervention messages. The newspaper articles were written specifically for this project and published in the local-language newspapers.

The format and content of each intervention strategy were pretested and implementation decided on that basis. For example, an impact study of the film revealed that an optimum way of showing this film would be to show it to groups of approximately 25 individuals and then initiate a discussion by inviting comments from the viewers to emphasize the salient points in the film. This was followed by a repeat showing if necessary.

As a form of incentive, and as an aid to intervention, medicines for common ailments were distributed to the individuals in the study sample. Dental extractions were performed in a field clinic at a central location. The visit to the clinic was used to reinforce the intervention message. On the basis of feedback information, the intervention programme was evaluated and restructured every year before a new follow-up began. Thus, intervention was a continuous process.

Analysis

The analysis compares two large cohorts followed prospectively in the Ernakulam district in different time periods by the same investigators; one control group and one intervention group. The control group was provided from an earlier 10-year follow-up study (1967–1977) of 10 287 individuals. The intervention group consisted of 12 212 individuals followed for five years (1977–1982). The major difference between the two studies was the adoption of the intervention programme in the later study. The 10-year, follow-up study differed in two other ways; its sample consisted of tobacco users as well as nonusers, and the first follow-up was conducted after three years, rather than after one year.

These two differences were neutralized by excluding a subset from the 10-year follow-up study data in the analysis. Thus, only those individuals in the control group practising some kind of tobacco habit found in the baseline survey were included in the analysis (6067). Moreover, only the first five years of the 10-year follow-up data on these individuals were analysed. Of the 6067 individuals in the baseline survey, 5126 (84.5%) were re-examined at least once in the subsequent five years (1967–1972). The mean follow-up period per person among these individuals was 4.7 years.

There was a three-year interval between the baseline examination and the first follow-up for the control group. Thus, there were four interviews and examinations in the control group compared to six in the intervention group in their respective five-year follow-up period. In order to keep the two groups comparable, the first two follow-ups of the intervention group were ignored in the analysis. Although 98% of the individuals were re-interviewed and re-examined at least once, only 93.4% (11 412) were included in the analysis. The mean follow-up period per person among these individuals was 4.8 years.

The response variable in this study, the change in tobacco habit, was defined as the stoppage of the tobacco habit at the time of the last interview and examination of the individual. The stoppage of the habit was defined as the complete stoppage of the tobacco usage at least six months prior to the date of interview. Those individuals who stopped their tobacco habit but restarted sometime later were not included in this category.

RESULTS

Table 1 compares the distribution of selected characteristics in the intervention and the control groups. Both groups represent samples of the population, which were ten years apart, and there was no specific attempt, such as by stratification, to ensure the comparability. In spite of this, the percentages in the two groups did not differ by any considerable amount. Some of the differences may reflect a temporal shift in the distributions. For example, a higher percentage of smokers in the intervention group compared to the control group (48% *versus* 36.1%) may reflect a growing popularity of smoking habits.

Some interesting relationships are apparent between the age, sex and type of tobacco habit in the intervention group (Tables 2 and 3). Women were essentially chewers only (93.2%), whereas males were mostly smokers (66.5%) (Table 2). Among men, chewers were much older than smokers; 66.5% of chewers, but only 8.4% of smokers, were 55

Table 1. Distribution of selected characteristics in the intervention and control groups

Characteristic	Intervention group		Control group	
	No.	%	No.	%
Total	11 412	100.0	5126	100.0
Age (years)				
15–34	3 356	29.4	1829	35.7
35–54	4 926	43.2	2185	42.6
55 and over	3 130	27.4	1112	21.7
Sex				
Men	8 021	70.3	3329	64.9
Women	3 391	29.7	1797	35.1
Tobacco habit				
Chewing	4 299	37.7	2349	45.0
Smoking	5 480	48.0	1853	36.1
Both	1 633	14.3	924	18.0
Habit duration (years)				
1–5	2 126	18.6	1100	21.4
6–10	2 928	25.7	1610	31.4
11 and over	6 358	55.7	2416	47.1
Oral lesion				
None	10 303	90.3	4572	90.2
Mild	764	6.7	381	7.4
Moderate	326	2.9	139	2.7
Severe	19	0.2	34	0.7

Table 2. Relationship between sex and the type of tobacco habit in the intervention study group

Habit	Men		Women	
	No.	%	No.	%
Chewing	1137	14.2	3162	93.2
Smoking	5330	66.5	150	4.4
Both	1554	19.4	79	2.3
Total	8021	100.0	3391	100.0

Table 3. Relationship between age, sex, and the type of tobacco habit in the intervention study group

Age (years)	Chewing		Smoking		Both		Total	
	No.	%	No.	%	No.	%	No.	%
Men								
15–34	43	3.8	2896	54.3	95	6.1	3034	37.8
35–54	338	29.7	1985	37.2	887	57.1	3210	40.0
55+	756	66.5	449	8.4	572	36.8	1777	22.2
Women								
15–34	263	8.3	44	29.3	15	19.0	322	9.5
35–54	1587	50.2	85	56.7	44	55.7	1716	50.6
55+	1312	41.5	21	14.0	20	25.3	1353	39.9

years or older (Table 3). Women smokers, although few in number, were somewhat younger than women chewers and women chewers were younger than men chewers. Similar relationships for the control group were described in earlier reports (Mehta *et al.*, 1969; Mehta *et al.*, 1971).

Table 4 shows the number and the percentage of the individuals reporting they had quit their tobacco habit (response rate), according to various characteristics. The response rate decreased with age in the intervention study group. It was higher among women than among men, among chewers than among smokers, among those without any oral lesions compared to those with some oral lesions, and among those with lower duration of tobacco habit. The direction of these differences was generally similar in the intervention and the control group.

Due to complex relationships between these variables, and the possibility of the presence of interaction effects between these variables and the intervention, a logistic regression model was fitted to study the effectiveness of the intervention (McCullagh & Nelder, 1983). The response variable was binary, 1 if the individual had given up the tobacco habit, 0 otherwise. The predictor variable of main interest was the study effect, 1 for the intervention group, 0 for the control group. Other variables such as age, sex, type of tobacco habit, duration of habit, and the grade of oral lesion were included as covariates. The GLIM package (Baker & Nelder, 1978) was used for model fitting, hypothesis testing, and prediction.

Table 4. Response rates according to selected characteristics

Characteristic	Intervention group		Control group	
	No.	%	No.	%
Age (years)				
15–34	239	7.1	65	3.6
35–54	475	9.6	81	3.7
55 and over	362	11.6	17	1.5
Sex				
Men	535	6.7	61	1.8
Women	541	16.0	102	5.7
Oral lesion				
None	991	9.6	159	3.5
Mild	68	8.9	4	1.0
Moderate	12	3.7	0	0.0
Severe	5	26.3	0	0.0
Tobacco habit				
Chewing	597	13.9	99	4.2
Smoking	418	7.6	56	3.0
Both	61	3.7	8	0.9
Habit duration (years)				
1–5	269	12.7	84	7.6
6–10	269	9.1	53	3.3
11 and over	540	8.5	26	1.1

The fitted model is displayed as Figure 1. In this model, all the main effects were highly significant. In addition, two-way interactions between the predictor variable and three covariates (sex, type of tobacco habit and duration of habit) were found to be highly significant. The model was found to be a good fit with the data through the analysis of scaled deviances (McCullagh & Nelder, 1983), as well as by looking at the differences between the observed and the predicted response probabilities.

The logistic model estimated the impact of intervention on the response odds, taking into account other covariates. It also estimated the relative contributions of the different levels of the covariates. Thus, the model showed that the odds of response for the age-group 35–54 years were 1.6 times greater than the corresponding odds for the age-group 15–34 years. Similarly, the odds ratio for the age group 55 years and above relative to the age-group 15–34 years was 2.1. For oral lesions relative to no oral lesion, the odds ratio was 0.89 for mild lesions, 0.48 for moderate lesions, and 1.7 (based on small numbers) for severe lesions.

Table 5 shows the odds ratio for sex, the type of tobacco habit, and the duration of the tobacco habit. These odds ratios were different for the intervention and the control groups owing to the presence of interaction effects. In the control group, the odds ratios for giving up the habit were high for women (*versus* men), for smokers (*versus* chewers), and for shorter duration of the habit (*versus* longer duration). The intervention tended to level these high odds ratios.

Fig. 1. Logistic regression model fitted to study the effectiveness of intervention

```
      ESTIMATE       S.E.       PARAMETER
 1   -5.987        0.5099       %GM
 0     ZERO        ALIASED      stud(1)
 2    3.468        0.5235       stud(2)
 0     ZERO        ALIASED      sex(1)
 3    3.302        0.4900       sex(2)
 0     ZERO        ALIASED      age(1)
 4   0.4885        0.9586E-01   age(2)
 5   0.7329        0.1198       age(3)
 0     ZERO        ALIASED      lesi(1)
 6  -0.1217        0.1313       lesi(2)
 7  -0.7379        0.2989       lesi(3)
 8   0.5252        0.5004       lesi(4)
 0     ZERO        ALIASED      hdur(1)
 9  -0.7581        0.2278       hdur(2)
10   -2.652        0.3550       hdur(3)
 0     ZERO        ALIASED      habi(1)
11    2.286        0.4799       habi(2)
12   0.7419        0.8045       habi(3)
 0     ZERO        ALIASED      stud(1).sex(1)
 0     ZERO        ALIASED      stud(1).sex(2)
 0     ZERO        ALIASED      stud(2).sex(1)
13   -2.537        0.5007       stud(2).sex(2)
 0     ZERO        ALIASED      stud(1).hdur(1)
 0     ZERO        ALIASED      stud(1).hdur(2)
 0     ZERO        ALIASED      stud(1).hdur(3)
 0     ZERO        ALIASED      stud(2).hdur(1)
14   0.3415        0.2454       stud(2).hdur(2)
15    2.013        0.3610       stud(2).hdur(3)
 0     ZERO        ALIASED      stud(1).habi(1)
 0     ZERO        ALIASED      stud(1).habi(2)
 0     ZERO        ALIASED      stud(1).habi(3)
 0     ZERO        ALIASED      stud(2).habi(1)
16   -2.145        0.4922       stud(2).habi(2)
17   -1.436        0.8202       stud(2).habi(3)
SCALE PARAMETER TAKEN AS        1.000

LINEAR PREDICTOR
%GM stud sex age lesi hdur habi stud.sex stud.hdur stud.habi
```

Table 6 shows the effect of intervention according to the types of tobacco habit and the duration of tobacco habit for men and women. These effects differed in various subgroups owing to the presence of interactions. Almost all odds ratios were considerably larger than 1.0, showing that there was a marked intervention effect on all categories of individuals. The odds ratios for women smokers, and smokers and chewers, were sometimes less than or close to 1, but these were based on very small numbers. The odds ratios were larger for men than for women, for chewers than for smokers, and for those with a larger duration compared to those with a shorter duration.

Another way of illustrating the impact of intervention is to display the response probabilities directly. Estimates of the response probability for some selected subgroups are

Table 5. Odds ratio for the response at different levels of covariates from the model

	Intervention group	Control group
Sex		
Women/men	2.1	27.1
Tobacco habit		
Smoking/chewing	1.2	9.8
Both/chewing	0.5	2.1
Habit duration (years)		
1–5/11 and over	1.9	14.1
6–10/11 and over	1.5	2.1

Table 6. Odds ratios in the intervention group relative to the control group (estimated from the logistic regression model)

Habit duration (years)	Chewing	Smoking	Both
Men			
1–5	32.1	3.8	7.6
6–10	122.7	14.4	29.2
11 and over	240.1	28.1	57.1
Women			
1–5	2.5	0.3	0.6
6–10	9.7	1.1	2.3
11 and over	19.0	2.2	4.5

Table 7. Impact of intervention on some selected subgroups

	Men, aged 35–54 years, tobacco users for 11 years or more, without any oral lesions			
	Smokers only		Smokers and chewers	
	Intervention	Control	Intervention	Control
No. of persons	1364	267	677	294
Estimated probability	7.1%	0.3%	3.3%	0.00%
Observed probability	7.0%	0.7%	3.5%	0.0%
	Women, aged 55 years and over, with a tobacco chewing habit without any oral lesions			
	1–5 years		11 years and over	
	Intervention	Control	Intervention	Control
No. of persons	58	23	1029	440
Estimated probability	26.5%	12.4%	16.0%	1.0%
Observed probability	30.2%	13.0%	14.6%	0.0%

shown in Table 7. The close agreement between the observed and estimated probabilities indicates a good fit. The response probabilities appeared to have a wide range. The model provided response probabilities for all possible subgroups in a similar way.

DISCUSSION

The results of the study clearly pointed out that the intervention was effective in terms of increasing the probability of individuals quitting their tobacco habit for almost all categories of people. The intervention effect was, however, different for different categories. It was higher for men, for chewers, and for those with a longer duration of the tobacco habit. This was due to the fact that the response probabilities for these categories of individuals were extremely low in the control group. Thus, the intervention seems to have pulled up the response probabilities for these 'hard core' subgroups and brought them up to levels somewhat comparable with those of other subgroups.

Although the results have been presented here in terms of the intervention effect, the comparison between the intervention group and the control group does not provide a simple comparison between intervention and no intervention. In the control group, individuals were interviewed about their tobacco habits, examined for the presence of oral cancer and precancerous lesions, explained the reasons for doing all this, and frequently advised by the dentist to discontinue practising their tobacco habit. All this constitutes a minimal intervention. In the intervention study, this later component was greatly enlarged and systematized. A social scientist was included in the team, specifically for imparting personal communication, and several available mass media were used. Thus, the intervention effect analysed here is really the effect of adding a systematic programme of behavioural intervention to an existing programme of oral examination by dentists and minimal intervention.

It is apparent from Table 4 that response probabilities were fairly large in certain subgroups of the control group (women, chewers, and those with a shorter duration of the habit). This was pointed out in an earlier report as well (Gupta *et al.*, 1980). This now does not appear to be very surprising; in the Multiple Risk Factor Intervention Trial (MRFIT) also, a large percentage of individuals (21 %) quit their smoking habit in the control (usual care) group without any active attempts at behavioural intervention. The control (usual care) group was, of course, interviewed and examined annually (Ockene *et al.*, 1982).

A rather unexpected finding from the logistic regression analysis was that the chewing habit appeared to be more difficult to give up than the smoking habit. The health effects of chewing habits are beginning to get some attention in the USA as well as internationally (IARC, 1985). The chewing habit is not only a risk factor for oral cancer, but also appears to be responsible for significant excess mortality (Gupta *et al.*, 1984). Thus, this finding, if true in general, would have important implications for public health policies. This finding from the model is a reversal of findings from the marginal analysis, but can be intuitively understood through the relationships between the age, sex, the type of tobacco habit, and the duration of tobacco habits, and thus, illustrates the importance of analysing the data through appropriate models.

The intervention and the control groups in the present study appeared to be comparable in most respects. The follow-up response, however, was much higher in the intervention group than in the control group. This was mainly due to an improved follow-up methodology after the experience of the 10-year follow-up study. The two studies, however, were 10 years apart, and the possibility cannot be ruled out that a part of the intervention study effect was partly due to some unknown variable which changed over the 10-year period, and was related to response probability as well. The chances of any such variable really existing and confounding the results to a significant extent, however, appear to be quite small.

ACKNOWLEDGEMENTS

This paper was written under a Takemi Fellowship awarded to the first author at the Harvard School of Public Health, Boston, MA, USA. The computing facilities were made available through a fellowship awarded to the first author by the Dana Farber Cancer Institute, Boston. The research and the data collection for this paper was done at the Tata Institute of Fundamental Research, Bombay, and was supported by funds from the National Institutes of Health under a PL–480 research agreement No. 01–022–N. The authors are grateful to Dr S. Baker for his kind assistance.

REFERENCES

Baker, R.J. & Nelder, J.A. (1978) *Generalized Linear Interactive Modelling (GLIM) System Release 3,* Oxford, Royal Statistical Society

Gupta, P.C., Bhonsle, R.B., Mehta, F.S. & Pindborg, J.J. (1984) Mortality experience in relation to tobacco chewing and smoking habits from a 10-year follow-up study in Ernakulam district, Kerala. *Int. J. Epidemiol.,* ***13,*** 184–187

Gupta, P.C., Mehta, F.S., Daftary, D.K., *et al.* (1980) Incidence rates of oral cancer and natural history of oral precancerous lesions in a 10-year follow-up study of Indian villagers. *Community Dent. Oral Epidemiol.,* ***8,*** 287–333

IARC (1985) *IARC Monographs on the Evaluation of the Carcinogenic Risk of Chemicals to Humans, Vol. 37, Tobacco Habits other than Smoking; Betel-quid and Areca-nut Chewing; and Some Related Nitrosamines,* Lyon

McCullagh, P. & Nelder, J.A. (1983) *Generalized Linear Models,* London, Chapman & Hill

Mehta, F.S., Pindborg, J.J., Gupta, P.C. & Daftary, D.K. (1969) Epidemiologic and histologic study of oral cancer and leukoplakia among 50 915 villagers in India. *Cancer,* ***24,*** 832–849

Mehta, F.S., Pindborg, J.J., Hamner, J.E., Gupta, P.C., Daftary, D.K., Sahiar, B.E., Shroff, B.C., Sanghvi, L.D., Bhonsle, R.B., Choksi, S.K., Dandekar, V.V., Mehta, Y.N., Pitkar, V.K., Sinor, P.N., Shah, N.C., Turner, P.S. & Upadhyay, S.A. (1971) *Report on Investigations of Oral Cancer and Precancerous Conditions in Indian Rural Populations 1966–1969,* Copenhagen, Munksgaard

Mehta, F.S., Gupta, P.C., Daftary, D.K., Pindborg, J.J. & Choksi, S.K. (1972) An epidemiologic study of oral cancer and precancerous conditions among 101 761 villagers in Maharashtra, India. *Int. J. Cancer,* ***10,*** 134–141

Mehta, F.S., Aghi, M.B., Gupta, P.C., Pindborg, J.J., Bhonsle, R.B., Jahawalla, P.N. & Sinor, P.N. (1982) An intervention study of oral cancer and precancer in rural Indian populations: A preliminary report. *Bull. World Health Organ.*, ***60,*** 441–446

Ockene, J.K., Hymowitz, N., Sexton, M. & Broste, S.K. (1982) Comparison of patterns of smoking behaviour change among smokers in the Multiple Risk Factor Intervention Trial (MRFIT). *Prev. Med.*, ***11,*** 621–638

World Health Organization (1984) Control of oral cancer in developing countries. Report of a WHO Meeting. *Bull. World Health Organ.*, ***62,*** 817–830

AUTHOR INDEX

SUBJECT INDEX

D

E

F

G

H

I

J

K

L

M

PUBLICATIONS OF THE INTERNATIONAL AGENCY FOR RESEARCH ON CANCER

SCIENTIFIC PUBLICATIONS SERIES

(Available from Oxford University Press)

No. 1 LIVER CANCER (1971)
176 pages

No. 2 ONCOGENESIS AND HERPES VIRUSES (1972)
Edited by P.M. Biggs, G. de-Thé & L.N. Payne
515 pages

No. 3 *N*-NITROSO COMPOUNDS - ANALYSIS AND FORMATION (1972)
Edited by P. Bogovski, R. Preussmann & E.A. Walker
140 pages

No. 4 TRANSPLACENTAL CARCINOGENESIS (1973)
Edited by L. Tomatis & U. Mohr,
181 pages

No. 5 PATHOLOGY OF TUMOURS IN LABORATORY ANIMALS. VOLUME 1. TUMOURS OF THE RAT. PART 1 (1973)
Editor-in-Chief V.S. Turusov
214 pages

No. 6 PATHOLOGY OF TUMOURS IN LABORATORY ANIMALS. VOLUME 1. TUMOURS OF THE RAT. PART 2 (1976)
Editor-in-Chief V.S. Turusov
319 pages

No. 7 HOST ENVIRONMENT INTER-ACTIONS IN THE ETIOLOGY OF CANCER IN MAN (1973)
Edited by R. Doll & I. Vodopija,
464 pages

No. 8 BIOLOGICAL EFFECTS OF ASBESTOS (1973)
Edited by P. Bogovski, J.C. Gilson, V. Timbrell & J.C. Wagner,
346 pages

No. 9 *N*-NITROSO COMPOUNDS IN THE ENVIRONMENT (1974)
Edited by P. Bogovski & E.A. Walker
243 pages

No. 10 CHEMICAL CARCINOGENESIS ESSAYS (1974)
Edited by R. Montesano & L. Tomatis,
230 pages

No. 11 ONCOGENESIS AND HERPES-VIRUSES II (1975)
Edited by G. de-Thé, M.A. Epstein & H. zur Hausen
Part 1, 511 pages
Part 2, 403 pages

No. 12 SCREENING TESTS IN CHEMICAL CARCINOGENESIS (1976)
Edited by R. Montesano, H. Bartsch & L. Tomatis
666 pages

No. 13 ENVIRONMENTAL POLLUTION AND CARCINOGENIC RISKS (1976)
Edited by C. Rosenfeld & W. Davis
454 pages

No. 14 ENVIRONMENTAL *N*-NITROSO COMPOUNDS — ANALYSIS AND FORMATION (1976)
Edited by E.A. Walker, P. Bogovski & L. Griciute
512 pages

No. 15 CANCER INCIDENCE IN FIVE CONTINENTS. VOL. III (1976)
Edited by J. Waterhouse, C.S. Muir, P. Correa & J. Powell
584 pages

No. 16 AIR POLLUTION AND CANCER IN MAN (1977)
Edited by U. Mohr, D. Schmahl & L. Tomatis
331 pages

No. 17 DIRECTORY OF ON-GOING RESEARCH IN CANCER EPIDEMIOLOGY 1977 (1977)
Edited by C.S. Muir & G. Wagner,
599 pages; out of print

No. 18 ENVIRONMENTAL CARCINOGENS. SELECTED METHODS OF ANALYSIS
Editor-in-Chief H. Egan
Vol. 1. ANALYSIS OF VOLATILE NITROSAMINES IN FOOD (1978)
Edited by R. Preussmann, M. Castegnaro, E.A. Walker & A.E. Wassermann
212 pages

SCIENTIFIC PUBLICATIONS SERIES

No. 19 ENVIRONMENTAL ASPECTS OF *N*-NITROSO COMPOUNDS (1978)
Edited by E.A. Walker, M. Castegnaro, L. Griciute & R.E. Lyle
566 pages

No. 20 NASOPHARYNGEAL CARCINOMA: ETIOLOGY AND CONTROL (1978)
Edited by G. de-Thé & Y. Ito,
610 pages

No. 21 CANCER REGISTF[illegible]TION AND ITS TECHNIQUES [illegible]78)
Edited by R. MacLennan, [illegible].S. Muir, R. Steinitz & A. Winkler
235 pages

No. 22 ENVIRONMF[illegible]TAL CARCINOGENS. SELECTED METH[illegible]S OF ANALYSIS
Editor-in-Chief H. F[illegible]an
Vol. 2. METHOD[illegible] FOR THE MEASUREMENT OF VINY[illegible] CHLORIDE IN POLY(VINYL C[illegible]LORIDE), AIR, WATER AND FOODST[illegible]FFS (1978)
Edited by D.[illegible] M. Squirrell & W. Thain,
142 pages

No. 23 PAT[illegible]OLOGY OF TUMOURS IN LABORA[illegible]RY ANIMALS. VOLUME II. TUMOU[illegible] OF THE MOUSE (1979)
Editor-ir[illegible]hief V.S. Turusov
669 pag[illegible]

No. 2[illegible] [illegible]NCOGENESIS AND HERPESVIR[illegible]ES III (1978)
Edi[illegible] by G. de-Thé, W. Henle & F. Rapp
Pa[illegible] 1, 580 pages
P[illegible] 2, 522 pages

[illegible]o. 25 CARCINOGENIC RISKS - [illegible]TRATEGIES FOR INTERVENTION (1979)
Edited by W. Davis & C. Rosenfeld,
283 pages

No. 26 DIRECTORY OF ON-GOING RESEARCH IN CANCER EPIDEMIOLOGY 1978 (1978)
Edited by C.S. Muir & G. Wagner,
550 pages; out of print

No. 27 MOLECULAR AND CELLULAR ASPECTS OF CARCINOGEN SCREENING TESTS (1980)
Edited by R. Montesano, H. Bartsch & L. Tomatis
371 pages

No. 28 DIRECTORY OF ON-GOING RESEARCH IN CANCER EPIDEMIOLOGY 1979 (1979)
Edited by C.S. Muir & G. Wagner,
672 pages; out of print

No. 29 ENVIRONMENTAL CARCINOGENS. SELECTED METHODS OF ANALYSIS
Editor-in-Chief H. Egan
Vol. 3. ANALYSIS OF POLYCYCLIC AROMATIC HYDROCARBONS IN ENVIRONMENTAL SAMPLES (1979)
Edited by M. Castegnaro, P. Bogovski, H. Kunte & E.A. Walker
240 pages

No. 30 BIOLOGICAL EFFECTS OF MINERAL FIBRES (1980)
Editor-in-Chief J.C. Wagner
Volume 1, 494 pages
Volume 2, 513 pages

No. 31 *N*-NITROSO COMPOUNDS: ANALYSIS, FORMATION AND OCCURRENCE (1980)
Edited by E.A. Walker, M. Castegnaro, L. Griciute & M. Börzsönyi
841 pages

No. 32 STATISTICAL METHODS IN CANCER RESEARCH
Vol. 1. THE ANALYSIS OF CASE-CONTROL STUDIES (1980)
By N.E. Breslow & N.E. Day
338 pages

No. 33 HANDLING CHEMICAL CARCINOGENS IN THE LABORATORY - PROBLEMS OF SAFETY (1979)
Edited by R. Montesano, H. Bartsch, E. Boyland, G. Della Porta, L. Fishbein, R.A. Griesemer, A.B. Swan & L. Tomatis,
32 pages

No. 34 PATHOLOGY OF TUMOURS IN LABORATORY ANIMALS. VOLUME III. TUMOURS OF THE HAMSTER (1982)
Editor-in-Chief V.S. Turusov,
461 pages

No. 35 DIRECTORY OF ON-GOING RESEARCH IN CANCER EPIDEMIOLOGY 1980 (1980)
Edited by C.S. Muir & G. Wagner,
660 pages; out of print

SCIENTIFIC PUBLICATIONS SERIES

No. 36 CANCER MORTALITY BY OCCUPATION AND SOCIAL CLASS 1851-1971 (1982)
By W.P.D. Logan
253 pages

No. 37 LABORATORY DECONTAMINATION AND DESTRUCTION OF AFLATOXINS B_1, B_2, G_1, G_2 IN LABORATORY WASTES (1980)
Edited by M. Castegnaro, D.C. Hunt, E.B. Sansone, P.L. Schuller, M.G. Siriwardana, G.M. Telling, H.P. Van Egmond & E.A. Walker,
59 pages

No. 38 DIRECTORY OF ON-GOING RESEARCH IN CANCER EPIDEMIOLOGY 1981 (1981)
Edited by C.S. Muir & G. Wagner,
696 pages; out of print

No. 39 HOST FACTORS IN HUMAN CARCINOGENESIS (1982)
Edited by H. Bartsch & B. Armstrong
583 pages

No. 40 ENVIRONMENTAL CARCINOGENS SELECTED METHODS OF ANALYSIS
Editor-in-Chief H. Egan
Vol. 4. SOME AROMATIC AMINES AND AZO DYES IN THE GENERAL AND INDUSTRIAL ENVIRONMENT (1981)
Edited by L. Fishbein, M. Castegnaro, I.K. O'Neill & H. Bartsch
347 pages

No. 41 *N*-NITROSO COMPOUNDS: OCCURRENCE AND BIOLOGICAL EFFECTS (1982)
Edited by H. Bartsch, I.K. O'Neill, M. Castegnaro & M. Okada,
755 pages

No. 42 CANCER INCIDENCE IN FIVE CONTINENTS. VOLUME IV (1982)
Edited by J. Waterhouse, C. Muir, K. Shanmugaratnam & J. Powell,
811 pages

No. 43 LABORATORY DECONTAMINATION AND DESTRUCTION OF CARCINOGENS IN LABORATORY WASTES: SOME *N*-NITROSAMINES (1982) Edited by M. Castegnaro, G. Eisenbrand, G. Ellen, L. Keefer, D. Klein, E.B. Sansone, D. Spincer, G. Telling & K. Webb
73 pages

No. 44 ENVIRONMENTAL CARCINOGENS. SELECTED METHODS OF ANALYSIS
Editor-in-Chief H. Egan
Vol. 5. SOME MYCOTOXINS (1983)
Edited by L. Stoloff, M. Castegnaro, P. Scott, I.K. O'Neill & H. Bartsch,
455 pages

No. 45 ENVIRONMENTAL CARCINOGENS. SELECTED METHODS OF ANALYSIS
Editor-in-Chief H. Egan
Vol. 6: *N*-NITROSO COMPOUNDS (1983)
Edited by R. Preussmann, I.K. O'Neill, G. Eisenbrand, B. Spiegelhalder & H. Bartsch
508 pages

No. 46 DIRECTORY OF ON-GOING RESEARCH IN CANCER EPIDEMIOLOGY 1982 (1982)
Edited by C.S. Muir & G. Wagner,
722 pages; out of print

No. 47 CANCER INCIDENCE IN SINGAPORE (1982)
Edited by K. Shanmugaratnam, H.P. Lee & N.E. Day
174 pages

No. 48 CANCER INCIDENCE IN THE USSR Second Revised Edition (1983)
Edited by N.P. Napalkov, G.F. Tserkovny, V.M. Merabishvili, D.M. Parkin, M. Smans & C.S. Muir,
75 pages

No. 49 LABORATORY DECONTAMINATION AND DESTRUCTION OF CARCINOGENS IN LABORATORY WASTES: SOME POLYCYCLIC AROMATIC HYDROCARBONS (1983)
Edited by M. Castegnaro, G. Grimmer, O. Hutzinger, W. Karcher, H. Kunte, M. Lafontaine, E.B. Sansone, G. Telling & S.P. Tucker
81 pages

No. 50 DIRECTORY OF ON-GOING RESEARCH IN CANCER EPIDEMIOLOGY 1983 (1983)
Edited by C.S. Muir & G. Wagner,
740 pages; out of print

SCIENTIFIC PUBLICATIONS SERIES

No. 51 MODULATORS OF EXPERIMENTAL CARCINOGENESIS (1983)
Edited by V. Turusov & R. Montesano
307 pages

No. 52 SECOND CANCER IN RELATION TO RADIATION TREATMENT FOR CERVICAL CANCER: RESULTS OF A CANCER REGISTRY COLLABORATION (1984)
Edited by N.E. Day & J.C. Boice, Jr,
207 pages

No. 53 NICKEL IN THE HUMAN ENVIRONMENT (1984)
Editor-in-Chief, F.W. Sunderman, Jr,
529 pages

No. 54 LABORATORY DECONTAMINATION AND DESTRUCTION OF CARCINOGENS IN LABORATORY WASTES: SOME HYDRAZINES (1983)
Edited by M. Castegnaro, G. Ellen, M. Lafontaine, H.C. van der Plas, E.B. Sansone & S.P. Tucker,
87 pages

No. 55 LABORATORY DECONTAMINATION AND DESTRUCTION OF CARCINOGENS IN LABORATORY WASTES: SOME *N*-NITROSAMIDES (1984)
Edited by M. Castegnaro, M. Benard, L.W. van Broekhoven, D. Fine, R. Massey, E.B. Sansone, P.L.R. Smith, B. Spiegelhalder, A. Stacchini, G. Telling & J.J. Vallon,
65 pages

No. 56 MODELS, MECHANISMS AND ETIOLOGY OF TUMOUR PROMOTION (1984)
Edited by M. Börszönyi, N.E. Day, K. Lapis & H. Yamasaki
532 pages

No. 57 *N*-NITROSO COMPOUNDS: OCCURRENCE, BIOLOGICAL EFFECTS AND RELEVANCE TO HUMAN CANCER (1984)
Edited by I.K. O'Neill, R.C. von Borstel, C.T. Miller, J. Long & H. Bartsch,
1013 pages

No. 58 AGE-RELATED FACTORS IN CARCINOGENESIS (1985)
Edited by A. Likhachev, V. Anisimov & R. Montesano
288 pages

No. 59 MONITORING HUMAN EXPOSURE TO CARCINOGENIC AND MUTAGENIC AGENTS (1984)
Edited by A. Berlin, M. Draper, K. Hemminki & H. Vainio
457 pages

No. 60 BURKITT'S LYMPHOMA: A HUMAN CANCER MODEL (1985)
Edited by G. Lenoir, G. O'Conor & C.L.M. Olweny
484 pages

No. 61 LABORATORY DECONTAMINATION AND DESTRUCTION OF CARCINOGENS IN LABORATORY WASTES: SOME HALOETHERS (1984)
Edited by M. Castegnaro, M. Alvarez, M. Iovu, E.B. Sansone, G.M. Telling & D.T. Williams
55 pages

No. 62 DIRECTORY OF ON-GOING RESEARCH IN CANCER EPIDEMIOLOGY 1984 (1984)
Edited by C.S. Muir & G.Wagner 728 pages

No. 63 VIRUS-ASSOCIATED CANCERS IN AFRICA (1984)
Edited by A.O. Williams, G.T. O'Conor, G.B. de-Thé & C.A. Johnson,
773 pages

No. 64 LABORATORY DECONTAMINATION AND DESTRUCTION OF CARCINOGENS IN LABORATORY WASTES: SOME AROMATIC AMINES AND 4-NITROBIPHENYL (1985)
Edited by M. Castegnaro, J. Barek, J. Dennis, G. Ellen, M. Klibanov, M. Lafontaine, R. Mitchum, P. Van Roosmalen, E.B. Sansone, L.A. Sternson & M. Vahl
85 pages

No. 65 INTERPRETATION OF NEGATIVE EPIDEMIOLOGICAL EVIDENCE FOR CARCINOGENICITY (1985)
Edited by N.J. Wald & R. Doll
232 pages

No. 66 THE ROLE OF THE REGISTRY IN CANCER CONTROL (1985)
Edited by D.M. Parkin, G. Wagner & C.S. Muir
155 pages

SCIENTIFIC PUBLICATIONS SERIES

No. 67 TRANSFORMATION ASSAY OF ESTABLISHED CELL LINES: MECHANISMS AND APPLICATIONS (1985)
Edited by T. Kakunaga & H. Yamasaki
225 pages

No. 68 ENVIRONMENTAL CARCINOGENS. SELECTED METHODS OF ANALYSIS VOL. 7 — SOME VOLATILE HALOGENATED ALKANES AND ALKENES (1985)
Edited by L. Fishbein & I.K. O'Neill
479 pages

No. 69 DIRECTORY OF ON-GOING RESEARCH IN CANCER EPIDEMIOLOGY 1985 (1985)
Edited by C.S. Muir & G. Wagner
756 pages

No. 70 THE ROLE OF CYCLIC NUCLEIC ACID ADDUCTS IN CARCINOGENESIS AND MUTAGENESIS (1986)
Edited by B. Singer & H. Bartsch
467 pages

No. 71 ENVIRONMENTAL CARCINOGENS. SELECTED METHODS OF ANALYSIS VOL. 8. SOME METALS: As, Be, Cd, Cr, Ni, Pb, Se, Zn (1986)
Edited by I.K. O'Neill, P. Schuller & L. Fishbein
485 pages

No. 72 ATLAS OF CANCER IN SCOTLAND 1975-1980: INCIDENCE AND EPIDEMIOLOGICAL PERSPECTIVE (1985)
Edited by I. Kemp, P. Boyle, M. Smans & C. Muir
282 pages

No. 73 LABORATORY DECONTAMINATION AND DESTRUCTION OF CARCINOGENS IN LABORATORY WASTES: SOME ANTINEOPLASTIC AGENTS (1985)
Edited by M. Castegnaro, J. Adams, M. Armour, J. Barek, J. Benvenuto, C. Confalonieri, U. Goff, S. Ludeman, D. Reed, E.B. Sansone & G. Telling
163 pages

No. 74 TOBACCO: A MAJOR INTERNATIONAL HEALTH HAZARD (1986)
Edited by D. Zaridze and R. Peto
(in press)

No. 75 CANCER OCCURRENCE IN DEVELOPING COUNTRIES (1986)
Edited by D.M. Parkin
339 pages

No. 76 SCREENING FOR CANCER OF THE UTERINE CERVIX (1986)
Edited by M. Hakama, A.B. Miller & N.E. Day
311 pages

No. 77 HEXACHLOROBENZENE: PROCEEDINGS OF AN INTERNATIONAL SYMPOSIUM (1986)
Edited by C.R. Morris & J.R.P. Cabral
668 pages

No. 78 CARCINOGENICITY OF CYTOSTATIC DRUGS (1986)
Edited by D. Schmähl & J. Kaldor
330 pages

No. 79 STATISTICAL METHODS IN CANCER RESEARCH, VOL. 3, THE DESIGN AND ANALYSIS OF LONG-TERM ANIMAL EXPERIMENTS (1986)
By J.J. Gart, D. Krewski, P.N. Lee, R.E. Tarone & J. Wahrendorf
220 pages

No. 80 DIRECTORY OF ON-GOING RESEARCH IN CANCER EPIDEMIOLOGY 1986 (1986)
Edited by G. Wagner & C. Muir
805 pages

No. 81 ENVIRONMENTAL CARCINOGENS. SELECTED METHODS OF ANALYSIS, VOL. 9, PASSIVE SMOKING (1986)
Edited by I.K. O'Neill, K.D. Brunnemann, B. Dodet & D. Hoffmann
(in press)

No. 82 STATISTICAL METHODS IN CANCER RESEARCH, VOL. 2 THE DESIGN AND ANALYSIS OF COHORT STUDIES (1986)
By N.E. Breslow & N.E. Day
(in press)

No. 83 LONG-TERM AND SHORT-TERM ASSAYS FOR CARCINOGENS: A CRITICAL APPRAISAL (1987)
Edited by R. Montesano, H. Bartsch, H. Vainio, J. Wilbourn & H. Yamasaki
(in press)

No. 84 THE RELEVANCE OF *N*-NITROSO COMPOUNDS TO HUMAN CANCER: EXPOSURES AND MECHANISMS (1987)
Edited by H. Bartsch, I.K. O'Neill & R. Schulte-Hermann
(in press)

NON-SERIAL PUBLICATIONS

(Available from IARC)

ALCOOL ET CANCER (1978)
By A.J. Tuyns (in French only)
42 pages

CANCER MORBIDITY AND CAUSES OF DEATH AMONG DANISH BREWERY WORKERS (1980)
By O.M. Jensen
145 pages

DIRECTORY OF COMPUTER SYSTEMS USED IN CANCER REGISTRIES (1986)
By H.R. Menck & D.M. Parkin
236 pages

IARC MONOGRAPHS ON THE EVALUATION OF THE CARCINOGENIC RISK OF CHEMICALS TO HUMANS

(English editions only)

(Available from WHO Sales Agents)

Volume 1
Some inorganic substances, chlorinated hydrocarbons, aromatic amines, N-*nitroso compounds, and natural products* (1972)
184 pp.; out of print

Volume 2
Some inorganic and organometallic compounds (1973)
181 pp.; out of print

Volume 3
Certain polycyclic aromatic hydrocarbons and heterocyclic compounds (1973)
271 pp.; out of print

Volume 4
Some aromatic amines, hydrazine and related substances, N-*nitroso compounds and miscellaneous alkylating agents* (1974)
286 pp.

Volume 5
Some organochlorine pesticides (1974)
241 pp.; out of print

Volume 6
Sex hormones (1974)
243 pp.

Volume 7
Some anti-thyroid and related substances, nitrofurans and industrial chemicals (1974)
326 pp.; out of print

Volume 8
Some aromatic azo compounds (1975)
357 pp.

Volume 9
Some aziridines, N-, S- *and* O-*mustards and selenium* (1975)
268 pp.

Volume 10
Some naturally occurring substances (1976)
353 pp.; out of print

Volume 11
Cadmium, nickel, some epoxides, miscellaneous industrial chemicals and general considerations on volatile anaesthetics (1976)
306 pp.

Volume 12
Some carbamates, thiocarbamates and carbazides (1976)
282 pp.

Volume 13
Some miscellaneous pharmaceutical substances (1977)
255 pp.

Volume 14
Asbestos (1977)
106 pp.

Volume 15
Some fumigants, the herbicides 2,4-D and 2,4,5-T, chlorinated dibenzodioxins and miscellaneous industrial chemicals (1977)
354 pp.

Volume 16
Some aromatic amines and related nitro compounds - hair dyes, colouring agents and miscellaneous industrial chemicals (1978)
400 pp.

Volume 17
Some N-*nitroso compounds* (1978)
365 pp.

Volume 18
Polychlorinated biphenyls and polybrominated biphenyls (1978)
140 pp.

Volume 19
Some monomers, plastics and synthetic elastomers, and acrolein (1979)
513 pp.

Volume 20
Some halogenated hydrocarbons (1979)
609 pp.

Volume 21
Sex hormones (II) (1979)
583 pp.

Volume 22
Some non-nutritive sweetening agents (1980)
208 pp.

IARC MONOGRAPHS SERIES

Volume 23
Some metals and metallic compounds (1980)
438 pp.

Volume 24
Some pharmaceutical drugs (1980)
337 pp.

Volume 25
Wood, leather and some associated industries (1981)
412 pp.

Volume 26
Some antineoplastic and immuno-suppressive agents (1981)
411 pp.

Volume 27
Some aromatic amines, anthraquinones and nitroso compounds, and inorganic fluorides used in drinking-water and dental preparations (1982)
341 pp.

Volume 28
The rubber industry (1982)
486 pp.

Volume 29
Some industrial chemicals and dyestuffs (1982)
416 pp.

Volume 30
Miscellaneous pesticides (1983)
424 pp.

Volume 31
Some food additives, feed additives and naturally occurring substances (1983)
314 pp.

Volume 32
Polynuclear aromatic compounds, Part 1, Environmental and experimental data (1984)
477 pp.

Volume 33
Polynuclear aromatic compounds, Part 2, Carbon blacks, mineral oils and some nitroarene compounds (1984)
245 pp.

Volume 34
Polynuclear aromatic compounds, Part 3, Industrial exposures in aluminium production, coal gasification, coke production, and iron and steel founding (1984)
219 pp.

Volume 35
Polynuclear aromatic compounds, Part 4, Bitumens, coal-tar and derived products, shale-oils and soots (1985)
271 pp.

Volume 36
Allyl compounds, aldehydes, epoxides and peroxides (1985)
369 pp.

Volume 37
Tobacco habits other than smoking; betel-quid and areca-nut chewing; and some related nitrosamines (1985)
291 pp.

Volume 38
Tobacco smoking (1986)
421 pp.

Volume 39
Some chemicals used in plastics and elastomers (1986)
403 pp.

Volume 40
Some naturally occurring and synthetic food components, furocoumarins and ultra-violet radiation (1986)
446 pp. (in print)

Volume 41
Some halogenated hydrocarbons and pesticide exposures (1986)
(in press)

Supplement No. 1
Chemicals and industrial processes associated with cancer in humans (IARC Monographs, Volumes 1 to 20) (1979)
71 pp.; out of print

Supplement No. 2
Long-term and short-term screening assays for carcinogens: a critical appraisal (1980)
426 pp.

Supplement No. 3
Cross index of synonyms and trade names in Volumes 1 to 26 (1982)
199 pp.

Supplement No. 4
Chemicals, industrial processes and industries associated with cancer in humans IARC Monographs, Volumes 1 to 29 (1982)
292 pp.

Supplement No. 5
Cross index of synonyms and trade names in Volumes 1 to 36 (1985)
259 pp.

INFORMATION BULLETINS ON THE SURVEY OF CHEMICALS BEING TESTED FOR CARCINOGENICITY

(Available from IARC)

No. 8 (1979)
Edited by M.-J. Ghess, H. Bartsch & L. Tomatis
604 pp.

No. 9 (1981)
Edited by M.-J. Ghess, J.D. Wilbourn, H. Bartsch & L. Tomatis
294 pp.

No. 10 (1982)
Edited by M.-J. Ghess, J.D. Wilbourn H. Bartsch
326 pp.

No. 11 (1984)
Edited by M.-J. Ghess, J.D. Wilbourn, H. Vainio & H. Bartsch
336 pp.

No. 12 (1986)
Edited by M.-J. Ghess, J.D. Wilbourn, A. Tossavainen & H. Vainio
385 pp.

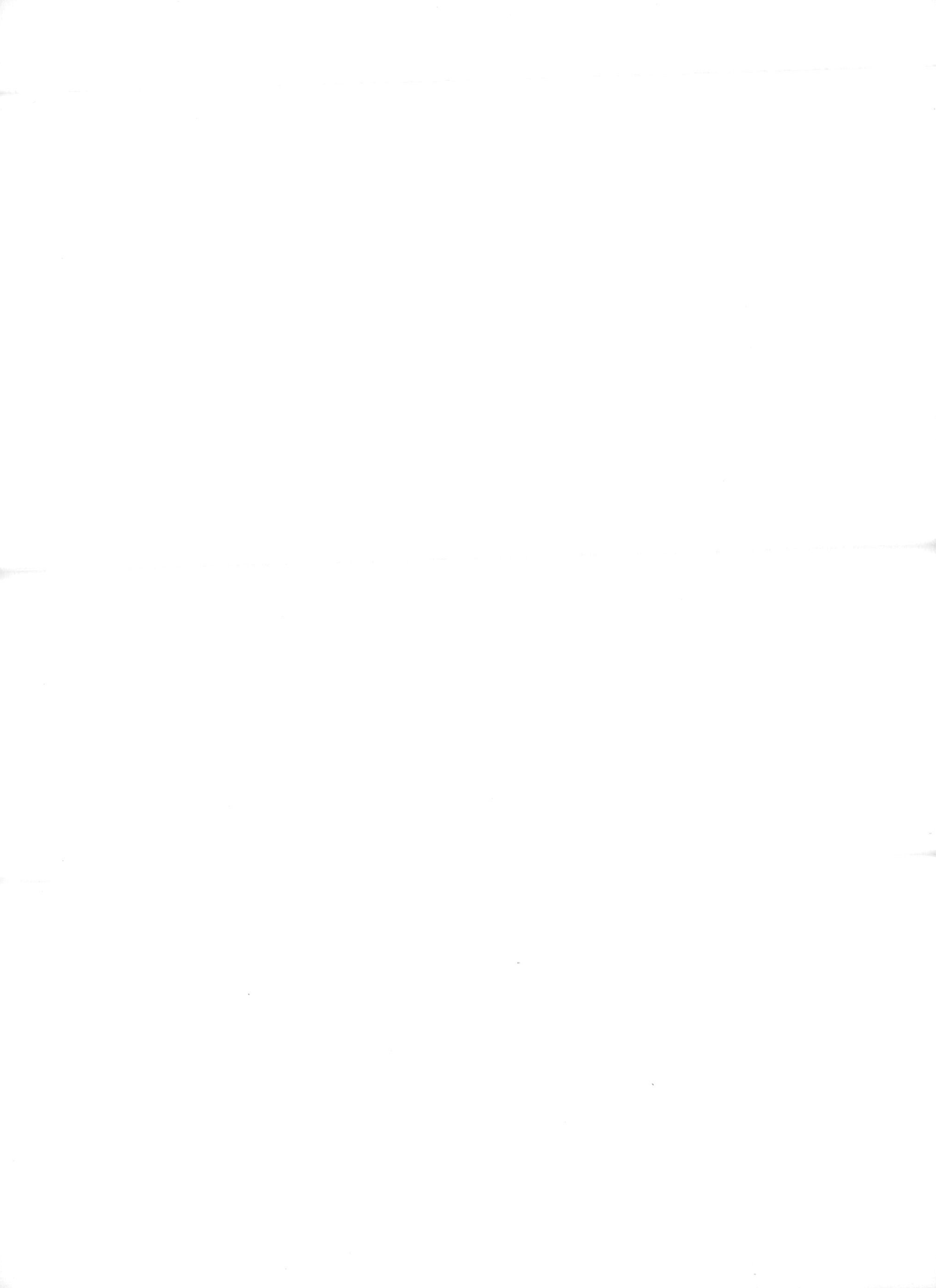

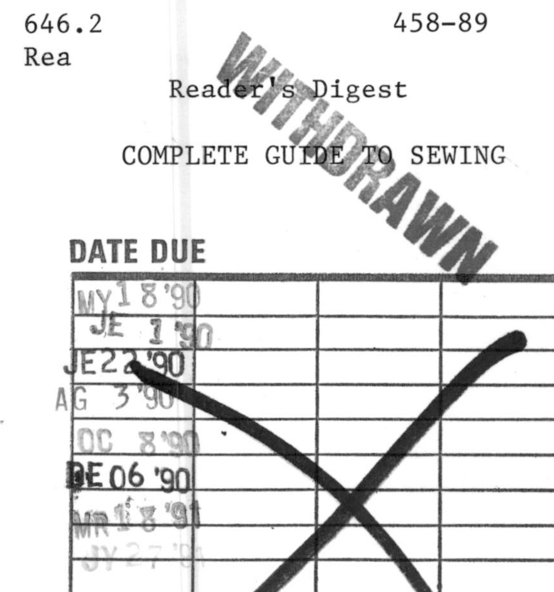

Reader's Digest

Complete Guide to Sewing

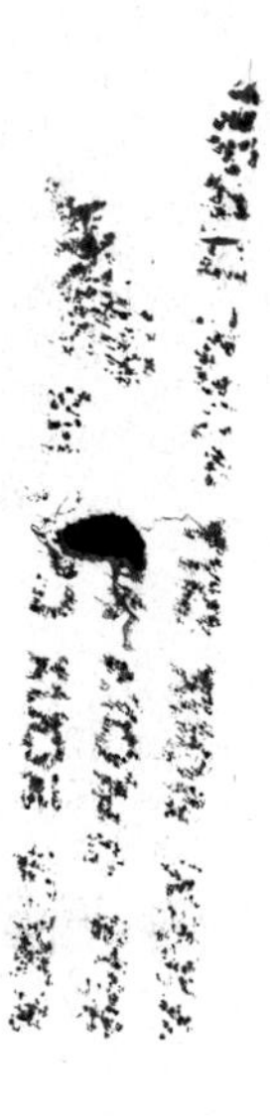

Reader's Digest

Complete Guide to Sewing

The Reader's Digest Association, Inc.
Pleasantville, New York / Montreal

How to use this book

Complete Guide to Sewing is designed to be useful not only for many years but, in several unusual ways, from the very first day.

Chapter title pages give a detailed, page-by-page list, actually a preview, of each chapter's contents.
Name tabs in the upper right-hand corners of facing pages identify the topic at hand, so you can tell at a glance, as you turn the pages, exactly where you are in the book.
Cross references at the tops of pages direct you to significant content elsewhere in the book that is related to those pages.
The index, though it is a traditional alphabetical listing in other ways, also has a special feature: When an entire section is devoted to a subject, the first entry for that subject appears in heavy type, followed by the section's page numbers.

This book was prepared with technical assistance from The Singer Company.

The credits and acknowledgments that appear on page 6 are hereby made a part of this copyright page.

Printed in the United States of America

Thirteenth Printing, March 1988

The Library of Congress has cataloged this work as follows:

Reader's digest complete guide to sewing. — Pleasantville, N.Y.: Reader's Digest Association, c1976.

528 p. : ill. (some col.); 23 x 29 cm.

Includes index.

1. Sewing. 2. Dressmaking. I. Reader's Digest Association. II. Title: Complete guide to sewing.

TT705.R38 646 75-32106
ISBN 0-89577-026-1 MARC

Contents

Complete Guide to Sewing

Editor:
Virginia Colton

Art director:
David Trooper

Associate art director:
Albert D. Burger

Associate editors:
Laura Dearborn
Susan C. Hoe
Therese L. Hoehlein
Mary E. Johnson
Gayla Visalli

Designers:
Larissa Lawrynenko
Virginia Wells
Lynn E. Yost

Copy editor:
Elizabeth T. Salter

Art assistants:
Lisa Grant
Juli Hopfl

Technical assistant:
Ben T. Etheridge

Photography:
W. A. Sonntag
Ernest Coppolino

Contributing artists:
Vicenta M. Aviles
Sylvia Bokor
Dominic Colacchio
Karen Coughlin
Susan Frye
Carmine Glielmi
Marilyn Grastorf
Hank Grindall
Rudie Hampel
Edward P. Hauser
George Kelvin
John A. Lind Corp.
Mary Jo Quay
Lorelle Raboni
Mary Roby
Jim Silks
Randall Lieu
Michael Vivo

Contributing photographers:
Joseph Barnell
Irving Elkin (cover)
Graphic Arts Department,
The Singer Company

The editors are grateful for the assistance of the individuals and organizations listed below

Contributing editors:
Peggy Bendel
Mary Anne Symons Brown
Hewitt McGraw Busse
Janet DuBane
Sharon S. Finkenauer
Nancy B. Greenspan
Marilyn Anne Speer

Technical assistance:
Education Department,
The Singer Company

Sewing machine consultant:
Joyce D. Lee

Research assistance provided by these manufacturers and organizations:

American Thread
The Armo Company
Div. of Crown Textile Mfg. Corp.
Belding Corticelli
B. Blumenthal & Co., Inc.
Brother International Corporation
Butterick Fashion Marketing Company
Century Ribbon Mills, Inc.
Coats & Clark Inc.
Colton Elastic
Div. of J.P. Stevens & Co., Inc.
DHJ Industries, Inc.
Elna Sewing Machines
Div. of White Sewing Machine Company
OY Fiskars AB
Hirschberg Schutz & Company, Inc.
Kirsch Company
Knitted Textile Association
Lily Mills Company
Logantex, Inc.
McCall Pattern Company
Maxant Button & Supply Co.
Montgomery Ward & Company
Moore Fabrics Company
Div. of Chicopee Mills, Inc.
Morse Electro Products Corp.
National Notion Association, Inc.
Necchi Sewing Machines
Manufacturing Company
C.M. Offray & Son, Inc.
Pellon Corporation
J.C. Penney Company, Inc.
Pfaff International Corporation
William Prym Inc.
Riccar American Company
The Risdon Manufacturing Company
Scovill Manufacturing Company
Sewing Notions Division
Sears, Roebuck and Co.
Simplicity Pattern Co. Inc.
Springs Mills, Inc.
Stacy Fabrics Corp.
Star Thread, Zippers & Tapes
American Thread
J.P. Stevens & Co., Inc.
Sublistatic Corporation of America
Swiss-Bernina, Inc.
Talon Division of Textron
Unique Invisible Zippers
Viking Sewing Machines
White Sewing Machine Company
J. Wiss & Sons Company
Wm. E. Wright Co.
YKK (USA), Inc.

Necessities of Sewing

Sewing tools

Measuring devices

Conversion to metric system. In anticipation of the change from inch-foot-yard to metric measurements, many measuring devices have been redesigned to show both. More such dual-purpose devices will appear in the future. Take care, in using any such device, that you do not interchange inch and centimeter measurements.

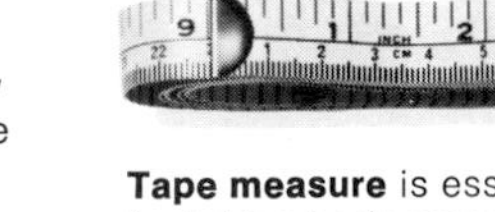

Tape measure is essential for taking body measurements. Best tape choice is flexible synthetic or fiberglass, which will not tear or stretch; 60″ length with measurements on both sides; made with metal-tipped (nonfraying) ends.

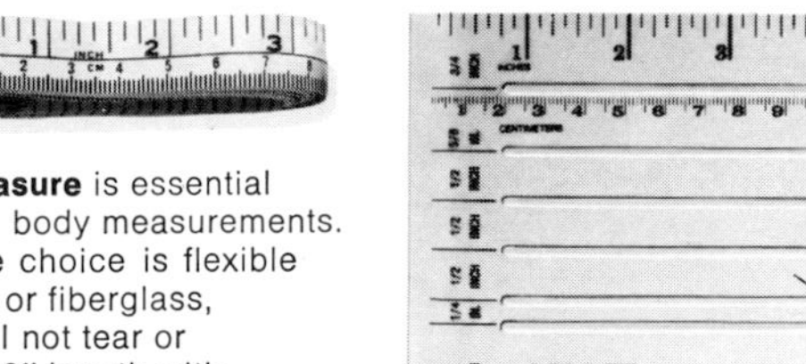

Transparent ruler lets you see what you measure or mark. Select one of flexible plastic (will measure slight curves), 12″ or 18″ long. Ruler is useful to check grainline of fabric; to mark buttonholes, tucks, pleats, bias strips; and as a guide for tracing wheel.

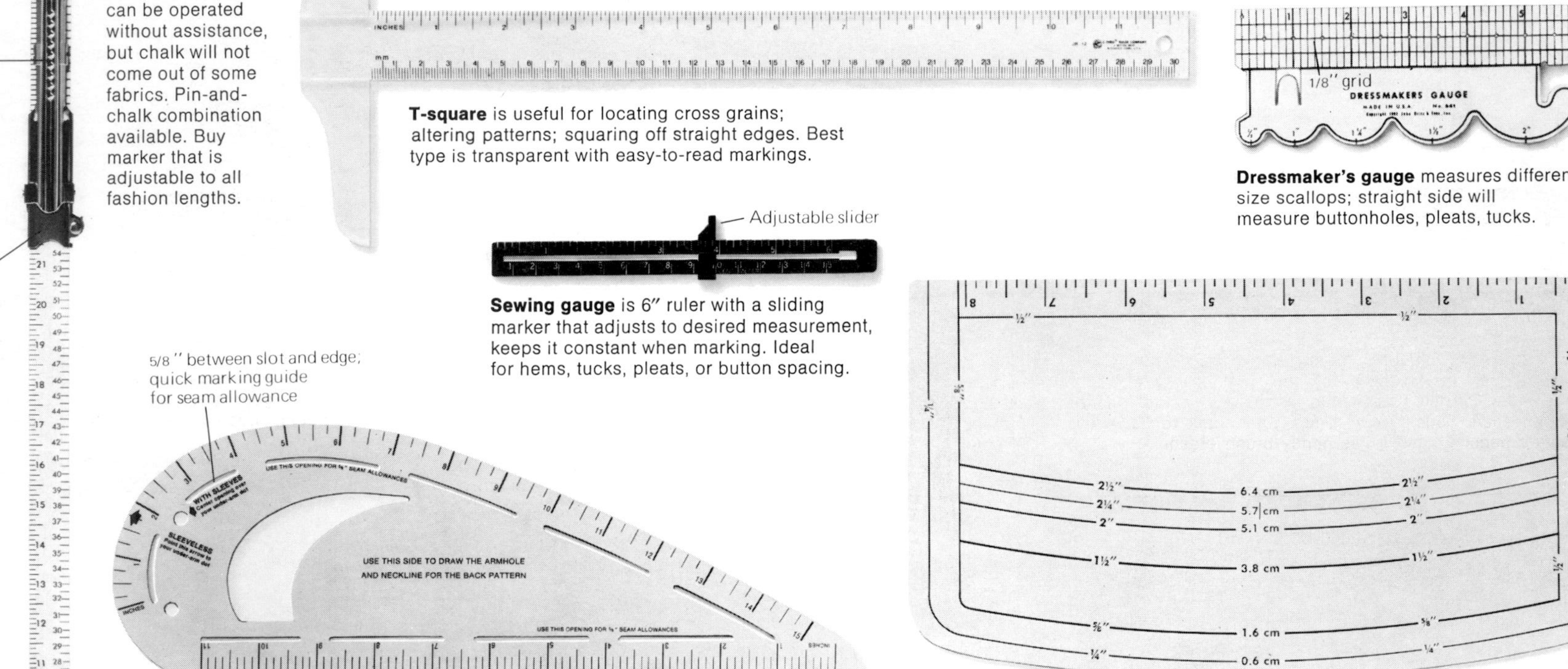

Skirt marker is an easy-to-use, accurate tool for marking hems. Of the various types, pin marker is most exact, but takes two people; chalk model can be operated without assistance, but chalk will not come out of some fabrics. Pin-and-chalk combination available. Buy marker that is adjustable to all fashion lengths.

T-square is useful for locating cross grains; altering patterns; squaring off straight edges. Best type is transparent with easy-to-read markings.

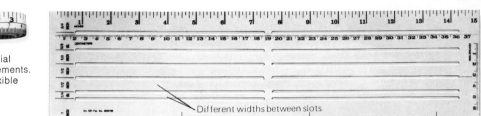

Dressmaker's gauge measures different size scallops; straight side will measure buttonholes, pleats, tucks.

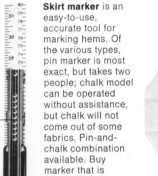

Sewing gauge is 6″ ruler with a sliding marker that adjusts to desired measurement, keeps it constant when marking. Ideal for hems, tucks, pleats, or button spacing.

French curve is useful when re-drawing construction lines on patterns, especially in curved areas, such as armholes, necklines, princess seams.

Hem gauge speeds marking of straight or curved hems; edge is turned and pressed in one step. Useful, too, for adjusting pattern lengths.

Yardstick is best device for taking long, straight measurements. Good also for checking grainlines, marking hems. Be sure surface of wood is smooth.

Cutting 89
Fabric-marking methods 94

Marking devices

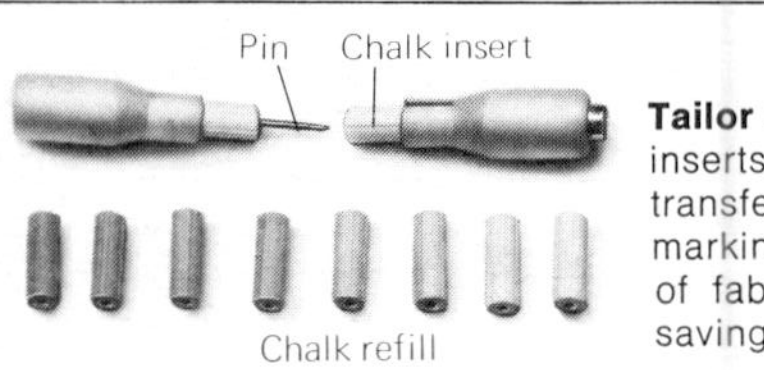

Tailor tacker with chalk inserts in various colors transfers construction markings to both sides of fabric in one time-saving operation.

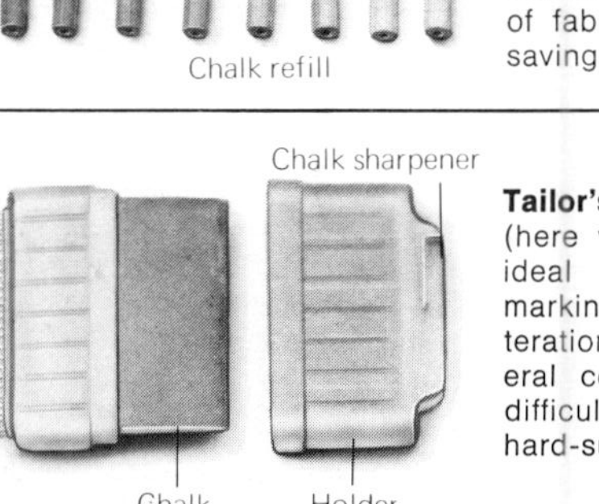

Tailor's chalk wedges (here with holder) are ideal for construction markings and fitting alterations; come in several colors. Wax type difficult to remove from hard-surfaced fabrics.

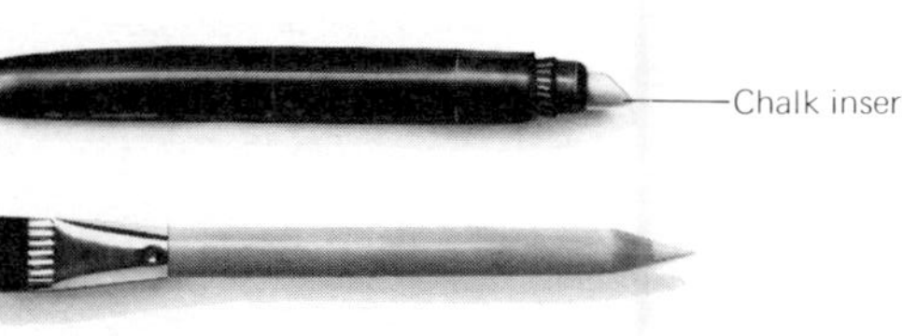

Chalk in pencil form is used like any pencil; makes a thin, accurate line, fine for marking pleats, buttonholes, and similar details. Chalk colors include white and pastel shades. Tailor's chalk pencil (top) comes with chalk refills; dressmaker's pencil (bottom) has handy brush eraser.

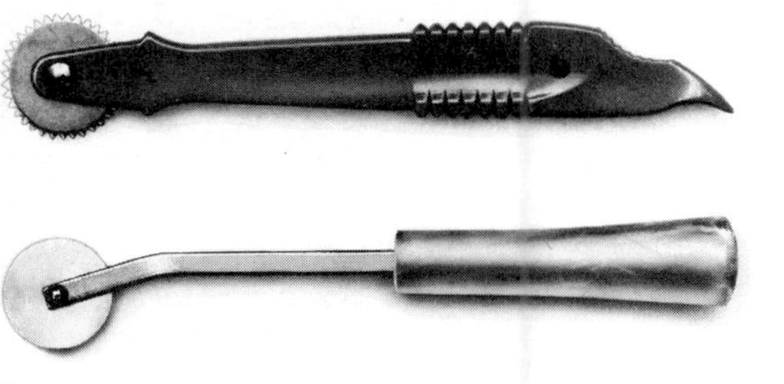

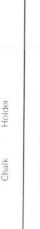

Tracing wheels are used with dressmaker's tracing paper to transfer pattern markings to fabric. Usual choice is serrated-edge wheel (top), suitable for most fabrics. Smooth-edged wheel (bottom) makes firmer markings on hard-to-mark fabrics; protects delicate, smooth ones.

Shears and scissors

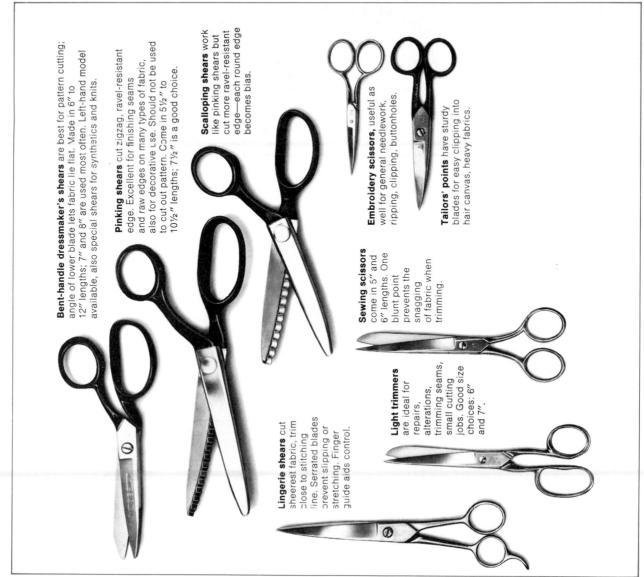

Bent-handle dressmaker's shears are best for pattern cutting; angle of lower blade lets fabric lie flat. Made in 6″ to 12″ lengths; 7″ and 8″ are used most often. Left-hand model available, also special shears for synthetics and knits.

Pinking shears cut zigzag, ravel-resistant edge. Excellent for finishing seams and raw edges on many types of fabric, also for decorative use. Should not be used to cut out pattern. Come in 5½″ to 10½″ lengths; 7½″ is a good choice.

Scalloping shears work like pinking shears but cut more ravel-resistant edge—each round edge becomes bias.

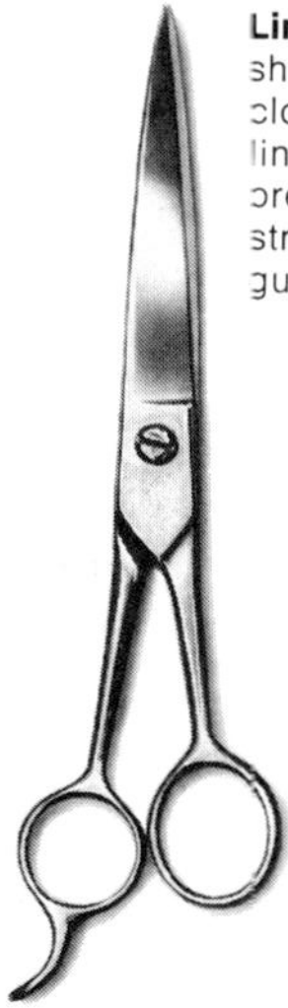

Lingerie shears cut sheerest fabric, trim close to stitching line. Serrated blades prevent slipping or stretching. Finger guide aids control.

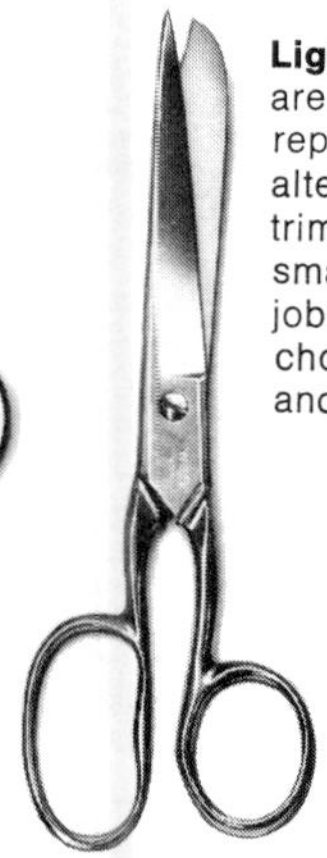

Light trimmers are ideal for repairs, alterations, trimming seams, small cutting jobs. Good size choices: 6″ and 7″.

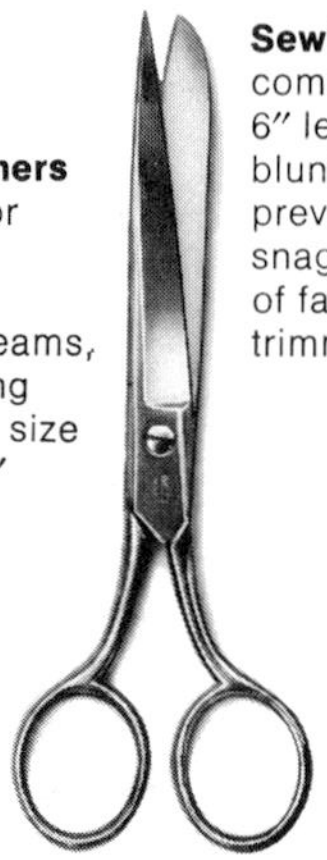

Sewing scissors come in 5″ and 6″ lengths. One blunt point prevents the snagging of fabric when trimming.

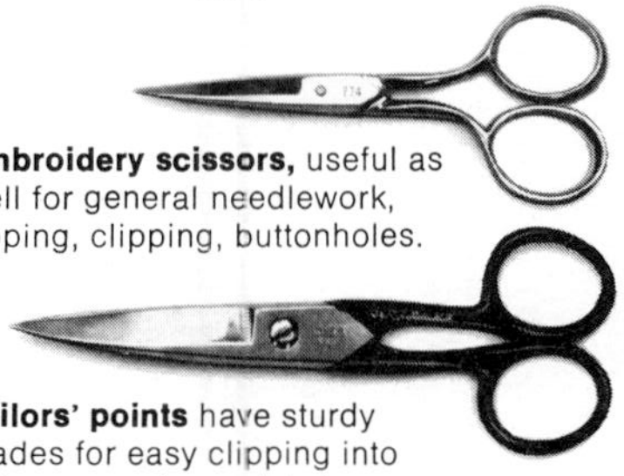

Embroidery scissors, useful as well for general needlework, ripping, clipping, buttonholes.

Tailors' points have sturdy blades for easy clipping into hair canvas, heavy fabrics.

Sewing supplies

Sewing machine 21-27

Thread

Thread for constructing a garment should be compatible with the fiber content and weight of the fabric. Interaction is best, where it is feasible, between thread and fabric of like sources—both synthetic, say, or both derived from animal or plant sources. Where exceptions are made, the reasons are practical; synthetic thread, for example, because of its stretchability, is best for any knit, regardless of fiber content. The chart below defines the most used thread types and gives recommendations for their use. Size numbers are given where they apply. The higher the number, the finer the thread; the median size is 50. Where letters denote size, A is fine, D is heavy. Use thread one shade darker than the fabric; for a print or plaid, the dominant color.

THREAD	FIBERS AND USAGE
Basting	**Cotton:** A loosely twisted thread used for hand basting. Loose twist makes it easy to break for quick removal from the garment. Available only in white —safest because there is no dye to rub off on fabric.
Button and carpet	**Cotton; cotton-wrapped polyester:** Tough, thick thread (size 16) used for hand-sewing jobs requiring super thread strength. Thread usually has "glazed" finish that makes it easier to slip through heavy fabric.
Darning cotton	**Cotton:** A very fine thread used for darning and mending. Strands can be separated, if desired, for work requiring even finer thread.
Elastic	**Nylon/cotton-wrapped rubber:** A thick, very stretchy thread used for shirring on sewing machine. Elastic thread is wound on bobbin only.
Embroidery floss	**Cotton; rayon:** Six thread strands twisted loosely together, made for decorative hand work. Strands can be separated for very fine work.
Extra-fine	**Cotton; polyester; cotton-wrapped polyester:** Thread (approximately size 60) used for lingerie or other work requiring a fine thread.
General purpose	**Cotton:** A medium thickness (size 50) is available in a wide range of colors (other sizes made in black and white only). Used for machine and hand sewing on light- and medium-weight cottons, rayons, and linens. Cotton thread is usually mercerized, a finishing process that makes it smooth and lustrous, also helps it to take dye better. The lack of give in cotton thread makes it an unwise choice for knits or other stretchy fabrics, as the stitches tend to pop.
	Silk: A fine (size A), strong thread for hand and machine sewing on silk

THREAD	FIBERS AND USAGE
General purpose (*cont.*)	and wool. Its fineness makes it ideal for basting all fabric types, as it does not leave holes from stitching or imprints after pressing. Because of its elasticity, silk is also suitable for sewing any type of knit. Recommended for tailoring because it can be molded along with the fabric in shaped areas.
	Nylon: A fine (size A), strong thread for hand and machine sewing on light- to medium-weight synthetics. Especially suited to nylon tricot.
	Polyester: An all-purpose weight (approximately size 50), suitable for hand and machine sewing on most fabrics, but particularly recommended for woven synthetics, also for knits and other stretch fabrics of any fiber. Most polyester threads have a wax or silicone finish to help them slip through fabric with a minimum of friction.
	Cotton-wrapped polyester: An all-purpose weight (approximately size 50) for hand and machine sewing on knits or wovens, of synthetic or natural fibers, or blends. Polyester core gives this thread strength and elasticity; cotton wrapping, a tough, heat-resistant surface.
Heavy-duty	**Cotton; polyester; cotton-wrapped polyester:** Coarse thread (approximately size 40) used where extra strength is required for hand or machine sewing of heavy vinyl, coating, or upholstery fabrics.
Metallic	**Metallized synthetic:** Shiny silver- or gold-colored thread, used for decorative stitching by hand or machine.
Quilting	**Cotton:** "Glazed" thread (size 40) used for hand or machine quilting.
Silk twist	**Silk:** Coarse thread (size D) used for topstitching and hand-worked buttonholes, also for decorative hand sewing and sewing on buttons.

Straight pins

Straight pins come in several lengths and thicknesses. Generally, the longer the pin, the thicker it is. Standard length for dressmaking is 1 1/16"; this type, known as a *seamstress*, or *silk*, pin, is suitable for light- to medium-weight fabrics. The 1" length, sometimes called a *pleating* pin, is extra-fine, suiting it for use on delicate fabrics. Long pins (1 1/4") are recommended for heavy materials; other lengths are available for special purposes, such as crafts. **Pin heads** are of three types: *flat, color ball* (glass or plastic), and *"T"*. The color ball has some advantage over the flat head in that it is easier to see and handle. A T-pin is convenient for heavy pile fabrics and loose knits; the head will not disappear into or slip through these fabrics. Standard pin point is sharp; ball-points are rounded to slip between yarns, which makes them a good choice for knits.

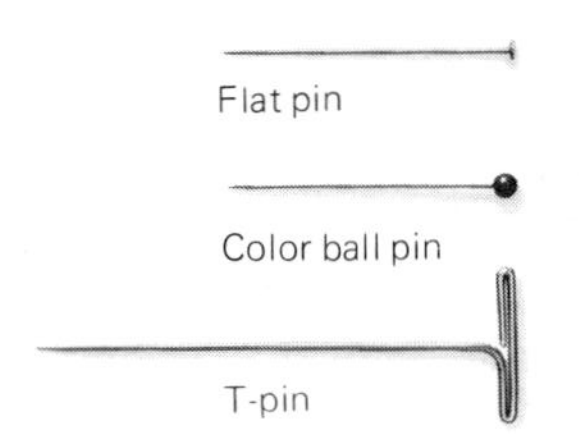

Metals of which straight pins are made

Brass:	**Steel:**	**Stainless steel:**
Soft metal; does not rust; usually nickel-plated;* retains sharp point for a long time.	Sturdy metal; can rust; usually nickel-plated;* least expensive; can be picked up magnetically.	Strong metal; does not rust; can also be picked up magnetically.

*Nickel plating sometimes leaves a black mark on fabric.

Hand-sewing techniques 122-136

Hand needles

Many types of needles are made for hand sewing, each for a specific purpose. These vary according to eye shape (long or round), length (in proportion to eye), and point (sharp, blunt, ball-point, or wedge). The chart below describes the basic types. Each embraces a range of sizes; the larger a number, the shorter and finer the needle. Examples are illustrated in comparable sizes to show the proportion from one type to another. For matching needle to job, consider the kind of work being done (some needles are named for their principal purpose, such as "crewel"), fabric structure (knitted or woven), weight, and thread thickness. Generally, a needle should be fine enough to slip easily through fabric, yet heavy enough not to bend or break. Long-eyed needles are designed to accommodate thick thread or several strands. Whatever the type, always work with a clean, well-pointed needle.

GENERAL HAND SEWING
This group of hand needles is used for general-purpose sewing. Most of them are sharp needles and each has a size range sufficient to accommodate most weights of fabrics.

Sharps (sizes 1–12) are the hand sewing needles in most common use. They are medium length and have a round eye. Suitable for almost all fabric weights.

Betweens (sizes 1–12) are also known as quilting needles. Their shorter length enables them to take fine stitches in heavy fabric.

Milliners (sizes 3/0–12) are longer than others in group, useful for basting.

Ball-points (sizes 5–10) resemble sharps except for the point, which is rounded to penetrate between knit yarns.

Calyx-eyes (sizes 4–8) are like sharps except thread is pulled into a slot rather than through an eye.

NEEDLECRAFT
This group of hand needles is used primarily for a variety of art and needlecraft purposes, such as embroidery, needlepoint, and decorative beading.

Crewels (sizes 1–10) are sharp, medium-length needles used primarily for embroidery work. Long eye allows several strands of embroidery floss to be threaded.

Chenilles (sizes 13-26) are sharp and heavy for use in embroidering with yarn.

Beading needles (sizes 10–15) are thin and long for beading and sequin work.

Tapestry needles (sizes 13–26) are heavy and have blunt points. Used mainly for needlepoint and tapestry work, they can also serve the purpose of a bodkin.

DARNING
These needles are used primarily for darning. They vary in length and diameter to accommodate most darning or mending jobs.

Cotton darners (sizes 1–9) are designed for darning with fine cotton or wool.

Double longs (sizes 5/0–9) are like cotton darners but longer and therefore able to span larger holes.

Yarn darners (sizes 14–18) are long and heavy, necessities for darning with yarn.

HEAVY-DUTY SEWING
These hand needles are ideal for heavy sewing jobs. Both the glover and sailmaker types have wedge-shaped points that pierce leather and leatherlike fabrics in such a way that the holes resist tearing.

Glovers (sizes 3/0–8) are short, round-eye needles with triangular points that will pierce leather, vinyl, or plastic without tearing them.

Sailmakers (sizes 14–17) are like glovers except that their triangular point extends part way up the shaft. Sailmakers are used on canvas and heavy leather.

Curved needles (sizes 1½"–3") are intended for use on upholstery, braided rugs, or lampshades—anywhere that a straight needle would be awkward. Some curved needles are double-pointed.

Sewing supplies

Machine bobbins 22-25
Using machine needles 26-27

Machine needles

Machine needles are selected according to weight and other fabric characteristics, as well as the thread type being used. In general, a needle should be fine enough to penetrate fabric without marring it, yet have a large enough eye that the thread does not fray or break. Needle sizes range from fine (size 9) for lightweight fabrics to heavy (size 18) for very heavy ones. Sizes 11 and 14 are used most often for general sewing. Most of the needles sold are made in a standard length that fits most modern machines. Check your machine instruction book. Needles do have different points, as explained below. Always replace dulled, bent, burred, or nicked needles; they can damage fabric.

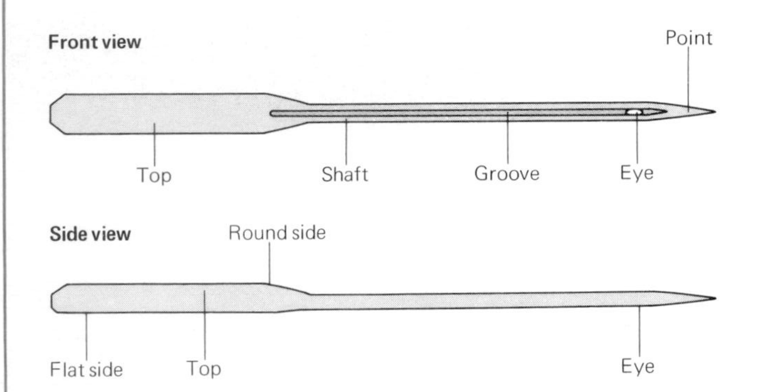

The illustrations at the left show both a front and a side close-up view of a machine needle. The thick or top portion is rounded on one side and flat on the reverse side, with the needle size usually etched into the rounded part. The thin or lower portion of the needle has a groove extending along the shaft from the rounded part to the eye. When a needle is inserted into any sewing machine, the rounded side should face the direction from which the needle is threaded. For example, if the needle is threaded from the front to the back, the rounded side should face front. This positions the groove toward the thread, permitting it to guide thread as it feeds through needle.

Specific sewing situations will require different needle points

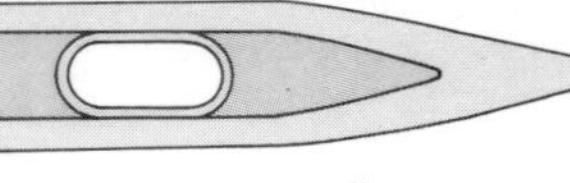

Regular sharp needle

Regular sharp needle is ideal for all *woven* fabrics because it helps to produce even stitching with a minimum of fabric puckering. A regular sharp-point needle is not generally advised for sewing on knits—it can cut the yarns and cause skipped stitches. Needles range from a fine size 9 to a heavy size 18. Also available is a twin needle version (with two points) for fancy topstitching.

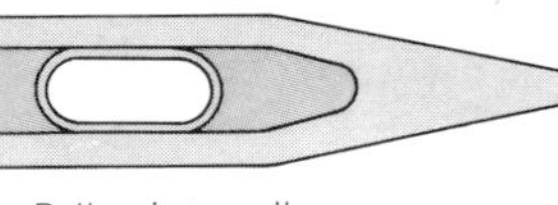

Ball-point needle

The slightly rounded ball-point is recommended for all knit and elastic fabrics because it pushes *between* fabric yarns instead of piercing them. Some modified types can also be used for wovens (follow the manufacturer's instructions). Available in sizes from 9 to 16, with point rounded in proportion to the needle size—points of larger sizes 14 and 16 being more rounded than those of sizes 9 and 11.

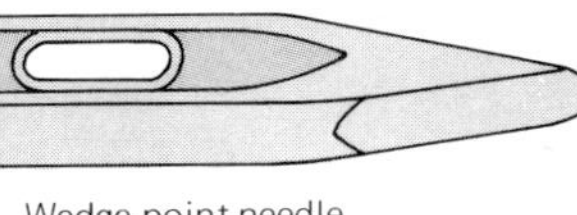

Wedge-point needle

The wedge-shaped point, designed for use on leather and vinyl, easily pierces these fabrics to make a hole that closes back upon itself. This avoids unattractive holes in the garment; also reduces the risk of stitches tearing the fabric. Wedge needles come in sizes 11 to 18. Size 11 is used for soft, pliable leathers; size 18 is suitable for heavy or multiple layers of leather.

Sewing aids

Of the many sewing aids made for home use, some, such as bobbins and pins, are necessities. Others, though not really necessary, are very handy for general sewing—a needle threader and thimble, for example. Still others, such as the loop turner, are needed only now and then for a special task, but are invaluable for that particular job. Then, too,

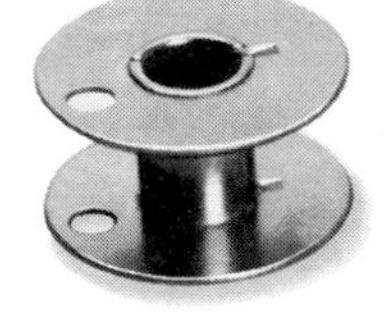
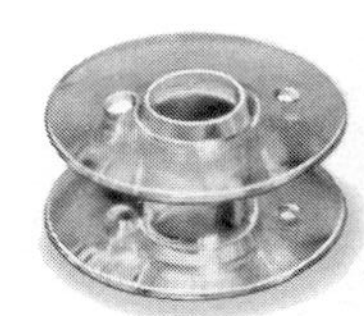
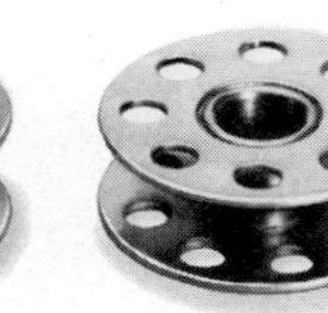
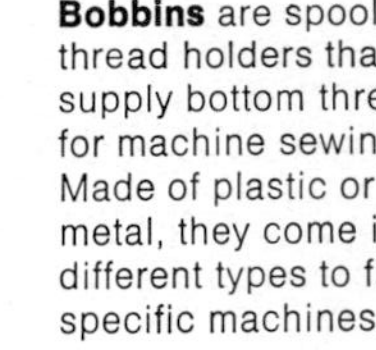

Bobbins are spool-like thread holders that supply bottom thread for machine sewing. Made of plastic or metal, they come in different types to fit specific machines.

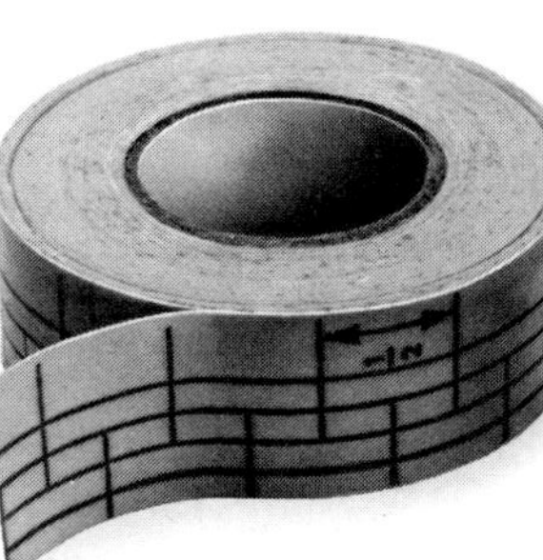

Self-stick sewing tape has measured markings on one side to use as a stitching guide; is especially useful for topstitching. Available in two types: one that separates into various widths, with stitching done next to tape; a second that can be stitched through.

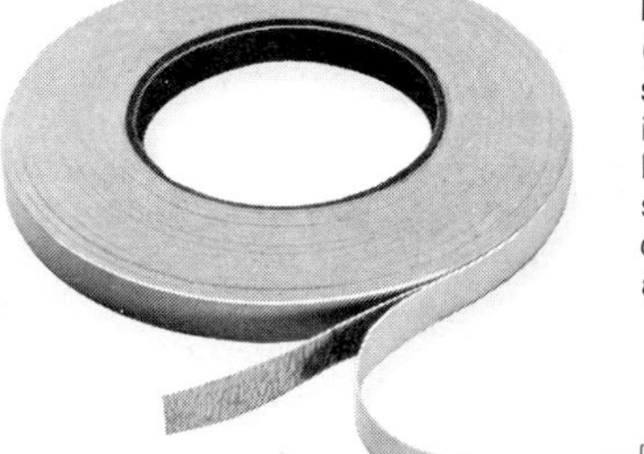

Double-faced tape (adhesive on both sides) will hold zipper in position or fabric layers together for stitching. *Do not sew over tape;* remove it after completing seam.

Protective paper peels off

there are the sewing aids, such as needle conditioners and scissors sharpeners, designed to help keep equipment in good working order. A sampling of such sewing aids is shown here; more are to be found on sewing counters, with new ones being invented every day. In buying sewing tools and supplies, it is wise to begin with a few basic ones, purchasing more as the need arises. In addition to aids specifically meant for sewing, other devices and some common household items can be used for sewing jobs. A magnet will pick up stray steel pins and needles. A fine crochet hook is helpful when tying short thread ends or for pulling snags to the wrong side of a knit. Tissue paper is useful in making pattern adjustments and also facilitates sewing slippery or very soft fabrics. Tweezers deftly remove tiny thread ends, tailor's tacks, and bastings. Other useful items include transparent tape to guide topstitching or hold pattern adjustments in place, a large safety pin used to draw elastic or cord through a casing.

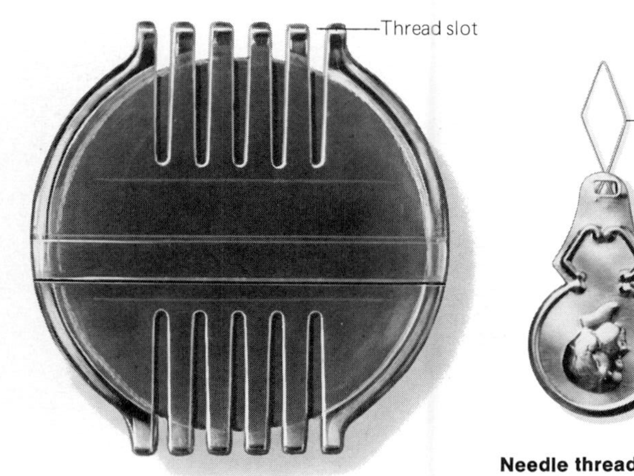

Beeswax is used to strengthen thread for hand sewing, reduce tendency to tangle and knot. Usually sold in container shown; to apply wax, thread is slipped through slots.

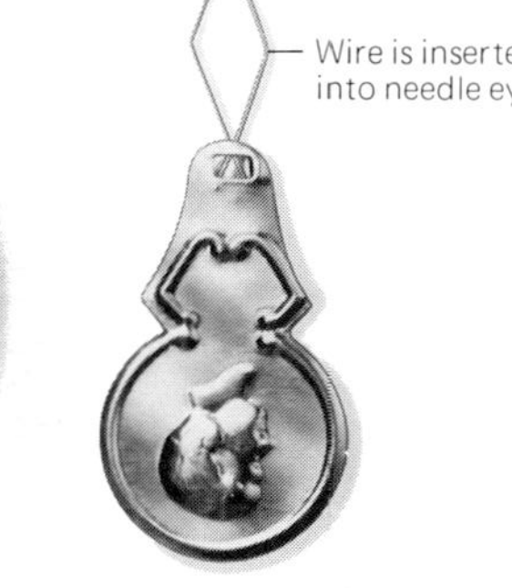
Wire is inserted into needle eye

Needle threader eases threading of hand or machine needles.

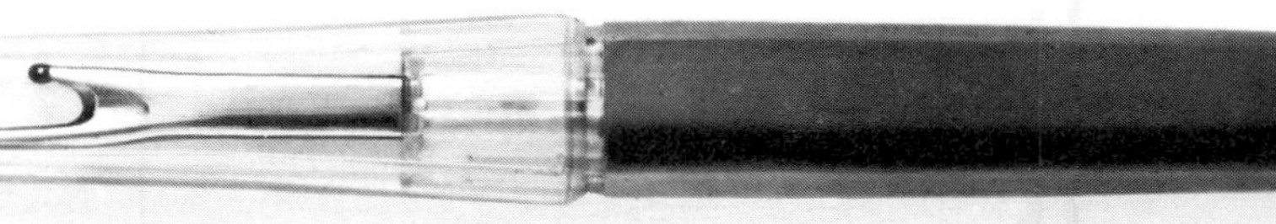

Seam ripper has sharp, curved edge for cutting seams open and a point for picking out threads. Can also be used for slashing machine-worked buttonholes. Use ripper carefully to avoid accidental cutting of fabric.

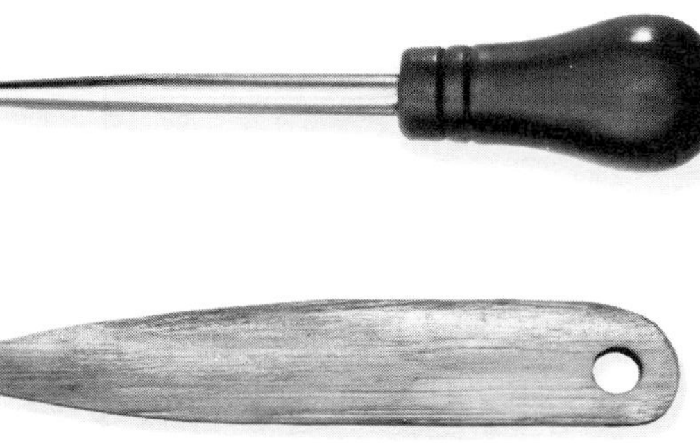

An awl or stiletto is a small, sharp instrument used to make the round holes needed for eyelets or keyhole buttonholes. For safety, tool should have snug-fitting cover.

Pointer and creaser is a flat wooden tool with a pointed end for pushing out corners, a rounded end to hold a seamline open for pressing.

Thimble protects middle finger while hand sewing. Comes in sizes 6 (small) to 12 (large) for snug fit.

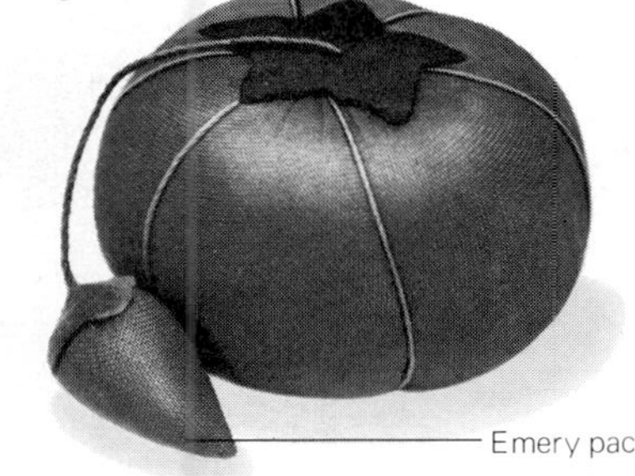
Emery pack

Pin cushion is a safe, handy place to store pins, keep them accessible. Some have an emery pack attached for cleaning both pins and needles.

Bodkin is a tool shaped like a long, blunt needle and used for threading elastic or cord through a casing. Can also be used to turn bias tubing. Bodkin types can vary; some have an eye through which elastic or cord can be threaded, others a tweezer or safety pin closure.

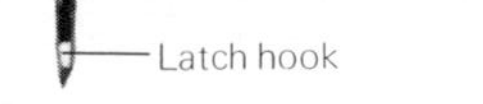
Latch hook

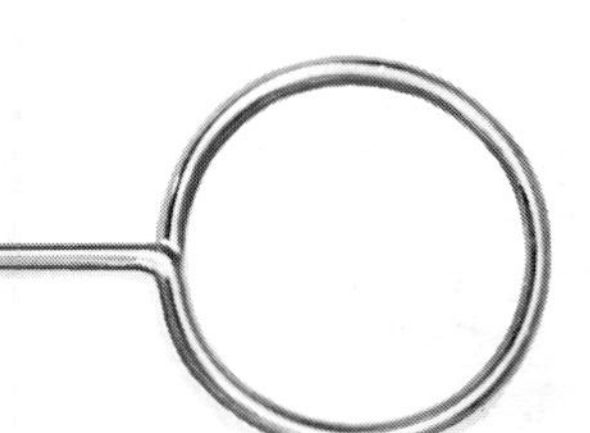

Loop turner is a long, wirelike tool with a hook at the end for grasping fabric when turning bias tubing to the right side.

Zippers and their application 316-329

Zippers

At first glance, zipper variety seems so great as to make selection difficult. Actually, it is narrowed down considerably by the very first step, the choice of *style*—the situation, location, type of opening, etc., for which the zipper is named. Another consideration is how conspicuous the zipper should be for the garment design. Zippers are made in three basic types, **conventional, invisible,** and **separating;** along with an illustration of each, the chart gives a description of styles within each group. Whatever zipper is selected, its weight should be compatible with that of the garment fabric. A zipper's weight is determined by its tape and structure (whether coil or chain). A *coil* is a continuous synthetic strand (nylon or polyester) twisted into a spiral and attached to a woven or knit synthetic tape. A *chain* consists of individual teeth, usually metal, attached to a cotton or cotton-blend tape. A coil, being lightweight and flexible, is ideal for light- to medium-weight fabrics. Although chains come in lightweight form too, they are slightly more rigid, which can cause buckling on a lightweight fabric, and thus are best used on medium to heavy fabrics. Zipper length is specified on the pattern envelope. Buy this length unless experience has shown the recommended lengths to be either too long or too short, in which case select the next appropriate length.

Chain construction

Synthetic coil construction

CONVENTIONAL ZIPPER	STYLE	WEIGHT	STRUCTURE	LENGTH
Conventional zippers, whether made with exposed teeth (chain) or coil, open at the top and are held together at the bottom. They come in more different styles than any other zipper type, each named for its most logical use. Some can be interchanged, however, if necessary. A neckline zipper, for example, can be shortened (see Zippers) and used as a skirt zipper. Size ranges given represent the overall output of all major manufacturers, and can vary within any single brand. Also, size increases do not necessarily come in 1″ increments; some styles increase in increments of 2″ or more. Depending on garment design, application may be by the centered, lapped, exposed, or fly method (see Zippers).	Neckline	Very light to medium	Coil or chain	4″–36″
	Skirt	Very light to medium	Coil or chain	6″–9″
	Dress	Very light to medium	Coil or chain	12″–14″
	Trouser	Medium to heavy	Chain	9″–11″
	Blue jean	Heavy	Chain	6″
	Decorative	Heavy	Chain	5″–22″
	Upholstery	Heavy	Chain	24″–36″

INVISIBLE ZIPPER	STYLE	WEIGHT	STRUCTURE	LENGTH
Invisible zippers are the newest type of zipper. As the name implies, they are structured differently from other zippers and are applied in a special way so that they disappear into a seam. When properly applied, neither the stitching nor the zipper teeth or coil is visible on the outside of the garment. Invisible zippers are used principally in skirts and dresses but they can go, in general, wherever a conventional zipper might be used, except in a trouser placket. Some manufacturers sell special zipper feet designed for application of their products. Some invisible zipper sizes are aggregates: e.g., 7″–9″ is one size.	No distinction of styles	Light to medium	Chain or coil	7″–22″

SEPARATING ZIPPER	STYLE	WEIGHT	STRUCTURE	LENGTH
Separating zippers are made to open at both top and bottom, permitting the zipper opening to separate completely. Although used mainly on jackets, they can really be applied to any garment with a completely opened front. It is possible also to get reversible separating zippers with pull tabs on both sides. Also, dual reversible and two-way zippers that zip from the top and from the bottom are available for jumpsuits and similar garments. A centered application is the method generally used.	Lightweight jacket	Medium	Chain	12″–24″
	Heavyweight jacket	Heavy	Chain	24″–26″
	Reversible	Medium to heavy	Chain	16″–22″
	Two-way	Medium to heavy	Coil or chain	20″–40″
	Dual-separating	Medium to heavy	Coil or chain	20″–60″

Sewing on buttons 351-352
Attaching fasteners 354-358

Buttons

Button buying involves both decorative and practical considerations. One overriding practical qualification: whether a button is washable or dry-cleanable. Buttons must be compatible with a

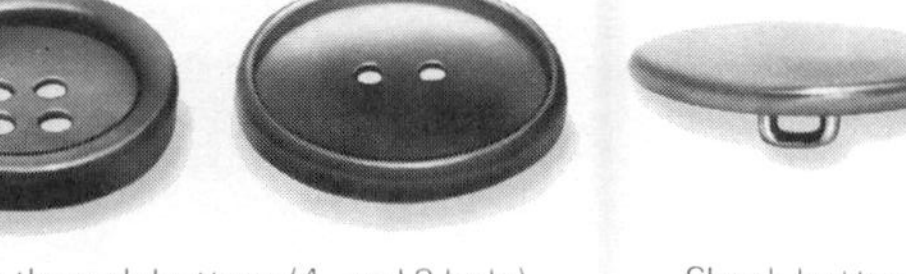

Sew-through buttons (4- and 2-hole) Shank button

garment's care requirements. Though made in many shapes and materials, buttons are basically of two types—**shank** and **sew-through.** The shank button has a solid top, with a shank beneath to ac-

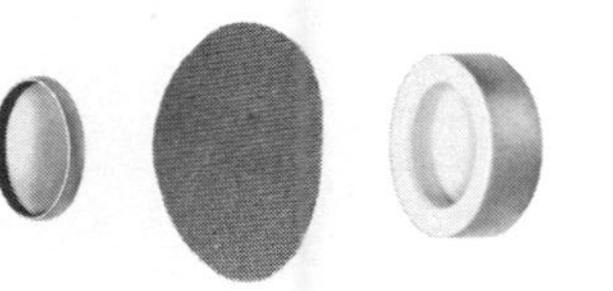

Metal pusher | Button back | Button shell | Cloth cutout | Holder

commodate thicker fabrics and keep the button from pressing too hard against the buttonhole. *Covered* shank buttons can be purchased within limits, but can be made to suit almost any need with do-it-yourself kits like the one shown here.

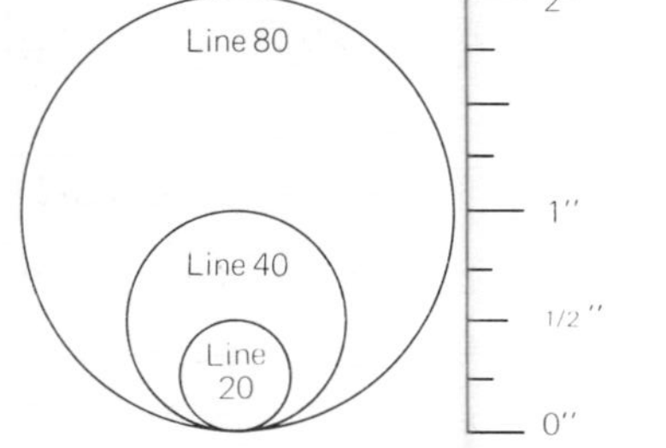

The sew-through button has holes, either two or four, through which the button is sewed. A thread shank can be added if necessary (see Fasteners). Buttons come from as small as ¼ inch to 2 inches or more in diameter, with most size increments in eighths of an inch. Size is based on a system of lines, equivalents for which are shown here.

Snaps

Ball Socket

Snaps are two-part (socket and ball) fasteners with limited holding power. Sizes range from fine (4/0) to heavy (4) in nickel or black-enamel finish and clear nylon.

Covered snaps are fabric-covered regular snaps, made for use on garment areas where they will be seen. Sizes are mostly heavy (2–4), the colors generally neutral.

Prongs

No-sew snaps are socket and ball fasteners that are not sewed to the garment but held in place by pronged rings. Holding power is good. Available in mostly heavy sizes.

Snap tape comes with regular or no-sew snaps attached to cotton or tricot tape. Permits multiple snap application at one time. Sold by the yard or in precut lengths.

Hooks and eyes

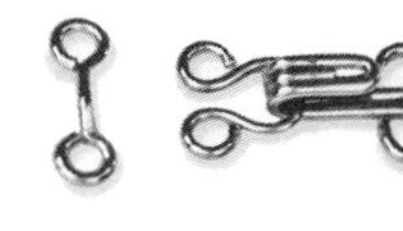

Hook and eye fasteners come with either straight eyes for lapped edges or loop eyes for meeting edges. Sizes from fine (0) to heavy (3) in nickel or black-enamel finish.

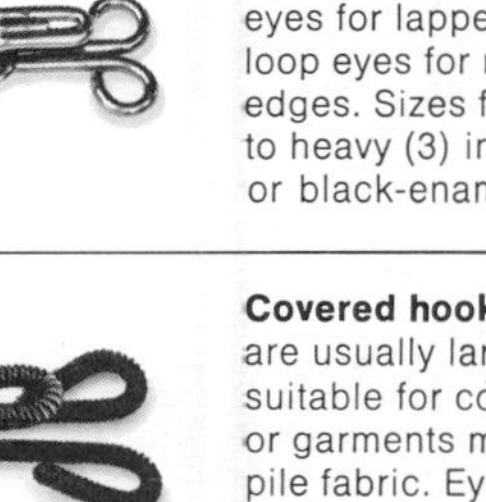

Covered hook and eye sets are usually large and suitable for coats, jackets, or garments made of deep pile fabric. Eyes are of the loop variety. Colors are mainly neutral.

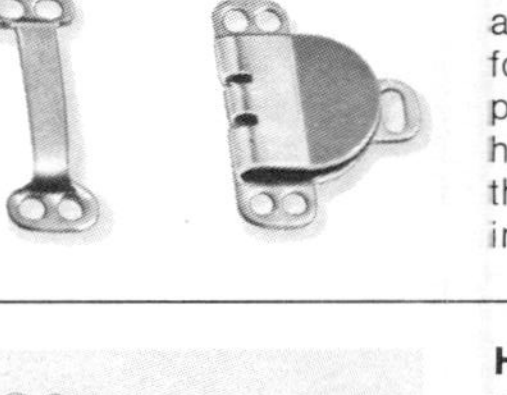

Waistband hook and eye sets are extra sturdy, ideal for waistbands on skirts or pants. Special design keeps hook from slipping off the straight eye. Available in nickel or black finish.

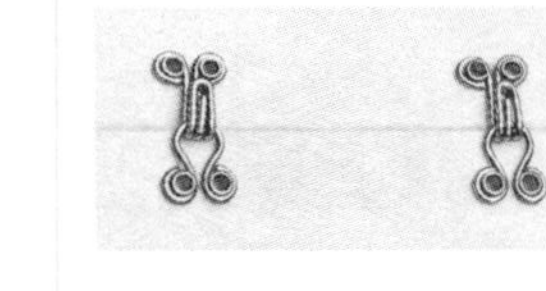

Hook and eye tape comes with medium hooks and loop eyes attached to cotton tape. Permits multiple hook and eye application at one time. Sold in neutral colors by the yard.

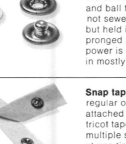

Eyelets

Eyelets are round metal reinforcements for holes that are made in belts and laced closures. They are easily applied with a special pliers, illustrated here (some pliers come with an interchangeable head that permits use also to attach no-sew snaps). Sold in packaged units; eyelets are available in nickel- and gilt-finish aluminum and enameled brass. Sometimes packaged with special pliers.

Nylon tape

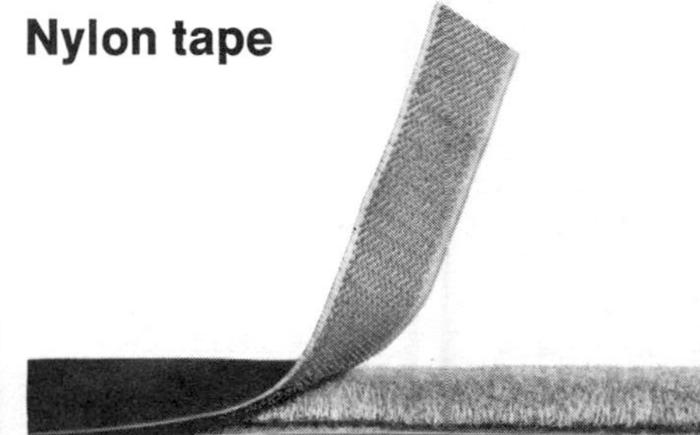

Nylon tape fastener is composed of two tape strips, one with a looped nap surface and the other with a hooked nap. When pressed together, surfaces grip and remain locked until pulled apart. Useful on garment details, such as cuffs and detachable trims; a good substitute for other closures in home decorating, as with upholstery. Tape comes in sew-on, iron-on, and stick-on forms.

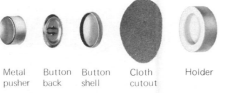

Sewing supplies

Tapes and trimmings used in construction

Bias tapes are fabric strips of varying widths, with prefolded edges. Suitable for curved hems, or as a casing. Double-fold type is folded in half (off center) for quick use as binding.

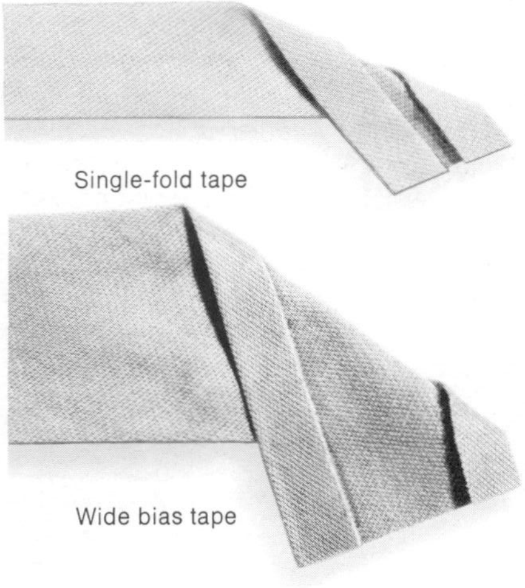

Single-fold tape

Wide bias tape

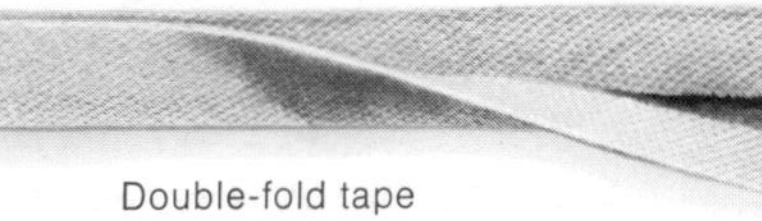

Double-fold tape

Seam binding, a straight tape used for finishing hem edges, comes in woven or lace form. Woven type is stable, and can also be used to stay seams. Lace has stretch, is ideal for knits.

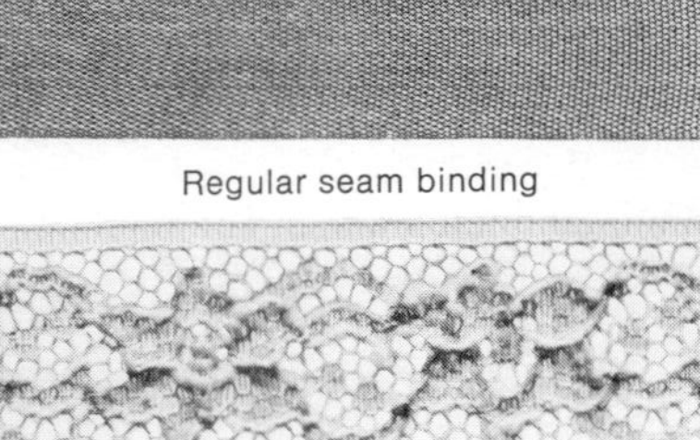

Regular seam binding

Lace seam binding

Hem facing is a wide, flexible tape cut to the width (approximately 2 inches) most often used for the job. Available in a bias strip with edges prefolded to the inside and in a more decorative lace construction. These prepackaged hem facings are useful when there is insufficient hem depth for a turned-up hem in a garment or a wish to eliminate bulk in a hem made from a heavy fabric. Bias hem facings can also be used as a wide casing or pressed in half for use as a binding. Both bias and lace types are available in an assortment of colors.

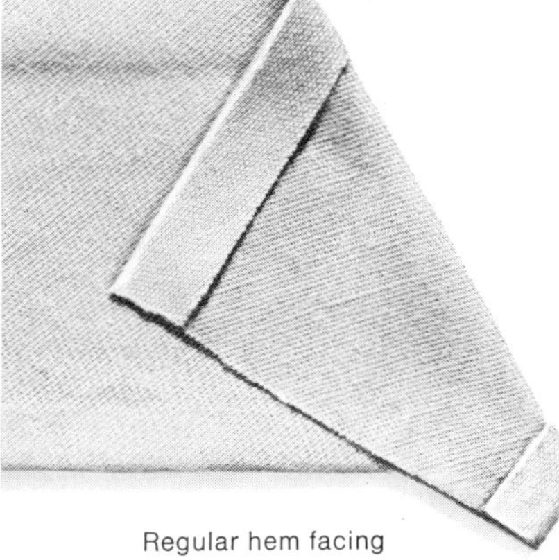

Regular hem facing

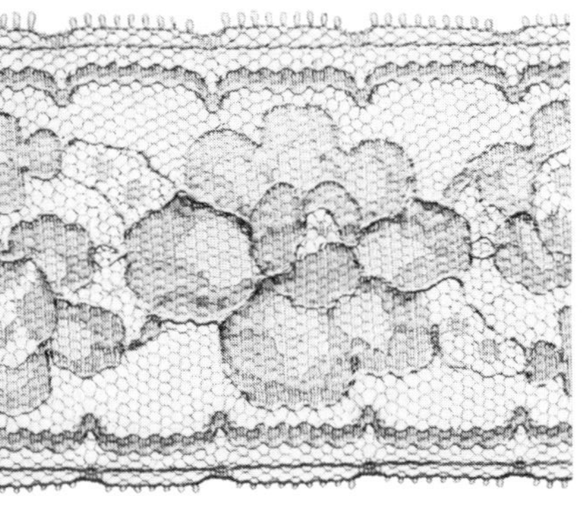

Lace hem facing

Twill tape is a woven stable tape used mainly for staying and strengthening seams, especially in tailoring. Usually made of cotton, twill tape comes in black and white, in widths of ¼, ½, ¾, and 1 inch.

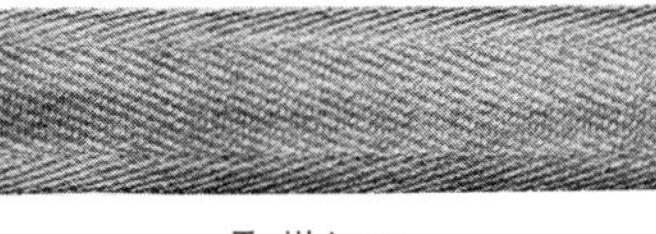

Twill tape

Grosgrain ribbon is both a practical and a decorative trim; its stability makes it ideal for finishing or staying a waistline. For firmer support, a slightly heavier, more rigid type is also available. Ribbons come in various colors and widths.

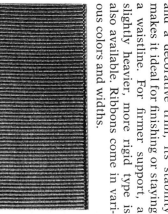

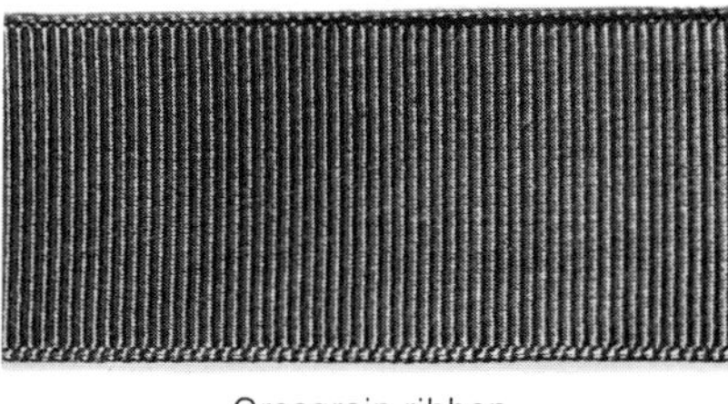

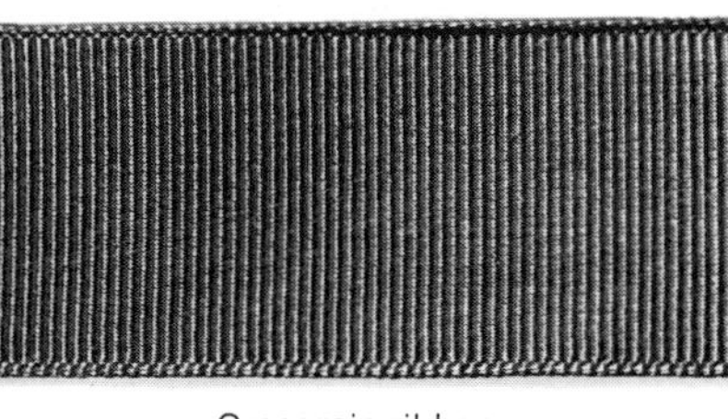

Grosgrain ribbon

Fold-over braid, too, is decorative as well as utilitarian. Both edges are finished; braid is folded in half, slightly off center, for easy application when binding or trimming an edge. Available in various colors and designs, usually by the yard.

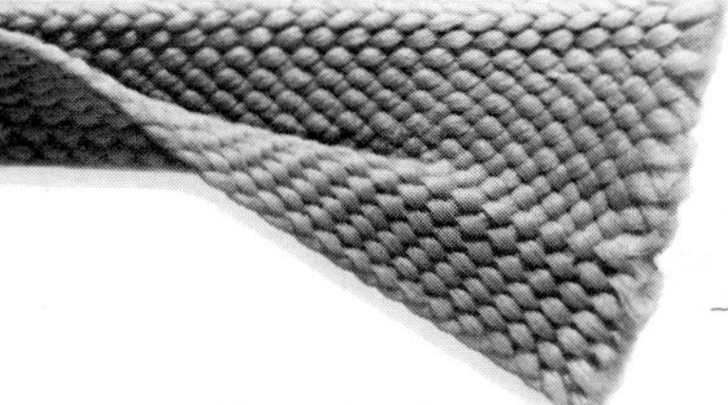

Fold-over braid

Horsehair braid, a stiffening made from transparent nylon strands, is used to finish the bottom of hems so as to emphasize the flare of the skirt; most often found on long evening wear. Available in ½ and 1 inch widths; wider braid may have a presewed ease thread along one edge.

Horsehair braid

Cable cord, which resembles string or twine, is usually made of cotton and can be used wherever a cordlike filler is needed, as in cording or corded buttonholes. Can also be inserted into bias tubing and used as a drawstring. It is usually sold by the yard in thicknesses ranging from approximately ¹⁄₁₆ to ½ inch.

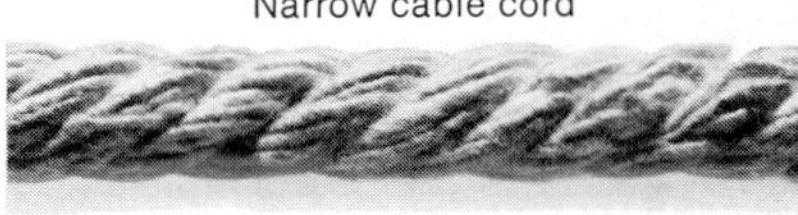

Narrow cable cord

Wide cable cord

Cording is a precorded decorative seam insertion used on garments or home decorating items, such as bedspreads. One edge is welted; the other acts as a small seam allowance. The most common type is made with a bias strip wrapped around cable cord. Welt sizes and colors are limited.

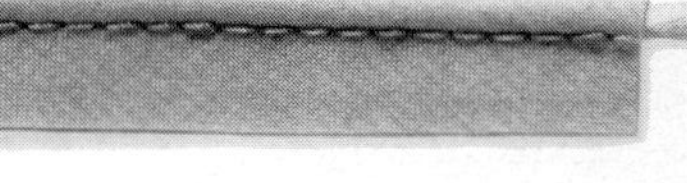

Cording

Ribbings are knitted, stretchy, decorative bands that are available in various widths and designs. The narrower ribbings are used as a quick finish and color accent for neck and wrist edges; the wider ones, as waistline insets or edgings. Some ribbings have small seam allowances constructed within the band to simplify application. Ribbings vary in amount of stretch; be sure that the stretch of the ribbing you wish to use is suitable to garment's need. Ribbings come in packaged quantities or by the yard.

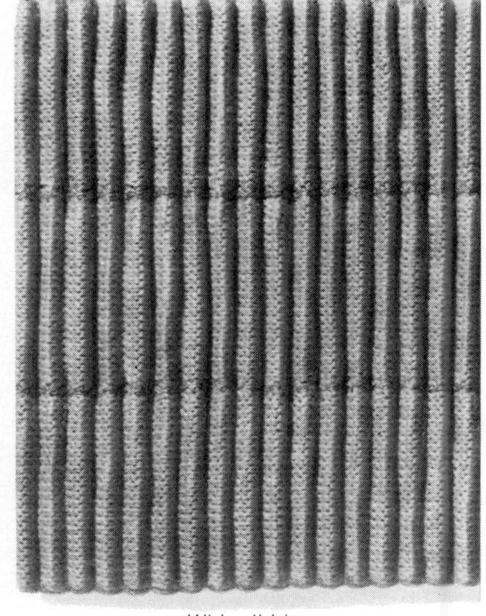

Wide ribbing

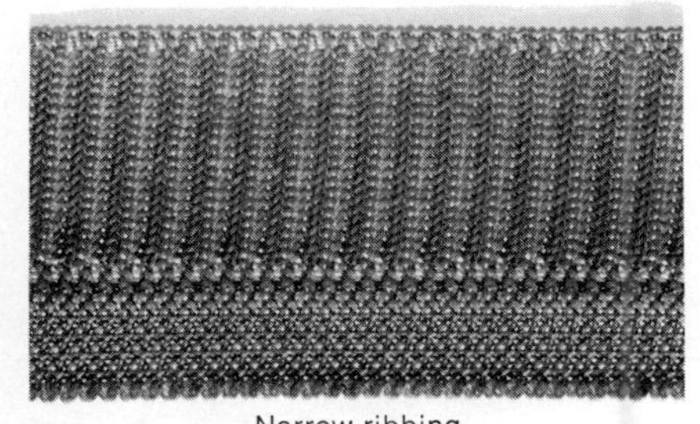

Narrow ribbing

Waistband stiffenings give rigid stability to waistlines; select one to suit need. *Belting,* a cardboardlike band, is the most frequently used insert for belts and waistbands; *professional waistbanding,* a non-roll, heat-set stiffener, can be used in place of interfacing; *men's waistbanding,* a preassembled waistband, finishes the inside of men's trousers.

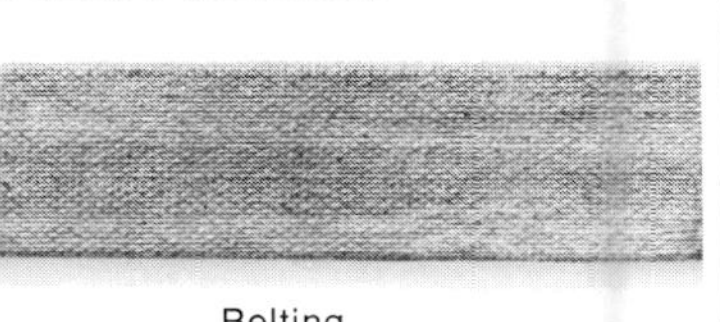

Belting

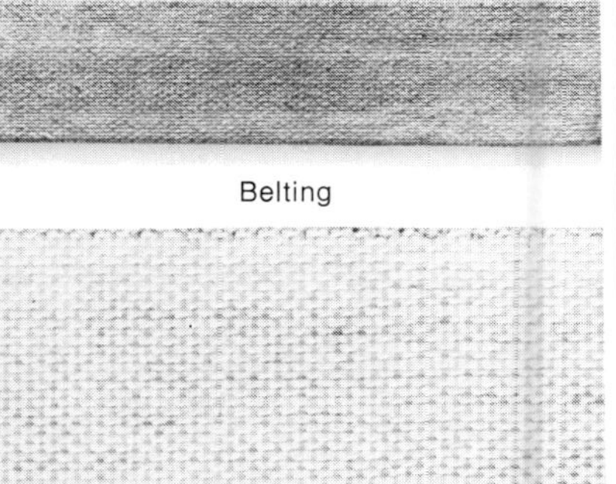

Professional waistbanding

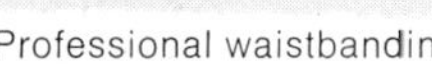

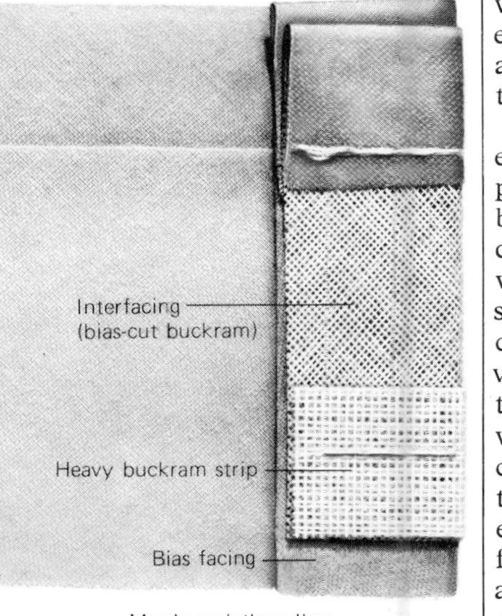

Men's waistbanding

Elastics

Most elastics are made from a rubber-core yarn covered with cotton, synthetic, or a blend of fibers. They may occur as a **single yarn** or as several yarns **braided, woven,** or **knitted** together. Single-yarn elastics can be used for hat bands, loop closings, or as elastic thread for shirring. Braided elastics can be identified by the lengthwise, parallel ridges that give these

Braided Woven Knitted

elastics a strong "grip." Because of its structure, braid narrows when stretched, and is recommended for casings rather than for stitching directly to a garment. Woven and knitted elastics are usually softer than braided elastics; their constructions enable them to maintain their original width when stretched. Woven and knitted elastics curl less than braided elastics and so can easily be stitched directly to a garment.

When selecting elastic, note that elastics are made and sold for special purposes, such as pajamas, lingerie, bra closures, etc. If a particular type cannot be found, look for an elastic with the features most suitable to the style and use of the garment. Consider construction (i.e., woven or braided), width, fiber content (especially important in swimwear—rayon stretches when wet), gripping power, weight compatibility. Look, too, for new elastic products, such as wide, colorful elastics that can serve as waistbands for skirts or pants. For best results, always use a ball-point sewing machine needle when sewing on the elastics.

Iron-ons and fusibles

Iron-ons are adhesive-backed fabrics that are pressed onto the garment fabric rather than stitched. They can be found in different forms and are used for different purposes. Some are available as interfacings (both non-woven and woven types); these are usually sold by the yard. Others come in the form of strips or patches for mending, repairing, or adding strength to such stress areas as knees or elbows. Some patch iron-ons are intended to be decorative; can serve as appliqués. Mending strips and patches are produced in precut lengths and/or shapes in a variety of fabrics, such as corduroy, twill, denim, knit, and muslin. Precut printed or embroidered designs are available for use as appliqués, or one can be cut from a plain strip or patch.

Iron-ons are recommended for use on fabrics that can withstand high iron temperatures (some require steam), but read package instructions and precautions. Pretest if possible.

There are also weblike bonding agents which, when melted between two layers of fabric, join them together. Used properly, they will hold a hem, facing, trim, or appliqué to a garment with no hand sewing. Fusing webs can also function as a lightweight interfacing between the garment and facing. These webs are not intended to form seams.

Fusing webs are sold by the yard, but they also come in packaged precut lengths and widths designed for specific areas, such as hems. They are recommended for all types of fabrics that can be *steam* pressed except sheers and a few synthetics. Check package instructions for recommendations, and be sure to pretest on a fabric scrap. Follow instructions carefully when applying web.

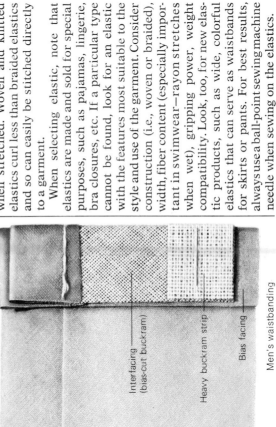

Sewing equipment

Pressing conveniences

Pressing is important at all stages of sewing to shape and set stitched lines. Steam iron and ironing board are essentials; the pieces of equipment shown here are useful additions. In any pressing procedure, follow these sound practices: (1) Press each stitched seam before crossing with another. First press over seamline (to embed stitches), then press open. (2) Use press cloth to prevent iron shine; dampen to produce more steam if needed. (3) Press with a gentle up-and-down motion. (4) Avoid pressing over pins and bastings. (5) To finger-press, run thumb along opened seamline.

A sleeve board provides two small, flat ironing surfaces on which seams and details of narrow garment sections (e.g., sleeves, pants legs) can be easily pressed. Also helpful when pressing hard-to-reach areas, such as necklines and sleeve caps. Below, sleeve is slipped over board, making its long seam easily accessible to the iron.

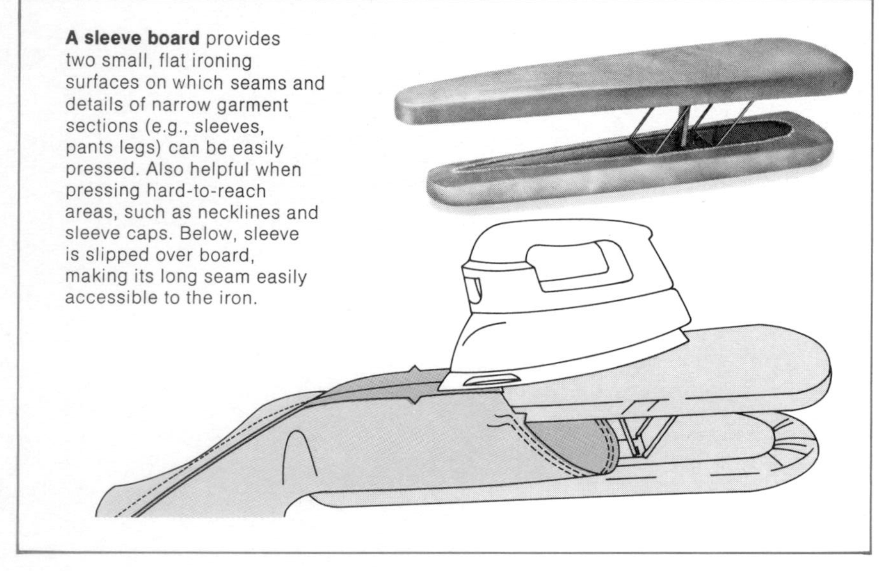

Tailor's ham, a firmly packed cushion, has rounded surfaces for pressing shaped areas, such as bust darts and curved seams. Below, princess line curve is molded as seam is pressed open. Covering is wool on one side, which holds steam as woolens are pressed; cotton on other for pressing all fabrics, especially at high temperatures.

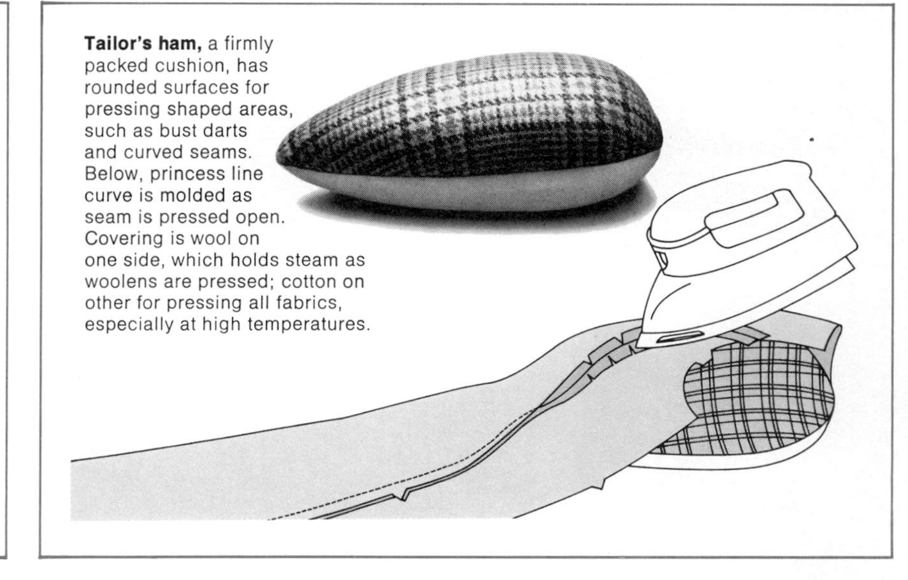

Press mitt, a padded glovelike cushion, is used as pressing surface for small garment areas; is especially handy where tailor's ham cannot reach. Comes with wool on one side, cotton on other, with pockets for slipping over hand. Mitt can also be used over sleeve board as shown below; provides rounded surface for molding sleeve cap.

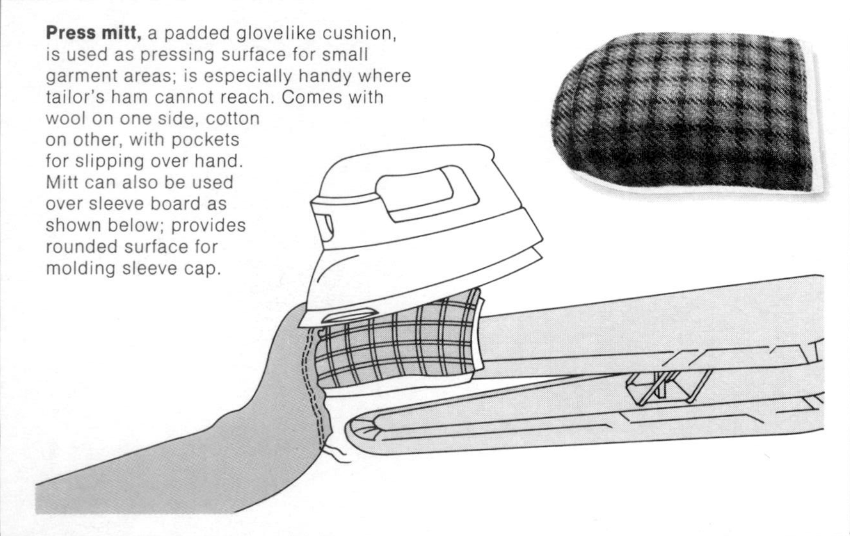

Seam roll, a firmly packed cylindrical cushion, is used primarily for pressing seams in very narrow areas, such as sleeves. As shown below, roll also allows seam to be pressed open with no marring of the surrounding fabric; bulk of garment falls away as seam of pants leg is pressed. Like the ham, roll is covered with wool on one side, cotton on the other.

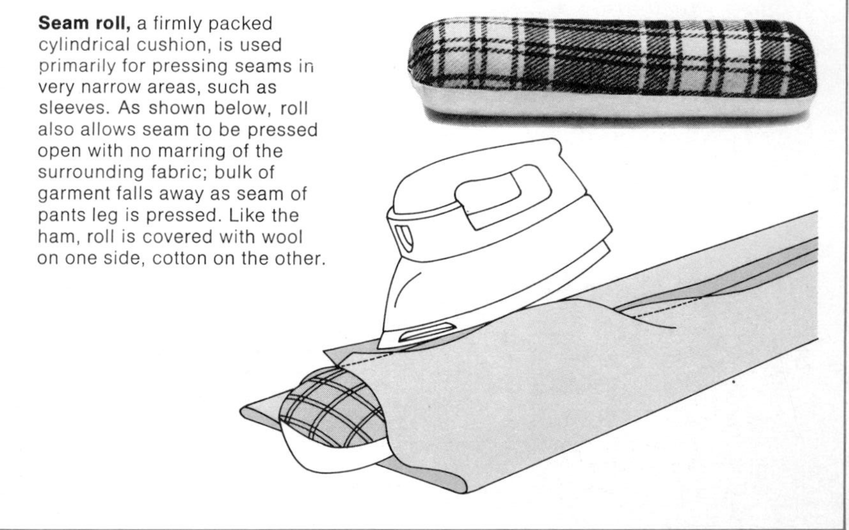

Tailor's board, a pressing tool made of hardwood, has a number of differently shaped edges and surfaces for pressing flat garment areas as well as points and straight and curved seams. Padded cover for board is available when soft edge in garment is desired.

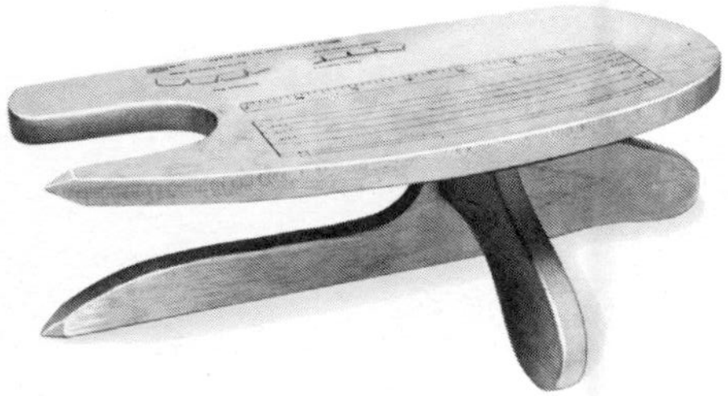

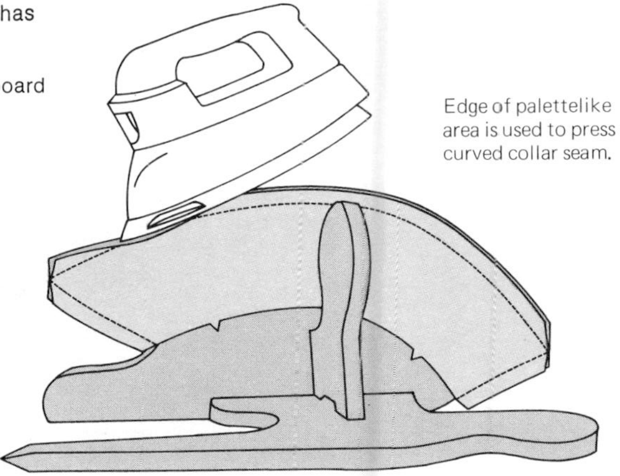

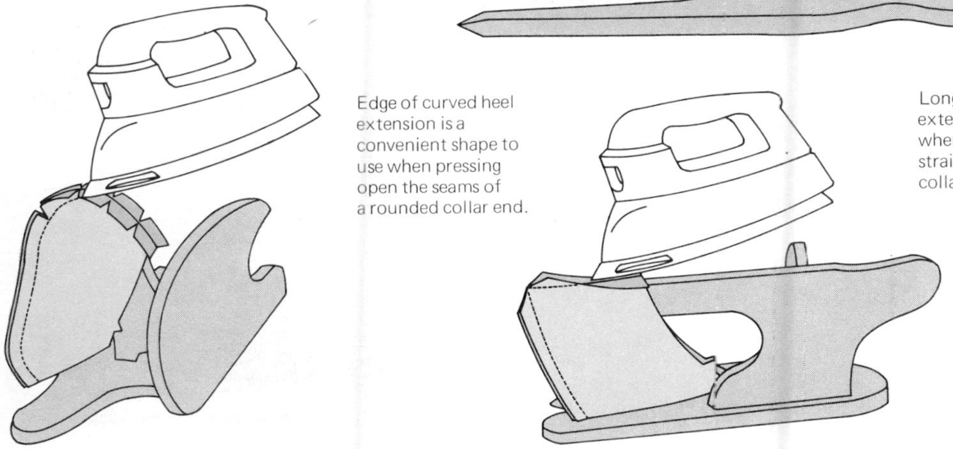

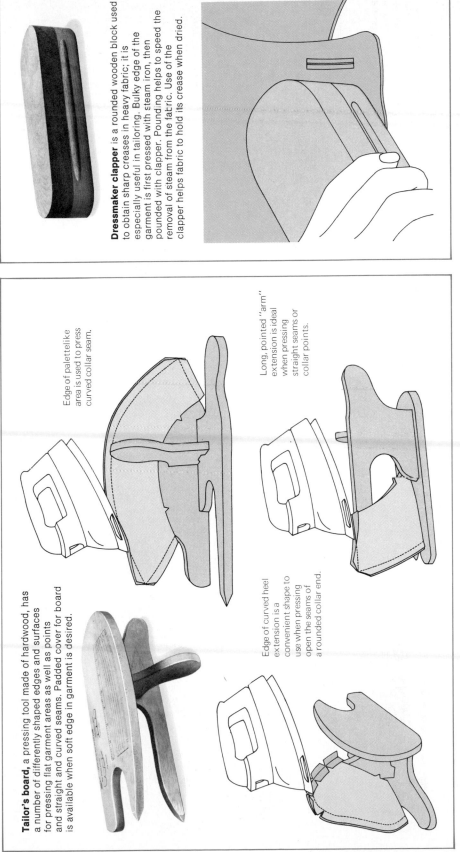

Edge of palettelike area is used to press curved collar seam.

Edge of curved heel extension is a convenient shape to use when pressing open the seams of a rounded collar end.

Long, pointed "arm" extension is ideal when pressing straight seams or collar points.

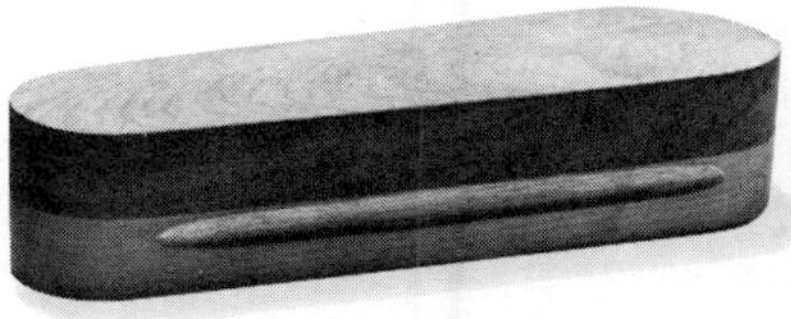

Dressmaker clapper is a rounded wooden block used to obtain sharp creases in heavy fabric; it is especially useful in tailoring. Bulky edge of the garment is first pressed with steam iron, then pounded with clapper. Pounding helps to speed the removal of steam from the fabric. Use of the clapper helps fabric to hold its crease when dried.

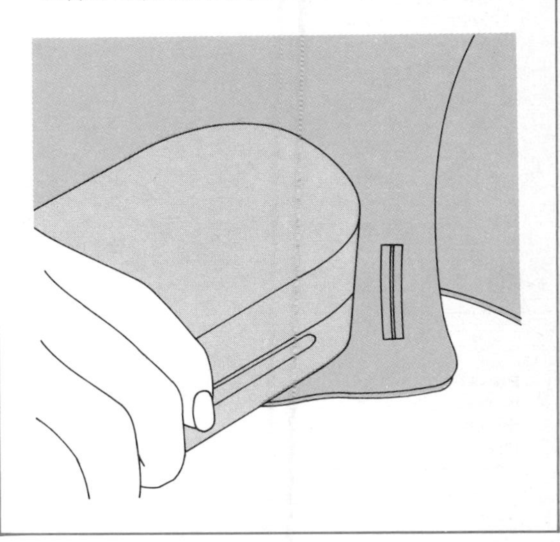

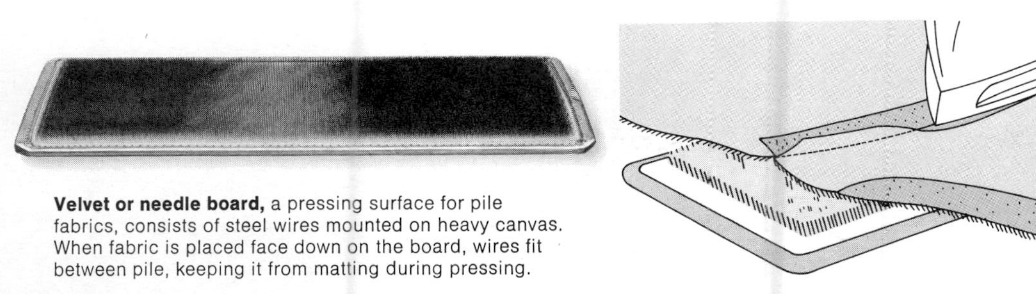

Velvet or needle board, a pressing surface for pile fabrics, consists of steel wires mounted on heavy canvas. When fabric is placed face down on the board, wires fit between pile, keeping it from matting during pressing.

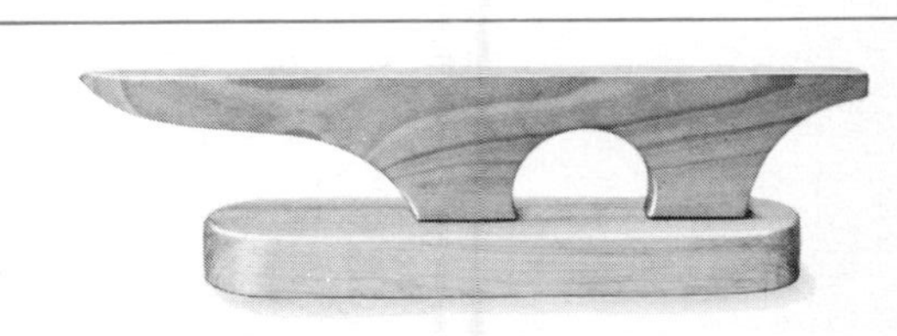

Point presser and pounding block is a wooden tool with a dual purpose: the straight point surface is used when pressing corners, points, and straight seams (see tailor's board); the block base works in the same way as the dressmaker clapper (above).

Sewing machine

General introduction

A basic requirement of all conventional sewing machines is a precisely timed movement of needle and shuttle hook to manipulate a top and bottom (bobbin) thread into a stitch (below, right). Tension discs and thread guides (see machine, right) help to control the flow of these threads.

Another important working relationship in stitch formation is the interaction between the needle, presser foot, and feed. While the presser foot holds the fabric, the needle passes through the fabric into the bobbin area to form stitches, and the feed moves the fabric for each stitch.

The functions described so far are necessary for straight stitches. They are also basic to zigzag and stretch stitches, but additional devices are needed for the formation of these. To create zigzag stitches, the needle must be able to move from side to side. For stretch stitches, the needle may also move from side to side, but it is the dual movement of the feed—forward and reverse—that makes stretch stitches unique. Capabilities such as these are built into the machine, with provision made for the user to activate them. On most models this is done by the manipulation of stitch length, width, and pattern selectors, and/or the insertion of special cams. With today's computerized sewing machines (not shown), stitch selection is achieved more simply by pressing a single button or a spot on a touch-sensitive panel.

A totally different sewing machine, the overlock (overedge, overcast, serger, or merrow) machine, forms overedge seams like those in ready-to-wear garments. It cannot perform all the functions of a conventional sewing machine, but its speed and professional results make it a useful sewing tool.

Basic parts and controls

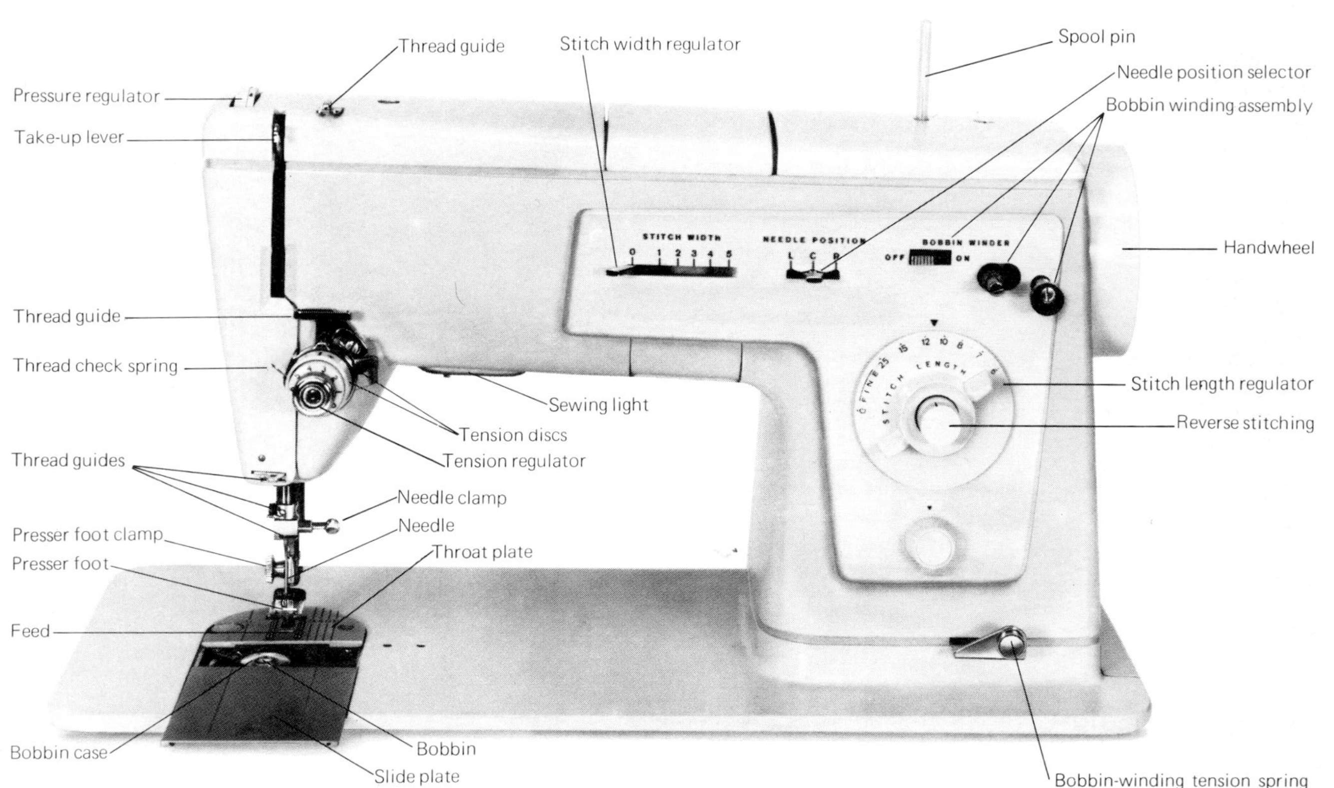

Timed sequence in stitch formation

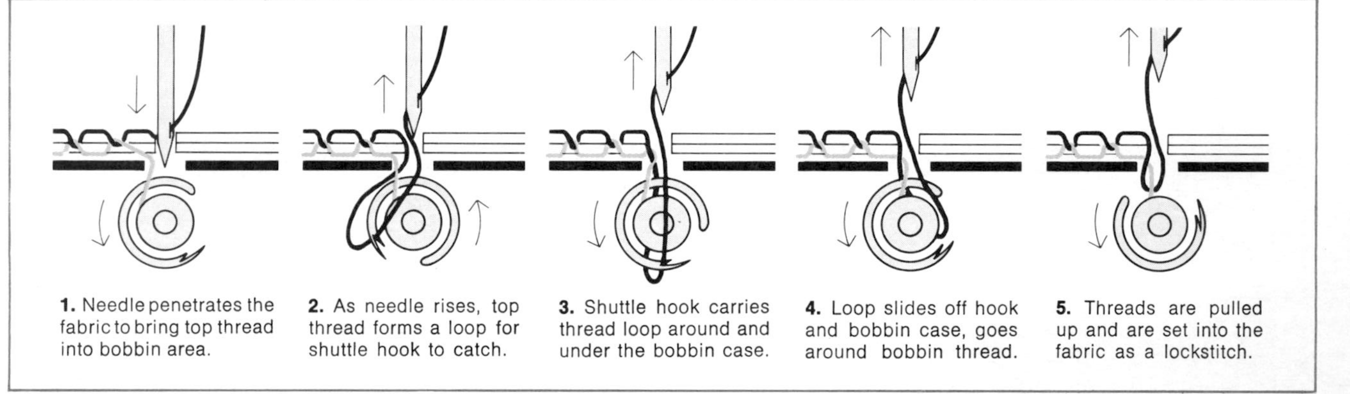

1. Needle penetrates the fabric to bring top thread into bobbin area.

2. As needle rises, top thread forms a loop for shuttle hook to catch.

3. Shuttle hook carries thread loop around and under the bobbin case.

4. Loop slides off hook and bobbin case, goes around bobbin thread.

5. Threads are pulled up and are set into the fabric as a lockstitch.

Upper threading

Though the parts involved differ in location and appearance, the upper threading progression for any machine is basically the same. As illustrated at the right, thread is fed from the **spool** through the **tension discs,** then to the **take-up lever,** and finally down to the **needle.** The number of thread guides between these points will vary with the machine. The part that differs the most from one machine to another is the **tension assembly** (three types are shown below).

Before threading any machine, remember to do two things: (1) raise the presser foot—this will allow the thread to pass between the tension discs; (2) bring the take-up lever to its highest point so needle will not come unthreaded when first stitch is started. The illustrations on this page will be useful as a general guide to upper threading; for specific instructions regarding your machine, refer to its instruction book.

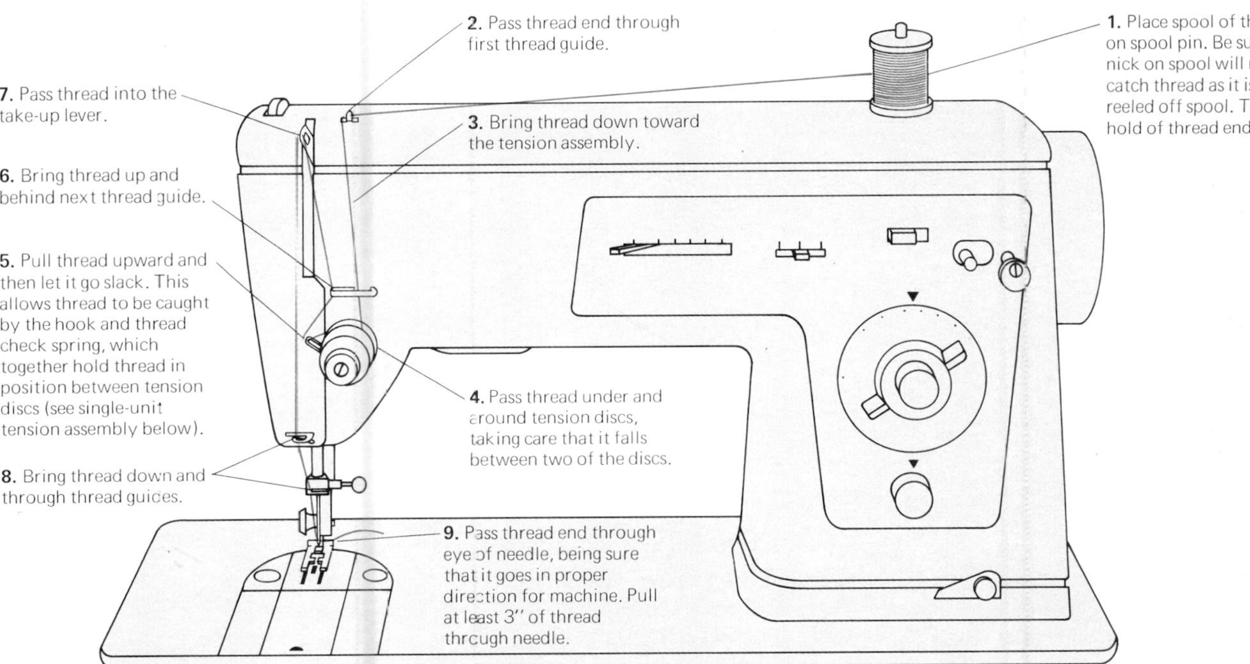
1. Place spool of thread on spool pin. Be sure nick on spool will not catch thread as it is reeled off spool. Take hold of thread end.
2. Pass thread end through first thread guide.
3. Bring thread down toward the tension assembly.
4. Pass thread under and around tension discs, taking care that it falls between two of the discs.
5. Pull thread upward and then let it go slack. This allows thread to be caught by the hook and thread check spring, which together hold thread in position between tension discs (see single-unit tension assembly below).
6. Bring thread up and behind next thread guide.
7. Pass thread into the take-up lever.
8. Bring thread down and through thread guides.
9. Pass thread end through eye of needle, being sure that it goes in proper direction for machine. Pull at least 3" of thread through needle.

Types of tension assemblies

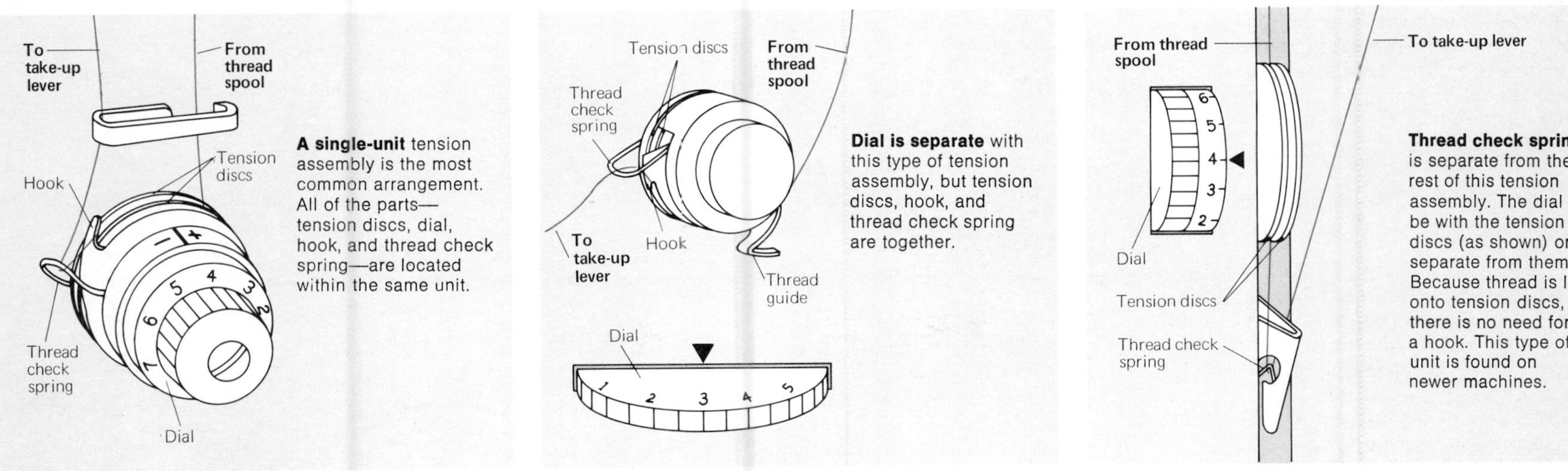
To take-up lever
From thread spool
Hook
Tension discs
Thread check spring
Dial
Tension discs
Thread check spring
From thread spool
To take-up lever
Hook
Thread guide
Dial

A single-unit tension assembly is the most common arrangement. All of the parts—tension discs, dial, hook, and thread check spring—are located within the same unit.

Dial is separate with this type of tension assembly, but tension discs, hook, and thread check spring are together.

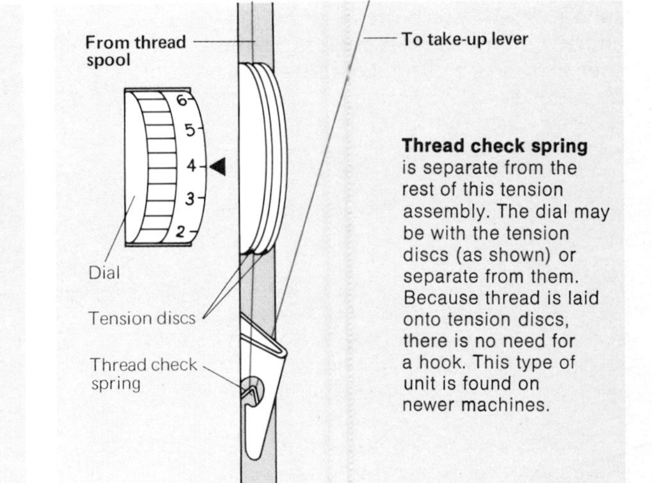
From thread spool
To take-up lever
Dial
Tension discs
Thread check spring

Thread check spring is separate from the rest of this tension assembly. The dial may be with the tension discs (as shown) or separate from them. Because thread is laid onto tension discs, there is no need for a hook. This type of unit is found on newer machines.

Sewing machine

Bobbin winding

The lower thread supply for any sewing machine is stored in the bobbin area, situated under the needle and throat plate and consisting of a small spool (the bobbin) and a case into which it fits. Both are precisely sized to fit each other and the machine. To play its part in stitch formation, the bobbin must be filled with thread, a procedure that differs with the type of sewing machine (see right). On some, the up and down action of the needle must be deactivated before the bobbin can be wound. This usually means loosening the flywheel. **To disengage needle,** hold the handwheel still and turn the flywheel toward you.

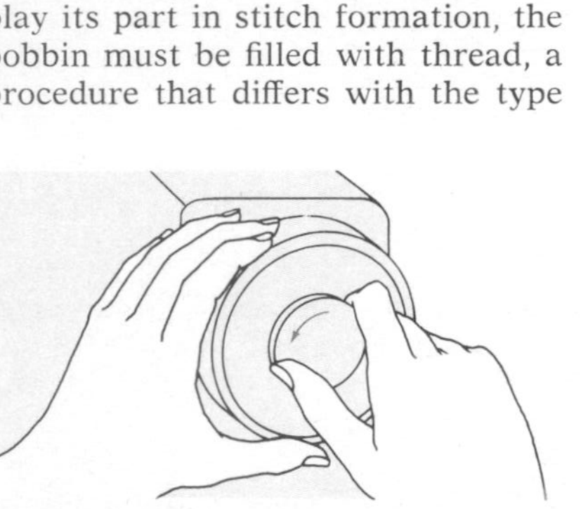

Disengaging needle

The thread should be wound evenly onto the bobbin. If it is not, there may be trouble in stitching, or unevenness in stitch tension. An uneven wind can sometimes be corrected by simply loosening or tightening the bobbin-winding tension spring. If this doesn't work, professional service may be needed.

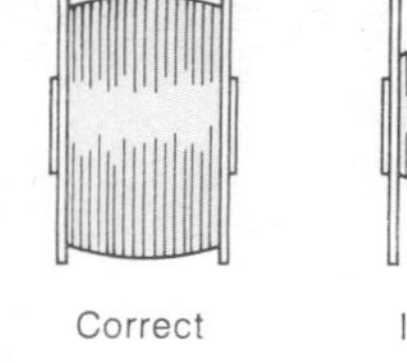

Correct

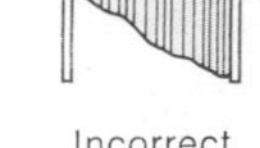

Incorrect

Methods of winding bobbins

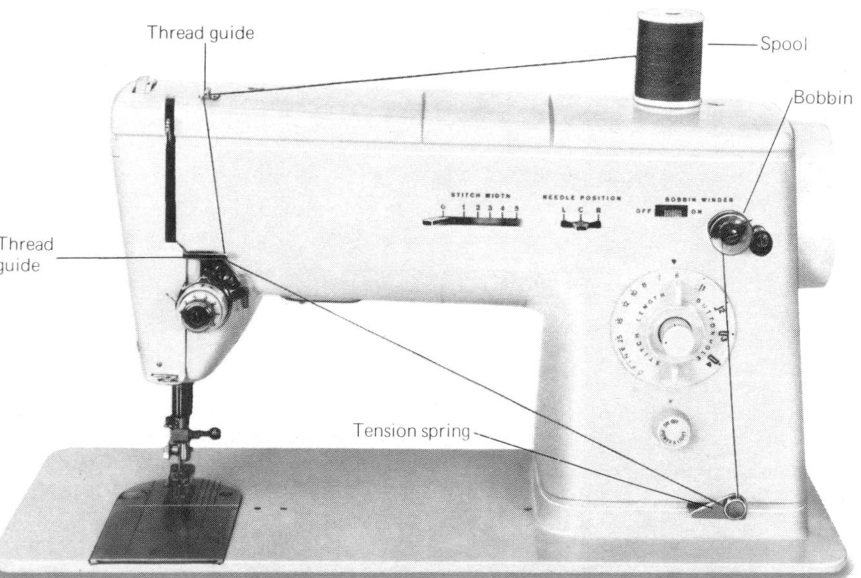

With bobbin-winding mechanisms outside the machine (this row and below left), the needle is first disengaged. On machine above, the thread feeds off the thread spool over through two thread guides, down through bobbin-winding tension spring, then up to bobbin.

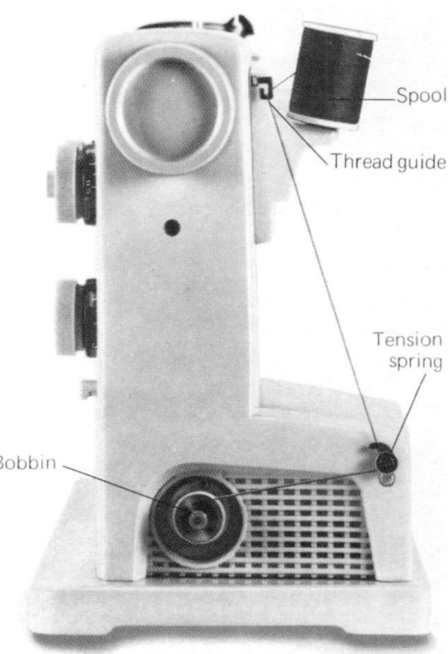

This bobbin is wound on side of machine. Thread goes from spool through thread guide and tension spring, then to bobbin.

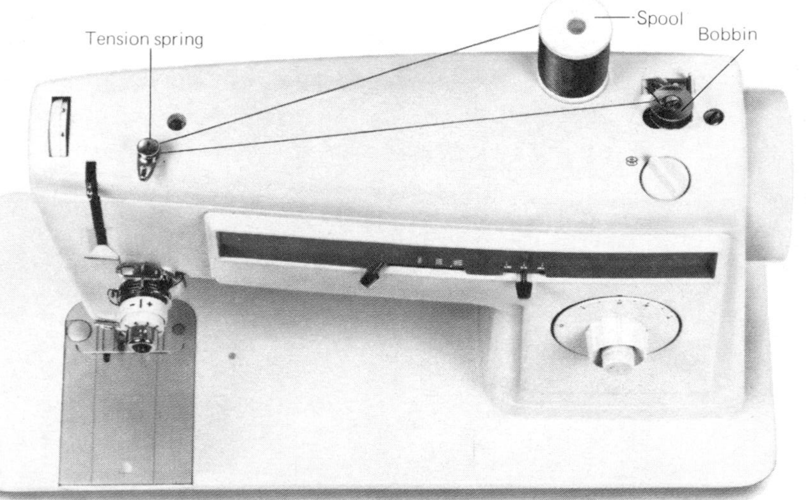

On the machine above, the bobbin is being wound on the top of the machine arm. The thread feeds from the spool over through the bobbin-winding tension spring, then onto the bobbin, which is in position on its spindle.

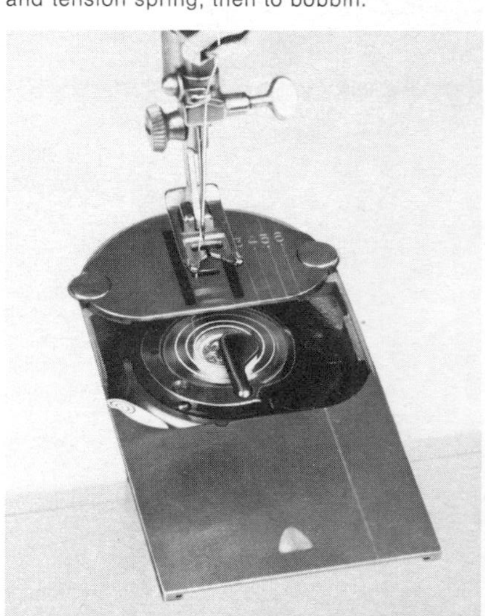

Bobbin winding inside the machine. With upper portion of machine threaded, bobbin rotates and fills as needle goes up and down.

Types of bobbins

Bobbins are made to exact size and other specifications to conform to the requirements of particular sewing machines. Use only the type recommended by the manufacturer of your machine (non-sewing machine companies also make bobbins). Replace any bobbin that is worn, cracked, or nicked; a damaged bobbin can cause sewing problems. A few extras are good to have on hand in any case.

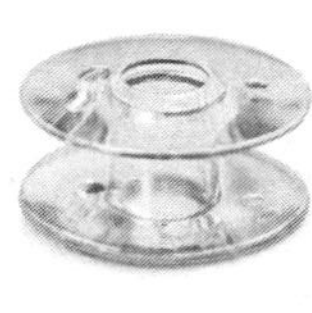

Most drop-in bobbins are made of clear plastic, but they can be of metal also. They are smooth-surfaced and their sides are usually rounder than those of other bobbin types.

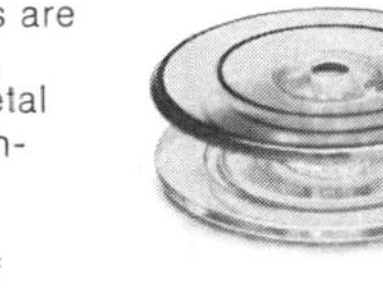

Special drop-in bobbins, made for machines that employ an inside-machine bobbin-winding mechanism, look like this. They are made of clear plastic; the top half is sometimes larger than the bottom half.

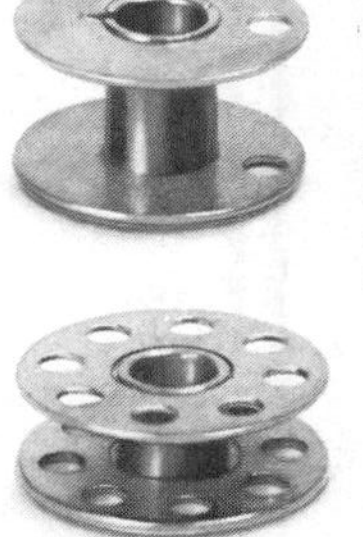

Removable-case bobbins may be made of plastic or metal. Their sides may be smooth-surfaced but some of the metal ones have several holes in each of the sides.

Bobbin removal

It is often necessary to remove a bobbin to either refill or replace it. Before removing a bobbin, bring needle and take-up lever to their highest positions, lift the presser foot, and, if necessary, remove the fabric beneath it. Then open the slide plate to gain access to the bobbin area. The photos below show the procedure for removing different bobbin types from their cases. Before removing any bobbin, it is best that the thread extending from the bobbin be cut short. This assures that a minimum of thread will be pulled out from under the bobbin case tension spring.

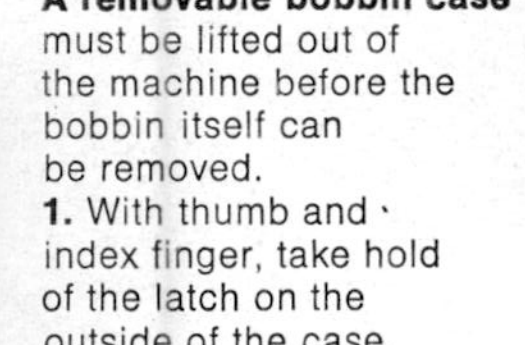

The most standard type of drop-in bobbin, as shown here, is merely lifted out of its built-in case.

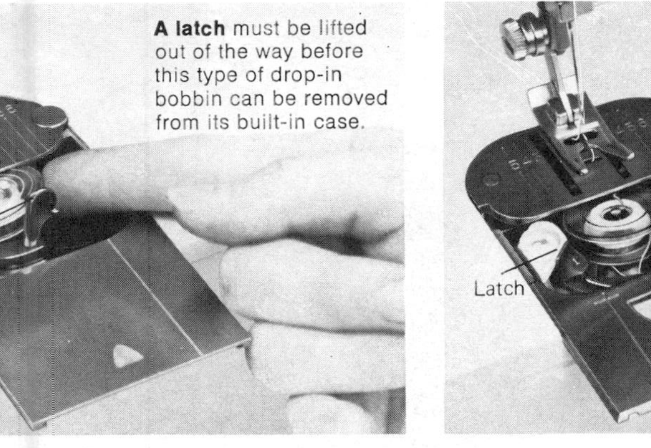

A latch must be lifted out of the way before this type of drop-in bobbin can be removed from its built-in case.

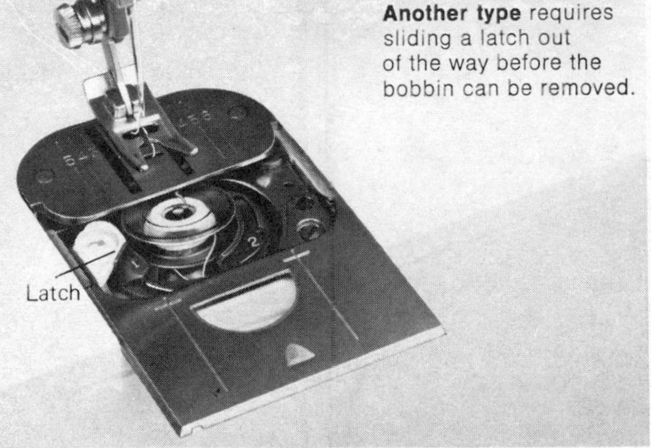

Another type requires sliding a latch out of the way before the bobbin can be removed.

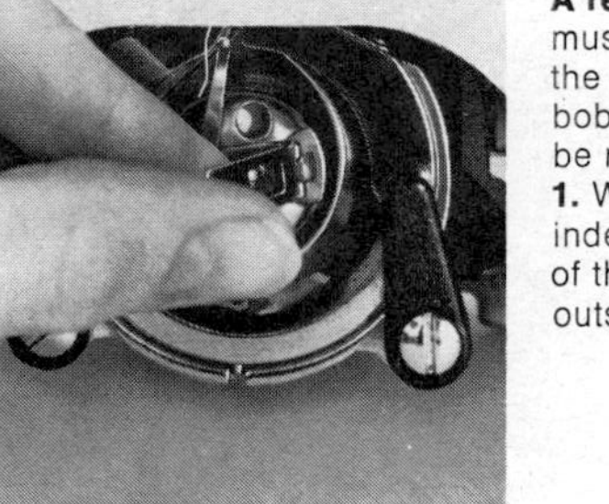

A removable bobbin case must be lifted out of the machine before the bobbin itself can be removed.
1. With thumb and index finger, take hold of the latch on the outside of the case.

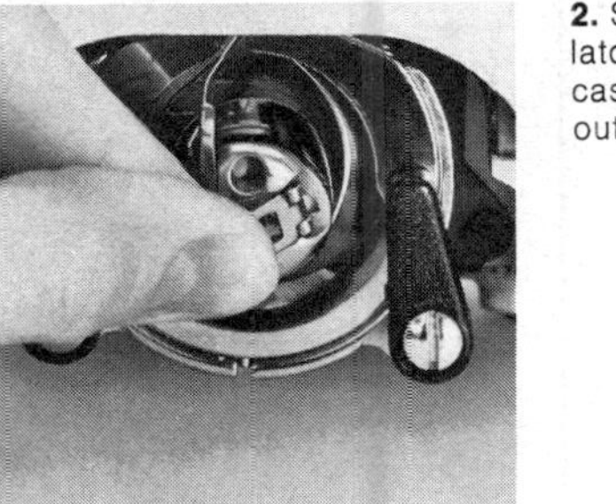

2. Still holding latch, pull the bobbin case and bobbin out of the machine.

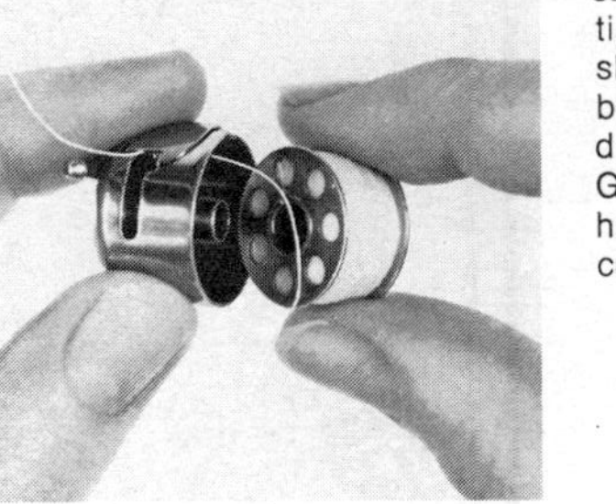

3. Release latch and tip the case over slightly, letting the bobbin slip some distance out of case. Grasp bobbin with other hand and pull it completely out of case.

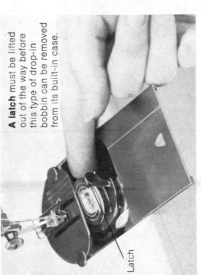

Sewing machine

Lower threading

Threading the lower portion of the machine involves threading the bobbin into its case. The way this is done depends upon the bobbin case itself. There are basically only two types of bobbin cases, built-in and removable, but within these types there are variations. Illustrated on these pages are examples of how various bobbin cases are threaded. Notice that built-in cases (this page) remain in the machine during threading and removable cases (opposite page) are taken out of the machine for threading.

For proper stitch formation, the flow of thread from the bobbin must be controlled. One way to control the flow is to force the thread to feed off the bobbin and through the slot opening of the bobbin case in a "V" direction. Another device, present on most bobbin cases, is the bobbin tension spring. Positioned over the slot opening of the bobbin case, this spring exerts pressure (tension) on the thread. The illustration below shows the direction the bobbin thread should take through the slot opening, under the tension spring. Some bobbin cases,

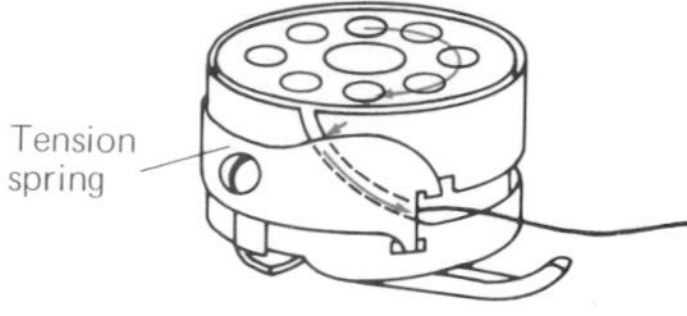

however, have neither a slot opening nor a tension spring; these employ other devices, such as a latch, to control the flow of bobbin thread. The illustrations on these pages are meant to serve as a general guide for threading the lower portion of the machine. For more precise instructions for your machine, consult the manufacturer's instruction book.

Threading built-in bobbin cases

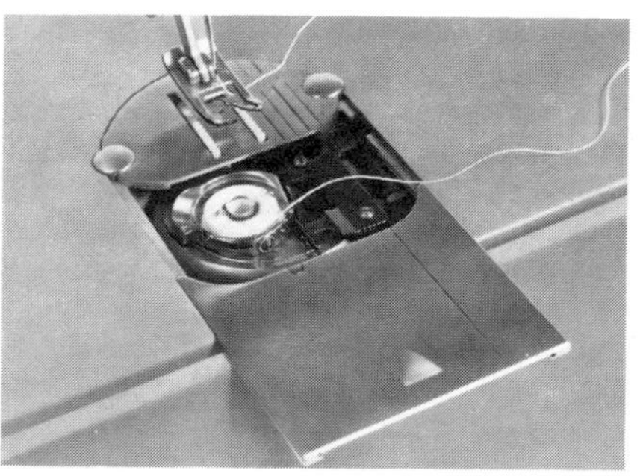

Standard built-in bobbin case. First, drop bobbin into case so that the thread feeds in the same direction as the slot.

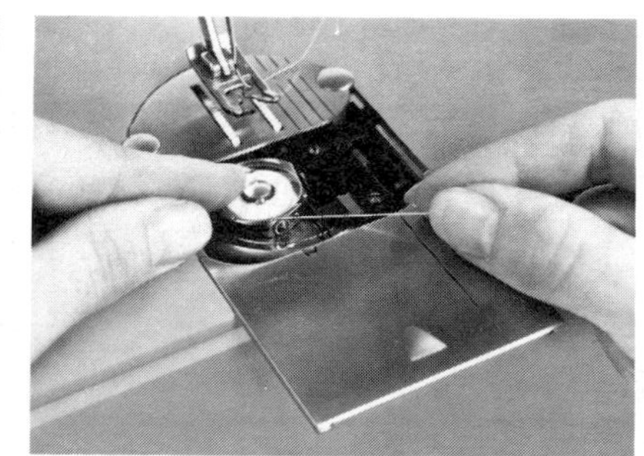

Exerting pressure on bobbin with one hand, grasp thread with the other hand and bring it to the opening of the slot.

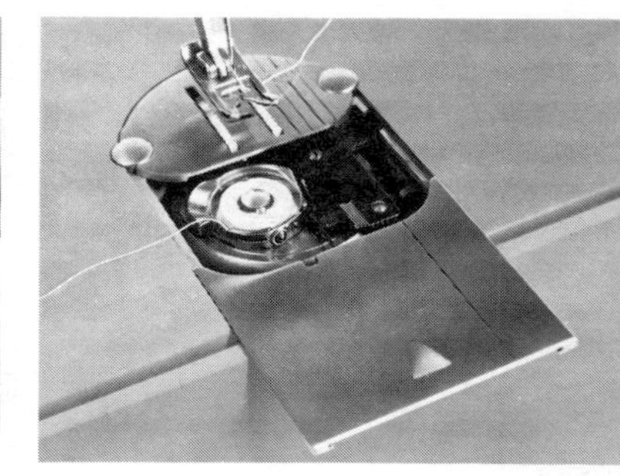

Still exerting pressure on bobbin, pull the thread back and under bobbin tension spring. Release thread and let go of bobbin.

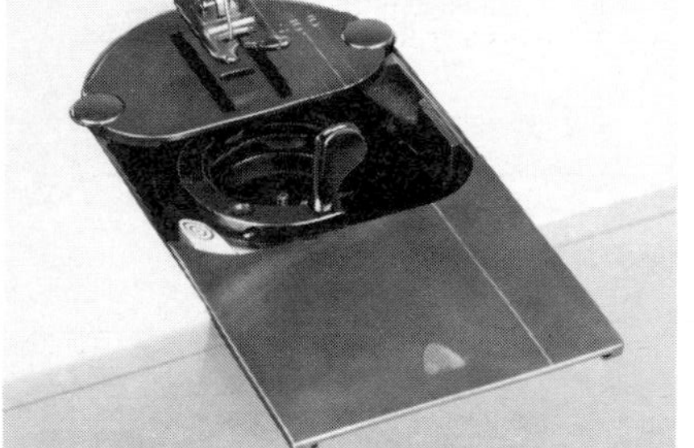

Case with latch but no threading points. With this type of bobbin case, you must first lift the latch up out of the way.

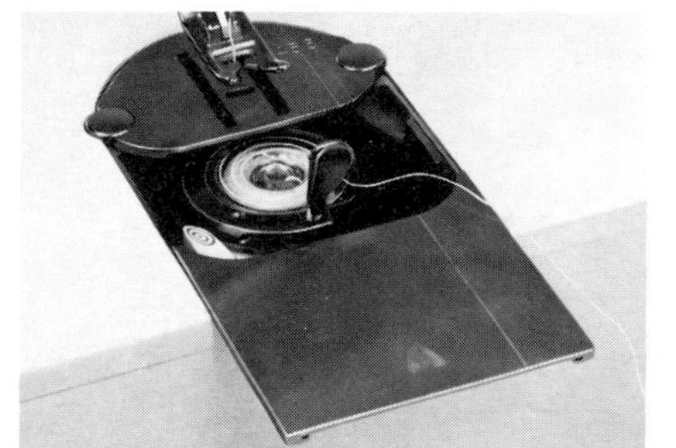

Then drop the bobbin into the case so that the thread is feeding off the bobbin toward the right-hand side of the latch.

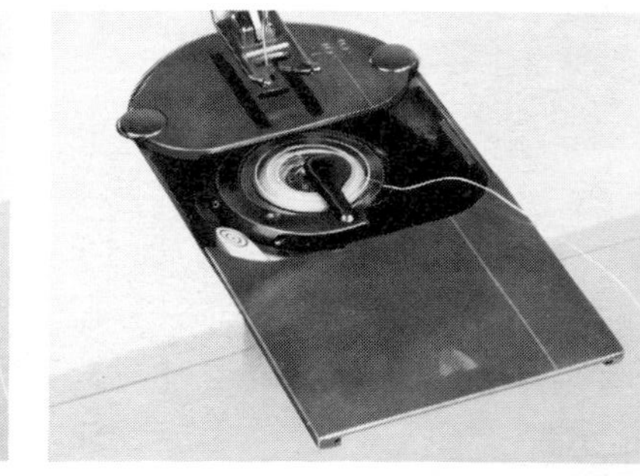

Then push the latch down. The pressure that the latch exerts on the bobbin acts as a "tension" for the bobbin thread.

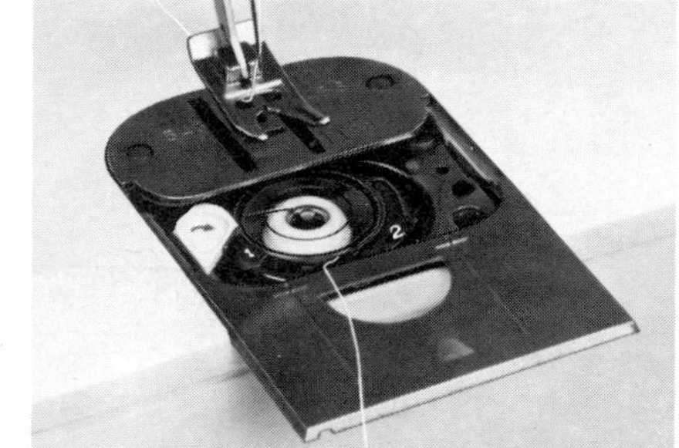

Case with latch and threading points. Push latch over out of the way and drop in bobbin (thread feeds in same direction as "finger").

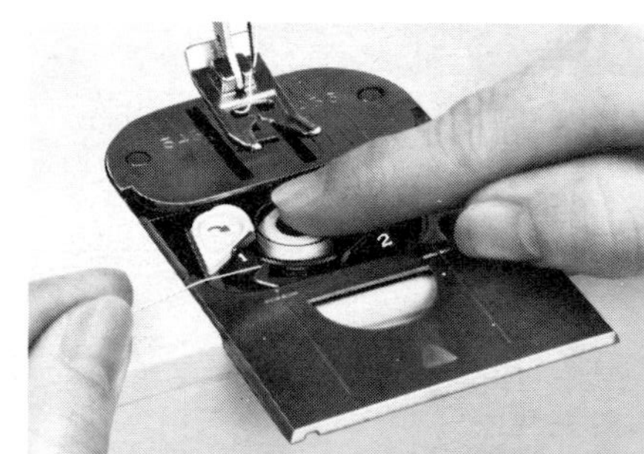

Slide latch back over bobbin. Hold bobbin; grasp thread with other hand and bring it to the "finger" opening, threading point 1.

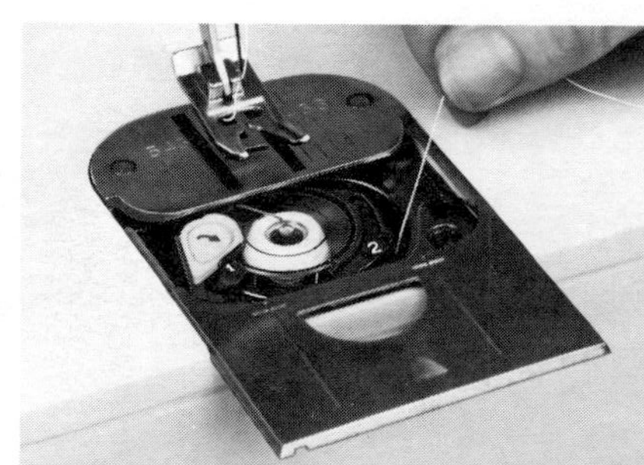

Pass the thread back and completely under the "finger" to threading point 2. Then release your hold on the thread.

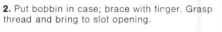

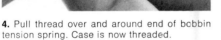

Threading a removable bobbin case

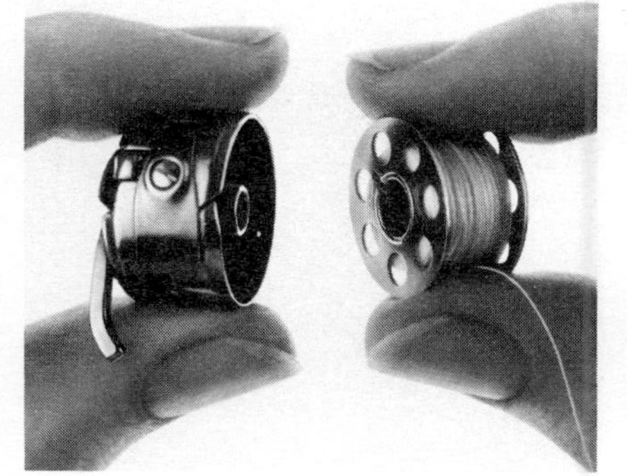
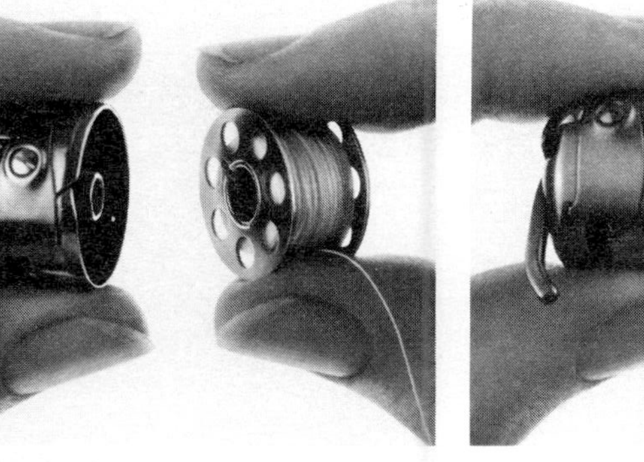

1. Hold case and bobbin as shown. Thread feeds off bobbin in same direction as slot.

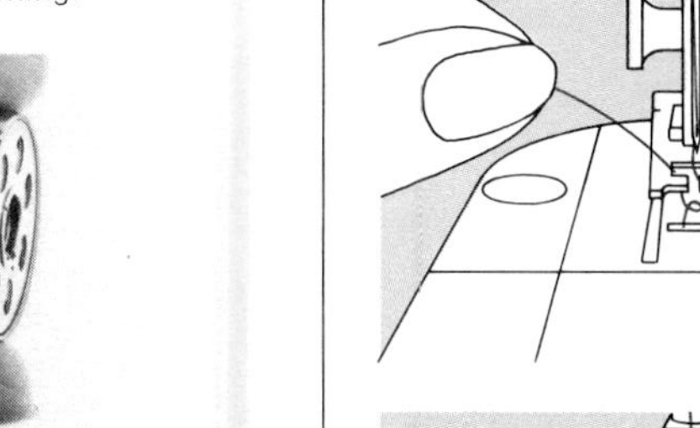

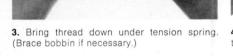

2. Put bobbin in case; brace with finger. Grasp thread and bring to slot opening.

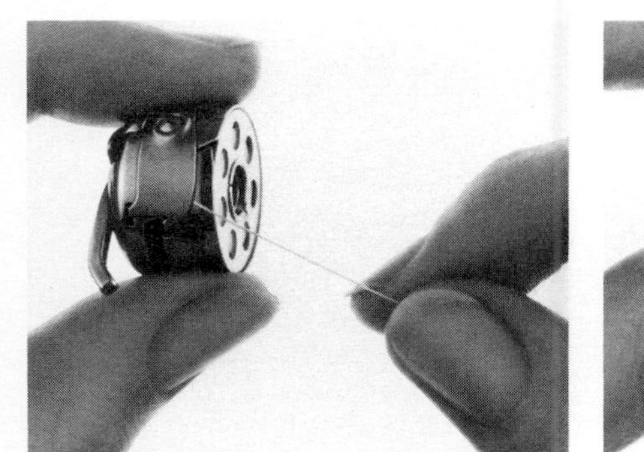

3. Bring thread down under tension spring. (Brace bobbin if necessary.)

4. Pull thread over and around end of bobbin tension spring. Case is now threaded.

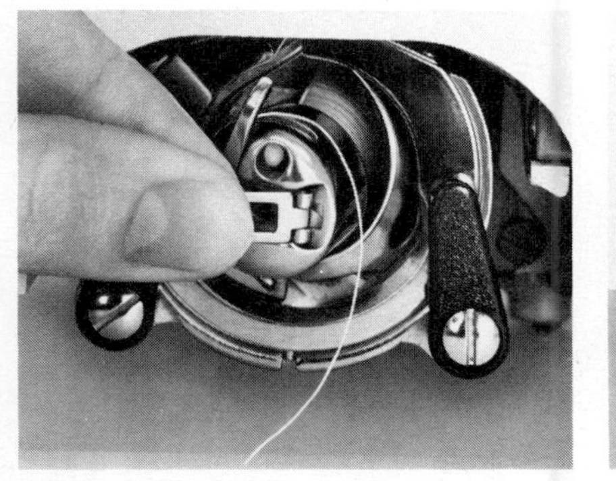

5. Grasp and pull out on the latch at the back of the bobbin case; bring case to machine.

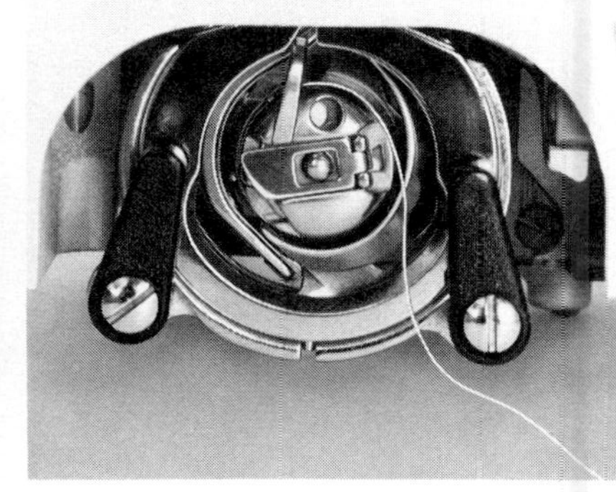

6. Insert the case into the machine, then release the bobbin case latch.

Raising the bobbin thread

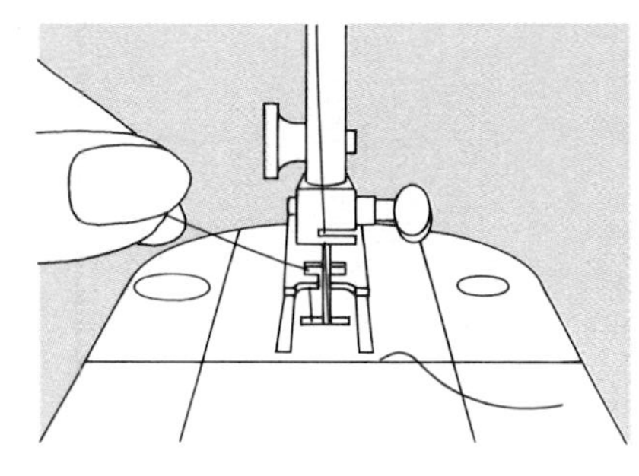

After the bobbin case has been threaded and, if necessary, inserted into the machine, close the slide plate and raise the bobbin thread as follows:

1. Holding the top thread with the left hand, turn the handwheel with the right hand until the needle is all the way down in the bobbin area.

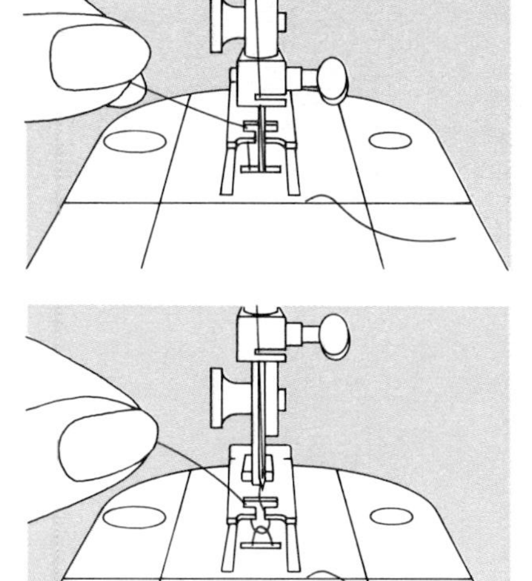
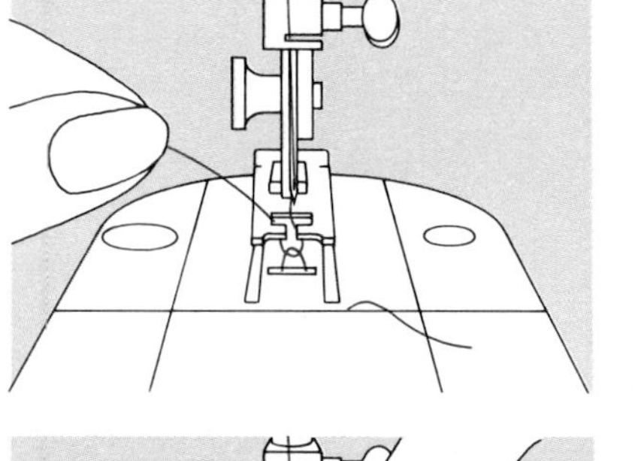

2. Still holding thread and rotating the handwheel, bring the needle up to its highest point. As the needle rises, a loop of bobbin thread will come up with it. Pull on the top thread to draw up more bobbin thread.

3. Release top thread, then pull on loop of bobbin thread to bring up free end of bobbin thread.

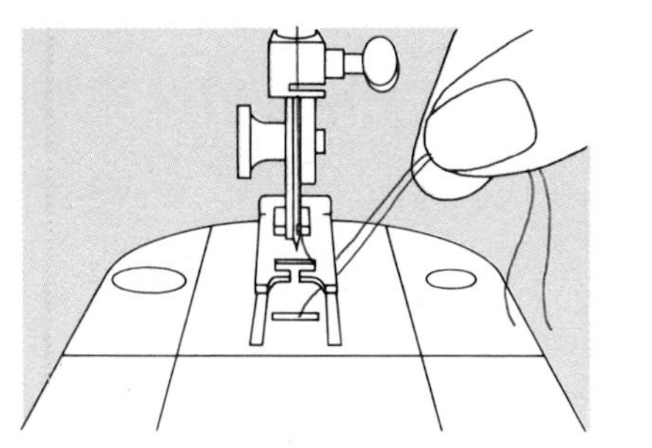
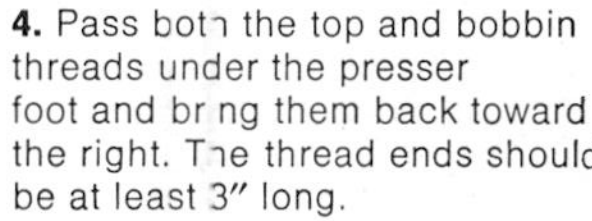

4. Pass both the top and bobbin threads under the presser foot and bring them back toward the right. The thread ends should be at least 3″ long.

Sewing machine

Needle sizes and types

Machine needles are made in different sizes and types to suit the varying needs of sewing. **Sizes** range from 9 (fine) to 18 (coarse). Coarser needles exist, but are harder to find. The higher the number, the coarser or thicker the needle. As a rule, the finer the thread and fabric weight, and the closer the fabric construction, the finer the needle should be. A second consideration is the **type of point.** Regular, sharp-pointed needles are used for most sewing. A ball-point is recommended for knits because its rounded point tends to slide between the yarns rather than pierce them. The third point type is the wedge, especially designed to penetrate leathers and vinyls so as to reduce the risk of splitting.

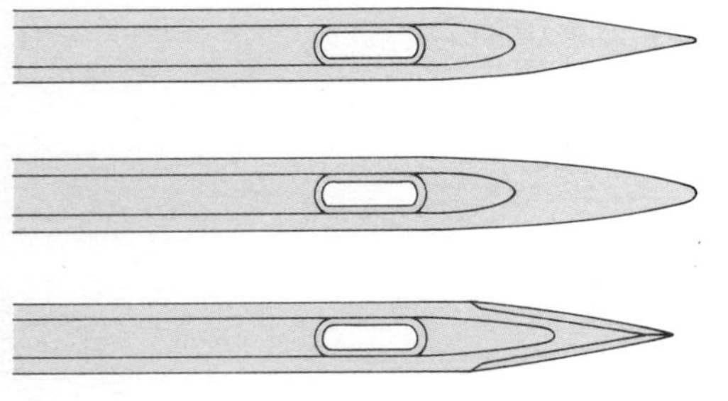

A sharp-point needle is the type used most often. Recommended for all types of woven fabrics, it commonly ranges from size 9 to 18.

A ball-point needle has a rounded point that makes it ideal for sewing on all types of knits. Sizes of these range from 9 to 16.

A wedge-point needle is expressly designed for use on leathers and vinyls. Needles of this type are available in sizes 11 to 18.

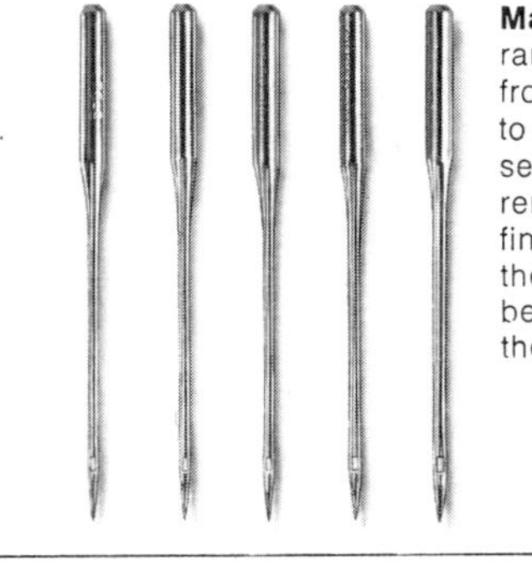

Machine needle sizes range, as a rule, from fine (size 9) to coarse (18). When selecting a needle, remember that the finer the weight of the fabric and thread being used, the finer the needle should be.

Twin and triple needles are used mainly for decorative stitching, and are usually a size 14. Additional spool pins are required for the multiple thread supply. Consult your sewing machine instruction book for their use, especially in zigzag stitching (you cannot always stitch full width).

Needle insertion

Besides choosing a needle that is the correct size and type for the fabric, it is also important that the overall size or conformation of the needle be correct for your sewing machine. Needles can differ in length, in the size of the shank (and the position of the shank, a consideration with twin or triple needles), and in the position and size of the scarf. All of these aspects of needle conformation can be critical in stitch formation. Most machine needles are interchangeable but it is important to follow the recommendations of the machine manufacturer. Or you can read the machine-needle package to see if that brand of needle will fit your machine.

Having chosen the proper needle, take care to insert it properly into the machine. The most universal method of **needle insertion** is explained below, but refer also to your machine instruction book. To remove a needle, reverse the insertion process. Check the needle condition at frequent intervals while sewing.

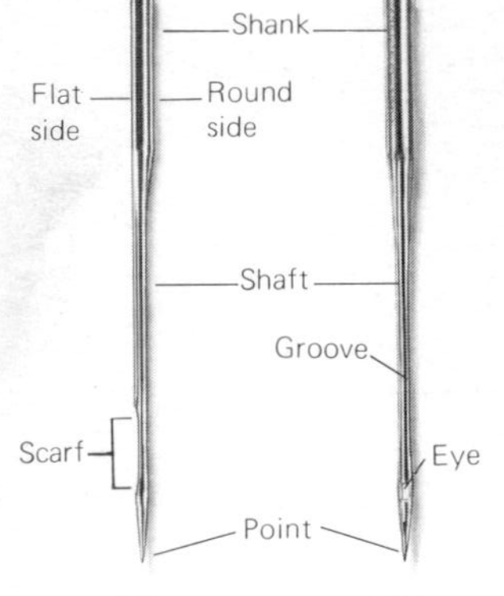

Side and front views of a machine needle are illustrated here. The upper part of a needle is called the *shank;* the lower part is the *shaft.* One side of the shank is *flat,* the other *rounded.* On the same side as the rounded part of the shank is the *groove* of the needle. The *eye* of the needle is just above the *point.* The *scarf* is an indentation behind the eye.

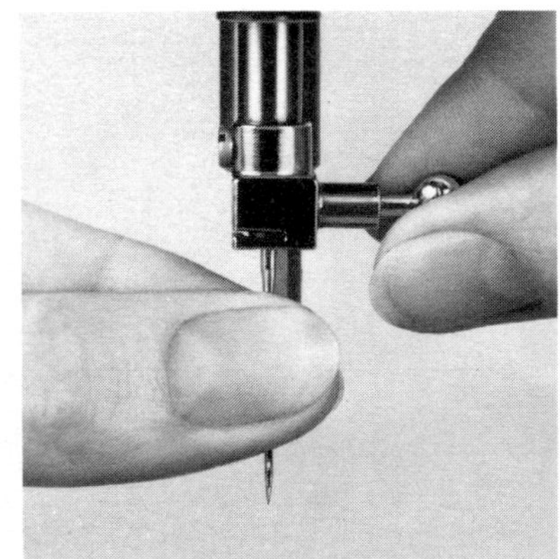

To insert a machine needle, first loosen the needle clamp screw. Then, with the flat side of the shank facing *away from* and the groove of the needle facing *toward* the last thread guide, push needle up into clamp as far as possible. Then tighten needle clamp screw. This procedure is correct for most machines, but it is wise to check the instruction book that accompanies your machine. To remove a needle, reverse the insertion process.

Needle faults

Many stitching problems are traceable to the needle. Listed below are the most common difficulties and remedies for them.

Needle is incorrectly inserted. If needle is not fully inserted into the needle clamp, or the groove is not positioned to the correct side, the result is usually skipped stitches or none at all.
Solution: Carefully re-insert needle.

Needle is wrong size for machine or fabric. If wrong size for machine, stitch formation is affected. If too fine a size for the fabric, thread might fray; if too coarse, needle might damage fabric. With either too fine or too coarse a needle, the stitches might look unbalanced.
Solution: Select needle of the proper conformation and size, and insert.

Needle is damaged or dirty. If needle has a burr on the point, eye, or groove, the thread might fray or break, or fabric might be damaged. A blunt needle can cause a thumping noise as it penetrates the fabric; it might also result in pulling on the fabric yarns or in skipped stitches. If the needle is bent, there might be skipped stitches, the fabric could be pulled to one side, or the needle might hit the throat plate and break. If the needle is dirty, it could cause skipped stitches.
Solution: Replace with a perfect needle.

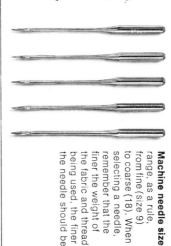

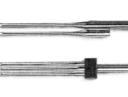

Needle/thread/stitch length selection

The table at the right is a guide to the recommended needle, thread, and stitch length combinations for most home sewing jobs. The selections are based on the following criteria.

Size of needle and thread depends fundamentally on the size of the fabric yarns—the finer the yarns, the finer both the needle and thread.

Needle type relates to fabric structure—sharp-point (regular) for wovens; ball-point for knits; wedge-point for leather and vinyl.

Thread type is chosen for its compatibility with the fabric's structure and fiber content (see Threads).

Stitch length for ordinary seaming depends on fabric *weight* (heaviness and density), *texture*, and *structure* (how the fabric is made). Of the three, weight is most important. As a general rule, the heavier the fabric, the longer the stitch; the lighter weight the fabric, the shorter the stitch. Within this rule, however, adjustments are made according to the other two characteristics, texture and structure. That is why the selection chart gives a *range* of stitch lengths for a specific fabric weight. Both velvet and crepe, for example, are classified as medium-weight, soft fabrics, with a recommended stitch length range of 10 to 12 stitches per inch. Because the crepe is less bulky, it needs a shorter stitch than a bulkier velvet. A relatively long stitch is recommended for such fabrics as leathers and unbacked vinyls. This is because the structure of such fabrics is susceptible to ripping, and the longer stitch length reduces this risk by making fewer needle holes.

Before starting any sewing project, it is wise to test and, if necessary, adjust the combination of needle, thread, and stitch length.

Fabric	Thread	Needle	Stitch length
Lightweight (soft) **Wovens:** Chiffon, organza, challis, crepe de Chine **Nets:** Fine lace; tulle **Knits:** Lingerie tricot, panné velvet	Silk, size A; nylon, size A; extra-fine (any fiber)	Size 9 or 11 regular for wovens and nets; size 10 or 11 ball-point for knits	10–15
Lightweight (crisp) **Wovens:** Lawn, dimity, voile, organdy, eyelet **Nets:** Some laces; coarser nets **Knits:** Ciré	Silk, size A; nylon, size A; mercerized cotton; extra-fine (any fiber)	Size 11 regular for wovens and nets; size 10 or 11 ball-point for knits	10–15
Medium-weight (soft) **Wovens:** Velvet, velveteen, gingham, chambray, batiste, crepe, corduroy **Knits:** Jersey, stretch terry, some double knits, some sweater knits	Polyester; cotton-wrapped polyester; mercerized cotton	Size 11 or 14 regular for wovens; size 10, 11, or 14 ball-point for knits	10–12
Medium-weight (crisp) **Wovens:** Brocade, shantung, faille, taffeta, peau de soie, chintz, piqué, percale, poplin, linen, some denims, some tweeds **Knits:** Some double knits, some bonded knits	Polyester; cotton-wrapped polyester; mercerized cotton	Size 11 or 14 regular for wovens; size 10, 11, or 14 ball-point for knits	10–12
Heavy (soft) **Wovens:** Fleece, velours, wide-wale corduroy, terry cloth, some coating fabrics, some fake furs **Knits:** Stretch velours, some fake furs, some sweater knits	Polyester; cotton-wrapped polyester; heavy-duty (any fiber)	Size 14 or 16 regular for wovens; size 14 or 16 ball-point for knits	10–12
Heavy (crisp) **Wovens:** Heavy suiting, burlap, ticking, canvas, upholstery fabric, double-faced wool, sailcloth, some denims, some gabardines, some coating fabrics, some tweeds **Knits:** Some jacquards, some double knits	Polyester; cotton-wrapped polyester; heavy-duty (any fiber)	Size 16 or 18 regular for wovens; size 14 or 16 ball-point for knits	8–12
Leathers and vinyls **Lightweight:** Kidskin, patent, capeskin, cobra, chamois, imitation leathers and suedes	Silk, size A; polyester; cotton-wrapped polyester	Size 11 or 14 leather (wedge-point)*	8–12
Medium-weight: Vinyls such as crinkle patent, embossed vinyl imitation reptile, imitation suedes, some genuine suedes	Silk, size A; polyester; cotton-wrapped polyester; mercerized cotton	Size 14 leather (wedge-point)*	8–12
Heavy: Cabretta, buckskin, calfskin, upholstery vinyl, some suedes	Polyester; cotton-wrapped polyester; heavy-duty (any fiber)	Size 14 or 16 leather (wedge-point)*	6–10

* If fabric is backed, a sharp-point can be used.

TOPSTITCHING RECOMMENDATIONS

Procedure and fabrics	Thread	Needle	Stitch length
Topstitching (straight) Wovens and knits, leathers and vinyls, all weights	Silk, size D (regular bobbin thread); cotton-wrapped polyester; mercerized cotton; heavy-duty (any fiber)	Size 16 or 18 regular for wovens; size 14 or 16 ball-point for knits; size 16 wedge-point for vinyls and leathers	6–12
Topstitching (zigzag) Wovens and knits, all weights	Polyester; cotton-wrapped polyester; mercerized cotton; heavy-duty (any fiber)	Size 14 or 16 regular for wovens; size 14 or 16 ball-point for knits	8–12 (length) 2–4 (width)
Topstitching (multi-needle) Wovens, light- and medium-weight	Polyester; cotton-wrapped polyester; mercerized cotton	Size 14 twin or triple	10–14

Sewing machine

Pressure and feed

As it is used here, pressure means the force exerted on the fabric as it is moved, by the action of the feed, under the presser foot. The two forces, pressure and feed, work together to produce properly stitched seams.

Pressure has several functions. It holds the fabric layers in such a way that they move evenly with one another. Another function of pressure is to hold the fabric taut; this helps to assure that stitches are properly set into the fabric, and thus that an even stitch tension is maintained.

Pressure also prevents fabric from (1) being pulled down into the bobbin area, and (2) hugging the needle, which can cause skipped stitches. The primary function of the feed, which is controlled by the stitch length regulator, is to move the fabric into position for each stitch. Feed also helps in holding the fabric layers taut during stitch formation.

Both the pressure and feed (stitch length) can be adjusted to suit fabric and sewing situation. As a rule, light pressure is used for lightweight fabrics, heavy for heavy fabrics. The length of the stitch depends on the job being done and the fabric being stitched (see pp. 27 and 30). For some sewing jobs, the action of the feed is totally eliminated—for example, when buttons are sewed on, so that there is no stitch length; or in free-motion stitching, in which stitch length is determined by how far you move the fabric. Both pressure and stitch length (feed) should be tested before the start of any sewing project. Some fabrics, such as piles and vinyls, because of their surfaces, are difficult to feed evenly. Pile fabrics tend to slip against each other, vinyls to stick together. Attachments are available to help solve feed problems posed by these and other materials (see p. 39).

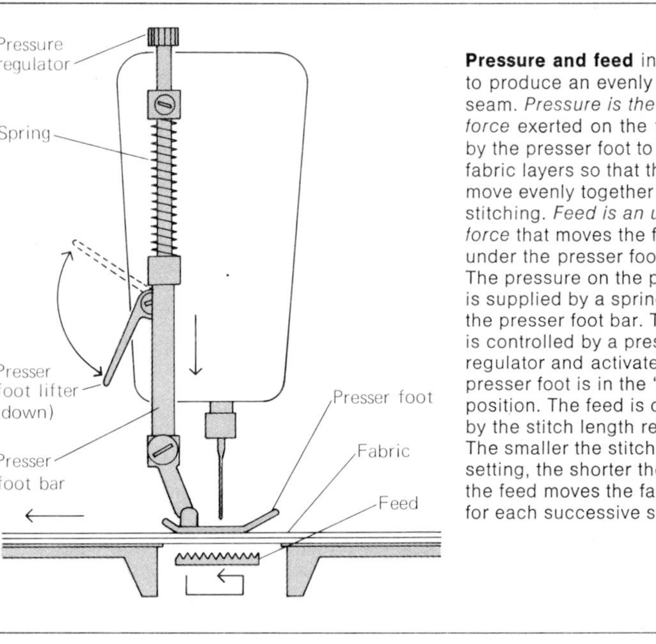

Pressure and feed interact to produce an evenly stitched seam. *Pressure is the downward force* exerted on the fabric by the presser foot to hold the fabric layers so that they move evenly together during stitching. *Feed is an upward force* that moves the fabrics under the presser foot.
The pressure on the presser foot is supplied by a spring on the presser foot bar. The spring is controlled by a pressure regulator and activated when the presser foot is in the "down" position. The feed is controlled by the stitch length regulator. The smaller the stitch length setting, the shorter the distance the feed moves the fabrics for each successive stitch.

Interaction of feed and pressure

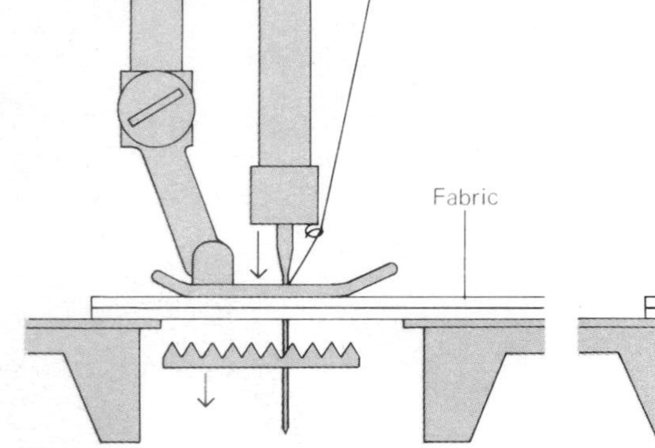

1. While needle and thread penetrate fabric, both feed and presser foot hold fabric taut. As needle descends, feed descends, leaving only the presser foot in contact with fabric.

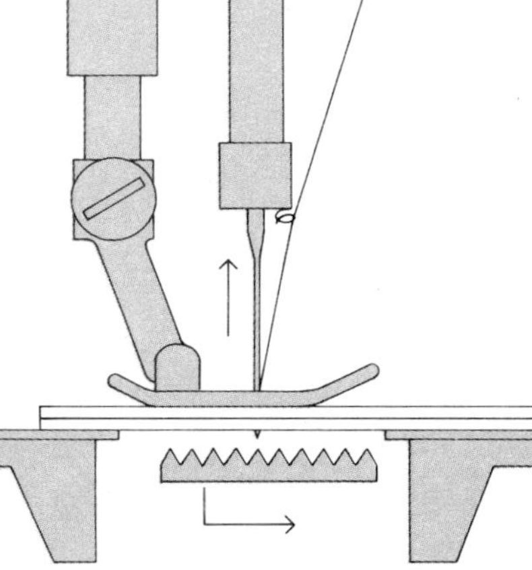

2. As the needle is coming up out of the fabric, the feed is moving forward. While this is happening, the presser foot continues to be in contact with the fabric.

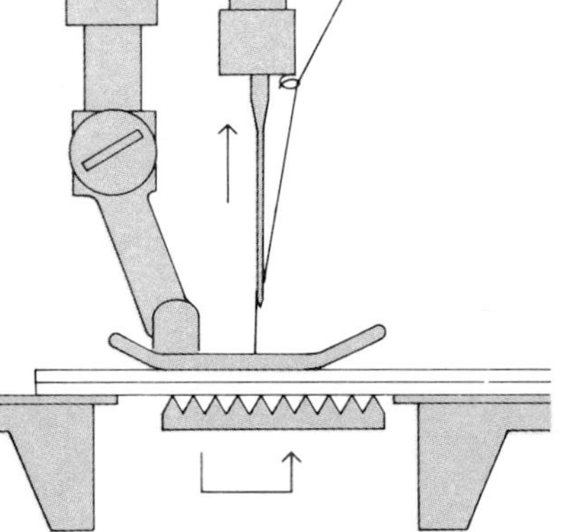

3. As the needle continues to move up, and to bring the stitch with it, the feed is also moving up toward the fabric. The presser foot continues to hold the fabric.

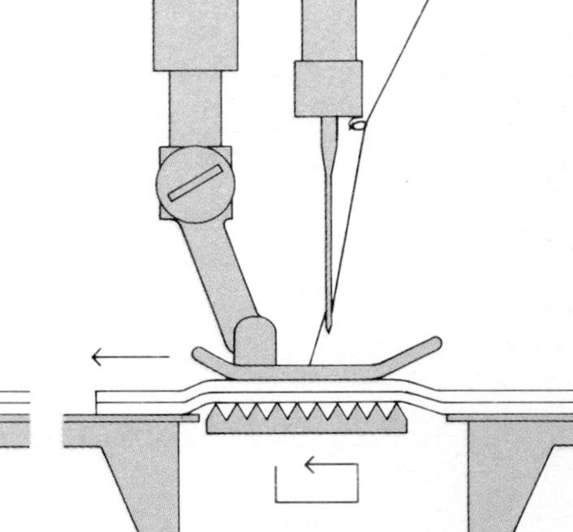

4. As the stitch is being set into the fabric, the feed comes up to help the presser foot keep the fabric taut and then to advance the fabric one stitch length.

Correct and incorrect pressure

The correct amount of pressure assures even feeding of fabric layers that are properly stitched and are undamaged in the process. The amount of pressure used will depend on the weight of the fabric. Generally, the lighter-weight the fabric, the lighter the pressure needed. With some fabrics, however, it is difficult to achieve a precise enough pressure to feed the fabric layers evenly. Examples are vinyls, pile fabrics, and plaid or stripe fabrics that are being matched. "Top feed" attachments are available to assist in the even feeding of such fabrics (see p. 39).

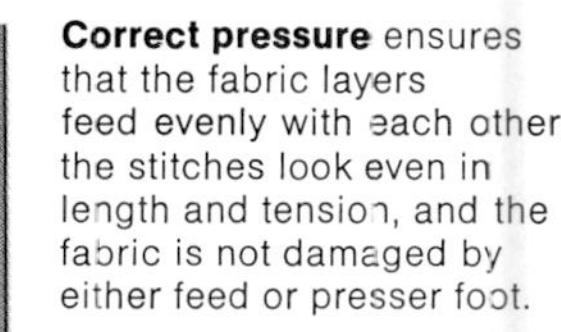

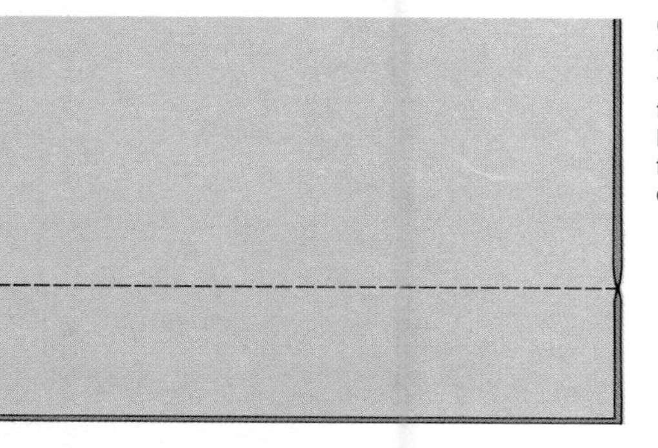

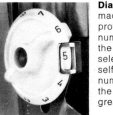

Correct pressure ensures that the fabric layers feed evenly with each other, the stitches look even in length and tension, and the fabric is not damaged by either feed or presser foot.

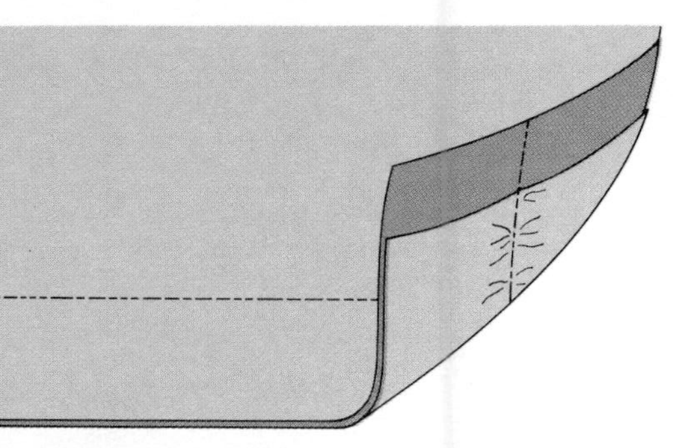

Too much pressure can have several results. Most often, the top layer slips while the bottom layer gathers up. Stitches could be uneven in length and tension. The feed could damage the bottom fabric layer. The combined action of presser foot and feed could mar the face side of the fabric layers.

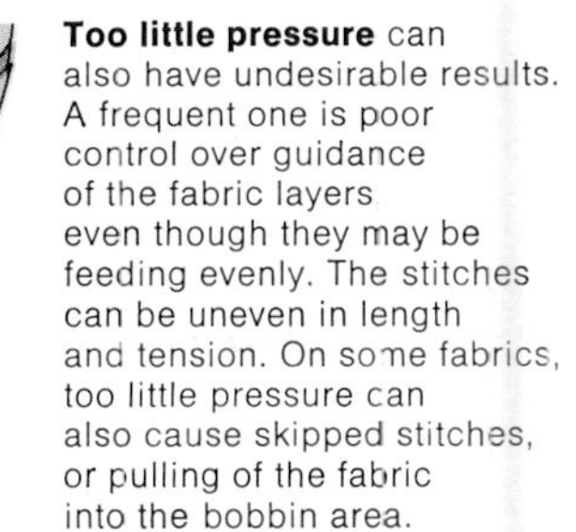

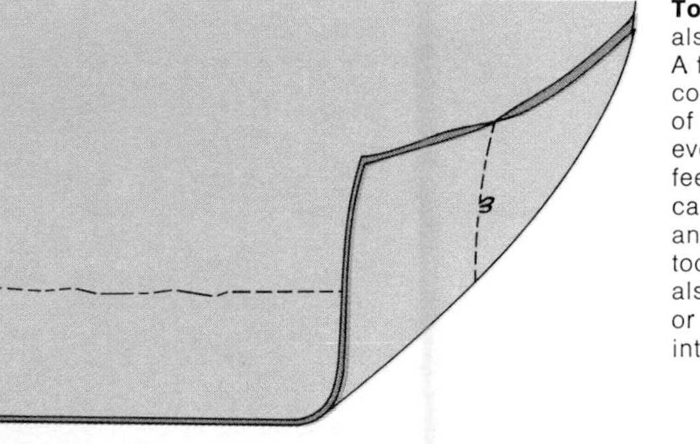

Too little pressure can also have undesirable results. A frequent one is poor control over guidance of the fabric layers even though they may be feeding evenly. The stitches can be uneven in length and tension. On some fabrics, too little pressure can also cause skipped stitches, or pulling of the fabric into the bobbin area.

Pressure regulators

The amount of force the presser foot exerts on the fabric is usually controlled by a pressure regulator. (On some machines, there is an automatic pressure adjustment mechanism.) This regulator is attached to a spring on the presser foot bar (see opposite page). Pressure is increased when the spring is compressed, decreased when it is elongated. Depending on the type of regulator, adjustments are made in several ways (see below).

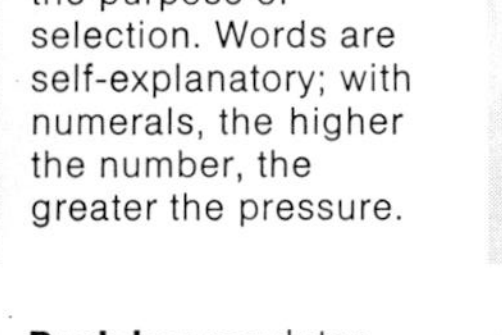

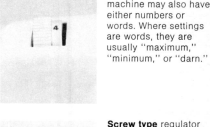

Dial on the side of machine arm will provide either numerals or words for the purpose of selection. Words are self-explanatory; with numerals, the higher the number, the greater the pressure.

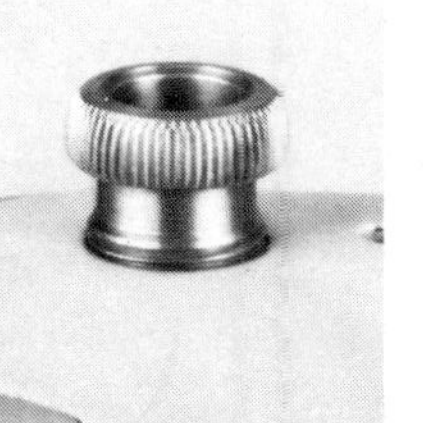

Dial on top of the machine may also have either numbers or words. Where settings are words, they are usually "maximum," "minimum," or "darn."

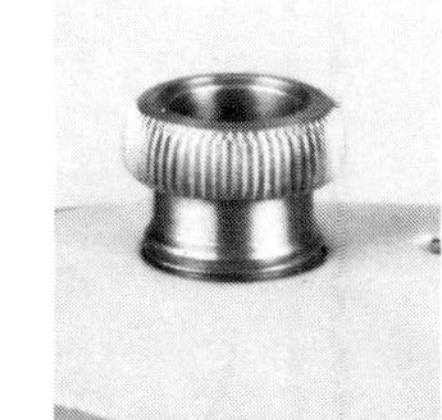

Push bar regulator has a lock-release collar around it. When *bar* is pushed down to increase the pressure, collar locks bar into place. When *collar* is pushed, the bar is released and pressure is decreased.

Screw type regulator is turned *clockwise* to increase pressure, *counterclockwise* to decrease pressure.

No-feed controls

The movement of the feed is important in almost all sewing, since it is the force that moves the fabric under the foot. In certain sewing situations, however, such fabric movement is undesirable. Examples of such situations are button sewing and free-motion sewing; for such techniques, the effect of the feed should be eliminated. Depending on the machine, this will be accomplished in one of two ways: (1) by dropping the feed, or (2) by covering the feed. Both methods are explained below.

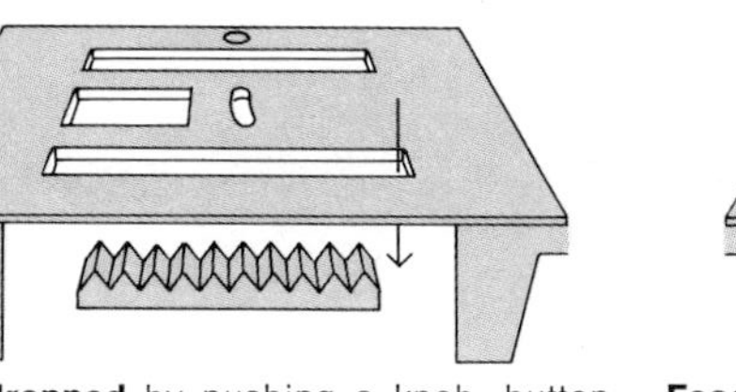

Feed is dropped by pushing a knob, button, or lever. This causes the feed to be brought below the level of the throat plate.

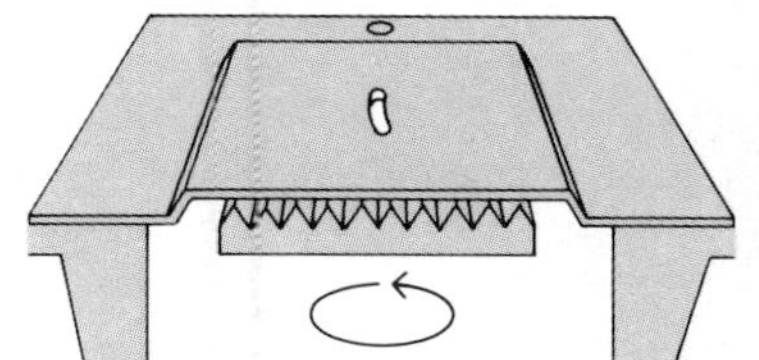

Feed is covered by means of a special throat plate, part of which is elevated above the level of a regular throat plate.

Stitch length in straight stitching

All sewing machines provide a stitch length regulator that permits changes in stitch length for different sewing situations. For seaming, the range is usually from 10 to 15 stitches per inch, depending on the fabric (see chart, p. 27). For temporary jobs, such as basting, or nonstructural details, such as topstitching, the stitches can be longer. (Very short stitches, 16 to fine, are used mainly for satin stitching, a zigzag stitch. For the meaning of length in zigzag stitching, see pages 32–33.) Most machines also have a reverse control, as part of the stitch length regulator or separate from it. When this is activated, the machine sews in reverse at approximately the same stitch length as it does when stitching forward.

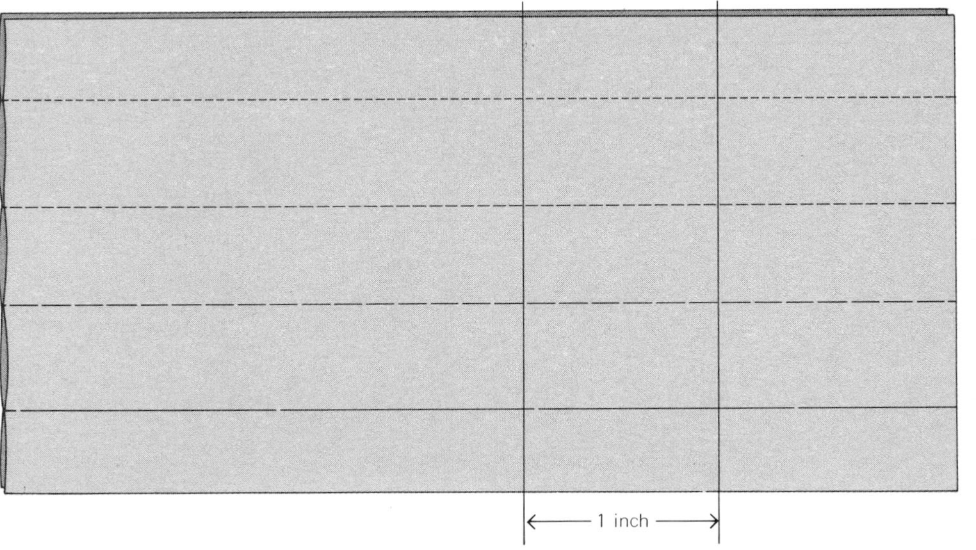

Fine stitch length ranges from 16 to 24 stitches per inch. Mainly used for seaming lightweight fabrics and for satin stitching.

Regular stitch length, ranging from 10 to 15 stitches per inch, is the length used for most sewing situations.

Basting stitches range from 6 to 9 stitches per inch. This stitch length is used for easing and gathering as well.

Longer basting stitches can be produced by some sewing machines. They can be as long as one stitch to every 2 inches.

Feed and stitch length

The major purpose of the feed is to move the fabric into position for each stitch. The distance that the feed moves the fabric is controlled by the stitch length regulator. When the regulator is set for a long stitch, the feed moves in a long elliptical path, advancing the fabric a considerable distance. When the control is set for a short stitch, the elliptical path of the feed is shorter, and the fabric is moved a shorter distance.

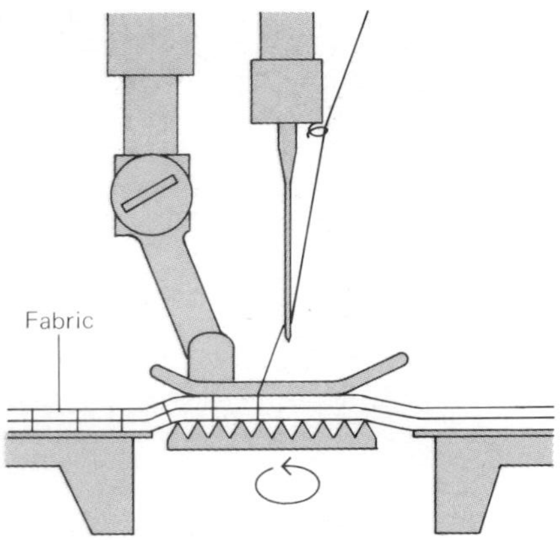

Fabric

The larger the elliptical path of the feed, the longer the stitch will be.

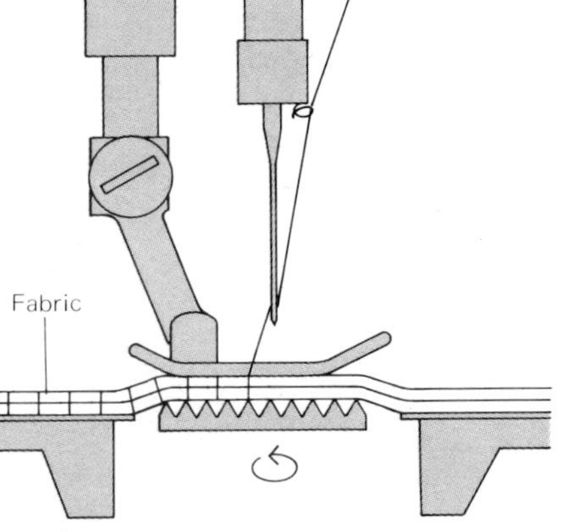

The smaller the ellipse formed by the feed, the shorter the stitch will be.

Stitch length regulators

The numbers on a stitch length regulator used to select stitch length may be based on either the inch or the metric system of measurement. In the inch system, numerals stand for number of stitches to an inch; those in the metric system, for the actual length of the stitch in millimeters. Both, however, are measuring the same stitch. If, for example, there are 12 stitches to a measured inch, each stitch will measure 2.1 millimeters.

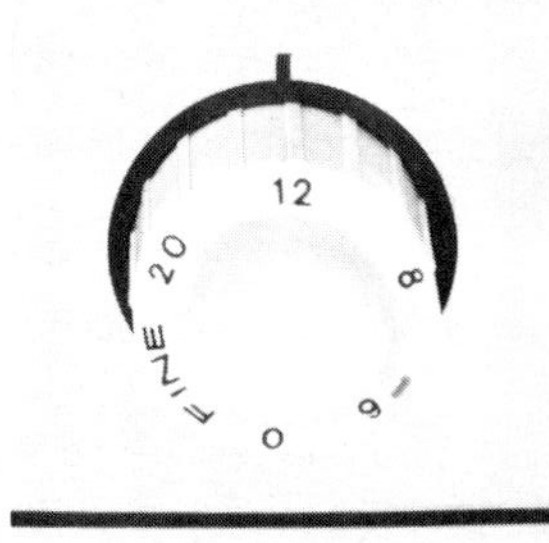

The inch system of measurement is the basis of this stitch length regulator. The reverse stitching control is not part of the dial shown here.

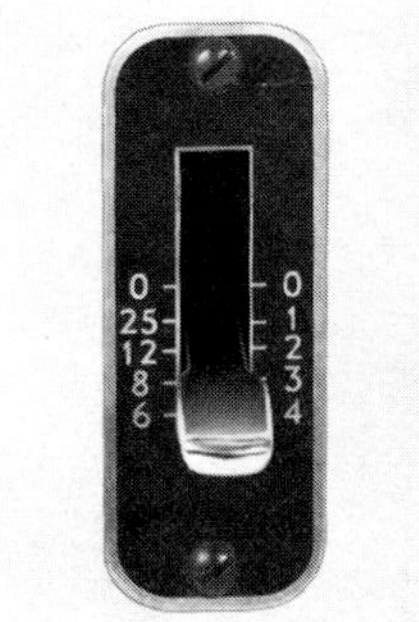

Both systems are used on this lever-type stitch length regulator. Stitches per inch are on the left and metric measurements are on the right.

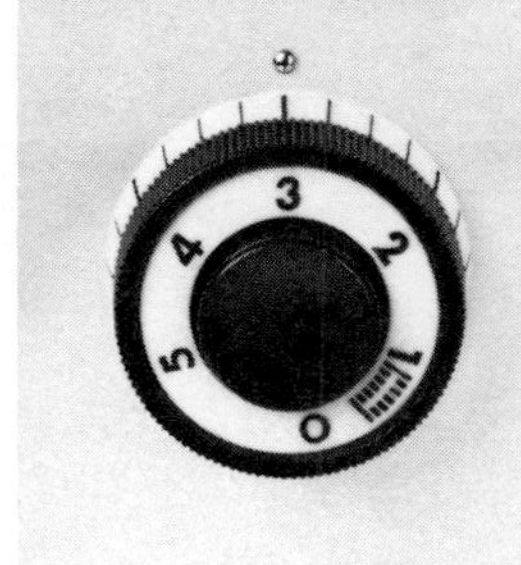

The metric system of measuring stitch length is used on this dial. The button in the center of the dial is the reverse stitching control.

Stitch tension

Every sewing machine has a tension control for the top thread; most machines also have one for the bobbin thread. These controls increase or decrease the pressure on the threads as they are fed through the machine. Too much pressure results in too much tension and too little thread for the stitch; too little pressure produces too little tension and too much thread. In general, too little thread causes fabric puckering and strained, easily broken stitches; too much produces a limp, weak seam. When pressure is correct on both threads, a balanced amount of each thread is used, and the connecting link of each stitch is centered between fabric layers. The link position is a good indicator of which thread tension is incorrect (see below). It can happen, however, that the link is in the right place, but either too much or too little of both threads has been used. To remedy this, adjust both tensions.

Test stitch tension before starting any sewing project. Use the same number and types of fabric layers as will be sewed, and the correct needle, thread, and pressure for them.

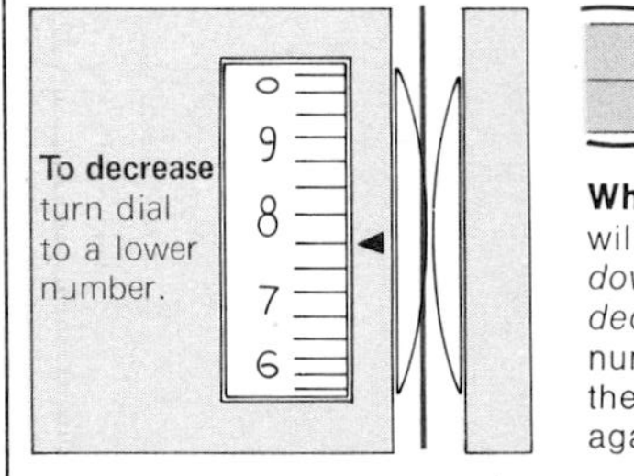

Correct tension: Link formed with each stitch will lie midway between fabric layers. Balanced amounts of both top and bobbin threads have been used for each stitch.

Top too tight: Links will fall toward top layer of fabric. This means that there is either too much tension on the top thread or too little on the bobbin thread.

Top too loose: Links are toward bottom fabric layer. This indicates either that the top tension is too loose or there is too much tension on the bobbin thread.

Top thread tension

The top thread tension control, situated on top of or close to the tension discs, bears numbers or symbols to indicate the amount of tension the dial is set for (see p. 21). Adjust this control with machine threaded and presser foot down (when foot is up, tension discs are open).

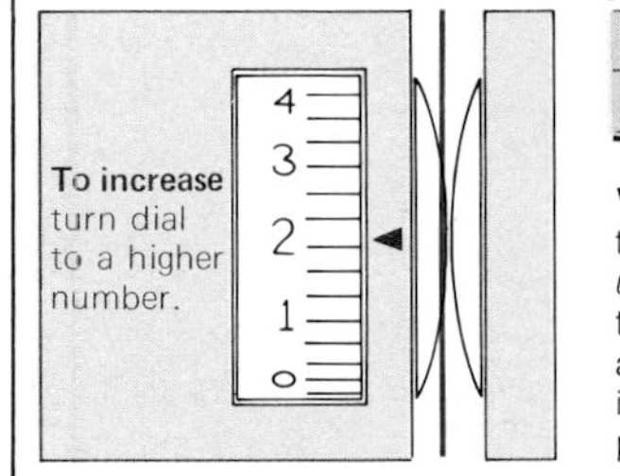

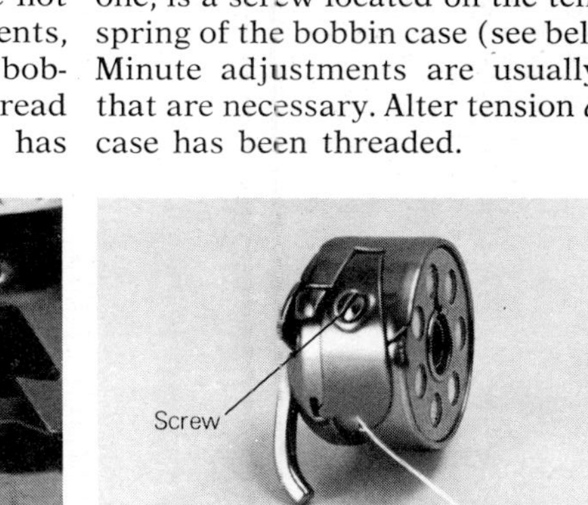

When top tension is too tight, link in stitch will fall toward top layer of fabric. To bring link *down,* toward the center of the fabric layers, *decrease* the top tension: Turn dial to a lower number (or into the minus range). This decreases the amount that the tension discs press against each other and the thread.

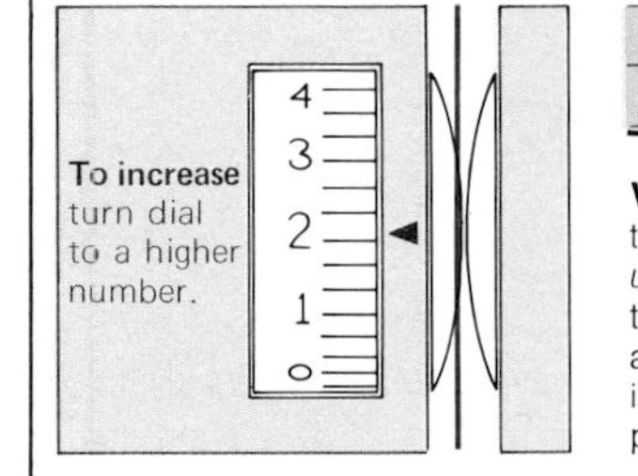

When top tension is too loose, the link will lie toward the bottom layer of fabric. To bring link *up,* toward the center of the fabric layers, *increase* the top tension: Gradually turn control to a higher number (or into the plus range). This increases the amount that the tension discs press against each other and the thread.

Bobbin thread tension

If stitch tension and balance are not corrected by top tension adjustments, it may be necessary to adjust the bobbin thread tension. The bobbin thread tension control, if the machine has one, is a screw located on the tension spring of the bobbin case (see below). Minute adjustments are usually all that are necessary. Alter tension *after* case has been threaded.

Screw

Most built-in bobbin cases have an adjustable tension screw. Using a screwdriver, turn the screw *clockwise to increase* and *counterclockwise to decrease* the tension.

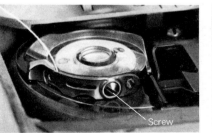

Screw

All removable bobbin cases have a tension screw. Like the screws in the built-in types, it is turned *clockwise to increase* and *counterclockwise to decrease* the tension.

Sewing machine

Zigzag stitching

Zigzag stitches are lockstitches with a side-to-side width (bight) as well as a stitch length. On non-computerized machines, stitch formation is dictated mainly by a **stitch pattern cam;** maximum pattern width is established by a **stitch width regulator.** Stitch length is selected as for straight stitching (see p. 30), and is the same for both stitch types at the same setting, but occurs to the eye as a *distance between points* rather than an actual stitch measurement (see top, right).

The cams, which may be either built-in or inserted, control stitch formation by means of indentations in their outer edges. A fingerlike follower, connected to the needle bar, tracks these indentations, moving the needle from side to side. The adjoining diagram illustrates the principle.

When cams are multiple, as they are with machines that offer several built-in stitch patterns (and with interchangeable cam stacks, which some machines provide), a **stitch pattern selector** positions the follower onto the appropriate cam.

The cams that produce zigzag stitch patterns are *single;* stretch stitching requires *double* cams (see p. 36).

Besides the controls mentioned, some machines have a **needle position selector,** which places stitches to the left or right of a normal (usually center) position—helpful in constructing hand-guided buttonholes, sewing on buttons, and positioning stitches closer to or farther from an edge.

A zigzag stitch has more give than a straight stitch, and so is less subject to breakage. Stitches lie diagonally across the fabric, so more thread is used, and the stress is not on a single line but apportioned across a span. In any zigzag stitching, always use a zigzag foot and throat plate.

The diagram shows, in simplified form, the inner workings of a zigzag stitch mechanism. As the *cam* rotates, a fingerlike *follower,* connected to the needle bar, rides along the cam and tracks its indentations. As the follower moves in and out, the *needle bar* is moved from side to side. (At the same time, the needle bar is also moving up and down in time with the shuttle hook to form lockstitches between the top and bottom threads.) With regard to controls activated by the user, the *stitch width regulator* establishes the maximum side-to-side motion; the *stitch length regulator* controls the distance the feed moves the fabric for each successive stitch. In machines with a number of built-in zigzag patterns, each formed by a different cam, a *stitch pattern selector* positions the follower onto the appropriate cam.

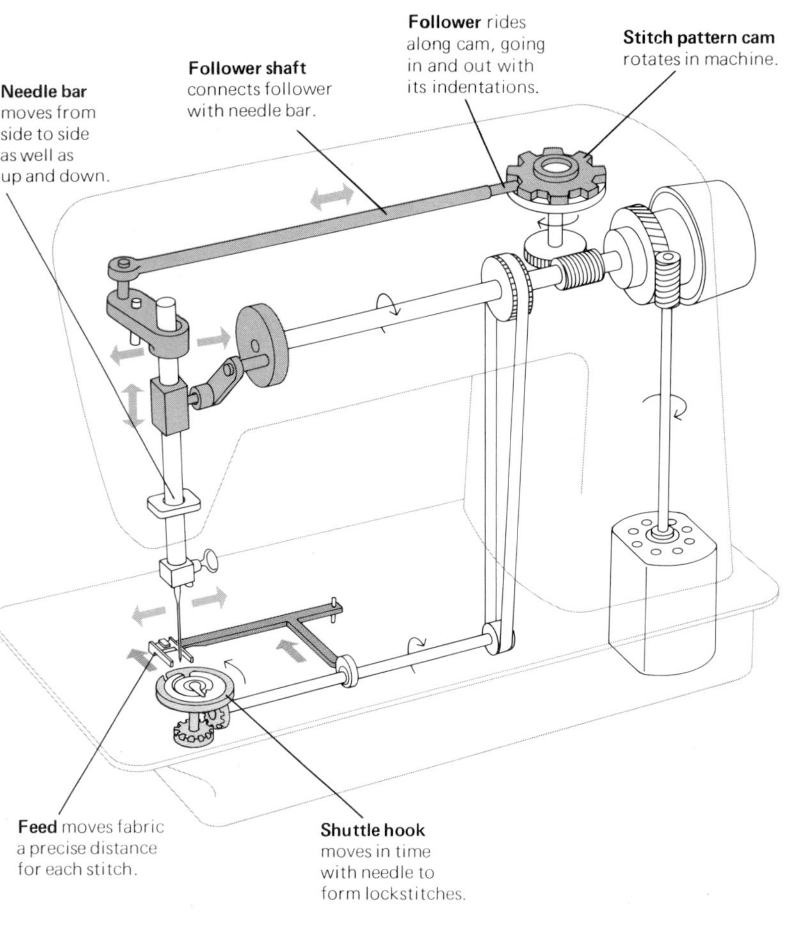
Needle bar moves from side to side as well as up and down.
Follower shaft connects follower with needle bar.
Follower rides along cam, going in and out with its indentations.
Stitch pattern cam rotates in machine.
Feed moves fabric a precise distance for each stitch.
Shuttle hook moves in time with needle to form lockstitches.

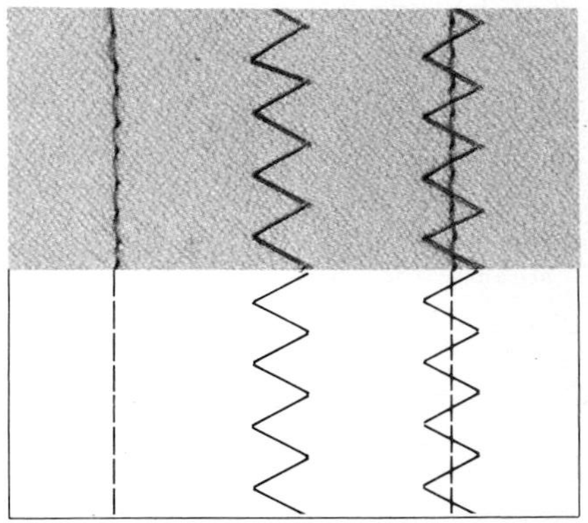

Stitch length is the distance between needle penetrations. It is the same for straight or zigzag stitches at the same setting, but penetrations for zigzag are from side to side.

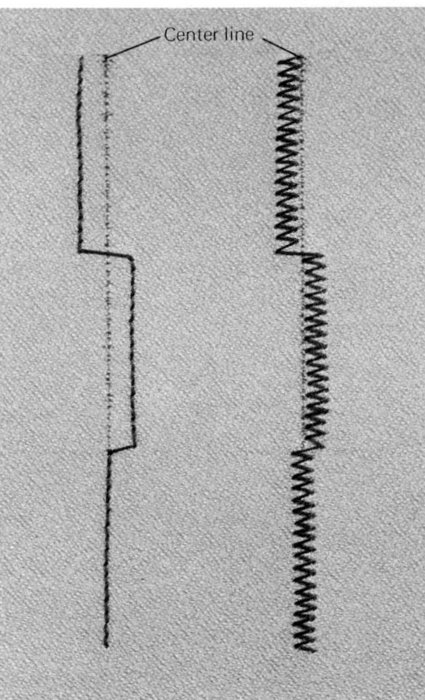
Center line

Needle position selector permits stitch patterns to be placed to a side (or sides) other than normal. In the example, center is normal position; stitches can go to left or right.

Length and width in zigzag stitching

A zigzag stitch can be varied in both length and width: *length* by the same stitch length regulator that controls straight-stitch length (see p. 30); *width* (how far the needle moves from side to side) by the stitch width regulator, with either symbols or numbers indicating the range. The higher the number, the wider the stitch; "O" setting produces a straight stitch.

The choices will depend on the fabric and the job. The stitch length rule in seaming (at a very narrow width setting) is usually the lighter the fabric, the shorter the stitch. In edge-finishing, the more fabric ravels, the wider the stitch should be. In decorative applications, the length and width are less crucial and can be set according to the desired effect.

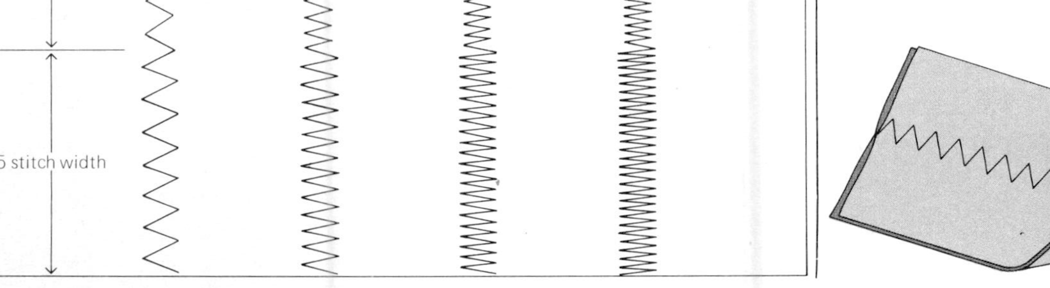

Tension in zigzag stitching

The tension of a zigzag stitch can be adjusted just like that of a straight stitch (see p. 31). In a balanced zigzag stitch, the interlocking link of the top and bottom threads falls at the corner of each stitch and midway between the fabric layers. When the tension (and, to some extent, the pressure) is incorrect, the stitch tends to draw up the fabric, particularly one that is lightweight or spongy. Pressure is important in stitch formation because it holds the fabric layers so that stitches can be properly set. A zigzag stitch used in construction should be properly balanced. In decorative uses, the top tension can be loosened so that the link falls toward the bottom layer, causing the resulting stitch pattern to be more rounded.

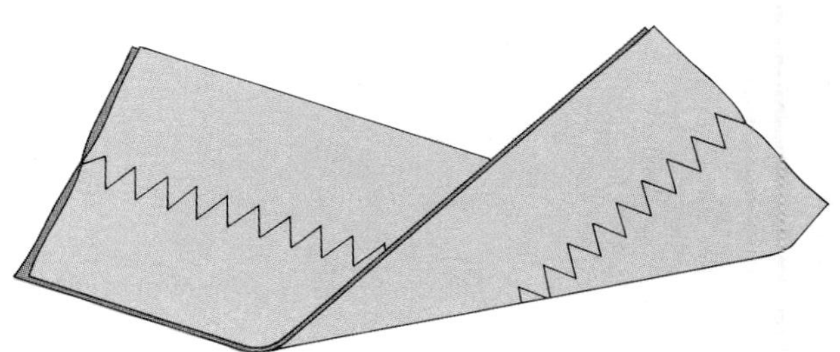

The correct tension places the link at the corner of each zigzag, and uses a balanced amount of both top and bobbin threads. Fabric lies flat; it has not been puckered by the zigzag stitching.

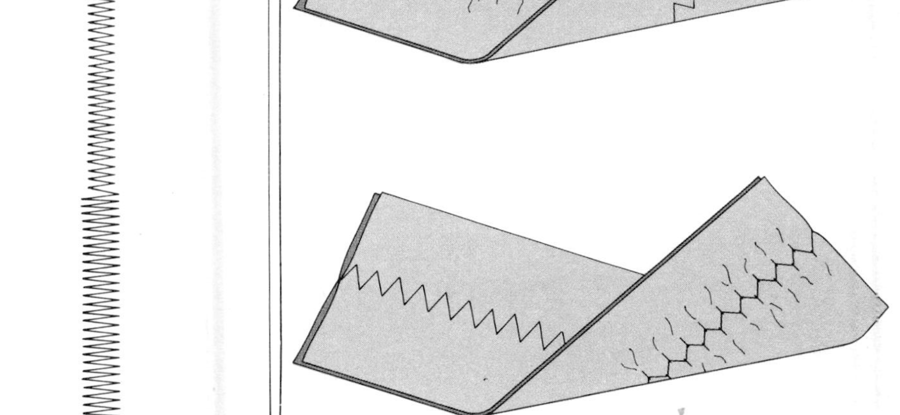

Too tight a top tension places the link toward the top fabric layer; the fabric might be puckered. To bring the link down toward middle of fabric layers, either decrease the top tension or, if machine permits it, increase the bobbin tension.

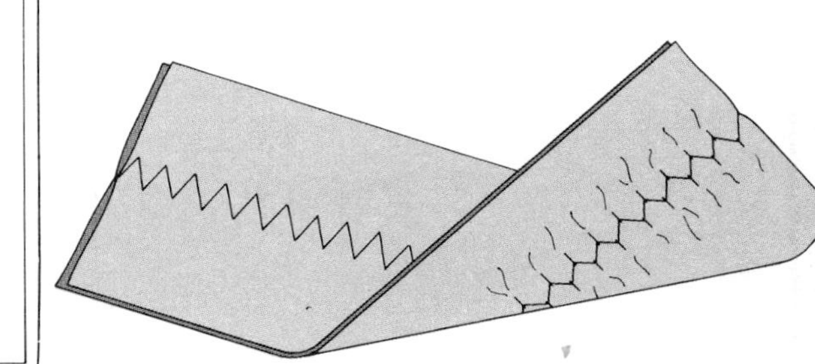

Too loose a top tension places the link toward the bottom fabric layer; also, the fabric might be puckered. To bring the link up toward the top fabric layer, either increase the top tension or, if machine permits it, decrease the bobbin tension.

Hemstitching 140
Shell tucks 165
Machine blind-hemming 294
Shell-stitched edge finish 314

Zigzag patterns that use straight stitches

In some of the patterns in this group, straight stitches are part of the design; an example is the blindstitch. Others, such as the multistitch, consist of straight stitches only, but in a zigzag configuration.

Length and width variations affect the practical uses of either type. For example, when the stitch length of the **blindstitch** is shortened, there are more zigzags per inch to catch the fabric more often, an important consideration in hemming. When the stitch is widened, the zigzags extend farther from the straight stitches to cover a wider span, good for heavier fabrics.

The **multistitch**, combining zigzag placement with the frequent "bites" of straight stitches in series, offers great flexibility and fabric control. Set narrow, it is excellent for edge-finishing fabrics that ravel; at a wider width, for mending, attaching elastic, stitching lapped and abutted seams.

Blindstitch pattern consists of several straight stitches followed by one zigzag. An important fact about the blindstitch: The zigzag always falls to the left of the straight stitches, so the edge to which the zigzag should go must be to the left of the needle. Length and width can be varied to suit the job. Use longer and narrower (near right) for delicate fabrics; shorter and wider (second row) for heavier fabrics. Used for blind hemming, seam finishing, double-stitched seams; decoratively, for hemstitching, shell-stitched edges (shown), and shell tucks.

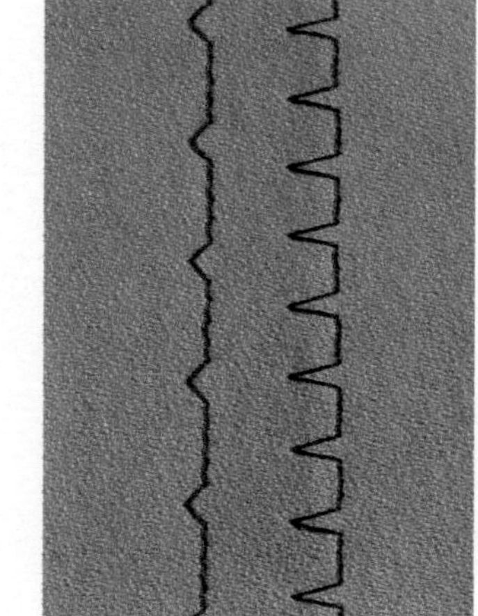

Blindstitch pattern set longer and narrower, shorter and wider;

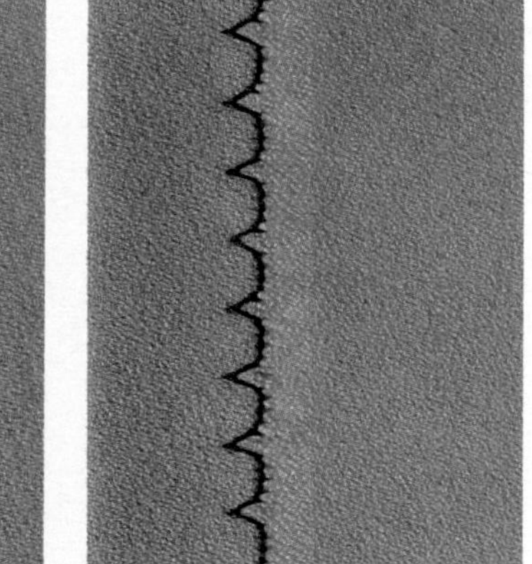

the blindstitch pattern shown as used for **hemstitching** application;

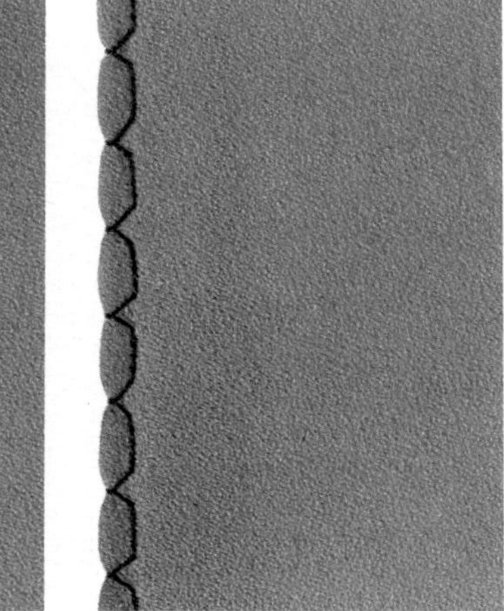

the blindstitch pattern used as a **shell-stitched** edge.

Multistitch pattern is a series of straight stitches placed in a zigzag design. The longer, narrower version (near right) is excellent for edge-finishing fabrics that ravel. Set shorter and wider (second row), the stitch is fine for mending. Pattern grows equally to the right and left of a center line. For a fagotted seam (shown), the two edges should be an equal distance from the center so that each stitch will catch an edge. The seamline should be at the pattern's center in a lapped seam; the meeting edges should be at the center in an abutted seam.

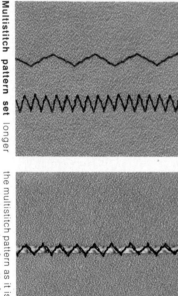

Multistitch pattern set longer and narrower, shorter and wider;

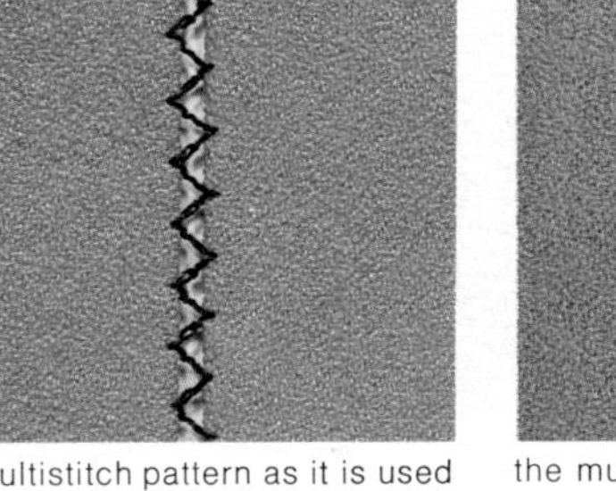

the multistitch pattern as it is used in stitching of a **fagotted seam;**

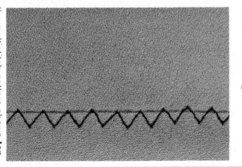

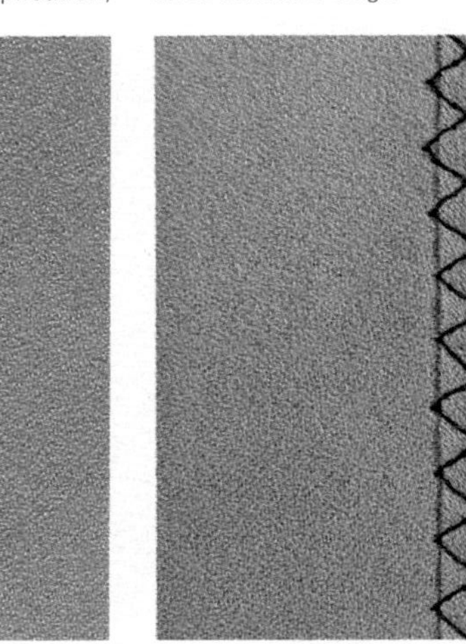

the multistitch pattern shown **top-stitching a bound edge.**

Decorative zigzag patterns

With decorative stitch patterns, it is useful to know whether one or both sides of the pattern are shaped. This helps in deciding which can be used for edgestitching or appliqué and how to place fabric under the foot.

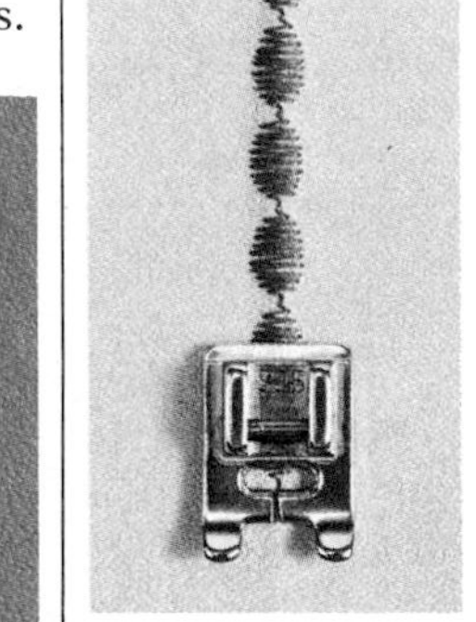

Both sides of most patterns are shaped. Patterns of this type are ideal as the center motif in a decorative panel. If the stitch width is narrowed, the pattern can be placed to the left or right of the center.

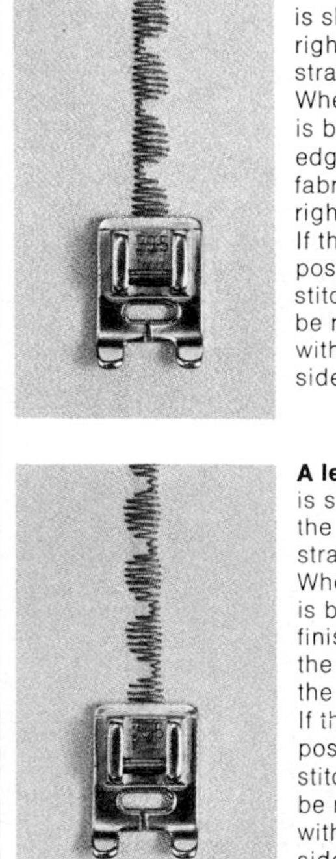

A right-sided pattern is shaped on the right side and straight on the left. When such a pattern is being used for edgestitching, place fabric edge to the right of the needle. If the needle position is changed, stitch width must be reduced to fit within the narrower side-to-side limits.

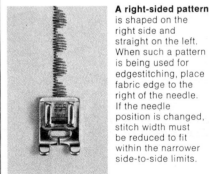

A left-sided pattern is shaped on the left side and straight on the right. When such a pattern is being used to finish an edge, place the fabric edge to the left of the needle. If the needle position is changed, stitch width must be reduced to fit within the narrower side-to-side limits.

Seams 149,151-153
Bound edges 302-303
Machine-worked buttonholes 343-344
Sewing on buttons 352

Using the plain zigzag stitch

As shown in the sample at the right, plain zigzag stitching can be both functional and decorative. First, a plain *satin stitch* decoratively finishes a raw edge. In the second example, an *abutted seam* is sewed with a zigzag stitch. The next two rows show *topstitching* with a zigzag—the first is stitched with a single needle, the second with a twin needle.

In the fifth example, machine *buttonholes* create finished openings for threading a ribbon. The ribbon is held in place by the zigzag stitches that are used to attach the *button*. Next, a length of *cord* is secured to fabric with zigzag stitching. The row to its right shows how, by changing the *needle position*, stitch groups can be placed on either side of a center. The final row is a *bound edge* finished with zigzag topstitching.

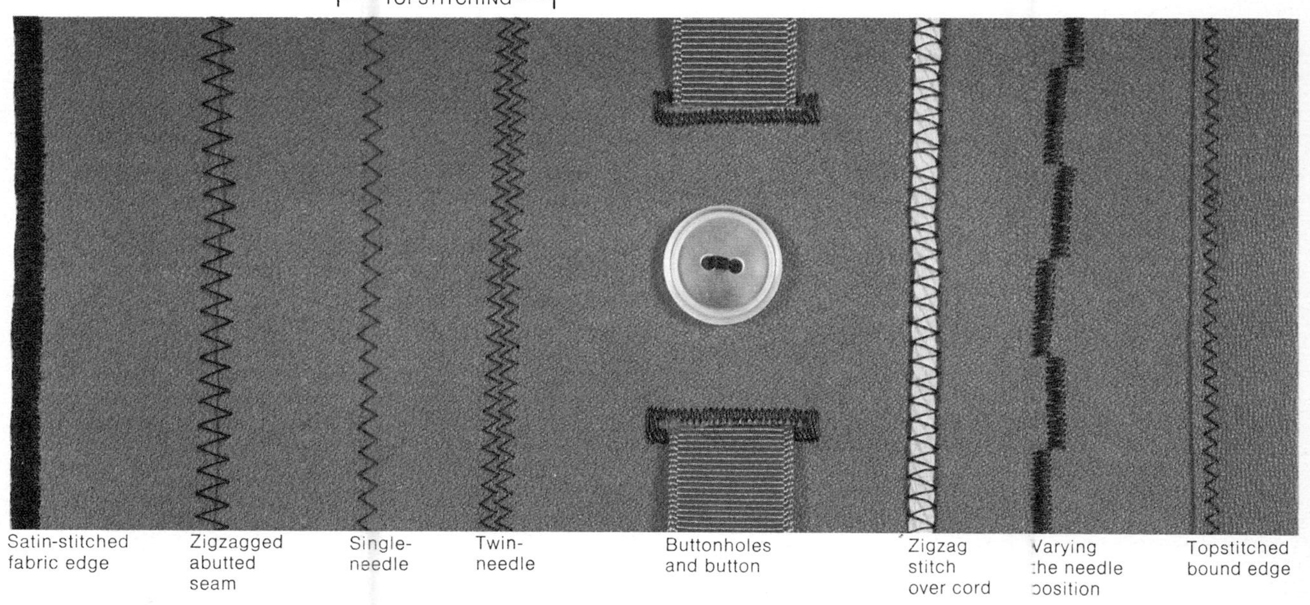

TOPSTITCHING

Satin-stitched fabric edge | Zigzagged abutted seam | Single-needle | Twin-needle | Buttonholes and button | Zigzag stitch over cord | Varying the needle position | Topstitched bound edge

Using patterned zigzag stitches

Though patterned zigzag stitches are most often used decoratively, they can be functional as well. Several patterns are used in this way in the sample at the right. To finish a raw edge, instead of the plain zigzag in the sample above, the choice is a *solid scallop*. Next to the edge finish, a *full-ball* motif is topstitched onto the fabric. In the third pattern, the *needle position* alternates to place groups of stitches to the left and right of a center line. The next row is a series of *arrowheads*. The two that follow are examples of zigzag/straight stitch patterns, the first the *multistitch* used on an abutted seam, the second a wavy motif that is topstitched onto the fabric with a *twin needle*. In the last example, slanted groups of narrow zigzag stitches are topstitched onto a *bound edge*.

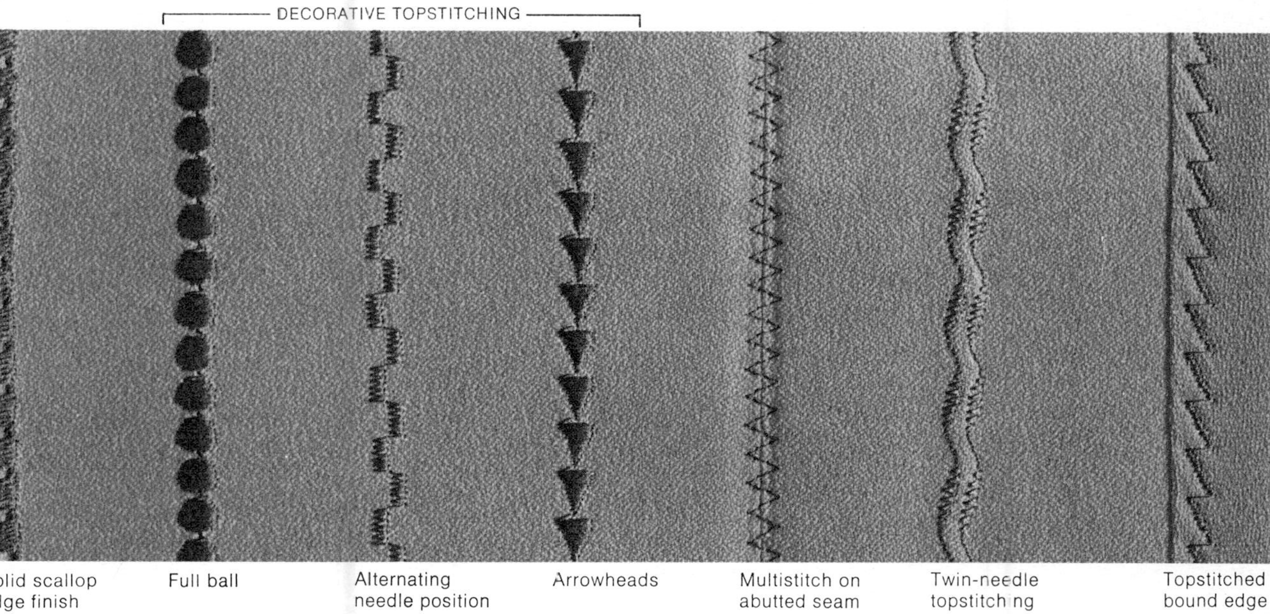

DECORATIVE TOPSTITCHING

Solid scallop edge finish | Full ball | Alternating needle position | Arrowheads | Multistitch on abutted seam | Twin-needle topstitching | Topstitched bound edge

Stretch stitching

Stretch stitches are produced by coordinated motions of needle and feed—that is, while the needle is moving as for straight or zigzag stitches, the feed is moving the fabric forward and backward according to the pattern's requirements. On non-computerized machines, pattern formation is cam-controlled. Because of the dual action, however, stretch stitch patterns have double (two-track) cams. The indentations on one track control the needle action; those on the other, the movement of the fabric by the feed. The diagram at right illustrates the basic principles by which stretch stitches are formed.

Stretch stitches require a **stitch pattern selector** to position the followers onto the appropriate cam tracks and, as a rule, **stitch width and length regulators** that permit the operator to control the stitch size.

The forward/backward feed action results, with most stretch stitches, in several stitches being formed in the same place. A typical straight stretch stitch consists of two stitches forward and one in reverse, or a total of three stitches in each place.

In any stitching, reverse stitches tend not to be exactly the same length as those sewed forward. In stretch stitching, where forward and reverse are used coordinately, this tendency can cause pattern distortion. To help correct it, many machines with stretch stitch capability are equipped with a **pattern balance control.**

Except for certain precise patterns, stitch tension is not as critical for stretch stitches as for straight or zigzag. If the tensions look too unbalanced, adjust them until stitches appear correct to the eye (see p. 31). Remember also to adjust the foot pressure as described on pages 28–29.

Stretch stitches are produced basically as shown in the diagram. As two-track *cam* rotates, a *follower,* connected to the needle bar, rides along one track to move the *needle bar* from side to side. Another follower, connected to the *feed,* simultaneously rides the other cam track to move the feed for forward and reverse stitches as required by the design. *Stitch pattern selector* positions followers onto appropriate cam tracks; *stitch width regulator* determines the maximum width of the pattern; *stitch length regulator* controls the stitch length. As these actions are taking place, the needle bar is moving up and down in time with the shuttle hook to form lockstitches between the top and bottom threads.

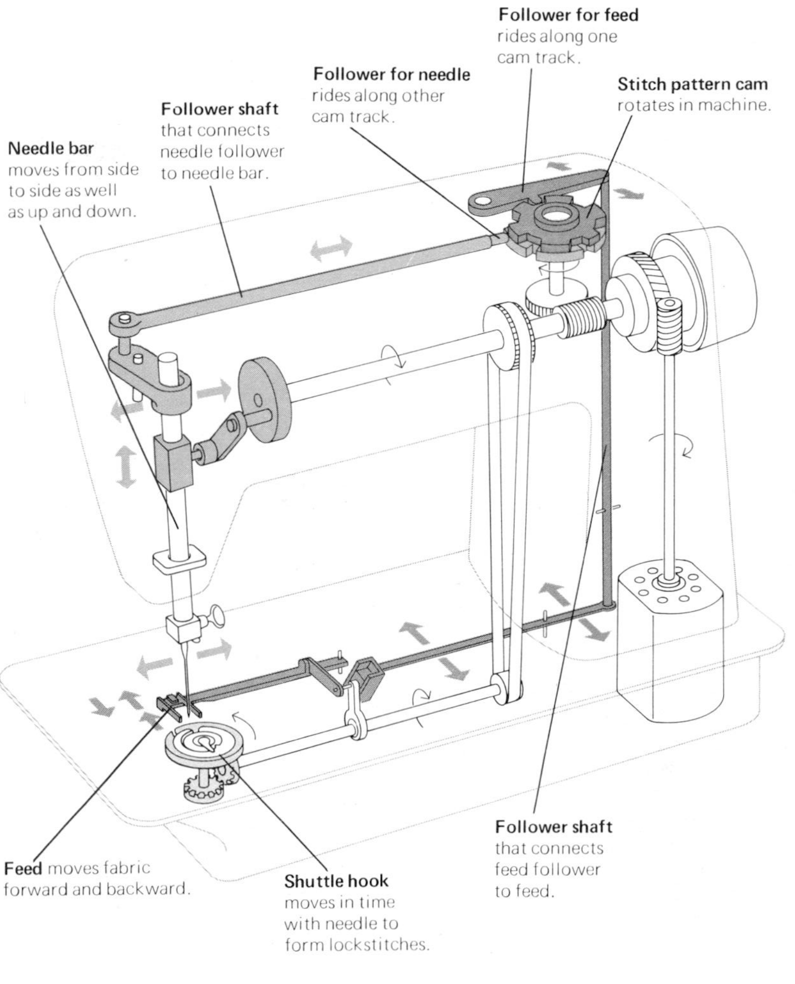
Follower for feed rides along one cam track.
Follower for needle rides along other cam track.
Stitch pattern cam rotates in machine.
Follower shaft that connects needle follower to needle bar.
Needle bar moves from side to side as well as up and down.
Follower shaft that connects feed follower to feed.
Feed moves fabric forward and backward.
Shuttle hook moves in time with needle to form lockstitches.

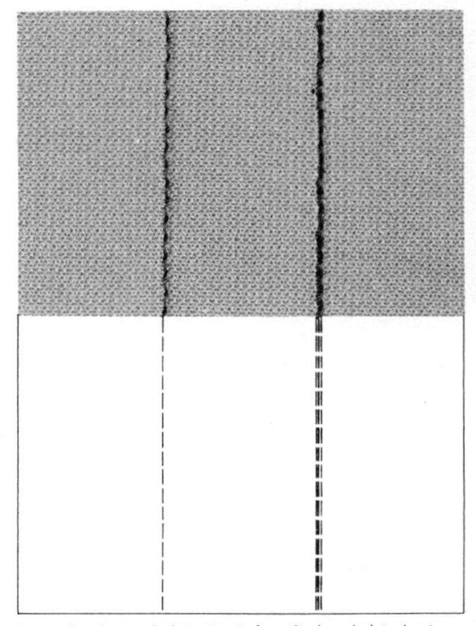

A typical straight stretch stitch, right, is two stitches forward and one reverse, putting three stitches in one place. Plain straight stitch, left, forms one stitch in each place.

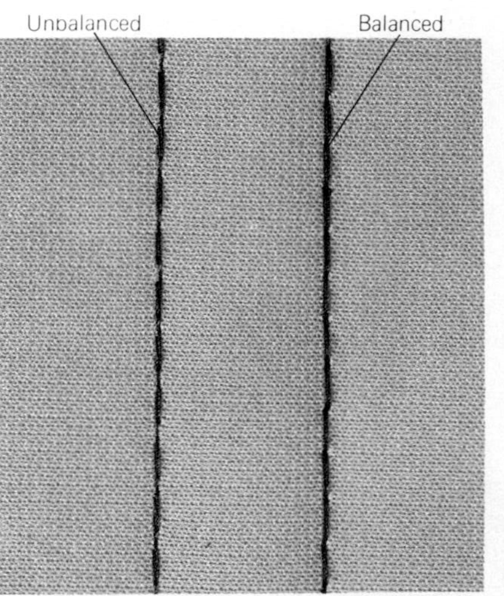
Unbalanced
Balanced

A pattern balance control (see machine booklet) helps to equalize slight length differences that can result between stitches sewed forward and backward in stretch stitch patterns.

Overedge seams 151
Topstitching 152
Abutted seams 153
Bound edges 302-303

Length and width in stretch stitching

Most stretch stitches look best sewed at the length and width recommended by the machine manufacturer, but they can usually be modified. Only certain patterns are approved for use, at "O" width setting, as a straight stretch stitch (see machine booklet). This is because, unlike others, they produce neither too much nor too little thread buildup in the seam.

Featherstitch set at recommended length and width; sewed at a longer stitch length and a narrower width; sewed at shorter stitch length but at a wider width; at recommended length, but "O" width (straight stretch stitch).

Alternatives to stretch stitches

Straight and zigzag stitches, used in a certain way, can sometimes substitute for stretch stitches. In some applications, they may even be better. A stretch stitch might, for example, be somewhat heavy for a very soft, lightweight stretchy fabric. The examples below show the plain and overedge stretch stitches used in seams and substitutes for them.

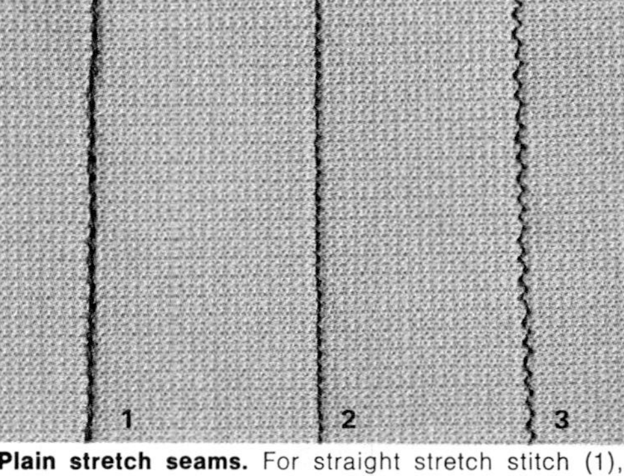

Plain stretch seams. For straight stretch stitch (1), substitute a short straight stitch (2), stretching fabric as you stitch; or (3) a narrow, short zigzag.

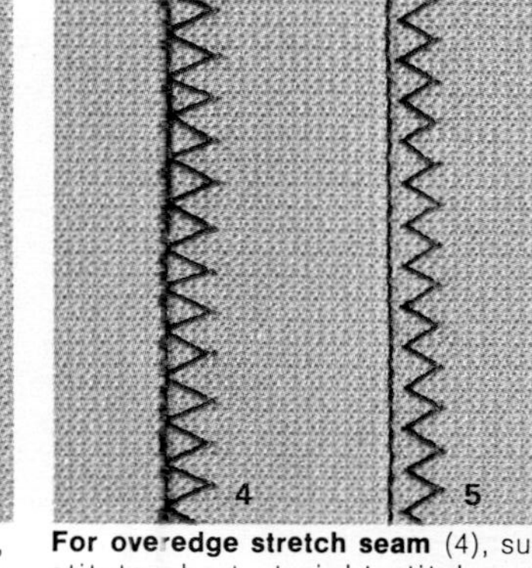
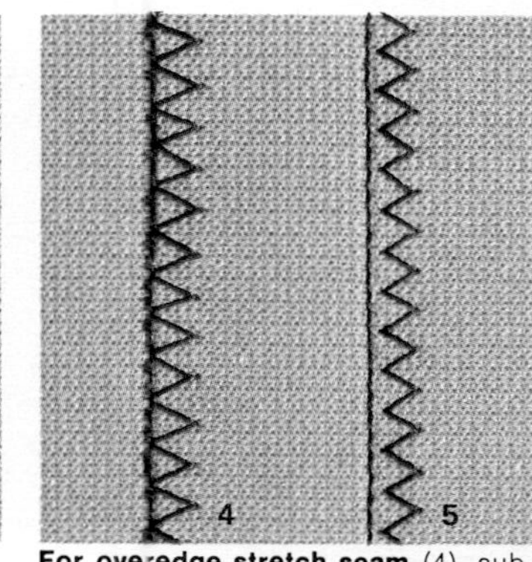

For overedge stretch seam (4), substitute short straight stitches on seamline (5), with zigzag next to that.

Using stretch stitches

As shown in the stitching sample at the right, stretch stitches can be decorative as well as functional, and some patterns can be both. The first row shows the *straight stretch* stitch, which is used for seaming. Next to that is a *rickrack* stitch, used most often for topstitching, but usable also on a lapped seam. The next example is the *featherstitch;* although topstitched onto this sample, this stitch is ideal for a fagotted seam.

The two rows that follow are stretch stitches used for *overedge stretch* seams. After these come three rows of decorative stitches, all *topstitched* here—the first two with a *single needle,* the third with a *twin needle.* A familiar motif, the Greek key, is next used to stitch an *abutted seam.* The final example is again topstitching, this time to a *bound edge.*

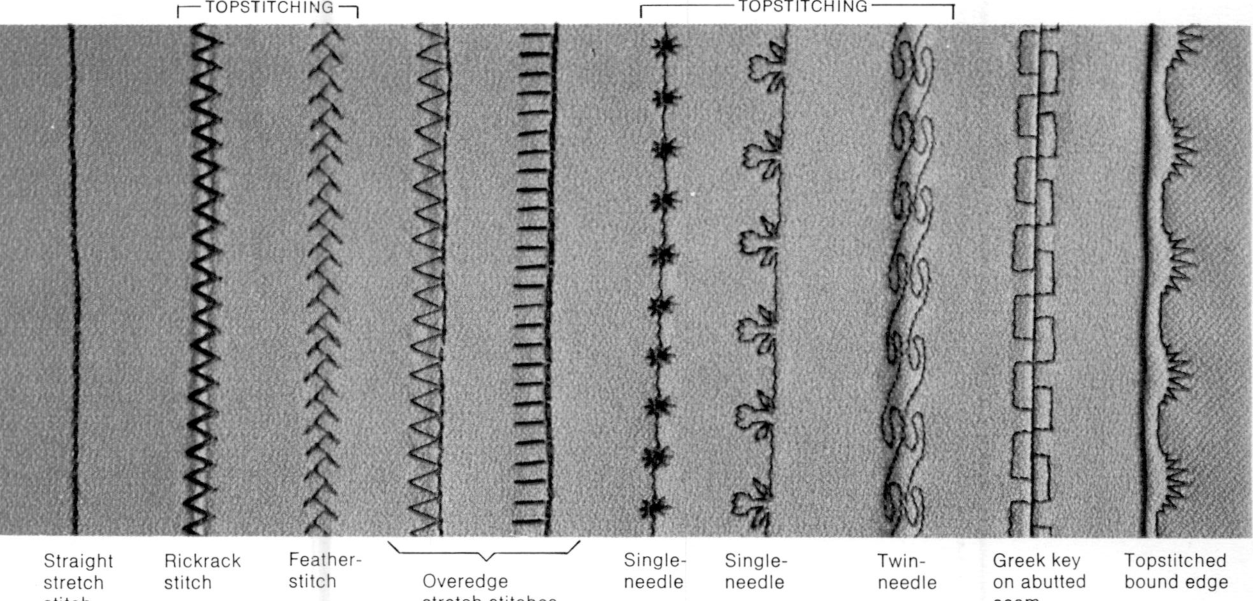

Sewing machine

Accessories

Shown below and opposite are additional accessories designed to increase a sewing machine's versatility and efficiency. Most of them take the form of variations on the presser foot, but the group also includes stitch pattern cams, special-purpose attachments, and stitching guides and gauges. The accessories illustrated are a representative collection of those that are available. The names given to them may vary. Also, some manufacturers may combine several features into one foot, e.g., a buttonhole foot that can also be used for stitching over cord. It should not be assumed that all the accessories shown are available for all machines, or that they are interchangeable from one machine to another. To learn what attachments are available for your machine, and how to use them, consult machine instruction book.

When using any type of presser foot, it is important to know what stitch can be sewed with it. This depends upon the needle hole. If it is small and round, the foot can be used only for straight stitching; if the hole is wide, the foot can be used for straight and zigzag stitching. The same is true for throat plates—use the straight stitch throat plate (small hole) for straight stitching, the zigzag throat plate (wide hole) for zigzag (and straight stitching as well). For multiple-needle work, foot and throat plate must have wide needle holes.

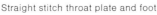

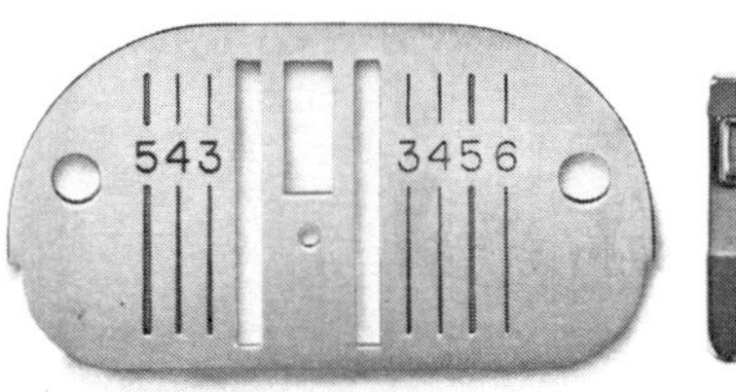

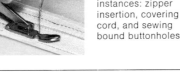

Straight stitch throat plate and foot

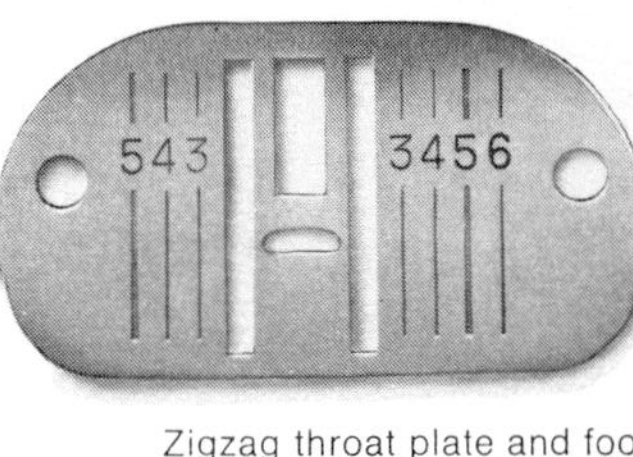

Zigzag throat plate and foot

Straight stitch foot is the best one to use when doing single-needle straight stitching. It is a narrow foot; one toe is slimmer than the other.

Zipper foot is used to stitch any seam with more bulk on one side than the other. Examples of such instances: zipper insertion, covering cord, and sewing bound buttonholes.

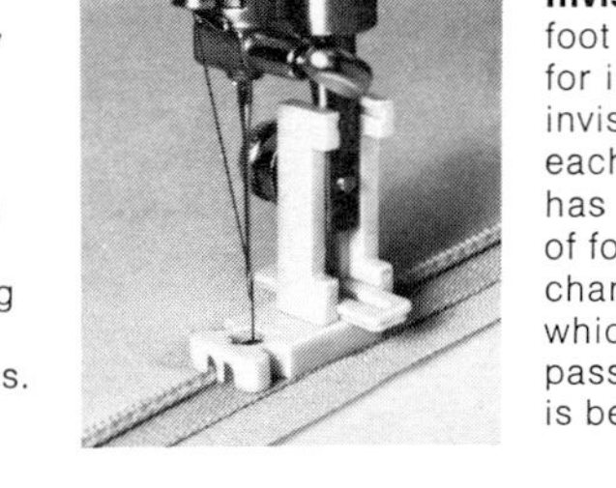
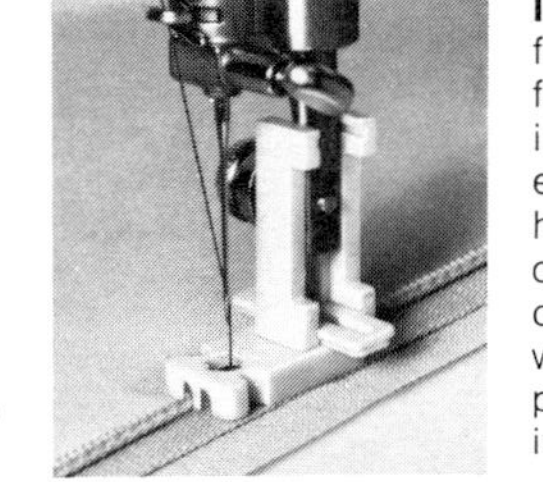
Invisible zipper foot is used only for insertion of invisible zippers; each zipper brand has its own. Bottom of foot has two channels through which zipper coils pass while zipper is being stitched.

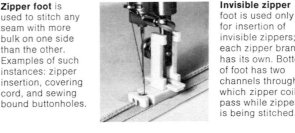

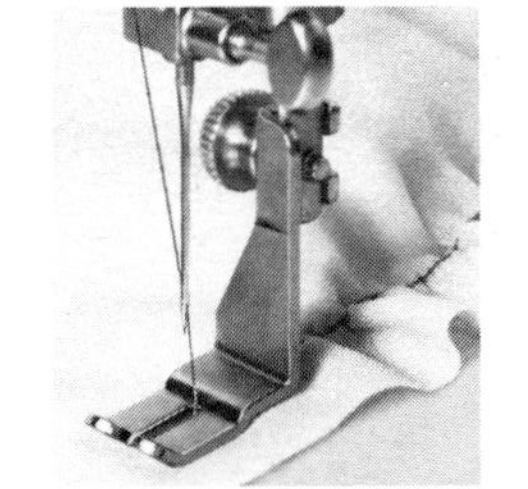
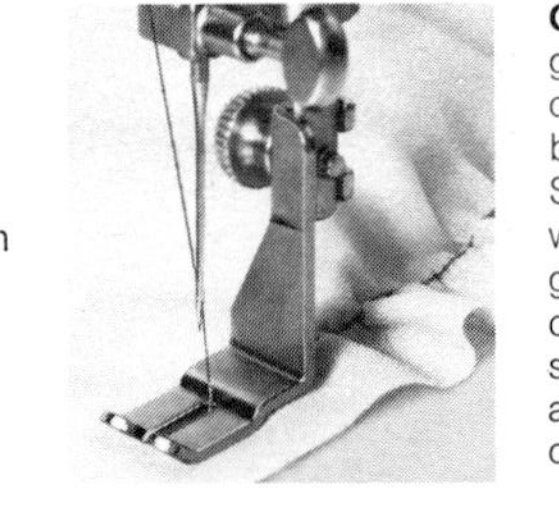
Gathering foot gathers up a length of fabric as it is being stitched. Some gathering feet will simultaneously gather one layer of fabric while stitching it to another flat piece of fabric.

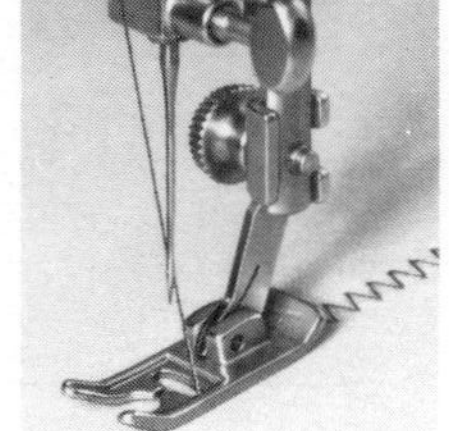
Zigzag foot, often referred to as an all-purpose foot is used primarily for plain zigzag stitching but can also be used for straight stitching.

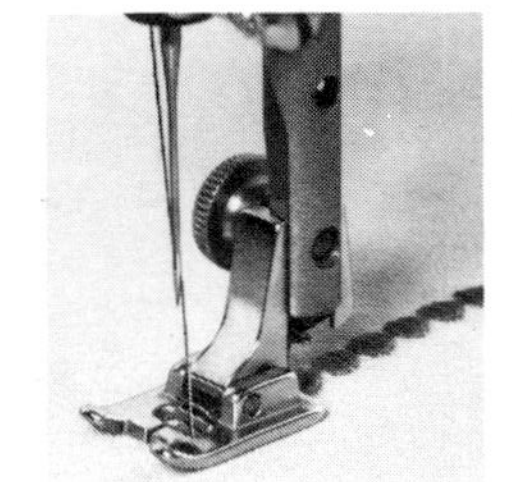
Embroidery foot is best for stitching decorative stitch patterns. Bottom of this foot is grooved to create a shallow "tunnel" that permits the dense stitching to pass easily under the foot.

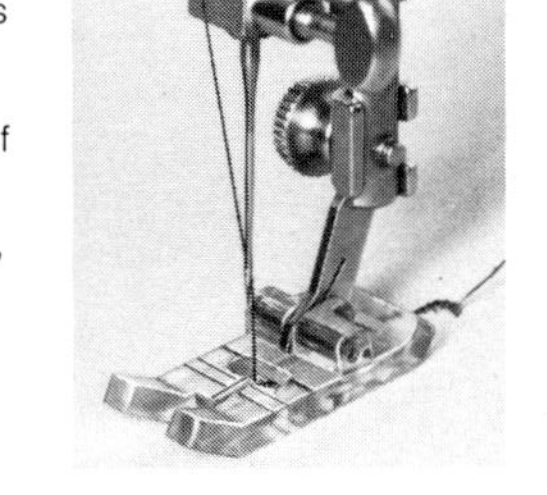
Buttonhole foot is used when stitching machine-worked buttonholes. It may be of metal or see-through plastic. Guidelines are usually etched into foot to help with stitch placement.

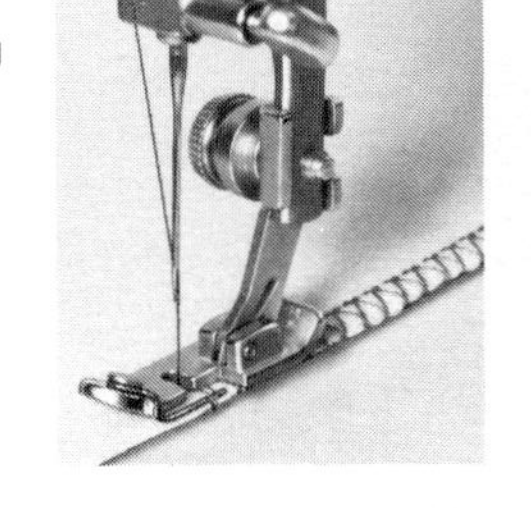
Overedge foot is designed to be placed along a fabric edge so that the stitches will fall over the edge of the fabric. A metal bar holds edge in place so stitches will set properly.

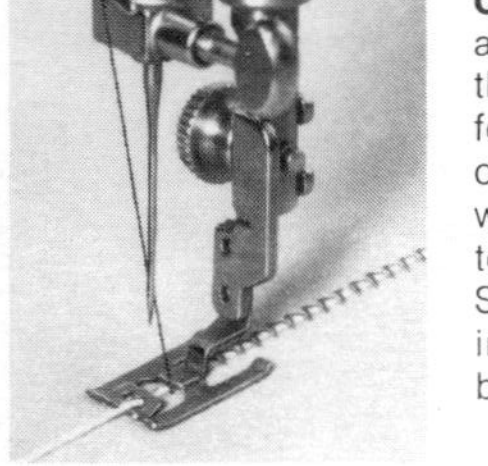
Cording foot has a built-in device that provides for a steady supply of cord to be fed with and attached to the fabric. Sometimes incorporated into buttonhole foot.

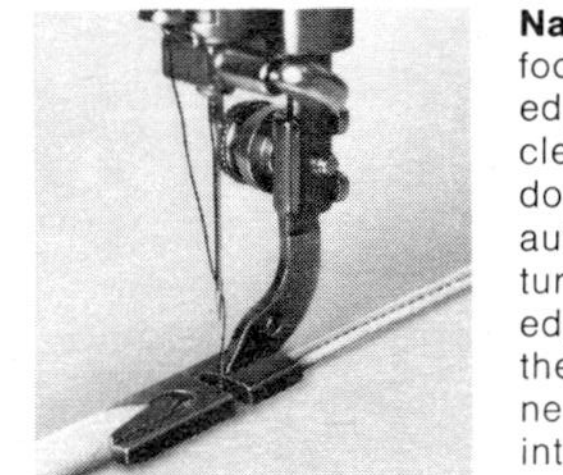
Narrow hemmer foot allows a raw edge of fabric to be clean-finished. It does this by automatically turning under the edge, which is then fed under the needle and stitched into place.

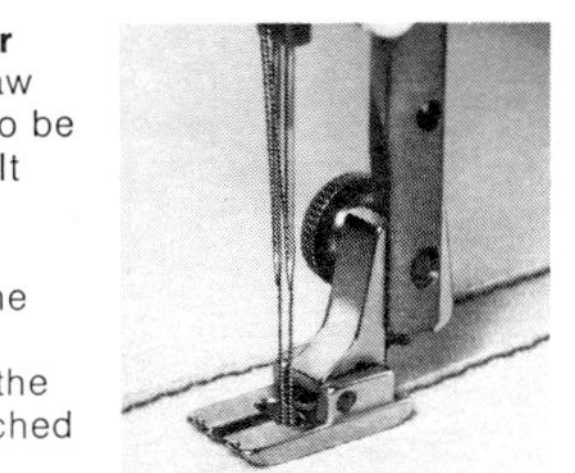
Pin tuck foot, with the aid of a twin needle, will form small pin tucks. These are sometimes called air tucks.

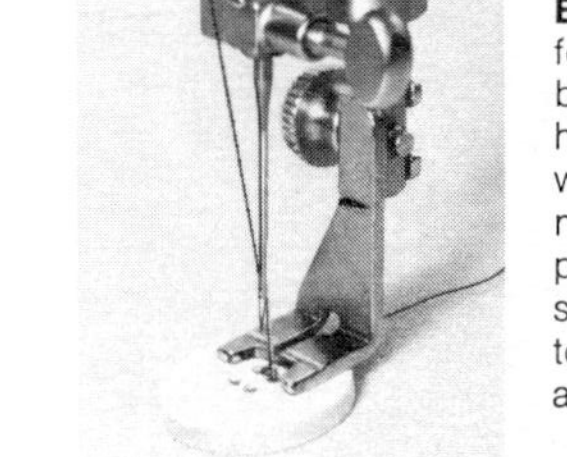
Button foot is used for sewing on buttons. Usually has a groove into which toothpick or needle is inserted, permitting the stitches also to be the basis of a thread shank.

Stitching accessories

The accessories described below are typical of auxiliary units that can increase a machine's stitching capabilities, or help to speed completion of large sewing jobs. The stitch pattern cams manipulate the action of the needle, and sometimes the feed, to produce intricate stitching designs. The chainstitch attachments permit stitch formation by the top thread alone (as compared to the usual machine stitch, the lockstitch, which uses both top and bottom threads for each stitch). The other attachments—the buttonholers, the ruffler, and the binder—utilize the machine's basic capabilities to complete particular jobs fast and accurately.

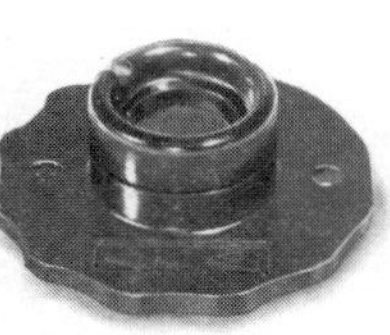

Stitch pattern cams, inserted into the machine, produce various stitch patterns.

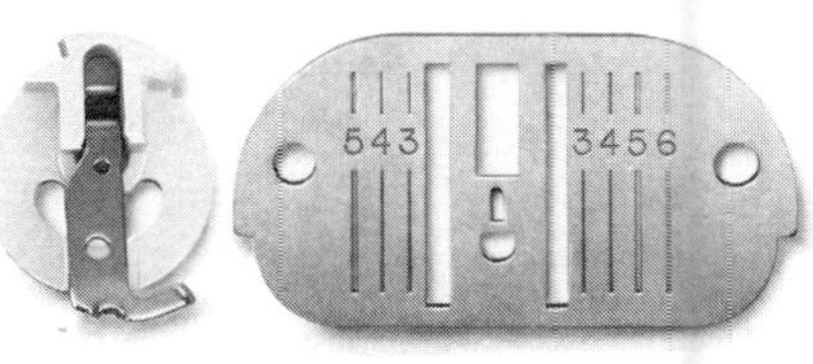

Chainstitch attachments permit just the top thread to form a continuous row of stitches.

Most buttonhole attachments require special cams to produce the buttonholes.

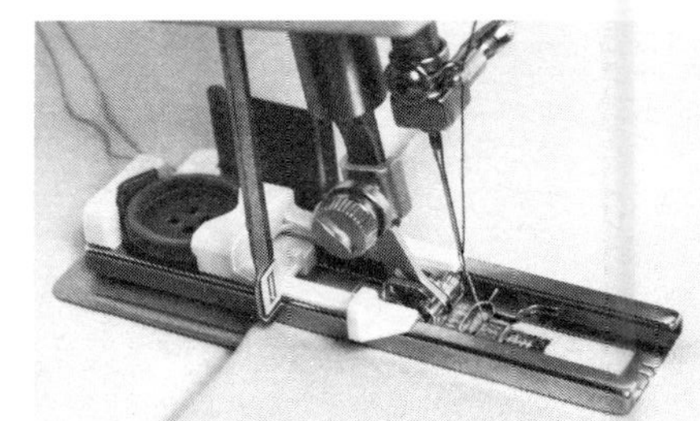

This buttonholer stitches buttonhole of the correct size for button in the attachment.

The ruffler attachment will quickly gather up a length of material. It is especially helpful with home decorating projects.

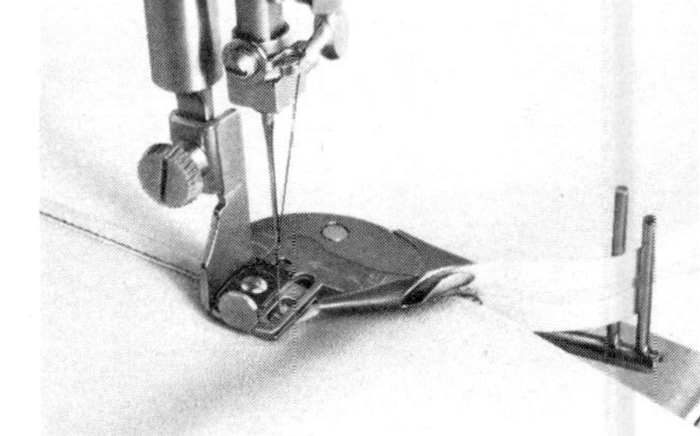

The binder positions the fabric and binding so that they can simultaneously be fed under the needle and stitched together.

Feed-related accessories

For proper stitching, fabric layers should move evenly together under the presser foot. Even feeding can be difficult, however, with some fabrics. To help with such feed problems, there are "top feed" assists that supply auxiliary grasping action on fabrics, especially the top layer.

For some sewing jobs, the action of the feed should be disengaged. Two such "no feed" situations are sewing on buttons and free-motion sewing.

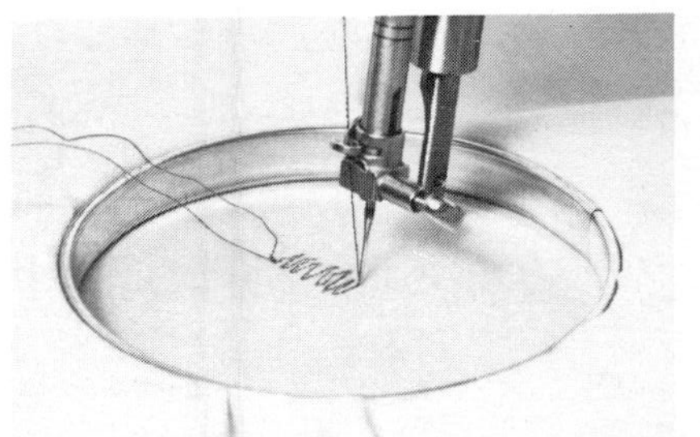

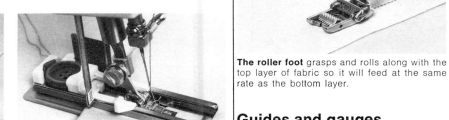

Hoop holds fabric taut for free-motion sewing. For this process, feed is disengaged.

The roller foot grasps and rolls along with the top layer of fabric so it will feed at the same rate as the bottom layer.

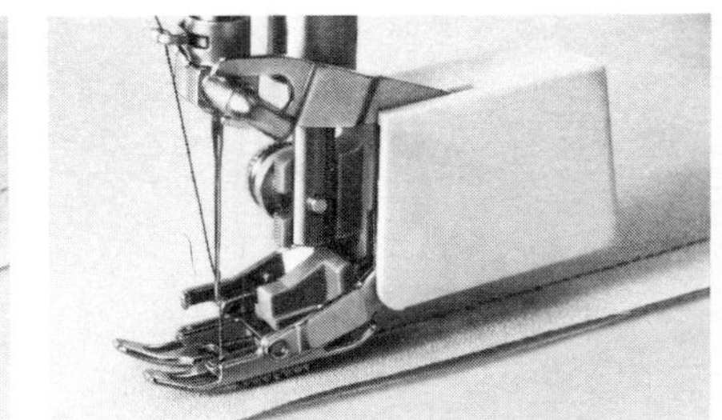

Another "top feed" assist attachment is synchronized with needle and feed to help both of the fabric layers to feed evenly.

Guides and gauges

Among the most useful supplements to the sewing machine are the gauges that help you to stitch a consistent distance from an edge or another line.

Another valuable aid is the guide that is used when blind-hemming by machine. It holds both garment and hem edge in place for stitching.

Seam gauge is attached to the machine bed, then adjusted to be a specific distance from needle.

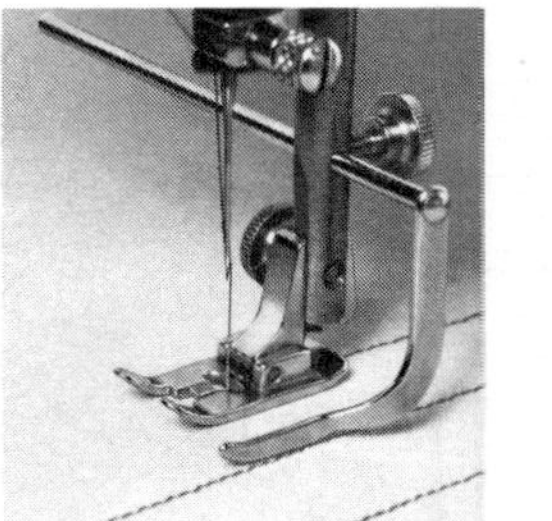
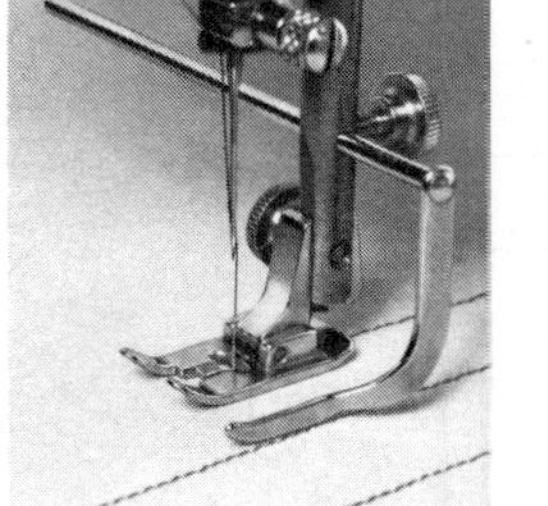

Quilter guide-bar extends out from foot to fall along a guiding line.

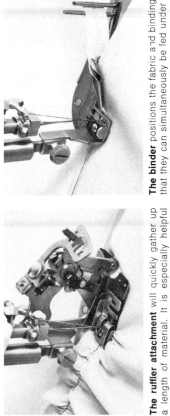

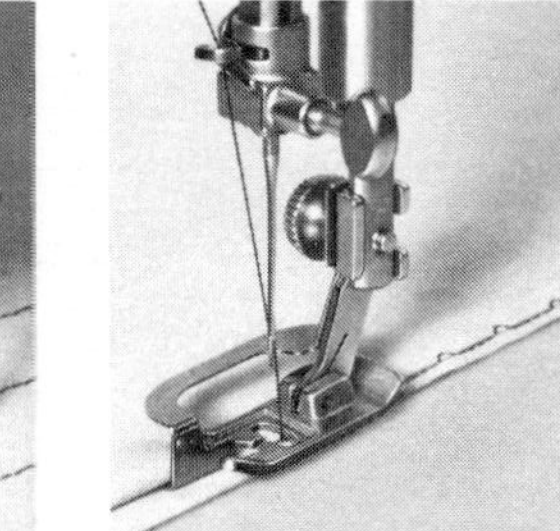

Blind-hemming guide is attached to foot to hold garment and hem in place.

Sewing machine

Solving common machine problems

BOBBIN (outside winding)

Does not wind
1. Make sure the thread is caught around the bobbin and in the proper direction. (If bobbin winds vertically, thread should be winding over top of bobbin from front to back; if it winds horizontally, thread should be coming in a clockwise direction around the bobbin back.)
2. Check to see that the bobbin is placed correctly on the winding spindle. (Some bobbin winders have a notch that must be fitted into a groove in the bobbin.)
3. Bobbin winding mechanism may not be set properly for winding. Check instruction booklet.
4. Rubber friction ring may be worn. It is replaceable. In the meantime, you can hold the bobbin winder spindle against the handwheel with a finger (if location of bobbin spindle makes this possible).

Winds unevenly
1. Thread may not be inserted in the thread guides and/or bobbin-winding tension spring.
2. You may be running the machine too fast.
3. The tension spring may need adjusting. With some models, you can do this yourself (see instruction booklet for further details); with other models service is required. **(S)** In the meantime, run the machine slowly and, using thumb and index finger, guide the thread from side to side.

During winding, needle moves up and down
1. Needle has not been disengaged. On most machines, this is done by turning the knob (flywheel) located in the center of the handwheel; on some machines, a lever must be released. See instruction booklet.
2. If knob or lever has been released, and needle still moves, the handwheel bearing probably needs oil. **(S)**
3. The problem need not cause immediate concern as it does the machine no harm (provided needle is undamaged and unthreaded).

BOBBIN (inside winding)

Does not wind
1. Power may not be on.
2. Check whether the thread has failed to catch, or perhaps the thread is broken.
3. Thread end may not be fastened to foot screw.
4. Winding mechanism may not be engaged.
5. Needle may not be threaded, or the machine may be threaded incorrectly.
6. Machine settings may be wrong for winding. Check machine instruction booklet.

Winds unevenly
1. Machine settings may not be correct.
2. Machine may not be threaded correctly.
3. Machine may be operating too fast.

Thread breaks
1. Machine may be operating too fast.
2. Settings may be incorrect.
3. Machine and/or needle may be threaded improperly.
4. Check for nicks on bobbin, throat plate, and/or needle. Replace damaged parts.
5. Needle may be hitting foot or throat plate.

Thread snarls during winding
1. Bobbin (two-piece type) may be improperly screwed together.
2. Winding procedure may be incorrect.
3. Machine settings and threading may be incorrect.
4. Thread end may not be caught properly. Start over, taking care to secure thread end properly when starting.

FABRIC

Layers feed unevenly
1. Presser foot pressure may be too heavy or too light.
2. You may need to stitch more slowly or apply surface tension.
3. It usually helps to place pins horizontally across the seam every 3 to 4 inches. It is best to remove each pin as you come to it, especially with heavy fabric; on medium to lightweight fabric, you can stitch over the pins.
4. With sticky or very lightweight fabrics, use tissue paper when stitching.
5. There are attachments that help maintain even feed on all fabric types, including piles and slippery materials.
6. For straight stitching, use both the straight stitch foot and throat plate if possible.

Does not feed in a straight line
1. Presser foot may be loose.
2. Presser foot could be bent. It may be possible to straighten it, but a new one is not expensive, and would probably be better.
3. Presser foot pressure may be too light or too heavy.
4. Needle may be bent.
5. There may be a defect in the machine feed. **(S)**
6. You may be pulling or pushing fabric to the point of interfering with machine feed.
7. For straight stitching, use both the straight stitch foot and throat plate if possible.

Puckers when stitched
1. Many fabrics pucker when stitched as a single layer.
2. If fabric is sheer, or very lightweight, the stitch length should not be too long. Also, pressure on the presser foot should be lessened.
3. If fabric is tightly woven or knitted, puckering is an indication that stitch length is too short.
4. Thread may be too thick for the fabric.
5. Needle may be too coarse for fabric.
6. Bobbin may be wound unevenly.
7. Stitch tension may be unbalanced.
8. If fabric is a lightweight stretchy knit, apply some surface tension.
9. If doing straight stitching, use both the straight stitch foot and throat plate.
10. If all adjustments fail, feed dog could be out of sync. **(S)**

Shows feed marks on the underside
1. Presser foot pressure may be too heavy.
2. If fabric still marks with pressure lessened, place tissue paper between the fabric and the feed.
3. The feed may be damaged or set too high. **(S)**

Is damaged (snagged or has holes around stitches)
1. Needle may be blunt or burred, too coarse for the fabric, or the wrong type of point for the fabric.
2. Check for a burr on the foot or feed or a nick in the throat plate—especially at needle hole. Replace damaged parts.

MACHINE

Motor does not run
1. Cord is not plugged in or is not plugged into a live outlet.
2. Power switch (present on some newer machines) is turned off.
3. Knee or foot accelerator may be jammed or improperly attached to power source.
4. If none of the foregoing solves the problem, there may be a loose or broken wire in the knee or foot accelerator, or other part of the electrical system. **(S)**

Motor runs, but handwheel does not turn
Thread or lint may be caught or tangled in the bobbin case area. It can usually be loosened by turning the handwheel back and forth a few times. If this does not work, remove the throat plate, bobbin, and case, and pick the thread or lint out with tweezers. When thread or lint has been removed, put a drop of machine oil in the bobbin case housing and run the machine for a few minutes without thread or fabric. This will loosen any remaining lint or other dirt. Clean oiled area with lint brush or cotton swab. To keep thread from jamming the bobbin, remove fabric immediately if machine stalls.

Motor runs, handwheel turns, but needle does not move
1. The needle may have been disengaged for bobbin winding and not tightened back to sewing position.
2. If needle has been tightened but still does not move, the motor belt is slipping because it is loose or worn. **(S)**

Motor, handwheel, and needle move, but fabric does not feed
1. Make sure the presser foot is down.
2. Check the stitch length regulator. It may be set at zero.
3. The pressure regulator may be at zero or "darn" position. It should be set for at least light pressure. If fabric is heavy, more pressure may be necessary for fabric to feed.
4. The feed dog may be in the lowered or "down" position.

Motor, handwheel, needle, and fabric move, but no stitch is formed
1. Thread may have come out of the needle.
2. Needle may be threaded in the wrong direction.
3. Needle may be inserted backward or may not be pushed all the way up into the clamp.
4. Needle may be the wrong length for the machine. Most fairly recent machines—manufactured over the past twenty years—take a standard-length needle (called a 15x1). Some older machines, however, require a special length. You must find a supplier for these.
5. Machine may be threaded incorrectly.
6. Bobbin may be empty.
7. Bobbin and/or case may be inserted incorrectly.
8. The timing of the machine might be off. **(S)**

Runs sluggishly
1. Bobbin winder may still be engaged.
2. Knee or foot control might be improperly positioned.
3. Machine may be in need of oiling and/or cleaning.
4. Motor belt may be worn. **(S)**
5. Electrical control may have a loose wire or need adjusting. **(S)**

Runs noisily
1. Machine probably needs oiling and/or cleaning.
2. The needle could be bent and hitting against foot or throat plate.
3. Bobbin and/or case may not be in tight enough.
4. Bobbin may be almost out of thread.

(S) signifies need for professional service.

Will not stitch in reverse
1. If machine is very old, it may not have this capability.
2. If it is a recent model, check the stitch control. It may be set for "stretch stitch" or "buttonhole"; sometimes these stitches cannot be reversed manually.

NEEDLE

Unthreads
1. Insufficient thread may have been pulled through the needle before the seam was started.
2. Machine may be out of top thread.

Breaks
1. You may be using the incorrect presser foot and/or throat plate for the stitch (e.g., using straight stitch foot and throat plate for a zigzag stitch).
2. Presser foot and/or throat plate may be loose or improperly fastened.
3. Needle might have become bent and hit the presser foot and/or throat plate.
4. Needle may be incorrectly inserted.
5. Needle might be too fine for the fabric being sewed and for the job being done.
6. You may have pulled too hard on fabric while stitching.
7. Check machine settings. They may be wrong or have been accidentally changed during stitching.
8. Needle may be defective.

PRESSURE REGULATOR

Hard to adjust
1. Presser foot may not have been lowered before change was made in the pressure setting.
2. Pressure regulator may be turned to its maximum. Try turning the other way. If this doesn't work, regulator may need a servicing. **(S)**

SLIDE PLATE

Falls off
1. Plate may have been inserted incorrectly.
2. The spring that holds plate in place may be bent or broken. If it is bent, you may be able to re-shape it. If broken, take it to a sewing machine dealer and order a new one.
3. Always remember to close the plate before lowering the machine into the cabinet.

STITCHES

Are uneven lengths
1. You might be pushing or pulling the fabric too much.
2. Pressure on the presser foot could be either too light or too heavy for the fabric.
3. There could be lint or other clog between the teeth of the feed dog.
4. The problem may actually be skipped stitches.

Have loops between them
1. If the loops are *large*, the machine is improperly threaded. Loops on the underside of fabric indicate that thread is not properly seated between the tension discs on the machine's upper portion. Loops on top of the fabric are the result of the bobbin thread's not being properly inserted into the bobbin case.
2. If loops are *small*, tensions are unbalanced. If loops are on the fabric's underside, tighten upper tension (or loosen lower if the instruction booklet specifies a way of doing it). If loops are on the top, loosen the upper tension (or tighten bobbin tension if this is possible).
3. Bobbin may be wound unevenly.
4. There may not be enough pressure to hold the fabric taut during stitch formation.
5. Problem could be timing, or some adjustment that would require a service call. **(S)**

Skip here and there
1. The most common cause of skipped stitches is the wrong type or size of needle for the fabric being sewed.
2. Needle may be blunt or bent.
3. Needle may be inserted backward or it might not be all the way up into the clamp.
4. Even if you detect nothing wrong with the needle, it may have accumulated lint or sizing from the fabric. This can happen with certain synthetics and permanent press fabrics, or in stitching through adhesives. Clean the needle, or change it.
5. There may be insufficient pressure on the presser foot.
6. Throat plate may be wrong for the purpose.
7. You may be stitching at an uneven speed.
8. While stitching, you may be pulling too hard on the fabric.

Break or "pop" in knit or other stretch fabric
1. Stretch fabrics require a "stretchable" thread. Use silk, synthetic, or cotton-wrapped synthetic.
2. If you are using one of these threads, and stitches still break, try stretching the fabric slightly as you stitch.
3. Stitch length and/or tension may be wrong.
4. If your machine has a stretch stitch, try that.

Zigzag stitches draw in the fabric, or cause it to ripple
1. Tension is probably too tight. Less tension is required for most zigzag stitching.
2. Fabric may be too sheer or lightweight for the width of your stitch. Use a backing fabric or narrower width.
3. Stitching may be too unbalanced.
4. Pressure may be too light or too heavy.
5. Zigzag may be totally wrong for the fabric. Try another type of stitch.

TENSION

Does not seem to hold an adjustment
1. A tension spring may be worn loose after many years of machine use. It is replaceable. **(S)** (One way to reduce wear on the tension spring is never to pull thread through the tension discs when presser foot is down.)
2. Timing could be off. **(S)**
3. Bobbin may be unevenly wound.

THREAD

Snarls at beginning of seam
1. Thread and/or fabric are probably pulled down into bobbin area. To release snarl, turn handwheel back and forth a few times to loosen caught material, then remove it and resume stitching. Snarls at the start can usually be prevented by placing needle in fabric before lowering presser foot and taking care to have both threads under the presser foot and drawn diagonally to the rear. Hold thread ends for the first few stitches. (On very soft or slippery fabrics, it is best not to backstitch.)
2. The machine may be improperly threaded.
3. You may be using the wrong throat plate, i.e., one with too large a hole for delicate or lightweight fabrics.

Snarls during stitching
1. Lint from the bobbin area may be caught in the stitching. Clean the bobbin area.
2. Bobbin thread may be running out. Replace with full bobbin.
3. Problem may be improper top or bottom threading and/or tension.
4. You may be using the wrong throat plate.
5. Timing may be off. **(S)**

Snarls at end of seam
1. Fabric and thread are being pushed into the bobbin area and are knotting. Turn the handwheel back and forth a few times to loosen; then remove snarl.
2. As a general rule, it is not good practice to stitch off the fabric—the threads can become knotted in the bobbin area.

Needle thread breaks
1. Usually this is caused by the needle being inserted backward or threaded backward.
2. Thread may be caught in the spool notch or it could be wrapped around the spindle.
3. There may be a rough or burred place on a thread guide, the presser foot, the needle eye, or throat plate hole. Replace damaged parts.
4. The needle may be blunt.
5. Needle may not be all the way up into the clamp.
6. Needle may be too fine for the thread, causing it to fray—often the case with silk buttonhole twist.
7. Thread might be old and dried out—silk and cotton tend to become brittle with age.
8. A knot may have formed in the thread, preventing it from traveling through one of the thread guides or the needle eye.

Bobbin thread breaks
1. Bobbin case may not be threaded properly and/or the case not inserted properly.
2. Bobbin may be too full.
3. Check for dirt or clog in the bobbin case.
4. Hole in the throat plate may be rough, making it necessary to replace the throat plate.
5. Bobbin tension may be too tight.
6. The bobbin or bobbin case could be damaged. **(S)**

Bobbin thread cannot be raised through hole in throat plate
1. Bobbin case may be improperly threaded, or it may not have been properly inserted.
2. Thread end coming out of bobbin case may not be long enough to pull up. Several inches should always be allowed.
3. Go through all threading and insertion steps more deliberately to be sure you are taking each one correctly. To raise bobbin thread, needle thread should be held taut, handwheel turned, then end of bobbin thread pulled free when loop appears.

(S) signifies need for professional service.

Sewing area

Providing the basic necessities

Fortunately for those who have little space to spare (which means most people), the necessities of sewing are actually very few, and can be accommodated in a relatively small area. The units illustrated below and on page 44 are doubly space-saving because they all serve more than one sewing purpose. And when they are closed, their sewing functions are concealed, and they become handsome additions to their surroundings. Each represents a type of convenience that is nationally available, as shown or in forms very similar.

To function efficiently, of course, the facilities that are provided must meet, or closely approximate, quite specific criteria.

Machine operation. The cabinet or other operating unit should be strong and steady, about 30 inches high, approximately 18 to 20 inches from front to back and 35 to 40 inches wide—enough space for machine and fabric.

Though a machine can simply rest on the surface, the ideal situation is like the one below, in which a recessed area is provided that exactly fits the base. If the cabinet also provides for machine storage, as this one does, so much the better. In the unit to its right on page 43, the machine fits conveniently on the lower shelf, and is concealed by the fold-down table when it is raised.

Fabric cutting and handling calls for a surface about 3 by 6 feet. If a working unit is built of components, like the one at the far right, the top can be made large enough for cutting. If a smaller surface must be used—or one not meant for cutting, such as a dining table or a bed—a cutting board is advisable. Besides providing efficiently for measuring, pinning, and cutting, the board will protect the surface beneath.

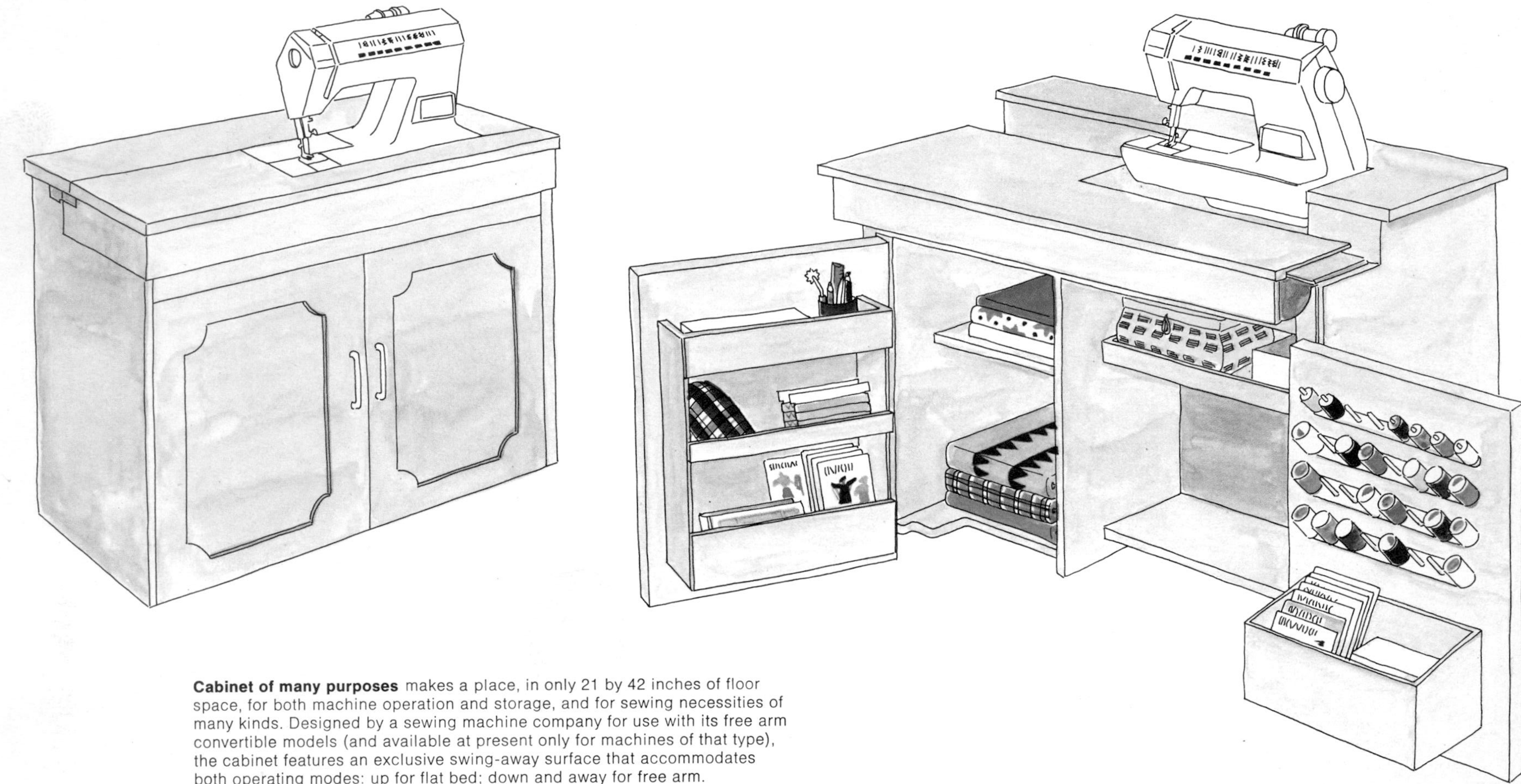

Cabinet of many purposes makes a place, in only 21 by 42 inches of floor space, for both machine operation and storage, and for sewing necessities of many kinds. Designed by a sewing machine company for use with its free arm convertible models (and available at present only for machines of that type), the cabinet features an exclusive swing-away surface that accommodates both operating modes: up for flat bed; down and away for free arm.

Sewing tools and supplies 8-17
Pressing equipment 18-19

Specialized storage. The important considerations here are appropriateness and accessibility. Broad shelves or shallow drawers are best for fabrics; patterns stay in better shape and are easiest to select if they are "filed" on end, with pattern numbers on top. Threads require spool holders, either built-in as in the cabinet on page 42, or the portable type that can be kept in a drawer or sewing box. Cutting and other sharp tools should be stored as you would good cutlery—so blades or points are protected, and you can reach what you need without risk or difficulty. Small items need organizing in a partitioned drawer or tray. Clear plastic units, preferably those that work like drawers, make it possible to see what is stored so you can pull out zippers or seam tapes without rummaging through the whole collection. If possible, separate books with vertical dividers.

Pressing equipment. Because pressing is important at every sewing stage, it is best if the board, iron, and special-purpose equipment are housed in or very near the sewing area. This is usually a question of available space; sometimes a closet can be partitioned to take the board and one of its shelves set aside for the rest. If the board must be kept elsewhere, look into the small portables you can set up on another surface.

Full-length mirror. Useful when taking measurements and at all fitting stages, a satisfactory mirror need not be expensive. Least conspicuous place for it: behind a closet door.

Dress form. To be truly useful, a dress form should be available for instant use. Check adjacent closets.

Lighting. Take advantage of natural daylight. Plan artificial light so that working areas are generously illuminated and shadow-free.

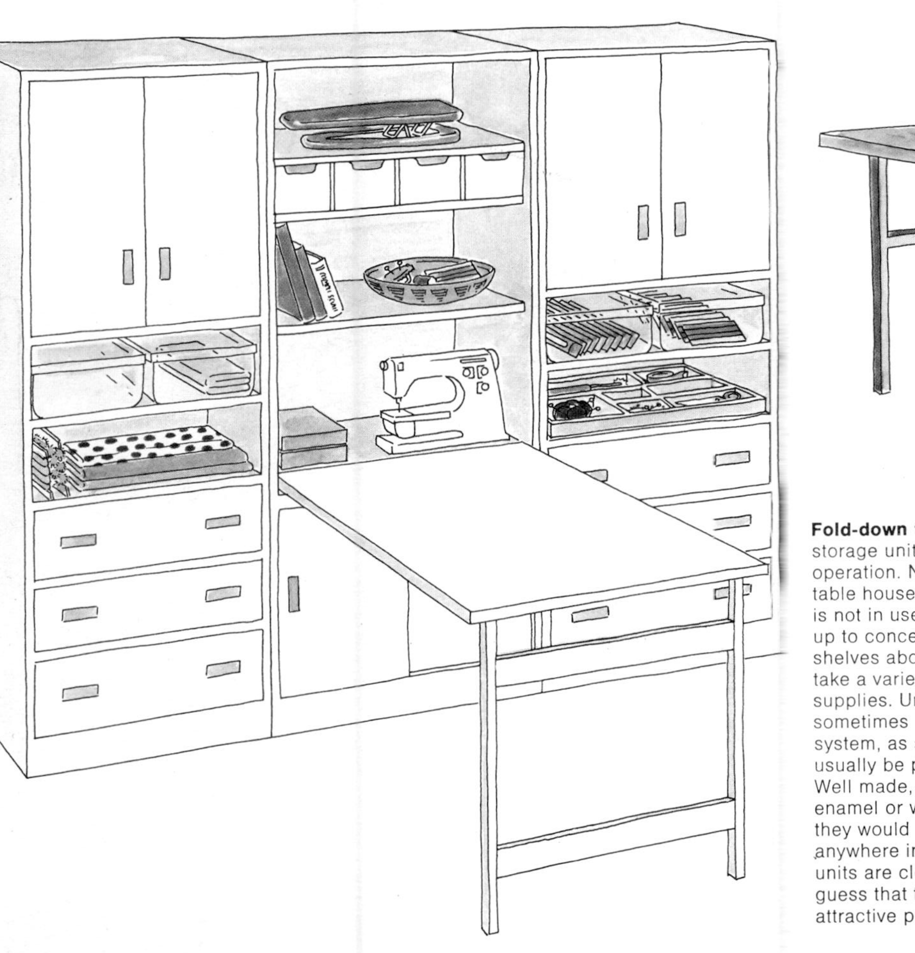

Fold-down table equips this storage unit for machine operation. Niche at far end of table houses machine when it is not in use; table folds back up to conceal it. Storage shelves above and cabinet below take a variety of tools and supplies. Units of this type are sometimes part of a modular system, as shown, but can usually be purchased separately. Well made, with handsome white enamel or wood grain finishes, they would be decorative assets anywhere in the house. When units are closed, no one would guess that they are anything but attractive pieces of furniture.

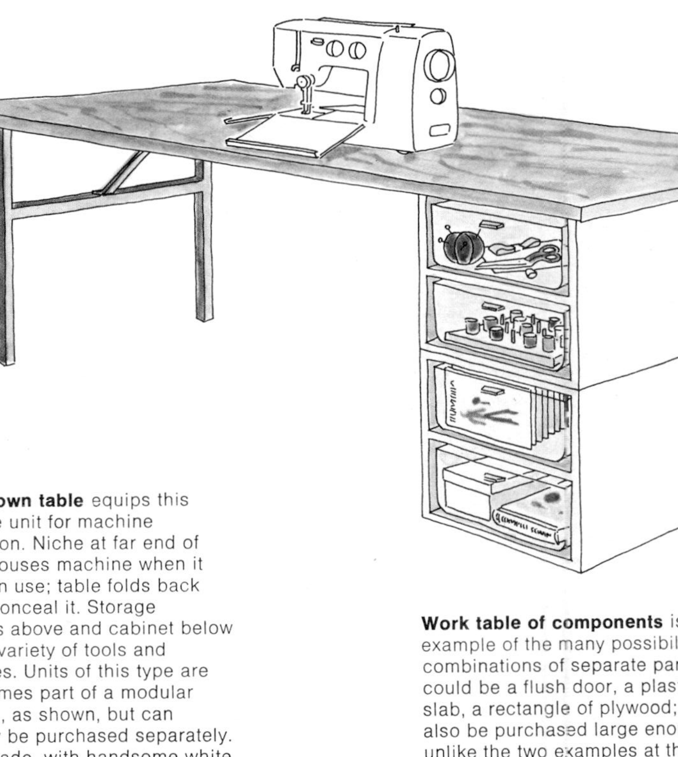

Work table of components is just one example of the many possibilities offered by combinations of separate parts. The top could be a flush door, a plastic-laminated slab, a rectangle of plywood; it could also be purchased large enough for cutting, unlike the two examples at the left. The storage units could also vary: both sides instead of one; stacked cubes as shown, a desk-type pedestal, or a modular base unit, perhaps bought unfinished and painted yourself. Legs, if they are used, should be well braced for steadiness.

Sewing area

Suiting storage to your needs

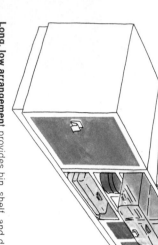

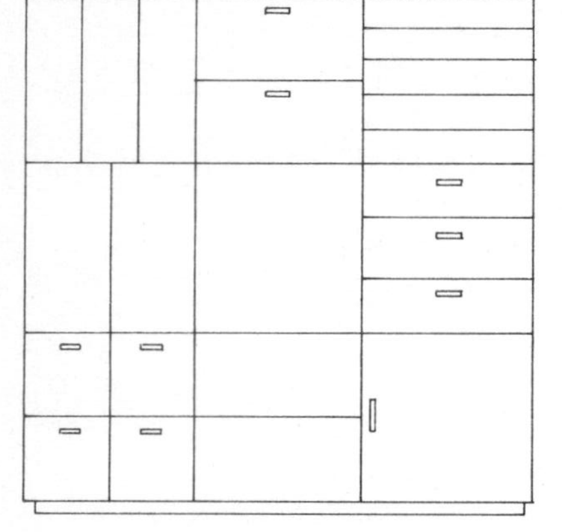

Sometimes supplementary storage is all a sewing area needs to function more efficiently. A practical solution is modular units based on the cube, and usually made of plastic, which can be chosen and arranged to suit your needs. Not all systems offer the same variations, but among the frequent possibilities are cubes with *dividers* that can be used horizontally or vertically; with *drawers* of different depths; with hinged *doors*.

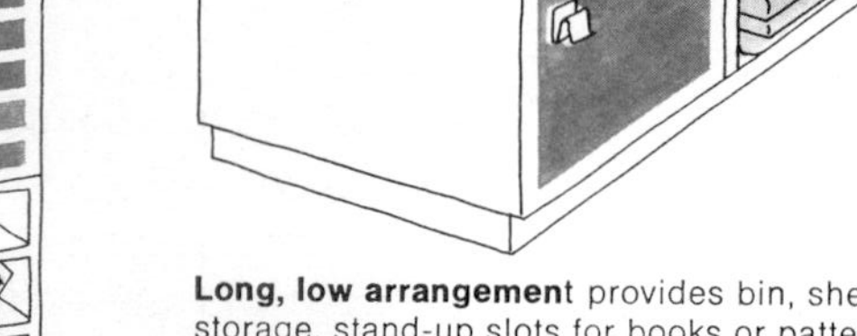

Long, low arrangement provides bin, shelf, and drawer storage, stand-up slots for books or patterns. Tops make a convenient surface for sorting and selecting.

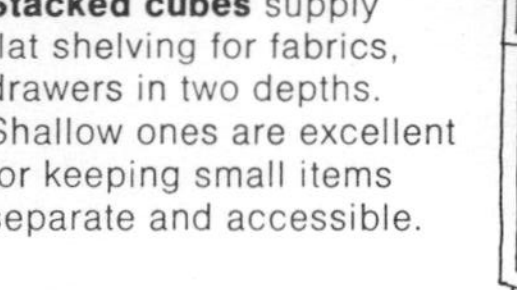

Stacked cubes supply flat shelving for fabrics, drawers in two depths. Shallow ones are excellent for keeping small items separate and accessible.

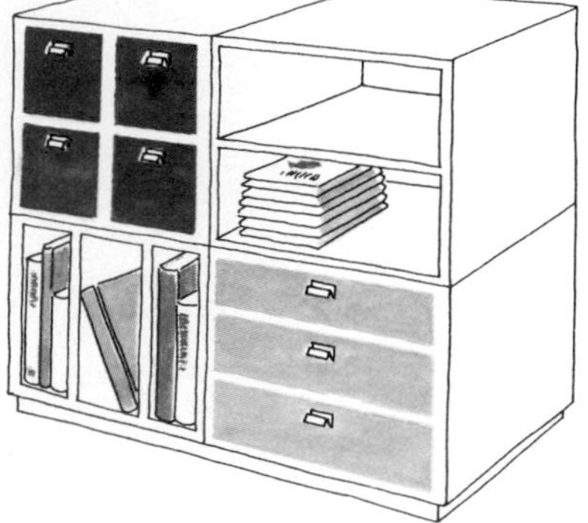

Cube combinations can be stacked to any desired height. If grouping will be free-standing, look for system that provides clips, pegs, or other means of holding the cubes together.

Unfinished furniture suppliers usually carry extensive lines of storage units, made to related heights, depths, and widths, that can be arranged in combinations like those on the left. The usual stacking procedure is shallower top units on deeper bases, similar in effect to a hutch cabinet. Though this method need not be followed, it is advisable, because it avoids the risk of the unit becoming dangerously top-heavy.

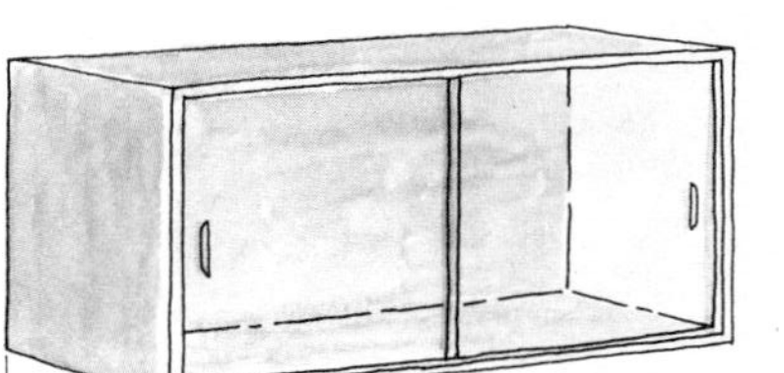

Glass sliding doors keep stored objects clean and visible.

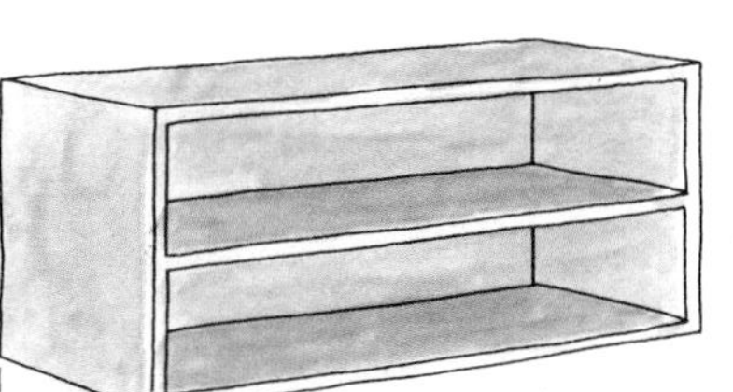

Horizontal divider creates flat, broad expanses for fabric.

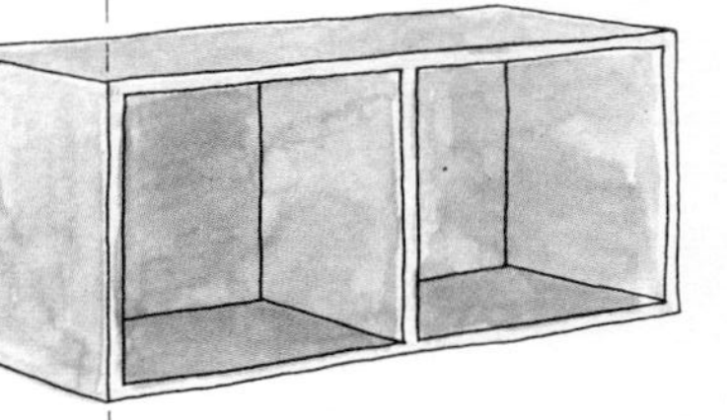

Vertical divider makes separate compartments for books, patterns.

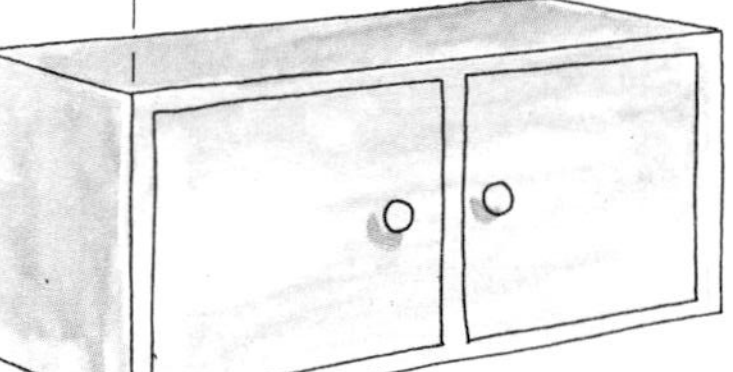

Opaque doors may be hinged, as shown, or the sliding type.

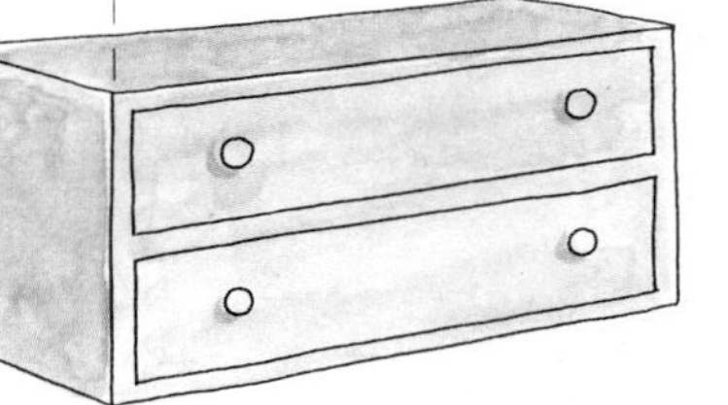

Drawers accommodate big items, can be divided for small ones.

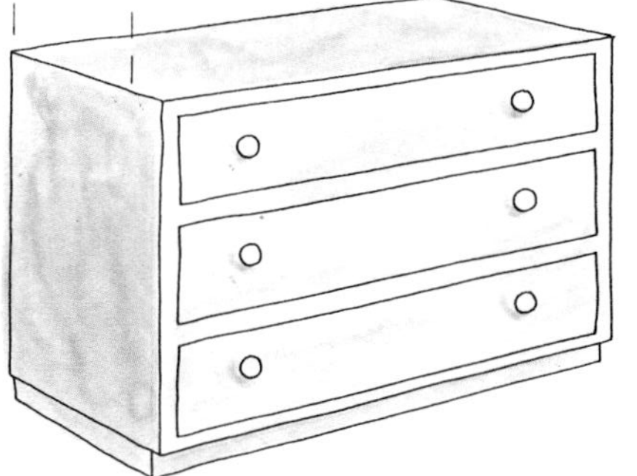

Deeper base units can be used alone or as a support for shallower top piece.

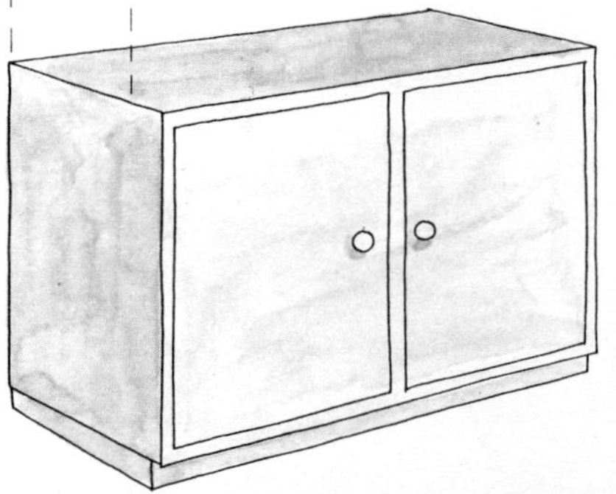

Hinged-door cabinet is another form of base unit, made to same dimensions.

Patterns Fabrics & Cutting

Pattern selection/size

Getting to know your figure 96-97
Basic pattern alterations 100-110

Recognizing your figure type

Feminine figures vary greatly in shape, so patterns are sized not only for different measurements but for figure types of varying proportions. To decide which type most closely approximates your own figure, first take your measurements (pp. 48–49). Next carefully appraise your silhouette, front and side, in a long mirror. (Wear undergarments or a bodysuit for both procedures.) You will then be ready to compare your figure with the standards.

Overall height is one indicator of figure type, but length of legs, and sometimes of neck, can make it deceptive. Far more important are length of torso and location within it of bust, waist, and hip levels. The figure-type drawings indicate the locations that are standard for each; the color bands, the total range spanned by all of the types. (All figures are drawn to the same height to make comparisons easier.) In comparing your figure to the standards, take special notice of differences in back neck to waist length, and shoulder to apex of bust.

Although figure types do not signify age groups, an age level may be implied and styles designed accordingly. It is best to stay within the size range of the figure type most like yours, but it is possible to choose from another and adjust the proportions (see Basic pattern alterations).

Bodice pieces from several figure types show how proportions compare. Note differences at shoulders and armholes, and in widths and back waist lengths.

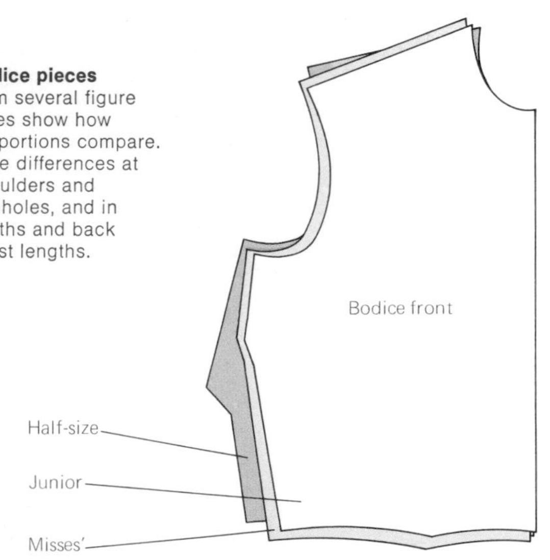

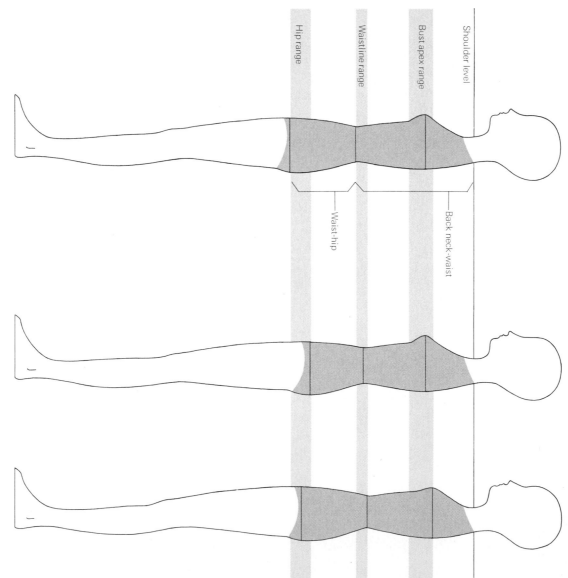

Shoulder level
Back neck-waist
Bust apex range
Waistline range
Waist-hip
Hip range

MISSES'
About 5′5″ to 5′6″ in height, well developed and proportioned. Taller, with longer back waist length, than all other figure types, except Women's. Hip is measured at 9″ below the waist. Statistically, this is considered to be the "average" figure.

MISS PETITE
About 5′2″ to 5′4″, with proportions similar to Misses', but shorter overall, with narrower shoulder. Hip measured 7″ below waist.

JUNIOR
About 5′4″, well developed, but shorter back waist length and higher bustline than Misses'. Hip is measured 9″ below waist.

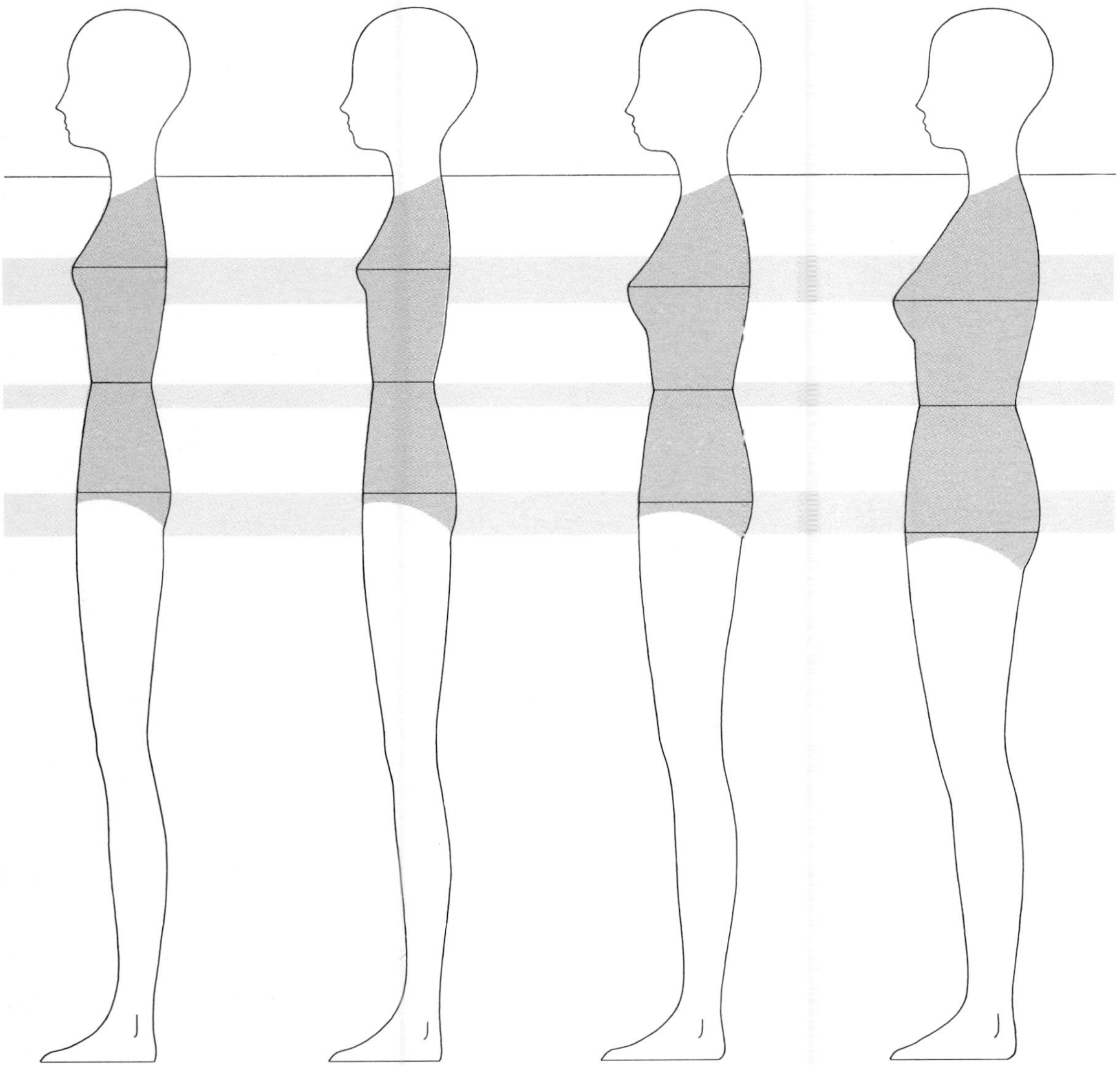

Size range charts

MISSES'

Size	6	8	10	12	14	16	18	20
Bust	30½	31½	32½	34	36	38	40	42
Waist	23	24	25	26½	28	30	32	34
Hip	32½	33½	34½	36	38	40	42	44
Back waist length	15½	15¾	16	16¼	16½	16¾	17	17¼

MISS PETITE

Size	6mp	8mp	10mp	12mp	14mp	16mp
Bust	30½	31½	32½	34	36	38
Waist	23½	24½	25½	27	28½	30½
Hip	32½	33½	34½	36	38	40
Back waist length	14½	14¾	15	15¼	15½	15¾

JUNIOR

Size	5	7	9	11	13	15
Bust	30	31	32	33½	35	37
Waist	22½	23½	24½	25½	27	29
Hip	32	33	34	35½	37	39
Back waist length	15	15¼	15½	15¾	16	16¼

JUNIOR PETITE

Size	3JP	5JP	7JP	9JP	11JP	13JP
Bust	30½	31	32	33	34	35
Waist	22½	23	24	25	26	27
Hip	31½	32	33	34	35	36
Back waist length	14	14¼	14½	14¾	15	15¼

YOUNG JUNIOR/TEEN

Size	5/6	7/8	9/10	11/12	13/14	15/16
Bust	28	29	30½	32	33½	35
Waist	22	23	24	25	26	27
Hip	31	32	33½	35	36½	38
Back waist length	13½	14	14½	15	15⅜	15¾

HALF-SIZE

Size	10½	12½	14½	16½	18½	20½	22½	24½
Bust	33	35	37	39	41	43	45	47
Waist	27	29	31	33	35	37½	40	42½
Hip	35	37	39	41	43	45½	48	50½
Back waist length	15	15¼	15½	15¾	15⅞	16	16⅛	16¼

WOMEN'S

Size	38	40	42	44	46	48	50
Bust	42	44	46	48	50	52	54
Waist	35	37	39	41½	44	46½	49
Hip	44	46	48	50	52	54	56
Back waist length	17¼	17 3/3	17½	17⅝	17¾	17⅞	18

JUNIOR PETITE
About 5′ to 5′1″, with fully developed figure. Shorter than Junior but with similar proportions. Hip is measured 7″ below waist.

YOUNG JUNIOR/TEEN
About 5′1″ to 5′3″, a developing figure with small, high bust, waist larger in proportion to it. Hip is measured 7″ below waist.

HALF-SIZE
About 5′2″ to 5′3″, larger waist, shorter back waist length, and narrower shculder than Misses'. Hip measured 7″ below waist.

WOMEN'S
About 5′5″ to 5′6″, similar to Misses' in height and proportions, but larger figure overall. Hip is measured at 9″ below waist.

Pattern selection/size

Taking measurements for fitting 100

Taking measurements

Measurements can be taken without assistance, but the task is easier when you have someone to help. For greatest accuracy, wear undergarments or a bodysuit when measuring; use a tape measure that does not stretch. Before starting, tie a string around your middle and let it roll to the natural waistline. Take vertical measurements first, then those "in the round." Pull the tape snug, but not too tight, always around the fullest part of each body area; be sure to keep the tape parallel to the floor. Record all measurements on a chart like the one on the opposite page. The dimensions listed there are sufficient for selecting pattern type and size. Others may be needed for garment fitting and alterations (see Fitting).

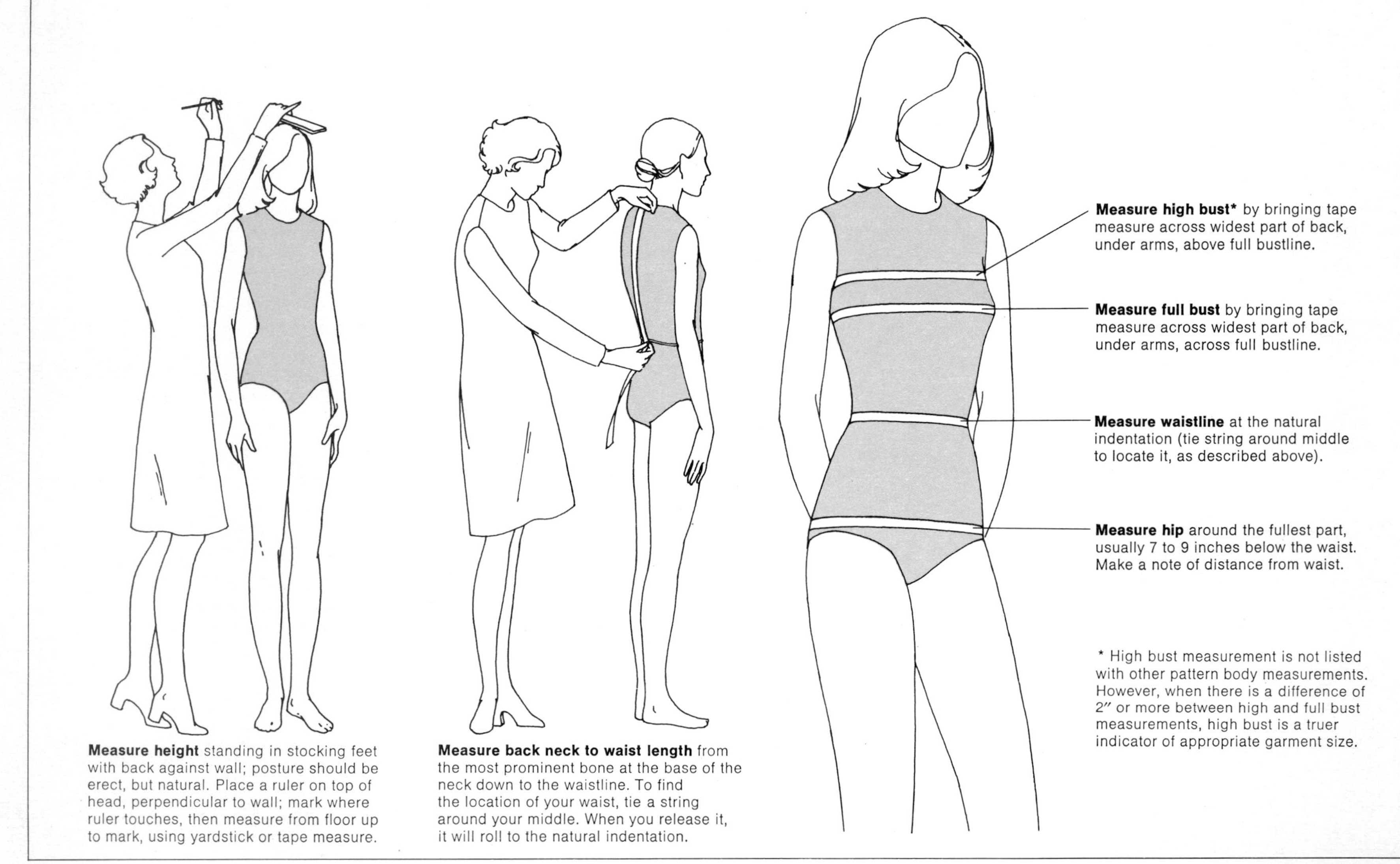

Measure high bust* by bringing tape measure across widest part of back, under arms, above full bustline.
Measure full bust by bringing tape measure across widest part of back, under arms, across full bustline.
Measure waistline at the natural indentation (tie string around middle to locate it, as described above).
Measure hip around the fullest part, usually 7 to 9 inches below the waist. Make a note of distance from waist.

Measure height standing in stocking feet with back against wall; posture should be erect, but natural. Place a ruler on top of head, perpendicular to wall; mark where ruler touches, then measure from floor up to mark, using yardstick or tape measure.

Measure back neck to waist length from the most prominent bone at the base of the neck down to the waistline. To find the location of your waist, tie a string around your middle. When you release it, it will roll to the natural indentation.

* High bust measurement is not listed with other pattern body measurements. However, when there is a difference of 2" or more between high and full bust measurements, high bust is a truer indicator of appropriate garment size.

Pattern size guidelines

After taking your measurements, and picking the figure type most like your own (pp. 46–47), you are ready to choose a pattern size according to the guidelines below. If your measurements do not correspond exactly to any one size, consider all pertinent factors and choose the size requiring the fewest major adjustments. Your pattern may—or it may not—be the same as your ready-to-wear size. It doesn't matter; ready-to-wear and pattern sizes have no necessary relation to one another. Pattern sizes, however, *do*—an important fact to remember. All commercial patterns are based on the same fundamental measurements, which makes sizes fairly consistent from brand to brand. Where differences occur, they are usually in shaping—variations in shoulder slope, dart contours and position, armhole curve, sleeve cap shape, and so on. These subtle differences often reflect fashion trends. They may incidentally cause certain pattern brands to fit some people better than others, but fundamentally the sizing is the same for all.

Dress, blouse, coat, or jacket size is selected according to full bust measurement. If your waist and/or hips do not correspond to the waist or hip allowances for this size, these areas are easily adjusted. An exception to this selection rule is made when there is a difference of more than 2 inches between the high and full bust measurements. Such a discrepancy indicates that the bust is full in relation to the body frame. Size in such cases should be chosen by the high bust measurement and the bust area should be adjusted (see Fitting).

Size for skirt or pants is determined by hip measurement. even if the hips are larger, proportionately, than the waist. When buying *wardrobe* patterns (those that include blouses, skirts, jackets, and so on), stay with the bust measurement.

Being one size on top and another on the bottom makes you one among many. Follow the recommendations above for each garment selection but, when possible, buy two sizes of the same pattern. Results will be the same, but alterations fewer.

When measurements fall between sizes, such additional factors as bone structure, fabric, and fit influence choice. The smaller size may be better if you are small-boned, the larger if you are large-boned. Stretchy fabrics allow some size leeway, those with considerable "give" often permitting the smaller size choice. Personal preference, too, may incline you toward a closer or looser fit.

Style may influence size choice, occasionally or often. Because the Misses' figure type comes the closest to average height and proportions, this range offers the widest selection of designs. If you find your taste and fashion preferences are not satisfied by the styles in your own group, you might consider choosing the nearest Misses' size and adjusting the pattern accordingly.

Measurement chart

When you have taken measurements and decided on a pattern size, a chart like the one below is well worth making. Keep it up to date by re-measuring every six months or so; changes may call for a different size. Enter your measurements in the first column, corresponding measurements for your pattern size in the adjoining column, differences (if any) in the third. Variances of ¼ inch or more in length, ½ inch or more in circumference, indicate a need for pattern adjustments (see Fitting).

MEASUREMENT	YOURS	PATTERN	DIFFERENCE
Height			
Back neck to waist			
High bust			
Full bust			
Waistline			
Full hip			
FOR PATTERN SIZE:			

Metric conversion

Anticipating a change to the metric system in this country, most pattern companies now list metric equivalents alongside inches in charts and direction sheets. In this system, a meter is the basic unit of measurement; any portion thereof is designated by a decimal. Thus, .01 meter is ¹⁄₁₀₀ of a meter, or one *centimeter* (the smallest unit for ordinary sewing purposes). The ruler below relates inch to metric measurements. As you see, there are just over 2½ centimeters (2.54, to be exact) to an inch. To arrive at an approximate conversion, merely multiply the number of inches by 2½.

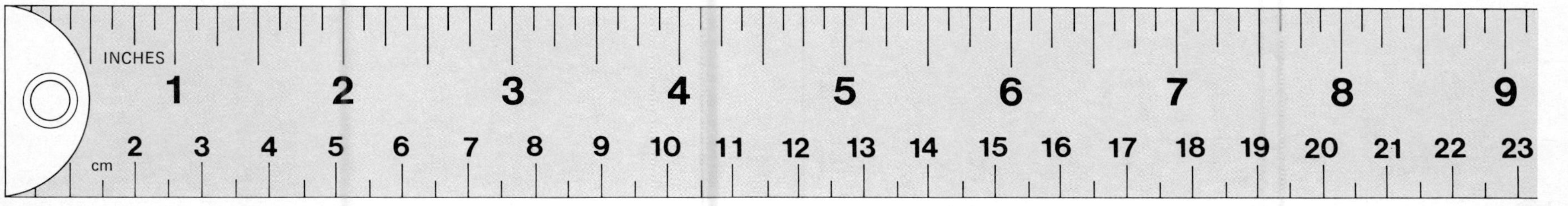

Pattern selection/style

Judging garment fit 97-99

Making design work for you

Combining style and fabric in a flattering fashion requires the artful use of four design elements—**line, detail, texture,** and **color.** While there is nothing mysterious about any of these, they each have the power to create illusion. By themselves or in combination, they can add to or diminish height, enlarge or reduce apparent figure size. Examples of the ways each element works are given here and on pages 52–53. Once you have some understanding of what they do, you must decide how you want to use them. This requires a realistic analysis of height and figure type (as explained on page 46) and some careful thought about what features you want to emphasize or divert attention from. There are few rules in this regard. The decisions are largely personal. For instance, if you are short, you might choose to emphasize your petiteness or aim for the illusion of greater height.

In general, *balance* is a desirable goal, and balance is achieved by minimizing or counteracting anything excessive. For example, wide hips might be balanced by a wide shoulder area in the garment. Basically, there are two approaches to balance—formal, in which the two halves of a design are identical, and informal, where the areas are visually in equilibrium, but not the same. The vertical lines on the opposite page are examples of formal balance; the diagonals, of informal.

An equally important goal is *harmony*—the esthetically pleasing relationship of all the elements that go into a fashion. Harmony is mainly a matter of appropriateness—a sense of what things belong together, and to the situation. This might best be made clear by some negative examples. One might be the cluttered look of too many garment lines combined with a busy print. A heavy tweed, ideal for a tailored skirt or suit, is cumbersome and inappropriate in a softly draped, flowing design.

No matter how carefully you plan choices in relation to what you conceive to be your best and worst features, two other influences are bound to affect your decisions. One is current fashion; the other, your personal preferences. The trick is to play those influences together to your advantage. Take color and texture, for example. If this season's featured color is unflattering to your figure, use it as an accent, preferably to call attention to one of your better features. If a popular color clashes with your eye color or skin tone, place it inside the garment as a lining. From the dominant trends in fashion, choose only those that you like and that suit you. Modify skirt width or length to your lines and liking; choose a less extreme version of a dress. Remember that what flatters is always more effective than what is simply new. When it comes to new styles, let this be your guide: Be extra analytical before buying a style sharply different from anything you've worn or tried on before.

If you find yourself confused by too many choices, scan your wardrobe for the garments you always feel good in, and for which you are often complimented. Stay within their limits of line, color, and texture—and you will never go wrong.

Silhouette (outside line)

The main lines of a garment are those that form its **silhouette**, or outside line. Basically, every silhouette is a variation of two familiar shapes—the rectangle and triangle. (To see the shape more clearly, squint when you look at a garment.) Variations on these basic shapes are created largely by relative closeness of fit, which falls generally into four categories—*fitted, semi-fitted, slightly fitted,* and *loosely fitted.* (The classification for a particular pattern is usually given on the envelope back.) A fitted garment emphasizes the figure's contours. The less fitted the shape, the less aware one is of the body and the more dominant the garment silhouette. The silhouette is dominant, too, when there are few seams or details to distract the eye, desirable if you wish to play up an interesting fabric. Fabric choice also affects silhouette; a crisp fabric, for instance, molds garment shape; a soft one tends to outline, and thus emphasize, body shape. Fashion, too, has its influence on silhouette. Whole eras have been symbolized by a particular garment shape. Memorable examples are the bustle and the leg-of-mutton sleeve.

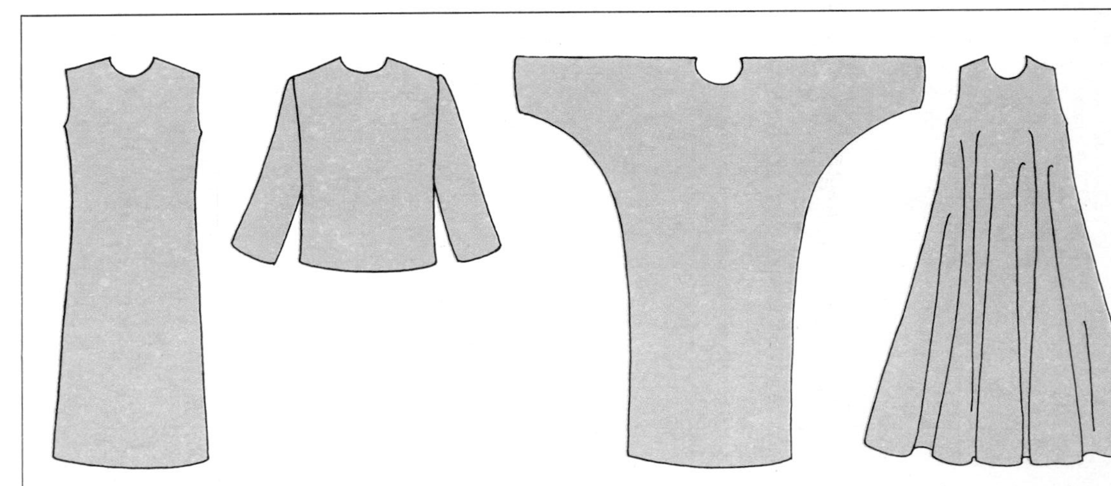

Rectangle is the basic silhouette when top and bottom are more or less equal in width. Narrow rectangle, left, is more slenderizing than wide or boxy one; box shape is excellent for diminishing height. Both shapes can be modified by seams, details, and fabric choice.

Triangle is the basic silhouette when garment is wider at top or bottom. Width at top helps to balance a wide hipline, also diminishes height. Broad base at bottom counteracts wide shoulders or top-heavy figure. Exaggerated, either one creates drama by deliberate imbalance.

Structural lines (inside)

Lines within a design add another dimension to silhouette. Skillfully used, they create pleasing illusion or diversion, help to establish balance or good proportion for the figure. Each kind of line—*horizontal, vertical, diagonal,* and *curve*—has its own way of influencing a look (see examples below). At times, a line's placement may be more significant than its character, because our eyes tend to move in a habitual direction, formed by the reading pattern followed since childhood—left to right, and top to bottom. Thus, if vertical and horizontal lines exist equally in the same design, the eyes will be drawn first to the horizontal.

There are some general principles regarding use of line: (1) The longer, wider, or more repetitious a line, the greater its influence in the total design. (2) Folds (pleats, for example) create lines, but at the same time add bulk. (3) The more lines there are in a fabric design (for example, a print), the fewer lines there should be in the garment.

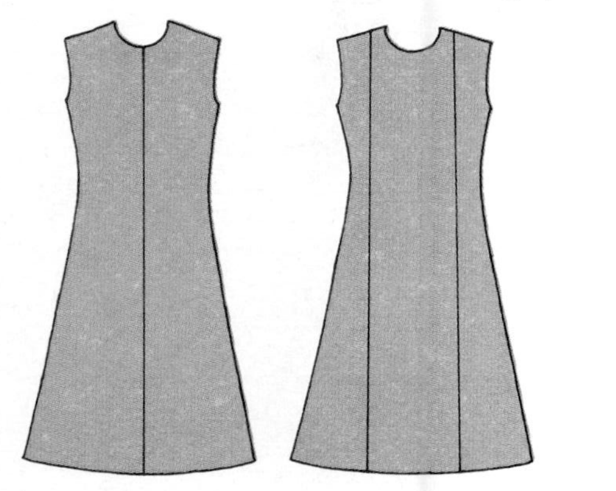

Verticals usually create the illusion of height and slimness. However, when repeated at even intervals, they can cause the figure to appear both wider and shorter, because the eye is drawn alternately from side to side.

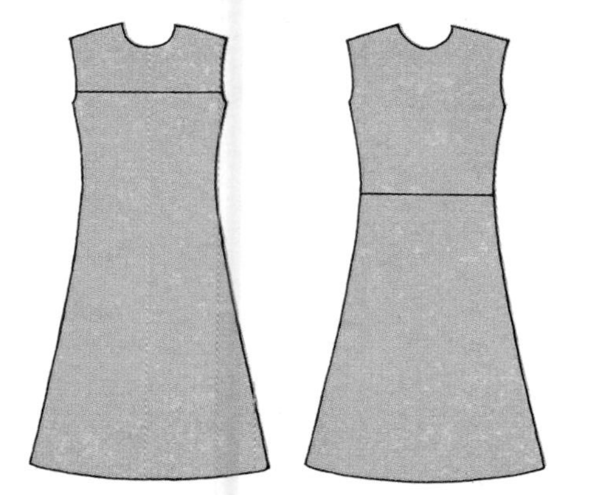

Horizontals tend to cut height, especially when used to divide a figure in half. One horizontal, however, used above or below the middle, makes a focal point of the smaller area, seeming to lengthen the longer one.

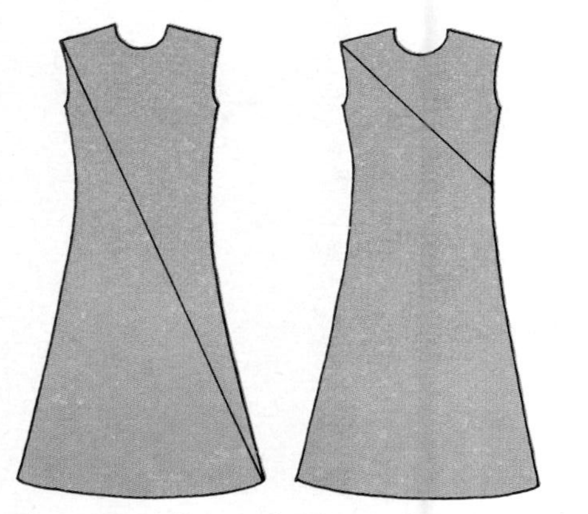

Diagonals may contribute to height or width, depending on their length and angle. A long diagonal creates a feeling of tallness. A short diagonal gives the impression of width and draws attention to the area in which it occurs.

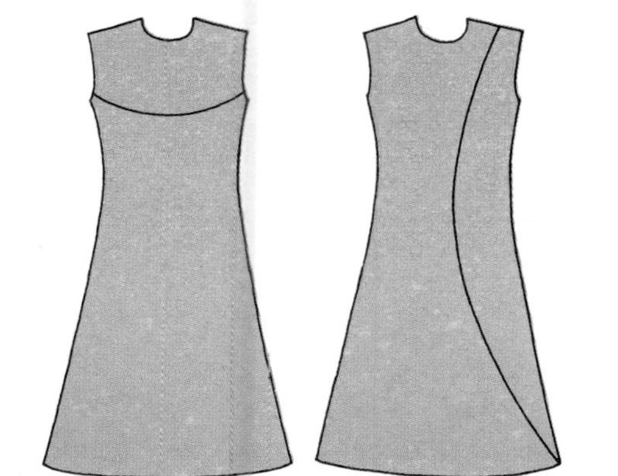

Curves produce the same effects as straight lines of similar length and placement, but more subtly. The visual impact is softer, more graceful. A curve also adds roundness and a look of greater weight wherever it occurs on the figure.

Details

Details such as sleeves, neckline, collar, and pockets, though they are subordinate to the silhouette and seams, can have just as strong an influence, depending on their shape and location. Among other things, they can serve to (1) echo and reinforce a silhouette, as bell-shaped sleeves would do on a tent dress; (2) add interest to a plain garment; (3) alter a garment's mood from, say, dressy to casual; (4) call attention to a good feature, perhaps also away from a less attractive one, as a ruffle framing a pretty face might divert the eye from very heavy hips. Often a detail can create different impressions at the same time, as illustrated by the collars below. The one on the left makes the neck seem longer, while at the same time adding width to the shoulder area and an impression of weight to the

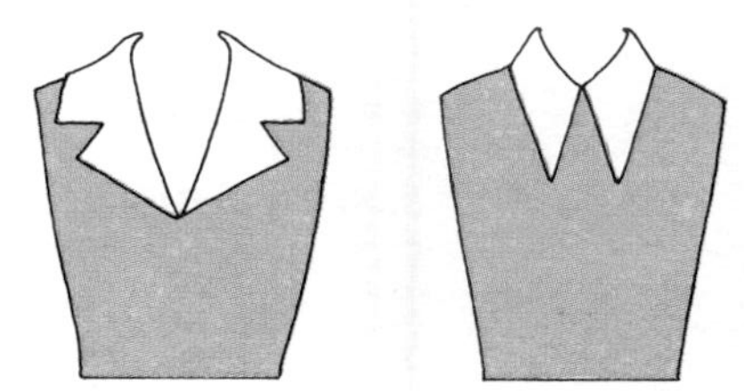

upper part of the body. The one on the right adds length to the face, but has little effect on height or neck length. Pockets at the hip always call attention to this area, but the overall illusion varies

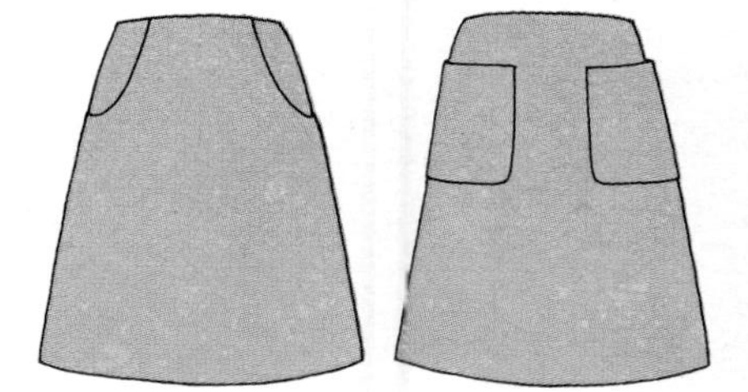

with their size and placement. Whatever the intended purpose of details, do not overdo them; too many cause confusion and diminish the effectiveness of each one. Take care, too, that such subsidiary features harmonize with the garment's silhouette and structural lines.

Pattern and fabric/creating illusions

Color and texture

Of the several elements that affect apparent figure size, **color** is one of the most influential. In general, warm, intense, and light colors advance, making the figure seem larger; cool, subdued, and dark colors recede, making it seem slimmer. To the right and below, paired illustrations show these contrasting principles at work.

Texture, too, has a definite effect on figure size. A shiny fabric, for example, makes the body appear larger; one with a matte finish is more slimming. The qualities characterized as "texture" include not only *light reflection* or sheen, but also *feel,* rough or smooth, *appearance,* and *"hand"*—the degree of stiffness or softness, weight and body that determines how a fabric drapes. Texture is important not only for its effect on the figure, but for its suitability to the style. For instance, tweed would not be appropriate for an evening dress but might be fine for a tailored floor-length skirt.

The best way to preview the effect of color and texture is to drape a length (at least 2 yards) over your body, and view it in a full-length mirror, preferably by natural light.

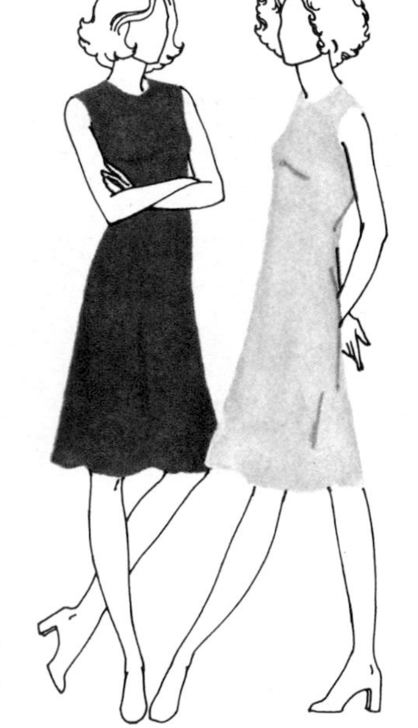

A dark color recedes, reducing apparent figure size; **a light color** advances, creating the opposite impression.

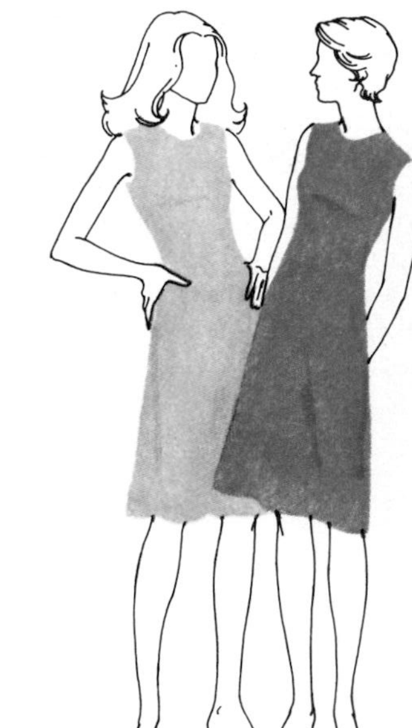

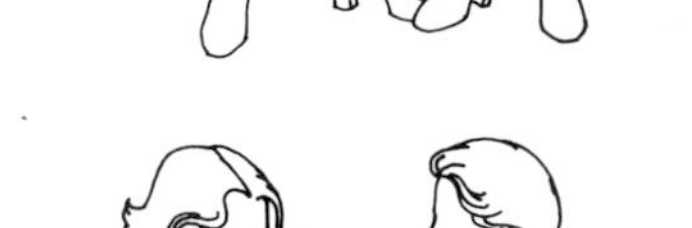

Warm colors—reds, yellows, and oranges—especially in bright or untempered tones, make a figure seem larger. **Cool colors**—blues, greens, violets—of comparable brightness or intensity have a slimming effect.

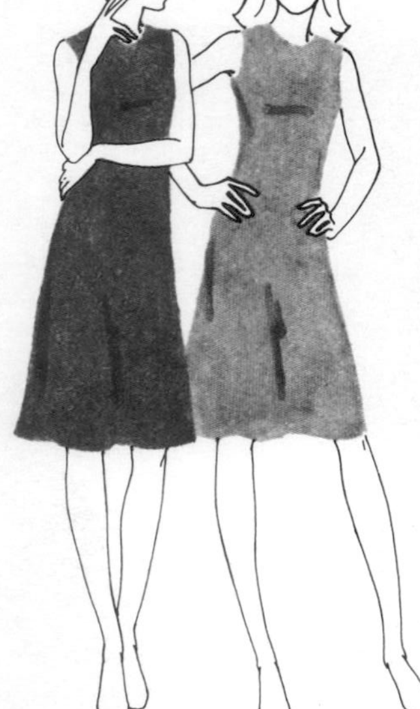

Bright or intense colors always make a figure appear larger than the same colors **subdued** (i.e., with gray added). If you want to look slimmer, use brights as accents rather than in large areas or as an entire garment.

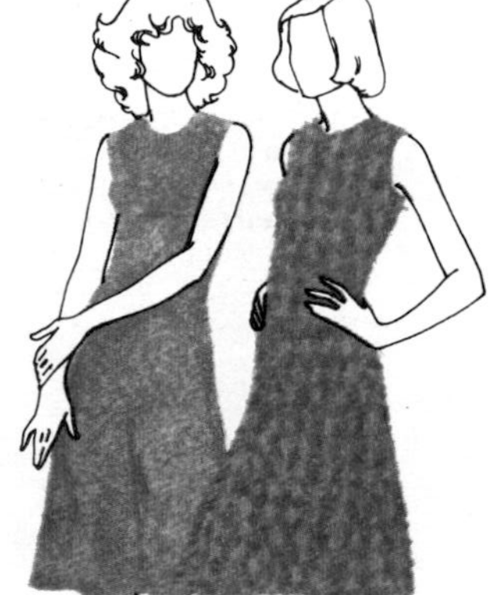

Pebbly or fluffy textures are bulkier than most **smooth** ones and so make figures look heavier. A petite person must be especially careful in choosing a rough texture lest it be overwhelming.

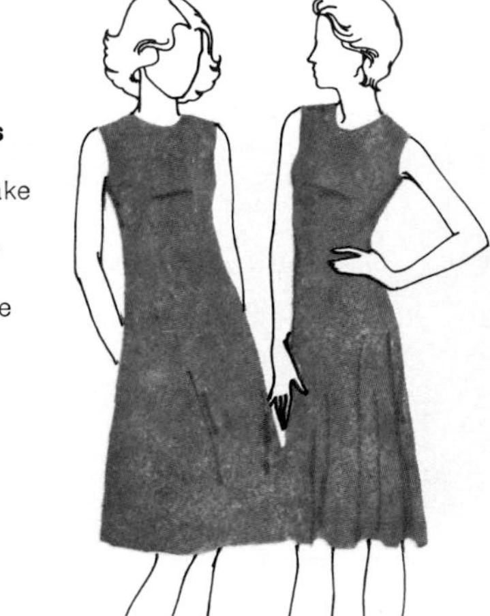

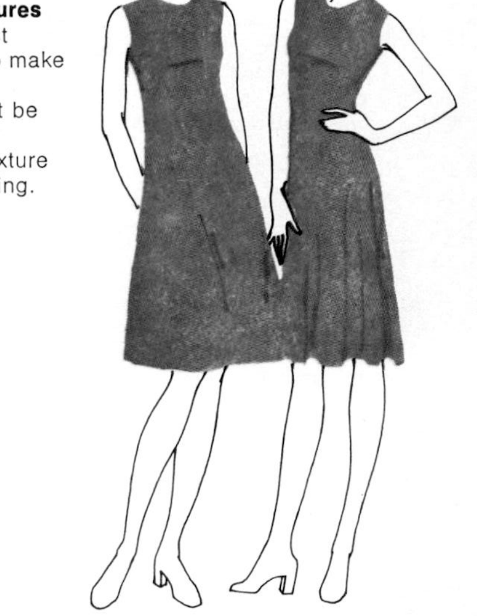

A stiff fabric in an unbroken garment line will conceal the figure but make it seem larger. The same silhouette in **soft, clinging fabric** is figure-revealing. Neither extreme is flattering to a figure less than perfectly proportioned. Moderately soft or crisp textures are better choices.

Proportion and scale

The space divisions and their relationships within a design are termed **proportions.** These divisions may be defined by inner design lines (as illustrated on page 51), or result from the ways in which color and texture are used (some examples are shown here). They always affect apparent height and figure size. While there are no exact rules about proportion ratios, it is generally agreed that the more interesting ones are those that are uneven—two to three, three to five, and so on.

When proportions are in a harmonious relation to each other and to the figure, they are said to be in **scale.** In fashion terms, this means that small prints, stripes, plaids, and details (collars, pockets, etc.) suit a petite figure best, and larger elements a larger figure. The principle is simply that too great a contrast of sizes has a jarring effect because the larger components overwhelm the smaller ones. Potential disproportions can be modified, however, by color choices. For example, a large plaid or floral will not seem as large in subdued tones and subtle combinations as the same motif would in vivid or contrasting colors.

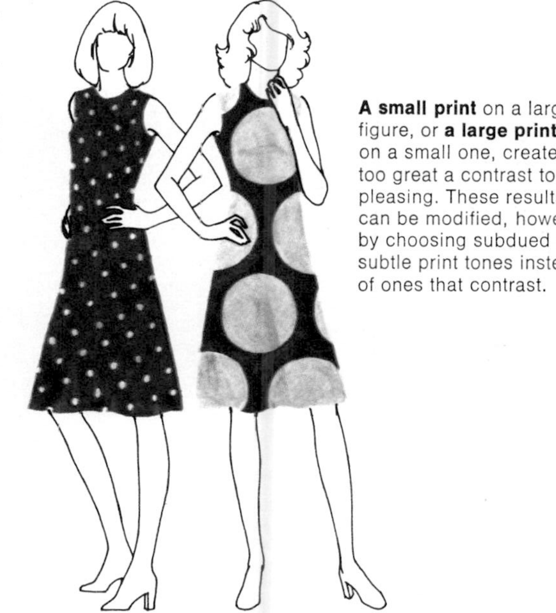

A small print on a large figure, or **a large print** on a small one, creates too great a contrast to be pleasing. These results can be modified, however, by choosing subdued and subtle print tones instead of ones that contrast.

Contrasting solids divide the figure horizontally at the point where colors meet. Watch proportions carefully when making such a division. For the slimmest, tallest look, stay with **one color.**

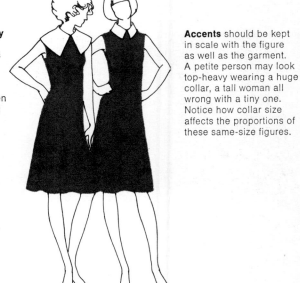

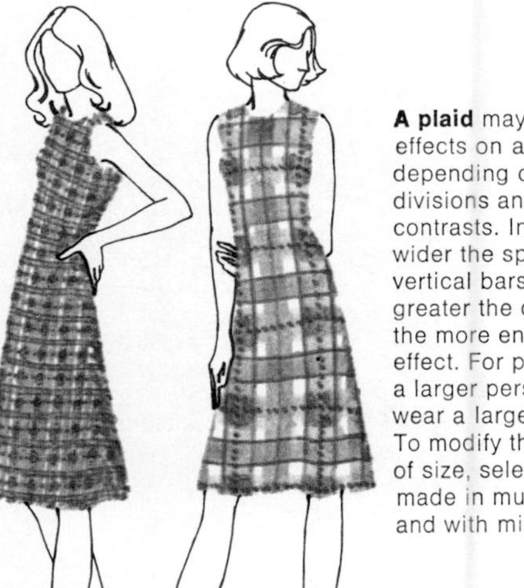

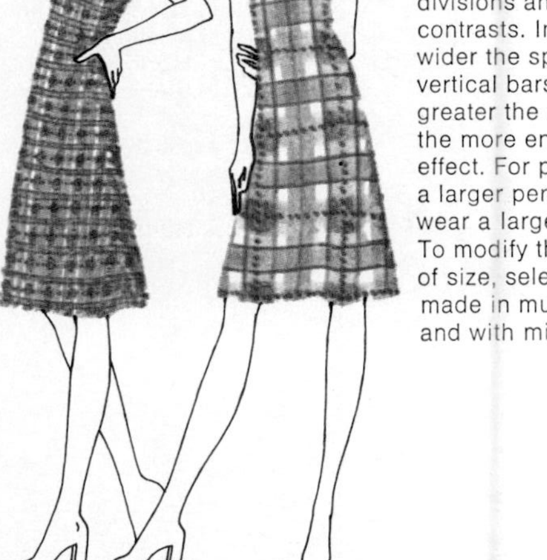

A plaid may have various effects on a figure, depending on its space divisions and color contrasts. In general, the wider the spaces between vertical bars, and/or the greater the color contrast, the more enlarging the effect. For proper scale, a larger person should wear a larger design. To modify the impression of size, select a plaid made in muted colors and with minimal contrast.

Stripes running vertically can make a figure look wider than similar stripes **horizontally** arranged, though the opposite is often assumed. The reasons: spacing between lines; amount of contrast in color divisions.

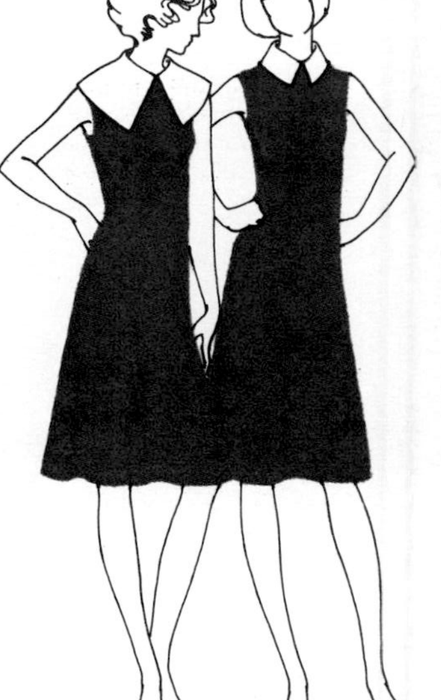

Accents should be kept in scale with the figure as well as the garment. A petite person may look top-heavy wearing a huge collar, a tall woman all wrong with a tiny one. Notice how collar size affects the proportions of these same-size figures.

Your pattern purchase

How to use a knit gauge 67

How to use pattern catalogs

A pattern catalog is a fashion directory where you can select the latest pattern designs, and also find information on suitable fabrics and accessories. Each catalog is organized according to a pattern company's notion of its customers' needs, but all contain a wide variety of timely fashions. For women, these are grouped by style types, such as dresses, sportswear, or lingerie, and further classified by figure types. For example, Junior dresses may be in one section, Half-size dresses in another. In addition, many catalogs contain sections for special categories, such as "easy-to-make" and "designer fashions." Patterns for children, boys, and men, for accessories, home furnishings, and crafts (including toys and costumes) are in separate divisions, usually after the women's styles.

Specific information relating to each pattern is printed alongside its illustrations. Some of the facts are pertinent to pattern selection, such as the types of styles and number of views to be found within the envelope. Also included are backviews, yardage requirements, notion needs, and fabric recommendations. This last is of special importance, particularly with regard to knits. "Recommended for knits" means that knits as well as woven fabrics are suitable for the design. "For knits only" means that wovens should not be used. Such a style has close fit and minimum shaping, relying on the stretchy fabric to mold to the figure. Other fabric limitations may be indicated, too, such as "Not suitable for plaids or stripes."

The newest fashions usually appear on the first few pages of the catalog. These patterns were developed for the time period specified on the cover. They reflect trends for the coming season, not only in styles, but in fabrics and accessories as well. The selections are thus current, available, and of course suitable for the fashions pictured.

A body measurement chart is located at the back of a company's catalog. It includes measurements for all figure types, and is a convenient reference, especially when you are sewing for someone else.

An index, usually on the last page, lists all the patterns in numerical order, and also the pages on which they appear. If you need to locate a certain pattern, and you know its number, the index is the fastest and easiest way to find it.

DRESSES
MISSES'
JUNIOR

DRESSES
WOMEN'S
HALF-SIZES

SEPARATES
PANTS, SKIRTS
BLOUSES
JACKETS
JUMPERS

ENSEMBLES
SUITS
COATS, CAPES

BRIDAL
EVENING
LINGERIE
SLEEPWEAR
MATERNITY

GIRLS'
CHILDREN'S
TODDLERS'
INFANTS'

MEN
TEEN-BOYS'
BOYS'

ACCESSORIES
HOME
FURNISHINGS
COSTUMES
SIZE CHART

Catalog tabs identify pattern types to be found within each section. The bulk of any book—about the opening two-thirds in most cases—is devoted to women's fashions, grouped by fashion images, figure types, and kinds of styles. Toward the back, you will find patterns for infants and children, men and boys, also accessories for the home and craft projects to the extent that an individual company makes patterns in these areas.

Pattern envelope front

The front of every pattern envelope bears the style number and illustrations of each fashion item and the variations on it that the envelope contains. Pattern price and size are usually included too. Before you buy, be sure the style and size are the ones you have requested. Most stores will neither exchange nor give refunds for patterns.

Once you have decided on the view you prefer, the sketch or photo can guide you toward an appropriate fabric type. The fabric illustrated may be crisp or soft, printed or plain, depending on what best suits the fashion. If you are considering a plaid, stripe, or obvious diagonal, look for a view showing such a fabric being used. It's your best assurance that the fabric is feasible.

Special-feature notices appear on some envelope fronts, calling attention to one or more desirable or unusual characteristics of the pattern. They may say, for example, that the pattern is easy to construct, slimming, or created by a well-known designer. If it is "for knits only," a knit gauge, for measuring knit stretchability, may appear on the front. (Some companies put it on the back.)

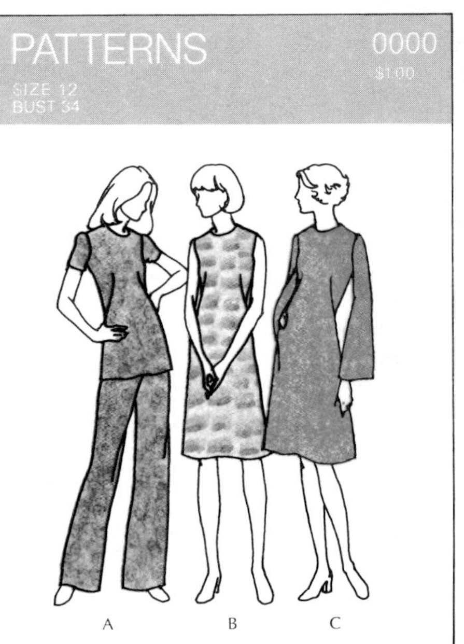

Pattern envelope front features a drawing, sometimes a photo, of each garment and any alternate views of it that the envelope contains. Illustrations can be used for guidance—garments are shown in fabrics chosen for their suitability to the design.

Buying extra yardage 68-69

Pattern envelope back

The envelope back supplies, in complete detail, all the information needed at the outset of a sewing project. A facsimile is shown at the right, with an explanation of the purposes each portion serves. What you see is typical of most pattern envelopes, though the arrangement of information may vary. As a rule, you should scan the entire envelope of each new pattern; every part tells you something important about that particular design. The most obvious feature, the yardage block, lists exact amounts of material needed for each view and every size in that pattern's range. Because space does not permit the inclusion of all fabric widths, those listed are for the fabric types most suited to the design. (If you plan to purchase fabric in a width that is not included, consult the conversion chart below for the approximate amount needed.) Fabric requirements are carefully calculated by experts to be economical yet adequate. Except when allowance must be made for special fabric, such as plaid, or for involved alterations, there is no need to buy more than is specified.

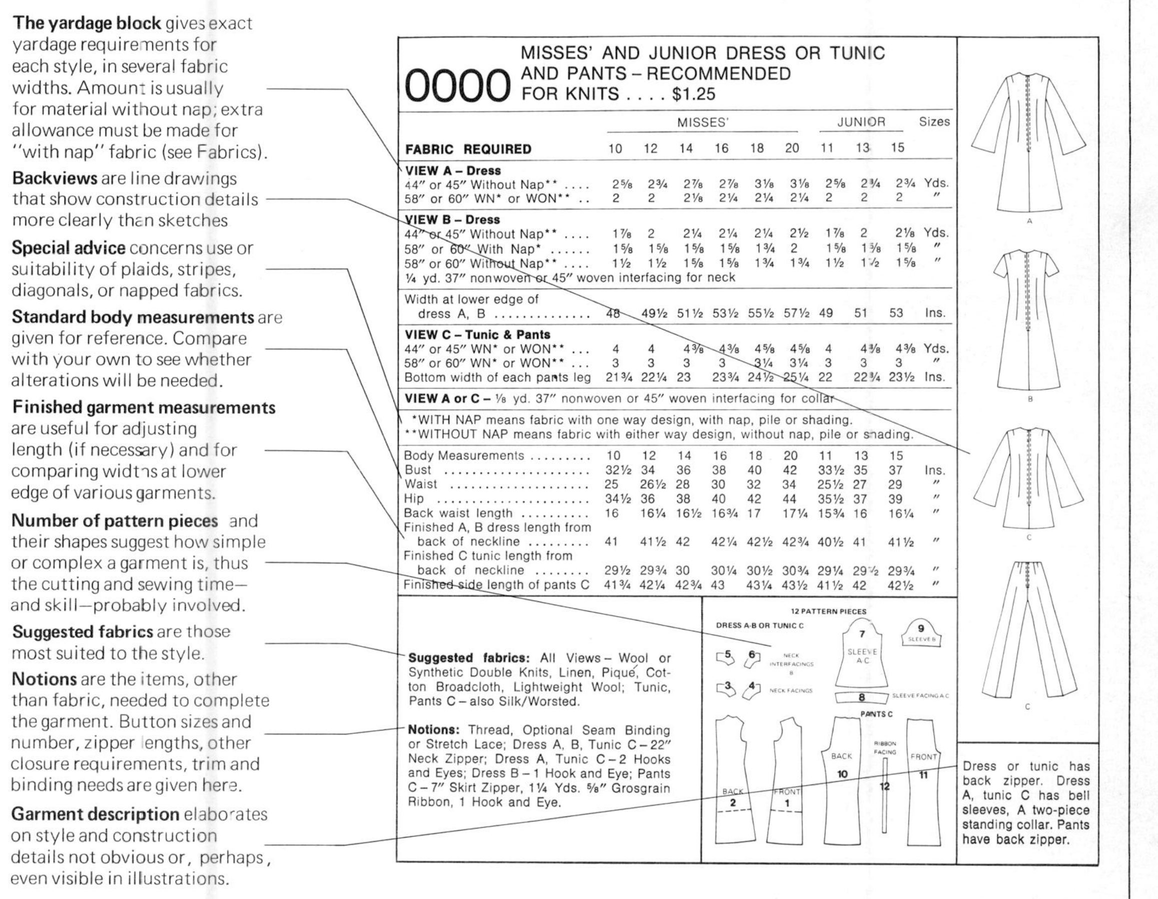

The yardage block gives exact yardage requirements for each style, in several fabric widths. Amount is usually for material without nap; extra allowance must be made for "with nap" fabric (see Fabrics).

Backviews are line drawings that show construction details more clearly than sketches

Special advice concerns use or suitability of plaids, stripes, diagonals, or napped fabrics.

Standard body measurements are given for reference. Compare with your own to see whether alterations will be needed.

Finished garment measurements are useful for adjusting length (if necessary) and for comparing widths at lower edge of various garments.

Number of pattern pieces and their shapes suggest how simple or complex a garment is, thus the cutting and sewing time—and skill—probably involved.

Suggested fabrics are those most suited to the style.

Notions are the items, other than fabric, needed to complete the garment. Button sizes and number, zipper lengths, other closure requirements, trim and binding needs are given here.

Garment description elaborates on style and construction details not obvious or, perhaps, even visible in illustrations.

0000 MISSES' AND JUNIOR DRESS OR TUNIC AND PANTS – RECOMMENDED FOR KNITS $1.25

FABRIC REQUIRED	MISSES' 10	12	14	16	18	20	JUNIOR 11	13	15	Sizes
VIEW A – Dress										
44" or 45" Without Nap**	2⅝	2¾	2⅞	2⅞	3⅛	3⅛	2⅝	2¾	2¾	Yds.
58" or 60" WN* or WON** ..	2	2	2⅛	2¼	2¼	2¼	2	2	2	"
VIEW B – Dress										
44" or 45" Without Nap**	1⅞	2	2¼	2¼	2¼	2½	1⅞	2	2⅛	Yds.
58" or 60" With Nap*	1⅝	1⅝	1⅝	1⅝	1¾	2	1⅝	1⅝	1⅝	"
58" or 60" Without Nap**	1½	1½	1⅝	1⅝	1¾	1¾	1½	1½	1⅝	"
¼ yd. 37" nonwoven or 45" woven interfacing for neck										
Width at lower edge of dress A, B	48	49½	51½	53½	55½	57½	49	51	53	Ins.
VIEW C – Tunic & Pants										
44" or 45" WN* or WON** ...	4	4	4⅜	4⅜	4⅝	4⅝	4	4⅜	4⅜	Yds.
58" or 60" WN* or WON** ...	3	3	3	3	3¼	3¼	3	3	3	"
Bottom width of each pants leg	21¾	22¼	23	23¾	24½	25¼	22	22¾	23½	Ins.
VIEW A or C – ⅛ yd. 37" nonwoven or 45" woven interfacing for collar										
Body Measurements	10	12	14	16	18	20	11	13	15	
Bust	32½	34	36	38	40	42	33½	35	37	Ins.
Waist	25	26½	28	30	32	34	25½	27	29	"
Hip	34½	36	38	40	42	44	35½	37	39	"
Back waist length	16	16¼	16½	16¾	17	17¼	15¾	16	16¼	"
Finished A, B dress length from back of neckline	41	41½	42	42¼	42½	42¾	40½	41	41½	"
Finished C tunic length from back of neckline	29½	29¾	30	30¼	30½	30¾	29¼	29½	29¾	"
Finished side length of pants C	41¾	42¼	42¾	43	43¼	43½	41½	42	42½	"

*WITH NAP means fabric with one way design, with nap, pile or shading.
**WITHOUT NAP means fabric with either way design, without nap, pile or shading.

Suggested fabrics: All Views – Wool or Synthetic Double Knits, Linen, Piqué, Cotton Broadcloth, Lightweight Wool; Tunic, Pants C – also Silk/Worsted.

Notions: Thread, Optional Seam Binding or Stretch Lace; Dress A, B, Tunic C – 22" Neck Zipper; Dress A, Tunic C – 2 Hooks and Eyes; Dress B – 1 Hook and Eye; Pants C – 7" Skirt Zipper, 1¼ Yds. ⅝" Grosgrain Ribbon, 1 Hook and Eye.

Dress or tunic has back zipper. Dress A, tunic C has bell sleeves, A two-piece standing collar. Pants have back zipper.

Fabric conversion chart*

	FABRIC WIDTHS							
	35"-36"	39"	41"	44"-45"	50"	52"-54"	58"-60"	66"
YARDAGE	1 ¾	1 ½	1 ½	1 ⅜	1 ¼	1 ⅛	1	⅞
	2	1 ¾	1 ¾	1 ⅝	1 ½	1 ⅜	1 ¼	1 ⅛
	2 ¼	2	2	1 ¾	1 ⅝	1 ½	1 ⅜	1 ¼
	2 ½	2 ¼	2 ¼	2 ⅛	1 ¾	1 ¾	1 ⅝	1 ½
	2 ⅞	2 ½	2 ½	2 ¼	2	1 ⅞	1 ¾	1 ⅝
	3 ⅛	2 ¾	2 ¾	2 ½	2 ¼	2	1 ⅞	1 ¾
	3 ⅜	3	2 ⅞	2 ¾	2 ⅜	2 ¼	2	1 ⅞
	3 ¾	3 ¼	3 ⅛	2 ⅞	2 ⅝	2 ⅜	2 ¼	2 ⅛
	4 ¼	3 ½	3 ⅜	3 ⅛	2 ¾	2 ⅝	2 ⅜	2 ¼
	4 ½	3 ¾	3 ⅝	3 ⅜	3	2 ¾	2 ⅝	2 ½
	4 ¾	4	3 ⅞	3 ⅝	3 ¼	2 ⅞	2 ¾	2 ⅝
	5	4 ¼	4 ⅛	3 ⅞	3 ⅜	3 ⅛	2 ⅞	2 ¾

Add additional ¼ yard for: Large difference in fabric widths; one-directional fabrics; styles with sleeves cut in one piece with body of garment.

* Courtesy of Cooperative Extension Service Rutgers University-The State University of New Jersey

To use the pattern envelope back as a shopping guide:
1. Read the section on "suggested fabrics" to see *what sort of fabrics* are most suitable to the style in the judgment of the pattern designer.
2. Check for fabric cautions or restrictions to be sure the fabric you have in mind is not "off limits."
3. Circle your size at the top of the yardage block. Run your eye down the left side until you find the view and the fabric width you have chosen; then glance across from left to right until you reach the vertical column under your size. The number you find there is the *yardage you will need* to buy. If your chosen fabric width is not among those that the envelope lists, check the conversion chart at the left for the approximate amount needed.
4. Look through the rest of the "yardage block" for the *interfacing, lining, and trim* requirements of your pattern, if any of these are needed.
5. Purchase all *notions* that are specified for your view. As for thread, you will usually need 1 small spool (125 yards) for skirt, pants, or simple top not requiring extensive seam finishing; 2 small spools or the equivalent (250 yards) for dress, coat, or suit.

The parts of a pattern

Pattern piece pointers 86
How to interpret cutting guides 86

Inside the envelope

Contents of all pattern envelopes are basically the same. The key element is the **tissue pattern,** each piece identified by name and number, and by view when pieces differ for, say, Views A and B. Because garments are usually identical on right and left sides, most pattern pieces represent half a garment section and are placed on folded fabric. The **direction sheet,** which you should turn to first, is a guide to pattern pieces needed for each view, and to cutting and sewing. Of the varied assistance it gives, the most directly useful parts are shown below: (1) **pattern piece diagram,** for identifying the pieces required for each view; (2) **cutting guides,** arranged by view, fabric widths, and pattern sizes; (3) step-by-step **sewing instructions.** The pattern in the example below is for an imaginary dress. Views A and B differ in sleeve length (short for A, long for B) and skirt style (narrower for A).

1. Pattern piece diagram
Silhouettes of all pattern pieces in envelope, for all garments and all versions of each. Key similar to one at right explains which pieces to use for which style.

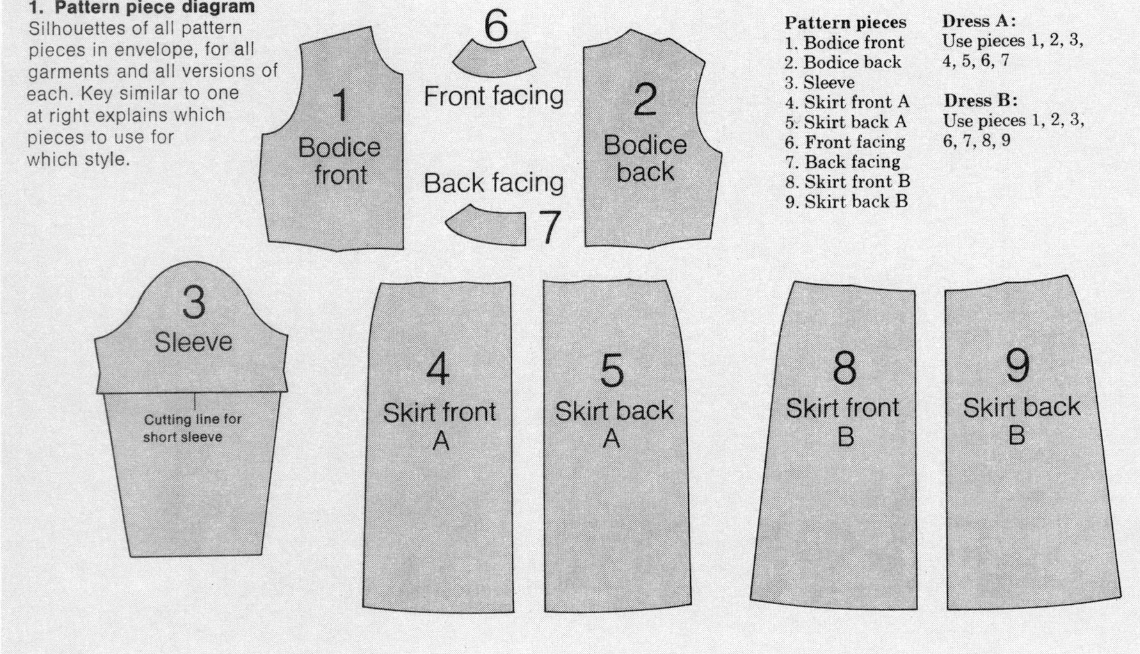

2. Cutting guides
Recommended layouts, given for different views, several fabric widths, and the pattern's entire size range. Illustration, for instance, pertains to Dress A, 44/45″ fabric, sizes 8–10–12.

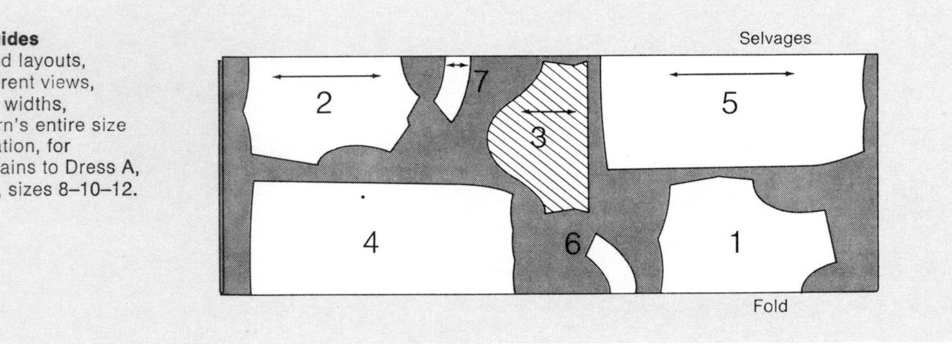

3. Sewing instructions
Step-by-step directions for constructing parts of garment in proper order; accompanying sketches illustrate technique. Shown, beginning steps in bodice construction.

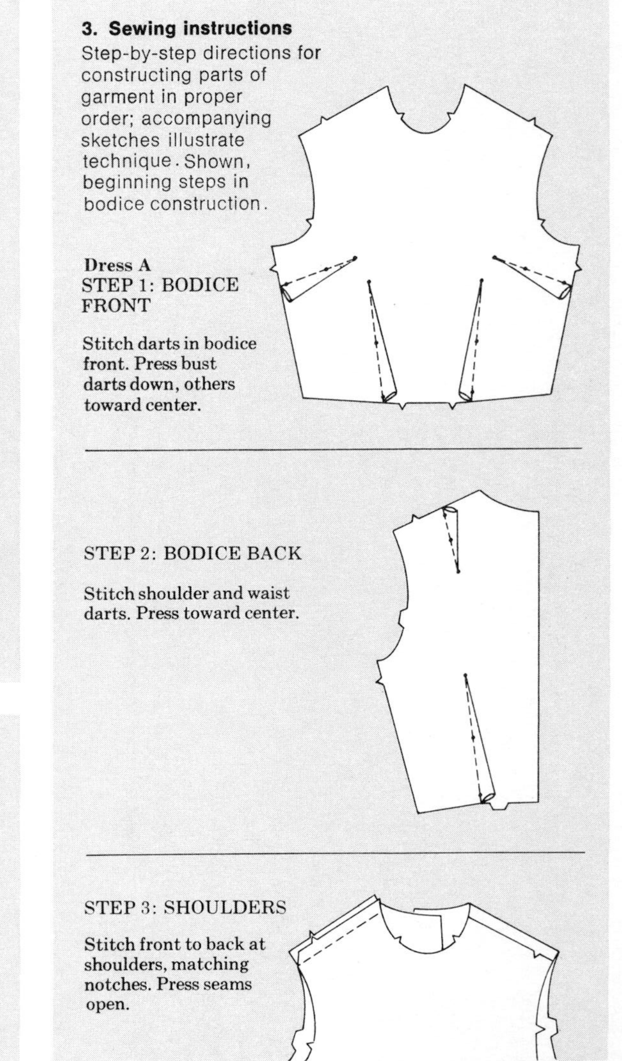

Dress A
STEP 1: BODICE FRONT

Stitch darts in bodice front. Press bust darts down, others toward center.

STEP 2: BODICE BACK

Stitch shoulder and waist darts. Press toward center.

STEP 3: SHOULDERS

Stitch front to back at shoulders, matching notches. Press seams open.

Transferring pattern markings to fabric 94
Directional stitching 144

What pattern markings mean

Every pattern piece bears markings that together constitute a pattern "sign language," indispensable to accuracy at every stage—layout and cutting, joining of sections, fitting and adjustment. Note all symbols carefully; each has special significance. Some pertain to alteration. The double line in the bodice piece below, for example, tells you to "lengthen or shorten here." Other marks are used for matching related sections. Piece numbers are even important, signifying the order in which sections are to be constructed. The markings defined below occur on most patterns. Less common ones—for pleats, gathers, buttonholes, pockets, etc.—are explained in sections on those subjects.

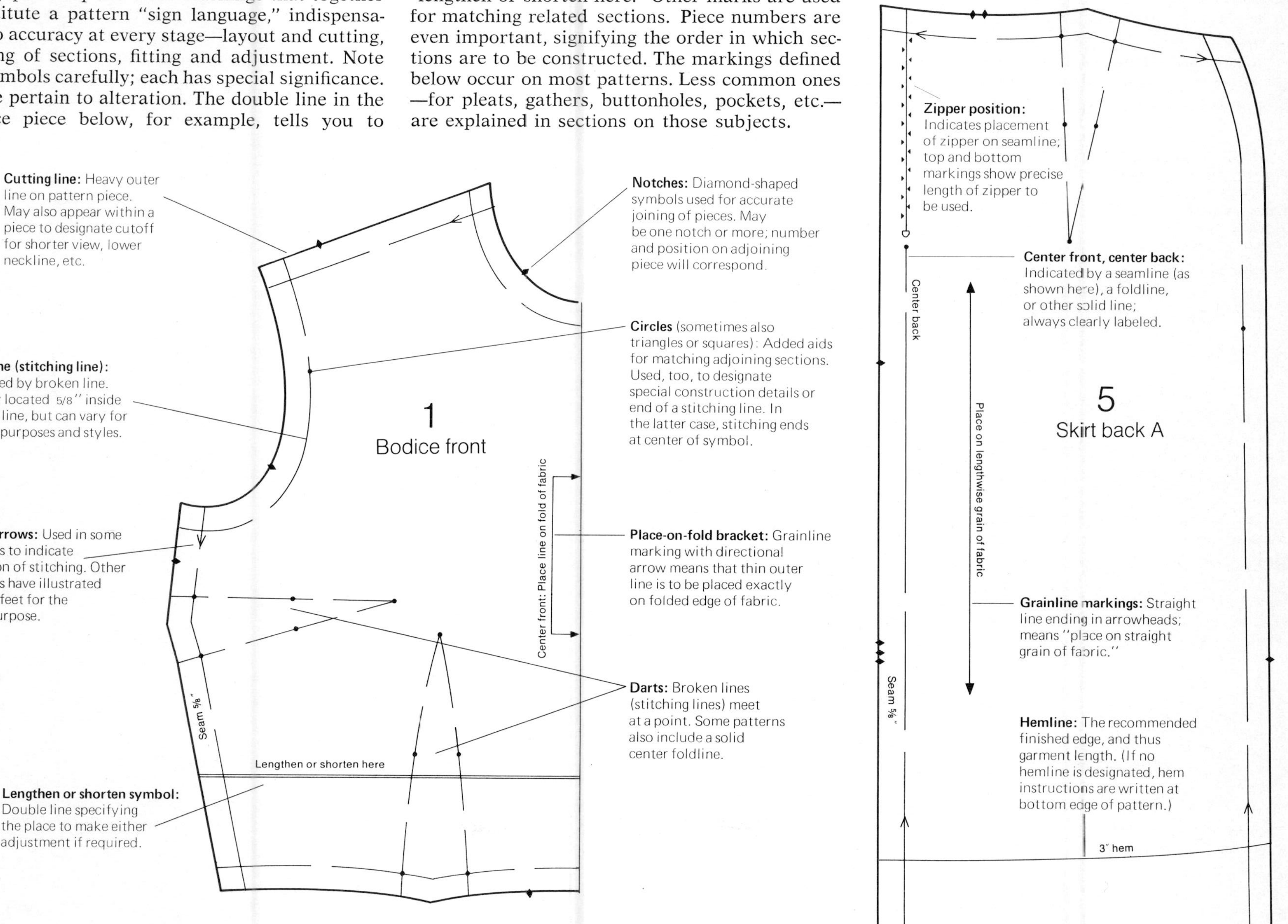

Cutting line: Heavy outer line on pattern piece. May also appear within a piece to designate cutoff for shorter view, lower neckline, etc.
Seamline (stitching line): Indicated by broken line. Usually located 5/8" inside cutting line, but can vary for certain purposes and styles.
Small arrows: Used in some patterns to indicate direction of stitching. Other patterns have illustrated presser feet for the same purpose.
Lengthen or shorten symbol: Double line specifying the place to make either adjustment if required.
1
Bodice front
Seam ⅝"
Lengthen or shorten here
Center front: Place line on fold of fabric
Notches: Diamond-shaped symbols used for accurate joining of pieces. May be one notch or more; number and position on adjoining piece will correspond.
Circles (sometimes also triangles or squares): Added aids for matching adjoining sections. Used, too, to designate special construction details or end of a stitching line. In the latter case, stitching ends at center of symbol.
Place-on-fold bracket: Grainline marking with directional arrow means that thin outer line is to be placed exactly on folded edge of fabric.
Darts: Broken lines (stitching lines) meet at a point. Some patterns also include a solid center foldline.
Zipper position: Indicates placement of zipper on seamline; top and bottom markings show precise length of zipper to be used.
Center front, center back: Indicated by a seamline (as shown here), a foldline, or other solid line; always clearly labeled.
Center back
Place on lengthwise grain of fabric
5
Skirt back A
Grainline markings: Straight line ending in arrowheads; means "place on straight grain of fabric."
Seam ⅝"
Hemline: The recommended finished edge, and thus garment length. (If no hemline is designated, hem instructions are written at bottom edge of pattern.)
3" hem

Fabric fundamentals

Natural and synthetic fibers

Fibers are the basic components of textile fabrics. Each has unique characteristics that it imparts to fabrics made from it. Although a fiber's character can be altered by yarn structure and by fabric construction and finishes, the original personality is still evident in the resulting fabric and central to its use and care.

Before this century, all fibers used for cloth were from natural sources. In recent years, a host of new, synthetic fibers have appeared, products of the chemistry laboratory. Whether a fiber is natural or synthetic has some bearing on its general characteristics. An overview and comparison of natural and synthetic fibers begins below. Consult charts here and on the opposite page for the properties and uses of individual fibers.

Natural fibers have the irregularities and subtleties inherent in natural things. These qualities contribute to the beauty of natural fabrics. Absorbency and porosity are also common to natural fibers, making them responsive to changes in temperature and humidity and comfortable to wear in a variety of climatic conditions. Less desirable is the fact that natural fibers, especially cotton and linen, have limited resiliency, so that fabrics made with them tend to wrinkle. This can be modified by wrinkle-resistant finishes, though at some sacrifice of comfort.

Cotton, linen, and wool occur as relatively short fibers (1½ to 20 inches long) called *staples.* Before fabric can be constructed, the staples must be twisted (spun) into continuous strands called yarns (see p. 60). When fibers are sorted for spinning, the longer and shorter lengths are usually separated. The longer staples make the best natural fabrics (identified as "combed" for cottons, "worsted" for wools). Such fabrics are supple and sleek and have a slight sheen. They are generally more expensive, but exceptionally durable.

Silk fiber is unreeled from the silkworm's cocoon into a long, continuous strand called a *filament.* The short strands left from this process are twisted together and used to produce rough-textured "spun silk."

All synthetic fibers begin as chemical solutions; forced through tiny holes into a chemical bath or air chamber, these harden into long ropes of fiber, also called filaments. Unless further treated (texturized or spun), these are smooth and slippery, which contributes to the tendency of many woven synthetics to unravel.

Synthetics are also highly resilient, and thus wrinkle resistant. On the other hand, almost all (except rayon) are low in porosity and absorbency, which makes them uncomfortable in hot or humid weather. Certain synthetics, nylon for one, are thermoplastic, that is, they can be molded under controlled conditions of heat and pressure, permitting the creation of interesting texture variations in the yarn or in the finished fabric.

One problem with synthetics is the array of terms used to identify them. This is less bewildering when you know the difference between a **generic** name for a fiber type, and a **trademark**—a particular company's name for that fiber. Orlon® and Acrilan®, for example, are registered trademarks (of different companies) for an acrylic. Any trademarked fiber may differ slightly from others in its group, but they all have the same chemical structure, and consequently similar characteristics.

Fiber blends are combinations of two or more different fibers. Usually the fiber present in the highest percentage dominates the fabric, but a successful blend will exhibit the desirable qualities of all.

You cannot always identify the fibers in a particular fabric from appearance alone. That is why it is so important to read all fabric information on the bolt or hang tag. The law requires uncut fabrics to be accompanied by a care label, in a form that can be sewed into the finished garment. Ask for it at time of purchase.

Natural fibers

Fiber and source	Characteristics	Typical fabrics and uses	Care
Cotton From seed pod of cotton plant	Strong, even when wet Absorbent Draws heat from body Tends to wrinkle Good affinity for dyes Shrinks unless treated Deteriorated by mildew Weakened by sunlight	Versatile fabrics in many weights and textures Used for summer wear, season-spanning garments, work clothes *Examples: Corduroy, denim, poplin, terry, organdy, seersucker*	Most cottons can be laundered, colorfast ones in hot water, others in warm or cold water Tumble-dry at hot setting Chlorine bleach can be used if care instructions permit Iron while damp
Linen From flax plant	Strong Absorbent Draws heat from body Wrinkles unless treated Poor affinity for dyes Some tendency to shrink and stretch Deteriorated by mildew	Fabrics usually have coarse texture and natural luster Weave weights vary from very light to heavy Used for spring and summer wear; also many household items	Usually dry-cleaned to retain the crisp finish Can be washed if softness is preferred Usually shrinks when washed
Silk From cocoons of silkworms	Strong Absorbent Holds in body heat Wrinkle-resistant Good affinity for dyes, but may bleed Resists mildew, moths Weakened by sunlight and perspiration	Luxurious, lustrous fabrics in many weights Used for dresses, suits, blouses, and linings *Examples: Brocade, chiffon, crepe, satin, tweed, jersey*	Usually dry-cleaned If washable, usually done by hand in mild suds Avoid chlorine bleach Iron at low temperature setting
Wool From fleece of sheep	Relatively weak Exceptionally absorbent Holds in body heat Wrinkles fall out Good affinity for dye Needs mothproofing Shrinks unless treated	Fabrics of many weights, textures, constructions Used for sweaters, dresses, suits, and coats *Examples: Crepe, flannel, fleece, gabardine, melton, tweed, jersey*	Usually dry-cleaned Many sweaters can be washed in tepid water and mild suds; do not wring Do not use chlorine bleach Some wools can be machine-washed; follow instructions

Synthetic fibers

Fiber and trademarks*	Characteristics	Typical fabrics and uses	Care
Acetate Ariloft[9] Celanese[5] Chromspun[9] Estron[9] Loftura[9]	Relatively weak Moderately absorbent Holds in body heat Tends to wrinkle Dyes well Resists pilling, shrinking, and moths Accumulates static electricity	Luxurious, silklike fabrics with deep luster and excellent draping qualities Used for lingerie, dresses, blouses, linings *Examples: Brocade, crepe, faille, satin, taffeta, lace, jersey, tricot*	Usually dry-cleaned If washable, can be done by hand or on gentle cycle of machine If tumble-dried, use low setting Iron at synthetic setting Affected by solvents containing acetone (e.g., nail polish remover)
Acrylic Acrilan[13] Bi-Loft[13] Creslan[2] Fina[13] Orlon[8] Zefran[7]	Low absorbency Holds in body heat Resists wrinkles Good affinity for dyes Resists mildew, moths Accumulates static electricity Tends to pill Heat-sensitive	Chiefly soft or fluffy fabrics, often with pile construction Often blended with other fibers Used for sweaters, dresses, and outerwear *Examples: Fake fur, fleece, double knit*	Some acrylics can be dry-cleaned but laundering is usually recommended Can be machine-washed (warm setting), tumble-dried Use fabric softener to reduce static electricity Often need no ironing if removed from drier before cycle stops
Glass Fiberglas[14]	Strong Nonabsorbent Resists wrinkles Low affinity for dyes Low abrasion resistance Undamaged by many chemicals, sunlight	Fabric types from sheer and lightweight to coarse and heavy Used principally for curtains, draperies, and upholstery	Hand laundering usually recommended Chlorine bleach can be used for white fabrics Ironing is not necessary as a rule
Metallic Lurex[7]	Weak Nonabsorbent Tarnishes unless coated properly Heat-sensitive	First made into yarns; these are usually coated with plastic, polyester, or acetate film and made into glittery fabrics	Launder or dry-clean according to care instructions Do not use high temperature for either washing or ironing
Modacrylic Acrilan[13] Elura[13] SEF[13] Verel[9]	Low absorbency Holds in body heat Resists wrinkles Resists moths, mildew Nonallergenic Very heat-sensitive Dries quickly Flame-resistant	Fabrics are chiefly deep-pile structures Used for coats, plush toys, carpets, and wigs *Example: Fake fur*	Deep-pile coats should be dry-cleaned For fabrics labeled washable, follow care instructions Avoid ironing; modacrylics melt at relatively low temperatures
Nylon Antron[8] Blue C[13] Caprolan[1] Celanese[5] Crepeset[3] Enkalure[3] Qiana[8] Zefran[7]	Strong Low absorbency Holds in body heat Resists shrinking, moths, and mildew Tends to pill Accumulates static electricity	Wide range of fabric textures and weights Often blended with other fibers Used for lingerie, linings, swimsuits, blouses, and dresses *Examples: Ciré, fake fur, satin, jersey*	Can be washed by hand or machine in warm water; use gentle machine cycle Use fabric softener to reduce static electricity Tumble- or drip-dry Iron at low temperature
Olefin Herculon[11] Marvess[15]	Holds in body heat Soil resistant Strong Heat-sensitive	Fabrics are usually bulky but lightweight, with a wool-like hand Used for outerwear filling and upholstery	Machine-wash, lukewarm water; use fabric softener in final rinse Tumble-dry, lowest setting Iron at lowest temperature setting, or not at all
Polyester Avlin[10] Blue C[13] Caprolan[1] Dacron[8] Fortrel[5] Kodel[9] Quintess[15] Trevira[12] Vycron[4] Zefran[7]	Strong Low absorbency Holds in body heat Resists wrinkling, stretching, shrinking, moths, and mildew Retains heat-set pleats Accumulates static electricity	Wide variety of fabrics in many weights and constructions Used for dresses, suits, sportswear, lingerie, linings, curtains, thread, filling for pillows *Examples: Crepe, double knit, lining*	Most polyesters are washable in warm water by hand or machine Tumble- or drip-dry Use fabric softener to reduce static electricity May need little or no ironing; use moderate setting for touch-ups
Rayon Avril[10] Beau-Grip[4] Coloray[6] Enkrome[3] Fibro[6] Zantrel[3]	Relatively weak Absorbent Holds in body heat Good affinity for dyes Wrinkles, shrinks, or stretches unless treated	Many fabric weights, textures silky to coarse Used for dresses, blouses, suits, linings, draperies *Examples: Butcher linen, matte jersey*	Many rayons must be dry-cleaned Some are washable in warm water, gentle machine cycle Iron while damp and at moderate setting
Spandex Lycra[8]	Strong Nonabsorbent Great elasticity Lightweight Light may yellow	Flexible, lightweight fabrics Often used with another fiber Used for swimwear, ski pants, foundations	Wash by hand, or by machine, using gentle cycle Avoid chlorine bleach Drip- or tumble-dry Iron at low temperature
Triacetate Arnel[5]	Relatively weak Resists wrinkling and shrinking Good affinity for dyes Retains heat-set pleats	Lightweight fabrics Used for sportswear and skirts where pleat retention is desirable *Examples: Sharkskin, tricot*	Hand- or machine-wash in warm water Drip-dry pleated garments; tumble-dry other styles Ironing usually required

*Fibers are those most widely used for fabrics; numbered names in fiber groups are representative trademarks of these companies: [1]Allied Chemical [2]American Cyanamid [3]American Enka Company [4]Beaunit Corporation [5]Celanese Corporation [6]Courtaulds North America [7]Dow Badische [8]E.I. DuPont de Nemours [9]Eastman Kodak Company [10]Avtex Fibers Inc. [11]Hercules [12]Hoechst Fibers [13]Monsanto [14]Owens-Corning Fiberglas Corporation [15]Phillips Fibers Corporation

Fabric fundamentals

The yarns that become fabrics

Yarns are continuous strands of fibers used in the making of woven and knit fabrics. There are two basic types, **spun** and **filament,** each with variations that give different characteristics to fabrics made of them.

A **spun yarn** is made by twisting together staples (short fibers). These can be products that occur naturally in this form, or synthetic filaments (usually long) cut to short lengths.

The spinning process consists of several steps that are basically the same for all fibers, with a few variations for fiber type and desired end product. Natural staples are first cleaned, sorted into matching lengths, and arranged in bunches—a process called *carding*. Sometimes the fibers are put through a second, more precise sorting called *combing*. In combing, the longest fibers are separated out and laid in parallel bunches; these become the combed cotton or worsted wool yarns that are the basis of high quality fabrics.

The final spinning steps are *drawing* (pulling staples lengthwise over each other) and *spinning* (twisting them together). The amount of twist affects fabric appearance and durability. A slack twist, for instance, is given to yarns intended for use in napped fabrics; a hard twist for smooth-surfaced fabrics, such as gabardine; maximum twist for crimped fabrics, such as crepe. In general, the harder the twist, the smoother and more durable the yarn.

A spun yarn variation is *ply yarn*—two or more single yarns twisted together. Another variation is *novelty yarn*. This can be either a single strand with varying amounts of twist, or ply yarn consisting of singles with different degrees of twist or different diameters. Examples are slub and bouclé. As a rule, novelty yarns are less durable than other types, because their uneven surfaces are subject to abrasion and snagging.

Filament yarn is the strand (several yards long) unreeled from a silkworm's cocoon or extruded from the chemical solution from which synthetic fibers derive. It is characteristically smooth, fine, and slippery. A single strand, or *monofilament*, is used for such fine fabrics as sheer curtaining and hosiery. Two or more twisted together are *multifilaments*. Fabrics constructed with these are stronger and more opaque than fabrics made of monofilaments.

A filament variation is produced by *texturizing*. In this process, a thermoplastic yarn is melted and heat-set to change its smooth surface to a coil, crimp, or loop shape. Such treatment increases the surface area, giving the yarns greater resiliency, bulk, elasticity, and absorbency. Stretch yarn is one result of texturizing.

There are special numbering systems to designate the thickness of single yarns. **Yarn count** applies to spun yarns; the higher the number, the *finer* the strand. **Denier** signifies thickness of a filament; the higher the number, the *coarser* the strand.

Spun yarn is composed of staples (short fiber lengths) twisted together into a continuous strand. The strand may contain one fiber type, or two or more fibers blended during the spinning process. The smoothest and strongest spun yarns are those made from longer staples that have been given a high degree of twist.

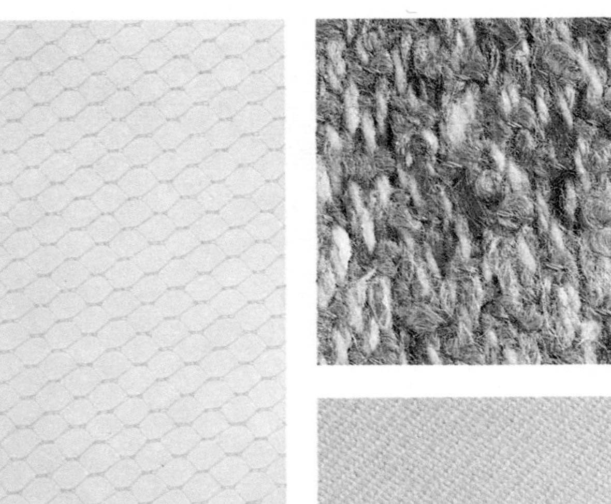

Filament yarn is a long, smooth strand unreeled from a silkworm's cocoon or extruded from a chemical solution (the source of man-made fibers). It may take the form of a monofilament (single strand), multifilaments (two or more strands twisted together), or staples (cut lengths to be made into spun yarn).

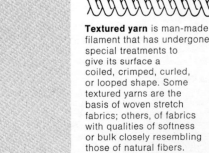

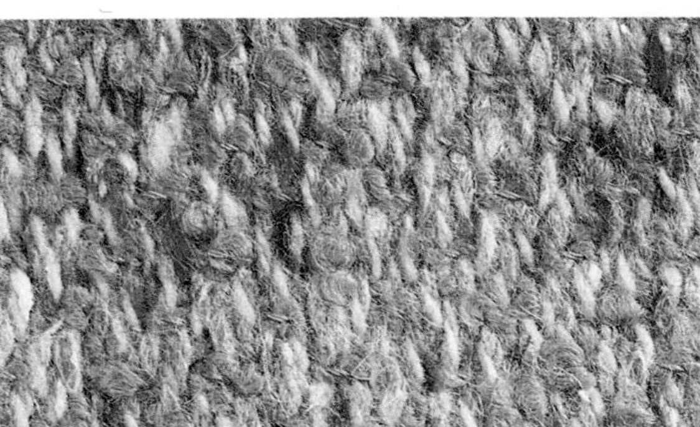

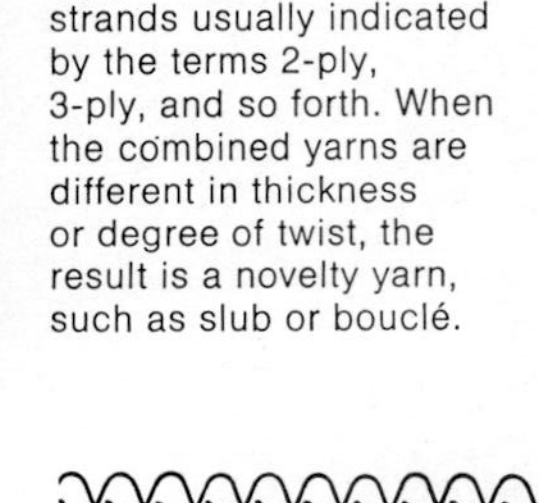

Ply yarn consists of two or more spun yarns twisted together, the number of strands usually indicated by the terms 2-ply, 3-ply, and so forth. When the combined yarns are different in thickness or degree of twist, the result is a novelty yarn, such as slub or bouclé.

Textured yarn is man-made filament that has undergone special treatments to give its surface a coiled, crimped, curled, or looped shape. Some textured yarns are the basis of woven stretch fabrics; others, of fabrics with qualities of softness or bulk closely resembling those of natural fibers.

Fabric structures

Woven fabric constructions

Woven fabrics are produced by the interlacing of yarns. *Warp* (lengthwise) yarns are first stretched onto a loom, and arranged so that they can be alternately raised and lowered by harnesses (movable frames). *Weft* (filling or crosswise) yarns are then inserted at right angles to the warp, by shuttles. Weave structures can be varied by rearranging the pattern in which warp and weft intersect.

There are three basic weaves, *plain, twill,* and *satin.* Most other types are variations on these three, except for patterned weaves. These are complex structures that require special devices attached to the loom (see examples of patterned weaves, p. 62).

Every woven fabric has a ribbon-like edge, or **selvage,** running lengthwise along each side. Always be sure that weft yarns are at right angles to the selvages; this indicates that fabric is *on grain,* an important consideration in cutting. Though rough-textured fabrics can be interesting, those with smooth, tightly twisted yarns and a high thread count (number of yarns per square inch of fabric) are the most durable.

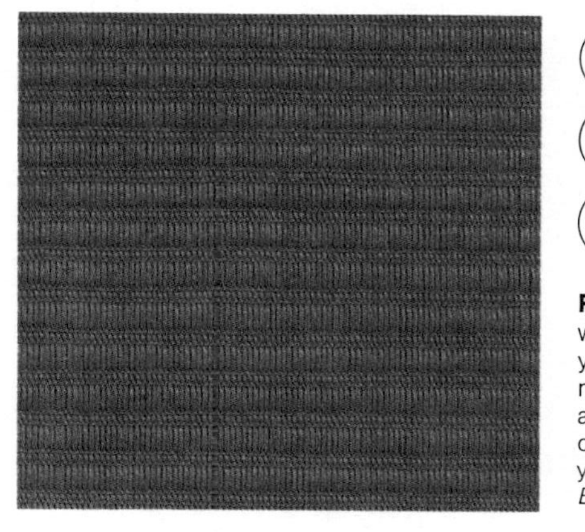

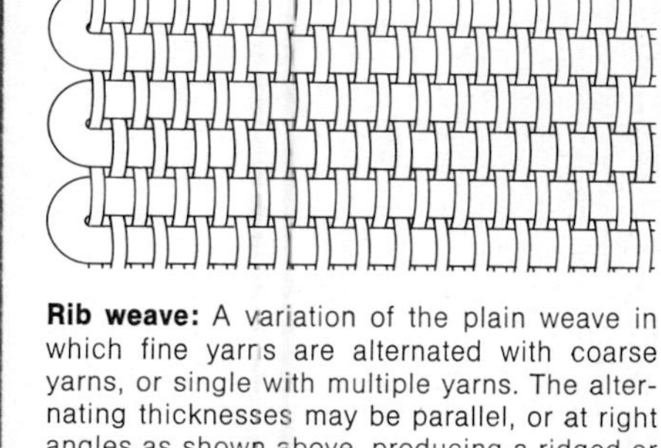

Rib weave: A variation of the plain weave in which fine yarns are alternated with coarse yarns, or single with multiple yarns. The alternating thicknesses may be parallel, or at right angles as shown above, producing a ridged or corded effect. Durability is limited because the yarns are exposed to friction.
Examples: Faille, ottoman, bengaline

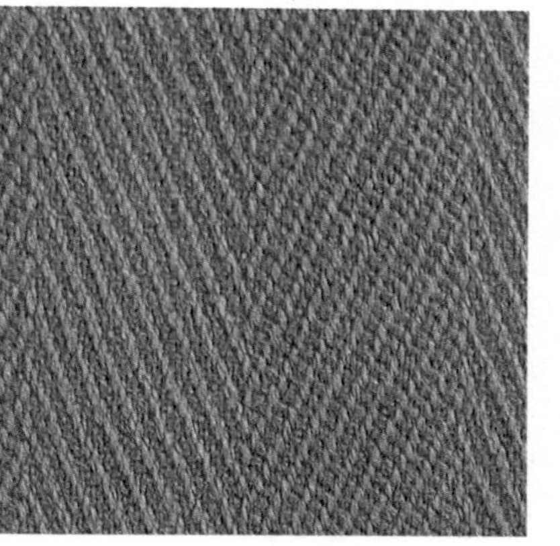

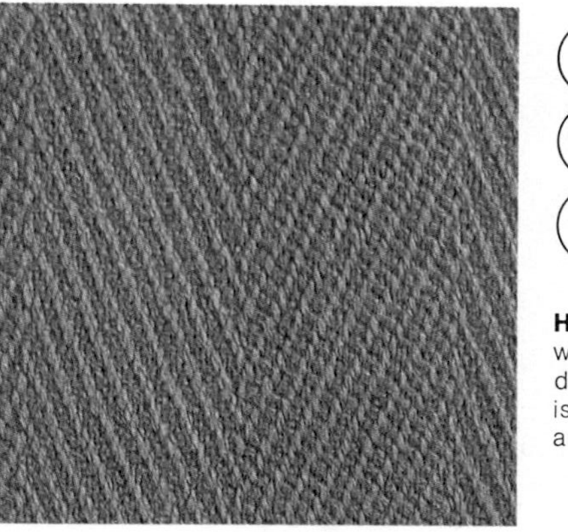

Plain weave: The simplest of the weave constructions, in which each filling yarn goes alternately over and under each warp yarn. Sturdiness varies with strength of the yarns and compactness of the weave structure. Plain weave is the basis for most prints.
Examples: Muslin, voile, challis, percale

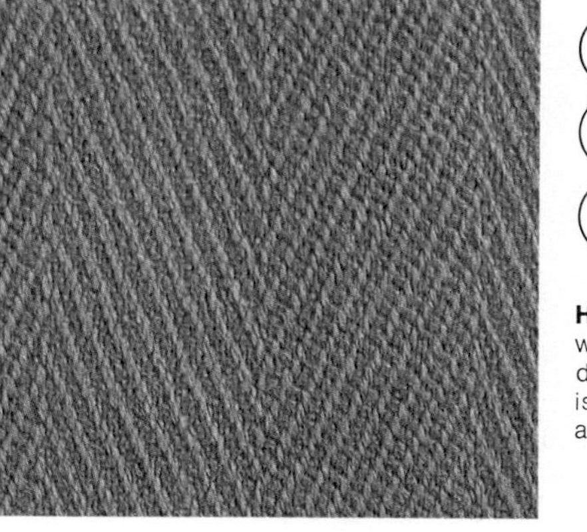

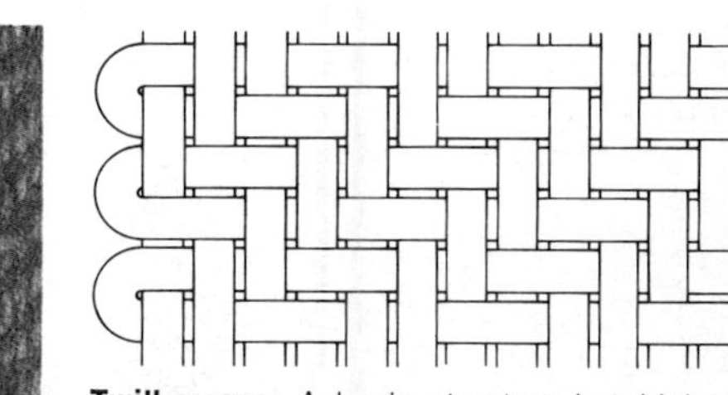

Twill weave: A basic structure in which weft yarn passes over at least two, but not more than four, warp yarns. On each successive line, the weft moves one step to the right or left, forming a diagonal ridge; the steeper the ridge, the stronger the fabric. As a rule, twills are more durable than plain weaves.
Examples: Denim, gabardine, serge

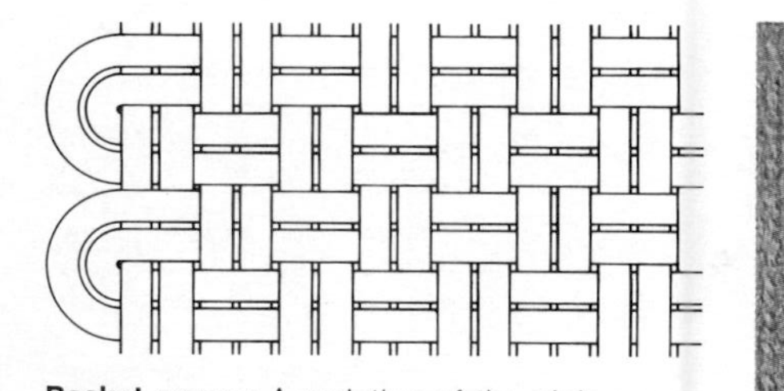

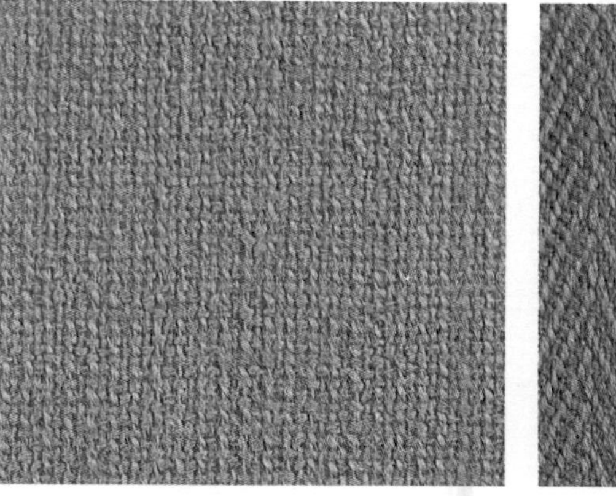

Basket weave: A variation of the plain weave in which paired or multiple yarns are used in the alternating pattern. The yarns are laid side by side without being twisted together. This makes the basket weave looser, less stable, often less durable than ordinary plain weaves.
Examples: Hopsacking, oxford shirting

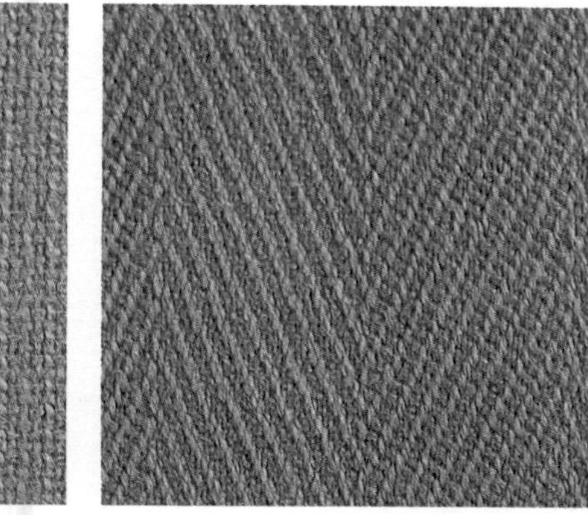

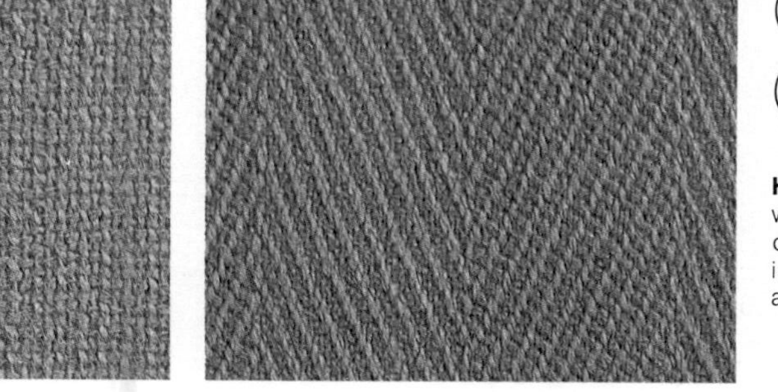

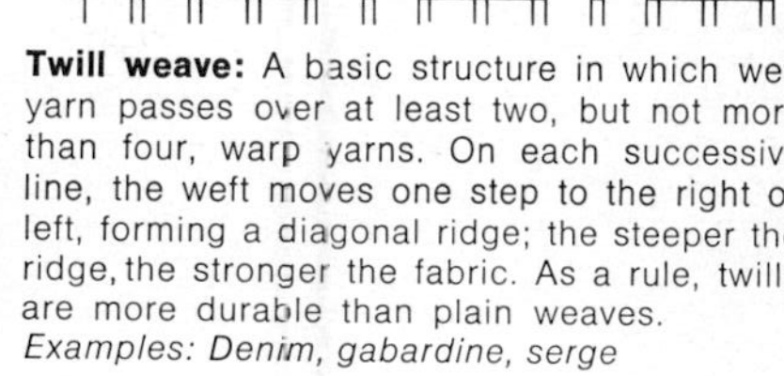

Herringbone weave: A variation of the twill weave in which the diagonal ridges switch direction to form a zigzag pattern. The design is more pronounced when contrasting colors are used for the ridges.

Fabric structures

Woven fabric constructions

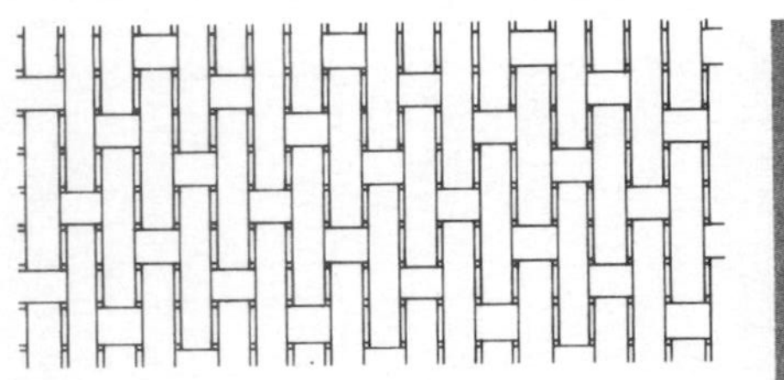

Satin weave: A basic structure in which a warp yarn passes over four to eight weft yarns in a staggered pattern similar to that of twill. Yarns exposed on the surface, called *floats*, give satin its characteristic sheen. **Sateen weave,** usually of cotton fiber, is a variation in which the floats are formed by weft yarns.
Examples: Peau de soie, crepe-back satin

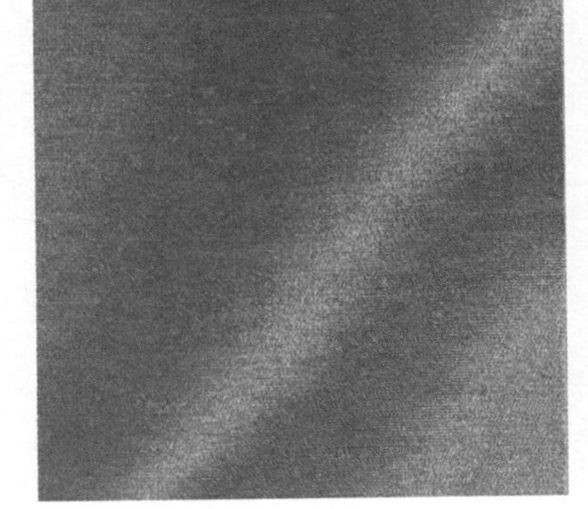

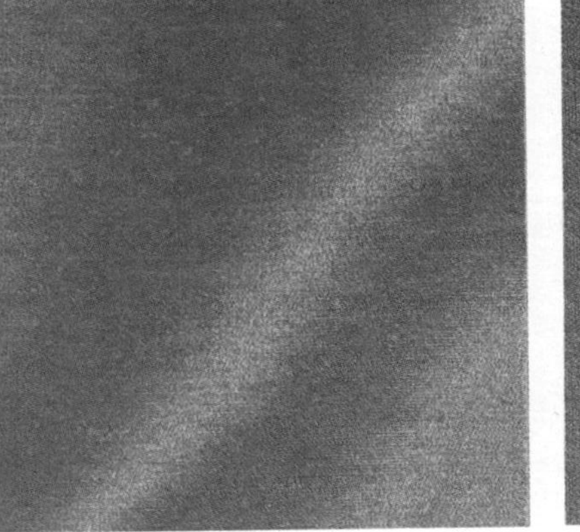

Dobby weave: A patterned structure, usually geometric in form, produced by a special attachment (dobby) on a plain-weave loom. The dobby raises and lowers certain warp yarns so that warp and weft interlace in a constantly changing pattern. Most familiar is the diamond shape, shown here.
Example: Bird's-eye piqué

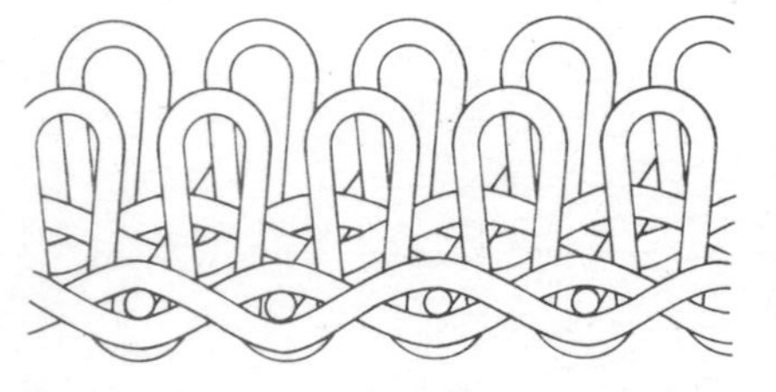

Pile weave: Here an extra filling or warp yarn is added to a basic plain or twill weave. By means of thick wires, the additional yarn is drawn into loops on the fabric surface. These loops can then be cut as for plush, sheared as for velvet, or left in loop form as for terry cloth.
Examples: Corduroy, velours, fake fur

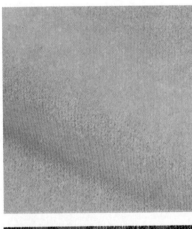

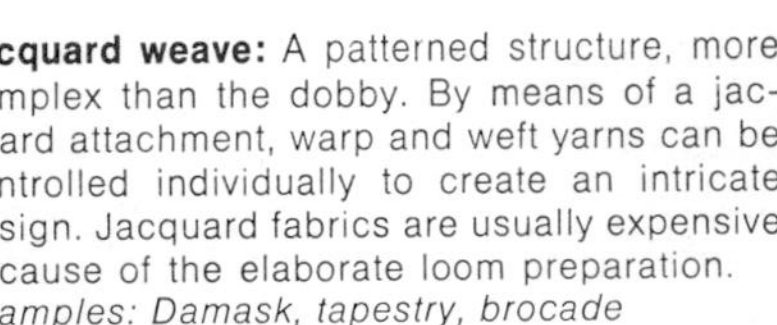

Jacquard weave: A patterned structure, more complex than the dobby. By means of a jacquard attachment, warp and weft yarns can be controlled individually to create an intricate design. Jacquard fabrics are usually expensive because of the elaborate loom preparation.
Examples: Damask, tapestry, brocade

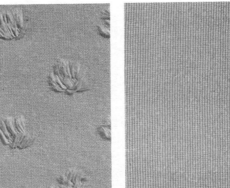

Swivel weave: To achieve this weave, an extra filling yarn is added to form a circle or other figure on the surface of a basic weave. Each swivel yarn is carried on the wrong side of the fabric from one design to the next, then cut when the fabric is completed.
Examples: Dotted swiss, coin-dot chenille

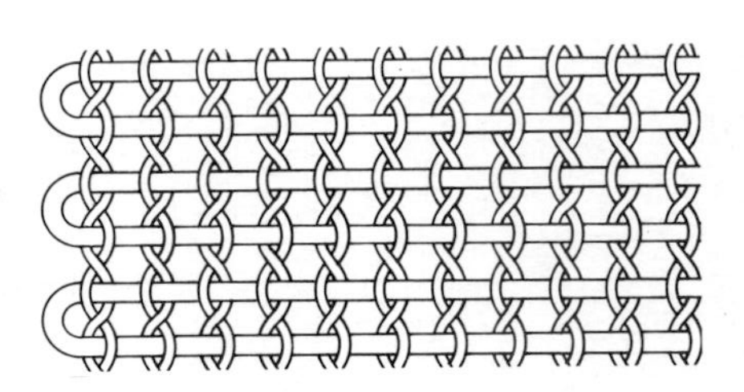

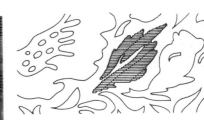

Gauze weave (also called leno weave): An open mesh structure produced by a *leno* attachment on the loom. The leno continuously changes the position of the warp yarns so that they become twisted in figure eight fashion around the filling yarns.
Example: Marquisette

Knit constructions

Knit fabrics are made up of a series of interlocking loops that result in a flexible construction. While all knits have stretch, they vary considerably in amount and direction of stretch. The influential factors in stretch are the yarn and the particular knit structure employed.

There are two basic knit structures, **weft** and **warp.** The first derives from age-old techniques of hand knitting. The second, a modern innovation, is the product of complex machines. Records show that the first knitting machine was invented in 1589. Today's advanced versions turn out an incredible range of fabrics from sheer lingerie knits to bulky sweater types, even piles and jacquard patterns.

Descriptions of knit variations are given at the right and on page 64. Relevant to them are the following terms: **Knit stitch** is a basic link in which a loop is drawn through the *front* of the previous one; **purl stitch,** a basic link in which a loop is drawn through the *back* of the previous one. All knit variations are achieved by changing the arrangement of these two basic stitches. **Ribs** (wales) are lengthwise rows of loops; **courses** are crosswise rows. These are comparable to warp and weft in woven fabrics. **Gauge** denotes the number of stitches per inch. Usually the higher the number, the finer the fabric.

Knit fabrics may be tubular or flat. Some flat types have perforated lengthwise edges comparable to selvages in woven fabrics. Complex stitches or special finishes sometimes obscure a knit structure, making it hard to tell whether a fabric is knitted or woven. To settle the question, pull a thread from one crosswise end. If loops show, the fabric is a knit; if a fringe appears, it is woven.

Warp knits

Warp knit fabric is constructed with many yarns that form loops simultaneously in the lengthwise (warp) direction. Each yarn is controlled by its own needle, and interlocked with neighboring yarns in zigzag fashion. This interlocking produces fabrics that are usually runproof and have limited stretchability, in varieties ranging from sheer laces to fake furs.

Because of their complex structures, warp knits can be produced only by machine. *Tricot* and *raschel* (shown below) are the most widely produced types. There are also *crochets* (similar to the hand work) and *simplexes* (double-knit tricots).

Warp knits are widely available, and comparatively low in cost—the machines used can produce up to 40 square feet of fabric per minute.

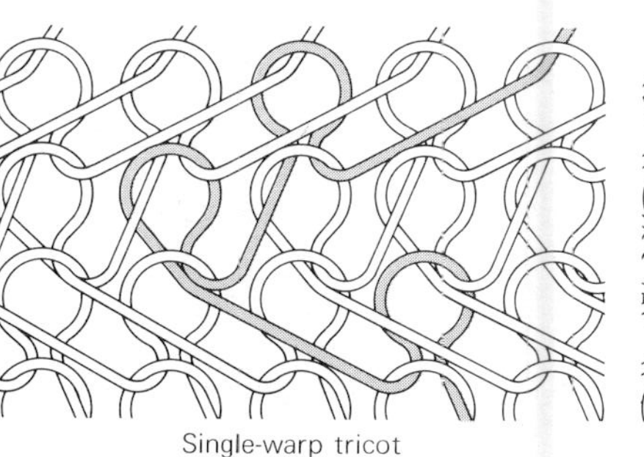

Single-warp tricot

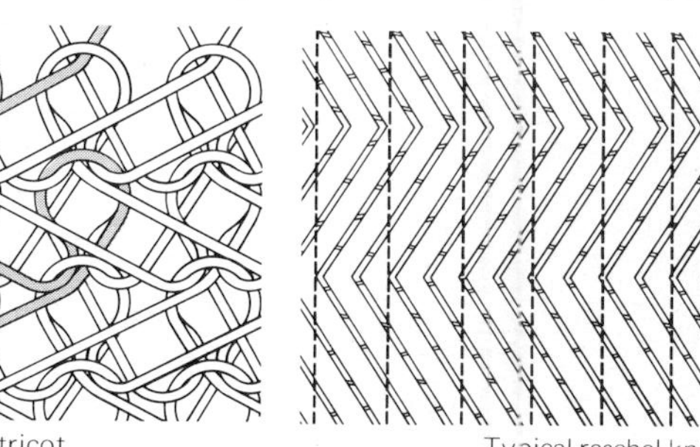

Double-warp tricot

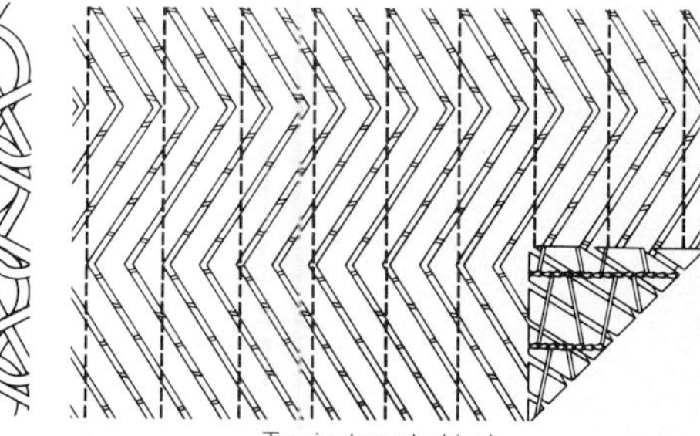

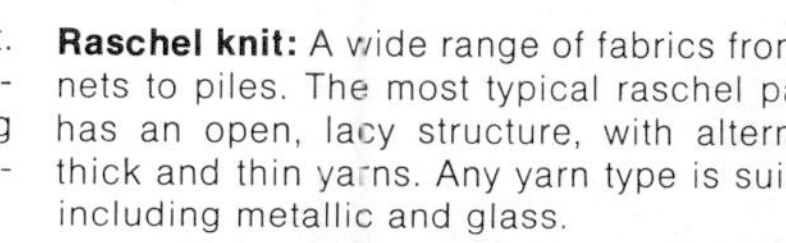

Typical raschel knit

Tricot knit: Fine ribs on the face, flat herringbone courses on the back. Can be single-, double-, or triple-warp construction. Technical differences are not discernible to the eye, but they do affect performance. Double- and triple-warp tricots are runproof; single-warp is not. Tricots are usually made with fine yarns, cotton or synthetic. They have a soft, draping quality and are suitable for linings, loungewear, lingerie, and dresses.

Raschel knit: A wide range of fabrics from fine nets to piles. The most typical raschel pattern has an open, lacy structure, with alternating thick and thin yarns. Any yarn type is suitable, including metallic and glass.

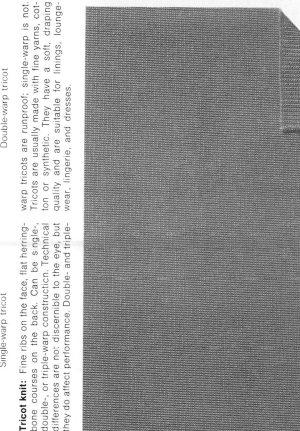

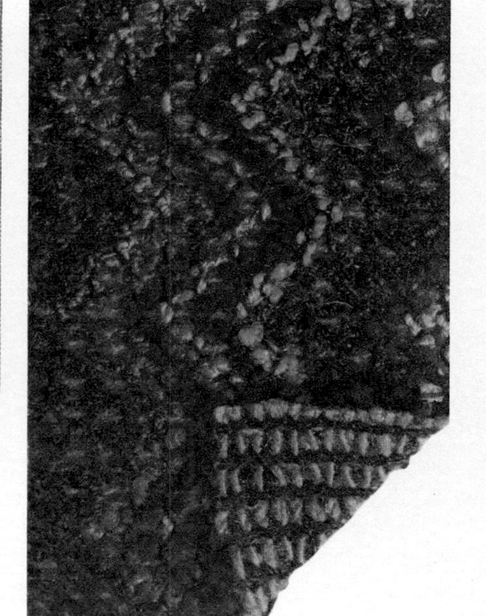

Fabric structures

Weft knits

Weft knit fabric is constructed with just one yarn that forms continuous rows of loops in the horizontal (weft) direction. Basically, the machine stitches are exactly like those done by hand, and fabric characteristics are similar. That is, the stretch is greater in width than in length, and a broken loop releases others in a vertical row, causing a run.

There are two distinct weft knit categories—*single* and *double*. Single knits have a moderate to great amount of stretch. Though very comfortable to wear, they may eventually sag in stress areas, such as seat or knees. Also, their edges tend to curl, creating difficulties in cutting and stitching. Double knits have body and stability similar to those of a weave.

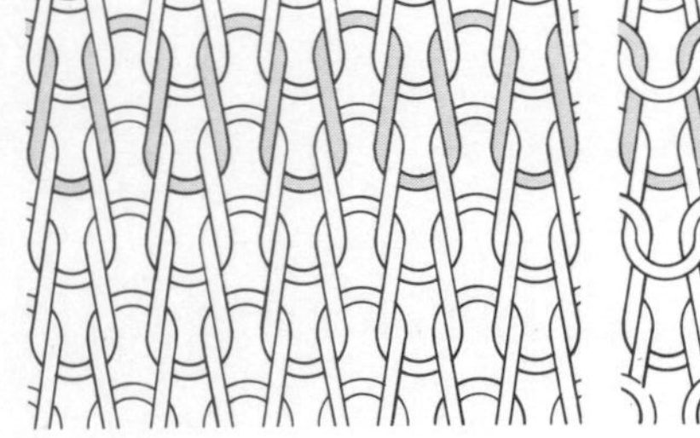

Plain jersey knit: A single construction in which all loops are pulled to the back of the fabric. The face is smooth, and it exhibits lengthwise vertical rows (wales); on the reverse side, there are horizontal rows of half-circles, which are characteristic of the purl stitch. Plain knits stretch more in width than in length.

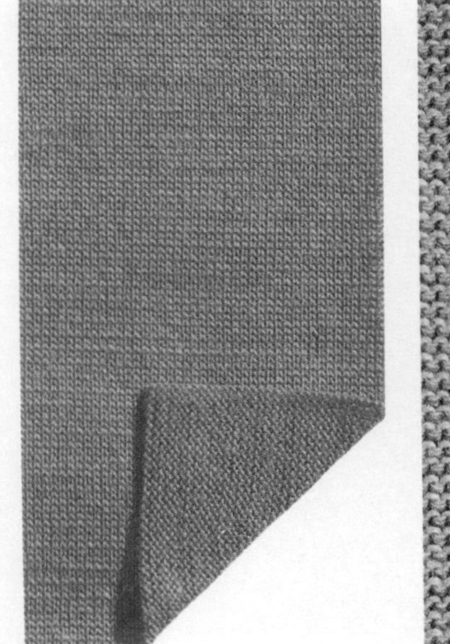

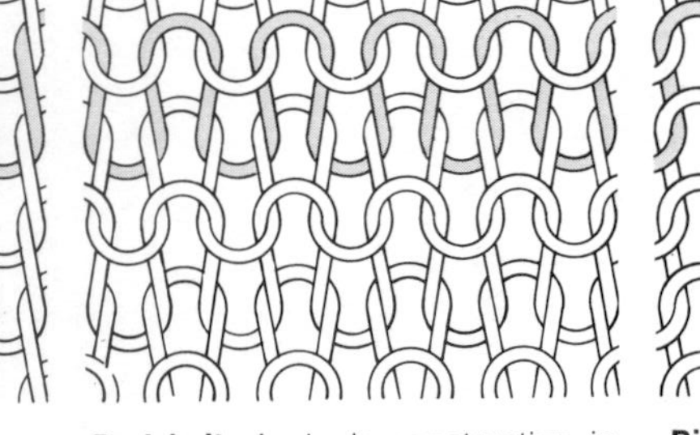

Purl knit: A single construction in which loops are pulled in alternate rows to the front and back of the knit, causing a purl stitch to appear on both sides of the fabric. Purl knits have nearly the same amount of stretch in both the lengthwise and the crosswise directions; this makes them ideal for infants' and children's wear.

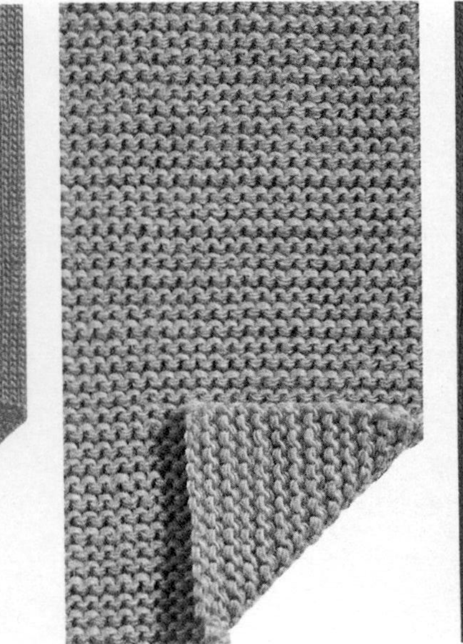

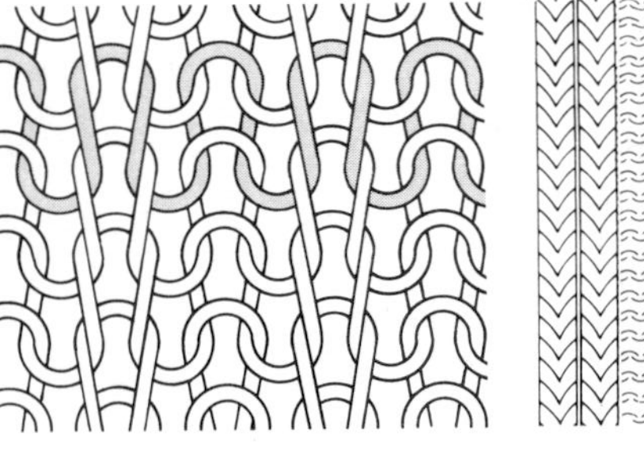

Rib knit: A single construction, with rows of plain and purl knit arranged so that the face and the reverse sides are identical. Rib knits have expansive stretch and strong recovery in the crosswise direction, which makes them especially suitable for cuffs and waistbands.

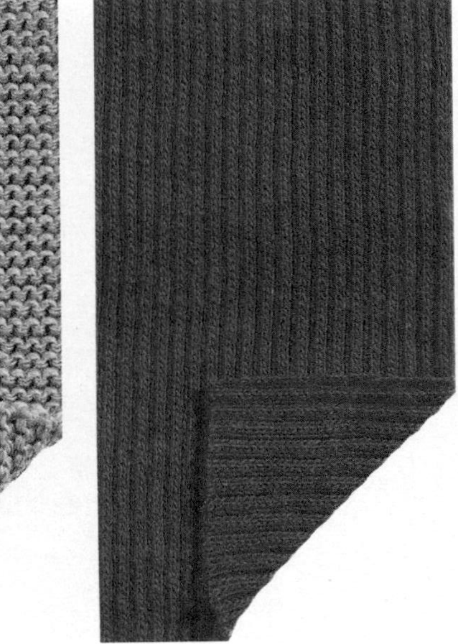

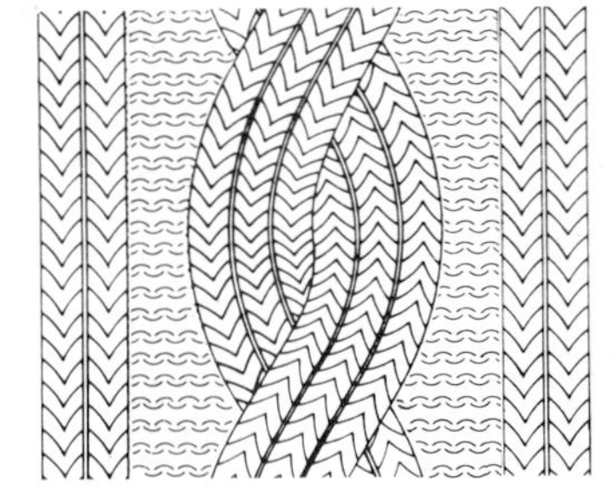

Patterned knits: Complex variations on the basic plain and purl knits. A cable knit is a typical example of a patterned knit.

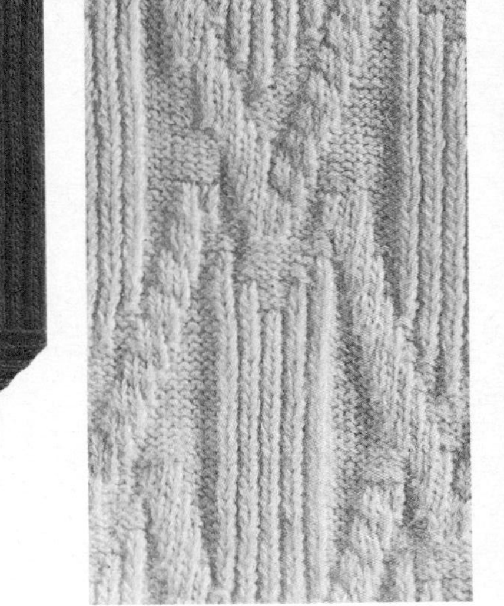

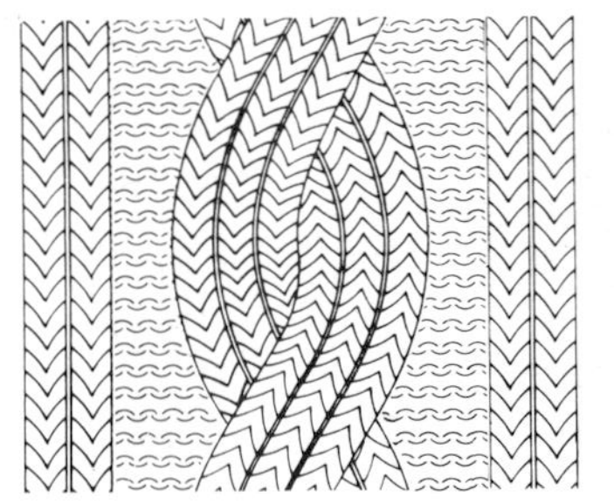

Double knit: Produced by two yarn-and-needle sets working simultaneously. Double knits have firm body and limited stretch capacity. Depending on the design, the face and back may look the same or different. Some complex double knits resemble the woven dobby and jacquard patterns.

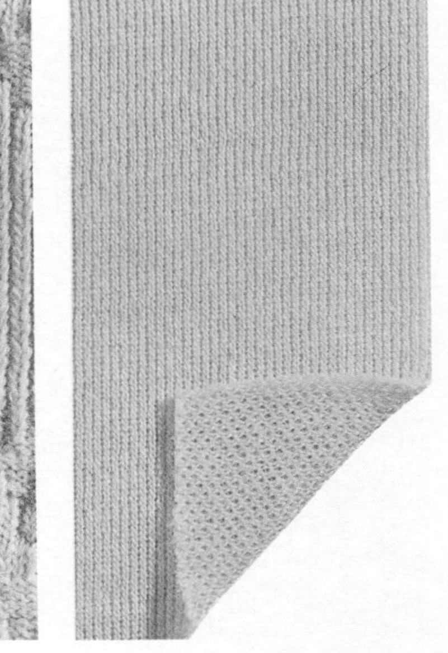

Other fabric constructions

There are several fabric constructions or processes that cannot be classified as knit or woven. Because practical applications are limited, these constitute only a small portion of all fabrics manufactured, but each has a significance worth noting.

An example is **felting,** one of the world's oldest methods of producing fabric. Some historians believe it might even have preceded weaving. Though of limited use for garments, it has wide applications for accessories and in household decor. **Netting** and **braiding,** too, are very old techniques. Both are used in lace-making. **Fusing, bonding,** and **laminating** are modern developments that use adhesives to interlock short fibers or glue fabrics together.

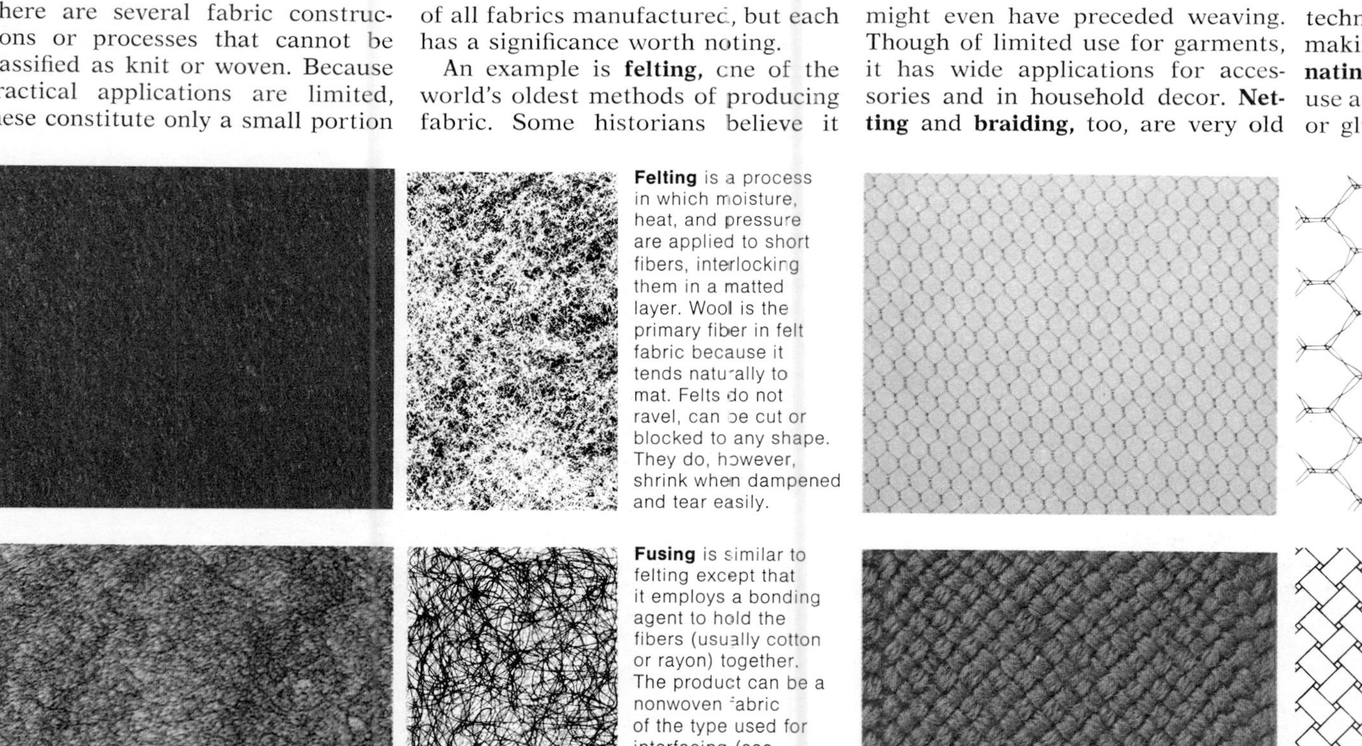

Felting is a process in which moisture, heat, and pressure are applied to short fibers, interlocking them in a matted layer. Wool is the primary fiber in felt fabric because it tends naturally to mat. Felts do not ravel, can be cut or blocked to any shape. They do, however, shrink when dampened and tear easily.

Fusing is similar to felting except that it employs a bonding agent to hold the fibers (usually cotton or rayon) together. The product can be a nonwoven fabric of the type used for interfacing (see p.76) or a web, which is itself a fusible bonding agent (see Fusibles).

Bonding is a process by which two or more fabrics are joined with an adhesive. The combination usually is a knit or loosely woven fabric backed by a lightweight lining. If one layer is a vinyl or foam, the product is called a **laminate.** All self-lined fabrics offer the advantages of dimensional stability, opaqueness, and body.

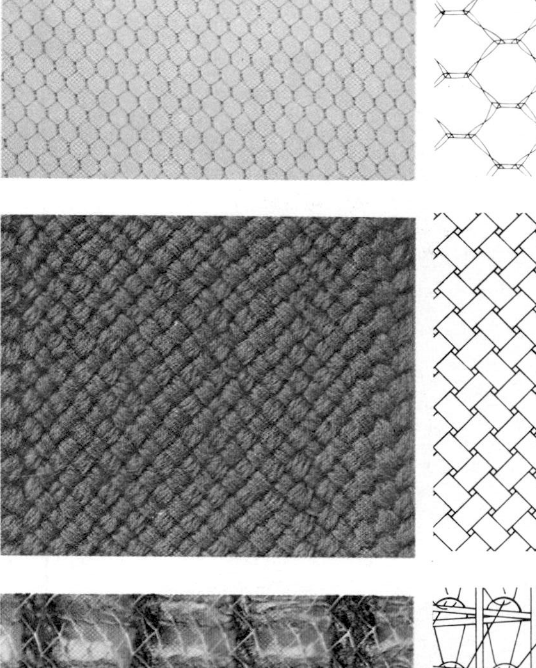

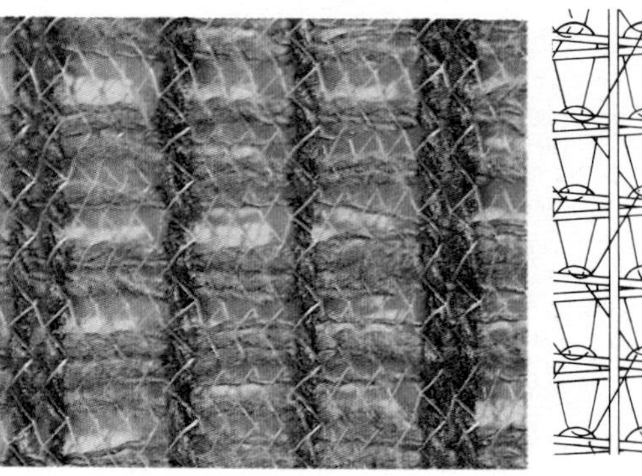

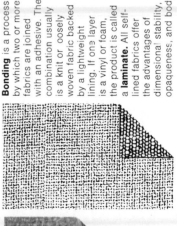

Netting is a fabric construction in which the yarns are held together by knots at each point where they intersect. This open-mesh structure can be varied to produce fabrics as heavy as fish net and as delicate as the mesh portion of a sheer lace. Many net fabrics, today, are made on tricot knit machines.

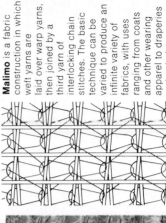

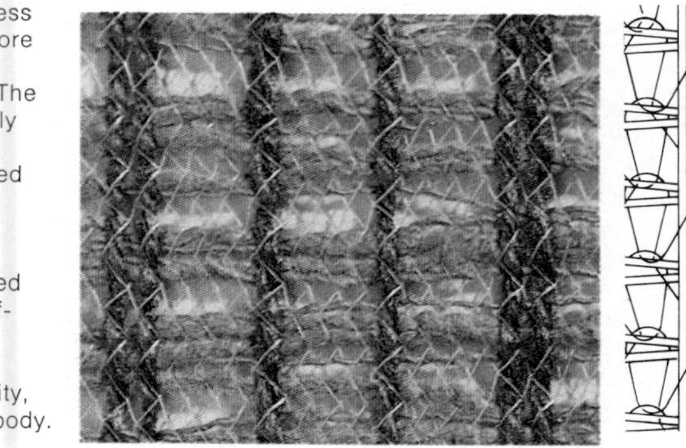

Braiding is a fabric construction in which three or more yarns from a single source are interlaced diagonally and lengthwise (just as in braiding hair). There are two forms, *flat* and *tubular.* Both yield a fabric that is narrow and flexible. Braiding is used primarily for garment trims, cords, and elastics.

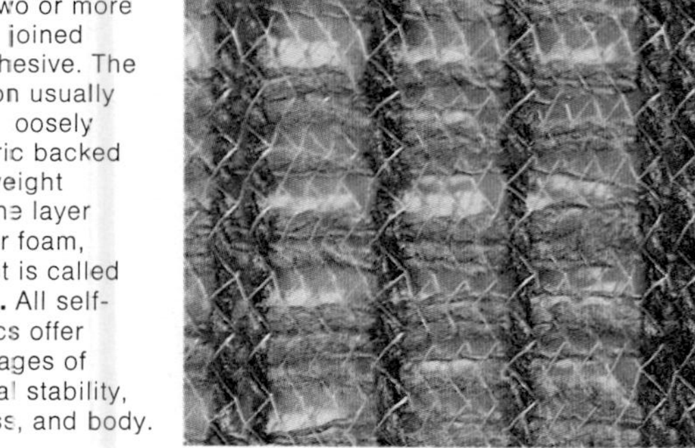

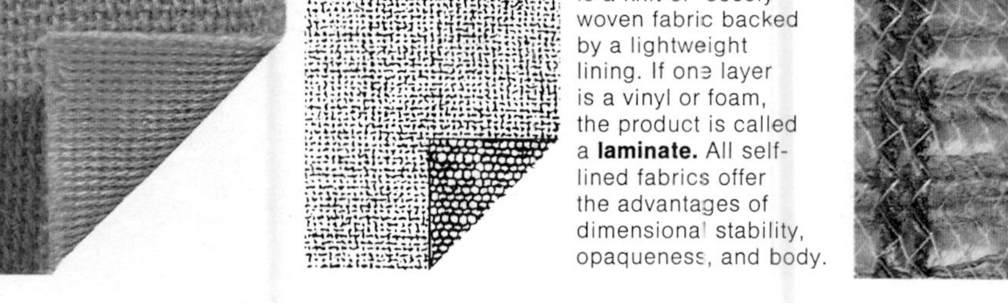

Malimo is a fabric construction in which weft yarns are laid over warp yarns, then joined by a third yarn of interlocking chain stitches. The basic technique can be varied to produce an infinite variety of fabrics, with uses ranging from coats and other wearing apparel to draperies and upholstery.

Fabric finishes

Types and purposes

Fabrics are given a variety of treatments, before, during, or after construction, designed to alter their performance and final appearance. Familiarity with these finishes will help you to select fabrics that meet your needs. To make understanding easier, these finishes are divided here into **functional** (affecting fabric behavior) and **decorative** (affecting a fabric's look or feel). The divisions, however, are not always so clear-cut. Napping, for instance, alters texture and adds warmth as well.

Functional finishes make a fabric more versatile or better suited to a specified need. Often, a single finish imparts more than one quality. Some side effects are desirable, others less so. Preshrinking, for example, makes a weave more compact and therefore more durable; a water-repellent finish tends to ward off stains and dirt as well as moisture. Treatment for wrinkle resistance, on the other hand, makes cotton less inclined to crease, but also less cool and comfortable.

Decorative finishes make fabric a pleasure to see and feel. Those described at the right are in wide commercial use. Not listed are hand techniques and those less significant in the fabric industry. Permanence, a major concern with color and texture, depends largely on quality of dye or technique used (see opposite page for ways to test quality). Commercial factors are influential, too. Fiber and yarn dyeing, for instance, are usually more permanent than piece dyeing, but less practical for meeting changing fashion needs.

To get maximum benefit from all finishes, care for a fabric as directed, and remember that the lasting potential of finishes is based on a garment's normal life expectancy.

Functional finishes—what to expect

Anti-bacterial: Resists many types of bacteria, including those in perspiration.
Anti-static: Does not accumulate static electricity, therefore does not cling.
Flame-resistant: Does not actively support a flame once its source has been removed. (Few textile fabrics can be made 100% fireproof.) By law, children's sleepwear fabrics must be treated for flame-resistance.
Mercerized (pertains to cottons and linens): Has greater strength and luster and better affinity for dye.
Mildew-resistant: Resists growth of mildew and other types of mold.
Mothproof: Resists attack by moths.
Permanent press (also called *durable press):* Sheds wrinkles from normal wear; requires no ironing when washed and dried according to care instructions; retains creases or pleats that have been heat-set. Has low abrasion resistance and should be laundered wrong side out for best results.
Preshrunk: Will not shrink more than the percentage indicated (usually 1% to 2%) if care instructions are followed.
Soil release (for permanent press fabrics): Permits removal of oil-based stains.
Stain- and spot-resistant: Resists water-based and/or oil-based stains (type or types should be specified on label).
Stiffened (permanent): Retains crisp finish through many washings (fiber structure has been permanently altered with chemicals).
Stiffened (temporary): Has body and crispness that may be lost in laundering but can be restored by adding starch (fabric has been sized, i.e., starched, to retain these attributes to time of purchase).
Stretch- and sag-resistant (pertains to knits): Maintains original dimensions through normal wear and many washings.
Wash-and-wear (also called *easy care* and *minimum care):* Requires little or no ironing after washing; resists and recovers from wrinkles caused by normal wear. Follow care instructions carefully; should not be twisted in washing; chlorine bleach may cause yellowing.
Waterproof: Is totally impervious to water under any and all conditions; pores of fabric are completely closed.
Water-repellent: Resists absorption and penetration of water, while remaining porous.
Wrinkle-resistant: Resists and recovers from wrinkles caused by normal wear.

Decorative finishing processes

COLOR

Bleaching: All natural color and staining are removed if the cloth is to be finished white, also before dyeing or printing.
Fiber (stock) dyeing: Natural fibers are dyed before spinning into yarn or matting into felt. A thorough and relatively permanent process.
Solution (dope) dyeing: Synthetic fibers are dyed in the liquid form before extrusion into filaments. Generally the most colorfast of the color treatments.
Yarn (skein) dyeing: Spools or skeins of yarn are immersed in a dye bath, permitting dye to penetrate to the core of the yarn. Permits the use of different colors to create a design such as a plaid or check. Gingham, for example, is a yarn-dyed fabric.
Piece dyeing: Fabric is dyed after construction. One common method is to unroll fabric, pass it through a trough containing dye solution, then re-roll it at the other end. The largest percentage of fabric by far is dyed this way because it allows for greater flexibility in manufacturing. Color is relatively fast if dyes used are those most suitable for the fiber.
Cross dyeing: There are three methods of cross dyeing: (1) Fabric is constructed with a combination of dyed and undyed yarns, then piece-dyed. (2) Fabric is constructed with undyed yarns of two different fibers, then piece-dyed in two different dye solutions, each with an affinity for one fiber. (3) Same as Method 2, but with two different dyes combined in a single dye bath. Many unusual effects—for example, frosty and iridescent—can be obtained with cross dyeing.

PRINT

Roller printing: Design is transferred to fabric by means of engraved copper cylinders, a different roller for each color. Fast and relatively inexpensive—thousands of yards per hour can be printed.
Screen printing: The dye is forced through screens with an impermeable coating on all areas not part of the design; a different screen is used for each color. Slower than roller printing but permits larger designs and brighter colors. Can be used successfully for knits.
Transfer printing: Design is first printed on paper, then transferred to fabric by means of heat under pressure. Quality of result is comparable to that of roller or screen printing, yet cost is about half. Can be used for knits.
Burnt-out printing: Fabric is "printed" with chemicals, which actually dissolve one of the fibers used in construction. Usual result is a raised motif on a sheer ground.
Discharge printing: Fabric is first dyed, then roller-printed with a chemical that bleaches out the design.
Duplex printing: Fabric is roller-printed on both sides, producing woven design effect.
Flocking: Fabric is roller-printed with an adhesive, then cut fibers are applied to the surface, resulting in textured pattern.
Resist printing: Resist paste (impervious to dye) is roller-printed on fabric. Fabric is next piece-dyed, then the paste removed, leaving light pattern on darker ground.
Warp printing: Warp yarns are roller-printed before weaving, then interlaced with plain weft yarns; design is usually mottled.

TEXTURE

Calendering: A pressing process in which fabric is passed between heavy rollers to make it smooth and glossy. Conditions of heat, speed, and pressure can be varied to achieve different effects.
Ciréing: Calendering variation in which wax or other sheen-producing substance is applied to fabric before contact with heated rollers. Final surface is superglossy.
Embossing: Calendering variation in which engraved and heated rollers form a raised design. Can be used for any fiber except wool; effect is permanent when the fiber is a thermoplastic, such as nylon, or when fabric has been treated with chemical resins.
Glazing: Calendering variation in which starch, glue, or shellac is applied to fabric before passing it over hot steel rollers that are moving faster than the fabric. Chintz is a glazed fabric.
Moiréing: Calendering variation in which two layers of fabric (usually rib weave of silk, acetate, or rayon) are passed over ridged rollers. Combination of moisture, heat, and intense pressure creates wavy bars that reflect light in differing ways.
Napping: A process in which the fabric surface is brushed to raise the fiber ends (yarn must be spun). The resulting texture is compact, soft, and warm. Fleece and flannel are examples of napped fabrics.
Plisséing: A treatment with caustic soda solution that shrinks fabric areas where it is applied, at the same time causing the dry areas to pucker. The result is a crinkled surface that may or may not be permanent.

Shopping for fabrics

Color and texture 52
Pattern envelope 54-55
Fabric grain and print alignments 84-85
Folding fabrics for cutting 87

Basic buying considerations

A successfully chosen garment fabric will complement the pattern design, flatter the wearer, perform according to expectations, and be of good quality for the money.

To determine a fabric's **suitability for a pattern,** check the pattern envelope. Illustrations on the front show fabrics appropriate for the design; the envelope back lists suggested fabrics chosen by the designer.

To find out whether a fabric is **becoming to you,** drape at least 2 yards of the material over yourself in front of a full-length mirror. In this way you can see the precise effect of color and texture on your skin tone and figure. (For guidance in the use of both color and texture, see Patterns.)

To predict a fabric's **probable behavior,** you must know its content and finishes, also how much it will shrink, and exactly how it should be cared for. The most reliable source of such information is the end-of-bolt label or the hang tag.

To **recognize quality,** or its opposite, you must become aware of the characteristics that signify excellence and those that disguise inferiority. The distinguishing features are often small and subtle, and detectable only to an experienced eye. There are some more obvious criteria, however, that can be used to advantage by novice and experienced shopper alike.

1. Weave should be firm. You can test this by scratching the surface; if the threads shift easily, the garment seams may be inclined to slip or develop holes around the stitching.

2. Weave should be uniform. Hold it up to the light and check for any unusually thick or thin areas. A fabric that has them would not wear evenly. The light test will also show up any weak spots or imperfections.

3. Filler yarns should meet selvages at right angles. Yarns at an oblique angle mean fabric is off-grain (see Cutting for test and remedy).

4. Dye color should be even and look fresh. If there is a creaseline, check whether color has rubbed off of it. This could indicate poor dye quality, and also pose a problem in cutting.

5. Print colors should be even, with no white (undyed) spots showing through them, except in areas that are clearly meant to be white.

6. A print that is geometric or otherwise symmetrical should meet the selvages at a right angle. An irregular print cannot be corrected.

7. No powdery dust should appear when fabric is rubbed between the fingers. Visible powder is an indication of too much sizing, a frequent device for concealing poor quality.

8. Fabric should shed wrinkles after crushing. If it does not, the garment will always look rumpled.

Special buying considerations

Extra thought must be given to the purchase of certain fabrics and materials because of special or unusual qualities. A review of this group begins here and goes through page 71.

Knits vary in stretchability. Just how much a knit stretches crosswise should be determined before purchase, because it is a factor in joining the right fabric to the right pattern. If the pattern you have chosen is marked "for knits only," it will probably supply a gauge like the one below, but for only one of three categories—slight, moderate, or super stretch. The purpose of the gauge is to help you tell whether a particular knit suits the pattern style.

This is how it works. Holding a 4-inch crosswise section of your knit against the gauge, stretch gently from the 4-inch mark to the outer limit of the ruler at the right. If the fabric stretches comfortably (that is, without distortion) to the designated point (or even beyond it), the knit has enough stretch for the pattern.

Notice, after ascertaining the fabric's stretch, whether it returns to its original dimensions. A knit that does not recover completely may sag or stretch out of shape in wearing.

Leather (the real kind) is usually sold by the square foot instead of the linear yard. Before purchase, therefore, you must calculate the footage requirements. Here is a conversion method, using 4 yards of 45-inch fabric as the example: (1) Calculate the number of square feet in 1 yard of the fabric width called for; in 1 yard of 45-inch fabric, the example chosen, there are 11¼ square feet. (2) Multiply the number of square feet by the number of required yards; in this case, 11¼ times 4, or a total of 45 square feet. (3) To this total, add an extra 15% for piecing and wastage; 45 times .15 equals 6.75; adding this amount to 45 gives you 51.75. You need 51¾ square feet of the leather.

In addition to footage, you should consider skin sizes, particularly the usable portions. If possible, compare these with the largest pattern pieces, taking into account any holes, scars, or irregular edges. To make the best use of usable areas, you might need to piece the leather or divide large pattern pieces into smaller sections.

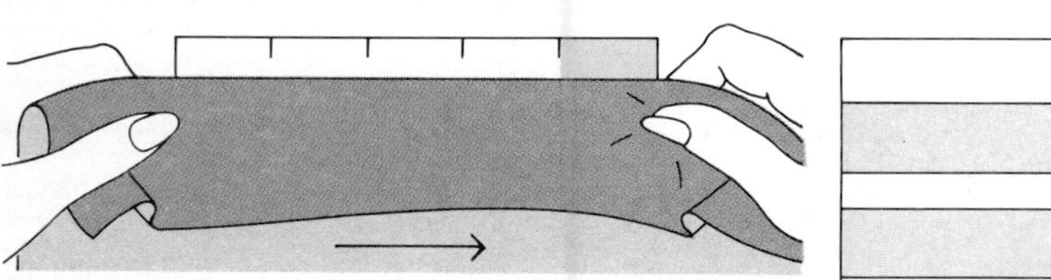

To use knit gauge, fold over a crosswise edge of the knit about 2". With left hand, brace knit against left edge of gauge. With right hand, take hold of knit at the 4" mark and gently stretch it to the mark it reaches comfortably.

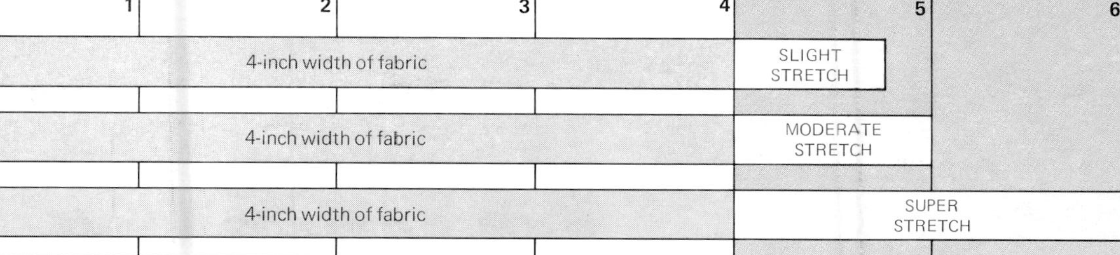

Shopping for fabrics

Working with plaids and stripes 90-91, 176-177;
diagonals and chevrons 92

Border prints, large-scale motifs 92, 120
Lace borders 312

Fabrics requiring special yardage

The construction or design of some fabrics imposes special yardage requirements. Such special needs may be specified on the pattern envelope; if it is not, you will have to do the calculating yourself. Examples of such fabrics are shown below and on the opposite page. Some fabrics could fall into more than one category. A large-scale print, for instance, might also be a one-way design. Consider all aspects in calculating yardage.

When **matching or design placement** is a factor, the length of one *repeat* should be added for each yard of fabric called for. (A repeat is the

Matching

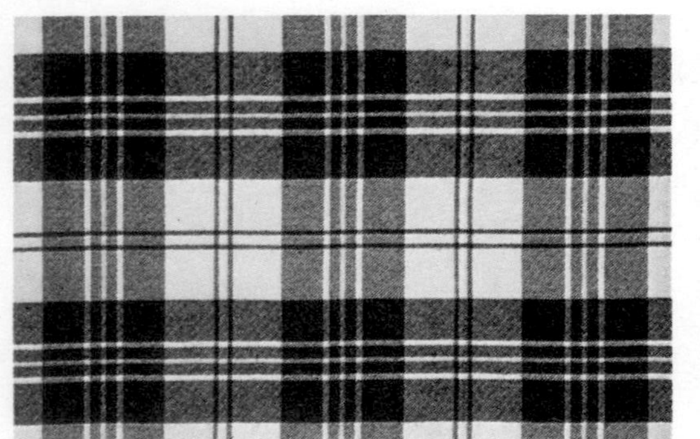

Plaids (multiple bands crossing at right angles; the repeat is a 4-sided area in which the design is complete): Require lengthwise centering and crosswise matching. Size of the repeat determines how much extra fabric is needed for matching. Uneven plaid takes still more yardage because it requires a one-way layout. These necessities apply also to geometric designs (a check, for example) where repeat is larger than ¼″.

Stripes (parallel bands of color in one direction only): Matching requirements depend on the direction of the lines and the pattern style. Extra yardage may be needed for horizontal (crosswise) stripes, or to match stripes in a chevron design (for details, see Cutting). No extra yardage is required for lengthwise stripes that will be used vertically on the figure.

Diagonals (lines that are woven or printed at an oblique angle to fabric selvage): Matching may or may not be possible, depending on the angle of the pattern seams. As a rule, extra yardage is needed only if the stripes are broad, or printed or woven in a variety of colors.

Special design placement

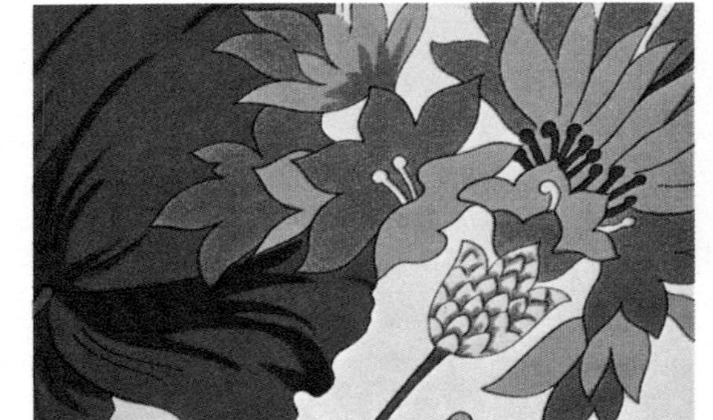

Large-scale prints (motifs 3″ or more wide or deep): Design must be balanced and motifs carefully placed on the figure (for details, see Cutting). Extra allowance must be made for matching if design is geometric (for example, polka dot or diamond). Additional yardage is needed if design is one-way.

Border print (marginal design along one selvage): No extra yardage is needed if the border is used vertically. Less than the specified amount may suffice if border is used horizontally (see Cutting). Choose a pattern that has a border-print view on the envelope, or calculate yardage by making a trial layout, aligning pattern pieces with the crosswise grain.

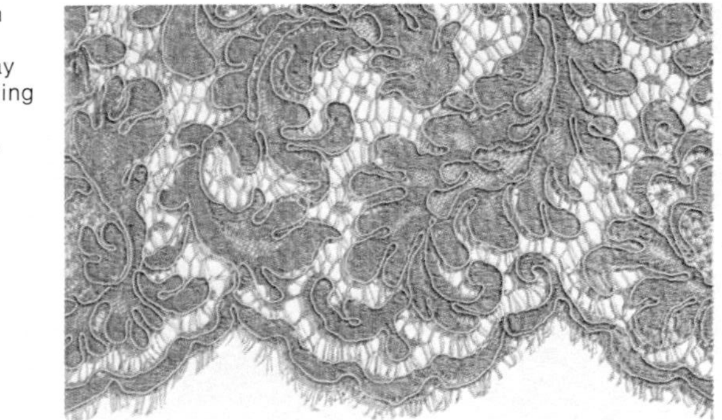

Lace (an openwork structure featuring flower or other motif on a net ground): A unique fabric because it has no grainline, making layout possibilities (and yardage needs) flexible. Thought must be given to placing motifs attractively on the figure, to matching them where possible, to laying them in one direction if necessary. Some laces have a scalloped edge that can be used at garment edges, such as sleeve or skirt hem, neckline or front opening.

One-way layout 90
Trial layout 93

area covered by one complete motif of the design.) For example, if 4 yards are required, and the repeat measures 2 inches, buy 4¼ yards.

If a **one-way layout** is necessary, the required yardage depends on the shapes of the pattern pieces. If top and bottom widths are approximately the same, no extra yardage should be necessary. When the top and bottom widths differ considerably (as in a widely flared skirt), a reasonable allowance is an extra ¼ yard for each yard of fabric specified. A more accurate approach, however, is a trial layout (see Cutting for procedure).

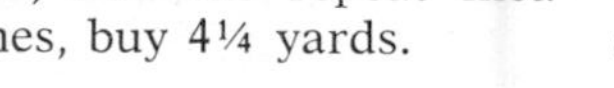

One-way layout

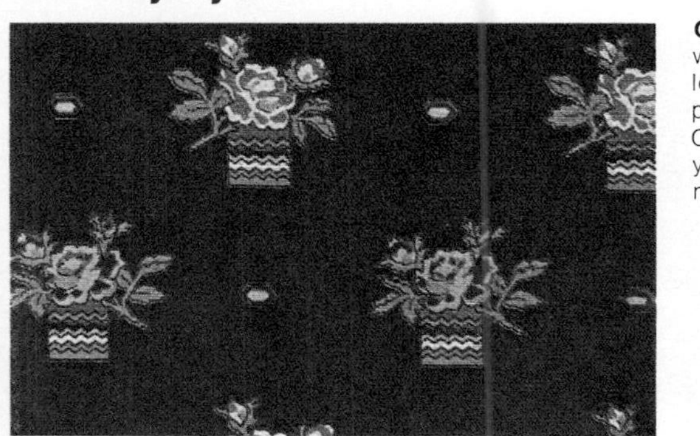

One-way design (printed or woven motifs not the same in both lengthwise directions; flower and paisley figures are often one-way): Check pattern envelope for nap yardage or estimate amount needed, using the criteria above.

Napped fabric (the surface of a plain or twill weave, or plain knit, has been brushed to create a soft, fuzzy texture; typical examples are fleece and flannel): Pattern pieces must be laid in one direction, usually with the nap running down.

Short-pile fabric (downy-textured surface less than ⅛″ deep, usually results from shearing pile yarns, as in velveteen): Cut with the nap running up for the richest color, with nap running down for a frosty effect.

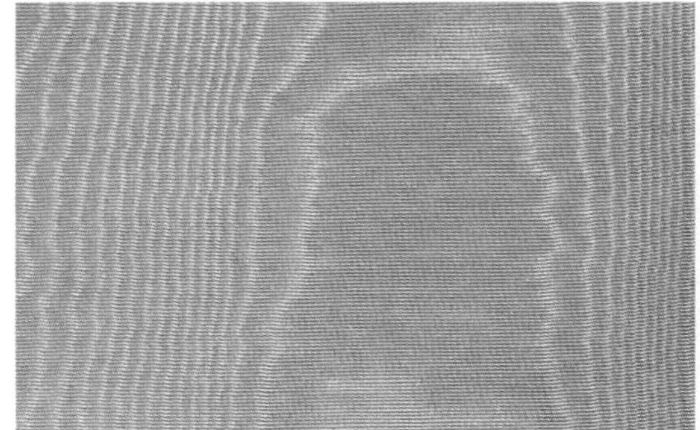

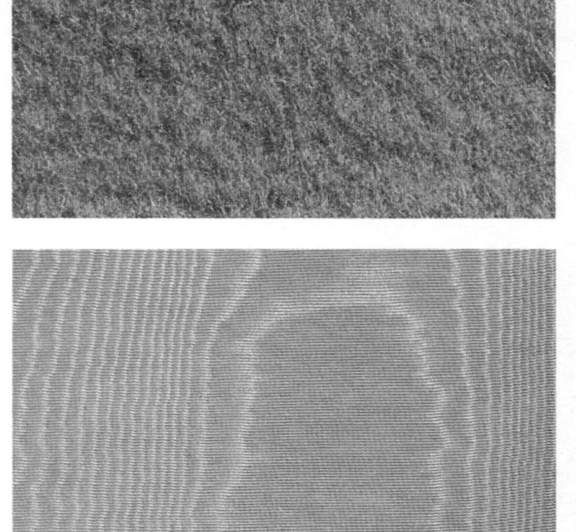

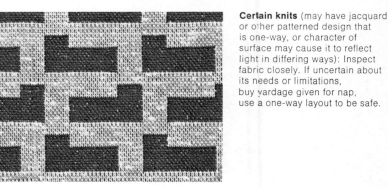

Moiré, satin, or iridescent (slick, shiny surface reflects light differently in each of the lengthwise directions): Can be cut in either direction, depending on the effect desired.

Deep-pile fabric (downy-textured surface more than ⅛″ deep, formed by extra warp or filling yarn, or by a special knit structure; plush and fake fur are examples): Almost always cut with the nap running down.

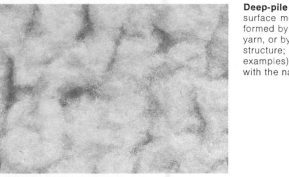

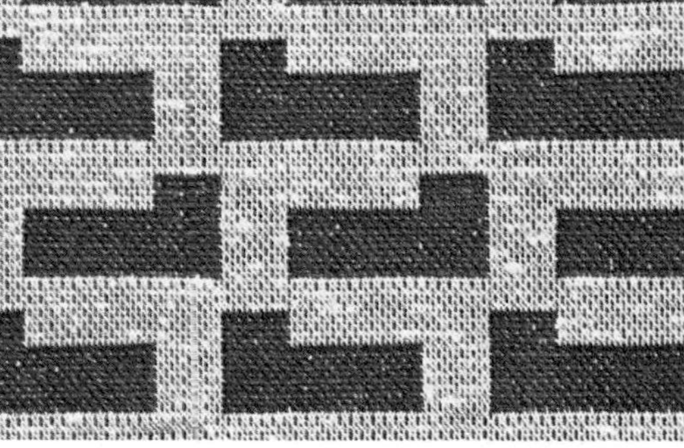

Certain knits (may have jacquard or other patterned design that is one-way, or character of surface may cause it to reflect light in differing ways): Inspect fabric closely. If uncertain about its needs or limitations, buy yardage given for nap, use a one-way layout to be safe.

Thread/needle/stitch length selection 26-27, 30-31

Special techniques: seaming 144, 149-152, 155-157; hems 302-303, 310-314; zippers 328

Special stitching and pressing needs

Because of their structure or finish, some fabrics call for special handling in stitching and pressing. A recognition of these unusual requirements is helpful in making sound fabric choices, especially when extra time or skill will be involved. You might consider, for instance, if you have the time to finish seams in a sheer garment, or the experience to handle a delicate brocade.

Awareness of special fabric characteristics can also guide you in establishing fabric/pattern relationships. Easing possibilities are limited in permanent press fabric, for example, making it a poor choice for a style with very full set-in sleeves.

Each fabric here and on the opposite page represents a group. Your selection could belong to more than one; an example is panne velvet with a stretch knit structure. Also, some judgment must always be made as to whether a fabric has all the characteristics of its category. Most crepes, for instance, are slippery, but not all. Any special techniques mentioned here are explained elsewhere in the book—see cross references above.

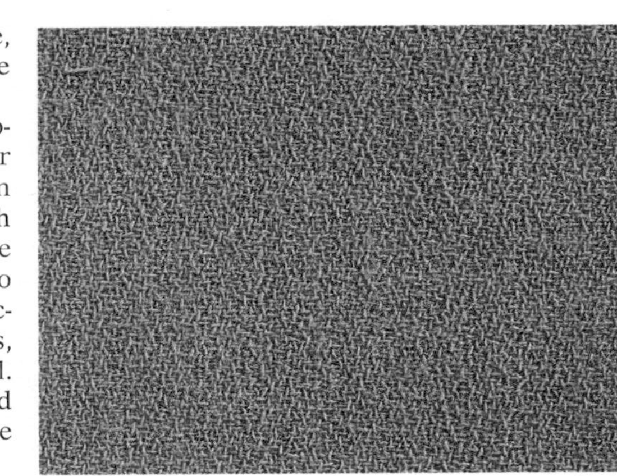

Crepe
Stitching: Stitch length and tension must be adjusted carefully to avoid puckering, usually to longer stitch and lessened tension. Most crepes have a tendency to slip and stretch. Tissue strips next to feed dog will solve the first problem; stabilizing of certain areas, such as shoulder and neckline, may be necessary to remedy the second.
Pressing: Steam causes some crepes to shrink or pucker; a fabric scrap should be pretested. A light touch is necessary to avoid overpressing.

Taffeta (brocade, satin)
Stitching: Can be stitched only once; removed stitches will leave holes. Should be handled as little as possible, because it wrinkles and soils easily. Also it does not ease well.
Pressing: May waterspot; use a *dry* iron at low temperature setting. Tip of iron should be used for opening seams, a press cloth and light touch for other areas; folded edges should not be flattened. Covering ironing board with thick pad or towel helps prevent flattening.

Sheers
Stitching: Inner construction of sheers must be neat because it shows through to the right side. Typically, French or other enclosed seam types are used. Soft sheers, such as chiffon, are inclined to slip or shift during stitching; they require tissue strips between the fabric and the feed dog.
Pressing: Soft sheers should be handled just like crepe. Crisp sheers rarely require any unusual pressing techniques.

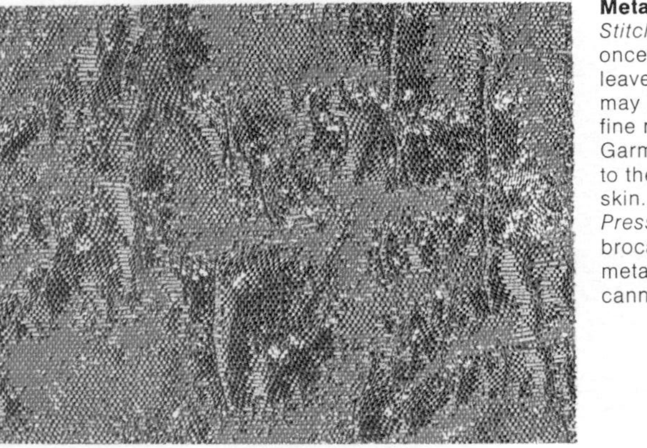

Metallic fabric
Stitching: Can be stitched only once; removed stitches will leave holes. Metallic threads may be cut by stitching; use fine needle and change it often. Garment may have to be lined to the edge to prevent scratching skin. Does not ease well.
Pressing: Same requirements as brocade. Steam may tarnish metallic yarns. Fullness of ease cannot be pressed out.

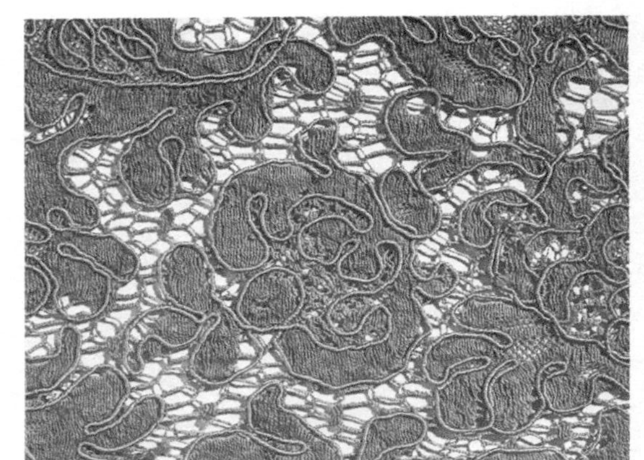

Lace
Stitching: Seams must be neatly finished as for all sheers, or the fabric should be underlined to conceal them. Seams can be made nearly invisible by the appliqué method. Edges, too, can be finished in this way.
Pressing: The same as for sheers, with care to avoid snagging.

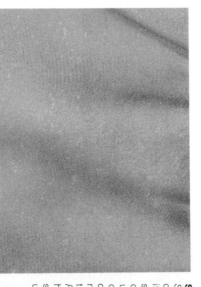

Special pressing equipment 19
Underlining sheers, laces 72-75
Lining a garment to its edge 81
Buttonholes for leather 340-342

Permanent press
Stitching: Tension and stitch length must be adjusted carefully to avoid puckering. Seams should be smooth before pressing. Difficult to ease; style chosen should have minimum fullness.
Pressing: Once pressed, crease and foldlines cannot be removed.

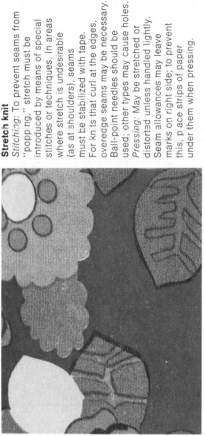

Velvet
Stitching: Can be stitched only once; removed stitches may leave holes. Should be stitched with fine needle, preferably in the direction of the nap.
Pressing: Must be pressed on wrong side of fabric, preferably with face against a needle board (see Pressing equipment). Use press cloth and low temperature setting; velvet can be melted by high temperatures. Steaming is an alternative technique.

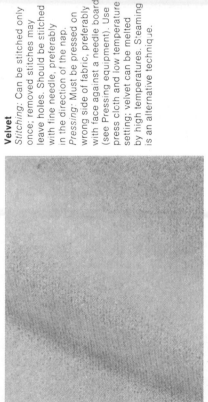

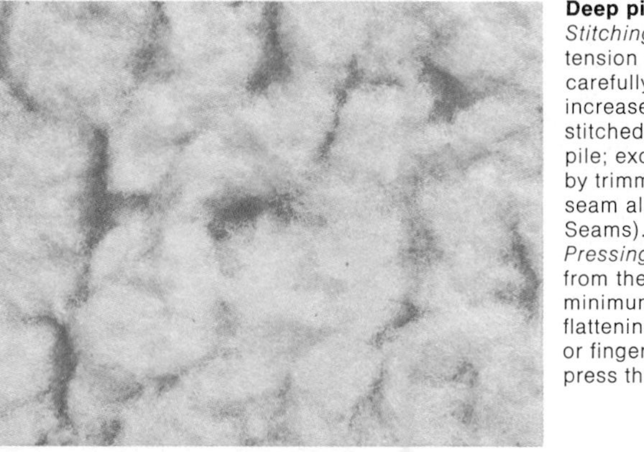

Deep pile
Stitching: Stitch length and tension should be adjusted carefully; usually pressure is increased. Seams should be stitched in the direction of the pile; excessive bulk is removed by trimming pile from the seam allowances (see Seams). Does not ease well.
Pressing: Must always be pressed from the wrong side with minimum pressure to avoid flattening pile. Tip of iron or fingers can be used to press the seams open.

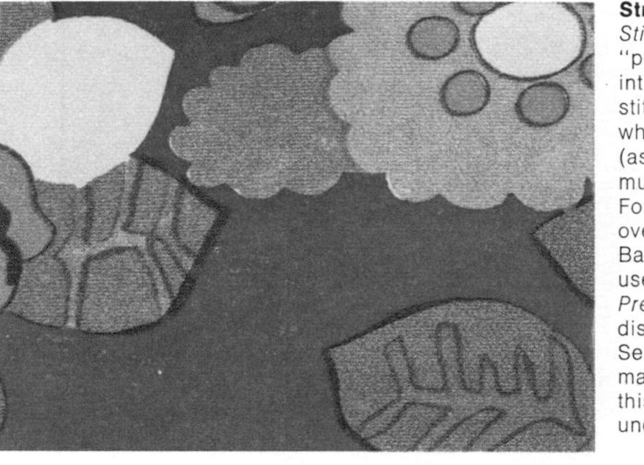

Stretch knit
Stitching: To prevent seams from "popping," stretch must be introduced by means of special stitches or techniques. In areas where stretch is undesirable (as at shoulders), seams must be stabilized with tape. For knits that curl at the edges, overedge seams may be necessary. Ball-point needles should be used; other types may cause holes.
Pressing: May be stretched or distorted unless handled lightly. Seam allowances may leave marks on right side; to prevent this, place strips of paper under them when pressing.

Leather
Stitching: Can be stitched only once; removed stitches will leave holes. Wedge-point needles should be used—they penetrate leather neatly and minimize tearing. To keep presser foot from sticking when topstitching, apply chalk or masking tape (pretest for satisfactory removal) over the area to be stitched.
Pressing: Seams should be pressed open, using fingers or dry iron set at low temperature. Adhesive may be needed to hold the seam allowances flat.

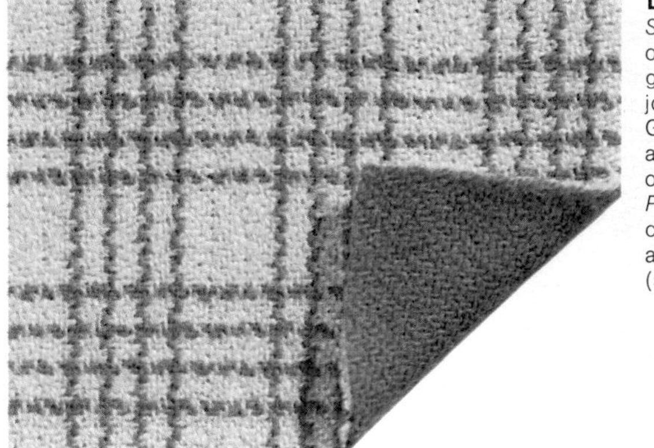

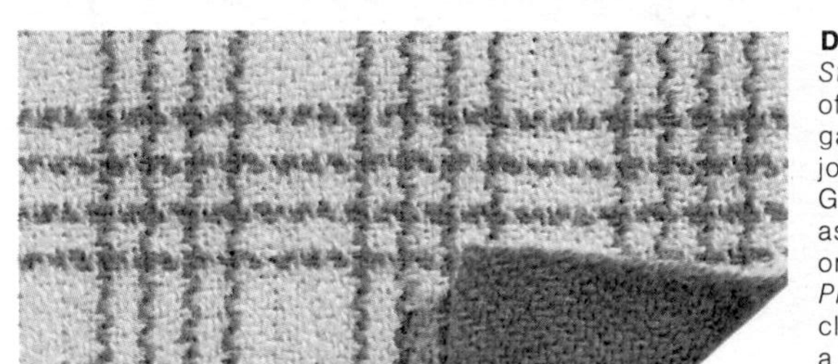

Double-faced fabric
Stitching: To take advantage of the reversible quality, garment sections are usually joined with flat-felled seams. Garment edges are finished, as a rule, with fold-over braid or a similar trim.
Pressing: A heavy-duty press cloth is needed to flatten seams; a clapper is useful as well (see Pressing equipment).

Underlying fabrics

Fabric types and selection

The underlying fabrics of a garment can be considered tools with which to build a better garment. Each of them —underlining, interfacing, interlining, and lining—has a specific function that influences the garment's finished appearance. This part of the book deals with the purpose, selection, and application of each of these fabrics. While all of the fabric types listed may not be used in a particular garment, the order of application is always underlining first, interfacing next, then interlining, finally lining.

Underlining is mainly intended to support and reinforce the garment fabric and the overall design. It also reinforces the seams. An additional benefit of underlining: it will give a degree of opaqueness to the garment fabric. This keeps the inner construction details and stitching from showing through to the outside of the garment.

Interfacing is also used to support the garment fabric and design. But, since it is usually a sturdier fabric than is used for underlining, its effect on the garment fabric is more apparent and definite. An interfacing can be applied to the entire garment but is usually applied only to parts.

Interlining is applied to a garment to supply warmth during wear.

Lining serves to give a neat finish to the inside of a garment and also contributes to the ease of putting the garment on and taking it off.

In considering which of the underlying fabrics are advisable or necessary for the garment you are constructing, it is much easier to decide about a lining or interlining than about underlining and interfacing. Linings and interlinings are, in effect, extras added to a garment for comfort and, in the case of linings, to conceal the inside of a garment. Neither of these helps in any way, however, to build in or maintain the shape of the garment. Underlining and interfacing do that.

	Purpose	Where used	Types	Selection criteria
Underlining	Give support and body to garment fabric and design Reinforce seams and other construction details Give opaqueness to garment fabric to hide the inner construction Inhibit stretching, especially in areas of stress Act as a "buffer layer" on which to catch hems, tack facings and interfacings, fasten other inner stitching	The entire garment or just sections	Fabrics sold as underlinings—can be light to medium in weight, with a soft, medium, or crisp finish Other fabrics, such as China silk, organdy, organza, muslin, batiste, lightweight tricot (for knits)	Should be relatively stable and lightweight Color and care should be compatible with garment Finish (e.g., soft, crisp) should be appropriate to desired effect
Interfacing	Support, shape, and stabilize areas, edges, and details of the garment Reinforce and prevent stretching	Entire sections, such as collars, cuffs, flaps Garment areas, such as the front, hem, neck, armhole, lapels, vents	Woven or nonwoven interfacings with or without fusing properties—can be light, medium, or heavy in weight	Should give support and body without overpowering the garment fabric Care and weight should be compatible with rest of garment Nonwovens are usually loftier than wovens Fusibles tend to add some rigidity to fabric
Interlining	Provide warmth	The body of a jacket or coat, sometimes the sleeves	Lightweight, warm fabrics, such as lamb's wool, felt, flannel, polyester fleece, lightweight blanket fabric	Light in weight Will provide warmth Not too bulky Care requirements should be compatible with rest of garment
Lining	Cover interior construction details Allow garment to slide on and off easily	Coats, jackets, dresses, skirts, and pants, in their entirety or just partially	Lightweight fabrics, such as sheath lining, silk, satin, sateen, crepe, batiste, taffeta, blouse fabrics	Should be smooth, opaque, durable Weight, color, and care should be compatible with the rest of garment An anti-static finish is desirable

There are two determining factors with underlining or interfacing: (1) how much shape or body is intended by the garment design; and (2) how much support is needed in order for the garment fabric to achieve that design. Generally speaking, the more structured and detailed a design is, the greater its need for an underlining and interfacing. The weight of the garment fabric is a factor, too. The lighter in weight or softer the fabric is, the more support it needs.

You should not, however, oversupport or undersupport any garment fabric in an attempt to achieve a certain garment design. Instead, choose another garment fabric more appro-

Garment fabric

Underlining. Applied before interfacing, interlining, lining.

Interfacing. Applied after underlining, but before interlining or lining.

Interlining. Applied after underlining and interfacing, but before lining.

Lining. Applied last, as the final, finishing touch.

Garment to which all four underlying fabrics could be applied has been chosen to show relation of these fabrics to one another and the order of their application. Regardless of number used, all fabrics should be draped together over your hand to see their combined effect.

priate to the needs of that particular design. A certain amount of judgment must always be exercised in the selection of a garment fabric to carry out a specific design. Some fabrics, even supported by both an appropriate underlining and interfacing, will still be too lightweight to sustain a very structured design. For certain designs, on the other hand, some fabrics may be too heavy. When any combination of fabrics will be used, always drape them over your hand to see their combined effect.

Underlining

Underlining is a lightweight fabric that is applied to the wrong side of the garment fabric primarily to give additional strength, support, and durability to the garment. Underlining also helps to maintain the shape of the garment and to reinforce its seams. Usually it will make the garment fabric opaque so that the inner construction details and stitching cannot be seen on the outside of the garment. Underlining fabrics are made from various fibers, finished in several different hands (soft, medium, and crisp), and available in a wide range of colors. There are also other fabrics, such as organza, tricot, and lightweight blouse and lining fabrics, that are not classified as underlinings but can serve the same purposes.

Underlinings are applied by two different methods; these are illustrated and explained on pages 74–75. Depending on the desired effect, either the entire garment or just some of its sections can be underlined. As illustrated at right, a fitted dress, which usually needs support and shaping in all of its sections, is most often completely underlined. As for the sheer blouse, however, its body needs the opaqueness given by an underlining but its soft, full sleeves are more effective if left unhampered by an underlining. Also, as with the seat of a skirt or the knees of pants, underlining may be applied to certain areas of a section for the purpose of reinforcing only the parts that take the greatest strain.

In deciding what underlining fabric is suitable, look for one that matches the garment fabric in *care requirements*, not necessarily fiber content. Since the main purpose of an underlining is to support and strengthen the garment fabric, be sure that the underlining gives no more than the garment fabric. Use a woven underlining with a woven garment fabric and cut out both on the same grain. Knits are not usually underlined but they can be if this is desired. A woven underlining cut on the straight grain will restrict the give of the knit; a woven underlining that is cut on the bias will allow the knit to give somewhat. To maintain most or all of the knit's give, use a lightweight tricot as an underlining and cut it out in the same direction as the knit garment fabric.

Choose a soft underlining if you want to maintain the softness of the garment fabric; a crisp underlining to give the garment fabric some crispness. Some garment designs may require more than one type of underlining. For example, a garment might need a crisp underlining to support its

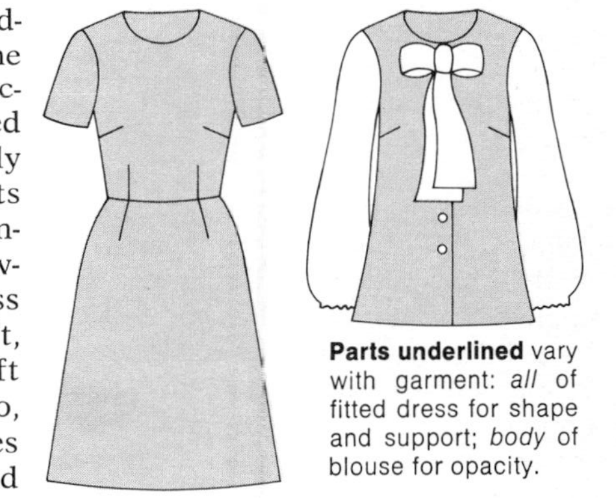

Parts underlined vary with garment: *all* of fitted dress for shape and support; *body* of blouse for opacity.

A-line skirt but require a soft underlining for its more fluid bodice.

As for the color of the underlining, choose one that will not show through enough to change the color impression of the garment fabric. As a final selection test, drape together all fabrics that will be used to see if they will function well together and complement the design of the garment.

Underlying fabrics

Hand basting 124-125
Darts 159-161

Methods of underlining

There are two methods of underlining a garment. In the first, the two fabric layers (underlining fabric and garment fabric) are always treated as though they were one layer. In the other method, the two fabrics are handled separately through the construction of darts and are then handled as one. With either method, it is necessary to re-position the underlining in relation to the face fabric before garment sections are seamed. The reason for the adjustment: a garment, on the body, is cylindrical; the underlining,

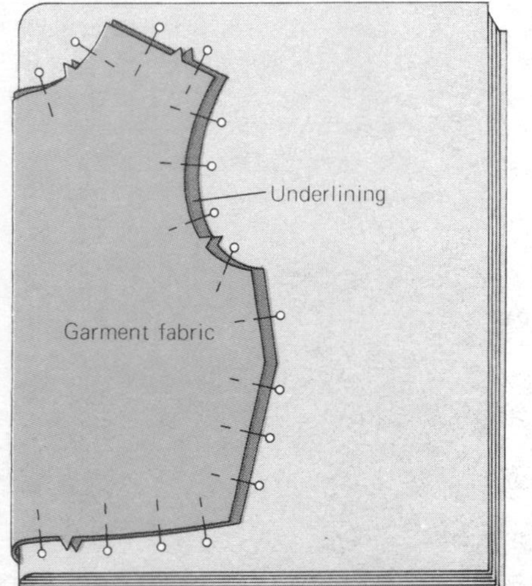

To re-position underlining, baste fabric layers together down center or one edge. Wrap fabrics around a thick magazine with underlining next to magazine. Smooth out fabrics; pin together, as they fall, along the edges.

because it will lie closer to the body, must be made into a slightly smaller "cylinder" than the one formed by the outer fabric. After re-positioning, the excess underlining is trimmed. New underlining seamlines must be marked (use seam gauge and chalk) to align with garment fabric seamlines.

Method 1: Treating two layers as one

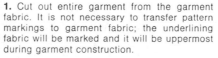

Of the two underlining methods, the technique shown and described below, in which garment and underlining fabrics are treated as one throughout, is used more often. When it is used, the underlining layer will reinforce all construction details, including darts, and will prevent them from showing through to the outside of the garment. Since the underlining will be uppermost during all construction steps, only that layer need be marked.

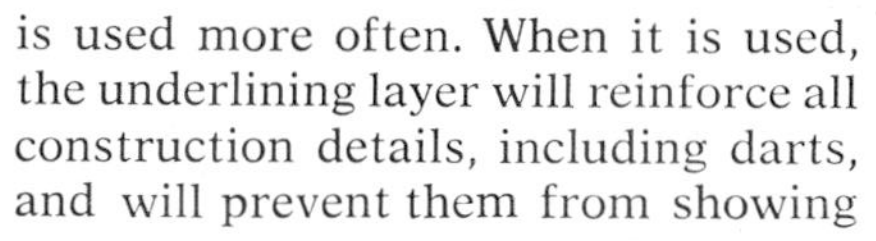

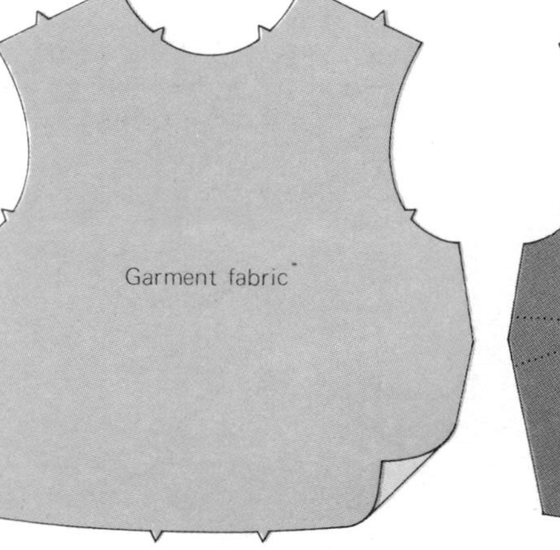

1. Cut out entire garment from the garment fabric. It is not necessary to transfer pattern markings to garment fabric; the underlining fabric will be marked and it will be uppermost during garment construction.

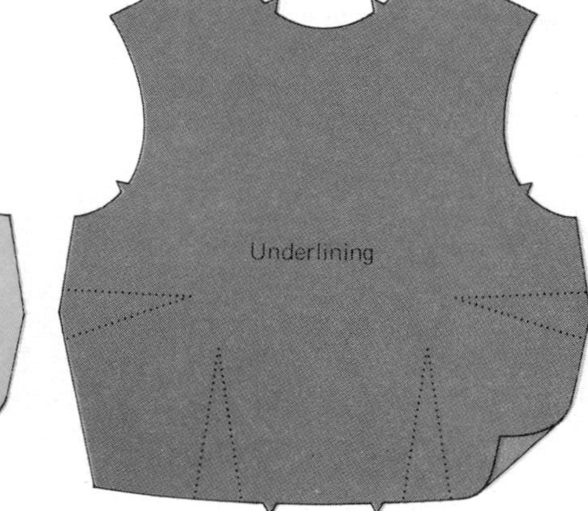

2. Remove pattern pieces from garment fabric sections. Decide which garment sections will be underlined and pin those pattern pieces to the underlining fabric. Cut out; transfer all pattern markings to the *right* side.

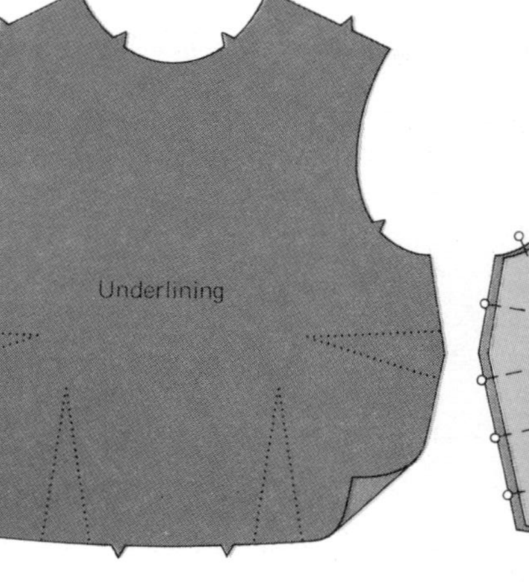

3. Wrong sides facing, center garment fabric over underlining. Baste fabrics together—down center of wide sections, along one edge of narrow pieces. Align basting with spine of magazine and re-position underlining (see left).

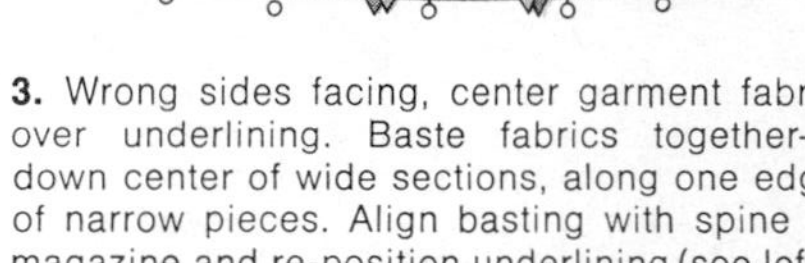

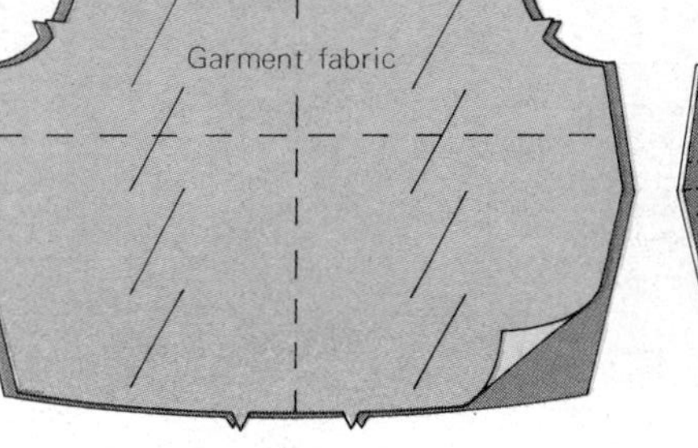

4. Remove fabric layers from magazine. With garment fabric uppermost, baste across center, then diagonal-baste a few rows within section. Remove pins; trim underlining at edges; mark new seamlines to match those on face fabric.

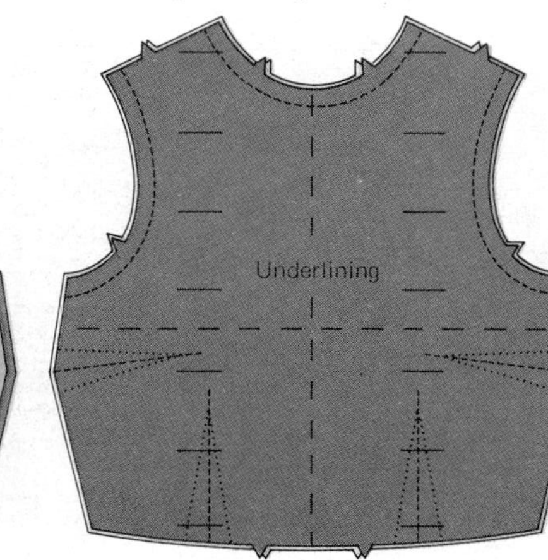

5. With underlining fabric uppermost, staystitch, where necessary, through both fabric layers. Machine-baste, through both fabrics, down center of each dart, starting 2 to 3 stitches beyond point of each dart.

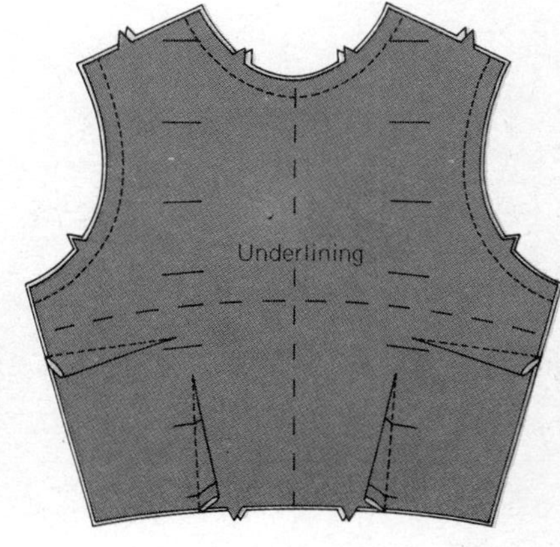

6. Fold each dart along its center. Match, pin, baste, and stitch each dart; remove hand bastings and the machine bastings that extend beyond dart points. Press each dart flat, then in the proper direction (see Darts).

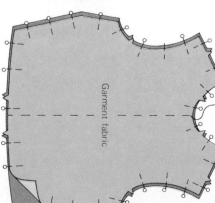

Machine pressure and tension 28-31
Fabric-marking methods 94
Directional and staystitching 144
Darts 159-161

Method 2: Handling layers separately

In this underlining method, the garment and underlining fabric layers are handled and sewed separately from the marking and staystitching through dart construction. (With this method, both layers must be marked.) The separately prepared layers are then basted to one another and handled as a single layer. The underlining layer will reinforce and prevent *seams* from showing through to the outside of the garment, but not the *darts*. Underlining by this method will, however, give a more finished look to the inside of the garment than will the method on page 74.

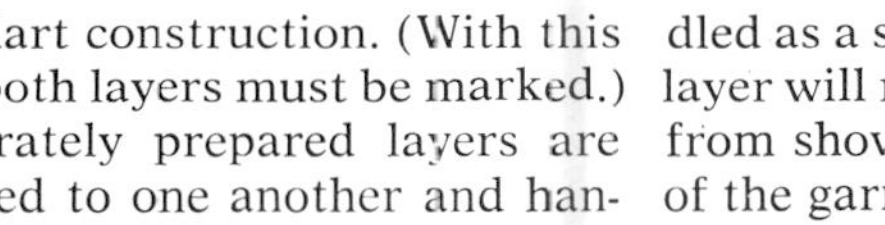
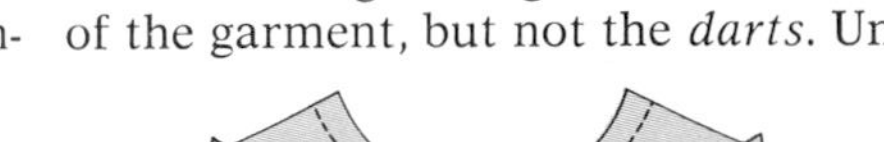
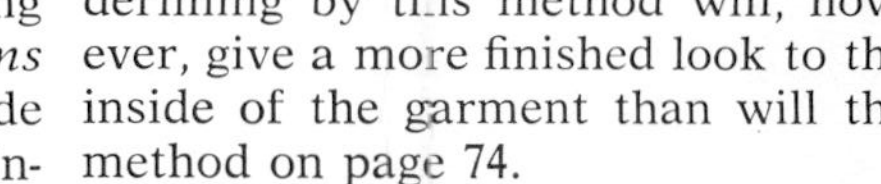

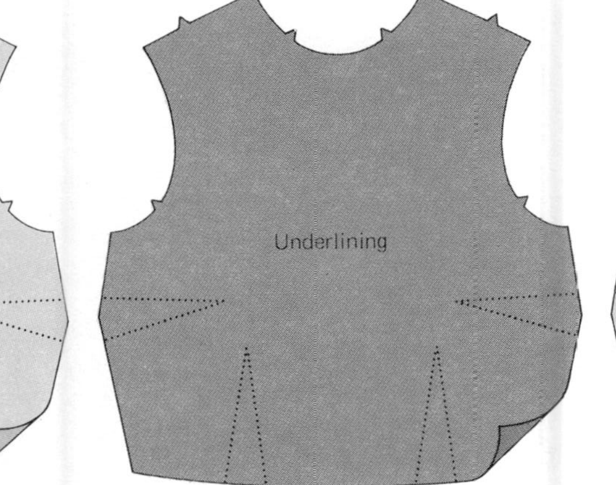

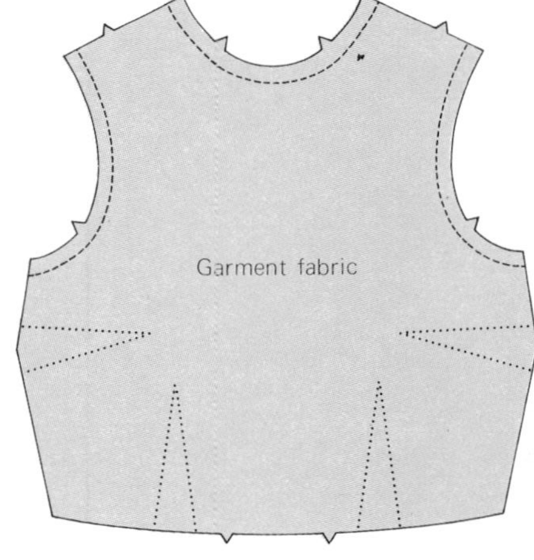

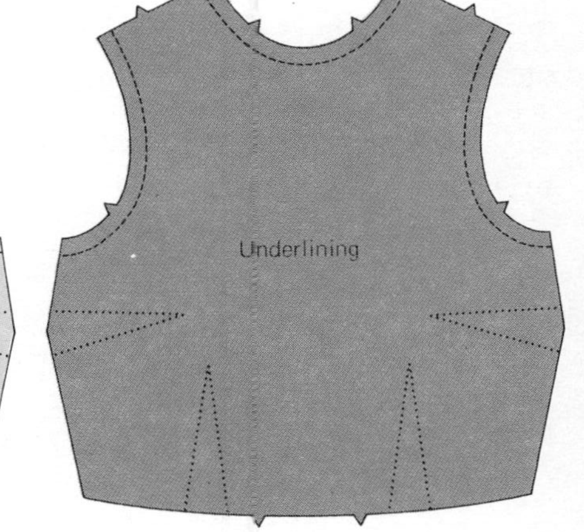

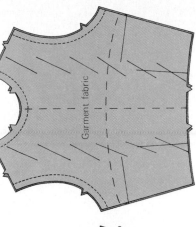

1. While pattern is still pinned to the cut garment fabric sections, transfer all the pattern markings to the *wrong* side. Method of marking will depend on the fabric (see Marking). Bodice above was marked with tracing wheel.

2. Remove pattern pieces from marked garment sections. Decide which garment sections are to be underlined and pin these pattern pieces to the underlining fabric. Cut out; transfer all pattern markings to the *wrong* side.

3. So that the edges will not stretch during handling, staystitch along the edges of each garment fabric section where necessary. Place stitching just inside the seamline and stitch directionally (see Directional stitching).

4. Also staystitch underlining sections as necessary to keep their edges from stretching in handling. Machine settings may need adjustment, since underlining fabric is usually lighter in weight than face fabric.

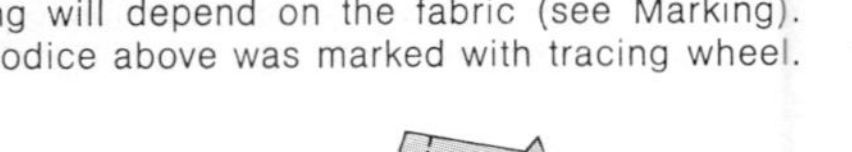

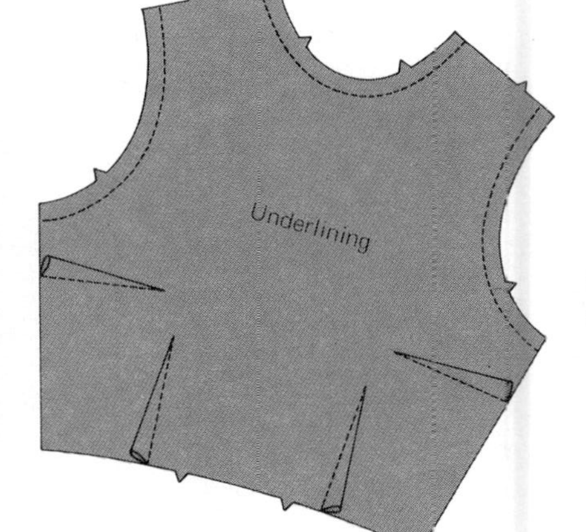

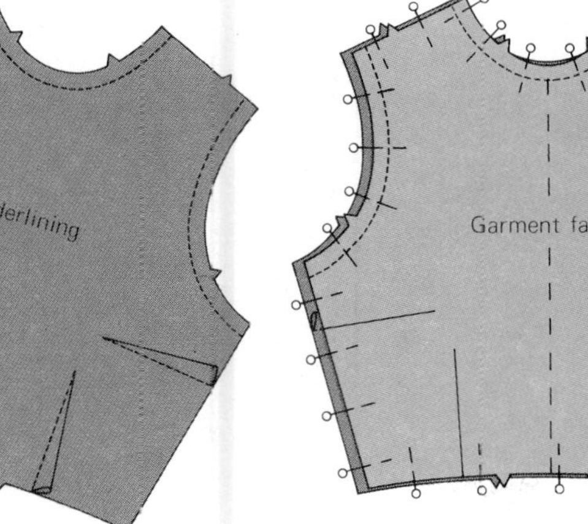

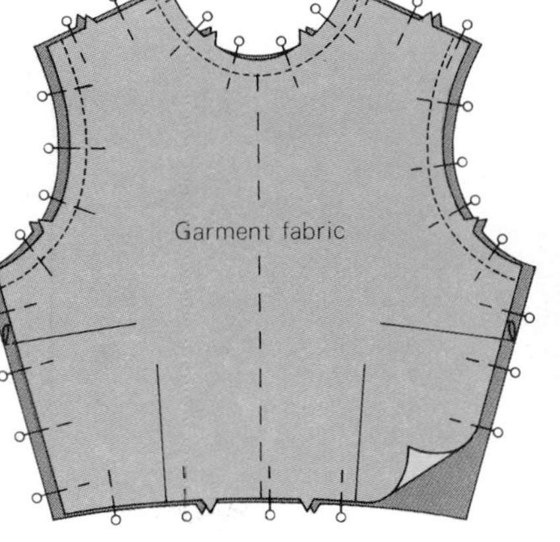

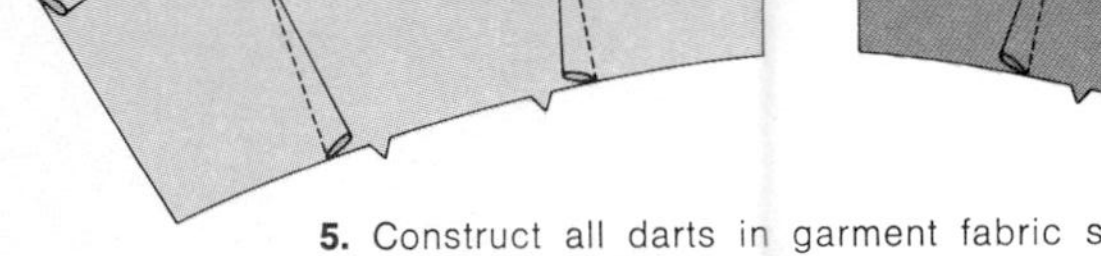

5. Construct all darts in garment fabric sections, then all darts in underlining sections. Press all darts flat as stitched. Press darts in garment fabric in proper directions (see Darts), corresponding darts in underlining fabric in opposite directions.

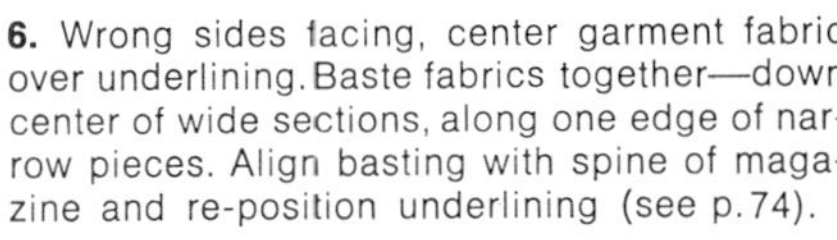

6. Wrong sides facing, center garment fabric over underlining. Baste fabrics together—down center of wide sections, along one edge of narrow pieces. Align basting with spine of magazine and re-position underlining (see p.74).

7. Remove garment sections from magazine. With garment fabric uppermost, baste across center, then diagonal-baste a few rows within section. Remove pins; trim away excess underlining; mark new underlining seamlines.

Underlying fabrics

Catchstitch (flat) 129
Darts 162
Tailoring 360-370
Sewing for men 388

Interfacings

An interfacing is a special type of fabric applied to the inside of a garment to give it shape, body, and support. In some instances, an entire garment will be interfaced; as a rule, however, interfacing is applied only to certain areas, such as collars, front or back openings, lapels, and hems, and to such details as pocket flaps.

Interfacings are made from many different fibers in several weights and degrees of crispness; they may be woven or nonwoven. A comparatively new category, fusible interfacings, instead of being stitched to the garment fabric, are ironed onto it. Fusibles, too, may be woven or nonwoven. The wide range makes it possible to choose an interfacing that will be compatible with any type of garment fabric. Two considerations are critical in selecting interfacing: (1) it should complement and reinforce the garment fabric without overpowering it; (2) though the two fabrics need not be identical in fiber content, it is always best that they should have the same care requirements.

The construction of an interfacing can differ from that of the garment fabric, that is, a nonwoven interfacing can be used with a woven garment fabric. There are characteristic differences, however, between woven and nonwoven interfacings that should be considered. Wovens are usually cut on the straight grain; nonwovens have no grain and so need not be cut in any particular direction. Nonwovens are more lofty than wovens. Both types are stable but there are "all-bias" nonwovens which have some give in all directions. If a degree of give is desired with a woven interfacing, it should be cut on the bias. With most fusibles, woven or nonwoven, there is no give once they are fused into place. Generally, a woven interfacing will shape better than a nonwoven. Of all the wovens, hair canvas shapes best.

Interfacings come in light, medium, and heavy weights. Weight should be compatible with but never overpower the garment fabric. With fusibles, remember that the adhesive tends to add some body to the garment fabric. Before making a final selection, drape over your hand all of the fabrics that will be sewed into the garment to see if they are suitably complementary.

Discussion of the different types of interfacings begins opposite and continues through page 79. For tailoring with hair canvas, see the Tailoring chapter; for tailoring with a fusible interfacing, see Sewing for men.

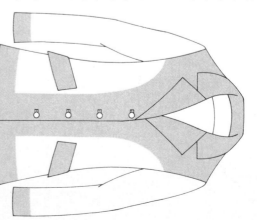

Interfacing is applied to certain parts of a garment, as illustrated by shaded areas above, to give the parts shape, body, and support.

Seams and darts in interfacing

A primary consideration in applying interfacings is how to form seams and darts in them without adding unnecessary bulk to the garment. Illustrated at the right are the three methods used for constructing seams and darts in nonfusible interfacings. (For detailed drawings of dart procedures, see Darts.) The method chosen depends on the weight of the interfacing. As a general rule, the heavier the interfacing, the greater the need to reduce its bulk. Bulk is reduced most by the **catchstitched seam,** in which interfacing is stitched to garment fabric. This seaming method is recommended for heavy, bulky interfacings. Less bulk is eliminated by either the **lapped** or the **abutted seam,** in which interfacing is seamed to interfacing. These are suitable for lighter-weight interfacings.

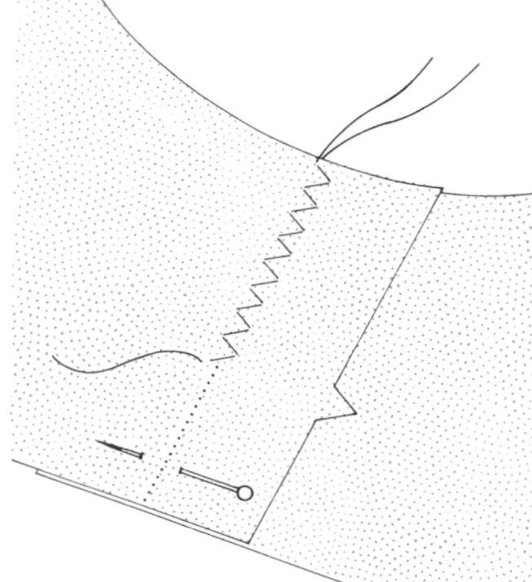

Lapped seam: Lap edges as shown, aligning their seamlines; pin in place. Stitch over seamline with wide zigzag stitch, or place row of straight stitching ⅛" on each side of seamline. Trim seam allowances.

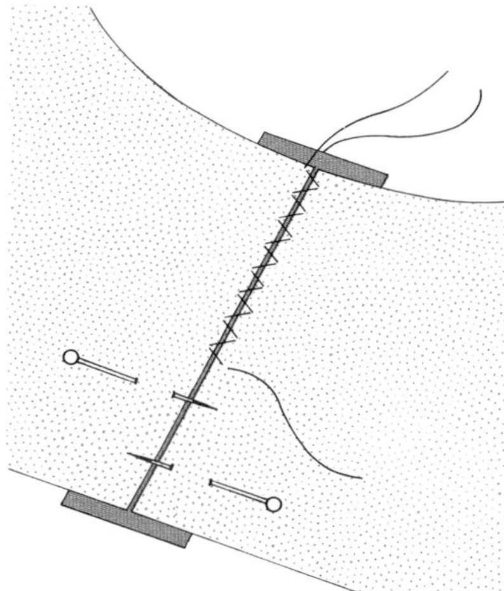

Abutted seam: Cut off seam allowances. Bring edges together; pin to an underlay of woven-edge tape. Stitch over seamline with wide zigzag stitch, or place straight-stitch row ⅛" on each side of seamline.

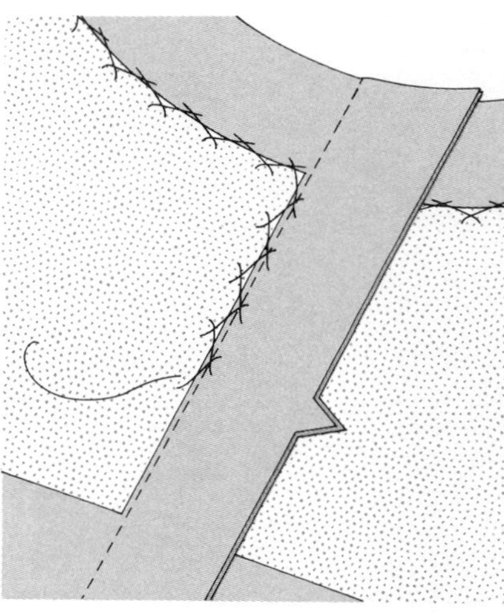

Catchstitched seam: Cut off seam allowances. Align interfacing edges with garment seamline; catchstitch interfacing to garment over seamline. If garment seam is stitched, lift seam allowances to align interfacing.

Light - to medium-weight interfacings

Lighter-weight interfacings comprise the largest group of interfacings. Made from a number of fibers, they can be either woven or nonwoven and are produced in several degrees of crispness. Choose an interfacing to conform to the care requirements of the garment fabric; it should not be heavier than the garment fabric but can be crisper. The procedure for applying this class of interfacings is illustrated and explained at the right. It is usually easier to construct and apply interfacing *as a unit* to a garment unit, as illustrated. If desired, however, the *parts* of a garment unit can be interfaced *separately* and the interfaced pieces then joined. Because these interfacings have relatively little bulk, they can be stitched into the garment seams and their seam allowances trimmed.

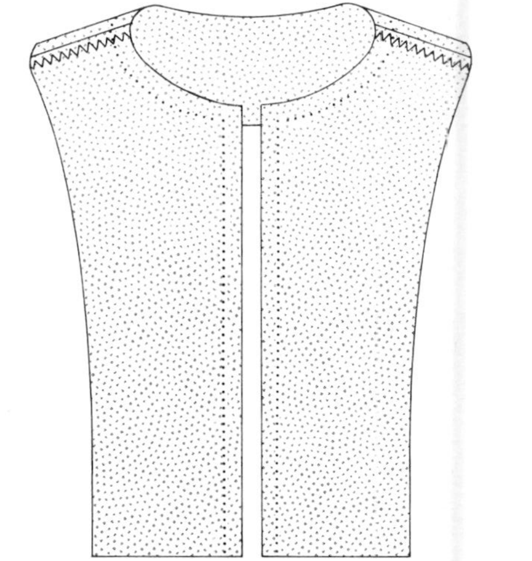

1. Cut out and mark the interfacing pieces. Using a **lapped** or **abutted seam** (see p. 76), join pieces to form a unit for each garment area that is to be interfaced.

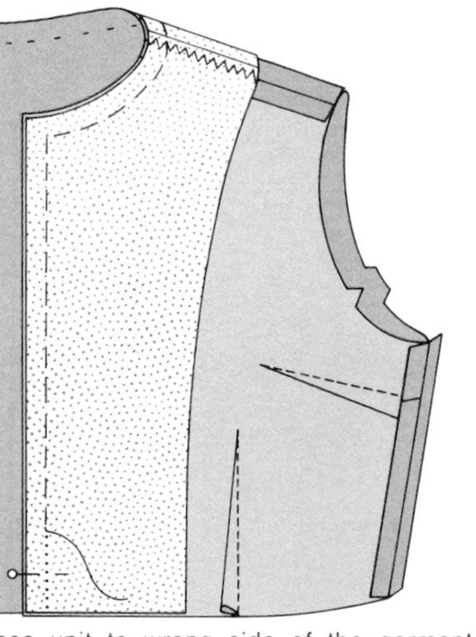

2. Place unit to wrong side of the garment area it is being applied to. Match seamlines and markings; pin unit in place; baste to garment just inside the seamlines.

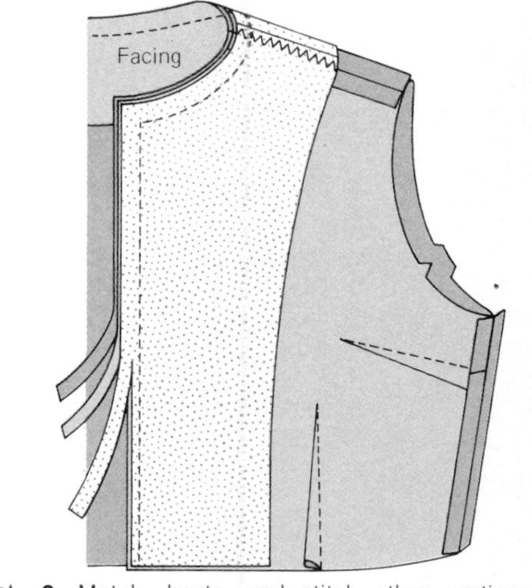

3. Match, baste, and stitch other sections, such as facing, to garment. Press. Trim and grade seams, trimming interfacing close to seamline. Continue with construction.

Heavy interfacings (catchstitched method)

Another category of interfacings consists of the heavy or bulky types. Most often used with the heavier fabrics typical of such garments as coats and jackets, these interfacings may be made from any of several fibers and can be either woven or nonwoven. This group also includes the hair canvases which, though not necessarily bulky, are rigid and should not be caught into garment seamlines. There are two different ways of applying these interfacings. The method at the right, the **catchstitched** method, is the one used most often. In this procedure, the seam allowances of the interfacing are cut off before it is applied. The second technique, the **strip** method, is explained on the next page. For the somewhat specialized interfacing techniques of tailoring, see the Tailoring chapter.

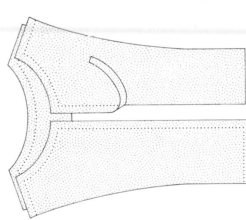

1. Cut out and mark the interfacing pieces. Trim away all of the seam allowances by cutting along the marked seamlines. *Do not join the pieces* to form units as in method above.

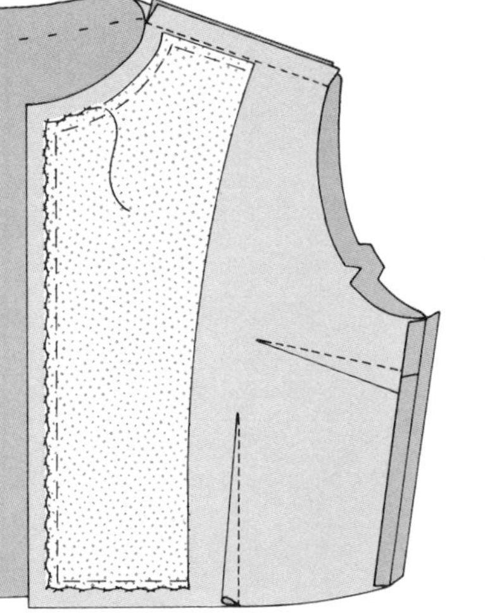

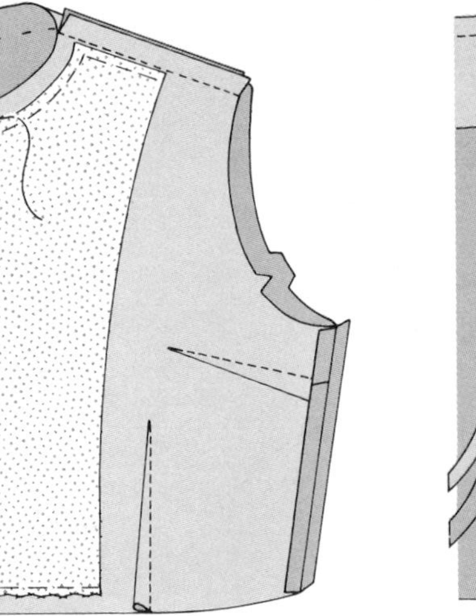

2. Align cut edges of interfacing to seamlines of section it is being applied to. Baste in place; catchstitch to garment over seamlines (see Catchstitched seam, p. 76).

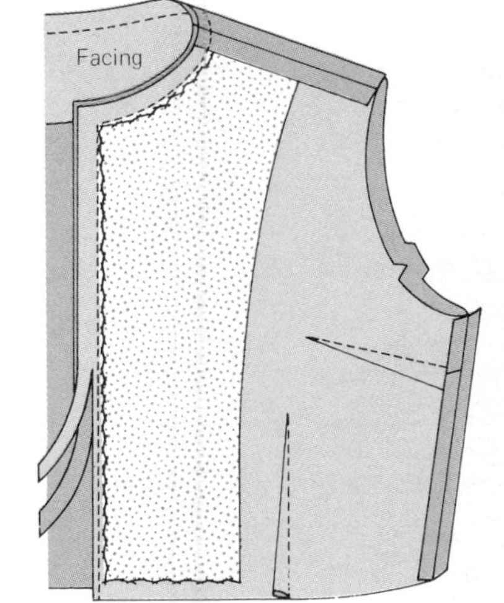

Match, pin, baste, and stitch other sections, such as the facing, to the garment. Press seams flat. Trim and grade seam allowances; continue with garment construction.

Underlying fabrics

Fabric-marking methods 94

Heavy interfacings (strip method)

Heavy or bulky interfacings can be applied to a garment by either of two methods. The first, the **catchstitched** method, is shown on the preceding page; the second, the **strip** method, is explained and illustrated here.

With the strip method, bulk is reduced by cutting off the seam allowances of the interfacing, and replacing them with strips of lightweight fabric, before the interfacing is applied to the garment. It is the lightweight fabric that is then caught into the garment seams and trimmed away after seaming. For the strips, you can use organza, lawn, or another similarly lightweight, stable fabric. The strip method is especially recommended for those interfacings that will ravel either during handling or while the garment is being worn. For a precise application, mark all seamlines on both interfacing and strips.

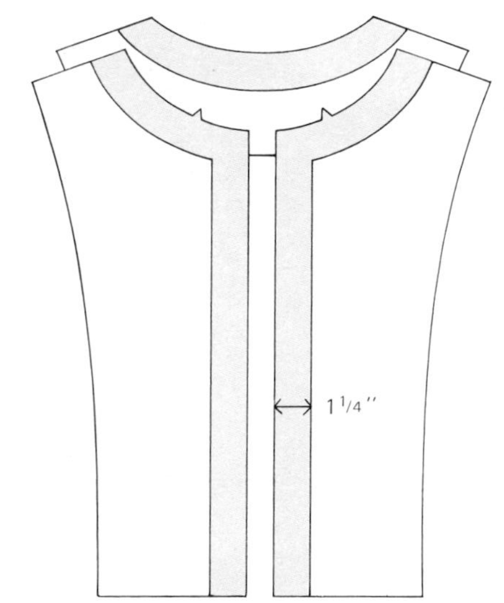

1. Cut strips of lightweight fabric, such as organza, 1¼" wide and the same shape as the edge being interfaced. Use the facing pattern pieces as a cutting guide for shape.

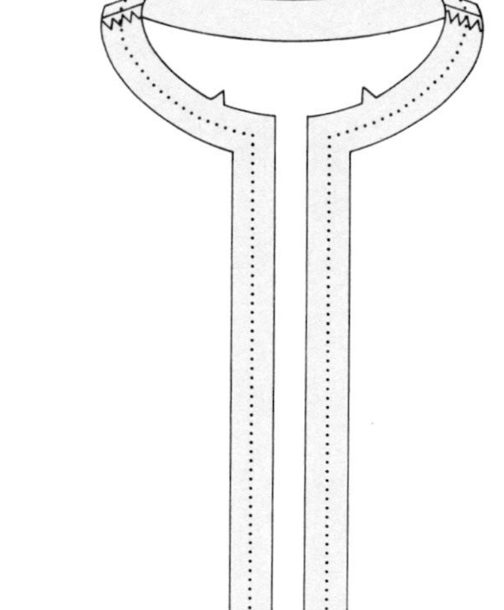

2. Before removing pattern, transfer seamline markings to strips. Join front and back sections at the shoulders, using either a lapped or an abutted seam (see p.76).

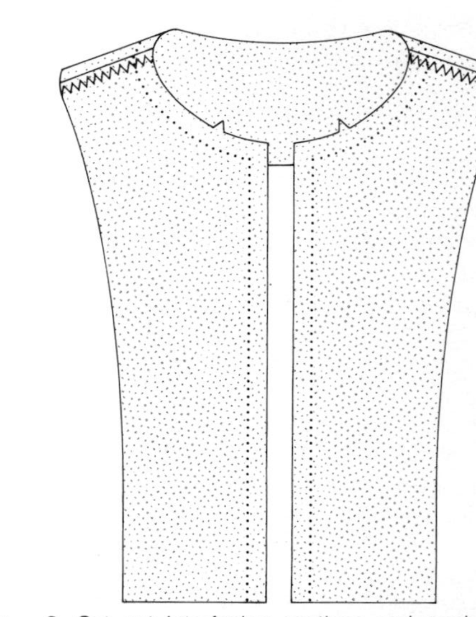

3. Cut out interfacing sections and mark all the seamlines; join front and back sections at the shoulders, using either a lapped or an abutted seam (see p.76).

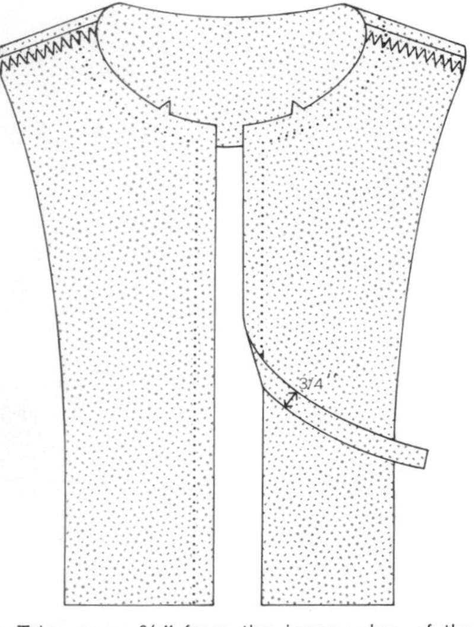

4. Trim away ¾" from the inner edge of the interfacing unit. This will place the cut edge of the interfacing approximately ⅛" beyond its original seamline.

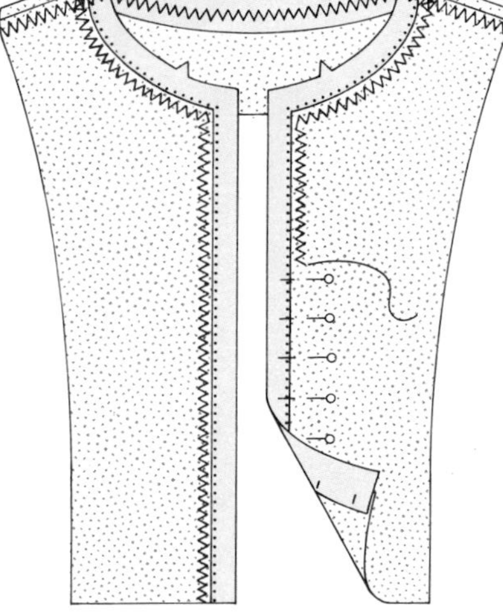

5. Position interfacing on strip unit so cut edge is ⅛" short of seamline; pin in place. Stitch along interfacing edge, using zigzag or two rows of straight stitching.

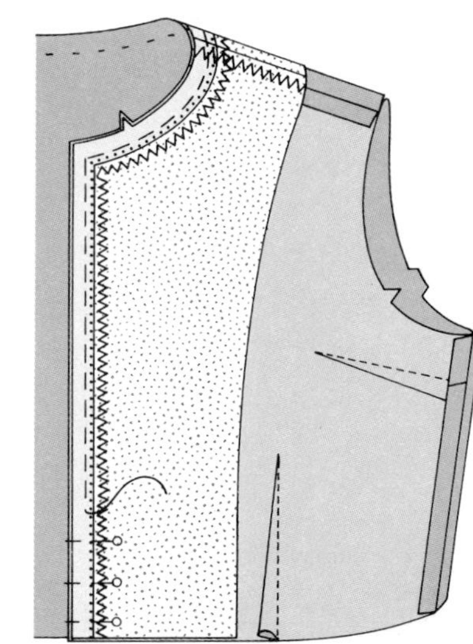

6. Place unit to wrong side of garment area that is being interfaced. Matching seamlines, markings, and cut edges, pin, then baste in place, inside the seamline.

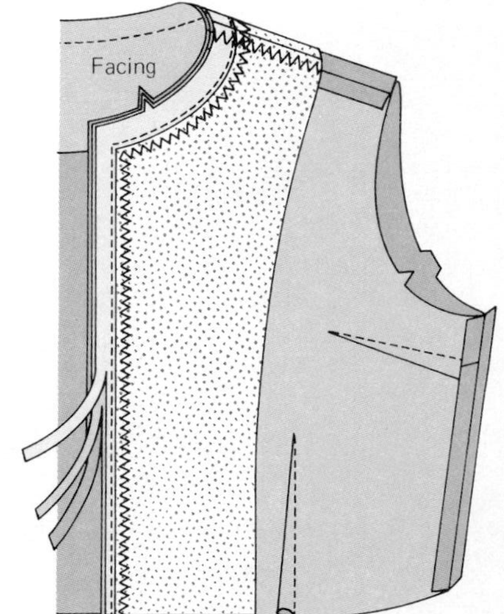

7. Match, baste, and stitch other sections, such as facing, to garment. Press. Trim and grade seams, trimming strip close to seamline. Continue with garment construction.

Fabric-marking methods 94 Catchstitch (flat) 129
Sewing for men 388

Fusible interfacings and their application

Fusible interfacings are those that are made with heat-sensitive adhesive on one side of the fabric. Like other interfacing types, they come in different weights and fibers and may be either woven or nonwoven. For a satisfactory bond, fusible interfacings depend upon a combination of heat and steam with a minimum of pressure. Refer to instructions that accompany the product and always test application of the interfacing to scraps of garment fabric before fusing it to the garment. In selecting a fusible interfacing, keep in mind that the adhesive tends to change the character of the garment fabric slightly by adding extra body and sometimes some rigidity to it. Illustrated and explained here is the basic application technique for fusible interfacings. For the use of fusible interfacings in tailoring, see the section on Sewing for men.

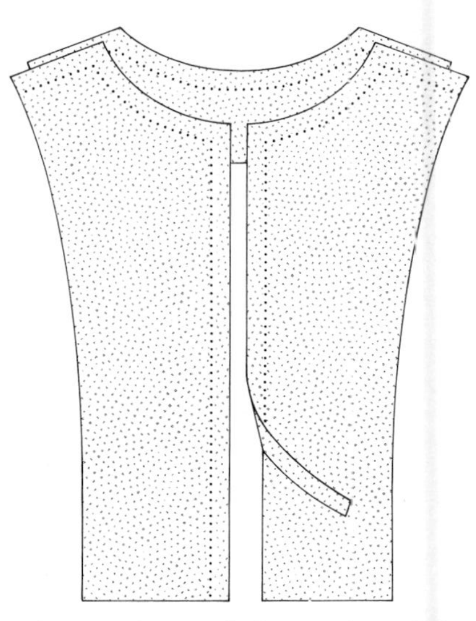

1. Cut out the interfacing sections. Before removing pattern pieces, mark all seamlines. Trim away all of the seam allowances (and center portion of darts, if they occur).

2. With adhesive side of interfacing toward wrong side of corresponding garment section, align cut edges of interfacing with garment seamlines. Fuse interfacing in place.

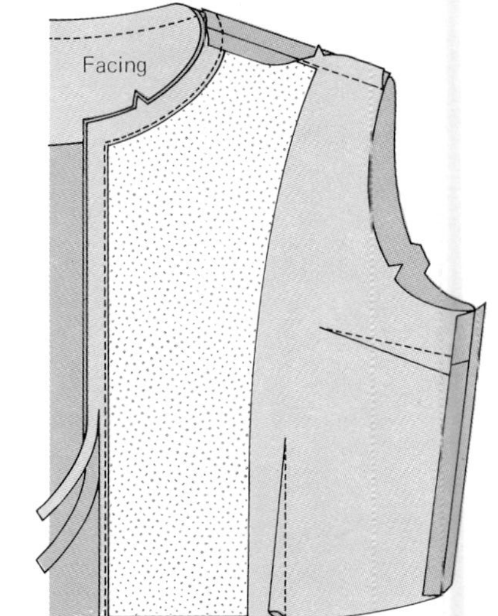

3. Match, pin, baste, and stitch other garment sections, such as facing, to garment. (Pull garment fabric through dart openings, if any, and stitch.) Press; trim.

Handling interfacing at a foldline

Sometimes one edge of an interfacing section will fall at a garment foldline rather than a seamline. This edge can be positioned to go right next to the foldline or it can extend approximately ½ inch beyond it. When interfacing extends beyond a foldline, the finished edge will be rounder than it is when interfacing stops at the foldline. Techniques for both kinds of placement are given below, first for a **one-piece collar** and then for an **extended facing.** (These same techniques can be applied to other situations in which an extension of the garment turns back on itself to finish the edge—for example, a hem.) The other edges of the interfacing are then secured according to the requirements of the interfacing type. Securing is no problem with fusible interfacing since it is all fused in place at once.

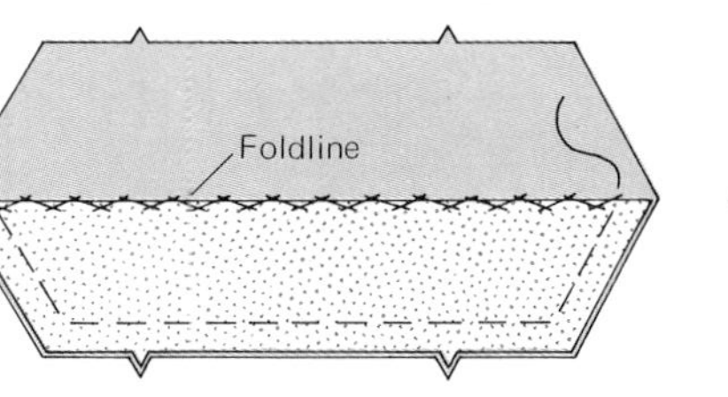

If constructing a one-piece collar in which the edge of the interfacing falls *along the foldline,* hold interfacing in place by catchstitching edge to collar over foldline.

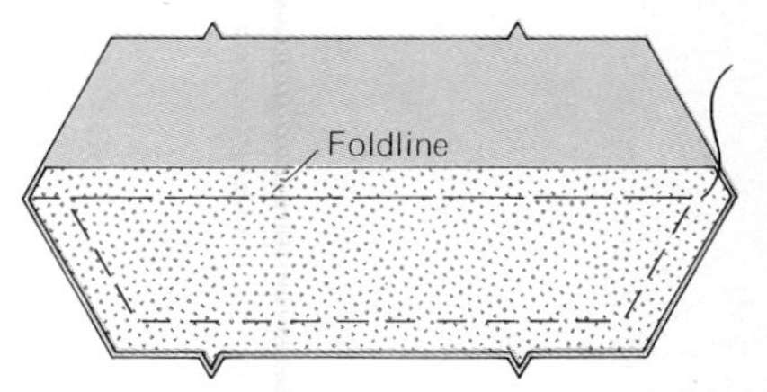

If interfacing will extend *beyond the foldline*, secure the interfacing to the collar along the foldline with very short stitches, spacing them approximately ½" apart.

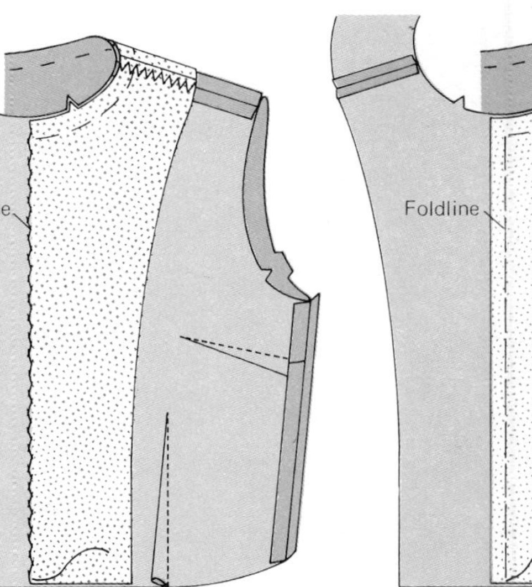

If garment has an extended facing and the edge of the interfacing is to fall *along the foldline,* hold interfacing in place by catchstitching edge to facing over foldline.

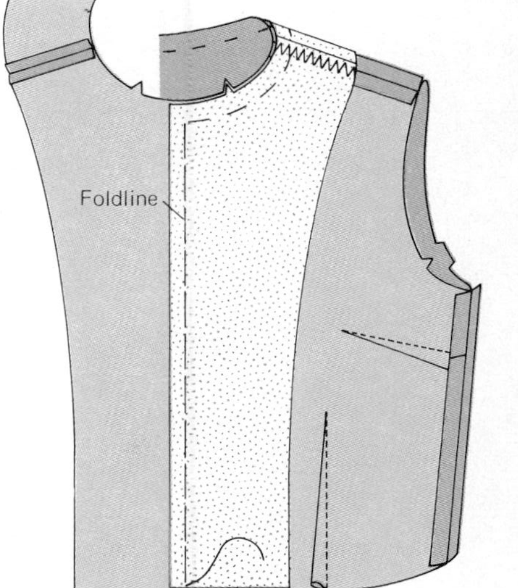

If interfacing will extend *beyond the foldline*, secure interfacing to garment along the foldline with very short stitches, spacing them approximately ½" apart.

Underlying fabrics

Sleeves 256-257 Hemming 290-297 Tailoring 378-381

Linings

A lining is applied to the inside of a garment to finish it and to hide the garment's inner construction. No matter what type of garment it is used in —dress, coat, jacket, pants—a lining is a luxurious as well as functional finishing touch. Most often made from a relatively slippery fabric, a lining can match or contrast with the color of the garment. It can even be made of a printed fabric, so long as it will not show through to the outside of the garment. Linings will add some degree of warmth to a garment as well as making it easier to put the garment on and take it off. Though lining fabrics are made from many different fibers, any specific choice should be limited to fabrics that are compatible with the care requirements of the rest of the garment. Also, a lining should be sufficiently opaque to conceal the garment's inner construction. Its qualities should be appropriate to the type of garment it is being applied to. For example, a winter coat lining should add considerable warmth to the garment. Further warmth can be achieved with the addition of a separate interlining (see p. 83). An interlining is built into some lining fabrics, for example, those that are quilted, eliminating the need for a separate one. These should be constructed and applied to the garment as a lining. A lining fabric should also be strong enough to stand up to the kind of strain and abrasion it will be subject to. A jacket or coat lining must withstand much more strain and abrasion than the lining of a loose-fitting dress. For one thing, a jacket or coat will be worn over other garments that might be abrasive in effect. Then, too, jackets and coats tend to be worn for more strenuous activities.

Application methods differ, the technique depending upon the type of garment the lining is being applied to The lining method shown below is for a **machine application** of a lining to a **jacket or coat.** It is appropriate for jackets and coats that have not been tailored; the amount of handling a garment receives during this application makes the method unsuitable for tailored garments. For the technique of applying a lining by hand, see the Tailoring chapter.

The procedures opposite are for lining a plain, **sleeveless vest or dress to its edges.** Page 82 shows a method of attaching a **free-hanging lining** to any dress, skirt, or pants that will be finished at the top edge by another garment section, such as a facing or waistband. A variation, the **skirt half-lining,** is dealt with there as well.

Machine application of lining to jacket or coat

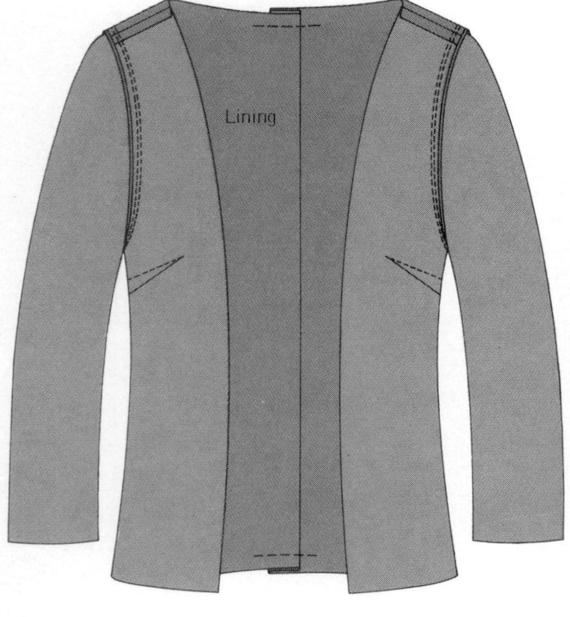

1. Join all lining sections to form a complete lining unit. Sew the sleeves into the armholes, using a double-stitched seam. If lining calls for a pleat down the center back, form the pleat and machine-baste across pleat top and bottom.

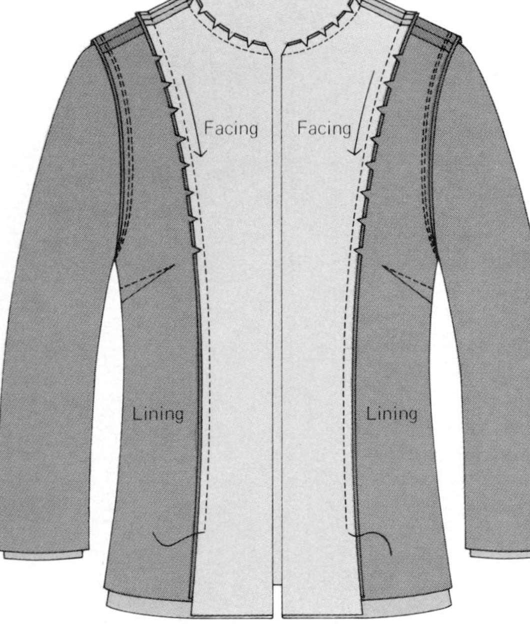

2. Right sides together, match, pin, and baste lining to facing edge. Facing side up, stitch in place. On each half, stitch from center back to a point twice the width of the hem from bottom edge. Trim, grade, clip seam; press toward lining.

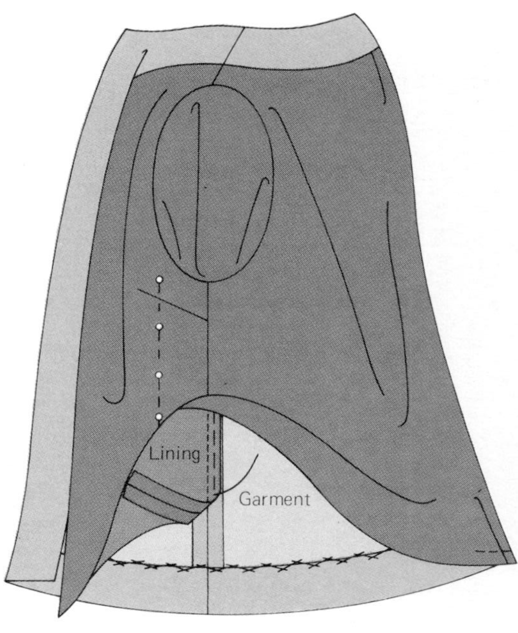

3. Turn garment right side out; hem garment. Pin lining to garment in front of both side seams. Lift lining up and baste each of its back side seam allowances to corresponding garment seam allowances to point 6″ above hem. Hem the lining.

Slipstitch (uneven) 132
Hemming 290-297

Centered zipper 318-319;
invisible 326-327

Lining a garment to its edge

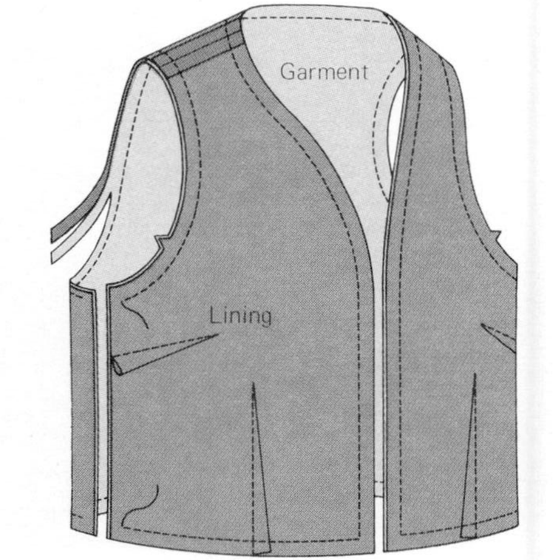

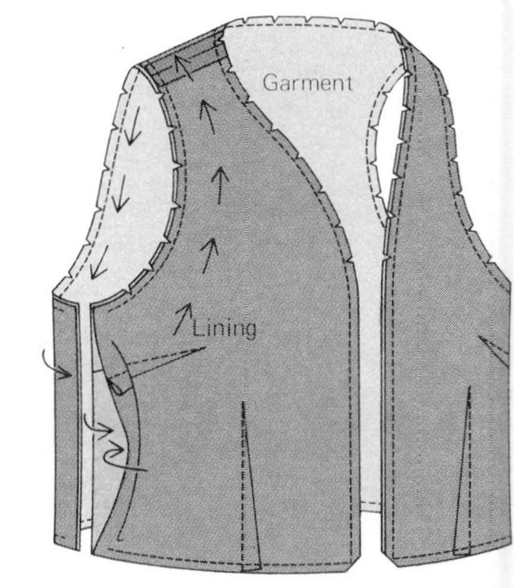

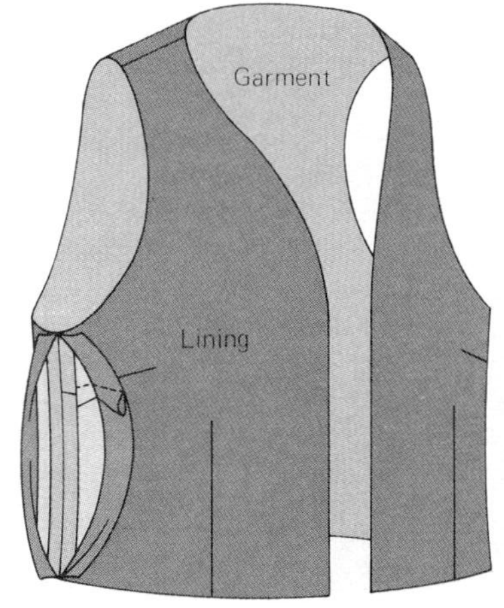

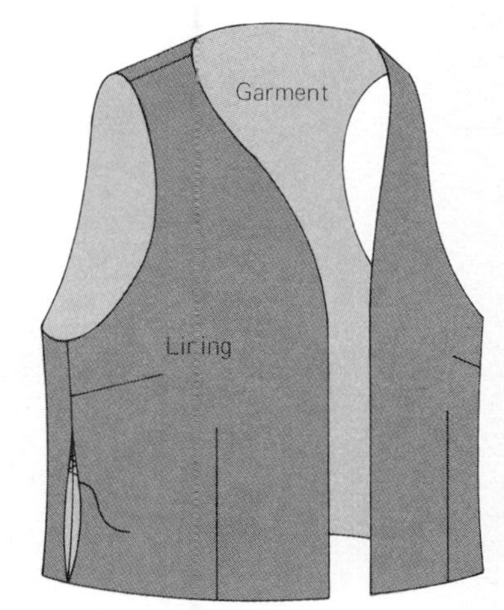

1. Construct garment and lining separately, leaving side seams open for both *vest* and *dress*; back seam as well on *dress*. Right sides facing, sew lining to garment: *vest*, all edges except side seams; *dress* at neck and armholes. Grade and clip or notch seams.

2. Press seams, then turn the garment to the right side. To turn a *vest*, pull each front through each shoulder, then pull both fronts out through one back side seam. To turn a *dress*, pull each back through each shoulder, then flip the front to the back.

3. Next, stitch the seams as follows: For the *vest*, stitch the side seams of the garment only; leave side seams of the lining open. For the *dress*, stitch the side seams of both the garment and lining. Press seams flat, then open. Seam-finish if necessary.

4. To finish *ves'*, slipstitch side seams of lining closed. To finish *dress*, stitch garment back seam and insert zipper; stitch lining back seam up to bottom of placket and slipstitch remainder to the zipper tapes; hem garment and lining separately.

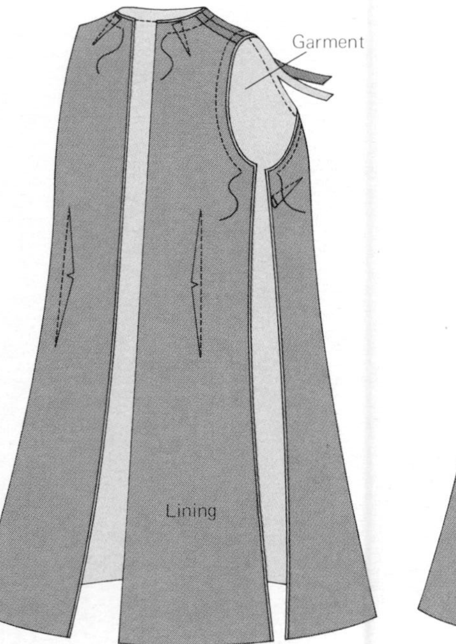

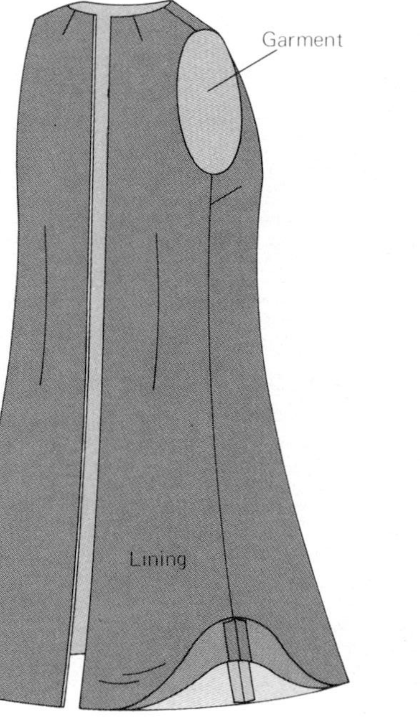

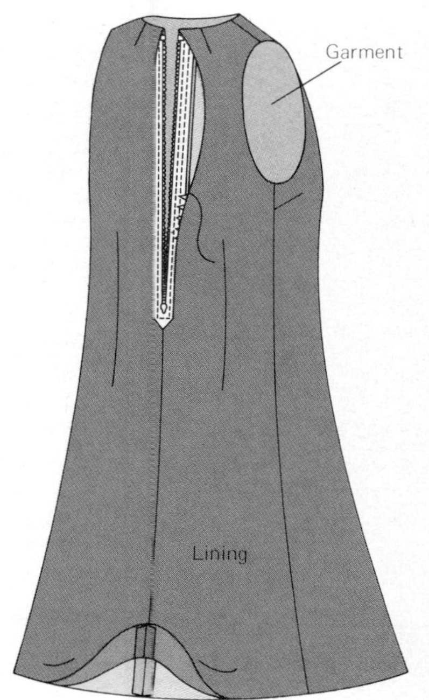

Slipstitch (uneven) 132

Seam finishes 149
Hemming 290-297

Applying a free-hanging lining

The lining method on this page is for attaching a free-hanging lining to a dress, skirt, or pants that will be finished at the top edge by another garment piece, such as a facing or waistband. Since garments of these types receive a good deal of strain during wear, choose a lining fabric that is relatively durable. Be sure that the care requirements of both lining and garment fabrics are compatible and that the lining fabric is of a color that will not show through to the outside of the garment. Use the garment's pattern pieces to cut out the lining; if you are making a half-lining, cut it to extend just below the seat area. The garment, before attaching the lining, should be finished through the stitching of the seams, darts, zipper, and sleeves. Sleeves may or may not be lined. If they are not being lined, apply a bias-bound seam finish to the lining armholes. When it is a sleeveless garment, the top and the armholes will be finished after the lining has been attached. The garment may or may not be hemmed.

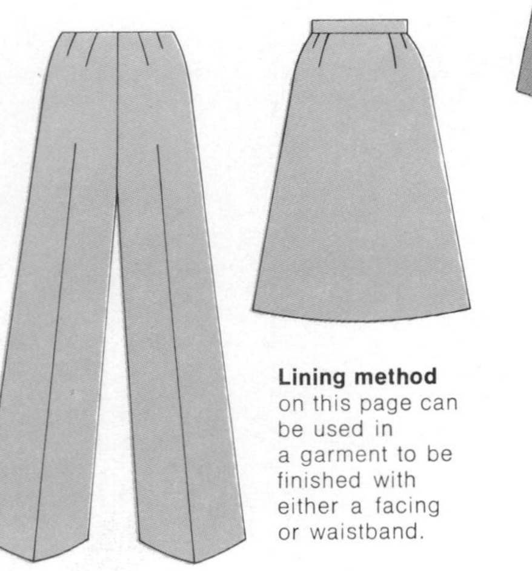

Lining method on this page can be used in a garment to be finished with either a facing or waistband.

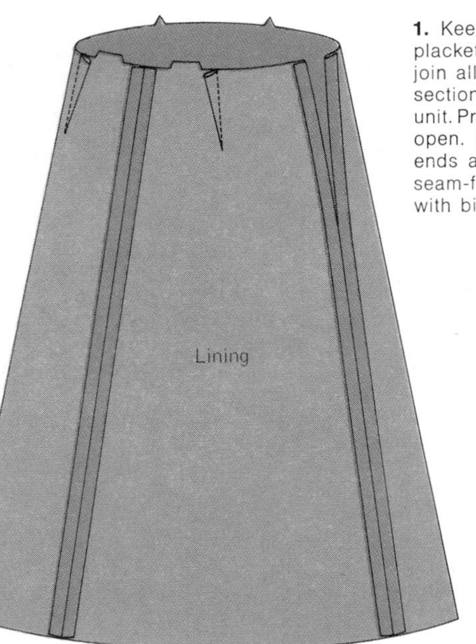

1. Keeping the placket area open, join all lining sections to form a unit. Press seams open. (If the lining ends at armholes, seam-finish edges with bias tape).

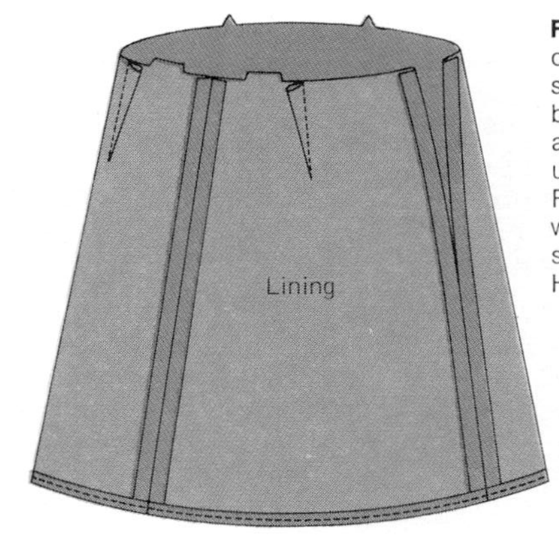

For skirt half-lining, cut the lining sections to just below the seat area and then form a unit as in Step 1. Finish lower edge with a turned-and-stitched hem (see Hemming).

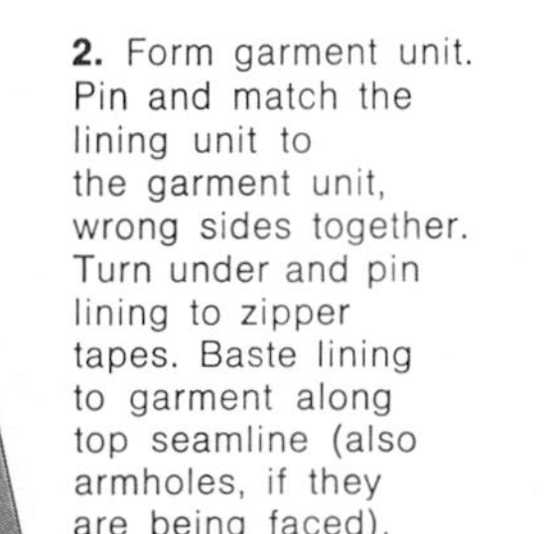

2. Form garment unit. Pin and match the lining unit to the garment unit, wrong sides together. Turn under and pin lining to zipper tapes. Baste lining to garment along top seamline (also armholes, if they are being faced).

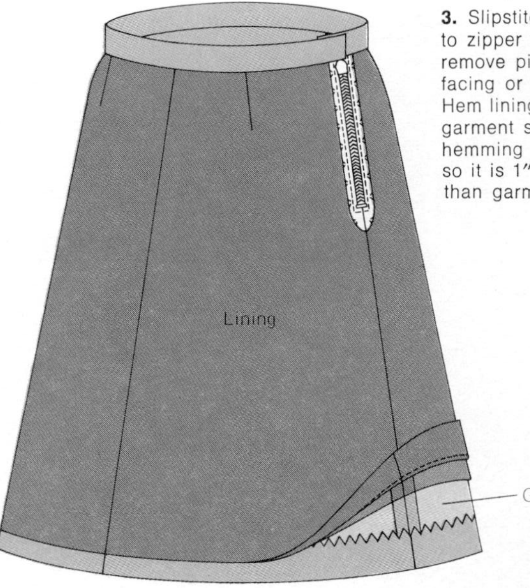

3. Slipstitch lining to zipper tapes; remove pins. Apply facing or waistband. Hem lining and garment separately, hemming lining so it is 1" shorter than garment.

Hand basting 124-125
Catchstitch (flat) 129
Lapped dart technique 162

Interlining

Interlining is a special type of underlying fabric whose main purpose is to insulate a garment, usually a coat or jacket, so it will keep the wearer warm. To do this, an interlining must have some insulating property built into it, as, for example, a napped or lofty fabric has. Interlinings should be lightweight but not thick; they should not add undue bulk or dimension to a garment. The most familiar interlining choices are lamb's wool and nonwoven polyester fleece. Other fabrics not classified as interlinings can serve the same purposes. Among them are felt, some pajama and nightwear fabrics such as plain and brushed flannels, and thin blanket fabrics. Then there are the fabrics sold and handled as linings that also work as interlinings. Examples are quilted, insulated, and fleece-backed linings. An interlining's care requirements should match those of the rest of the garment, though interlined garments are best dry-cleaned. Choose a color that will not show through to the outside of the garment. Be sure, when you plan to interline, that there is adequate wearing ease to accommodate the added thickness; keep this ease in mind while fitting the garment. Because of the ease problem, sleeves are not usually interlined; they can be if ease is sufficient. Use lining pattern pieces to cut interlining.

There are two methods of interlining. The first is to **apply the interlining to the lining,** in a way similar to the underlining method on page 74, then apply lining to garment. The other is to **apply interlining to garment** and then line the garment. See page 80 for basic lining methods.

Applying interlining to lining

Apply each section of the interlining to corresponding section of lining fabric. Interlining is trimmed away at the hemline. Sew lining unit together as though the two fabrics were one. Machine-baste through both fabrics just inside neck and front seamlines. Trim interlining close to all seamlines.

Applying interlining to garment

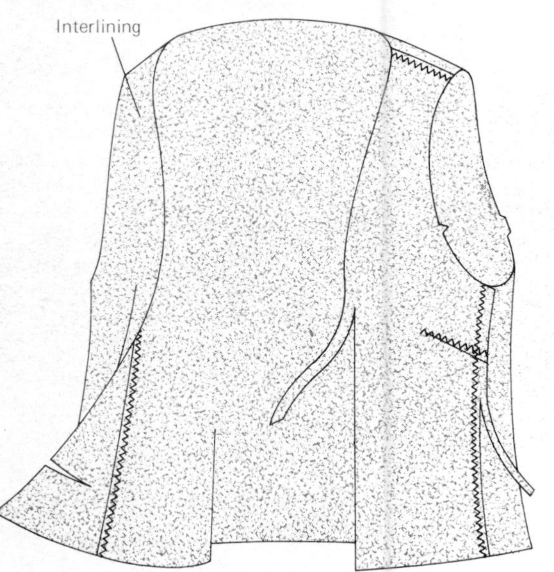

1. Stitch the interlining sections together, lapping seams and darts (see p. 76). Trim away the interlining along the lower edge at a depth that is equal to twice the width of the garment's hem. Trim away neck and front seam allowances.

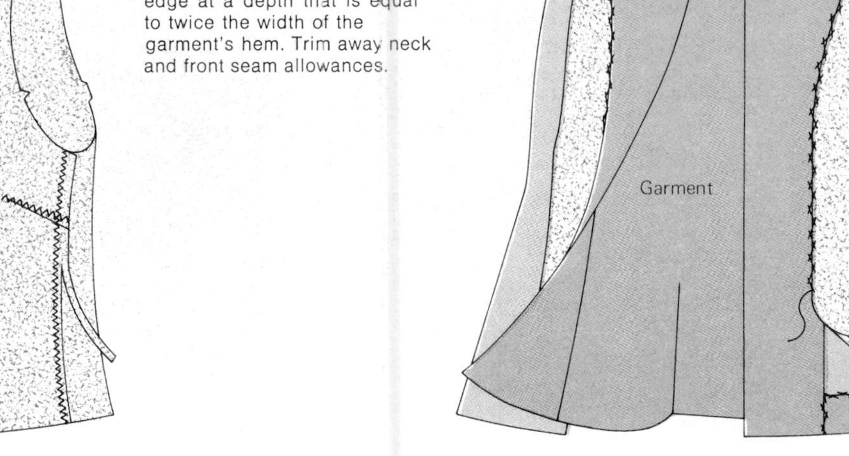

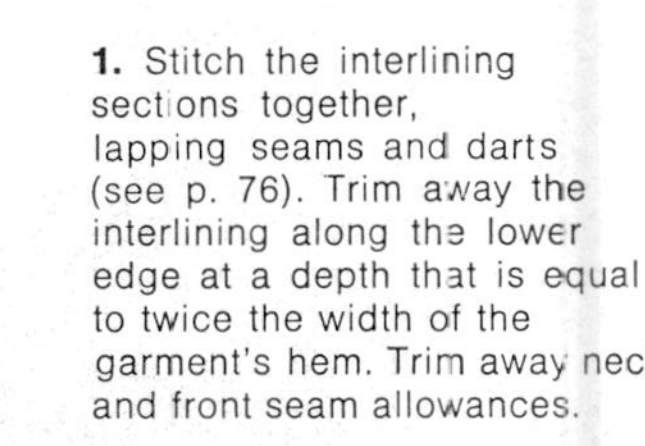

2. Next pin and match the interlining unit to the wrong side of the garment, lapping the neck and front edges over the right side of the facing. Baste unit to garment inside the armhole seamlines; trim; diagonal-baste to garment side seam allowances. Catchstitch neck and front edges to facing.

Cutting preliminaries

Preparing woven fabrics for cutting

Proper fabric preparation is an essential preliminary to cutting. It is helpful, before undertaking these procedures, to understand the basic facts of fabric structure. In weaving, fixed or *warp* yarns are interlaced at right angles by filler or *weft* yarns. A firmly woven strip, called *selvage,* is formed along each lengthwise edge of the finished fabric. Grains indicate yarn direction—*lengthwise,* that of the warp; *crosswise,* that of the weft. Any diagonal that intersects these two grainlines is *bias.* Each grain has different characteristics that affect the way a garment drapes. Lengthwise grain, for instance, has very little give or stretch. In most garments, the lengthwise grain runs vertically (that is, from shoulder to hemline). Crosswise grain has more give and thus drapes differently, giving a fuller look to a garment. As a rule, crosswise grain is used vertically only to achieve a certain design effect, as in border print placement (see Unusual prints, p. 92). Bias stretches the most. A bias-cut garment usually drapes softly. It also tends to be unstable at the hemline.

Straightening fabric ends. This first step must be taken with every fabric so that it can be folded evenly, also checked for grain alignment. Three methods are shown at right; each is suitable for different kinds of fabric. *Tearing* is the fastest, but appropriate only for firmly woven fabrics; other types may snag or stretch. *Drawing a thread* is slower, but the most suitable for loosely woven, soft, or stretchy fabrics. *Cutting on a prominent line* is a quick, simple method for any fabric that has a strong woven linear design.

Checking fabric alignment comes next. During manufacture, the fabric may have been pulled *off-grain,* so that grainlines are no longer at perfect right angles. A garment made with such fabric will not hang correctly, so re-alignment must be done before cutting (see opposite page). Bear in mind that not every off-grain fabric can be corrected, especially those that have water repellent or permanent press finish, or a bonded backing.

Preshrinking is advisable if shrinkage possibilities are unknown, if two or more different fabrics are being used for a washable garment, or if maximum shrinkage is expected to be more than one percent. To preshrink washable fabric, launder and dry it, using the same methods to be used for the garment (follow fabric care instructions). To preshrink drycleanable fabric, (1) dampen fabric (see first re-aligning step opposite); (2) lay on flat surface to dry (do *not* hang it up); (3) press lightly on wrong side. *One caution:* This process may cause some fabrics to waterspot or become matted. It is wise to pretest a scrap. If both shrinking and grain adjustment are necessary, preshrink first, then re-align grain.

Press fabric that is wrinkled or has a creaseline, testing to see if the crease can be removed. If it cannot, or a faded streak shows up along the fold, this area must be avoided in layout and cutting (see Folding fabrics, p. 87).

Warp

Weft

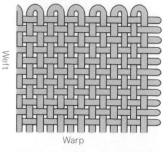

Woven fabric: Basically two sets of yarns, *warp* and *weft,* interlaced at right angles.

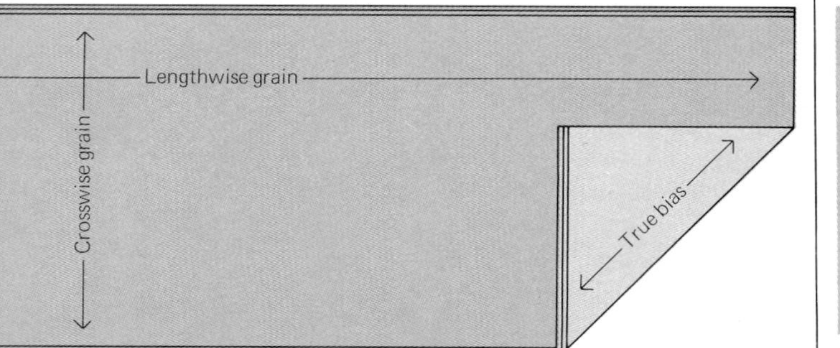

Selvage is formed along each lengthwise edge. **Lengthwise grain** parallels selvage; **crosswise grain** is perpendicular to it. **Bias** is any diagonal that intersects these grains; **true bias** is at a 45° angle to any straight edge when grains are perpendicular.

Straightening ends

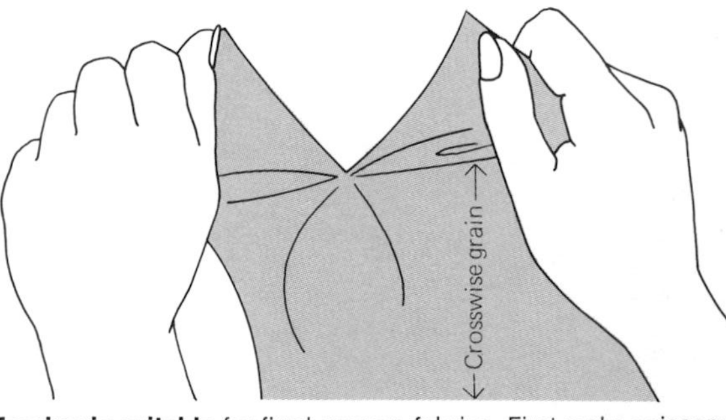

Tearing is suitable for firmly woven fabrics. First make scissors snip in one selvage; grasp fabric firmly and rip across to opposite selvage. If strip runs off to nothing part way across, repeat, beginning farther from edge.

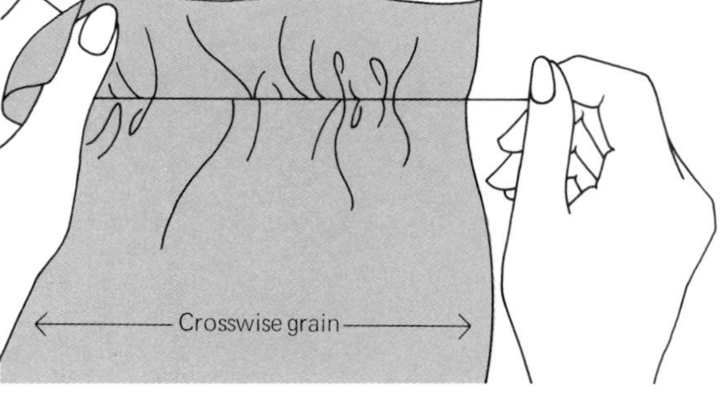

A drawn thread is better for soft, stretchy, or loose weaves. Snip selvage; grasp one or two crosswise threads and pull gently, alternately sliding thread and pushing fabric until you reach other selvage. Cut along pulled thread.

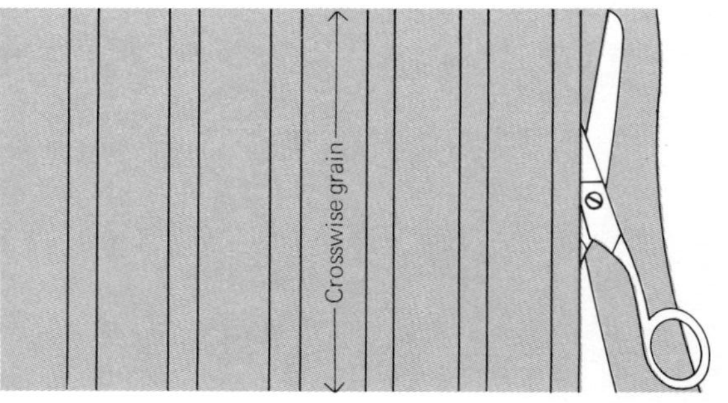

Cutting on a prominent fabric line is limited to fabrics with a woven stripe, plaid, check, or other linear design. For *printed* designs of this type, use first or second methods (tearing or drawn thread), whichever is appropriate.

Re-aligning grain

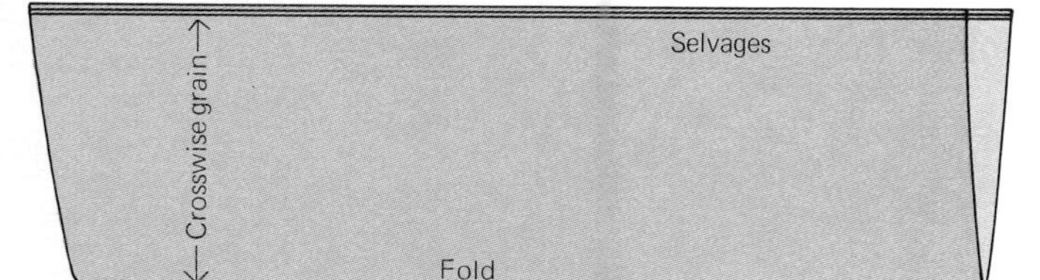

After straightening ends, fold fabric lengthwise, bringing selvages together and matching crosswise ends. If fabric edges fail to align on three sides (as shown), or if edges align but corners do not form right angles, fabric is skewed or *off-grain* and must be re-aligned before cutting.

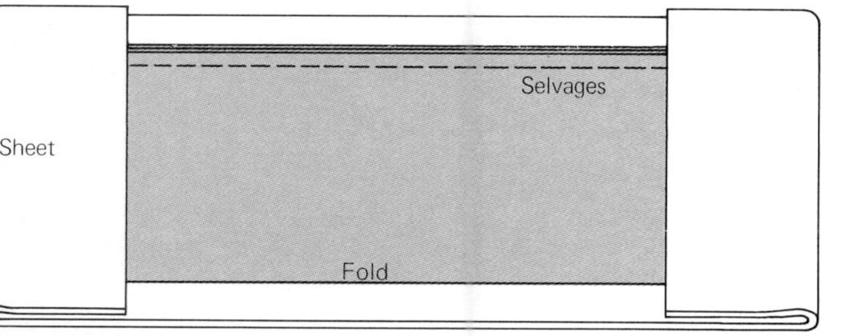

Dampening fabric is first step in re-aligning it. This relaxes finish, making fabric more pliable. Fold fabric lengthwise, matching selvages and ends; baste edges together. Enclose in a damp sheet (as shown) and leave several hours; or moisten fabric itself, using sponge or spray bottle. Pretest small area; if water damages fabric, omit this step.

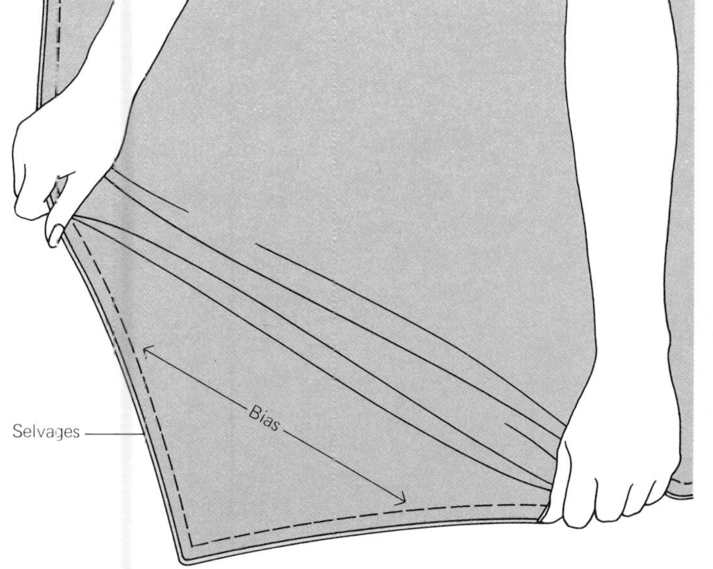

Next, fabric is stretched on the bias. This is usually sufficient to put it back in proper shape. Pull gently, but firmly, until fabric is smooth and all corners form right angles (easier to accomplish if two people work together). Use caution; too much stretching can cause further distortion. Lay fabric on a flat surface to dry, then press if necessary.

Selvage

An off-grain print makes fabric seem crooked even if grainlines are true. This cannot be corrected. Avoid such fabrics by carefully examining print before purchase.

Preparing knits for cutting

Knits are structured differently from wovens but prepared for cutting in much the same way, except for straightening of ends. Since there are no selvages, and threads cannot be pulled, you must rely on your eye to tell whether a knit is even. If the design is boldly structured, cut along a prominent line; otherwise follow the procedures below.

Knit fabrics come in two forms, *flat* and *tubular*. Some flat knits have perforated lengthwise edges, which are comparable to the selvages on wovens. These should not be used, however, as a guide for aligning fabric; they are not dependably straight.

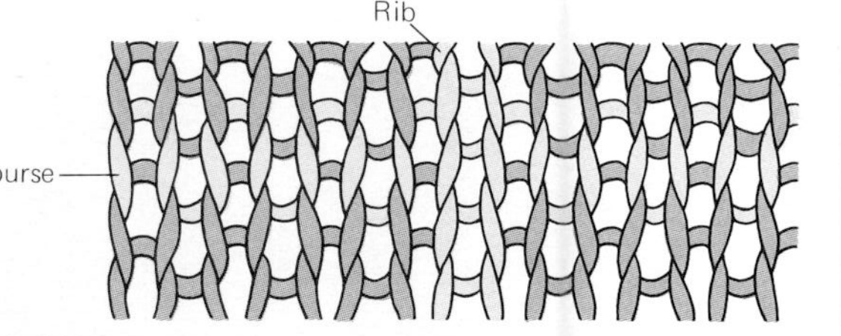

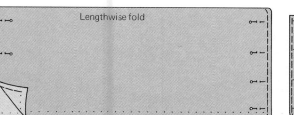

Knit fabric is formed by interlocking loops of yarn called *ribs*, which can be compared to the lengthwise grain in woven fabrics. The rows of loops at right angles to ribs, called *courses*, are comparable to crosswise grain of woven.

Lengthwise fold

To straighten ends of a flat knit, baste with contrasting thread along one course at each end of fabric. Fold fabric in half lengthwise; align markings and pin together. (For alternative method, see Folding knits for cutting, p. 87.)

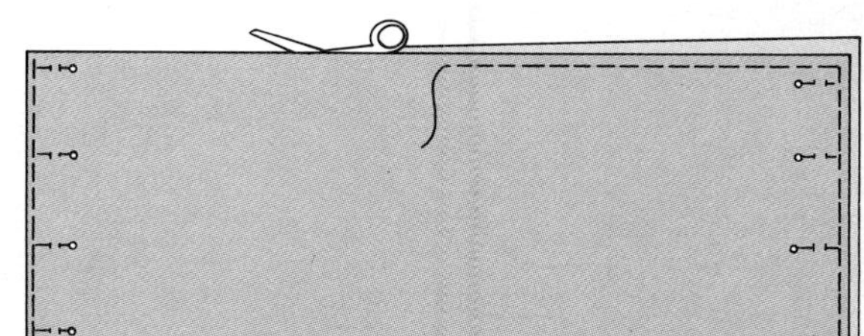

Straighten ends of a tubular knit same as flat knit, then cut open along one rib. If edges curl, press lightly, then baste together. Only exception is a narrow tube (usually 18″ wide); this is used as is, without lengthwise seams.

Cutting preliminaries

Parts of a pattern 56-57
Pattern alterations 100-110

Pattern piece pointers

1. Assemble all pieces needed for your view.
2. Return to the envelope any pattern pieces that are not needed; they could cause confusion.
3. Cut apart small pieces, such as facings and pockets, if printed on one sheet of tissue.
4. *Do not trim* extra tissue margin that surrounds cutting lines; this is useful for alterations.
5. Determine how many times each piece is to be cut (such information is on the tissue itself).
6. Press pattern pieces with warm iron, if exceptionally wrinkled; otherwise smooth with hands.
7. Alter pattern, if necessary (see Fitting chapter). Be certain that any alterations made are visible on both sides of the pattern tissue.
8. Check overall garment length; change if desired.
9. Consider possible style changes. You may wish to re-locate or eliminate pockets, create a more convenient opening, eliminate or add a seam (see Cutting basic design changes, p. 93). All such remodeling must be decided upon before cutting.

Identifying right side of fabric

Right side or *face* of fabric should be identified before cutting. Often it is obvious, but sometimes careful examination is needed to tell right side from wrong. One means of identification is the way fabric is folded—cottons and linens are right side out, wools wrong side out. If fabric is rolled on a tube, face is to the inside. Here are some additional clues: **Smooth fabrics** are shinier, slicker, or softer on the right side. **Textured fabrics** are more distinctly so on the face. For example, slubs may be more outstanding, a twill (diagonal weave) better defined. Such fabrics often have small irregularities, such as extra thick nubs, on the wrong side. **Fancy weaves,** such as brocade, are smoother on the right side, floats usually loose and uneven on the back. **Printed designs** are sharper on the right side, more blurred on the back. The **selvage** is smoother on the right side. Some knits roll toward the right side when stretched crosswise.

The fabric face is generally more resistant to soil and abrasion but you can use the wrong side out if you prefer its look. When there is no visible difference between sides, make one the back and mark it with chalk to avoid confusion.

Selecting pattern layout

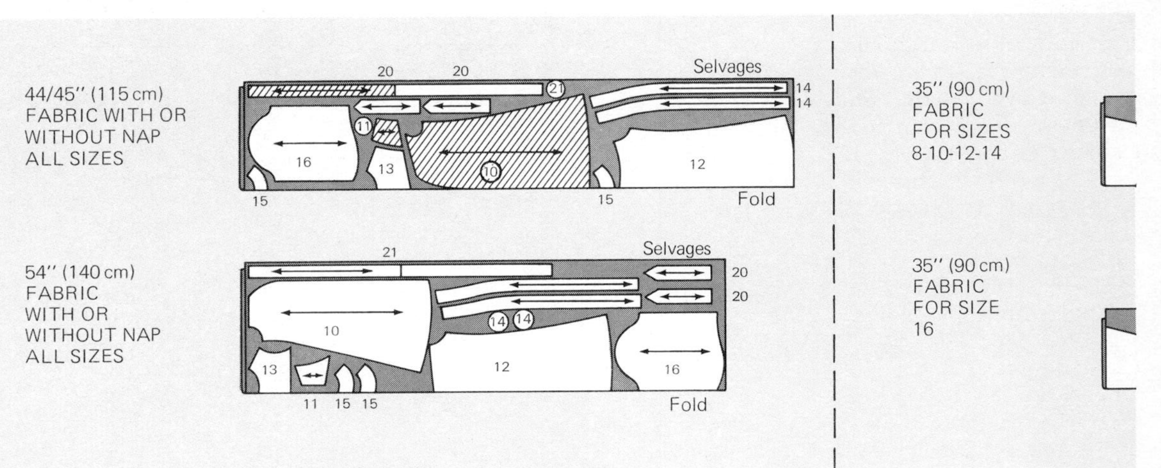

To find correct pattern layout, look for view that corresponds to your choice, then for fabric width and size that match yours. Circle this view so you won't confuse it with other views as you work. If there is no layout for your fabric width, or if you are combining views, a trial layout may be necessary (see Trial layout, p. 93, for procedure).

How to interpret cutting guides

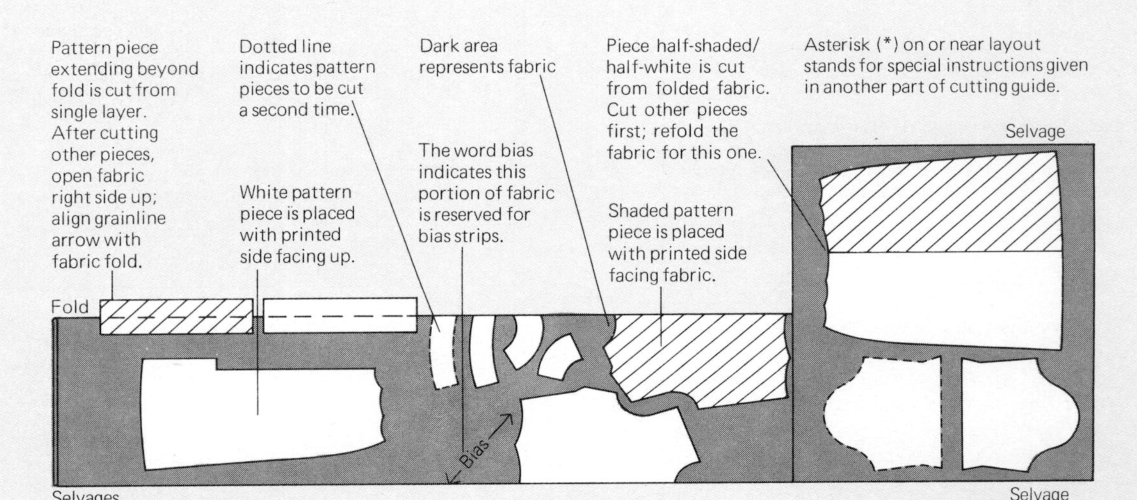

Pattern piece extending beyond fold is cut from single layer. After cutting other pieces, open fabric right side up; align grainline arrow with fabric fold.
Dotted line indicates pattern pieces to be cut a second time.
White pattern piece is placed with printed side facing up.
Dark area represents fabric
The word bias indicates this portion of fabric is reserved for bias strips.
Piece half-shaded/ half-white is cut from folded fabric. Cut other pieces first; refold the fabric for this one.
Shaded pattern piece is placed with printed side facing fabric.
Asterisk (*) on or near layout stands for special instructions given in another part of cutting guide.
Fold
Bias
Selvages
Selvage
Selvage

Cutting layout above is representative of types to be found in any pattern guide sheet. To make the drawing more informative, all possible variations are included; the average actual layout is usually much simpler. Every pattern company provides, in its instruction sheets, a key to the use of its particular layouts. Consult this before proceeding.

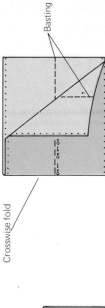

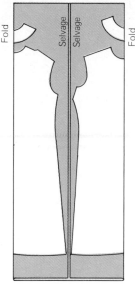

Folding fabrics for cutting

The first step in following a cutting layout is to determine how fabric should be folded, if at all. Precision is vital here. Where selvages meet, they should match exactly. (Shifting of slippery or soft fabric can be prevented by pinning selvages together every few inches.) If the material was folded at the time of purchase, make sure the foldline is accurate and re-press it if necessary. Also test to see if fold can be removed—a permanent crease must be avoided in cutting. (A double lengthwise fold, right, is one way around the problem.) When no fold is indicated, lay fabric right side up.

It does not matter whether right or wrong sides are together, except in these instances: Fold *right sides* together when layout calls for partial lengthwise fold. Fold *wrong sides* together of all napped fabrics, designs to be matched, prints with large motifs, and fabric to be marked with tracing paper (see Marking methods, p. 94).

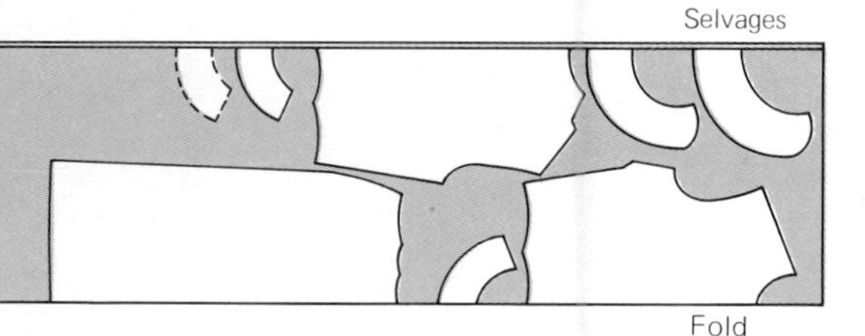

Standard lengthwise fold: Made on lengthwise grain with selvages matching along one edge (the way fabric often comes from the bolt). The fold most often encountered in layout guides, it is convenient and easy to manage.

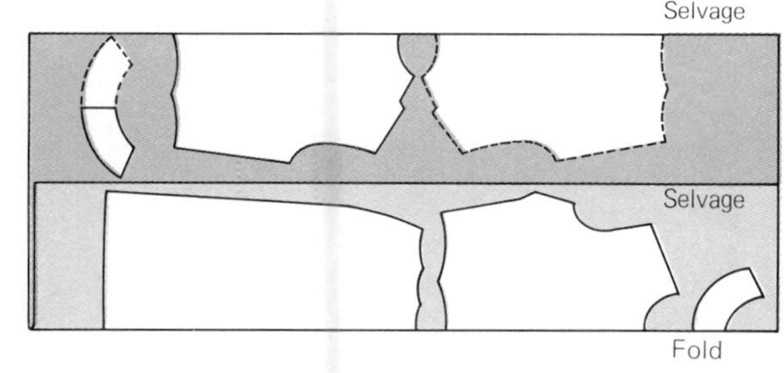

Partial lengthwise fold: Made on lengthwise grain with one selvage placed a measured distance from fold; balance of fabric is single layer. Width of double portion is determined by widest pattern piece to go in this space. Care must be taken to maintain uniform distance from selvage to fold.

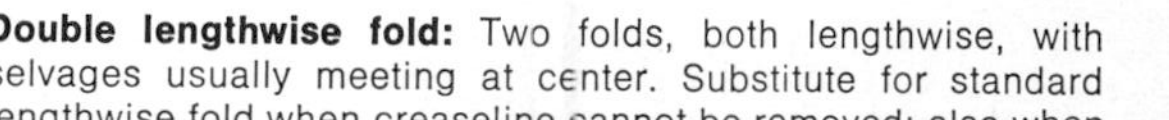

Double lengthwise fold: Two folds, both lengthwise, with selvages usually meeting at center. Substitute for standard lengthwise fold when creaseline cannot be removed; also when both front and back pieces are to be cut on fold. Keep distance consistent from each fold to selvage.

Crosswise fold: Made on crosswise grain with selvages matching along two edges. Generally used when the lengthwise fold would be wasteful of fabric, or to accommodate any unusually wide pattern pieces. *Not* to be used for napped or other one-way fabrics (see Cutting directional fabrics, p. 90).

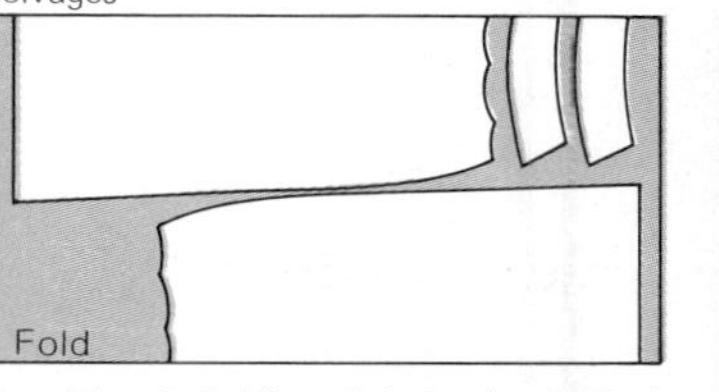
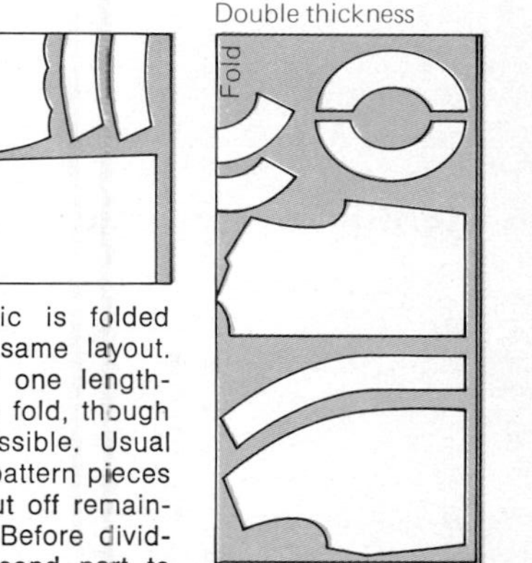

Combined folds: Fabric is folded two different ways for same layout. Most often consists of one lengthwise and one crosswise fold, though any combination is possible. Usual procedure is to lay out pattern pieces for one portion, then cut off remaining fabric and re-fold. Before dividing fabric, measure second part to be sure there is enough length.

Folding a knit

There are two ways to fold knit accurately. You can (1) match crosswise basting used for straightening ends (see Preparing knits for cutting, p. 85) or (2) mark a lengthwise rib, as at right. Should knit be too fine for either method, fold it as evenly as you can, making sure ribs are not twisted along foldline. If fabric already has a crease, check it for accuracy; re-press if necessary; also make sure crease can be removed. Special care must be taken with knit fold—it acts as a guide for straight grain when pattern is pinned.

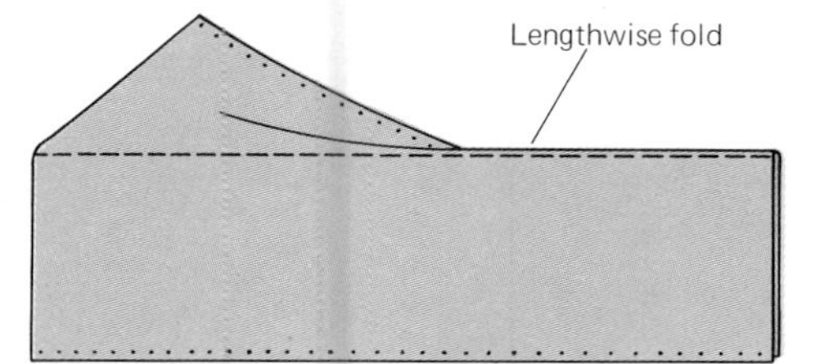

Before folding knit lengthwise, baste along one rib near center of fabric, using contrasting thread; fold on baste line. If knit has perforated edges, these need not match.

When folding knit crosswise, baste first as for lengthwise fold, then fold fabric, aligning the baste marks. Pin along basting through both layers of fabric.

Basic cutting procedure

Pinning

For pinning pattern to fabric, the general order is *left to right* and *fold to selvages*. For each pattern piece, pin fold or grainline arrow first, then corners, and finally edges, smoothing pattern as you pin. *Place pieces as close together as possible*, overlapping tissue margins where necessary. Each layout is designed to use fabric economically. Even small changes may result in the pieces not fitting into the space apportioned to them.

The efficient way to place pins is diagonally at corners and perpendicular to edges, with points toward and inside cutting lines. (On delicate fabrics, and leather and vinyl, in which pins could leave holes, pin within seam allowances.) Use only enough pins to secure foldlines, grainline arrows, corners, and notches—too many pins can distort fabric, making it difficult to cut accurately. A few more than usual may be needed for slippery or soft fabrics. A firm hand on the pattern while cutting gives adequate fabric control.

Do not allow fabric to hang off the edge of the cutting surface. If it is not large enough to accommodate all fabric at once, lay out and pin one portion at a time, carefully folding up the rest.

Before starting to cut, lay out *all* illustrated pieces, then re-check your placements. Cutting is a crucial step, not to be done in haste. If underlining, lining, or interfacing are to be cut using garment pattern pieces, cut garment first; remove pattern and re-pin to each "under" fabric.

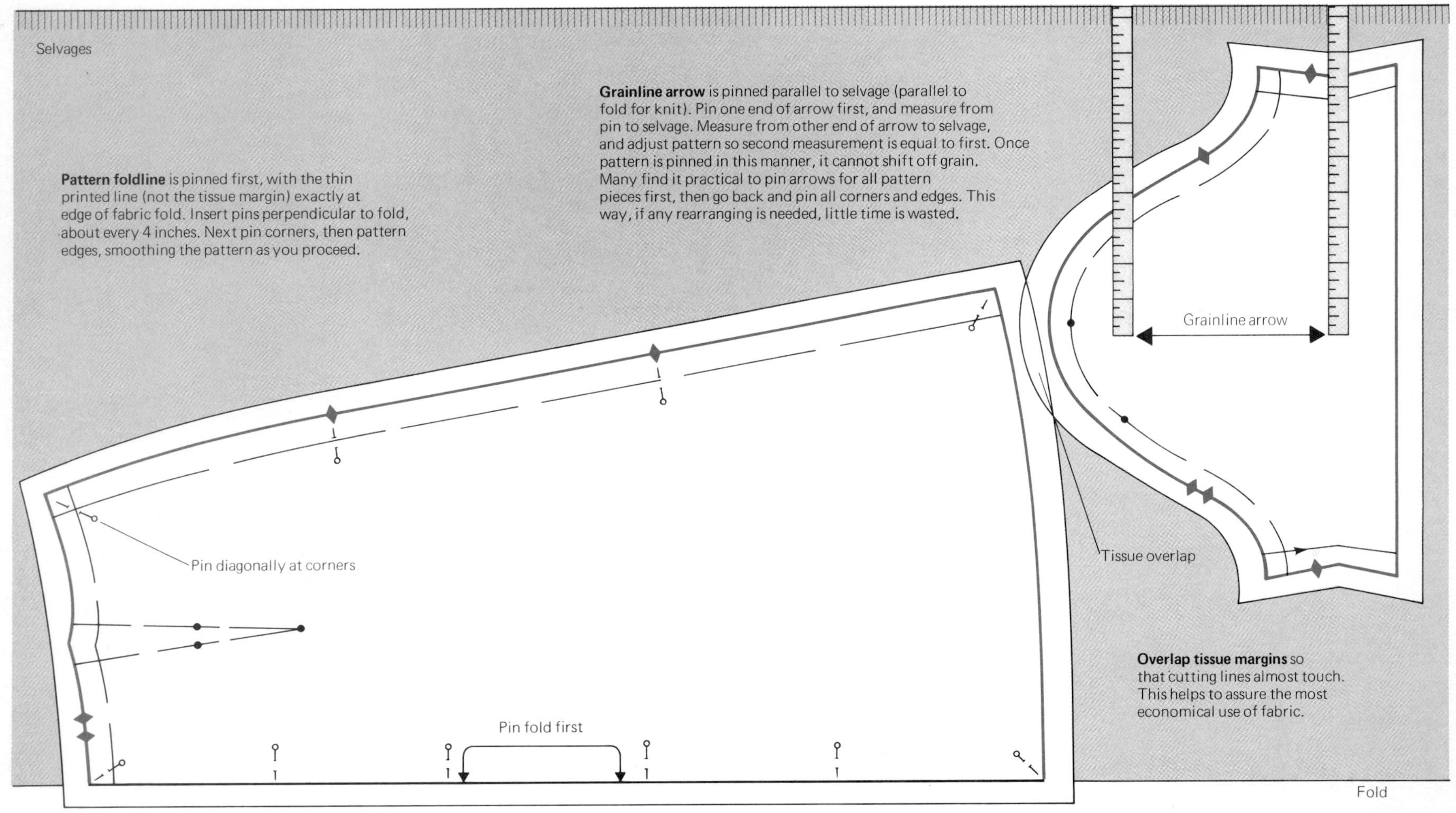

Pattern foldline is pinned first, with the thin printed line (not the tissue margin) exactly at edge of fabric fold. Insert pins perpendicular to fold, about every 4 inches. Next pin corners, then pattern edges, smoothing the pattern as you proceed.

Grainline arrow is pinned parallel to selvage (parallel to fold for knit). Pin one end of arrow first, and measure from pin to selvage. Measure from other end of arrow to selvage, and adjust pattern so second measurement is equal to first. Once pattern is pinned in this manner, it cannot shift off grain. Many find it practical to pin arrows for all pattern pieces first, then go back and pin all corners and edges. This way, if any rearranging is needed, little time is wasted.

Overlap tissue margins so that cutting lines almost touch. This helps to assure the most economical use of fabric.

Cutting

For accurate cutting results, always keep fabric flat on the cutting surface, and use the proper shears and techniques as described below. Bent-handle shears help in keeping fabric flat. These are available in four blade types—*plain, serrated, pinking,* and *scalloping.* Plain and serrated blades can be used interchangeably, but serrated blades are designed to grip knits and slippery fabrics. Pinking and scalloping shears should be used only for seam finishing, never to cut out a garment; they do not produce a precise edge, and they also obscure notches. A 7- or 8-inch blade will suit most cutting situations; a 9-inch length is better for heavy fabrics. Be sure that blades are sharp; dull ones will chew fabric. If the scissor action is stiff, cutting control may be difficult. One remedy is to adjust the blade screw slightly; another, to apply greaseless lubricant. Electric scissors can be substituted for standard ones, and are just as efficient, once you acquire the knack of using them.

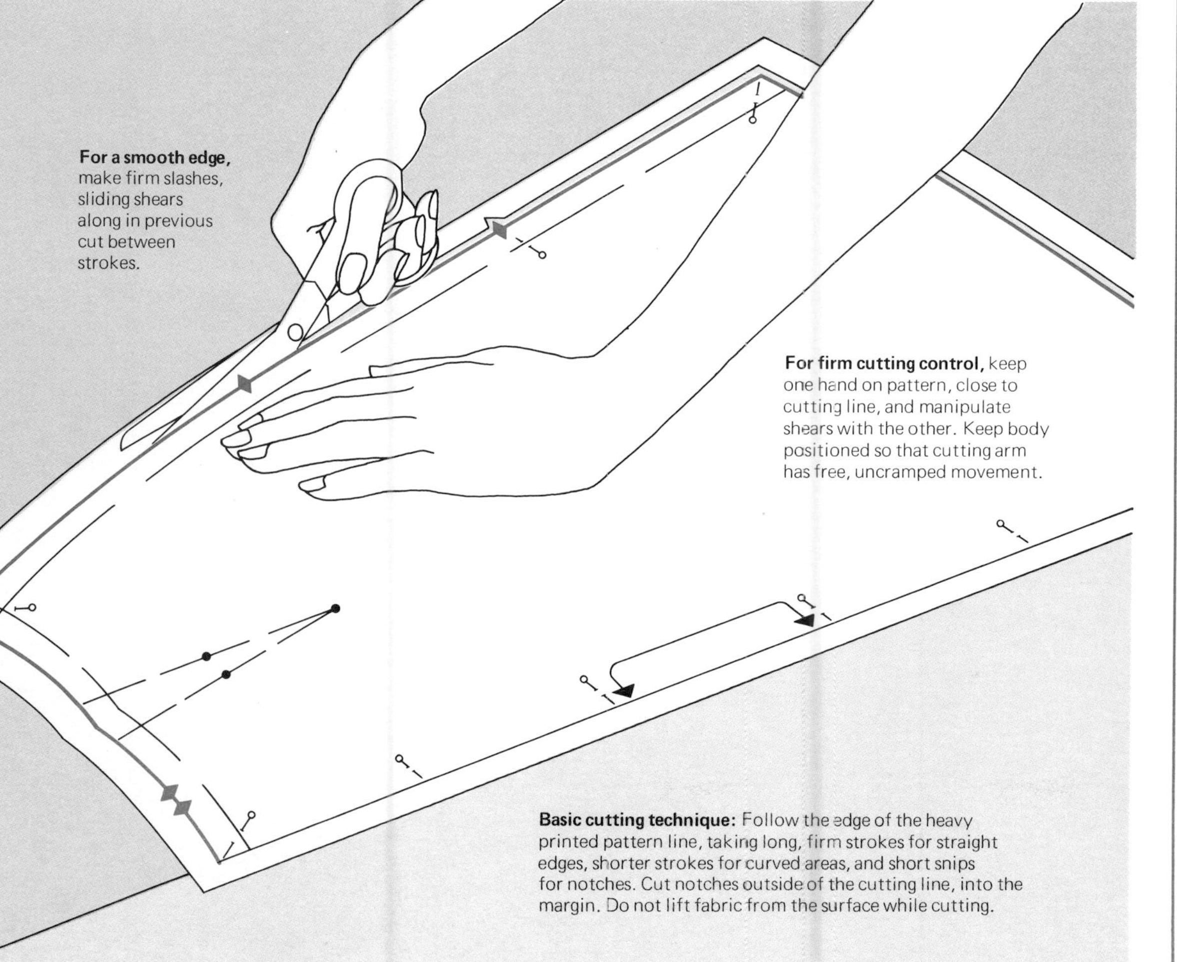

For a smooth edge, make firm slashes, sliding shears along in previous cut between strokes.

For firm cutting control, keep one hand on pattern, close to cutting line, and manipulate shears with the other. Keep body positioned so that cutting arm has free, uncramped movement.

Basic cutting technique: Follow the edge of the heavy printed pattern line, taking long, firm strokes for straight edges, shorter strokes for curved areas, and short snips for notches. Cut notches outside of the cutting line, into the margin. Do not lift fabric from the surface while cutting.

Special cutting tips

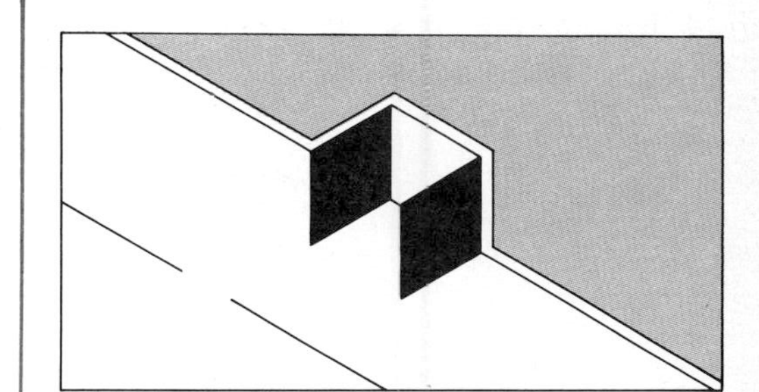

Cut double or triple notches as single units, snipping straight across from point to point—simpler and more convenient than cutting each one individually.

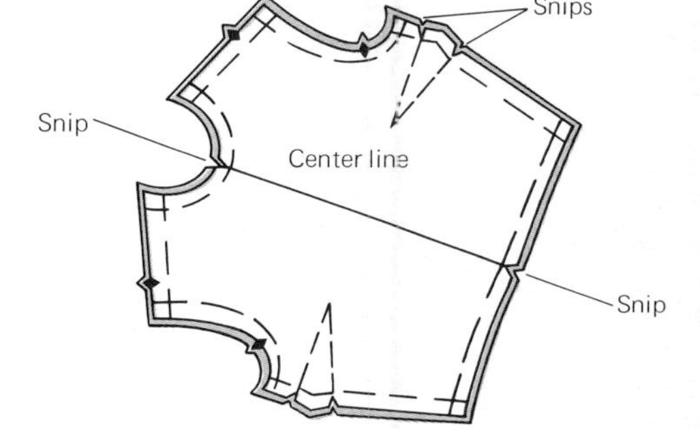

Identify garment center lines with small snip into each seam allowance at top and bottom edges; do same for any adjoining piece, such as collar. Snips are useful, too, to identify dart lines, especially when pin/chalk marking method is used (see p. 94).

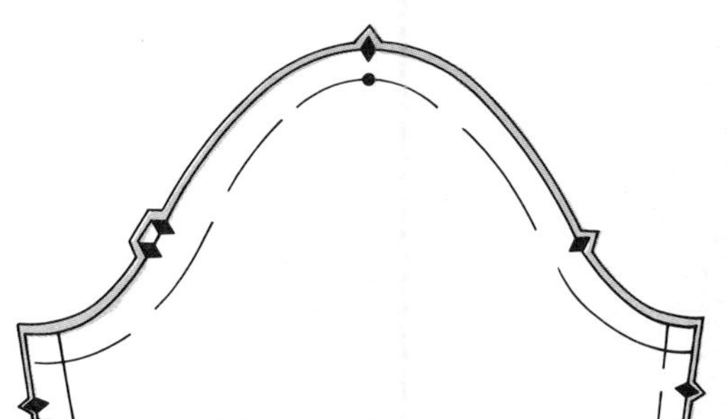

Identify top of sleeve cap by cutting a notch just above large circle on the pattern. Such a notch is easier to see when setting in the sleeve.

Cutting special fabrics

Plaid proportions 53

Yardage for plaids and stripes 68-69
Yardage for one-way layout 69

General recommendations

Certain fabrics involve special considerations in pattern selection and layout. Guidelines for the handling of such fabrics begin here and continue through page 92. A fabric can fall into one of the problem categories, or more than one. A plaid, for example, might also be a directional fabric.

Directional fabrics are so called because they must be laid in one direction for cutting; they are described as "with nap" on pattern envelope and guide sheet. Included in this category are truly napped fabrics (with pile or brushed surfaces); designs that do not reverse (one-way designs); and surfaces that reflect light in varying ways (shaded). Satins and iridescents are examples of the last. To determine if a fabric is a directional type, fold it crosswise, right sides together, then fold back a part of the top layer along one selvage. If the opposing layers do not look exactly the same, the fabric is a "nap" for cutting purposes.

To test a napped fabric (one with pile or brushed surface) for direction, run a hand over it. It will feel smooth with nap running down, rough with nap running up. In deciding which direction to use, consider the following: *Short naps* (such as corduroy) can be cut with nap running up for rich color tone or down for a frosty effect. The same is true of *shaded* fabrics. *Long piles* or shags should be cut with nap running down for better appearance and wear. *One-way designs* are cut according to the natural bent of the design, or the effect desired.

Because all pattern pieces must be laid in one direction (see illustration, above right), a crosswise fold cannot be used. If such a fold is indicated, fold fabric as specified, with wrong sides together; cut along foldline and, keeping wrong sides together, turn the top layer so nap faces in the same direction as it does on the layer beneath.

Plaids, most stripes, and other geometrics as well are, for the most part, the same for cutting purposes. What differences occur are due to proportions within the design (see details opposite). These fabrics are usually more effective and easier to handle in a simple style. A good pattern choice is one that shows a plaid or stripe view on the envelope. *Avoid* any pattern designated "not suitable for plaids or stripes"; stay away, too, from princess seams and long horizontal darts.

Directional fabrics

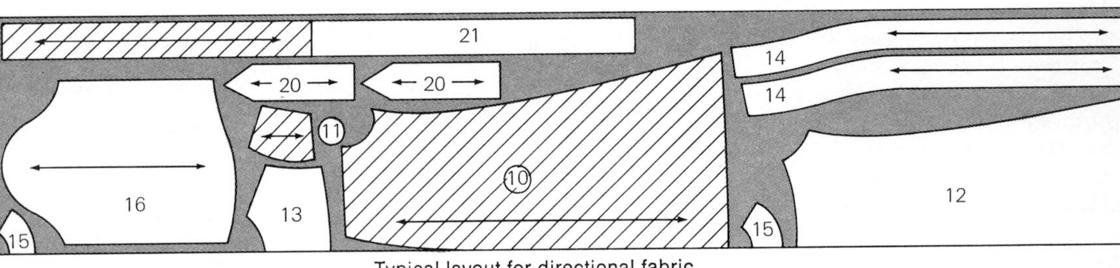

Typical layout for directional fabric

Laying out pattern on plaids and stripes

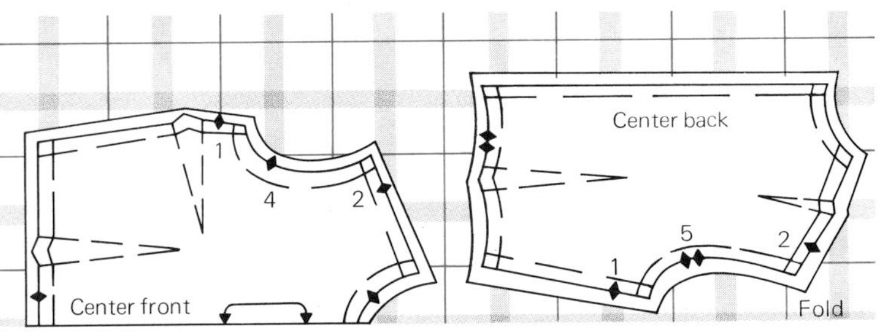

Centering is the first consideration when laying pattern on plaid, stripe, or comparable geometric design. Decide which lengthwise bar or space is to be at garment center. Fold fabric exactly in half at this point for pattern piece that is to be cut on a fold; for other sections, align point with the center seamline (or center line for piece with extended facing). Centers must be consistent for bodice and skirt, sleeve and collar—all major garment sections.

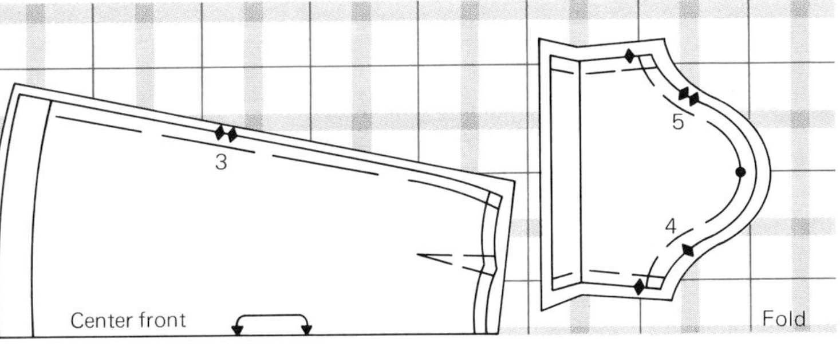

Placement of dominant crosswise bars is the second consideration when planning a layout in plaid or crosswise stripes. As a rule, the dominant stripes should be placed directly on, or as close as possible to, the garment edges, such as hemline and sleeve edge. (Exceptions are A-line or other flared shapes. In these cases, place the least dominant color section at hem edge so the curved hemline will be less conspicuous.) Avoid dominant stripes, too, at the waist and across the full part of bust or hip.

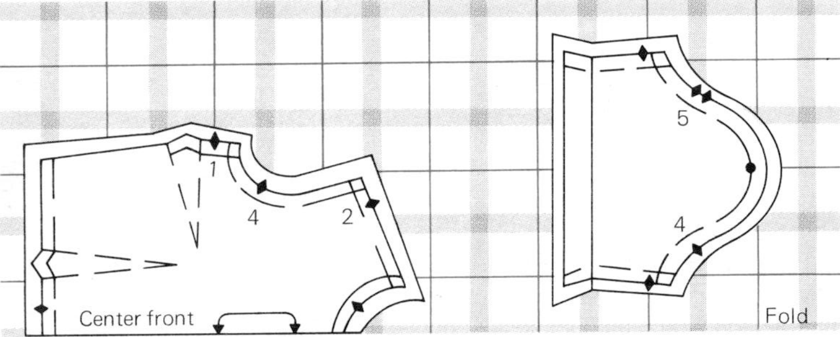

Crosswise matching of major garment sections is accomplished by placing corresponding notches on identical crossbars (lines that will be horizontal). To match sleeve and garment front, for example, place front armhole notches of both sleeve and garment on the same crossbars. *Do all matching at seamlines—not at cutting lines.* It may or may not be possible to match such diagonals as darts, shoulder seams, and pants inseams. This depends on angle of stitch line and particular fabric design.

Even and uneven plaids

A plaid is a design of woven or printed color bars that intersect at right angles. The arrangement of these bars may be even or uneven, as illustrated at right; which it is should be determined before fabric is purchased because this affects pattern choice as well as layout necessities.

A four-sided area in which the color bars form one complete design is called a *repeat.* To tell whether a plaid is even or uneven, fold a repeat in half, first lengthwise, then crosswise. A plaid is *even* when color bars and intervening spaces are identical in each direction; it is *uneven* if they fail to match in one or both directions. Stripes also may be even or uneven; each type is handled by the same methods as a corresponding plaid. The exception is a diagonal stripe, discussed on page 92.

Even plaids, either square or rectangular, are the easiest to work with, though a rectangular plaid is somewhat more difficult to match where seaming is bias. An even plaid is suitable for a garment with a center opening or center seams, also for one cut on the bias (see Chevron, p. 92).

Uneven plaids require extra thought and care in layout planning and have fewer style possibilities.

When plaid is uneven crosswise, pattern pieces must be laid in one direction, like napped fabrics.

When plaid is uneven lengthwise, the repeats do not have a center from which the design can be balanced out in both directions, and so the design goes around the body in one direction only. A type of balance can be established, however, by placing a dominant vertical bar or block at centers front and back. *Avoid* designs with center seams or kimono or raglan sleeves. An exception can be made to these precautions when a plaid fabric that is uneven lengthwise is reversible. In this case, the pattern should have center seams, or they must be created (see Design changes, p. 93). Plan the layout so that the design reverses itself to each side of the center seams. This is accomplished by cutting each garment section twice, with printed side of pattern facing up, and using wrong side of fabric for half the garment.

When plaid is uneven in both directions, the same considerations apply as for plaids that are uneven lengthwise, plus the need to lay all pattern pieces in one direction as for napped fabrics.

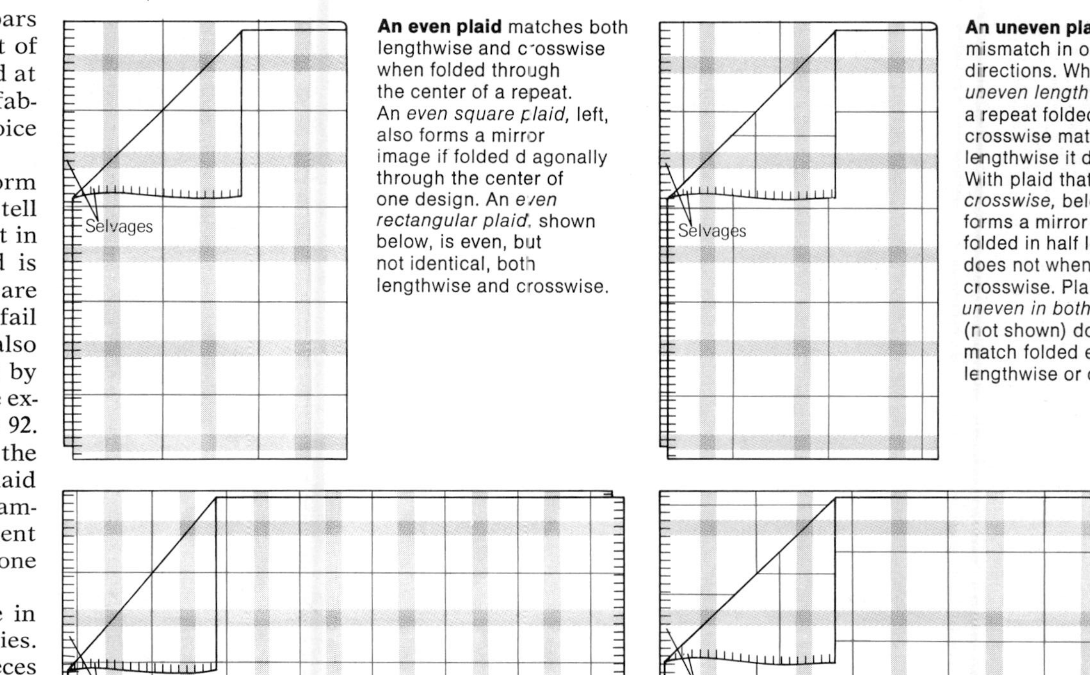

An even plaid matches both lengthwise and crosswise when folded through the center of a repeat. An *even square plaid,* left, also forms a mirror image if folded diagonally through the center of one design. An *even rectangular plaid,* shown below, is even, but not identical, both lengthwise and crosswise.

An uneven plaid may mismatch in one or both directions. When plaid is *uneven lengthwise,* left, a repeat folded in half crosswise matches; folded lengthwise it does not. With plaid that is *uneven crosswise,* below, repeat forms a mirror image when folded in half lengthwise; does not when folded crosswise. Plaid that is *uneven in both directions* (not shown) does not match folded either way—lengthwise or crosswise.

Cutting plaids

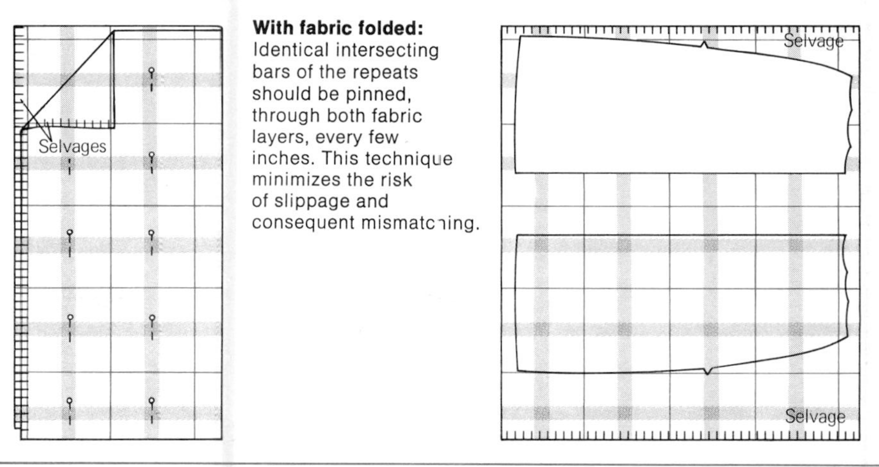

With fabric folded: Identical intersecting bars of the repeats should be pinned, through both fabric layers, every few inches. This technique minimizes the risk of slippage and consequent mismatching.

With a single layer, cutting is more accurate than with folded fabric but it takes more time. With fabric right side up, pin and cut each pattern piece once. To cut second piece, remove pattern and lay garment section right side down against remaining fabric; match bars lengthwise and crosswise; pin. For pattern piece to be cut on a fold, use method for folded plaid.

Cutting special fabrics

Diagonal weaves 61
Yardage for diagonals and unusual prints 68-69
Trial garment / large scale print 120

Diagonals

Of the woven diagonals (twill weaves), some have barely perceptible ribs, as typified by gabardines; ribs of others are bold, as in the example below. The first type is handled like any plain weave. The latter group, which also includes diagonally printed stripes, requires careful pattern selection. *Avoid* any pattern designated "not suitable for obvious diagonal fabrics," and designs with center seams, long diagonal darts, gored skirt sections, collar cut on a fold, or a V-neckline.

An exception to the above limitations can be made for an obvious diagonal fabric that is reversible. Here the wrong side of the fabric is used for half the garment; diagonals are then balanced in *chevron* or V-shaped seams. Chevrons can also be created by cutting a plaid, stripe, or other geometric on the bias. To work this way, a design must be even lengthwise (see test below).

Diagonals should be cut from a single layer—each pattern piece pinned once with printed side up, once with printed side down. *Exception* is a chevron of reversible fabric. Here all garment sections are cut with pattern pieces face up and half of the *fabric* sections reversed for the left side.

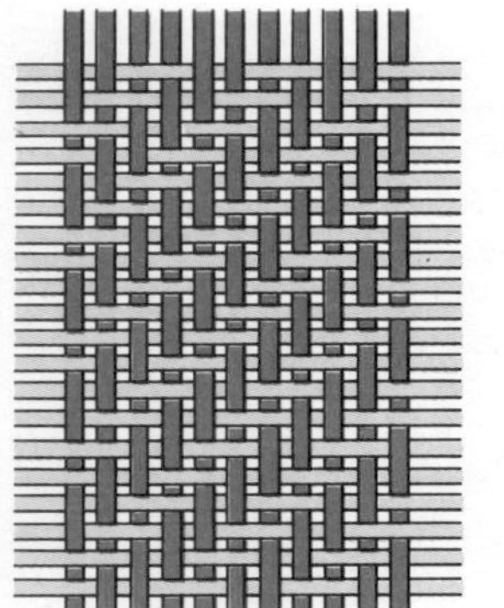

A woven diagonal may form an obvious "stripe" on the bias. Such fabric requires careful pattern selection.

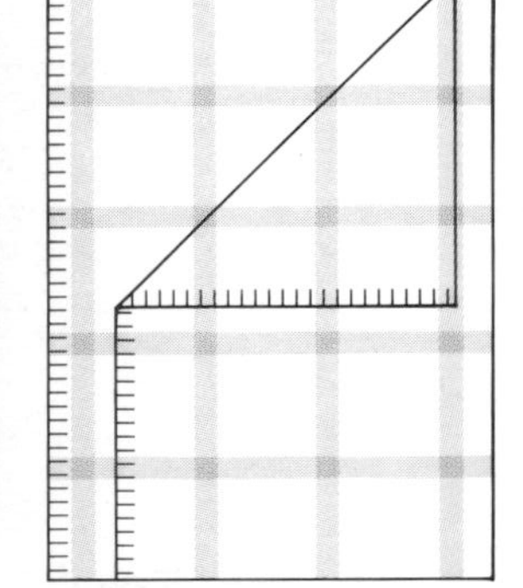

To test for chevron possibility, fold fabric lengthwise; turn a corner back diagonally through center of repeat.

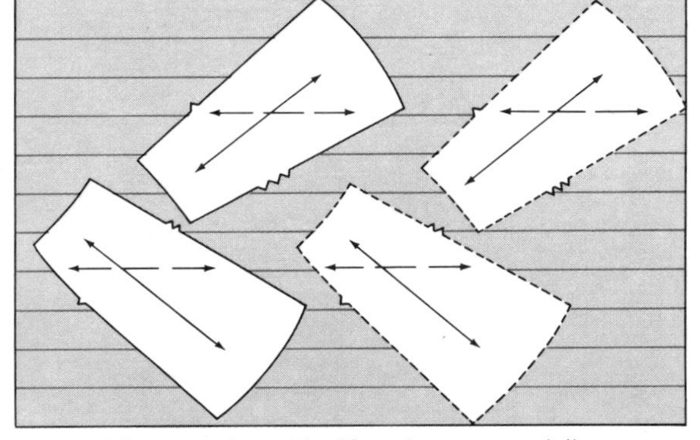

To cut stripe or plaid on the bias, draw new grainline arrows at 45° angle to original ones (unless already provided). Cut each garment section individually, following centering and matching principles on pages 90 and 91.

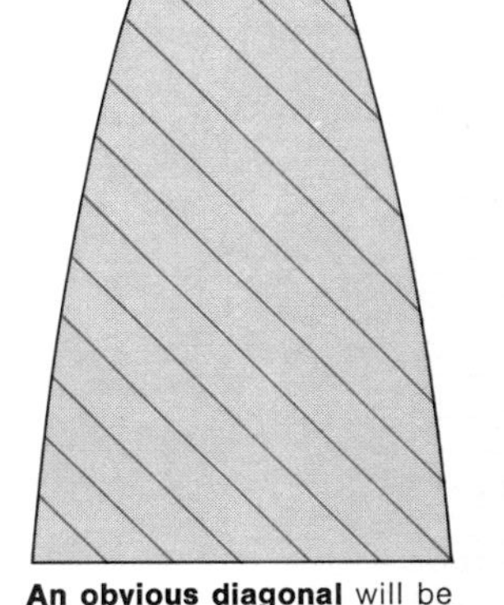

An obvious diagonal will be most successful in a pattern design that involves few seams or structural details.

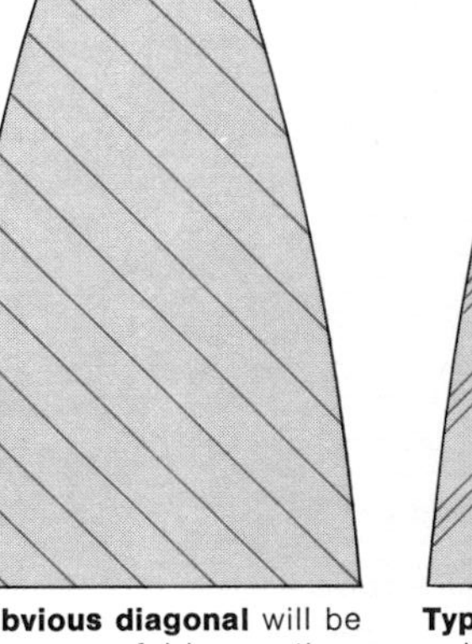

Typical chevron shape is V pointing up at center, down at sides. Chevron above is made with stripe cut on bias.

Unusual prints

Fabric with a large motif requires careful placement, and sometimes matching, of the design. A precise motif, such as a diamond, must be centered and matched just like a plaid. A random one, paisley for instance, need not be matched, but should be balanced. Whatever the design, seams and intricate details should be as few as possible. To decide placement, drape fabric over your figure before a full-length mirror and try various approaches. If the garment has center seams, motifs might be placed opposite one another an equal distance from the center. As a rule, though, the asymmetrical balance illustrated at the right is more pleasing. In any case, do not place motifs directly on the full part of bustline or buttocks. Another point to remember: a large scale print is often a one-way design, in which case pattern pieces must be laid out as for directional fabrics (see p. 90).

Border print fabric is one with a marginal design running lengthwise along one edge. It can be used in two ways. One is to run the border vertically, placing it to each side of center front and/or center back seams. The other, more usual way is to place the border at the garment hem, as shown at right. For the latter, major garment sections are cut on the crosswise grain (with new grainline arrows drawn perpendicular to the original ones). If the garment being cut this way has no waistline seam, its entire length must fit on the fabric width, leaving little or no hem allowance. One solution is to place hemline at the selvage, omitting hem altogether. Or you can leave a small allowance at the selvage for stitching on a hem facing (mandatory if there is printing on selvage). *Avoid* A-line or gored skirts for horizontal border; it cannot be matched on bias-cut seams.

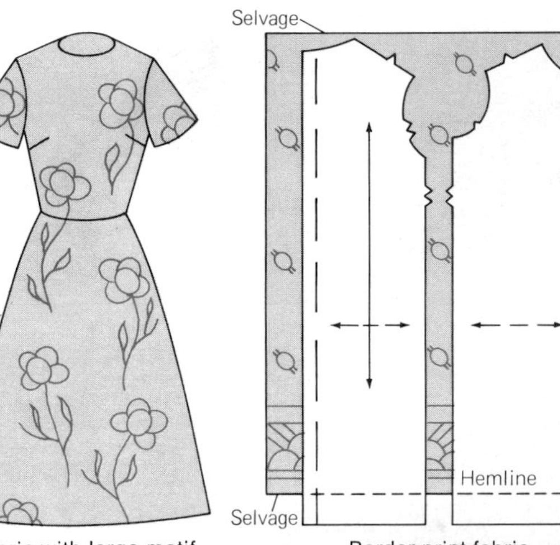

Fabric with large motif

Border print fabric

Special cutting techniques

Types of shears 9
Stitching sheer fabrics 156

Professional tips

Listed below are supplements to basic pinning and cutting techniques, ideas based on experience.

1. To keep fabric from slipping, and also protect the cutting surface, cover cutting area with felt or a folded sheet. A useful alternative is a cutting board (a sewing aid available at notion counters). Fabric can be pinned directly to it to prevent slippage.
2. For better control and more comfortable cutting, have cutting surface accessible from at least three sides. If this is impossible, separate pattern sections so that you can turn pieces around if necessary.
3. For bulky fabrics, which are often difficult to pin, or delicate fabrics that could be marred by pins, consider pin substitutes, such as upholstery weights, masking tape, or aerosol pattern holder.
4. Heavy or bulky fabric can be cut more accurately if you cut through one layer at a time.
5. When cutting from a single layer, cut each pattern piece once with printed side up, once printed side down, to obtain right and left sides for garment.
6. A very thin or slippery fabric, such as chiffon or lightweight knit, will shift less if you pin it to tissue paper (the same tissue can be used later to facilitate stitching). Such fabrics are also easier to cut with serrated scissors, which grip the fabric.
7. For fewer seams to finish, place the edge of any pattern piece that corresponds to straight grain, directly on a selvage. If selvage is tight and tends to pull, clip into it every two to three inches.
8. Use each pattern piece the correct number of times. Such items as cuffs often require more than two pieces.
9. Keep shears sharp by cutting nothing but fabric with them (paper dulls the blades).
10. Sharpen slightly dull scissors by cutting through fine sandpaper. Take very dull ones to a professional.
11. Save fabric scraps left from cutting; they are often usable for small items, such as buttonhole patches, and for testing stitches and pressing techniques.

Trial layout

Should you need to establish a layout not provided in the cutting guides, the simplest approach is to choose the one closest to your requirements and follow it closely, making changes as needed. At first, pin only foldlines or grainline arrows, so pieces can be shifted with minimal re-pinning.

If none of the layouts even approximate your needs, proceed as follows: Fold fabric with standard lengthwise fold (see p. 87). Without pinning, lay out all pattern pieces, first the major garment sections, then smaller pieces. Experiment with various pattern arrangements and, if necessary, different fabric folds, until everything fits satisfactorily; then pin all pattern pieces.

To determine a yardage requirement if none is available, there is a way to make an experimental layout prior to fabric purchase. Simply fold a bed sheet to desired fabric width and proceed as above, then measure the amount of sheeting used.

Cutting basic design changes

Some characteristic of a fabric, such as its bulk or design, may suggest a change in basic pattern style. For example, a coat of heavy fabric would have sharper edges without facing seams. Or you might want to change some pattern feature, such as the location of an opening. As a rule, seams that are added or eliminated should correspond to the fabric straight grain; if they do not, garment grainlines may be altered. Remember that a change in one section can affect the treatment of an adjoining one. For instance, a facing seam might have to be eliminated along with a bodice seam.

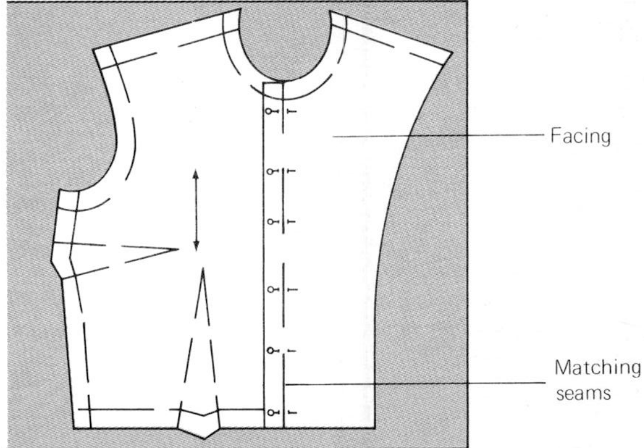

Eliminate a seam by placing pattern seamline on fabric fold. Such a change is recommended when fabric will be more attractive with fewer seams (e.g., a plaid or large print). Method is applicable only to seams that coincide with straight grain. If zipper opening is eliminated by this step, decide where to re-locate it before proceeding.

Fold
5/8" seam allowance
Pattern foldline

Create a seam by adding a ⅝" seam allowance to the pattern foldline. This technique can be used to provide a more convenient opening, or to balance an uneven plaid or obvious diagonal when fabric is reversible. The new seam must fall on the straight grain. Pattern piece need not be cut near fabric foldline, but if it is, the fold must be slit.

Facing
Matching seams

Eliminate a facing seam by pinning garment and facing patterns together with seamlines matching; both seams must coincide with straight grain. This produces an extended facing, as shown above. Especially recommended for bulky fabric. Seam that joins two facing pieces can be eliminated the same way (such seam need not be on straight grain).

Uneven basting 124
Simplified tailor's tacks 135
Tailor's tacks 136
Machine tailor's tacks 142

Marking methods

Marking—the transfer of significant pattern notations to fabric—is done after cutting and before removing pattern. The symbols selected for transfer are those that make clear *how* and *where* garment sections are shaped and joined and details are placed. Usually included are dart, tuck, gathering, and pleat lines, large dots and squares, center front and back locations, buttonhole and other detail placements. It is helpful to mark seamlines that are intricately shaped; *all* seamlines, if you are inexperienced. When garment is to be underlined, usually only the underlining is marked.

Common marking methods and their typical uses are discussed below. You must decide which is most suitable for each situation. In general, any device can be used provided it makes a precise, clear mark without disfiguring the material. *Always pretest a fabric swatch* to be sure marks show up clearly and can later be removed.

Tracing paper and wheel is a fast method that works best on plain, opaque fabrics. It is less satisfactory for multicolored fabrics, and not recommended for sheers, because marking shows through to the right side. It is preferred to other methods for its convenience, but the wheel can rip tissue, thus limiting the reusability of a pattern.

While tracing, keep cardboard under fabric to prevent marring of the surface beneath. Use serrated wheel for most fabrics, smooth wheel for those that are delicate, hard to mark, or napped. With fabric folded wrong sides together, both layers can be marked at once, using double-faced paper or two sheets back to back. With fabric right sides together, layers are marked one at a time.

Tailor's chalk is also a quick marking device. Only dots are registered, but these can be connected, if desired, after pattern is removed. For this use ruler and chalk, regular or wax type. The first tends to rub off easily; the wax type is more durable, but cannot be removed from some fabrics.

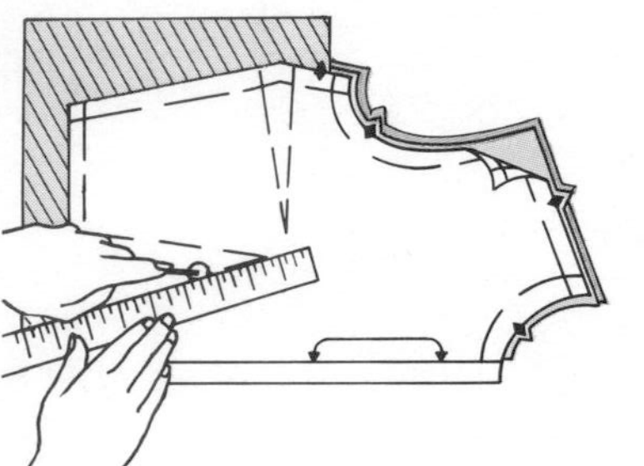

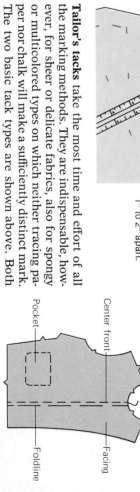

To trace marks, place waxed side of dressmaker's tracing paper against *wrong side* of fabric. (It may be necessary to move a few pins.) Trace markings with wheel, taking short, firm strokes; use ruler as guide for straight lines.

Traced marks should be precise, in a color that contrasts, but not drastically, with fabric. Use cross hatches (X's) to indicate pattern dots. Individual dots can also be recorded, using dull pencil or stick.

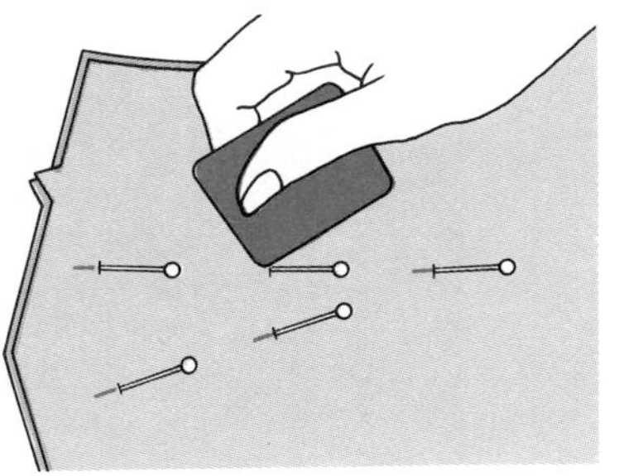

Chalk marking: First push pin through each symbol, and both fabric layers, forcing pinheads through tissue. Remove pattern. Make chalk dot at each pin, on wrong side of each fabric layer.

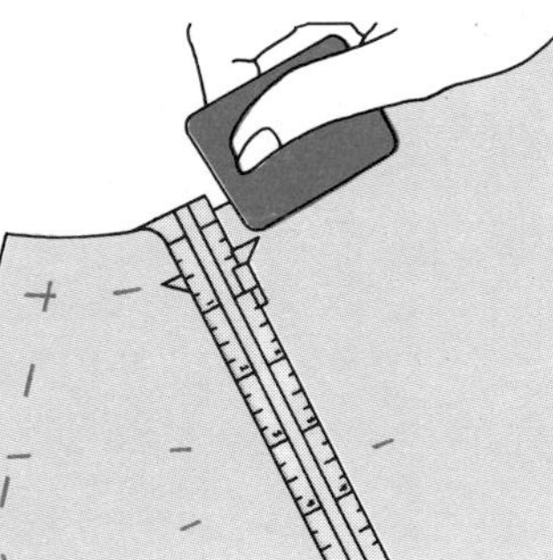

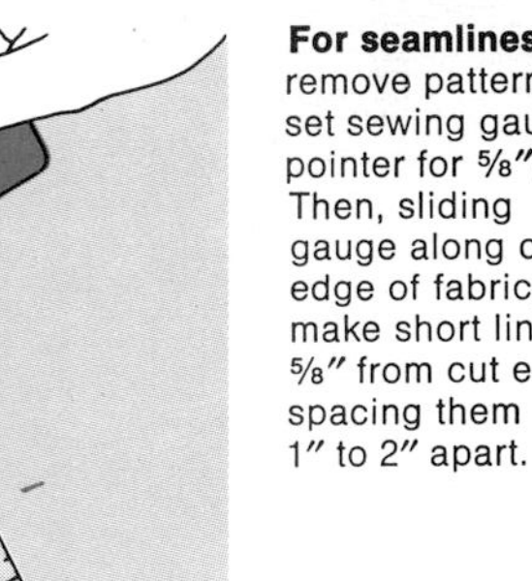

For seamlines, remove pattern; set sewing gauge pointer for ⅝″. Then, sliding gauge along cut edge of fabric, make short lines ⅝″ from cut edge, spacing them 1″ to 2″ apart.

Tailor's tacks take the most time and effort of all the marking methods. They are indispensable, however, for sheer or delicate fabrics, also for spongy or multicolored types on which neither tracing paper nor chalk will make a sufficiently distinct mark. The two basic tack types are shown above. Both are made by hand. A third version, **machine tailor's tacks,** shown and described in Machine stitch section, is particularly useful for multiple markings, such as pleat lines. If many tacks must be made on one garment, it is helpful to use a different color thread for each pattern symbol—one for darts, another for seamlines, and so on.

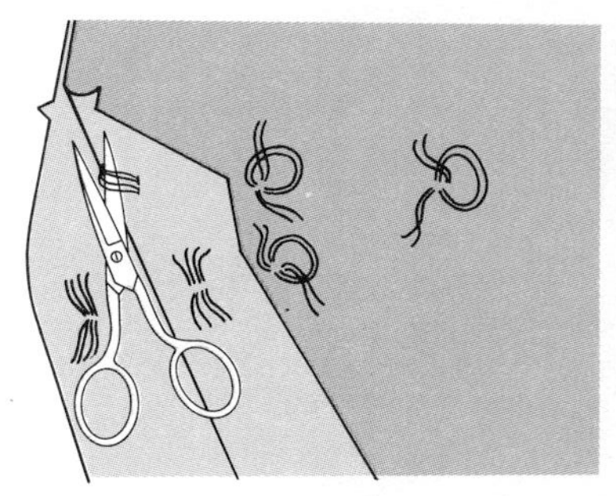

Tailor's tacks: Used to transfer individual markings to doubled fabric. When completed, tacks are cut apart between the fabric layers. (See Hand stitches for detailed instructions.)

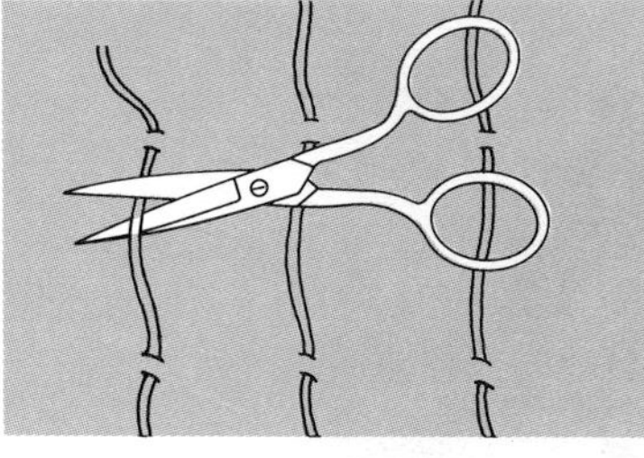

Simplified tailor's tacks: Uneven basting used to mark single fabric layer. Very useful for marking fold, center, and pleat lines. (See Hand stitches for instructions.)

Thread tracing is a practical way to transfer markings, such as pocket placement symbols, which must show on the right side. Markings are first transferred with tracing paper, then re-traced with hand or machine basting, depending on the fabric.

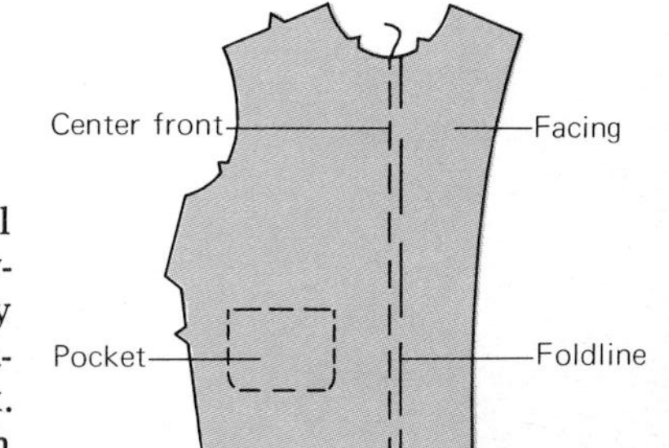

Thread tracing: With tracing paper and wheel, trace symbol onto wrong side of garment section. Remove pattern; then go over marking with uneven basting or straight-stitch machine basting. Use a contrasting thread color.

Portfolio of Fitting Methods

Fitting

Fitting techniques

Standard figure types 46-47

A look at fitting methods

Made as they are for millions of people, patterns naturally have their fit limitations. Chances are a pattern will fit you well in some places and less well in others. The trick in making fashions that fit is learning where you and the pattern part company. Once you learn what the differences are, the pattern alterations are, in fact, simple.

To help you know what type of alterations you need and the complexity you can expect with each, we have grouped the alterations into two types.

The first group is **basic pattern alterations.** These are the alterations that are concerned primarily with bringing the paper pattern measurements closer to your own. To make them, you work with some of your own body measurements plus the measurements printed on the back of the pattern envelope, and in some cases, actual measurements of the printed pattern. This group of alterations includes basic length and width changes as well as positioning of darts.

Advanced pattern alterations, the second group, are made with the aid of a *fitting shell.* A fitting shell is made from a basic pattern, in an inexpensive test fabric, such as muslin, for the express purpose of checking the specifics of fit: location of grainlines, darts, and seams; drape of the garment; sleeve fit, etc. Completed shell adjustments are recorded on a *master pattern,* which is used with each new pattern, making it easy to locate areas requiring alteration.

Preliminary pattern alterations are not the only means to a good fit, however. There are other helpful tests and adjustment methods to use as you sew. The **try-on session,** midway through construction, is a useful technique for making simple adjustments before you have finished sewing (pp. 118–119). A **test garment** can make a very practical contribution, and we explain how to use such a trial run to best advantage (p. 120).

As you gain experience with fitting, you will find that it becomes second nature. You will also learn which steps, if any, you wish to take for individual garments—some garments are worth the trouble, some may not be. Be selective in this decision, though. Even if it is not a "special" garment, it may not really be wise to skip fitting steps on something you will wear constantly.

Getting to know your figure

If your pattern selection meant compromising on a measurement or two, as it usually does, you will alter the pattern accordingly. Before you think about pattern alterations, however, consider how well you know your figure. You should know it well enough to analyze its relation to a standard pattern figure. To help you, we show below the ways people and patterns can differ: in proportion, in contours, in posture, and in symmetry.

If you haven't already done so, now is the time to make an honest appraisal of your figure. The better you know your own body, the easier it will be to achieve the desired fit. It can be difficult to be honest about our own shortcomings. It is sometimes easier to see what is right than what is wrong. Then too, many women think of their figure as a fixed thing, forgetting that the process of maturing tends to change the human form.

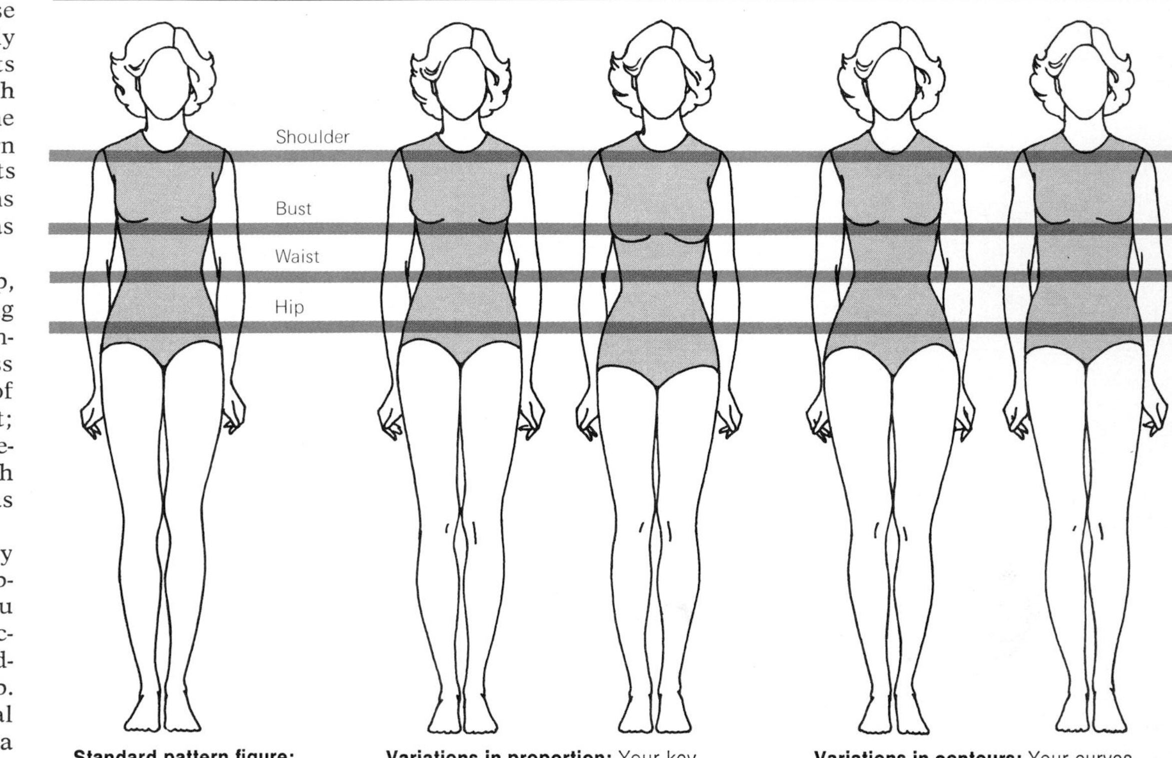

Standard pattern figure: The figure for which any pattern is sized is an imaginary one. It has perfect posture, symmetrical features, and unvarying proportions and contours. Your own figure is almost sure to differ in some way from this ideal standard.

Variations in proportion: Your key features—bust, waist, hips—may fall higher or lower along your height than those of the pattern's standard. Hem lengths are also a question of personal proportions, whatever the current fashion. Altering a pattern to suit your proportions is a simple process of taking measurements and adjusting lengths and widths.

Variations in contours: Your curves, bulges, and hollows may not only differ from the pattern's standard, but also change with time. Weight gained or lost, physical maturing, and foundation garments (or their absence) all affect contours. Fitting a pattern to your personal contours may call for adjusting the darts and curved seams that shape a garment to the figure.

There are several ways to do an objective job of self-appraisal. A good start is taking accurate, if unflattering, figure measurements. They can provide the basis for comparison with patterns, as recommended on page 101. The fitting shell also points out areas in need of attention (see page 111). Another way to recognize potential fitting problems is to trade a fit analysis with a friend, or make it a mother/daughter project.

If you are working alone, try to "depersonalize" the figure checking process. One way to cultivate detachment: blot out your face in your mind's eye as you study your reflection in the mirror. This focuses your attention on the details of the fit, rather than on the overall impression, and seems to make honesty easier to achieve. Another approach: study photographs of yourself wearing home-sewed garments, covering the face as you do.

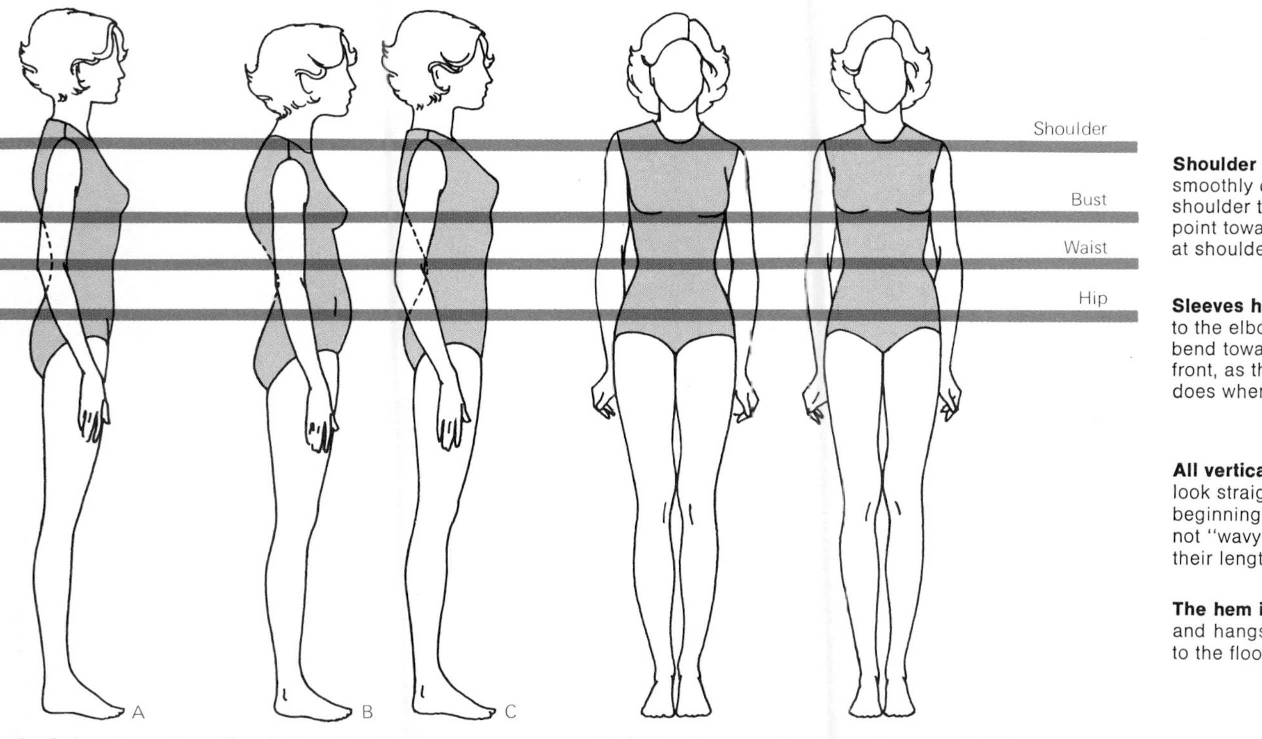

Variations in posture: Standard posture is shown in A; B and C are two common variations that cause fitting problems. Test your posture by standing against a wall. If shoulders, shoulder blades, and hips touch, your posture is standard (A). When just the shoulder blades touch (B), there's a tendency to slump and be round-shouldered. When just the shoulders touch (C), the posture is super-erect and square-shouldered. Pattern alterations at shoulder seams, bodice back, and abdomen are usually needed with the B or C postures.

Variations in symmetry: Almost everyone's left side is different from her right. When a figure is noticeably asymmetrical, garments hang differently, or wrinkle more, on one side than the other. Of the uneven figure features that lead to fitting problems, these are the most common: one shoulder is higher or slopes more than the other; one hip is higher than the other; one side of the waist curves more than the other. In order to achieve a good fit, seams and darts in the affected areas may have to be adjusted.

What is good fit?

The goal of any pattern alteration is to make the pattern fit better, but before you alter, you must decide what you *mean* by good fit. In making this judgment, there are four main factors to consider: **appearance, comfort, design,** and **fabric.**

For a good **appearance,** all darts and seams must fall in the proper places, as shown below. Overall, your garment should have a smooth look—no pulls or wrinkles, no sagging or baggy areas.

Shoulder seams rest smoothly on the shoulder tops, point toward and end at shoulder joint.

Sleeves hang straight to the elbow, then bend toward the front, as the arm does when relaxed.

All vertical seams look straight from beginning to end, are not "wavy" along their length.

The hem is even and hangs parallel to the floor.

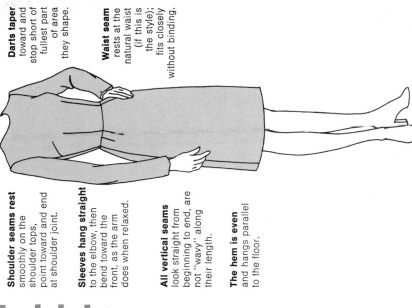

Darts taper toward and stop short of fullest part of area they shape.

Waist seam rests at the natural waist (if this is the style); fits closely without binding.

Fitting techniques

Design considerations in fashion sewing 50-53

What is good fit?

Because it depends on so many variables—the individual figure, the designer's intent, the probable wearing situations—good fit is hard to define. It is possible, however, to describe and evaluate some of the factors involved in good fit so that you can decide for yourself what kind of fit you want in the garments you sew. As explained on page 97, **appearance** is one of the important considerations; others are **comfort, design,** and **fabric.**

Comfort, of course, is of primary importance. The most attractive garment in your closet will hang there forever unless it feels good when you wear it. Of course, some garments, by definition, are more comfortable than others; but you should be able to sit, bend, walk, and reach in any garment without straining its seams or feeling restricted. The main contributor to comfort is *wearing ease,* which is explained fully on page 101.

The **design** of a garment may be based on either a close fit, as illustrated below, or a loose fit, as shown on the opposite page. It is important to keep in mind the look the designer was aiming for when you fit individual garments. The photographs and illustrations in the pattern catalog and on the envelope of your pattern selection can be valuable guides in this respect. In addition, certain features of a garment are clues to a *close* fit: a sil-

CLOSE-FITTING DESIGNS tend to stay fairly near the figure, sometimes hugging it more in certain areas. With styles of this sort, it is important not to overfit; this can result in strained seams and wrinkles. How close is too close depends somewhat on your figure. A trim fit usually flatters a slender figure, a looser fit is kinder to a figure that is fuller.

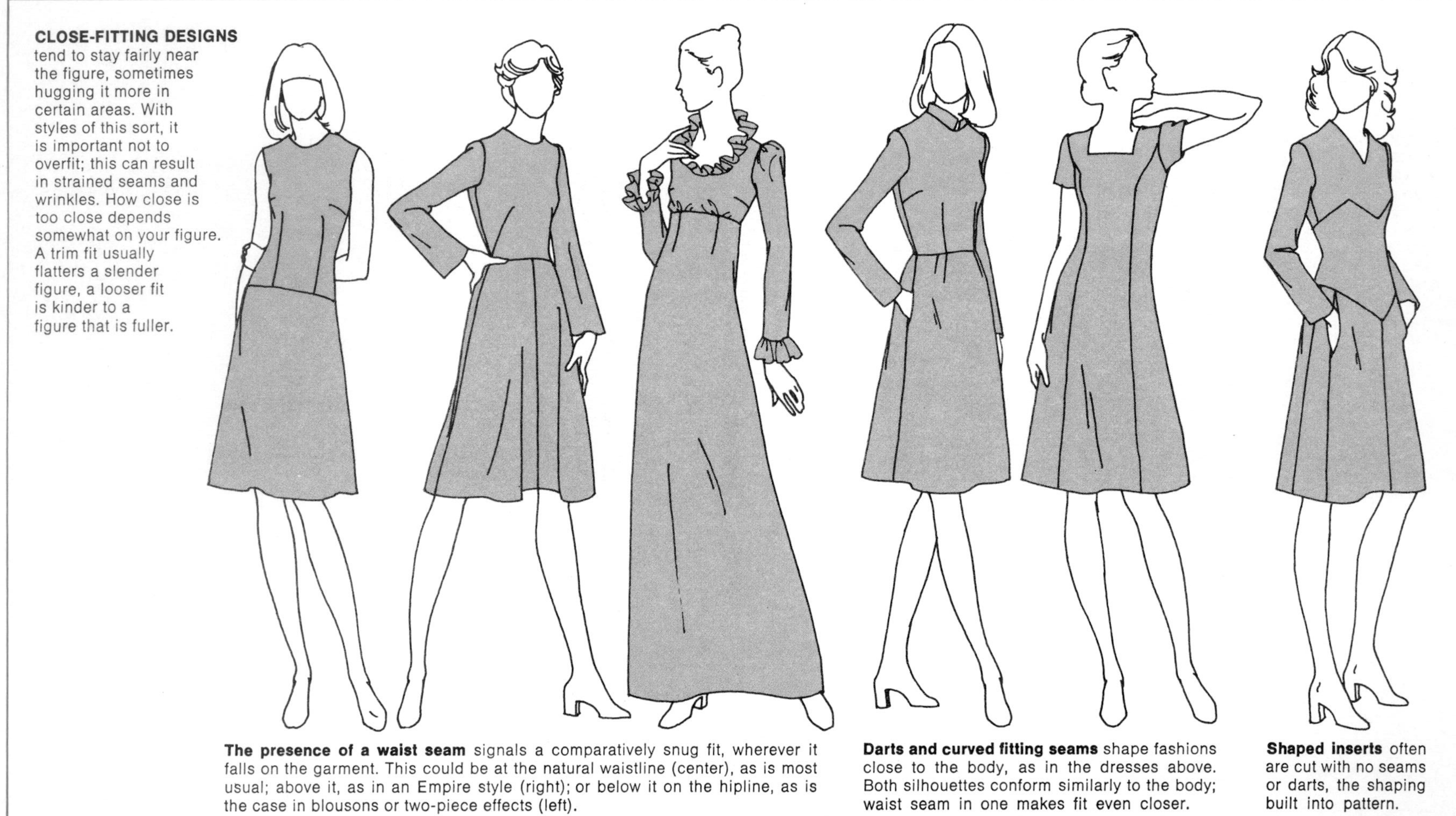

The presence of a waist seam signals a comparatively snug fit, wherever it falls on the garment. This could be at the natural waistline (center), as is most usual; above it, as in an Empire style (right); or below it on the hipline, as is the case in blousons or two-piece effects (left).

Darts and curved fitting seams shape fashions close to the body, as in the dresses above. Both silhouettes conform similarly to the body; waist seam in one makes fit even closer.

Shaped inserts often are cut with no seams or darts, the shaping built into pattern.

houette that defines the form and, within it, such details as a waist seam; darts and curved seams; shaped inserts; sometimes bias-cut sections. A *loose* fit is often signaled by such design devices as a silhouette that camouflages the details of the figure beneath; within the silhouette, fullness controlled softly by gathers, shirring, release tucks, or unpressed pleats rather than by darts and fitted seams. Bear in mind that some parts of a garment may be close-fitting and other parts soft and loose. The classic shirtdress, made with a gathered or pleated skirt, is an example. Even on loose-fitting garments, some parts of the garment may be fitted to the body, as is the waistband on a full, gathered skirt, or the shoulder seam on a smock.

Fabric is crucial to good fit—recommendations on the pattern envelope are to be taken seriously. Styles for "stretch knits only" are relying on some "give" in the fabric. Those calling for thick fabrics are usually designed a bit larger to accommodate the bulk; the same style in a thinner fabric would probably be too big. When fabric types are interchangeable—soft or crisp, for example—remember that the style will look very different according to which you use. Also, be aware of the "clinging" tendency of some fabrics; these define body shape even if a garment is loose-fitting.

LOOSE-FITTING GARMENTS may be designed to have a sweep of fullness, as are the cape, caftan, and tent dress; or with softening influences—blouson top, billowing sleeve, dirndl skirt, shirred yoke. To fit a smaller figure, some fullness can be altered out so the design won't collapse. Larger figures might need to add to all but the fullest designs to achieve the intended draping.

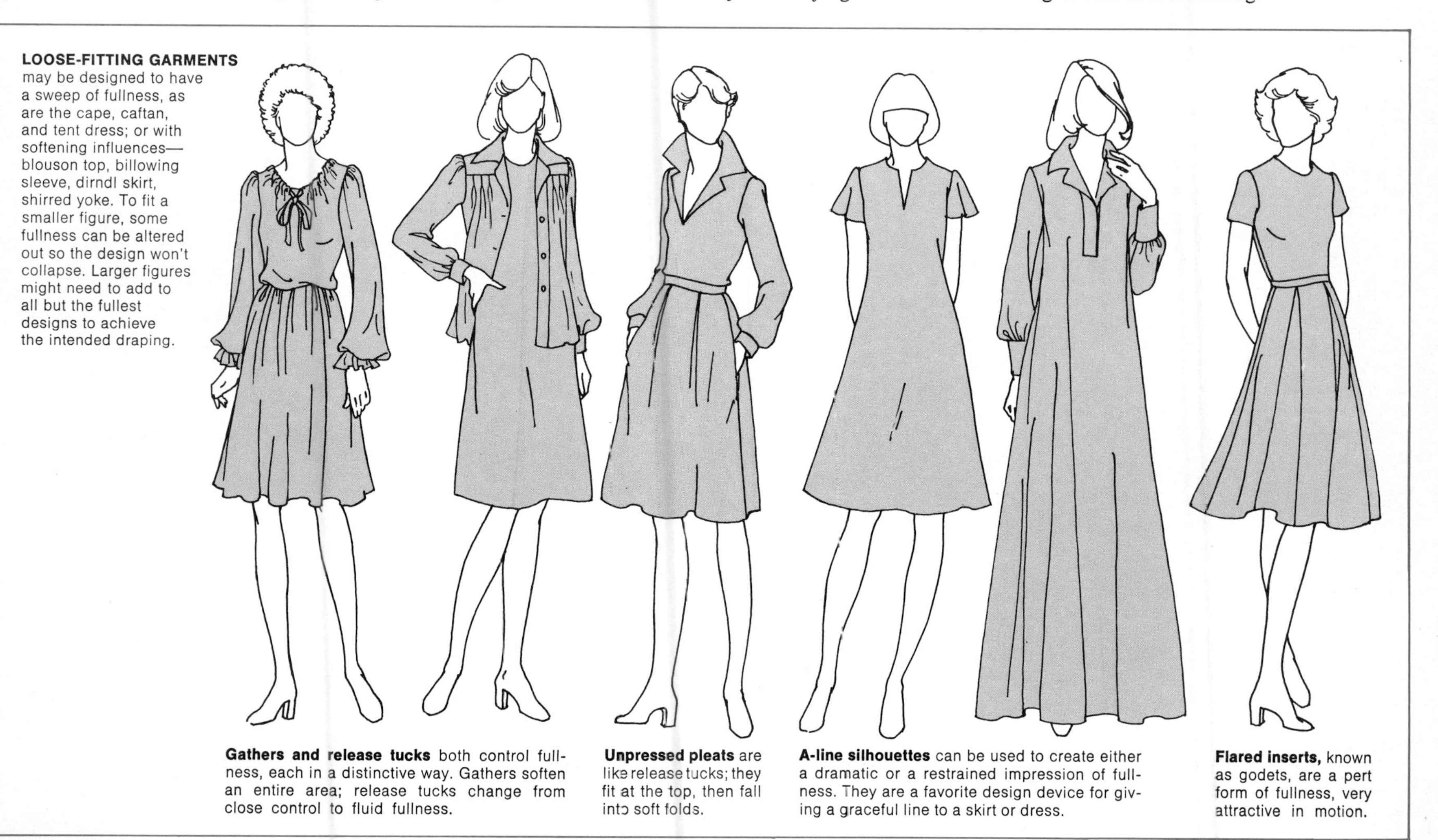

Gathers and release tucks both control fullness, each in a distinctive way. Gathers soften an entire area; release tucks change from close control to fluid fullness.

Unpressed pleats are like release tucks; they fit at the top, then fall into soft folds.

A-line silhouettes can be used to create either a dramatic or a restrained impression of fullness. They are a favorite design device for giving a graceful line to a skirt or dress.

Flared inserts, known as godets, are a pert form of fullness, very attractive in motion.

Measurements in pattern size selection 48-49

Basic pattern alterations

Most of the corrections needed to bring patterns closer to individual body measurements can be done right on the pattern. What follows is an easy three-step method for making these basic alterations. If you need further alterations, use this method as the starting point for later construction of a fitting shell (see p.110).

The first step is **taking key figure measurements.** Some of these are additional to the measurements taken to determine pattern size. For this procedure you will need a tape measure, some string to mark the waist, and a friend to help. The second step is **comparing your measurements with the pattern's** to find the places that need alteration. The final step is **making the alterations.** Those covered on pages 102 to 110 are the most frequent, involving changes in length and width.

This method assumes selection of blouse and dress patterns according to bust measurement, a basis that works well for most women. When it does, bust alterations will usually be simply a matter of re-positioning darts. If, however, the bust is disproportionately large in comparison with the other standard body measurements, or if bra cup size is a "C" or larger, you may find it easier to stay with the pattern size that accords with your other measurements and enlarge the bust area (see p. 105). The bodice should fit satisfactorily in the back and chest/shoulder area. The high bust measurement (pp. 48–49) is often a clue to situations where this choice is appropriate. Pants patterns should be selected by hip measurement and the waistline and length altered if necessary.

One thing to keep in mind when doing pattern alterations is the need to keep the design lines intact. For example, if you measure less than the pattern and have to alter, don't take away too much or the style could be lost. It is generally better to allow yourself too much fabric than too little, because it is easier to take in than it is to add on. You can also lose style lines by adding too much, particularly if a garment is intricately seamed. If you discover that you need a great many pattern alterations, it would seem sensible to question the accuracy of the size you have chosen. Perhaps another size, or a comparable size in another figure type, will fit with fewer alterations.

One: Taking key measurements

Careful and honest measuring is essential. For the most reliable results, stand naturally and wear your customary type of undergarments. If you recently took some of the measurements described below in the course of selecting your pattern size, note them again (no need to re-measure). You may want to record your measurements for future reference. If you do, don't forget to check them every six months or so, or if you gain or lose weight, to see if there have been any significant changes.

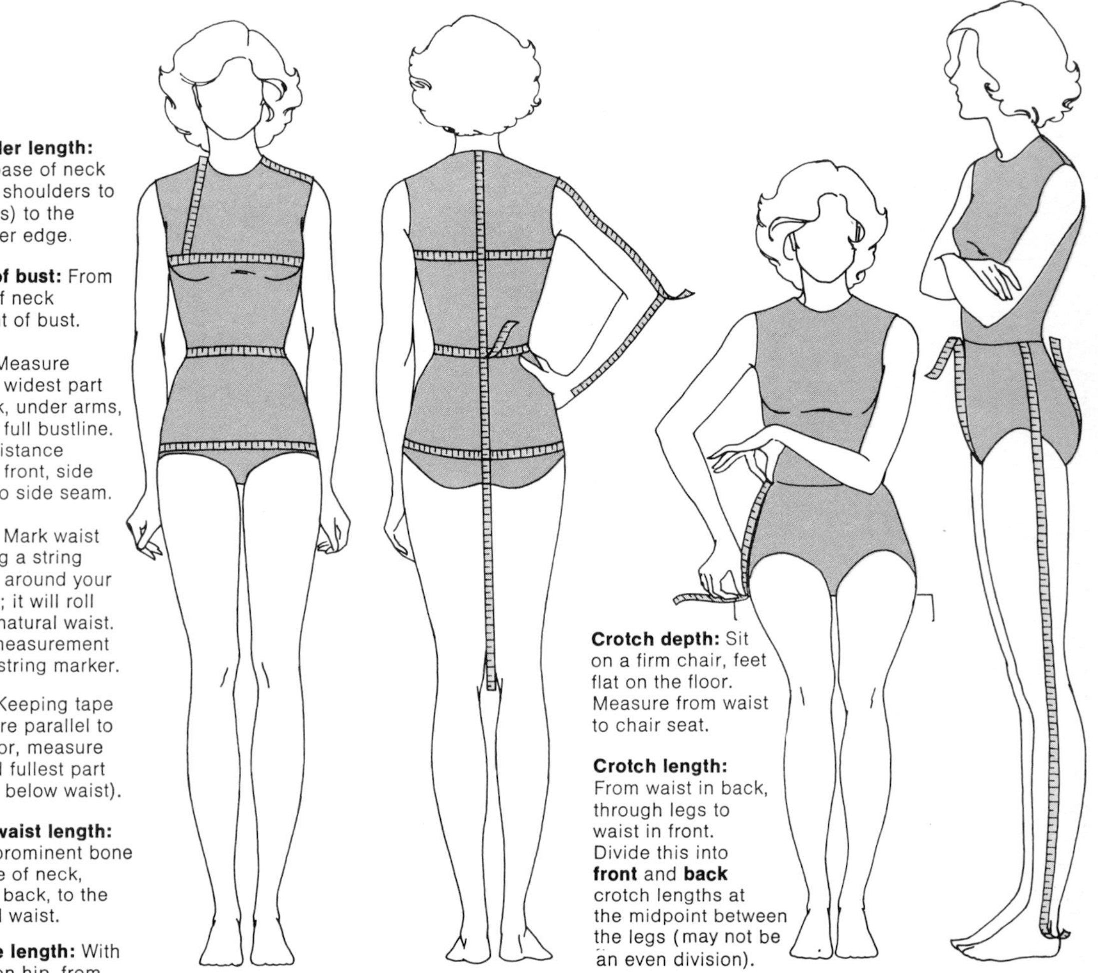

Shoulder length: From base of neck (shrug shoulders to find this) to the shoulder edge.

Apex of bust: From base of neck to point of bust.

Bust: Measure across widest part of back, under arms, across full bustline. Note distance across front, side seam to side seam.

Waist: Mark waist by tying a string snugly around your middle; it will roll to the natural waist. Take measurement at the string marker.

Hips: Keeping tape measure parallel to the floor, measure around fullest part (7″–9″ below waist).

Back waist length: From prominent bone at base of neck, center back, to the natural waist.

Sleeve length: With hand on hip, from the shoulder joint to the wrist bone. For **elbow dart placement,** note length from shoulder to elbow.

Finished length: For *dresses*, measure from base of neck at center back to the hem. For *skirts*, subtract back waist length from finished dress length. For *blouses*, use back waist length plus a tuck-in allowance.

Crotch depth: Sit on a firm chair, feet flat on the floor. Measure from waist to chair seat.

Crotch length: From waist in back, through legs to waist in front. Divide this into **front** and **back** crotch lengths at the midpoint between the legs (may not be an even division).

Finished length (pants): Measure from waist to hem, at the side of the leg. May be more or less than pattern, depending on curve of hips.

Two: Comparing measurements

To decide when and where you need pattern alterations, you must compare your personal figure measurements with the corresponding measurements on the pattern. In some cases you will measure the pattern itself; in others, the relevant measurements will appear on the pattern envelope. Take into consideration what you learned in your figure analysis (pp. 96–97). This, combined with your measurements and an idea of the kind of fit you wish to achieve, will show you where to alter.

Remember that your measurements are not supposed to exactly match those of the paper pattern. No garment can or should fit as closely as the tape measure, for you need enough room in any garment to sit, walk, reach, and bend. The chart below gives the *least* amounts a pattern should measure over and above your figure in six crucial places. This extra amount is called **wearing ease**, which should be distinguished from design ease. Design ease is the designed-in fullness that will cause some styles to measure considerably larger, overall or in particular areas, than your figure plus the applicable minimums given in the chart. You cannot know how much design ease has been included in a pattern, but you will be sure of keeping it, and therefore of retaining the style lines of the garment, if you take care to include wearing ease in your alterations. There are exceptions to the wearing ease estimates below: a pattern designed for stretchy knit will provide less wearing ease; strapless garments will also be given less; larger figures may need more than the suggested minimum for a truly comfortable fit. Fill in your own measurements on the chart and use them when altering the paper pattern. When comparing your measurements with those on the back of the pattern envelope, make no allowance for wearing ease.

MEASUREMENT	YOURS	PLUS EASE: AT LEAST	TOTAL	PATTERN MEASURE	CHANGE + −
Bust		3″			
Waist		3/4″			
Hip		2″			
Crotch depth		1/2″			
Front crotch length		1/2″			
Back crotch length		1″			

Compare **bust, waist, hip,** and **back waist length** measurements given on the pattern envelope with your own (without any allowance for wearing ease).

Measure the pattern's **shoulder seam** and compare it with your **shoulder length.** The two should match closely. For a dropped shoulder seam or yoke, measure pattern at shoulder markings. If the neckline sets below the neck base, the pattern will specify by how much; add this amount to the shoulder seam before making the length comparison.

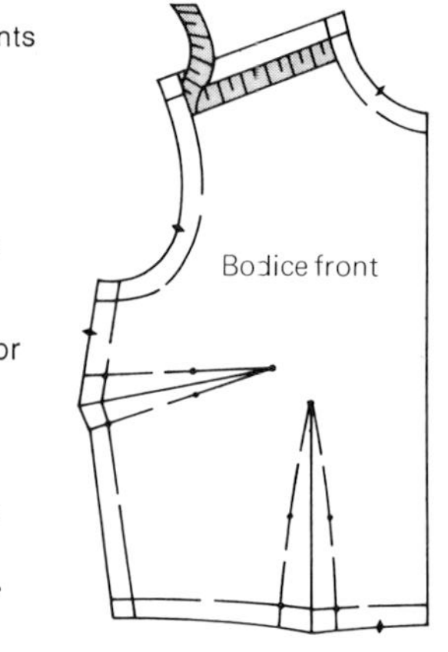

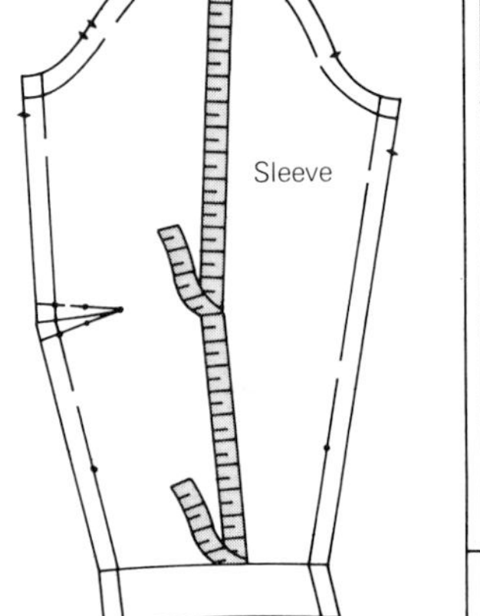

To check **bust dart placement,** measure pattern from neck seam (where it meets shoulder seam) toward the dart point to determine where pattern locates apex of bust. Then, using your body measurement, compare actual apex of bust to location on pattern. Bust darts should point toward the apex of your bust but end an inch from it. If the neckline sets below the neck base, the pattern will tell you by how much; add this amount when measuring.

To compare **sleeve lengths,** measure the pattern down the center. (On fitted sleeves, this will not be a straight line.) For **elbow dart placement,** note how far from the shoulder the darts occur. This will tell you whether to alter sleeve length above or below darts, or both. The elbow dart points to the elbow when it is bent. If there are two, the elbow goes between; if three, the center one points to the elbow. If there is a cuff, allow for its finished width when comparing. Extra length must be allowed, too, for a very full sleeve.

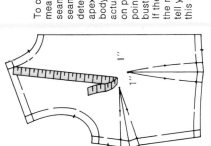

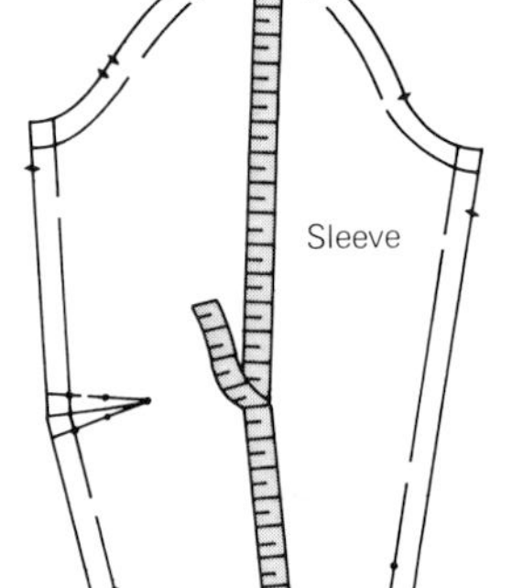

If the garment's **finished length** is given on the pattern envelope, use it for comparison with the length you need or want. If it is not given, measure all patterns except pants patterns at center back, pants pattern along side seam, to determine pattern's finished length.

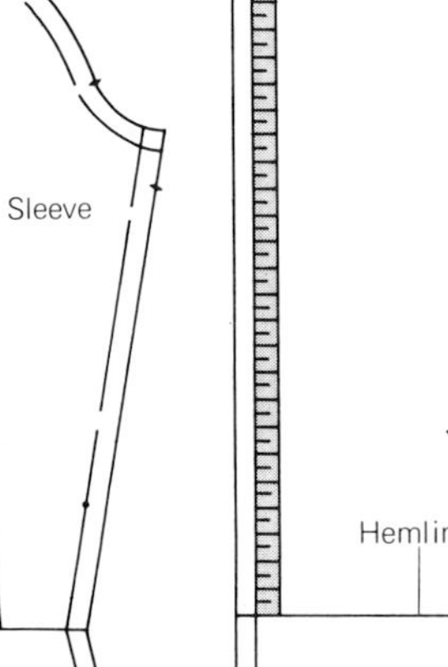

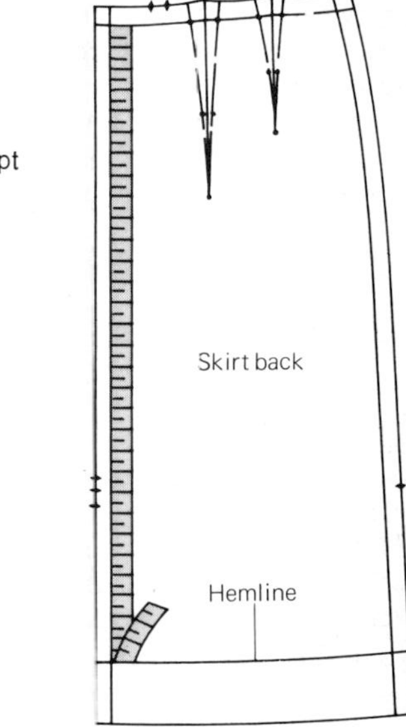

To find **crotch depth** of a pants pattern, draw a line (if there is none on pattern) at right angles to the grain from the side seam to the crotch point at the inseam. Do this on front and back pattern pieces. Measure from the waist seam to this line, along the side seam, for pattern crotch depth.
For **front and back crotch lengths,** measure the crotch seam on the pattern and compare result with your measurements. (The pattern should be longer for a comfortable fit.)
Stand the tape measure on edge to measure accurately around curves of pattern.

Basic pattern alterations

Three: Making the alterations

When you have compared your figure measurements to those of the pattern, as described on the preceding page, and decided where and how much you will need to alter, you are ready to make the basic pattern alterations. The steps for specific individual alterations are described in detail on the following pages. To insure accuracy in any of these alterations, follow these basic principles whenever you work with pattern pieces.

1. Press the paper pattern pieces with a warm, dry iron to remove wrinkles before making any alterations on the pattern.

2. All pattern pieces must be flat when any alteration is completed. Sometimes a pattern piece must be cut and spread; this can cause bubbles. The bubbles must be pressed flat before the pattern is laid onto the fabric for cutting.

3. Pin the alterations in first, check them with a tape measure or ruler for accuracy, then tape the change in place.

4. If it is necessary to add length or width, use tissue paper to accomplish the increase.

5. Take any necessary tucks **half** the depth of the required change. Remember that the total amount that is removed by a tuck will always be twice the depth of that tuck.

6. When an alteration interrupts a cutting or stitching line, draw a new line on the pattern that is tapered gradually and smoothly into the original line. This will keep your alteration from being obvious in the finished garment.

When several alterations will have to be made, the *length* alterations should always come first. This is the only way to make certain that any width alterations you may later make will be at the correct place on the pattern. Length alterations should be attended to in the following order: above the waist, below the waist or overall length, then the sleeve. Your next area of attention should be *dart placement*. When you are satisfied that your darts are pointing in the proper direction and are the correct length, you are ready to move on to any *width* adjustments that are needed. Width adjustments should be made first at the bust, then at the waist, then at the hip. Other specialized alterations take place after all basic length and width changes have been made.

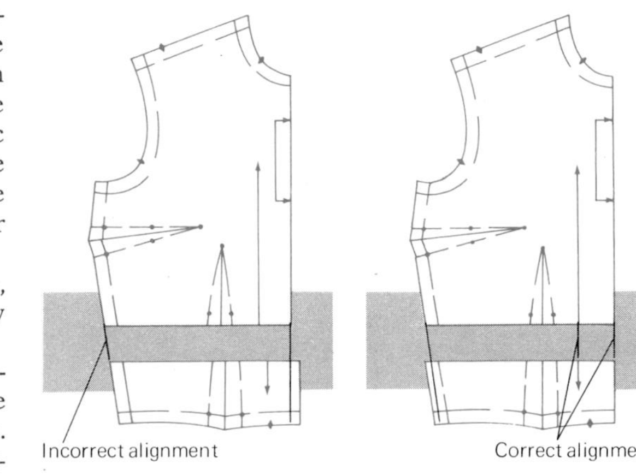

Grainlines and "place on the fold" lines must be straight when any alteration is completed. Note grainline indication on original pattern piece and take care to preserve it on the altered piece. To re-draw a "place on the fold" line, align a ruler with the intersection of seamline and foldline at top and bottom of pattern piece; draw a new line.

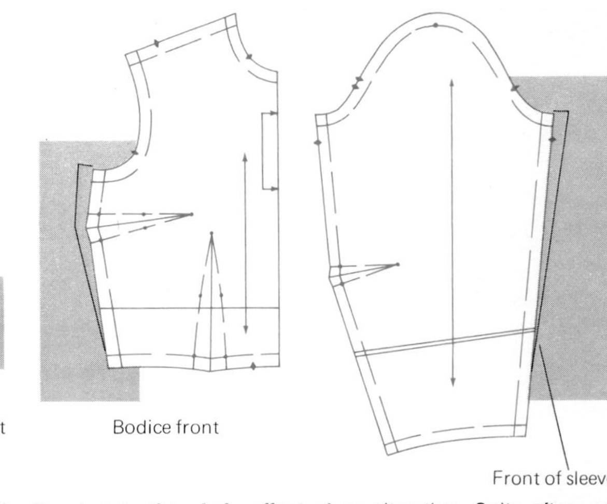

Be alert to the chain effect of an alteration. Quite often, an alteration in one pattern piece calls for a corresponding alteration elsewhere, or for a matching alteration on pieces that join the changed one, so seams will match. This is particularly important at the armhole. If you add to the side seam of a bodice, be aware of the effect on the sleeve seam.

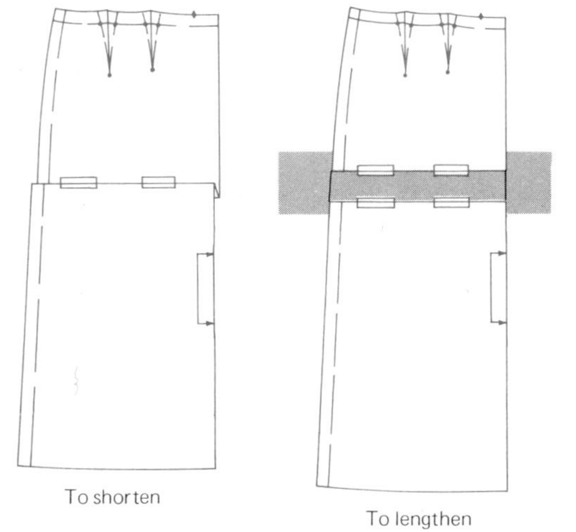

For length alterations, use the printed line labeled "lengthen or shorten here" for any length alterations required in the body of the garment. Skirt or pants can be altered at both the alteration line and the lower edge if a large amount is being added or removed. Apportioning the alteration in this way retains the garment shape.

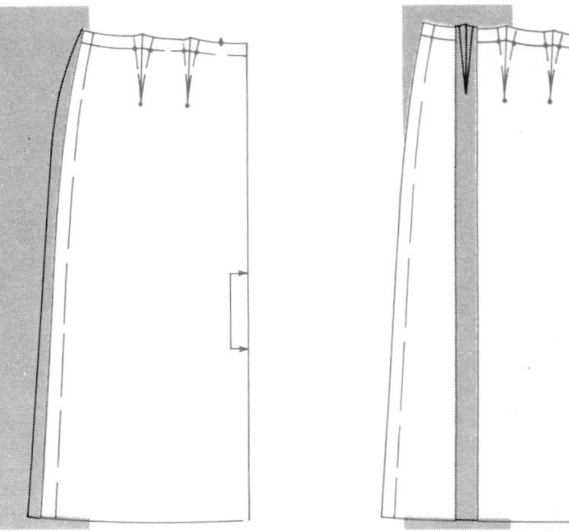

For width alterations, remember that you can usually add or subtract up to 2″ at seams. Divide the required change by the number of seams and add or subtract the resulting figure at each seam. If more than 2″ is to be altered, a technique known as "cutting and spreading" puts the enlargement or reduction exactly where it is needed.

Length alterations (increasing)

DRESSES AND SKIRTS

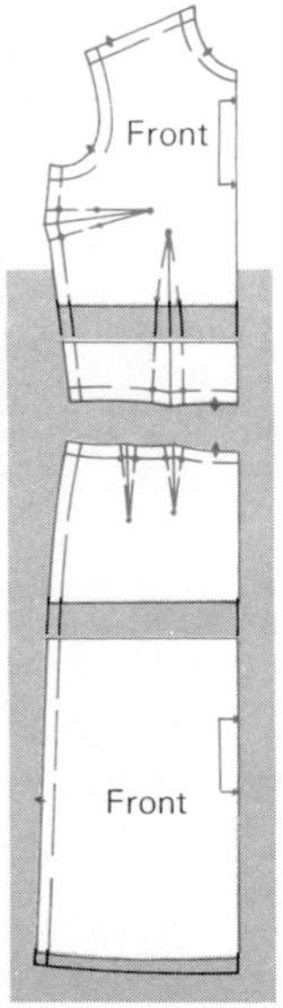

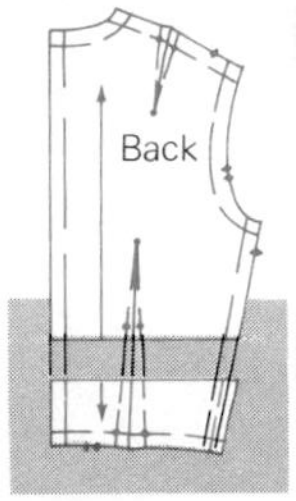

Front
Back
Front

Fitted: When altering back waist length, alter bodice front to match. To keep skirt shape, cut and spread at alteration line. More length may be added at lower edge if needed.

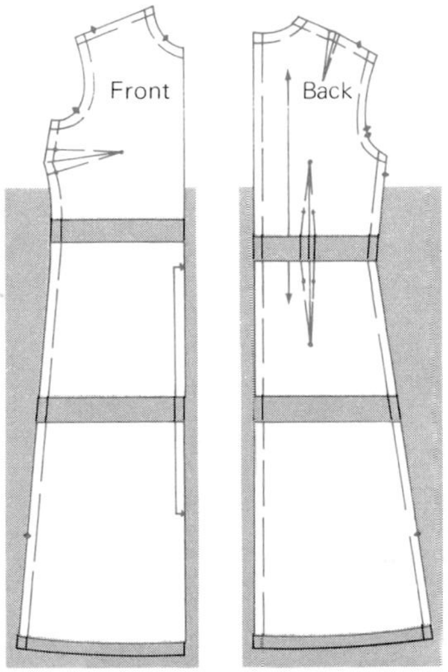

Front
Back

A-line: Add length above waist mark at center back to alter the waist length; below the waist mark to alter the finished length. Make the same alterations front and back.

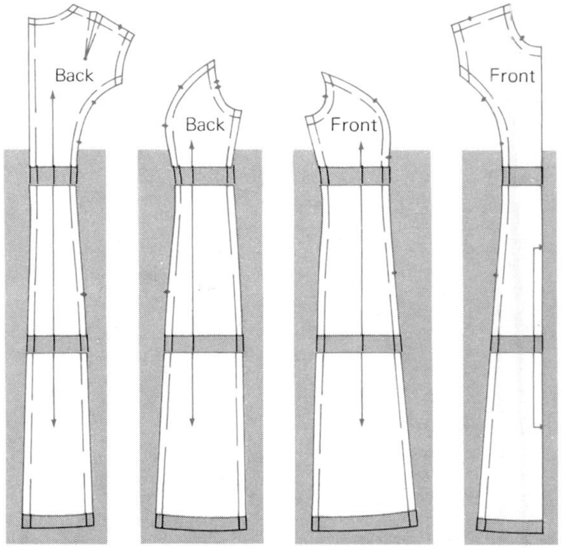

Back
Back
Front
Front

Princess: Add length above the waist mark at center back to alter the back waist length; below the waist to alter the finished length. Alter all the panels to match. If no additional length is needed at center front, taper to nothing from side seams to center front.

SLEEVES

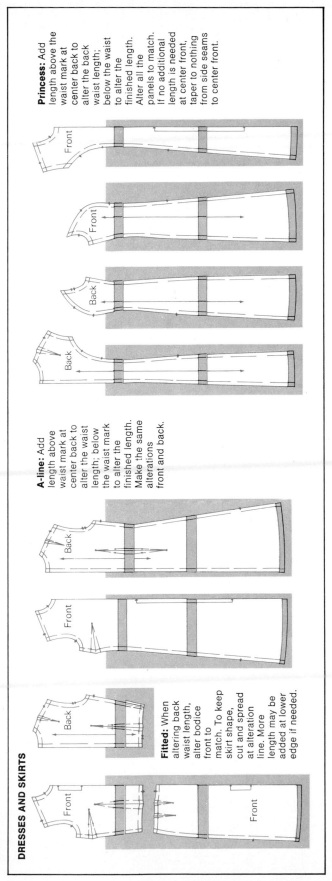

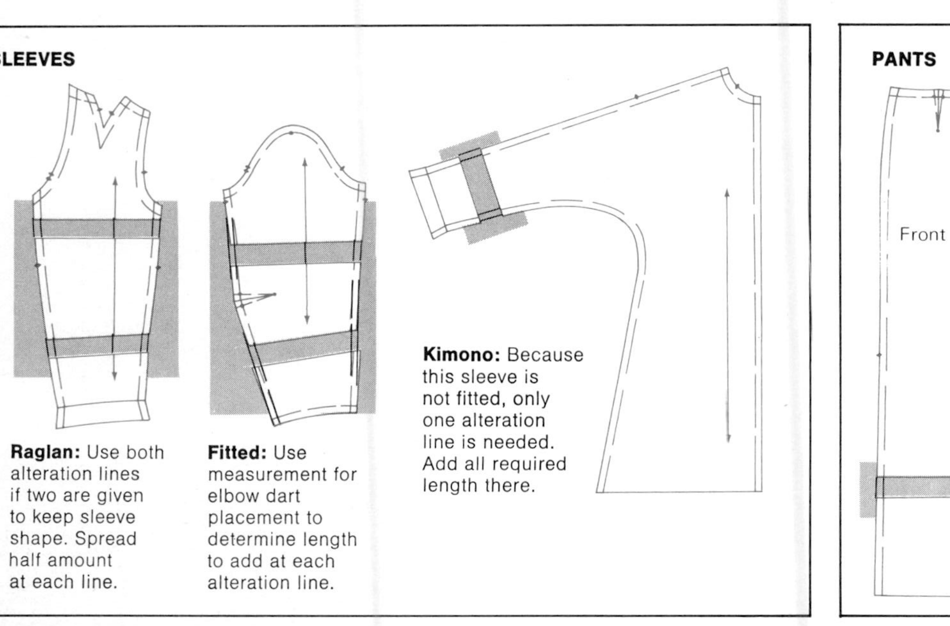

Raglan: Use both alteration lines if two are given to keep sleeve shape. Spread half amount at each line.

Fitted: Use measurement for elbow dart placement to determine length to add at each alteration line.

Kimono: Because this sleeve is not fitted, only one alteration line is needed. Add all required length there.

PANTS

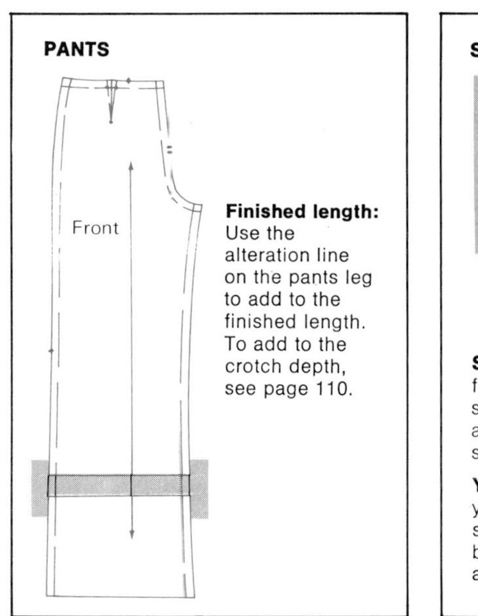

Finished length: Use the alteration line on the pants leg to add to the finished length. To add to the crotch depth, see page 110.

SHOULDER

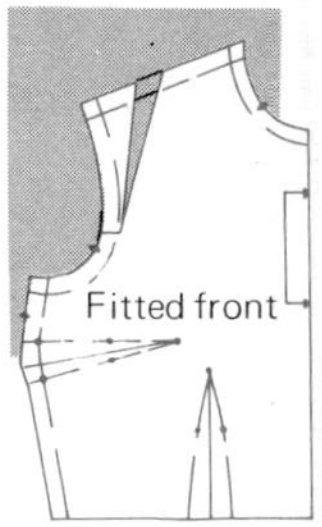

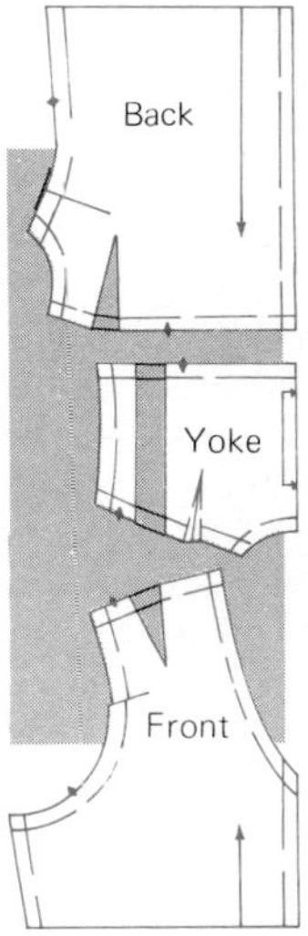

Fitted front
Back
Yoke
Front

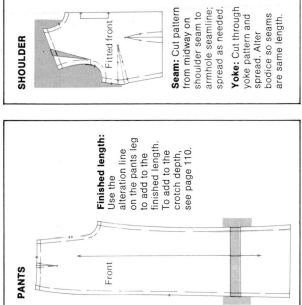

Seam: Cut pattern from midway on shoulder seam to armhole seamline; spread as needed.

Yoke: Cut through yoke pattern and spread. Alter bodice so seams are same length.

Basic pattern alterations

Length alterations (decreasing)

DRESSES AND SKIRTS

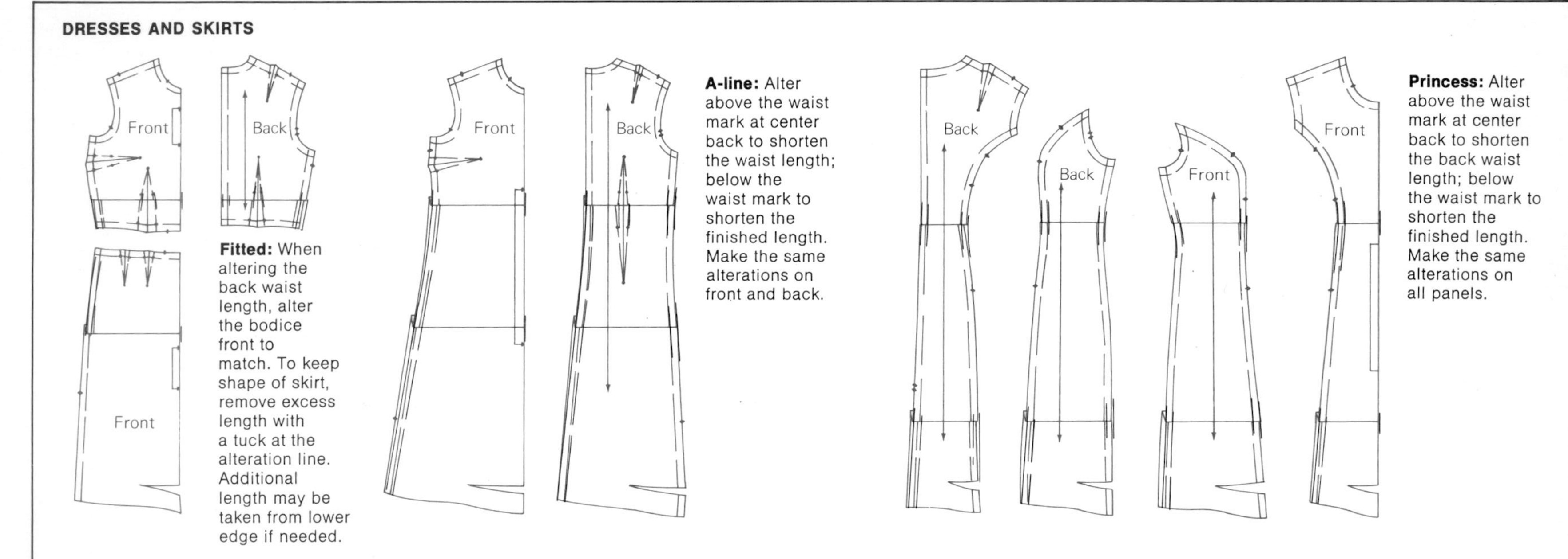

Fitted: When altering the back waist length, alter the bodice front to match. To keep shape of skirt, remove excess length with a tuck at the alteration line. Additional length may be taken from lower edge if needed.

A-line: Alter above the waist mark at center back to shorten the waist length; below the waist mark to shorten the finished length. Make the same alterations on front and back.

Princess: Alter above the waist mark at center back to shorten the back waist length; below the waist mark to shorten the finished length. Make the same alterations on all panels.

SLEEVES

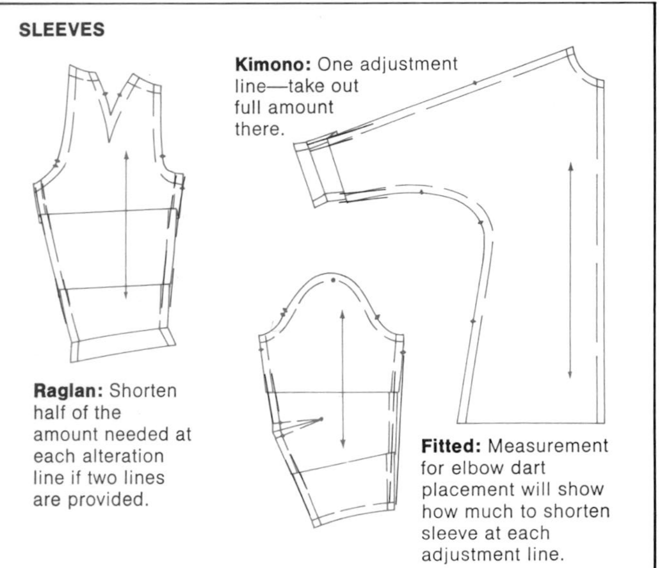

Raglan: Shorten half of the amount needed at each alteration line if two lines are provided.

Kimono: One adjustment line—take out full amount there.

Fitted: Measurement for elbow dart placement will show how much to shorten sleeve at each adjustment line.

PANTS

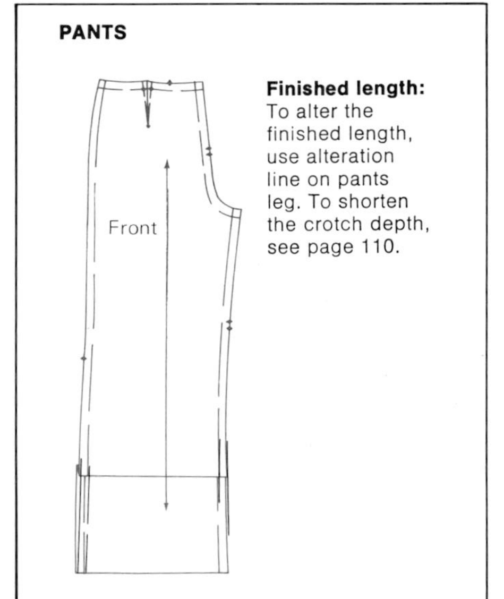

Finished length: To alter the finished length, use alteration line on pants leg. To shorten the crotch depth, see page 110.

SHOULDER

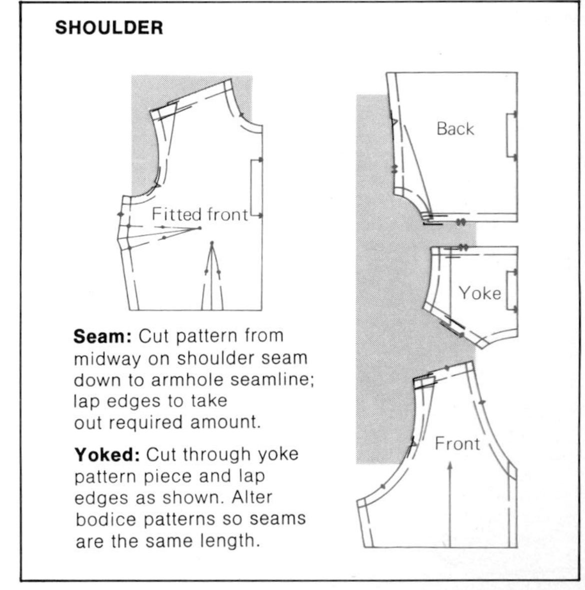

Seam: Cut pattern from midway on shoulder seam down to armhole seamline; lap edges to take out required amount.

Yoked: Cut through yoke pattern piece and lap edges as shown. Alter bodice patterns so seams are the same length.

Raising bust darts

To raise bust darts slightly, mark the location of the new dart point above the original. Draw new dart stitching lines to new point, tapering them into the original stitching lines.

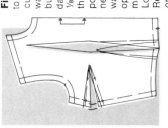

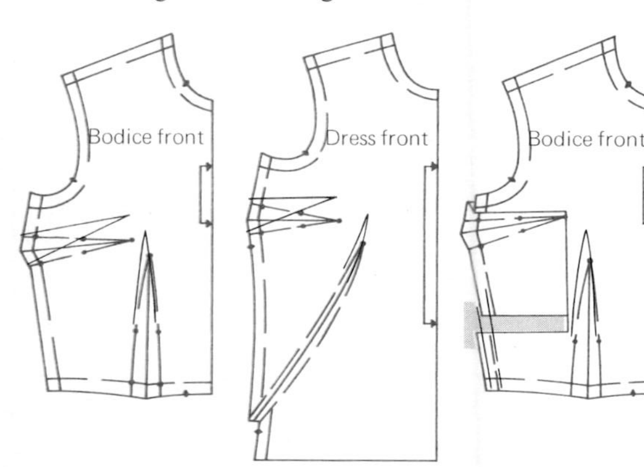

An alternative method, especially useful when an entire dart must be raised by a large amount, is to cut an "L" below and beside the dart as shown at right above. Take a tuck above the dart deep enough to raise it to the desired location.

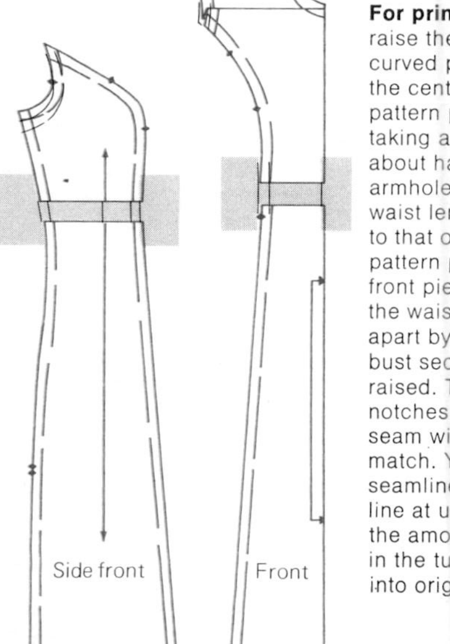

For princess styles, raise the most curved portion of the center front pattern piece by taking a tuck just about halfway down armhole seam. To keep waist length equal to that of back pattern pieces, cut front pieces above the waist; spread apart by the amount bust section was raised. The underarm notches at the side seam will no longer match. You must lower seamline and cutting line at underarm by the amount removed in the tuck; taper into original lines.

Lowering bust darts

To lower bust darts slightly, mark the location of the new dart point below the original. Draw new dart stitching lines to new point, tapering them into the original stitching lines.

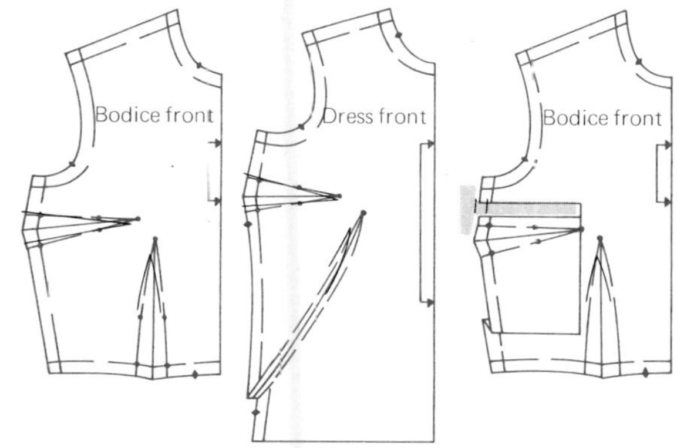

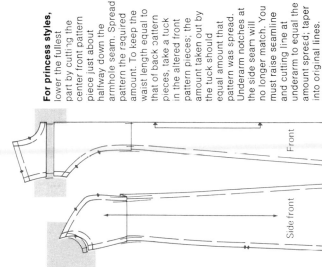

An alternative method, especially useful when the entire dart must be lowered by a large amount, is to cut an "L" above and beside the dart as shown at the right above. Take a tuck below the dart deep enough to lower it to the desired place.

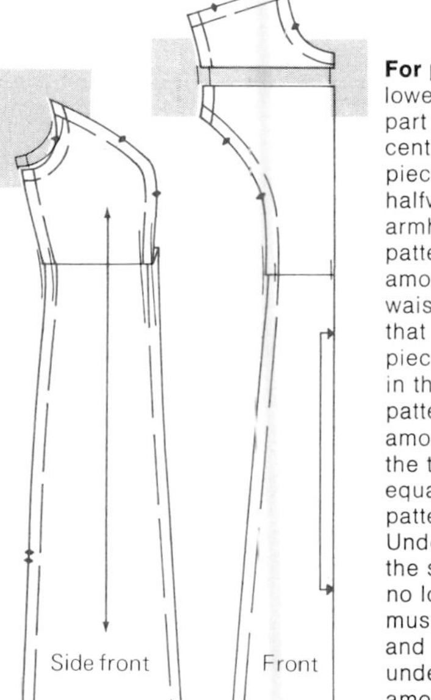

For princess styles, lower the fullest part by cutting the center front pattern piece just about halfway down the armhole seam. Spread pattern the required amount. To keep the waist length equal to that of back pattern pieces, take a tuck in the altered front pattern pieces; the amount taken out by the tuck should equal amount that pattern was spread. Underarm notches at the side seam will no longer match. You must raise seamline and cutting line at underarm to equal the amount spread; taper into original lines.

Enlarging the bust area

Additions of up to 2 inches can be made at the side seams. Apportion the amount equally and taper to nothing at armhole and waistline. For larger additions, cut and spread as explained below.

Fitted: Cut pattern from waist to shoulder seam, cutting along foldline of waist dart and through mark for bust apex. Also cut side bust dart on foldline to within ⅛" of bust point. Spread the vertical cut at the bust point by half the amount needed. (Do not spread at waist or shoulder.) This will open up the underarm cut, making bust dart deeper. Locate dart point within cuts. Re-draw darts, tapering into original stitching lines.

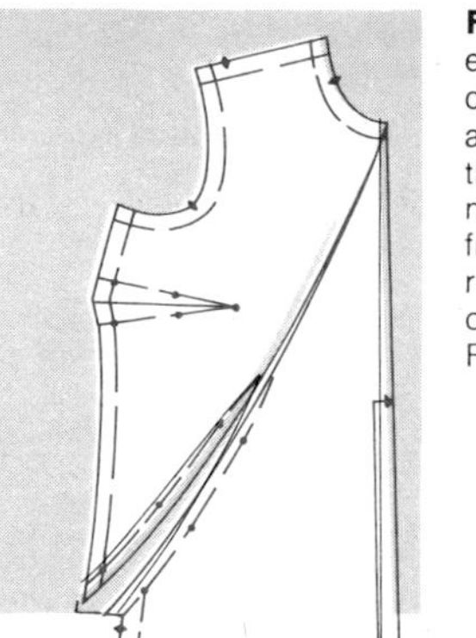

French dart: Draw a line extending foldline of dart to center front. Cut on this line and spread pattern apart half the total amount needed. Keep neck edge on original center front. Locate dart point and re-draw darts, tapering into original stitching lines. Re-draw center front line.

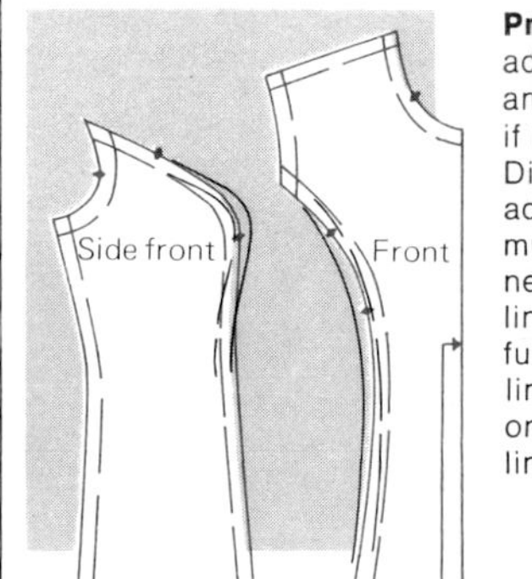

Princess seam: Up to 2" can be added this way; remember that an additional 2" can be added, if necessary, at side seams. Divide total inches to be added by 4 to determine how much to add to each seam. Mark new stitching and cutting lines outside the old ones at fullest part of curve. Re-draw lines, tapering them into original cutting and stitching lines at armhole and waistline.

Basic pattern alterations

Width alterations: increasing the waist

In general, to increase at the waist, you add one-fourth the total amount at each of the side seams, front and back. So as not to distort side seams when adding large amounts, distribute some of the increase over any darts or seams that cross the waistline. (Note exception for circular skirt.)

PANTS

When increasing the waist by a large amount, add to front and back crotch seams, as well as side seams. Note: Taper to nothing at curve of crotch seam.

WAISTBAND

Enlarge a waistband (of pants or skirt) by the same amount and in the same places that the garment was enlarged. This is usually at the side seam marks. Cut and spread the pattern the amount needed.

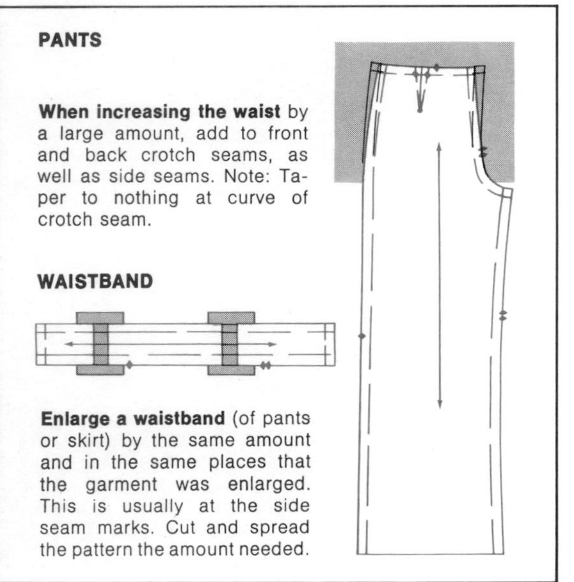

DRESSES

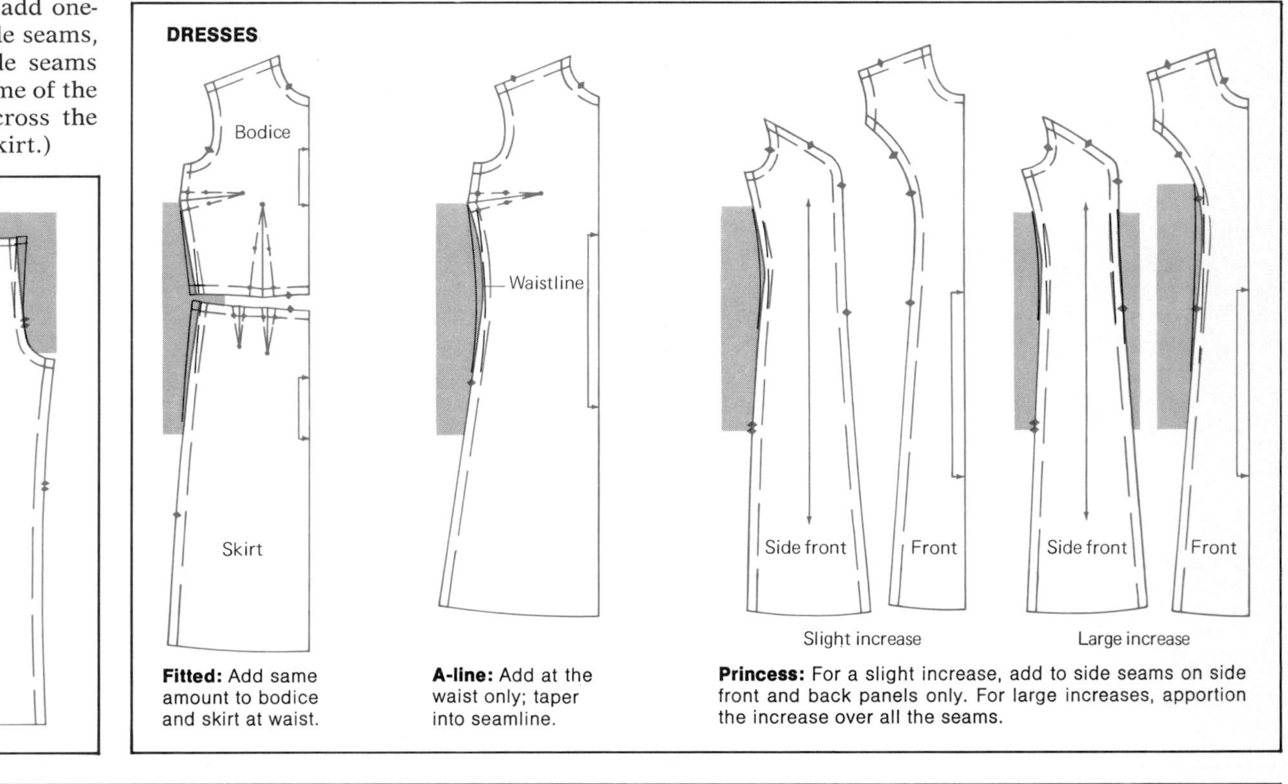

Slight increase

Large increase

Fitted: Add same amount to bodice and skirt at waist.

A-line: Add at the waist only; taper into seamline.

Princess: For a slight increase, add to side seams on side front and back panels only. For large increases, apportion the increase over all the seams.

SKIRTS

Gored: Slight increases are made at the side seams only; there is no change on the center front and back panels. To make a large increase, apportion the increase over all of the seams.

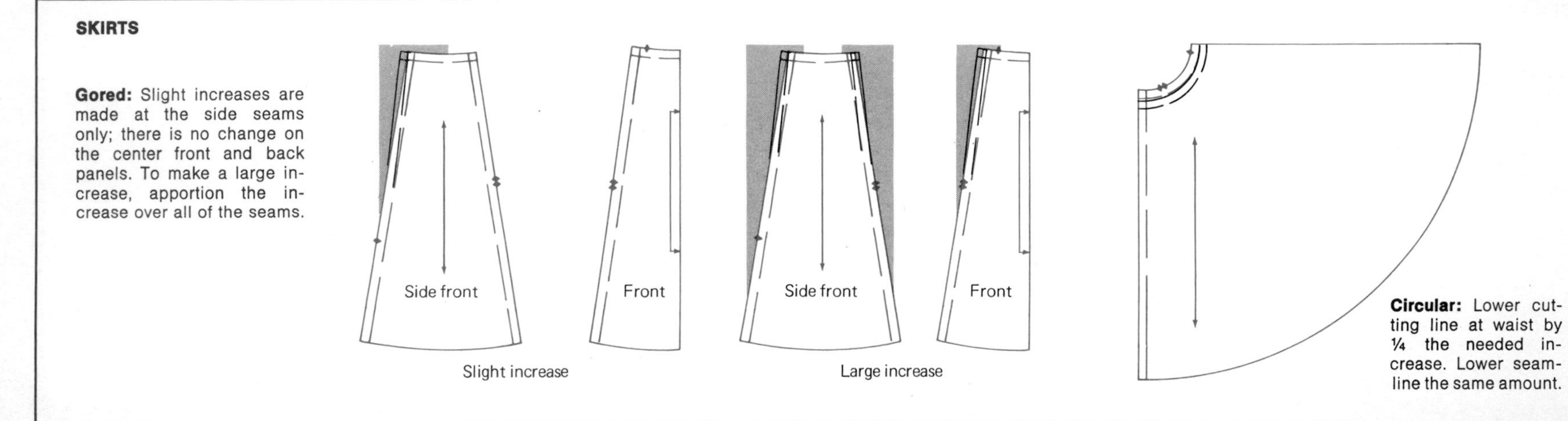

Slight increase

Large increase

Circular: Lower cutting line at waist by ¼ the needed increase. Lower seamline the same amount.

Width alterations: decreasing the waist

Generally speaking, to decrease at the waist, you take away one-fourth the total reduction at each of the side seams, front and back. If the decrease is larger, distribute some of it over any darts or seams that cross the waistline. (Note the exception for a circular skirt.)

PANTS

When decreasing the waist of pants by a large amount, alter front and back crotch seams. Note: Taper smoothly into original cutting line.

WAISTBAND

Decrease a waistband (of pants or skirt) by the same amount and in the same places that the garment was decreased. This is usually at the side seam marks. Tuck out amount to be reduced.

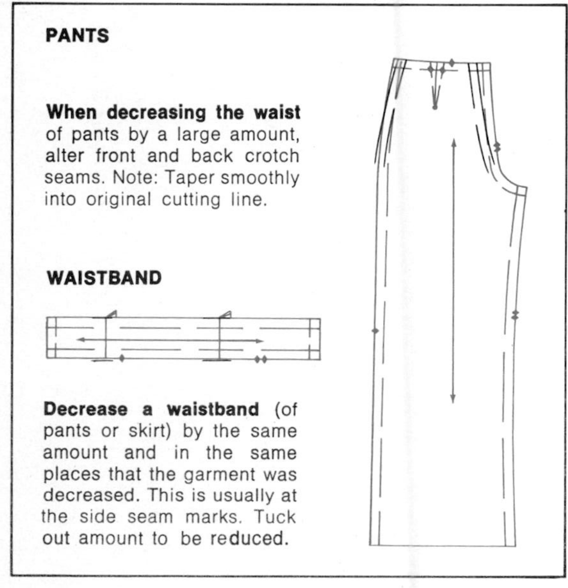

DRESSES

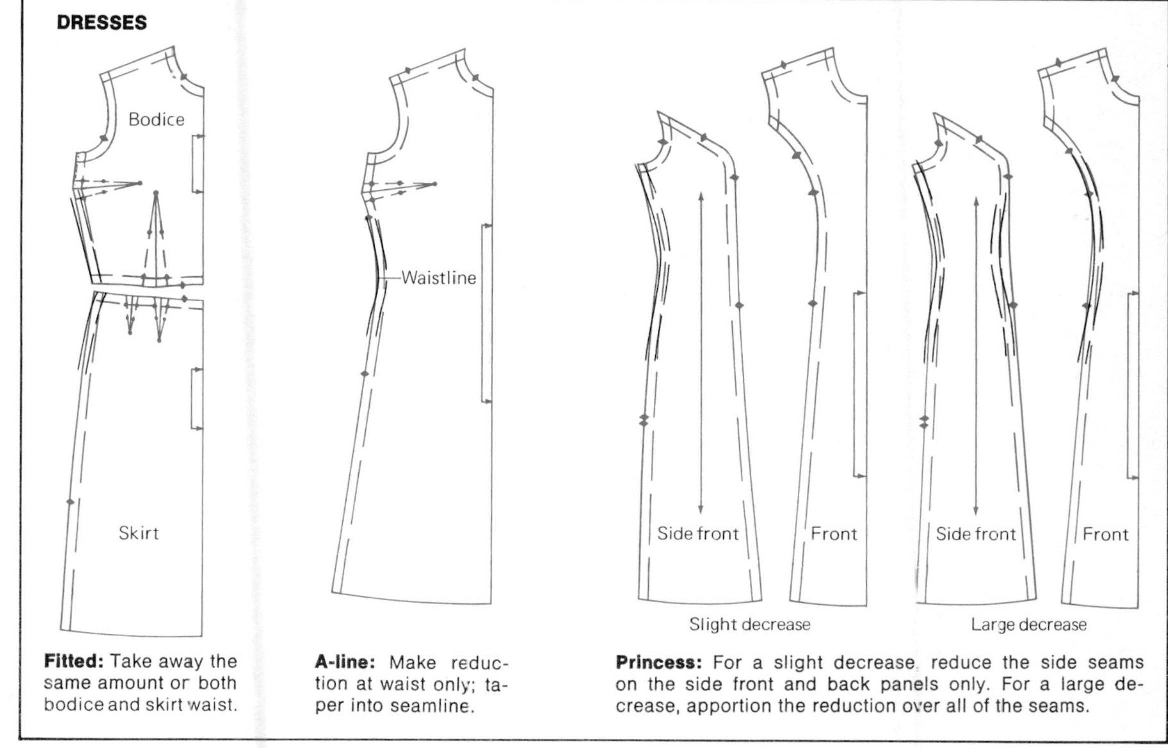

Fitted: Take away the same amount or both bodice and skirt waist.

A-line: Make reduction at waist only; taper into seamline.

Princess: For a slight decrease, reduce the side seams on the side front and back panels only. For a large decrease, apportion the reduction over all of the seams.

SKIRTS

Gored: Slight decreases are made at the side seams only; there is no change on the center front and back panels. For a large decrease, apportion the reduction over all of the seams.

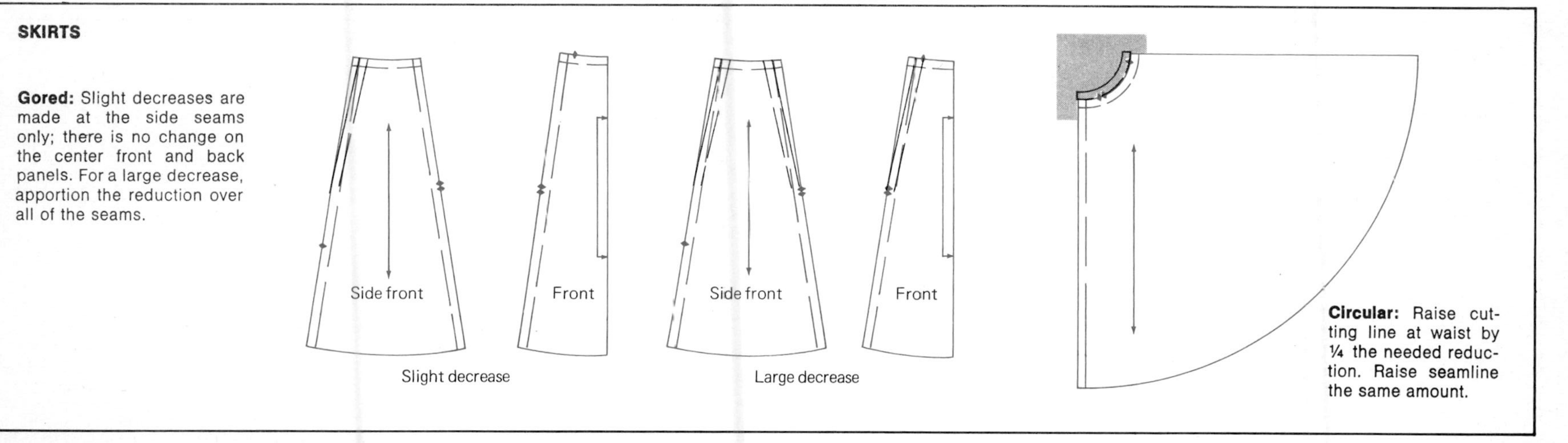

Circular: Raise cutting line at waist by ¼ the needed reduction. Raise seamline the same amount.

Width alterations: increasing the hipline

To add **2 inches or less** to the hipline, enlarge pattern at side seams; add one-fourth the total amount needed at each of the side seams, front and back. If adding **more than 2 inches,** distribute it more evenly over the garment by means of the "cut and spread" methods shown on this page.

PANTS

If hip measurement is followed when pants patterns are purchased, only a slight alteration should be necessary. Add to the hipline at side seams, tapering to the original cutting line at waist and thigh.

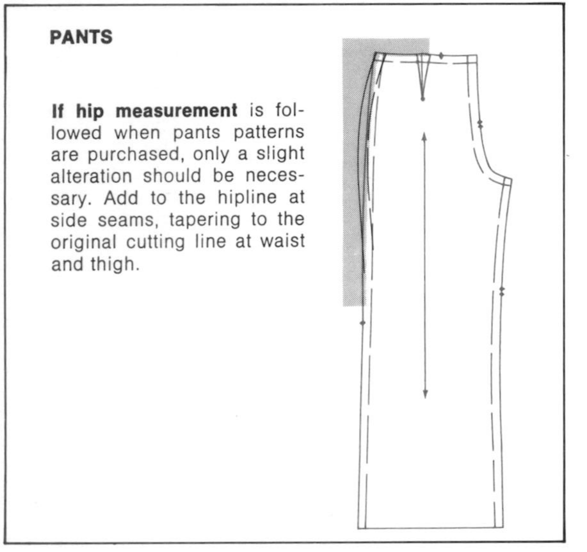

DRESSES

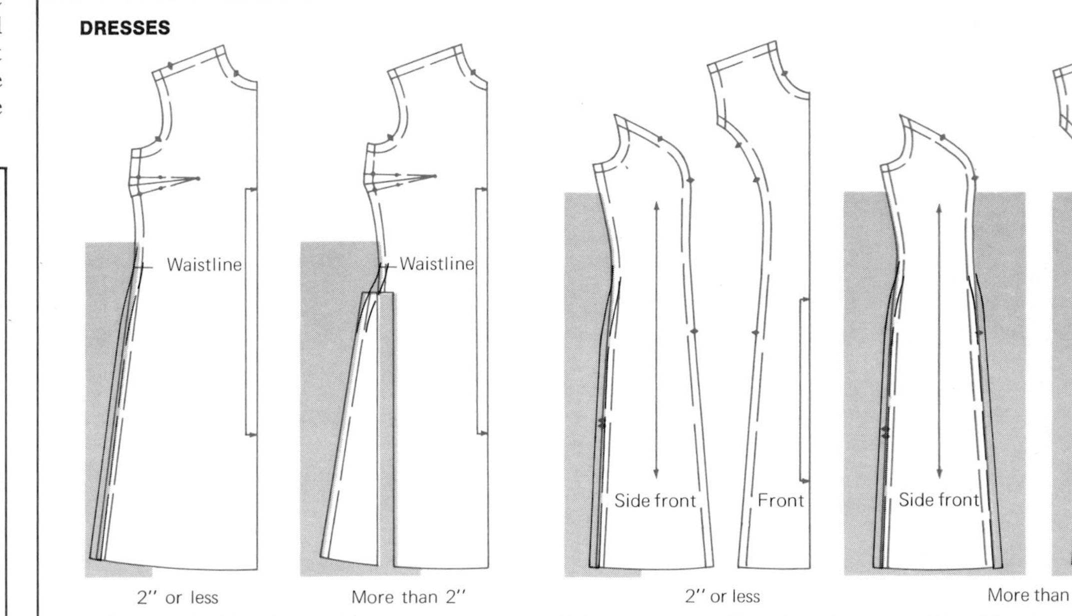

2″ or less More than 2″

A-line: Up to 2″, add at side seams. More than 2″, slash pattern parallel to grainline; spread ¼ amount needed, front and back.

2″ or less More than 2″

Princess: To add 2″ or less, increase at the side seams, making no change on the front and back panels. To add more than 2″, apportion the increase over all of the seams.

SKIRTS

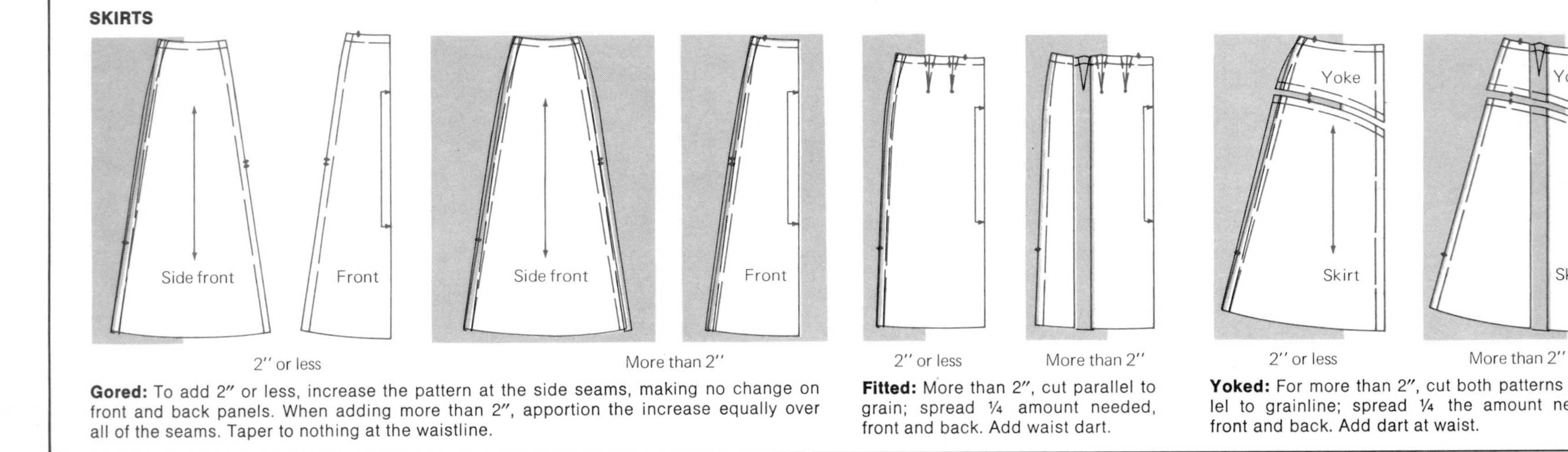

2″ or less More than 2″

Gored: To add 2″ or less, increase the pattern at the side seams, making no change on front and back panels. When adding more than 2″, apportion the increase equally over all of the seams. Taper to nothing at the waistline.

2″ or less More than 2″

Fitted: More than 2″, cut parallel to grain; spread ¼ amount needed, front and back. Add waist dart.

2″ or less More than 2″

Yoked: For more than 2″, cut both patterns parallel to grainline; spread ¼ the amount needed, front and back. Add dart at waist.

Width alterations: decreasing the hipline

In most cases, to decrease at the hipline, you take away one-fourth of the total reduction at each of the side seams, front and back. The new cutting lines taper from waist to hem. It is usually not wise to try to remove more than an inch unless there are many seams; style lines would be lost.

PANTS

If the hip measurement is followed when pants patterns are purchased, only a slight alteration should be needed. Decrease the hipline at the side seams, front and back, tapering into the original cutting line at the waistline.

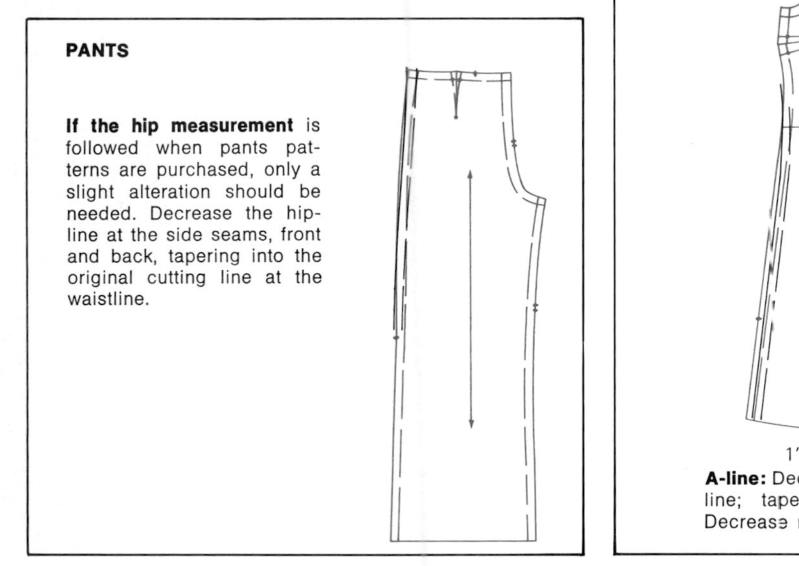

DRESSES

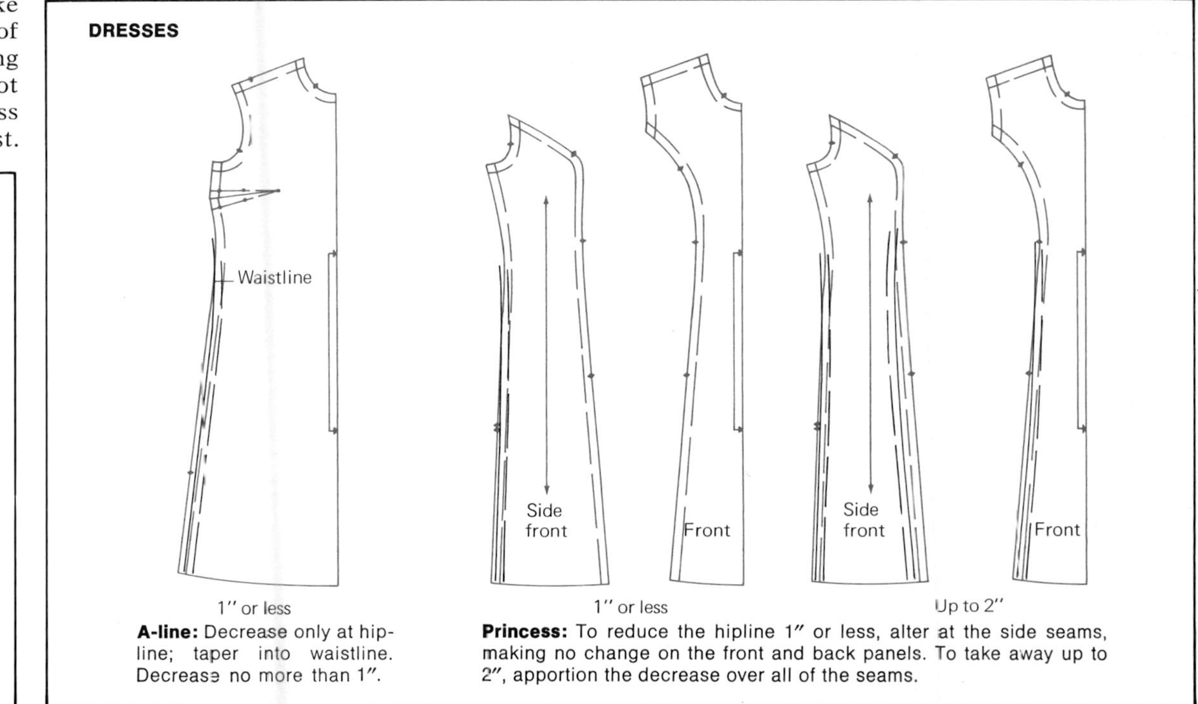

A-line: Decrease only at hipline; taper into waistline. Decrease no more than 1″.

Princess: To reduce the hipline 1″ or less, alter at the side seams, making no change on the front and back panels. To take away up to 2″, apportion the decrease over all of the seams.

SKIRTS

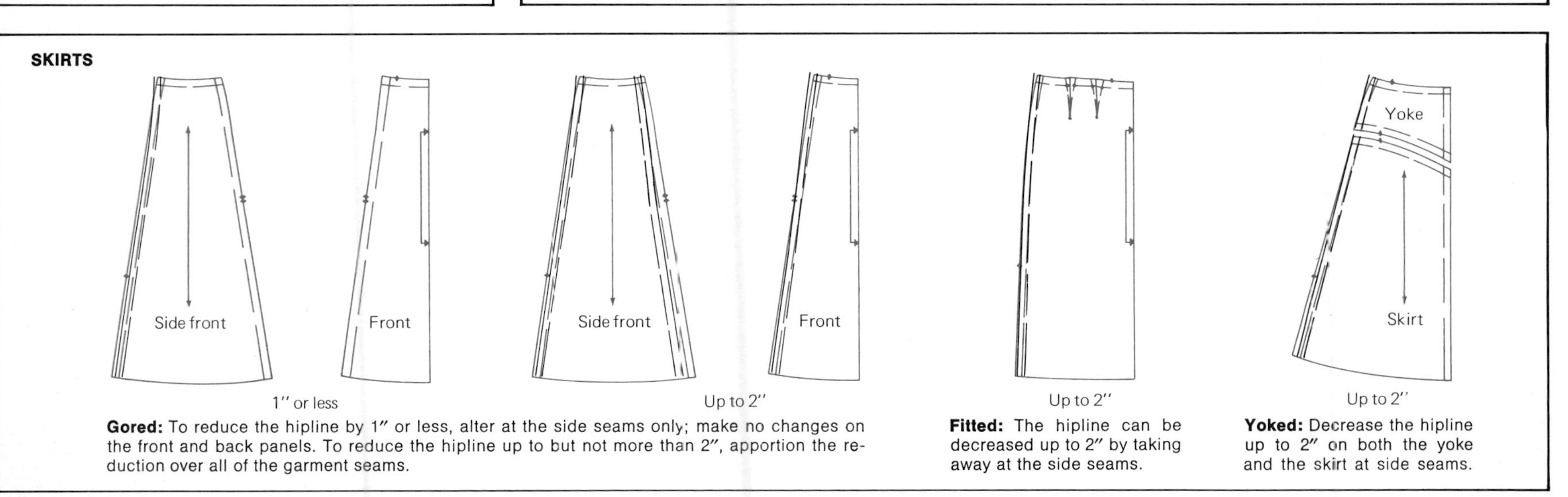

Gored: To reduce the hipline by 1″ or less, alter at the side seams only; make no changes on the front and back panels. To reduce the hipline up to but not more than 2″, apportion the reduction over all of the garment seams.

Fitted: The hipline can be decreased up to 2″ by taking away at the side seams.

Yoked: Decrease the hipline up to 2″ on both the yoke and the skirt at side seams.

Basic pattern alterations

Adjusting the pants crotch seam

Good fit in pants depends primarily on how the torso portion is fitted—the legs rarely need special attention. See page 100 for instructions on taking body measurements. **Width** alterations for waist and hip have been discussed in the preceding pages. The other two measurements that are vital to good torso fit are **crotch depth** and **crotch length.** One or both may need altering.

The crotch **depth** is the measurement of the distance from your waist to the bottom of your hips, taken when you are sitting. This measurement indicates whether any adjustments are needed in the area between your waist and the top of your legs. Consequently, any alterations to the crotch depth will affect both crotch seam and side seam.

The crotch **length** is the actual length of the crotch seam, taken between the legs, from waist at center front to waist at center back. This measurement takes into account any extreme stomach or hip contours, and it affects only the crotch seam —not the side seam. It is important to apportion the total crotch length into what is needed at front and at the back. For example, if you have just a protruding derriere, you would want all the additional length in the back where it is needed, not half in front and half in back.

The crotch length can be altered either at the crotch point, which is at the intersection of the crotch seam and the inseam, or it can be altered along the crotch seam itself. When the length is altered at the crotch **point,** an additional change occurs—either an increase or a decrease in the width of the pants leg at the top of the thigh. Which it is depends on whether the crotch seam is lengthened or shortened. In most instances, this is an advantage. Use the crotch **seam** method of altering the crotch length if only stomach or derriere is a problem. This method adds or takes away fullness exactly where it is needed on the front or back. It is possible to alter at both the point and along the seam for very rounded or flat stomach or derriere.

When both crotch depth and crotch length alterations are needed, **alter the crotch depth first.** A crotch depth alteration will change the crotch length. It is necessary to re-measure the pattern's crotch seam before determining how much (if any) additional altering the crotch length will need.

Altering crotch depth

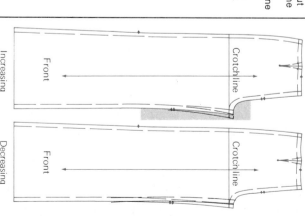

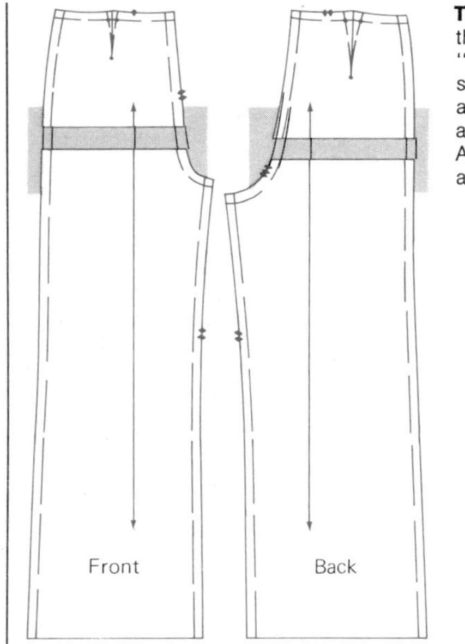

To increase: Cut the pattern on the "lengthen or shorten here" line and spread full amount needed. Alter pants front and back alike.

Front
Back
Decreasing
Decreasing

To decrease: Take a tuck on the "lengthen or shorten here" line. Make the tuck half as deep as the total amount needed. Alter pants front and back alike.

Altering crotch length

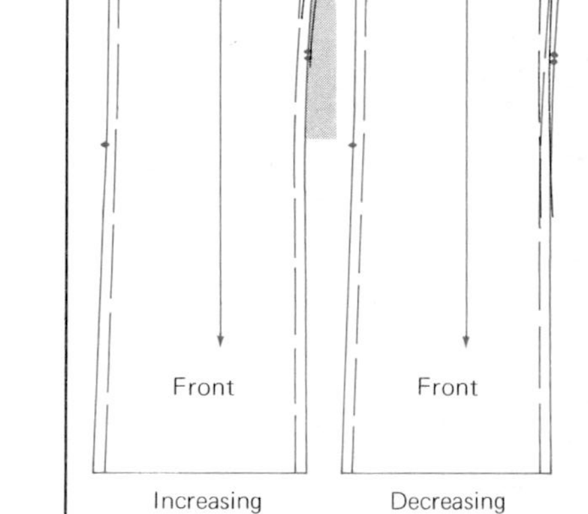

CROTCH POINT METHOD: Draw a crotch line as shown (if not on pattern). This line starts at the side seam and ends at the crotch point; it is at right angles to the grainline.

To increase the crotch length, extend line at crotch point the amount needed; draw new cutting lines at inseam and crotch.

To decrease the crotch length, shorten line at crotch point as needed; draw new cutting lines at inseam and crotch.

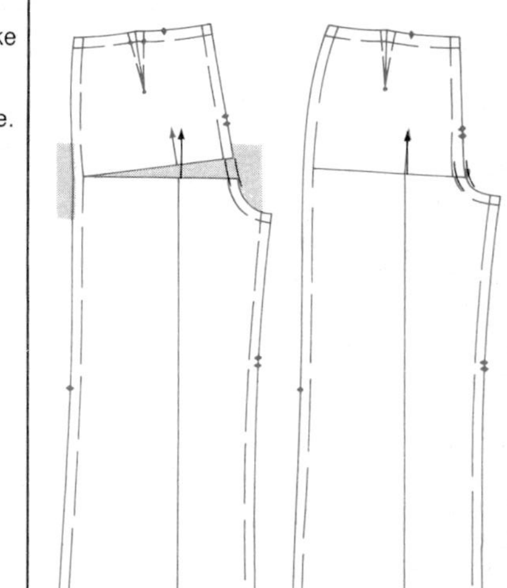

CROTCH SEAM METHOD: Cut and spread to add length; take a tuck to decrease length.

To increase the crotch length, cut the pattern on alteration line to (not through) the side seam. Spread as needed, tapering toward side seam.

To decrease the crotch length, fold the pattern on the alteration line to take away the amount needed at the crotch seam. Taper the fold so that no change is made in the side seam.

Fitting shell and master pattern

Layout and cutting 84-94
Fabric-marking methods 94
Uneven basting 124

A method for advanced alterations

If you need more than the basic pattern alterations, or if you want additional knowledge of fitting techniques, you will want to make a fitting shell and master pattern. A **fitting shell** is made from a basic pattern—it may be a dress, pants, or just a bodice—sewed in inexpensive fabric and used exclusively for solving fitting problems. After the shell has been altered to fit you perfectly, all the adjustments you have made are transferred to the shell's paper pattern. The adjusted shell pattern then becomes your **master pattern.** This method takes some time and patience, but your master pattern can save considerable time and trouble whenever you sew. By using it with each new style you make, you can check for potential fitting problems before cutting the pattern in fabric, avoiding costly waste of fabric and time.

To make a fitting shell and master pattern, you will need the following supplies.

Pattern: The classic fitting shell is a closely fitted sheath. Most pattern companies offer just such a style for use in fitting. The purpose of such a dress is not to actually wear it, but to use it to fit body areas as closely as possible. The master pattern that you develop from it can be used to alter virtually every pattern you sew. If your fitting problems occur in the bust or shoulder area only, use just the bodice for your shell. Another possibility is to make the shell from your favorite pattern—the one that you sew again and again—and use your master pattern for this style. If you want a pants shell, choose a straight-leg style with a waistband and darts. Once the waist and hips have been fitted, the shell can be used with any pants style, no matter how full the legs.

Fabric and notions: A fitting shell is often called a "muslin," this being the traditional fabric for this use. You may prefer another fabric. Gingham is good and the woven checks help to keep grainlines straight. An old bedsheet will do, or fabric leftovers, so long as they are firmly woven and of medium weight. Of course, you must be sure your fabric is grain-perfect.

In addition, you will need any zippers called for by your pattern and, if your shell is a skirt or pants, some grosgrain ribbon to use as a firm, nonstretchy trial waistband.

How to make the shell

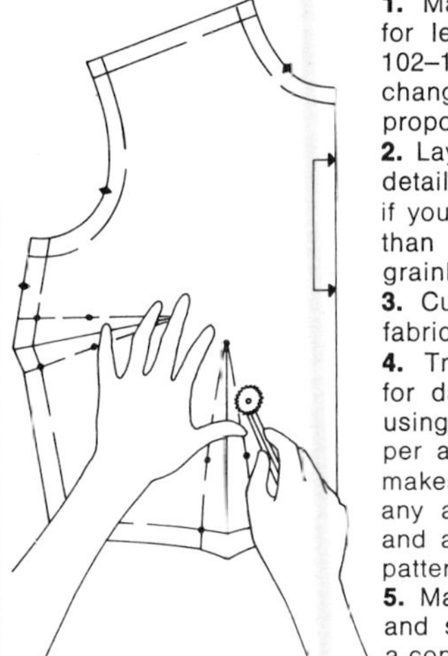

1. Make any basic alterations for length and width (see pp. 102–110) to take care of major changes and bring pattern into proportion with your figure.
2. Lay out the pattern, omitting details like facings, collars, etc., if you are using a pattern other than the classic shell. Keep grainlines accurate.
3. Cut out the pattern, saving fabric scraps for later use.
4. Transfer all stitching lines for darts and seams to fabric, using dressmaker's tracing paper and a tracing wheel. This makes it easier to keep track of any adjustments in your shell, and aids in altering the master pattern as well.
5. Mark center front on bodice and skirt with hand basting in a contrasting thread color.
6. Sew the shell together, following the pattern instructions; use a long machine stitch for easy removal (a chain stitch, if available, is ideal). For the dress shell, eliminate the sleeves for the first fitting—put them in after shoulders have been adjusted. Omit waistband from pants or skirt—use a length of grosgrain instead.
7. Staystitch armholes and neckline on the stitching line; clip the seam allowances and press to wrong side.
8. Baste all of the hems in place.

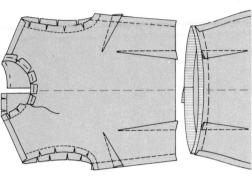

Judging the fit

Wearing shoes and appropriate undergarments, try on your shell, right side out. Be very critical about the fit; this is the time to settle all fitting problems, however troublesome they might be. Naturally you will track down the cause of every wrinkle and see to the adjustment that makes it disappear. Remember, too, to give your shell the comfort test: sit, reach, bend, and walk to find out whether and where there are any strained seams. Be sure to study your own backviews as well (another person is helpful here) and try to think objectively about the way the shell fits your figure.

To adjust the shell, first locate your fitting problems among those shown on the pages that follow. The solutions include explanations of how to adjust the shell as well as how to transfer the adjustment to the master pattern. Resolve *all* your fitting problems on the shell before putting *any* on the master pattern. This may take more than one fitting session and require taking out and re-stitching seams and darts. If this seems time-consuming, remember it will save you many hours in future sewing. Keep track of all adjustments. Fit your shell from the top down, because a single adjustment on top might solve the problems below.

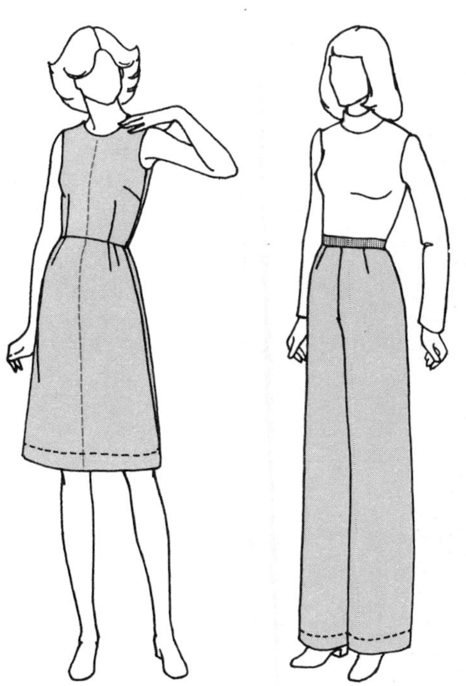

Fitting shell and master pattern

Neckline alterations

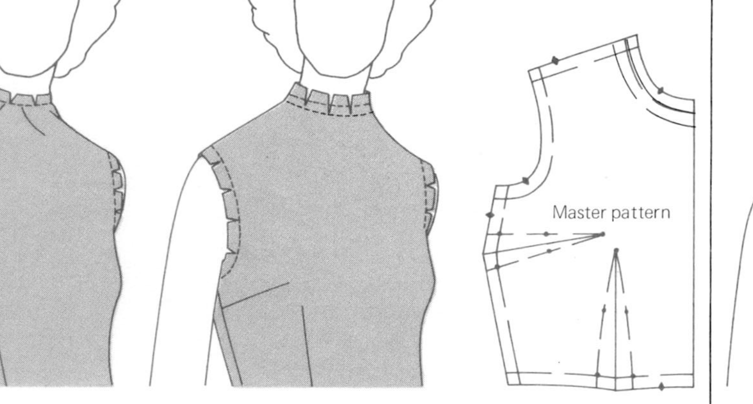

The neckline binds.
Solution: Lower the seamline to the neck base; clip the seam allowance until neckline feels comfortable.
Alteration: Draw cutting and stitching lines in new lowered position on the bodice front and back. Alter the neckline facings to match.

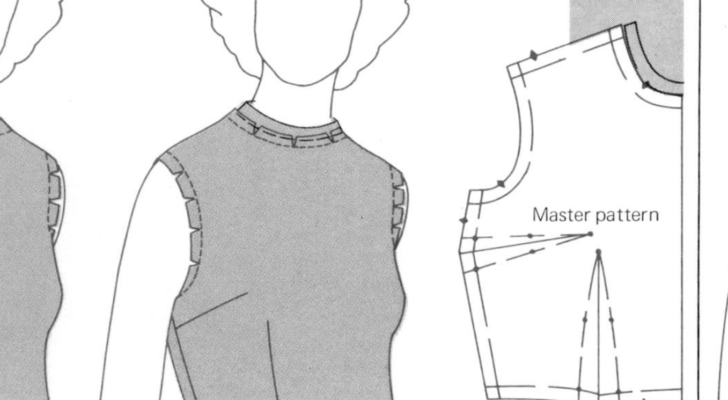

The neckline gapes.
Solution: Raise the seamline to the neck base with a self-fabric bias strip.
Alteration: Draw cutting and stitching lines in new raised position on the bodice front and back. Alter the neckline facings to match.

Shoulder alterations

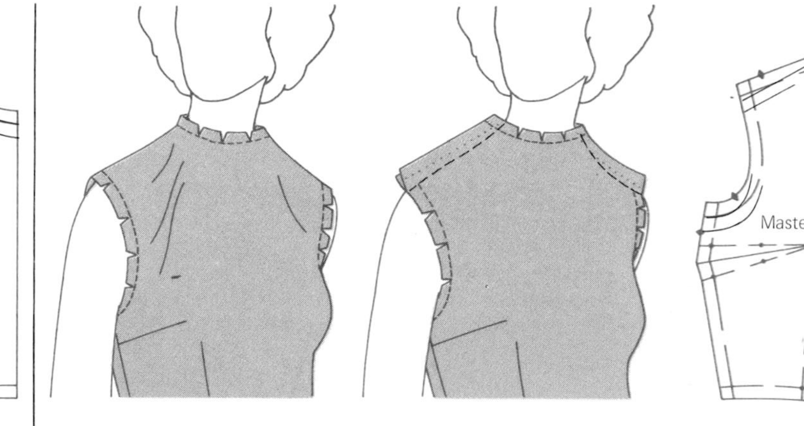

Shell wrinkles above the bust dart at the armhole and below the shoulder in the back. This occurs when shoulders slope more than pattern; one shoulder may slope more than the other.
Solution: Open up the shoulder seam; take out excess fabric by stitching seam deeper. Taper to original seamline at neckline. Re-draw armhole to keep its shape.
Alteration: Draw new cutting and stitching lines for shoulder seams and armholes, lowering armhole at underarm by an amount equal to that removed at shoulder.

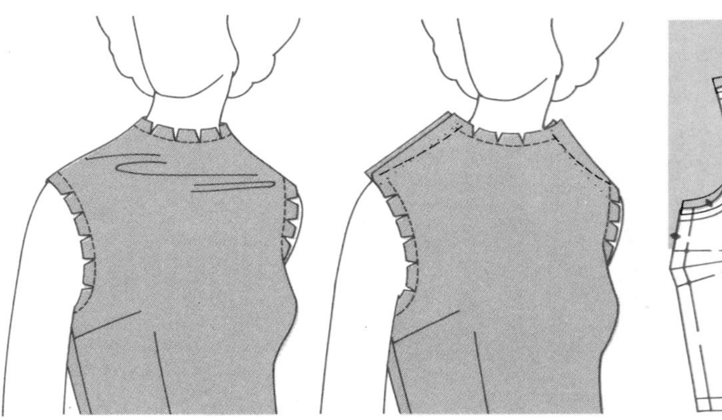

Shell feels tight and wrinkles through the shoulders in front and back. This occurs when shoulders slope less than pattern.
Solution: Release the shoulder seams and re-stitch a narrower shoulder seam to gain additional space. Taper to original seamline at neckline. Re-draw the armhole to keep its original shape.
Alteration: Draw new cutting and stitching lines for shoulder seams and armholes, raising armhole at underarm by an amount equal to what was added at shoulder.

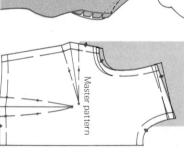

Bust adjustments

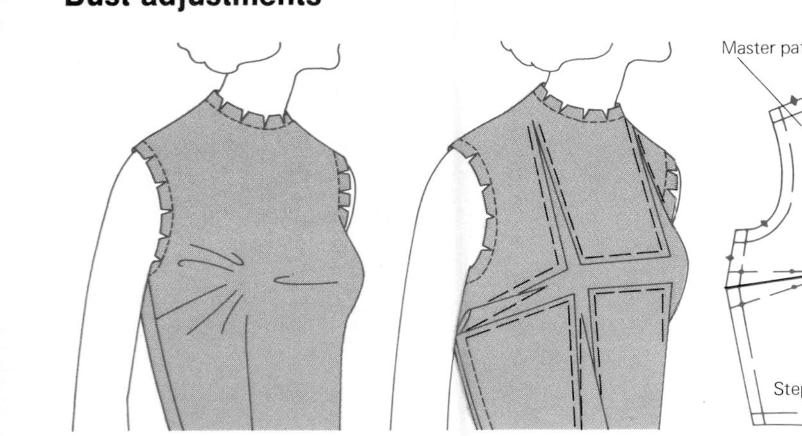

Bodice too tight across bustline. Shell wrinkles under dart and the grain may be pulled up in front.
Solution: Release the bust darts, then cut the fabric through the center of each dart to the center front and to the shoulder, respectively, crossing the apex of the bust. Spread each cut until bodice fits smoothly, filling in open spaces with scraps. Re-stitch darts, using original stitching lines.
Alteration: On lines drawn through the centers of the bust darts, cut the pattern and spread it the amount needed for one side—half the total amount. Locate original point of dart within each slash and re-draw dart stitching lines, starting at original stitching line at base. Restore grainline and "place on fold" line.

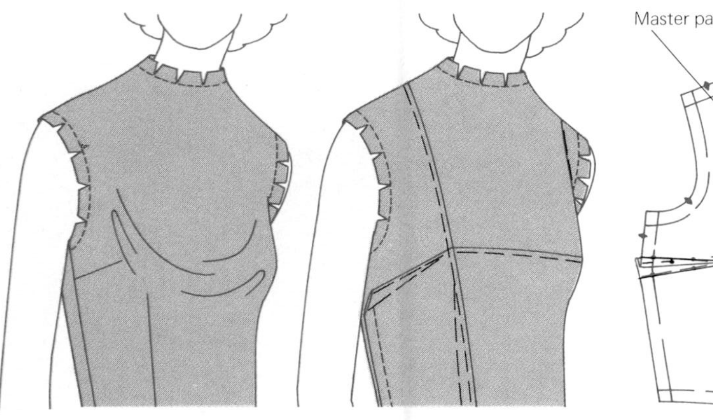

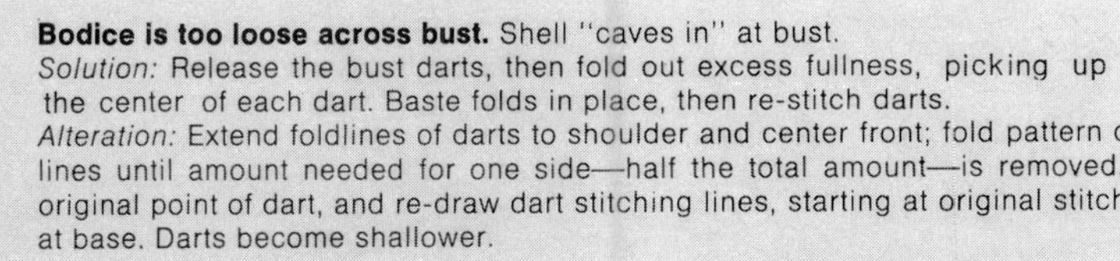

Bodice is too loose across bust. Shell "caves in" at bust.
Solution: Release the bust darts, then fold out excess fullness, picking up through the center of each dart. Baste folds in place, then re-stitch darts.
Alteration: Extend foldlines of darts to shoulder and center front; fold pattern on these lines until amount needed for one side—half the total amount—is removed. Locate original point of dart, and re-draw dart stitching lines, starting at original stitching line at base. Darts become shallower.

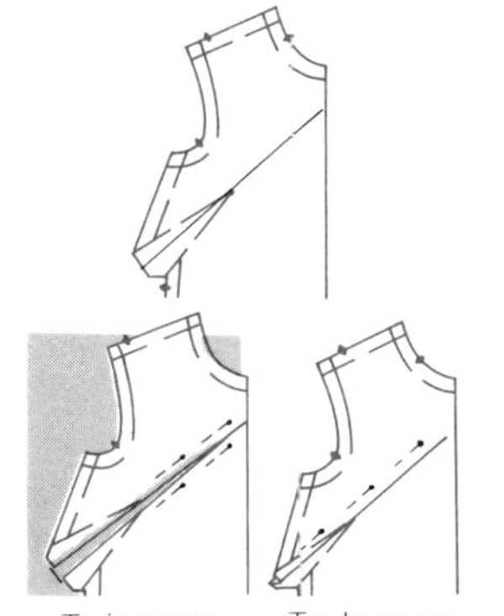

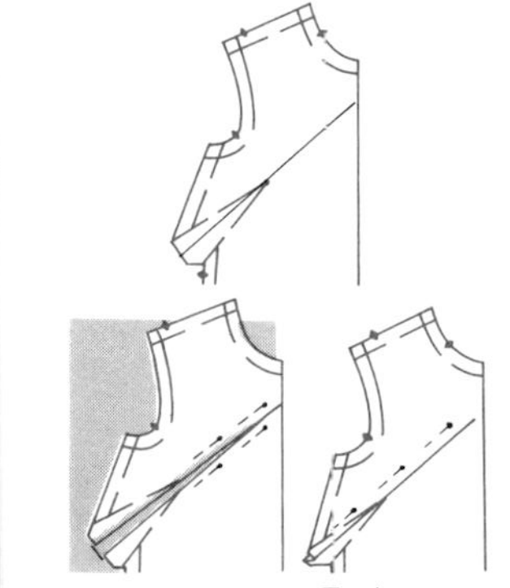

French dart alteration: On a line drawn through the center of the bust dart, cut and spread (or fold out) ½ total amount needed. Keep neck edge on original center front.

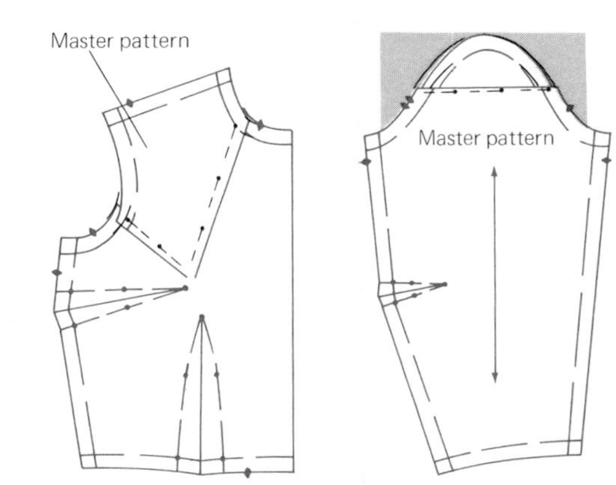

Armholes and/or neckline gape because of full bust.
Solution: Remove excess fabric by folding out fullness from gaping area to bust point as shown above. (Since this makes the armholes smaller, you will need to remove extra ease in the sleeve cap by taking a tuck ¼ as deep as the alteration dart at the armhole.)
Alteration: Cut pattern from armhole and/or neckline to bust point, and lap the cut edges to remove excess. (Remove excess ease from the sleeve cap with a tuck, as shown.)

Fitting shell and master pattern

Shoulder and back adjustments

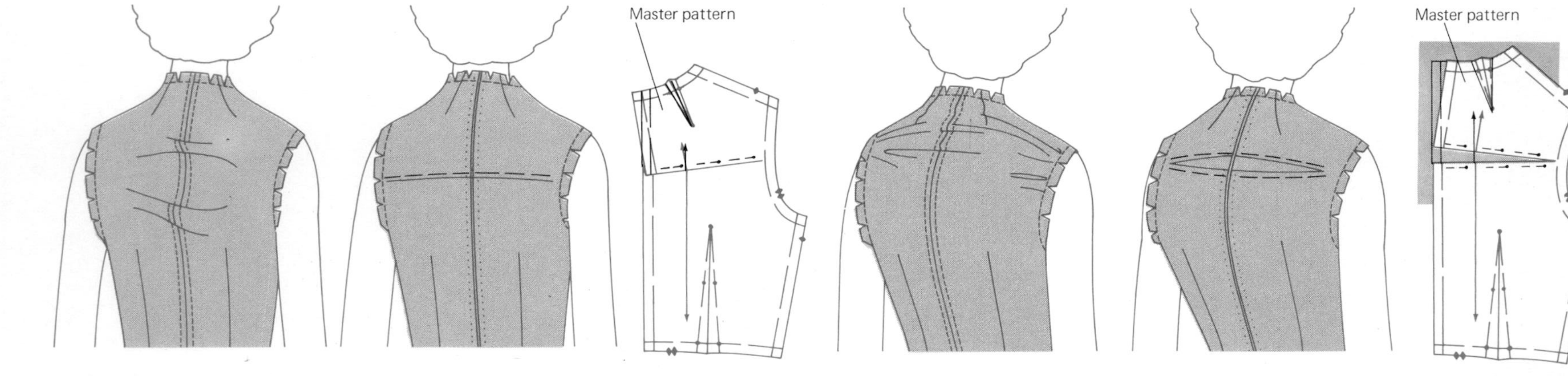

Shell wrinkles across shoulder blades because posture is very erect.
Solution: Baste a tuck across the shoulder blades, tapering to nothing at the armholes. (Note: This requires removal and subsequent replacement of the zipper.) Also, let out the neckline or shoulder darts, making them shorter if necessary.
Alteration: Take an identical tuck in back bodice pattern. Straighten the center back cutting line and make the neckline dart shallower (or omit it) to compensate for the amount taken away when straightening the center back line.

Shell pulls across the shoulders from slumping posture (round shoulders).
Solution: Cut shell across the back where it is strained; do not cut through armhole. Spread slash open until back fits smoothly; fill in with fabric scraps. (Note: This procedure requires removal and subsequent replacement of the zipper.)
Alteration: Cut and spread the pattern same as the shell. Straighten the center back cutting line and deepen the neckline dart (or create one) to compensate for the amount added when straightening the center back line.

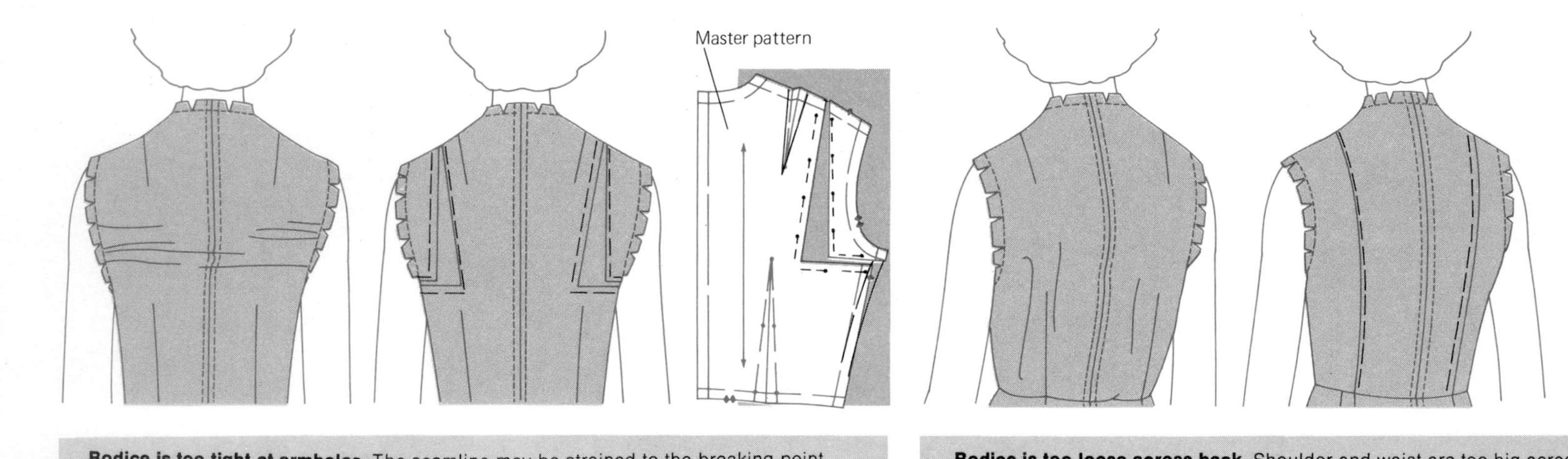

Bodice is too tight at armholes. The seamline may be strained to the breaking point.
Solution: Relieve the strain by cutting an "L" from the side seam (do not cut through the armhole seam) to the shoulder seam. Spread slash open until back fits smoothly; fill in with fabric scraps.
Alteration: Cut and spread pattern the same as shell. Deepen shoulder dart to remove any excess in shoulder seam. Re-draw side seam, tapering from new position at underarm to original position at waistline. Add same amount to sleeve seams.

Bodice is too loose across back. Shoulder and waist are too big across the back.
Solution: Remove excess fabric by basting a continuous waist-to-shoulder dart.
Alteration: Take a tuck from waist to shoulder, incorporating waist and shoulder darts. This is called a *fitting tuck* (it will not appear on a final garment). Because waist and shoulder darts must be retained in the pattern for fitting body contours, restore the darts lost in the fitting tuck to their original position, making them shallower, if necessary, so waist and shoulder seams will match.

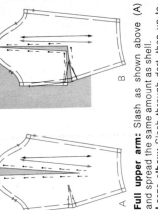

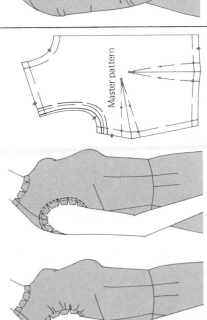

Armholes

Armholes are too low.
Solution: Raise the underarm curve by basting in place a self-fabric bias strip.
Alteration: Draw new cutting and stitching lines to raise the underarm curve on front and back bodice patterns. Curve on sleeve at underarm must be raised by the same amount so that sleeve can be easily set into armhole.

Armholes are too high.
Solution: Relieve the strain by clipping into the seam allowance; mark a new stitching line for the armhole seam.
Alteration: Draw new cutting and stitching lines to lower the underarm curve on front and back bodice patterns. Curve on sleeve at underarm must be lowered by the same amount so that sleeve can be easily set into armhole.

Sleeves

Take horizontal tuck across sleeve cap ¼ as deep as total taken from fitting shell.

Sleeves are too loose.
Solution: Take a tuck down the top of the sleeve to remove the excess, tucking the entire length if the whole sleeve is too big. If it is only the upper arm that is too large, taper the tuck to nothing at the elbow.

Alteration: If you have taken in the sleeve along its entire length, take a tuck down the center of the pattern, keeping it parallel to the grainline. The tuck will remove some ease from the sleeve cap, so you must alter the armhole by raising the underarm curve (the notches on sleeve and armhole will no longer match). If only the upper arm needed adjustment, see the drawing at the far right above. Underarm curve must be raised in this situation as well.

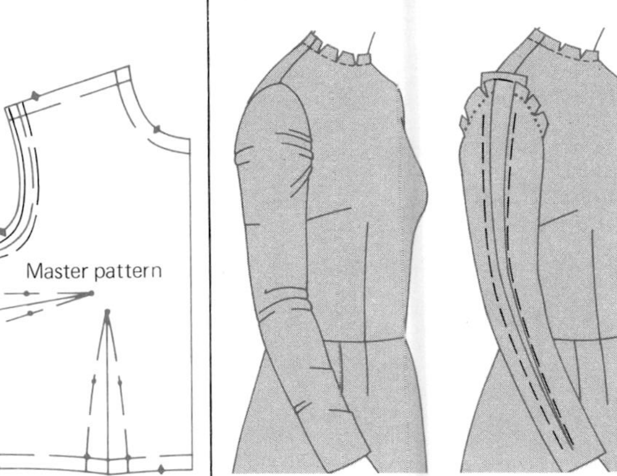

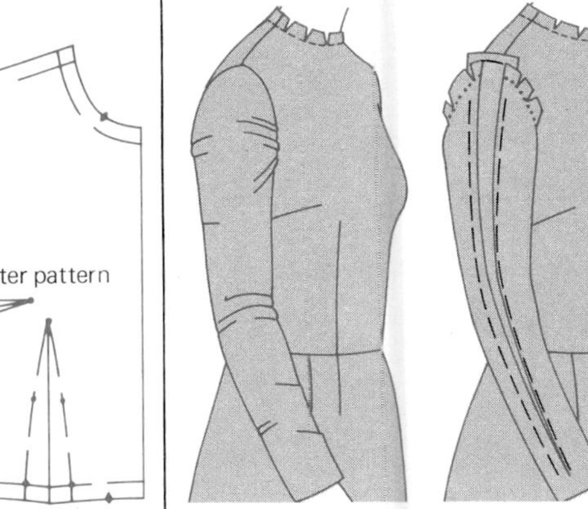

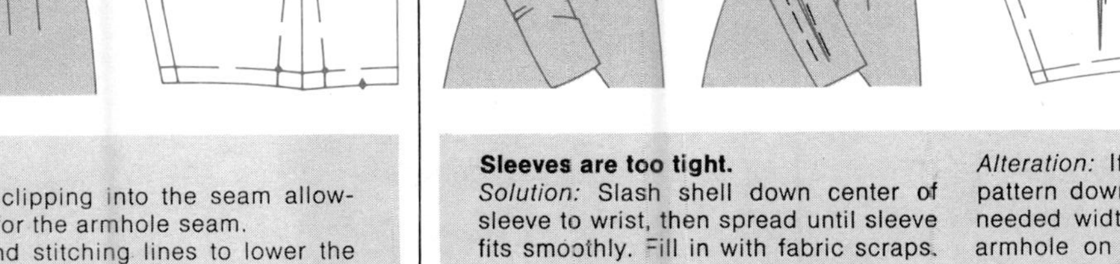

Full upper arm: Slash as shown above (A) and spread the same amount as shell.
Large elbow: Slash through dart, then up toward sleeve cap, and spread amount needed as shown above (B); re-draw seam and dart.

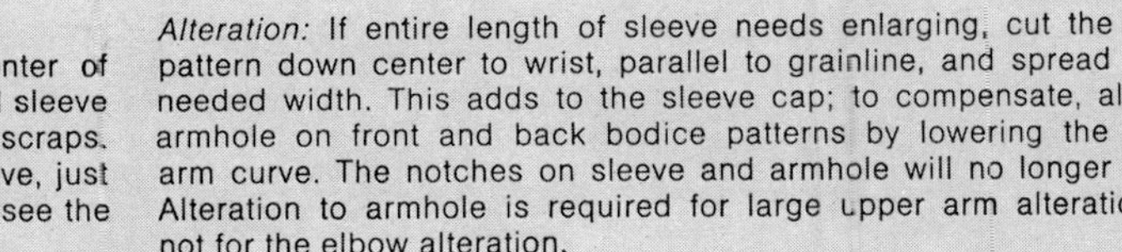

Sleeves are too tight.
Solution: Slash shell down center of sleeve to wrist, then spread until sleeve fits smoothly. Fill in with fabric scraps. You may enlarge the entire sleeve, just the upper arm, or the elbow (see the drawing at the right).

Alteration: If entire length of sleeve needs enlarging, cut the sleeve pattern down center to wrist, parallel to grainline, and spread to add needed width. This adds to the sleeve cap; to compensate, alter the armhole on front and back bodice patterns by lowering the underarm curve. The notches on sleeve and armhole will no longer match. Alteration to armhole is required for large upper arm alteration, but not for the elbow alteration.

Fitting shell and master pattern

Skirt or pants front

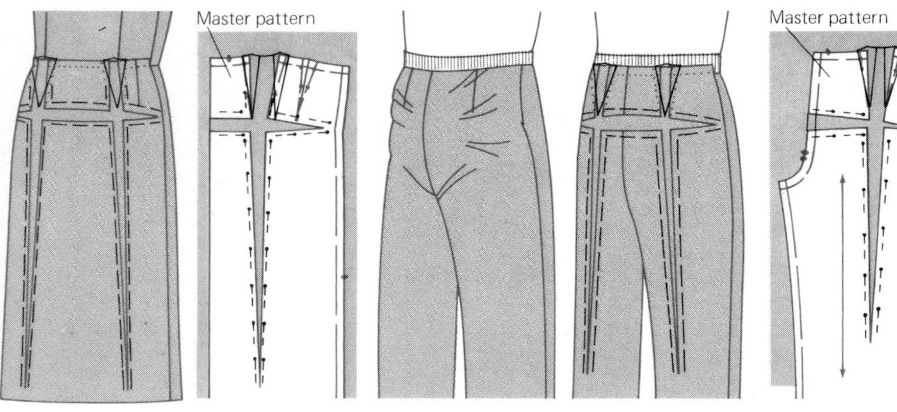

Shell is too tight across abdomen. Strain may cause skirt hem to pull up, pants to wrinkle at crotch.
Solution: Release the darts nearest center front. Enlarge the area over the abdomen and make the darts deeper by cutting through the center of the released waistline darts to within 1″ of the hem edge (or to knee on pants). Cut again from side seam to side seam just below the dart points. Spread cuts the amount needed, keeping center front line straight; fill in spaces with fabric scraps. Pin darts back in, using the original stitching lines. (Darts will be much deeper; if they are very deep, make two darts instead of one.)
Alteration: Carefully transfer the changes to master pattern by cutting and spreading it to match shell.

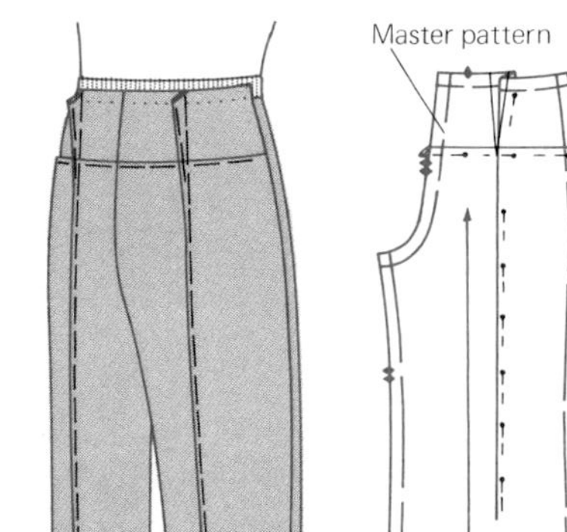

Shell "caves in" at abdomen. If abdomen is very flat, the skirt may droop in front; pants may wrinkle.
Solution: Release darts nearest to center front. Reduce the fabric over the abdomen and make the darts shallower by taking a tuck through the center of the dart that tapers to within 1″ of hem edge (or to knee on pants). Take another tuck from side seam to side seam, just below dart points. When satisfied that enough excess has been removed, baste the tucks in place and pin the darts back in (if they were not eliminated in tuck), using original stitching lines. Darts will be shallower.
Alteration: Carefully transfer changes by tucking pattern to match shell. Taper horizontal tuck to nothing at side seams. Re-draw darts, using original stitch lines.

Skirt or pants side seam

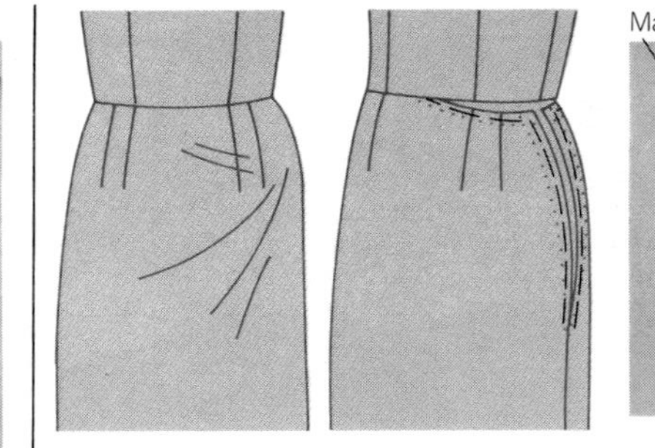

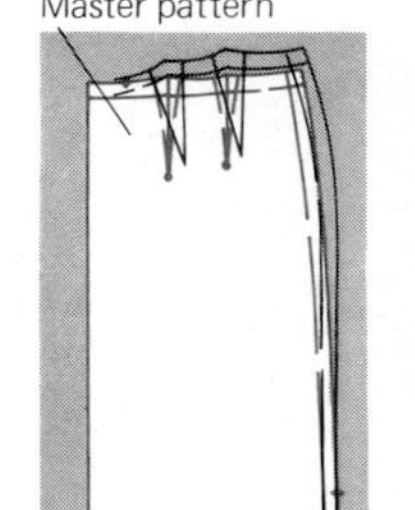

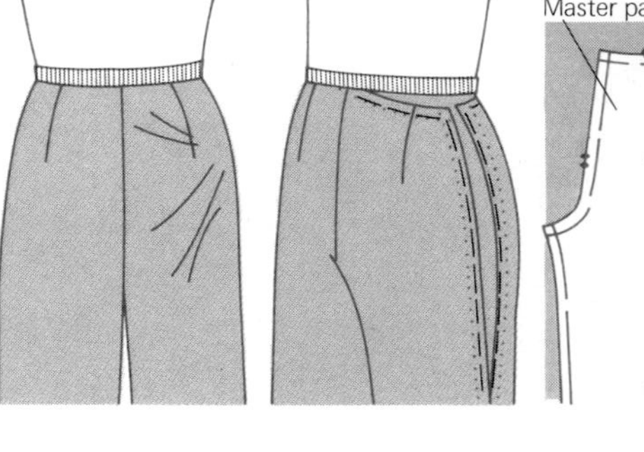

Shell pulls on one side of the body because one hip is higher or larger than the other.
Solution: For a slight adjustment, let out the waist and side seams and fit the darts to the figure contours. Do this in front and back. For a major adjustment, cut and spread the shell across the hipline as shown below. Do this in addition to the dart and seam adjustments described for slight adjustment.
Alteration: Transfer the shell changes by drawing new cutting and stitching lines. Label the alteration as for right or left side. For a major alteration, make a separate pattern piece for the affected side.

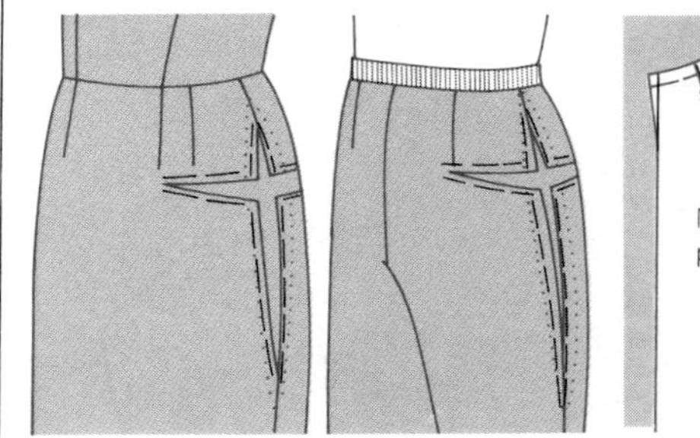

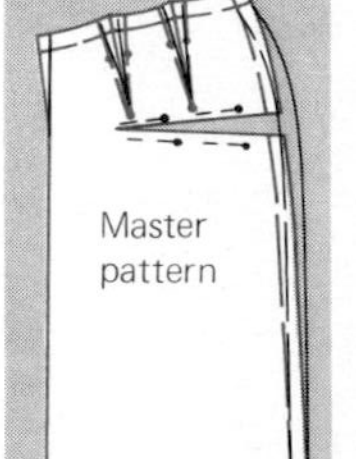

Skirt or pants back

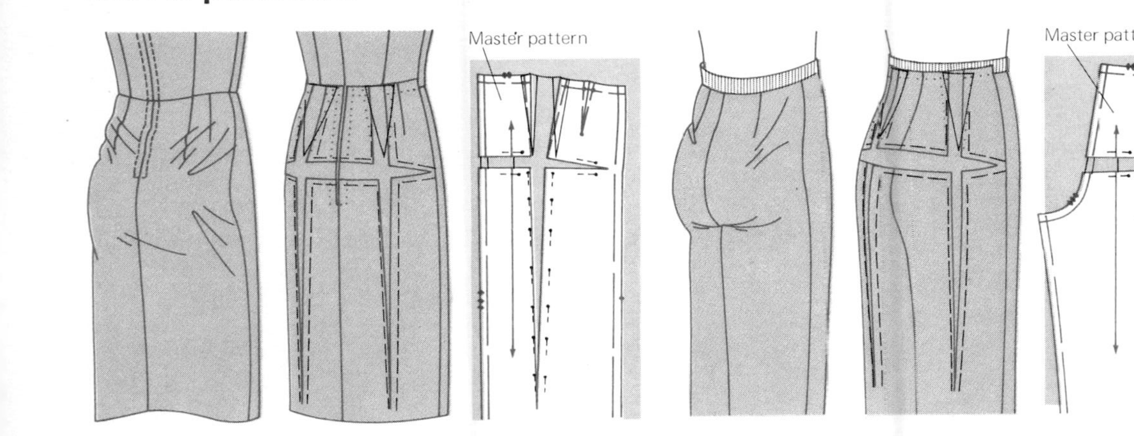

Shell is too tight in back only. Skirt may be wrinkled below the waist; pants wrinkle at the crotch.
Solution: Release the darts nearest center back. Enlarge the area over the buttocks and make the darts deeper by cutting through the center of the released waistline darts to within 1″ of the hem edge (or to knee on pants). Cut again from side seam to side seam just below the dart points. Spread cuts the amount needed, keeping center back line straight, and fill in the spaces with fabric scraps. Pin the darts back in, using the original stitching lines. (Darts will be much deeper; if they are very deep, make two darts instead of one.)
Alteration: Carefully transfer changes to the master pattern by cutting and spreading it to match shell.

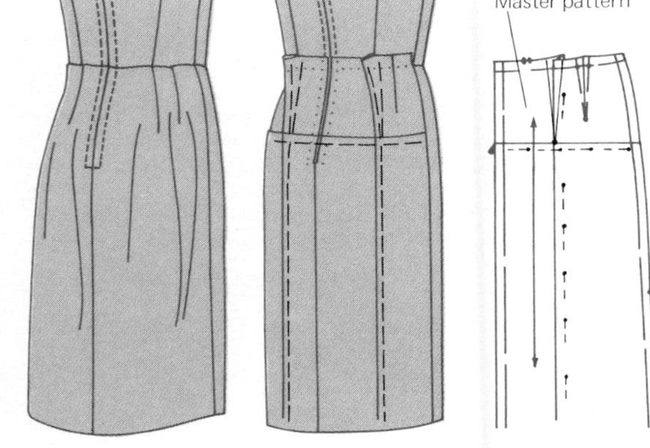

Shell is too loose in back only. Skirt will collapse in the back and the hem may droop. Pants are inclined to wrinkle from sagging at the crotch.
Solution: Release darts nearest center back. Reduce the amount of fabric over the buttocks and make the darts shallower by taking a tuck through the center of the dart that tapers to within 1″ of hem edge (or to knee on pants). Take another tuck from side seam to side seam, just below dart points. When satisfied that enough excess has been removed, baste tucks in place and pin darts back in (if not eliminated in the tuck), using original stitching lines. Darts will be much shallower.
Alteration: Carefully transfer the changes by tucking pattern to match shell. Re-draw darts.

Pants legs

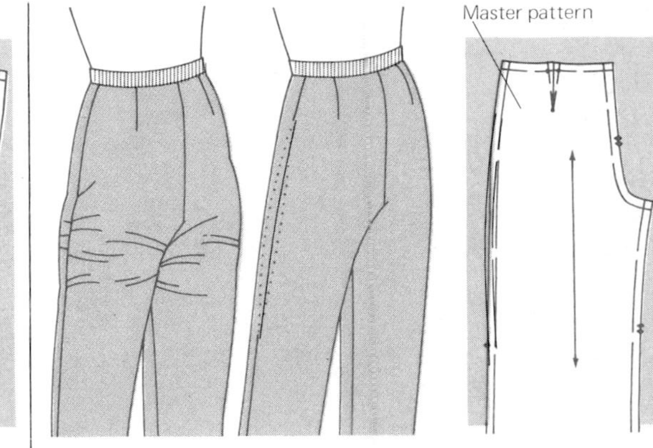

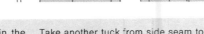

Pants legs are too tight at thigh.
Solution: Let out side seams until shell fits smoothly; taper addition to nothing at hip and knee.
Alteration: Transfer the changes made in the shell by drawing new cutting and stitching lines on the pants back and front patterns. Divide increase equally among front and back side seams.

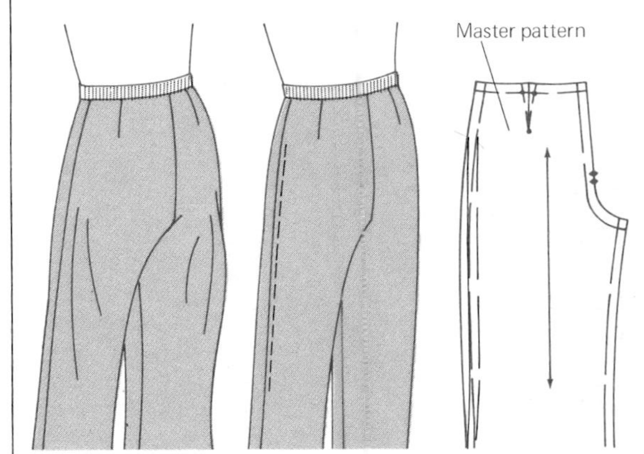

Pants legs are too loose at thigh.
Solution: Take in side seams until shell fits smoothly; taper reduction to nothing at hips and knee.
Alteration: Transfer the changes made in the shell by drawing new cutting and stitching lines on the pants back and front patterns. Divide the reduction equally among front and back seams.

Fitting shell and master pattern

How to use the master pattern

When the shell has been adjusted to solve all fitting problems to your satisfaction, you are ready to transfer the adjustments to the pattern pieces from which the shell was made. The adjusted pieces are your master pattern. For future reference, note on the master pattern each amount you have added or taken away. When adding to the pattern, use tissue paper and transparent tape.

Label any asymmetrical pattern alterations as to whether they are for the right or the left side. Later, you can cut out on the line for the larger side and, with dressmaker's carbon paper and tracing wheel, mark the differing stitching lines for each side. If this is impractical, as it will be when one hip is much higher than the other, make separate patterns for right and left sides and cut pattern pieces from single layers of fabric.

Back your altered master pattern with non-woven, iron-on interfacing; this will make it durable. Keep your fitting shell and try it on from time to time. If you find you need to make new adjustments because of figure changes, you can easily alter your master pattern.

To use the master pattern with other patterns, follow this two-step suggestion. First place the master pattern under related pieces of the new pattern and check for **length** adjustments. Align the new pattern with the master at shoulders or underarm if a bodice or a dress, at waistline if a skirt or pants. Make all of the needed length adjustments. Then put the new pattern over the master again and match up the waistlines. Check for **width** adjustments at bust, waist, and hip. Also make sure that **darts** are correctly positioned. Other specialized alterations, such as high hip, gaping neckline, etc., should be noted at this time.

The basic fitting sheath, although it consists of a separate bodice and straight skirt, can be used to check the fit of almost any style of garment. For example, if you want to test the fit of a dress that has no waistline seam, lap the waist seamlines of the master bodice and skirt (keeping a straight line at center front), then lay the new pattern on top of the master. If your new pattern has a shoulder yoke, lap the seamlines of the bodice and yoke and pin in place; then slip master pattern underneath and see where alterations will be needed.

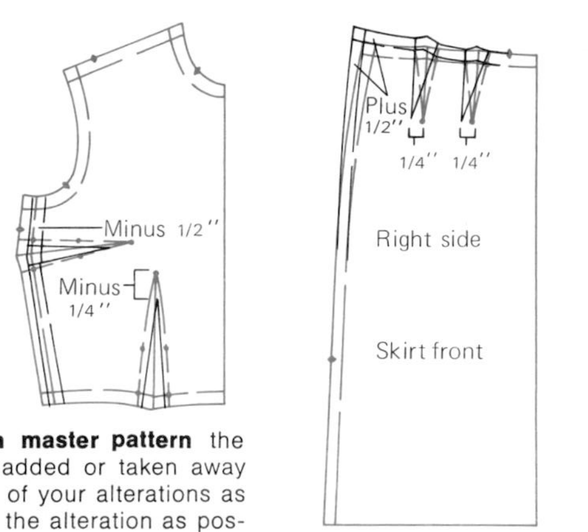

Note on master pattern the amount added or taken away by each of your alterations as close to the alteration as possible. This will be useful for future reference, and avoid any possible confusion about the nature and extent of individual alterations.

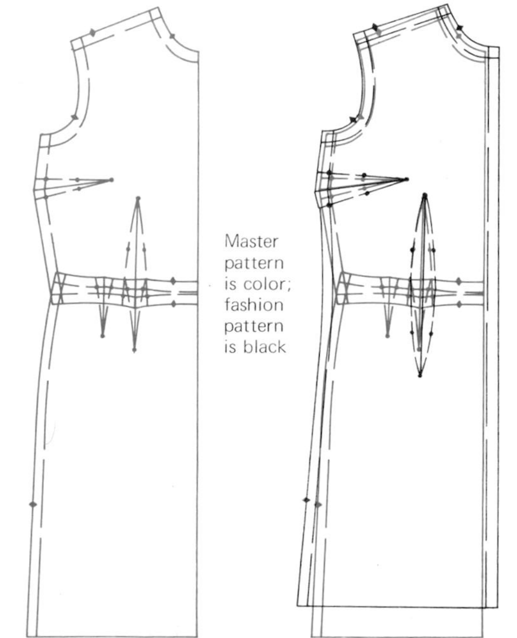

Master pattern is color; fashion pattern is black

Using the master with other patterns is a very simple procedure. Simply slip master pattern piece underneath the appropriate piece from new pattern; match up center fronts or center backs and other key points. You will be able to see clearly where the new pattern requires alteration.

The try-on fitting

It is wise to try on any garment as soon as the major seams have been stitched. Some fine adjustments can only be seen when fabric and pattern meet. This is a good time, too, to make minor seam and dart adjustments that may still be needed.

Schedule a try-on fitting when back and front have been joined at sides and shoulders; underlining and interfacing are in place. Staystitch armholes and necklines so they won't stretch; expect these openings to be snug because of extended seam allowances. Pin up hems. Lap and pin openings.

Try on pants and skirts before the waistband is attached. Staystitch at waist to prevent stretching.

To get a clear and accurate picture of fit, wear appropriate shoes and undergarments. Remember also to try your garment on right side out.

Machine-baste sections together for this fitting. It will be easier to make changes. If your fabric is too delicate for machine stitching, pin-baste instead, placing the pins a few inches apart on the right side along stitching lines.

If your fabric has worked up somewhat differently than the fabric the designer had in mind, you may have to take in or let out some seams. Work from the shoulders down, adjusting darts, if you must, along the way. Pin in place all patch pockets, flaps, etc., to check their positions.

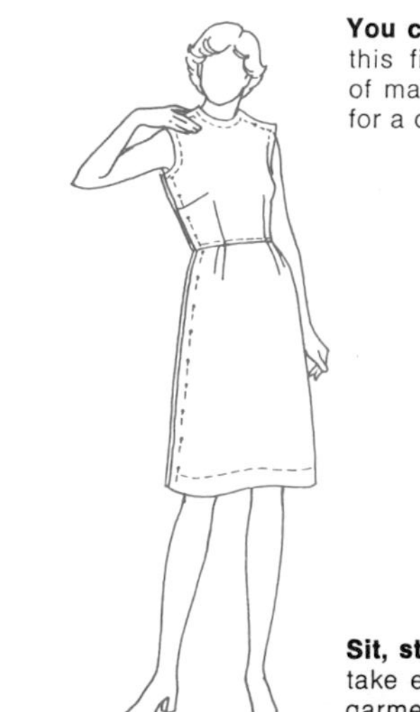

You can pin- or machine-baste for this fitting if there is a possibility of many changes. Pinning is better for a delicate fabric.

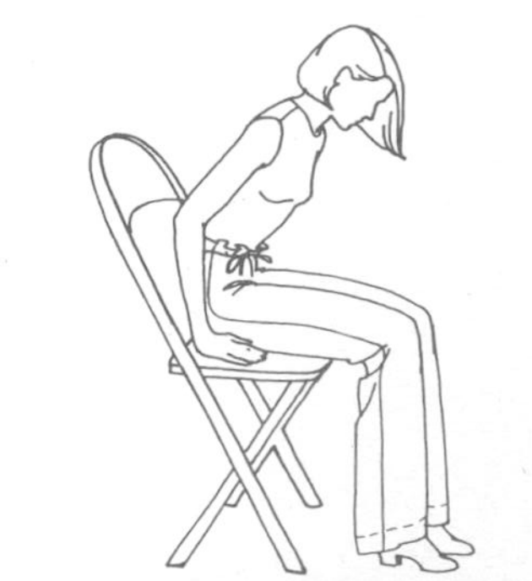

Sit, stand, walk, bend, and reach—take every relevant position in your garment to thoroughly test its fit.

Finer points (to adjust in try-on fitting)

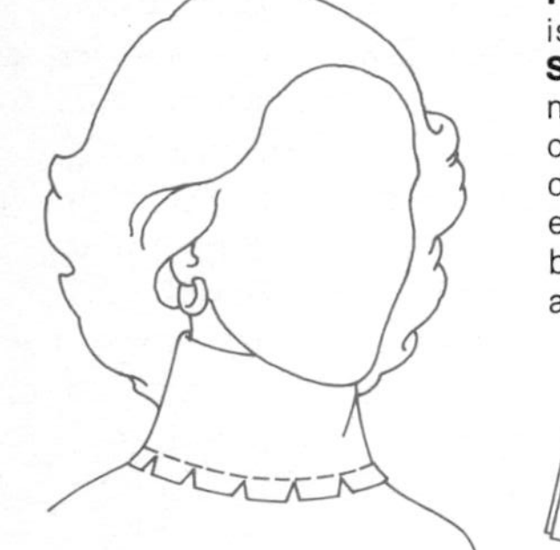

Problem: A stand-up collar is too high.
Solution: Adjust the collar, not the neckline. If the collar is shaped, re-stitch a deeper seam along the top edge. If collar is a folded bias band, take deeper seam at neckline edge of collar only.

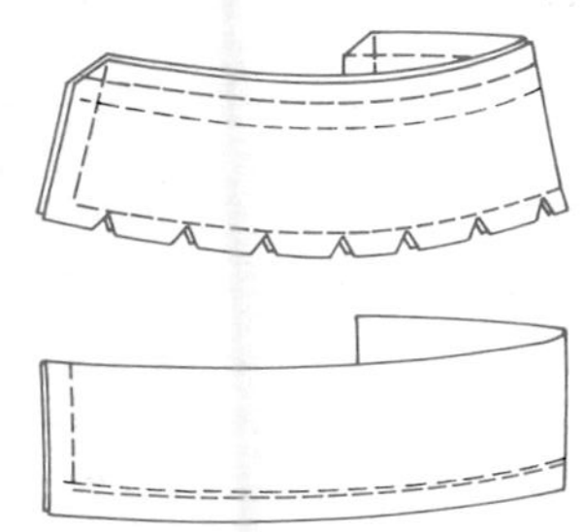

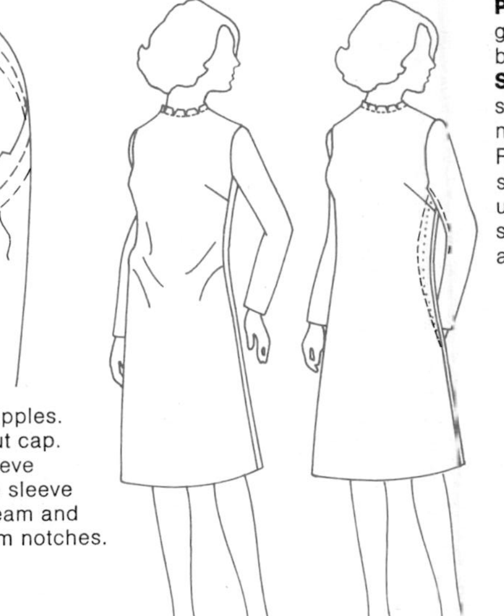

Problem: Toc much ease in sleeve cap; material ripples.
Solution: Remove s eeve from garment; smooth out cap. Easestitch ⅛″ from seamline, within cap area (sleeve cap seam allcwance now measures ¾″). Re-baste sleeve to armhole, aligning new ease line with armhole seam and maintaining ⅝″ seam allowance between underarm notches.

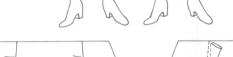

Problem: A stretchy knit garment ends up too big through the middle.
Solution: Take in side seams for a closer (but not too close) fit. Remember to deepen seam allowance on sleeve underarm seams so that sleeve and bodice armholes will match.

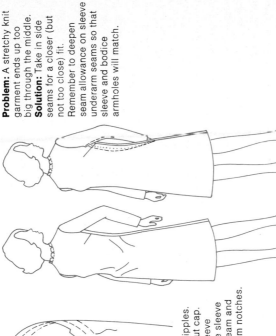

Problem: A low U- or V-shaped neckline gapes.
Solution: Lift bodice front at shoulder near neck to remove excess fabric between bust apex and shoulder. Taper adjustment to nothing at the armhole. Alter the neckline facing to match.

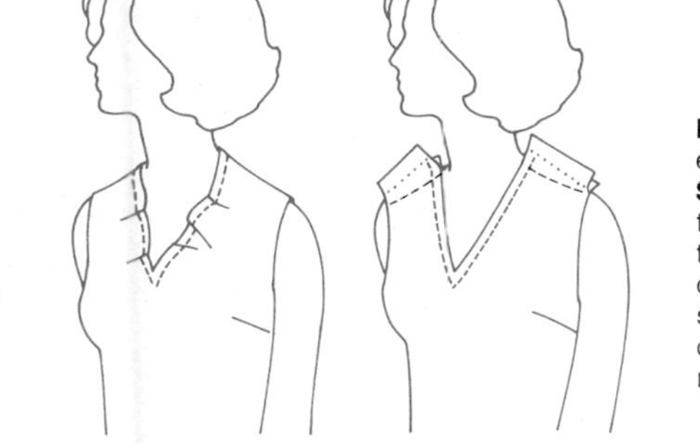

Problem: Wrinkling on either side of darts.
Solution: Darts may be too straight to conform to your figure. Re-stitch da'ts, curving them slightly inward. Taper carefully to points. Darts may need shortening.

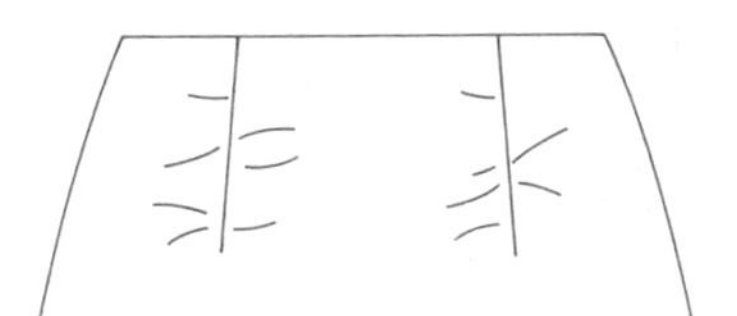

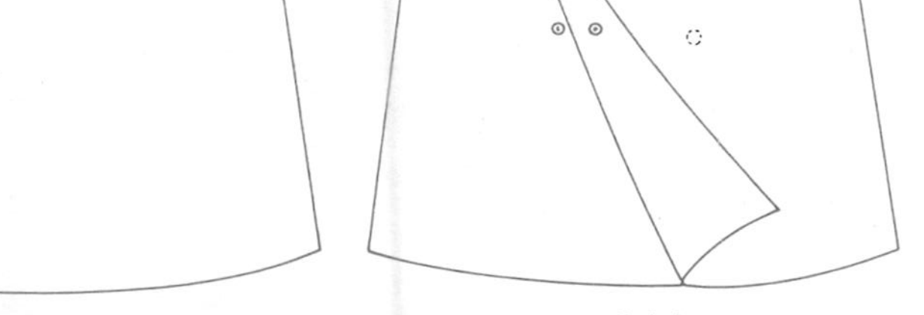

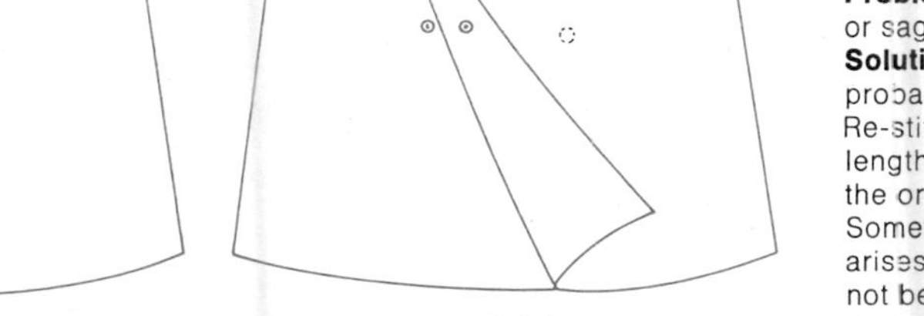

Problem: Front opening, or lapped edge on wrap skirt, sags slightly.
Solution: First try re-pinning the hem. If unevenness is extreme, or if it is back fold that sags, try correcting by raising waist seamline in sagging areas until hem is even. A third possibility: support the sagging edge with concealed snaps (particularly good if fabric must be matched crosswise).

Problem: Fabric bulges or sags below the dart.
Solution: Darts are proɔably too short. Re-stitch to a longer length, maintaining the original width. Sometimes this problem arises when dart has not been tapered smoothly to point in stitching. Re-stitch.

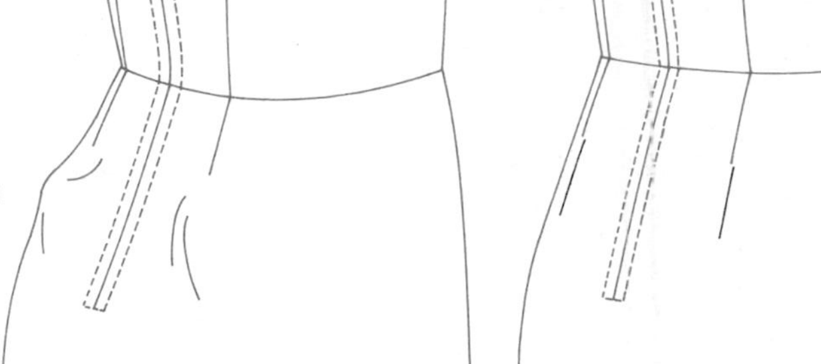

The test garment

When to make a test garment

If you approach a new sewing project with any uncertainty, it can be well worth the time it takes to make up the pattern you have chosen in a less expensive fabric than the one you plan to use. This test garment can prevent costly mistakes and disappointments in the actual garment.

Several considerations may suggest the advisability of a test garment. Perhaps the **fabric** is an expensive or unusual one, such as a beaded knit or bridal lace. Or it may require special treatment during sewing. Leathers and vinyls, for example, show pin and needle marks, which makes it impossible to fit them after cutting. Still another difficulty may be the design—a large scale or border print, or an intricate plaid. By penciling the motif onto a test fabric, you can determine design placement before cutting the real fabric.

Sometimes the **pattern** is the problem. It may be a more intricate style than you are accustomed to, or a silhouette you have never worn. A test garment lets you practice new or complicated techniques in advance, check the suitability of the style to your figure, and make sure of the accuracy of any pattern alterations you have made.

Choose a test fabric as close as possible in weight and draping properties to your final fabric—except if the garment is to be underlined. When this is the case, construct your mock-up of underlining fabric, make your adjustments in it, then take it apart for use as a sewing guide.

On test garments, you can eliminate facings, collars and pockets, and, if you are fairly sure of their fit, the sleeves. If you like the garment in the substitute fabric, you can finish it later.

An intricate style can pose problems of many kinds. In this hypothetical dress design, not only do the parts go together in an unusual way, but welt seaming is featured throughout. A test garment would give advance practice in all steps, avoiding costly mistakes in cutting and sewing actual fabric.

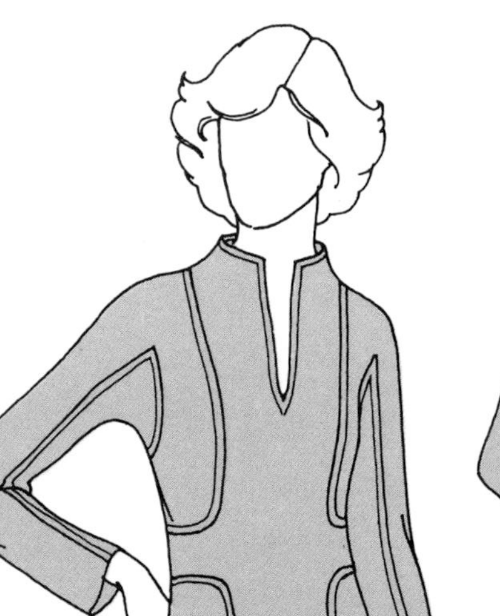

Fashion trends often incorporate design variations, such as this unusual sleeve. Those who shy away from such patterns because they seem too advanced should welcome the idea of practice garments.

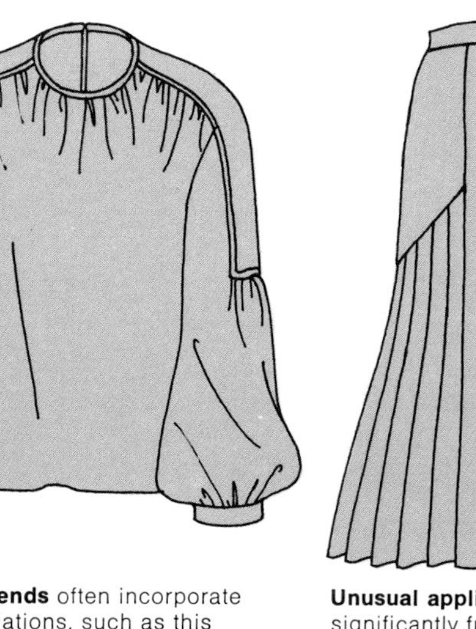

Unusual applications can deviate significantly from standard techniques, as in this pleated skirt. Your test fabric in such a situation should fold, hang, and otherwise perform as much like the final fabric as possible.

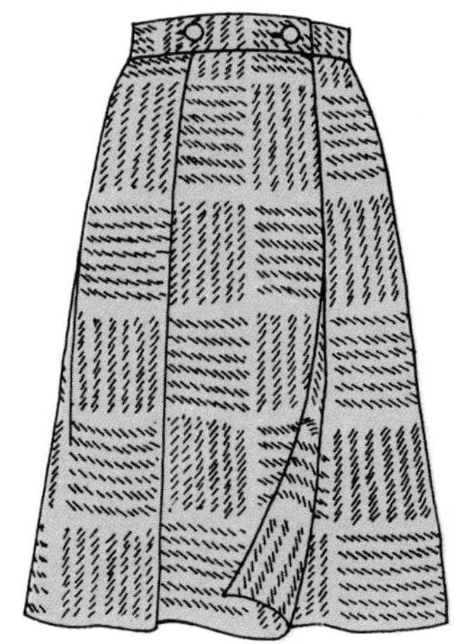

Top-quality fabrics assure the effectiveness of garments with simple lines. You can feel more confident cutting into such luxurious material if you have solved all fit problems beforehand on an inexpensive fabric.

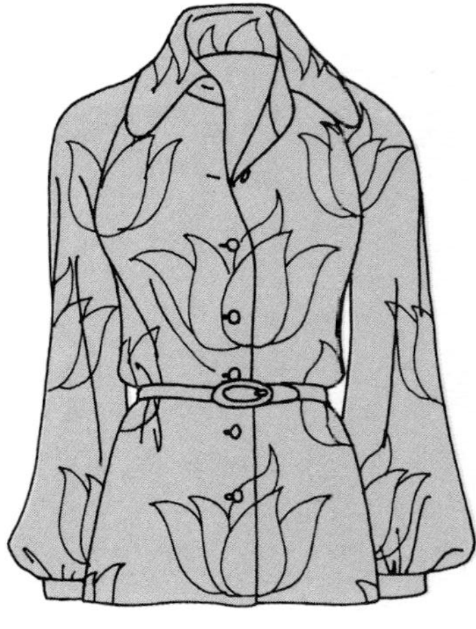

Large-scale prints call for very careful placement if they are to be striking in the way the designer intended, and flattering to the wearer. When the motif must also be matched, as it is here, a practice garment is almost indispensable.

Construction Basics

Hand sewing techniques

General suggestions

Though precise recommendations vary from one procedure to another, there are general principles that apply to hand sewing of any kind.

Threading tips: Cut thread at an angle, using sharp scissors. Never break or bite thread—this frays the end, making it difficult to pass through the eye of the needle.

To thread a needle, hold the needle in the left hand and the thread end in the right between thumb and index finger. Pass thread end through the needle eye and, with the same motion, transfer the needle to right thumb and index finger. Then, with left hand, draw thread end out from the eye about one-third of the way down the remaining thread supply.

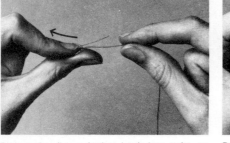

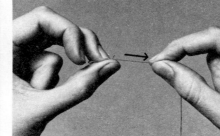

Hand-sew with a comparatively short thread. For permanent stitching, use a working length of 18 to 24 inches; for basting, the thread can be longer. (Working length is from needle eye to knot.) Except for buttons, snaps, and hooks and eyes, you will seldom need a double thread.

Needle choice: Select a hand needle that is suitable to the thread and fabric, and comfortable for you. A fine needle is best: short for short, single stitches, such as padding stitches; longer for long or multiple stitches, such as basting.

Thread color and type: For basting and thread marking, use white or a light-colored thread that contrasts with the fabric. Dark thread can leave marks on a light-colored fabric. For permanent hand stitching, thread can match or contrast as you prefer.

Silk thread is the easiest to use for hand sewing, and is especially good for basting because it will not leave an impression after pressing. Cotton, synthetic, and cotton/synthetic threads are acceptable. Silk twist is used for buttonholes and buttons, and also for some decorative hand sewing.

Twisting and knotting can be a problem in hand sewing—with any thread, but particularly with those that are made entirely, or partly, of synthetic fibers. To keep the problem to a minimum, use a short length of thread, and do not pull tightly on the thread. It is also helpful to thread the needle with the end cut from the spool and to wax the thread before starting to sew. When twisting does occur, allow the thread to untwist itself in this way: First let the thread dangle, with the needle end down, then slide your fingers gently down the thread.

Securing stitching at beginning and end

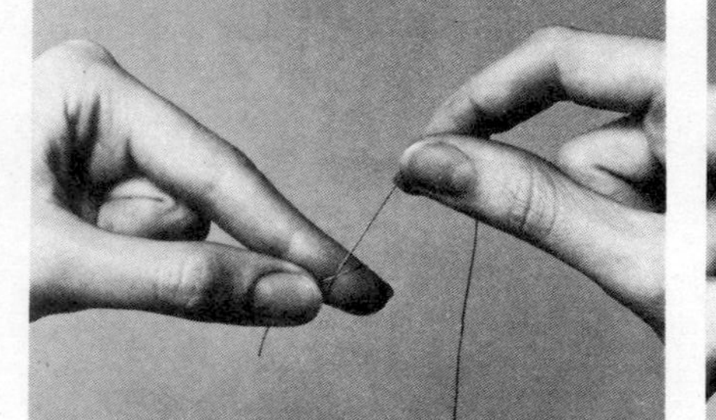

To tie a knot in a thread end, first hold end between thumb and index finger while bringing supply thread over and around finger.

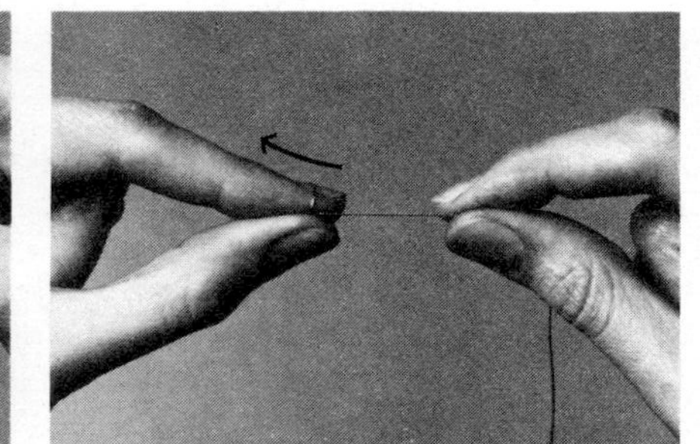

Holding supply thread taut, slide index finger along thumb toward palm. This will cause the thread end to twist into the loop.

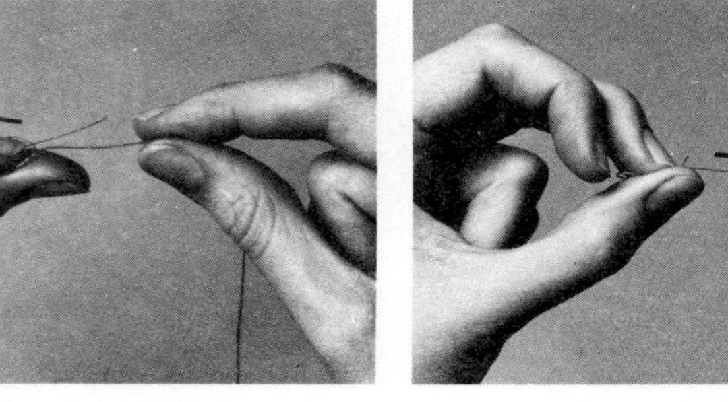

Slide index finger farther back into palm so that the loop will slide off finger. Hold open loop between tip of index finger and thumb.

Bring middle finger down to rest on and hold the open loop. Pull on supply thread to make loop smaller and form the knot.

Knot at beginning: Most hand stitching is secured at the beginning with a knot at the end of the thread. In basting, the knot can be visible; in permanent stitching, it should be placed out of sight against an inside layer. At the left is shown a step-by-step procedure for tying a knot. The usual way is to thread the needle with one end, then knot the other.

Backstitching can also be used to secure the beginning as well as the end of a row of stitches. Sometimes it is even preferable to a knot, especially in garment areas where a knot could leave an indentation after pressing. A typical instance is in tailoring, where a thread knot within a section that has been padstitched would show on the right side.

The shorter the backstitch, the more secure it will be. In general, use a short backstitch to secure permanent stitches and a long backstitch to secure those that will be removed, such as basting. For a very secure finish, use a backstitch in combination with a loop, as shown below.

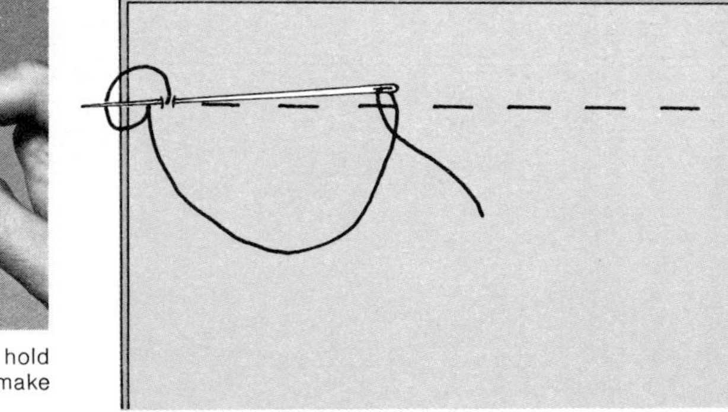

To secure thread at the end of a row of stitching, bring needle and thread to the underside. Take one small stitch behind thread, catching only a single yarn of the fabric. Pull needle and thread through, leaving a small thread loop. Take another short backstitch in the same place, but pass needle and thread through loop of first stitch. Pull both stitches close to fabric; cut thread.

Glossary of hand stitches

Arrowhead tack / Backstitch

ARROWHEAD TACK see **Tacks** (construction)

BACKSTITCH
One of the strongest and most versatile of the hand stitches, the backstitch serves to secure hand stitching and repair seams; for hand-understitching, topstitching, and handpicking zippers. Though there are several variations, each is formed by inserting needle behind point where thread emerges from previous stitch. **The beginning or end** of a row of hand stitching can be secured with a backstitch. Fasten permanent stitching with a short backstitch; use a long backstitch to secure stitches that will be removed. A more secure finish combines the backstitch with a loop through which the stitch is fastened.

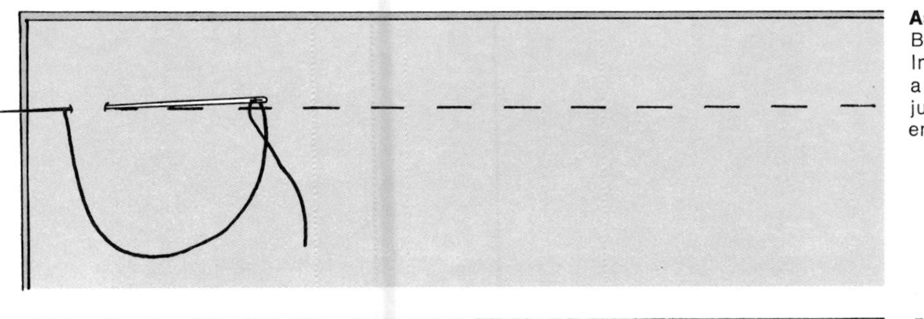

As a beginning or end in hand stitching: Bring needle and thread to underside. Insert needle through all fabric layers a stitch length *behind* and bring it up just in *back* of point where thread emerges. Pull thread through.

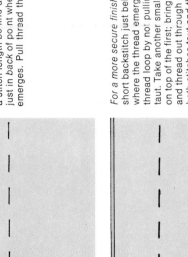

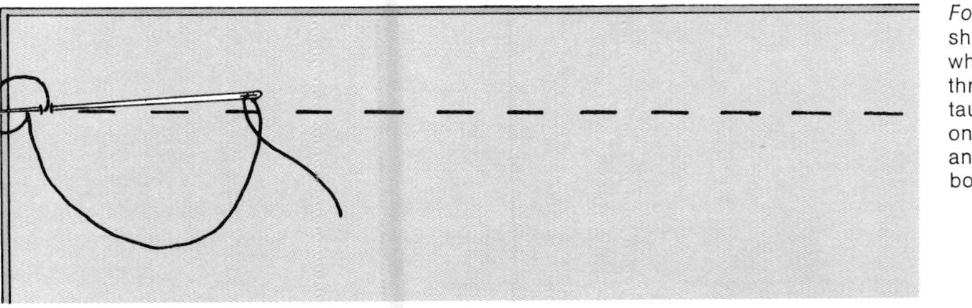

For a more secure finish, take a very short backstitch just behind the point where the thread emerges, but leave a thread loop by not pulling the stitch taut. Take another small backstitch on top of the first; bring the needle and thread out through the loop. Pull both stitches taut and then cut thread.

Even backstitch is the strongest of the backstitches. The stitches look much like machine stitching; that is, they are even in length with very little space between them. Stitch is used mainly to make and repair seams.

Even backstitch: Bring needle and thread to upper side. Insert needle through all fabric layers approximately $\frac{1}{16}$" to $\frac{1}{8}$" (*one-half* a stitch length) behind the point where the thread emerges, and bring needle and thread out the *same* distance in front of that point. Continue inserting and bringing up needle and thread one-half a stitch length behind and in front of the thread from the previous stitch. From top side, finished stitches look similar to straight machine stitching.

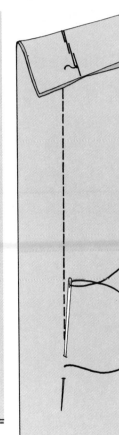

Half-backstitch is similar to the even backstitch except that length of stitches and space between them are equal. Although not as strong as the even backstitch, this stitch can be used to repair a seam.

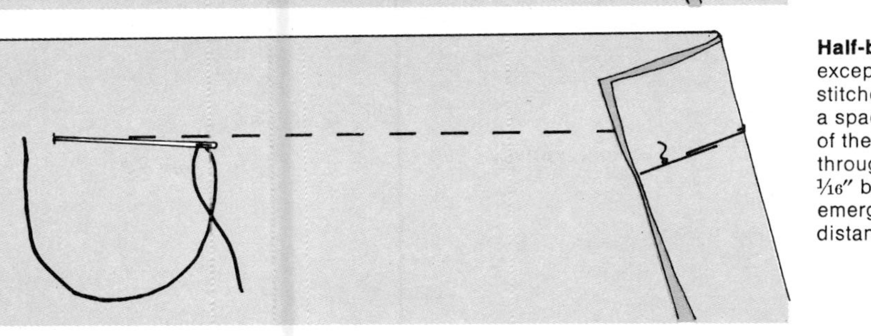

Half-backstitch: Similar to even backstitch except that, instead of finished stitches meeting on top side, there is a space between them equal to the length of the stitches. Needle is inserted through all fabric layers approximately $\frac{1}{16}$" behind the point where the thread emerges, but is brought out *twice* this distance ($\frac{1}{8}$") in front of that point.

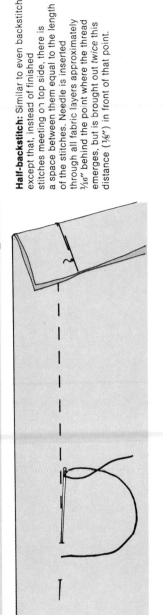

Glossary of hand stitches

Hand understitching 147
Hand-picking zippers 319, 323

Backstitching / Basting

Prickstitch is a much more decorative backstitch than the even or the half-backstitch. Seen from the top side, the stitches are very short, with long spaces between them. This stitch is mainly used to hand-pick a zipper.

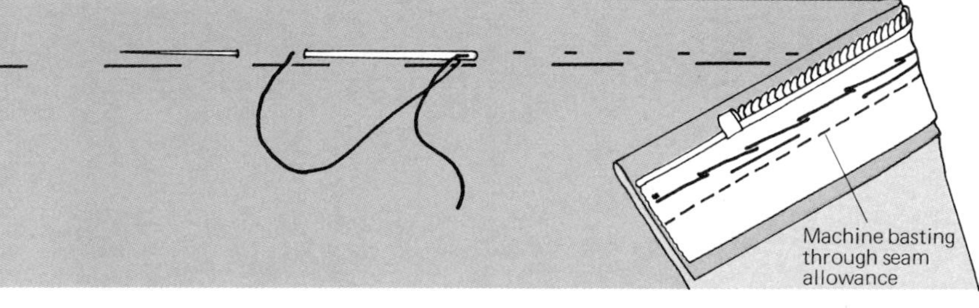

Prickstitch: Similar to half-backstitch except that the needle is inserted through all fabric layers *just a few fabric threads* behind and then brought up approximately ⅛″ to ¼″ in front of the point where thread emerges. Finished stitches on the top side are very short, with ⅛″ to ¼″ space between them.

Pickstitch can look like any of the backstitches; the only difference is that the stitch is not taken through to the underlayer of fabric. Primarily a decorative backstitch, it is ideal for topstitching and hand-understitching, where only the top part of the stitch should be seen.

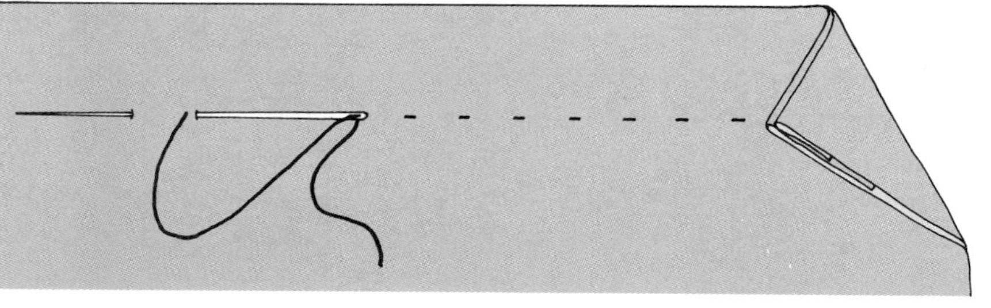

Pickstitch: Any of the backstitches but *made without catching underlayer* of fabric. When the underlayer is not caught, underpart of stitch becomes invisible.

BAR TACK see **Tacks** (construction)

BASTING
Hand basting is used to temporarily hold together two or more fabric layers during fitting and construction. **Even basting** is used on smooth fabrics and in areas that require close control, such as curved seams, seams with ease, and set-in sleeves.

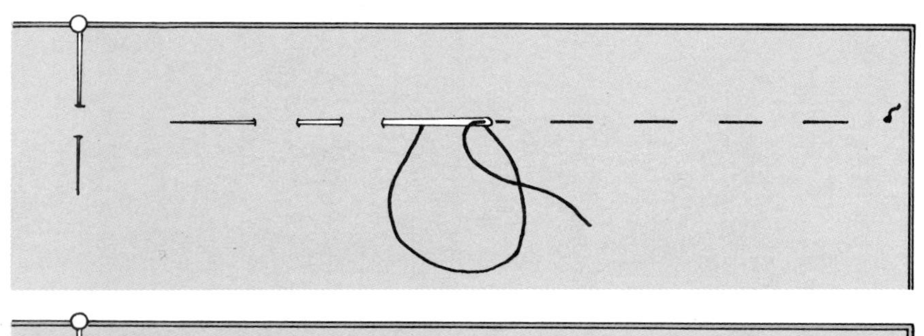

Even basting: Short (about ¼″) temporary stitches, taken the *same distance* apart. Working from right to left, take several evenly spaced stitches onto the needle before pulling it through.

Uneven basting is used for general basting, for edges that require less control during permanent stitching, and for marking (marking stitches can be long and spaced far apart).

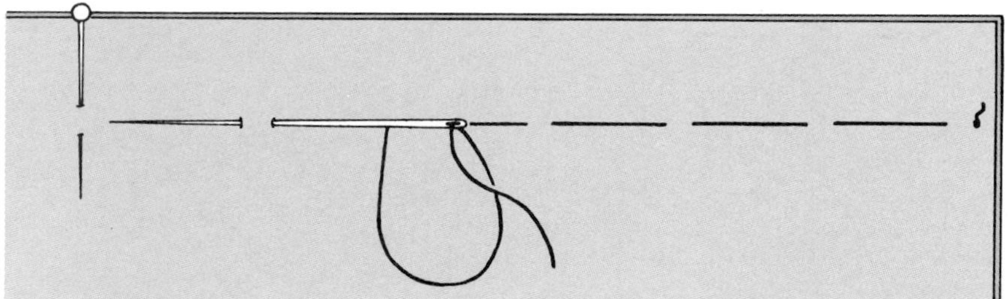

Uneven basting: Like even basting, these are short temporary stitches, about ¼″ long, but taken about 1″ apart.

Basting / Blanket stitch

Diagonal basting consists of horizontal stitches taken parallel to each other and producing diagonal floats in between. It is used to hold or control fabric layers within an area during construction and pressing. Short stitches, taken close together, give more control than do longer stitches taken farther apart. The *short* diagonal basting is used to hold seam edges flat during stitching or pressing; the *long* diagonal basting, for such steps as holding underlining to garment fabric during construction.

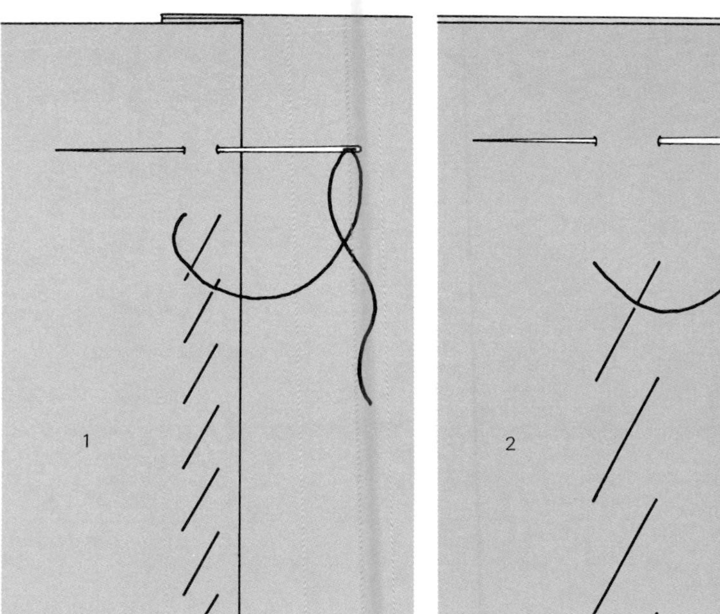

Diagonal basting: Small stitches, taken parallel to each other, producing diagonal floats in between. When making the stitches, the needle points from right to left. For greater control, take short stitches (1), spaced close together. Where less control is needed, stitches can be longer (2), with more space in between them.

Slip basting is a temporary, uneven slipstitch that permits precise matching of plaids, stripes, and some large prints at seamlines. It is also a practical way to baste intricately curved sections, or to make fitting adjustments from right side.

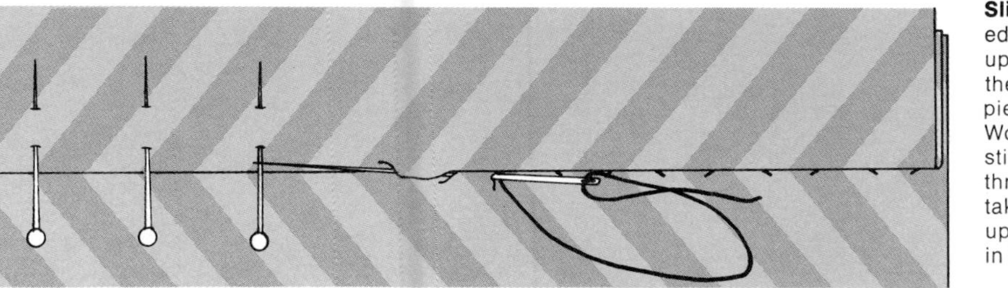

Slip basting: Crease and turn under one edge along its seamline. With right sides up, lay the folded edge in position along the seamline of the corresponding garment piece, matching the fabric design; pin. Working from right to left and using stitches ¼" in length, take a stitch through the lower garment section, then take the next stitch through fold of upper edge. Continue to alternate stitches in this way, removing pins as you go.

BLANKET STITCH

Traditionally an embroidery stitch, the blanket stitch can also be used in garment construction. It often serves, as in the illustration, to cover fabric edges decoratively. Another use is in construction details. A bar tack is formed, for example, by working the stitch over threads.

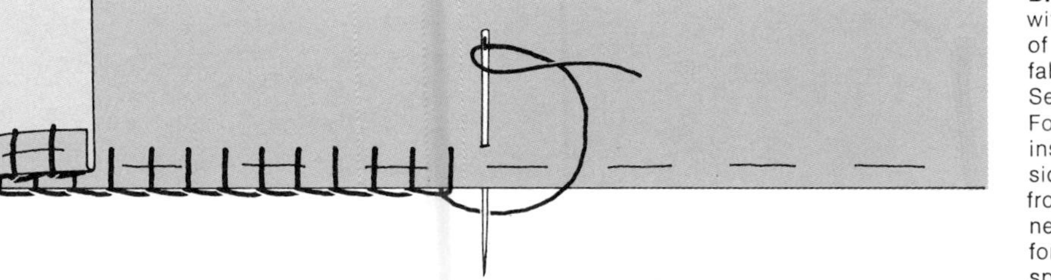

Blanket stitch: Work from left to right, with the point of the needle and the edge of the work toward you. The edge of the fabric can be folded under or left raw. Secure thread and bring out below edge. For the first and each succeeding stitch, insert needle through fabric from right side and bring out at edge. Keeping thread from previous stitch *under* point of needle, draw needle and thread through, forming stitch over edge. Stitch size and spacing can be the same or varied.

Glossary of hand stitches

Blanket-stitch tack / Chainstitch

BLANKET-STITCH TACK — see **Tacks** (construction)

BLIND-HEMMING STITCH — see **Hemming** (blind)

BUTTONHOLE STITCH
A "covering" stitch used as a decorative finish and in the making of hand-worked buttonholes.

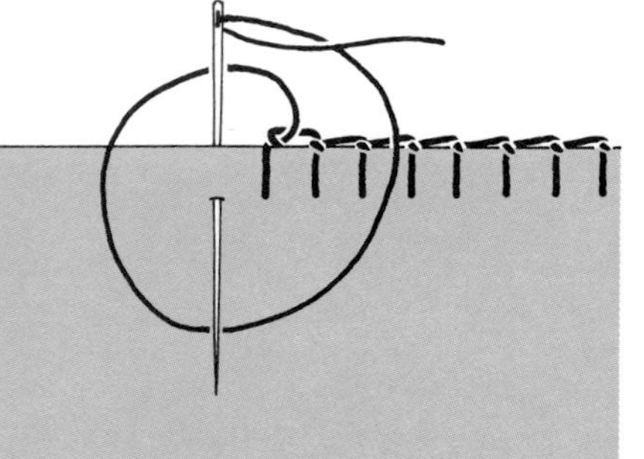

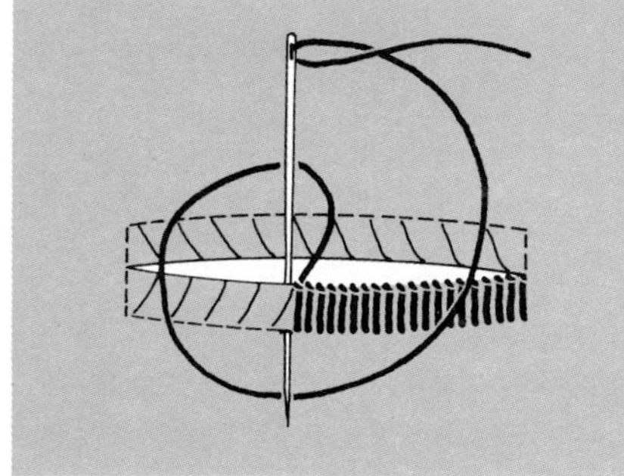

Buttonhole stitch: Work from right to left, with point of needle toward you but edge of fabric away from you. Fasten thread and bring out above the edge. For first and each succeeding stitch, loop thread from previous stitch to left, then down to right. Insert needle from underside, keeping looped thread *under* both *point and eye* of needle. Pull needle out through fabric, then *away* from you to place the purl of the stitch on the fabric's edge. Stitch depth and spacing can be large or small, depending on fabric and circumstance.
For hand-worked buttonholes: Follow basic directions for buttonhole stitch, making stitches ⅛" deep with no space between.

CATCHSTITCH — see **Hemming** (blind and flat)

CATCHSTITCH TACK — see **Tacks** (construction)

CHAINSTITCH
A continuous series of looped stitches that form a chain. Can be used decoratively, as illustrated at right, on clothing, linens, lingerie. Takes a more functional form in the thread chain shown and described below.

Chainstitch: Work from right to left. Fasten thread and bring up to right side. For each stitch, loop the thread up and around; insert needle just behind where thread emerges and bring it up, over the looped thread, a stitch length in front of that point. Pull thread through, to the left, to form looped stitch.

A thread chain can serve as a belt carrier, thread eye, or button loop, or as an alternative to the French tack. It can be as long as needed. The chain may be fastened to lie flat against the garment, or given a looped shape by making the chain longer than the distance between the markings that indicate its beginning and end.

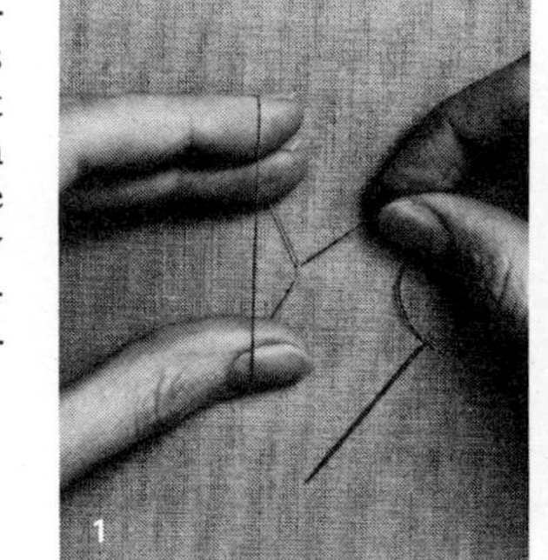

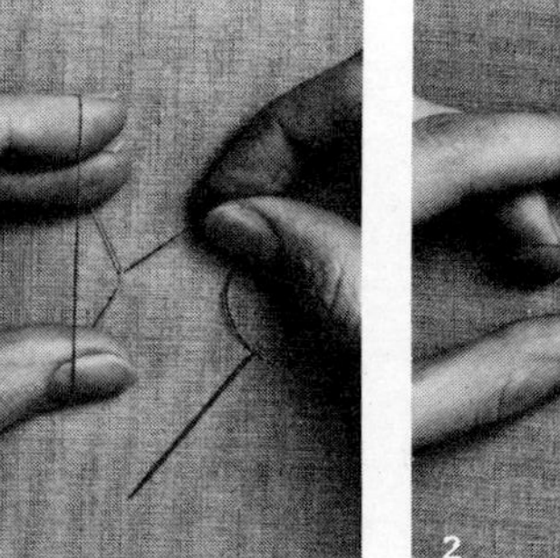

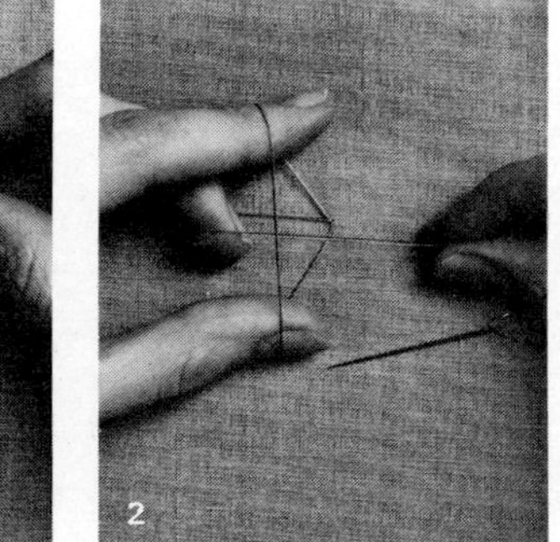

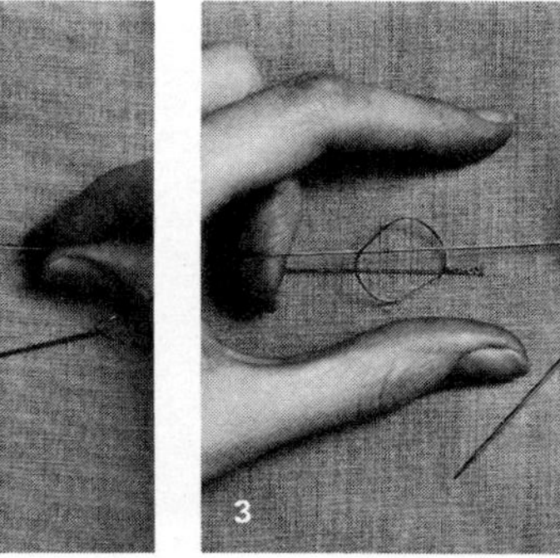

Thread chain: Mark on garment where chain begins and will be fastened. At beginning mark, take a small stitch and draw thread through, leaving a 4" to 5" loop. Hold loop open with thumb and first two fingers of left hand; hold supply thread with right thumb and index finger (1). Reach through and grasp supply thread with second finger of left hand to start new loop (2). As you pull new loop through, the first loop will slide off other fingers and become smaller as it is drawn down to fabric (3). Position new loop as in 1; continue chaining to desired length. To secure, slip needle through last loop and fasten.

Cross stitch / Fagoting stitch

CROSS STITCH
Horizontal stitches, taken parallel to each other, whose floats cross in the center to form X's. Can be used decoratively or constructively, either in a series, as shown at the right, or as a single cross stitch.

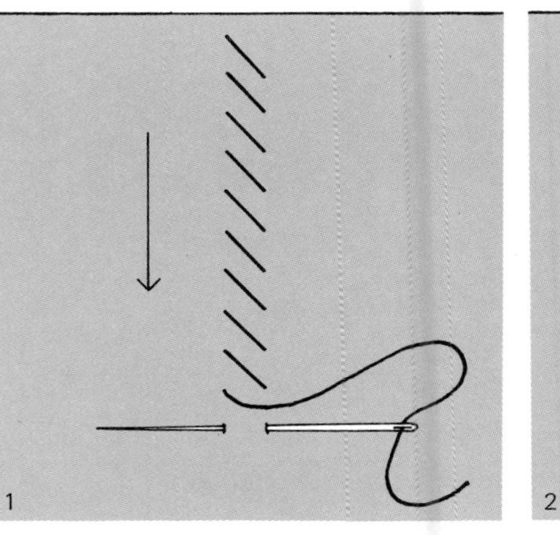

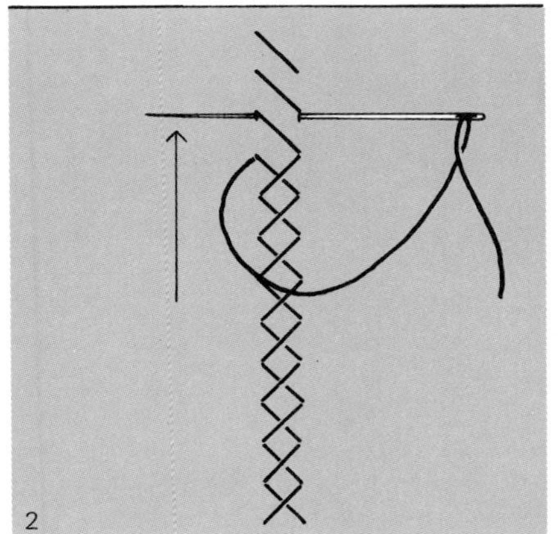

Cross stitch: Working from top to bottom (1) with needle pointing left, make row of small horizontal stitches spaced as far apart as they are long. Pull the thread firmly but not taut. This produces diagonal floats between stitches. When the row is finished, *reverse direction*, working stitches from bottom to top (2), still with needle pointing left. Thread floats should cross in the middle, forming "X's".

CROSS-STITCH TACK — see **Tacks** (construction)

DIAGONAL BASTING — see **Basting**

EVEN BACKSTITCH — see **Backstitch**

EVEN BASTING — see **Basting**

EVEN SLIPSTITCH — see **Slipstitch**

FAGOTING STITCH
A decorative stitch used to join two fabric sections, leaving a space in between. As a rule, fagoting should be used only in those areas where there will be little strain, such as yoke sections or bands near the bottom of a skirt. Fabric edges must be folded back accurately so as to maintain the position of the original seamline, which, after fagoting, should be at the center of space between folded edges.

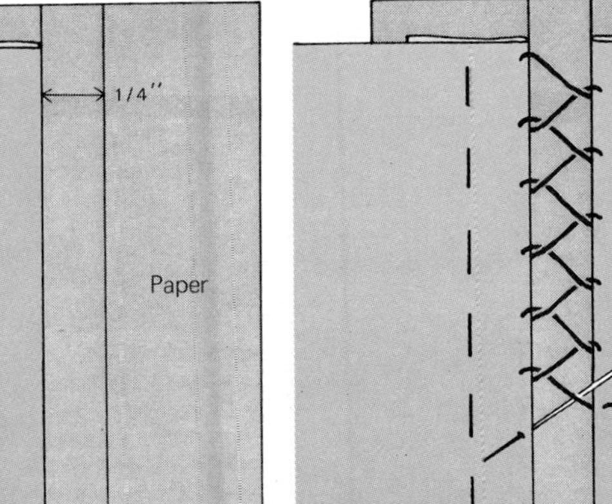

Fagoting stitch: On paper, draw parallel lines to represent width of opening between folded-back fabric edges (usually ¼"). Fold each seamline back by half this measurement, then pin and baste each edge to paper along parallel lines. Fasten thread and bring up through one folded edge. Carry thread diagonally across opening and insert needle up through opposite fold; pull thread through. Pass needle *under* thread, diagonally across opening, and up through opposite fold. Continue in this way along entire opening, spacing stitches evenly. When finished, remove paper and press seam.

Glossary of hand stitches

Featherstitch / Hemming stitches

FEATHERSTITCH
Primarily decorative, the featherstitch is made up of a series of stitches taken on alternate sides of a given line.

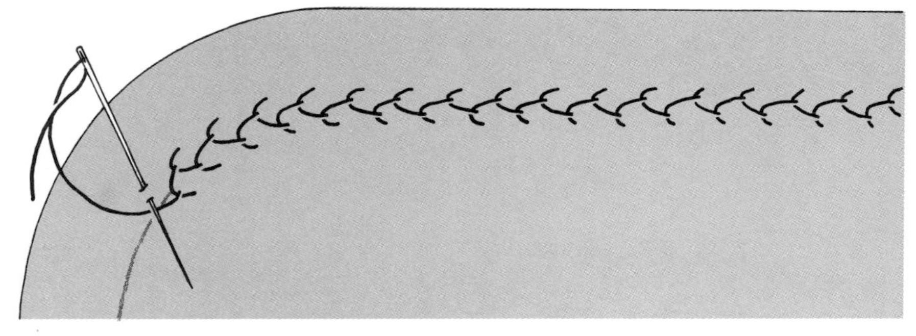

Featherstitch: Mark line stitching is to follow on right side of fabric. Fasten thread on underside of stitch line and bring up to right side of fabric. For first and each succeeding stitch, pass needle and thread diagonally *across* line to *opposite* side. Holding thread in place, and with needle pointing down and diagonally toward line, take a small stitch above thread, bringing point of needle out *on top* of thread. Draw on stitch so it is taut but loose enough that thread under it curves slightly. Continue making stitches on opposite sides of line, keeping stitch length, spacing, and needle slant the same.

FRENCH TACK see **Tacks** (construction)

HALF-BACKSTITCH see **Backstitch**

HEAVY-DUTY TACK see **Tacks** (construction)

HEMMING STITCHES
Used to secure a hem edge to a garment. Depending on the situation, the choice will be either a *flat* or *blind* hemming technique.

HEMMING STITCHES, FLAT
These stitches pass over the hem edge to the garment.

Slant hemming stitch. Quickest, but least durable because so much thread is exposed and subject to abrasion.

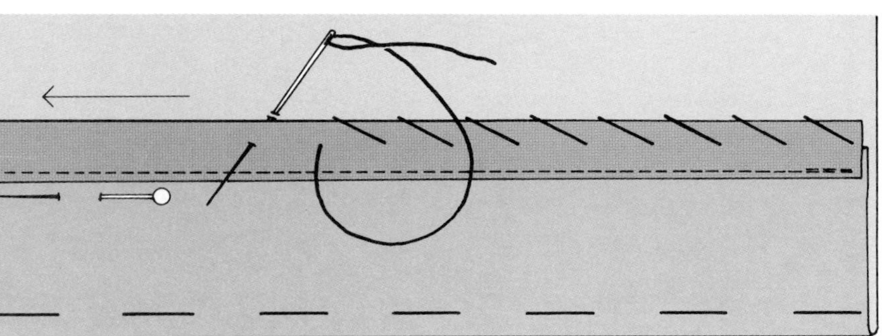

Slant hemming stitch: Fasten thread on wrong side of hem, bringing needle and thread through hem edge. Working from right to left, take first and each succeeding stitch approximately ¼″ to ⅜″ to the left, catching only one yarn of the garment fabric and bringing the needle up through edge of hem. This produces long, slanting floats between stitches.

Vertical hemming stitch. A durable and stable stitch best suited for hems whose edges are finished with woven-edge or stretch-lace seam tape. Very little thread is exposed, reducing the risk of fraying and breaking.

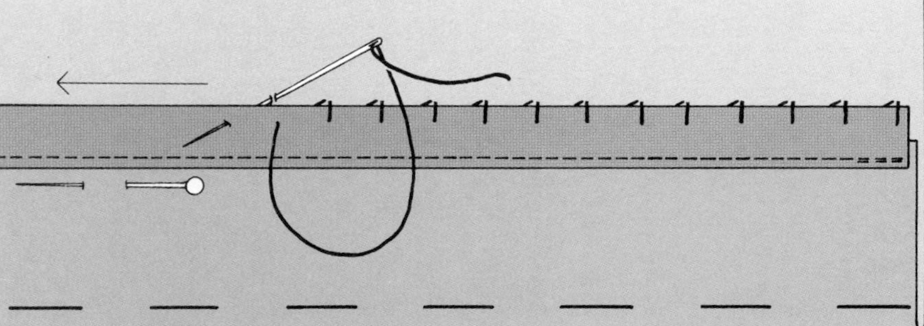

Vertical hemming stitch: Stitches are worked from right to left. Fasten thread from wrong side of hem and bring needle and thread through hem edge. Directly *opposite* this point and beside the hem edge, begin first and each succeeding stitch by catching only one yarn of garment fabric. Then direct the needle down diagonally to go through the hem edge approximately ¼″ to ⅜″ to the left. Short, vertical floats will appear between the stitches.

Hemming stitches

Uneven slipstitch is a durable and almost invisible stitch suitable for a folded hem edge. The stitches are slipped through the fold of the hem edge, minimizing the possibility of the thread's fraying or breaking.

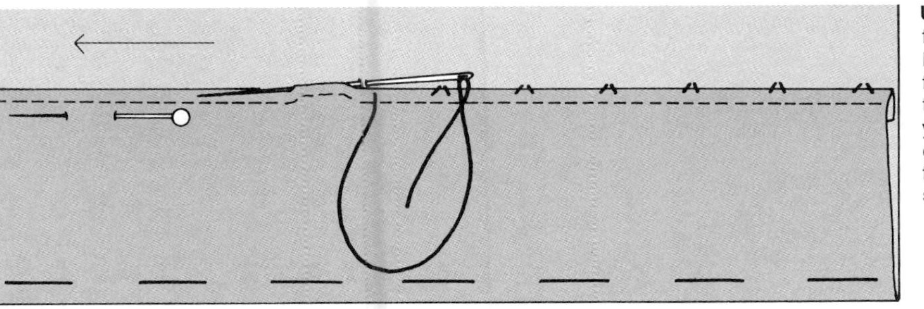

Uneven slipstitch: Stitches are worked from right to left. Fasten thread, bringing needle and thread out through fold of hem. Opposite, in the *garment*, take a small stitch, catching only a few yarns. Opposite that stitch, in the *hem* edge, insert needle and slip through fold for about ¼″. Continue alternating stitches in this fashion.

Flat catchstitch is a strong hemming stitch particularly well suited to a stitched-and-pinked hem edge. Take special note of the direction for working and of the position of the needle. Notice, too, that with each stitch, the thread crosses over itself.

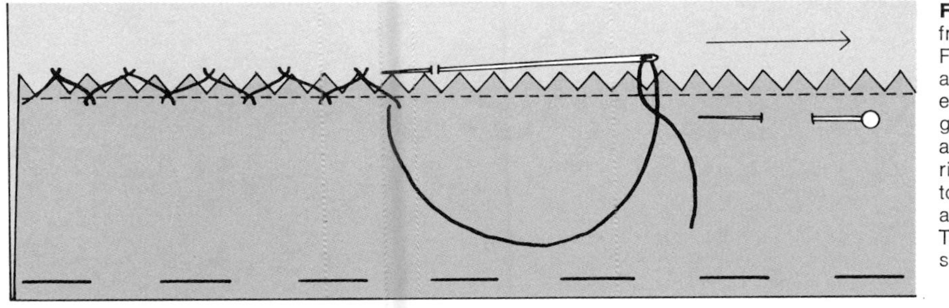

Flat catchstitch: Stitches are worked from left to right with needle pointing left. Fasten thread from wrong side of hem and bring needle and thread through hem edge. Take a very small stitch in the garment fabric directly above the hem edge and approximately ¼″ to ⅜″ to the right. Take the next stitch ¼″ to ⅜″ to the right in the hem. Continue to alternate stitches, spacing them evenly. Take special care to keep the stitches small when catching the garment fabric.

HEMMING STITCHES, BLIND

These stitches are taken *inside*, between the hem and the garment. In the finished hem, no stitches are visible and the edge of the hem does not press into the garment.

Blind-hemming stitch is a quick and easy stitch that can be used on any blind hem.

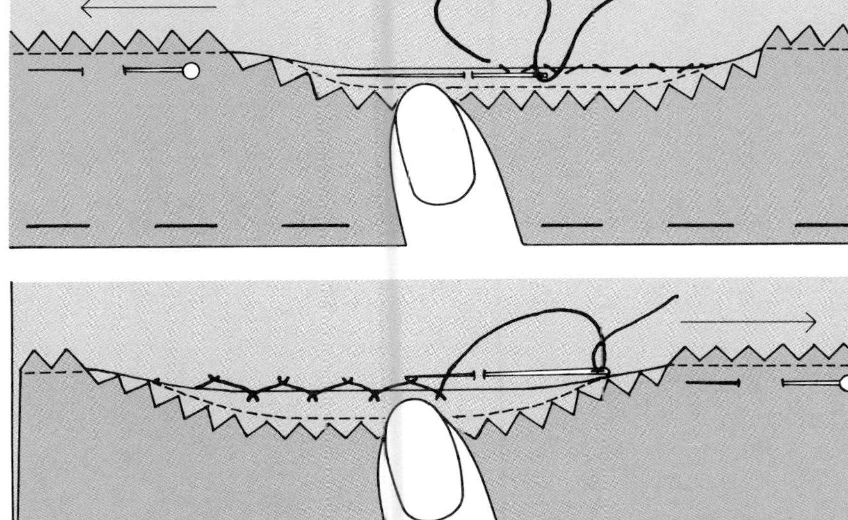

Blind-hemming stitch: Work from right to left with needle pointing left. Fold back the hem edge; fasten thread inside it. Take a very small stitch approximately ¼″ to the left in the garment; take the next stitch ¼″ to the left in the hem. Continue to alternate stitches from garment to hem, spacing them approximately ¼″ apart. Take care to keep stitches small, especially those taken on garment.

Blind catchstitch is the same stitch as the catchstitch used for flat hemming except that it is done between the hem and the garment. This stitch is a bit more stable and secure than the blind-hemming stitch, and is particularly good for heavy fabric.

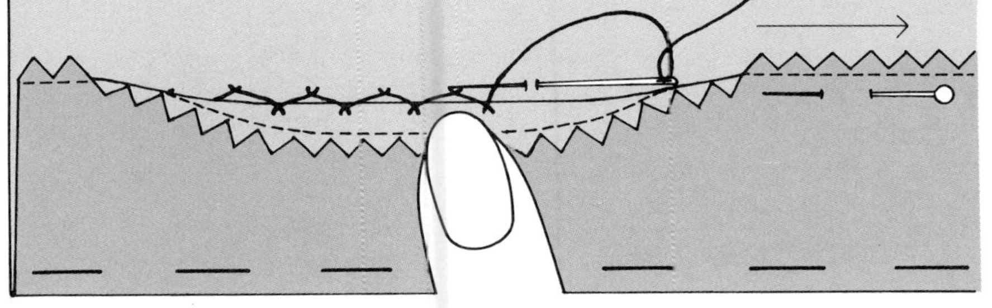

Blind catchstitch: Work from left to right with needle pointing left. Fold back hem edge; fasten thread inside it. Take a very small stitch about ¼″ to the right in the garment; take the next stitch ¼″ to the right in the hem edge. Continue to alternate stitches from garment to hem, spacing them approximately ¼″ apart. Keep stitches small, especially when stitching on the garment fabric.

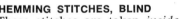

Glossary of hand stitches

Hemstitching / Overhand stitch

HEMSTITCHING
This is an ornamental hem finish, traditionally used for linens and handkerchiefs. Hem edge is folded under and basted in place, then several threads are pulled from the fabric directly above this edge. Exact number drawn depends on fabric's coarseness, but space they leave should be ⅛ to ¼ inch. Each stitch must group an equal number of lengthwise threads.

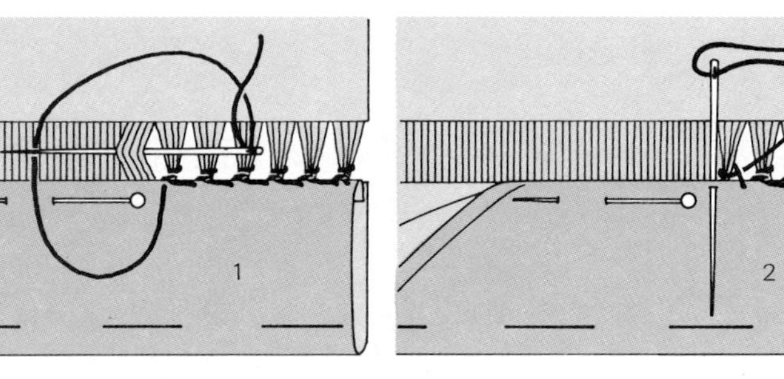

Hemstitching: Working on wrong side and from right to left, fasten thread; pull up through folded hem edge. Slide needle under several lengthwise threads; loop thread to left *under* point of needle (1). Pull thread through to left and draw it down firmly near the hem edge. Then take a stitch through garment and hem edge, catching only a few fabric threads (2). Repeat until edge is finished. Keep the number of lengthwise yarns the same in each group.

Double hemstitching is done by applying duplicate rows of hemstitching on both sides of drawn threads. While stitching second edge, be sure to maintain the thread groupings established by the first row of stitching.

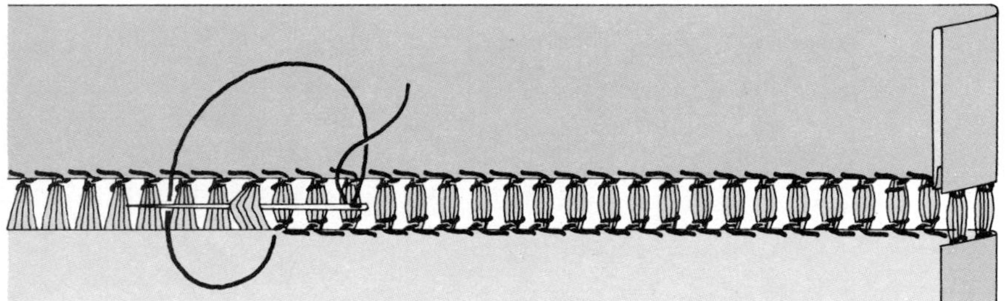

Double hemstitching: When one edge has been finished as described above, turn work and make duplicate stitches along opposite edge of drawn threads. Take care to retain thread groups that were established on the first edge.

OVERCAST STITCH
This is the customary hand stitch for finishing the raw edges of fabric to prevent them from raveling. In general, the more the fabric ravels, the deeper and closer together the overcast stitches should be.

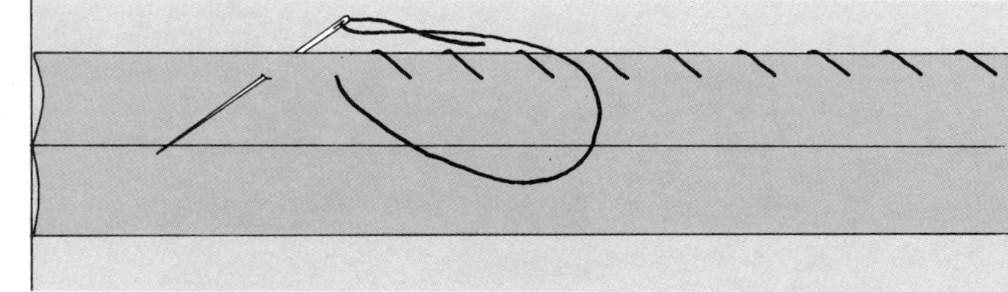

Overcast stitch: Working from either direction, take diagonal stitches over the edge, spacing them an even distance apart at a uniform depth.

OVERHAND STITCH
These tiny, even stitches are used to hold together two finished edges, as, for example, when attaching lace edging or ribbon to a garment.

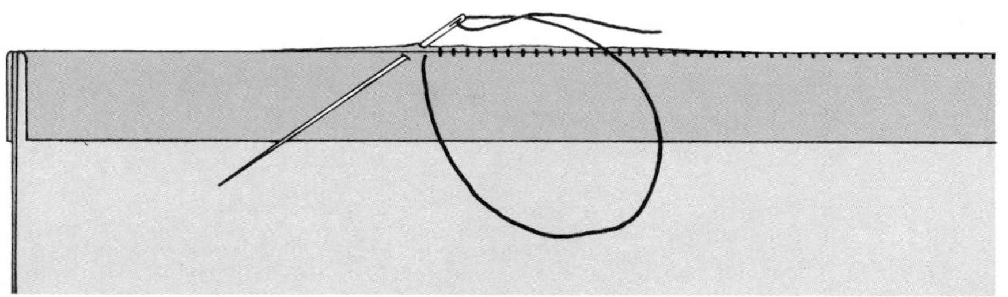

Overhand stitch: Insert needle diagonally from the back edge through to the front edge, picking up only one or two threads each time. The needle is inserted *directly behind* thread from previous stitch and is brought out a *stitch length away*. Keep the stitches uniform in their size and spacing.

Tucks 165 Gathering 179
Tailoring 366-370

Padding stitch / Running stitch

PADDING STITCHES

Padding stitches are used, primarily in tailoring, to attach interfacing to the outer fabric. When the stitches are made *short* and close together, they are also helping to form and control shape in certain garment sections, such as a collar or lapel. *Longer* padding stitches are used just to hold interfacing in place; they are like diagonal basting except that they are permanent and the stitches are shorter (see Tailoring).

Chevron padding stitches are formed by making each row of stitches in the opposite direction from the preceding one; that is, work from top to bottom on one row, then, without turning fabric, work next row bottom to top.

Parallel padding stitches are formed by making each row of stitches in the same direction.

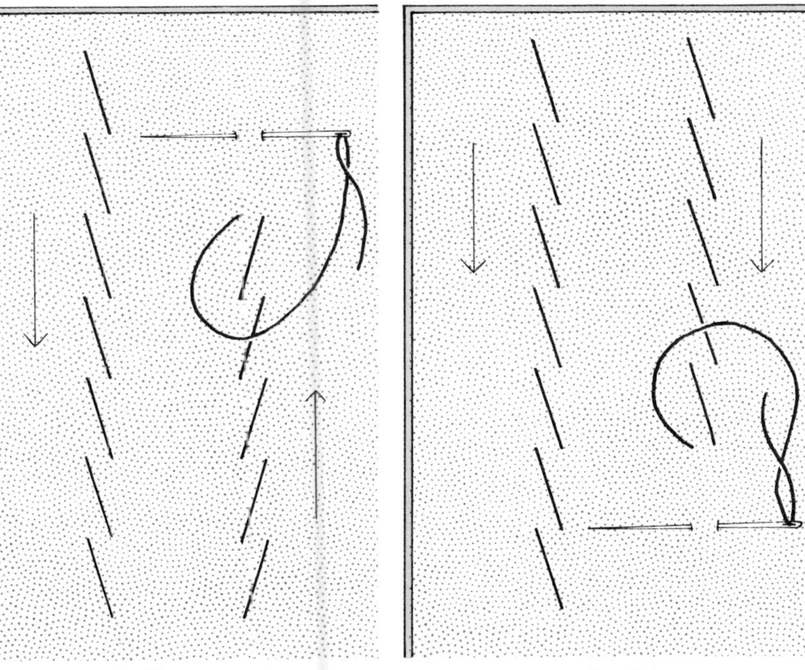

Chevron Parallel

Chevron padding stitches: Working from top to bottom, make a row of short, even stitches from right to left, placing them parallel to each other and the same distance apart. Without turning the fabric, make the next row of stitches the same way except work them from bottom to top. Keep alternating the direction of the rows to produce the chevron effect.

Parallel padding stitches: These stitches are made the same way as the chevron padding stitches except that all rows are worked in the same direction.

PICKSTITCH

see **Backstitch**

PLAIN-STITCH TACK

see **Tacks** (construction)

PRICKSTITCH

see **Backstitch**

RUNNING STITCH

A very short, even stitch used for fine seaming, tucking, mending, gathering, and other such delicate sewing. The running stitch is like even basting except that the stitches are smaller and usually permanent.

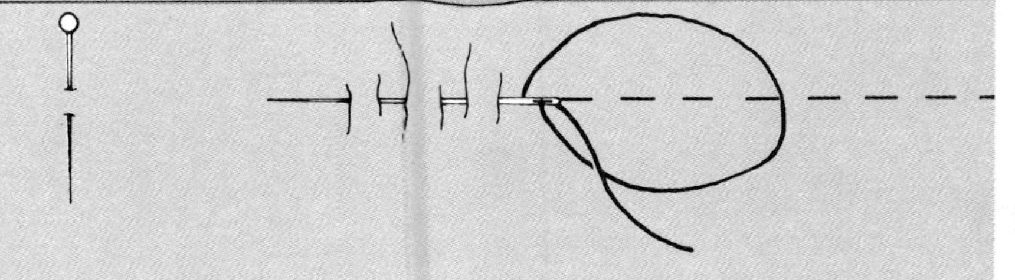

Running stitch: Working from right to left, weave the point of the needle in and out of the fabric several times before pulling the thread through. Keep stitches and the spaces between them small and even.

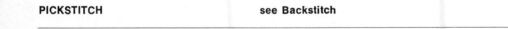

Glossary of hand stitches

Saddle stitch / Slipstitch

SADDLE STITCH
This is a variation of the running stitch, but the stitches and spaces between them are longer, generally ¼ to ½ inch. Used primarily for hand topstitching and intended to be a strong accent, the saddle stitch is usually done with buttonhole twist, embroidery floss, or tightly twisted yarn, often in a contrasting color.

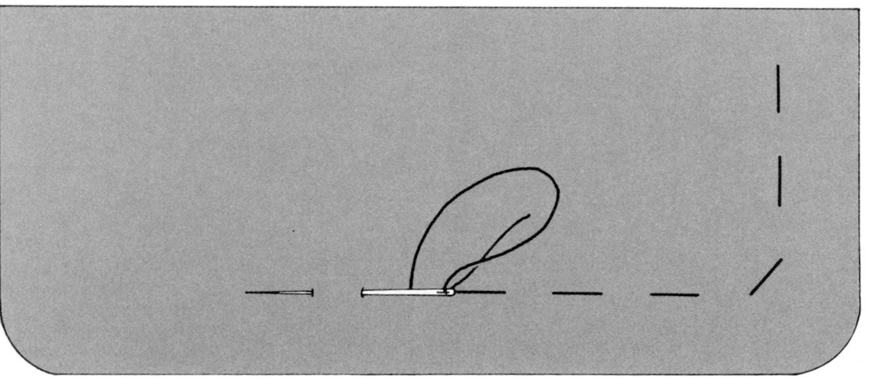

Saddle stitch: Fasten thread and bring the needle and thread through to right side of fabric. Working from right to left, take a stitch ¼″ to ½″ long, leave a space the same length, then take another stitch. Continue taking stitches in this way, making them equal in length and in intervening space.

SIMPLIFIED TAILOR'S TACKS see **Tacks** (construction)

SLANT HEMMING STITCH see **Hemming** (flat)

SLIP BASTING see **Basting**

SLIPSTITCH
This is a nearly invisible stitch formed by slipping the thread under a fold of fabric. It can be used to join two folded edges, or one folded edge to a flat surface.
Even slipstitch is used to join two folded edges. It is a fast and easy way to mend a seam from the right side, especially one that would be difficult to reach from the inside.

Uneven slipstitch is used to join a folded edge to a flat surface. Besides being a flat hemming stitch, it is useful for attaching patch pockets, trims, and coat and jacket linings, as well as for securing the edges of a facing to zipper tapes.

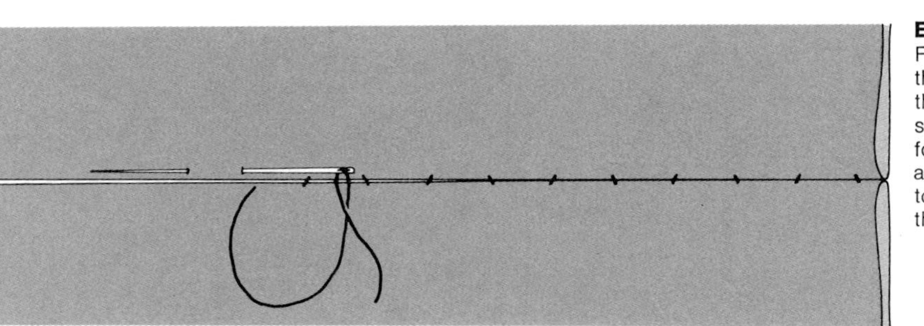

Even slipstitch: Work from right to left. Fasten thread and bring needle and thread out through one folded edge. For the first and each succeeding stitch, slip needle through fold of opposite edge for about ¼″; bring needle out and draw the thread through. Continue to slip the needle and thread through the opposing folded edges.

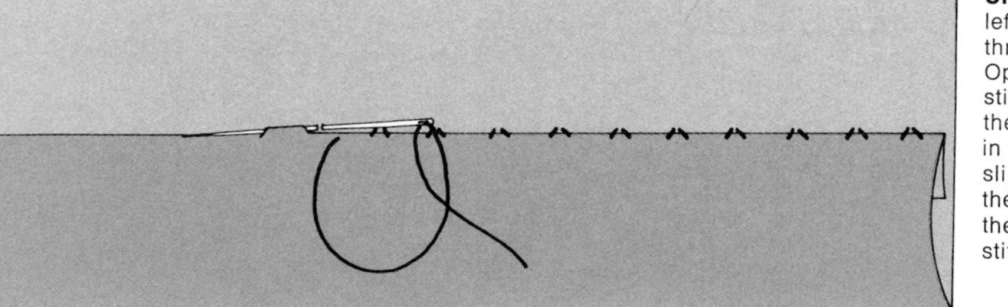

Uneven slipstitch: Work from right to left. Fasten thread and bring needle and thread out through the folded edge. Opposite, in the *garment*, take a small stitch, catching only a few yarns of the garment fabric. Opposite this stitch, in the *folded edge*, insert needle and slip it through the fold for about ¼″; then bring the needle out and draw the thread through. Continue alternating stitches from garment to fold.

Tacks

TACKS
Certain hand stitches done during construction or for marking.

TACKS, CONSTRUCTION
Stitches used to join areas that must be held together without a seam, or as a reinforcement at points of strain.
Arrowhead tack is a triangular reinforcement tack done from the right side at such points of strain as the ends of a pocket.

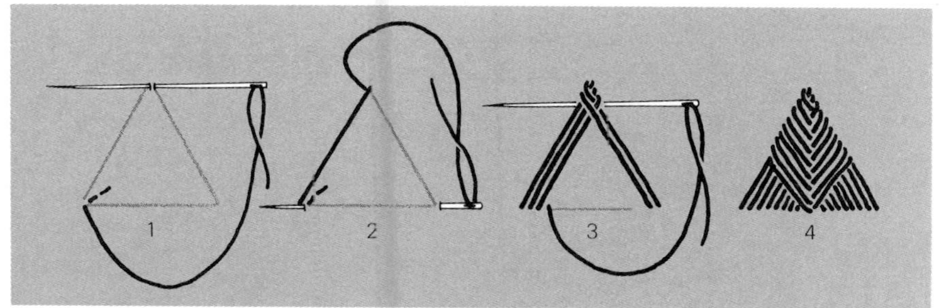

Arrowhead tack: Using chalk or thread, mark triangular arrowhead shape on right side of garment. Take two small running stitches *within* triangle and bring needle and thread out at lower left corner. At upper corner, take a small stitch from right to left (1). Draw thread through and insert needle at right corner, bringing it out at left corner barely *inside* previous thread (2). Draw thread through and repeat, using marked lines as guides and placing threads side by side until triangle is filled (3) and (4).

Bar tack is a straight reinforcement tack used at such points of strain as the ends of a hand-worked buttonhole or the corners of a pocket.

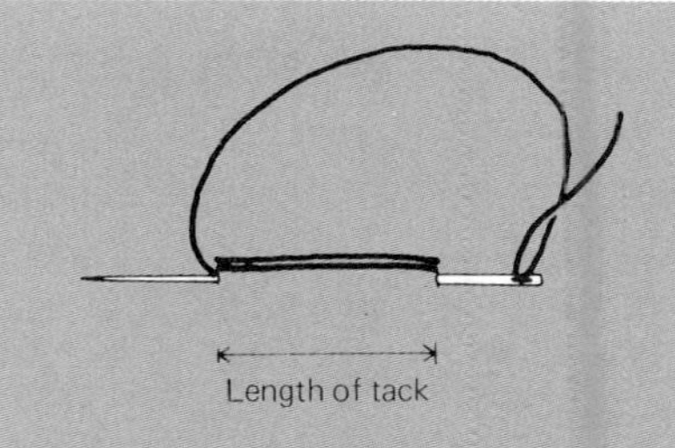

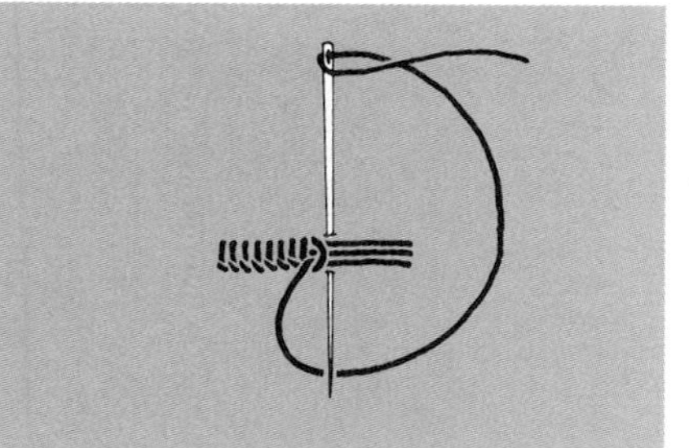

Bar tack: Fasten thread and bring needle and thread through to right side. Take two or three long stitches (the length that the bar tack is to be) in the same place. Catching the fabric underneath, work enough closely spaced blanket stitches around the thread to cover it. (For basic blanket stitch, see p. 125.)

Blanket-stitch tack is formed between two garment sections, as for example, a facing and a garment front. The blanket stitch is used, but differently from the way it is employed to cover an edge. In tacking applications, it catches and joins *two* fabric layers and there is *more space* (about 1 to 2 inches) between the stitches.

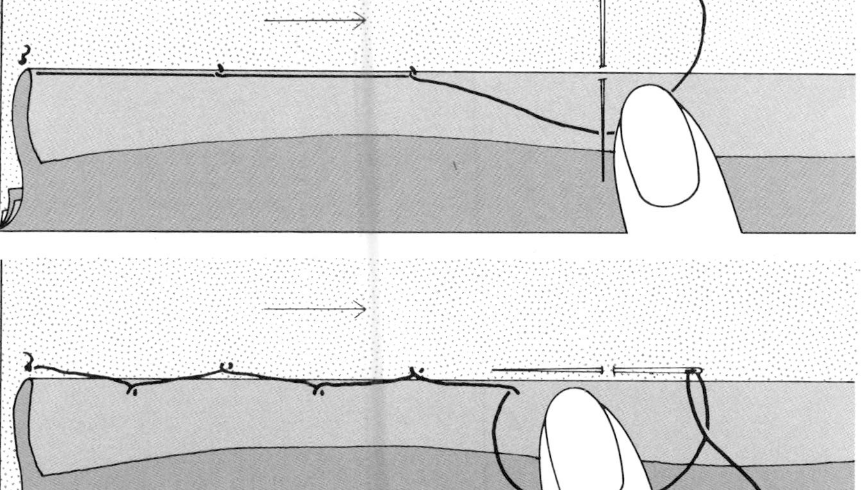

Blanket-stitch tack: Work from left to right, with facing folded back and needle pointing toward you. Fasten thread in facing. One to two inches to right, with needle passing over supply end of thread, take a small vertical stitch in interfacing or underlining, then through facing. Draw needle and thread through. Repeat at 1″ to 2″ intervals, allowing a slight slack between stitches.

Catchstitch tack is similar to blind hemming using a catchstitch. When used to tack, the stitches are more widely spaced, approximately ½ to 1 inch apart, and they are used to hold such garment sections as a facing to a front section.

Catchstitch tack: Work from left to right, with facing folded back and needle pointing left. Fasten thread in facing. One to two inches to right, take a small stitch in the interfacing or underlining. Pull needle and thread through. Take the next short stitch 1″ to 2″ to the right in the facing. Repeat sequence, allowing a slight slack between stitches.

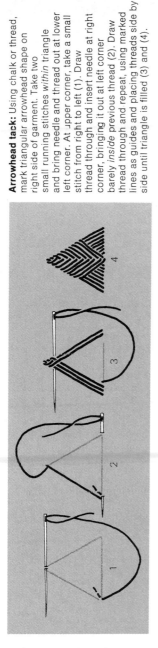

Glossary of hand stitches

Tacks

Cross-stitch tacks. Used to tack folds in place, such as those found at the shoulder or center back of a jacket or coat lining. Both decorative and functional, such tacks provide a degree of flexibility not possible with machine stitching.
Single cross-stitch tack is used in such areas as a facing edge, where only one spot needs to be tacked. Usually stitched several times.

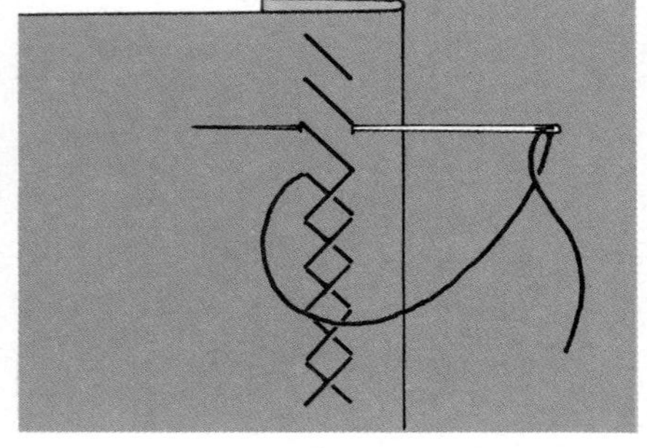

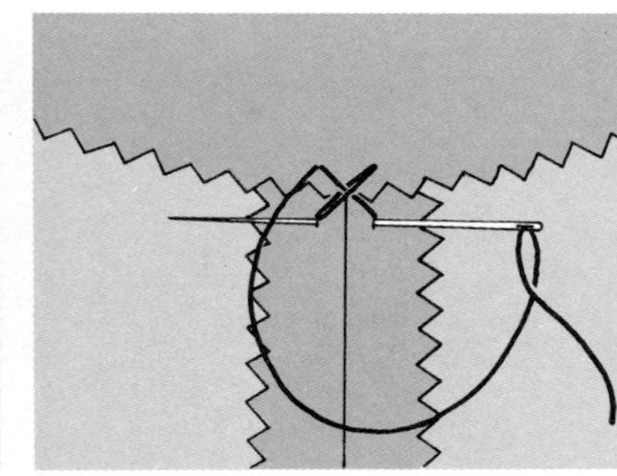

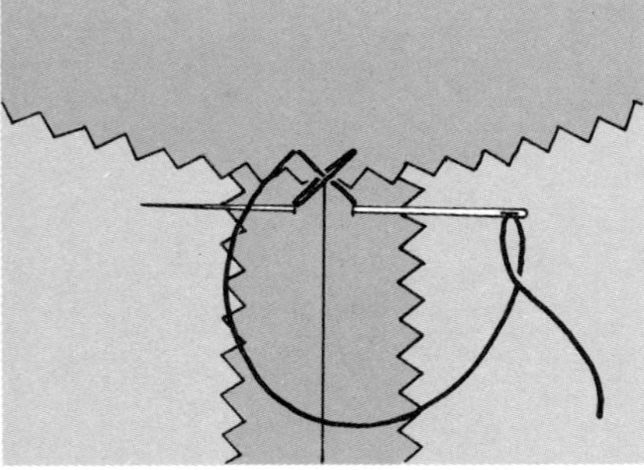

Cross-stitch tacks: Pin or baste fold in position; tack in place with a series of cross stitches. Length to be tacked will be indicated on pattern.
Single cross-stitch tack: Make a cross stitch over edge to be tacked (here a neck facing edge at shoulder seam), then make two or three more cross stitches, in the same place, over the first. (For basic cross stitch, see p.127.)

French tack is made similarly to the bar tack. It is used to link two separate garment sections, such as the bottom edge of a coat to the bottom edge of its lining, while still allowing a certain amount of movement to the two sections that are linked.

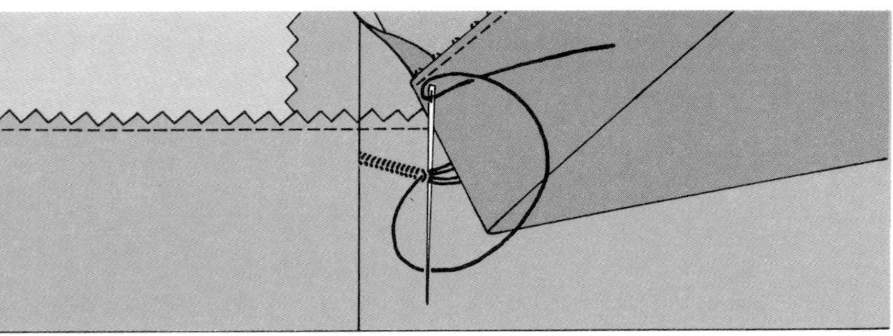

French tack: Take a small stitch through top of garment hem edge, then another small stitch directly opposite in the lining, leaving a 1" to 2" slack in the thread between stitches. Take similar stitches several times in the same places. Then work closely spaced blanket stitches over the threads. (For basic blanket stitch, see p.125.)

Heavy-duty tack is a very sturdy tack that is used for joining areas of a heavy garment.

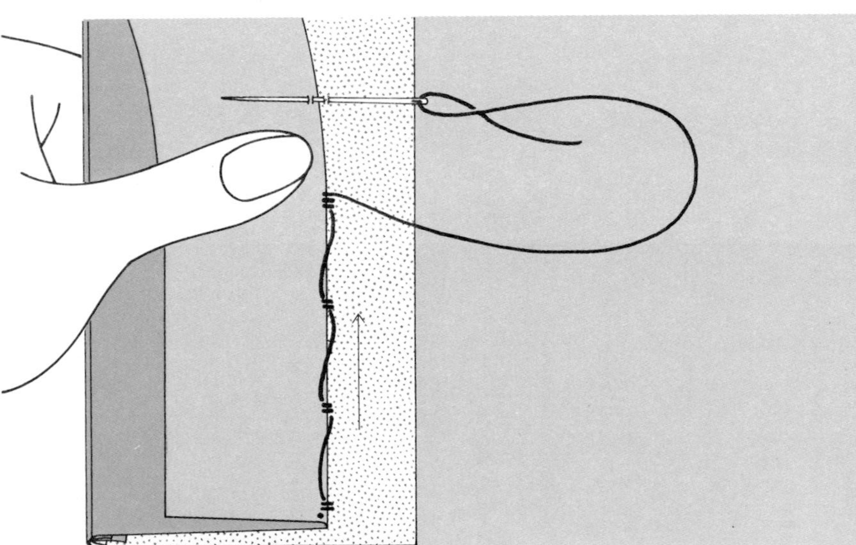

Heavy-duty tack: Work from bottom to top, with the facing folded back and the needle pointing from right to left. Fasten thread in facing. Take a short stitch, catching only a few threads of interfacing or underlining and then facing. Draw needle and thread through; take one or two more stitches above first. Do not pull thread taut. Make the next and each succeeding set of stitches 1" to 2" above the set just completed.

Tacks

Plain-stitch tack is used for tacking together sections of lightweight garments. It is like the blind-hemming stitch except that the stitches are spaced farther apart.

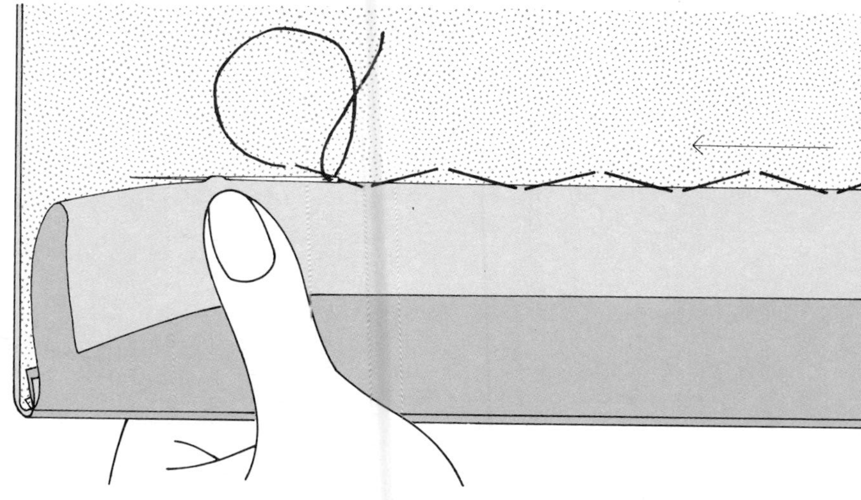

Plain-stitch tack: Work from right to left, with facing folded back. Fasten thread in facing. Take one short horizontal stitch ½″ ahead in the interfacing or underlining; then, ½″ to 1″ ahead of this stitch, take another short horizontal stitch in facing. Pull needle and thread through and repeat. Do *not* pull thread taut.

TACKS, MARKING

Marking tacks are used to transfer construction details and matching points from the pattern to cut fabric sections. As alternatives to chalk or tracing paper, they can be more time-consuming, but there are certain situations where marking tacks are necessary (see Marking).

Simplified tailor's tacks are basically uneven basting stitches. They are best confined, as a general rule, to marking single layers of fabric; are especially well suited to such markings as fold or center lines.

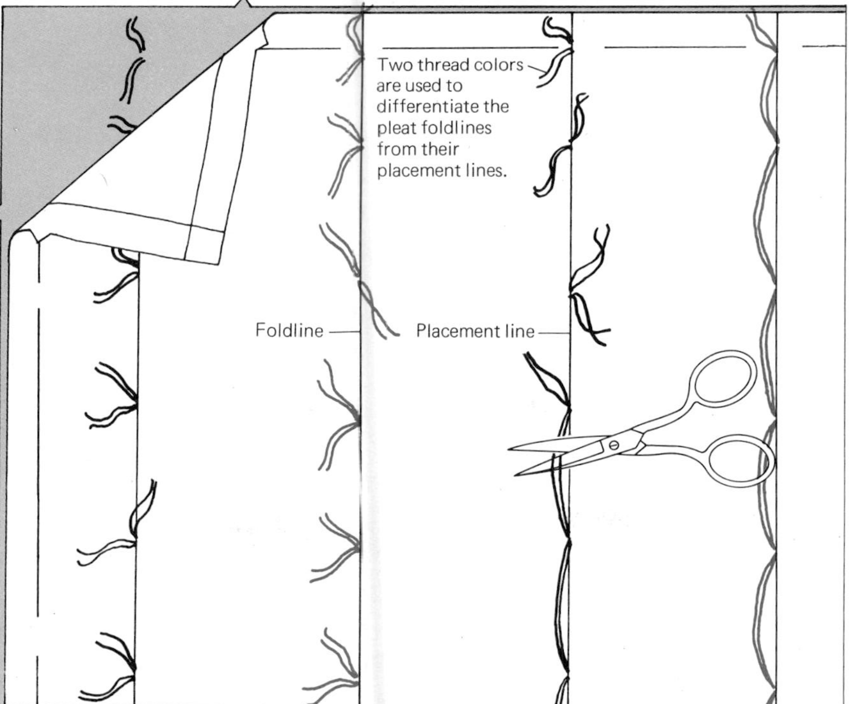
Two thread colors are used to differentiate the pleat foldlines from their placement lines.
Foldline
Placement line

Simplified tailor's tacks: Using a long length of double unknotted thread, take a small stitch on pattern line through pattern and fabric. Pull needle and thread through, leaving a 1″ thread end. Take similar stitches about every 2″ to 3″, leaving thread slack in between. Cut threads at center points between stitches and gently lift pattern off fabric, taking care *not* to pull out thread markings.

Glossary of hand stitches

Fabric-marking methods 94

Tacks / Whipstitch

Tailor's tacks are used to transfer individual pattern symbols, such as dots, to double layers of fabric.

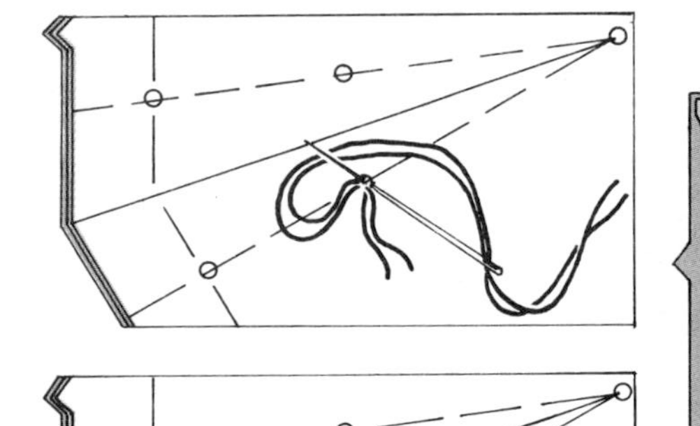

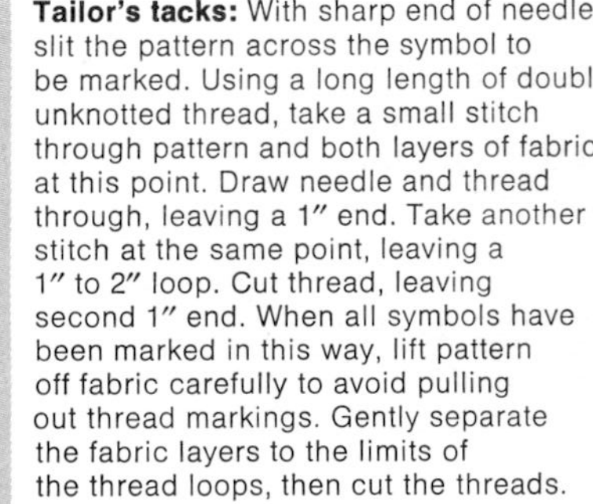

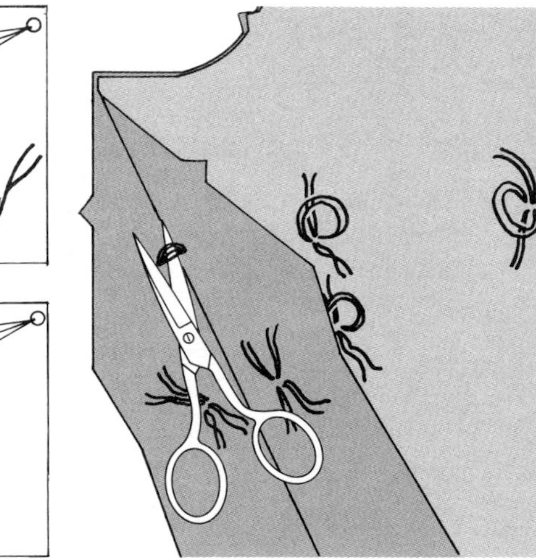

Tailor's tacks: With sharp end of needle, slit the pattern across the symbol to be marked. Using a long length of double, unknotted thread, take a small stitch through pattern and both layers of fabric at this point. Draw needle and thread through, leaving a 1″ end. Take another stitch at the same point, leaving a 1″ to 2″ loop. Cut thread, leaving second 1″ end. When all symbols have been marked in this way, lift pattern off fabric carefully to avoid pulling out thread markings. Gently separate the fabric layers to the limits of the thread loops, then cut the threads.

THREAD CHAIN	see **Chainstitch**
TOPSTITCHING	see **Backstitch, Saddle stitch**
UNDERSTITCHING	see **Backstitch**
UNEVEN BASTING	see **Basting**
UNEVEN SLIPSTITCH	see **Slipstitch**
VERTICAL HEMMING STITCH	see **Hemming** (flat)

WHIPSTITCH
This is a variation of the overhand stitch, the main difference being the angle at which the needle is held. Though generally used to join two finished edges, it can also hold a raw edge neatly against a flat surface.

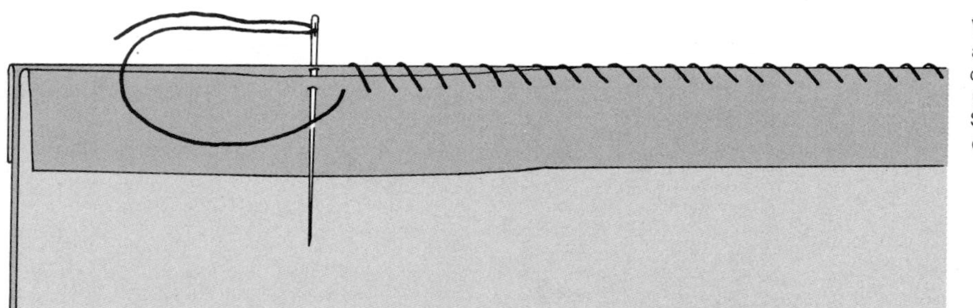

Whipstitch: Insert needle at right angle and close to the edge, picking up only a few threads. Slanted floats will be produced between the tiny stitches. Space between stitches can be short or long, depending on the circumstances.

Machine facsimiles of hand stitches

Arrowhead tack / Basting

ARROWHEAD TACK see **Tacks** (construction)

BACKSTITCH
Used to secure the beginning and end of a row of machine stitching. Backstitching eliminates the need to tie thread ends, but it should not be used to secure stitching in such areas as the tapered end of a dart because reversing the stitching direction can sometimes distort the fabric.

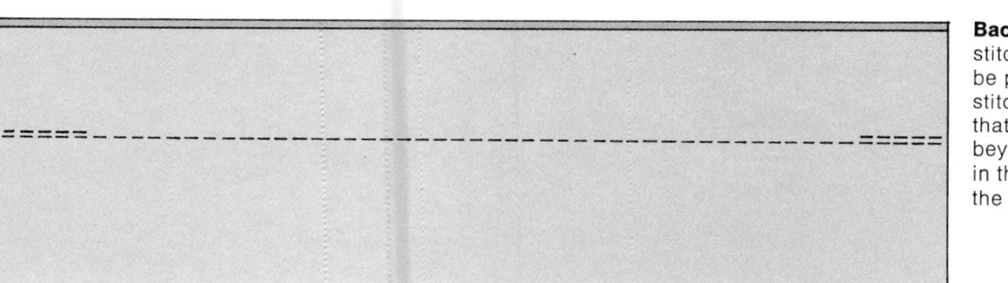

Backstitch: Made by utilizing the reverse stitching mechanism, the backstitch can be produced by any machine. Position these stitches on top of, or just inside, those that form the seam. Avoid backstitching beyond the cut edge; this can result in the fabric's being pulled down into the hole of the throat plate.

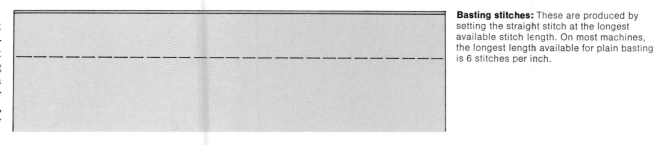

Tying thread ends is another way of securing threads at the ends of a row of machine stitching. Although not as strong as backstitching, it is a neater finishing technique and is especially useful in securing such decorative work as topstitching.

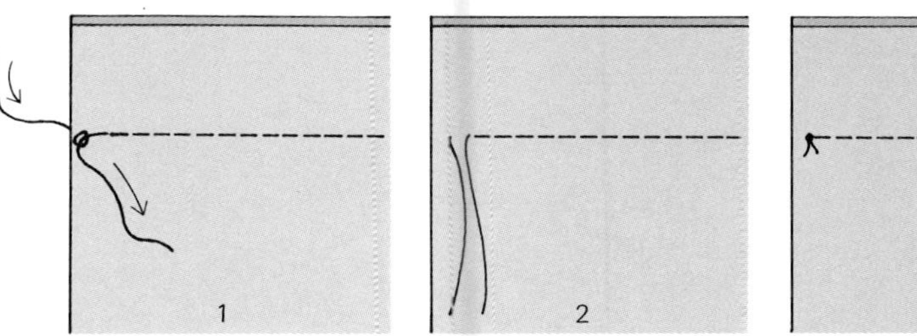

To tie thread ends, you must first bring the lower thread through to the other side of the fabric. Pull on upper thread to start lower thread (1), then pull it through completely (2). Tie threads together, using a square knot; trim away excess thread ends (3).

BAR TACK see **Tacks** (construction)

BASTING
Machine basting is a long straight stitch used to hold fabric layers together during fitting or permanent machine stitching. The longer basting stitches can sometimes be used as a marking device. Machine basting or marking should not be used, however, on fabrics that will be damaged by the piercing of the needle.

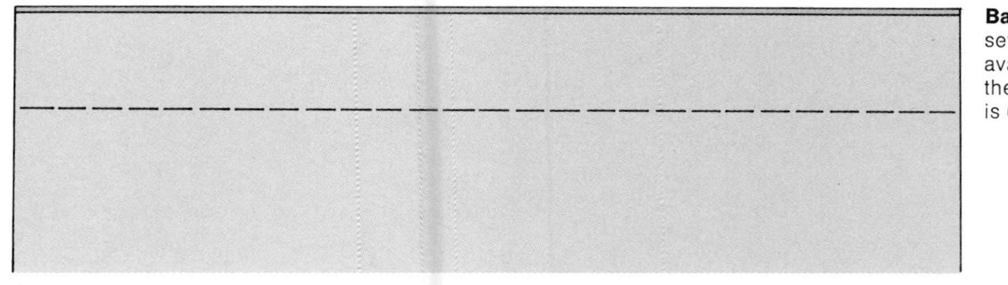

Basting stitches: These are produced by setting the straight stitch at the longest available stitch length. On most machines, the longest length available for plain basting is 6 stitches per inch.

A longer basting stitch is available on some more elaborate machines by the use of a built-in mechanism or insertion of a separate stitch-pattern cam.

Blind-hemming stitch / Buttonhole stitch

BLIND-HEMMING STITCH
Referred to as the blindstitch, this zigzag stitch pattern is used primarily for blind hemming by machine (see Hems). It can also be used to stitch seams, and as a seam finish (see Seams), and to produce the effect of hand-prickstitching in a machine zipper application (see Zippers).

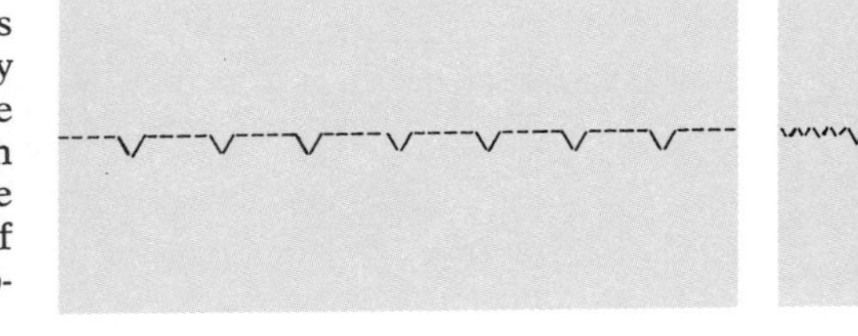

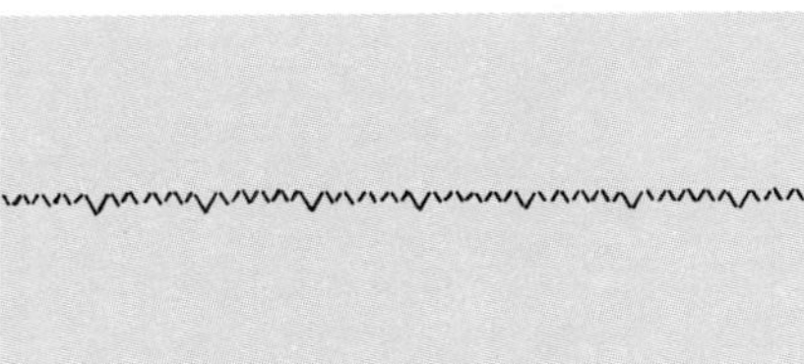
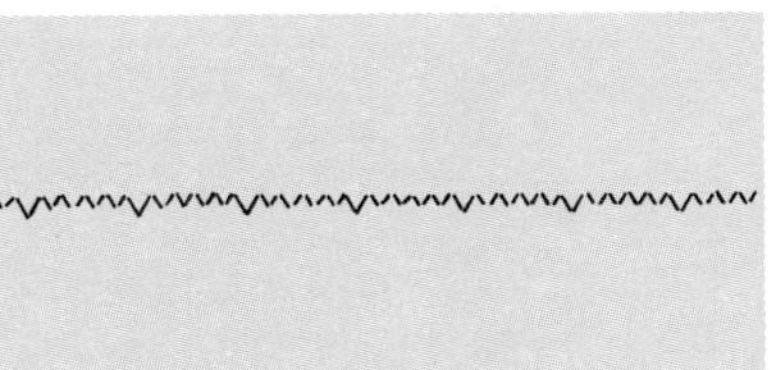
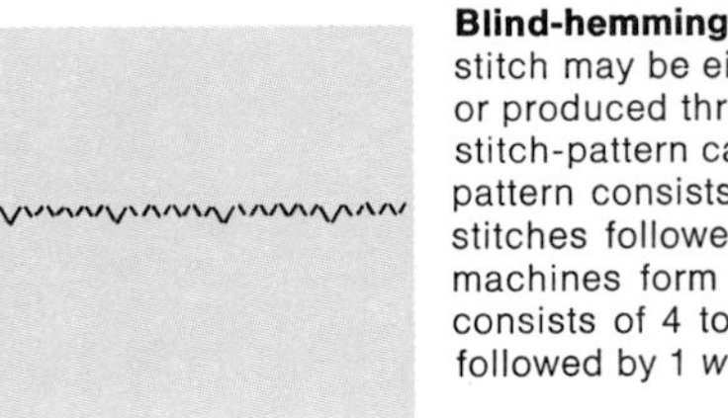
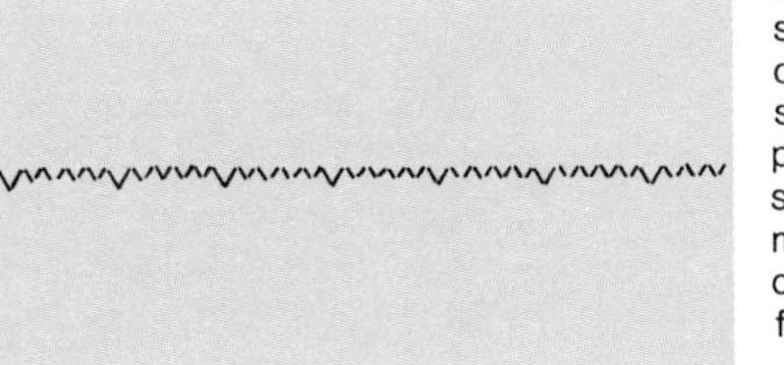
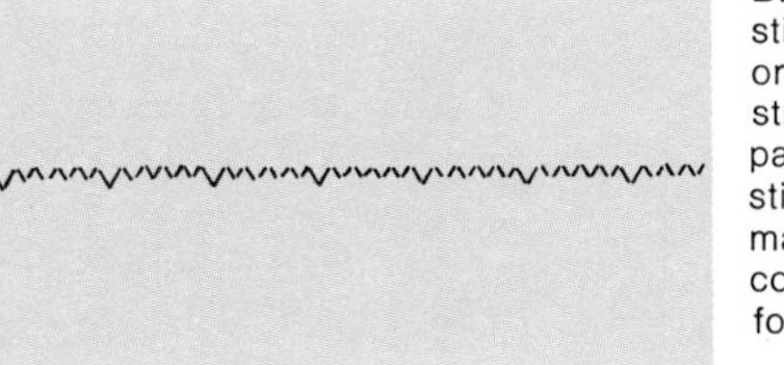
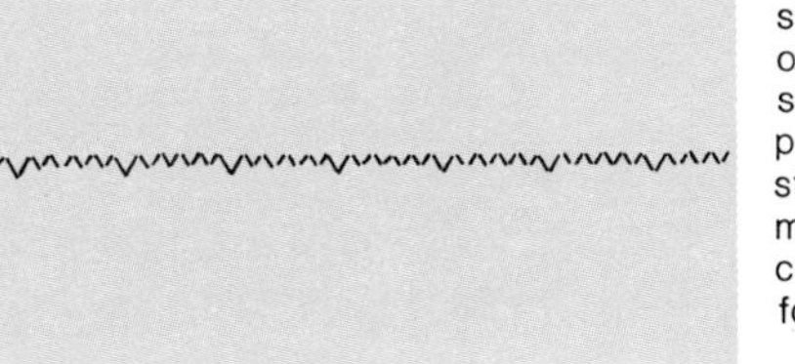
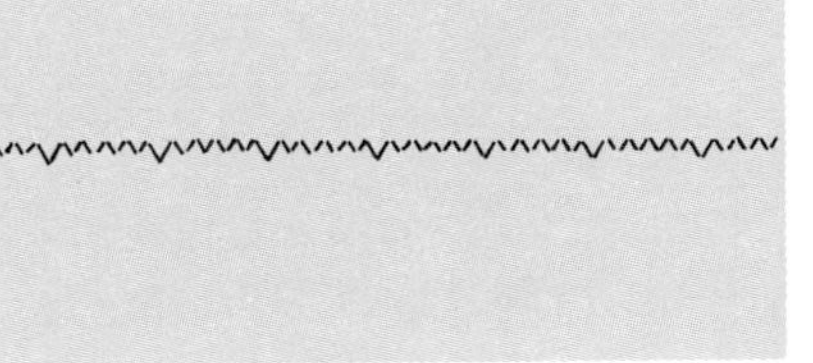

Blind-hemming stitch (blindstitch): This stitch may be either built into the machine or produced through the insertion of a stitch-pattern cam. As a rule, the stitch pattern consists of 4 to 6 straight stitches followed by 1 zigzag, but some machines form a blindstitch that consists of 4 to 6 *narrow* zigzag stitches followed by 1 *wider* zigzag.

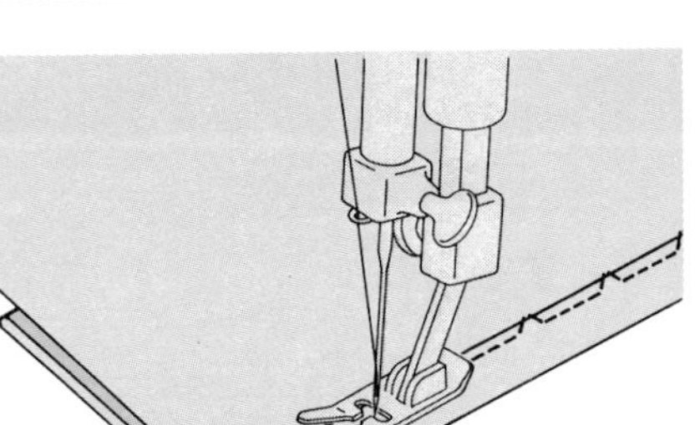

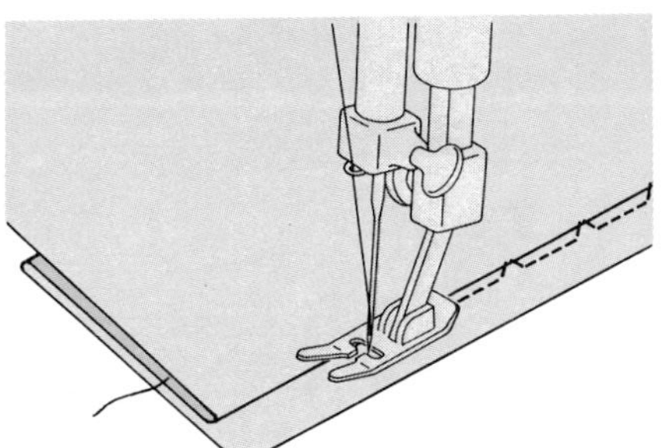
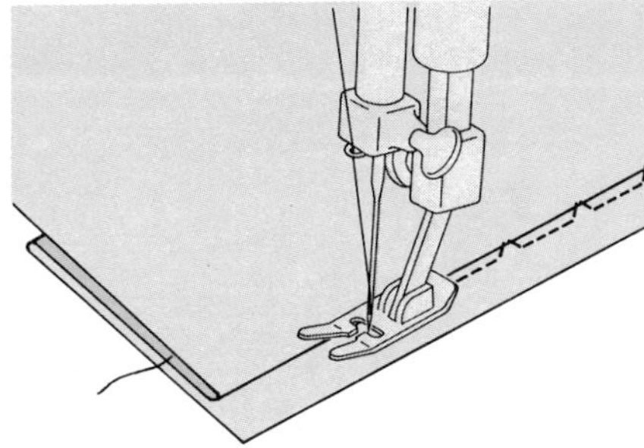
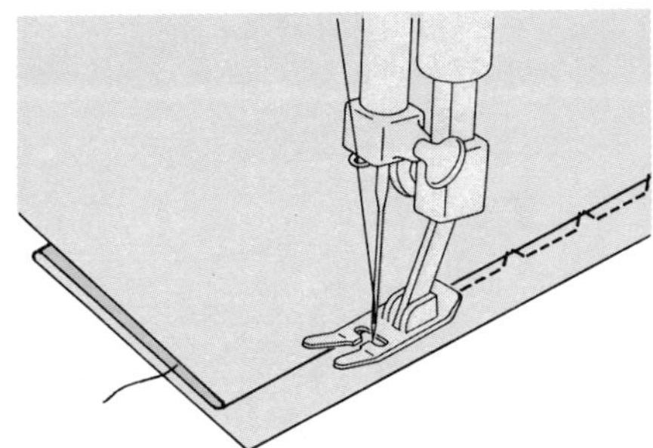

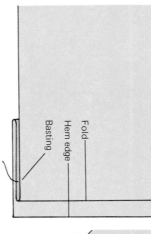

To blind-hem by machine, first fold up hem allowance and hand-baste in position ½″ below hem edge. With wrong side up, fold hem allowance under and position beneath foot with fold slightly to the left of the center of the foot and the hem edge to the right of foot. Stitch so that the straight stitches are formed on the hem edge and the zigzag stitch bites into the fold. The stitch length and width, and the positioning of the garment, should be tested before hem is stitched.

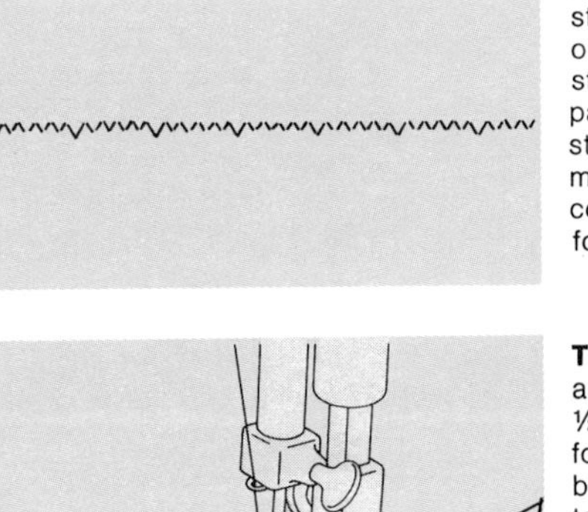

A prickstitch effect on a zipper placket is achieved by using the blindstitch in place of topstitching in the last step of a zipper application. Fold zipper placket under, letting one seam allowance extend. Using zipper foot positioned to the right of the needle, place placket under foot with fold toward the left. Stitch, placing the straight stitches on the seam allowance and letting zigzag catch the fold. It is best that seam allowance be wider than normal (⅞″) and zigzag stitch as narrow as possible. Test before applying to garment.

BUTTONHOLE STITCH
Machine stitching of buttonholes, whether automatic or manual, generally requires a zigzag stitch. (For single exception, see explanation at right.) All machine buttonholes have two straight sides with bar tacks at ends. Bar tacks are usually straight, as in buttonhole being formed here, but some machines or attachments produce round or keyhole ends.

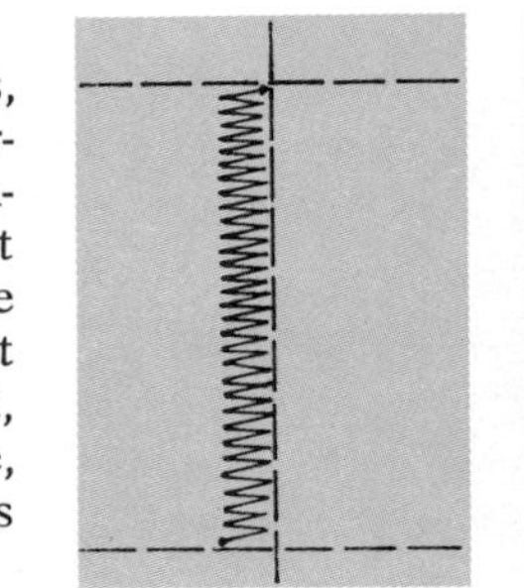
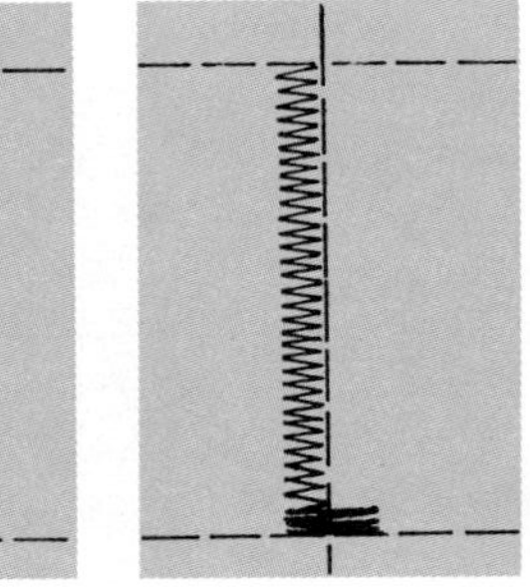
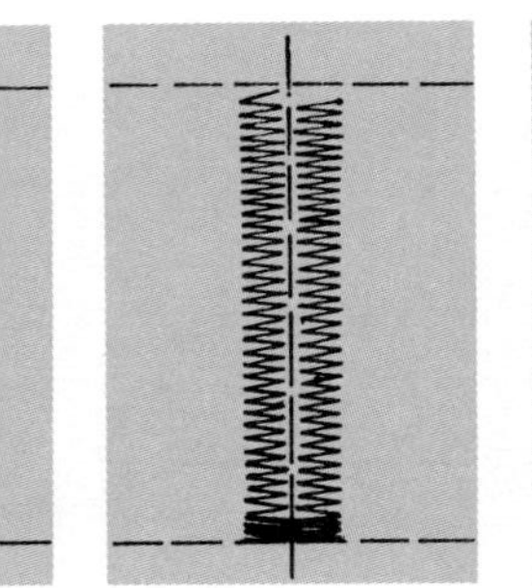
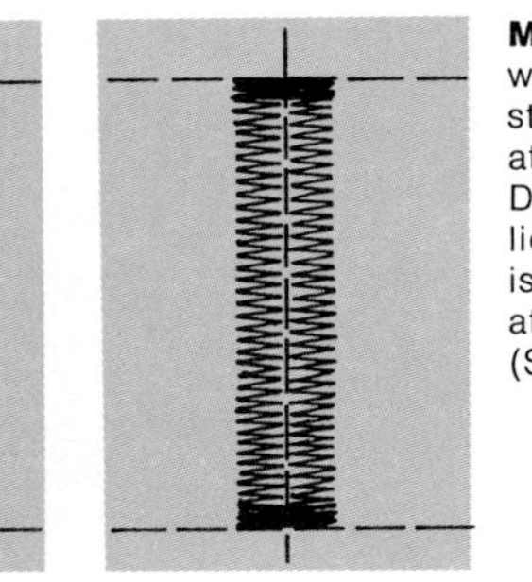

Machine-worked buttonholes are made with a zigzag stitch (except those made with straight-stitch machines in which an attachment jogs *fabric* from side to side). Differences in how a buttonhole is formed lie in the mechanism by which buttonhole is produced (built-in or a separate attachment) and which steps are automatic. (See Machine-worked buttonholes.)

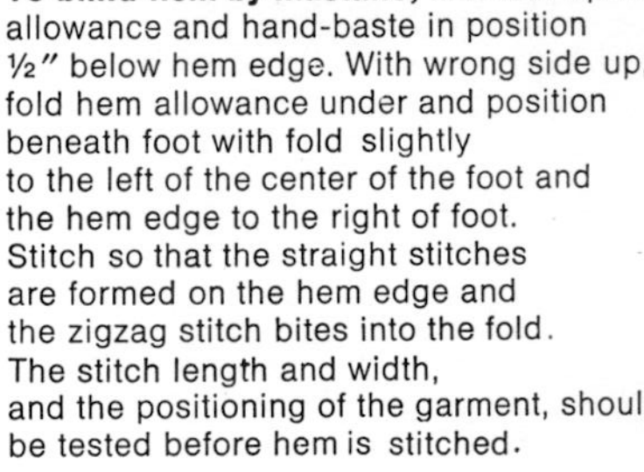
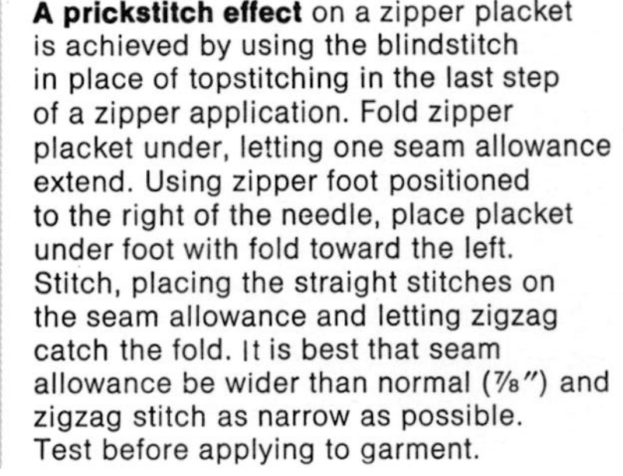
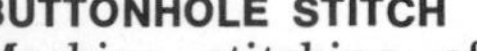

Chainstitch / Fagoting stitch

CHAINSTITCH

A series of interlocking stitches made from a single thread (needle thread), the chainstitch can be used for seaming and also as a thread chain for belt carriers and French tacks. When used to stitch on fabric, it looks like ordinary straight stitching from the top side and a series of interlocking loops on the underside. Unless secured, the stitches can easily be removed by pulling on the thread end. Because of this characteristic, the chainstitch can also be used as a temporary seaming stitch.

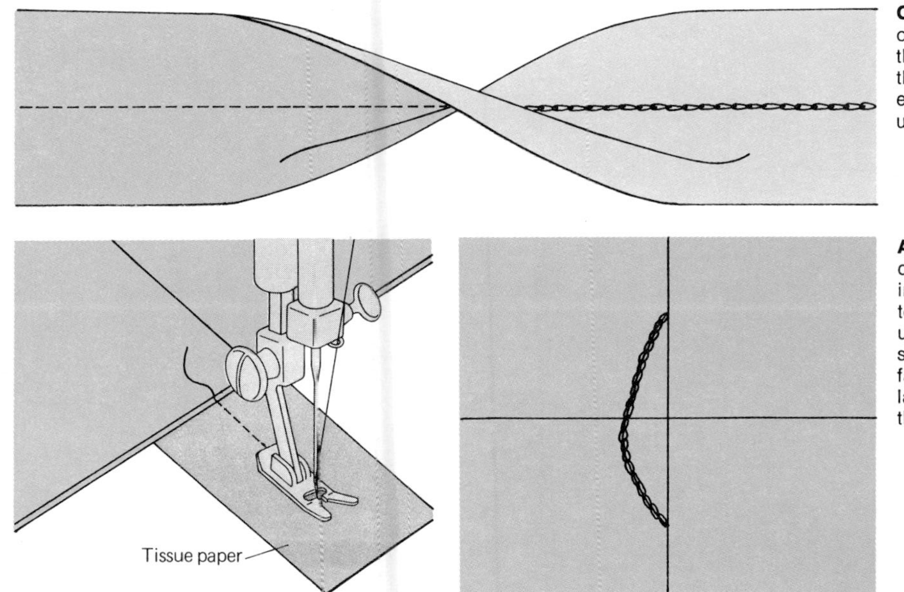

Chainstitch: This stitch is available on only a few machines. It is achieved through the use of special machine fittings that allow the needle thread to form the entire stitch (the bobbin thread is not used in the making of a chainstitch).

A thread chain is the most common use of the machine chainstitch. Start the chain in the garment, then stitch off the garment to the length required. (Sometimes an underlay of tissue paper is required when stitching off garment.) Cut thread. To fasten, bring cut thread end through the last loop; remove tissue and fasten the end in the garment by hand.

FAGOTING STITCH

This is a stitch that is used for decorative joining of garment sections, leaving a space between the edges. The fabric edges must be folded back and positioned accurately to ensure that the original seamline, after fagoting, falls at the center of the space between the edges. Suitable for fagoting: any stitch pattern that stitches equal distances to the right and left of the center of the foot. Fagoting should not be applied to garment areas that must withstand strain during wear.

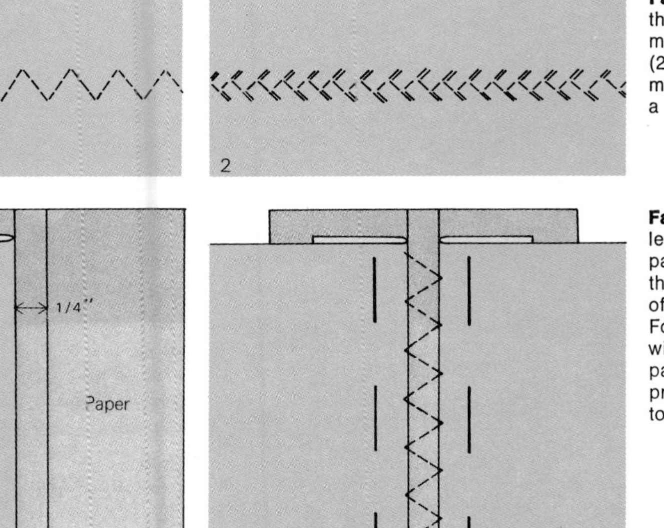

Fagoting stitches: Two stitch patterns that are well suited to fagoting are the multistitch zigzag (1) and the featherstitch (2). These may be either built into the machine or produced by means of a separate cam inserted in the machine.

Fagoting: First test to determine stitch length and width. On paper, draw two parallel lines to represent the width of the stitch (this will also be width of space between the two folded edges). Fold back each seamline by half this width, then pin and baste each edge to paper along lines. Center opening under presser foot and stitch, being sure to catch each folded edge in stitching.

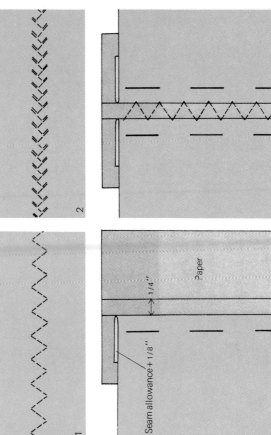

Machine facsimiles of hand stitches

Seam finishes 148-149
Overedge seams 151

Featherstitch / Overcast stitch

FEATHERSTITCH

A decorative as well as functional stretch stitch that can be used for fagoting, embroidery, or quilting. Most often, it is the featherstitch, set at a 0 stitch width, that is used for the straight stretch stitch.

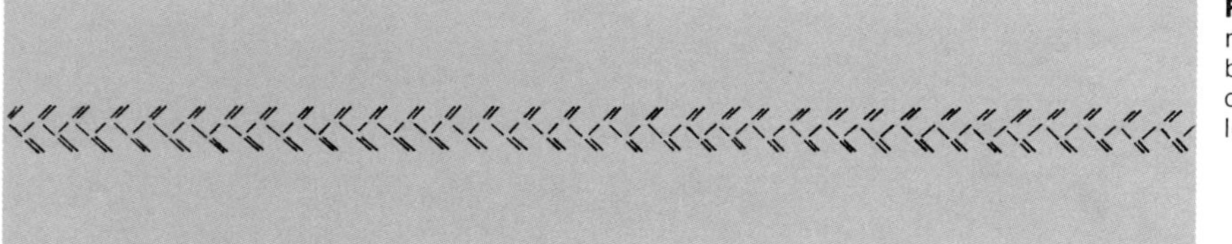

Featherstitch: Stretch stitch available on more elaborate machines. May be either built in or produced by insertion of a separate stitch-pattern cam. Stitch length and width usually adjustable.

FRENCH TACK

see **Tacks** (construction)

HEMSTITCHING

Decorative hemming process characterized by threads drawn out above hem allowance. Exact number of yarns drawn will depend on coarseness of fabric, but, in general, space of the drawn work is ⅛ to ¼ inch. The blindstitch, as shown in the drawings at the right, is the stitch most often used to fasten the hem edge.

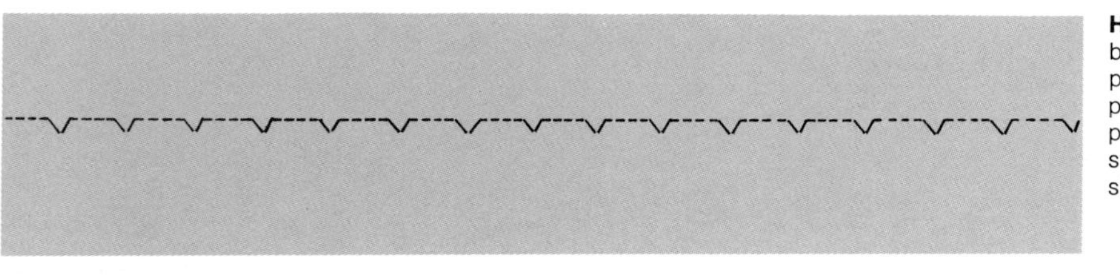

Hemstitching: Done most often with the blindstitch, which may be built in or produced by means of a separate stitch-pattern cam. The straight stitches are placed on the drawn threads; zigzag swings over to catch the fabric. Adjust stitch length and width to suit fabric.

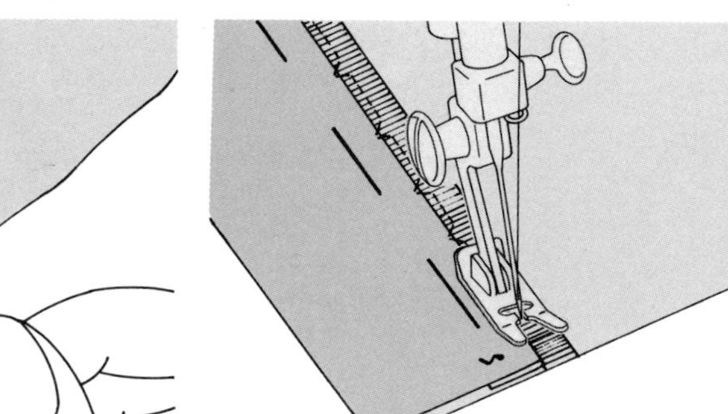

To hemstitch, first fold up hem allowance, then fold under hem edge and baste in place. Draw out yarns above hem edge. With hem allowance up, blindstitch in place, letting the straight stitches stitch on the threads and the zigzag stitch catch the hem edge. Other machine stitches suitable for hemstitching are the Paris point stitch and the Turkish hemstitch. Formation of these usually requires insertion of a separate stitch-pattern cam.

OVERCAST STITCH

Zigzag and other overedging stitches that will form stitches over the edge of the fabric can be used as overcast stitches. The most basic applications are formation of narrow seams and finishing of seams.

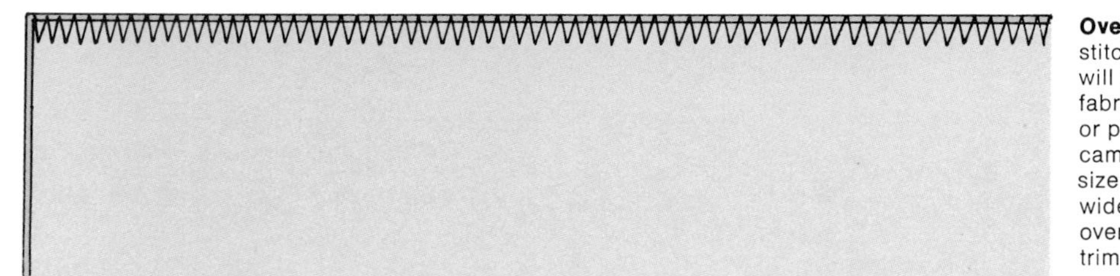

Overcast stitch: Basically the zigzag stitch, but can be any machine stitch that will form stitches over the edge of the fabric. These may be built into the machine or produced by means of stitch-pattern cams. Stitch length and width can range in size from short and narrow to long and wide. Position fabric so stitches will form over the edge; or stitch and then trim away excess fabric.

Tailoring 370

Overhand stitch / Prickstitch

OVERHAND STITCH see **Overcast stitch**

PADDING STITCHES

Stitches used to hold interfacing to such garment parts as undercollar and lapel of a tailored garment. Machine padding stitches show on outside of sections they are applied to.

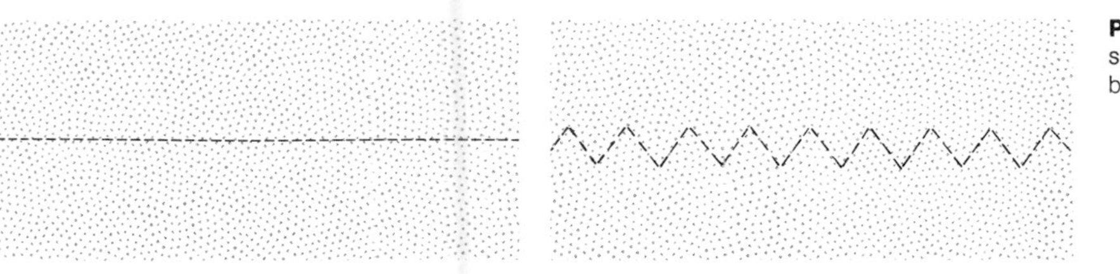

Padding stitches: Either plain straight stitch or multistitch zigzag stitch can be used for machine padding.

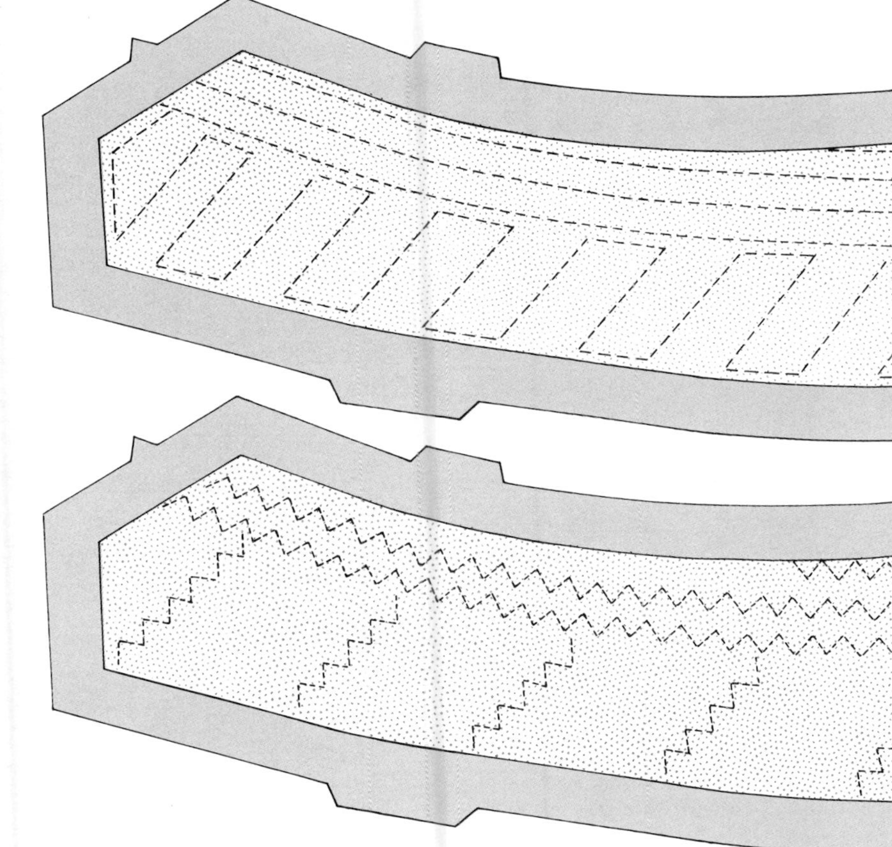

The straight stitch is available on all types of sewing machines.

The multistitch zigzag stitch may be built in or produced through the use of a separate stitch-pattern cam.

PRICKSTITCH see **Blind-hemming stitch**

Machine facsimiles of hand stitches

Fabric-marking methods 94

Tacks

TACKS, CONSTRUCTION
Arrowhead tack. A decorative triangular tack used to reinforce small areas of strain.
Bar tack. A straight tack used for reinforcement at such small areas of strain as the ends of a pocket.

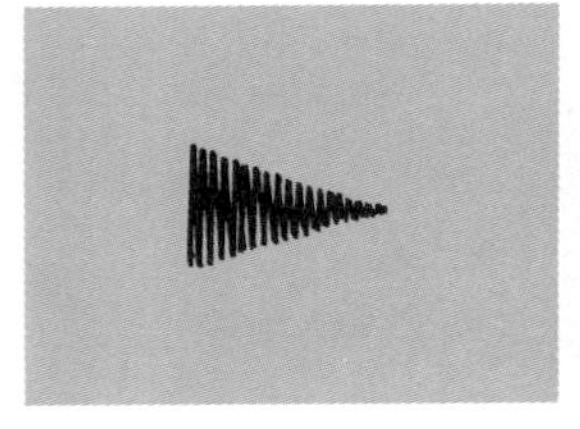

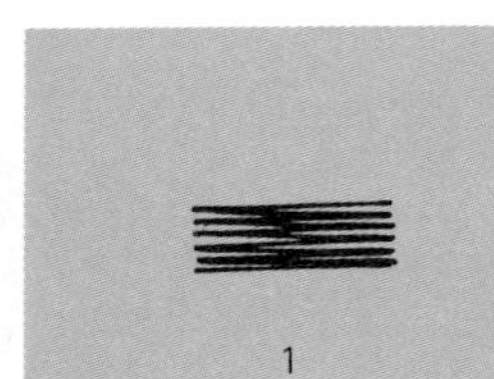
1

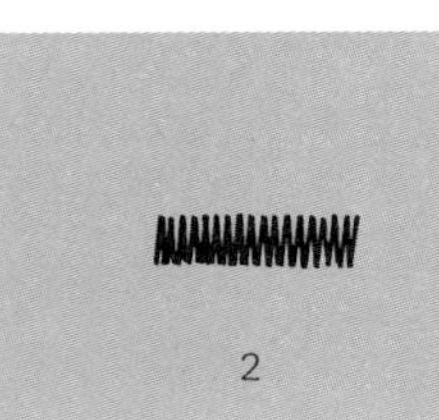
2

Arrowhead tack: This tack is basically an individual unit of the arrowhead stitch pattern. The stitch pattern may be built into the machine or require use of a separate stitch-pattern cam.
Bar tack: This type of tack can be made with a wide zigzag stitch set at a very fine stitch length (1); or a medium-width zigzag set at a fine stitch length (2).

French tack. Free-swinging tack used to hold together two separate garment sections while allowing each to move somewhat independently of the other.

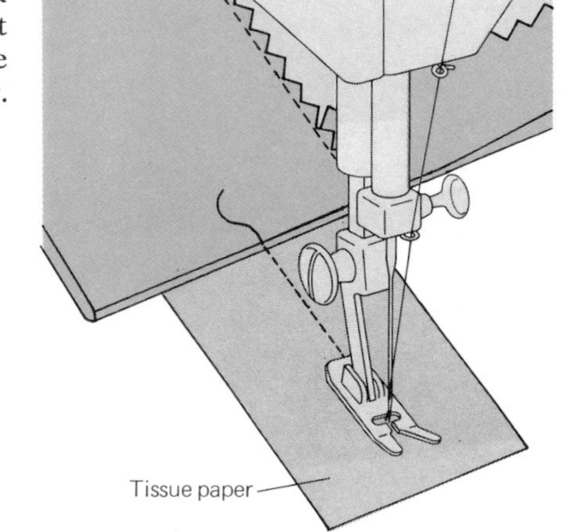

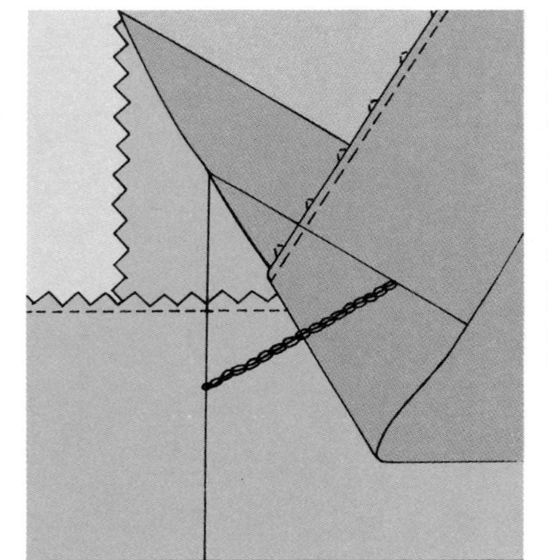

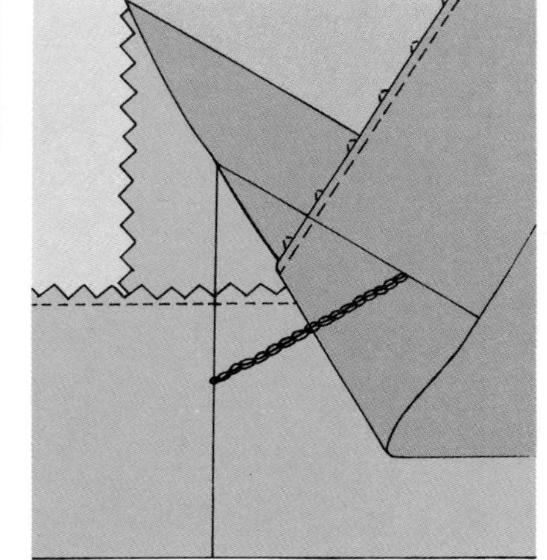

French tack: This tack is made with the chainstitch. A chainstitch capability is available on only a few machines that are equipped with special machine fittings which permit the needle thread alone to make the entire stitch. Start the chain in one garment edge, then chainstitch off the garment to the desired length. It is sometimes recommended that an underlay of tissue be used when chaining off the garment. To secure stitches, cut thread and bring through last loop; remove paper and hand-fasten the free end of the chain to the other garment edge.

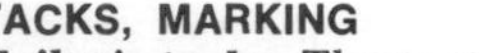

TACKS, MARKING
Tailor's tacks. These stitches, like the hand-made tailor's tack that they derive from, are used to transfer pattern markings to fabric sections.

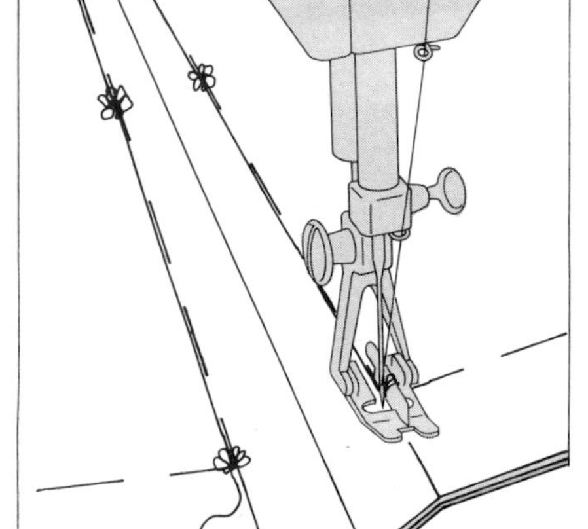

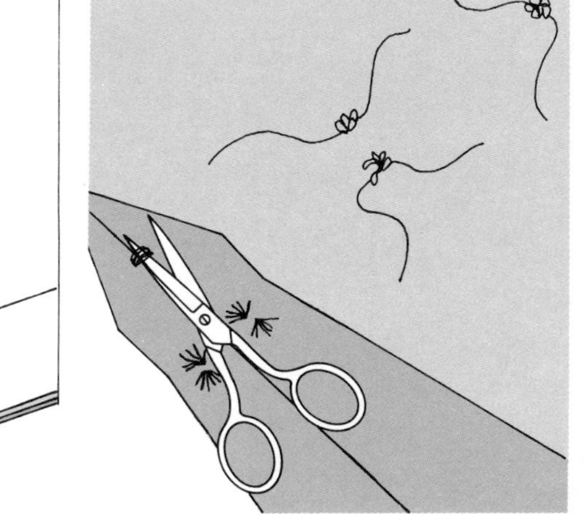

Tailor's tacks: Basically a wide zigzag stitch, this tack also relies on a special machine foot with a raised bar that allows the stitches to be held in an upright position. Very little tension is used. To tack, set machine for a very fine stitch length, or drop feed altogether. Stitch several times in the same place, then slide tack backward off the bar of the foot. To remove paper pattern, cut top thread between tacks. Gently pull the fabric sections apart to the limits of thread loops and cut the threads.

Thread chain / Whipstitch

THREAD CHAIN   see **Chainstitch**

TOPSTITCHING

Machine stitches done from the right side of garment for decorative or functional reasons, sometimes both.

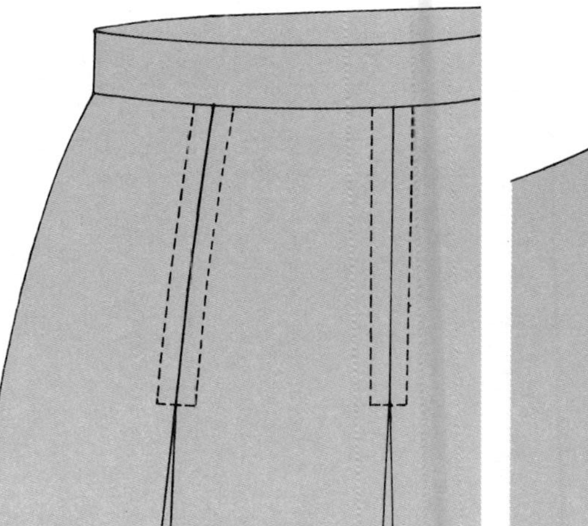

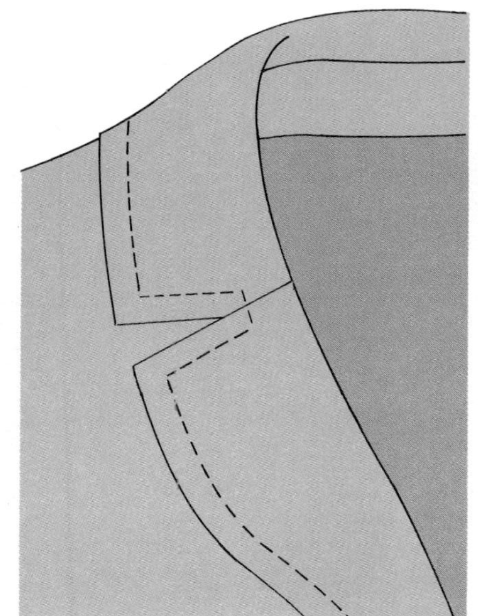

Topstitching: Most often it is the plain straight stitch, set at a longer-than-usual stitch length, that is used for topstitching, but in some situations a zigzag can be appropriate. The thread can be ordinary sewing thread or a heavier thread, such as silk twist. A double thickness of regular thread can also be used in the needle. Thread color can match or contrast, according to effect desired.

UNDERSTITCHING

A line of straight stitching applied along certain seamlines, such as neckline facing seams, to keep facing and seam allowances lying flat in a particular direction.

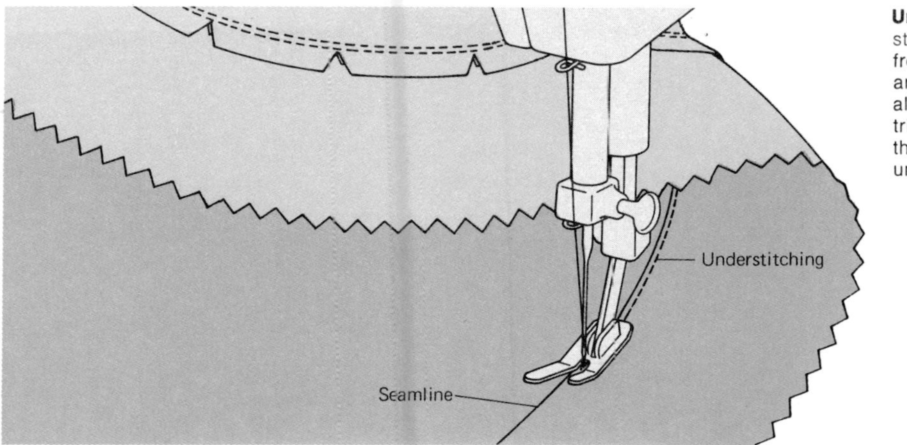

Understitching: This technique uses the straight stitch. The stitching is done from the right side, close to the seamline, and through all fabric layers and seam allowances. The seam allowances are first trimmed, graded, and clipped or notched, then pressed to the side where the understitching will be placed.

WHIPSTITCH   see **Overcast stitch**

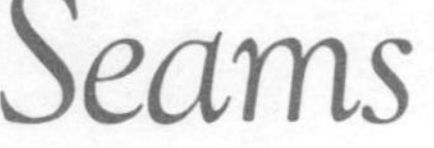

Grain in fabric 84-85

Directional stitching

Directional stitching is the technique of stitching a seam or staystitching a seamline in a particular direction. Its purpose is to support the grain and to prevent the fabric from changing shape or dimension in the seam area. The need for directional stitching arises especially with curved or angled edges, or when constructing garments from loosely woven or dimensionally unstable fabrics.

Stitching should be done with the grain whenever possible. An easy way to determine the correct stitching direction is to run your finger along the cut fabric edge. The direction in which the lengthwise and crosswise fabric yarns are pushed together is **with the grain.** The direction in which they are pushed apart is **against the grain.** In general, if you stitch from the wider part of the garment to the narrower, you will be stitching with the grain. On edges where the direction of the grain changes, as a long shaped seam, stitching should be done in the direction that stays longest with the grain. Illustrations at right show typical examples of grain direction on various garment sections. Also, stitching direction is sometimes indicated on the pattern seamline.

With the grain   Against the grain

Necklines are treated somewhat differently from the norm because the grain, over an entire neck edge, changes direction several times. It is advisable to staystitch each neck edge in two stages, according to the changes of grain direction peculiar to each. When seaming these edges, however, it is inconvenient—and unnecessary—to change stitching direction to follow the grain, especially if edges have been staystitched. Proper pressure and stitch tension will help to maximize the total effect of directional stitching.

The exception to the principles of directional stitching occurs with pile fabric. It is more important to stitch in the direction of the pile than that of the grain. For example, a skirt cut with the pile running down should be stitched accordingly, from waist to hemline.

Staystitching is a row of directional stitching, placed just inside certain seamlines, to prevent them from stretching out of shape during handling and garment construction. It also helps to support the grain at the seamline. The most important seamlines to staystitch are those that are curved or angled, as at a neckline or armhole. When working with a loosely woven or very stretchy fabric, it is advisable to staystitch all seamlines.

Staystitching is done immediately after removing the pattern from the cut fabric sections, and before any handling, such as pinning, basting, or fitting. It is done through a single layer of fabric, using a regular stitch length and matching thread, usually ½ inch from the cut edge. (On placket seamlines, place staystitching ¼ inch from cut edge.) Stitch with the grain whenever possible and change direction whenever necessary.

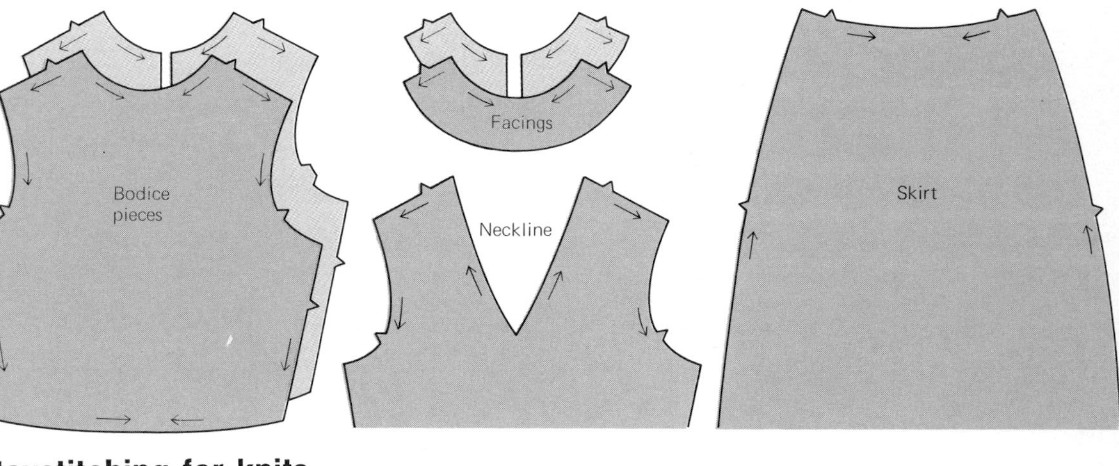

Staystitching for knits

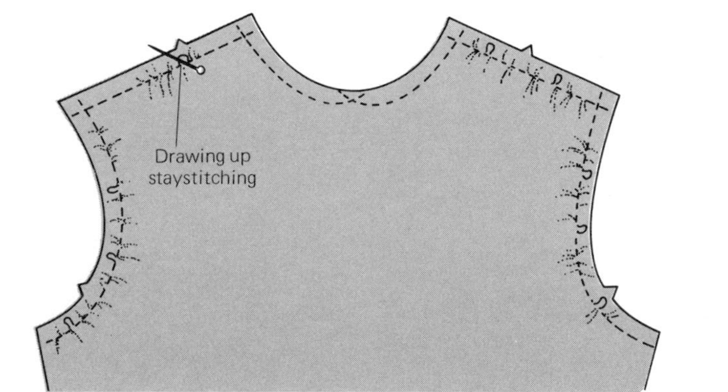

Staystitching for a knit is just as important as for a woven fabric, even though there is no grain direction. The principal purpose is to prevent stretching. After staystitching, lay pattern on top of each fabric section to see if it is the correct size and shape. If knit has stretched slightly, pull staystitching up gently with a pin at 2" intervals until fabric shape matches pattern. If knit was pulled in too much, clip staystitching in a few places.

Pressing 18-19
Thread/needle/stitch length selection 26-27
Machine pressure and tension 28-31
Hand basting 124

Forming a seam

The seam is the basic structural element of any garment and so must be formed with care. The machine should be adjusted correctly to the fabric for stitch length, tension, and pressure. Thread should be properly matched to fabric. Most often, right sides of fabric are placed together; however, in some instances wrong sides are together. Although ⅝″ is the standard seam width, always check your pattern for required width in special seaming situations. Seams should be backstitched at the beginning and end for reinforcement.

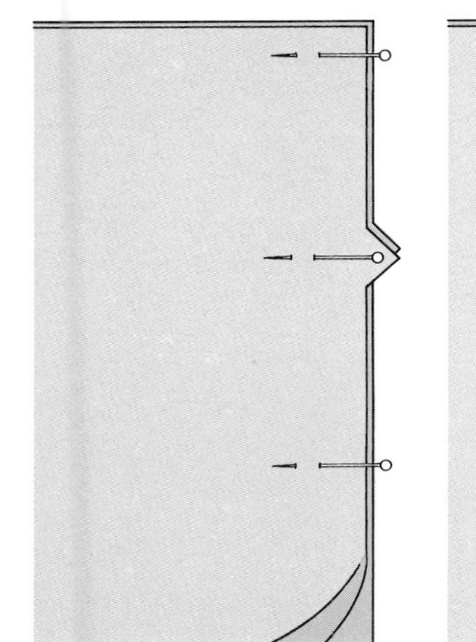

1. Pin-baste seam at regular intervals, matching notches and other markings along seamline. Place pins perpendicular to seamline with tips just beyond seamline and heads toward seam edge.

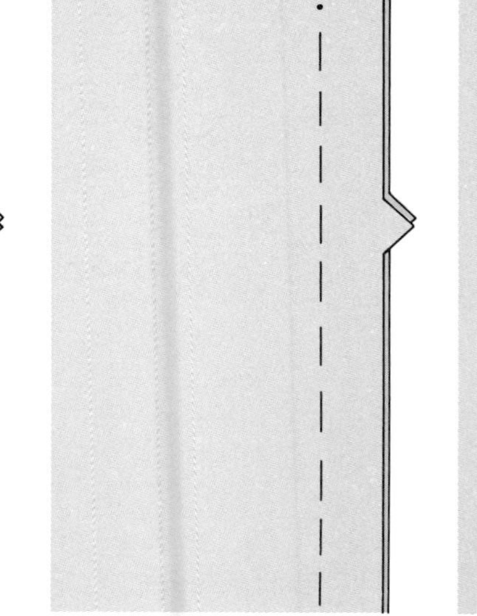

2. Hand-baste close to the seamline, removing pins as you baste. As your skill increases, it may not always be necessary to hand-baste; with many simple seams, pin-basting will be sufficient.

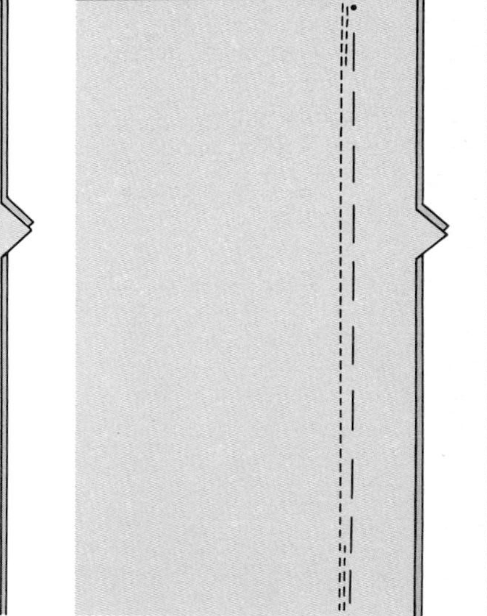

3. Position needle in seamline ½″ from end; lower presser foot. Backstitch to end, then stitch forward on seamline, close to but not through the basting. Backstitch ½″ at end. If seam was pin-basted, remove pins as you stitch. Clip threads close to stitching.

4. Remove thread basting. Unless instructions specify another pressing method, seams are first pressed flat in the same direction as they were stitched, then pressed open. Some seams may need clipping or notching before being pressed open.

Keeping seams straight

Needle hole
3/8″ 1/2″ 5/8″ 3/4″
5 4 3 3 4 5 6
5/8″ crossline
Fabric edge

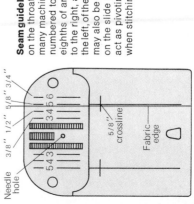

Seam guidelines are etched on the throat plate of many machines. These lines, numbered to indicate eighths of an inch, extend to the right, and sometimes the left, of the needle. There may also be crosslines on the slide plate, which act as pivoting guides when stitching corners.

Needle hole
5/8″
Seam and hem guide
Fabric edge

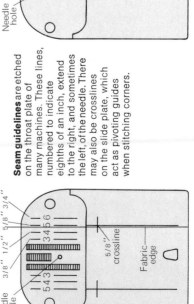

A separate gauge, attached to the machine, is a good substitute for the etched guidelines. Very helpful for stitching curves.

Needle hole
5/8″
5/8″
Tape
Fabric edge

Masking or adhesive tape, placed at a distance of ⅝″ from the needle hole, will provide the necessary guidance on a machine that has neither etched guidelines nor a separate gauge.

Seams

Plain seams

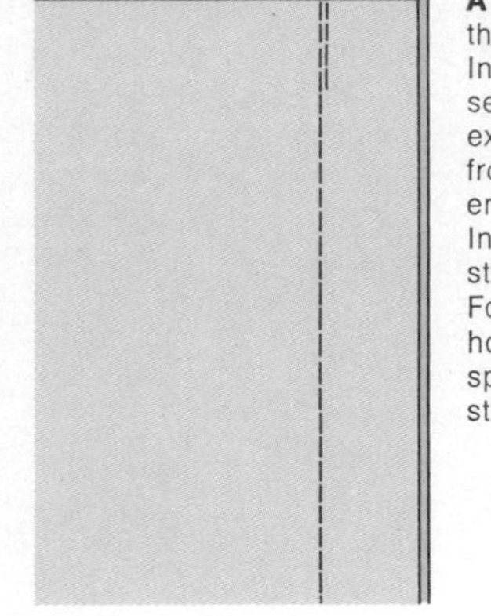

A straight seam is the one that occurs most often. In a well-made straight seam, the stitching is exactly the same distance from the seam edge the entire length of the seam. In most cases, a plain straight stitch is used. For stretchy fabrics, however, a tiny zigzag or special machine stretch stitch may be used.

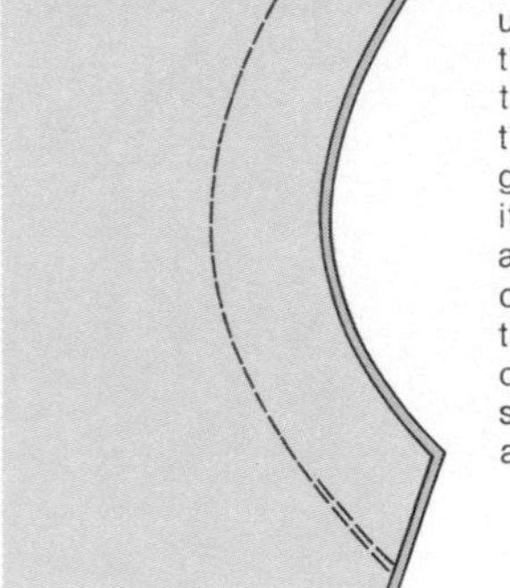

A curved seam requires careful guiding as it passes under the needle so that the entire seamline will be the same even distance from the edge. The separate seam guide will help greatly; it should be placed at an angle so that the edge closest to the needle does the guiding. To get better control, use a shorter stitch length (15 per inch) and slower machine speed.

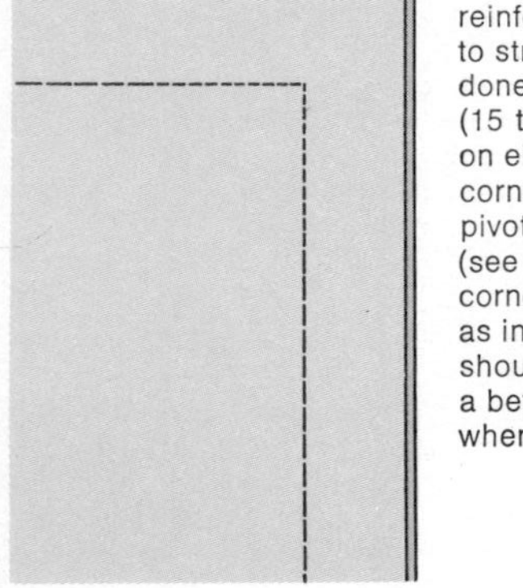

A cornered seam needs reinforcement at the angle to strengthen it. This is done by using small stitches (15 to 20 per inch) for 1″ on either side of the corner. It is important to pivot with accuracy (see top right). When cornered seams are enclosed, as in a collar, the corners should be blunted so that a better point results when the collar is turned.

How to make cornered seams

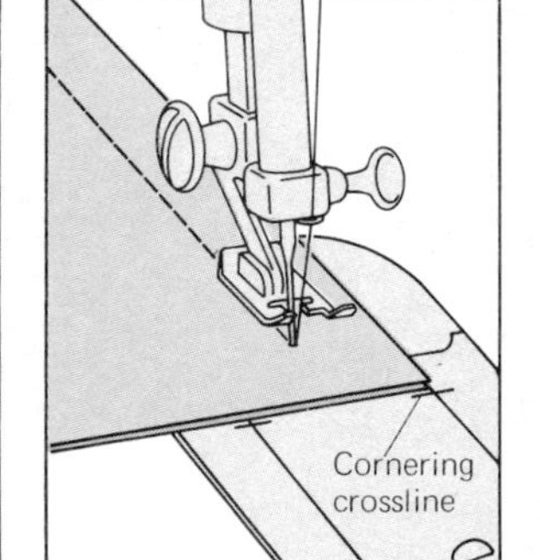

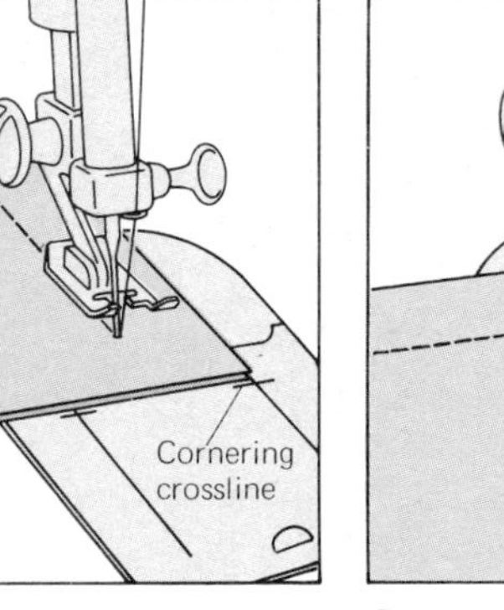

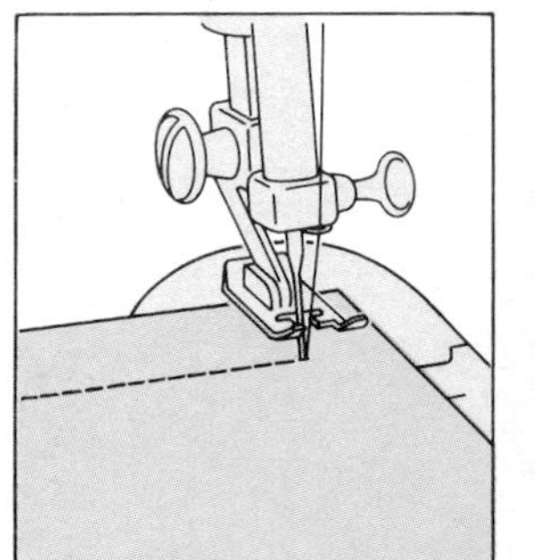

To stitch a cornered seam, line up edge of fabric with ⅝″ guideline on throat plate. Stitch seam toward corner, stopping with needle in fabric when edge reaches cornering crosslines on slide plate. Raise presser foot.

Pivot fabric on the needle, bringing the bottom edge of fabric in line with the ⅝″ guideline on machine.

Lower foot and stitch in the new direction, keeping edge of fabric even with the ⅝″ guideline.

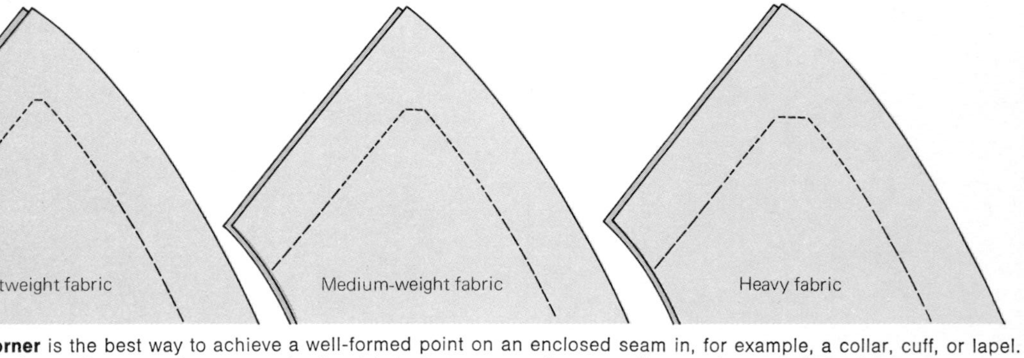

Blunting the corner is the best way to achieve a well-formed point on an enclosed seam in, for example, a collar, cuff, or lapel. Take one stitch diagonally across the corner of a fine fabric, two on a medium one, three on heavy or bulky fabric.

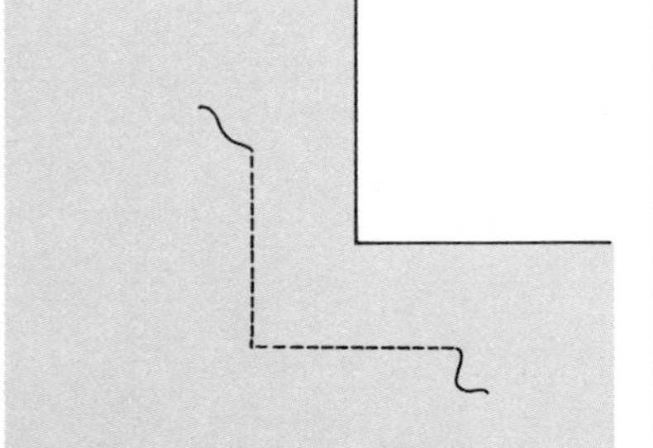

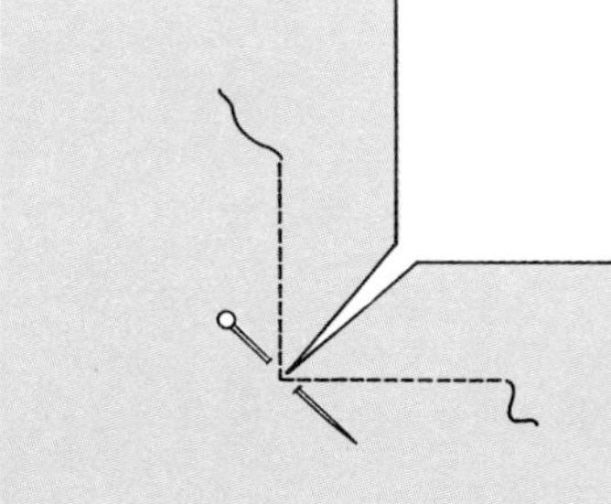

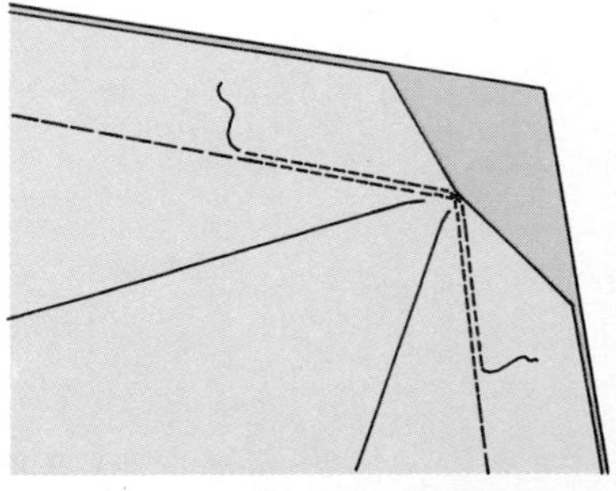

To join an inward corner with an outward corner or straight edge, first reinforce the inward angle, stitching just inside the seamline 1″ on either side of corner.

Insert a pin diagonally across the point where stitching forms the angle. Clip exactly to this point, being careful not to cut past the stitches.

Spread the clipped section to fit the other edge; pin in position. Then, with clipped side up, stitch on the seamline, pivoting at the corner.

Pressing 18-19 Hand pickstitch 124
Princess seam 158

Additional seam techniques

Depending on their location or shape, some seams may require you to take subsequent steps, other than pressing, if they are to have the desired professional look. The range of supplementary procedures is shown below. In some situations, one extra step will suffice; in others, however, it will take several—or even, as in the case of a faced neckline seam, *all* of them—to make a seam lie flat and smooth. When more than one technique is involved, this is the appropriate progression: (1) trim, (2) grade, (3) clip or notch, (4) understitch. A good sharp pair of small scissors is indispensable for most of the processes. In undertaking any of them, consider the fabric type carefully. One that doesn't ravel can be trimmed closer than one that does. Keep clipping or notching to a minimum on loosely woven fabric. Remember, the thicker the fabric, the greater the need to reduce bulk.

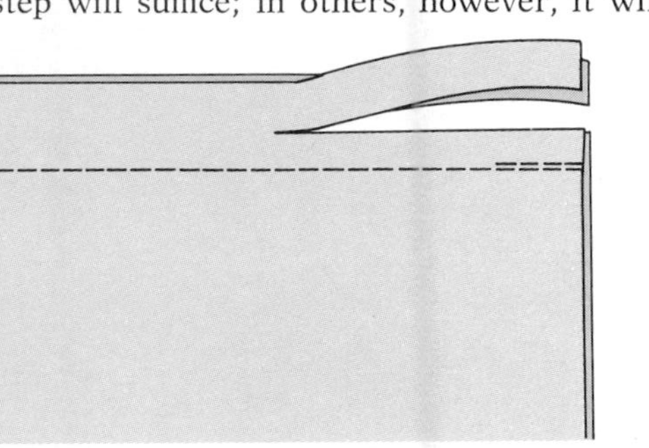

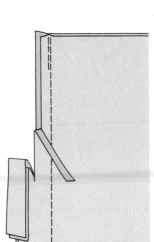

Trimming means cutting away some of the seam allowance. It is done when the full width of the seam allowances would interfere with fit (as in an armhole) or with further construction (as in a French seam). It is the preliminary step to grading (see the next drawing); seams are first trimmed to half their width before grading.

Grading (also called blending, layering, or beveling) is the cutting of seam allowances to different widths, with the seam allowance that will fall nearest the garment side cut the widest. It is recommended that seams be graded when they form an edge or are enclosed. The result is a seam that lies flat without causing a bulky ridge.

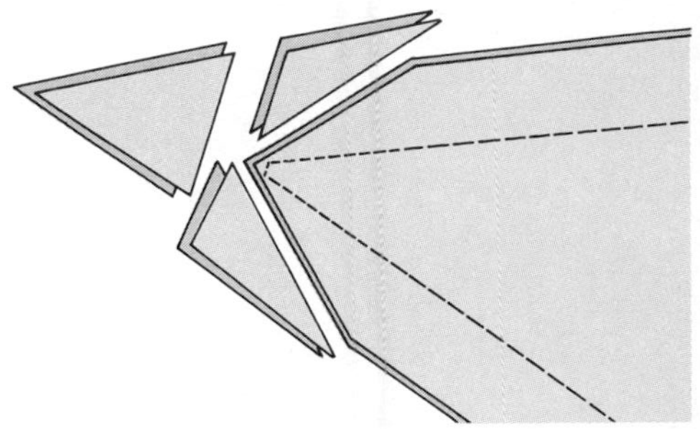

To trim a corner of an enclosed seam, first trim the seam allowances across the point close to the stitching, then taper them on either side. The more elongated the point, the farther back the seam allowance should be trimmed, so that when point is turned, there is no danger of seam allowances overlapping and causing bulk.

Clipping and notching are used on curved seams to allow them to lie smooth. *Clips are slits* cut into the seam allowance of convex, or *outward,* curves that permit the edges to spread. (With either technique, hold scissors points just short of seamline to avoid cutting past the stitching.) *Notches are wedges* cut from seam allowance of concave, or *inward,* curves; space opened by removal of fabric lets edge draw in. When clips and notches face one another, as in a princess seam (see next sketch), they should be staggered to avoid weakening seam.

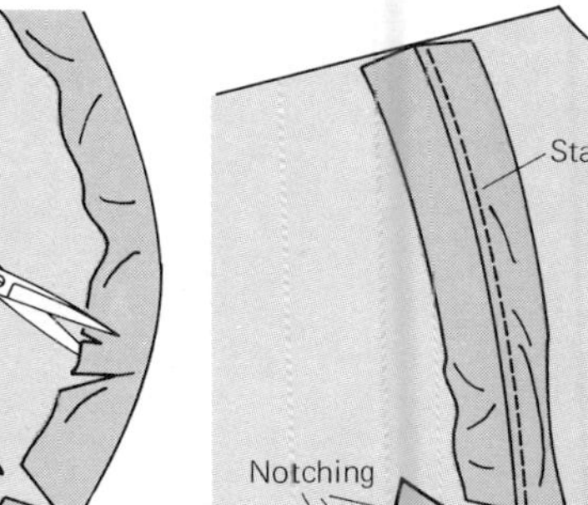

Joining inward and outward curves: This s handled in a special way. First staystitch outward curve and clip seam allowance *to* stitching, not through it. With clipped edge on top, stitch seam. Notch inward curve to make seam lie smooth. Press seam open over tailor's ham.

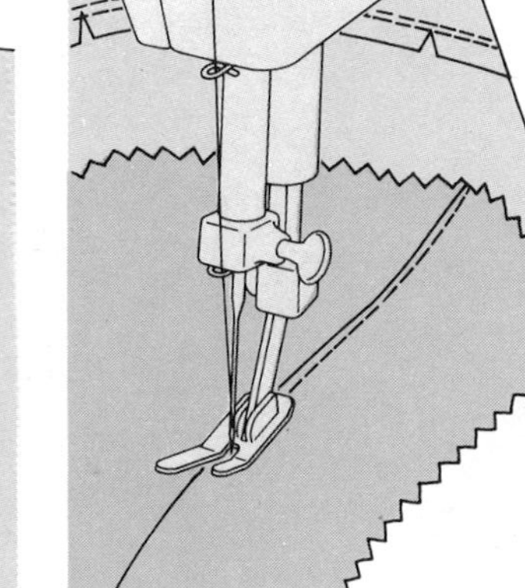
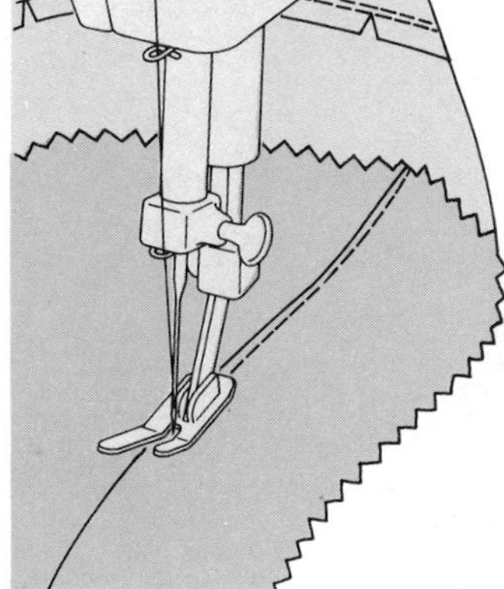
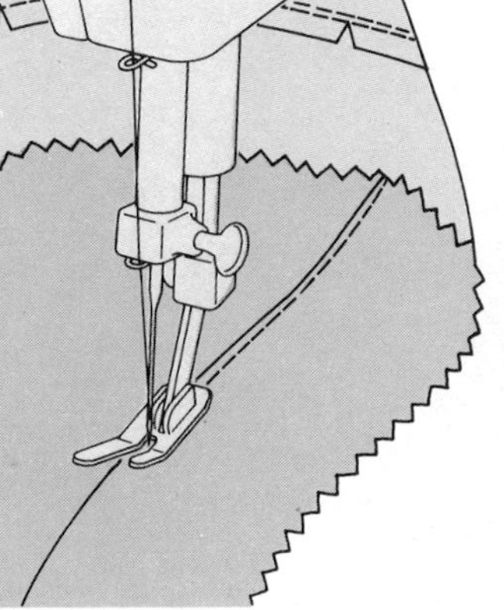

Understitching keeps a facing and its seamline from rolling to garment right side; it is done after seam allowances have been trimmed and graded, then clipped or notched. Working from the right side, stitch through facing and seam allowances, staying close to seamline.

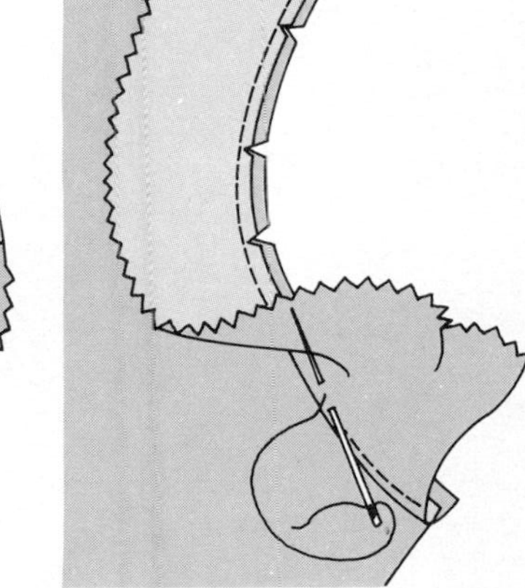

Hand understitching is desirable on a fine fabric or when machine stitching could distort a tailored shape. Use hand pickstitch; stitch through facing and seam allowances, as with machine understitching. Advisable on tailored collar because fabric control is more precise.

Seam finishes

Zigzag stitching 32-37
Overcast stitch 130

When and how to apply them

A seam finish is any technique used to make a seam edge look neater and/or keep it from raveling. Though not essential to completion of the garment, it can add measurably to its life. Less tangibly, finished seams are a trim professional touch, in which you can take pardonable pride.

Three considerations determine the seam finish decision: *(1) The type and weight of fabric.* Does it ravel excessively, a little, or not at all? *(2) The amount and kind of wear—and care—the garment will receive.* If a garment is worn often, then tossed into the washer, the seams need a durable finish. On the other hand, if the style is a passing fad, or will be worn infrequently, you may elect not to finish the seam edges. *(3) Whether or not seams will be seen.* An unlined jacket warrants the more elaborate bias-binding finish. A lined garment requires no finishing at all, unless the fabric has a tendency to ravel a great deal.

Plain straight seams are finished after they have been pressed open. Plain *curved* or *cornered* seams are seam-finished right after stitching, next clipped or notched, then pressed open.

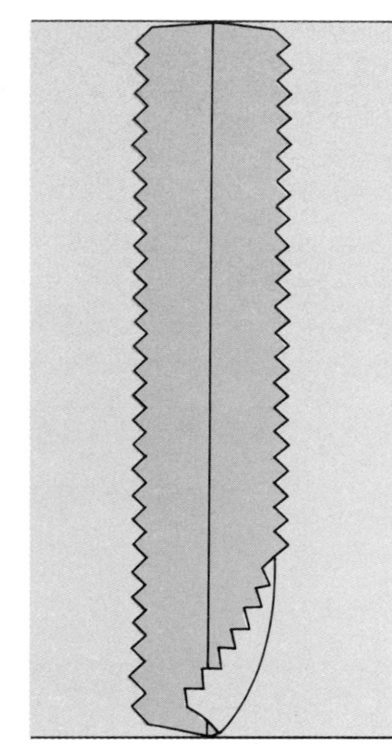

Pinked: Cut along edge of seam allowance with pinking shears. For best results, do not fully open shears nor close all the way to the points. If fabric is crisp and lightweight, it is possible to trim two edges at once, before pressing seam open. Otherwise do one edge at a time. Pinking is attractive, but will not of itself prevent raveling.

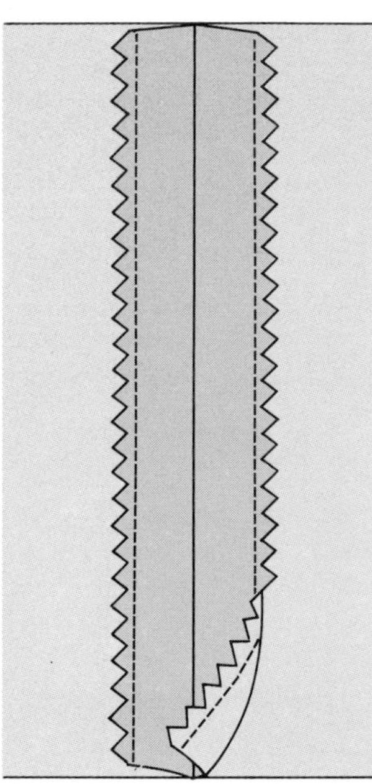

Stitched-and-pinked: Using a short stitch, place a line of stitching ¼″ from edge of seam allowance, then pink edge. This finish can be used where pinking is desired, and it will minimize raveling.

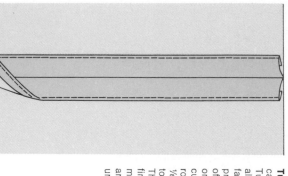

Turned-and-stitched (also called clean-finished): Turn under edge of seam allowance ⅛″ (¼″ if fabric ravels easily); press. Stitch along edge of fold. It may be helpful, on difficult fabrics or curved edges, to place a row of stitching at the ⅛″ or ¼″ foldline to help turn edge under. This is a neat, tailored finish for light- to medium-weight fabrics, and is suitable for an unlined jacket.

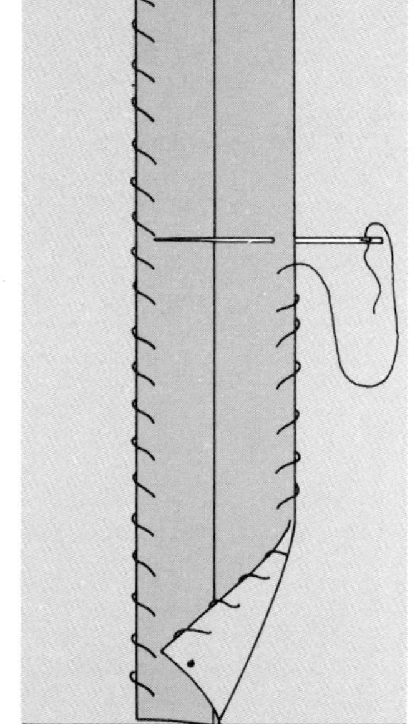
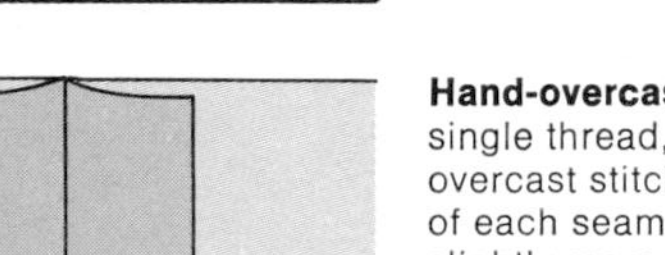

Hand-overcast: Using single thread, make overcast stitches at edge of each seam allowance slightly more than ⅛″ in depth and spaced ¼″ apart. Do not pull thread too tight. Use this method when a machine finish is impractical or a hand finish is preferred.

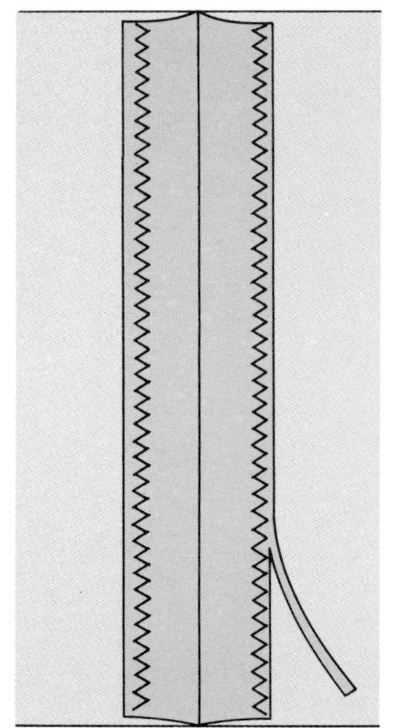

Zigzagged: Set stitch for medium width and short (about 15) length. Then stitch near, but not on, the edge of seam allowance. Trim close to stitching. This is one of the quickest and most effective ways to finish a fabric that ravels. It *can* be used for a knit, but special care must be taken not to stretch the seam edge, or it will ripple.

Bias tapes 16
Cutting and joining bias strips 298-299

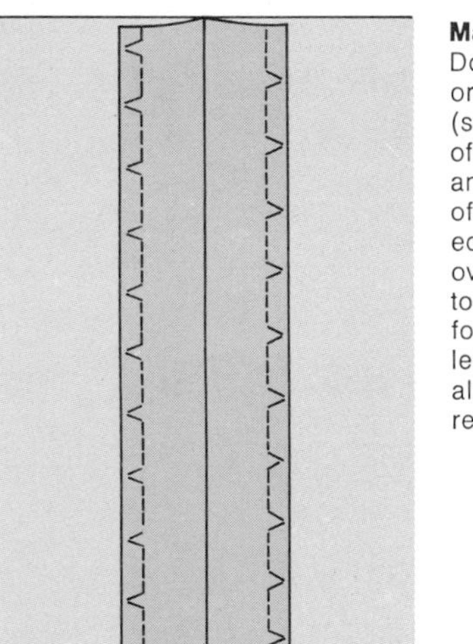

Machine-overedged: Done with overedge or blindstitch setting (special stitch pattern of 4–6 straight stitches and 1 zigzag). Point of zigzag should fall on edge of fabric. If using overedge, position fabric to right of the needle; for blindstitch, to the left. This method is an alternative to the regular zigzag.

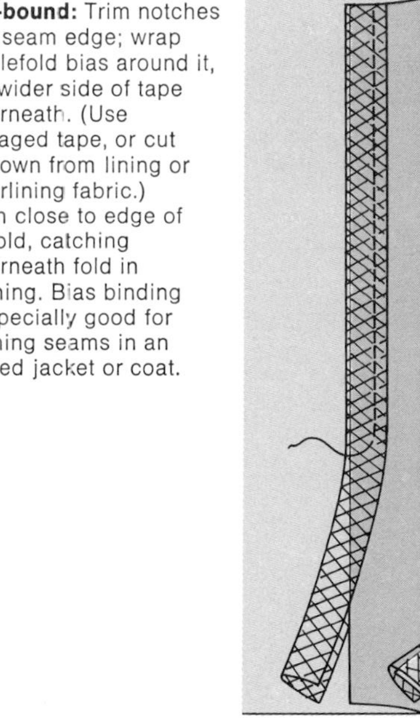

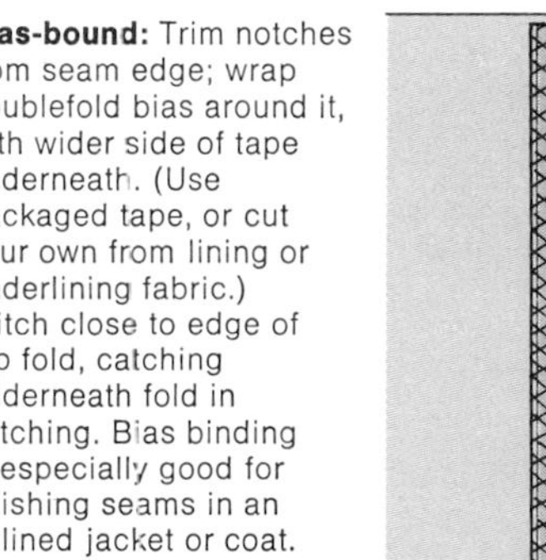

Bias-bound: Trim notches from seam edge; wrap doublefold bias around it, with wider side of tape underneath. (Use packaged tape, or cut your own from lining or underlining fabric.) Stitch close to edge of top fold, catching underneath fold in stitching. Bias binding is especially good for finishing seams in an unlined jacket or coat.

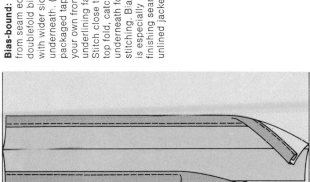

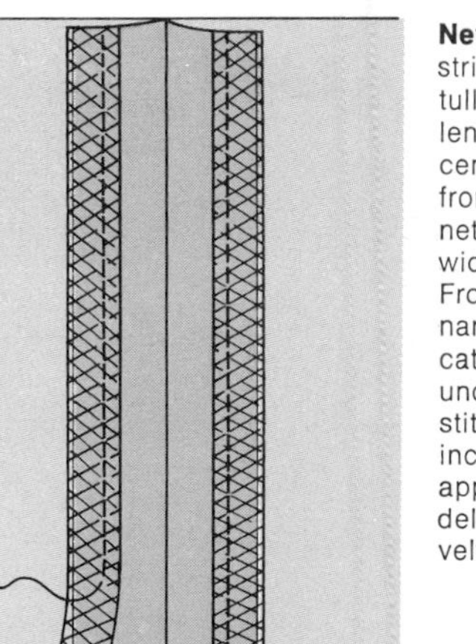

Net-bound: Cut ½″-wide strips of nylon net or tulle; fold in half lengthwise, slightly off center. Trim notches from seam edge and wrap net around edge with wider half underneath. From top, edgestitch narrow half of binding, catching wider half underneath in the stitching. This is an inconspicuous and appropriate finish for delicate fabrics, such as velvet or chiffon.

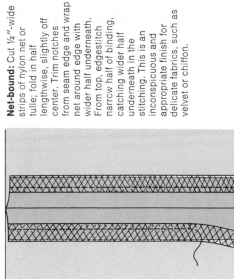

Hong Kong: An alternative to the bias-bound finish, this is especially suitable for heavy fabrics. Proceed as follows:
1. Cut 1½″-wide bias strips from a lightweight material that matches garment. Or, use single- or double-fold bias tape and press it open.

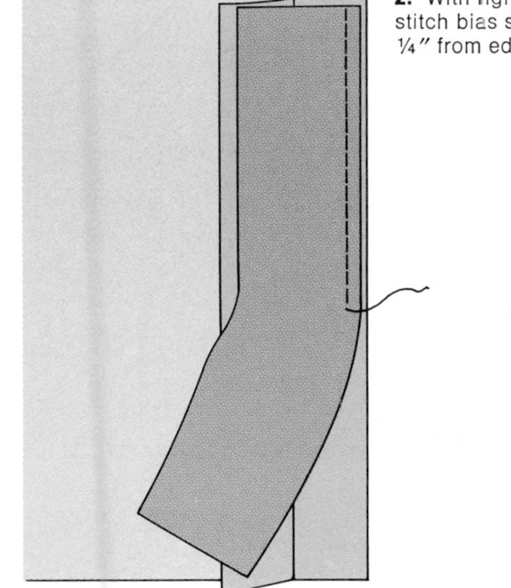

2. With right sides together, stitch bias strip to seam allowance ¼″ from edge.

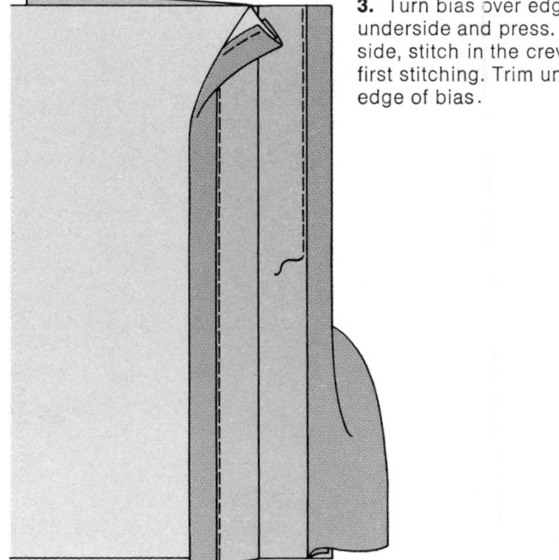

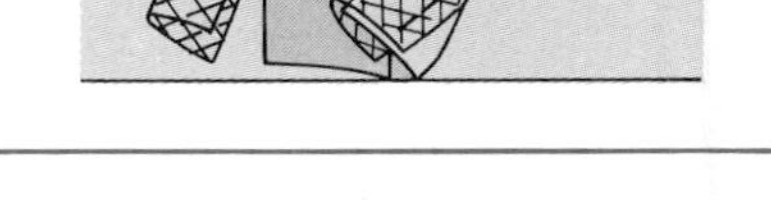

3. Turn bias over edge to the underside and press. From the right side, stitch in the crevice of the first stitching. Trim unfinished edge of bias.

Self-finished seams

Self-enclosed seams

Self-enclosed seams are those in which all seam allowances are contained within the finished seam, thus avoiding the necessity of a separate seam finish. They are especially appropriate for visible seams, such as occur with sheer fabrics and in unlined jackets. Also, they are ideally suited to garments that will receive rugged wear or much laundering. Proper trimming and pressing are important steps if the resulting seams are to be sharp and flat rather than lumpy and uneven.

Precise stitching is essential, too. See topstitching of seams for helpful suggestions.

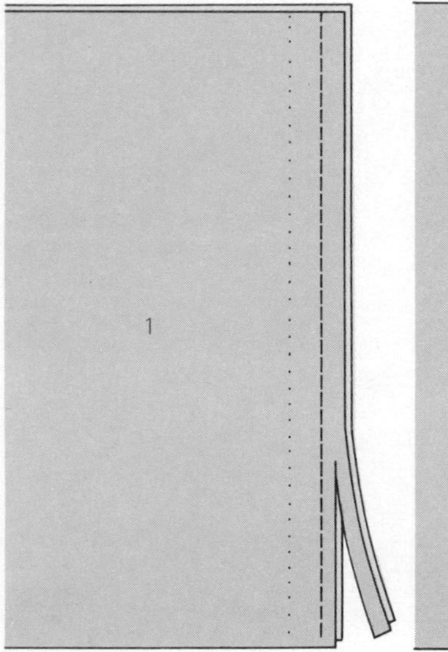

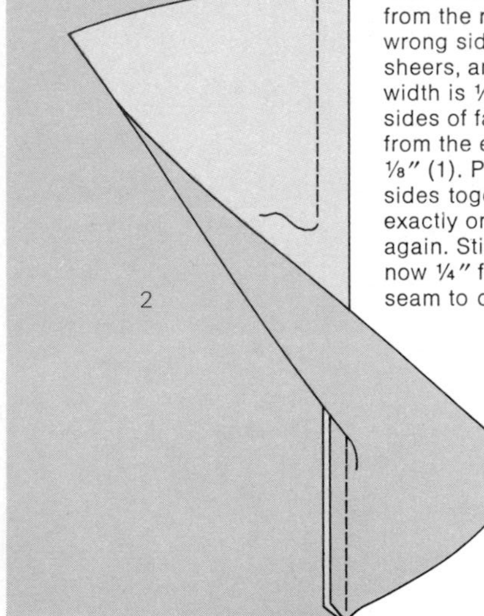

The French seam is stitched twice, once from the right side and once from the wrong side. It is the classic seam for sheers, and looks best if the finished width is $\frac{1}{4}''$ or less. With wrong sides of fabric together, stitch $\frac{3}{8}''$ from the edge. Trim seam allowances to $\frac{1}{8}''$ (1). Press seam open. Fold right sides together, with stitched line exactly on edge of fold, and press again. Stitch on the seamline, which is now $\frac{1}{4}''$ from the fold (2). Press seam to one side.

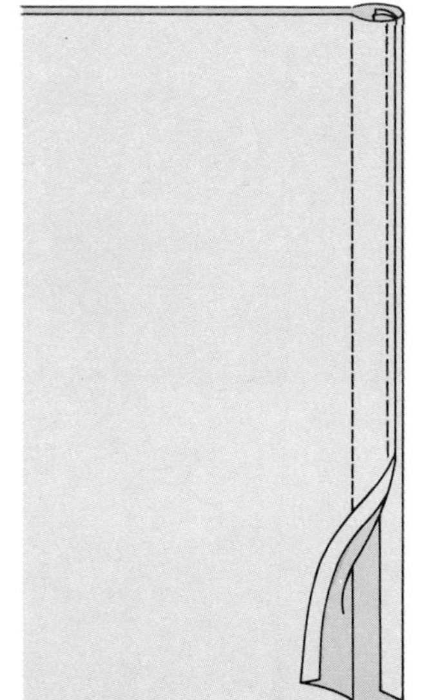

The mock French seam can be used in place of the French seam, especially on curves, where a French seam is difficult to execute. With right sides of fabric together, stitch on the seamline. Trim seam allowances to $\frac{1}{2}''$. Turn in the seam edges $\frac{1}{4}''$ and press, matching folds along the edge. Stitch these folded edges together. Press seam to one side.

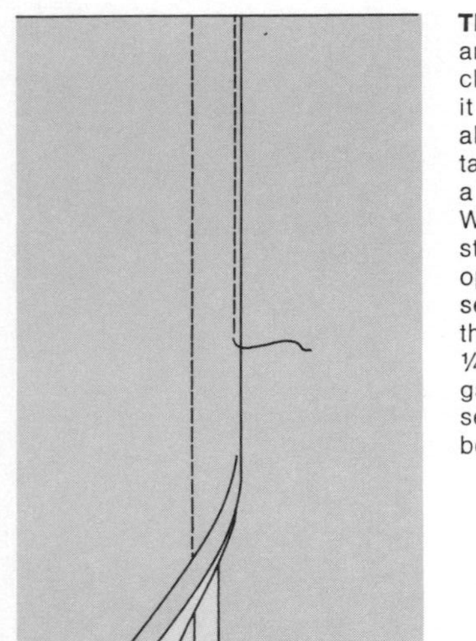

The flat-felled seam is very sturdy, and so is often used for sports clothing and children's wear. Since it is formed on the right side, it is also decorative, and care must be taken to keep widths uniform, within a seam and from one seam to another. With wrong sides of fabric together, stitch on the seamline. Press seam open, then to one side. Trim the inner seam allowance to $\frac{1}{8}''$. Press under the edge of outer seam allowance $\frac{1}{4}''$. Stitch this folded edge to the garment. Be careful to press like seams in the same direction (e.g., both shoulder seams to the front).

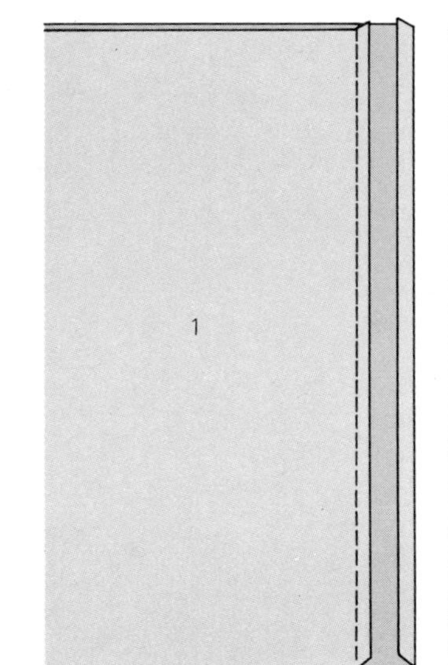

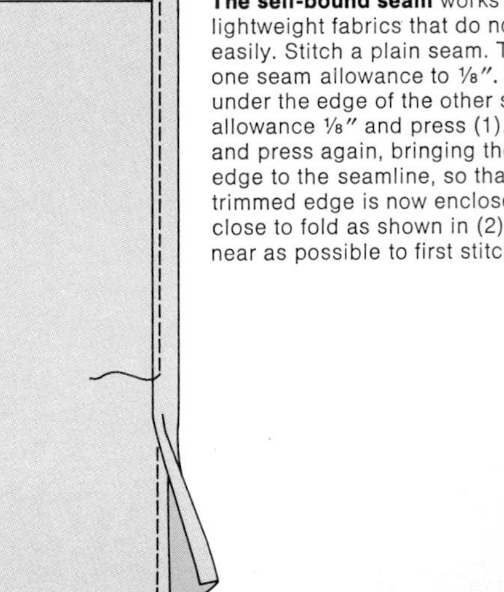

The self-bound seam works best on lightweight fabrics that do not ravel easily. Stitch a plain seam. Trim one seam allowance to $\frac{1}{8}''$. Turn under the edge of the other seam allowance $\frac{1}{8}''$ and press (1). Turn and press again, bringing the folded edge to the seamline, so that the trimmed edge is now enclosed. Stitch close to fold as shown in (2), as near as possible to first stitching.

Cable cord 16
Zigzag stitching 32-37

Overedge seams

Overedge seams are very narrow, never more than ¼ inch wide, and are used when a seam should be flexible or have minimum bulk. Seam allowances are either finished by the seam stitches themselves when the seam is stitched, or subsequently by an additional row of stitches. A plain zigzag stitch, or a variation of it, is used for most overedge seams. Some seams are trimmed to the finished width before they are constructed, some after they are constructed. Test stitch length and width so stitches will not draw up fabric. Follow pattern seamlines so that the size of the garment is maintained.

The hairline seam can be used for collars, cuffs, and facings in sheer fabrics. This seam is stitched with a narrow zigzag, then trimmed close to the stitching so that no seam allowances show through. To give it more weight, filler cord may be added during the stitching.
Set machine for narrow and short zigzag stitch. Unwind sufficient cord that there will be no strain on it.
Lead cord under stitching (consult machine manual for exact instructions).
Stitch along the seamline, covering cord in the process. Trim seam allowances. Turn to right side. Work seam to the edge and press.

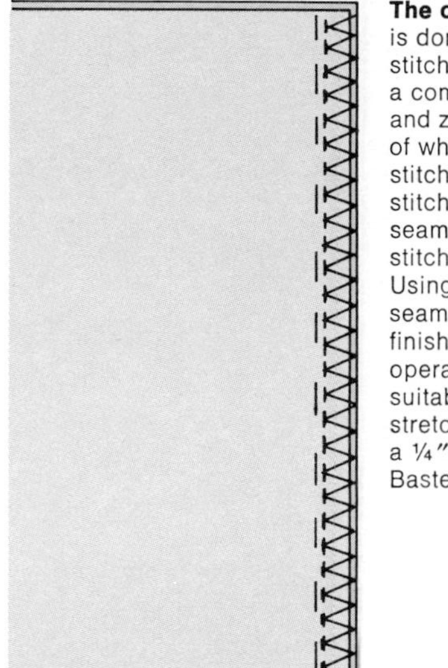

The zigzag seam is similar to the hairline, but the stitch is wider. Its principal use is with fur and fake fur fabrics, where the stitch will disappear into the fabric. Trim seam allowances to ⅛″ for short pile, ¼″ for a long pile fabric. (Cut through the skin or backing only, not the fur.) Mark notches on new seam edges with chalk. Baste seam. Stitch, using a plain zigzag (medium width and short length for short pile; wide width and regular length for longer pile). From right side, with a pin, gently pull free any hairs caught in the stitching. Finger-press the seam to one side.

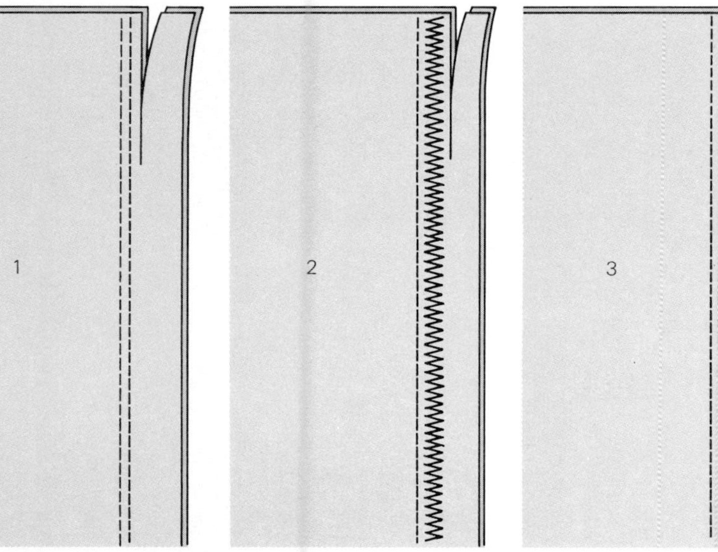

A double-stitched seam is especially good for knits, such as tricot or soft jersey, where edges tend to curl. Stitch a plain seam with straight or straight-stretch stitch. Machine-stitch a second row ⅛″ from the first, using one of the following: a straight stitch (1), a zigzag (2), a blindstitch or other overedge stitch (3). Trim seam allowances close to the stitching. Press seam to one side.

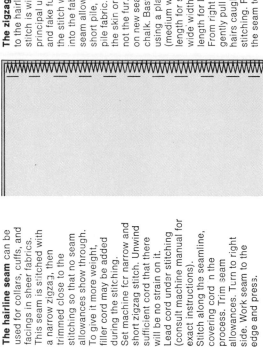

The overedge-stitch seam is done by using a special stitch pattern that is a combination of straight and zigzag stitches, some of which are stretch stitches. The straight stitches fall on the seamline; the zigzag stitches go over the edge. Using this type of stitch, seams can be joined and finished in one stitching operation. They are suitable for knit or stretch fabric. Start with a ¼″ seam allowance. Baste and then stitch seam.

Decorative and special seams

Chart (topstitching) 27
Machine accessories 38-39
Hand basting 124-125
Fagoting stitches 127, 139

Topstitching seams

Seams are topstitched from the right side, with usually one or more seam allowances caught into the stitching. Topstitching is an excellent way to emphasize a construction detail, to hold seam allowances flat, or to add interest to plain fabric.

There are two main considerations when topstitching. The first is that normal stitching guides will not, as a rule, be visible, so new ones have to be established. A row of hand basting or tape, applied just next to the topstitching line, can help. The presser foot is also a handy gauge. Another useful device is a quilter guide-bar positioned along a line parallel to the topstitching line.

The other consideration with topstitching is how to keep the underlayers flat and secure. *Even* basting will hold pressed-open seam allowances; *diagonal* basting will hold those that are enclosed or pressed to one side. Grading and reducing seam bulk will contribute to a smooth top side.

A long stitch is best when topstitching. Use buttonhole twist or single or double strands of regular thread. Adjust needle and tension accordingly.

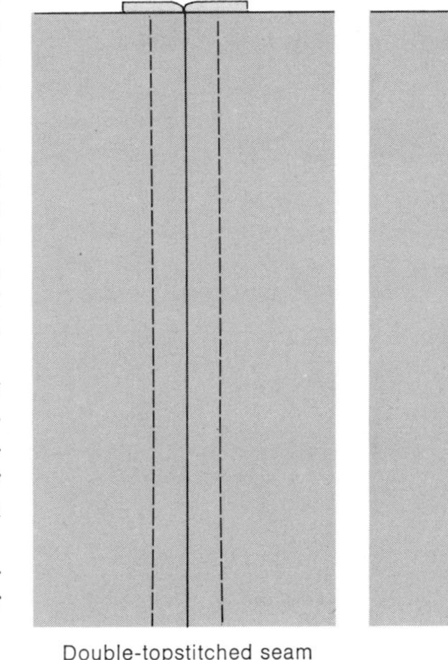
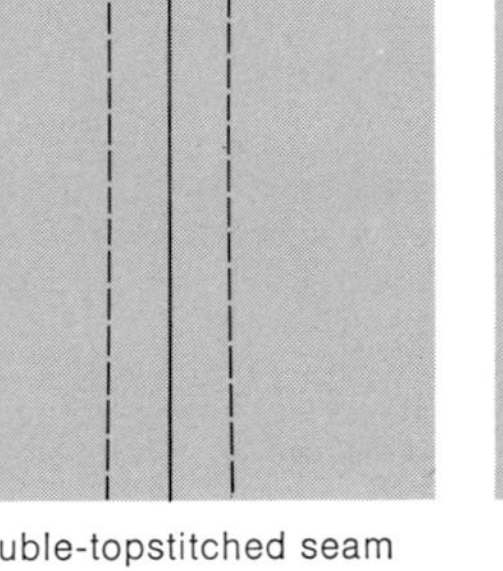
Double-topstitched seam

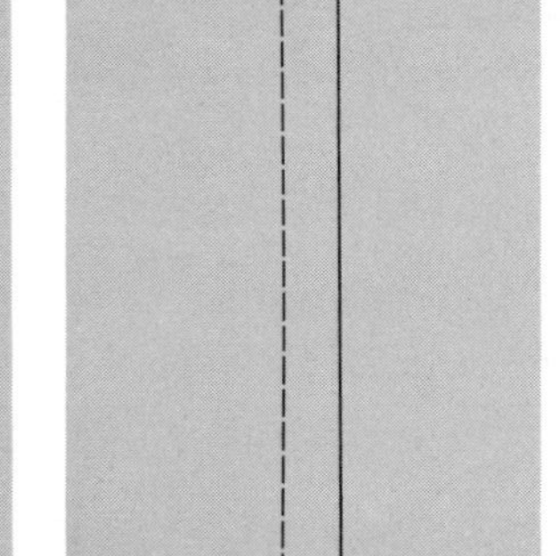
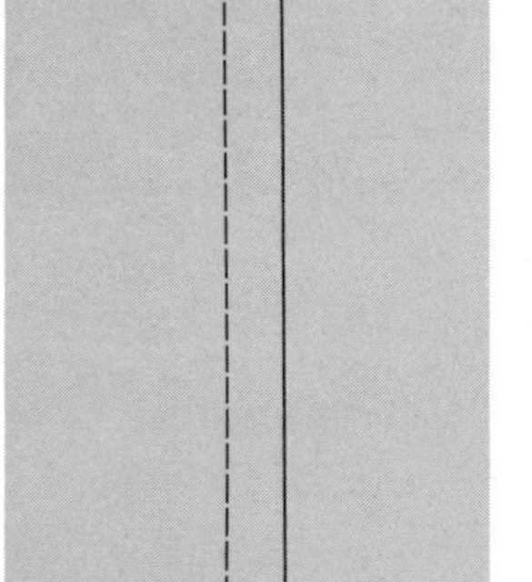

Welt seam

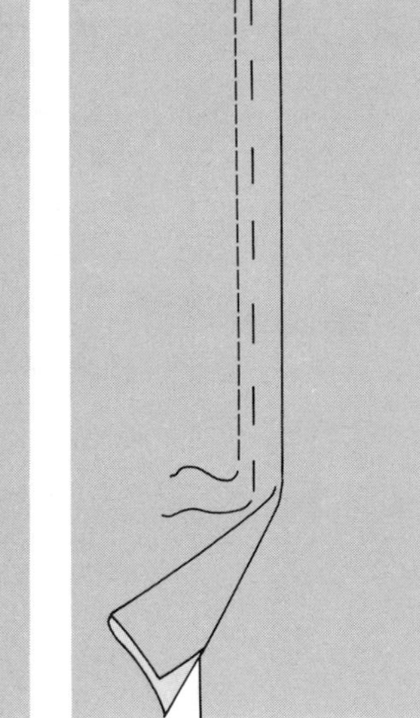
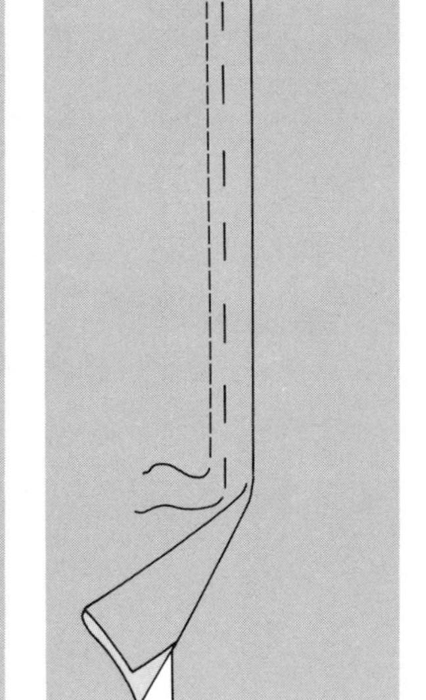
Tucked seam

Double-topstitched seam: Press plain seam open. Topstitch an equal distance from each side of seamline, catching seam allowances into stitching.
Welt seam: Stitch a plain seam and press both seam allowances to one side; trim inside seam allowance to ¼″. Topstitch, catching wider seam allowance.
Tucked seam: Fold under one seam allowance; press. With folded edge on top, match seamlines and baste through all thicknesses. Stitch ¼″ to ⅜″ from fold. If seam is curved, first staystitch top seam allowance, clip or notch, and press to wrong side. Then baste in position; topstitch close to fold.

Slot seam: Machine-baste on the seamline, leaving long threads at each end. Clip bobbin thread every fifth stitch (1). Press seam open. Cut a 1½″-wide underlay of same or contrasting fabric. Center it under seam and baste. Topstitch an equal distance from the center on each side. Pull out basting threads (2).

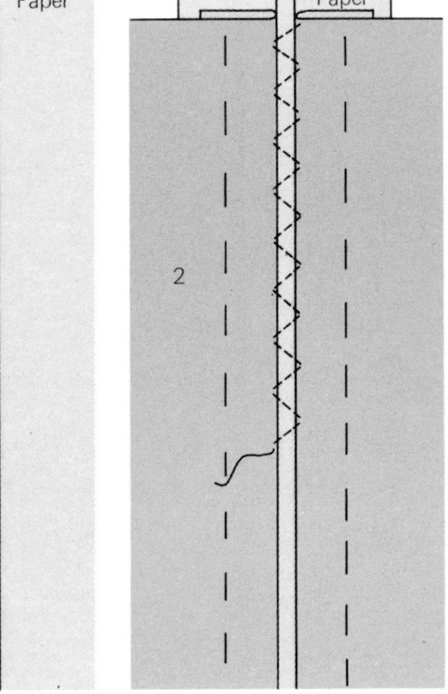

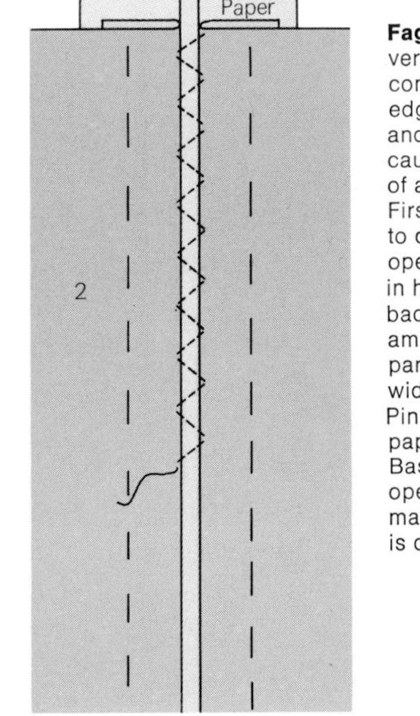

Fagoted seam: Machine version of openwork consists of two folded edges, positioned parallel and apart, with each edge caught by the outer points of an even zigzag stitch. First make a test stitch to determine width of opening. Divide this width in half; fold each seamline back by this halved amount. On paper, draw parallel lines to represent width between folded edges. Pin re-folded fabric to paper along parallel lines. Baste (1). Stitch, centering opening under foot and making sure that each edge is caught in stitching (2).

Cord and cording 16
Making cording 300

Seaming interfacings

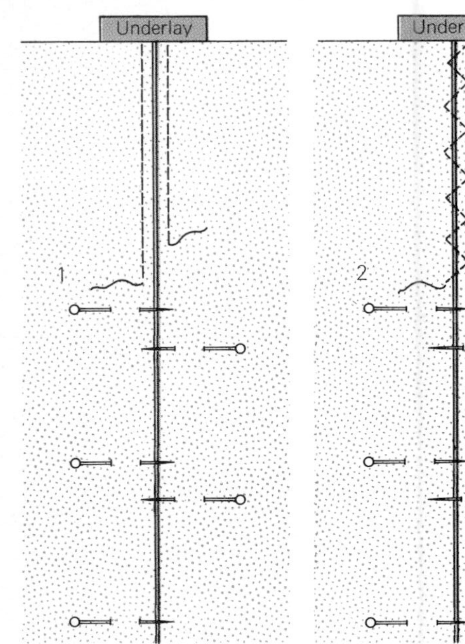

Abutted seams are one way of eliminating bulk from interfacing seams. Trim off seam allowances, bring two edges together, and pin or baste them to an underlay of seam binding or twill tape cut slightly longer than seams. With a short stitch length, stitch (1) ⅛″ from each edge with straight stitches, or (2) through center of seam with wide zigzag. For zigzag, abutted edges should be aligned with center of presser foot so stitches catch both sides equally.

Lapped seams are also used to eliminate bulk, especially on interfacing and interlining. Mark seamlines. Lap one edge over the other with seamlines meeting in the center. Place a row of straight stitching on either side of seamline (1), or stitch with wide zigzag through center (2). Trim both seam allowances close to stitching.

Corded seams

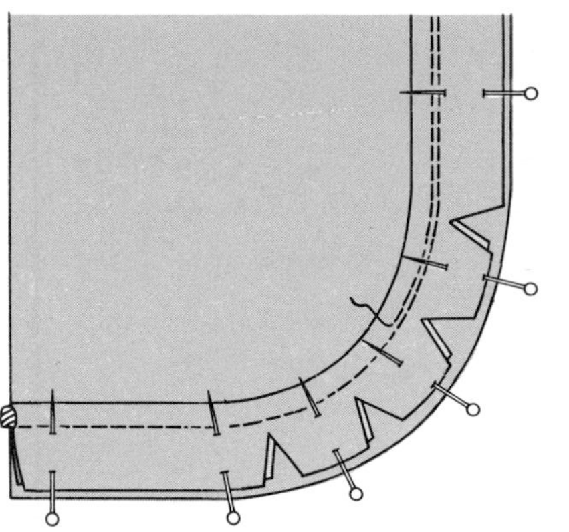

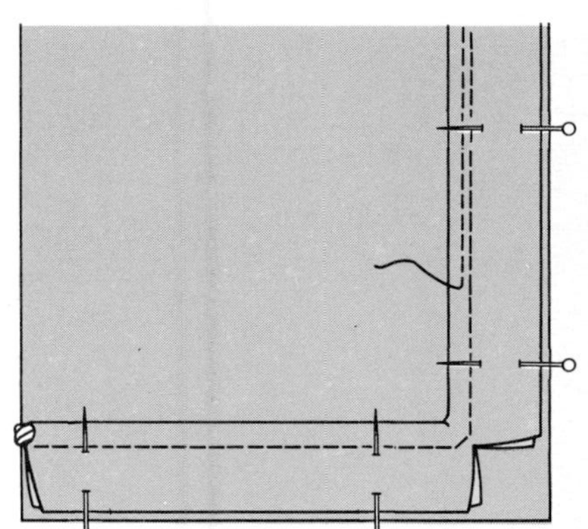

A corded seam is used in both dressmaking and home decorating. You can buy covered cording, or make your own cording. To insert cording in a seam: (1) Pin or baste cording to right side of one seam allowance, aligning cording stitch line with seamline, and having raw edge of cording toward raw edge of garment seam. With zipper foot to right of needle, stitch, placing the stitching just to the left of the cording stitches. (2) Place seam allowances with right sides together and cording in between. Using the original line of stitching as a guide, stitch through all layers, crowding the stitches between cord and first stitching. Press; trim and grade seam as necessary. When stitching corded seams, it is important that each successive row of stitching be placed slightly closer to the cording. In this way you can be sure no stitching will show on the right side.

To apply cording to a curved seam: Pin cording to right side of one seam allowance, matching cording stitch line and seamline. Around curve, clip or notch seam allowance of cording almost to stitching. Stitch as in Step 1 above, using a shorter stitch length around curve. Stitch seam as in Step 2 above. Trim cording seam allowance to ⅛″; trim, grade, and clip remaining seam allowances. Press. Turn right side out.

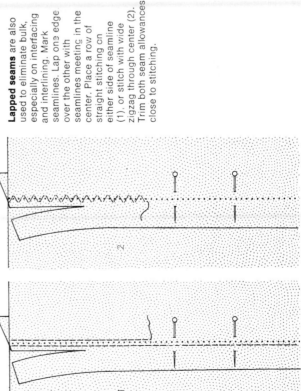

To apply cording to a square corner: Pin cording to right side of one seam allowance, matching cording stitch line and seamline. At corner, clip seam allowance of cording almost to stitching. Stitch as in Step 1 above, using a short stitch length at corner. Stitch seam as in Step 2 above. Cut diagonally across corner close to stitching. Trim cording seam allowance to ⅛″; trim and grade the remaining seam allowances.

Special seaming situations

Threads 10
Stitch length selection 30-31
Bias in fabrics 84-85
Gathering 178

Cross seams

Seams that cross, as they do at a waistline, shoulder, or underarm, should be pressed and seam-finished before joining. To make sure that the seamlines of cross seams will align after they are joined, and that all of the seam allowances will be caught flat in the stitching, pin through both seamlines with a fine needle; then pin through both seam allowances on each side of the matched seamlines. When the seam is stitched, trim seam allowances diagonally, as shown, to reduce bulk.

Bias to bias

When joining two bias edges, first baste and then stitch, being careful not to stretch fabric. To reduce the risk of stitches breaking under strain during wear, use a shorter-than-usual stitch and a thread with give. If it is a lengthwise seam, fasten basting with a long backstitch and cut, leaving several inches of thread. Allow basted piece to hang overnight so it can stretch to its "wearing" length before seaming. The loose basting lets fabric slip along thread as it stretches.

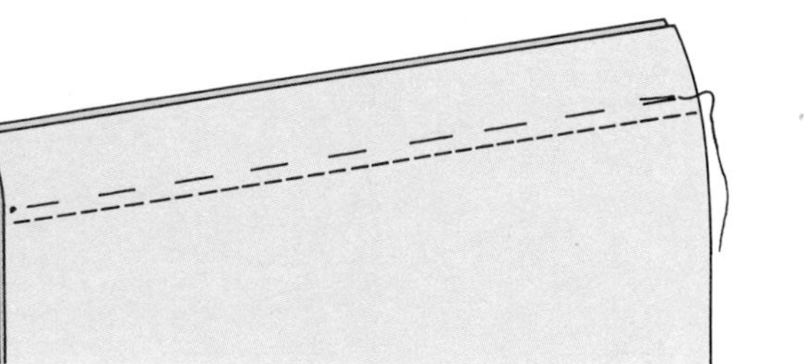

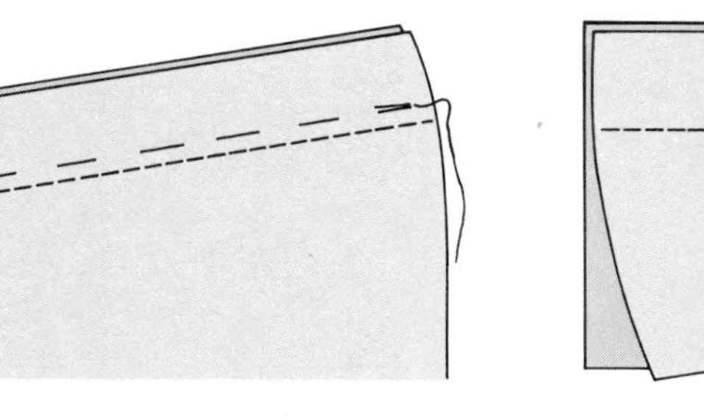

Bias to straight

When joining a bias to a straight edge, take special care not to stretch the edge that is bias, or the seam will not lie smooth (that is, it will ripple). Handling the bias edge gently, pin-baste it to the straight edge, placing pins perpendicular to the seamline at intervals of about every 3 to 4 inches. Stitch the seam with the bias edge on top, removing the pins as you stitch. Bear in mind that plaids cannot be matched if one fabric edge is bias and the other straight.

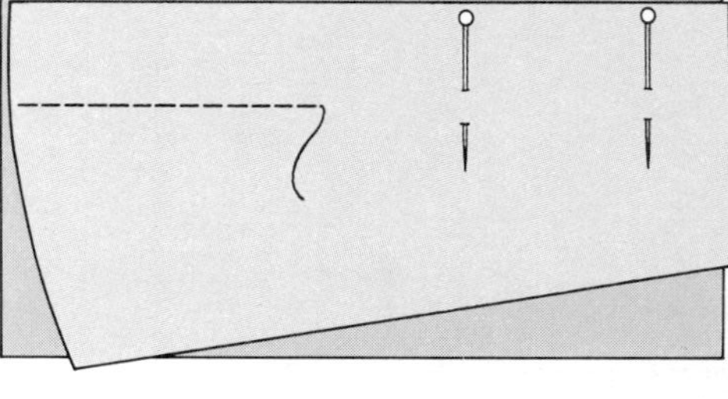

Seams with fullness

When two seams to be joined are uneven in length, the longer edge must be drawn in to fit the shorter. This is done, depending on the degree of adjustment, by **easing** or **gathering:** easing for slight to moderate fullness; gathering for a larger amount. It is important to recognize the difference between the two seams when finished. An *eased* seam has subtle shaping but is smooth and unpuckered. It may or may not call for control stitching. A *gathered* seam requires control stitching and retains more fullness. In both cases, the key to success is even distribution of fullness.

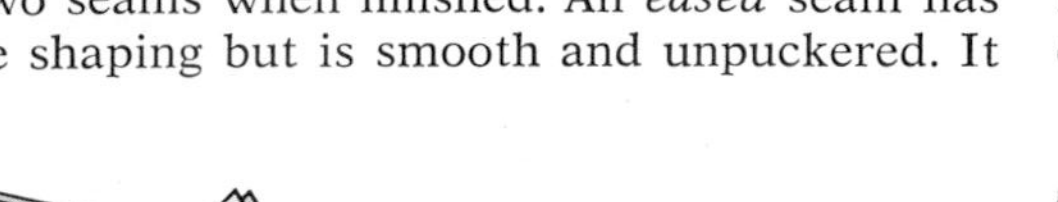

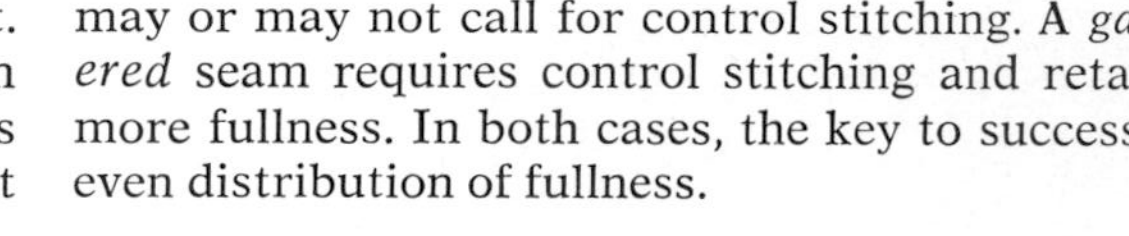

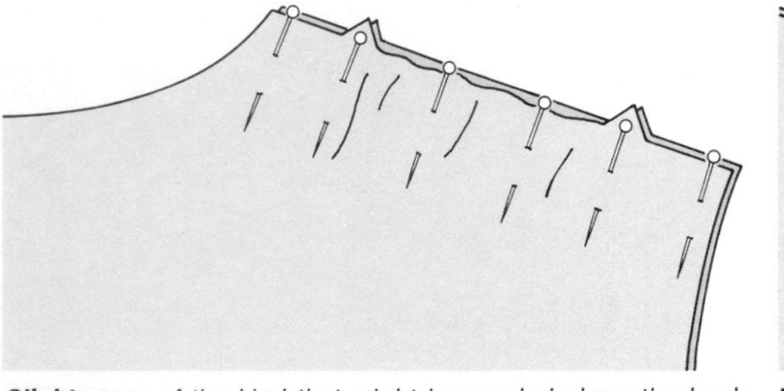

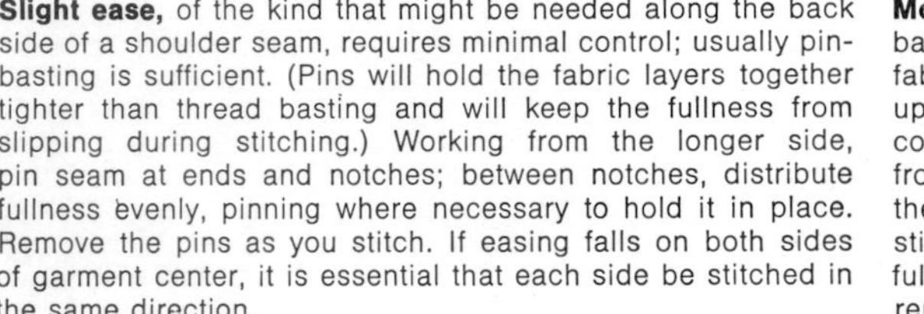

Slight ease, of the kind that might be needed along the back side of a shoulder seam, requires minimal control; usually pin-basting is sufficient. (Pins will hold the fabric layers together tighter than thread basting and will keep the fullness from slipping during stitching.) Working from the longer side, pin seam at ends and notches; between notches, distribute fullness evenly, pinning where necessary to hold it in place. Remove the pins as you stitch. If easing falls on both sides of garment center, it is essential that each side be stitched in the same direction.

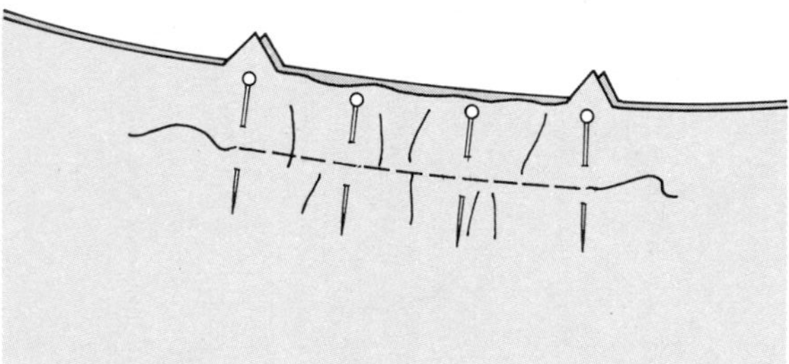

Moderate ease is controlled by a dual process of machine-basting, then pinning. Test stitch length on a single layer of fabric. Stitch should be long enough so fullness can be drawn up easily on the bobbin thread, but not too long, or it will not control the fullness evenly. Machine-baste a thread's width from seamline in area of longer piece that is to be eased in; then pin seam at ends and notches. Draw fabric up on ease-stitching, distributing fullness evenly. Pin as needed to hold fullness. With seam still pinned, baste. Stitch, eased side up, removing pins as you stitch.

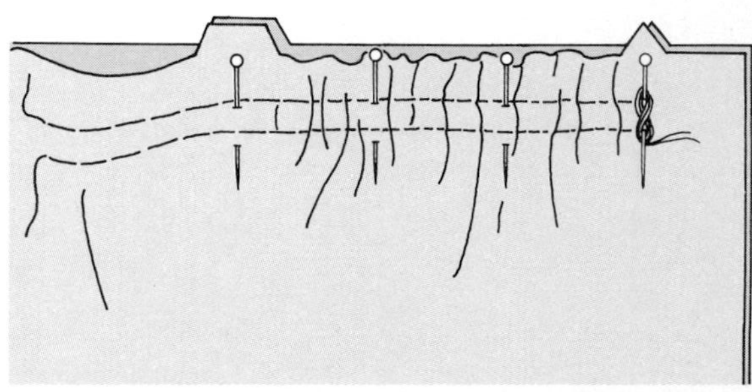

Gathering is the process of drawing fullness into a much smaller area by means of two rows of machine-basting. From the right side, stitch one basting line just next to the seamline; stitch the second ¼" away in the seam allowance. (See Gathering pages for details.) If seams intersect the gathered area, begin and end gathering stitches at seamlines. Pin seam edges together at matching points, such as notches. Draw up bobbin threads, distributing fullness evenly. Wind drawn threads around a pin to secure gathers. Pin-baste and stitch seam with gathered side up.

Tapes (woven edge, bias, twill) 16
How to preshape tape 299

Taped seams

Tape is sometimes added to a seam to keep it from stretching, or to strengthen it. The purpose, in any particular instance, depends on the type of seam and the fabric. While the seams most often taped are those at waistline, shoulder, and neckline, taping is advisable for any seam where there is likely to be strain. An example is the underarm curve of a kimono sleeve. When very little give is wanted in the seam, use firm tape, such as woven-edge or twill (¼ to ½ inch wide). If a seam should have give, yet hold its shape, use ½-inch bias tape. It is recommended that all tapes be preshrunk before application. As a general rule, tape should not extend into cross seams; that adds too much bulk. Cut tape the seam length less seam allowances, and position it so that ends stop at cross seamlines. Whenever possible, stitch with the tape side up, to ensure that tape is caught in the seam.

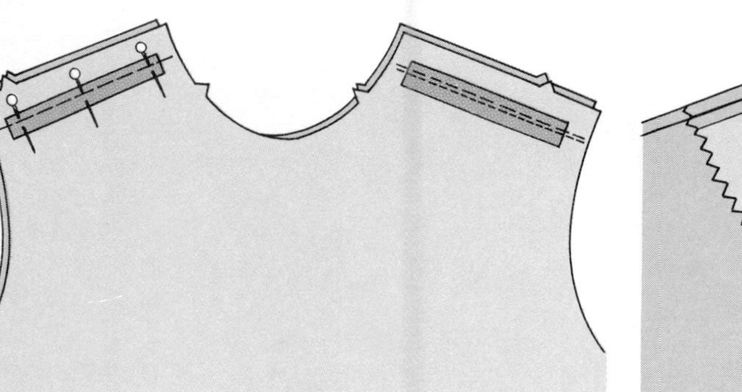

Tape at the shoulder (or other straight seam) should be attached to just one side of the seam, usually the back. Using the pattern as a guide, cut woven-edge or twill tape (¼″, ⅜″, or ½″ width) just long enough to fit between neck and armhole seams. Baste tape to seamline, positioning it ⅛″ into seam allowance. Stitch with tape side up.

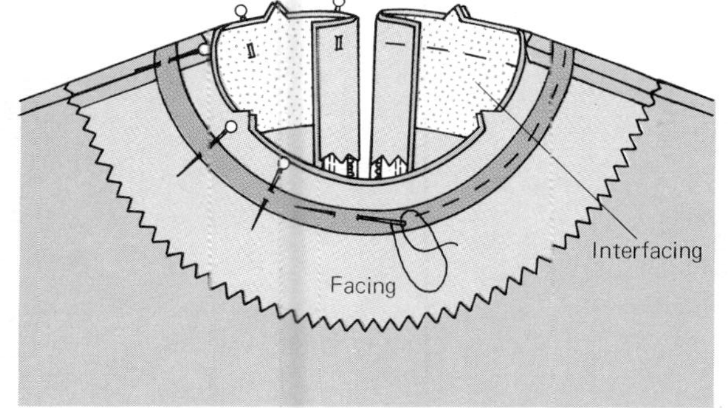

Tape at the neckline (or any curved area) is easier to apply if preshaped into a curve (see How to preshape tape). Use ¼″ twill tape; it shapes more easily than other firm types. Baste interfacing and facing to neck. Center tape over the neck seamline, on top of the facing. With tape side up, baste, then stitch through all layers.

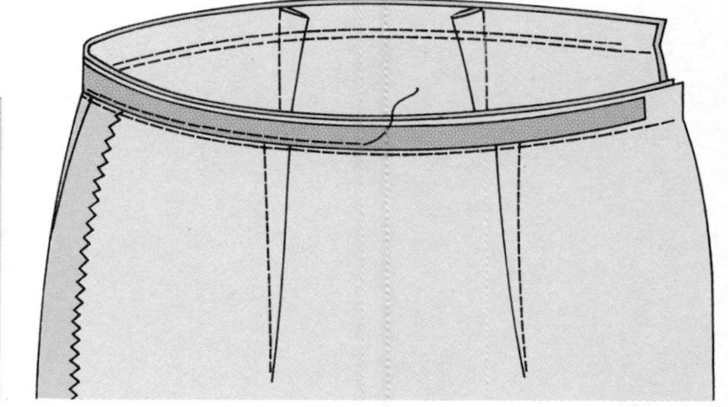

Tape at the waistline is applied to the skirt, after waist seam is stitched. Position tape close to seamline; stitch along edge closest to the seamline. Trim seam allowances even with outer edge of tape. Here tape serves three purposes: keeps the waist from stretching; strengthens the seam; and minimizes raveling of seam allowances.

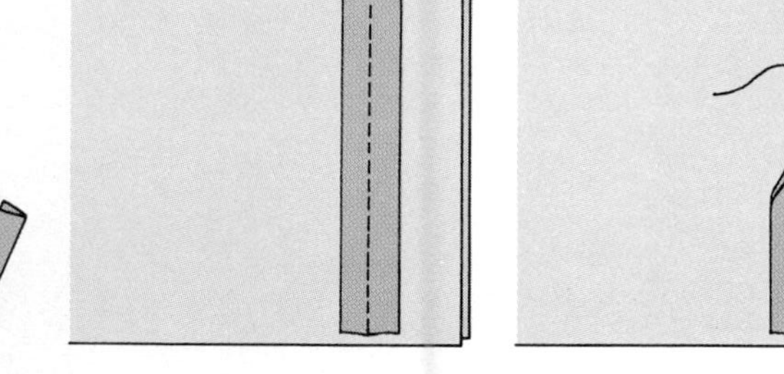
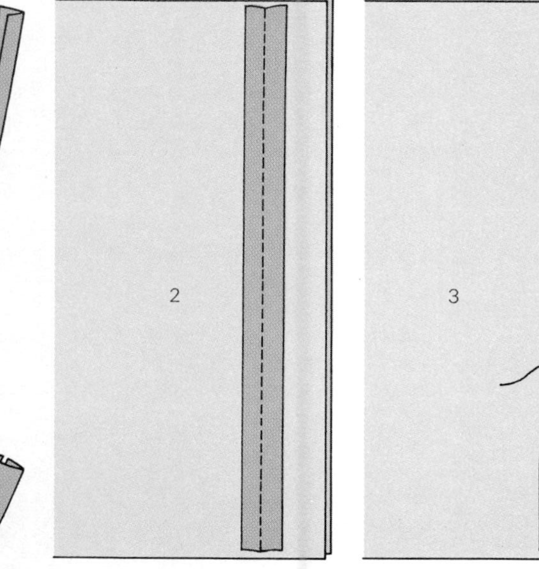

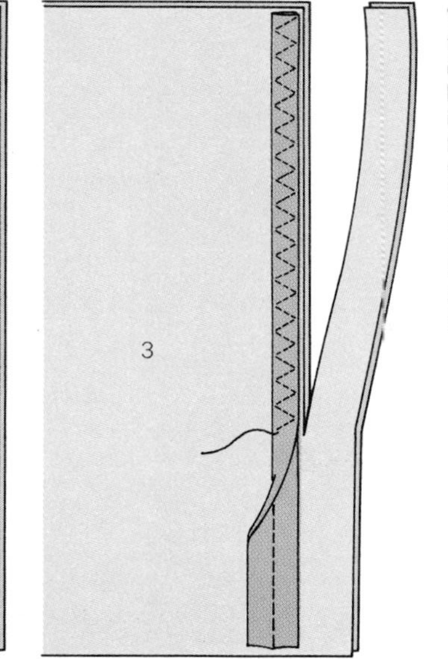

Taping with bias is advisable for raschel and other open-structured or stretchy knits. Use rayon bias tape, cut in half lengthwise (1). Place the fold exactly on seamline. Open the tape; baste and stitch through crease and seamline (2). If the seam is to be overedged, re-fold tape and zigzag or overedge stitch through tape and both seam allowances. Trim close to the stitching (3).

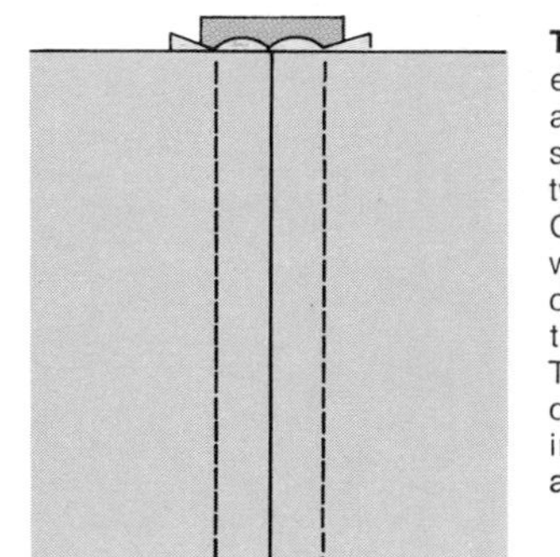
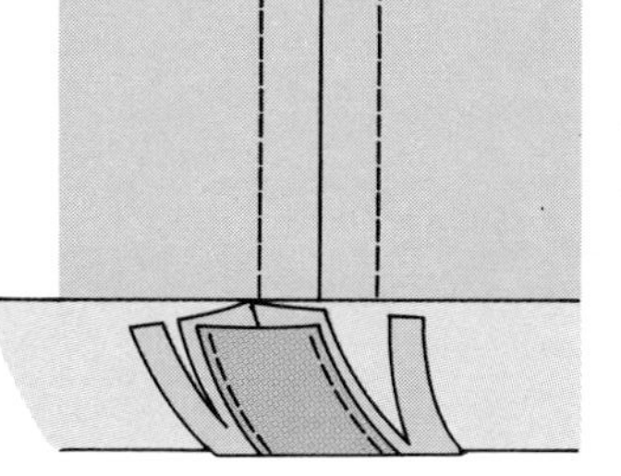

Tape under a topstitched seam, especially when garment is a knit, will contribute stability and support. Use twill tape, here ¾″ wide. Center it over the seam on the wrong side. Baste each edge of the tape through both the seam allowance and garment. Topstitch ¼″ to each side of the seam. Tape will be caught in the stitching. Trim seam allowances even with the tape.

Seaming special fabrics

Machine pressure and tension 28-31
Machine accessories 38-39
Tying thread ends 137

Sheers, knits, and vinyls

Sheers and laces: Because construction details in sheers and laces show through (unless the garment is underlined), seams should be narrow and inconspicuous. Traditional seams for these fabrics are the French and mock French seams; double-stitched seams are a good choice for a very textured sheer, such as heavy lace; hairline seams are appropriate for collars, cuffs, and similar garment parts. Pin, or hand-baste with silk thread, in the seam allowance only. Stitch with a fine needle (#11 for most sheers, #9 for chiffon) and use silk or extra-fine lingerie thread. Use the straight stitch throat plate if possible; it has a small hole and fabric is less likely to be dragged into it. Pressure and tension should generally be decreased slightly and a shorter stitch used. The roller foot is ideal for laces since it will not snag the fabric.

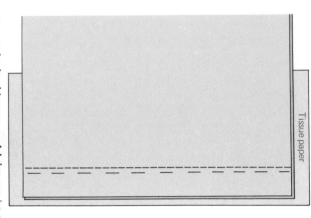

Tissue paper under hard-to-manage fabrics can be an aid to stitching. It (1) assists the fabric to feed through the machine more easily; (2) helps keep the fabric from being dragged into the hole of the zigzag throat plate; (3) prevents marring by the feed dog. Baste a strip of tissue paper to one side of the seam. With tissue paper next to the feed dog, stitch the seam. To remove paper, pull it away first from one side of stitching, then from the other.

Knits: Seam choice for a particular knit is based on two considerations—the amount of stress on the seam, and the degree of stretch in the fabric. Amount of stress is determined by the location of the seam (side, crotch, shoulder, neck) and by the fit of the garment—tighter fit requires stronger seams. Degree of stretch can be classified as *minimum, moderate, or maximum.*

Generally, seams in knits should be constructed with "give" so the seam will not break when the fabric is stretched. The exception is seams that will be stayed with a separate strip of fabric; the stay counteracts the "give." To achieve the desired combination of stretch and strength, the right **thread, needle,** and **stitch pattern** must be chosen. Synthetic threads, such as polyester or polyester/cotton, are very strong and have a certain amount of stretch, and thus are excellent choices for knits; silk also has natural stretch and recovery. A ball-point needle, by going between yarns instead of cutting through them, reduces the risk of damage.

The stitch pattern is determined by the machine; study your manual for special stretch stitches and uses. A straight stitch works perfectly well even on stretchy knits if the proper thread is used and the fabric is stretched slightly during stitching in the following way: hold the fabric in front of the presser foot with one hand and, with other hand behind the presser foot, gently stretch the fabric as it passes under the needle. Test seam on scrap fabric; if seam allowance becomes narrower, the seam may need to be stitched at ½-inch guideline. When stitching is completed, the seam should be smooth and even. If the fabric has stretched too much, the seam will look wavy and distorted; if stretched too little, it will look puckered or gathered.

A zigzag stitch is, in itself, a "stretchier" stitch than the plain straight stitch, so the fabric need not be stretched during stitching. Care must be taken when zigzag stitching lightweight fabrics to see that they are not pulled into the hole in the throat plate. Use of tissue paper plus holding the fabric taut will help.

Knits have varying degrees of stretchability and this amount should be determined before cutting and sewing any knit (also before deciding on a particular pattern). There are roughly three stretch categories, classified according to how much 4 inches of knit fabric will stretch crosswise without distortion: 4 inches of a *minimum* stretch knit will stretch to 4¾; of a *moderate* stretch knit, to 5; of a *maximum* stretch knit, to 6.

Minimum stretch knits are used primarily for comfort in wear. They can be stitched the same way as wovens, as long as the correct thread and a ball-point needle are used. Use the stretch-as-you-stitch technique for *moderate stretch* knits. In most cases, seam allowances need not be finished. However, if the raw edges tend to roll, an overedge seam is advisable. *Maximum stretch* knits must be stretched during stitching. Since the edges tend to curl, an overedge seam is usually best.

Some knits have poor recovery; that is, they do not spring back to their original shape after stretching. For the most part, it is better to avoid such knits. However, should you already have purchased one, use lightened pressure to help minimize stretching while sewing, and tape crosswise seams (especially shoulder and waist) to prevent their stretching during wear.

Vinyls and smooth leathers comprise a group of "slick" fabrics that show puncture marks from pins and needles. They also tend to stick to the presser foot when stitched slick side up. To ensure that puncture marks do not blemish the finished garment, pin or baste only in seam allowances or hold edges together with paper clips; stitch seams only after fit of garment is satisfactory. The tendency of these materials to stick to the machine foot can be inhibited by coating their sewing surface with baby oil, talcum, cornstarch, or chalk spot remover. Test on a scrap of the material to be sure that whatever you use will come off satisfactorily. Masking tape can also be used if it can be removed with no ill effects.

There are special wedge-shaped needles that make it easier to sew vinyls and leathers. Stitch length should be between 8 and 12, and seams should not be backstitched—tie off thread ends instead. Press seams open with fingers, then flatten with a pounder. Use rubber cement to hold seam allowances flat, or topstitch on either side of seam.

Thread/needle/stitch length selection 26-27
Hand basting 124

Pile fabrics

The range of pile fabrics encompasses short-to-long pile lengths as well as sparse-to-dense pile coverage; backing fabric may be either woven or knitted. In most instances, the pile, not the backing fabric, is the major concern when stitching. So as not to distort the pile, stitch seams in the direction of the pile. Since most piles slip and feed unevenly, care must be taken to exert the proper amount of pressure on fabric while stitching. Avoid too much pressure, however; it can mar the pile. Basting and top feed assists will help layers feed evenly. The longer or denser the pile, the greater the need to reduce bulk from seams. This can be done by shaving pile from seam allowances (illustrations below) or by narrowing the seam allowance and using an overedge seam. Be sure to pull pile from stitching before shaving pile or trimming seam (see right). If fabric is a knit, and some give should be built into the seam, either use a zigzag stitch, or stretch the fabric slightly while using a straight stitch. Finish all seam edges. Avoid stretch stitches; the forward-reverse motion involved can distort the pile and its direction.

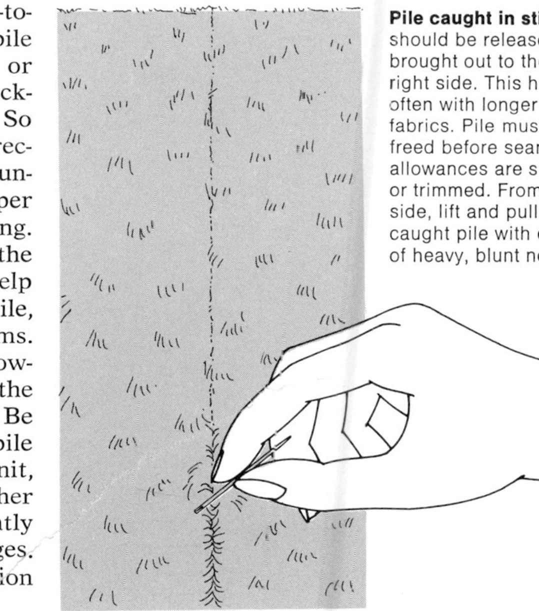

Pile caught in stitching should be released and brought out to the right side. This happens often with longer pile fabrics. Pile must be freed before seam allowances are shaved or trimmed. From right side, lift and pull out caught pile with eye end of heavy, blunt needle.

Short pile can be trimmed from seam allowances before seaming. Be sure to fit the garment first—seamlines cannot be let out once pile has been shaved off. To shave pile, hold scissors close to and parallel with backing fabric. Cut with short, even strokes. Take care not to shave pile past ⅛″ inside the seamline.

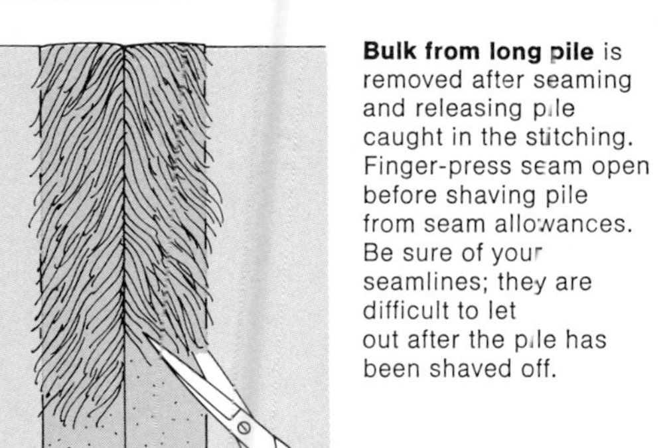

Bulk from long pile is removed after seaming and releasing pile caught in the stitching. Finger-press seam open before shaving pile from seam allowances. Be sure of your seamlines; they are difficult to let out after the pile has been shaved off.

Joining unlike fabrics

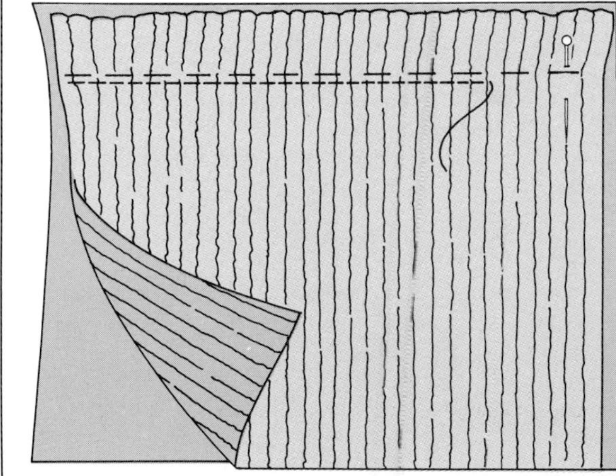

Knit to woven: When a knit garment section is joined to one that is woven, the knit section will usually be smaller than the woven. To ensure balanced distribution of the two in relation to each other, first divide and pin-mark both edges into eighths. Then, with right sides together, match sections at pin marks and baste the two together. Stitch with knit side uppermost, stretching the knit to fit the woven.

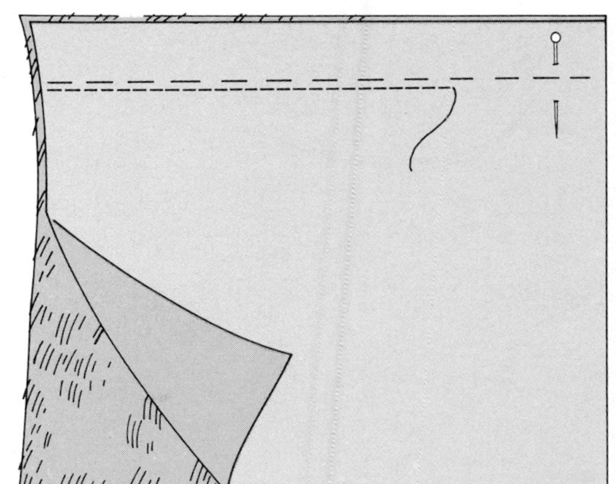

Pile to smooth: There may be difficulty, when stitching a pile fabric to one with a smooth surface, in getting the two surfaces to feed evenly with each other. This slippage can be minimized by hand-basting the two edges together with short, even stitches. Then, exerting appropriate pressure on the fabrics, stitch, in the direction of the pile, with the smooth-surfaced fabric uppermost as you stitch.

Shaping devices

Pressing 18-19
Fabric-marking methods 94

Princess seams

Princess seams are shaped seams designed to fit the body's contours. Beginning at shoulder or armhole, front or back, and running lengthwise, they may go just to the waistline seam or extend all the way to the hem. A typical princess seam will curve *outward* to accommodate the fullest part of the bust or back, then *inward* to conform to the waist, and finally *outward* again to fit over the hips. Careful checking of fit, pattern adjustments, and marking are necessary if the curves of the seam are to follow the contours of the body. Proper use of clipping and notching will permit the curves to lie smoothly against the body. Pressing should be done over a tailor's ham; its rounded shape helps retain and mold curves as seam is pressed.

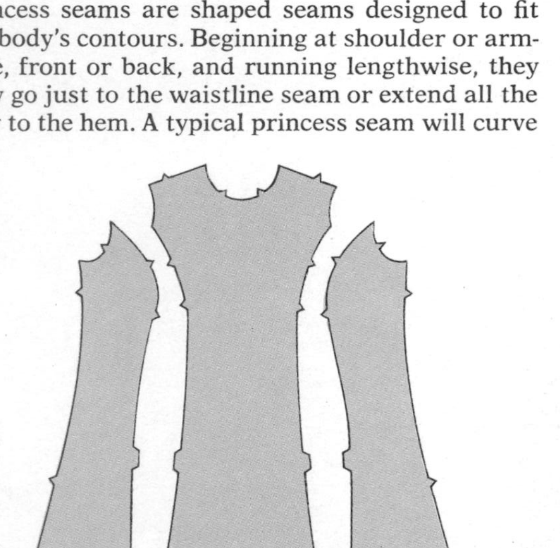

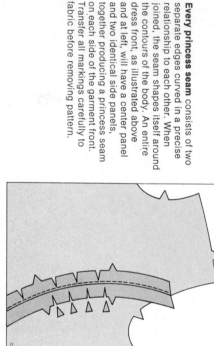

Every princess seam consists of two separate edges curved in a precise relationship to each other. When joined, the seam shapes itself around the contours of the body. An entire dress front, as illustrated above and at left, will have a center panel and two identical side panels, together producing a princess seam on each side of the garment front. Transfer all markings carefully to fabric before removing pattern.

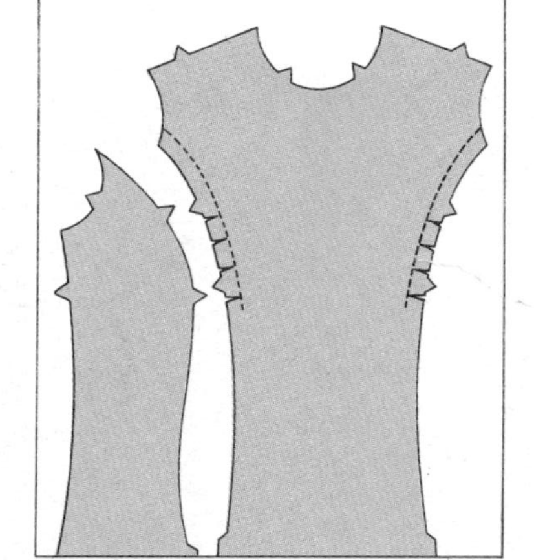

1. Place a row of reinforcement stitches just inside the seamlines of the center panel, from the top edge to just below bottom notch. Clip between notches.

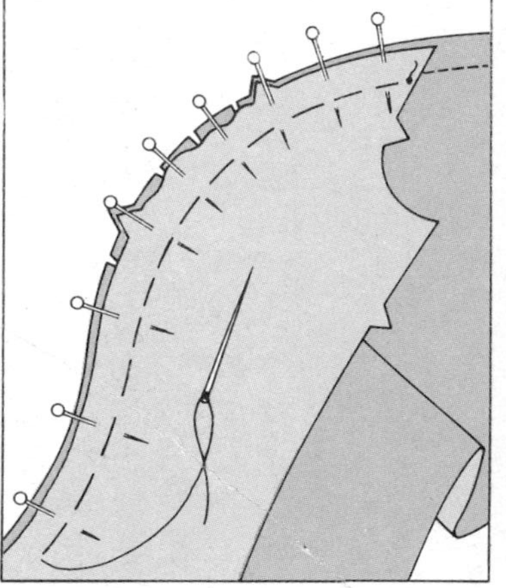

2. With side panel on top, match and pin the seamline, spreading the clipped edge to fit. Make additional clips if necessary. Baste in place.

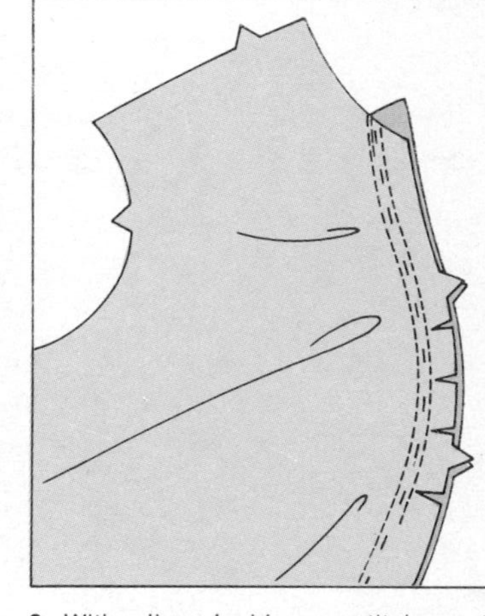

3. With clipped side up, stitch on the seamline, beyond the ends of the clips, being careful to keep the underside smooth. Backstitch at both ends of seam.

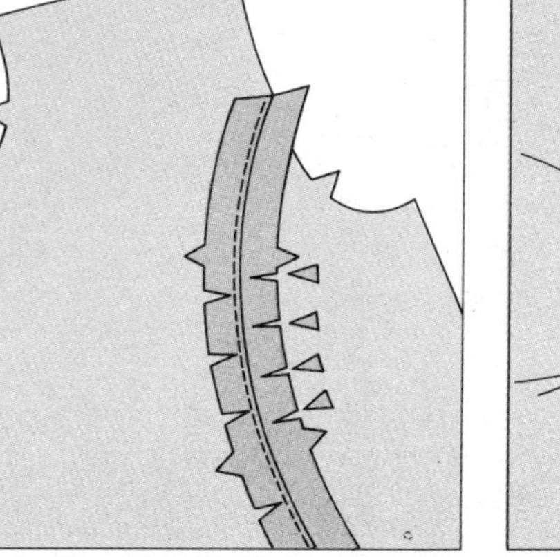

4. Remove basting and finger-press the seam open. Notch out fullness from the inward curve. Wherever possible, stagger positioning of clips and notches.

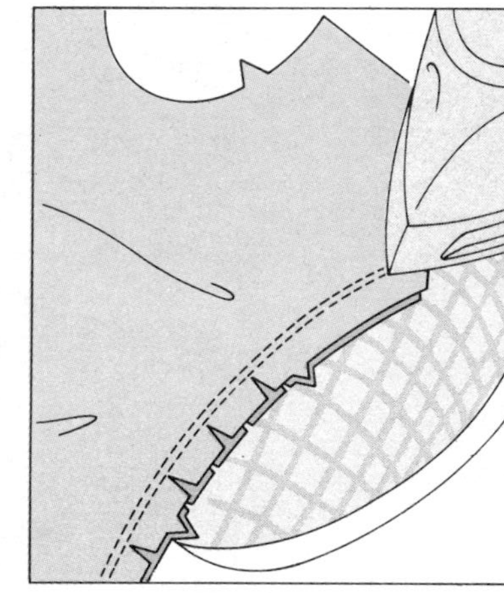

5. Close seam and place over a tailor's ham. With tip of iron, press seam flat. Do not press into the body of the garment, especially in the curved areas.

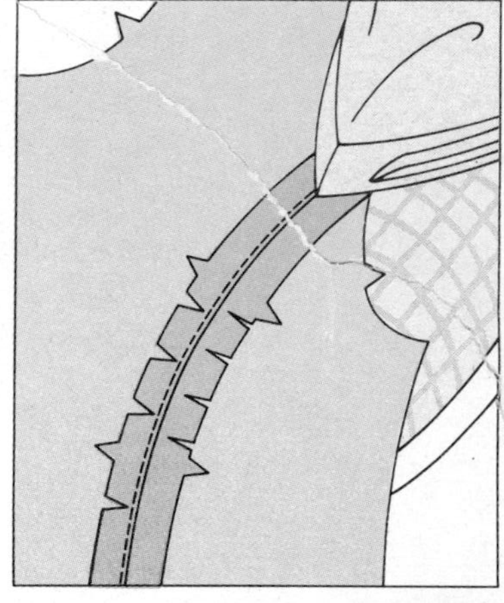

6. Press the seam open over a tailor's ham. Re-position the seam whenever necessary to keep the curve of the ham matched to the curve of the seam.

Darts

Darts are one of the most basic structural elements in dressmaking. They are used to build, into a flat piece of fabric, a definite shape that will allow the fabric to conform to a particular body contour or curve. Darts occur most often at the bust, back, waist, and hips; accuracy in their position and in their fit is important if they are to gracefully emphasize the lines in these areas. Important, too, is precise marking of construction symbols. Choose a marking method that is suitable to the fabric in hand. Stitching direction is from the wide end of the dart to the point. Knot thread ends at the point to secure them. Backstitching can be used as a reinforcement at the wide end but should not be used at the point.

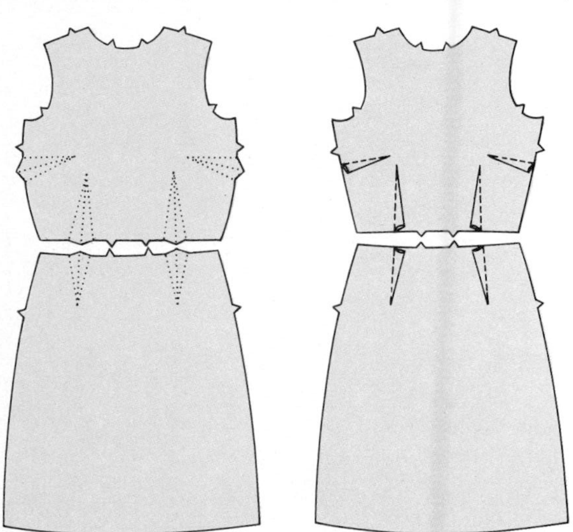

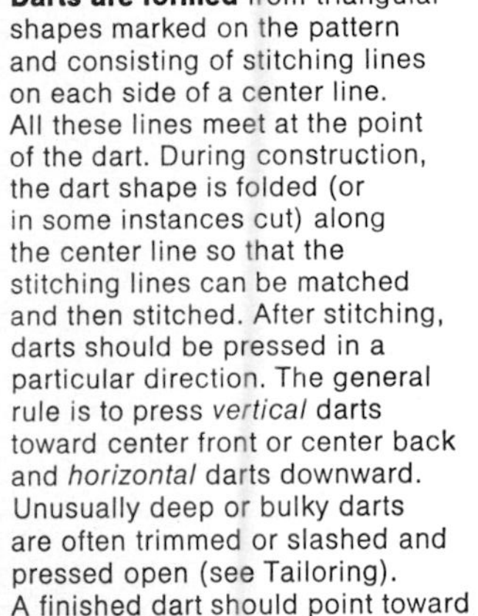

Darts are formed from triangular shapes marked on the pattern and consisting of stitching lines on each side of a center line. All these lines meet at the point of the dart. During construction, the dart shape is folded (or in some instances cut) along the center line so that the stitching lines can be matched and then stitched. After stitching, darts should be pressed in a particular direction. The general rule is to press *vertical* darts toward center front or center back and *horizontal* darts downward. Unusually deep or bulky darts are often trimmed or slashed and pressed open (see Tailoring). A finished dart should point toward the fullest part of the body contour to which it is conforming.

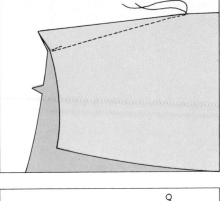

1. Before removing pattern, transfer the markings to wrong side of fabric. Tailor's tacks are shown here, but method will depend on fabric being marked.

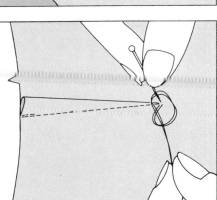

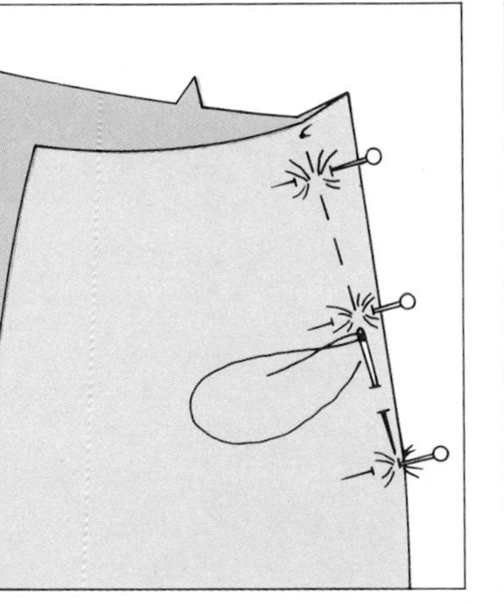

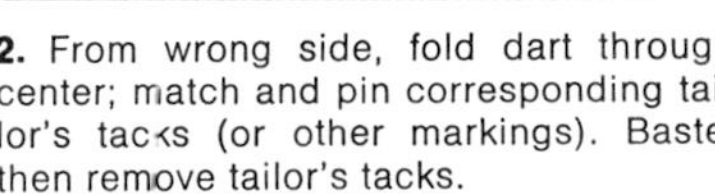

2. From wrong side, fold dart through center; match and pin corresponding tailor's tacks (or other markings). Baste; then remove tailor's tacks.

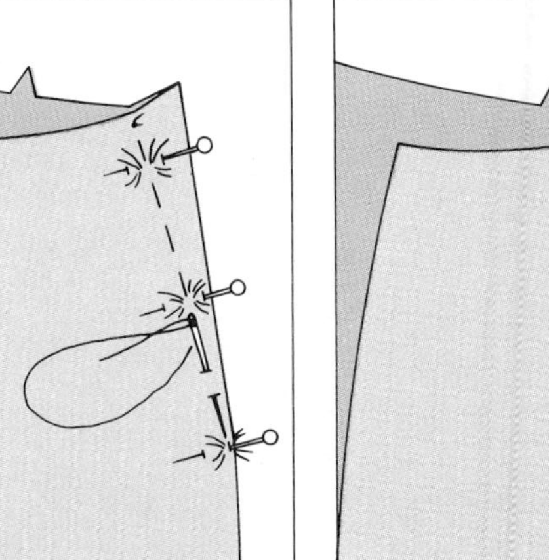

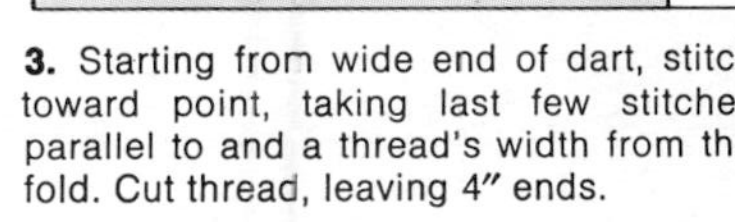

3. Starting from wide end of dart, stitch toward point, taking last few stitches parallel to and a thread's width from the fold. Cut thread, leaving 4" ends.

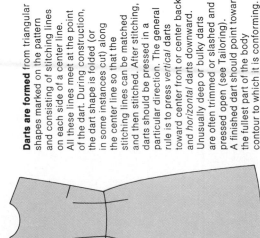

4. With thread ends together, form knot (do not pull tight). Insert pin through knot, then into point of dart. Tighten knot, letting pin guide it to dart point.

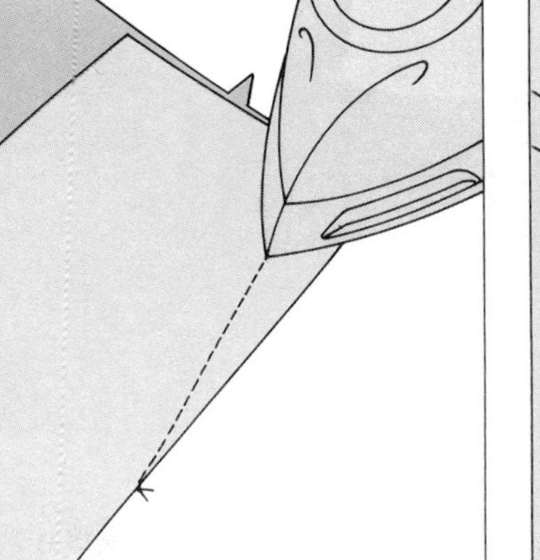

5. Extend dart and press it flat as it was stitched. Press toward the point, being careful not to go beyond it—this could crease the garment.

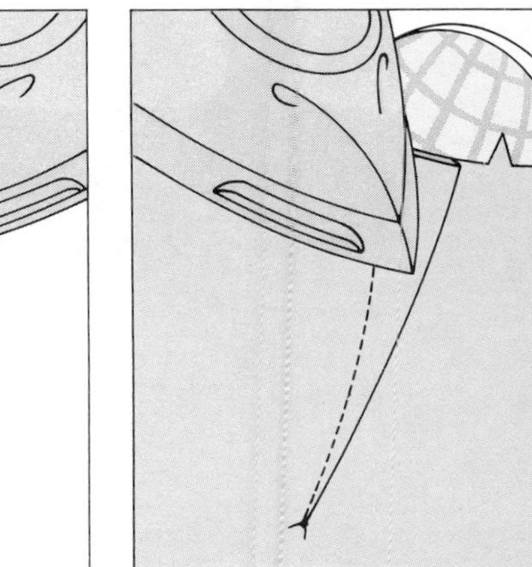

6. Place dart, wrong side up, over tailor's ham. Press according to direction it will take in finished garment, being careful not to crease rest of garment.

Shaping devices

Pressing 18-19
Fabric-marking methods 94

Contour dart and French dart

A contour dart is a long, single dart that fits at the waistline and then tapers off in two opposite directions to fit either both the *bust* and *hip* (front contour dart) or the fullest part of both the *back* and the *hip* (back contour dart). In effect, it takes the place of two separate waistline darts, one of them tapering toward the bust or back and the other toward the hip.

A French dart extends diagonally from the side seam in the hip area to the bust. The diagonal line can be straight or slightly curved. French darts are found on the front of a garment, never the back.

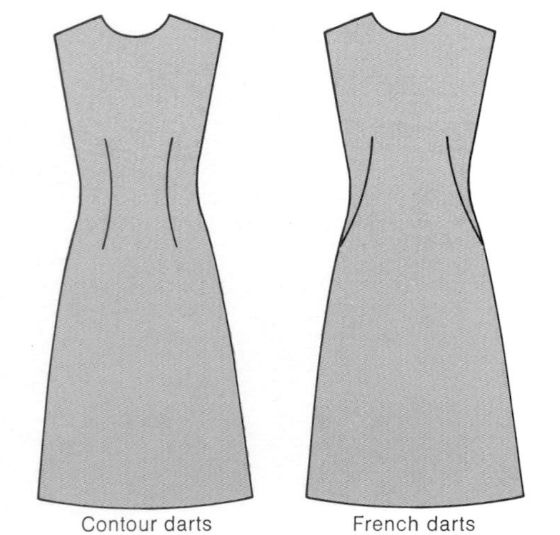

Each of these darts is constructed in a special way. The contour dart is stitched in two separate steps and directions. The shape of the French dart necessitates its being cut open *before* seaming so that the two stitching lines can be accurately matched. For both the contour and French darts, all the stitching, fold, or slash lines, as well as all matching points, should be clearly marked. Because their lines are usually more complex than those of the simple dart, they are best marked with tracing wheel and dressmaker's carbon. If you must mark some other way, be sure that the shape of the lines is clearly indicated. Clipping is another essential in these darts. It will relieve strain at the waist and other curved sections, permitting the dart to be shaped and lie smooth.

Constructing a contour dart

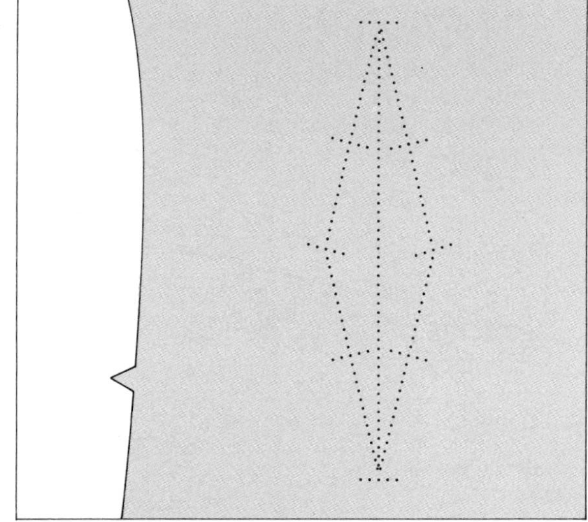

1. Transfer construction symbols to wrong side of fabric. Tracing wheel is good for this purpose, but test it first for legibility of markings and effect on fabric. Mark the stitching lines, center line, and all matching points.

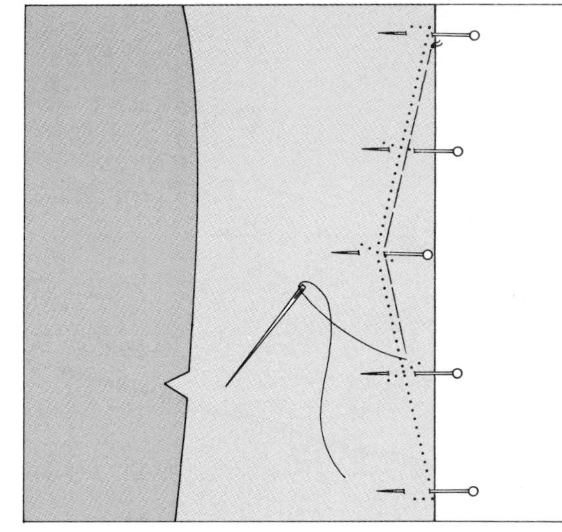

2. Working from wrong side, fold dart along center line. Match and pin stitching lines, first at the waist, then at both points, then at other matching points in between. Baste just inside the stitching line; remove pins after basting.

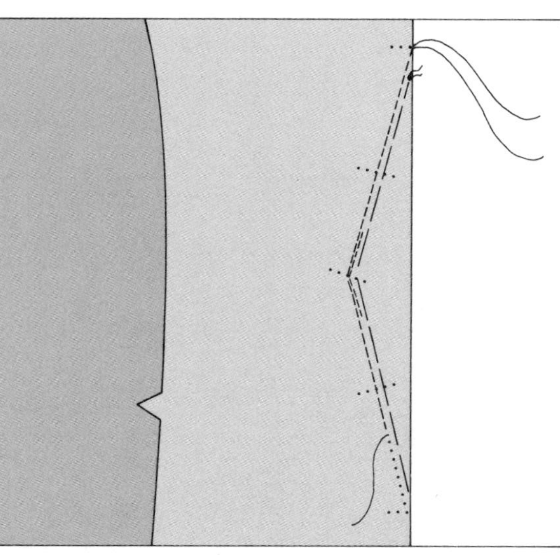

3. A contour dart is stitched in two separate steps, beginning each time at the waist and stitching toward the point. Instead of backstitching, overlap the stitching at the waist. Tie thread ends at both points of the dart (see Step 4, p.159).

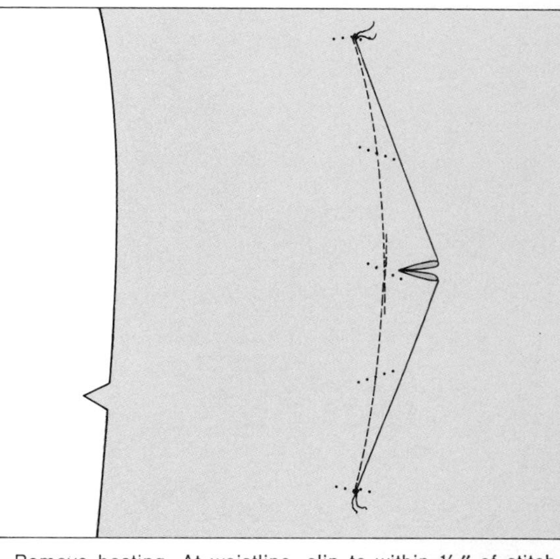

4. Remove basting. At waistline, clip to within ⅛" of stitching. (Clip will relieve the strain and allow the dart to curve smoothly past waist.) Press dart flat as it was stitched; then press it toward the center of garment.

Constructing a French dart

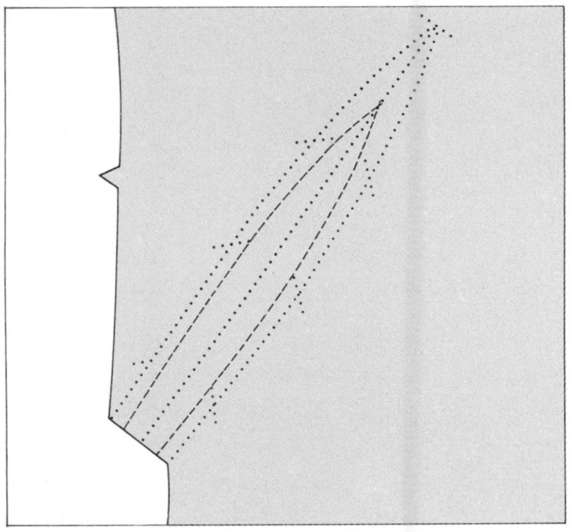

1. Transfer pattern markings to wrong side of fabric. Staystitch ⅛″ inside each stitching line. Start each line of staystitching from the seamline end of the dart and taper both to meet approximately 1″ from point of dart.

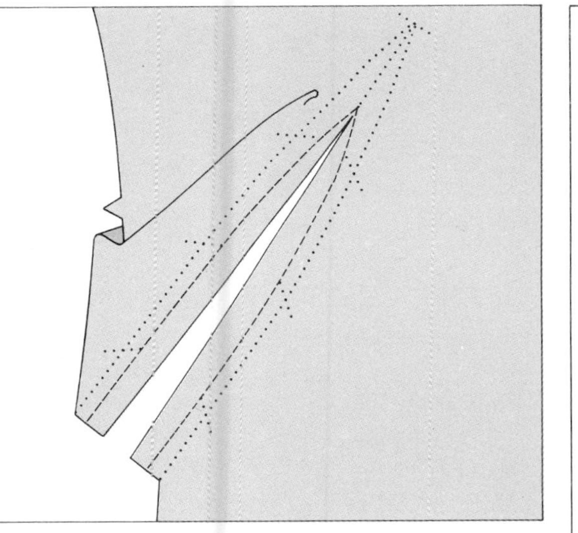

2. Slash through the center of the dart to where the rows of staystitching intersect. (This will not be necessary on those French darts in which part or all of the center portion is removed when the garment section is cut out.)

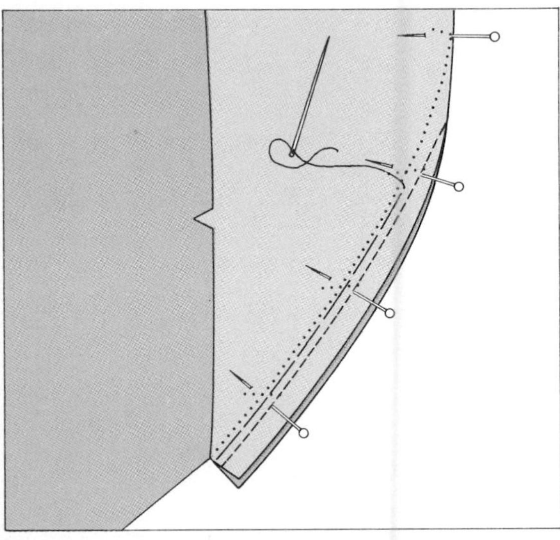

3. With right sides together, match and pin the stitching lines. It may be necessary to ease the lower edge to the upper edge in order to get the points to match accurately. Baste along stitching line; then remove pins.

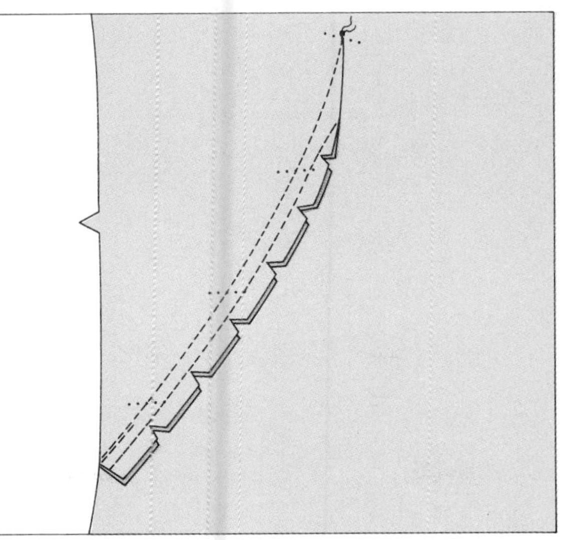

4. Stitch dart from end to point, knotting thread ends (Step 4, p. 159). End can be backstitched. Remove bastings. Clip seam allowances to relieve strain and let dart curve smoothly. Press flat as stitched, then downward over a tailor's ham.

Continuous-thread darts

A continuous-thread dart is one that is stitched so as to leave no thread ends to be tied at the point. Stitching *direction* is from point to end, the opposite of the usual way. This dart is used mainly where a thread knot would detract from the look of a garment—in sheer fabrics, for example, or when the dart fold is to be on the outside of the garment.

Each continuous-thread dart requires a special re-threading of the machine, in which the bobbin thread is passed through the needle and tied to the upper thread, creating one continuous strand. This strand is then wound back onto the top spool until the knot, and enough thread to stitch one dart, has been pulled through the top threading points.

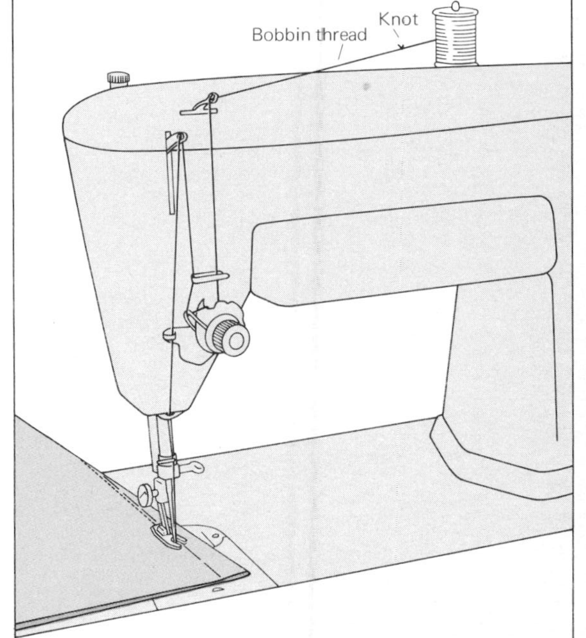

Special threading for each continuous-thread dart: First thread machine as usual and pull bobbin thread up through throat plate. Then unthread needle and pass bobbin thread through needle eye in direction opposite to way needle was originally threaded. Tie bobbin and upper threads together with as small a knot as possible. Re-wind top thread back onto spool, allowing knot, and enough bobbin thread to stitch one full dart, to pass through top threading points.

Darts in interfacing

Pressing 18-19 Fabric-marking methods 94
Catchstitch (flat) 129

Abutted dart

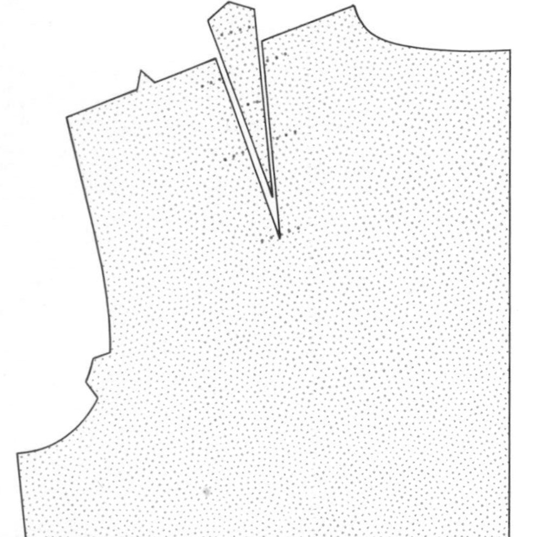

An abutted dart is a special type of dart that is used in such fabrics as interfacing to eliminate unnecessary bulk. The first step is to mark, with tracing wheel and carbon paper, the stitching lines and matching points of the dart. Then cut out center of dart along both stitching lines.

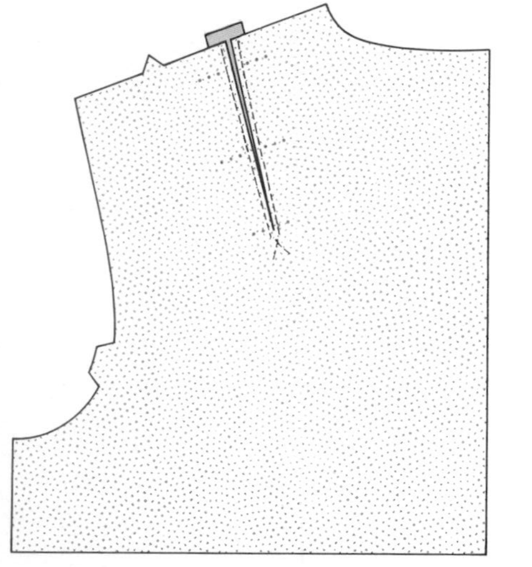

Bring cut edges together and baste in place to an underlay of woven-edge tape or a 1″-wide strip of lightweight fabric. Cut underlay slightly longer than dart. With straight stitching, stitch ⅛″ to each side of abutted line; if using zigzag stitch, center over the abutted line. Press.

Lapped dart

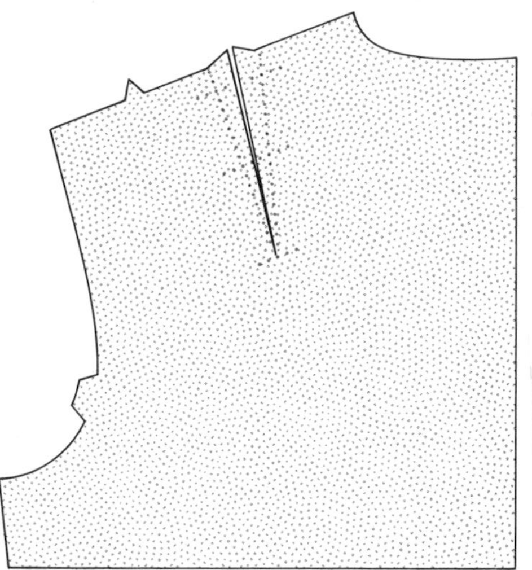

A lapped dart is another special dart type used to eliminate unnecessary bulk from interfacing. Mark, with tracing wheel and carbon paper, the matching points and the center and stitching lines. Slash along center of dart to the point, being careful not to cut beyond the point.

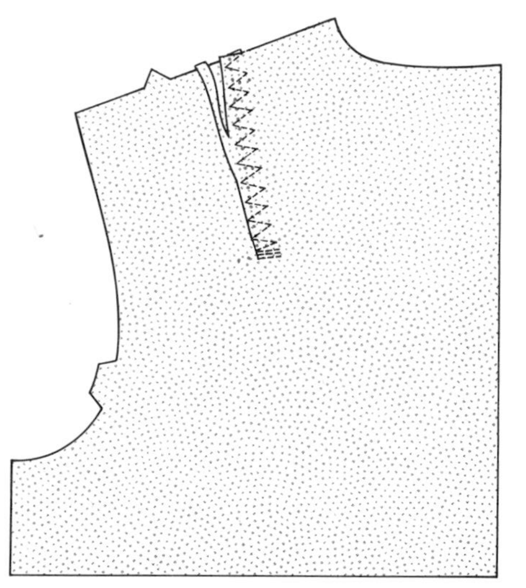

Lap edges so the stitching lines meet; baste in place. Center the presser foot over the stitching line and stitch, using a short, wide multistitch zigzag or plain zigzag stitch. If using a straight stitch, place a row ⅛″ to each side of stitching line. Trim excess fabric and press.

Catchstitched dart

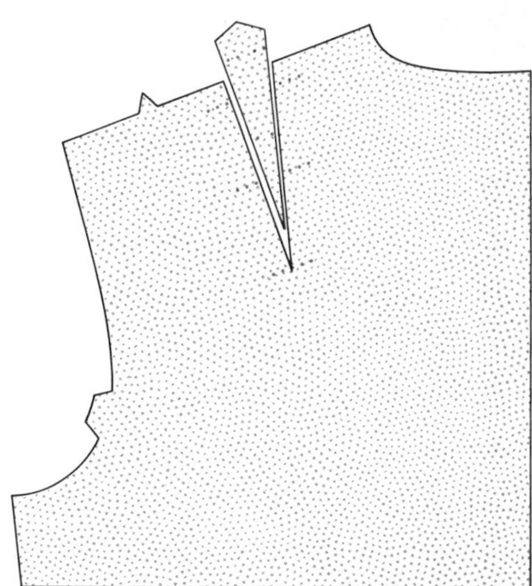

A catchstitched dart is an effective way to eliminate the bulk of an interfacing dart that is aligned with a dart in the garment. Using tracing wheel and carbon paper, mark the dart stitching lines and matching points. Cut along both stitching lines to remove center portion of dart.

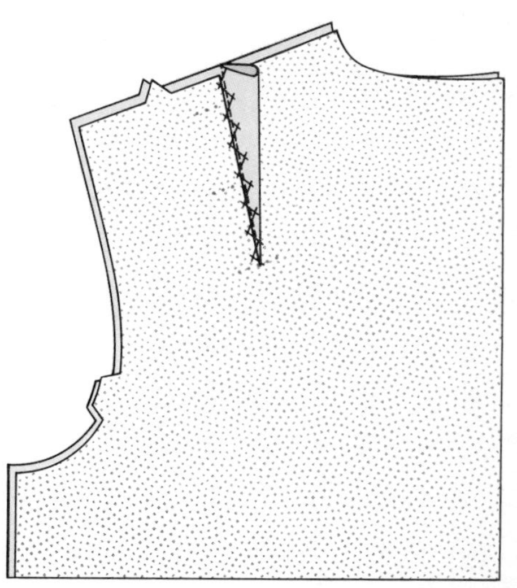

Position the open interfacing dart over the stitched garment dart. Pull garment dart up through the two cut edges. Pin edges of interfacing alongside the stitching lines of the garment dart. Catchstitch each edge to the garment dart over its stitching line. Press.

Darts in underlined garments

Underlining 74-75

Construction methods

Darts in garments that are underlined can be handled in two ways. The first method is to construct each dart through both garment and underlining fabrics as if the two fabrics were one. The other method is to stitch garment darts and underlining darts separately. The first, stitching both darts as one, is the method most often used. It is especially recommended for sheer fabrics because the dart does not show through to the outside. The second method, stitching darts separately, is suitable for very heavy or bulky fabrics. Whichever method is used, each dart is constructed according to its type (see pp.159–161). There is one slight difference in French dart construction when the dart is to be underlined as one with the garment fabric. The two rows of staystitching for the basic French dart (see p.161), if stitched from point of intersection to end of dart, will serve to hold fabrics together in this area; a row of machine-basting from point of dart to staystitching intersection will secure the center (see right). Balance of construction would then proceed as usual.

Darts stitched through two layers

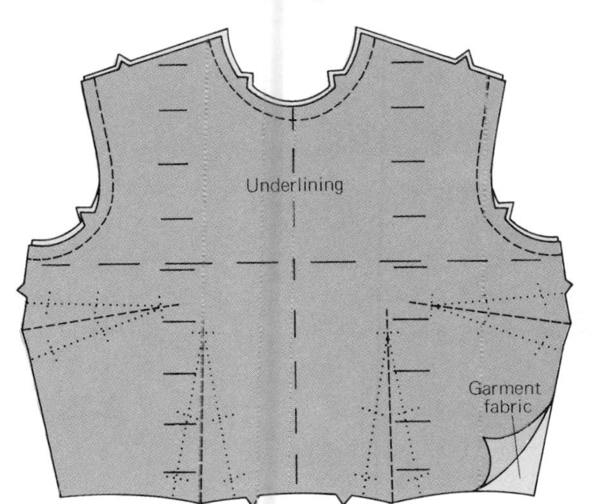

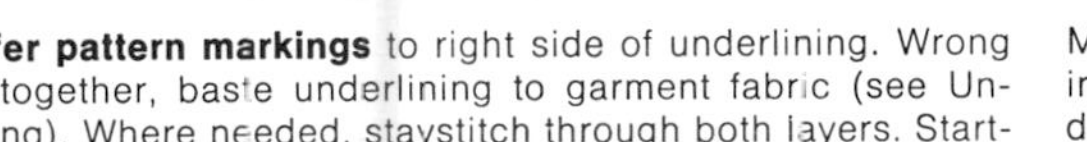

Transfer pattern markings to right side of underlining. Wrong sides together, baste underlining to garment fabric (see Underlining). Where needed, staystitch through both layers. Starting just beyond point, machine-baste down center of darts.

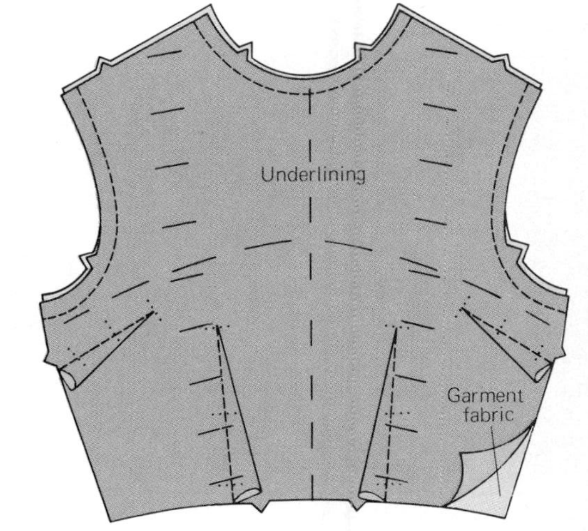

Match, baste, and stitch each dart. Remove machine basting beyond point. Press darts flat and then in correct wearing direction. Basting that is holding layers together should remain during further garment construction.

Darts stitched separately

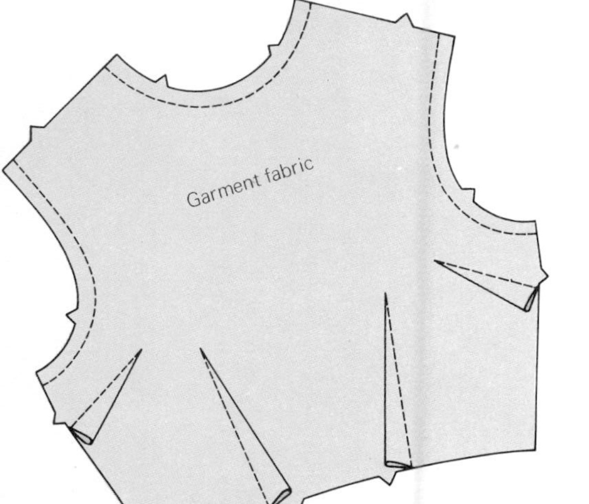

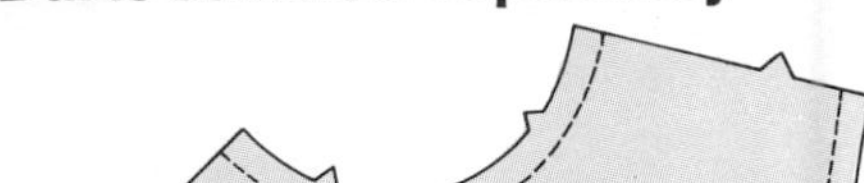

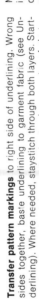

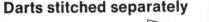

When stitching underlining and garment darts, mark both fabrics on wrong side and staystitch each layer individually. Stitch all darts; press flat as stitched. Then press each garment dart in its correct direction; press corresponding underlining dart in opposite direction.

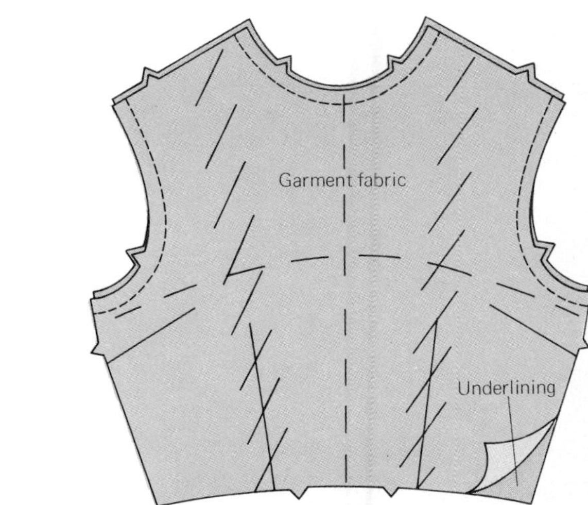

With wrong sides together, baste underlining to garment fabric (see Underlining). Because of shaping built in by darts, it may be necessary to place the layers over a tailor's ham for basting. When layers are joined, continue garment construction, handling both layers as one.

Tucks

Pressing 18-19 Machine accessories 38-39
Fabric-marking methods 94

Basic tucks

A tuck is a stitched fold of fabric that is most often decorative in purpose, but it can also be a shaping device. Each tuck is formed from two stitching lines that are matched and stitched; the fold of the tuck is produced when the lines come together. A tuck's width is the distance from the fold to the matched lines. The width can vary, as can the space between tucks. Tucks that meet are called **blind tucks;** those with space between them are **spaced tucks.** A very narrow tuck is a **pin tuck.** Most tucks are stitched on the straight grain, parallel to the fold, and so are uniform in width. Some, such as the curved dart tuck, are stitched off-grain and their width consequently varies.

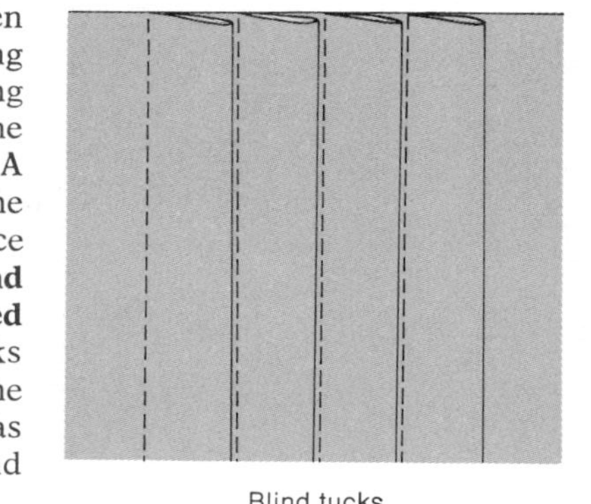

Blind tucks

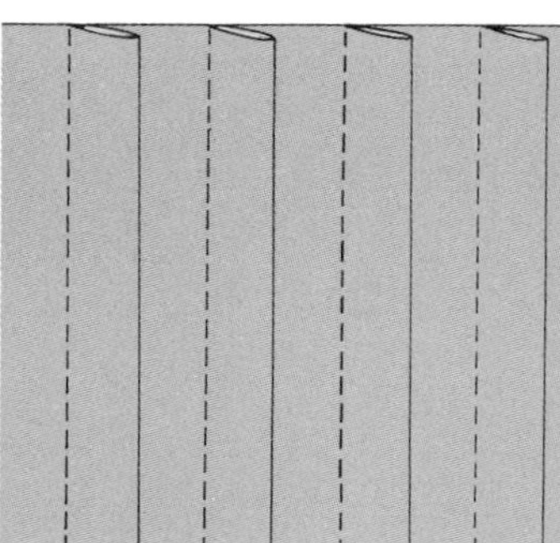

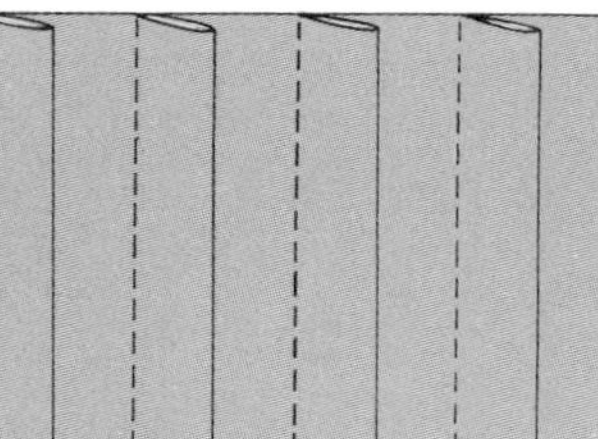

Spaced tucks

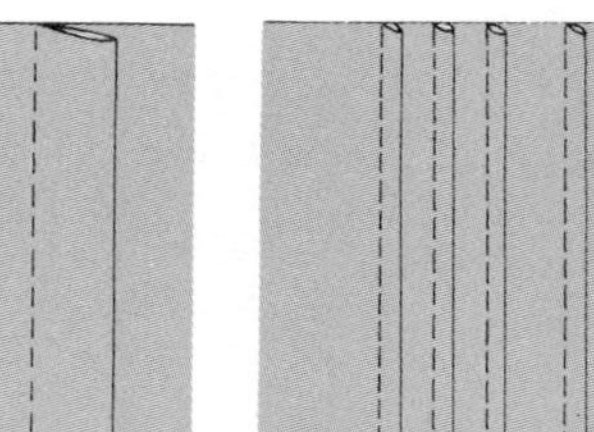

Pin tucks

How to make a tuck

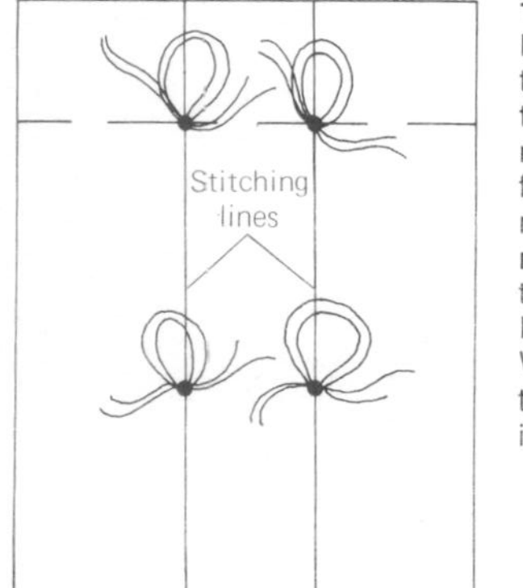

1. Mark the stitching lines of each tuck. If a tuck is to be made on the *outside* of garment, mark the *right* side of fabric; if on the *inside*, mark on *wrong* side. Use marking method suitable to fabric and to tuck location (see Marking). Width of tuck is one-half the distance between its stitching lines.

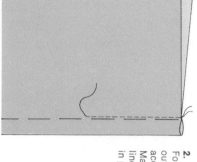

2. Remove pattern. Fold tuck to inside or outside of the garment, according to design. Match the stitching lines and baste in place. Stitch tuck.

Useful gauges

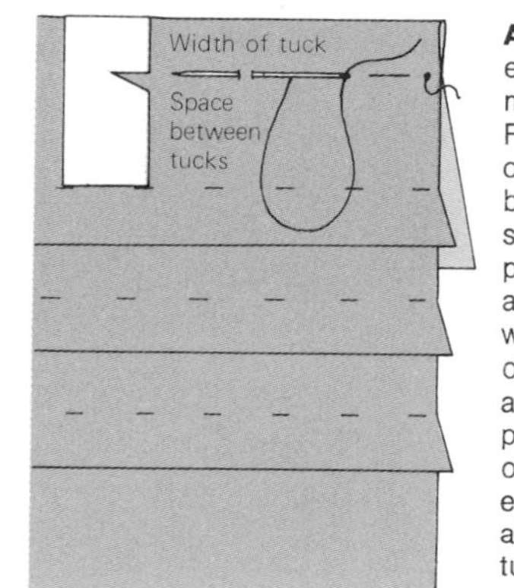

A cardboard gauge can eliminate the need for marking stitching lines. First determine *width* of tuck and *space* between stitching lines of successive tucks. Cut a piece of cardboard as long as the sum of these two widths; from one end mark off the tuck width and make a notch. Lower edge is placed along stitching line of previous tuck; upper edge is at fold; notch is at the stitching line of tuck being formed.

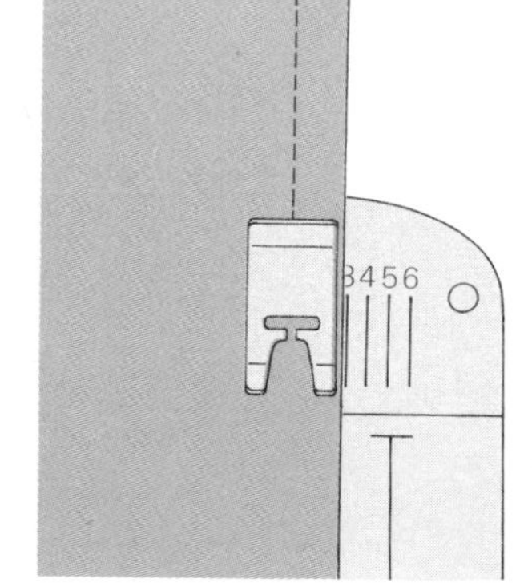

Throat plate markings on machine are helpful gauges for precise stitching of tucks that range from ⅜″ to ⅝″, and sometimes ¾″, in width. For instance, you can stitch a ⅜″ tuck by keeping the fold of the tuck on the 3 mark. Other aids to stitching to a precise width are the edge of the presser foot (for narrow tucks); a separate seam gauge; or a quilter guide-bar (for wider tucks).

Pressing tucks

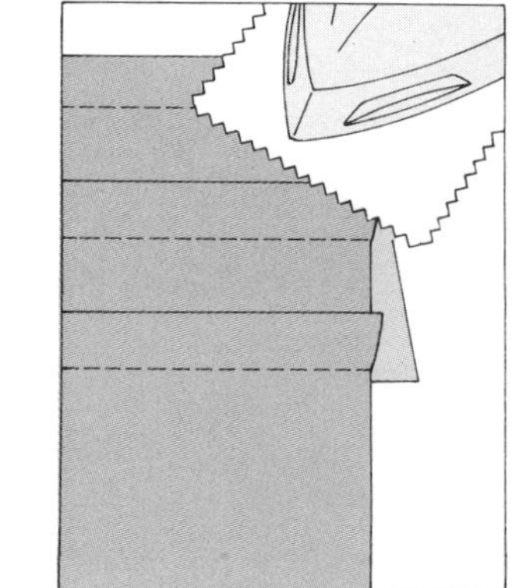

1. Press each tuck flat as it was stitched. If pressing from right side, be sure to use a press cloth so as not to mar the fabric.

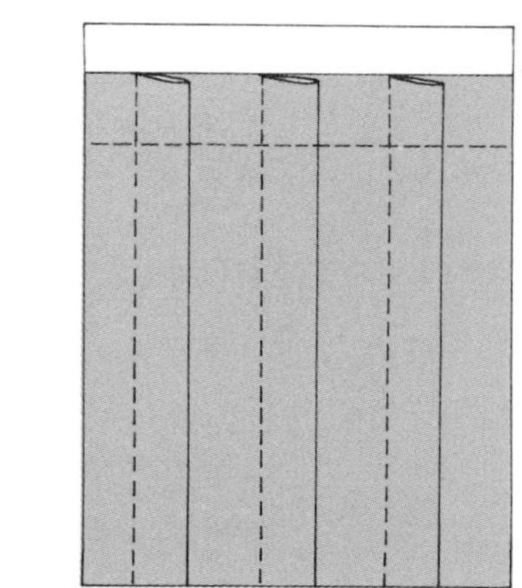

2. Then press all tucks in the direction in which they will be worn. To keep the ends of all tucks in position during balance of garment construction, staystitch across them as shown.

Special kinds of tucks

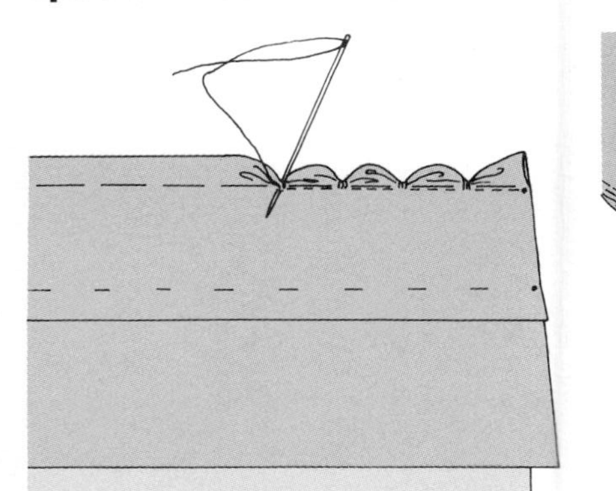

To form a shell tuck by hand, baste, then sew a narrow tuck. Use a running stitch, but every ½″ take a few overhand stitches in place to scallop tuck. Or machine-stitch tuck; then do overhand stitches, passing thread through tuck between scallops.

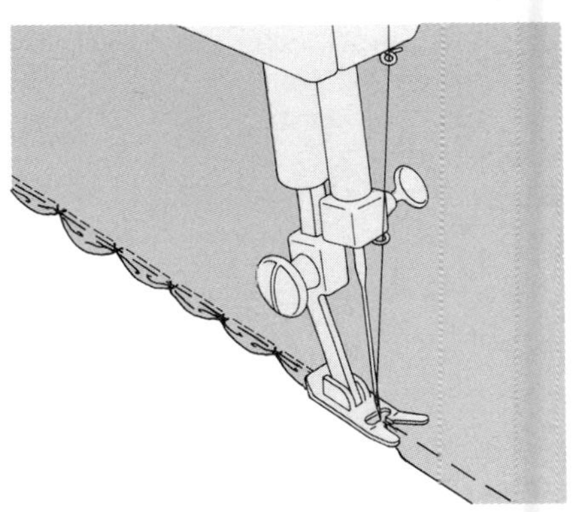

To form a shell tuck by machine, first baste a ⅛″ tuck. Set machine for the blindstitch. Place tuck under foot with fold to left of needle so that the zigzag stitch will form over the fold and scallop the tuck. Pretest for proper stitch length, width, and tension.

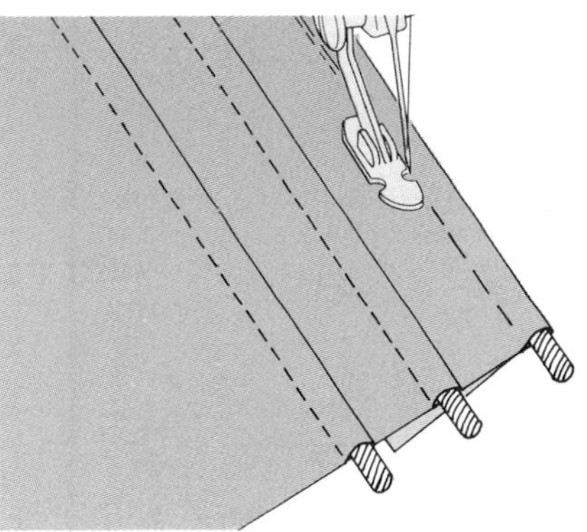

To make a corded tuck, fold the tuck, positioning cord inside along the fold. Baste. Using a zipper foot, stitch close to cord. Test this procedure before tucking garment to make sure that the size of the cord is right for the width of the tuck.

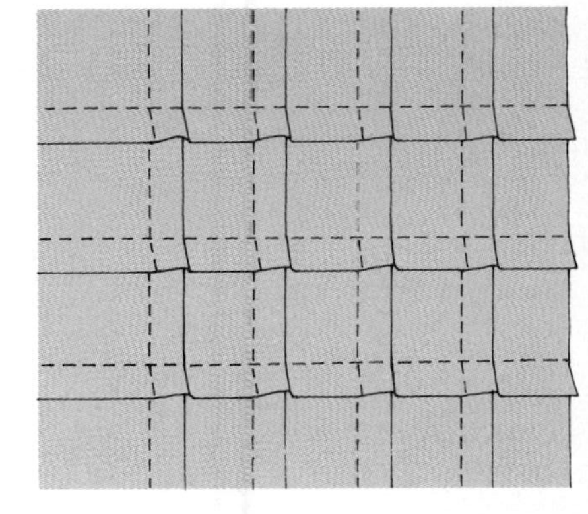

To form cross tucks, first stitch all the lengthwise tucks and press them in one direction. Then form the second, or crossing, set of tucks at right angles to the first, taking care to keep the first set of tucks facing downward as you stitch.

Additional techniques

Tucks can be added to any plain garment before it is cut. Tuck fabric first, then strategically position pattern over tucks and cut out section. Required extra fabric width is equal to twice the width of a tuck times the total number of tucks being added to the garment piece.

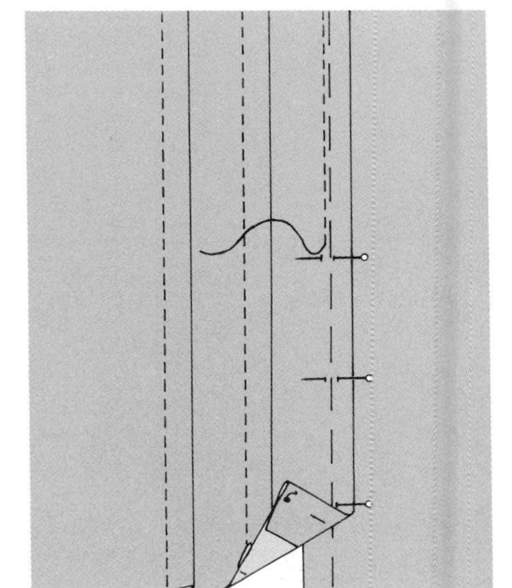

Piece fabric widths if one is not sufficient for all tucks. Fold under and baste a tuck at end of one piece, letting a ⅝″ seam allowance extend underneath. Lap this tuck, along its stitching line, ⅝″ beyond edge of other fabric piece. Pin and stitch.

Dart or released tucks

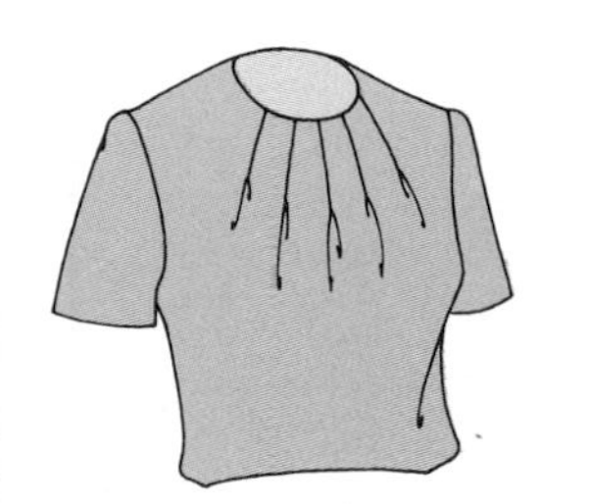

Dart tucks, sometimes also called released tucks, are used to control fullness and then release it at a desired point, such as the bust or hips. They can be formed on the inside or outside of the garment; fullness can be released at either or both ends. Sometimes the tuck is stitched across the bottom. Dart tucks may be stitched on the straight grain, or, in some instances, the stitching lines may be curved to build in a certain amount of shaping. Care must be taken, especially when stitching lines are curved, to match them accurately. Reinforce the stitches by tying threads or backstitching. Press carefully to avoid creasing folds.

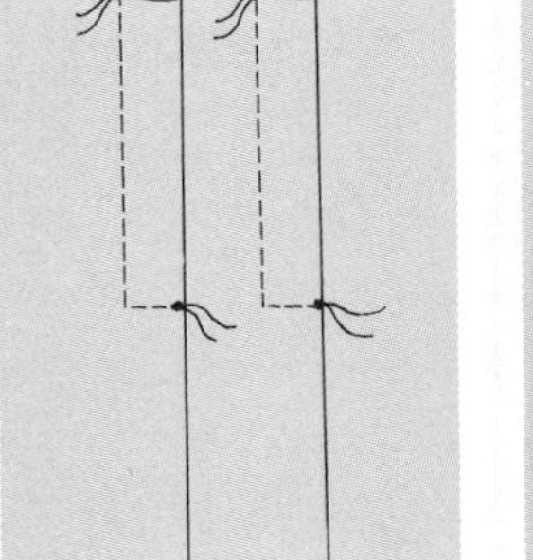

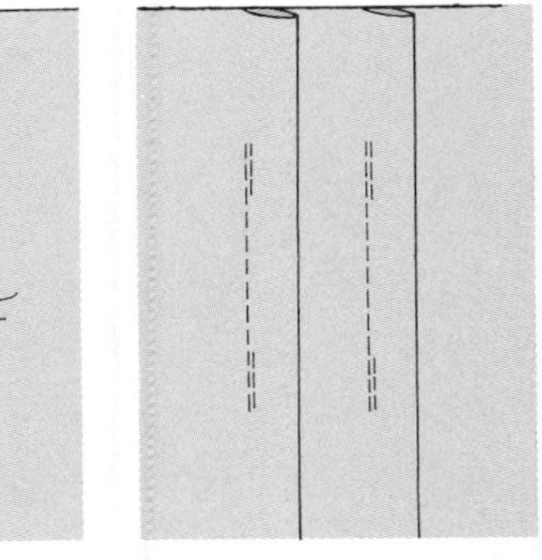

Pleats

Grain in fabrics 84-85

General information

Pleats are folds in fabric that provide controlled fullness. Pleating may occur as a single pleat, as a cluster, or around an entire garment section. Basically, each pleat is folded along a specified line, generally called the **foldline,** and the fold aligned with another line, the **placement** line (see illustrations at right). Patterns will vary as to what these lines are actually called and how or whether they appear on the pattern.

Most pleats are formed by folding a continuous piece of fabric onto itself. The exception is a pleat with a separate underlay stitched at the back. Pleats can be folded in several different styles (see below), the most common being the **side (knife) pleat, box pleat,** and **inverted pleat. A pleat with an underlay** is always an inverted pleat. Such variations as **accordion** and **sunburst pleats** are difficult to achieve at home and are best done by a commercial pleater. Pleat folds can be soft or sharp, depending on how they are pressed, but any pleat will hang better if it is folded on the straight grain, at least from the hip down.

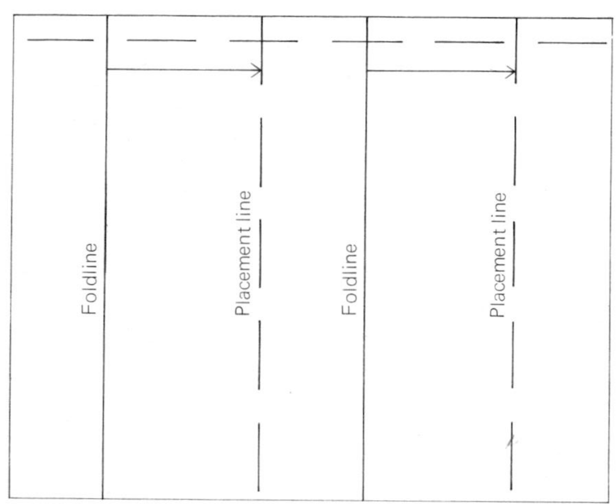

Though pattern markings vary, each pleat requires a foldline and a placement line or other marking to which it is brought. Arrows showing folding direction may also appear. Sections to be pleated are usually cut as a single layer.

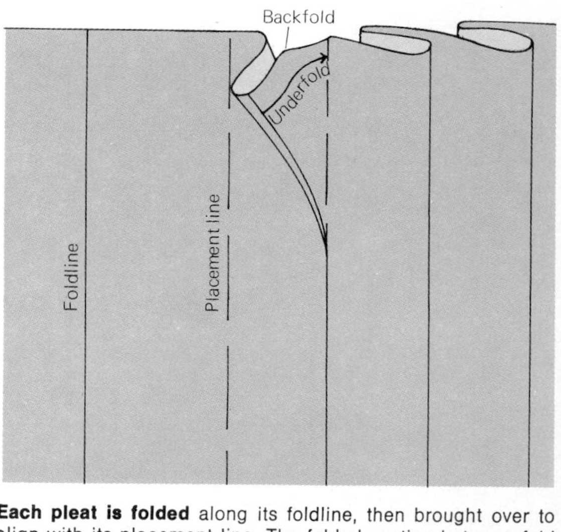

Each pleat is folded along its foldline, then brought over to align with its placement line. The folded section between fold and placement lines is called the pleat **underfold;** its fold is referred to as the **backfold** of the pleat.

Types of pleats

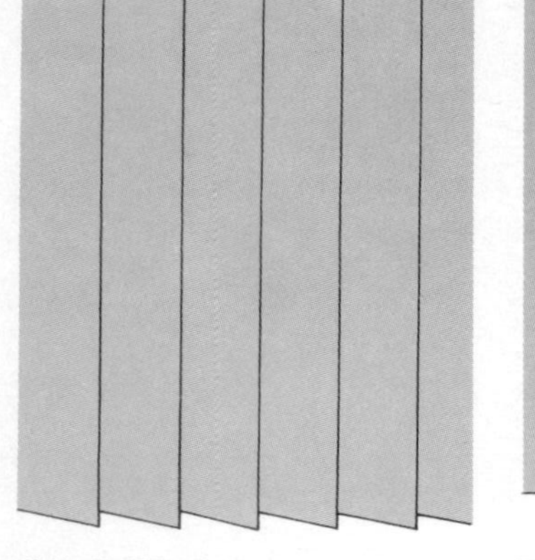

Side (knife) pleats have one foldline and one placement line; all the folds are turned in the same direction. Some garments may have one cluster facing one way and another facing the opposite way.

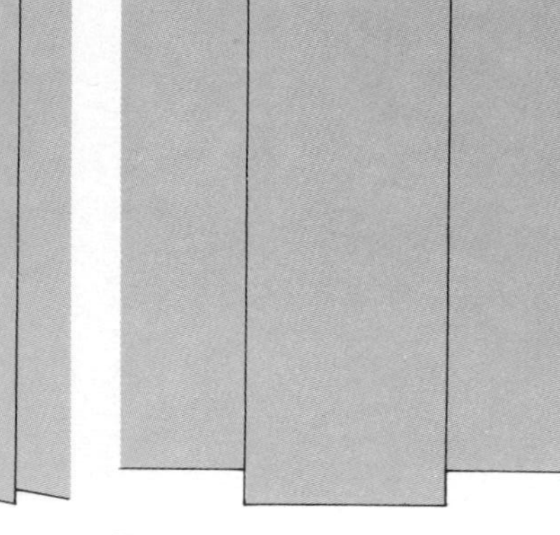

Box pleats have two foldlines and two placement lines; the two folds of each pleat are turned away from one another. The backfolds in box pleats are facing and may or may not meet—it is not necessary.

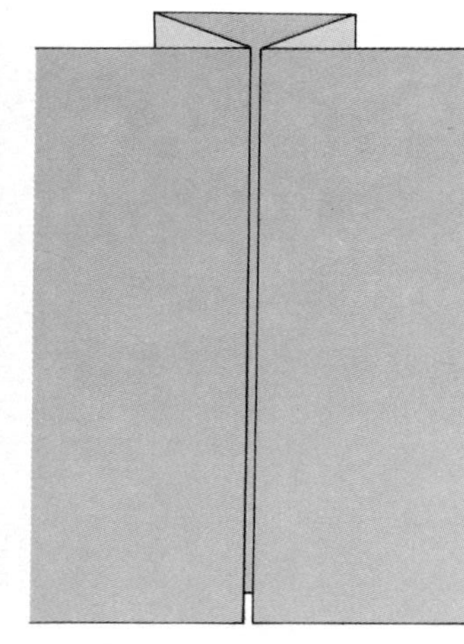

Inverted pleats have two foldlines and a common placement line. The two folds of each pleat are turned toward each other and in this case they must meet. The backfolds face away from each other.

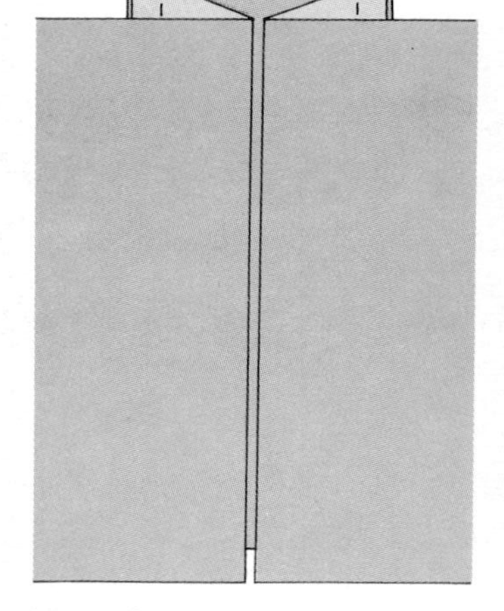

Pleat with separate underlay: An inverted pleat in appearance, but constructed with a separate underlay that forms underside of pleat. In place of usual two backfolds, there are two seams.

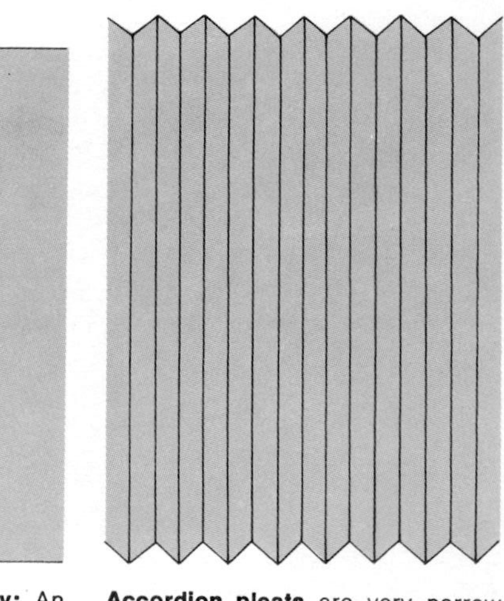

Accordion pleats are very narrow pleats of uniform width resembling the bellows of an accordion. Front folds stand slightly away from the body, giving flared effect. Best done by a commercial pleater.

Fabric considerations

Almost any type of fabric can be pleated provided the right pleating techniques and finishes are employed. These are some of the considerations to bear in mind when choosing a fabric for pleating.

Pleat folds may be either soft or sharp. The fabric best suited for sharply folded pleats is one that will crease easily, is smooth and crisp, light to medium in weight, and firmly woven. Gabardine is a typical example. The fabric can be made of almost any fiber. Some synthetics, such as the acrylics, will resist creasing enough to make pleating difficult, but not impossible. Knitted fabrics, too, are generally difficult to crease, especially the heavier, bulkier knits.

Consider, too, whether the garment will be laundered or dry-cleaned. Either cleaning process can remove sharp pleats, but when a garment is professionally dry-cleaned it is automatically re-pressed in the process. Laundering at home will necessitate re-forming and pressing the pleats yourself each time the garment is washed. This should not discourage use of a fabric you like; if each fold is **edgestitched** (see p.171), the folds will stay in shape and in place through any type of cleaning. **Topstitching** can be used to keep pleats in position in the hip-to-waist area (see pp.170–171).

Another possibility is to have the fabric, or the finished garment, professionally pleated. Commercial pleaters can apply a finish that makes pleats truly permanent. Elaborate pleats, such as accordion pleats, can only be made successfully by a professional pleater. Consult pleaters in your locality for the types of pleats they offer, the cost, and the amount and type of fabric required. Ask, too, if the fabric will need to be prepared in any way. You can also buy prepleated fabric, though only in certain pleat styles.

For soft, unpressed pleats, almost any fabric is suitable. The best choices are those that are fluid and will fall into graceful folds. Any material that cannot be sharply pleated is a likely candidate for soft pleats. With thick, spongy fabrics, soft pleats are usually the only possibility.

To be sure a fabric will pleat as you want it to, it is wise to make several test pleats before pleating the garment, perhaps edgestitching or topstitching as well, to see whether these techniques will help.

Pleat size and fabric weight should also be coordinated. Lightweight fabrics usually pleat well into any size and type of pleat. Heavier fabrics should generally be limited to pleats that are not too deep and have ample space between them.

Pleats hang better and hold their shape longer if they are folded on the straight, preferably lengthwise grain, at least from the hip down. If the garment is shaped to fit the body from the hip up, it will be impossible to maintain the straight grain in this area. Before cutting the garment out, be sure to position the fabric on grain. Take special care to square the grain of a woven stripe or plaid so that the fabric's horizontal lines will square with its vertical lines after the pleats are formed. If the fabric is a printed stripe or plaid, be sure that it is printed on grain; if it is not, do not use the fabric for pleating. When marking pleat lines, it is sometimes better to use the pattern just to locate these lines and then, with the pattern removed, baste-mark the lines, following the grain with your eye.

An exception to the use of the lengthwise grain would be a fabric with a border print along one selvage. To achieve the desired effect, it may have to be positioned on the crosswise grain. It might also be possible to pleat a plaid on the crosswise grain, which could reduce the fabric requirement.

Underlinings are generally not recommended for a pleated garment, especially if it is being pleated all around. This is because it is extremely difficult to keep the fabric layers together along all of the folds. If an underlining should be necessary, carefully match and baste it to the fashion fabric along all of the pleat lines before folding. It will be a further help if all of the folds are edgestitched after the pleats have been formed. If there are only one or two pleats in the entire garment, edgestitching may be unnecessary.

A pleated garment may be lined, but the lining itself should not be pleated and should in no way interfere with the movement of the pleats. To retain the desired swing, the lining can be a half lining, that is, one that extends to just below the fullest part of the hips. It could also be a full-length lining, extending to the bottom of the garment, but with side seams left open far enough up to allow movement. If there are no pattern pieces for the lining, you can make it yourself in two ways. With one method, you first pleat the pattern and then cut out the lining from the pleated-down pattern, following the shape of its outer edge. The other way is to use a plain A-line skirt pattern to cut out the lining pieces. Bottom edge can be hemmed or seam-finished. The turned-and-stitched finish (see Seam finishes) is usually sufficient.

Pleat finishes

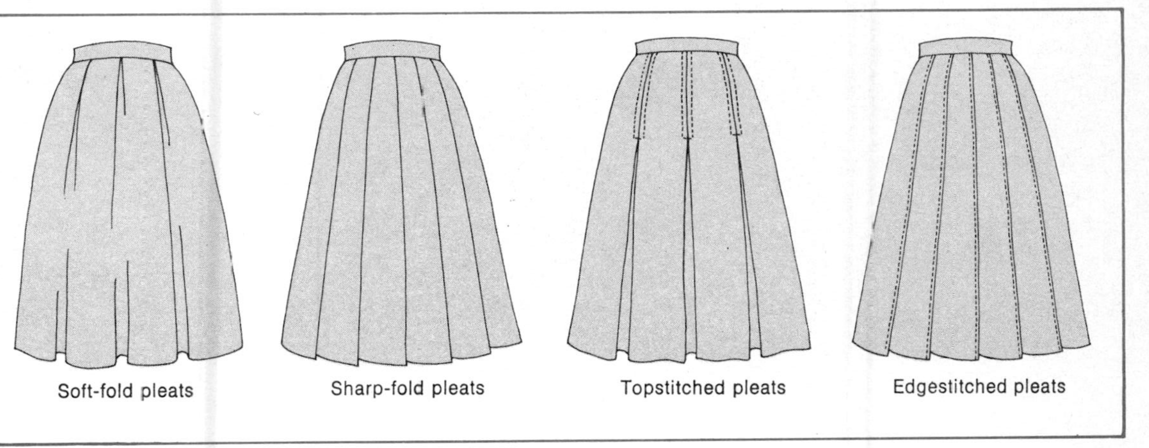
Soft-fold pleats · Sharp-fold pleats · Topstitched pleats · Edgestitched pleats

Pleats

Pressing 18-19
Simplified tailor's tacks 135

Pleating methods

Pleats can be formed from either the right side or the wrong side of the fabric. The method will depend on the fabric, the type of pleat being formed, and the pattern being used. If the fabric has a definite motif that must be followed in order to achieve a particular effect, it is best to mark and form the pleats from the right side. If the pleat is a type that is to be stitched on the inside from the hip to the waist, it will be easier to mark and form the pleats from the wrong side. Some patterns may also have certain seaming requirements that will make it necessary to match and stitch the pleats from the wrong side. This will be the case, for example, when you are constructing a pleat with a separate underlay.

In pressing pleats, use a press cloth whenever possible. If soft pleats are desired, press lightly if at all; if pleats will be sharp, use steam to help set the creases. If you want sharper pleats, dampen press cloth, press, then allow pleats to dry thoroughly before moving them. To help maintain folds during further construction, do not remove the bastings holding pleats until necessary.

Pleats formed from the right side

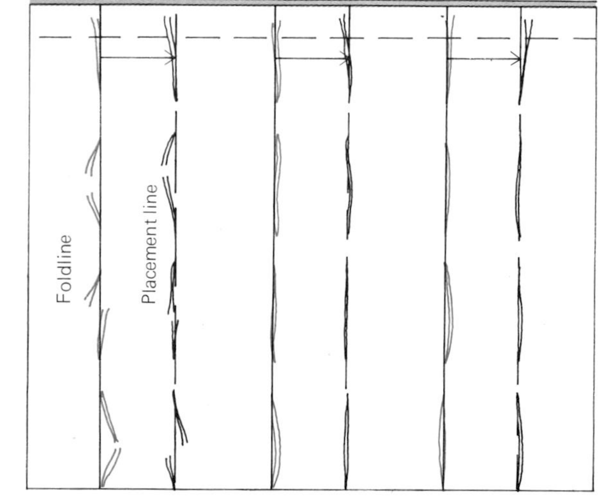

1. With pattern pinned to right side of fabric, mark each fold and placement line with simplified tailor's tacks. Use one thread color for foldlines, another for placement lines. Take small stitches every 3", leaving thread loose between them. Before removing pattern, clip thread between stitches.

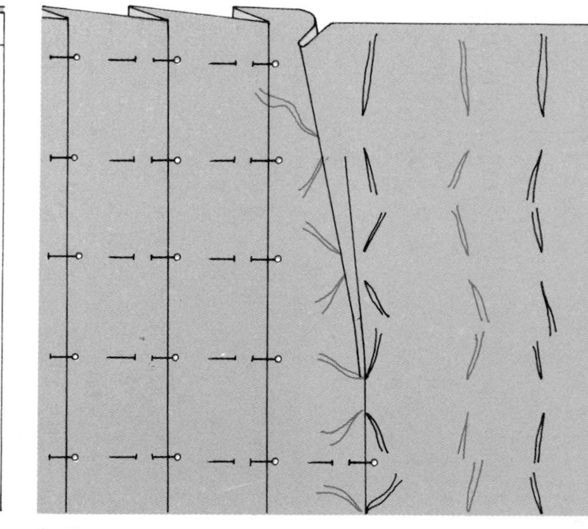

2. Remove pattern carefully to avoid pulling out thread markings. Working from right side, fold fabric along a foldline; bring fold to its placement line. Pin pleat through all thicknesses in the direction it will be worn. Do the same for each pleat, removing thread markings as you pin.

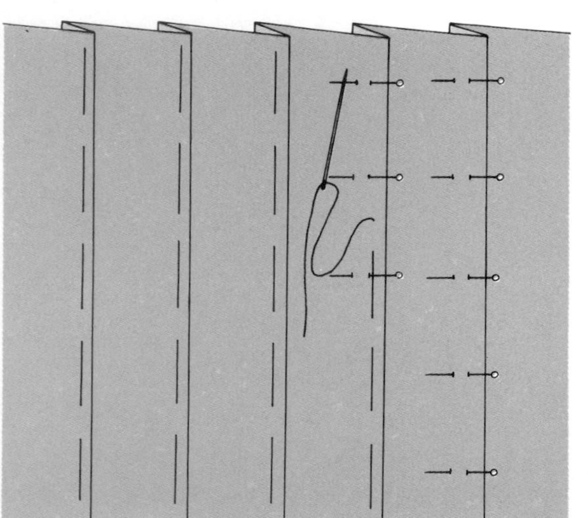

3. Baste each pleat close to the foldline through all thicknesses. Remove pins as you baste. Baste with silk thread; it leaves the fewest indentations in the fabric after pressing. This basting should be retained as far into further garment construction as possible.

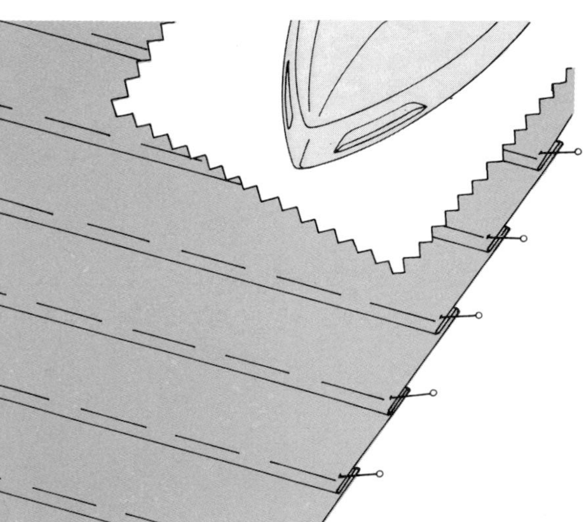

4. With fabric right side up, position a group of pleats over ironing board. (Support rest of garment during pressing.) Using a press cloth, press each pleat. For soft pleats, press lightly; for extra sharp pleats, dampen the press cloth and let pleats dry before moving them.

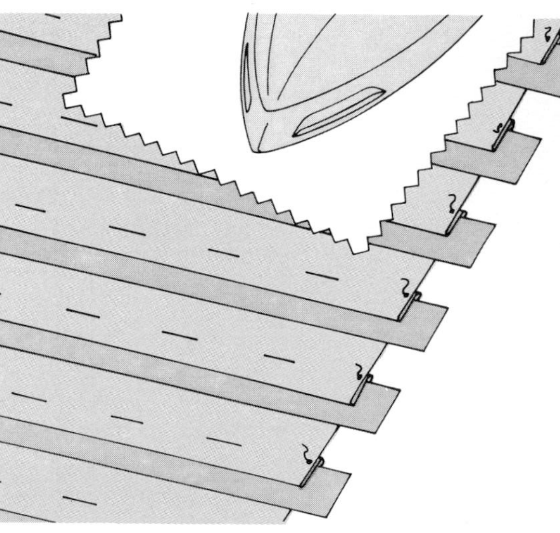

5. With garment wrong side up, press pleats again, using press cloth. If backfolds leave ridges during pressing, remove them by first gently pressing beneath each fold; then insert strips of heavy paper beneath folds and press again. Ridges can also be pressed out from the right side.

Pressing 18-19
Fabric-marking methods 94

Pleats formed from the wrong side

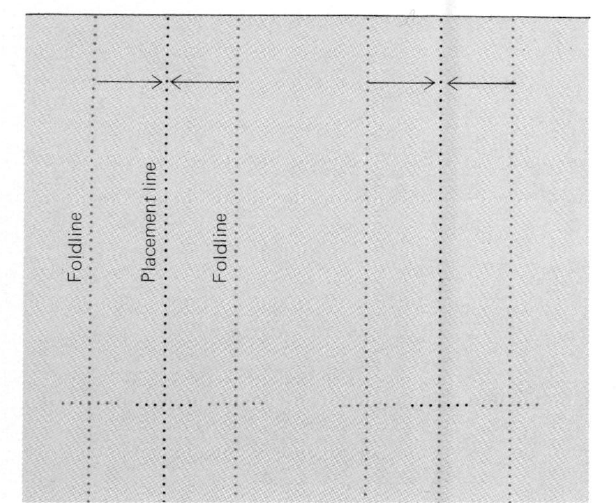

1. Before removing pattern, mark, on the wrong side of fabric, all foldlines and placement lines. Choose a method of marking that will show on but not mar the fabric (tracing paper is illustrated). Use one color (thread or tracing paper) to mark foldlines; another to mark placement lines.

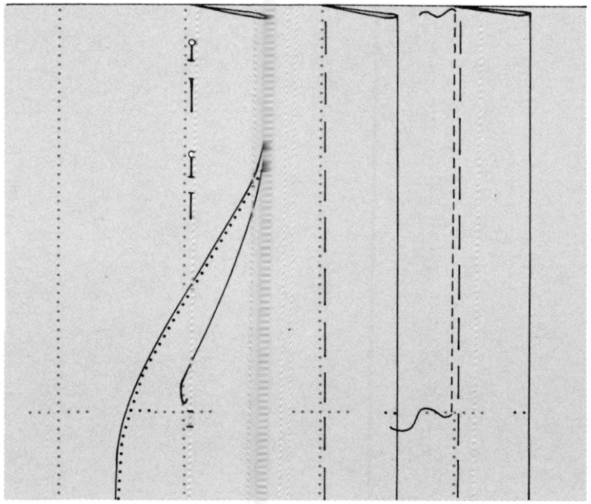

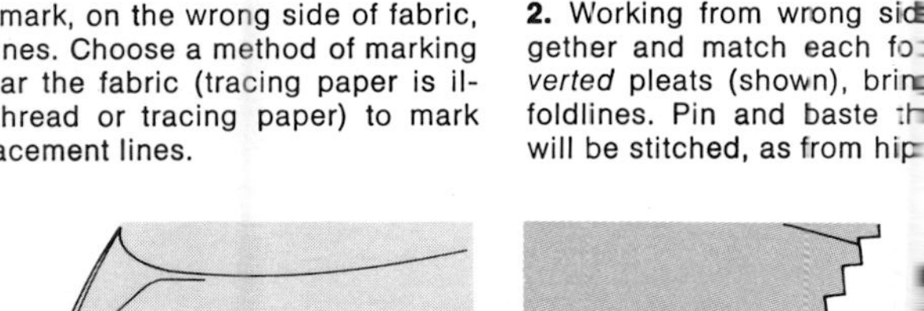

2. Working from wrong side, if *side* or *box* pleats, bring together and match each foldline to its placement line; if *inverted* pleats (shown), bring together and match each set of foldlines. Pin and baste through both thicknesses. If pleats will be stitched, as from hip to waist, do this now.

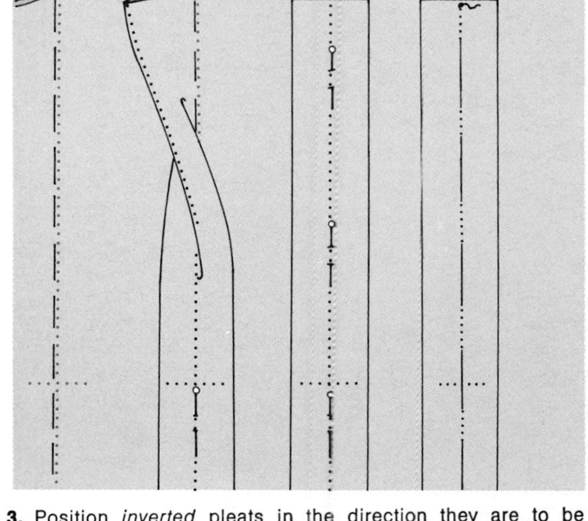

3. Position *inverted* pleats in the direction they are to be worn. This is done by spreading open the underfold of each pleat and aligning placement line to matched foldlines. Pin, then baste in place with silk thread, through all thicknesses the entire length of each pleat.

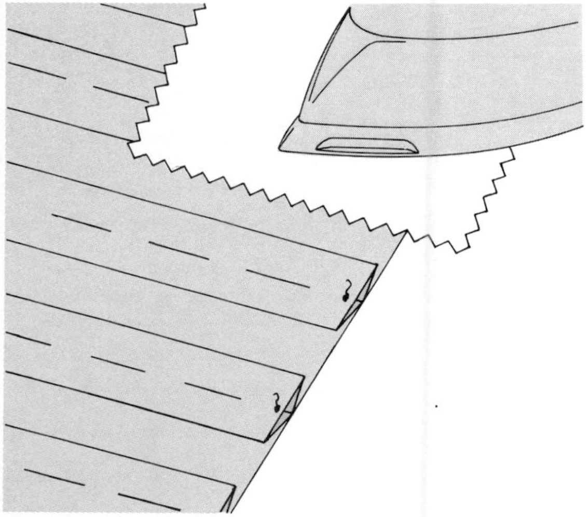

4. With wrong side up, using a press cloth, press all of the pleats in the direction they will be worn. When they are *side* pleats, all of the backfolds should be turned in one direction; the backfolds of *box* pleats will be facing each other; *inverted* pleats are pressed as shown above.

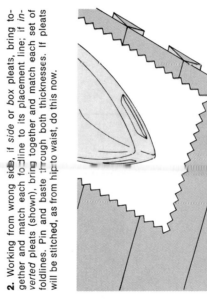

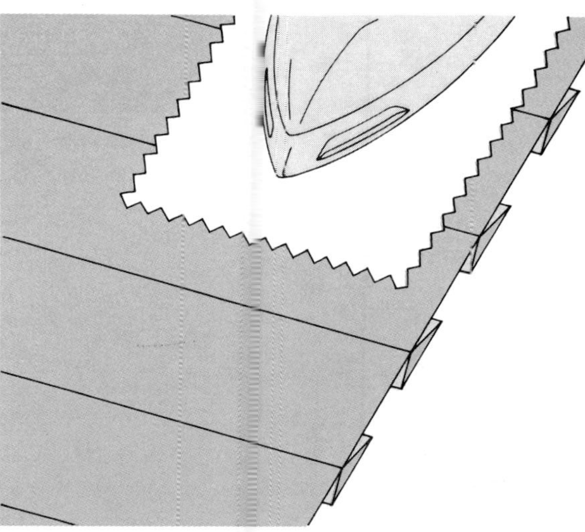

5. Turn garment to right side and, using a press cloth, press again. Be sure that all the pleats are facing in the direction that they will be worn. The basting that is holding the pleats in position should be left in place as long as possible during the balance of garment construction.

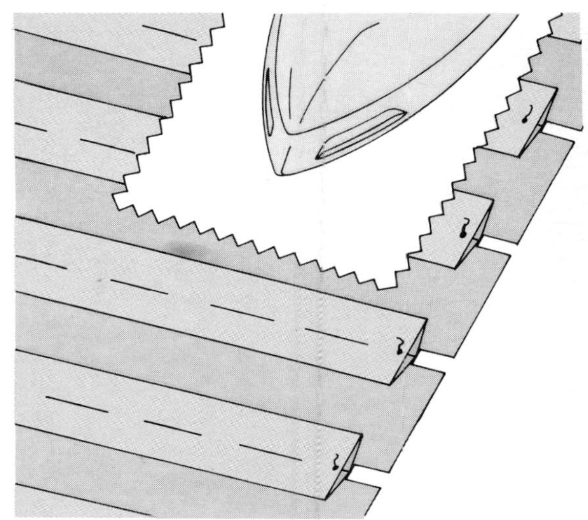

6. To remove ridges that may have been formed by the backfolds, turn garment to wrong side and press again, but using these techniques: First press gently under each fold; then insert strips of heavy paper under the folds and press again. These procedures can also be used on right side.

Pressing 18-19
Hemming 290-295

Pleat with separate underlay

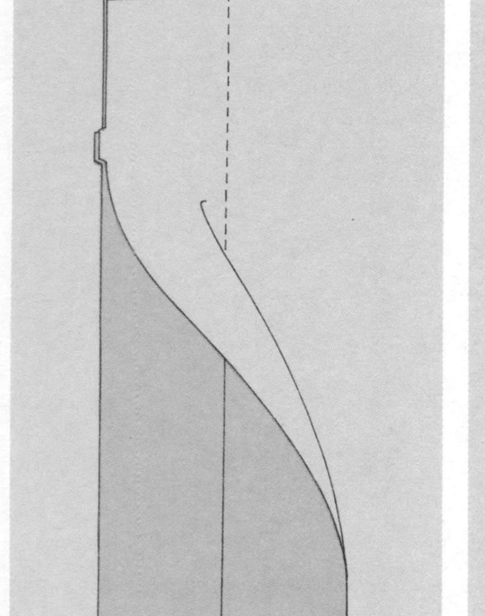

To form a pleat with a separate underlay, first bring together and match foldlines. Baste. If the foldlines are to be partially stitched together, do this step next; then remove basting from stitched area only. Press pleat extensions open along foldlines.

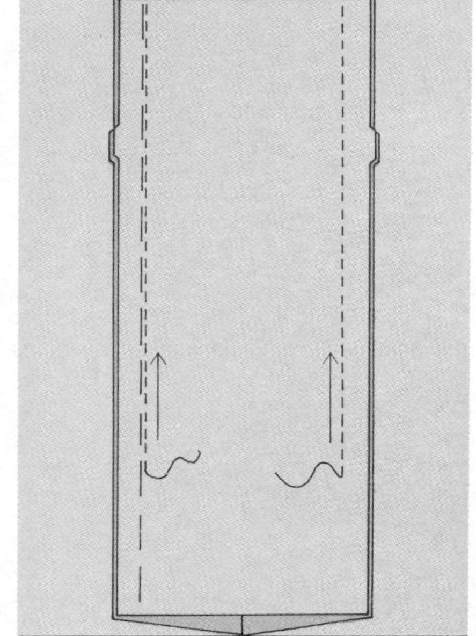

With right sides together, position pleat underlay over the pleat extensions, matching markings; baste along each seam. Beginning 6" up from the hem edge, stitch each side of the pleat underlay to each pleat extension. Remove bastings and press seam flat as stitched.

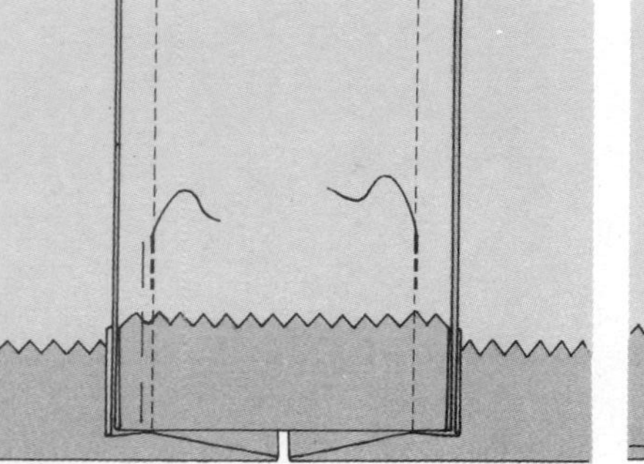

Remove bastings holding foldlines together. Hem skirt and pleat extensions separately from underlay. After hemming, match, rebaste, and stitch the unstitched part of the underlay to the pleat extensions. Stitch from hem edge up to previous stitching.

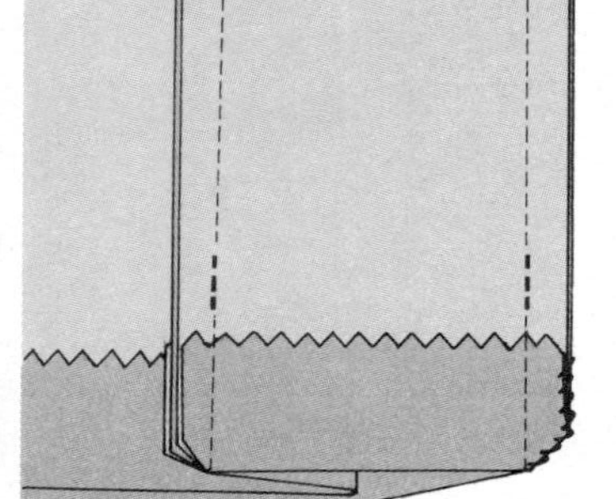

Press seams flat as stitched. Finish seam allowances of underlay and extension so their edges will not show beyond hem edge: First trim diagonally across the corners of all seam allowances; then whipstitch together each set of seam allowances within the hem area.

Topstitching and edgestitching pleats

Topstitching and edgestitching are two valuable techniques for helping pleats to lie and hang as they should. **Topstitching,** though primarily decorative, serves also to hold pleats in place in the hip-to-waist area. It is done through all thicknesses of the pleat. **Edgestitching** is applied along the fold of a pleat both to maintain the fold and to give it a sharper crease. It is done after the hem is completed. When using either of these techniques, stitch from the bottom of the garment up toward the top. When applying both techniques to the same pleat, edgestitch first.

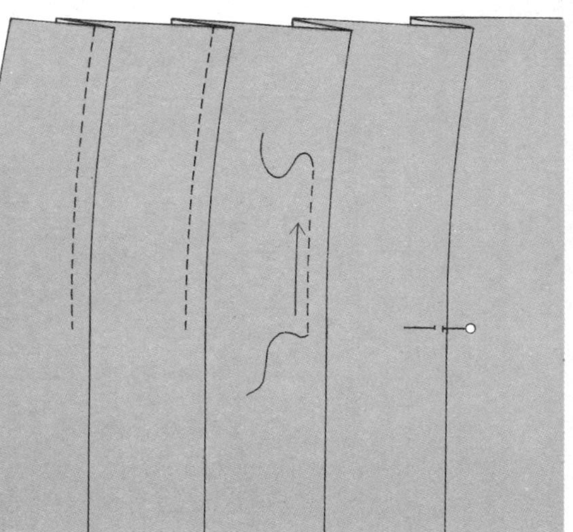

To topstitch side pleats in the hip-to-waist area, first pin-mark each pleat at the point where the topstitching will begin. Then, with the garment right side up, stitch through all thicknesses, along the fold, from the pin to the top of pleat. Bring thread ends to underside and tie.

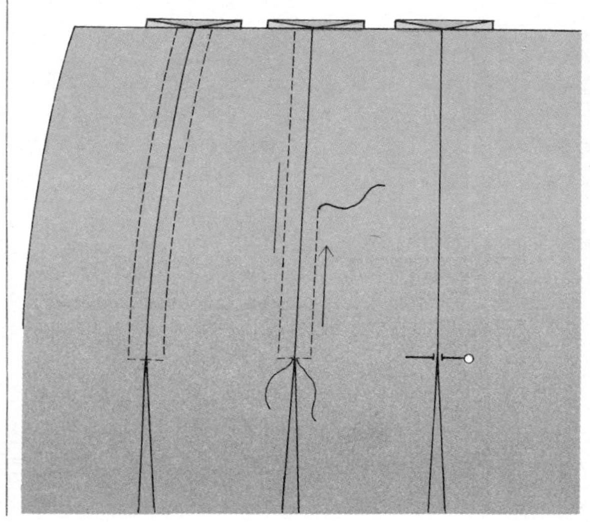

Topstitch inverted pleats on both sides of the matched foldlines. Pin-mark each pleat where the topstitching will begin. With garment right side up, insert needle between foldlines at marked point. Take two or three stitches across the pleat, pivot, then stitch along foldline to waist. Beginning again at the mark, stitch across pleat in opposite direction, pivot, then stitch to the waist. Bring all threads through to the underside and tie.

Tying thread ends 137
Turned-and-stitched seam finish 148

To edgestitch pleat folds, extend the pleat and stitch, through the two thicknesses as close to the fold as possible. Stitch from the finished hem edge up. Bring thread ends through to underside and tie. Both folds can be edgestitched, as shown, or just outer or inner folds if that is more suitable.

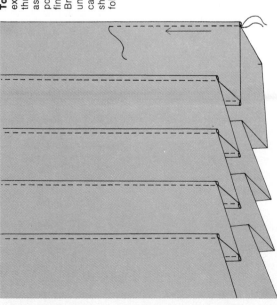

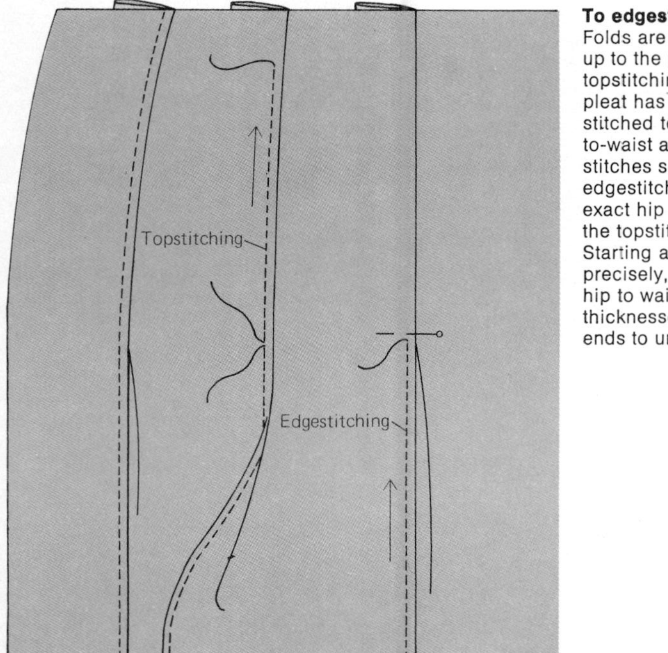

To edgestitch *and* topstitch: Folds are first edgestitched up to the point where the topstitching will begin. If pleat has already been stitched together in the hip-to-waist area, remove a few stitches so that the edgestitching can extend to exact hip point where the topstitching will begin. Starting at that point precisely, topstitch from hip to waist through all thicknesses. Bring all thread ends to underside and tie.

Staying pleats

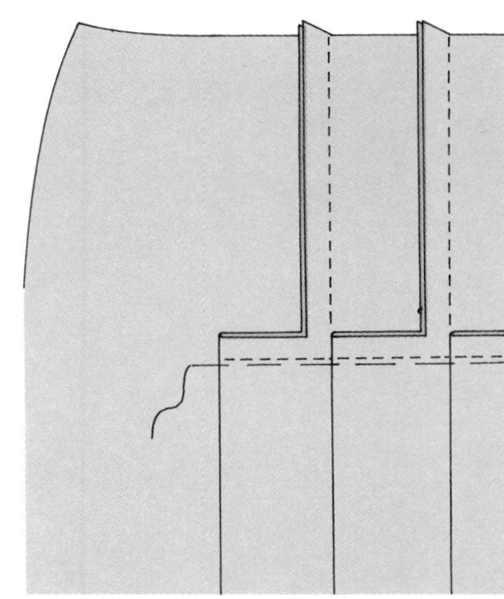

Separate stay can be added to give support to stitched-down pleats in which top part of underfold has been eliminated by pattern piece. Seam each pleat down, then across underfold; baste in wearing direction.

Cut stay as wide as garment part and deep as area to be stayed plus seam allowances; turn-and-stitch lower edge. Baste in place at top; slipstitch lower edge to tops of underfolds (other edges will be caught in seams).

Self-stay can be formed on a stitched-down inverted pleat. First stitch down pleat. Then, in two steps, stitch across both sides of underfold. Slit along backfolds to stitching; trim fabric behind to 5/8" from stitching, as shown.

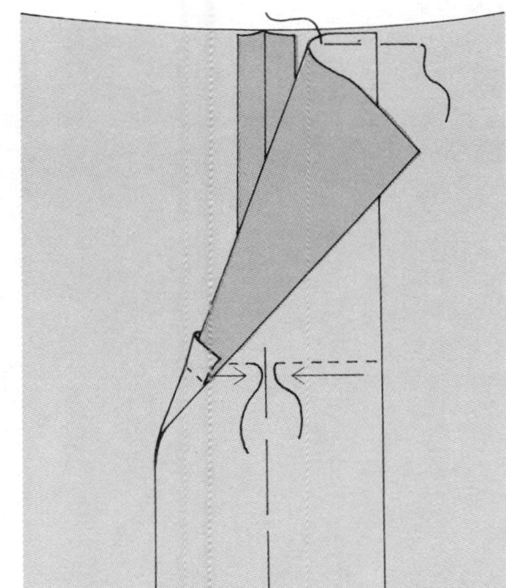

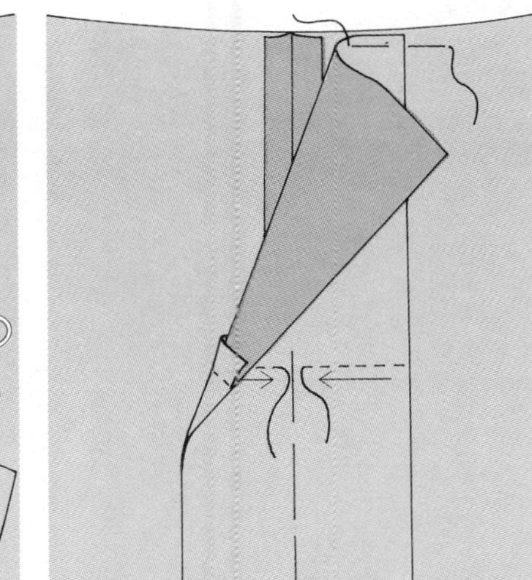

Bring the top of the trimmed underfold back up to top edge of garment. Carefully align this self-stay with the rest of the pleat and baste it in place along top. This top edge will be caught into the seam.

Hemming 290-295

Hemming pleated garments

Depending upon the type of pleats, the hem in a pleated garment is done sometimes before and sometimes after pleats are formed. **Hemming before pleating** is easier, but it is appropriate only when the pleats are all-around and straight, or when the top portion does not require seaming or extensive fitting. If shortening should be needed after hemming, garments pleated as described can be raised from the top without distorting the pleats. The amount that can be *added* after hemming is very limited; only half the width of the top seam allowance is available for the purpose.

Hemming after pleating is the more common order of procedure and is necessary when there is only a single pleat or a cluster; when the pleat is formed with a separate underlay; or when, on an all-around-pleated garment, the pleats are seamed or fitted at the top. Sometimes, especially with heavier fabrics, it may be helpful to press in the pleat folds to within 8 inches of the hem edge, hem, then press in the pleat folds the rest of the way.

Seams within a hem are treated in different ways according to where the seam is—that is, whether at a flat part or at the backfold of the pleat—and whether the seam is stitched before or after hemming (see below). Most seams are stitched before hemming, but, in some cases, such as a garment that is hemmed before pleating, or a pleat formed with a separate underlay, there will be one or two seams to be stitched after hemming.

Handling seam allowances in hem area

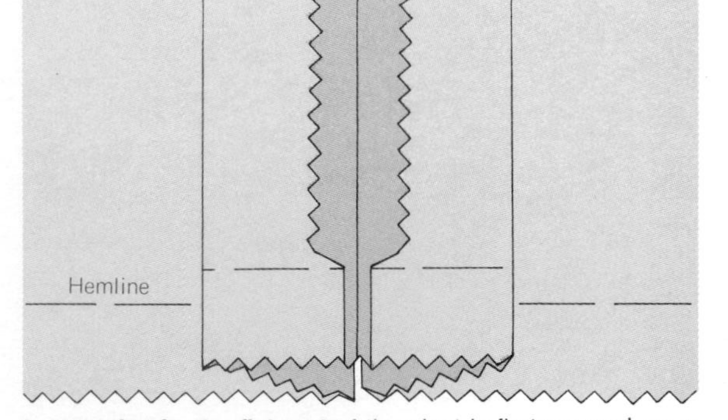

A seam that is at a flat part of the pleat is first pressed open and then trimmed to half its width from the hem edge to the hemline. This is a grading technique that will eliminate unnecessary bulk from the hem in this area.

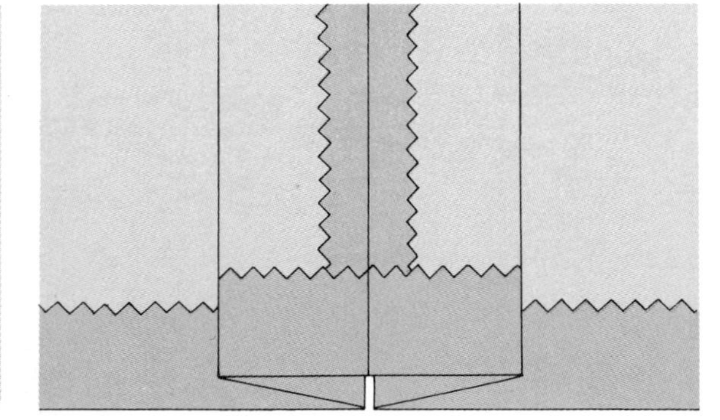

Finish the hem edge and stitch the hem in place, using a method that is suitable to the fabric (see Hemming). When turning up hem, make certain that seamlines are matched and seam allowances are in the pressed-open position.

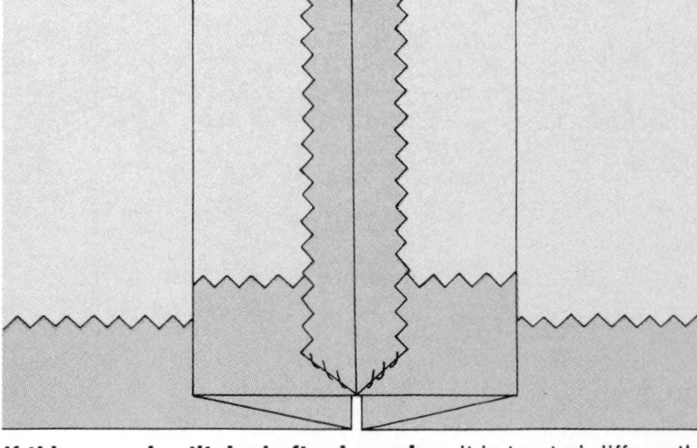

If this seam is stitched after hemming, it is treated differently. First press seam open, then trim diagonally across each corner at the bottom of the seam allowances. Whipstitch these trimmed edges flat to the hem.

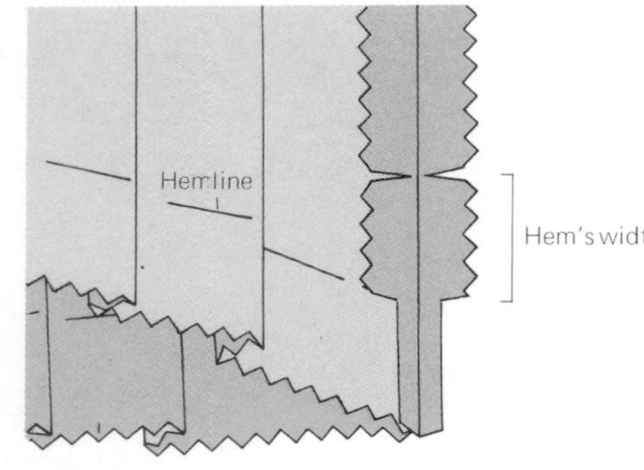

A seam that is at the backfold of a pleat is also first pressed open and trimmed to half width from hem edge to hemline. Then, so seam allowances can turn in different directions, clip into them a hem's width above hemline.

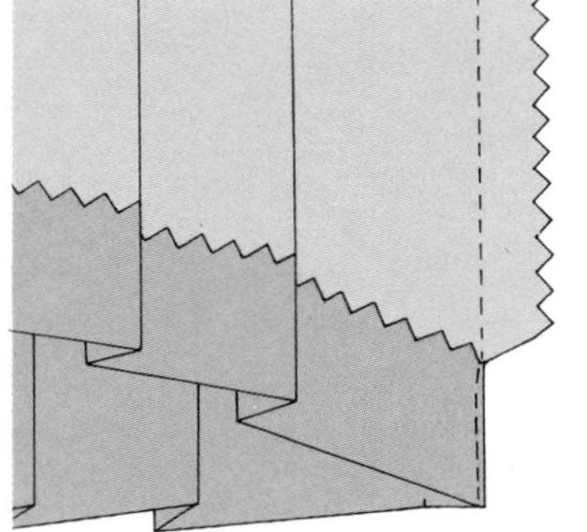

Finish the hem edge and stitch hem in place, using a suitable hemming method. To keep backfold creased, edgestitch close to the fold, from the hemline up to meet the seam at the point where it was clipped. Secure thread ends.

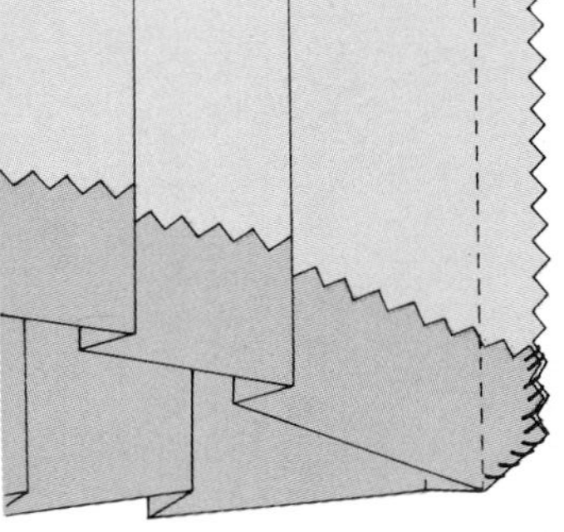

If this seam is stitched after hemming, first press seam flat as stitched. Then trim diagonally across both corners at bottom of seam allowances. Whipstitch together the trimmed edges, then rest of hem area seam allowances.

Adjusting fullness within hem

The amount of fullness in a pleated hem can be reduced or increased by re-stitching the seam (or, proportionately, the *seams*) within the hem area.

To reduce fullness, re-stitch a *deeper* seam, wider at hem edge and meeting original seam at hemline. Remove original stitches from altered part of seam; press; trim new seam allowances.

To increase fullness, re-stitch a *shallower* seam, narrower at hem edge and meeting original seam at hemline. Remove original stitches from altered part of seam; press; trim new seam allowances.

In either case, do not alter the original seamline so much that you distort the shape and hang of the hem. The altered seam is pressed open or flat according to where it falls on the pleat.

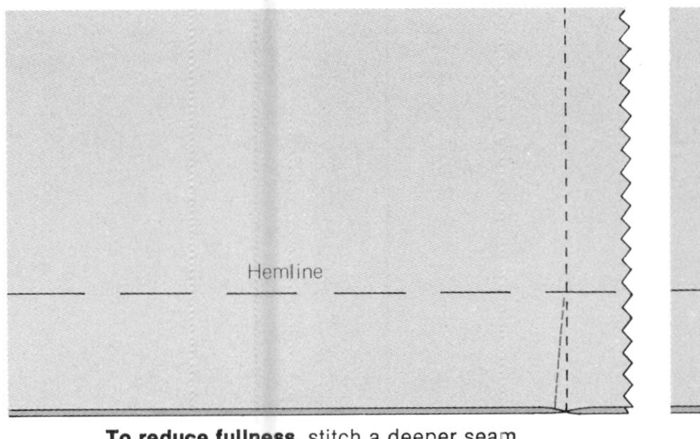

To reduce fullness, stitch a deeper seam.

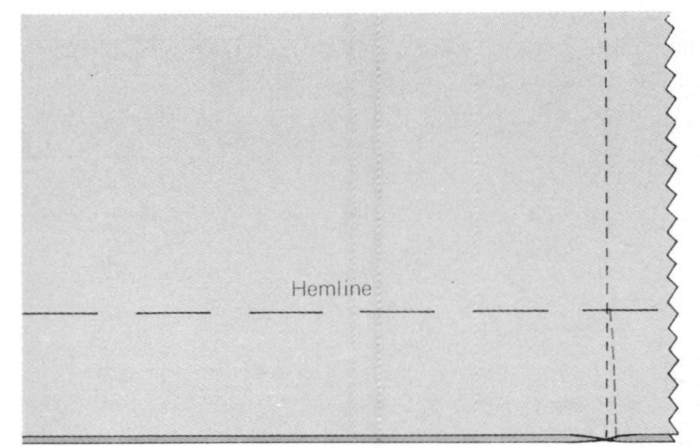

To increase fullness, stitch a narrower seam.

Plackets in pleated garments

The placket seam is usually the last seam to be formed in a garment that is pleated all around. It is at this point that the zipper should be installed. The pleats around the zipper can then be formed. Proper positioning of this final seam is important in order for the zipper to be as inconspicuous as possible. If the pleats are **box or inverted,** try to position the placket seam down the center of the pleat underfold; then install the zipper by either the centered or invisible zipper method (both described in Zipper section). If the garment is **side-pleated,** try to position the seam where the pleat backfold will fall; then insert the zipper by means of the special lapped application that is shown and described below.

For box or inverted pleats, position final seam down center of underfold and use either the centered or invisible zipper application. With inverted pleats, the folds will conceal the zipper placket; box pleats may not.

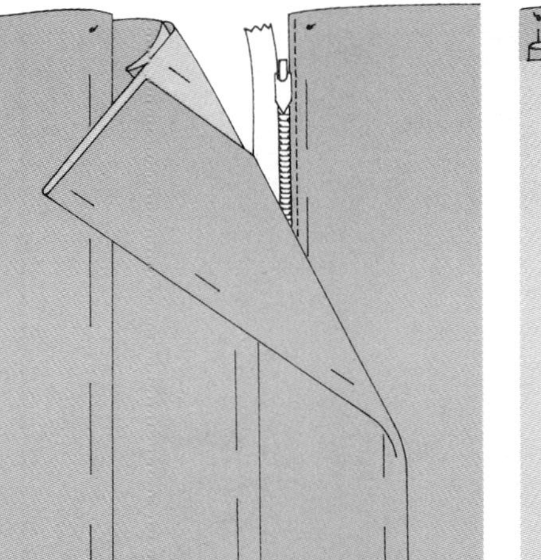

For side (knife) pleats, stitch the final seam at the pleat backfold, leaving top part open for zipper. Clip into the left seam allowance; turn it to wrong side of garment and baste in place, as shown.

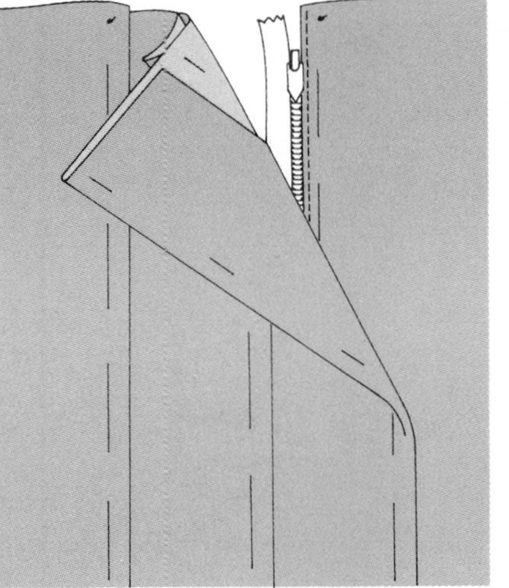

Turn garment to right side; position closed zipper under basted seam allowance with the folded edge close to the teeth and top stop just below top seamline. Baste. Then, using a zipper foot, stitch close to fold.

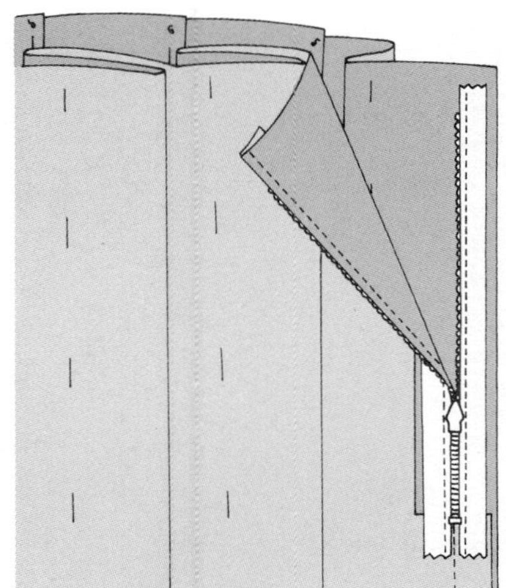

Turn garment to wrong side; extend unclipped seam allowance. Place other half of zipper face down on the seam allowance with the teeth ⅛" beyond the seamline. Baste, then open zipper and stitch to seam allowance.

Pleats

Altering pleated garments

Alterations in a pleated garment will be fewer, and easier to make, if the pattern is selected by hip measurement. Overall width or length adjustments, if needed, are best made in the pattern before the garment is cut out. Slight fitting modifications, such as tapering a garment to improve fit from hip to waist, are taken care of in the garment itself after it has been test-fitted.

A width alteration in a garment with all-around pleats must be divided and applied equally to each of the pleats. With side (knife) or box pleats, this involves moving both the fold and placement lines; with inverted pleats, only the foldlines. For a garment with a single pleat or a cluster, it is easier to alter the *unpleated* part of the garment. In order for pleats to hang properly, grainline must be maintained from at least the hip down. (It is often impossible to keep the grain perfect above the hip because of the shaping involved.)If the fabric you are using has a definite vertical design, as a plaid would have, it is necessary to position width alterations to conform to it.

Length adjustments

Length alterations are best made on the pattern, along the lengthening/shortening line specified on the pattern piece (see drawing below). This is the point where the designer feels a change will least affect the garment's shape. Length can also be adjusted at the hemline in hemming. After hemming, length can be changed slightly by lowering or raising the garment at the top seamline.

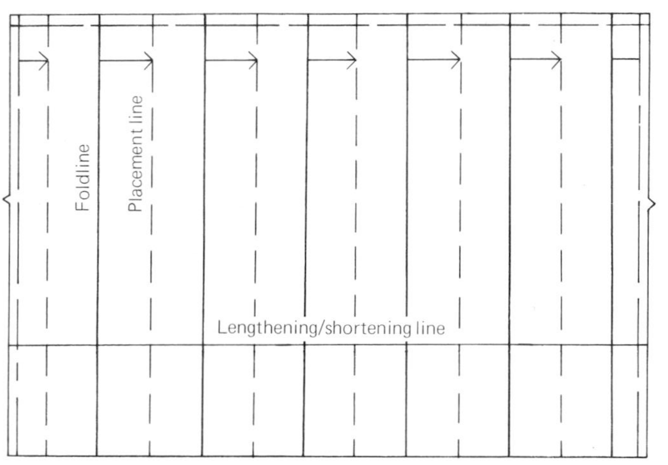
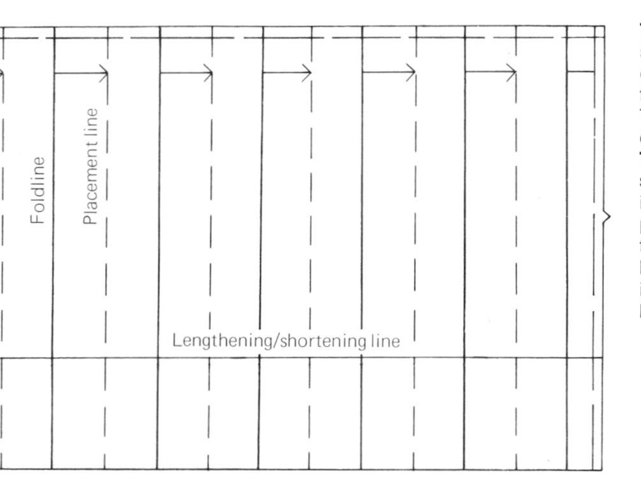

To lengthen, cut pattern along the lengthening/ shortening line. Tape tissue paper to one edge, then spread the two cut pattern edges apart the amount that the pattern is to be lengthened. Tape in place. Re-draw all the pleat, seam, and cutting lines affected by the alteration.
To shorten, measure up from the lengthening/ shortening line the amount the pattern is to be shortened. Draw a line across pattern parallel to, and the measured distance from, the adjustment line. Fold pattern on adjustment line. Bring fold to the drawn line and tape in place. Re-draw the pleat, seam, and cutting lines that were affected by the alteration.

Width adjustments in pattern

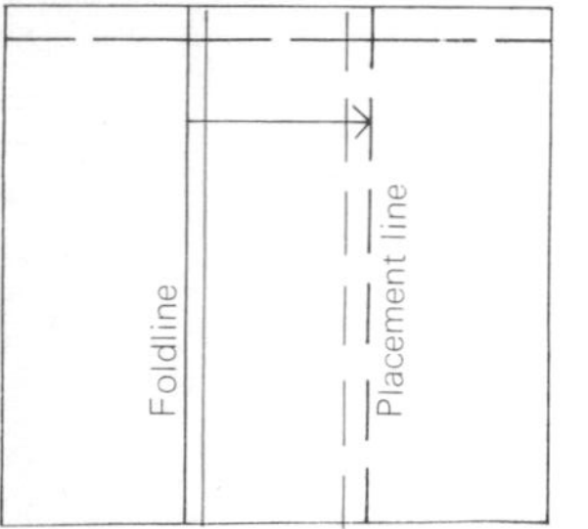

Side (knife) pleats are altered by re-positioning both the fold and the placement lines.
To increase garment width, re-draw both lines so pleat is *narrower.*

To decrease garment width, re-draw both lines so the pleat is *wider.*

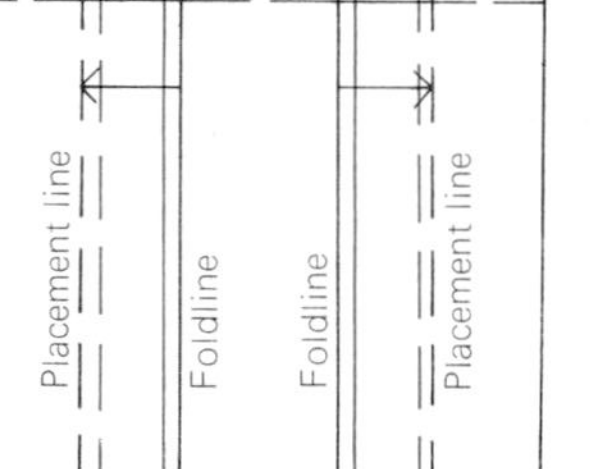

Box pleats are altered by re-positioning both foldlines and both placement lines.
To increase garment width, re-draw the lines so the pleat is *narrower.*

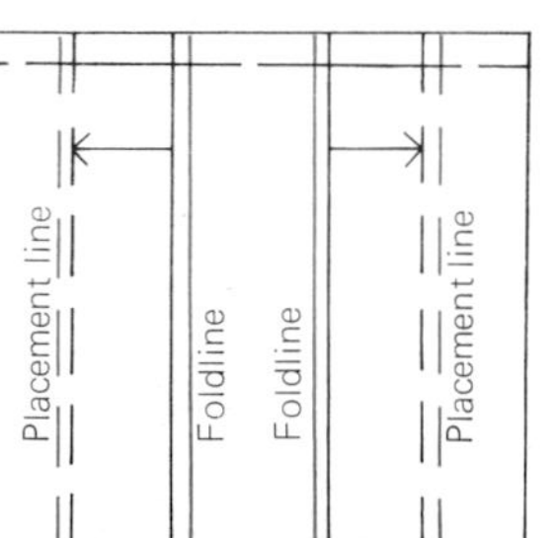

To decrease garment width, re-draw a *wider* pleat.

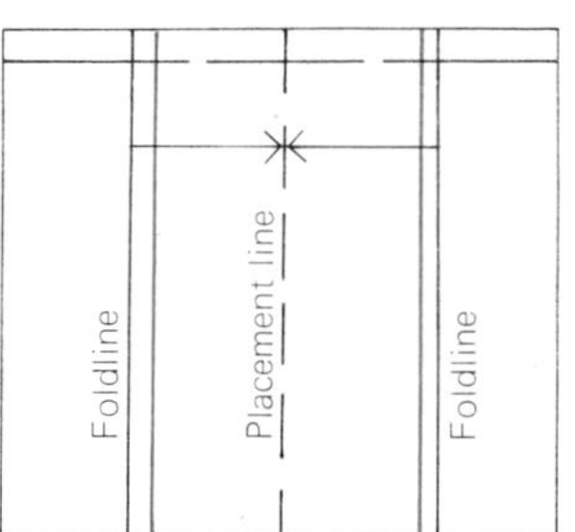

Inverted pleats are altered by re-positioning the *foldlines only.*
To increase garment width, re-draw each foldline *inside* the original.

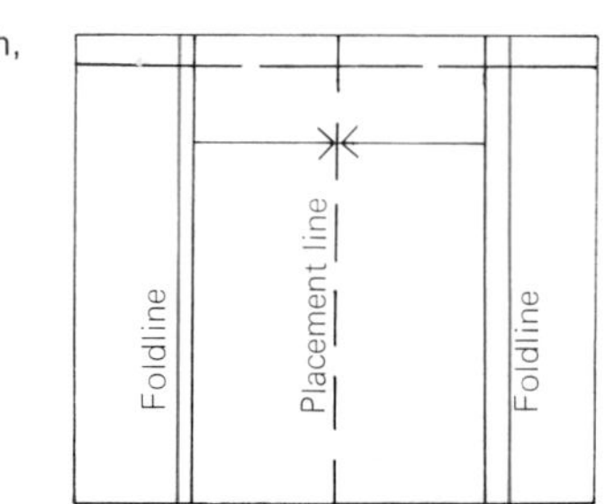

To decrease garment width, re-draw each foldline *outside* the original.

Width adjustments in hip-to-waist area

Sometimes a pleated garment will need alteration from hip to waist only. This is best done in the fabric after pleats have been basted in place. Try the garment on to determine how much it must be taken in or let out. Remove garment and release basting in hip-to-waist area. Divide total amount of alteration by the number of pleats and alter each pleat by the fractional amount (see below).

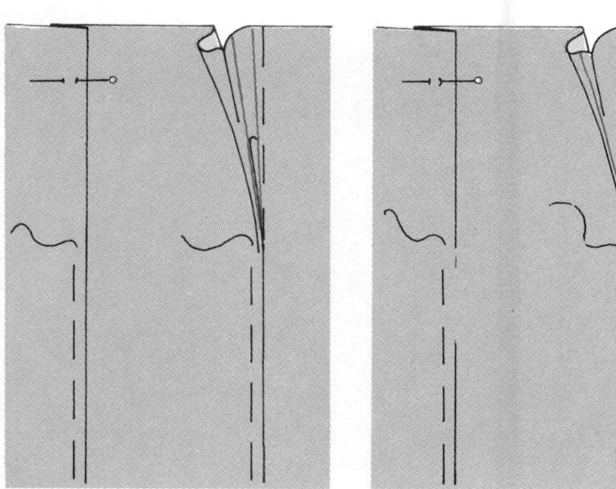

Pleats only folded: Re-fold all pleats by the same amount, *narrower to increase* and *deeper to decrease* garment width.

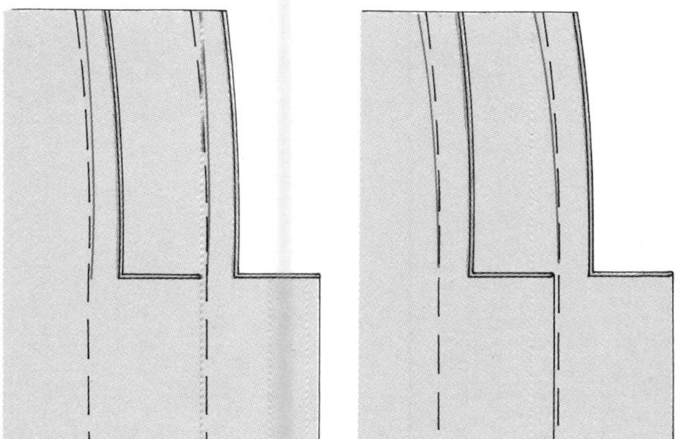

Pleats to be seamed: Re-position all seams equally *inside* originals to *increase* and *outside* to *decrease* garment width.

To correct hang

If pleats overlap at bottom, lower skirt from top (no more than half the seam allowance). Re-fit pleats at top if necessary; mark new top seam. If pleats still overlap, overall width must be adjusted (see below).

If pleats spread open at the bottom edge, raise garment from top to correct the hang. Re-fit the pleats at the top if necessary; mark new seamline. If this proves inadequate, re-adjust overall garment width (see below).

Adjusting overall garment width in fabric

Overall garment width can, if necessary, be adjusted in the fabric after all pleats have been basted in place. The technique is similar to width adjustment in patterns in that pleats are made narrower (to increase) or wider (to decrease). It differs in that, along with a uniform width adjustment from the hip down, the garment can easily and accurately be tapered through the hip-to-waist area as well. For side or box pleats, adjustment is made equally on fold and placement lines. With inverted pleats, only the foldlines are altered. Maintain the original grainline from the hip down.

1. Making sure that all pleat lines are still marked, release one pleat. Re-pin this pleat on marked lines but extend it out from the garment.

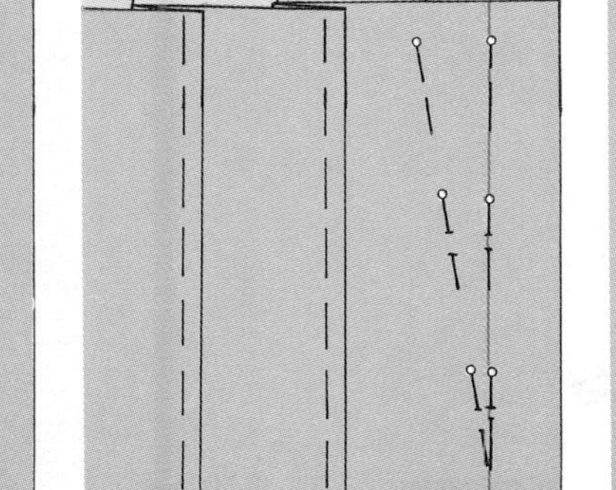

2. Put garment on; take in or let out extended pleat at hip, tapering to waist, until garment fits comfortably. Remove garment.

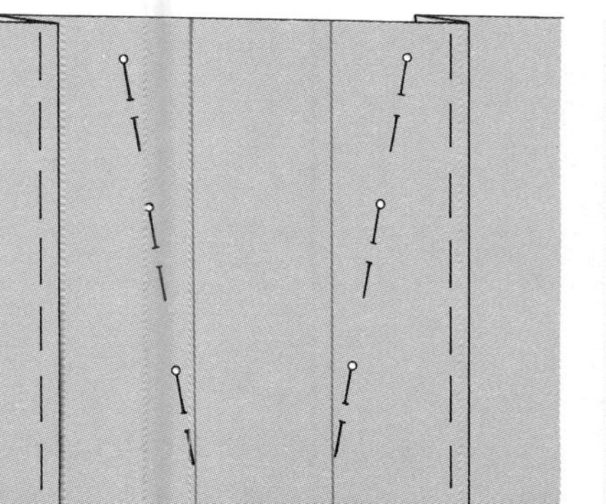

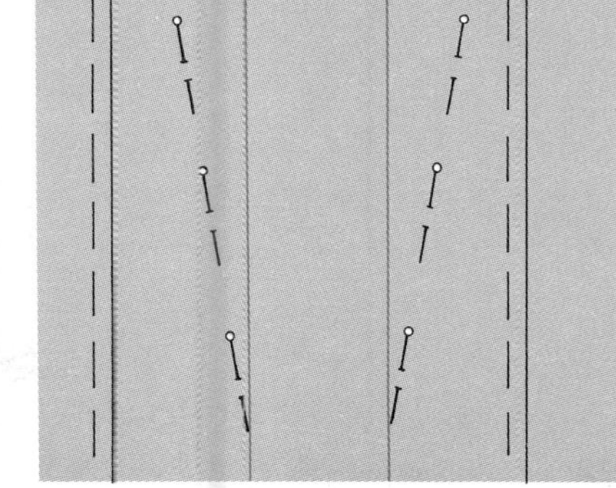

3. Leaving garment pinned, pin-mark both new pleat lines; release pleat. Measure between old and new lines at a few points; double measurement for total at each point.

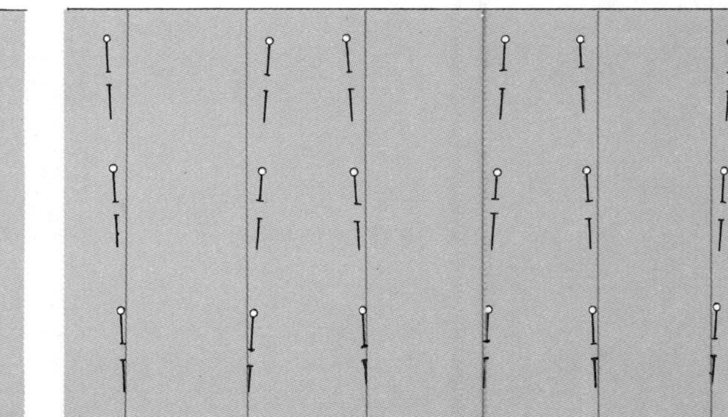

4. Divide amount of total change at each point by the number of pleat lines to be changed. Alter each line by that amount at the same points. From hip down, the new line should remain parallel with the original; from hip up it will probably be tapered.

Pleating according to a plaid or stripe

An all-around-pleated skirt in a plaid or striped fabric must often be made without a pattern. The reason: the vertical bars in a particular fabric will rarely correspond to the pleat lines on a pattern. A patternless pleated skirt is not difficult to make, but it does require understanding of basic pleating principles and methods. It also requires you to calculate the fabric requirements for your size (see opposite page) and for the pleat style you choose. As an example of the pleating possibilities one fabric can offer, we have pleated the same even-plaid fabric (shown unpleated at the right) in three different ways to emphasize different blocks.

There are only two limitations to pleating according to fabric. You must keep repeats consistent and folds at a depth that will hang satisfactorily—not so deep as to be lumpy; not so shallow that the pleats will not swing gracefully. Wearing ease at the hip is usually about 3 inches, but this can be modified slightly to accommodate the fabric design. Keep in mind, also, that an uneven plaid is suitable for side pleats only.

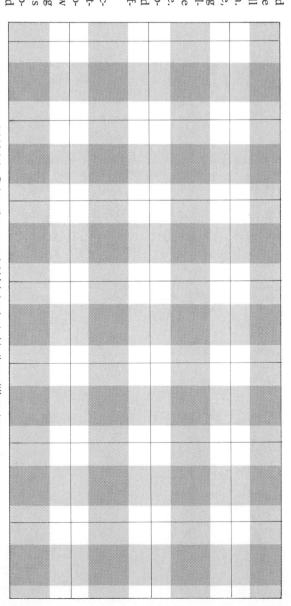

Above, a typical even-plaid fabric. Below, the same plaid fabric pleated in three different ways.

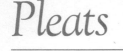

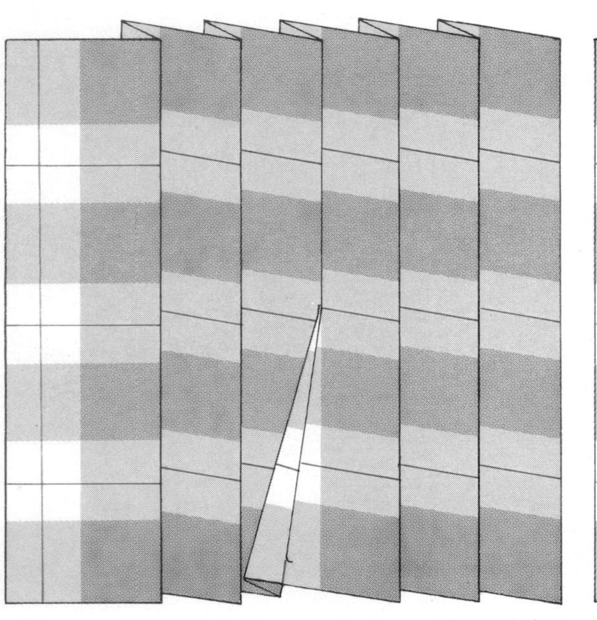

1. The even-plaid fabric in the example above, side-pleated so as to emphasize the vertical rows of darker blocks.

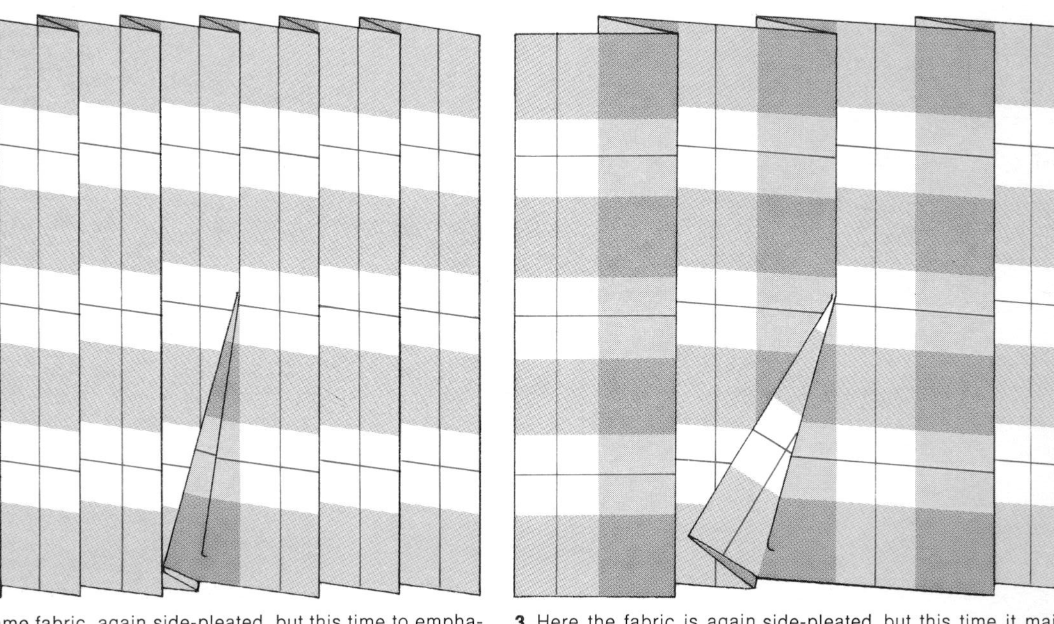

2. The same fabric, again side-pleated, but this time to emphasize the horizontal rows of the fabric.

3. Here the fabric is again side-pleated, but this time it maintains the original motif of the fabric.

Taking your body measurements 100
Slip-basting 125
Centered zipper 318-319
Invisible zipper 326-327

Estimating amount of fabric needed

Fabric needs for an all-around-pleated plaid skirt depend mainly on **width of fabric, desired skirt length,** and **hip measurement.** Fabric width and hip measurement are simple, but skirt length takes some figuring. It is the *finished length* plus *top seam and hem allowances.* You will probably need two to three lengths for one skirt. To each extra length, you must add a full horizontal motif to allow for matching. Based on the premise that the unpleated circumference should be about two and one-half to three times the hip measurement, minimum requirements are *two* lengths of 54-inch-wide fabric and *three* of 36- or 45-inch-wide fabric. For 36-inch hips, for example, 108 inches would be roughly sufficient. To achieve it, you would have to join *two* skirt lengths of 54-inch or *three* of 36- or 45-inch fabric. Larger hips might require another whole length, though all of it might not be used.

Waistline
Hemline
Total length

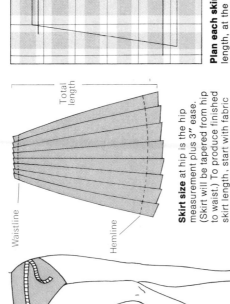

Skirt size at hip is the hip measurement plus 3" ease. (Skirt will be tapered from hip to waist.) To produce finished skirt length, start with fabric lengths equal to the length finished skirt will be plus top seam and hem allowances.

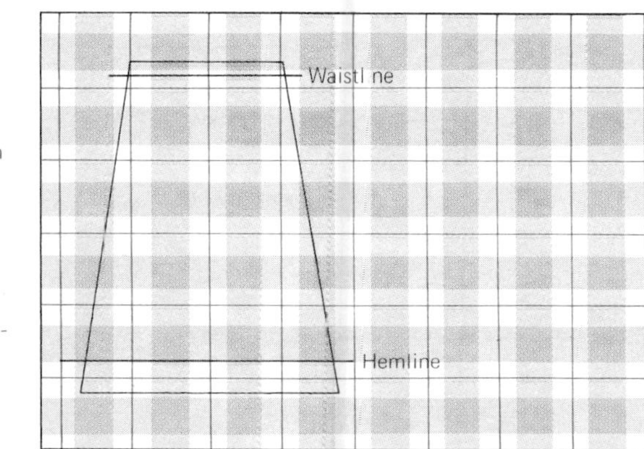

Plan each skirt length so that the hemline is located, on each length, at the same dominant horizontal motif or stripe. When cutting out additional lengths, be sure to include an additional horizontal motif to allow for matching all the lengths horizontally to the first length.

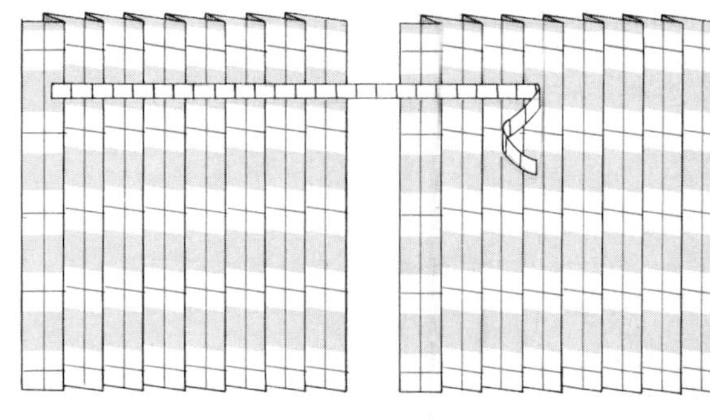

Cut lengths to match horizontally *and* repeat vertical progression exactly; slip-baste lengths together. Locate seams, especially placket seam, at center of underfold for inverted or box pleats (zipper, centered or invisible); at backfold for side pleats (special lapped application, p.173).

Single or cluster pleats

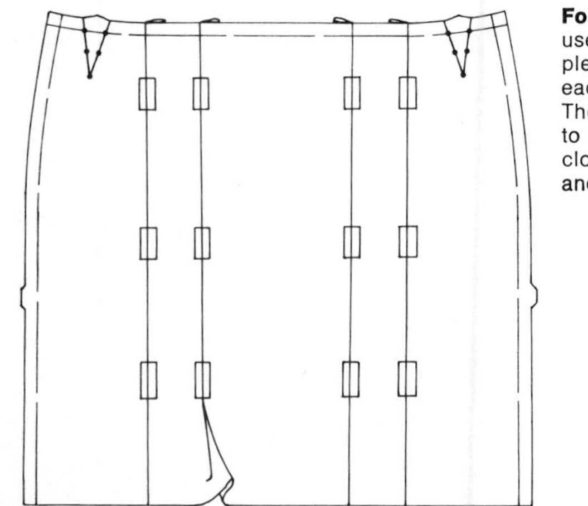

For a single pleat or cluster, use the pattern, as follows: First pleat pattern, pinning or taping each pleat along its entire length. Then pleat fabric according to its lines, conforming as closely as possible to type, size, and number of pleats in pattern.

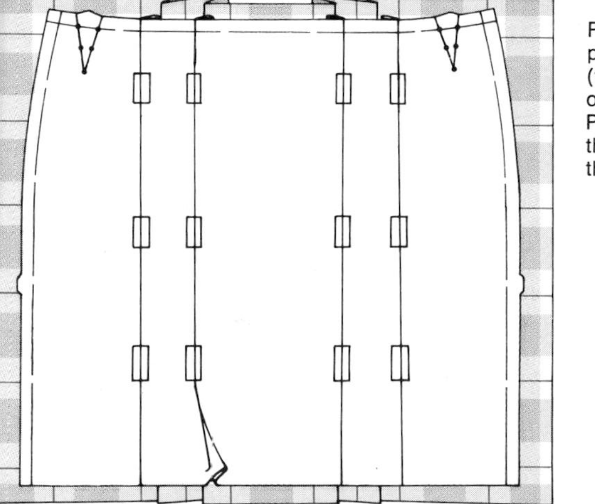
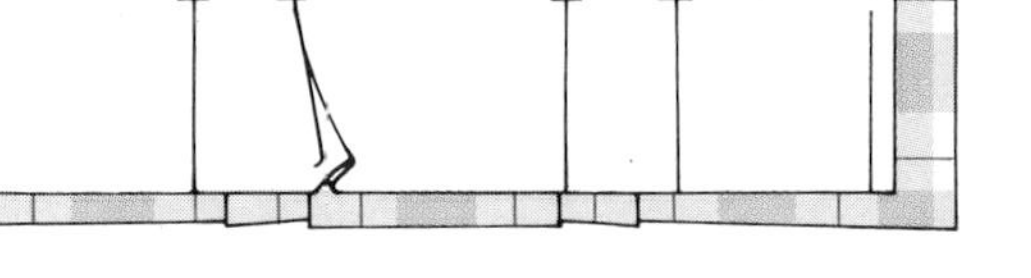

Position pleated portion of pattern over the pleated fabric (the two should be the same, or very nearly the same, in area). Pin the pattern to the fabric, then cut out garment piece along the outside cutting lines.

Gathering

Thread selection 10
Stitch length selection 30-31
Grain in fabrics 84-85
Seam finishes 148-149

General information

Gathering is the process of drawing a given amount of fabric into a predetermined, smaller area, along one or several stitching lines, to create soft, even folds. Fabric is usually gathered to one-half or one-third the original width; the effect may be soft and drapey or crisp and billowy, depending on the fabric. Gathering most often occurs in a garment at waistline, cuffs, or yoke, or as ruffles. Gathering is done after construction seams have been stitched, seam-finished, and pressed. Because gathers fall best on the lengthwise grain, the rows of stitching should run *across* the grain. Stitch length for gathering is longer and tension is looser than usual; it is advisable to pretest both on a scrap of your fabric. Suitable stitch lengths vary from 6 to 12 stitches per inch, shorter for sheer or light fabrics and longer for thick, heavy materials. The shorter the stitch length, the more control you have over the gathers, no matter what the fabric. In gathering, it is the bobbin thread that is pulled, and a looser upper tension makes it easier to slide the fabric along the thread. For heavy fabrics or extensive gathering, use an extra-strength thread in the bobbin.

Basic procedure

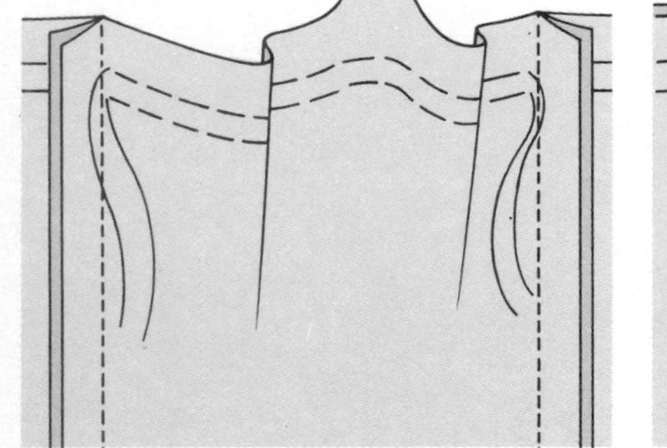

1. Working on the *right* side of the fabric, stitch two parallel rows in seam-allowance, one a thread width above seamline, the other ¼" higher. Leave long thread ends. Break stitching at seams, as illustrated; it is difficult to gather through two thicknesses.

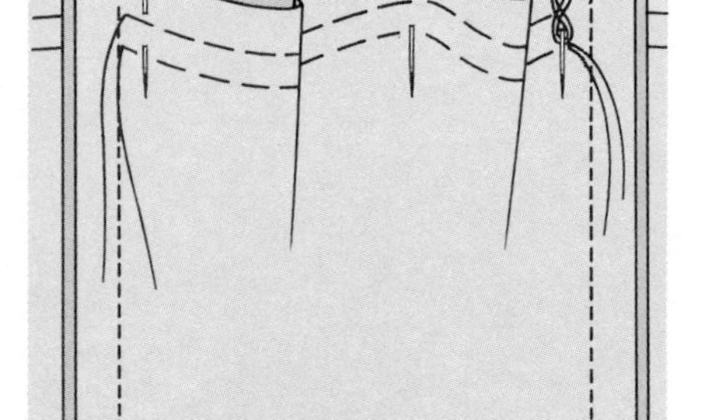

2. Pin the stitched edge to the corresponding straight edge, right sides together, matching notches, center lines, and seams. Anchor bobbin threads (now facing you) at one end by twisting in a figure 8 around pins. Excess material is now ready to gather.

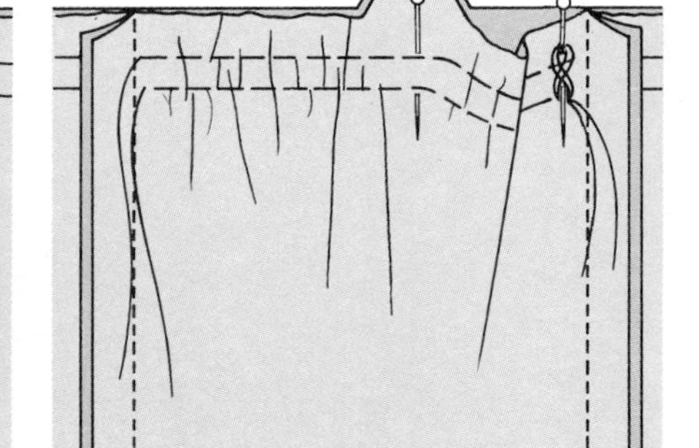

3. Gently pull on the bobbin threads while, with the other hand, you slide the fabric along the thread to create uniform gathers. When this first gathered section fits the adjoining edge, secure the thread ends by winding them in a tight figure 8 around a pin.

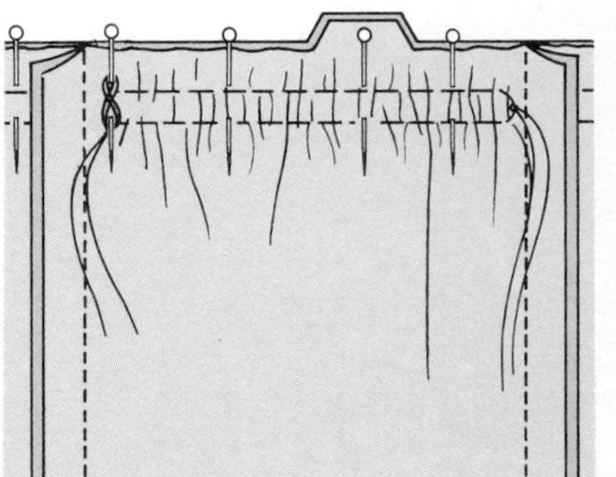

4. To draw up the ungathered portion, untie the bobbin threads and repeat the process from the other end. When the entire gathered edge matches the straight edge, fasten the thread end. Adjust gathers uniformly and pin at frequent intervals to hold folds in place.

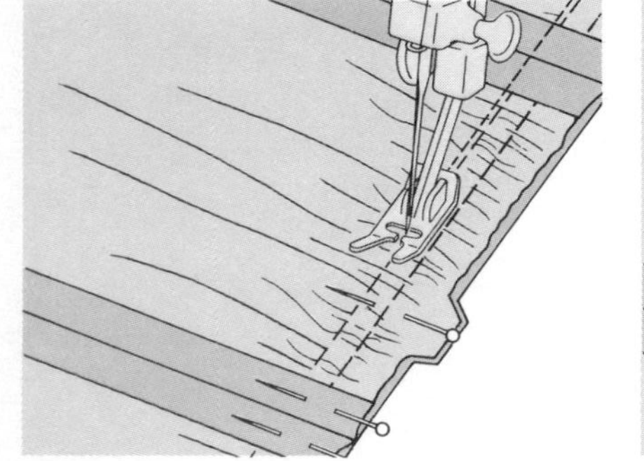

5. Before seaming gathered section, be sure machine is set to stitch length suitable to fabric and tension is balanced. With gathered side up, stitch seam on seamline, holding fabric on either side of needle so that gathers will not be stitched into little pleats.

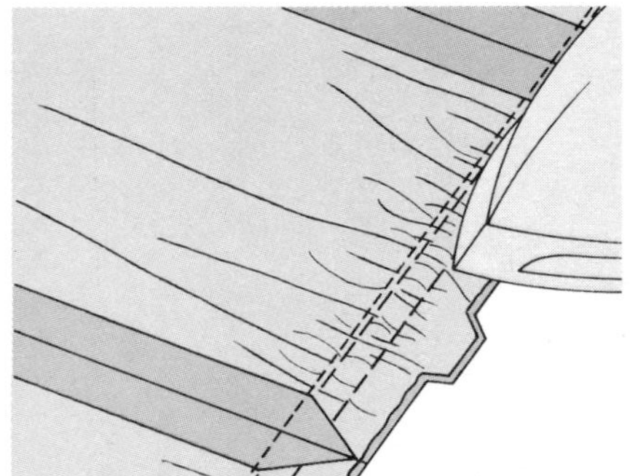

6. Trim any seam allowances, such as side seams, which are caught into the gathered seam. Press seam as stitched, in the seam allowances, using just the tip of the iron. Seam-finish the edge with a zigzag or overedge stitch, *or* apply a stay (opposite page).

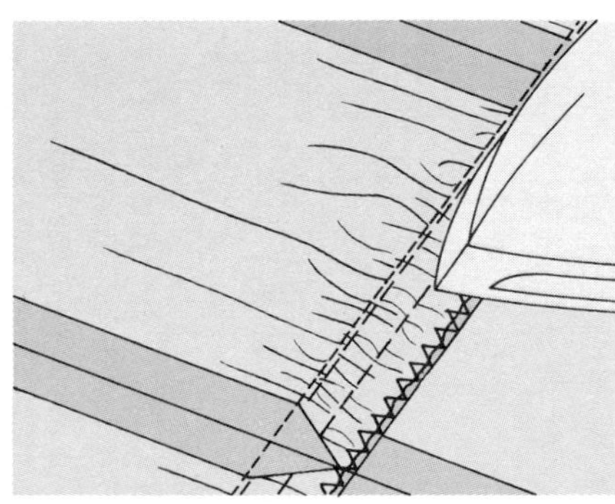

7. Open garment section out flat and press seam as it should go in finished garment—toward bodice if a waistline seam, toward shoulder if a yoke seam, toward wrist if a cuff. Again, work with just the tip of the iron, pressing flat parts only, taking care not to crease folds.

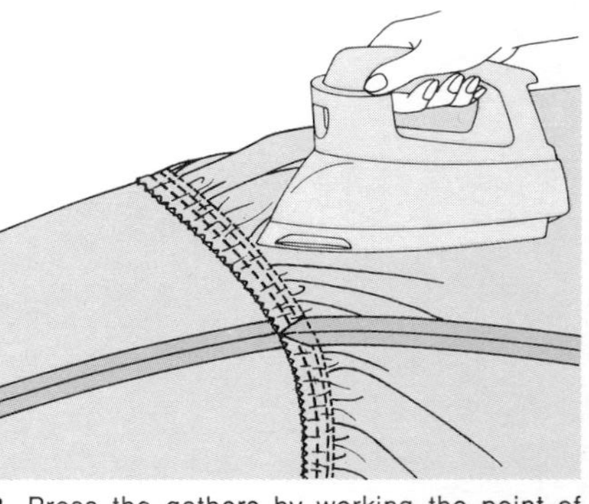

8. Press the gathers by working the point of the iron into the gathers toward the seam. Press from the wrong side of the fabric, lifting the iron as you reach the seam. Do not press *across* the gathers; this will flatten and cause them to go limp.

Zigzag stitching 32-33
Machine attachments 38-39
Uneven basting 124
Running stitch 131

Other methods of gathering

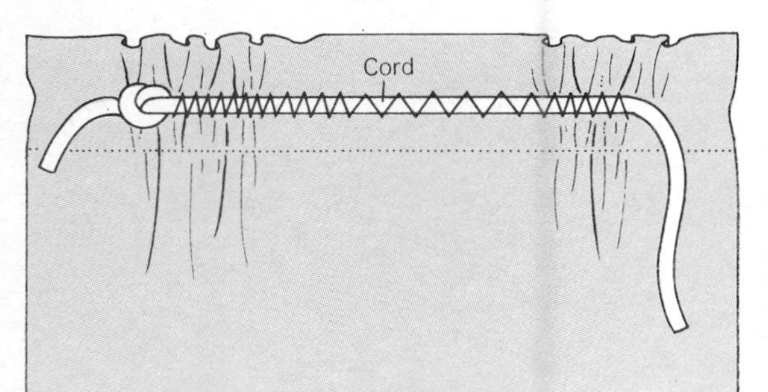

Zigzag stitching over a thin, strong cord is useful when a long strip or a bulky fabric is to be gathered. Place cord ¼″ above seamline; use widest zigzag stitch over cord to hold it in place. Pull on cord to form gathers.

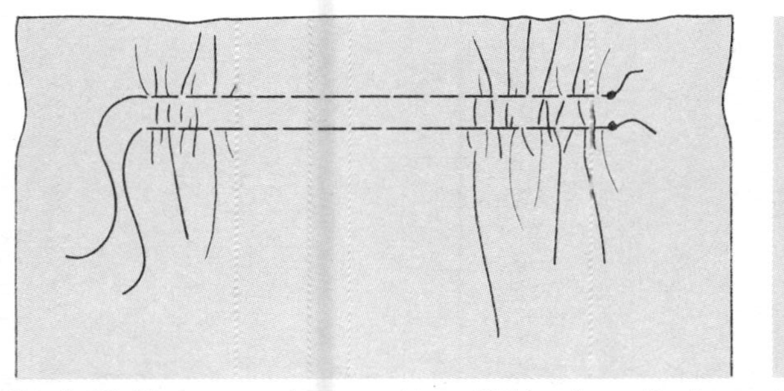

Hand stitching can replace machine stitching for gathering small areas or very delicate fabrics. Using small, even running stitches, hand-sew at least two rows for best control. To gather, gently pull unknotted ends of threads.

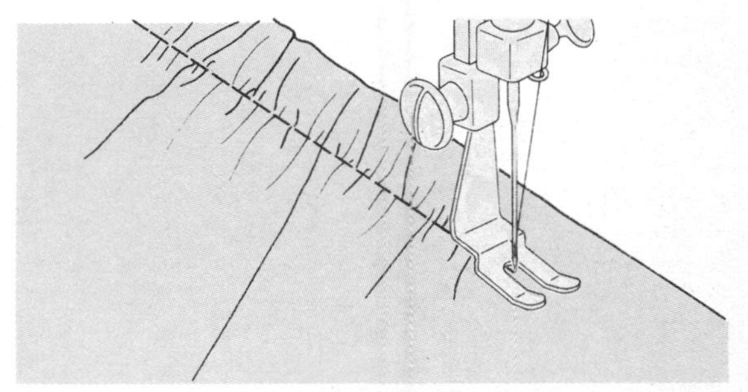

A gathering foot automatically gathers with each stitch machine takes. The longer the stitch, the more closely the fabric will be gathered. Determine amount of fabric needed by measuring a sample before and after gathering.

Staying a gathered seam

A gathered seam often needs a stay to prevent stretching or raveling, to reinforce or to add comfort, and to give a professional look to the inside. Stay can be woven seam binding, twill tape, or narrow grosgrain ribbon. With gathered edge of seam up, place stay on seam allowances so that one edge is right next to permanent stitching. Straight-stitch close to lower edge, through all thicknesses. Trim seam allowances even with the top edge of the stay. If fabric frays readily, zigzag-stitch seam allowances to the stay. Press seam and stay in correct direction (Step 7, opposite page).

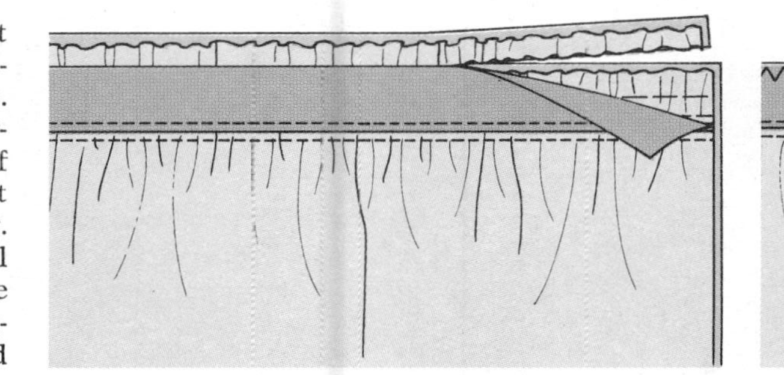

Do not trim seam to be stayed until tape is stitched on.

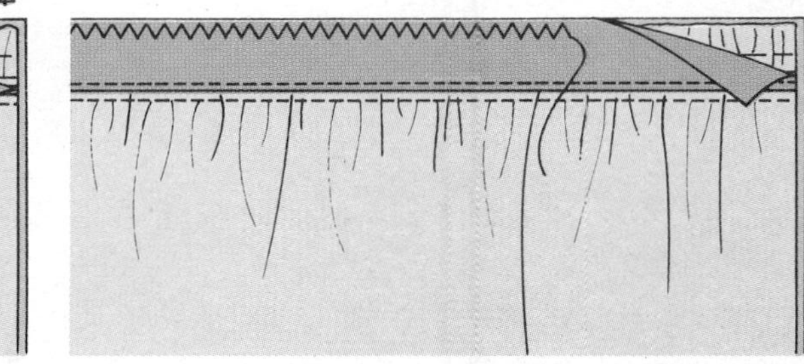

Stitch along top edge of stay if the fabric frays easily.

Joining one gathered edge to another

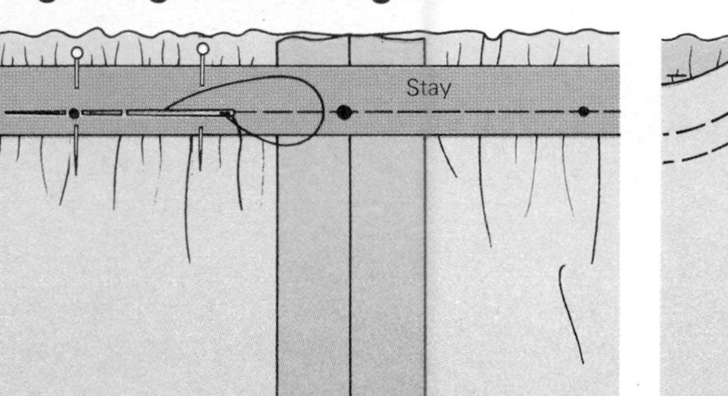

1. Cut a stay to match length finished seam is to be. Transfer pattern markings to stay and pin to wrong side of one section, matching markings. Gather section and baste to tape.

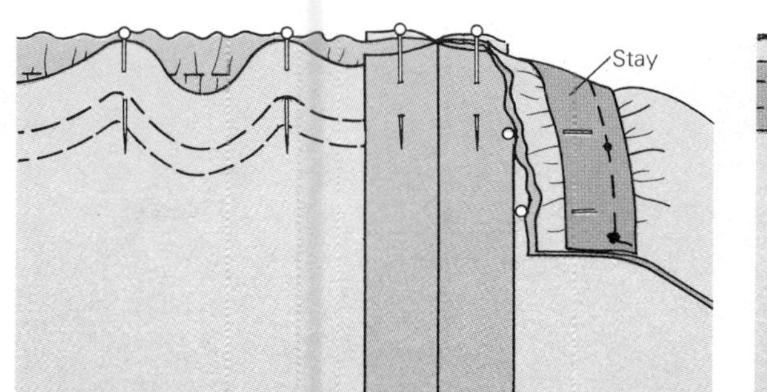

2. Pin ungathered section to section gathered in Step 1, right sides together, matching all markings. Gather second section to fit first one, and baste in place.

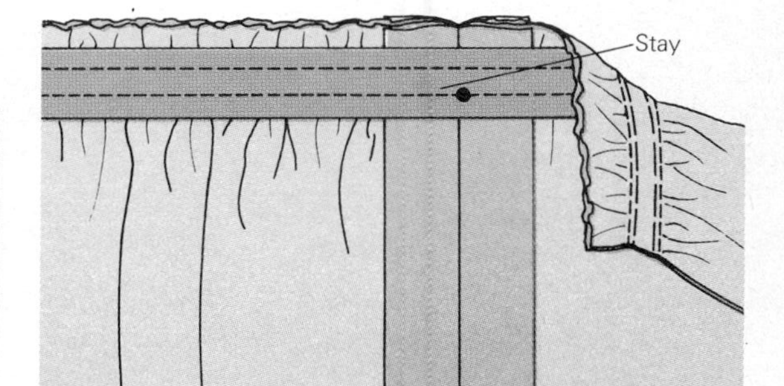

3. Stitch through all layers, including stay tape, on seamline. Stitch a second row ¼″ into seam allowances. Press seam allowances in one direction with stay uppermost.

Shirring

Stitch length 30-31; width 32-33 Tying thread ends 137
Pin tucks 164

General information

Shirring is formed with multiple rows of gathering and is primarily a decorative way of controlling fullness. In contrast to gathering, in which fullness is controlled within a seam, the fullness in shirring is controlled over a comparatively wide span. Lightweight fabrics are the most appropriate for shirring; they may be either crisp or soft. Voiles, batistes, crepes, and jerseys are excellent choices. No-iron fabrics are good because it is difficult to press shirring without flattening it. Your pattern should specify the areas to be shirred; these can range from a small part, such as a cuff, to an entire garment section, such as a bodice. Rows of shirring must be straight, parallel, and equidistant. They may be as close together as ¼ inch or as far apart as an inch or so, depending on personal preference and pattern specifications. Width to be shirred is determined by the pattern.

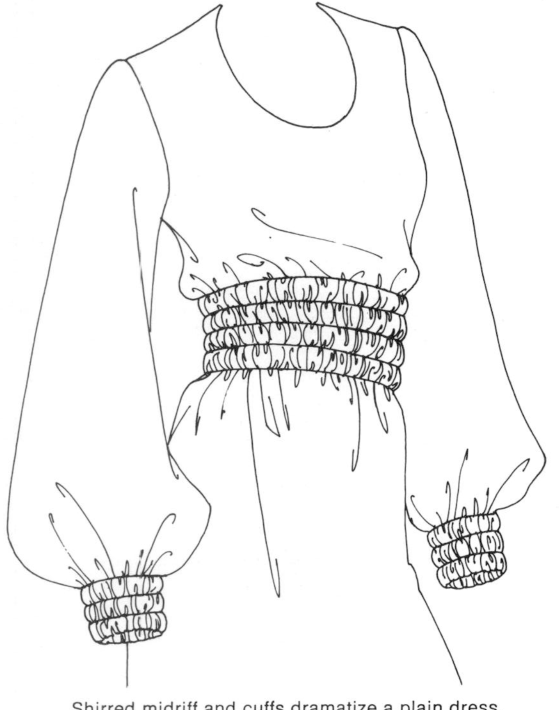

Shirred midriff and cuffs dramatize a plain dress.

Basic procedure

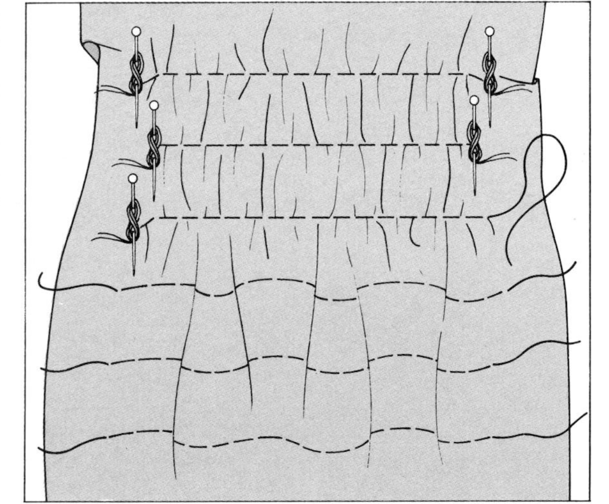

1. Stitch repeated rows of gathering stitches over section to be shirred, spacing rows an equal distance apart. Gather each row separately by pulling on bobbin thread. Measure first row when it is shirred and make sure that all subsequent rows are gathered to the same length.

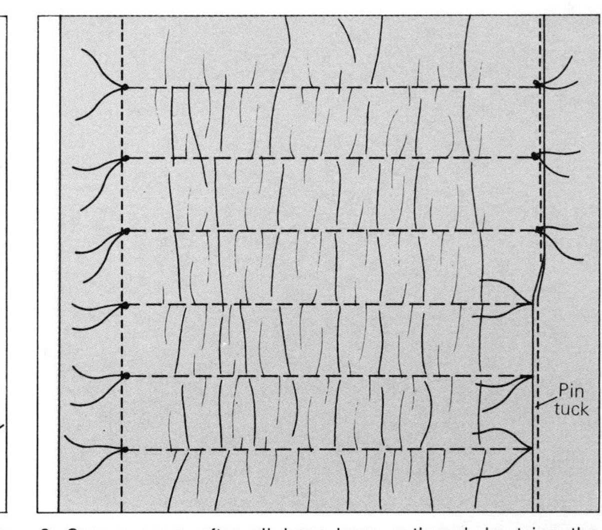

2. Secure rows, after all have been gathered, by tying the thread ends on each row; then place a line of machine stitching across the ends of all rows. **If ends of shirred area will not be stitched into a seam,** enclose the thread ends in a small pin tuck to hold them securely.

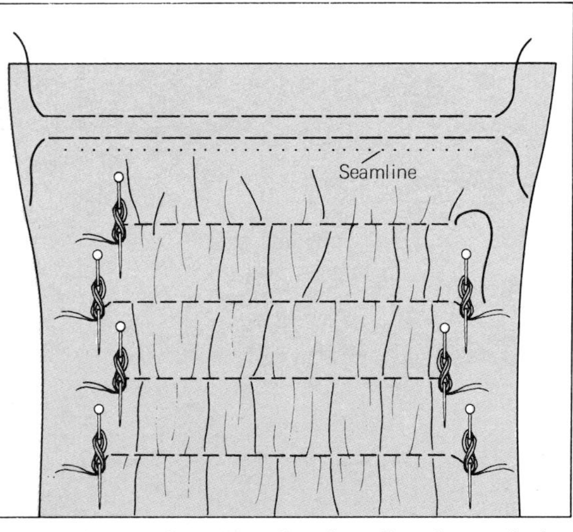

If shirring is to be joined to a flat piece, first place gathering stitches in seam allowance, one row just inside seamline and a second ¼″ above. Stitch rows for shirring, and shirr to desired width. Gather and attach seam as specified in basic procedure for gathering (p.178).

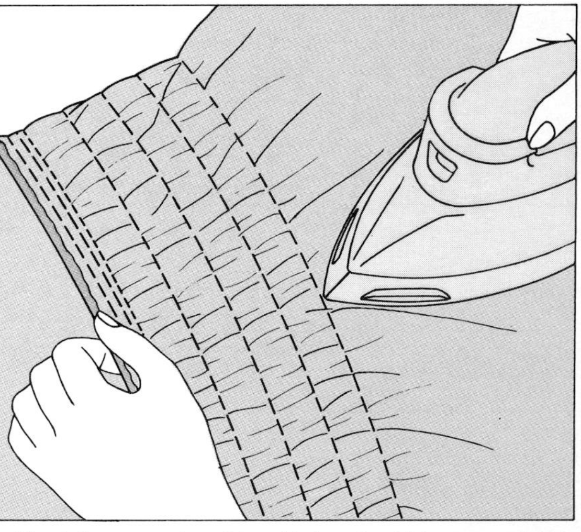

3. The fullness produced by shirring should be pressed with great care; if it is not, the weight of the iron will flatten the folds and ruin the intended effect. Press on the wrong side, into the fullness, with just the point of the iron. Do not press into the shirred area itself.

Elastic thread 10
Cord 16
Machine attachments 38-39
Slipstitch (uneven) 132

Staying a shirred area

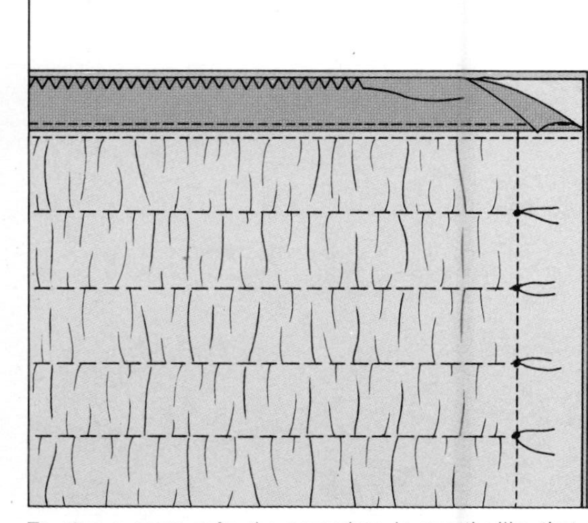

To stay a seam only, the procedure is exactly like that for a gathered seam (p.179). Position stay tape over shirred side of untrimmed seam allowance, keeping edge just next to seamline. Stitch lower edge of tape; trim seam allowances even with top edge, then zigzag through all layers.

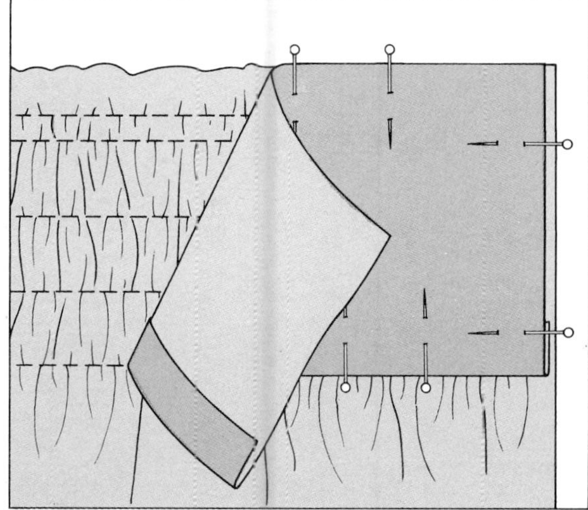

To stay a seam and a section, cut stay fabric the same width and ½″ deeper than shirred section. Pin stay to wrong side of shirred area, turning under lower edge and keeping seam edges even; baste. Stitch stay into seams when garment sections are joined; tack lower edge to last row of gathering.

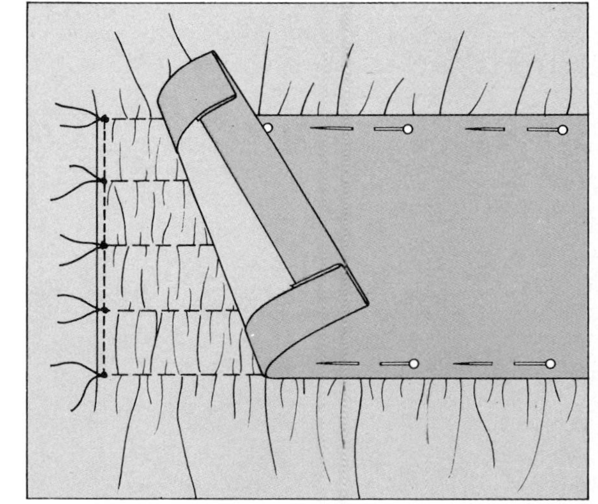

To stay a shirred section, cut a strip of self-fabric 1″ wider and deeper than shirring. Turn in raw edges ½″ on all sides; pin in place to the wrong side of shirred area. Hand-sew the stay in place with small, invisible stitches. A stay will protect the shirred area from strain.

Elasticized shirring

This stretchy, flexible form of shirring hugs the body neatly, yet expands and contracts comfortably with body movements. It is easily done by using elastic thread in the bobbin and regular thread in the needle. Wind the elastic thread on the bobbin by hand, stretching it slightly, until the bobbin is almost full. Set the machine to a 6–7 stitch length, and test the results on a scrap of your fabric. Adjust stitch length and tension if necessary. Sometimes, to get the desired fullness, the bobbin (elastic) thread must be pulled after stitching as in gathering. Mark the rows of shirring on the right side of the garment. (Or, after marking the first row, you can use the quilter guide-bar to space the other rows.) As you sew, hold the fabric taut and flat by stretching the fabric in previous rows to its original size. To secure ends, draw the needle thread through to the underside and tie. Run a line of machine stitching across all the knots or hold them with a narrow pin tuck at each end of the shirred section.

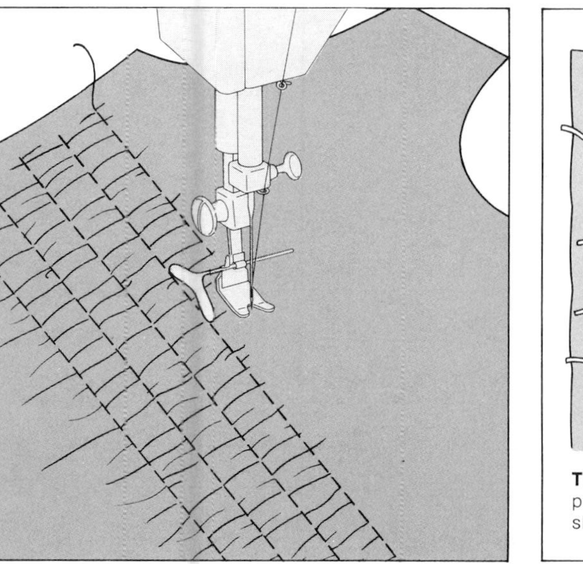

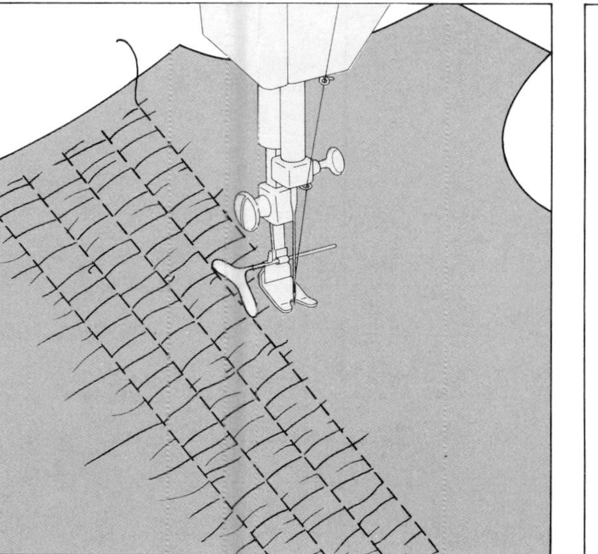

Shirring with cord

This technique is essentially gathering with cord (see p.179) but in multiple rows. Cord is placed directly on shirred lines; ends are secured by knotting.

Smocking

Thread selection 10
Hand needles 11
Grain in fabrics 84-85
Hand-sewing techniques 122

General information

Smocking consists of fabric folds decoratively stitched together at regular intervals to create a patterned effect. The folds may be pulled in when the stitching is done, or the fabric may be first gathered into folds and then smocked (see **Gauging,** below). The best fabric choices for smocking are those that are lightweight and crisp, but almost any fabric can be smocked. You will need two and one-half to three times the desired finished width; patterns specify fabric required.

The smocked section is done before the garment is constructed. Popular areas for smocking in garments are yokes, bodices, pockets, sleeves, and waistlines. All smocking is based on a grid of evenly spaced dots (see **Stitching guide,** below); the variety among stitches is achieved by the differing points at which dots are joined. If a fabric such as gingham is being used, its pattern can serve in place of the grid. A decorative thread, such as six-strand embroidery floss or silk buttonhole twist, is favored for this technique; the colors can be chosen to match or complement the fabric. It will take long crewel needles to reach the span required by some of the stitch patterns. Smocking can be simulated by means of the decorative stitches provided by today's sewing machines.

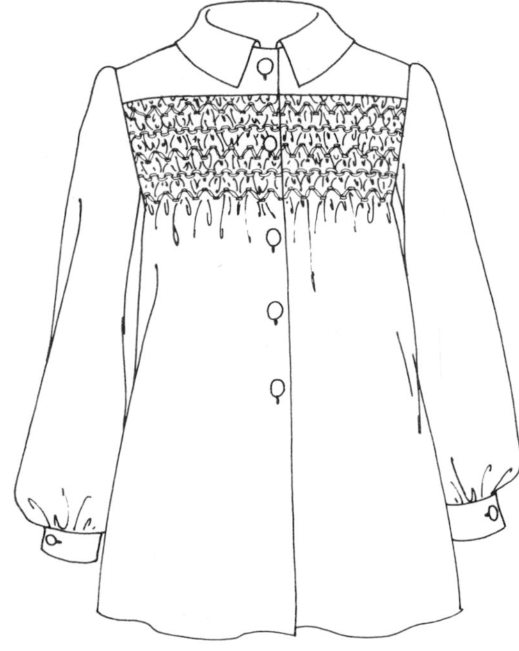

Typical use of smocking shows decorative effect.

Stitching guide

The stitching guide or pattern may be purchased as an iron-on transfer, or you can make your own dot pattern with a very hard-leaded pencil. Rows of dots should align with the fabric grain.

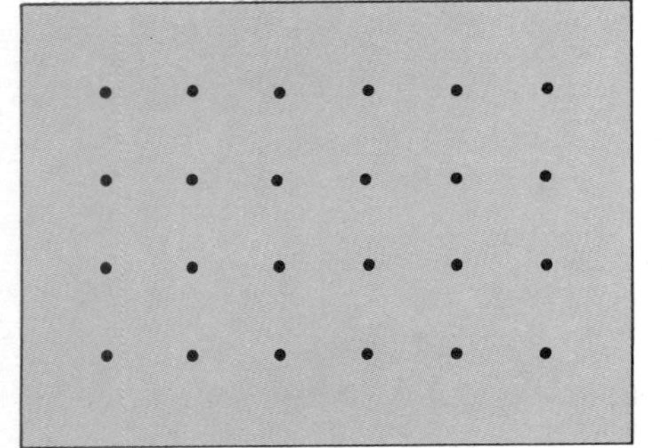

Mark the dots to guide stitching on *right* side of fabric.

Gauging (advance gathering)

Taking small stitches under dots, as shown, baste along each row. Leave one end loose; draw up two rows at a time to desired width. Dots will appear at tops of folds to indicate smocking stitch points.

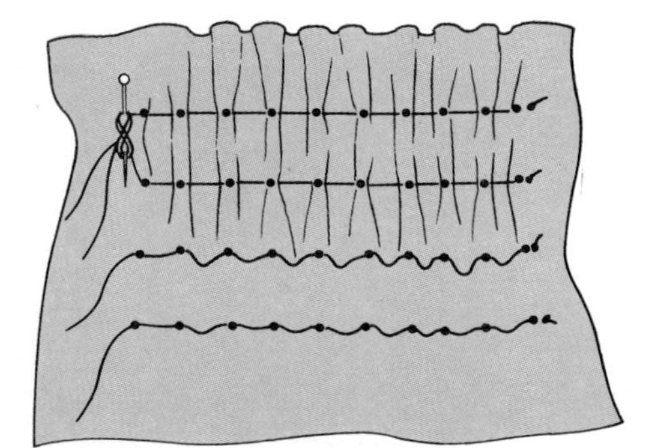

Smock at dots; when finished, remove gathering stitches.

Cable stitch

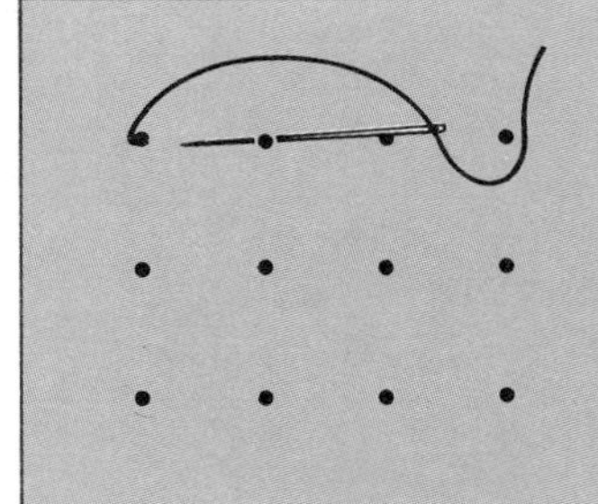

Bring the needle from underside through first dot. Keeping thread *above* needle, take a short stitch through fabric under the second dot and draw fabric up.

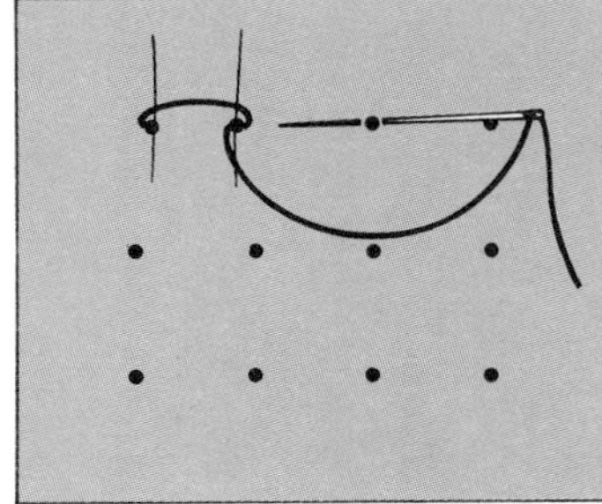

Keeping thread *below* needle, take a short stitch under third dot. Draw up fabric. To keep folds even, always pull thread at right angle to stitch.

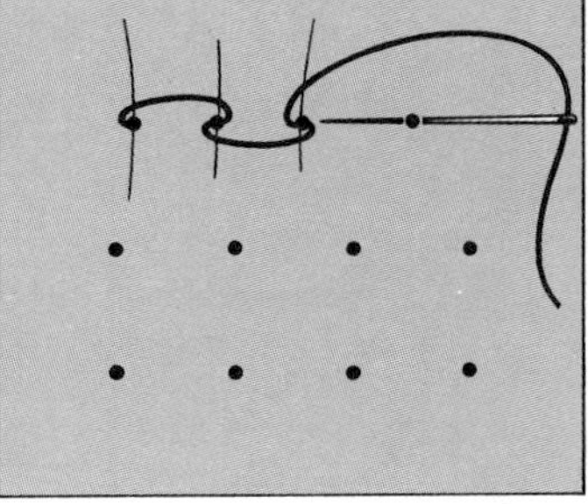

On fourth dot, keep thread *above* needle. Alternate in this way until the row is finished. Try to keep folds even when drawing up stitch.

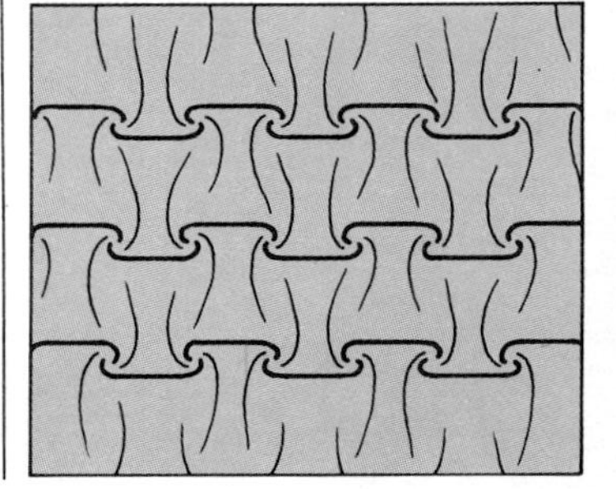

Repeat the identical procedure for each subsequent row, alternating thread above and below needle in matching pattern dots. This will make rows exact duplicates, as this pattern requires.

Honeycomb stitch

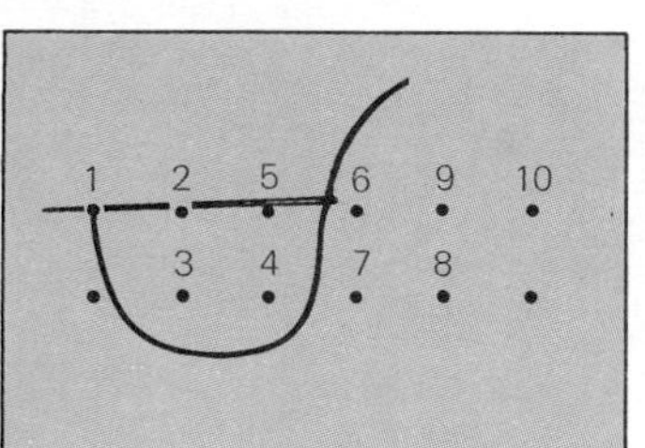

Work from left to right with needle pointing left. Bring the needle out at 1, then take a small stitch at 2 and another at 1; pull thread taut.

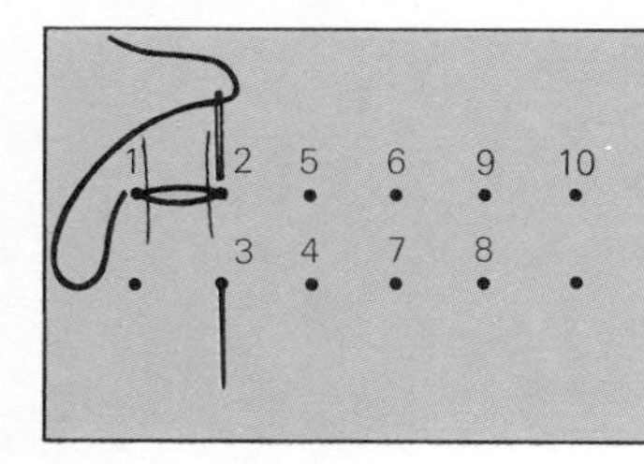

Re-insert needle at dot 2 and bring it out at dot 3 in row below (two rows are worked together for this design). Thread will be underneath the fold.

Repeat first stitch procedure by taking a small stitch at dot 4 and another at dot 3. Pull the thread taut. Then re-insert the needle next to dot 4.

Pass the needle up from dot 4 to dot 5 in the upper row, and continue to repeat pattern until the whole row is done. End in the bottom row.

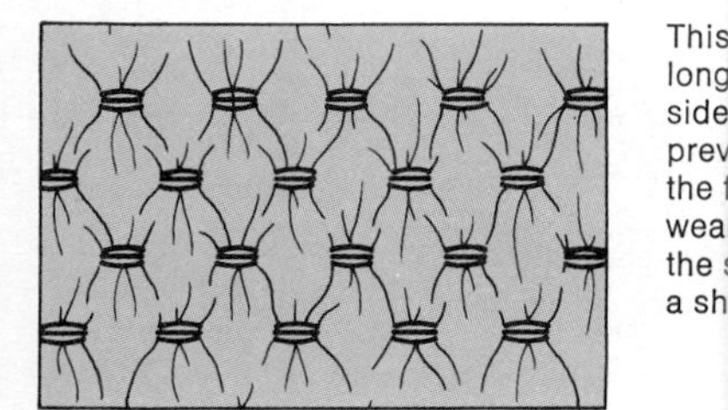

This stitch produces long floats on wrong side. A stay will prevent snagging of the floats during wear. Apply the stay the same as for a shirred section.

Wave stitch

Bring the needle from the underside through dot 1. Keeping thread *above* the needle, take a stitch at dot 2. Pull thread tight to complete stitch.

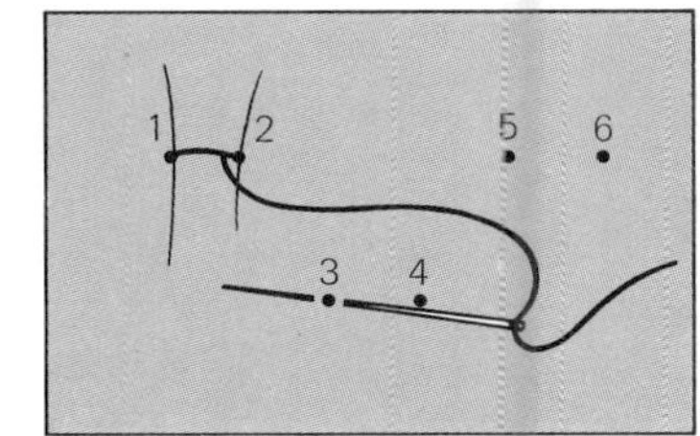

Take next stitch at dot 3 in second row (in this design, two rows are worked together); draw the thread through.

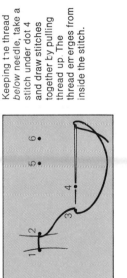

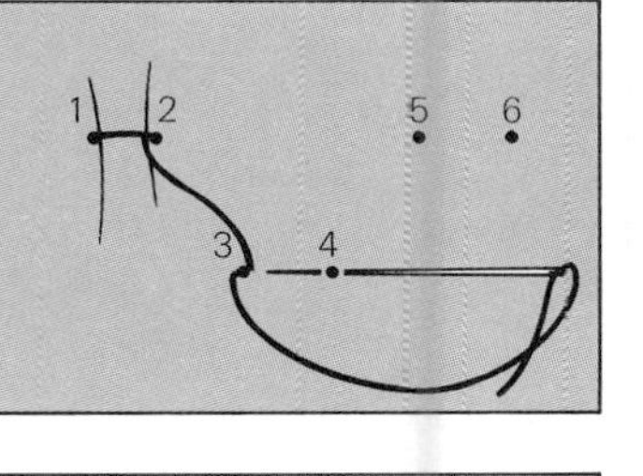

Keeping the thread *below* needle, take a stitch under dot 4 and draw stitches together by pulling thread up. The thread emerges from inside the stitch.

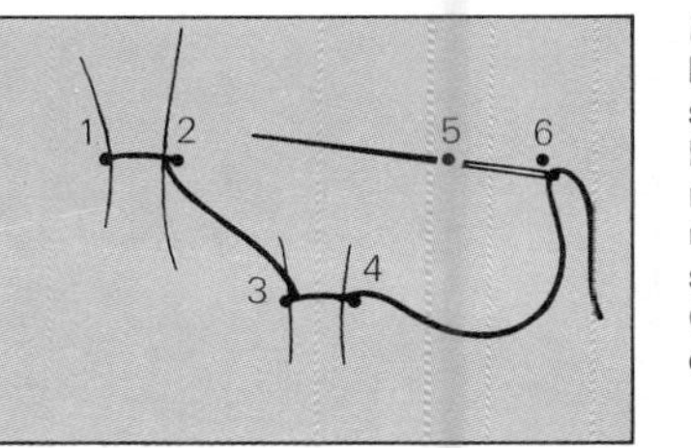

Return to first row by taking complete stitch at dot 5. Keep thread *above* needle when picking up dot 6. Draw stitches together. Continue to end of that row.

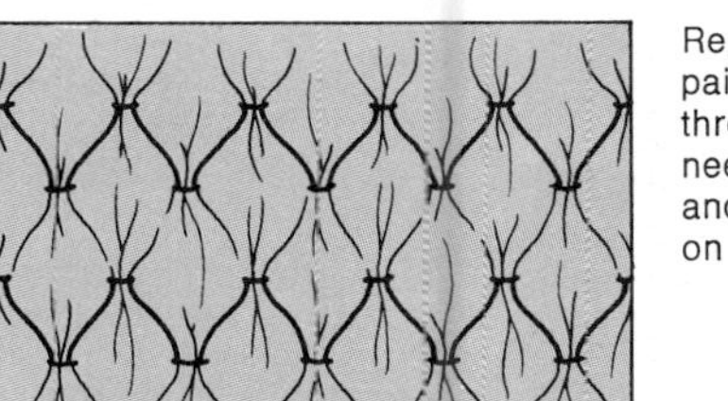

Repeat for all pairs of rows, with thread *above* the needle on upper rows and *below* needle on lower rows.

Smocked effect by machine

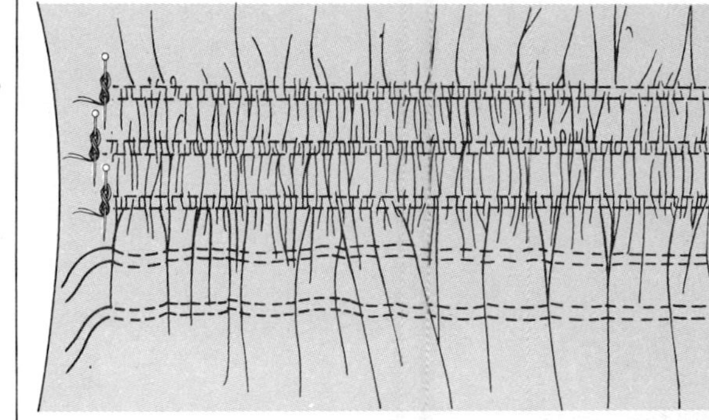

1. Place rows of gathering stitches in groups of two, ¼″ apart. Repeat paired rows as required by size of smocked area, spacing them ¾″ apart. Gather each group.

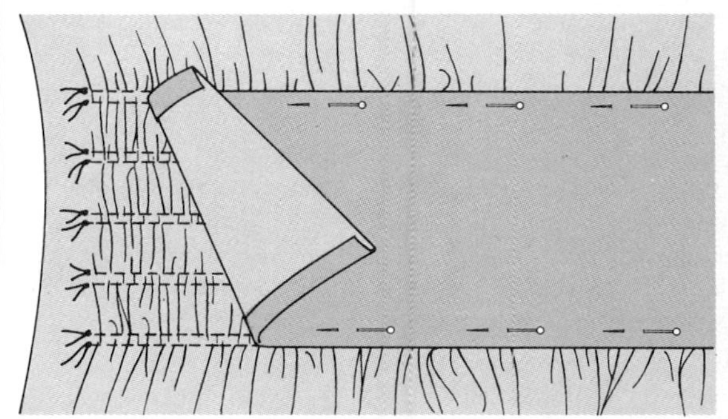

2. Cut an underlay 1″ wider than the shirred area; fold under *long* raw edges ½″ and pin or baste to wrong side. Test decorative machine stitches for maximum width of ¼″.

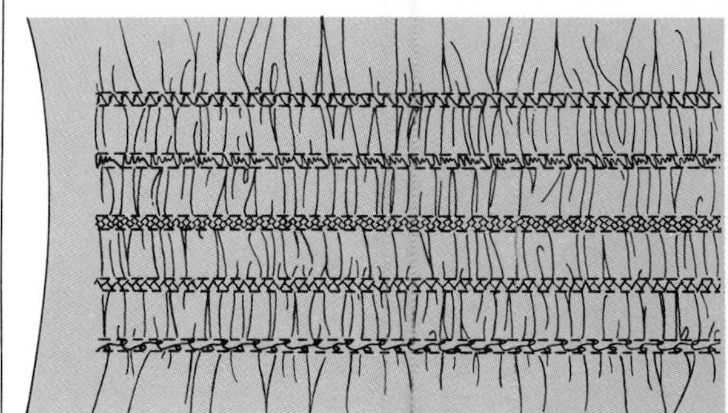

3. With garment right side up, place decorative stitching between the ¼″ rows of shirring. Striking effects can be created using different patterns and thread colors.

Ruffles

Grain in fabrics 84-85
Cutting and joining bias strips 298-299

Types of ruffles

A ruffle is a strip of fabric cut or handled in such a way as to produce fullness. Though primarily decorative, ruffles may also serve a practical purpose, such as lengthening a garment. Ruffles are of two types, **straight** and **circular,** which differ in the way they are cut. The straight ruffle is cut as a *strip* of fabric; the circular ruffle is cut from a *circle.* With the straight ruffle, both edges are the same length and the fullness is produced through

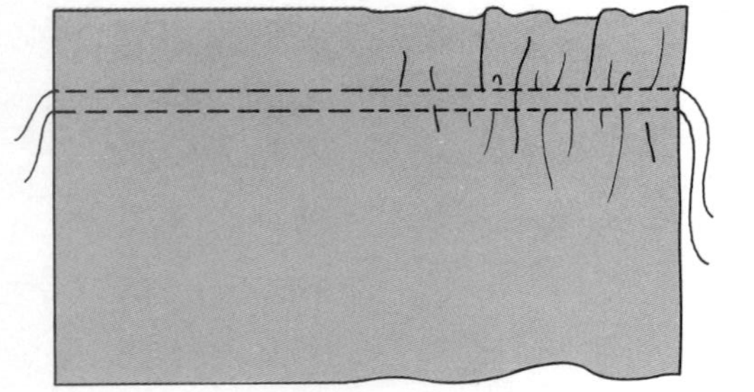

Straight ruffles are gathered to produce fullness.

gathering, sometimes pleating. For the circular ruffle, a small circle is cut from the center of a larger one and the inner edge forced to lie flat, producing fullness on the outer, longer edge. Soft,

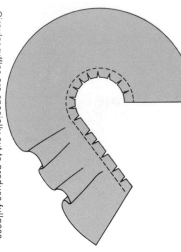

Circular ruffles are specially cut to produce fullness.

lightweight fabrics ruffle best. A general rule for deciding the proper relation between ruffle width and fullness: the wider the ruffle (or the sheerer the fabric) the fuller the ruffle should be.

Straight ruffles

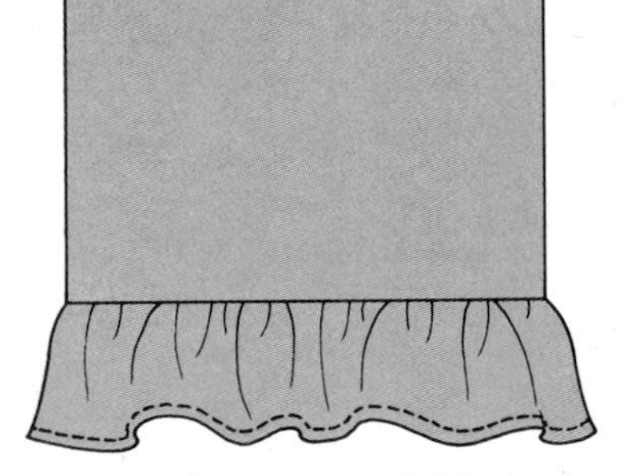

A plain ruffle has one finished edge (usually a small hem); the other edge is gathered to size and then sewed into a seam or onto another unfinished edge.

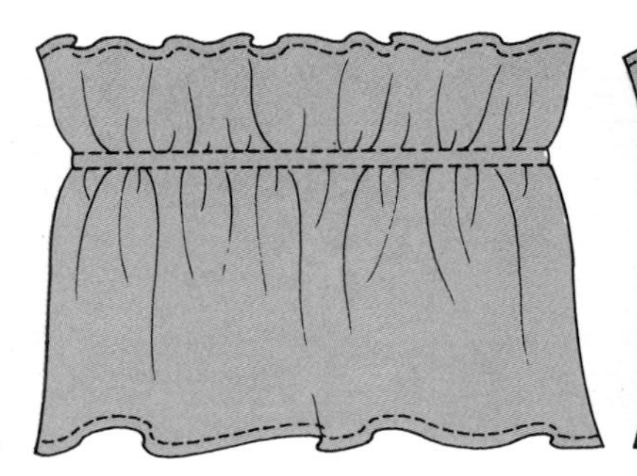
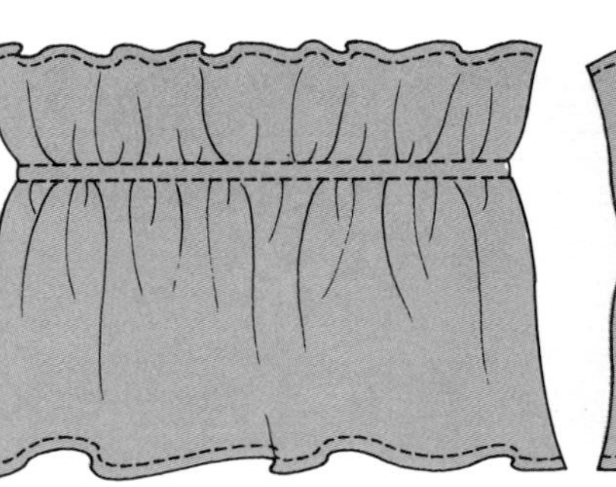

A ruffle with a heading has both edges finished or hemmed. It is gathered at a specified distance from the top edge to give a gracefully balanced proportion.

A double ruffle is gathered in the center, halfway between the two finished edges. It is then topstitched through the center to the garment section.

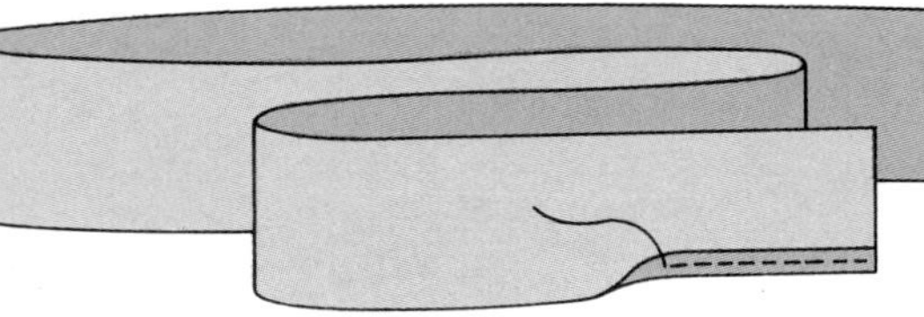

Single-layer ruffles are made from one layer of fabric and the edges finished with either a narrow machine or a hand-rolled hem. The edges can also be finished with decorative stitching, if appropriate to design of finished garment.

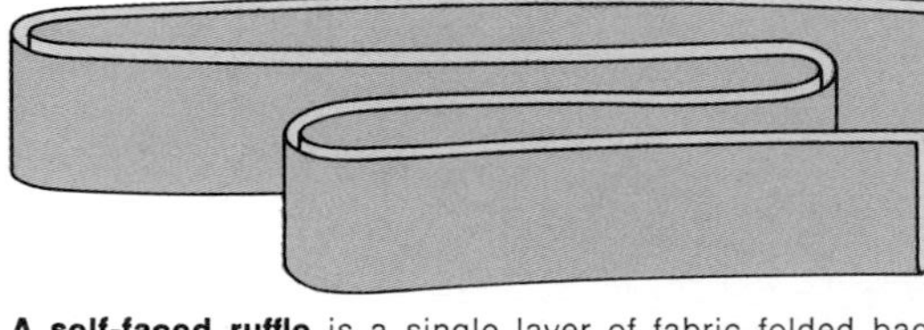

A self-faced ruffle is a single layer of fabric folded back on itself. It is used when both sides of a ruffle will be visible, or to give added body to sheer or flimsy fabrics. It creates a luxurious appearance wherever it is used.

Determining length and piecing

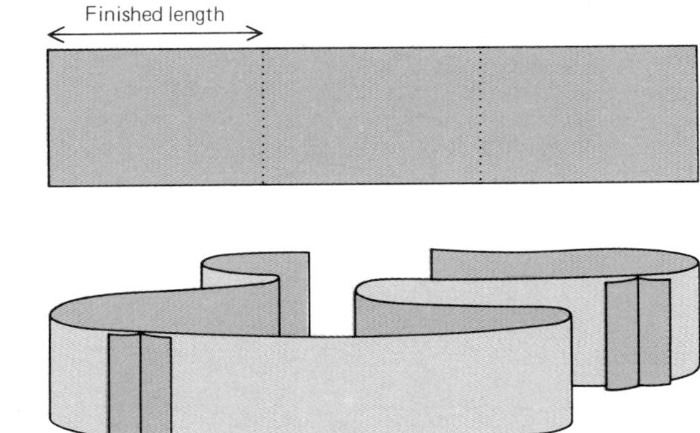

To determine length of fabric needed for a ruffle, allow about three times the finished length for a fully gathered ruffle, twice the length for a ruffle that is slightly gathered. Straight ruffles are usually cut on either the crosswise or the bias grain.

Piecing of fabric strips is frequently necessary to achieve required length. Seam strips with right sides together, making sure sections match in pattern and direction of grain. On ruffles for sheer curtains, strips can be cut along the selvage to get maximum length without piecing and to avoid the necessity of hemming.

Decorative machine stitching 32-37
Machine attachments 38-39
Hand-rolled hem 314

Single-layer straight ruffles

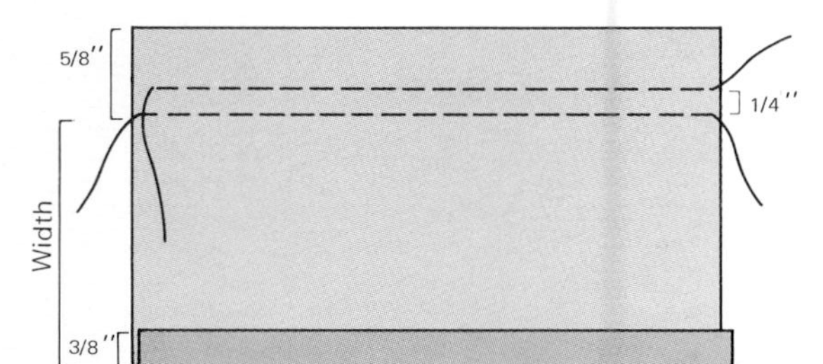

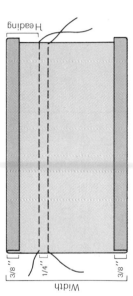

Plain ruffles can be any width. Cut strip to desired finished width plus 1". This allows for 5/8" seam allowance and 3/8" hem. Make hem first (see Hemming, below). Then place two rows of gathering stitches, 1/4" apart, inside seam allowance. Pull bobbin threads to gather to desired length.

Ruffles with headings require a fabric strip 3/4" wider (for hems) than the finished width. Make a 3/8" hem on each edge (see Hemming, below). Determine width of heading; place first gathering row that distance from one edge. The second row is placed 1/4" below. Gather to size.

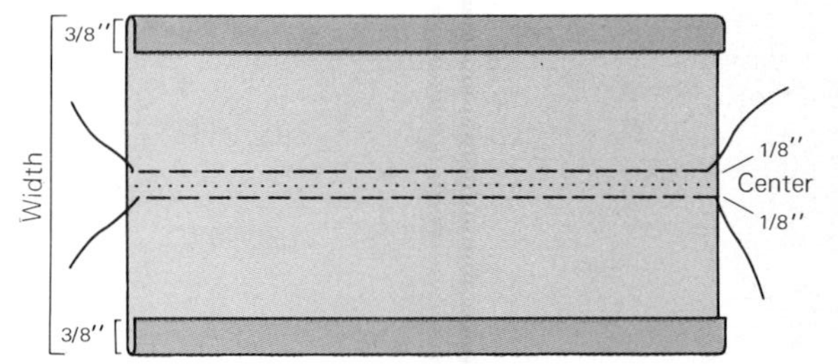

Double ruffles require strips 3/4" wider than ruffle is to be. Make a 3/8" hem on each edge (see Hemming, below). Place gathering rows at the center of the strip, one 1/8" below and the other 1/8" above the center line. Stitch so bobbin thread is on right side of ruffle; this makes gathering easier to do.

Hemming single-layer ruffles

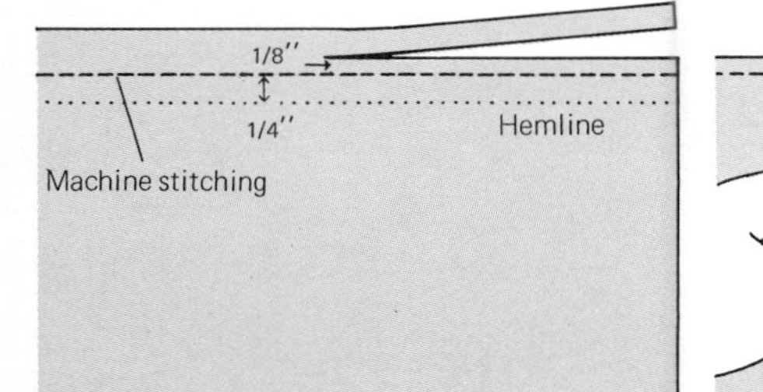

To hem edge by hand, first machine-stitch 1/4" above marked hemline. Trim hem allowance to 1/8". Fold hem to wrong side, turning just far enough that the stitch line shows.

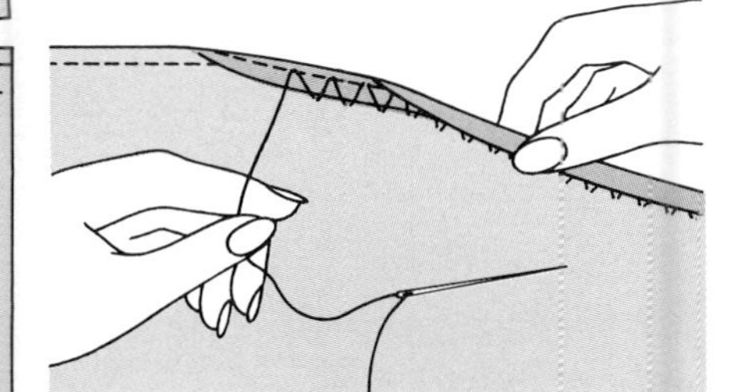

Working right to left, take small stitch through fold; then, 1/8" below and beyond that stitch, catch a few threads of ruffle. Pull thread to roll hem to wrong side.

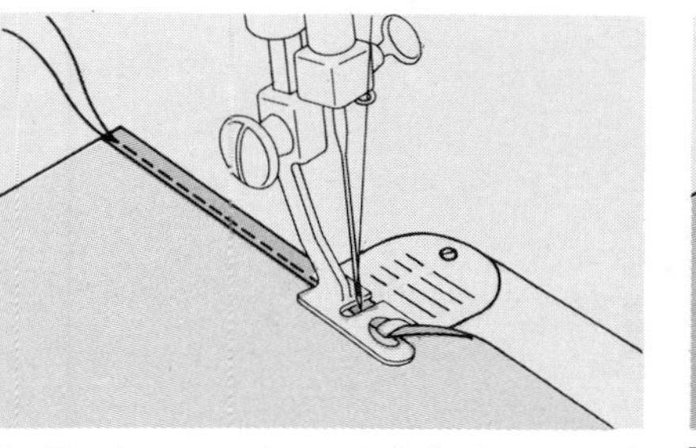

Machine hems can be made to look very much like hand-rolled hems with the help of a hemmer foot attachment. Check machine instruction book for specific directions.

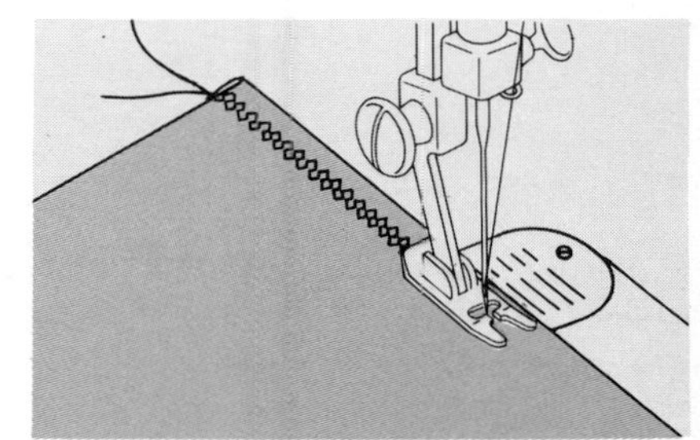

Decorative machine stitching can be applied along the raw, unturned edge as a substitute for a hem. Or it can be placed on a turned-back hem edge to both hold and finish it.

Self-faced ruffles

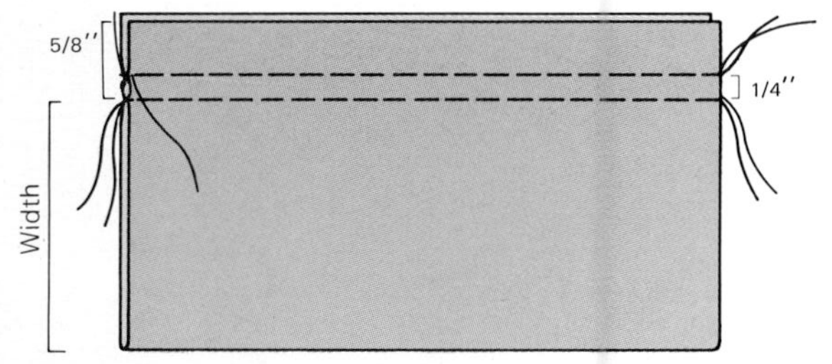

Plain ruffles to be self-faced require a double width of fabric folded in half, wrong sides together. Cut strip twice as wide as ruffle is to be, plus 1 1/4" (5/8" seam allowance on each layer). After folding strip, stitch gathering rows and pull threads as for single-layer type.

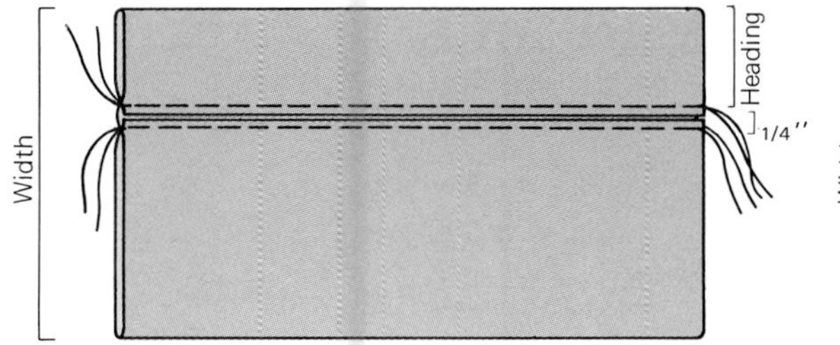

Ruffles with headings require a fabric strip double the intended width. Fold fabric wrong sides together, so edges meet on underside at desired depth of heading. Pin-baste edges. Then, where edges meet, sew two rows of gathering stitches, 1/4" apart, each holding a raw edge in place.

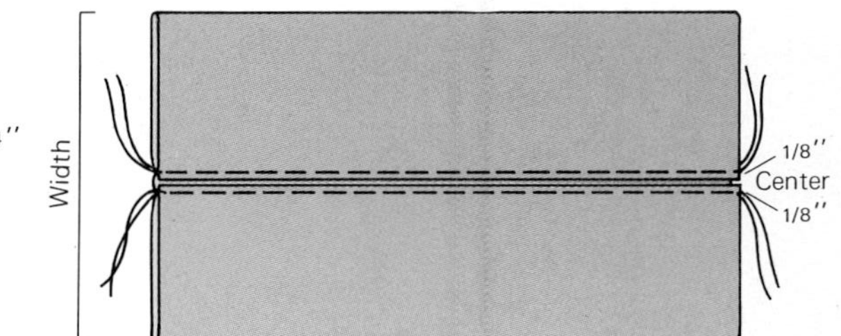

Double ruffles that are to be self-faced require strips exactly twice the desired finished width. Fold fabric, wrong sides together, so edges meet at center line. Pin-baste. Stitch gathering rows 1/4" apart (1/8" from each edge). Have bobbin thread on right side; it aids gathering.

Ruffles

Gathering 178-179
Collars 214

Stitching a plain ruffle into a seam

To sew a ruffle into a seam, first hem or face the ruffle strip; next pin the ungathered strip to one garment section; then gather the ruffle to fit and permanently stitch it in place. The adjoining garment section is sewed on over the ruffle. Special care must be taken with the ruffle seam allowance so that its extra fullness does not cause bulk in the completed seam. The seam allowance should be pressed flat before the second garment section is attached; after attaching, the seam should be carefully graded, clipped, and notched. The finished seam should be pressed so that the seam allowance of the ruffle is not pressed back onto the ruffle, where it would distort the hang of the ruffle. It would also necessitate extra pressing, which could flatten out the fullness.

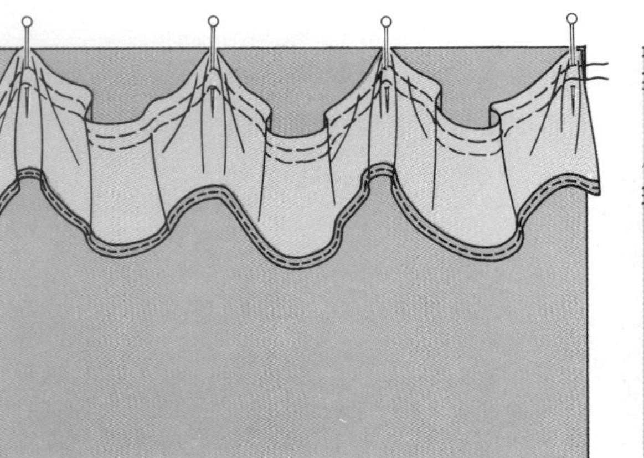

1. Pin-mark the prepared ruffle strip and the garment edge to which it will be joined into an equal number of parts. Right sides together, match and pin ruffle to garment at markings. Gather ruffle to fit edge, distributing fullness evenly.

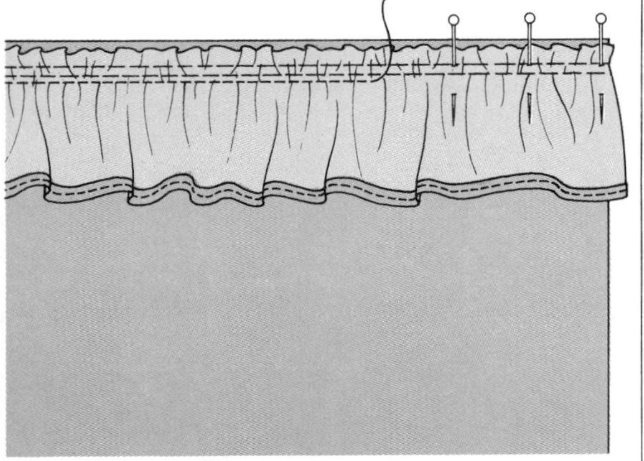

2. When ruffle is gathered to size and pinned in place, stitch it to garment section on seamline. Stitch with ruffle up, and, as you stitch, hold work in such a way that the gathers are not sewed into little pleats.

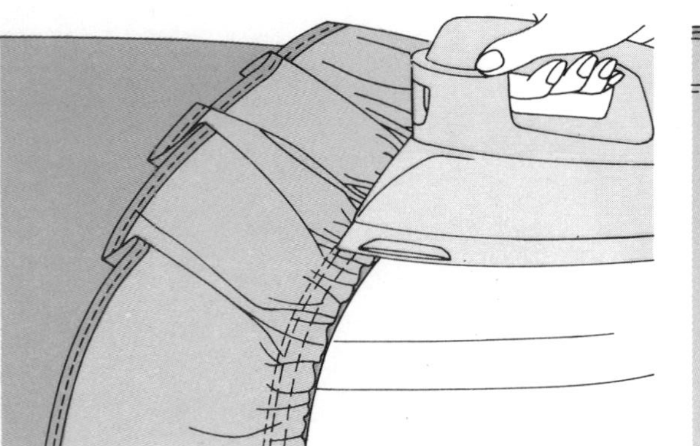

3. Press seam before joining to second garment section to prevent lumps or uneven stitching. Using just the point of the iron, press ruffle edge flat within the *seam allowance only*—do not let the iron go beyond the stitch line.

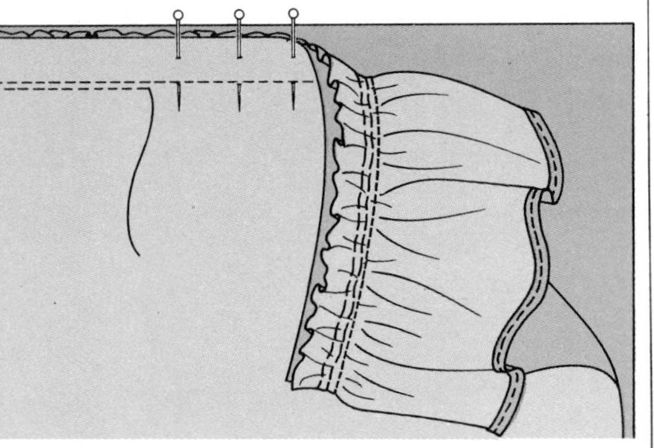

4. Pin edge with ruffle attached to second seam edge, right sides together, so ruffle is between the two garment sections. Stitch a thread width from first seam so no stitching will show on right side of garment or ruffle.

Stitching a ruffle to curves or corners

Ruffles must frequently be sewed into curved seams or sharp corners, a situation that occurs often in collars. In such cases, the ungathered ruffle must be pinned to the garment piece with extra fullness provided at the curve or corner. This allows for the greater distance the ruffle's outer edge must span. After stitching, the fullness in the seam allowance should be carefully graded and notched out.

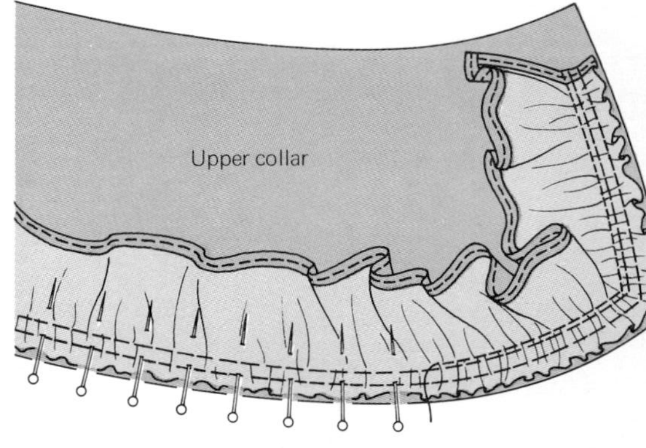

When attaching a hemmed ruffle, remember that the right side of the ruffle must show on the completed garment. If the garment piece is a collar, have right side of ruffle against right side of upper collar as you stitch.

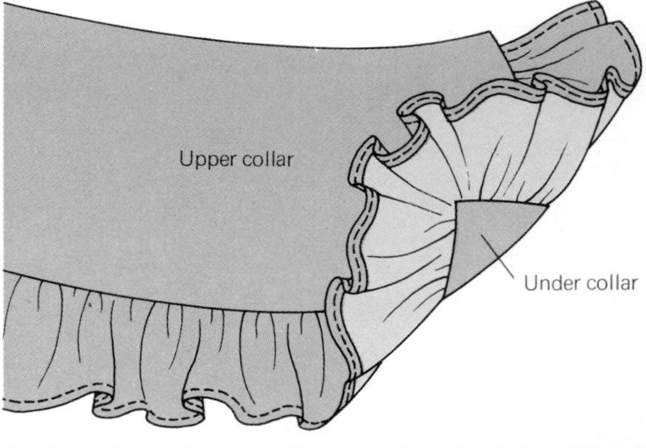

As the under and upper collar are being joined, the ruffle will be between the two garment sections. The final stitching should be slightly outside any other stitching so that no previous thread lines will show on finished collar.

Slipstitch (uneven) 132
Reducing seam bulk 147
Bias strips 298-299

Stitching a plain ruffle to an edge

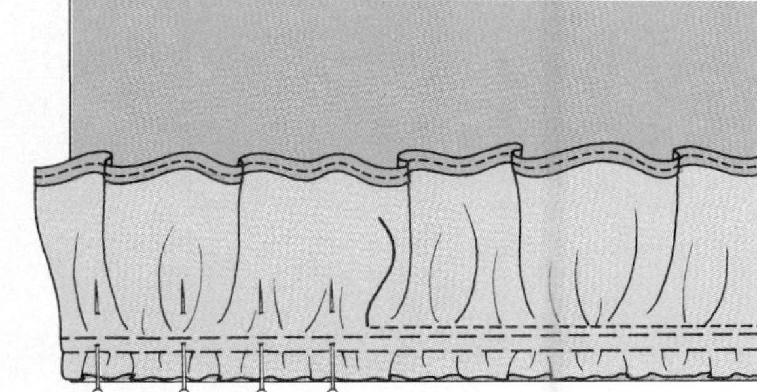

To attach a ruffle to a straight edge, pin the ungathered strip to the straight edge, gather it to fit, then permanently stitch in place. Trim the seam allowance *of the ruffle only* to ⅛", leaving other seam allowances intact.

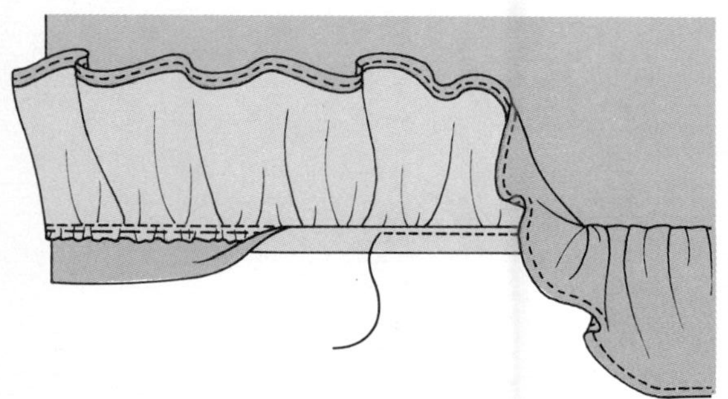

Fold untrimmed seam allowance under ⅛", then fold again so that cut edge of ruffle is enclosed and inside fold of seam allowance is on seamline. Pin in place and topstitch along edge at stitch line through seam allowances only.

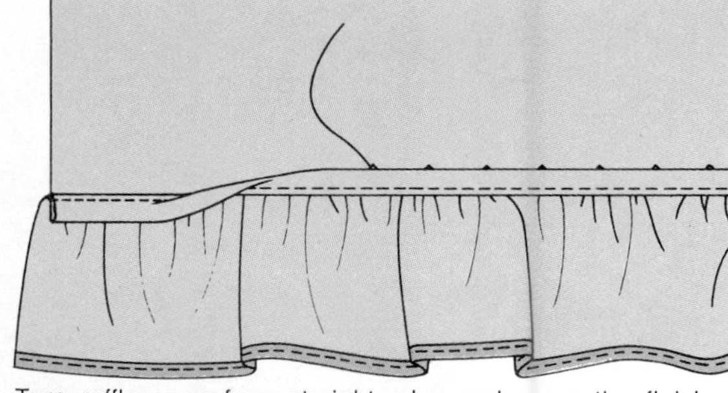

Turn ruffle away from straight edge and press the finished seam allowance toward garment so ruffle will hang properly. To be sure seam allowance will stay in that position, slipstitch the finished edge to the garment.

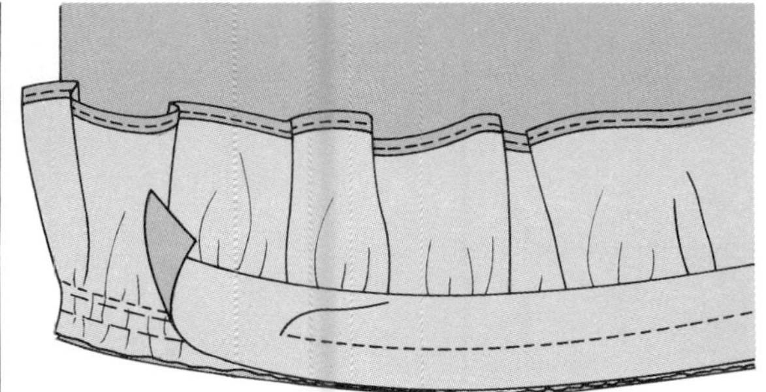

To stitch a ruffle to a curved edge, proceed as for gathering ruffle to edge; baste in place. Place right side of a 1¼"-wide bias strip to wrong side of ruffle, raw edges even. Stitch through all thicknesses on seamline.

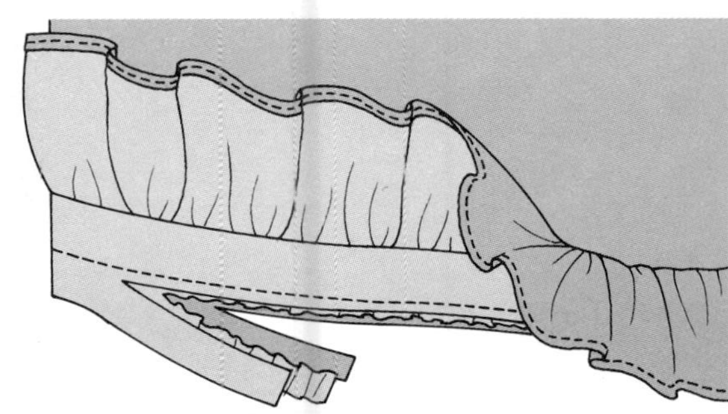

Trim and grade seam allowances, removing as much of the bulk of the ruffle seam allowance as possible. Bias strips are recommended here because they shape around curves better than the straight seam allowance could.

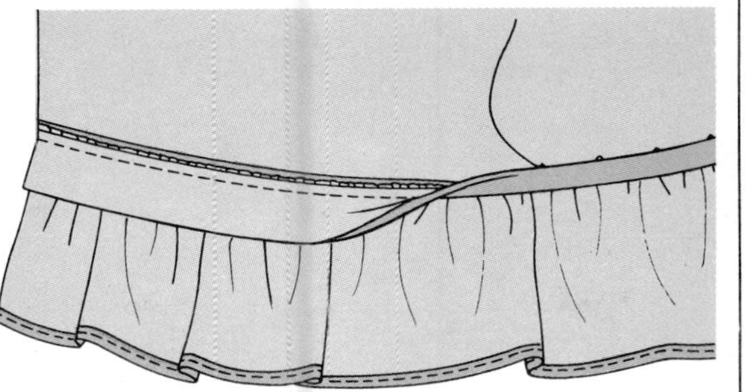

Turn ruffle away from edge and seam allowance toward garment so that ruffle is in proper position. Press seam allowance flat. Turn under remaining raw edge of bias strip ¼" and slipstitch to garment.

Attaching headed or double ruffles

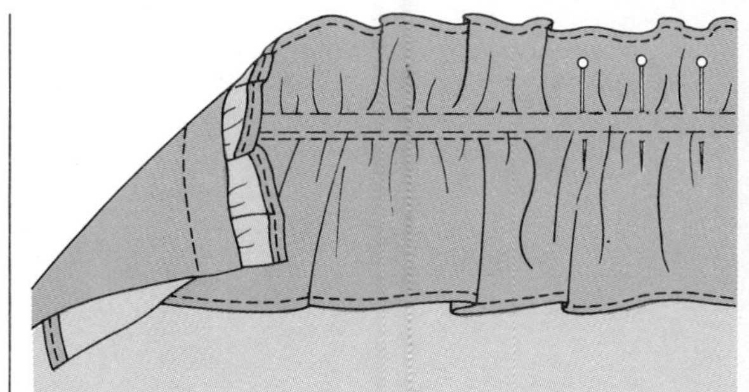

If ruffle is at an edge, place wrong side of ungathered ruffle against wrong side of garment, matching bottom row of gathering stitches to seamline on garment. Gather ruffle to fit; stitch, with the ruffle up, along the seamline.

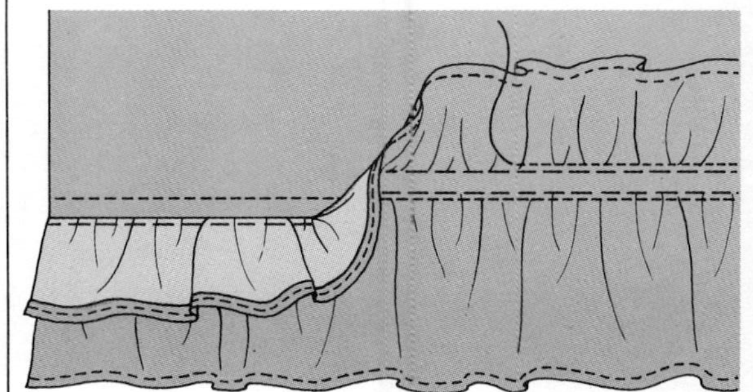

Trim seam allowance of garment to ¼". Turn ruffle to outside of garment and topstitch in place along top row of gathering stitches. The seam allowance will be completely enclosed by the second line of stitching.

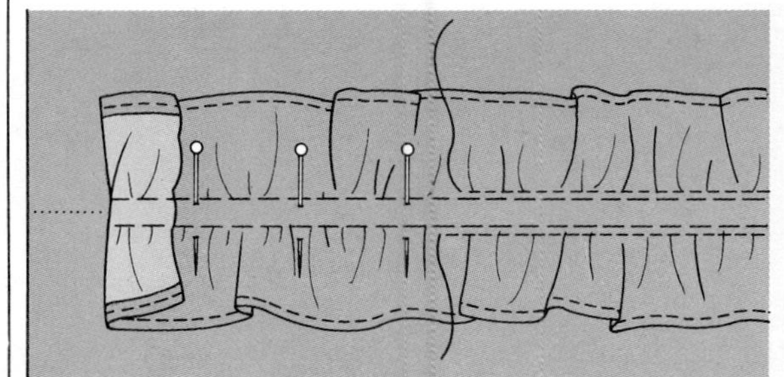

If ruffle is not at an edge, first mark desired location for ruffle on right side of garment. Pin ungathered ruffle to garment, gather to fit, and topstitch to garment. Use gathering stitches as a guide, stitching just alongside them.

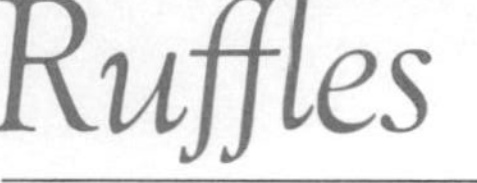

Ruffles

Grain in fabrics 84-85

Circular ruffles

The deep fullness and the fluid look characteristic of circular ruffles are created by the way the fabric is cut rather than by means of gathering stitches. Circular ruffles can be used anywhere that gathered ruffles would be suitable; they are especially effective at necklines and when made of sheer, filmy fabrics. To make circular ruffles, a paper pattern is essential. Measure the length of the edge to which ruffle will be attached; this will be the circumference of the inner circle. Next, decide the width of the ruffle; this will be the distance between the inner and outer circles.

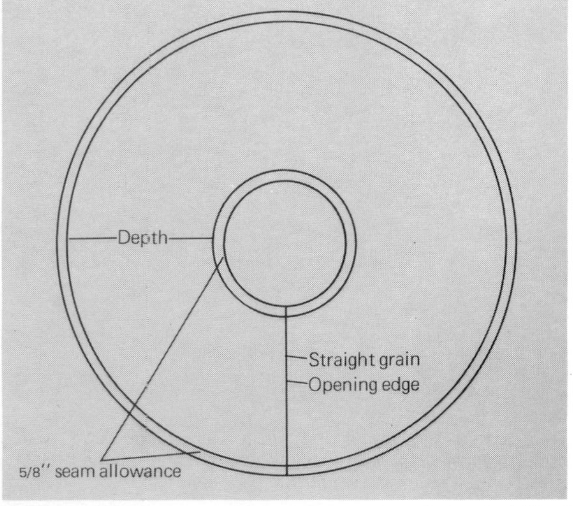

On paper, draw inner circle first. Draw outer circle at width of ruffle. Add ⅝″ at edge of each circle.

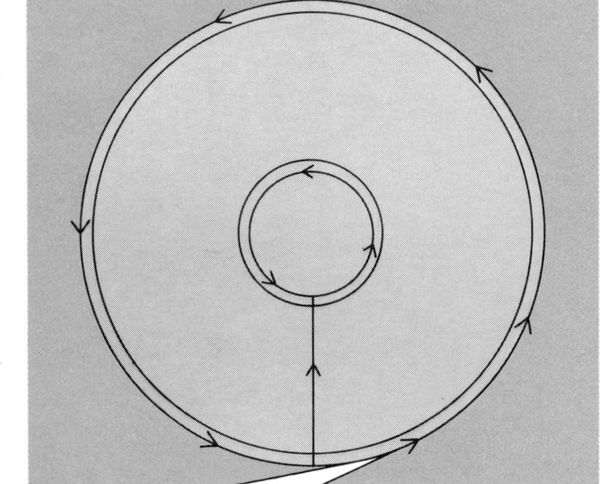

Cut fabric along outermost circle first. Then cut on grainline to the innermost circle and cut it out.

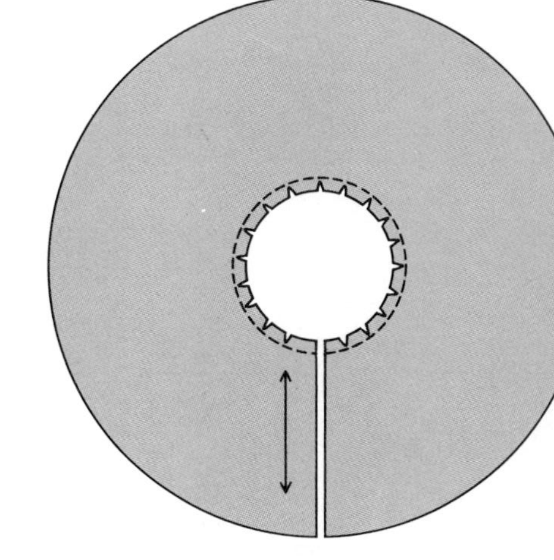

Staystitch inner circle on seamline. Clip seam allowance repeatedly until inner edge can be pulled out straight.

Piecing to achieve length

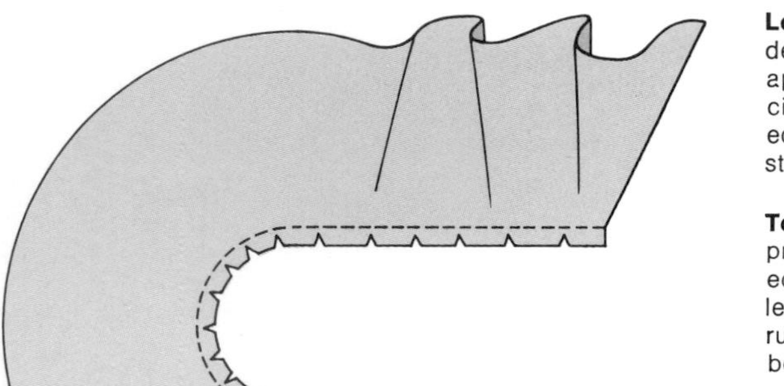

Long ruffles may require piecing. Circumference of inner circle determines length you get from each piece (circumference is approximately three times the diameter). Cut out as many circles as needed to reach desired length. Staystitch all inner edges and clip seams so circles can be pulled flat. Lay stretched circles end to end to calculate length.

To join pieces, simply seam the adjoining straight ends and press seams open and flat. Sew together enough circles to equal or exceed the length of the edge to be joined. Excess length can be trimmed from either or both ends of the pieced ruffle. For self-faced ruffles, be sure to cut out twice the number of circles needed for each ruffle's full length.

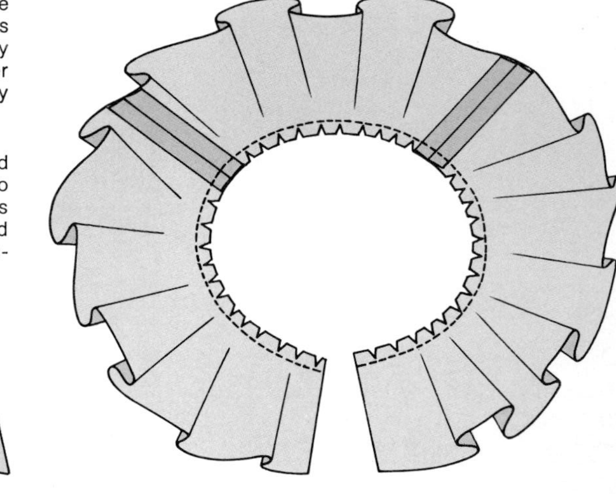

Neckline finishes 193-195

Finishing outer edge

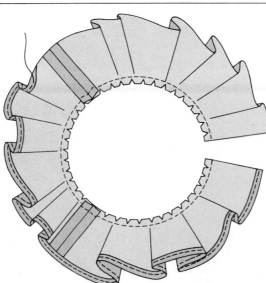

Single-layer circular ruffles are finished on outer edge, before attaching, with a narrow hem or decorative stitching. This creates a definite "right" and "wrong" side.

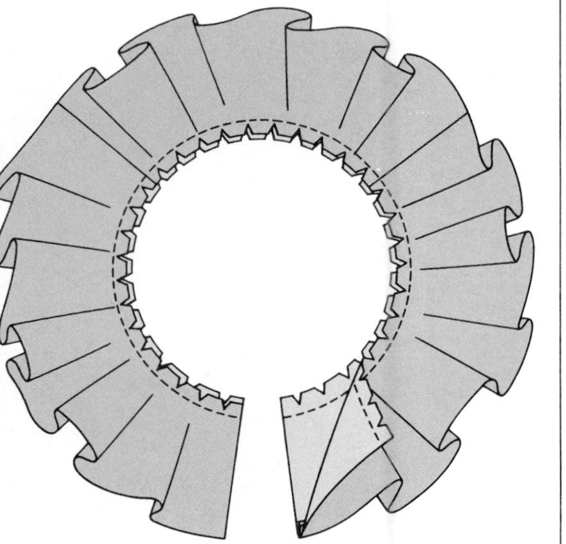

Self-faced circular ruffles require duplicate circles, or two identical pieced strips. With right sides together, stitch along outer edge. Trim seam and turn to right side.

Attaching to a garment

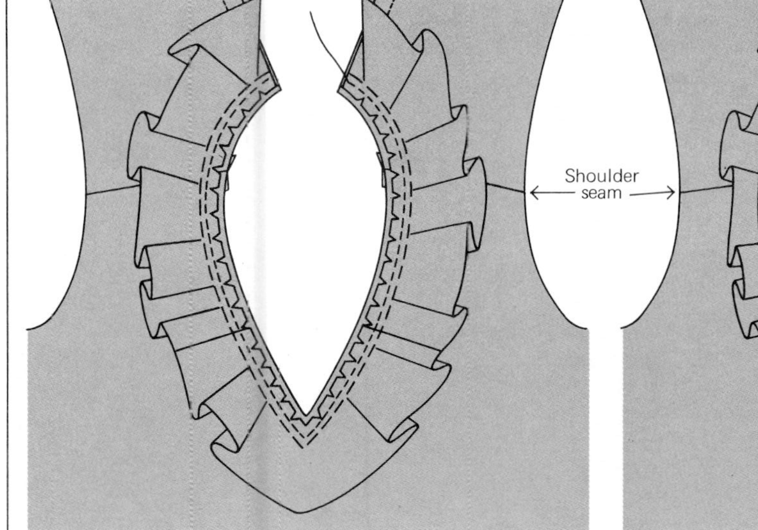

1. Place wrong side of ruffle against right side of garment with ruffle seam allowance flat and smooth (additional clips may be required). Baste layers together.

2. Join facing sections and seam-finish outer edge. Match facing to garment edge, seams and notches aligned. Baste, then stitch, reinforcing point with short stitches.

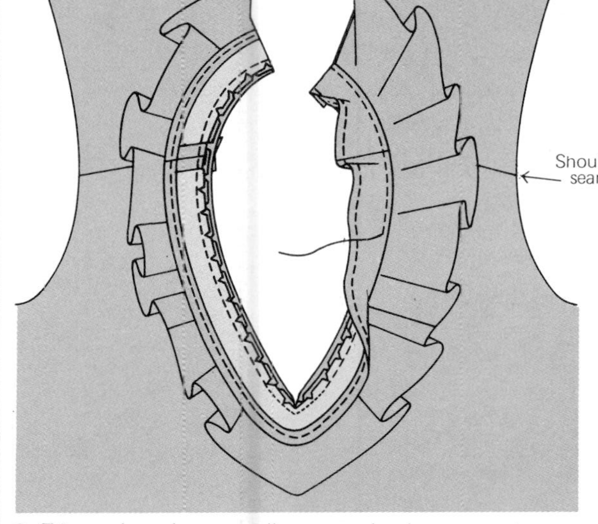

3. Trim and grade seam allowances, leaving garment seam allowance the widest. Clip seam allowances to stitching. Understitch to keep facing from rolling to right side.

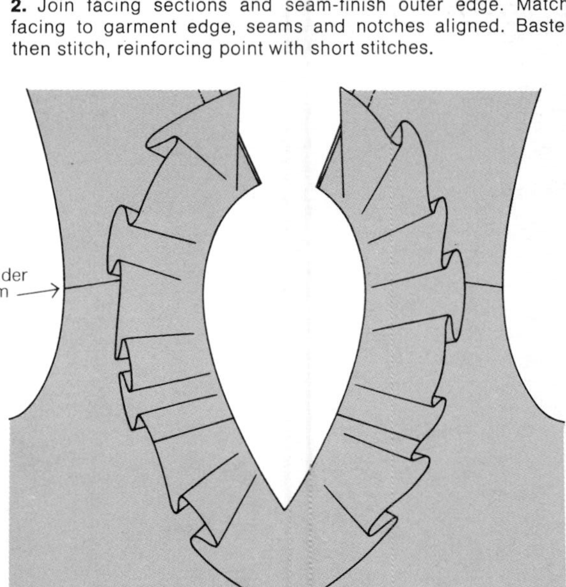

4. Turn facing to inside, finish ends and tack to zipper. Turn ruffle away from garment when pressing neckline seam; do not press ruffle flat onto garment.

Ruffles

Finishing ends

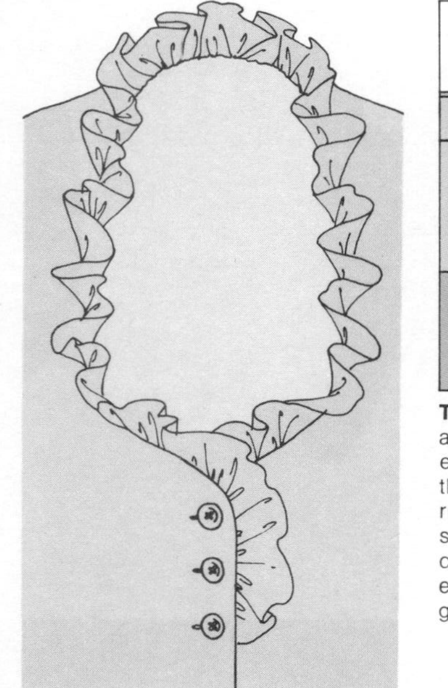

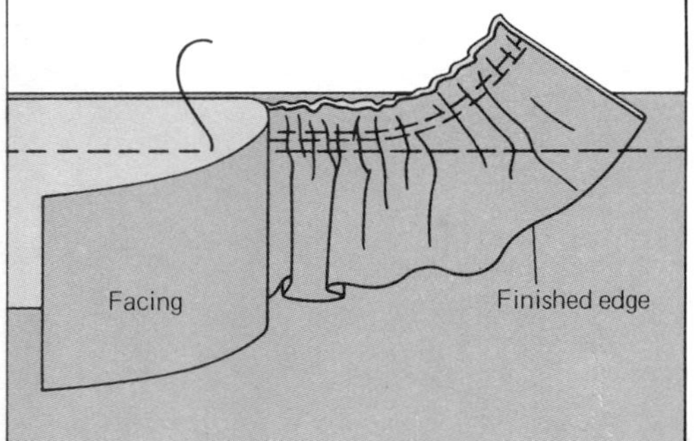

Tapering ends into the garment seamline is a common method for finishing off ruffles, especially when the ruffle does not continue the full length of the seam. Position the ruffle on the seam, drawing it beyond the seam allowance until the outer finished edge crosses the seamline where the ruffle will end. Only this outer edge will be visible on garment as ruffle ends slant inward.

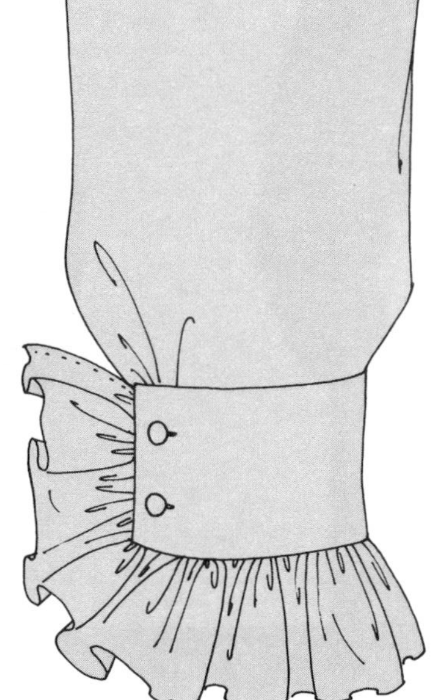

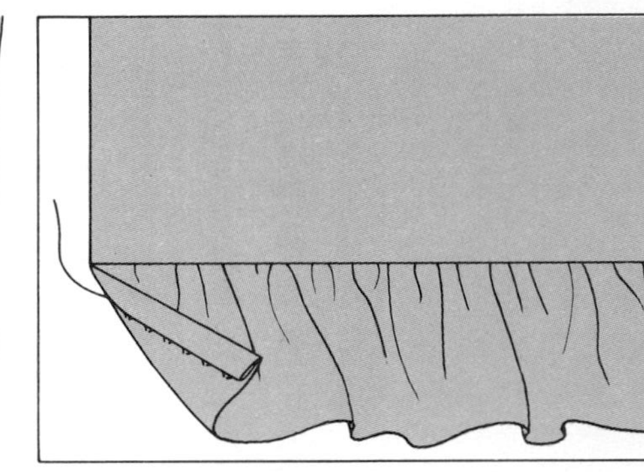

Tiny hems are used to finish a ruffle edge not caught into a seam, as might be the case at a cuff. In such instances, attach ruffle on its normal seamline; at end of ruffle, turn fabric to wrong side and slipstitch in place with tiny hand stitches. In cases where the flat ends of two ruffles meet, fold ends under and seam together by hand.

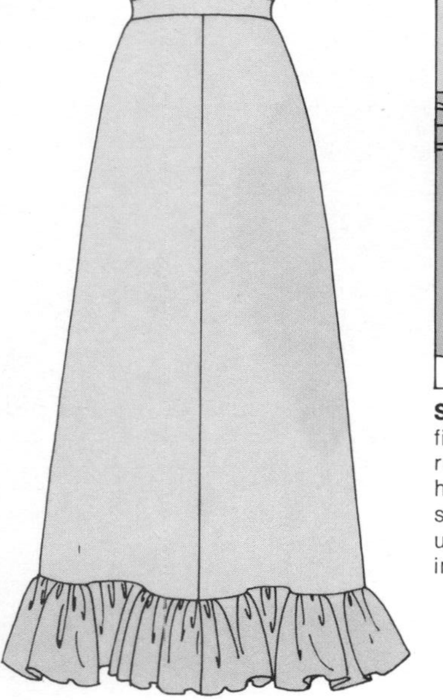

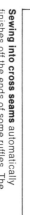

Sewing into cross seams automatically finishes off the ends of some ruffles. The ruffle is usually attached first, then handled as a continuation of the straight seam being joined. Fold seam allowances under at bottom edge and hand-tack them in place to finish off the hem edge.

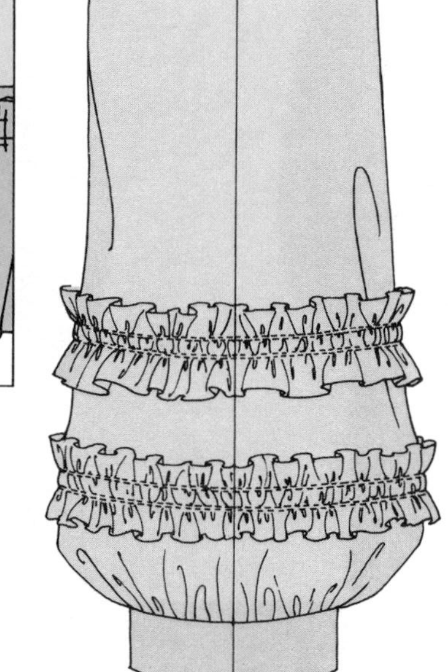

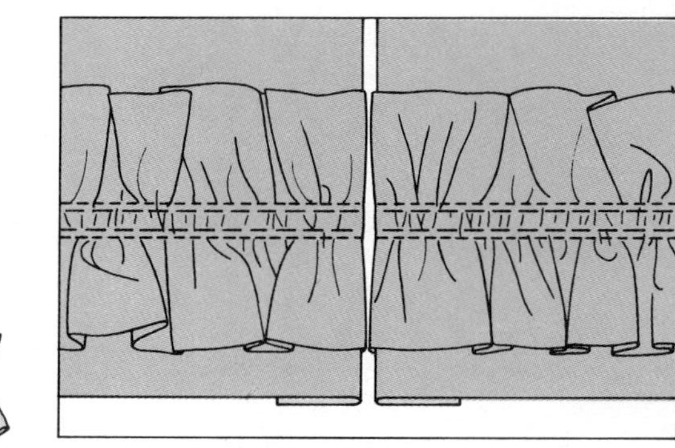

Ruffles not applied to an edge are almost always incorporated into a cross seam. Before stitching the cross seam, make sure the gathering or topstitching rows are aligned with one another so that the ruffles match perfectly when the seam is completed.

Necklines & Collars

Neckline finishes

Interfacing 72-73, 76-79

Neckline facings

A facing is the fabric used to finish raw edges of a garment at such locations as neck, armhole, and front and back openings. There are three categories of facings: shaped facings, extended facings (essentially shaped facings), and bias facings.

A facing is shaped to fit the edge it will finish either during cutting or just before application. A **shaped facing** is cut out, using a pattern, to the same shape and on the same grain as the edge it will finish. A **bias facing** is a strip of fabric cut on the bias so that it can *be* shaped to match the curve of the edge it will be applied to. After a facing is attached to the garment's edge, it is turned to the inside of the garment and should not show on the outside.

In order to reduce bulk, both shaped and bias facings can be cut from a fabric lighter in weight than the garment fabric. Because the extended facing is cut as one with the garment, garment and facing fabric are always the same. The illustrations at the right show some examples of neckline shaped facing pieces and a bias facing.

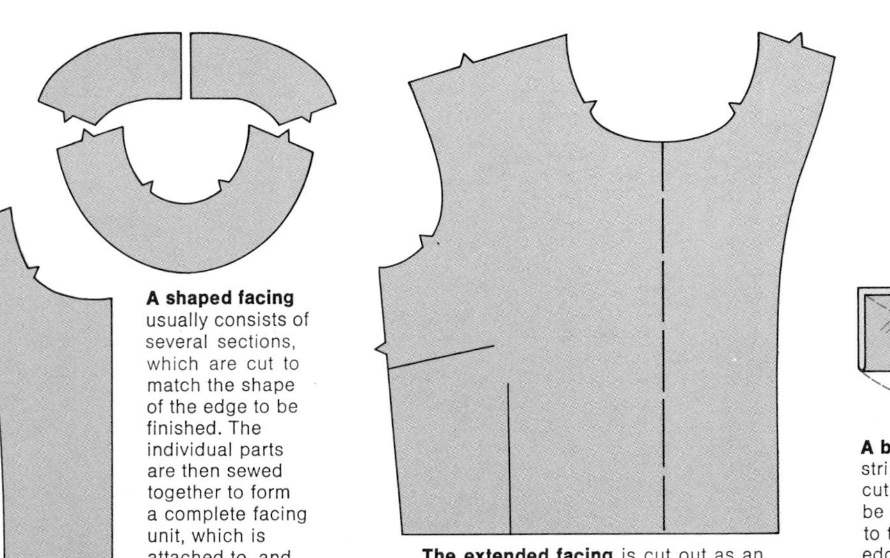

A shaped facing usually consists of several sections, which are cut to match the shape of the edge to be finished. The individual parts are then sewed together to form a complete facing unit, which is attached to, and serves as a finish for, the raw edge.

The extended facing is cut out as an extension of the garment; it is then folded back along the edge it finishes.

A bias facing is a narrow strip of lightweight fabric cut on the bias so it can be shaped to conform to the curve of the edge it will finish. Less bulky and conspicuous than a shaped facing.

Interfacing necklines

Depending on pattern and fabric, it may be necessary or desirable to interface a garment neckline before applying the facing. Interfacing will help to define, support, and reinforce the shape of the neck. The type of interfacing is dictated by the garment fabric; the method of application will depend on both the pattern instructions and the type of interfacing selected. If the pattern does not include separate pattern pieces for cutting out the interfacing, use the facing pattern pieces, but trim away ½ inch from the outer edges of the interfacing so that this edge will not extend beyond the completed facing (see below).

When it is an extended facing, the inner edge of the interfacing may either meet the garment foldline or extend ½ inch beyond it into the facing portion. If edge and foldline meet, catchstitch the edge to the garment foldline; if the edge extends, match the garment and interfacing foldlines and stitch the two together along the fold, using very short stitches approximately ½ inch apart. If a zipper will be inserted, reduce the bulk of the interfacing by trimming it away at the placket seamline. If the zipper has been applied, trim the interfacing as close to the placket seamline as possible (see below). Topstitching on zipper determines how far *in* the interfacing can extend.

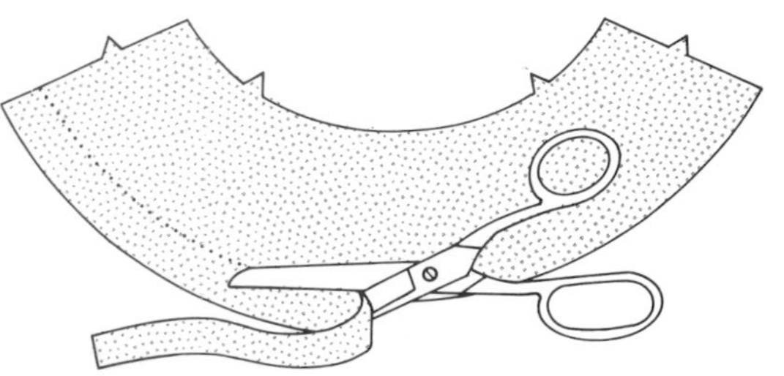

If the facing pattern was used to cut out interfacing pieces, trim ½" from the outer edge of each.

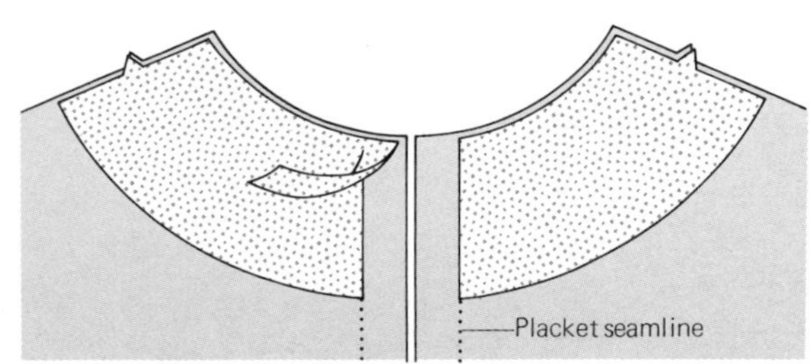

If zipper has not been applied to the garment, trim away the unnecessary interfacing along the placket seamline.

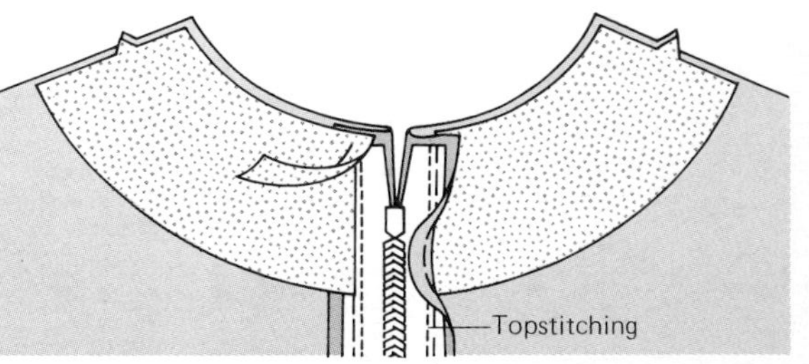

If zipper has been applied, trim interfacing along placket topstitching; position cut edges under seam allowances.

Construction of shaped neckline facings

Shown and explained below are the three most typical examples of shaped neckline facings. Although they look different, they are similarly constructed. If interfacing is being used at the neckline, apply it to the garment before attaching the facing. If any alterations have been made in the garment that affect the edges to be faced, be sure to alter facing and interfacing accordingly.

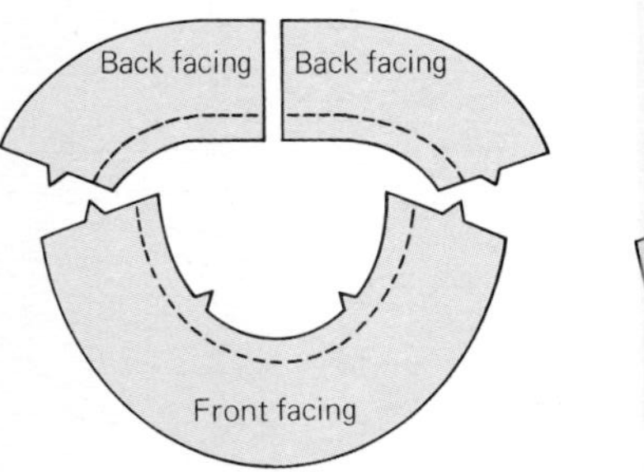

Round neck facing pieces

1. To help maintain the shape of the facing, staystitch ⅛″ inside the neck seamline of each facing section. With an extended facing, staystitch inside the garment neck seamline as well. Lay the pattern pieces back onto the fabric sections to check whether the staystitched edges have retained their original measurements. If section is shorter, clip and release a few stitches; if longer, pull up on several of the stitches.

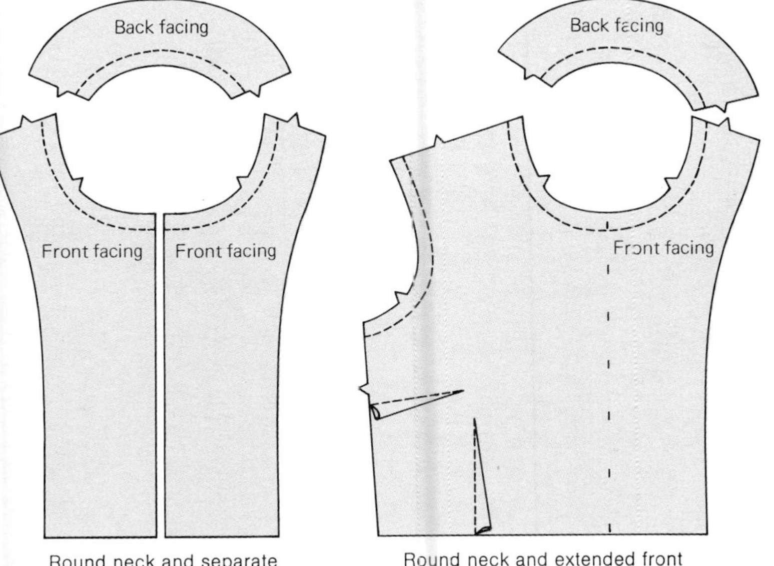

Round neck and separate front facing pieces

Round neck and extended front facing unit

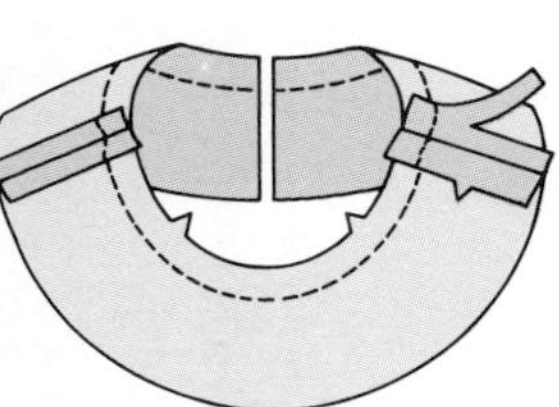

Round neck facing unit

2. With right sides together and the markings matched, seam the front facing sections to the back facing sections at shoulders. Press seams flat as stitched, then open. Trim the seam allowances to half-width; seam-finish if necessary, using a hand overcast stitch. A complete extended facing unit will consist of two garment fronts with each of their extended facings seamed, at the shoulders, to the back neck facing section.

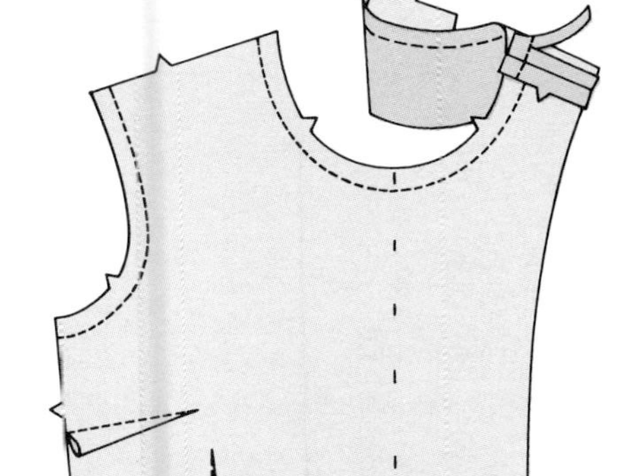

Round neck and separate front facing unit

Round neck and extended front facing unit

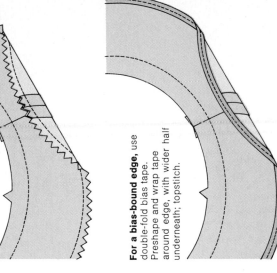

3. Keeping seam allowances open, apply a finish suitable to the fabric along the outer, unnotched edge of the facing unit. Some of the possible finishes are shown below. (Also see Seam finishes.)

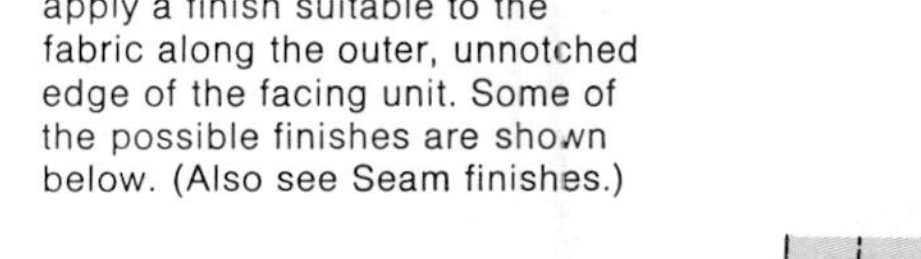

A turned-and-stitched finish is best for lightweight fabrics. Turn edge of facing under ¼″; press. Stitch close to the folded edge.

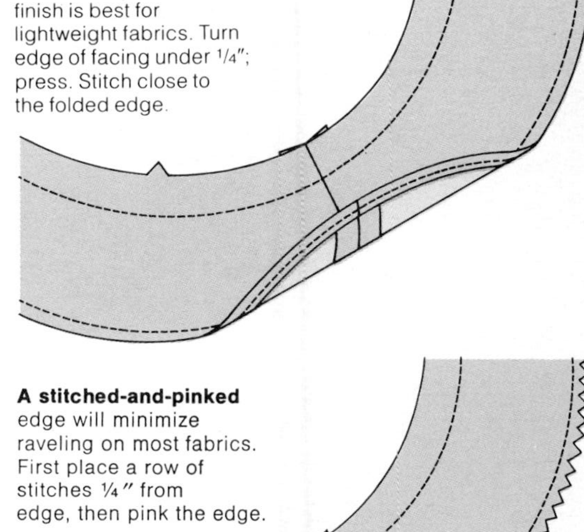

A stitched-and-pinked edge will minimize raveling on most fabrics. First place a row of stitches ¼″ from edge, then pink the edge.

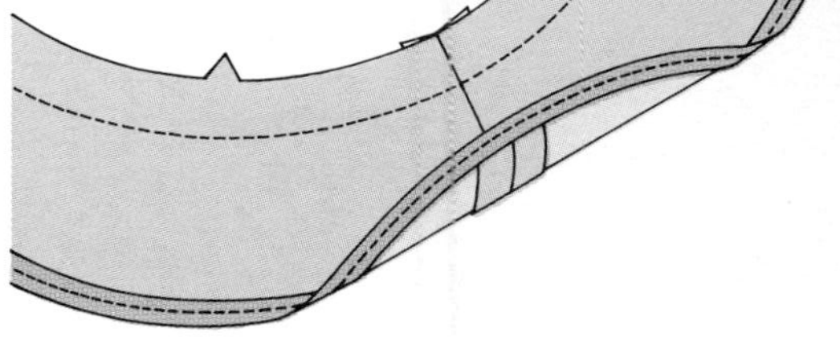

For a bias-bound edge, use double-fold bias tape. Preshape and wrap tape around edge, with wider half underneath; topstitch.

Neckline finishes

Pressing 18-19
Reducing seam bulk 147
Centered zipper 318-319; lapped 322-323; invisible 326-327

Applying shaped facing to neckline with zipper

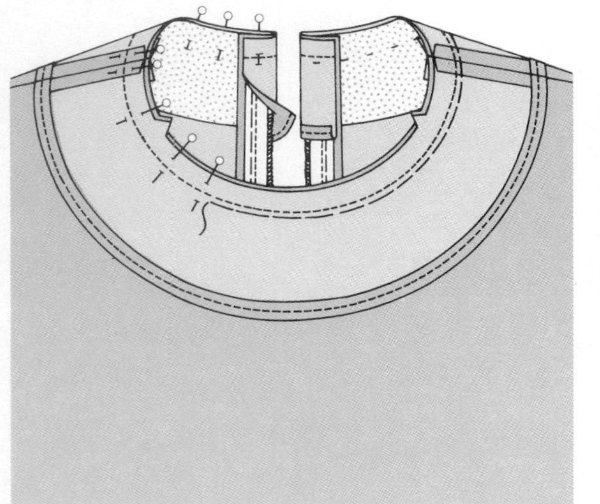

1. Right sides together, matching notches, markings, and seamlines, pin facing to neck. **If zipper has been inserted,** open zipper and wrap ends of facing to inside around each zipper half. Baste facing to garment along neck seamline.

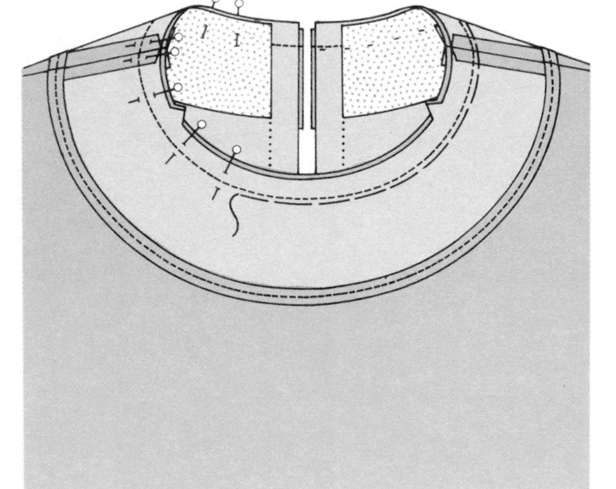

If zipper has not been inserted, facing ends can be handled in two ways. To use the **first method,** shown above, keep center back seam allowances of both facing and garment extended; then pin and baste them together in this position.

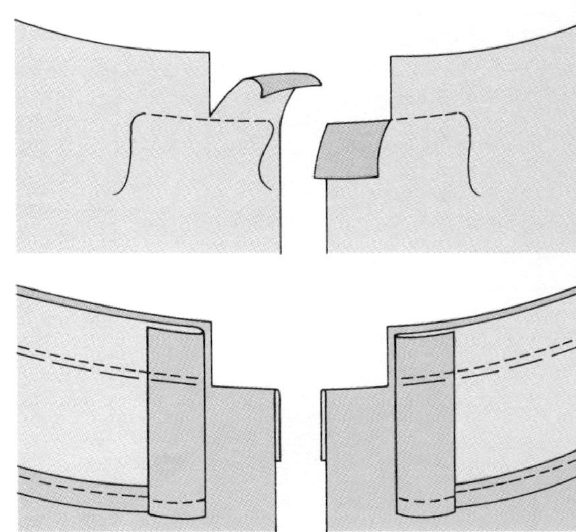

To use **second method,** reinforce neck seamline for ½″ on each side of center back seam. Clip seam allowance along center seamline to reinforcement stitches; fold ends down to inside of garment. Fold facing seam allowances back; baste.

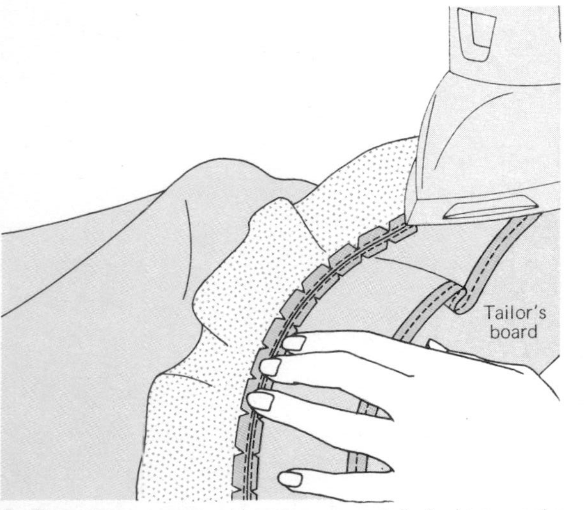

4. Place seam, wrong side up, over a tailor's ham or the curved edge of a tailor's board. Using the tip of the iron, press seam open. Press carefully to prevent the seam edges from making an imprint on right side of garment.

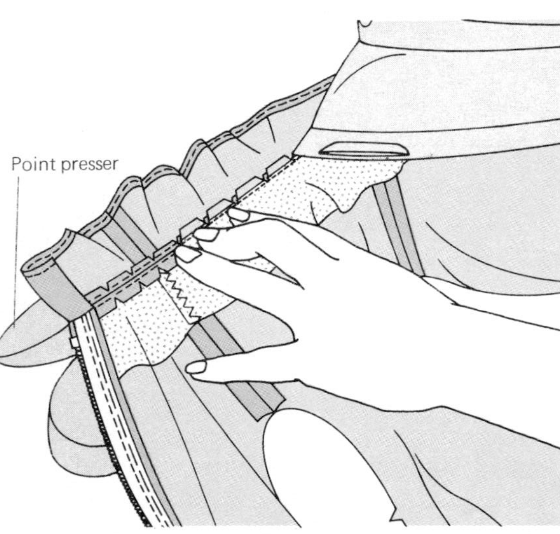

From the wrong side, with the facing extended away from the garment, place seam over a point presser. Press all seam allowances toward the facing. Press carefully so as not to crease either the facing or the garment.

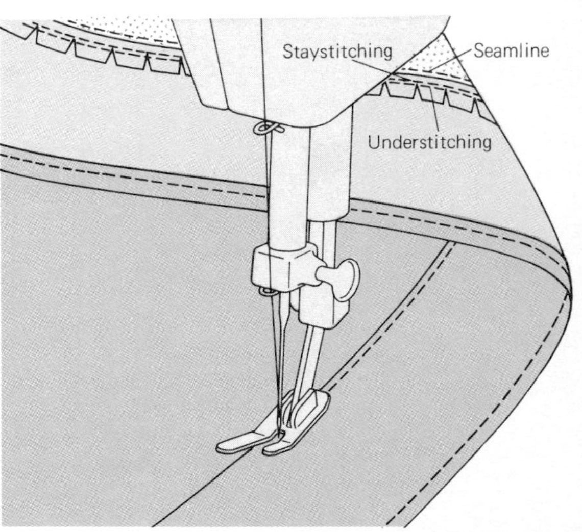

5. To keep facing from rolling to outside of garment, the seam should be understitched. With facing and seam allowances extended away from garment, stitch from right side close to neck seamline, through facing and seam allowances.

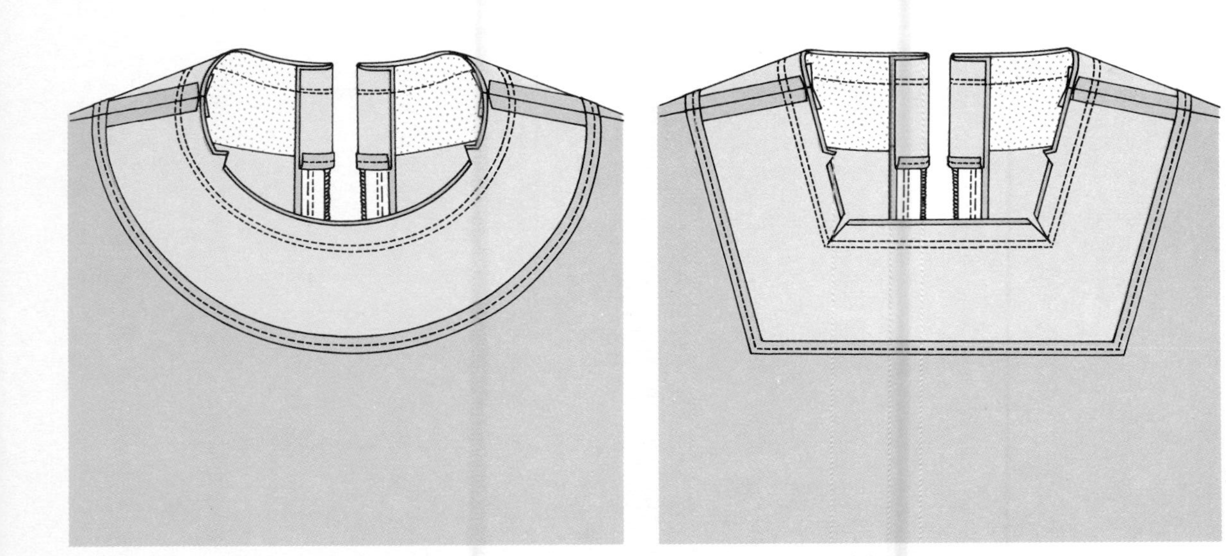

2. With facing side up, stitch facing to garment along the neck seamline; secure stitching at both ends. Check to be sure that the neck seamlines will align with each other when the zipper is closed. Remove bastings. Press seam flat.

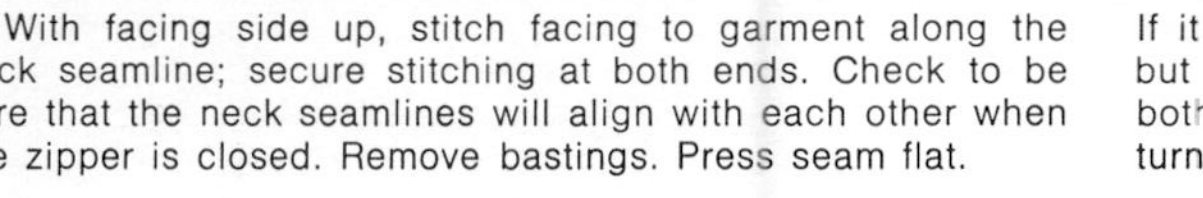

If it is a **square neckline,** apply the facing in the same way but reinforce the corners by using short stitches for 1″ on both sides of each corner. To relieve strain when facing is turned to inside of garment, clip into the corners.

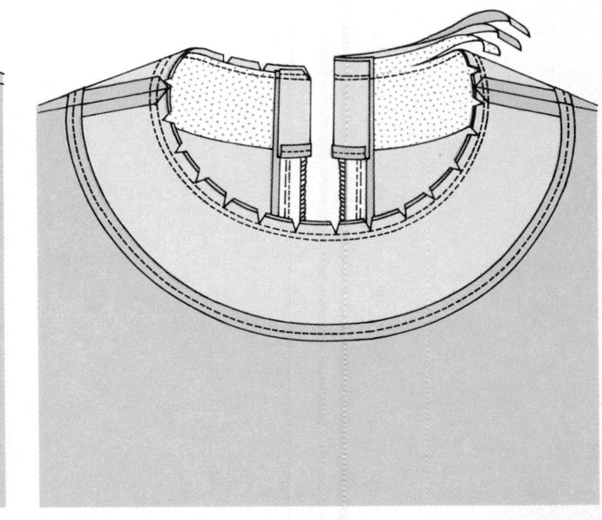

3. Trim and grade seam allowances, making garment seam allowance the widest. Trim diagonally across center back seam allowances and cross-seam allowances at shoulders. Clip curved seam allowances. If not already in, insert zipper.

6. Turn facing to inside of garment, allowing seamline to roll inside slightly. Align facing and garment seamlines and center markings, then press along neck edge. To hold edges in place, it may be helpful to diagonal-baste along neck edge.

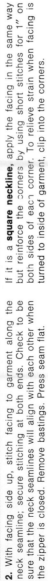

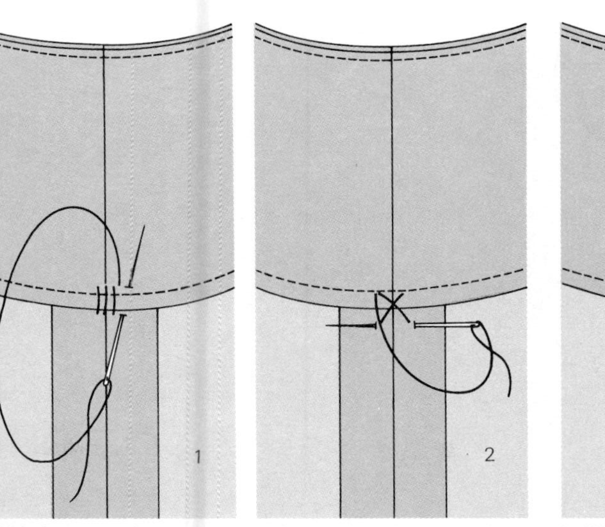

7. With facing and garment seamlines aligned at shoulders, tack facing in place. Use either several closely spaced whipstitches (1) or a cross-stitch tack (2), catching only facing edge and seam allowances of garment.

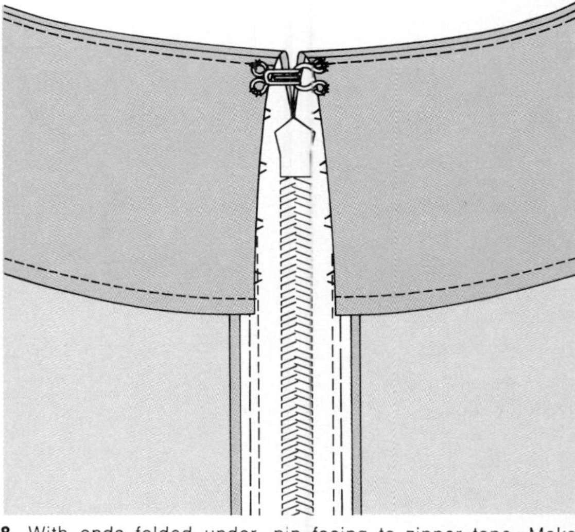

8. With ends folded under, pin facing to zipper tape. Make sure that the facing will not be caught in the zipper. Open zipper and slipstitch facing to zipper tape. Close zipper and attach fastener at top of placket.

Pressing 18-19 Bound and machine-worked buttonholes 330-346

Applying shaped facing to neckline and garment opening

Some designs require facing of both the neck *and* a front or back opening. The facing used for the opening may be a separate piece or an extended facing. Buttonholes are the usual closure. Bound buttonholes are constructed *before* facing is applied; machine buttonholes, *after* application.

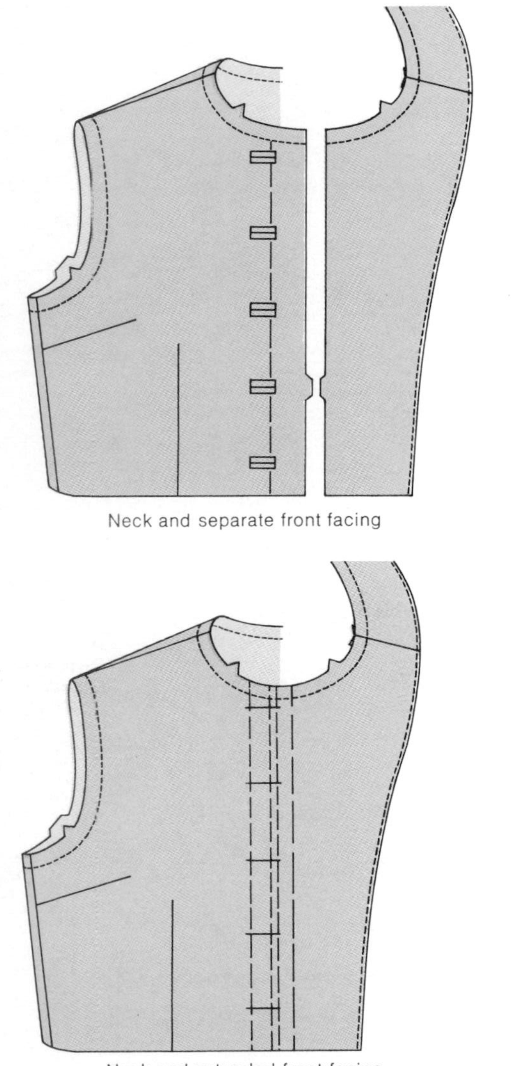

Neck and separate front facing

Neck and extended front facing

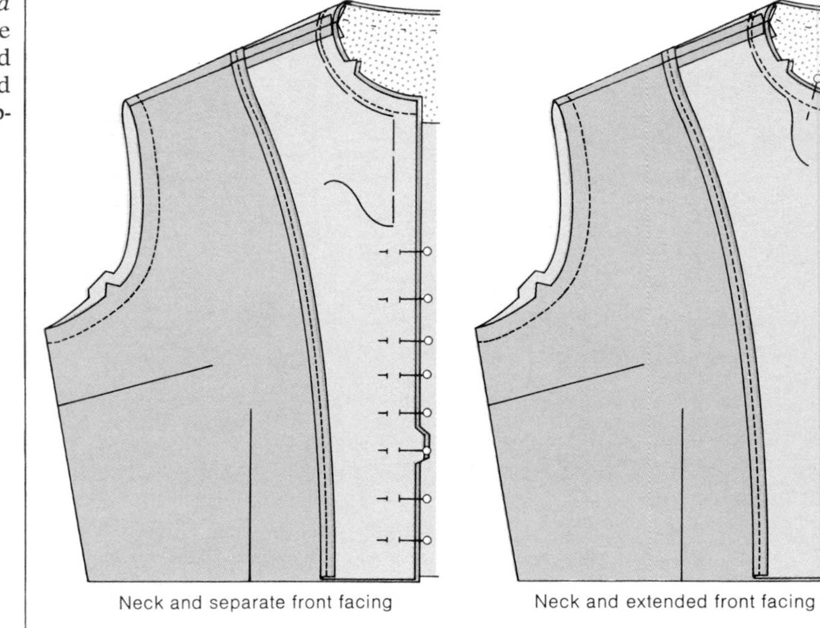

Neck and separate front facing

Neck and extended front facing

1. With right sides together, matching markings and notches, pin and baste the facing to the garment along the neck seamline. When it is a **separate front facing,** pin and baste down the opening edge. With an **extended facing,** the facing has been folded back onto the garment, producing a fold rather than a seam. In this situation, there is no need to match, pin, and baste.

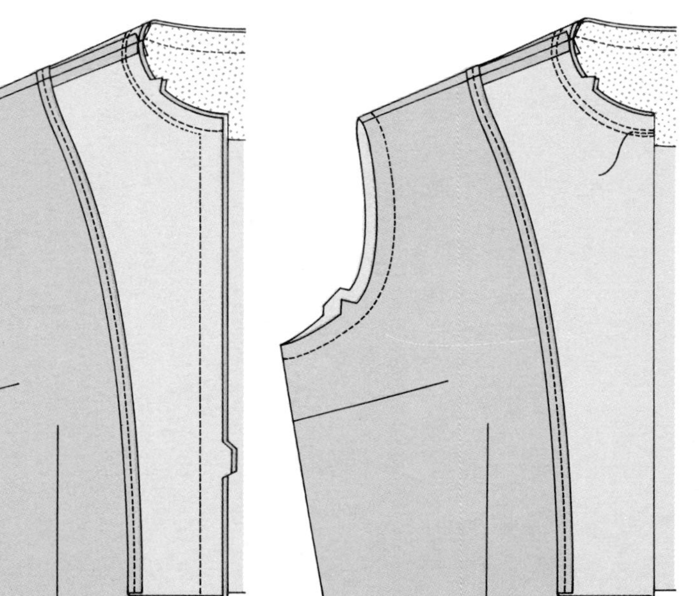

Neck and separate front facing

Neck and extended front facing

2. Stitch facing to garment along the seamline. With the **separate front facing,** it may be advisable to stitch directionally, starting at center back and stitching to lower edge of front facing on each side. Reinforce corners formed by the neckline and opening edge seamlines, by taking small stitches for 1″ on both sides of each corner. With the **extended facing,** just the neck seamline is stitched; backstitch at both ends to secure stitching. After appropriate stitching, remove bastings and press the seam flat as stitched. Do not press the fold of an extended facing.

Cross-stitch tack (single) 134
Whipstitch 136
Reducing seam bulk 147

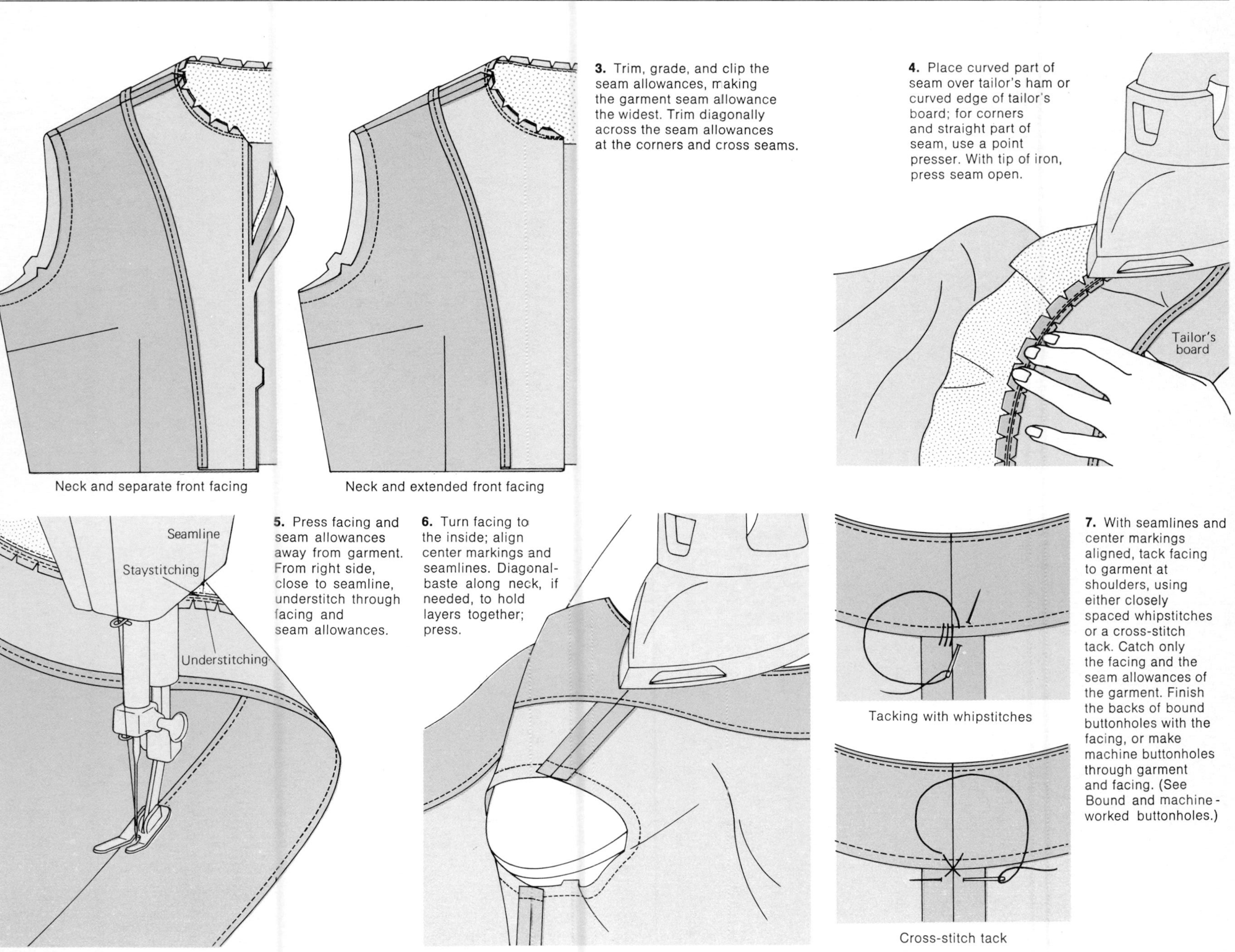

Neck and separate front facing

Neck and extended front facing

3. Trim, grade, and clip the seam allowances, making the garment seam allowance the widest. Trim diagonally across the seam allowances at the corners and cross seams.

4. Place curved part of seam over tailor's ham or curved edge of tailor's board; for corners and straight part of seam, use a point presser. With tip of iron, press seam open.

5. Press facing and seam allowances away from garment. From right side, close to seamline, understitch through facing and seam allowances.

6. Turn facing to the inside; align center markings and seamlines. Diagonal-baste along neck, if needed, to hold layers together; press.

Tacking with whipstitches

Cross-stitch tack

7. With seamlines and center markings aligned, tack facing to garment at shoulders, using either closely spaced whipstitches or a cross-stitch tack. Catch only the facing and the seam allowances of the garment. Finish the backs of bound buttonholes with the facing, or make machine buttonholes through garment and facing. (See Bound and machine-worked buttonholes.)

Pressing 18-19
Cross-stitch tack (single) 134
Whipstitch 136
Reducing seam bulk 147

Combination facings

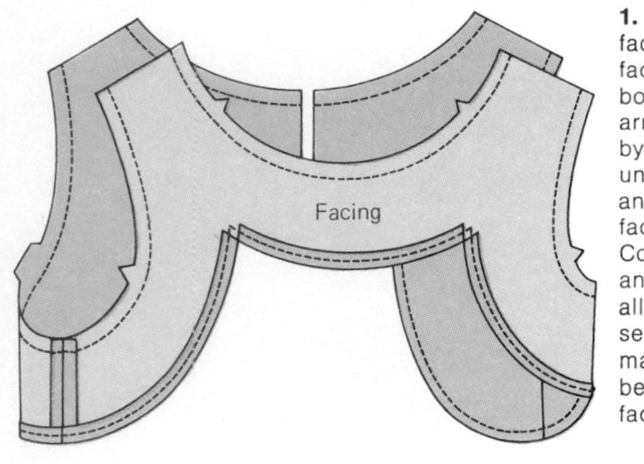

1. A combination facing is a shaped facing in which both the neck and armholes are finished by the same facing unit. Staystitch neck and armholes of both facing and garment. Construct facing unit and garment, leaving all the shoulder seams open. Zipper may be inserted before or after the facing is applied.

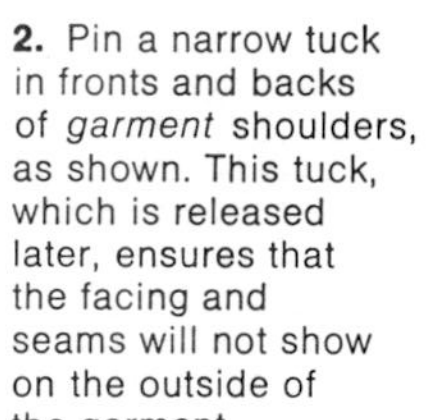

2. Pin a narrow tuck in fronts and backs of *garment* shoulders, as shown. This tuck, which is released later, ensures that the facing and seams will not show on the outside of the garment.

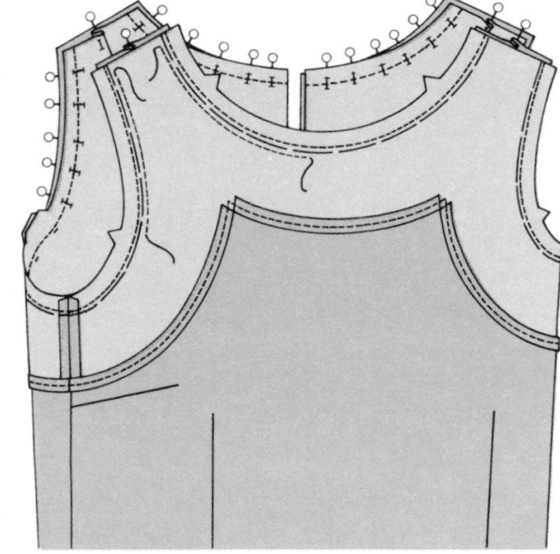

3. Right sides together, pin and baste facing to garment along the neck and armhole seamlines of the *facing*. (For facing treatment at zipper placket, see p. 194.) Facing side up, stitch facing to garment, starting at shoulder seamlines.

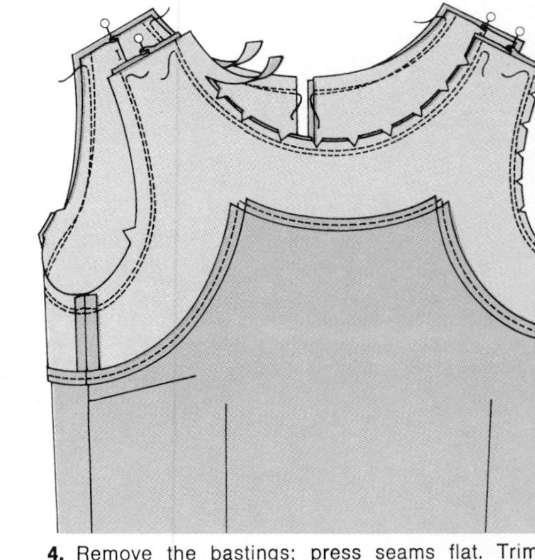

4. Remove the bastings; press seams flat. Trim, grade, and clip seam allowances. Trim cross-seam allowances diagonally. Place seams over curved part of tailor's board and press all seams open. Then press all seam allowances toward facing.

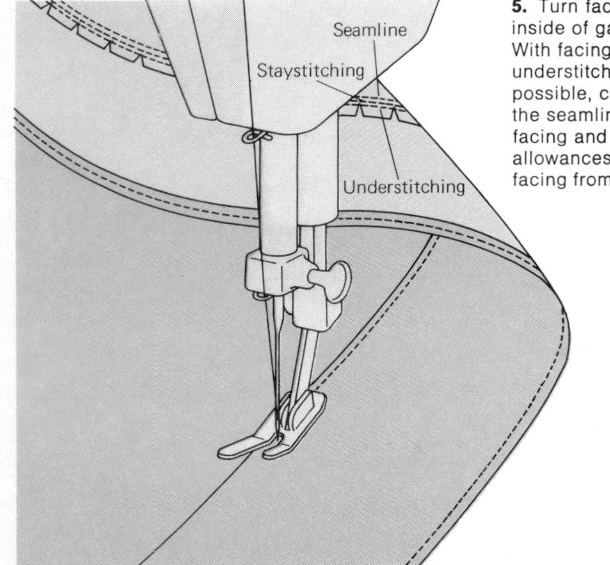

5. Turn facing to the inside of garment. With facing side up, understitch, where possible, close to the seamline through facing and seam allowances. Press facing from inside.

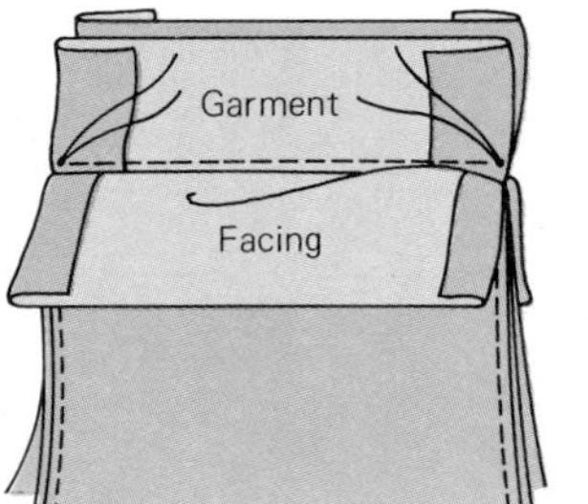

6. Release tucks at shoulders. With neck and armhole seam allowances folded back and the facing out of the way, baste and stitch the garment shoulder seams. Tie thread ends. Press seams flat, then open; push through opening.

7. Trim facing seam allowances at the shoulders to ¼″. Turn under and slipstitch together, over garment seams.

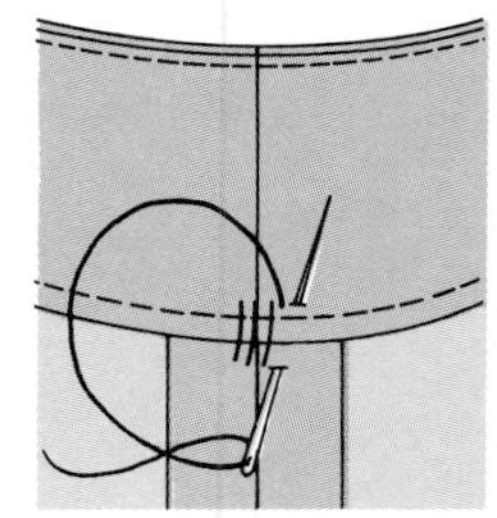
Tacking with whipstitches

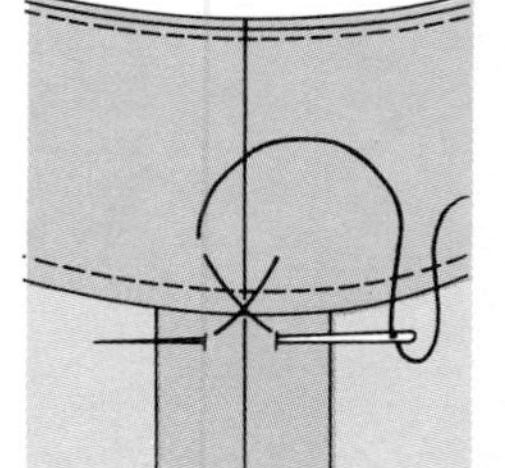
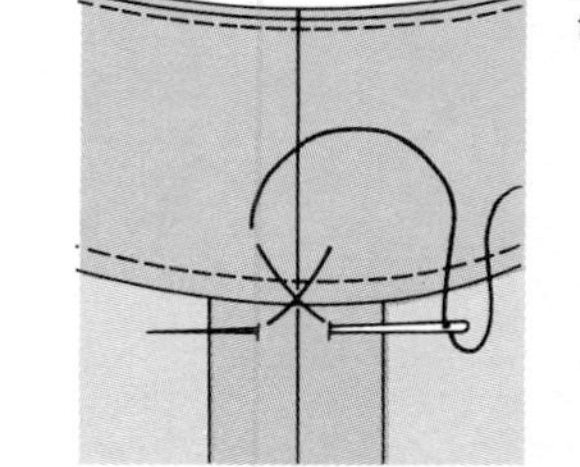
Cross-stitch tack

8. Press facing shoulder seams. With side seams aligned, tack the facing to garment seam allowances, using either a few closely spaced whipstitches or a cross-stitch tack. At zipper placket, slipstitch the turned-under facing ends to the zipper tapes. Attach fastener at top of placket.

Slipstitch (uneven) 132
Cutting and piecing bias strips 298-299

Centered zipper 318-319;
lapped 322-323; invisible 326-327

Constructing and applying a bias facing

A bias facing is a narrow rectangular strip of lightweight fabric, cut on the bias so that it can be shaped to conform to the curve of the edge it will be sewed to and finish. This shaping is done with the aid of a steam iron. For details, see Step 1. The bias facing is often used instead of a shaped facing on garments made of sheer or bulky fabrics. A conventional shaped facing, because of its width, might be too conspicuous on a garment made from sheer fabric; a shaped facing cut from garment fabric might be too bulky when the fabric is thick or heavy.

The finished width of a bias facing is generally from ½ to 1 inch. The *cut* width of the strip, however, must be twice the finished width plus two seam allowances. (The strip is folded in half lengthwise. The folding automatically gives the facing one finished edge.) The total length needed equals the length of the seamline of the edge being faced plus 2 inches for ease and finishing. It may be necessary to piece bias strips to obtain the required length.

The zipper should be inserted in the garment before applying a bias facing.

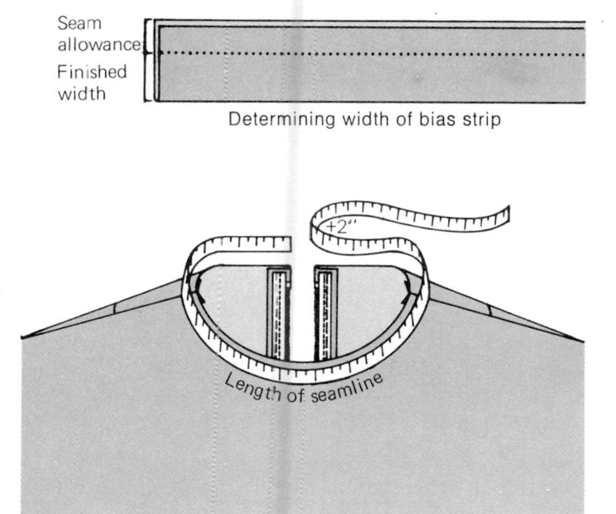

Determining width of bias strip

Determining length of bias strip

Length and width. Bias strip should be twice the desired finished width plus two seam allowances, each the same width as the garment seam allowance. Length equals length of edge being faced plus 2″ for ease and finishing.

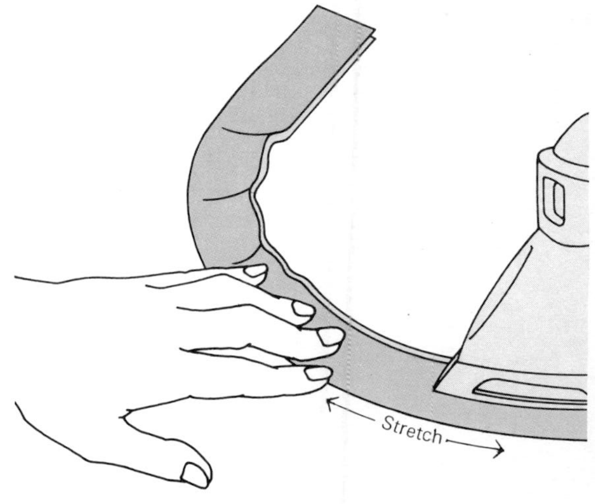

1. Cut out strip; fold it in half lengthwise. Using a steam iron, press strip flat. Shape by pressing again, stretching and curving folded edge to mold raw edges into curve that matches edge being faced. Keep raw edges even.

2. With all edges even, pin and baste facing to right side of garment. If edges of facing are slightly uneven from the shaping, trim and even them before pinning to garment. Stitch along seamline. Remove bastings and press.

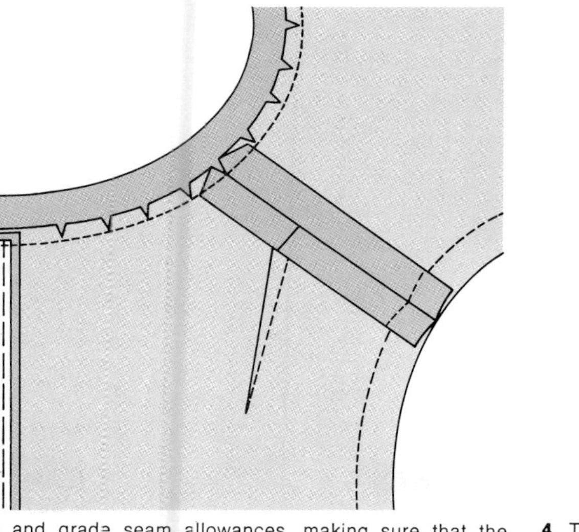

3. Trim and grade seam allowances, making sure that the garment seam allowance is the widest. Clip seam; trim ends of bias to ¼″. Extend facing up and away from garment and press along seamline. Fold ends of facing to inside.

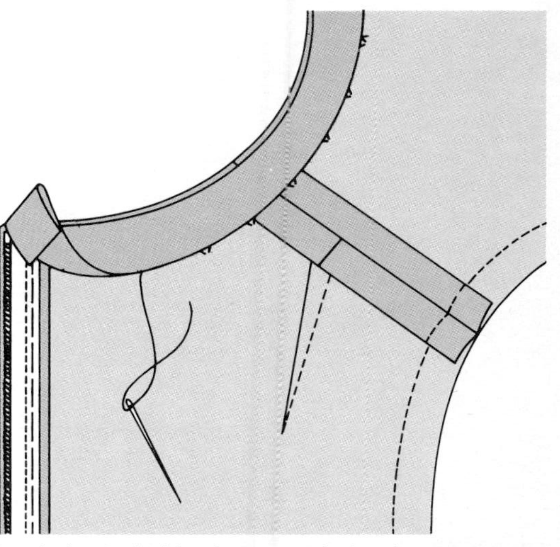

4. Turn facing to inside of garment, letting the seamline roll slightly beyond the edge. Pin in place along folded edge. Slipstitch edge and ends of facing to inside of garment. Remove pins. Press. Attach fastener at top of placket.

Neckline finishes

Corded seams 153
Bias strips 298-299
Making cording 300

Corded necklines

The application of cording, made from self or contrasting fabric, gives a decorative finish to a neckline edge. There are two application methods. The first, used most often, is to stitch the cording to the garment and then apply a separate facing. The second requires a specially constructed cording that is made with knit fabric and is a combination cording and facing. Another variable concerns the way the ends are finished; this will depend on whether or not the neckline has a placket opening. If cording is applied to a neckline that does not have a placket, the finished neckline must be large enough to slip easily over the head.

In most cases a narrow cord is used as filler for the cording, but a wider cord can be used. If a woven fabric is used to cover the cord, cut it on the bias; knit fabric can be cut crosswise or bias. If applying cording to a *neckline that will be faced,*

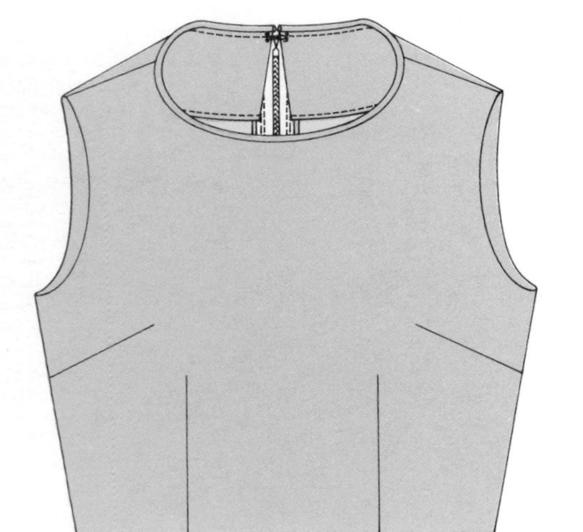

cut fabric for cording wide enough to encase the cord plus two seam allowances. When using the *special knit combination* cording and facing, cut the fabric wide enough to encase the cord plus 1 inch. The length of cording needed for any application, regardless of placket presence or absence, is the length of the neck seamline plus 1¼ inches. Before applying any cording, finish all garment details that fall within the neck seamline.

Application of cording to faced neckline

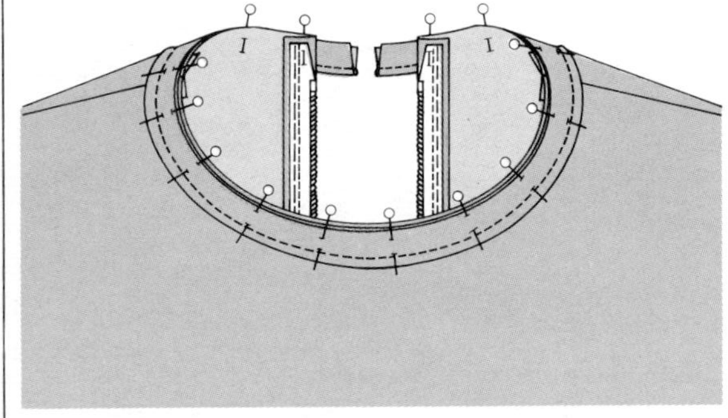

1. With zipper open, pin the cording to right side of garment, with cord just outside seamline and the cording stitch line just inside seamline. Leave excess cording at ends.

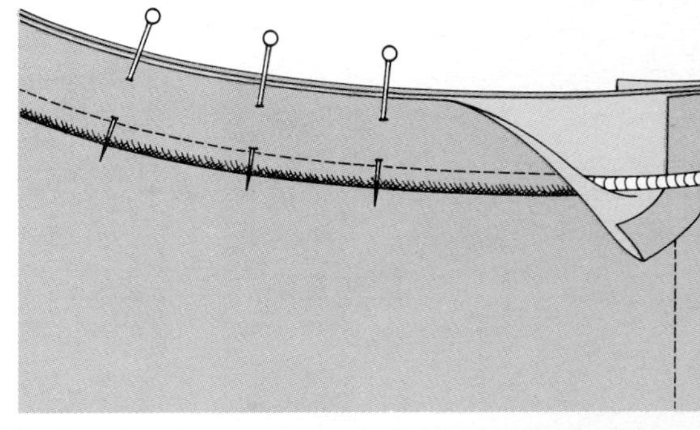

2. At ends, release enough of stitching holding cord to open fabric, then cut cord even with placket edges. Trim fabric ends to ¼"; fold in, even with cord; re-wrap around cord.

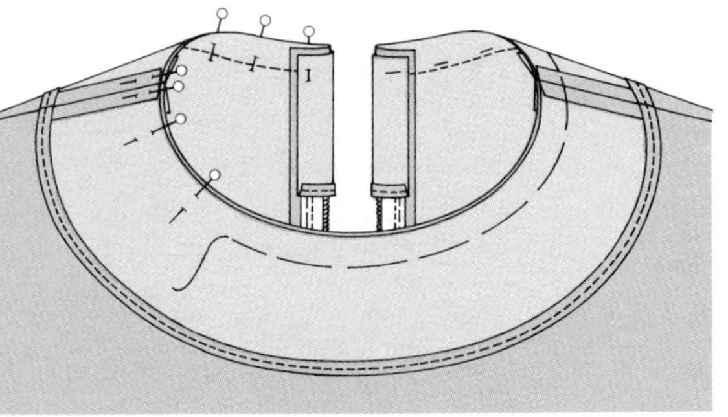

4. Remove bastings. Construct facing unit (p. 193). With right sides together, pin and baste facing to garment. Wrap ends of facing around zipper halves to inside of garment.

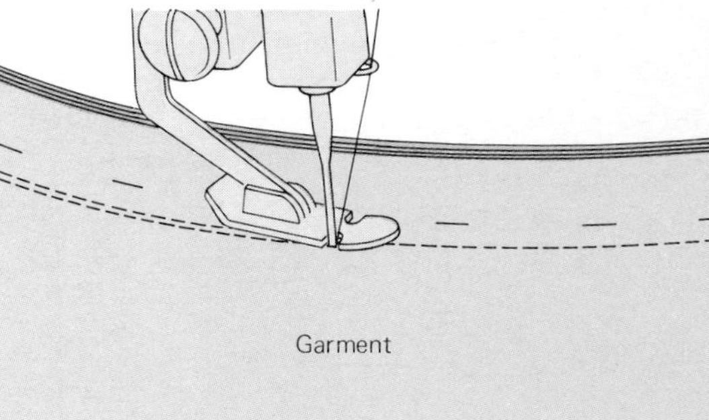

5. With wrong side of garment up, stitch facing to garment along seamline. Crowd stitching between cord and the row of stitching from Step 3. Secure thread ends. Remove bastings.

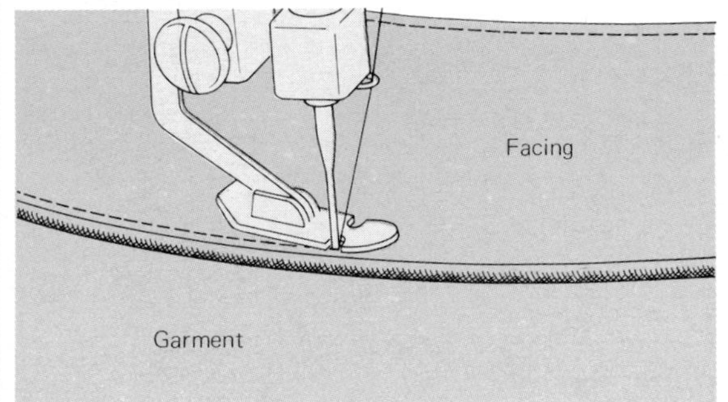

7. Extending facing and seam allowances away from garment, understitch along neck seamline. Use zipper foot; stitch from right side of facing, through all seam allowances.

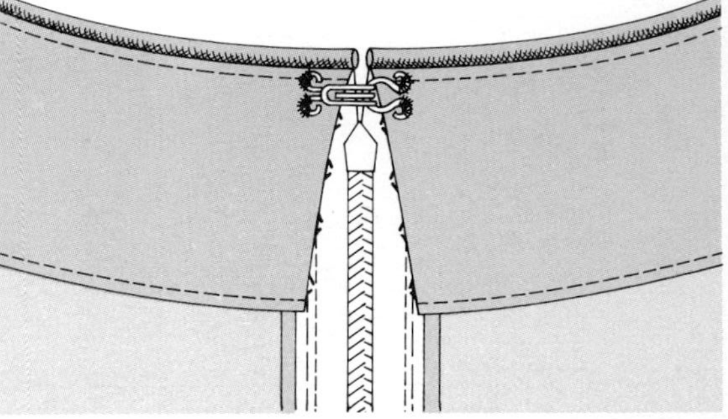

8. Turn facing to inside and press. Tack facing to garment at shoulders. Tack fabric at ends of cording closed. Slipstitch facing ends to zipper tapes. Attach fastener at top.

Slipstitch (uneven) 132
Trimming and grading seams 147
Seam finishes 148-149
Fasteners 354-357

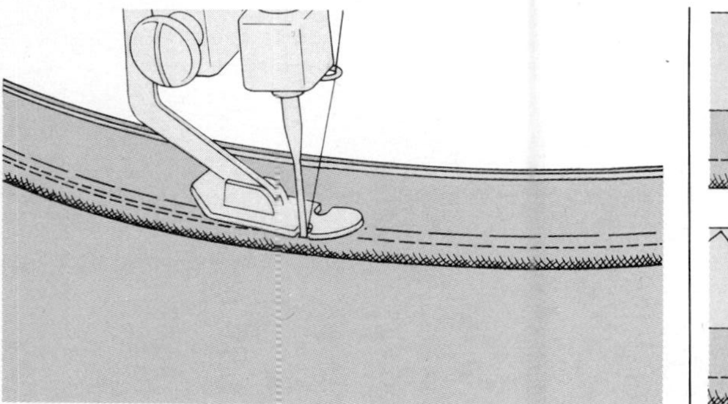

3. Baste cording to garment; remove pins. Using a zipper foot adjusted to right of needle, stitch cording to garment. Stitch between cord and the stitching encasing the cord.

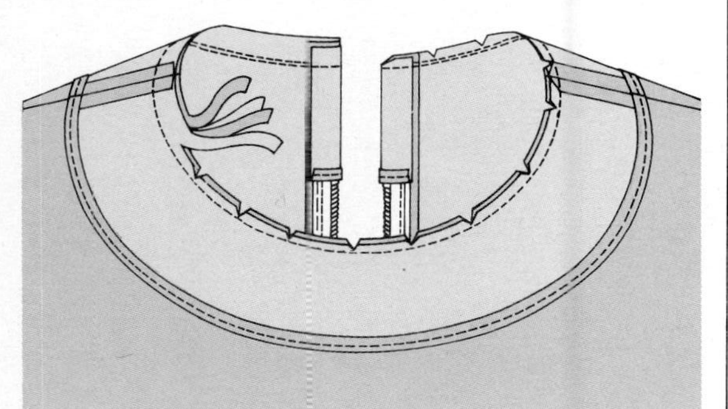

6. Press seam flat. Trim, grade, and clip the seam allowances. Trim diagonally at cross seams and corners. Press seam open, then press facing and seam allowances away from garment.

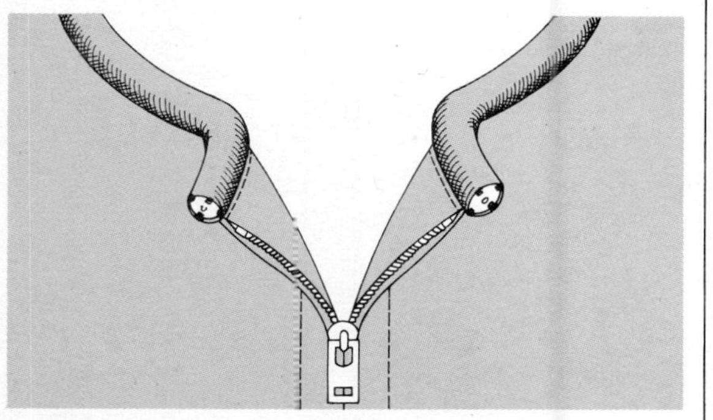

If heavy cord has been used, instead of tacking the fabric closed at ends, attach a large snap to ends of cording. This will serve as a finish and as a fastener for neckline as well.

Special application (knit cording)

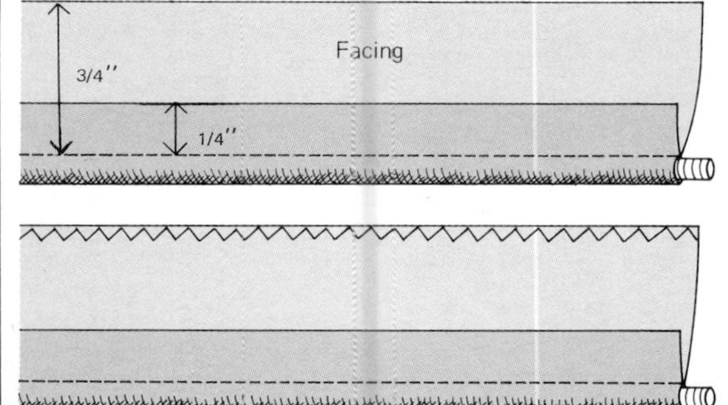

1. Wrap strip around cord as shown (for size of strip, see p. 200). Using a zipper foot, stitch close to cord. Seam-finish "facing" edge. Trim garment seam allowance to ¼".

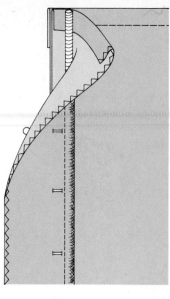

2. Pin the ¼"-wide side of cording to right side of garment, aligning its edge with garment edge, its stitch line along garment seamline. Treat ends as in Step 2, opposite page.

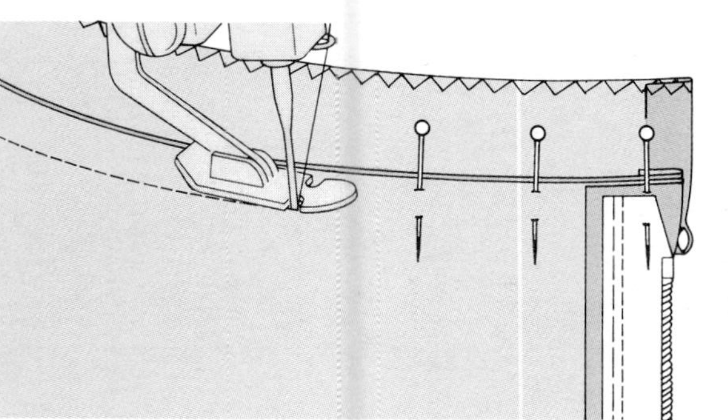

3. With wrong side of garment up, and the zipper foot adjusted to right of needle, stitch cording to garment on the ¼" seamline. Remove pins as you stitch.

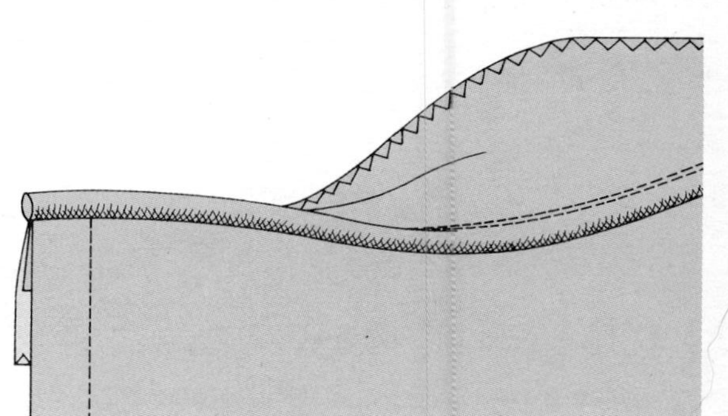

4. Turn cording to inside of garment; press. Sew fabric closed at ends of cording. Tack cording to garment at shoulders and zipper; attach fastener.

Cording necklines without plackets

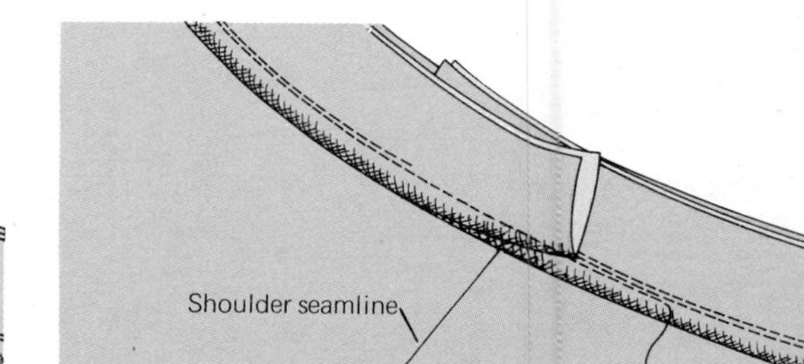

To cord a neckline with no placket opening, apply cording as required by its type, but allow the ends to overlap at a shoulder seamline. Release stitching at each end and trim cord to shoulder seamline. Overlap ends, easing empty part of casing away from seamline. Stitch across ends through all layers. Turn cording to inside and tack.

Neckline finishes

Bound and banded necklines

The illustrations below are designed to show how finished bound and banded necklines differ from each other and from a plain faced neckline. The essential difference lies in where the upper edge of the finish falls; this is dictated by where and in what manner the finish is stitched to the neckline.

Supposing all four necklines were based on the same simple jewel neckline, as these are, the *uppermost edge* of the **faced, bound** and **shaped-band** necklines would be at the same level; the *seamline* of the **strip band** would be at this level, but its uppermost edge would be above. With a plain **faced** neckline, the facing is stitched to the neck seamline, which becomes the finished edge when the facing is turned to the inside. With a **bound** neckline, the original seam allowance is trimmed from the garment, permitting the binding to be attached some distance away and its upper edge ultimately to fall where the original seamline was. **A shaped band** is an additional, but integral, part of the garment; its upper edge forms the finished neckline edge without changing the location. A **strip band** is an extension above the original neckline, very much like most collars are.

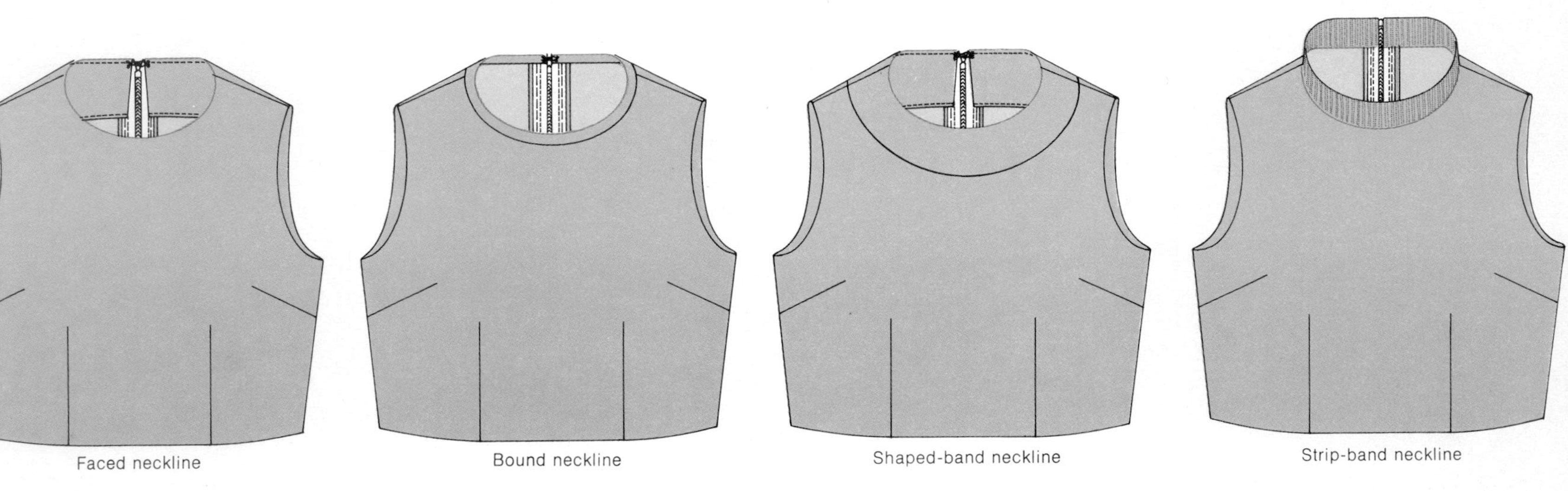
Faced neckline
Bound neckline
Shaped-band neckline
Strip-band neckline

Bound necklines

A neck edge can be finished by binding it with a strip of self or contrasting fabric. The finished width of the binding, which should be no more than 1 inch, is the same as the width of the seam allowances used in application. If finished width is to be 1 inch, the seam allowances are also 1 inch, which places the seamline 1 inch below the cut edge. **If pattern is not designed for binding,** cut away the original seam allowance so that the top edge of the bound neckline finish will fall along the original seamline. The actual width of the strip will depend on whether it is to be a *single- or double-layer binding*. The **length needed** is the length of the seamline plus 2 inches. Cut strip on the grain with the most stretch—bias for woven fabrics, crosswise for knits.

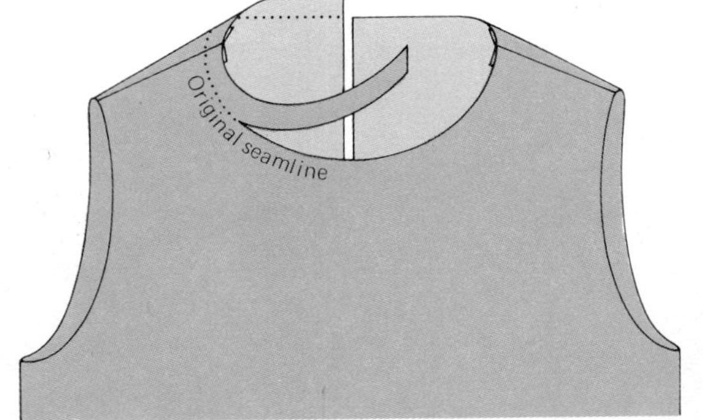

If your pattern is not designed for a bound neckline finish, trim away the seam allowance. This permits the top edge of the finished neckline to fall along the original *seamline*.

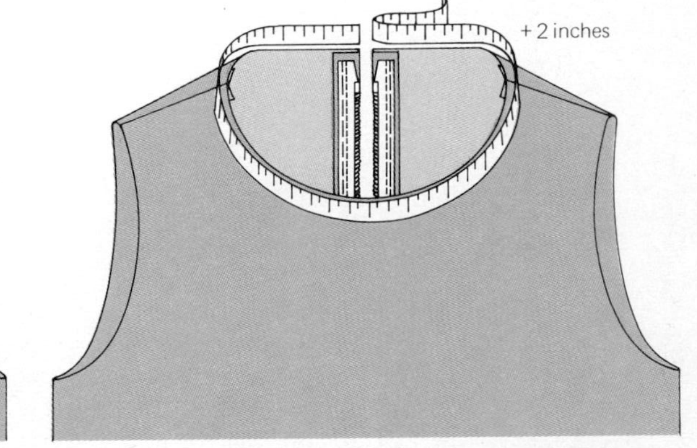

The length of the binding strip equals the length of the garment seamline plus 2″ for ease and for finishing the ends. Take this measurement after the zipper has been inserted.

Slipstitch (uneven) 132
Fasteners 354-355

Applying a single-layer binding

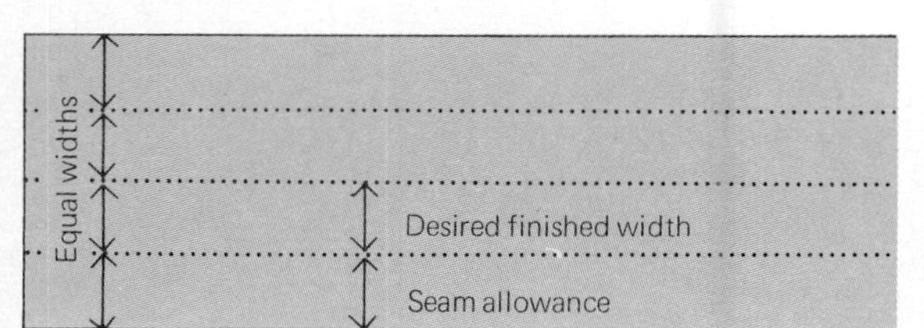

1. For a single-layer binding, cut strip four times the desired finished width and the length of the neck seamline plus 2". Have seam allowance widths the same as finished width.

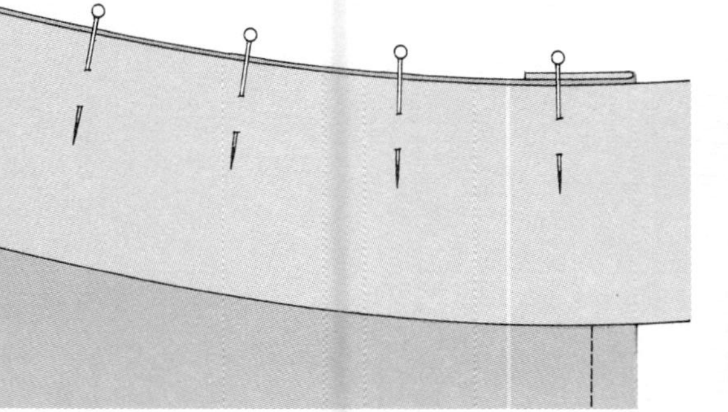

2. Open zipper. With right sides together and edges even, pin the binding to the garment along the seamline. Stretch binding if necessary to fit smoothly around curves.

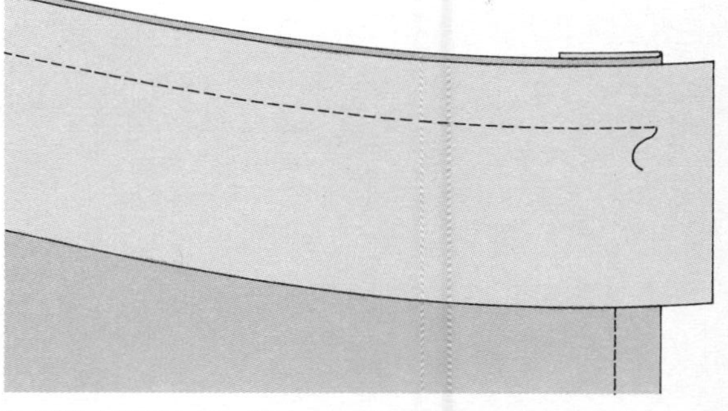

3. With binding up, stitch to garment along the seamline, removing pins as you stitch. Secure thread ends. Press flat. Trim excess binding at ends to ½".

4. Fold ends of binding back, even with placket edges. Trim across corners and cross-seam allowances. Bring binding up over the seam allowances to inside of garment. Press.

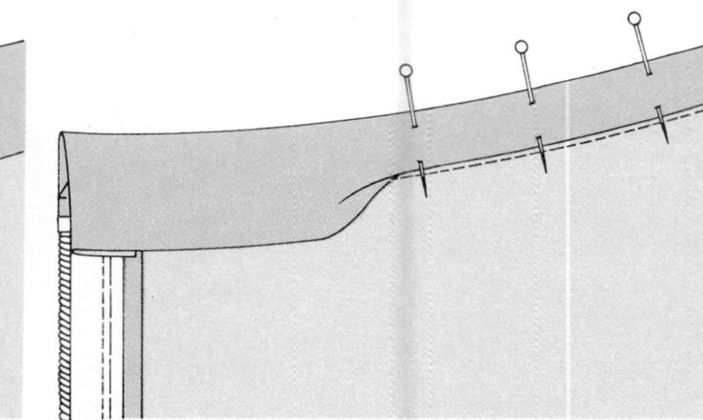

5. If binding strip is made of a **woven** fabric, turn under the raw edge along the seamline. Press with fingers to shape the binding to the curve; pin in place.

If it is a **knit** binding, let the raw edge lie flat, extending to the inside of the garment. Pin binding in place, but from the *right side,* through all thicknesses, along seamline.

6. With bindings of **woven** fabric, slipstitch ends of binding closed. Slipstitch folded edge to garment along entire neck seamline. Stitches should not show to right side.

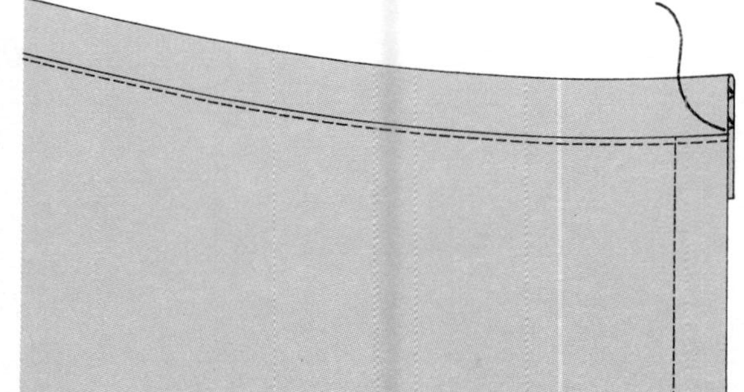

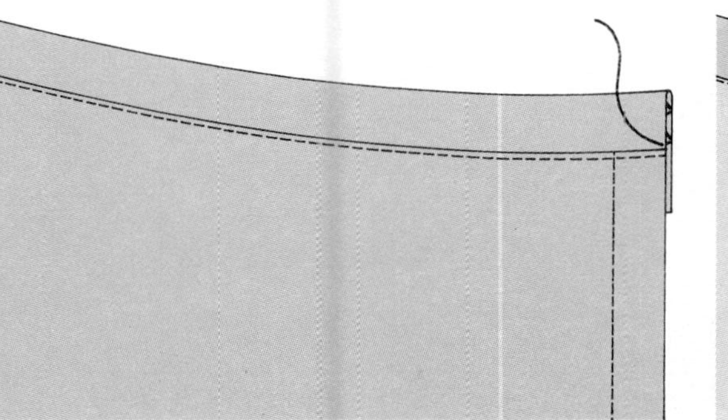

On **knit** bindings, slipstitch ends closed. Then, from right side of garment, stitch in seam groove through all thicknesses; remove pins as you stitch. Trim off excess binding.

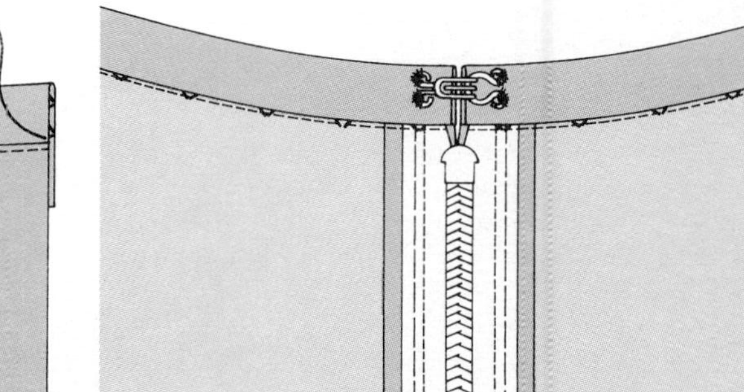

7. From inside, press the neck edge. Close zipper and attach a hook and round eye to binding ends. The ends of the binding should meet when hook and eye are fastened.

Neckline finishes

Pressing 18-19 Slipstitch (uneven) 132
Fasteners 354-355

Applying a double-layer binding

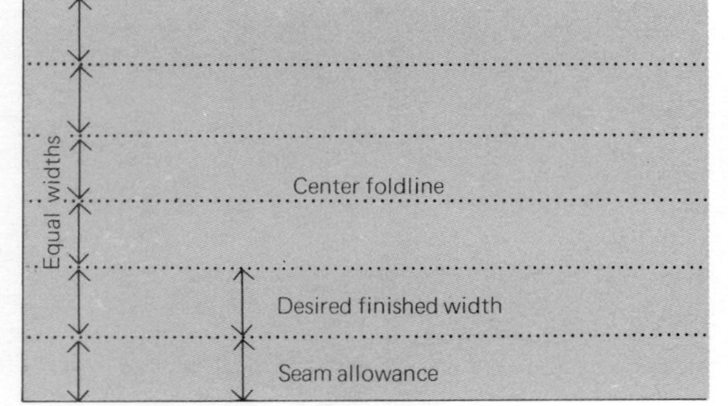

1. For a double-layer binding, cut the strip six times the desired finished width and the length of neck seamline plus 2". Have seam allowance widths the same as finished width.

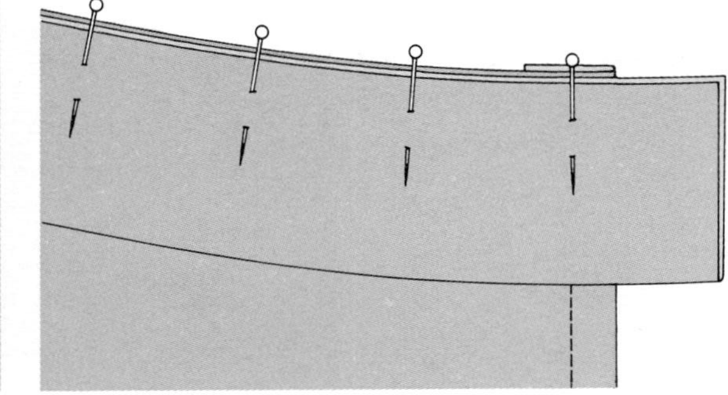

2. Open zipper. Wrong sides together, fold binding strip in half lengthwise. Keeping all edges even, pin to garment along seamline. Stretch binding to fit around curves.

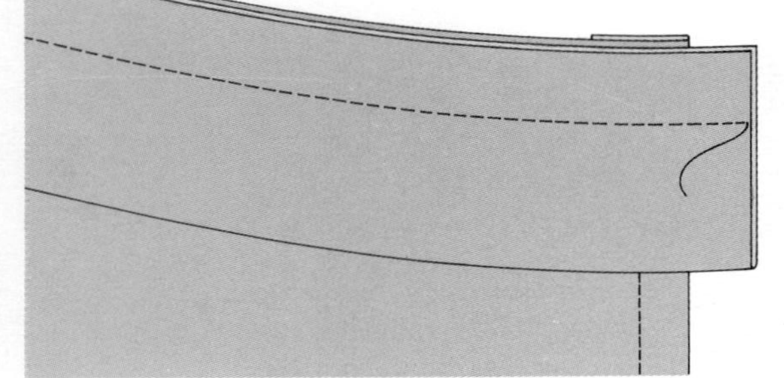

3. With binding up, stitch to garment along the seamline, removing pins as you stitch. Secure thread ends. Press flat. Trim excess binding at ends to ½".

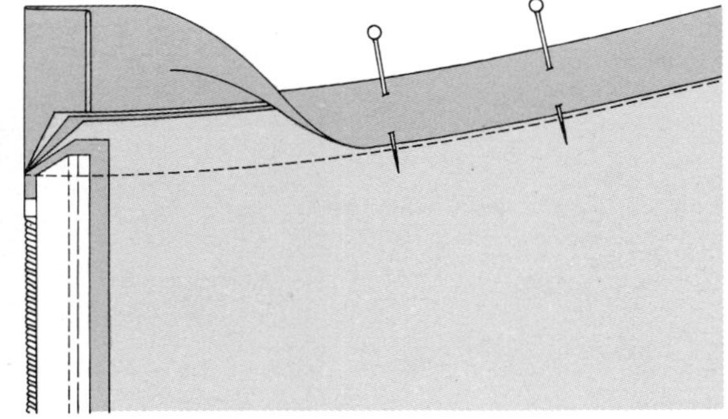

4. Fold ends of binding back, even with placket edges. Trim across corners and cross-seam allowances. Bring binding up over seam allowances to inside of garment. Pin in place.

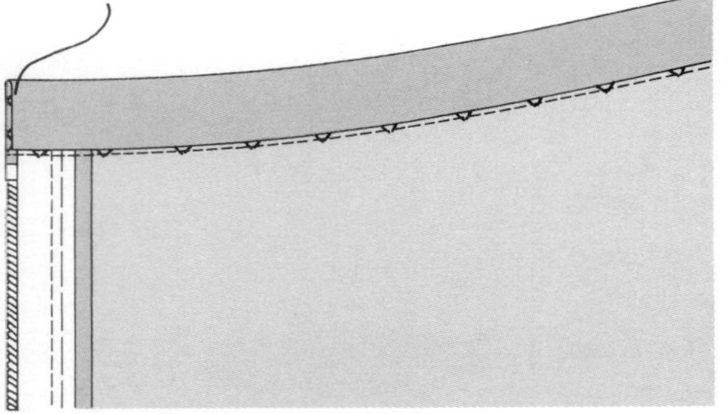

5. Slipstitch ends of binding closed. Then slipstitch the folded edge of binding to garment along the entire neck seamline. Stitches should not show to right side of garment.

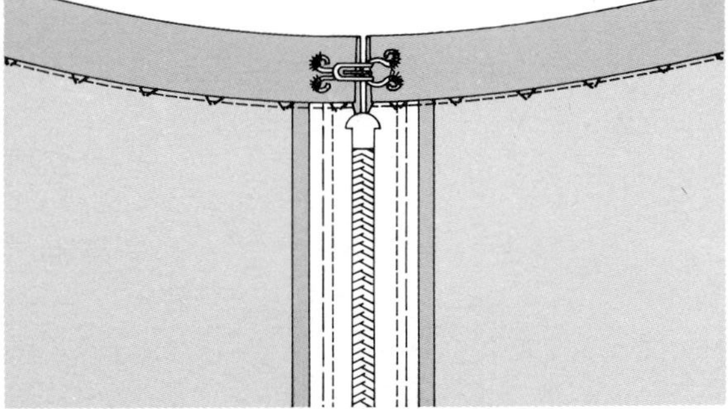

6. From the inside, press the neck edge. Close zipper and attach a hook and round eye to binding ends. The ends of the binding should meet when hook and eye are fastened.

Binding a neckline without placket

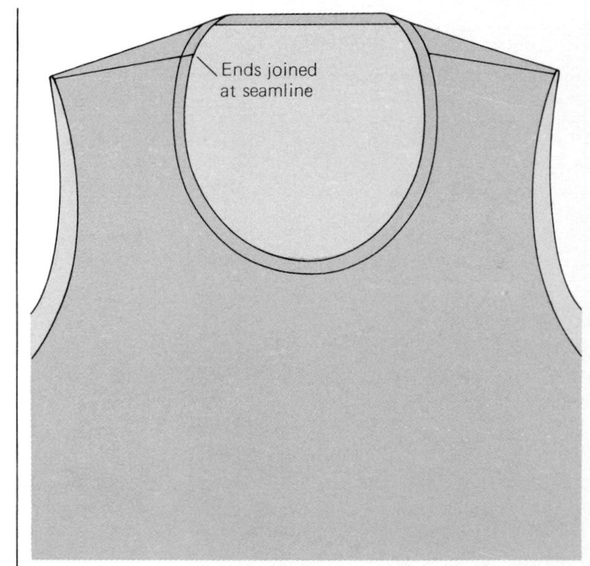

Single- or double-layer binding may be used. The only difference from the basic applications is in the handling of the ends, and that they be joined at a garment seamline.

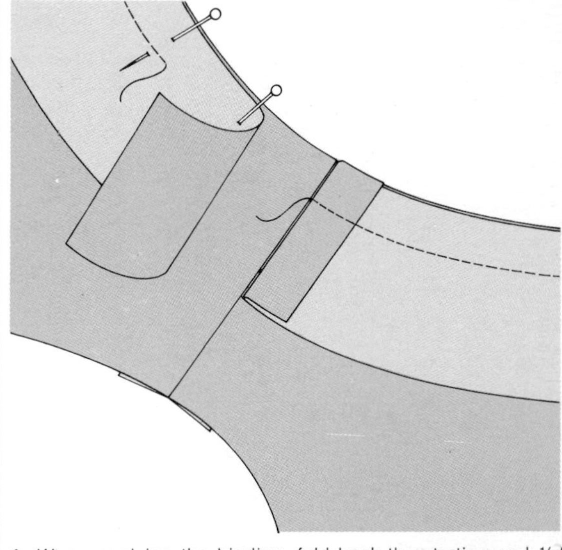

1. When applying the binding, fold back the starting end ½" and align the fold with the garment seamline. Pin binding in place and stitch to within 3" of starting point.

Prepackaged binding

Some prepackaged tapes can be used to bind neckline edges. The two most often used for this are **double-fold tape** and **fold-over braid.** Both have finished edges. Also, both are folded off-center so that, when positioned properly, both edges will be caught in the same stitching. These tapes can also be preshaped to match the curve they will be applied to. Other prepackaged tapes can also be used, provided they have finished edges, are folded off-center, and can be satisfactorily shaped.

When **shaping tape** to fit an inward curve, which necklines generally are, stretch the open edges while easing in the folded edge. To shape an outward curve, do the reverse: stretch the fold while easing in the open edges.

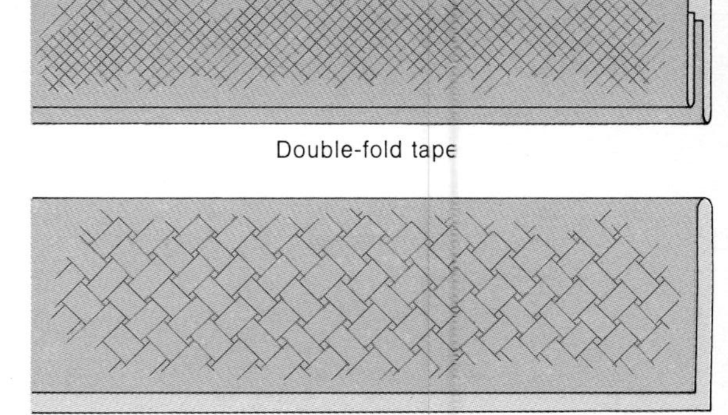

Double-fold tape

Fold-over braid

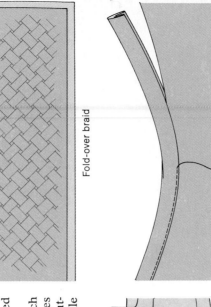

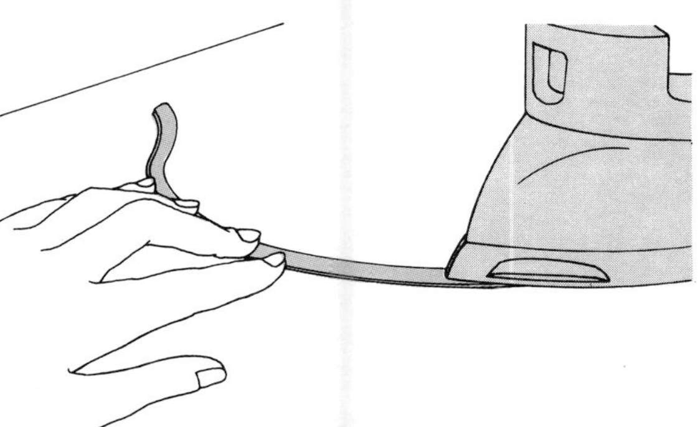

1. These bindings should be shaped to match the curve of the neck edge before application to garment. With your hand and a steam iron, mold the binding into the proper curve.

2. Wrap shaped binding around neck edge with wider half to inside of garment and the fold along the neck edge. Topstitch along outer edge of narrower half, handling ends as below.

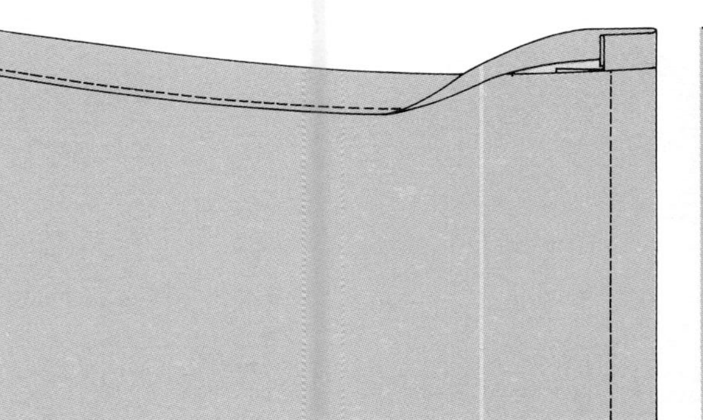

If neckline has a placket opening, fold ends back even with edges of placket. Then topstitch binding to neckline and attach fastener at ends (see Step 6, opposite page).

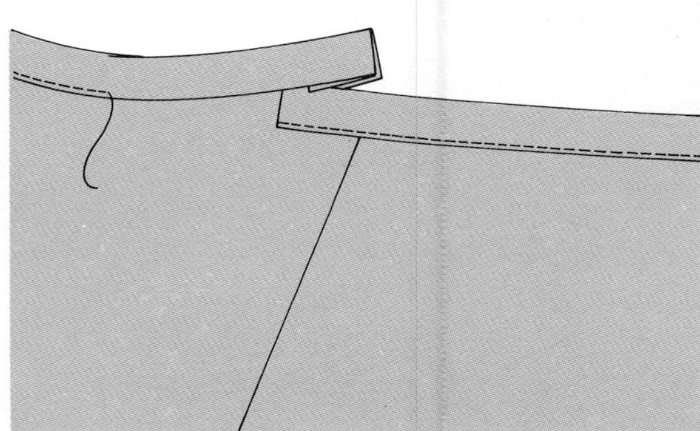

If there is no placket, place the starting end ½″ ahead of a garment seamline. Stitch to within 3″ of start. Fold second end under to align with seamline, and complete stitching.

2. Trim away excess binding at this end to ½″ beyond fold of starting end. Lap this end over the beginning fold and stitch the rest of the way across, through all thicknesses.

3. When the binding is turned up, the end folded first will be on top. Slipstitch ends together as they lie. Finish according to binding type (single- or double-layer).

Neckline finishes

Shaped bands and strip bands

Another way to finish a neckline is with a separate fabric band. The two basic types are the **shaped band** and the **strip band.** The shaped band, which is cut to a precise shape according to a pattern, has two main parts: the band and its facing (sometimes an extended facing). The strip band is a strip of fabric folded in half lengthwise; it is shaped to conform to the neckline curve either before or during application. Suitable only for knit fabrics with stretch, how a strip band is applied depends on the amount of stretch in the fabric and also on the size of the neckline (see pp. 208–209).

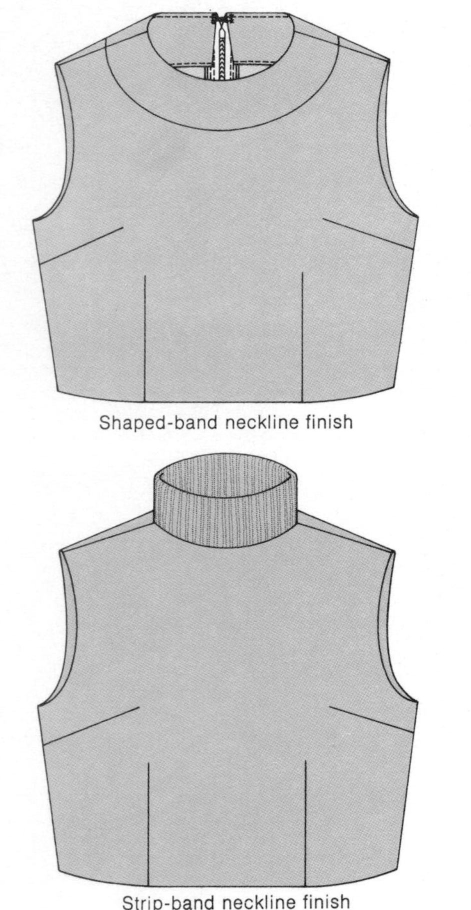

Shaped-band neckline finish

Strip-band neckline finish

Shaped-band neckline finish

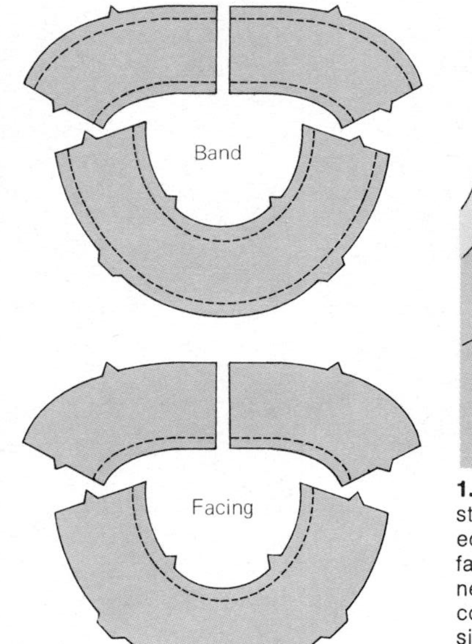

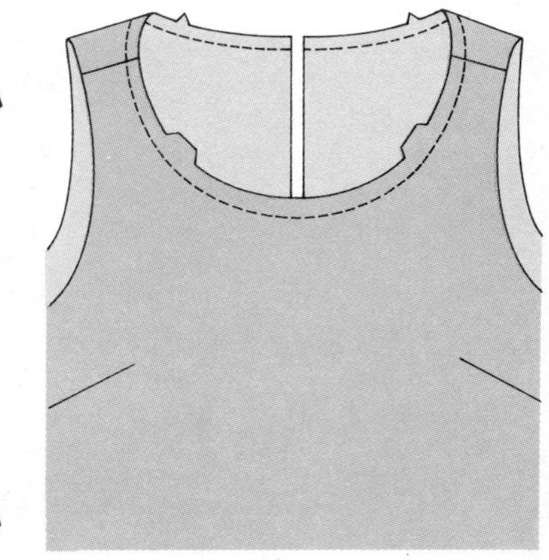

1. To help maintain their shapes, apply staystitching along the neck and outer edges of the band, the neck edge of the facing, and the top edge of garment. If neckline is a V or square, reinforce the corners with short stitches for 1″ on both sides of corners, then clip into the corners. Do not insert zipper.

2. Select an interfacing appropriate to the garment fabric and apply it to the band. Interfacing illustrated is a fusible. With right sides together, match and then seam the band sections to form complete band. Press seams flat, then open. Trim seam allowances to half-width. Construct facing unit as described on page 193.

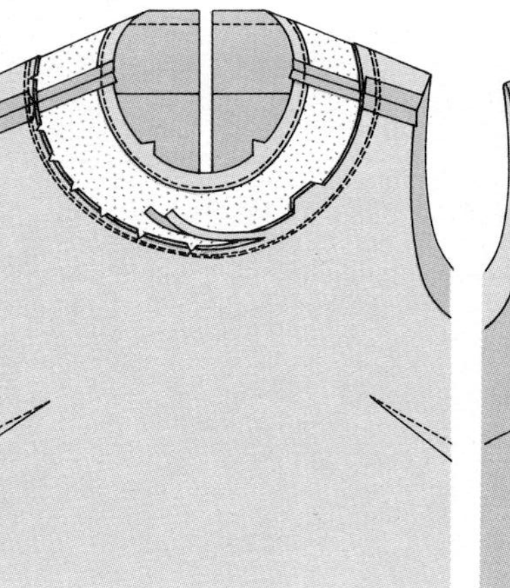

3. With right sides together, matching all markings, notches, and cross seamlines, pin and baste the band to the garment. Stitch along seamline. Remove the bastings and press seam flat. Trim, grade, and notch the seam allowances. Press the seam open; then press the seam allowances and the band up, away from the rest of the garment.

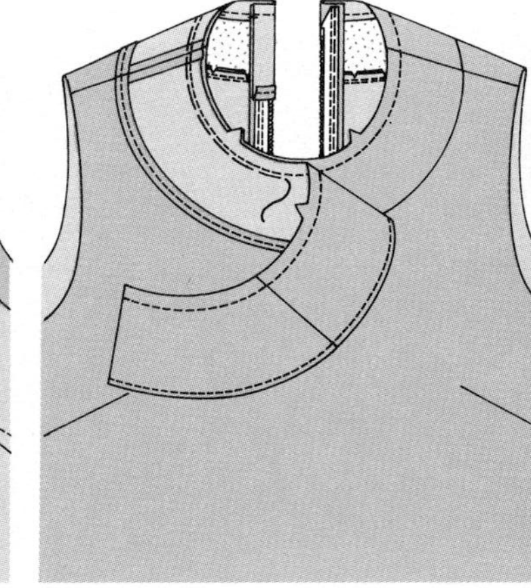

4. Insert the zipper, positioning the top stop ½″ below neck seamline, being sure to match the cross seams within the placket. Open zipper. With right sides together, and matching all markings, notches, and seamlines, pin and baste the facing to the band along neck edge. Stitch. Remove bastings and press the seam flat.

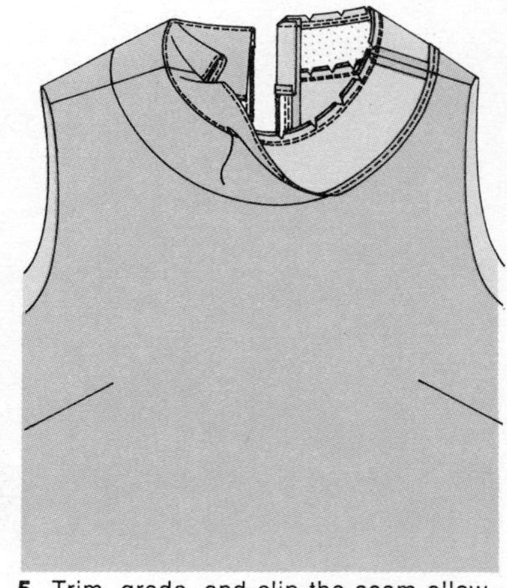

5. Trim, grade, and clip the seam allowances. Press seam open, then press seam allowances and facing away from garment. With facing right side up, understitch along seamline through all layers. Turn facing to inside; secure it to garment at shoulder seams and slipstitch the ends of facing to zipper tapes. Attach appropriate fastener at top.

Placket bands

The **placket band** is a variation of the shaped band, in that it is cut from a pattern and applied in a similar way. Both a type of garment opening and its finish as well, it is most often straight, which permits both the band and its facing to be cut out as one piece. Such a facing is an extended facing.

Sometimes the unit will be a **combination neck and placket band,** as in the second illustration below. When this is the case, it is applied by a combination of techniques from those used for the neckline shaped band, on the opposite page, and the placket band, shown and explained at the right.

Straight placket band

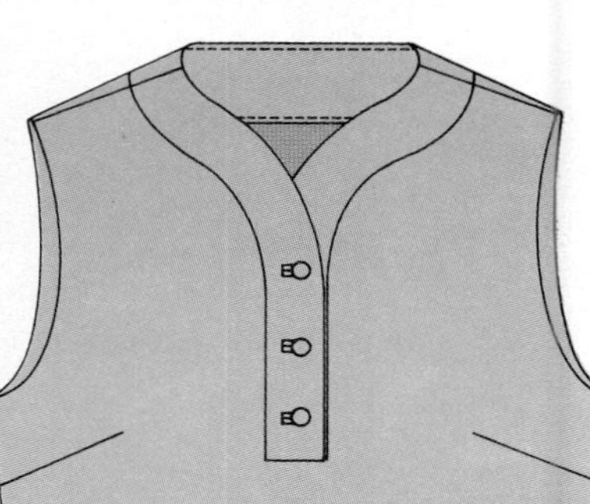

Combination neck and placket band

Straight placket band

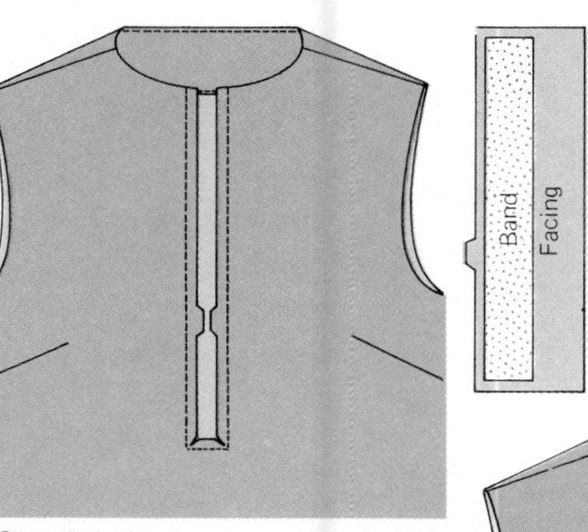

1. Staystitch the opening a thread width from the seamline, using shorter, reinforcement stitches at corners and across the bottom. Clip into corners.

2. Apply interfacing to wrong side of each placket band. Placket band illustrated is interfaced with a fusible interfacing; facing is an extended facing. If bound buttonholes are planned, construct them in the right-hand placket band at this point.

3. For each band, fold right side of band to right side of facing. Pin and baste along upper edge, then stitch across tc intersecting seamline. Press seam flat as stitched. Trim and grade seam; trim diagonally across corner. Press seam open.

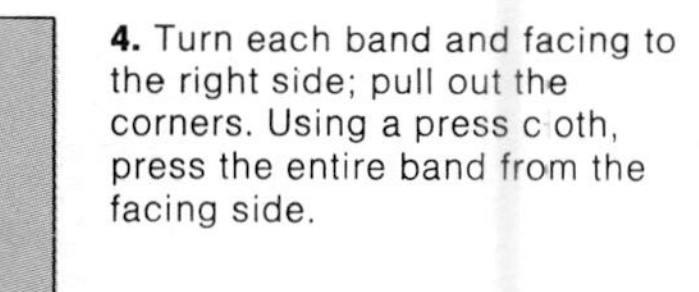

4. Turn each band and facing to the right side; pull out the corners. Using a press cloth, press the entire band from the facing side.

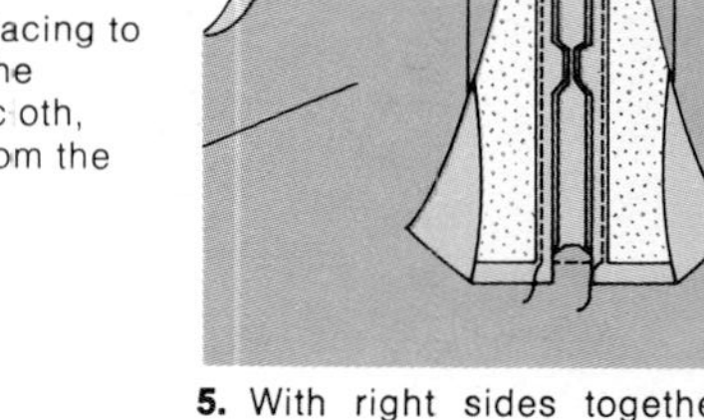

5. With right sides together, matching markings, notches, and seamlines, pin and baste each band to the garment. With band side up, stitch in place. Press.

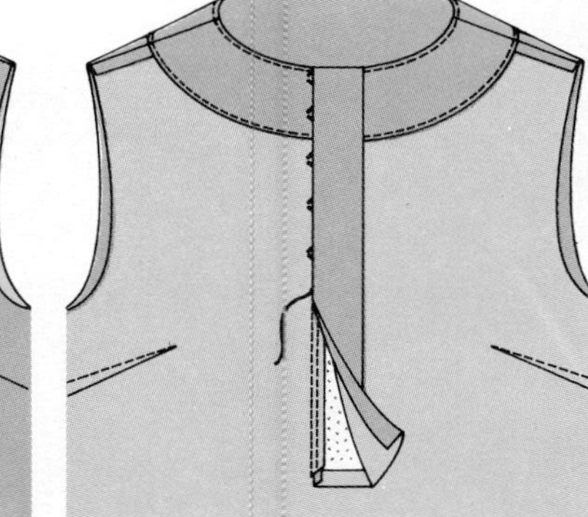

6. Trim and grade seam allowances. Press seams open, then toward bands. Finish backs of bound buttonholes. Turn under edge on each facing; slipstitch to band.

7. With right sides together, match, pin, and stitch lower edge of left-hand band to garment at end of placket. Press seam flat, then downward.

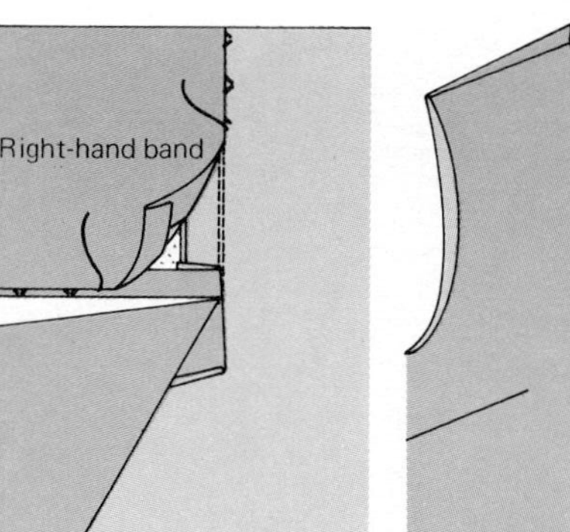

8. At lower end of right-hand band, trim and turn in seam allowances; slipstitch them together. Press flat. Apply machine buttonholes now if they are being used.

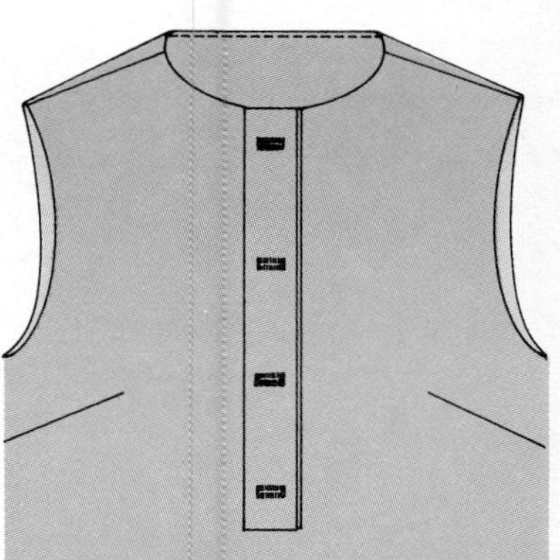

9. Match center lines and lap right-hand band over left. Sew buttons to left band.

Neckline finishes

Strip bands

Strip bands are a suitable neckline finish only for knit fabrics that stretch. In recognition of the wide variations in the stretchiness of knits, two application techniques have been devised. The first is for knits with **limited stretch,** e.g., most double knits; the second is for **very stretchy** knits, such as sweater knits. Bands cut from slightly stretchy (limited stretch) knits are shaped to match the curve of the neck *before* being applied. If the neckline is high, it may be necessary to insert a zipper (see pp. 210–211). If it is a wide or low neckline that allows enough leeway for the garment to be easily put on or taken off, as the elongated neckline at right would do, a zipper is not needed. Stretchy knit bands, which are ideal for higher necklines, are shaped to the neck edge *during* application. In these cases, a zipper is optional.

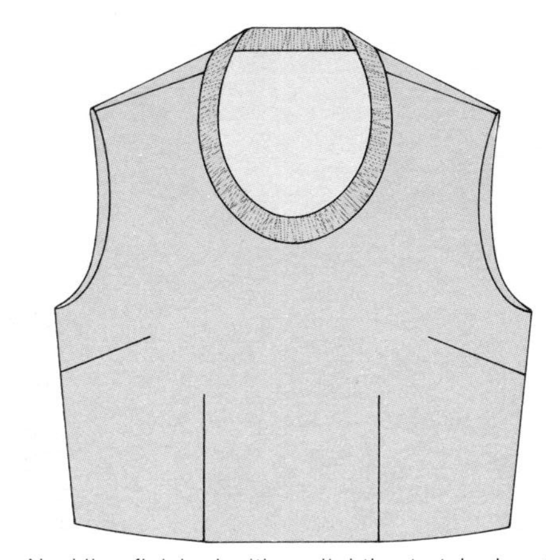
Neckline finished with a slightly stretchy band

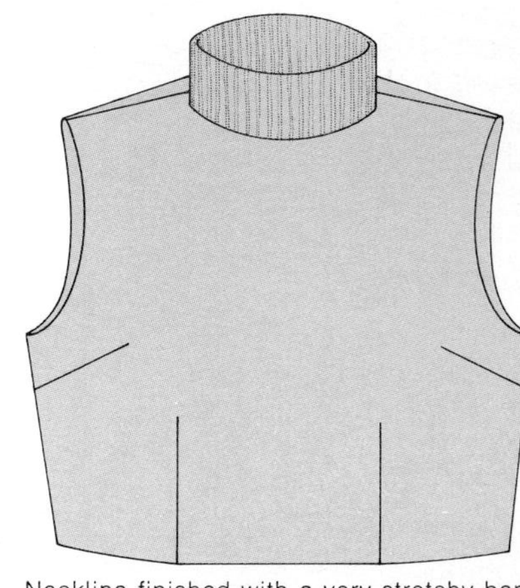
Neckline finished with a very stretchy band

Basic application of a limited-stretch strip band

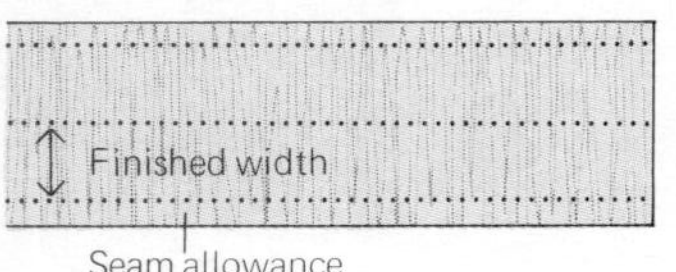

1. Cut strip twice the desired finished width plus two seam allowances. Length is equal to the length of neckline seam plus two seam allowances. Cut on crosswise grain.

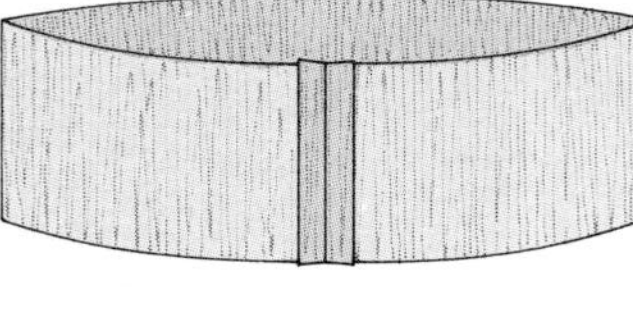
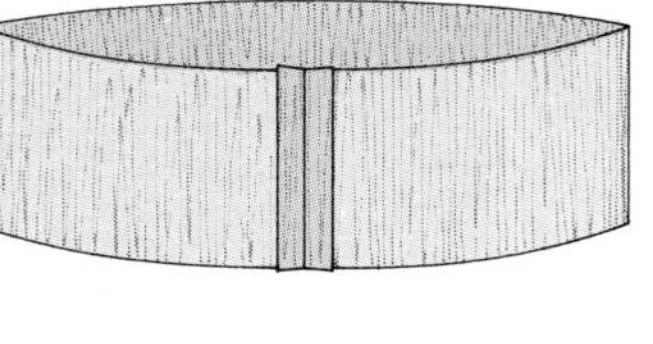

2. Form a closed circle by seaming ends of band together. Trim and press open. An overedge seam can also be used. Form all bodice seams that intersect the neckline.

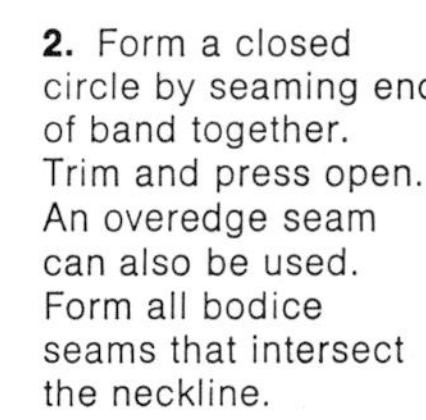
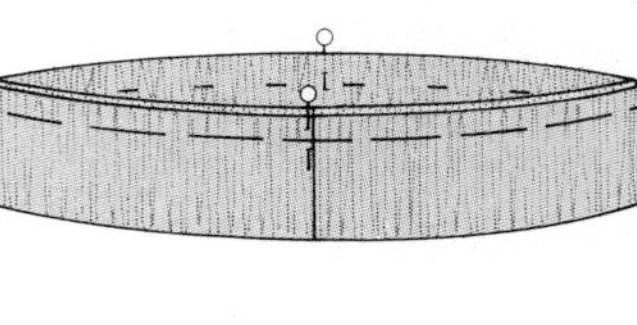

3. Fold strip in half lengthwise, with its wrong sides together and edges even. Baste edges together. Pin-mark center back (the seam) and center front (at opposite halfway point in band).

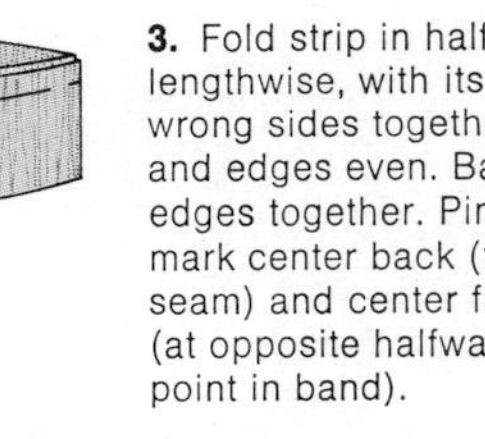

4. On a piece of muslin or heavy paper, draw exact shape of the entire neckline seam. Mark on it center front and back. Pin this guide to ironing board.

5. Pin band to guide, matching center front and back markings. Shape band so that curve of its neck seamline matches drawn guideline. Shape with the aid of a steam iron, stretching the cut edges and allowing the folded edge to ease itself into shape. Pin in place while shaping. Allow band to dry before removing it. If shine develops on top surface, use this side as underside. Remove bastings.

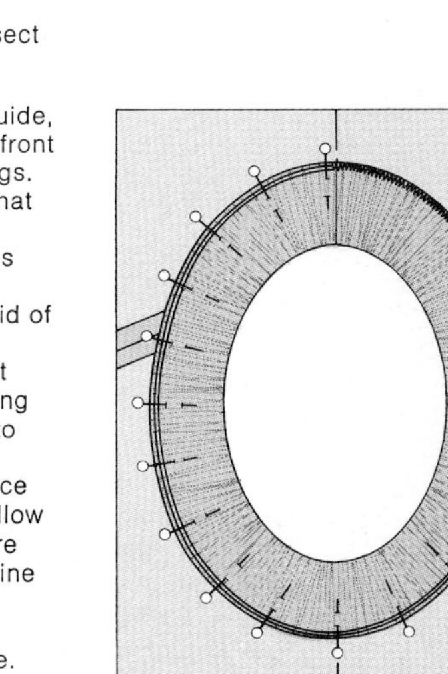
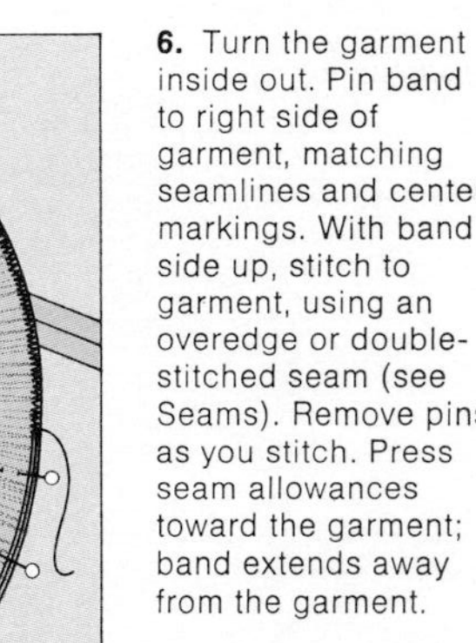

6. Turn the garment inside out. Pin band to right side of garment, matching seamlines and center markings. With band side up, stitch to garment, using an overedge or double-stitched seam (see Seams). Remove pins as you stitch. Press seam allowances toward the garment; band extends away from the garment.

Ribbing 17
Overedge seams 151

Stretchy strip bands

A stretchy knit strip band can be cut from the same fabric as the garment or cut from a purchased banding called "ribbing." Ribbing is a stretchy knit fabric that is sold either by the yard or in packaged quantities cut and finished to a specific width. Whichever you choose, the knit should be stretchy but have the ability to recover (return to its original shape after having been stretched). Most typical of the necklines to which stretchy bands can be applied successfully are the **crew neck,** the **mock turtleneck,** and the **turtleneck.** The width of the band will be determined by the neckline type. Examples of suitable finished widths are 1 inch for a crew neck, 2 inches for a mock turtleneck, and 4 inches for a turtleneck (2 inches when it is turned back on itself). Most prepackaged ribbings are a precise width and can be used only at that width. If you are cutting the band yourself, cut it twice the finished width plus two seam allowances. Then fold it in half lengthwise, producing one finished edge. The length of the band is determined by (1) the stretch and recovery capabilities of the knit; (2) measurements at the parts of the body it must first pass over and then fit snugly (that is, it must slip over the head but hug the neck); (3) the tension required for a suitably close fit during wear.

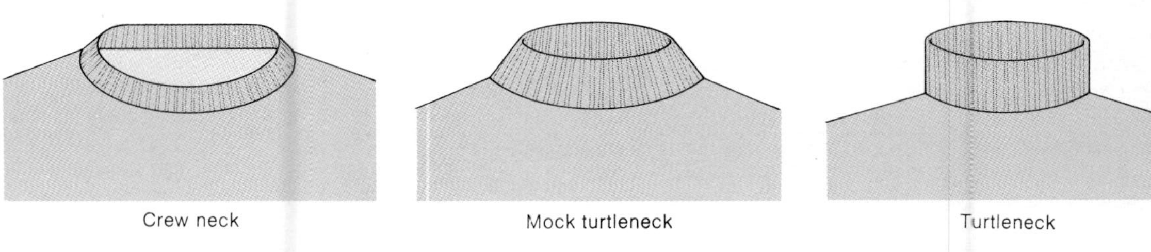
Crew neck
Mock turtleneck
Turtleneck

To give an example, a turtleneck band applied to a neckline without a zipper must have the right combination of stretch and recovery, and be of sufficient length, to pass over the head, yet hug the neck when worn. Generally such a band is cut from 2 to 4 inches shorter than the neck seamline. If the neckline has a zipper opening, the band can be very nearly the same length as the neckline because it will only have to hug the neck.

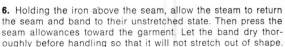

Basic application of a stretchy strip band

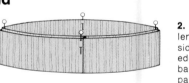

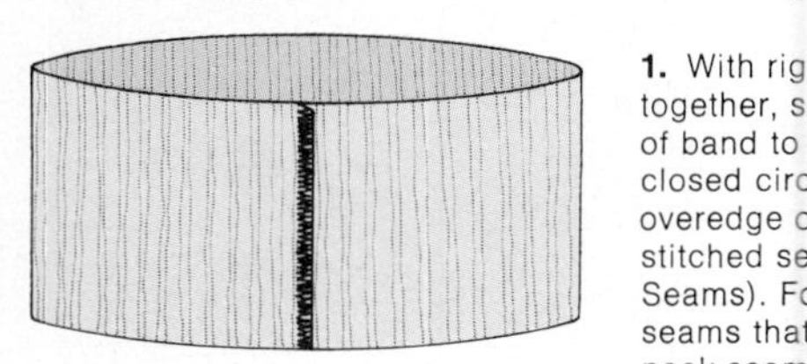
1. With right sides together, seam ends of band to form a closed circle. Use overedge or double-stitched seam (see Seams). Form bodice seams that intersect neck seamline.

2. Fold band in half lengthwise, wrong sides together and edges even. Divide the band into four equal parts; mark with pins. One mark, the center back, is at the seam formed in Step 1.

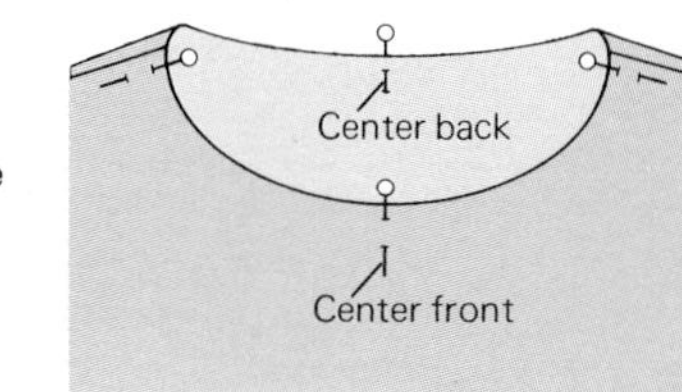

3. To ensure equal distribution of band over garment edge, divide the garment's neckline into four equal parts. Two marks are at center front and back, others are halfway between.

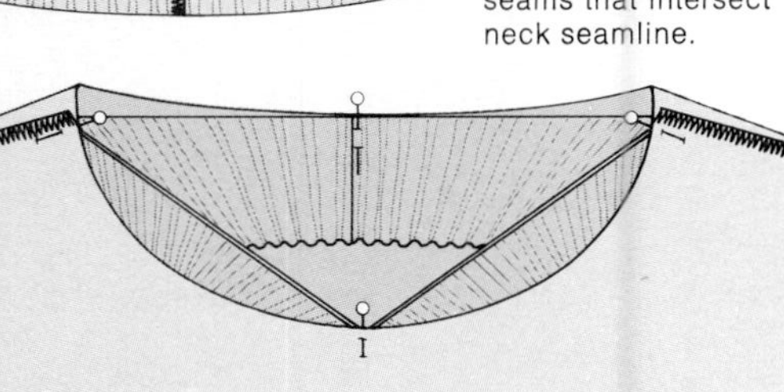
4. Turn the garment inside out. Place band to right side of garment, matching pin marks and neck seams. Stretch band to fit garment neckline; pin in place. Take care to keep raw edges of band and garment even.

5. With band side up, stitch band to garment, using either an overedge or double-stitched seam (see Seams). Stretch the band so that it lies flat against the garment's edge; do not stretch the garment. Remove pins as you stitch.

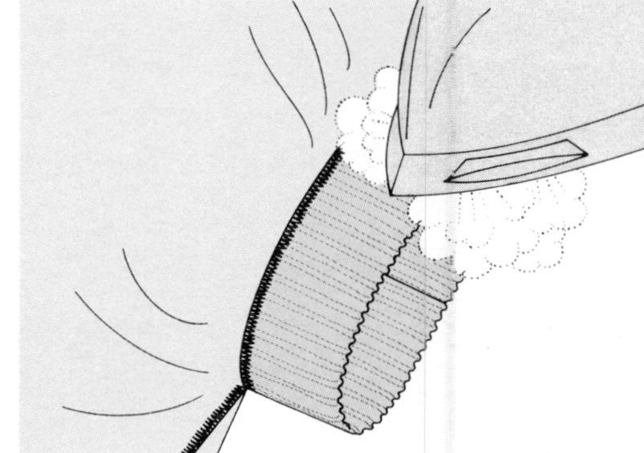
6. Holding the iron above the seam, allow the steam to return the seam and band to their unstretched state. Then press the seam allowances toward the garment. Let the band dry thoroughly before handling so that it will not stretch out of shape.

Neckline finishes

Zippers in strip-band necklines

If necessary, a zipper can be added to a strip-band neckline. This is done by applying the band to the garment, according to the type of fabric it is cut from, while making allowances for the insertion of the zipper. Follow one of the band applications from pages 208–209, but allow for the exceptions explained in the zipper methods on these two pages. Techniques described here will place the zipper between the two layers of the band. If you use a single-layer prepackaged ribbing, the top of the zipper is finished differently. Use the exposed zipper method if garment has no placket seam; centered zipper method if there is a seam.

Exposed zipper application

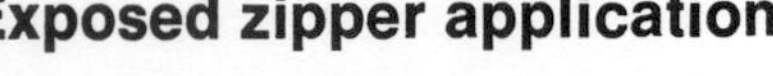

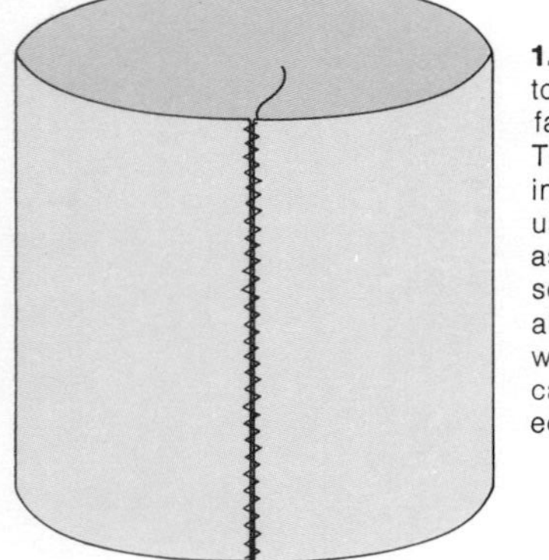

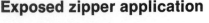

1. Cut band according to type of neckline and fabric (see pp. 208–209). Temporarily seam band into closed circle, using an abutted seam, as follows: trim away seam allowances, then abut seamlines and join with a zigzag stitch, catching both of the edges in the stitching.

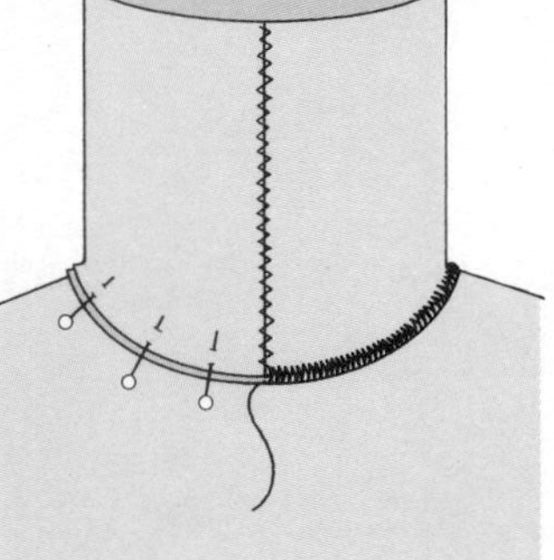

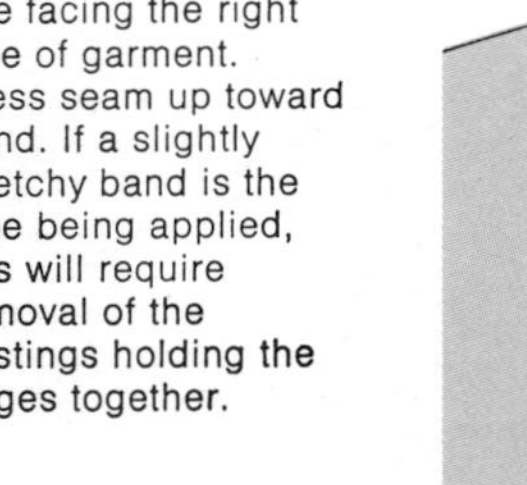

2. Apply band to garment, using appropriate method (see p. 208 or 209), except stitch only one band edge, the one facing the right side of garment. Press seam up toward band. If a slightly stretchy band is the type being applied, this will require removal of the bastings holding the edges together.

3. To locate center of placket, lightly press a crease, from the right side, along the center back of the garment. To determine how long placket opening should be, place zipper along crease, with top stop just below the foldline of band (the top of placket), and insert a pin just below the bottom stop to mark bottom of placket.

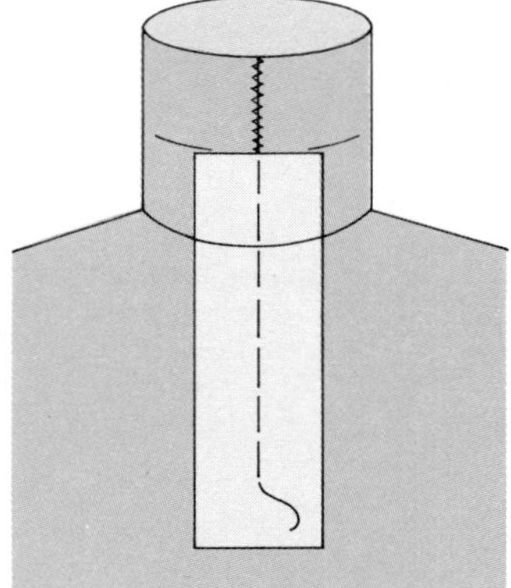

4. Cut a piece of stay fabric 3″ wide and 2″ longer than placket opening. Draw a line or press a crease in stay fabric the length of the placket opening. Center this line over crease in garment; pin and baste in place along line.

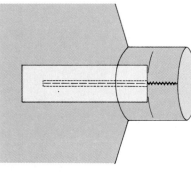

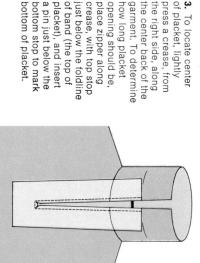

5. Sew stay fabric to garment by stitching ⅛″ from both sides of centered lines and across the bottom of the placket.

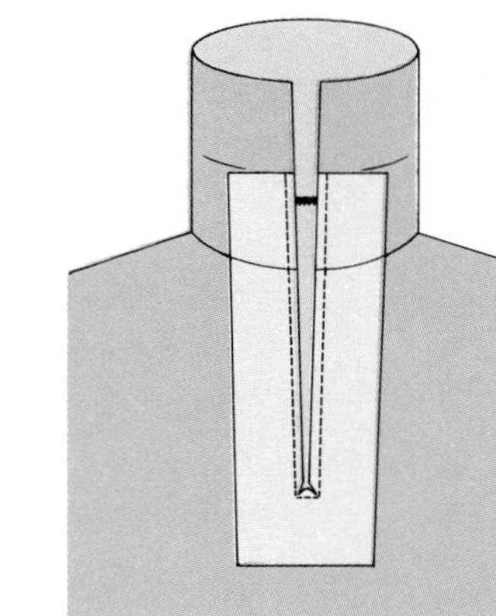

6. Slash through and remove stitching of the abutted seam in the band and cut along the centered lines to within ½″ from end of placket. Then cut to the stitching at each corner, forming a wedge at bottom.

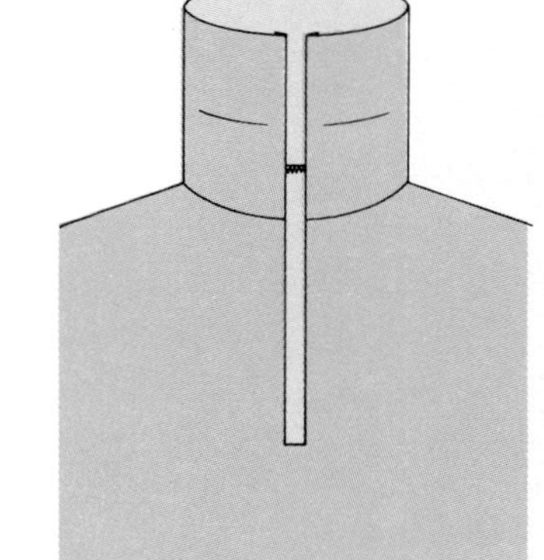

7. Turn all the stay fabric to inside of garment; press so that none of it shows on the right side of the garment.

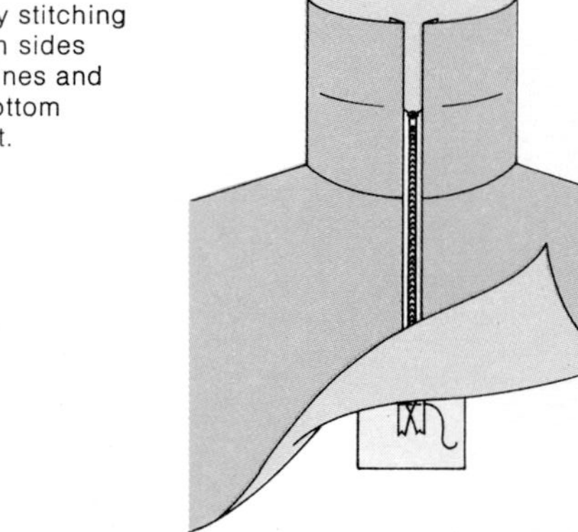

8. Position zipper under opening with top stop at fold of band and bottom stop at the end of placket opening; pin. Slip-baste zipper to edges of opening. Lift garment up to expose the wedge and bottom of zipper. Using a zipper foot, stitch across base of wedge, through the wedge, stay fabric, and zipper tapes.

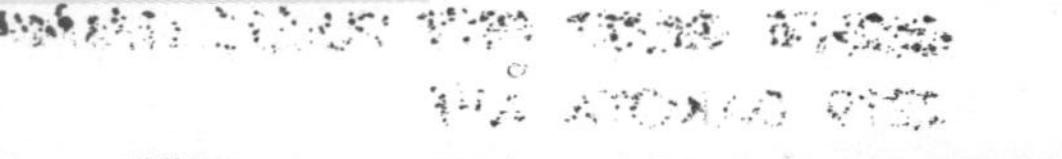

Prepackaged ribbing 17
Catchstitch (flat) 129
Centered zipper application 318-319

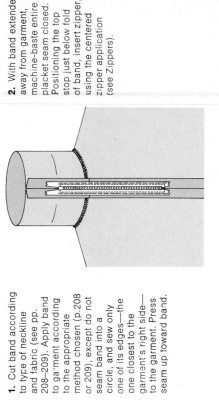

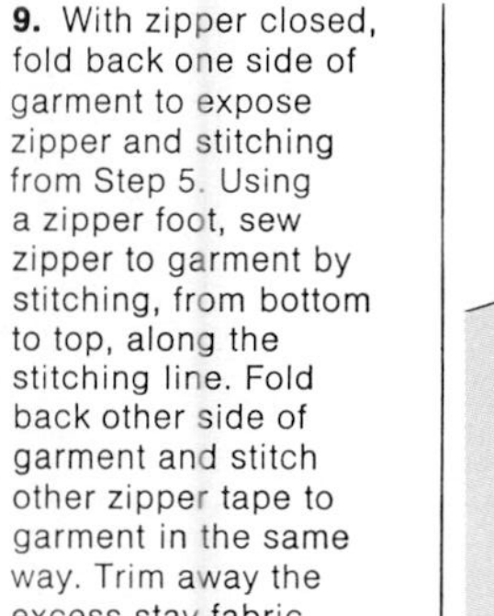

9. With zipper closed, fold back one side of garment to expose zipper and stitching from Step 5. Using a zipper foot, sew zipper to garment by stitching, from bottom to top, along the stitching line. Fold back other side of garment and stitch other zipper tape to garment in the same way. Trim away the excess stay fabric.

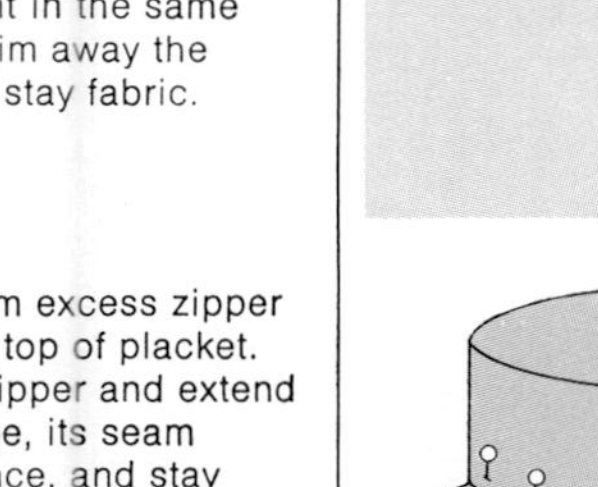

10. Trim excess zipper tape at top of placket. Open zipper and extend one tape, its seam allowance, and stay fabric. Fold free half of band down to right side of band, matching ends. Pin in place and stitch along zipper stitching line. Repeat process for other half of zipper.

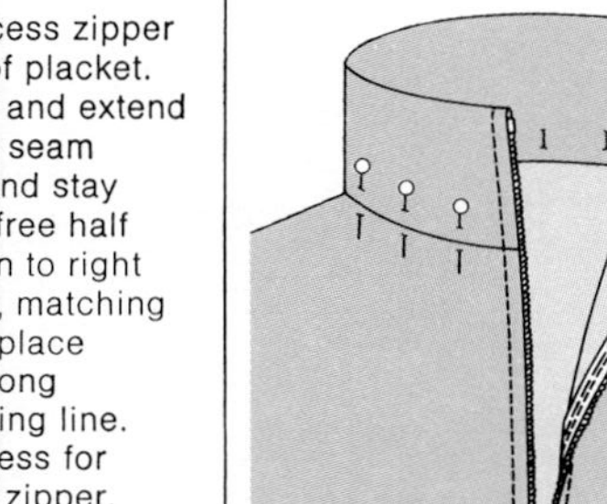

11. Turn band to inside of garment and match neck seamlines of band and garment; pin in place from right side. Stitch from the right side, in the seam groove, removing pins as you stitch. Use a straight stitch for this, stretching the fabric, if necessary, as you stitch.

Centered zipper application

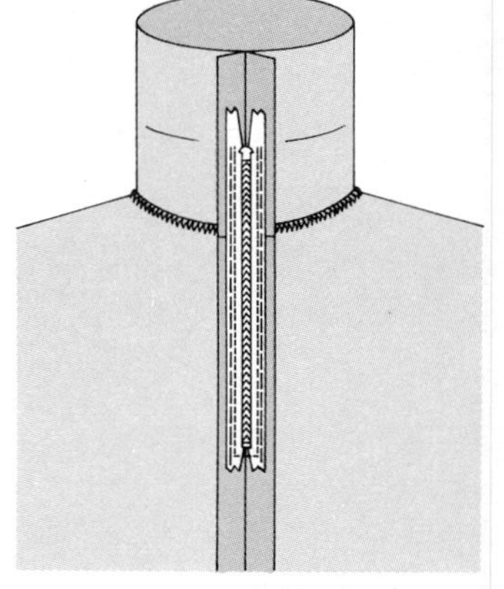

1. Cut band according to type of neckline and fabric (see pp. 208–209). Apply band to garment according to the appropriate method chosen (p.208 or 209), except do not seam band into a circle, and sew only one of its edges—the one closest to the garment's right side—to the garment. Press seam up toward band.

2. With band extended away from garment, machine-baste entire placket seam closed. Positioning the top stop just below fold of band, insert zipper, using the centered zipper application (see Zippers).

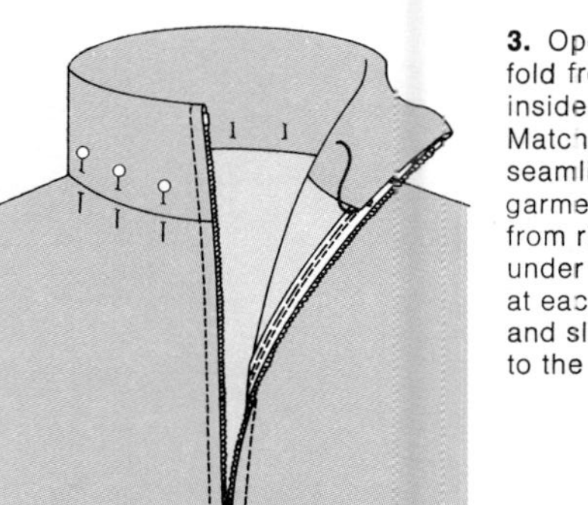

3. Open zipper and fold free half of band to inside of garment. Match the neck seamlines of band and garment; pin in place from right side. Fold under edges of band at each zipper tape and slipstitch them to the tapes.

4. Stitch from the right side, in the seam groove, through all layers; remove pins as you stitch. Use a straight stitch for this, stretching the fabric, if necessary, as you stitch.

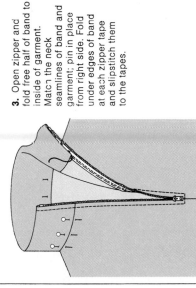

Prepackaged ribbing

Many of the prepackaged ribbings usable for strip-band necklines have only a single layer. Because of this, the part of the zipper that extends into the band cannot be stitched between layers, as was specified in the two preceding zipper applications. When positioning a zipper for a neckline that has a single-layer band, place its top stop at the top edge of the band and turn under the upper ends of the tapes. Then apply the zipper, catching the turned-under tapes in the stitching (1). To finish the zipper within the band area, and ensure that it will lie flat against the band, catchstitch the edges of the zipper tape to the band (2).

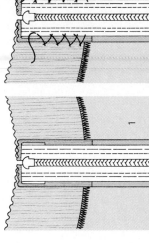

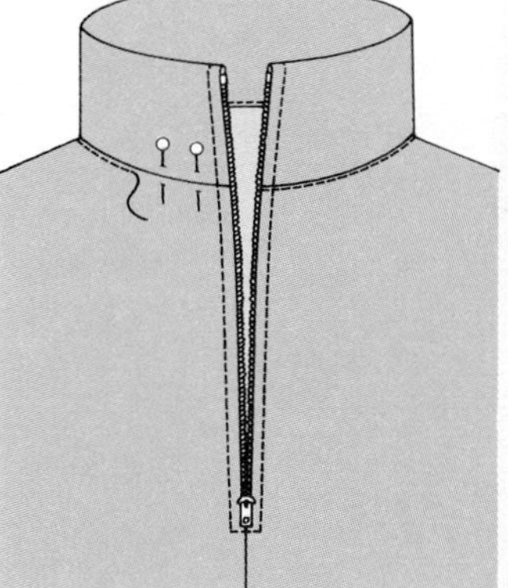

Collars

Types of collars

Though they come in many shapes and sizes, all collars are basically one of three types: **flat, standing,** or **rolled.** And different as they may be in other respects, collars are alike in one way that is important to understand. Each has a top and bottom portion, usually called the *upper* and *under collar,* sometimes the *collar* and *collar facing.* It does not matter how the outer edge of a collar is shaped; this shape does not affect its basic construction. The curve of the inner edge, however, is important. It is the relation of the curve at this edge to the neckline curve that determines the collar's type. The more alike the two curves are, the less the collar will stand up from the neck edge (flat collar). The more these curves differ, the more the collar will stand up (standing collar). If the curves differ slightly, the collar will stand up to some extent, then fall (rolled collar).

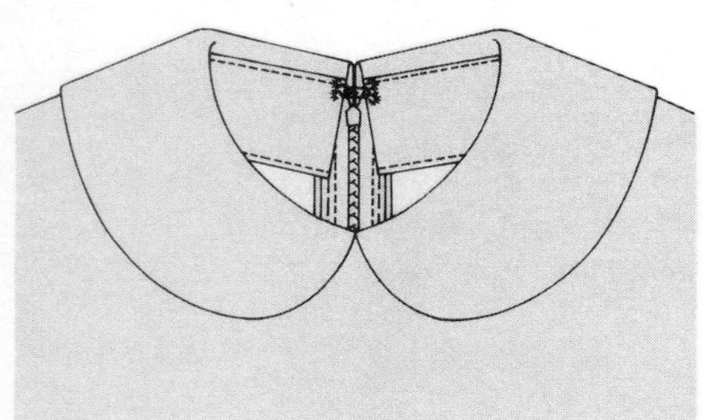

A flat collar emerges from the neck seamline to lie flat against the garment, rising only slightly above the garment's neck edge. A typical example is the Peter Pan collar. Flat collars occur most often in untailored garments, such as dresses, and in children's wear.

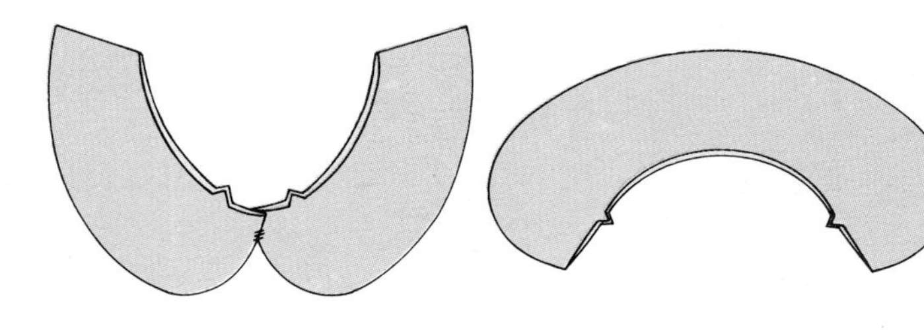

A complete flat collar may consist of two separate units or one continuous unit. When a collar has two units, one is intended for the right-hand portion of the neck, the other for the left-hand portion. The construction of a flat collar is explained on page 214; its application is described on page 215.

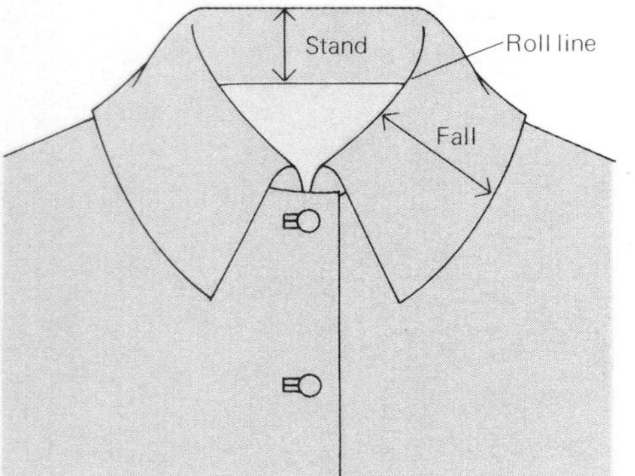

A rolled collar first stands up from the neck edge, then falls down to rest on the garment. The line at which the collar begins to fall is called the *roll line.* The positioning of this line determines the extent of the stand, and thus the fall, of the collar. Examples of the rolled collar, other than the one shown, are the notched and the shawl collars.

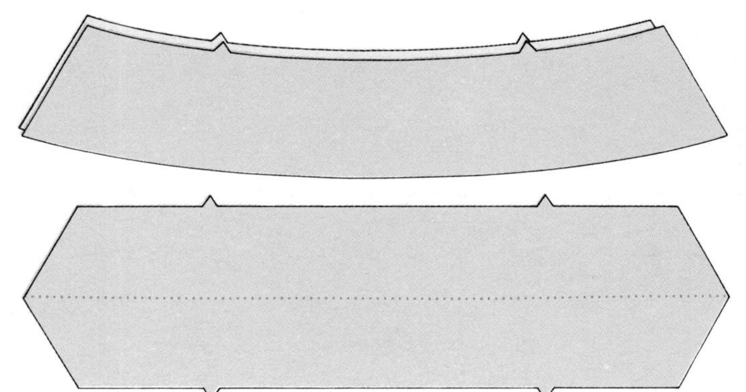

Rolled collars are usually constructed from separate upper and under collars. Some, however, are constructed from one piece that, when folded back onto itself, forms the entire collar. Either type may or may not have a seam at the center back. Construction and application methods for the rolled collar are on pages 216–224.

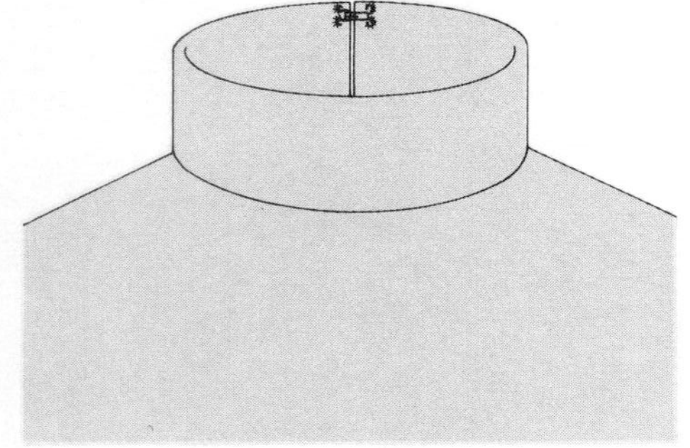

A standing collar extends above the neck seamline of the garment either as a narrow, single-width band or as a wider, double-width band that will fold back down onto itself. Most standing collars are straight, but they can be curved so that they stand up at a slight angle. Shirt collar with a stand is a variation of the standing collar.

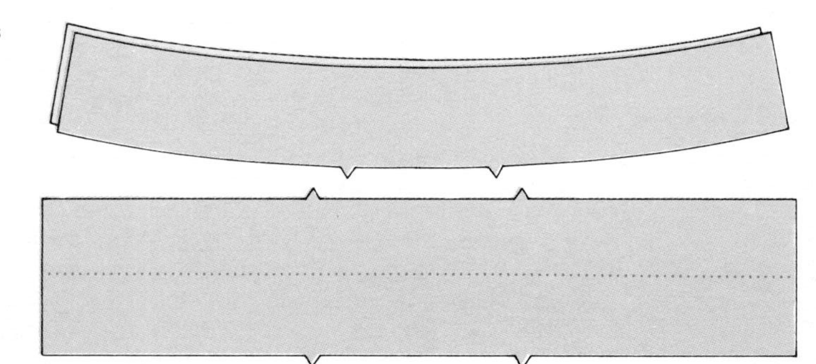

A standing collar may be either rectangular or slightly curved in shape. Some have a separate upper and under collar; others are formed from one piece that folds back on itself to form the entire collar. The methods for construction and application of standing collars are detailed on pages 225–228.

Interfacing 72-73, 76-79
Fabric-marking methods 94
Tailoring 363-374
Sewing for men 388

Interfacings

Interfacing is an important part of any collar because it helps to define and support the collar's shape. On collars that will not be tailored, any type of interfacing is usable, fusible or nonfusible, so long as its weight is compatible with that of the garment fabric. If a collar is to be tailored, the best interfacing choice is an appropriate weight of either a fusible or a nonfusible hair canvas. For general guidance in the selection of interfacings, see the section on Interfacing.

This part of the book deals with collars that will not be tailored. For techniques of tailoring collars with a nonfusible interfacing, see Tailoring; to tailor collars with fusible interfacing, see Sewing for men. As a general rule, interfacing is applied to the wrong side of the under collar; there are exceptions to this, however, and these are clarified as they arise in the collar construction methods that follow. Basic methods of applying interfacing to an under collar are given below.

Where to apply the interfacing

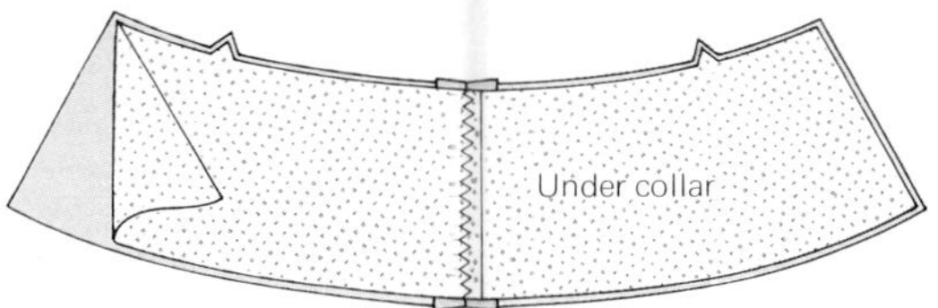

Interfacing is generally applied to the wrong side of the under collar. Some exceptions to this rule are discussed in connection with the adjoining three illustrations.

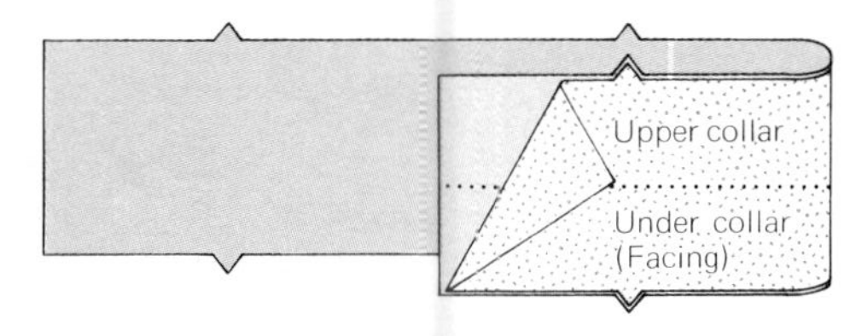

If constructing a standing collar in which both parts of the collar are one piece, interfacing can be applied to *wrong side of entire piece* if garment fabric is not too bulky.

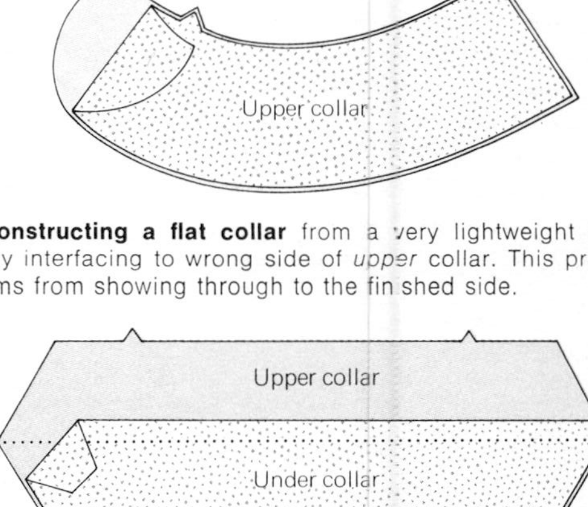

If constructing a flat collar from a very lightweight fabric, apply interfacing to wrong side of *upper* collar. This prevents seams from showing through to the finished side.

With a one-piece rolled collar, interfacing is applied to wrong side of the under collar area but, if you prefer, it can *extend ½" beyond foldline* into the upper collar.

Interfacing applications

The method chosen for the application of interfacing depends upon the type of interfacing being used. Shown at the right are the methods appropriate for lighter-weight and heavy conventional interfacings, and for fusibles. Some general rules, however, apply to them all. (1) Transfer all pat-

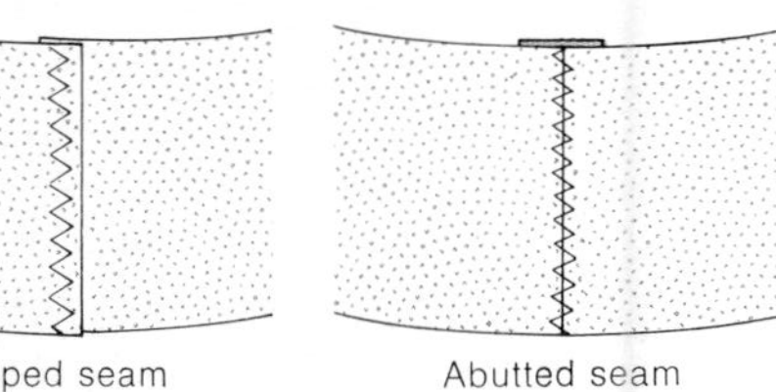

Lapped seam Abutted seam

tern markings to the interfacing. (2) If there is a center back seam, and the interfacing is a nonfusible, join the interfacing, before application, with either a lapped or an abutted seam (see Seams in interfacing). (3) Reduce bulk at corners by trimming across them $\frac{1}{16}$ inch inside the seamline. For techniques to use on collars that are to be tailored, see Tailoring (nonfusible interfacings) and Sewing for men (fusible interfacings).

Lighter-weight interfacings: Transfer markings. Form seam if necessary. Trim across corners $\frac{1}{16}''$ inside seamline.

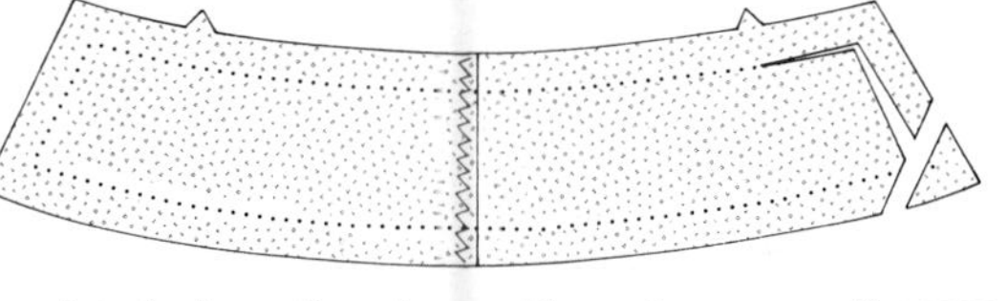

Heavy interfacings: Transfer markings. Form seam if necessary. Trim away all seam allowances and across corners.

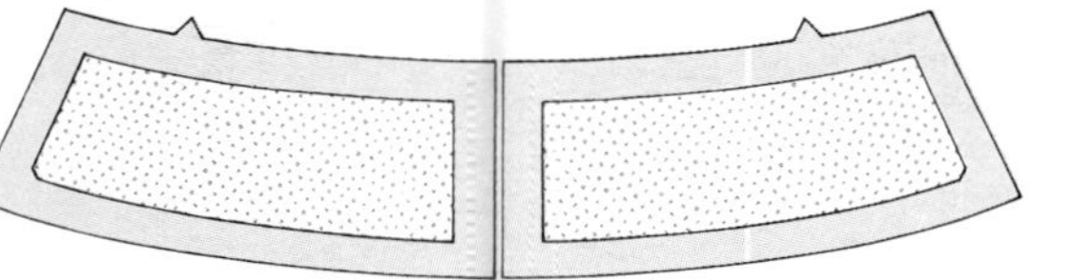

Fusible interfacings: Transfer markings. Trim all seam allowances and corners. Fuse to wrong side of under collar.

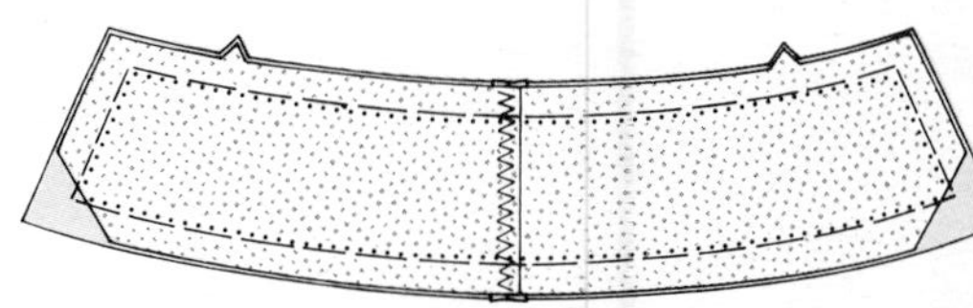

With the interfacing to the wrong side of the under collar, match, pin, and baste inside the seamline.

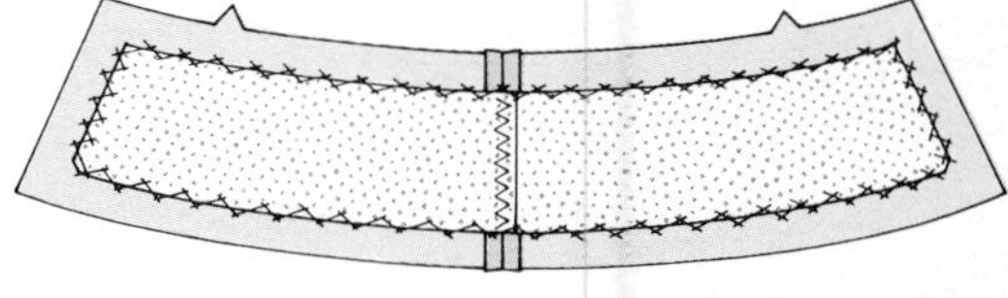

Match and baste the interfacing to wrong side of under collar. Catchstitch to under collar over all the seamlines.

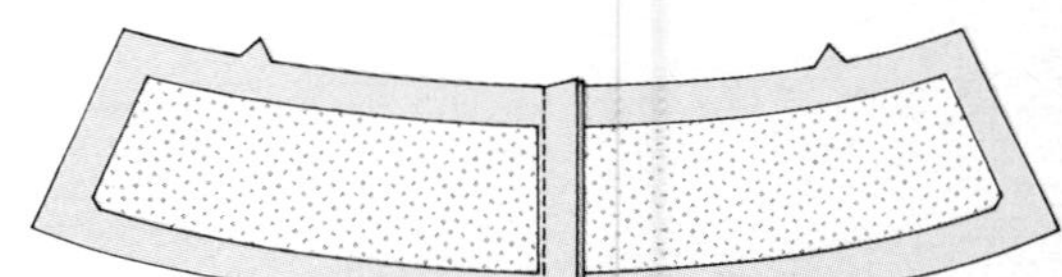

If necessary, form center back seam in garment fabric (do not catch interfacing in seam). Press seam flat, then open.

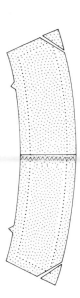

Flat collars

Pressing 18-19
Interfacing 72-73, 76-79
Diagonal basting 125
Seams 146-147

General information

Flat collars are the easiest type to construct and apply. One of the most familiar forms is the Peter Pan collar, being made and applied on these two pages. It is made up of two separate collar units, one applied to the left-hand portion of the neck and the other to the right-hand portion. The techniques used here can be followed for any kind of flat collar, including those that consist of only one unit, which spans the entire neck edge. A zipper is the usual garment closure; insert it before applying the collar. If bound buttonholes will be used, construct them before applying the collar and finish their backs after application; make worked buttonholes after applying collar.

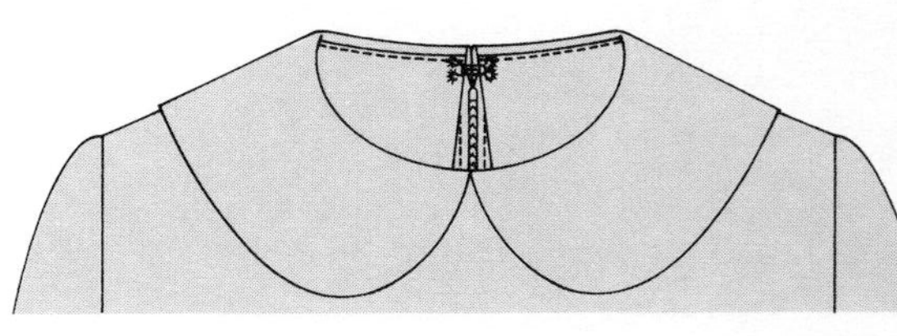

Construction of a flat collar

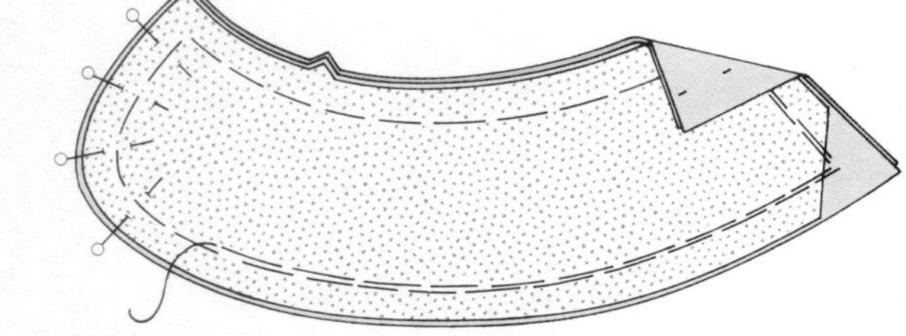

1. Apply interfacing to wrong side of each under collar. Right sides together, match, pin, and baste each upper collar to each under collar, leaving neck edges open.

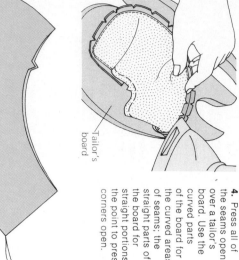

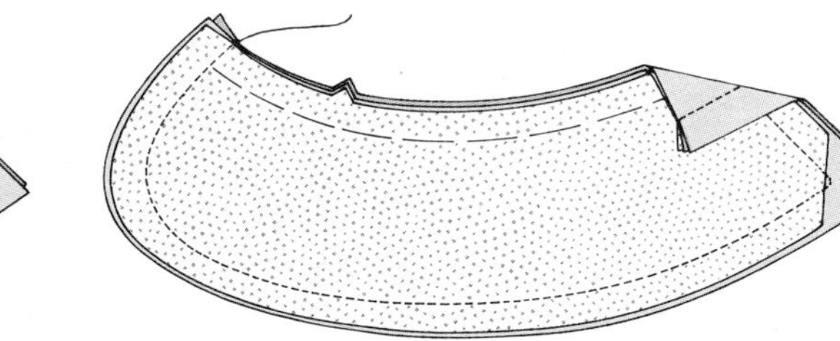

2. Stitch each unit along outer seamline, again leaving neck edges open. Use short reinforcement stitches at corners; stitch across corners to blunt them (see Seams). Press.

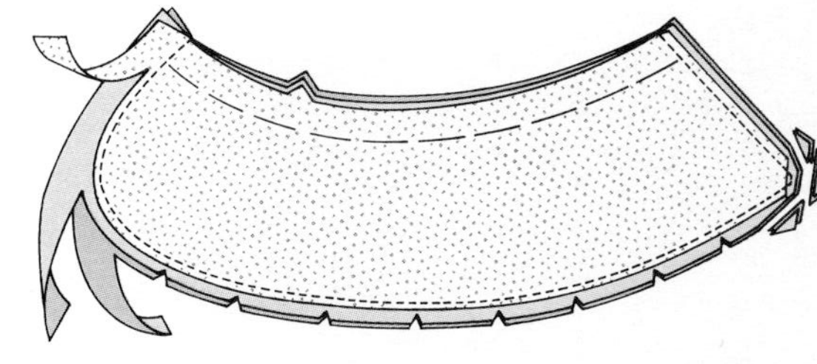

3. Trim and grade seam allowances; trim across corners and taper seam allowances on both sides of each; notch or clip the curved seam allowances (see Seams).

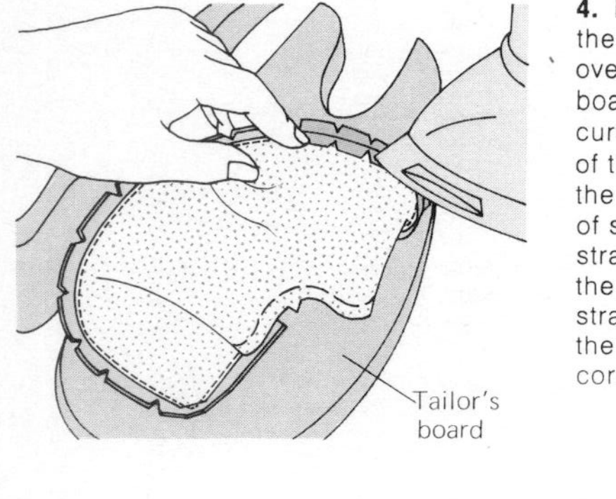

4. Press all of the seams open over a tailor's board. Use the curved parts of the board for the curved areas of seams; the straight parts of the board for straight portions; the point to press corners open.

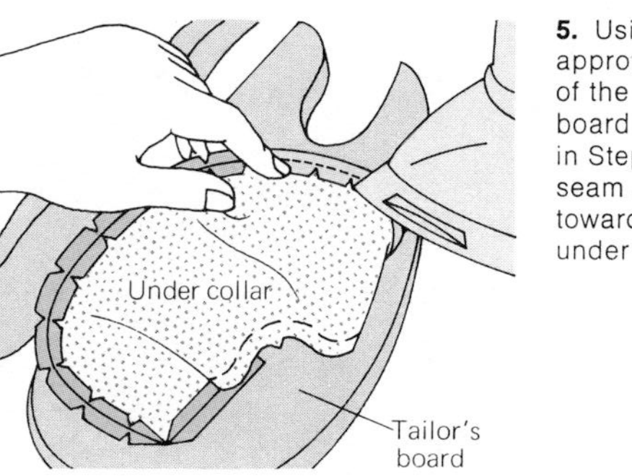

5. Using the appropriate parts of the tailor's board as explained in Step 4, press seam allowances toward the under collar.

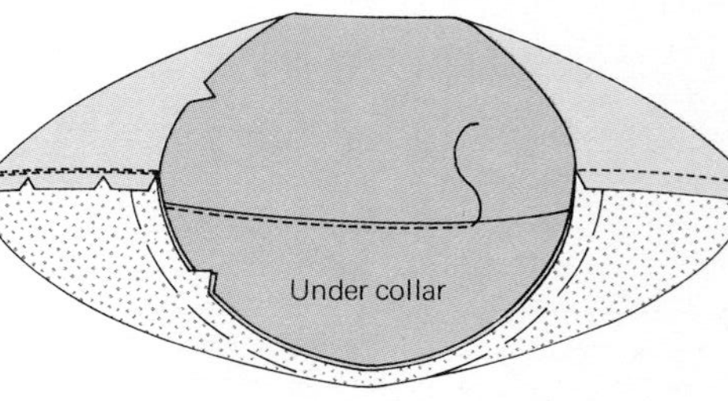

6. If desired, understitch the outer edge of each collar unit. With under collar right side up, understitch along the seamline, catching the seam allowances underneath.

7. Turn collar units right side out. To pull out corners, push a needle, threaded with a double, knotted length of thread, out through corner point. Pull on thread.

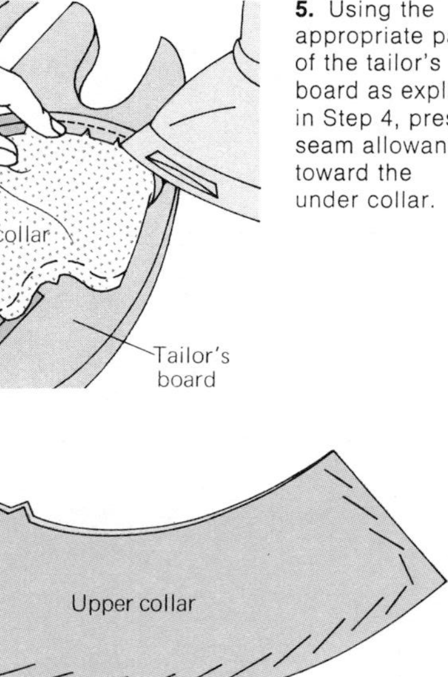

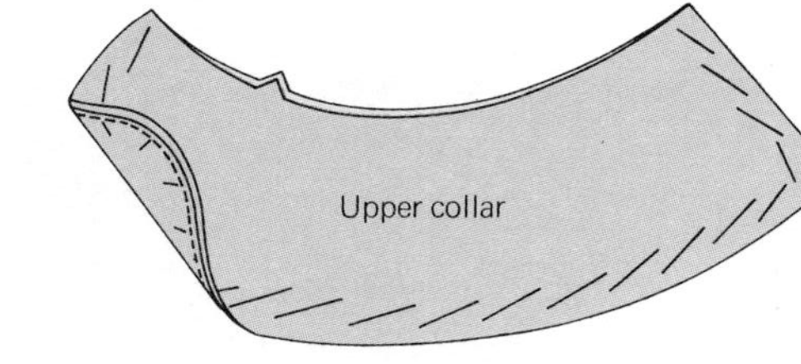

8. With the fingertips, work each outer seamline slightly toward the under collar side; hold edges in place with diagonal basting. Using a press cloth, press collar.

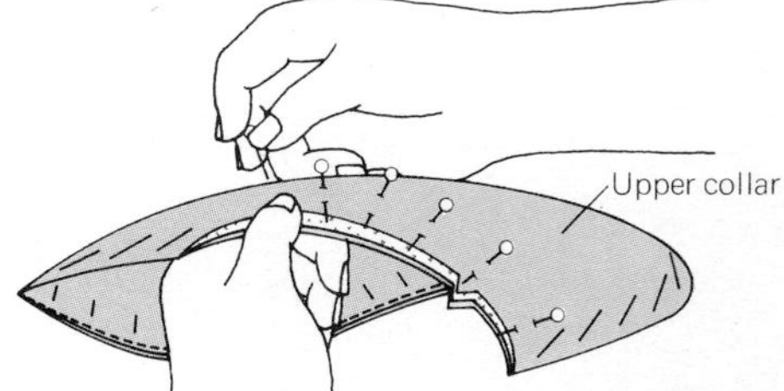

To form a slight roll, hold each collar unit, as shown, over hand, upper collar on top. Pin neck edges together as they fall; baste together along seamline of under collar.

Slipstitch (uneven) 132
Cross-stitch tack (single) 134
Fasteners 354-355

Applying a flat collar

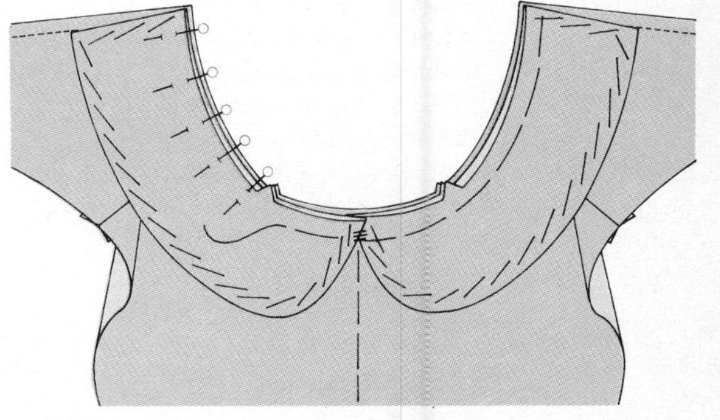

1. Before applying the collar, staystitch the neckline and form all seams and darts that intersect the neck seamline. Apply interfacing to the garment if necessary.

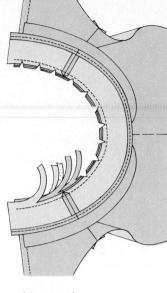

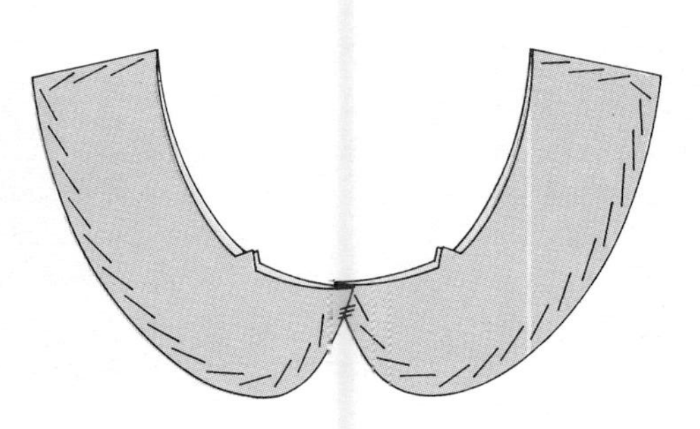

2. If collar consists of two units, as this Peter Pan flat collar does, align and join the two where their neck seamlines meet (seam allowances may overlap).

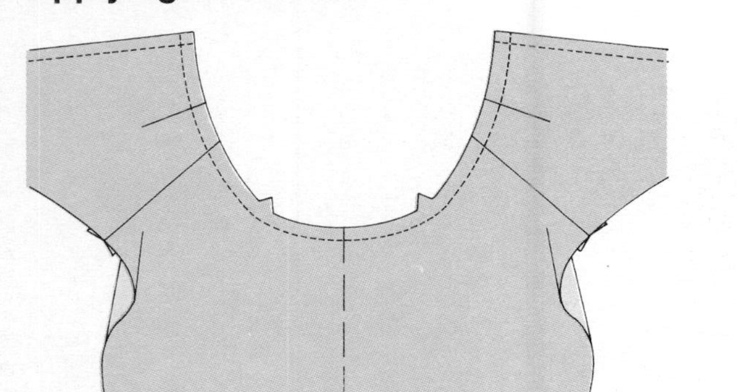

3. Match, pin, and baste the collar to the garment along the neck seamline. Be sure that the point at which the two units are joined falls at the garment center.

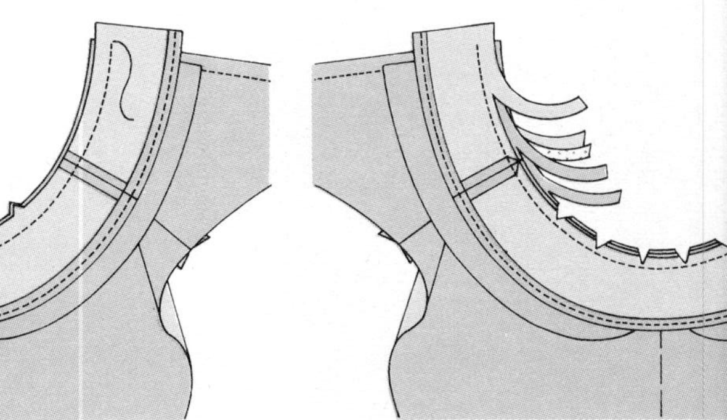

4. Form facing unit (see p.193). With the right side of facing toward upper collar, match, pin, and baste unit to collar and garment at neck seamline (ends will extend at placket).

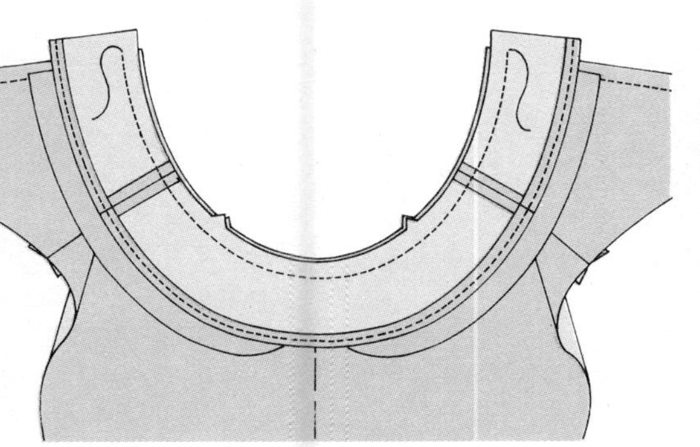

5. Facing side up, stitch facing and collar to garment at neck seamline; secure stitching. Be sure ends of seamline align when zipper is closed. Remove bastings; press.

6. Trim and grade the seam allowances, making the garment seam allowance the widest. Trim diagonally across the cross-seam allowances. Notch or clip the seam allowances.

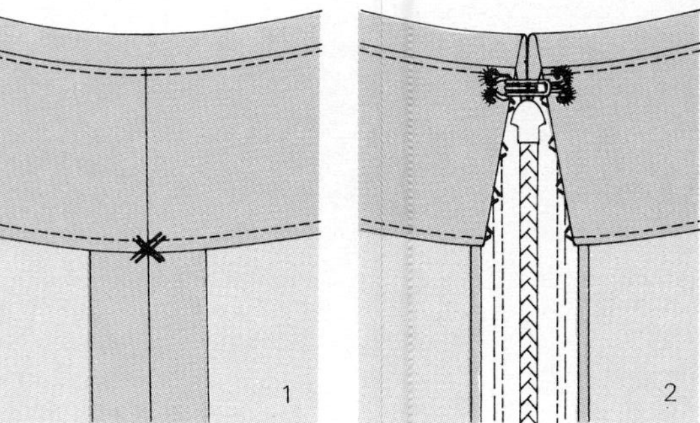

7. Place seam over a tailor's board. Press the entire seam open, running tip of iron between facing and collar seam allowances.

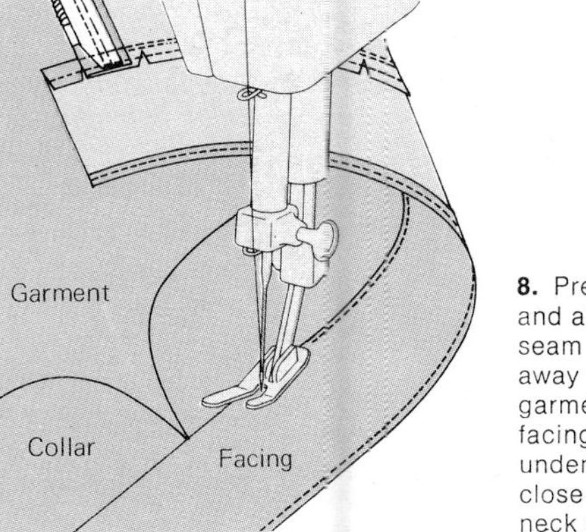
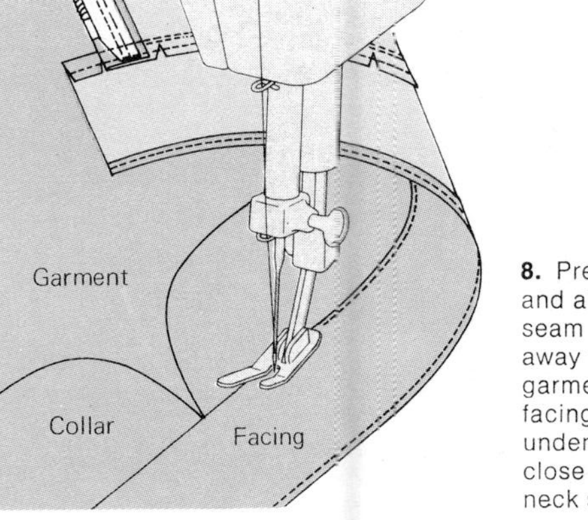

8. Press facing and all the seam allowances away from the garment. With facing side up, understitch close to the neck seamline.

9. Press facing to inside of garment. Tack facing edge in place at shoulder seamlines (1). Turn facing ends under at zipper and slipstitch in place; attach fastener (2).

Rolled collars

Interfacing 72-73, 76-79 Tailoring 363-374 Sewing for men 388

General information

Rolled collars are differentiated from flat collars by a **roll line** that breaks the collar into **stand** and **fall** areas. The position of the roll line determines the location and size of both stand and fall. Typical examples of rolled collars are illustrated below, the second being the classic notched collar. Another is the shawl collar (pp. 222–224).

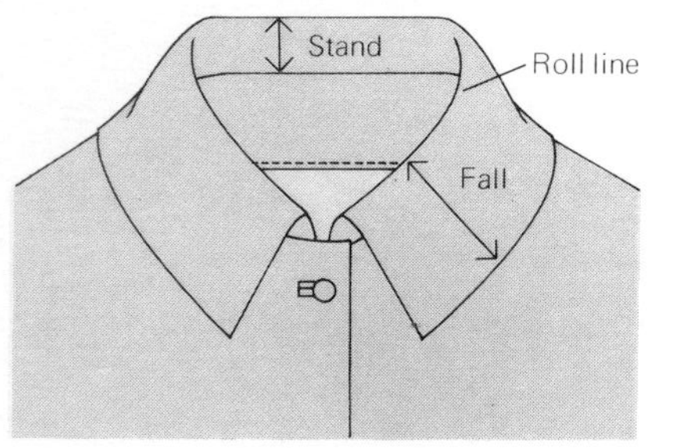

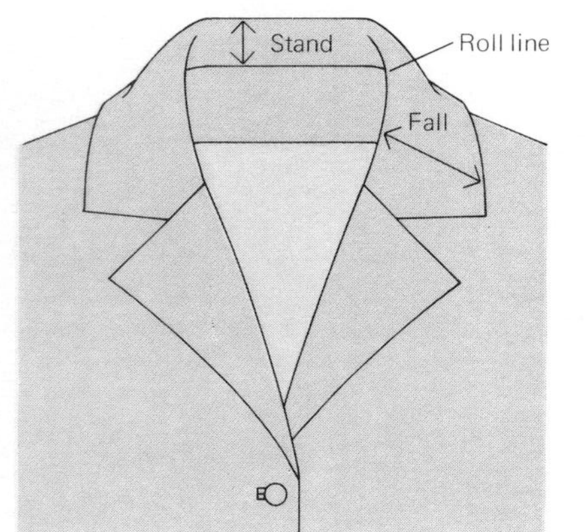

Methods are given on these two pages for the construction of both the two-piece form of the rolled collar (upper and under collars separate) and the one-piece (upper and under collars set apart by a fold). Methods of application appear on pages 218–221; the choice of method depends upon the weight of the garment fabric and whether or not there is a back neck facing. Tailoring details are given in two sections. To tailor a collar with nonfusible hair canvas, see Tailoring; with fusible interfacing, see Sewing for men.

Construction of a two-piece rolled collar

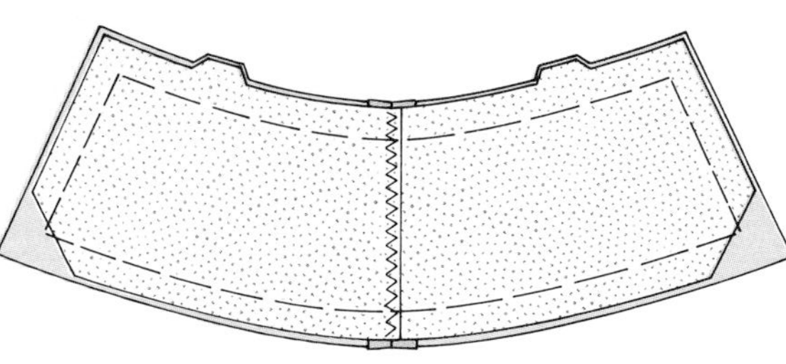

1. Apply interfacing to wrong side of under collar. If there is a center back seam: for the garment fabric, use a plain seam trimmed to half-width and pressed open; for the interfacing, use a lapped or abutted seam.

2. Right sides together, match, pin, and baste the upper collar to the under collar along the outer seamline, leaving the neck edges open. If necessary, slightly stretch the under collar to fit the upper collar.

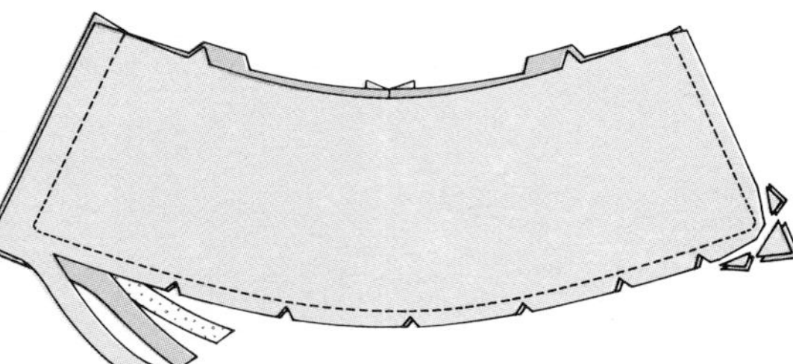

4. Trim and grade the seam allowances, making the seam allowance nearest the upper collar the widest. Trim across corners and taper seam allowances on both sides of corners. Notch or clip curved seam allowances (see Seams).

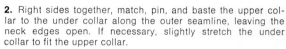

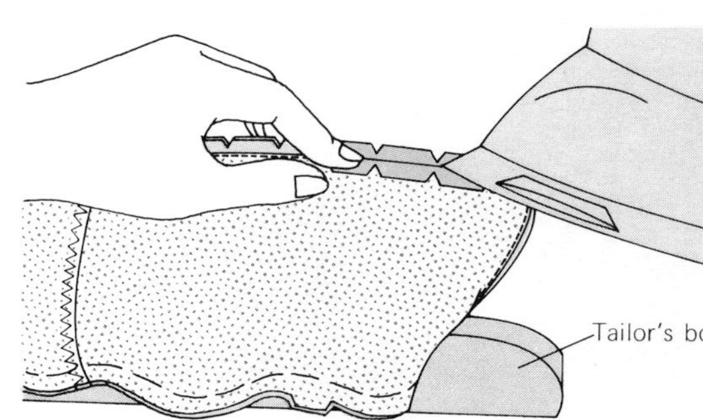

5. Press the entire seam open over a tailor's board. Use the curved edges of the board for the curved areas of the seam; the straight edges of the board for the straight portions; the board's point for the corners.

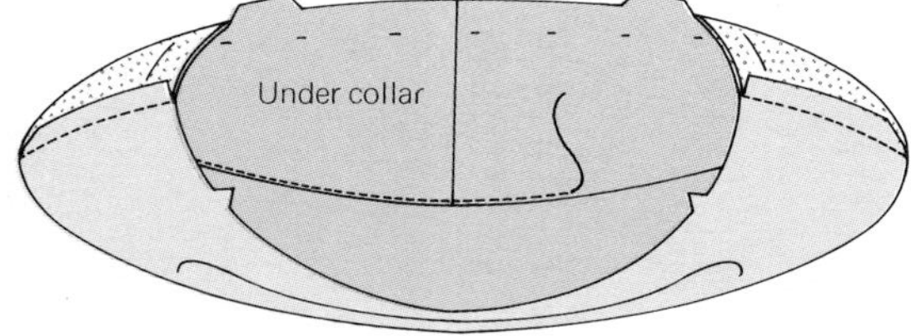

7. If necessary, understitch the outer seamline. With the under collar side up, understitch close to the seamline, catching all of the seam allowances underneath. Turn collar right side out; to pull out corners, see Step 7, page 214.

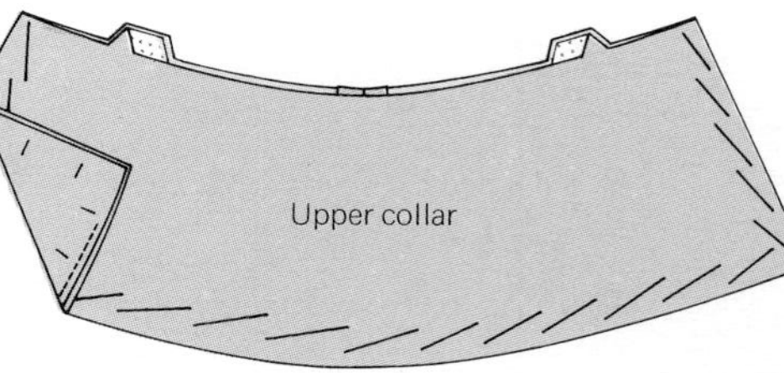

8. Work the outer seamline slightly toward the under collar side so that it will not show from the upper side. Hold outer edges in place with diagonal basting; leave neck edges open. Using a press cloth, press the collar.

Pressing 18-19
Diagonal basting 125
Seams 146-147

3. Stitch upper collar to under collar along outer seamline, leaving neck edges open. Use short reinforcement stitches at corners; stitch across corners to blunt them (see Seams). Remove bastings from outer seamline; press.

6. Press all of the seam allowances toward the under collar, again placing the curved, straight, and cornered parts of the seam over the appropriate parts of the tailor's board. Take care not to crease the rest of the collar.

9. Mold collar, over pressing ham, into shape intended by pattern. Pin and baste through all layers along roll line. Steam collar; let dry. Remove from ham; pin and baste neck edges together as they fall. Remove diagonal bastings.

Construction of a one-piece rolled collar

In one-piece rolled collars, the upper and under collars are areas defined at their "outer edges" by a fold rather than separate pieces joined by a seam. One half of the collar piece is designated the upper collar, the other half the under collar. (There are some one-piece collars that begin, literally, as two pieces because of a center back seam; when it is joined, the two form the one piece.) The fold between the upper and under collar areas makes the construction of a one-piece rolled collar different from that of the two-piece version, the one-piece collar being formed when the two halves are folded together and seamed at the sides. The application of both collars, however, is the same (see pp. 218–221).

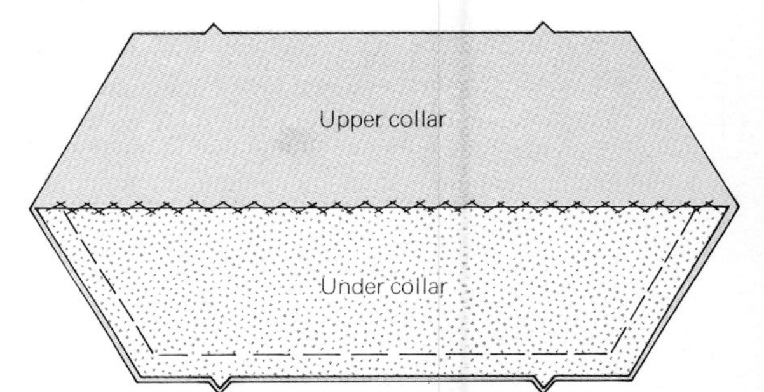

1. Apply interfacing to the under collar area. If edge of interfacing meets the foldline, catchstitch in place over the foldline; if edge extends beyond the foldline, hold in place along foldline with small stitches spaced ½" apart.

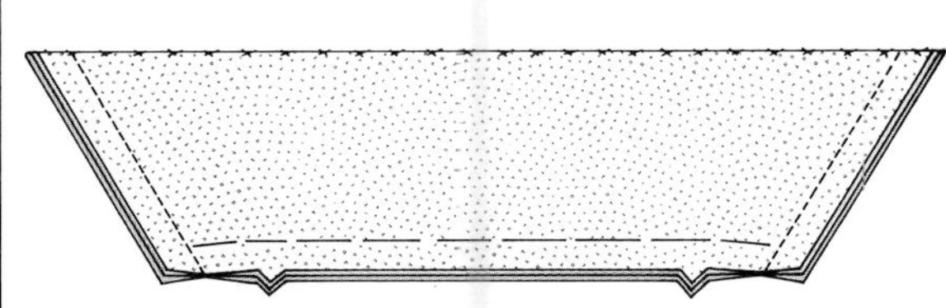

2. Fold collar in half along the foldline so that the right sides of the upper and under collars are facing. Match, pin, and baste along the side seams; stitch along the seamlines and secure stitching at ends. Remove bastings from side seams.

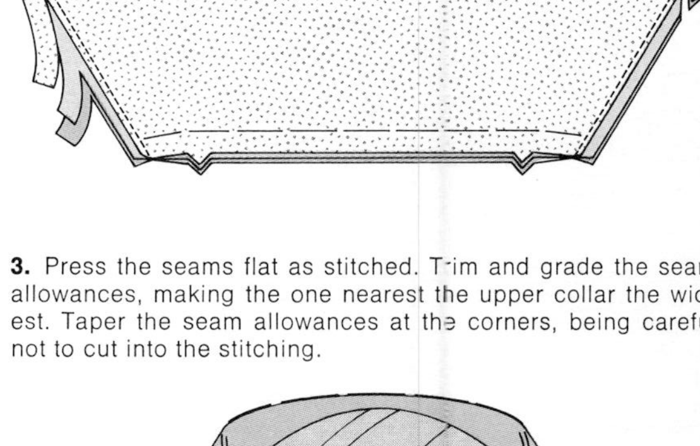

3. Press the seams flat as stitched. Trim and grade the seam allowances, making the one nearest the upper collar the widest. Taper the seam allowances at the corners, being careful not to cut into the stitching.

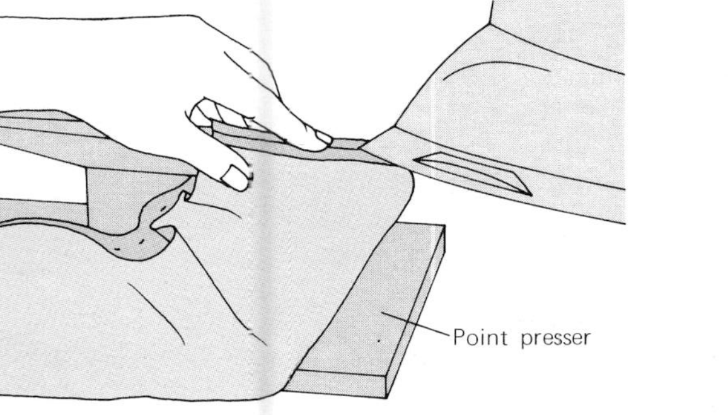

4. Using a point presser, press the seams open, then press all the seam allowances toward the under collar. Turn the collar right side out; to pull out the corners, see Step 7, page 214. Using a press cloth, press the collar.

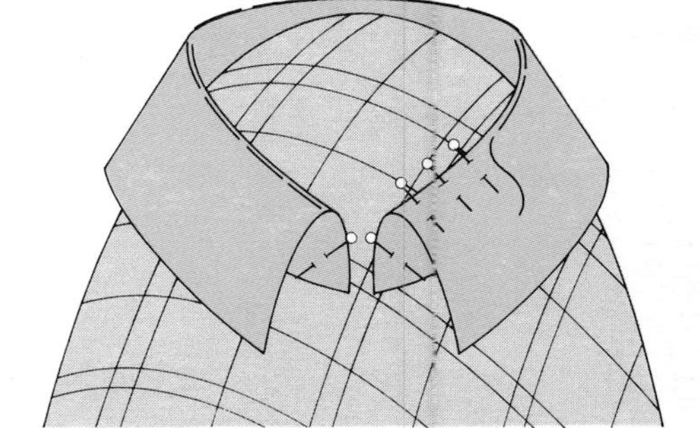

5. Mold collar, over a pressing ham, into the shape intended by the pattern. Pin and baste through all layers along the roll line. Steam collar; let it dry. Remove from ham; pin and baste neck edges together as they fall.

Rolled collars

Applying a rolled collar (light- to medium-weight fabrics)

This method of collar application can be used if the garment fabric is light to medium in weight. With this method, both the upper and under collars are sewed to the garment at the same time that the facing is being attached to the garment. If the garment needs interfacing, apply it before attaching the collar. If bound buttonholes are being used, construct them before applying the collar; finish their backs (or construct worked buttonholes) after the collar and facing have been applied to the garment. Construct the collar according to one of the methods from pages 216–217.

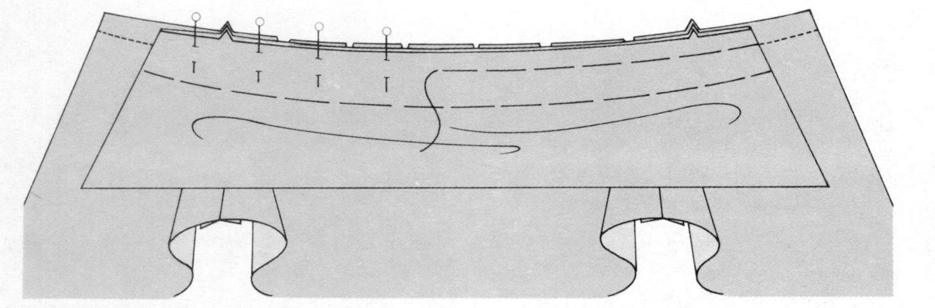

1. Staystitch garment neck edges and form all seams and darts that intersect neck seamline. With under collar toward right side of garment, match, pin, and baste collar to garment, clipping garment seam allowance, if necessary, so collar will fit easily.

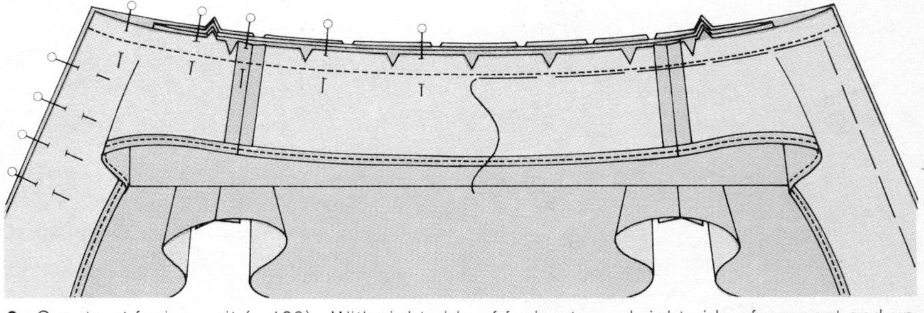

2. Construct facing unit (p.193). With right side of facing toward right side of garment and upper collar, match, pin, and baste facing through collar and garment at neck and garment opening. Clip facing seam allowance at neck, if necessary, so facing fits easily.

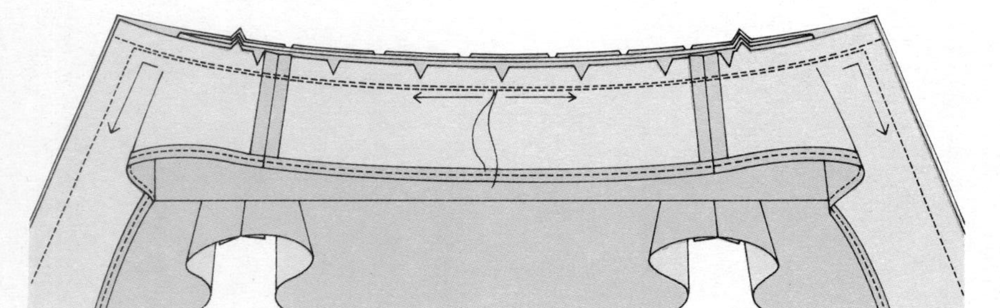

3. Facing side up, stitch facing and collar to garment. Stitch each side directionally, from center back to the bottom of the garment opening. Use shorter reinforcement stitches for 1″ on both sides of each corner. Remove bastings. Press seam flat as stitched.

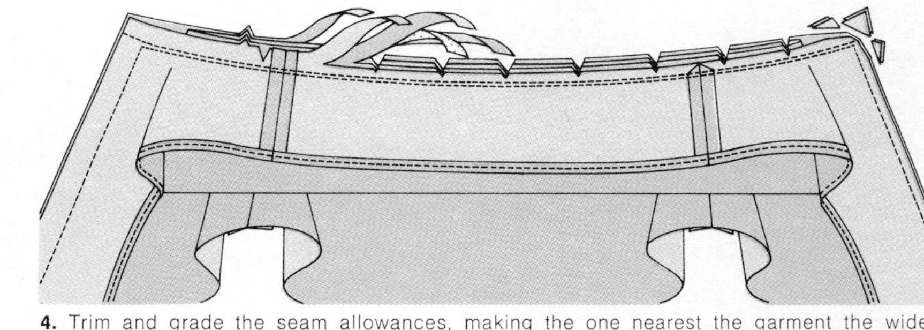

4. Trim and grade the seam allowances, making the one nearest the garment the widest. Trim diagonally across the cross-seam allowances and corners; taper the seam allowances on both sides of each corner (see Seams). Notch or clip the curved seam allowances.

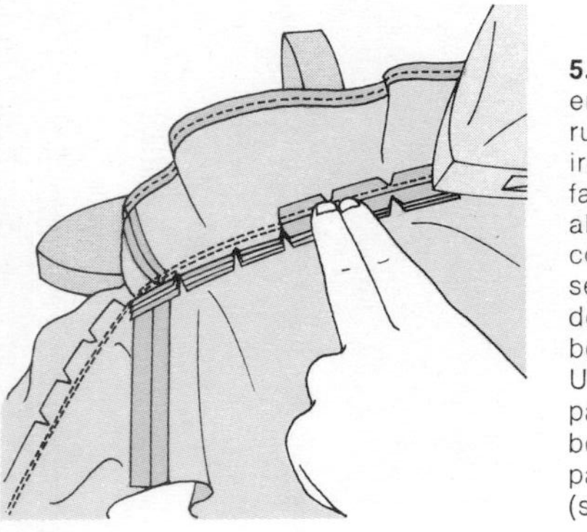

5. Press the entire seam open, running tip of iron between the facing seam allowance and collar or garment seam allowance, depending on area being pressed. Use appropriate parts of tailor's board for various parts of seam (see Pressing).

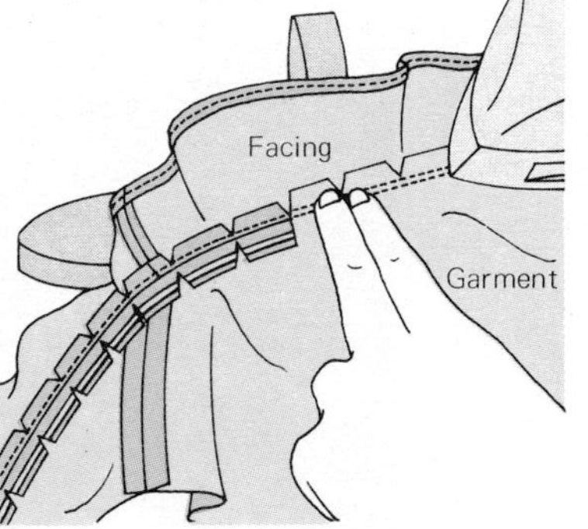

6. Still using the tailor's board, press all the seam allowances toward the facing.

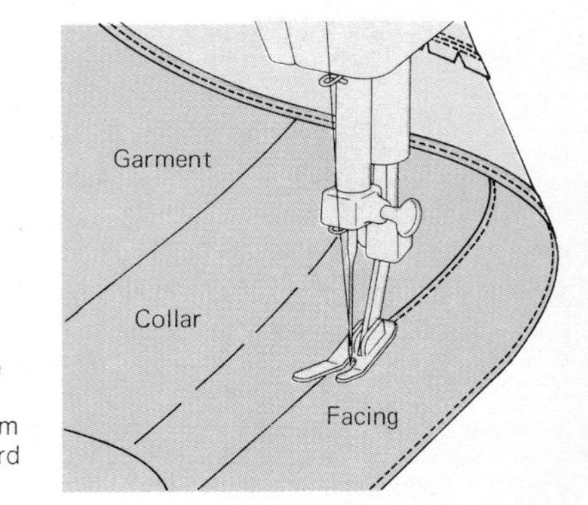

7. Understitch the neck and garment opening seamlines where necessary. Facing side up, stitch close to seamline, through all the seam allowances. Press facing to inside of garment; tack at shoulder seams.

Plain-stitch tack 135
Bound and worked buttonholes 330-348

Applying a rolled collar (heavy or bulky fabrics)

This is the method to use if the garment fabric is bulky or heavy. In this technique the under collar is sewed to the garment and the upper collar to the facing. The resulting seams are then pressed open and allowed to fall onto each other as they will. Attaching the collar in this manner causes the bulk at the neckline to be divided between the two seams. If necessary, interface the garment before attaching collar. If bound buttonholes are being used, construct them before applying the collar; finish their backs (or construct worked buttonholes) after collar and facing have been applied.

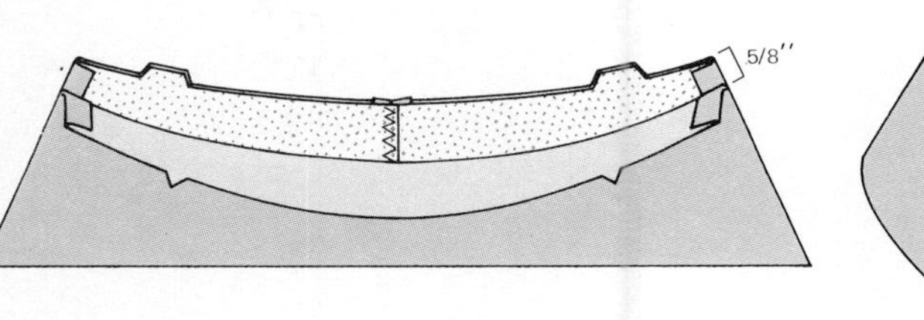

1. Construct the collar, following the appropriate construction method from pages 216–217 but ending stitching at the sides ⅝" from the neck edge.

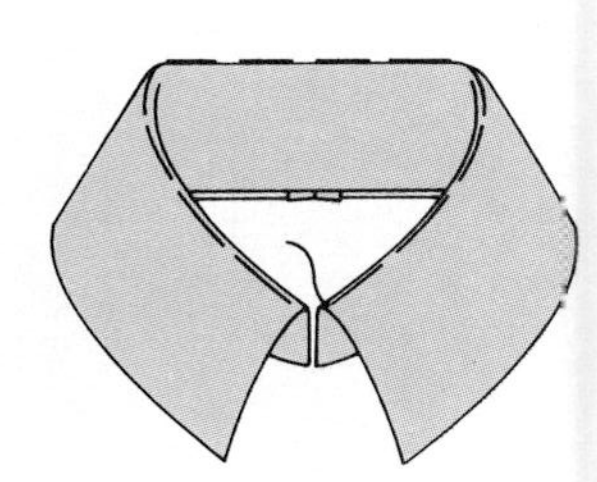

2. Mold the collar as in Step 9 or 5, page 217, but do not baste neck edges together.

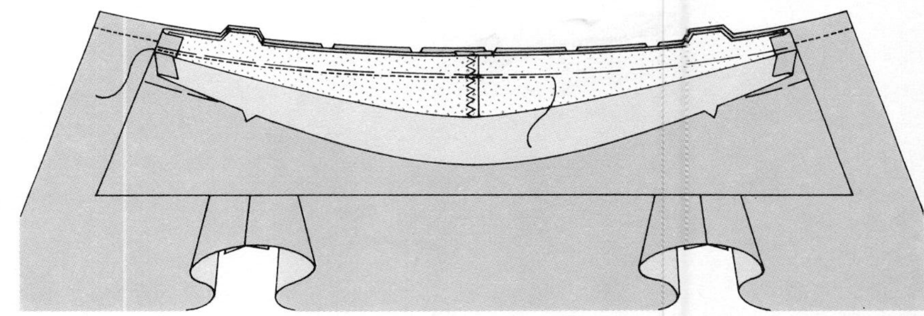

3. Staystitch garment neck edge; form all seams and darts that intersect neck seamline. Right sides together, match, pin, and baste under collar to garment; clip garment seam allowance if necessary for collar to fit. Stitch along seamline; secure stitching. Press.

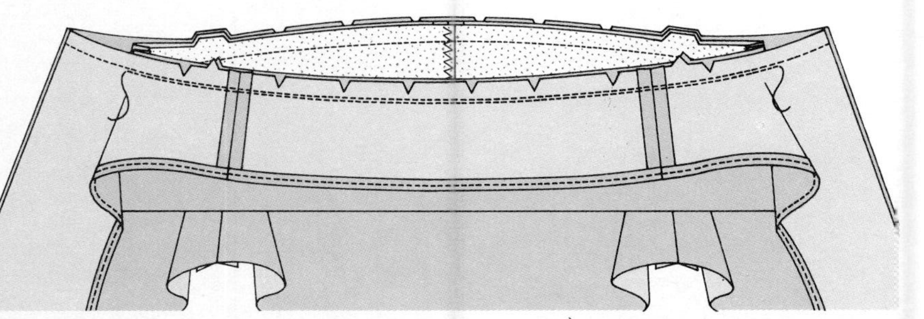

4. Construct facing unit (p.193). With right sides together, match, pin, and baste facing to upper collar only; clip facing seam allowance if necessary for facing to fit. Upper collar side up, stitch facing to upper collar; secure stitching. Remove bastings.

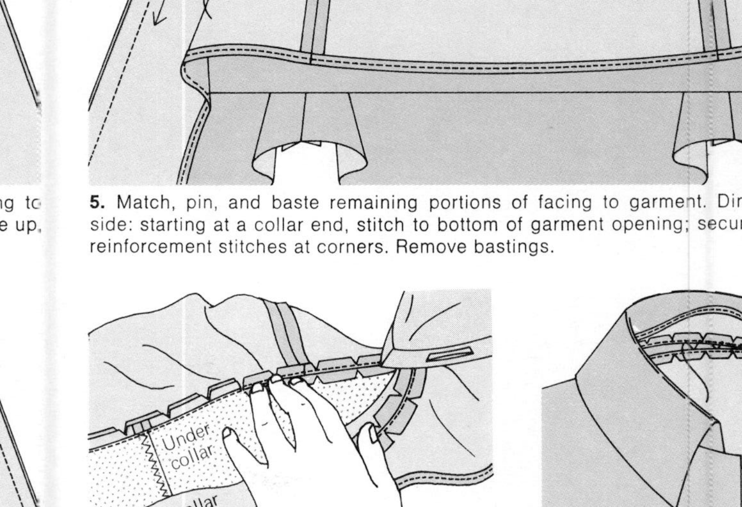

5. Match, pin, and baste remaining portions of facing to garment. Directionally stitch each side: starting at a collar end, stitch to bottom of garment opening; secure stitching. Use short reinforcement stitches at corners. Remove bastings.

6. Press all seams flat; trim. Trim across corners and taper seam allowances on both sides of each corner. Grade seam allowances beyond the collar ends to the bottom of each opening side. Notch or clip all seam allowances.

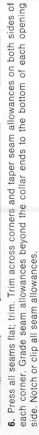

7. Using a tailor's board, press all seams open; then press the seams beyond collar and along garment opening toward facing.

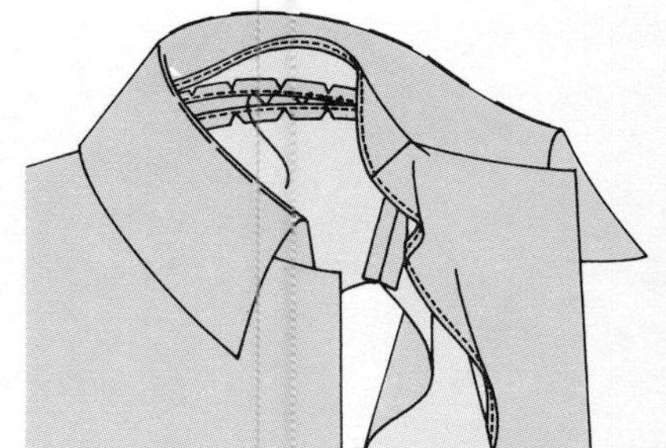

8. Turn facing to inside. Allow neck seamlines of collar to fall as they may; pin, then tack in place with plain-stitch tack.

Interfacing 72-73, 76-79
Reducing seam bulk 147

Applying a rolled collar to garment without back neck facing

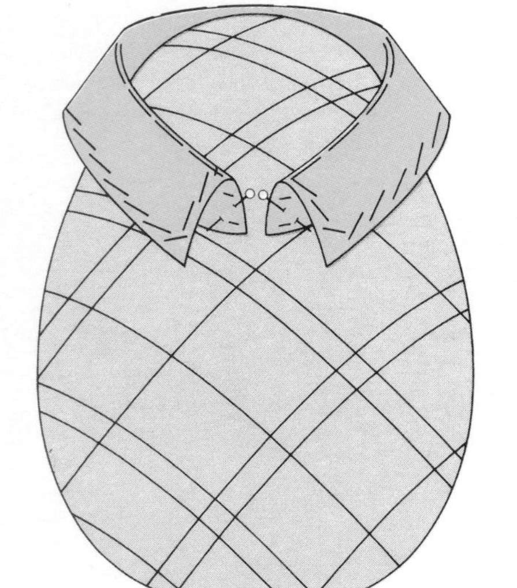

1. Construct the collar, following appropriate method from pages 216–217. Mold the collar over a pressing ham as in either Step 9 or Step 5 on page 217. Remove collar from ham as directed but do not baste neck edges together.

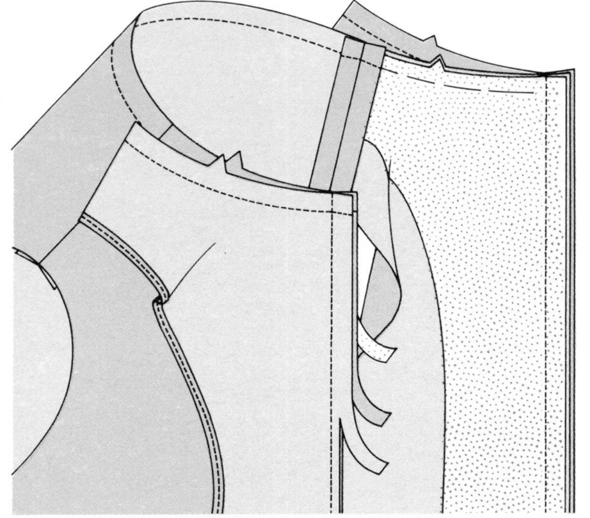

2. Staystitch garment and facing; form all seams and darts that intersect garment neck seam. Interface garment; construct bound buttonholes. Sew facing to garment at opening edges. Press seams flat; trim and grade; press seams open.

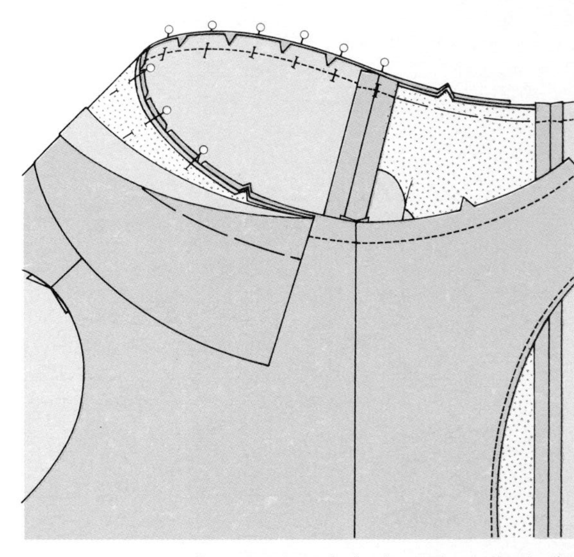

3. Right sides together, match and pin the under collar to the garment neck seamline from one shoulder to the other, clipping the seam allowance of the garment where necessary so that the collar will fit smoothly.

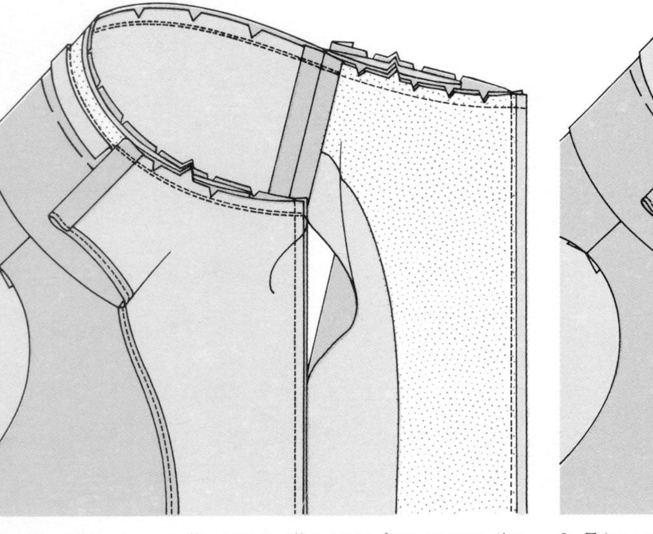

7. Keeping the upper collar seam allowance free across the back, stitch the facing and collar to the garment along the neck seamline. Secure stitching at both ends. Remove all of the bastings; press the seam flat.

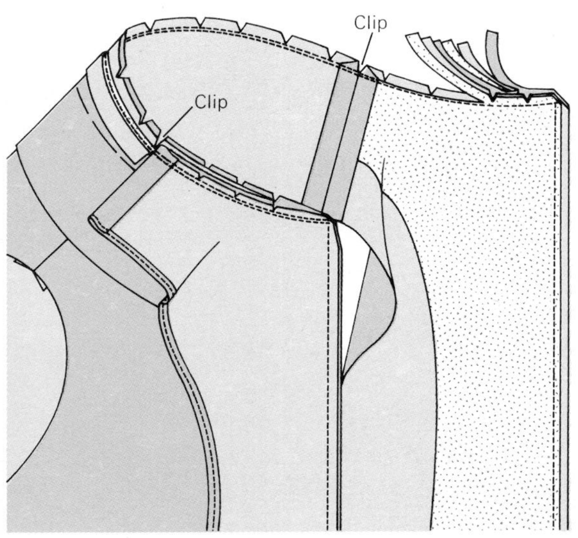

8. Trim and grade seam allowances, making seam allowance of garment the widest. Trim across corners and taper seam allowances on both sides of each corner; at both shoulders, clip into all seam allowances. Clip or notch curved areas.

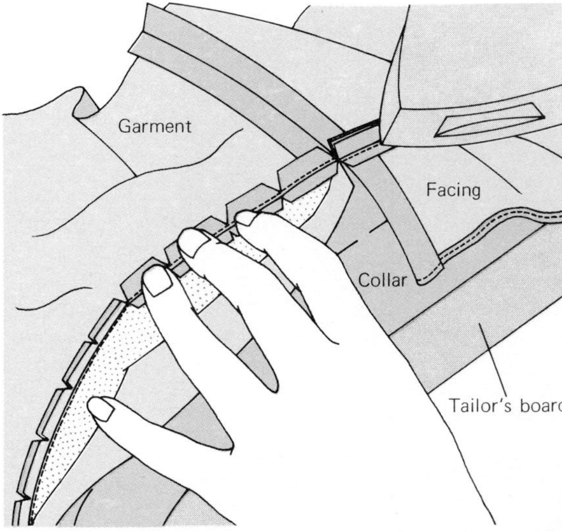

9. Using a tailor's board, press the entire seam open, pressing between the facing and the collar or garment from each shoulder to front edge; between under collar and garment across the back neck from shoulder to shoulder.

Pressing 18-19

Slipstitch (uneven) 132
Bound and worked buttonholes 330-348

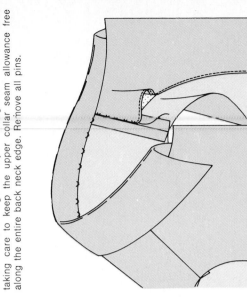

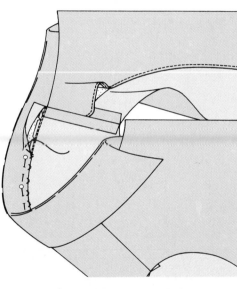

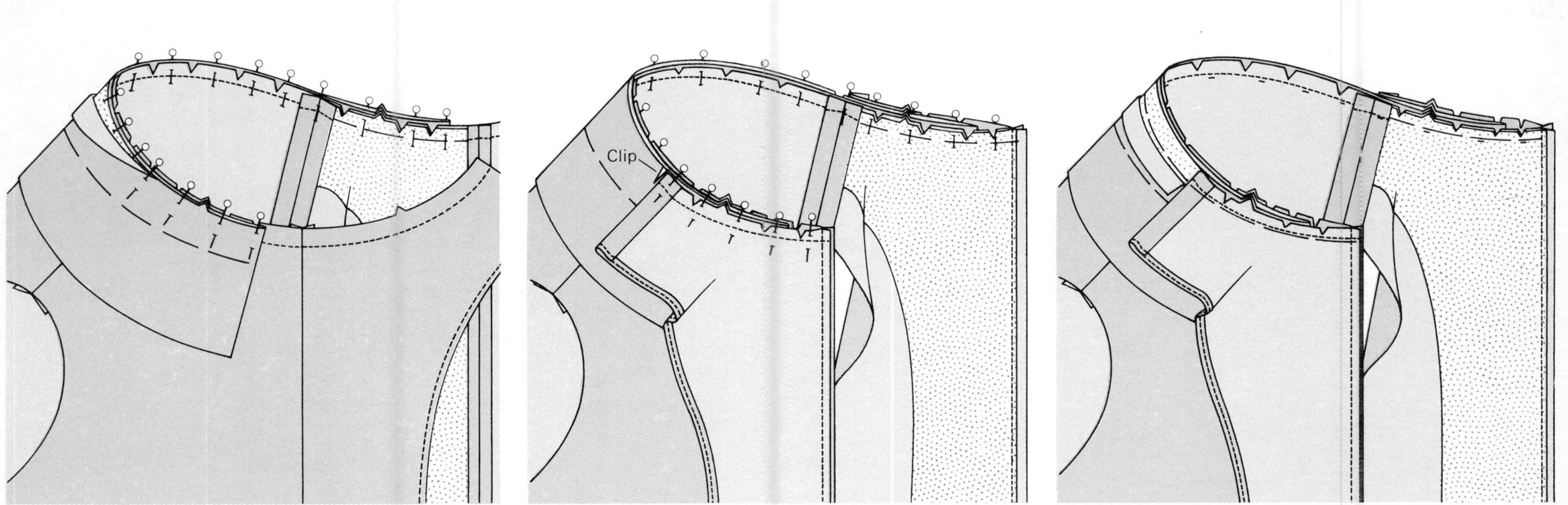

4. Match and pin both the under collar and the upper collar to the garment neck seamline from each shoulder to corresponding end of collar. Clip the garment seam allowance if this is necessary for the collar to fit.

5. At both shoulders, clip upper collar to seamline. Right sides together, match and pin facing to garment and collar along neck seamline, clipping facing seam allowance if necessary. Fold back facing ends at shoulder seamlines.

6. Fold back the free portion of the upper collar seam allowance. Baste through all layers along the neck seamline, taking care to keep the upper collar seam allowance free along the entire back neck edge. Remove all pins.

10. Place seam over a point presser and press the front parts of the seam down, toward the garment; the back portion of the seam up, toward the collar. Press seams at opening edges toward facing; turn facing to inside of garment.

11. Let collar fall into position along its roll line; smooth the upper collar over the under collar. Turn under the free upper collar seam allowance; pin, then slipstitch in place along the garment neck seamline. Press.

12. Slipstitch turned-under ends of facing in place along garment shoulder seamlines; press. If necessary, finish the backs of bound buttonholes (or construct worked buttonholes). Remove bastings from collar at roll line.

Rolled collars

Pressing 18-19 Interfacing 72-73, 76-79 Staystitching 144

Shawl collar

The shawl collar is like the standard notched collar in that the completion of both these collar styles involves the formation of lapels (see illustration below and on p. 216). The shawl is different from the notched collar in that its upper collar and lapels are cut from a single pattern piece; this eliminates the need for the seam between collar and lapels that is characteristic of a notched collar. The outer edge of a shawl collar is usually an unbroken line, but on some patterns this edge will be scalloped or notched to give the impression of a notched collar. As a general rule, the shawl collar is attached to a wrapped-front garment that is held together by a tie belt rather than by buttons or some other kind of fastener.

Pattern pieces for a typical shawl collar are shown here. Notice that the upper collar, lapels, and front facing are cut from the same pattern piece. The under collar and back neck facing are separate pattern pieces.

Constructing and applying a shawl collar

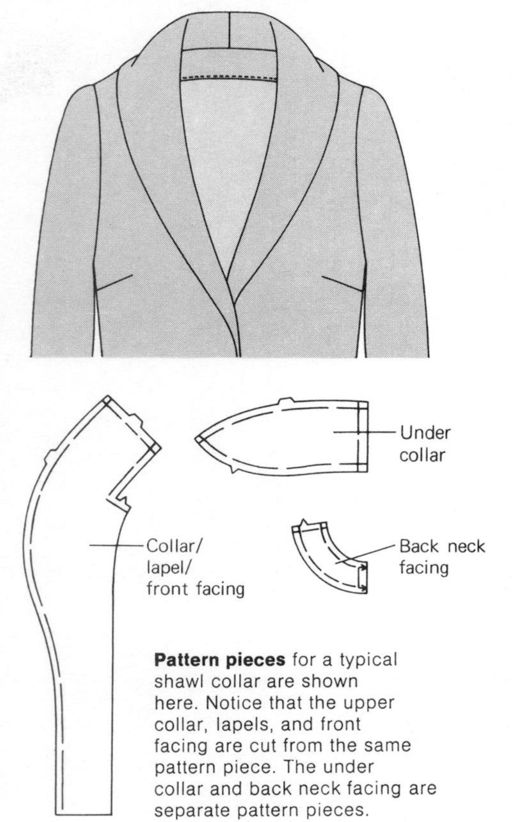

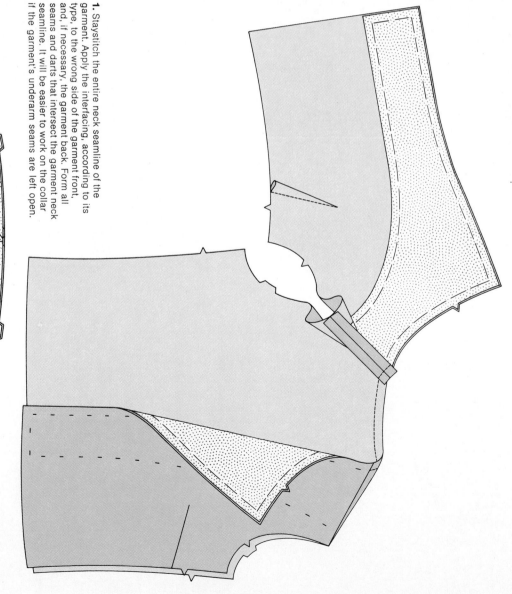

1. Staystitch the entire neck seamline of the garment. Apply the interfacing, according to its type, to the wrong side of the garment front, and, if necessary, the garment back. Form all seams and darts that intersect the garment neck seamline. It will be easier to work on the collar if the garment's underarm seams are left open.

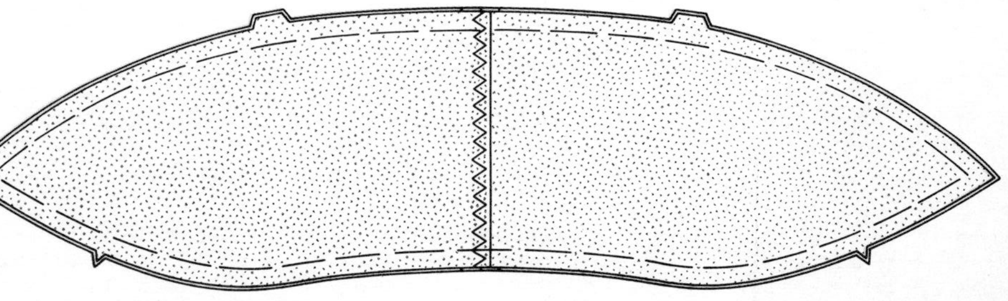

2. Form the center back seam in the under collar. Press seam flat, trim to half-width, then press open. Apply interfacing to wrong side of under collar (see p.213).

Catchstitch (flat) 129
Whipstitch 136
Seams 146-147
Seam finishes 148-149

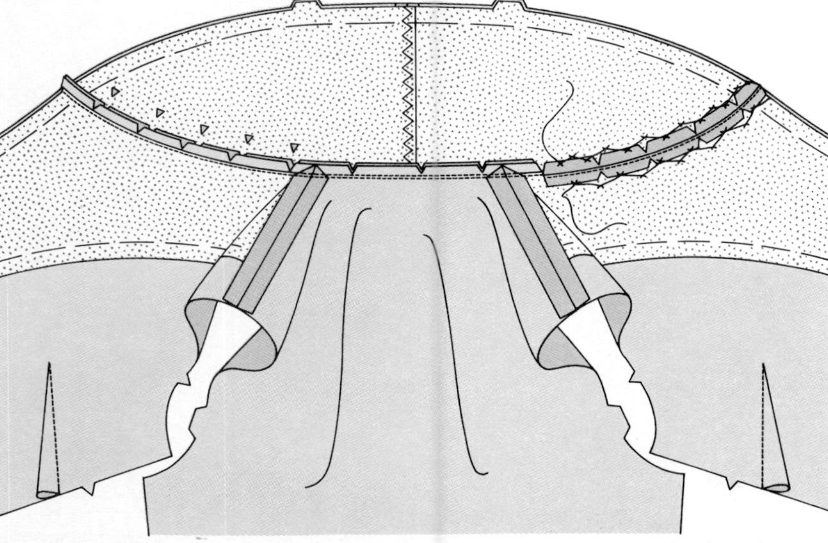

3. Right sides together, match and pin under collar to garment along neck seamline; clip garment seam allowance if necessary for collar to fit smoothly. Baste along neck seamline. Garment side up, stitch under collar to garment. Remove bastings; press seam flat.

4. Trim seam allowances to 3/8"; diagonally trim the cross-seam allowances. Finger-press seam open; clip the garment seam allowance and notch the under collar seam allowance until they both lie flat. Press seam open; catchstitch over both edges to hold seam open.

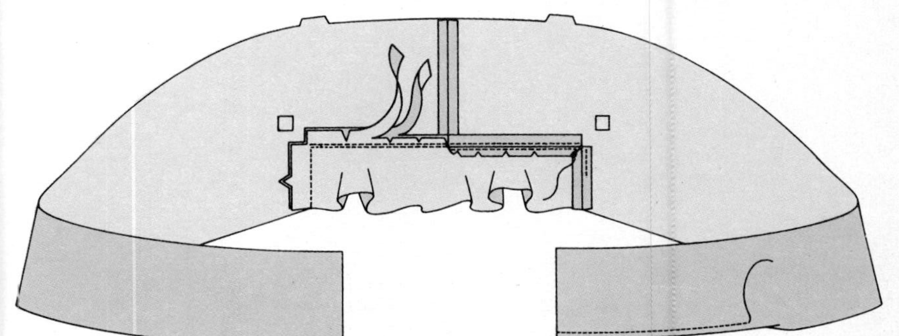

5. Staystitch neck seamline of the collar/lapel/front facing pieces and reinforce corners with short stitches. Seam the two pieces together. Press seam open, then flat; trim to half-width. Clip into both corners. Staystitch neck seamline of back neck facing piece.

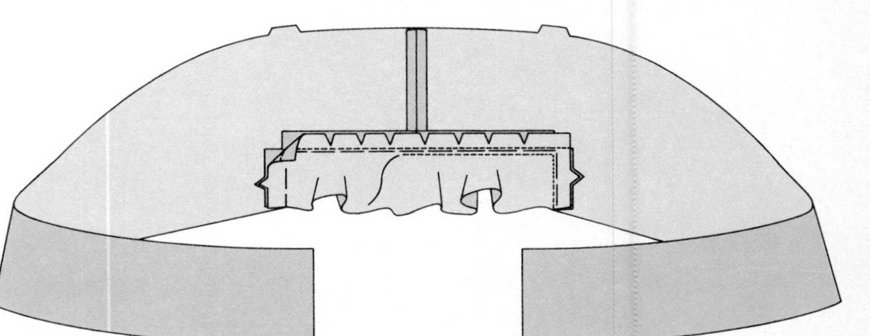

6. Match and baste the back neck facing to the collar/lapel/front facing; clip back neck facing seam allowance where necessary and spread collar/lapel/front facing at corners. Collar/lapel/front facing side up, stitch the seam, reinforcing and pivoting at corners.

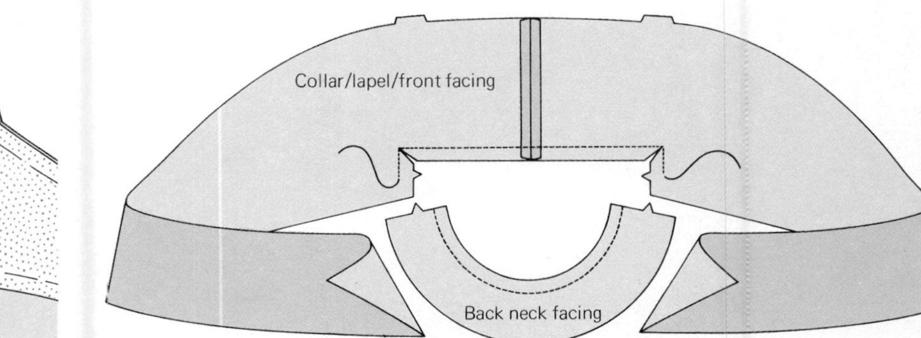

7. Press seam flat, trim to 1/4", then press seam open. Notch out both corners of the back neck facing seam allowance; whipstitch these edges together. If necessary, apply a seam finish to the outer, unnotched edge of the entire unit.

(Continued next page)

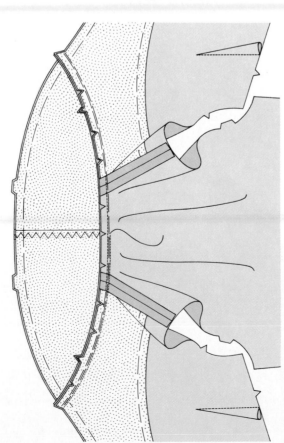

Diagonal basting 125
Plain-stitch tack 135
Understitching 147

Constructing and applying a shawl collar

8. With right sides together, match and baste the collar/lapel/facing unit to the under collar. Stitch the seam directionally, from center back down on each half. Press seam flat; trim. Clip into seam at both ends of lapel roll line. Grade seam *above* the clips, making seam allowance of collar/lapel/facing unit the widest; grade seam *below* clips so that the garment seam allowance is the widest. Clip and notch the seam; press open. Press seam above clips at roll line toward the under collar; press the seam below these clips toward the facing.

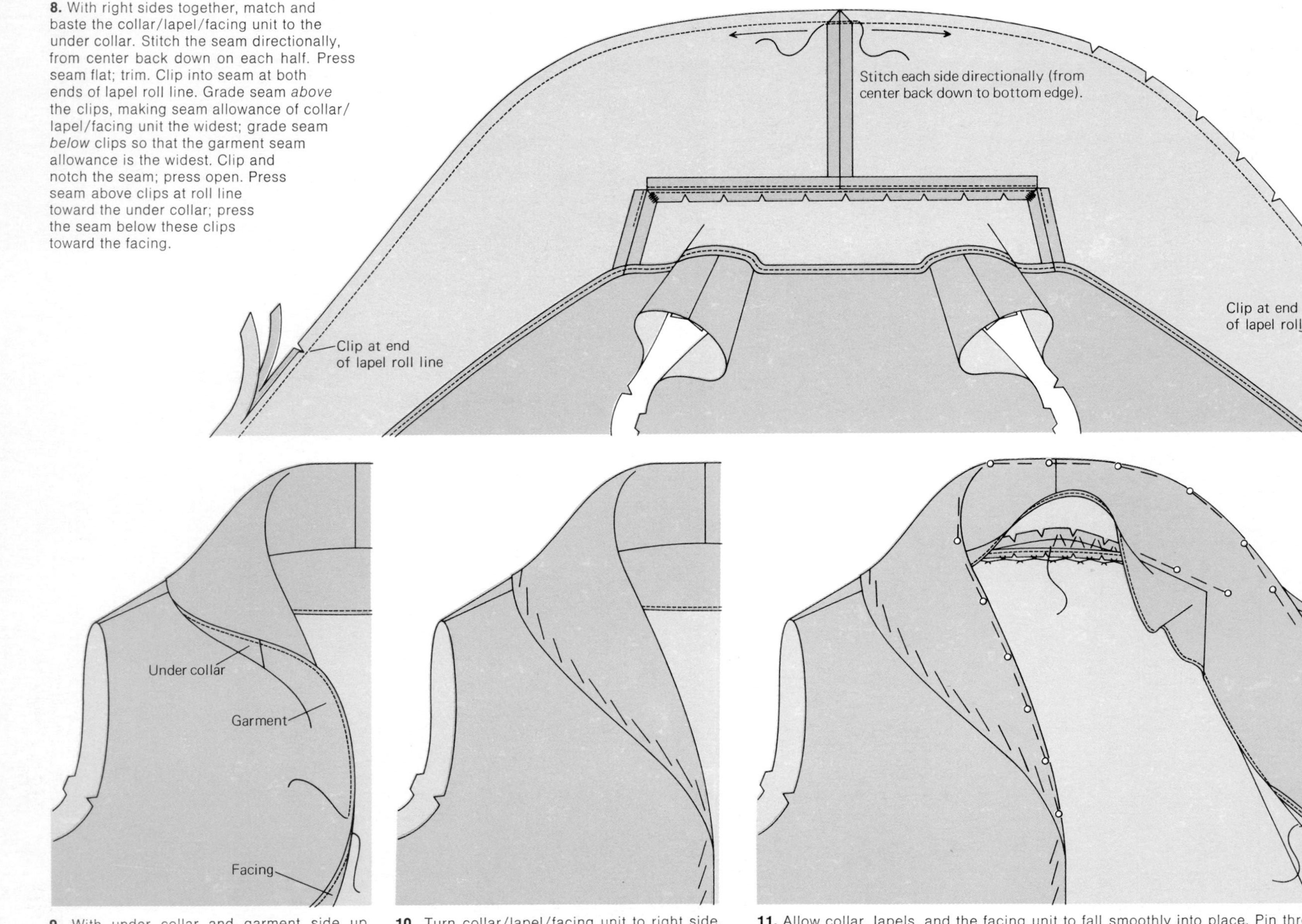

9. With under collar and garment side up, understitch outer edge of collar and lapels. With facing side up, understitch each edge of garment opening below the lapels.

10. Turn collar/lapel/facing unit to right side. Roll outer edge of collar and lapels toward under collar; roll edges of garment opening toward facing. Diagonal-baste along edges.

11. Allow collar, lapels, and the facing unit to fall smoothly into place. Pin through all layers along the roll line and just above the back neck seamline. Lift up back neck facing and, using a plain-stitch tack, stitch facing and garment neck seamlines together as they fell. Remove pins. Tack lower edges of facing to garment.

Standing collars

Pressing 18-19
Interfacing 72-73, 76-79
Stitching cornered seams 146
Reducing seam bulk 147

General information

Standing collars extend up from the neck seamline and are of two types: (1) the **plain standing collar,** also called the band or Mandarin collar; (2) the **turn-down standing collar,** sometimes known as the turtleneck or roll-over collar. The basic difference between the two is their initial width, the turn-down collar being twice as wide as the band style so that it can turn back down onto itself.

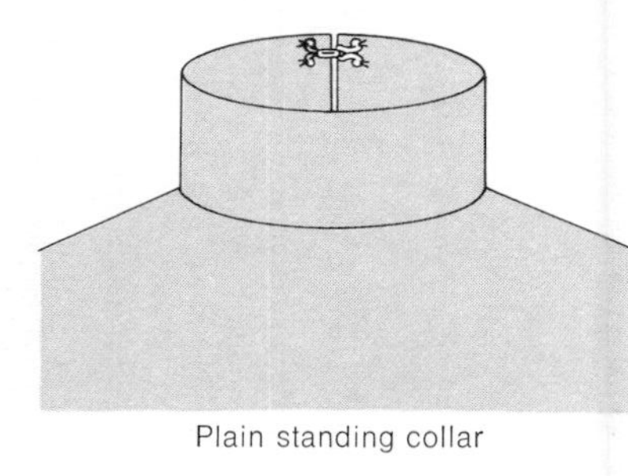

Plain standing collar

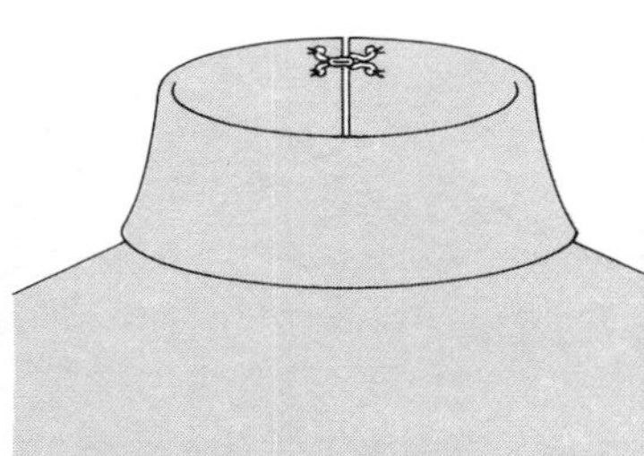

Turn-down standing collar

Standing collars are either rectangular or curved. Those that are rectangular, which either type can be, may be constructed from either one or two pieces. If a collar is curved, as only the plain collar can be, it will consist of two pieces. Names given to the parts of a standing collar vary. The parts of the collars shown on the next few pages have been identified as either *collar* or *facing*. Sometimes only the collar is interfaced; if it is a one-piece unit, secure interfacing at foldline (see Interfacings). Both collar and facing can be interfaced if desired. Such interfacing decisions depend on the weight of the garment fabric. For a variation of the standing collar, a shirt collar with a stand, see pages 227–228.

Constructing a one-piece collar

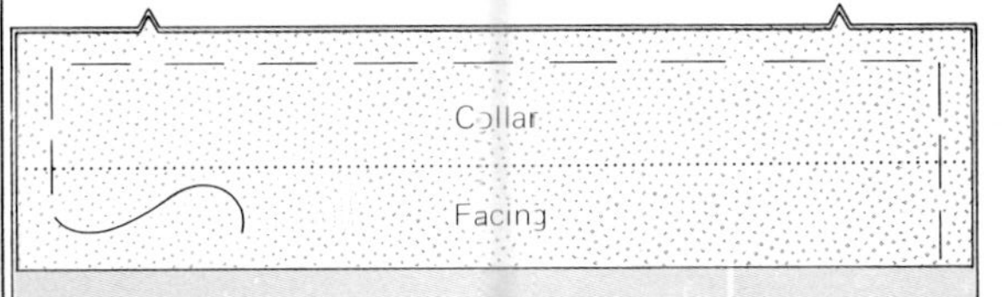

1. Interfacing for plain band collar is trimmed along neck seamline of facing, then applied to wrong side of collar and facing. (If garment fabric is bulky, interface collar only.)

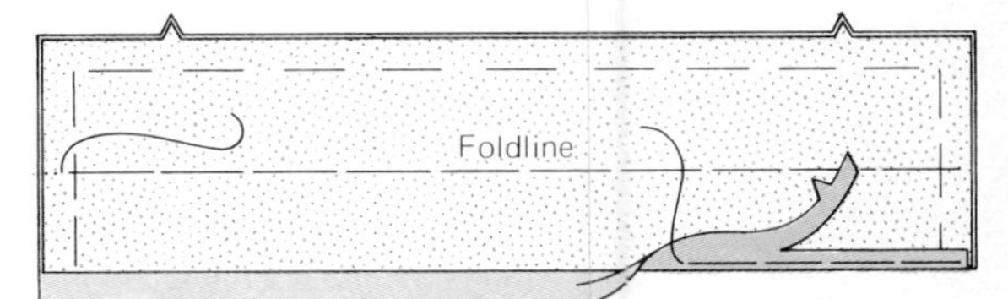

2. If necessary, baste interfacing in place along foldline. Fold up facing edge along its neck seamline; baste in place along seamline. Press; then trim to ¼″.

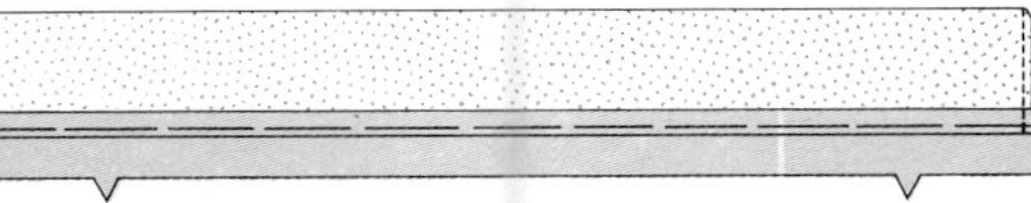

3. Fold section along its foldline with right sides of collar and facing together. Match and stitch together along side seams. Press flat; trim and grade seam allowances.

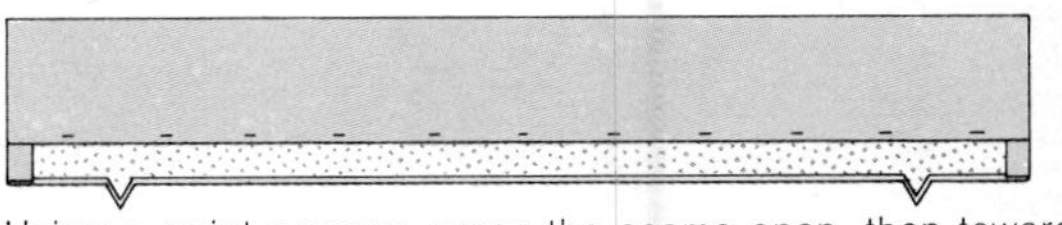

4. Using a point presser, press the seams open, then toward the facing. Turn collar right side out. Using a press cloth, press the collar. Remove bastings at foldline.

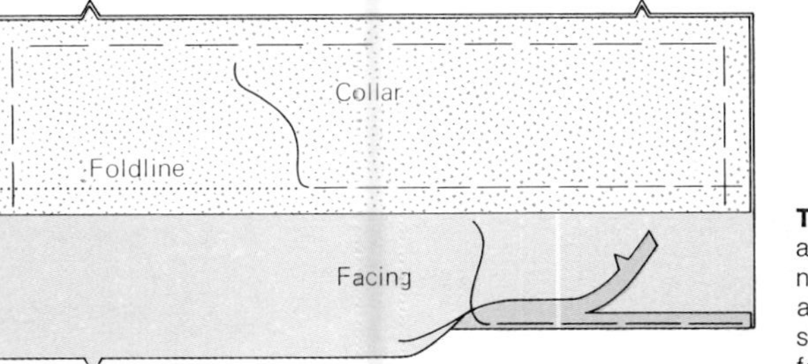

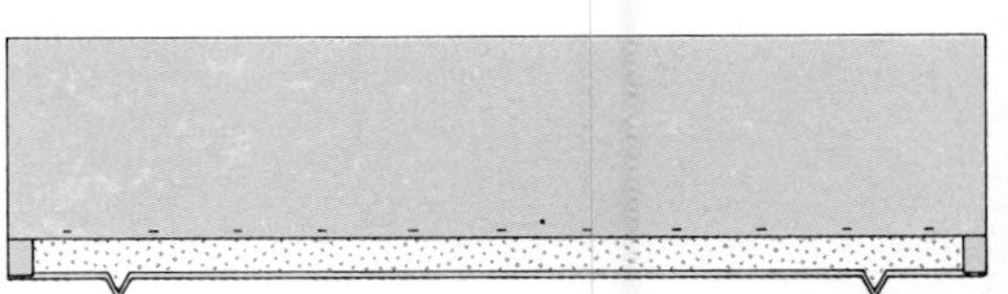

Turn-down collar is cut twice as wide as it would be if it were a plain band collar. So that the finished turn-down collar will not be too stiff or bulky, apply interfacing to the collar portion and ½″ into the facing area. Hold in place at the foldline with short stitches, spaced ½″ apart. Proceed with construction, following Steps 2, 3, and 4 above.

Constructing a two-piece collar

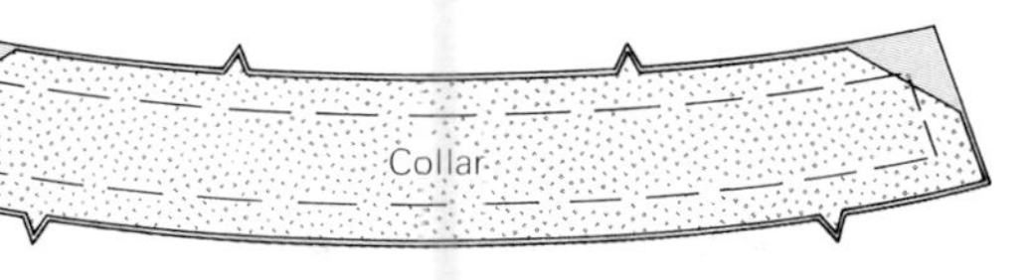

Whether the two-piece collar is curved, as shown, or rectangular in shape, the construction procedure is the same. **1.** Apply interfacing to the wrong side of the collar section.

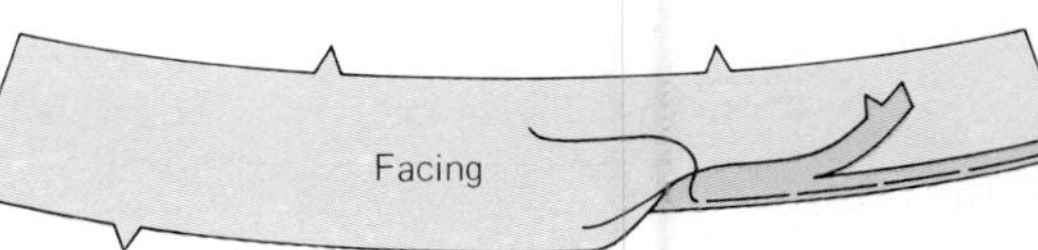

2. Fold up the facing's edge along its neck seamline and toward the wrong side of the facing. Baste in place near fold. Press; then trim to ¼″.

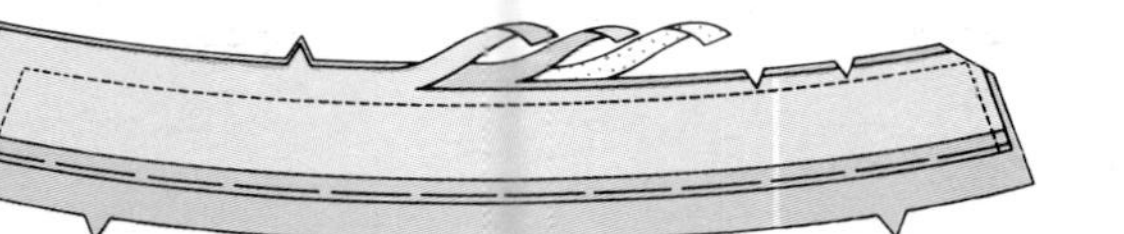

3. With right sides together, match, baste, and stitch collar to facing along the side and upper seamlines. Press seams flat. Trim, grade, and notch or clip seam allowances.

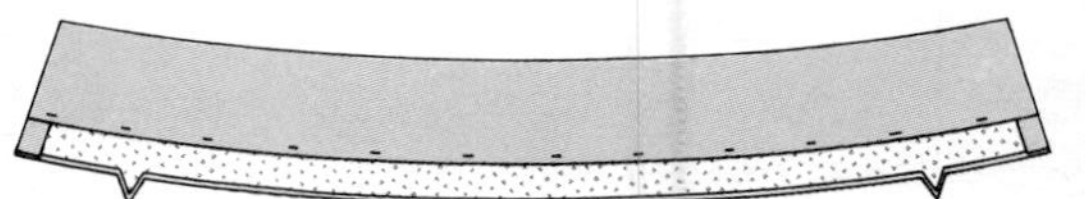

4. Press seams open, then toward the facing. Understitch the upper seamline if necessary. Turn collar right side out. Using a press cloth, press the collar.

Standing collars

Pressing 18-19
Slipstitch (uneven) 132
Reducing seam bulk 147
Fasteners 354

Applying a standing collar to a garment

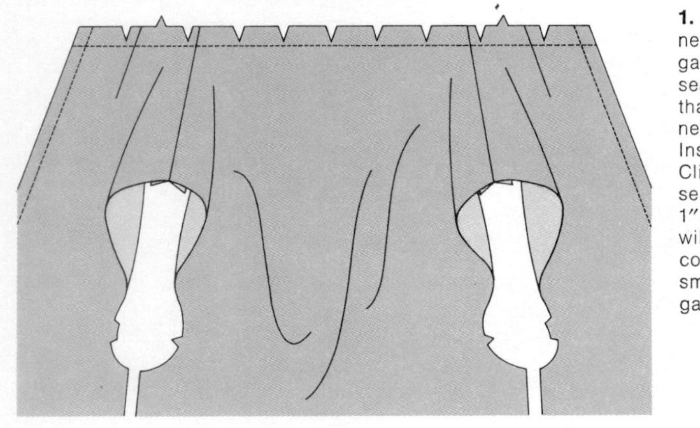

1. Staystitch the neck seamline of the garment. Form all seams and darts that intersect the neck seamline. Insert the zipper. Clip into the neck seam allowance at 1″ intervals; this will permit the collar to fit smoothly onto the garment.

2. With right sides together, match, pin, and baste the edge of the collar to the garment along the neck seamline. Stitch the seam and secure stitching at both ends.

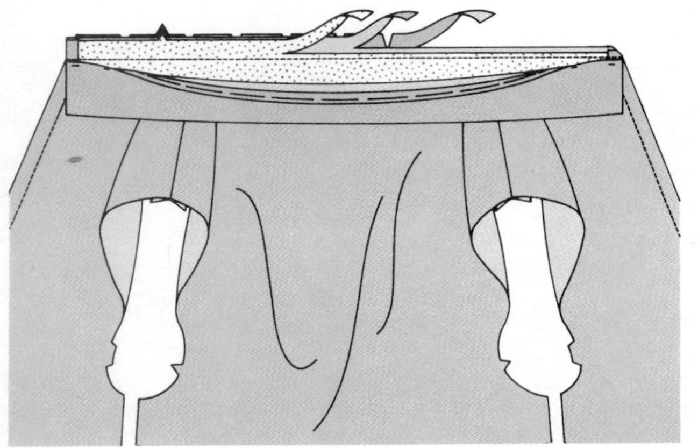

3. Press seam flat. Trim and grade seam allowances, making the collar seam allowance the widest. Trim diagonally across the corners and cross-seam allowances.

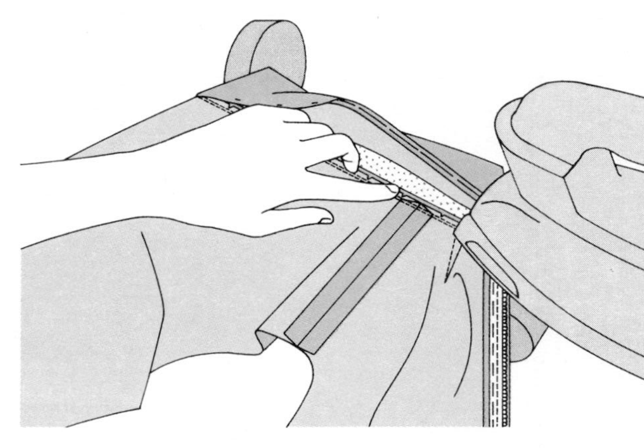

4. Using the curved edge of the tailor's board, press the seam open, then press it up, toward the collar.

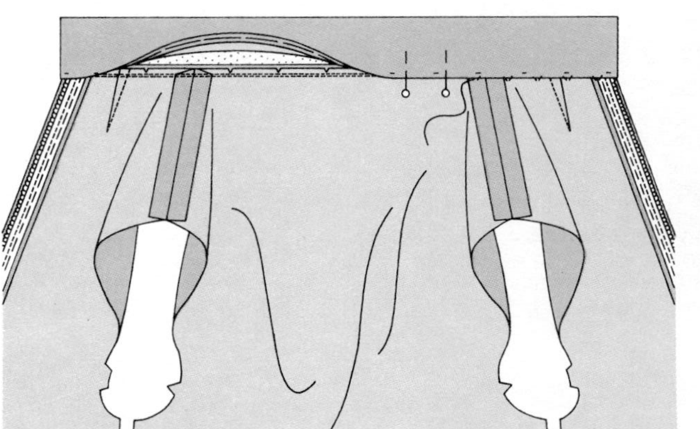

5. Bring the facing edge down to align with the neck seamline; pin in place. Slipstitch facing to garment along the neck seamline, removing pins as you stitch. Remove bastings at facing edge and press neckline seam.

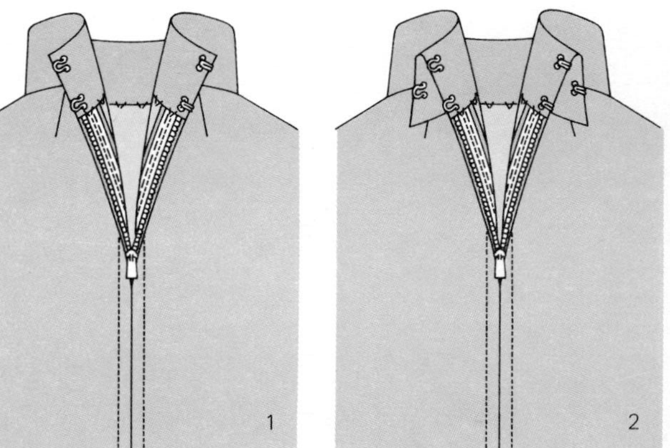

6. Attach fasteners so that the ends of collar meet when fastened. With a plain standing collar (1), sew two sets to the inside of collar, placing one set at neck, the other at the top of collar. For a turn-down collar (2), attach two sets as for the plain collar but sew another set to the center of the turned-down portion.

Shirt collar with a stand

A shirt collar with a stand is commonly found on men's shirts but can also be used for jackets and for women's wear. This type of collar can be thought of as having two sections, *collar* area and *stand* area. The stand may be cut as a separate piece or it may be an extension of the collar. Whether the stand is cut as one with the collar or separately, the collar unit is applied to the garment the same way as any other standing collar.

As a rule, it is the under collar that is interfaced, but if the fabric is very lightweight or sheer, interfacing can be applied to the upper collar; this will prevent the seams from showing through to the finished side of the collar. It is always advisable to interface the stand. If the stand area is an extension of the collar, the interfacing is applied to *both* under collar and stand in a single piece. The usual garment closure is buttonholes. Since a buttonhole is generally constructed in the collar stand after it has been applied to the garment, it may be more convenient to construct all of the buttonholes for both the garment and the stand after applying the collar.

Topstitching of the collar and stand is optional, but it is usually necessary if the placket of the garment has been topstitched.

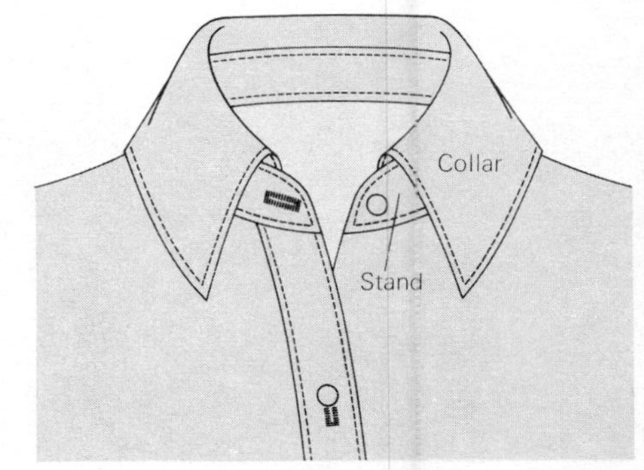

Constructing a shirt collar with a separate stand

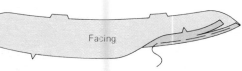

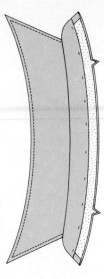

1. Interface the under collar (and stand if it was cut out as part of under collar). Baste upper collar to under collar along side and upper seamlines. (If stand's facing was cut out as part of upper collar, handle neck edge as in Step 5.)

2. Stitch the seam. Use shorter stitches at the corners; stitch across corners to blunt them. Press seam flat. Trim, grade, and clip the seam allowances. Trim across corners and taper seam allowances on both sides of corners.

3. Press seam open, then toward the under collar. Turn the collar to the right side; pull out the corners (see Step 7, p. 214). Press collar from the under collar side. If desired, topstitch along the outer finished edges.

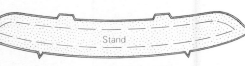

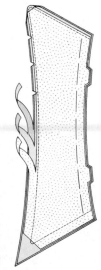

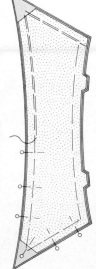

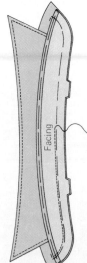

4. Apply the interfacing to the wrong side of the collar stand. (If the collar stand was cut out as a continuation of the collar, the stand was interfaced in Step 1 when the interfacing was applied to the under collar.)

5. Fold up the stand's facing edge along its neck seamline and toward the wrong side of the facing. Pin, then baste in place close to the fold. Remove pins. Press; then trim the seam allowance to ¼″.

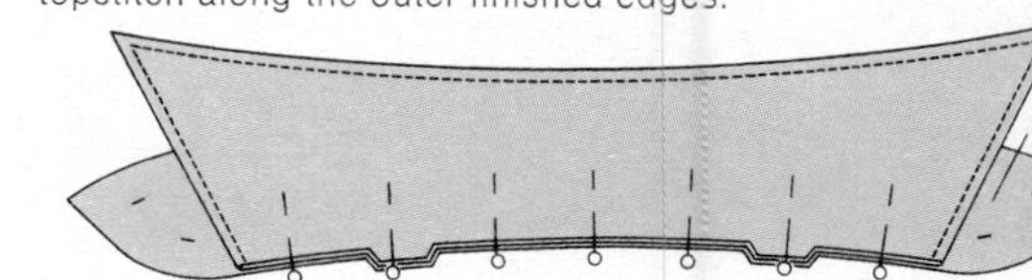

6. With the right side of the under collar toward the right side of the stand, match and pin the collar to the stand along the lower edge of the collar. The stand will extend beyond the ends of the collar.

7. With the right side of the upper collar toward the right side of the stand's facing, match and pin the facing to the collar and the stand. Baste through all thicknesses along seamline; remove pins. Stitch entire seam; remove bastings.

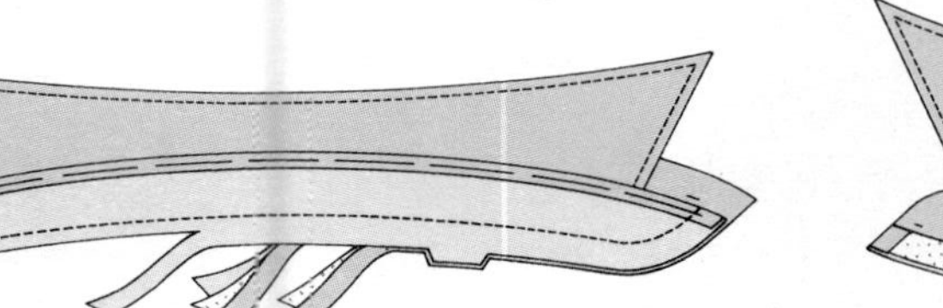

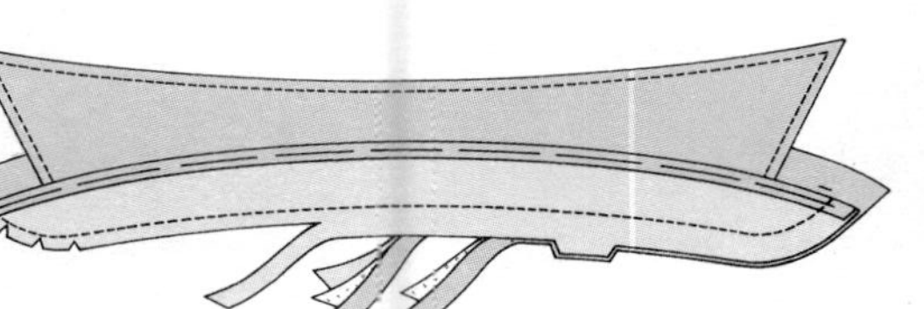

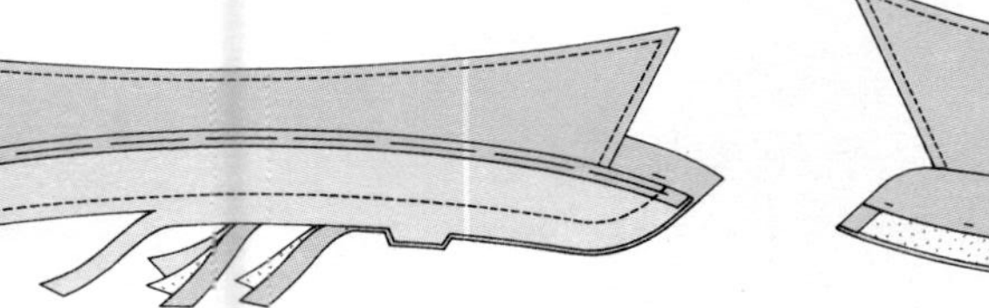

8. Press seam flat. Trim and grade the seam, making the facing seam allowance the widest. Notch and clip the curved seam allowances. Press the seam open, guiding point of iron between the facing and upper collar seam allowances.

9. Turn stand and facing to the right side. Using a press cloth, press the seam, facing, and stand down, away from the collar. If necessary, diagonal-baste through all thicknesses to hold them in place during pressing.

Pressing 18-19
Slipstitch (uneven) 132
Reducing seam bulk 147
Topstitching 152

Applying a shirt collar with a stand to a garment

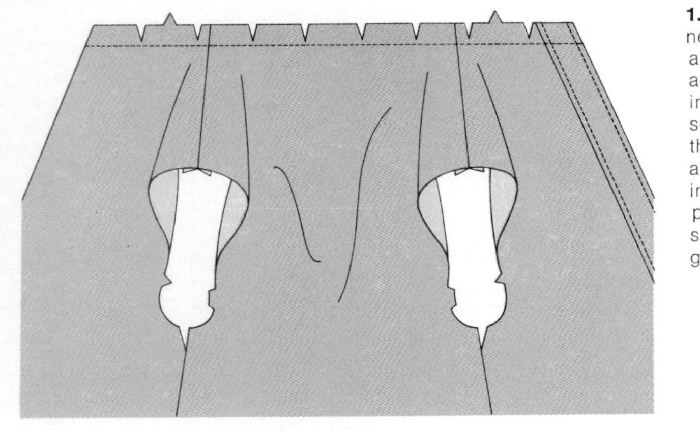

1. Staystitch garment neck seamline and form all seams and darts that intersect the neck seamline. Clip into the neck seam allowance at 1" intervals; this will permit collar to fit smoothly onto the garment.

2. With right sides together, match and pin the stand to the garment along the neck seamline. Stitch the seam; secure the stitching at both ends.

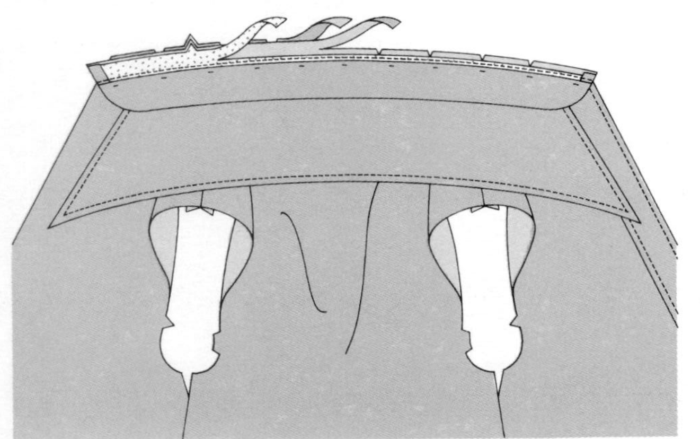

3. Press seam flat. Trim and grade the seam allowances, making the seam allowance of the stand the widest. Clip or notch seam if necessary.

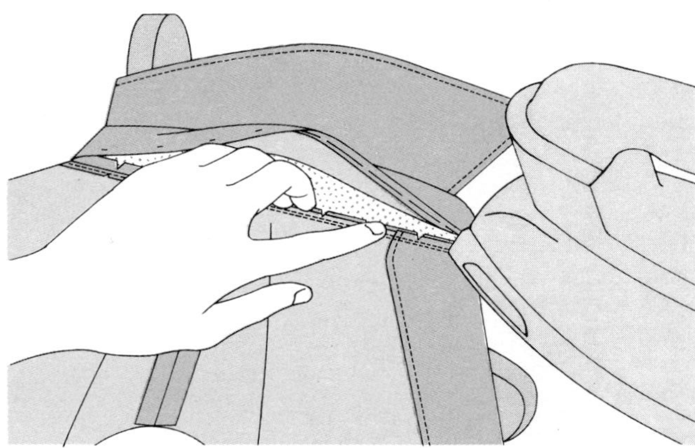

4. Using the curved part of a tailor's board, press the seam open, then up, toward the collar.

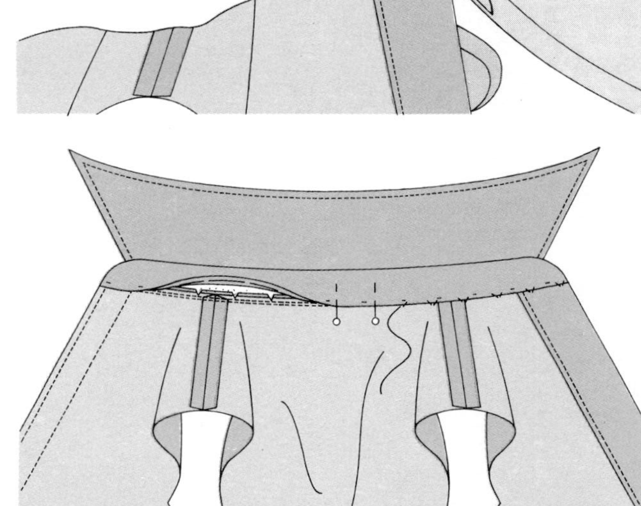

5. Bring the facing edge down to align with the neck seamline; pin in place. Slipstitch facing to garment along the neck seamline. Remove pins and all bastings.

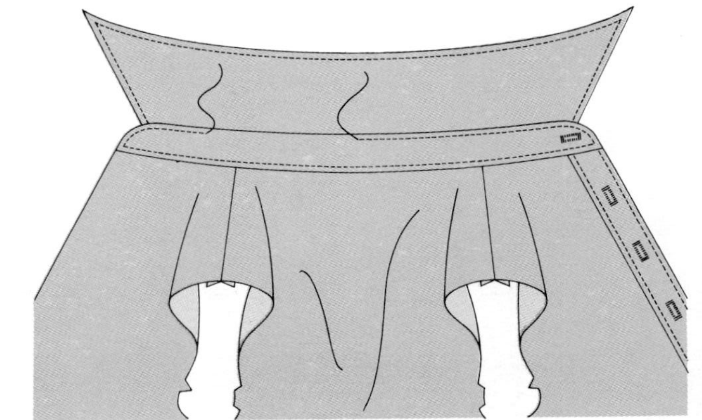

6. From the facing side, press the neckline seam. If desired, topstitch along all edges of the stand. Start and end topstitching on upper edge of stand at center back. Bring threads to the inside and tie. Construct buttonhole in the stand (and buttonholes in garment if postponed until this stage).

Waistlines Waistbands & Belts

Waistline joinings

Zigzag stitching 32-37
Fitting techniques 103-120

General information

Waistline seams that join the top and the bottom of a garment may be located almost anywhere on the body between the hip and the bust. A garment waistline may fall, as many do, at the natural waistline, but it may also lie just underneath the bust, as it does in an Empire style, or be placed on the hips, as it is in a dropped-waist style. The waistline may be either closely or loosely fitted.

Some waistlines are formed not with an actual seam but by means of an attached casing or an insert of fabric or ribbing. The basic procedure for constructing a joining, an insert, or a casing remains the same regardless of location or fit.

Waistline seams are not always straight horizontal seams; they may be curved or angled sharply toward the bust or hips. It is generally best to fit the bodice and skirt individually to the body before joining them with the waist seam.

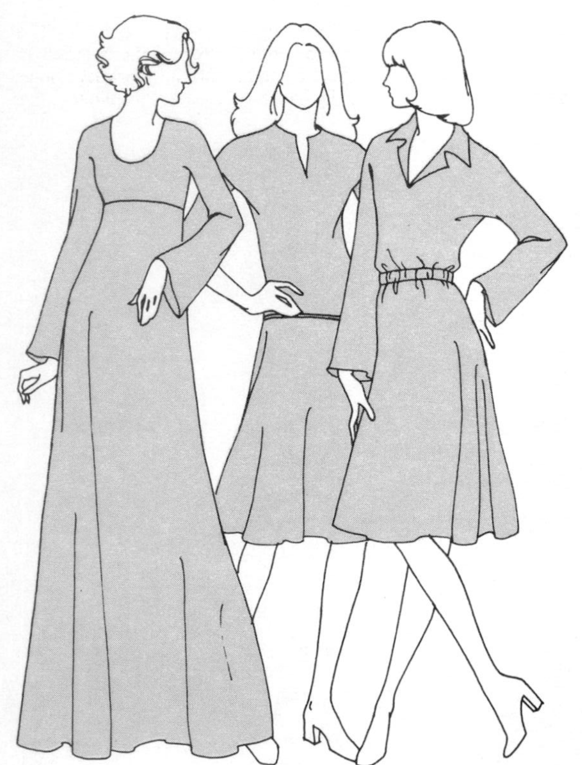

Preparation

Before the waistline seam is sewed, the following steps must be completed: (1) waistline edges on both bodice and skirt staystitched; (2) all darts, tucks, or pleats made; (3) all vertical seams stitched, seam-finished, and pressed open; (4) skirt waistline seam easestitched. Do the last step, easestitching, from the right side on the skirt waist seamline, breaking stitching at side seams and leaving 3-inch thread ends. If bodice ease is called for, follow pattern instructions. If zipper placket intersects the waistline, zipper can be inserted only after forming waist seam.

Joining a bodice to a fitted skirt

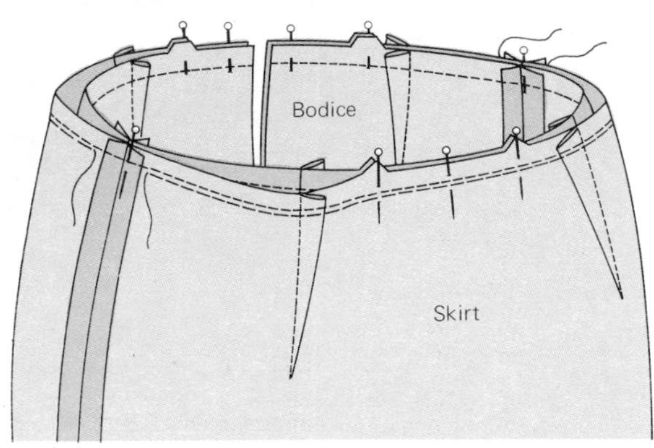

1. Turn the skirt to the wrong side and the bodice to the right side. Slip the bodice into the skirt (work is done with bodice inside skirt, their right sides together). Align and pin cut edges, carefully matching side seams, center front and back, all notches. The skirt may be slightly larger than the bodice; easestitching will correct this.

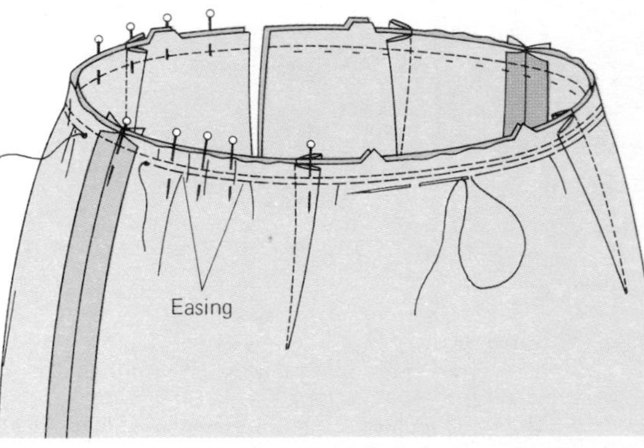

2. Pull on bobbin threads of easestitching until each skirt section exactly fits corresponding bodice section. Secure ease threads by knotting. Distribute fullness evenly, avoiding gathers, tucks, or any fullness within 2″ of either side of center front and back. Pin at frequent intervals; baste. Try on garment and make necessary adjustments.

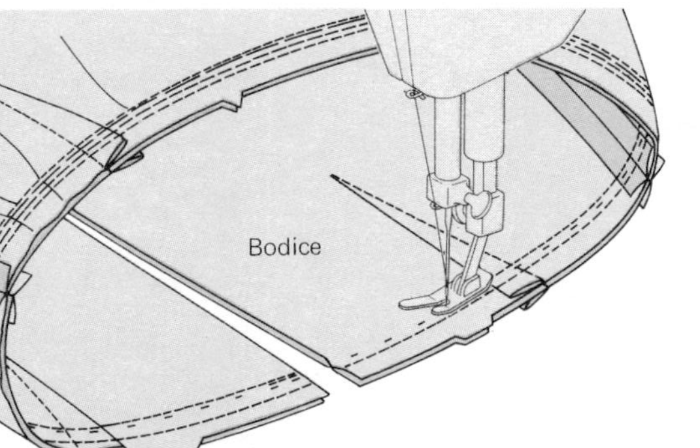

3. Stitch the waistline seam from placket edge to placket edge. Reinforce seam by beginning and ending it with backstitching. The garment is easiest to handle at this point if bodice is placed inside the skirt as it was for pinning and basting, and the seam stitched from the inside, along the bodice seamline, as illustrated.

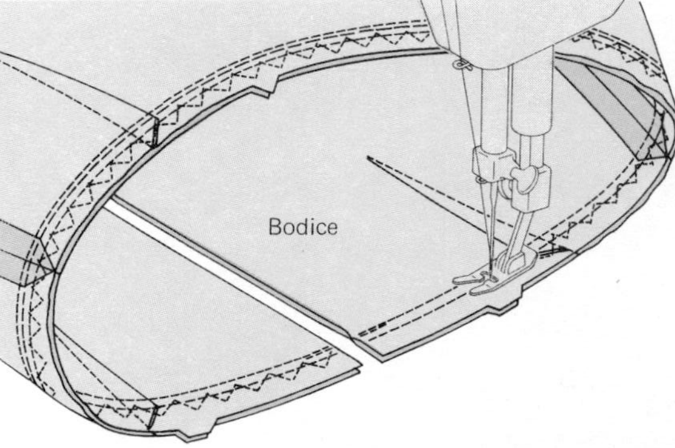

4. Trim ends of darts and cross-seam allowances. Remove bastings. Press seam as stitched. Finish seam in one of the two following ways: stitch seam allowances together with a zigzag or multistitch zigzag; or apply a waistline stay. Pull the bodice out of the skirt and press the seam again, with both seam allowances directed toward the bodice.

Joining a bodice to a gathered skirt

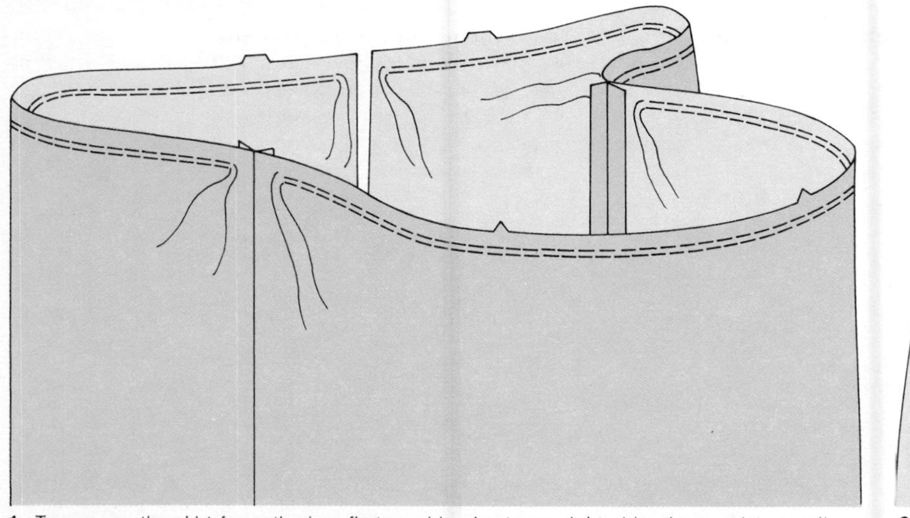

1. To prepare the skirt for gathering, first machine-baste on right side along waist seamline. Section stitching so that it begins and ends at the center back and side seams, at least ⅝″ away from the vertical seamlines. This assures that the bulk of vertical seam allowances will not be caught in the gathers. Leave thread ends at least 3″ long. Place a second row of gathering stitches ¼″ away from the first in the seam allowance.

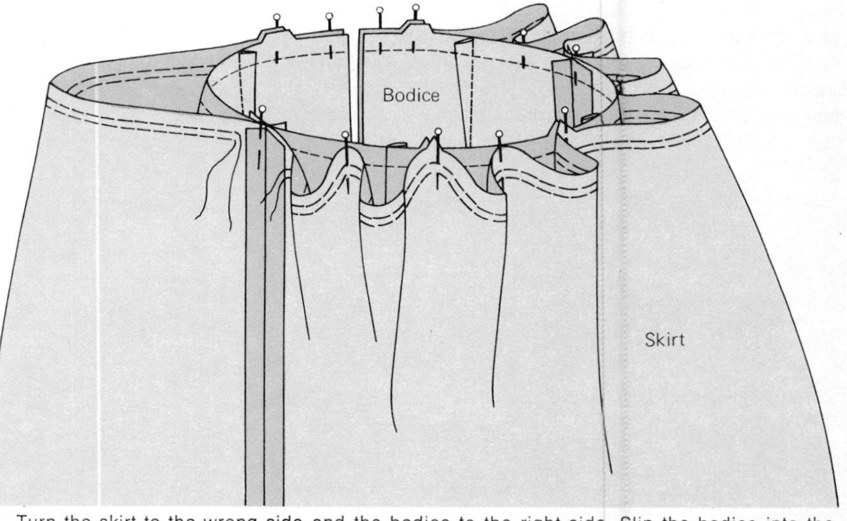

2. Turn the skirt to the wrong side and the bodice to the right side. Slip the bodice into the skirt so that their right sides are together. With raw edges even, pin the two sections together at center front and back, side seams, and notches. Pin again at points midway between those already pinned, carefully apportioning the fabric. If the skirt has a great deal of fullness, the fabric may need further dividing and pinning.

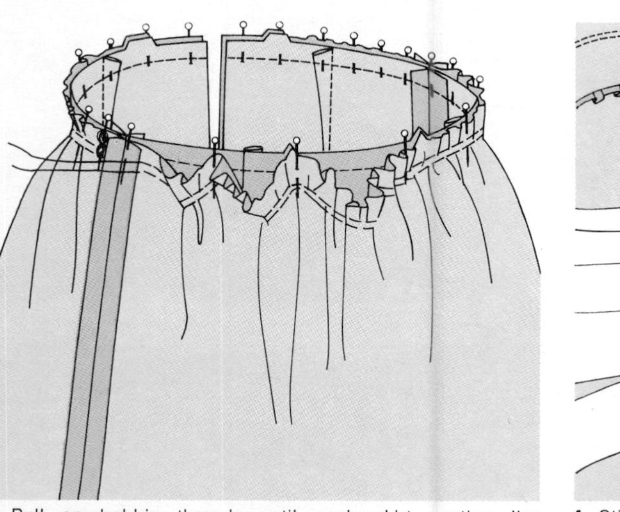

3. Pull on bobbin threads until each skirt section lies flat against corresponding bodice section. Knot threads or wrap them around vertically placed pins to secure. Distribute fullness evenly so that no tucks are visible. Pin at frequent intervals. If desired, baste the waistline seam and try on garment for final fitting before stitching.

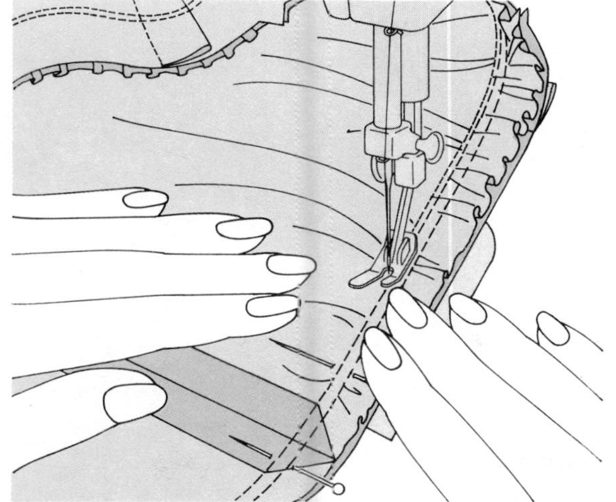

4. Stitch the waistline on the skirt side, from opening to opening. This seam is easiest to handle with the skirt inside the bodice. Work slowly, feeding fabric through the machine carefully and keeping any pleats or tucks from being caught in the seam. Trim darts and cross-seam allowances. Remove any gathering threads visible on the right side.

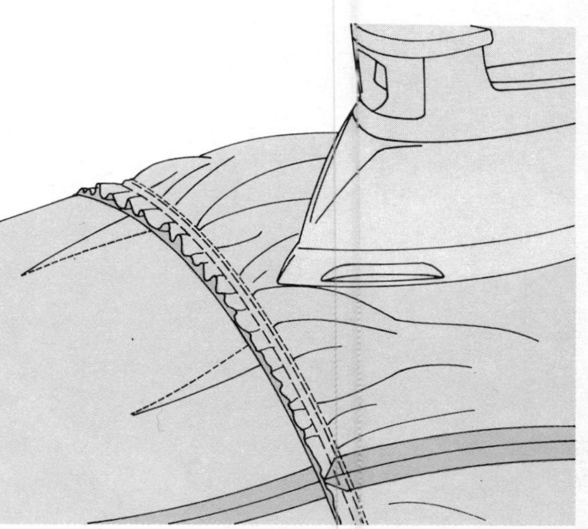

5. Press seam as stitched, then pull bodice up out of skirt. To avoid flattening gathers, press up into them with the tip of the iron. Press the seam allowances flat from the bodice end, taking care to touch the iron to the seam edge only. To finish seam, stitch raw edges together with the zigzag or multistitch zigzag, or apply a waistline stay.

Waistline joinings

Applying a waistline stay

Waistline seams should be stayed to prevent stretching. The stay may be applied either before or after zipper insertion. A stay applied *before* zipper insertion is machine-stitched to the skirt seam allowances and the ends caught into the zipper seam. A stay that is applied *after* zipper insertion is tacked to darts and seams by hand and fastens separately behind the zipper (see bottom row of illustrations). This second type of stay keeps the garment from riding up at the waistline and relieves stress on the zipper in that area. It is particularly useful for delicate or stretchy fabrics and for dresses that have no separate waistline seam or whose styling calls for skirt fabric heavier than the bodice fabric. The stay should be made of a firmly woven tape or ribbon, such as cotton twill tape, good quality seam binding, or grosgrain ribbon. Its width can vary from ½ inch to 1 inch, the wider width recommended for the stay that fastens separately. Preshrink whatever material is used as a stay.

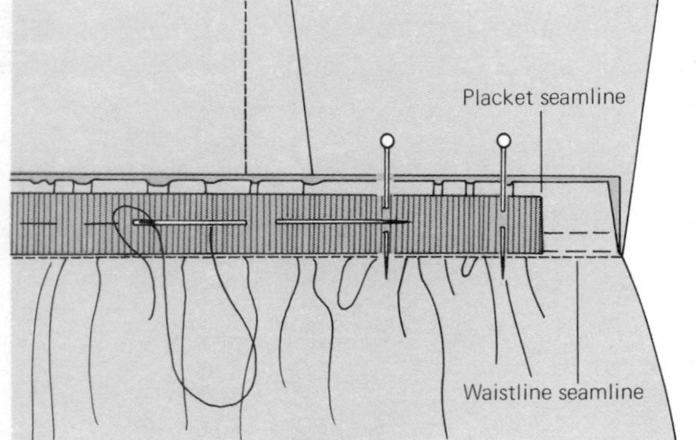

To stay a waistline before inserting a zipper: Measure the garment's waistline from placket seamline to placket seamline; cut stay to this measurement. Pin and baste it to the seam allowances on the skirt side, with ends at placket seamlines and the edge along the waist seamline.

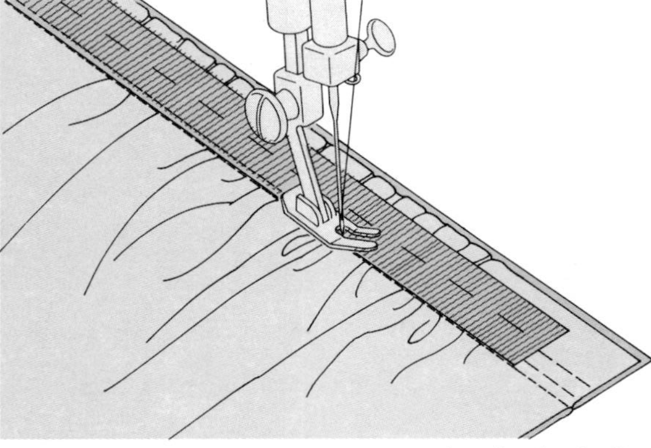

Holding stay and seam allowances together, let the bodice fall inside the skirt so that the right sides of the bodice and skirt are together. With the garment in this position, machine-stitch the stay, through both seam-allowance layers, just above the stitched seam.

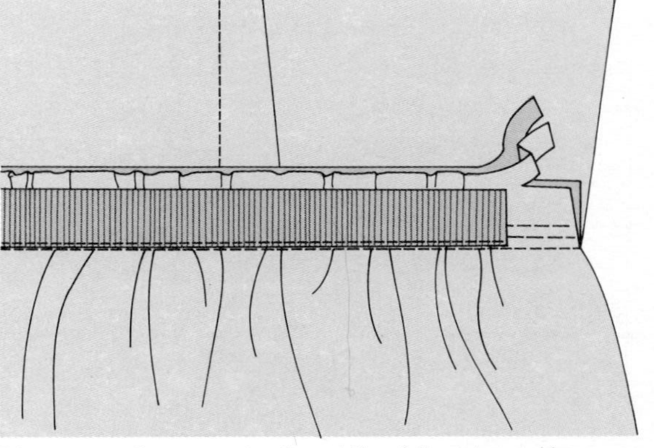

Trim seam allowances to the width of the stay, taking care not to cut the stay. If the fabric is bulky, trim the skirt seam allowance narrower than that of the bodice. If the fabric frays easily, apply a suitable seam finish through the stay and both of the seam allowances. Press toward bodice.

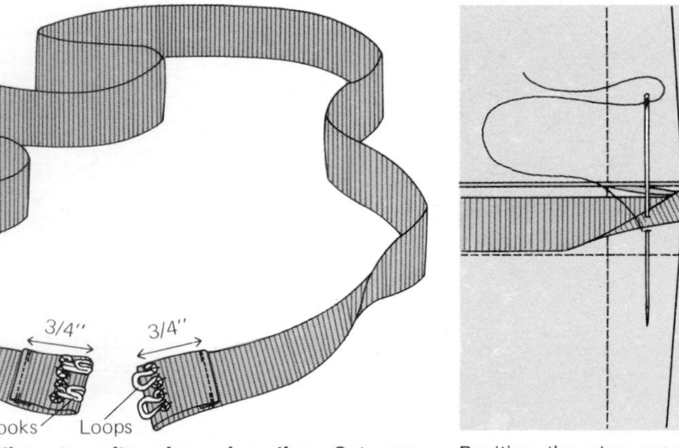

To apply a waistline stay after zipper insertion: Cut grosgrain ribbon the length of the waistline seam plus 2". Finish ends by folding them back 1", then turning raw edges under ¼" and machine-stitching in place. Sew hooks and round eyes to ends, with loops extending beyond edge.

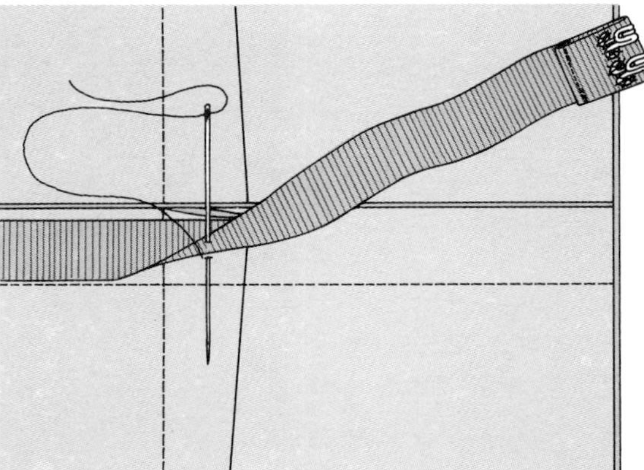

Position the stay over the waistline seam and pin its center to the seam allowance at center front. With this as the starting point, pin the stay to side seams and darts. Hand-tack the stay securely at these points. Be sure that the stitches go through both waistline seam allowances, as well as darts or vertical seam allowances, but do not show on the right side. If the garment has no center front seam, tack the stay to just the waist seam allowances at that point. Leave at least 2" of stay free at each side of the zipper so it can be fastened easily before the zipper is closed.

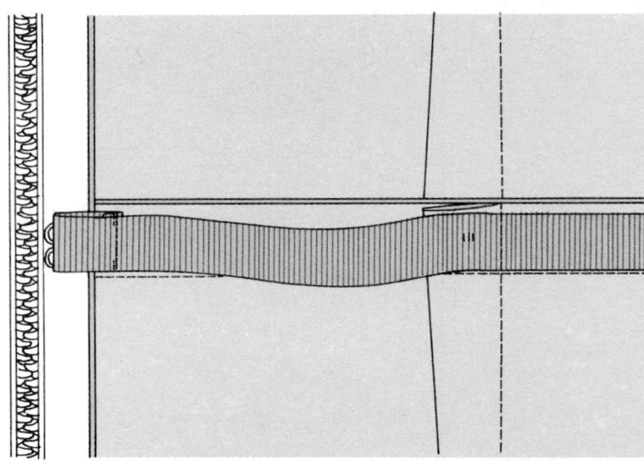

Zigzag stitching 32-37
Seams in knits 156

Inset waistlines

A waistline inset can be made of fabric or ribbed stretch banding. On a fabric inset, there are two waistline seams to sew; each should be stayed (see opposite page), or the inset faced, with the facing serving as a stay. Ribbed stretch banding pulls the waistline to size while providing comfortable fit; it is sewed in differently from a fabric inset. The amount of banding depends on its stretchability and whether or not the garment has a zipper. If there is no zipper, the banding must slip over the shoulders. With a zipper, the banding need only fit snugly around the waist without undue stretching. When measuring the amount needed to encircle the waist, allow ½ inch for joining seams if banding must be pieced or joined, and 1¼ inches for seam allowances if there will be a zipper. For a garment with no zipper, seam the banding into a circle. Place right sides together and join ends with a ¼-inch seam. If banding is to be used double, seam first, press open; fold banding with seam allowances inside.

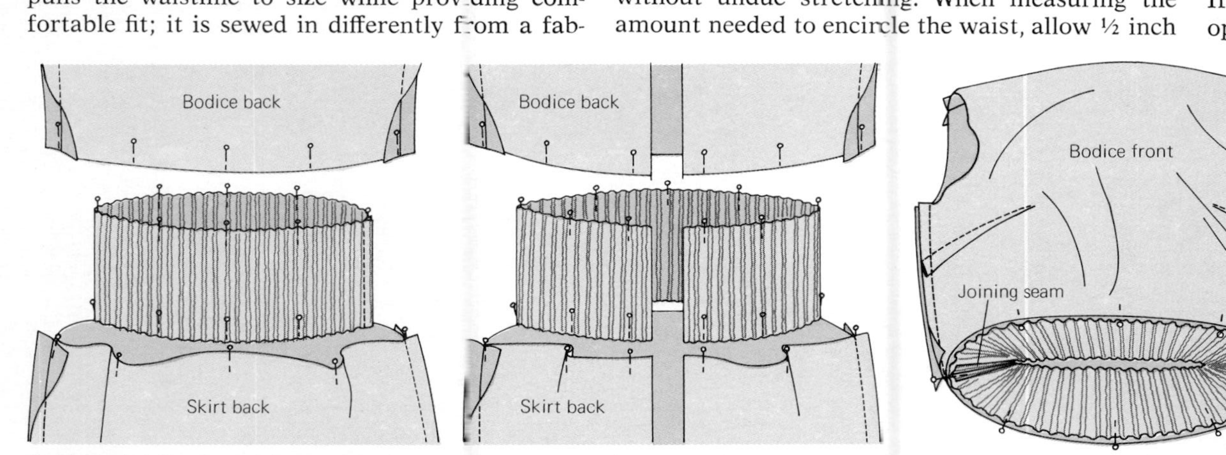

1. Divide banding into eight equal sections; mark divisions with pins. Pin-mark the bodice and skirt into eighths also. For accuracy, pin-mark first at side seams, center fronts and backs, then halfway between these points. **If a zipper is to be inserted,** leave the ⅝″ seam allowances out of sectioning: place a pin ⅝″ from each end of banding, then divide the area between the two pins into eighths.

2. With right sides together, pin the banding to the bodice, matching pin markings. If banding has been sewed into a circle, match the joining seam to a bodice construction seam (either the left side seam or center back seam). **If there is to be a zipper,** pin free ends of banding to placket openings, with raw edges of banding matched to raw edges of bodice. Banding may have to be stretched slightly.

3. Stitch the seam from the banding side, stretching each section of banding to fit the corresponding bodice section. Finish the seam with a second row of stitching or a zigzag stitch, ¼″ away from the first row of stitching, within the seam allowance. Trim seam close to second stitching.

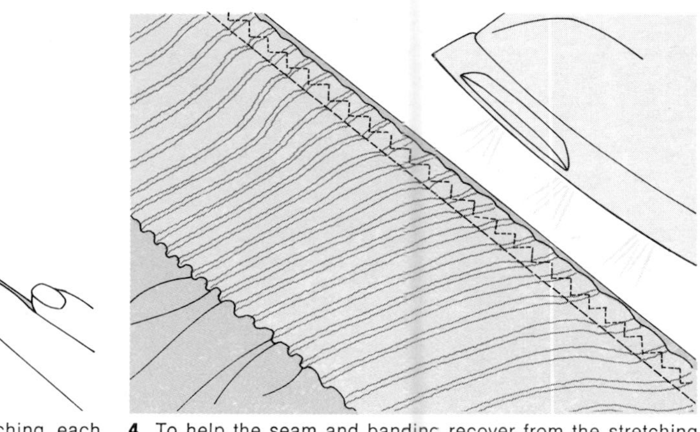

4. To help the seam and banding recover from the stretching that had to be done when the seam was stitched, steam the seam from both the banding and bodice sides. Hold the iron above the fabric and allow the steam to penetrate the seam for a few seconds. Let area cool before continuing.

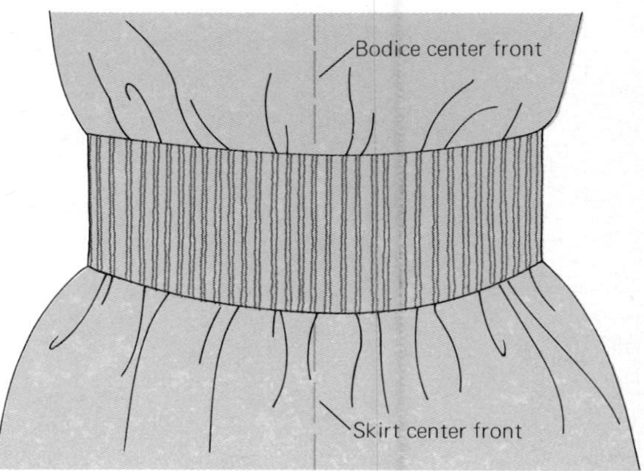

5. To attach the banding to the skirt, repeat steps 2 to 4. Pin carefully so that the ribs of the inset run vertically. This is easily done by following one rib down from bodice center front to skirt center front. **If a zipper is to be inserted,** carefully match the cross seams of the inset.

Waistline casings

Packaged bias tapes 16
Zigzag stitching 32-37

Types of casings

A casing is a fabric "tunnel" made to enclose elastic or a drawstring. When the elastic or drawstring is drawn in, the effect is similar to that of a conventional waistline joining or waistband, but far easier to construct. Waistline casings are practical because they can be adjusted easily to changes in waist measurement—merely tighten or loosen the drawstring or elastic. Replacement of drawstring or elastic is equally simple.

All casings should be at least ¼ inch wider than the elastic or drawstring they are to enclose, to allow for its free movement through the fabric tunnel. There are two types of casings, fold-down and applied. A **fold-down casing** is formed by turning an extension at the garment edge to the inside and stitching it in place. This casing is ideal for pull-on pants and skirts, especially those made of knit fabrics. An **applied casing** consists of a separate strip of fabric that is stitched to the area to be drawn up, on either the outside or the inside of the garment. If the casing is inside but the drawstring is to be tied on the outside, provision must be made to lead the drawstring outside. This can be done with buttonholes or with openings in the garment seam; either must be planned and constructed before the casing is applied.

A *heading* can be formed on either type of casing, provided it occurs at an edge. Simply allow enough extra width for the desired heading, stitch the casing as directed, then stitch a second row at the proper depth for the casing (see illustration below right). When the casing is drawn up, it will gather the heading automatically. A *shirred* effect can be achieved by stitching several additional rows on an extra-wide casing and threading elastic or drawstrings through each of the channels.

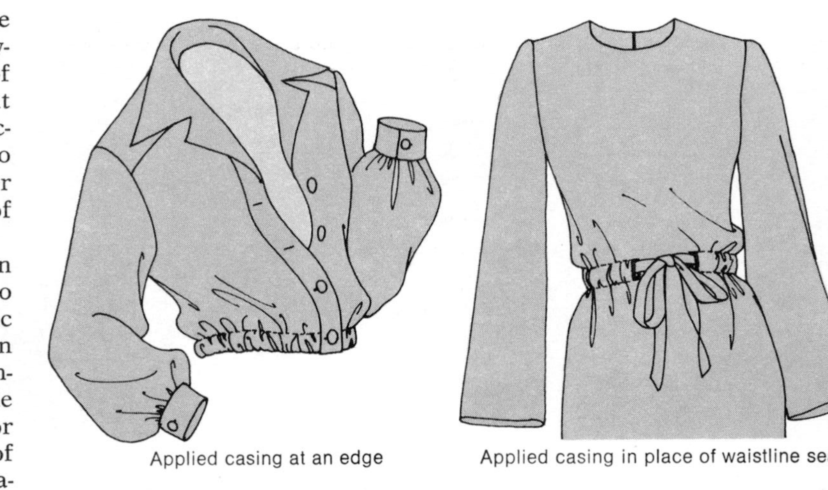

Applied casing at an edge

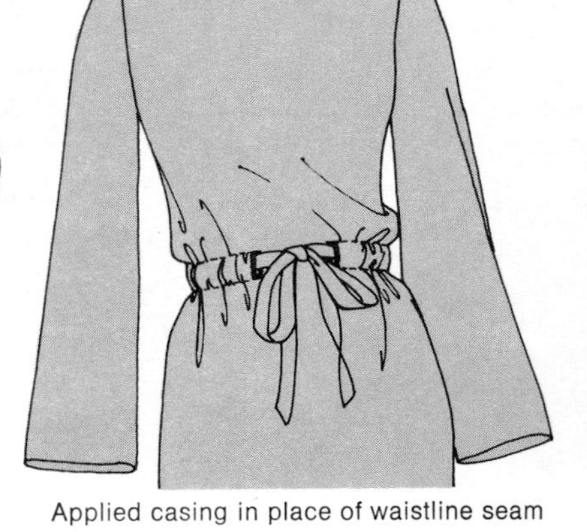

Applied casing in place of waistline seam

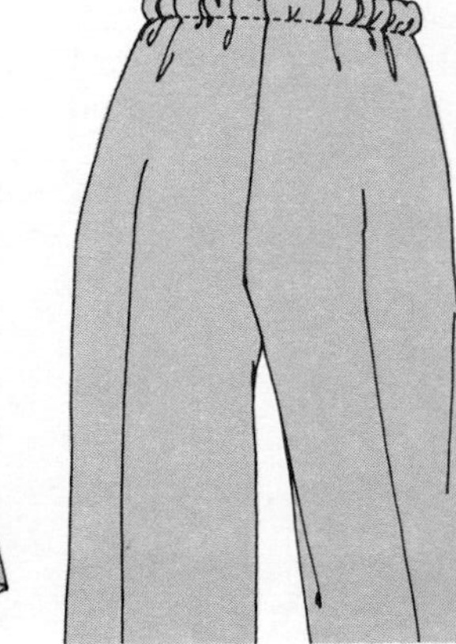

Fold-down casing

Fold-down casings

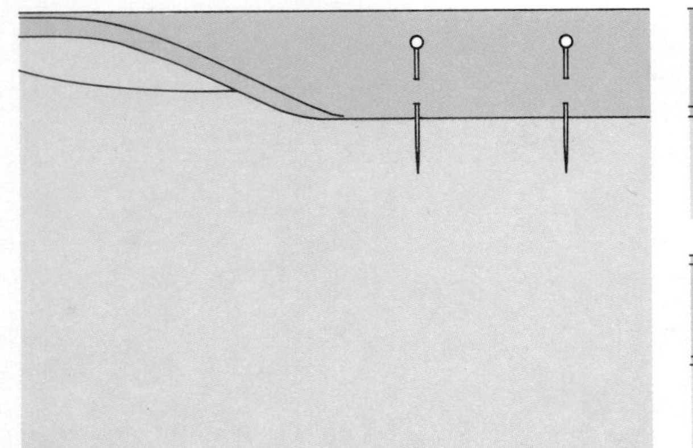

A fold-down casing is best suited to straight edges but can be used on a curved edge if kept very narrow. It is appropriate at the waistline of skirts, pants, and blouses. To make the casing, turn garment edge under ¼" and press. Turn casing to wrong side the desired depth and pin in place.

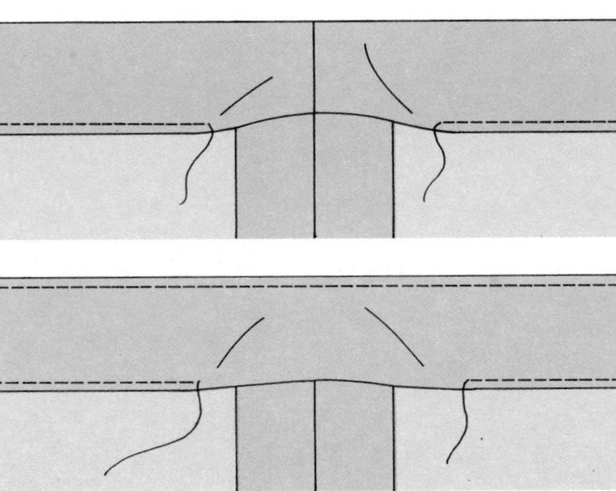

Machine-stitch lower edge of casing in place (on knits, use a small zigzag stitch for elasticity). On a closed circle, leave a small opening for threading elastic or drawstring (not needed if ends are open). If casing will have no heading, place second row of stitching close to top fold.

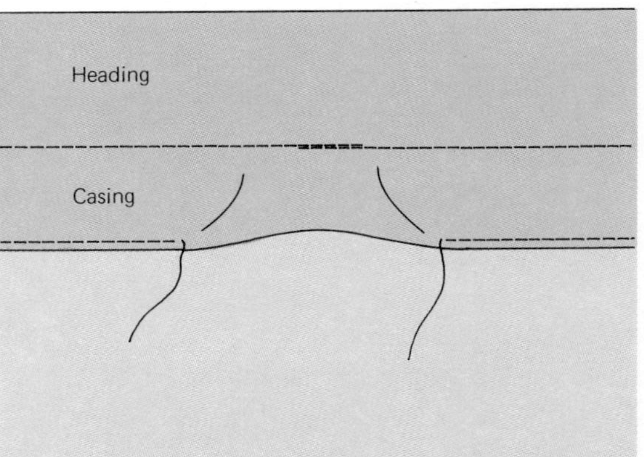

For a casing with a heading, follow preceding steps, except make casing wider and omit edgestitching along top fold. Then measure up from lower stitching the desired width of casing and machine-stitch a second row (no opening needed in this row). Backstitch (or overlap) ends to secure.

Applied casings

An applied casing may be sewed onto a one-piece garment that has no waistline seam; in effect, it substitutes for the seam by providing some fit at the waistline. The applied casing may also act as a facing for the top edge of pants and skirts and the lower edge of blouses and jackets. It may be sewed to either the inside or the outside of a garment. If it is sewed outside, the casing may be made either of the garment fabric or of a contrasting trim. A casing sewed inside is usually made of a lightweight lining fabric or a prepackaged bias tape to reduce unnecessary bulk. If an inside casing has a drawstring that is to be led to the outside, it is necessary to provide buttonhole or in-seam openings. An applied casing is most easily shaped to a garment if casing is cut on the bias.

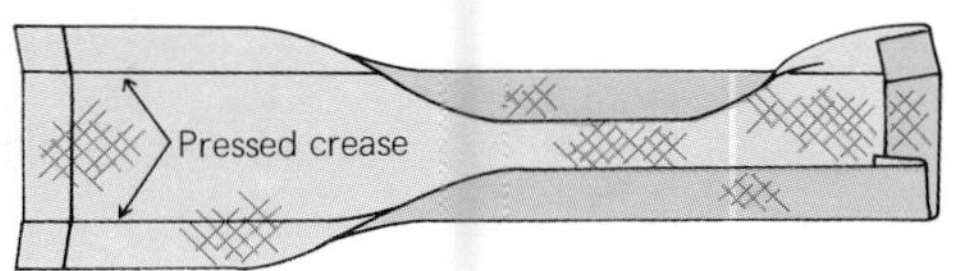

To prepare casing from fabric, first determine the width that the finished casing should be. It must be equal to the width of the elastic or drawstring plus ¼-inch ease for freely threading the elastic or drawstring through the casing. In addition to these finished width requirements, ¼-inch seam allowances are required on the edges; for this, allow an additional ½ inch in your width calculation. Length is determined by the circumference of the garment at the place where the casing will be applied plus ½ inch for finishing ends. Determine true bias of the fabric, then pencil the dimensions of the casing onto the fabric to ensure accurate cutting. After cutting the casing, fold under and press ¼ inch to the wrong side on all edges. Press ends under before pressing down sides.

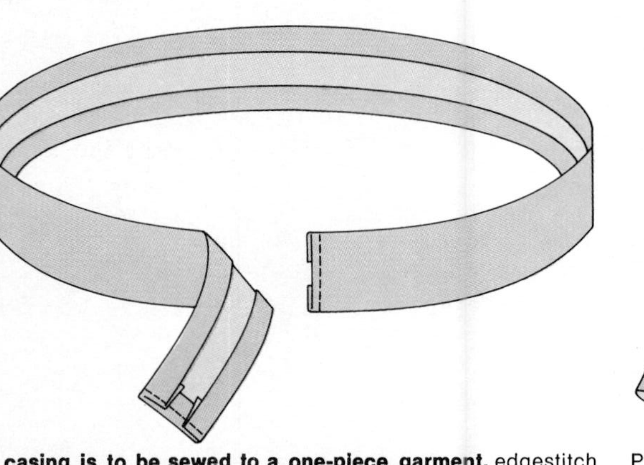

If casing is to be sewed to a one-piece garment, edgestitch both ends (turned under in preparation described above).

Pin casing to garment with lower edge on waistline marking, on inside or outside of garment as pattern instructs.

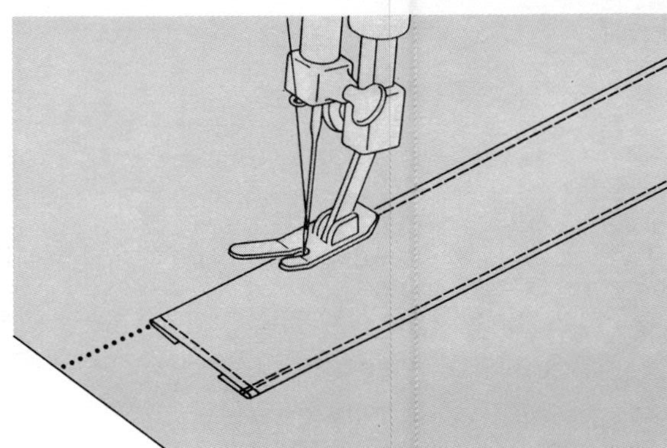

Edgestitch casing to garment on long sides. Backstitch at both ends of stitch lines to strengthen. Press casing flat.

If casing will also serve as facing, first trim seam allowance at garment edge to ¼″. With right sides together and starting at a vertical seam, pin casing to garment.

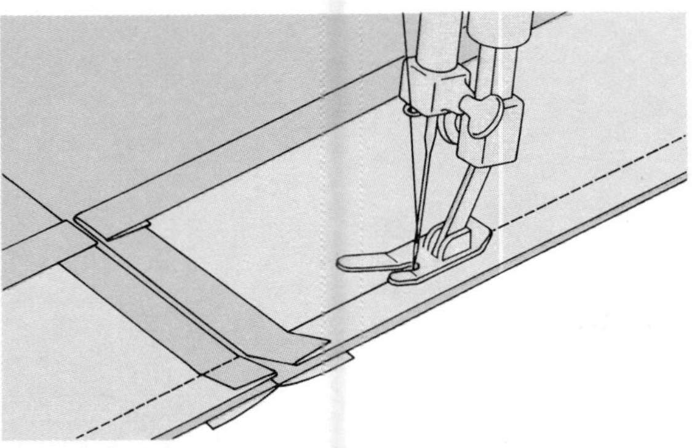
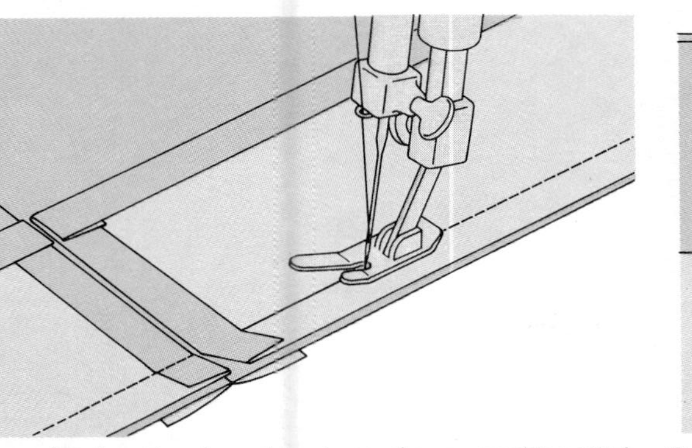

With ends of casing turned back as shown, machine-stitch along pressed crease of casing, which is ¼″ from cut edge. Overlap stitching at ends for reinforcement.

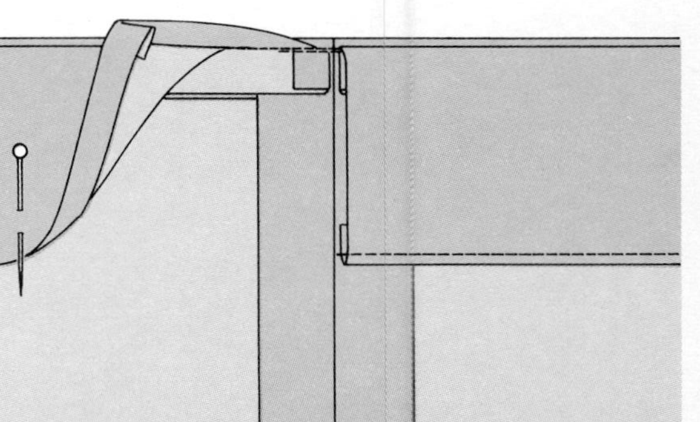

Turn casing to wrong side of garment, letting garment edge roll slightly inside. Pin casing in place. Edgestitch along lower edge, again overlapping stitching. Press flat.

Waistline casings

Catchstitch (flat) 129
Slipstitch (even) 132
In-seam buttonholes 338
Worked buttonholes 343-347

Threading elastic and drawstrings

Casings are threaded with elastic or drawstrings that, when drawn or tied, fit snugly around the body. Elastic for this purpose should be a firm, flat type or non-roll waistband elastic. The exact length depends upon the elastic's stretchability, but it should be slightly less than the measurement of the body at the casing position plus ½ inch for lapping. Drawstrings may be cord, fabric tubing, braid, leather strips, ribbons, even scarves. Elastic can be combined with fabric or ribbon tie ends to give comfort and a pretty finish; the length of the ribbon ends depends upon the type of tie desired. If the area behind the drawstring opening needs reinforcement, you can fuse a patch of interfacing, about 1 inch wide and slightly longer than the opening, to it.

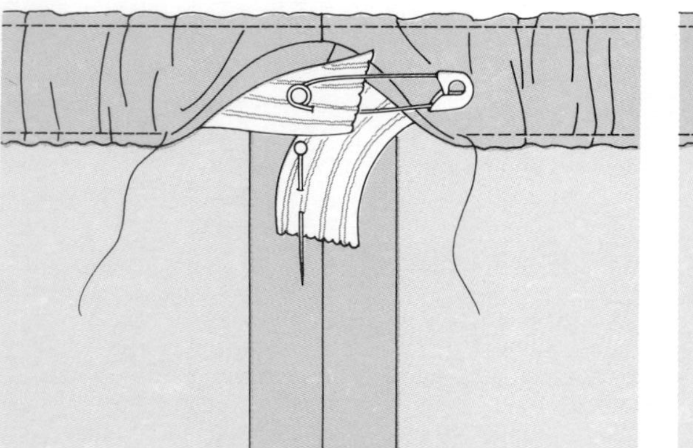

To insert elastic into a casing, attach a safety pin to one end of the elastic; secure other end to garment so it will not be pulled through the casing as the pin is worked around the waistline. Take care not to twist the elastic.

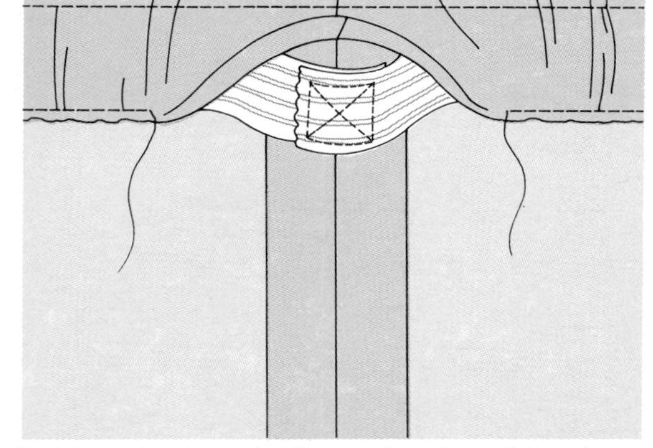

To join ends of elastic, first overlap them ½″ and pin. Stitch a square on the overlapped area, crisscrossing it for strength. Or make several rows of zigzag stitching on all sides of this area. Pull joined ends inside casing.

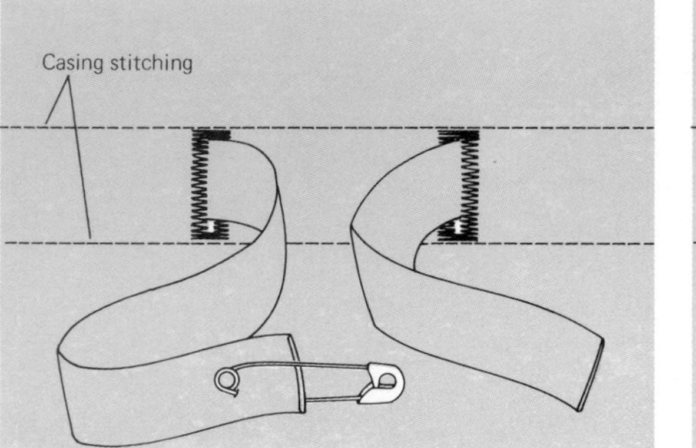

A drawstring can be threaded through a casing with the help of a safety pin. If it is an inside casing, the drawstring can be led in and out through two vertical buttonholes, worked on the garment before the casing is applied.

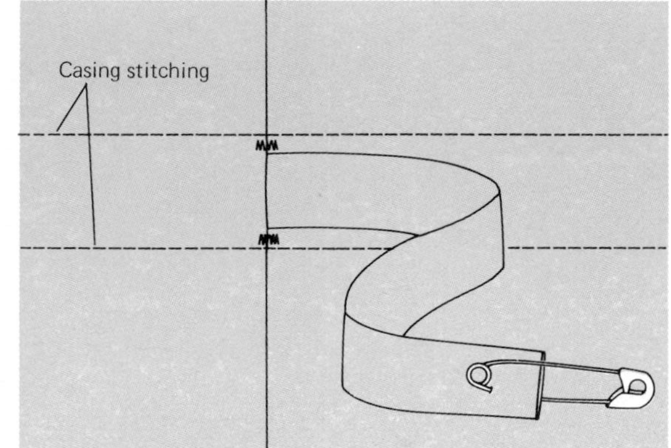

A drawstring can also be led through an inside casing by way of in-seam openings. Simply leave openings in seams the width of the drawstring; reinforce with bar tacks at ends or small squares of seam binding stitched into seam.

Finishing a full casing

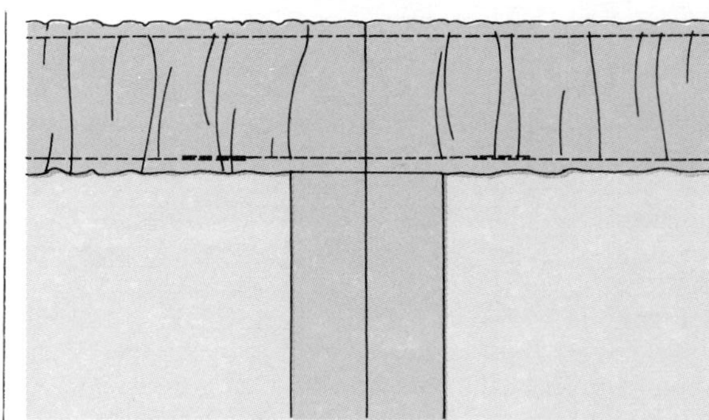

On a fold-down casing, close the opening by edgestitching. Keep area flat by stretching the elastic slightly as you sew. Take care not to catch the elastic in the stitching.

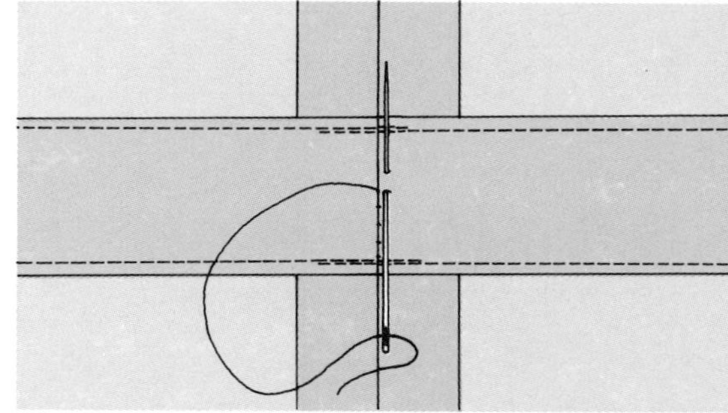

To finish an inside applied casing, slipstitch the ends of the casing together by hand. Make certain that the drawstring or elastic is not caught in the stitching.

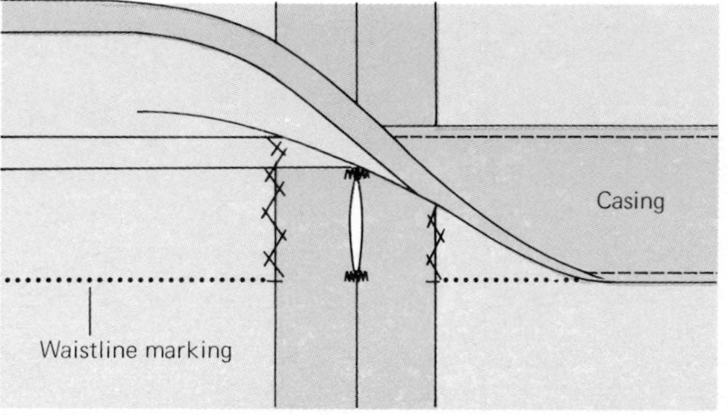

To hold seam allowances flat in an in-seam opening, catchstitch them to the garment. Be sure to do this before the casing is applied, taking care that the catchstitches do not show on outside of the garment.

Elastics 17
Zigzag stitching 32-37

Whipstitch 136
Centered zipper 318; invisible 326

Finishing a partial casing

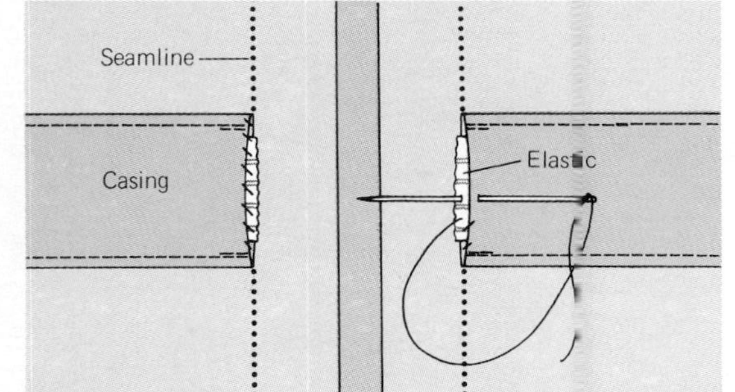

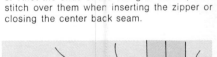

If a centered zipper is used with a casing, casing should stop at zipper seamlines. Apply casing; insert elastic or drawstring; tack ends of elastic to ends of casing.

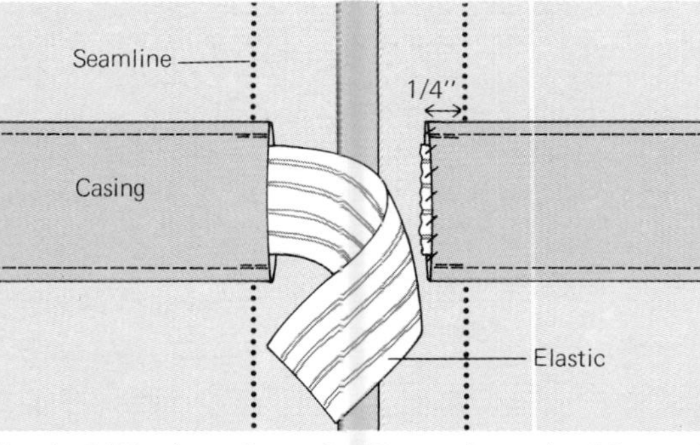

If an invisible zipper is used with a casing, extend the casing ¼″ beyond zipper seamlines as it is applied. Sew ends of elastic or drawstring to ends of casing.

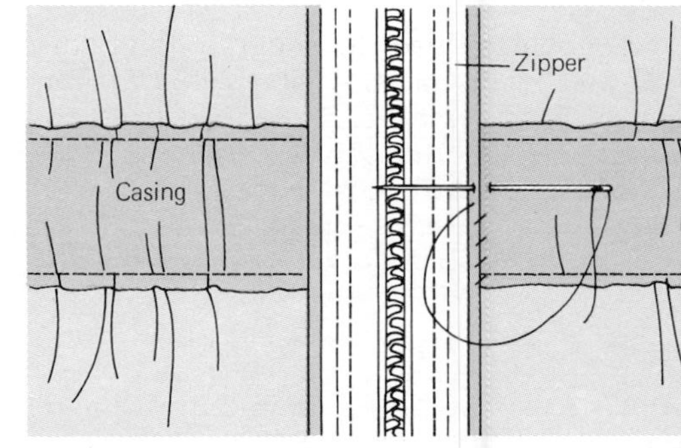

Insertion of either zipper will secure ends of casing and elastic or drawstring. To finish, press zipper seam allowances flat over casing; whipstitch to casing as shown.

Mock casings

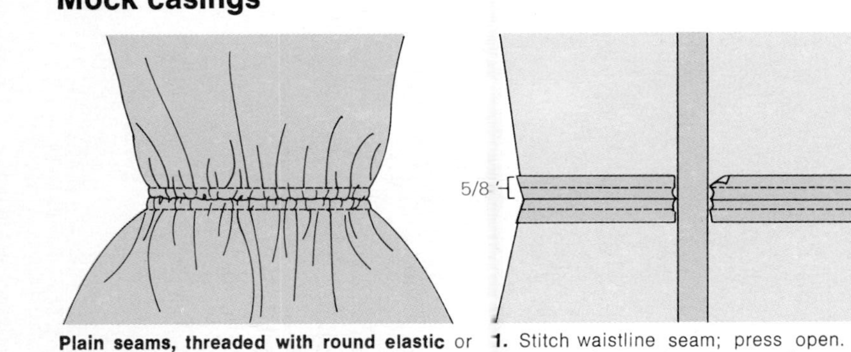

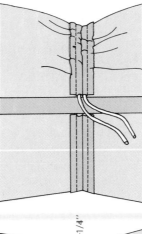

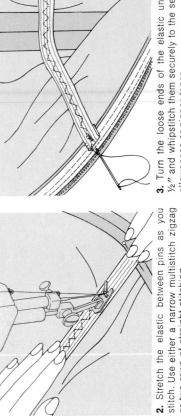

Plain seams, threaded with round elastic or fine strong string, can substitute for conventional casing. Effect resembles shirring.

1. Stitch waistline seam; press open. Form "casings" by stitching seam allowances to garment ¼″ on each side of seamline.

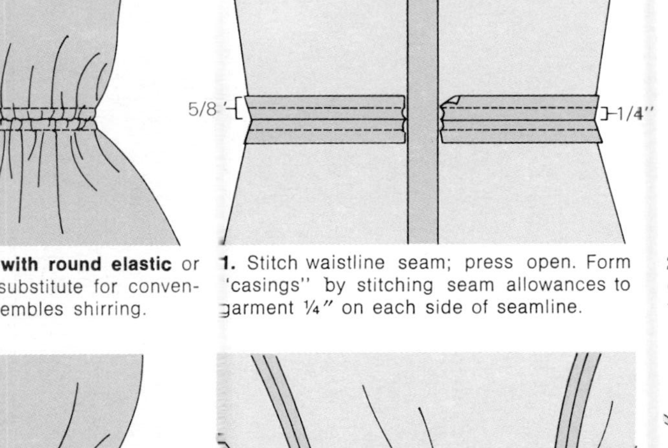

2. Using a tapestry needle, thread string or elastic through the casings. Adjust the shirring to the desired waist measurement.

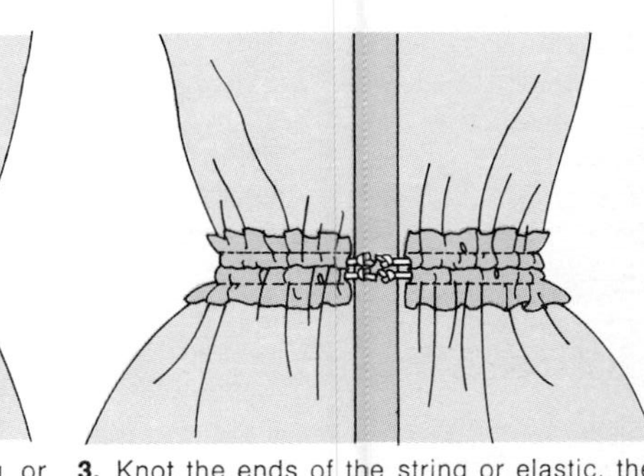

3. Knot the ends of the string or elastic, then stitch over them when inserting the zipper or closing the center back seam.

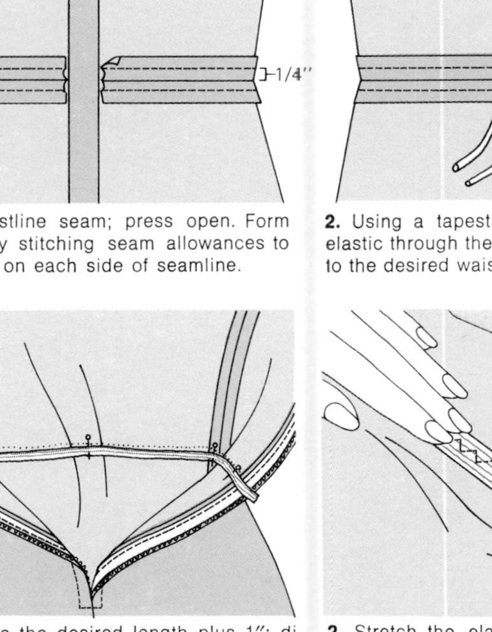

Narrow elastic can be stitched to the wrong side of a garment that has no waist seam. The result is very similar to that of a casing.

1. Cut elastic the desired length plus 1″; divide it and waistline into eighths. Pin elastic in place, with ½″ ends at openings.

2. Stretch the elastic between pins as you stitch. Use either a narrow multistitch zigzag or two rows of straight stitching.

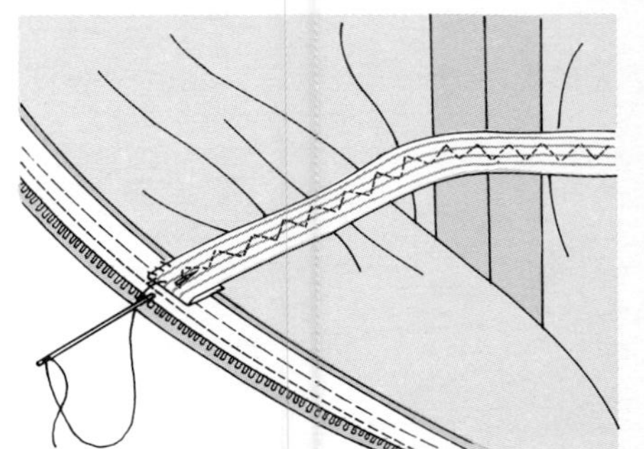

3. Turn the loose ends of the elastic under ½″ and whipstitch them securely to the seam allowances or zipper tapes.

Waistbands and facings

Wearing ease 101 Waistline alterations 106-107 Seams with fullness 154

General information

There are several ways to finish the waistline edge of a garment. The straight waistband is the most familiar finish, but a contour waistband, stretch waistband, or facing may be used. The pattern will specify a waistline treatment, but a different finish can often be substituted if desired.

Straight and contour waistbands are stable, inflexible finishes. They are made to fit the body's waist measurement plus some allowance for wearing ease. Straight waistbands are rectangular in shape and should be no wider than 2 inches. Contour waistbands are wider than 2 inches and are shaped to accommodate the difference in girth between the waist and rib cage or waist and hips.

Stretch waistbands are flexible and can be used on knit or woven fabrics. They can be made of a combination of fabric and elastic or of a decorative elastic. If a stretch waistband is to be used on a garment without a zipper, the hips should be no more than 10 inches larger than the waist; if the difference is greater, the garment will not pull over the hips and still fit the waist snugly.

A facing provides a clean, smooth finish that does not extend above the waistline edge. Made of a lightweight fabric, it can help reduce bulk.

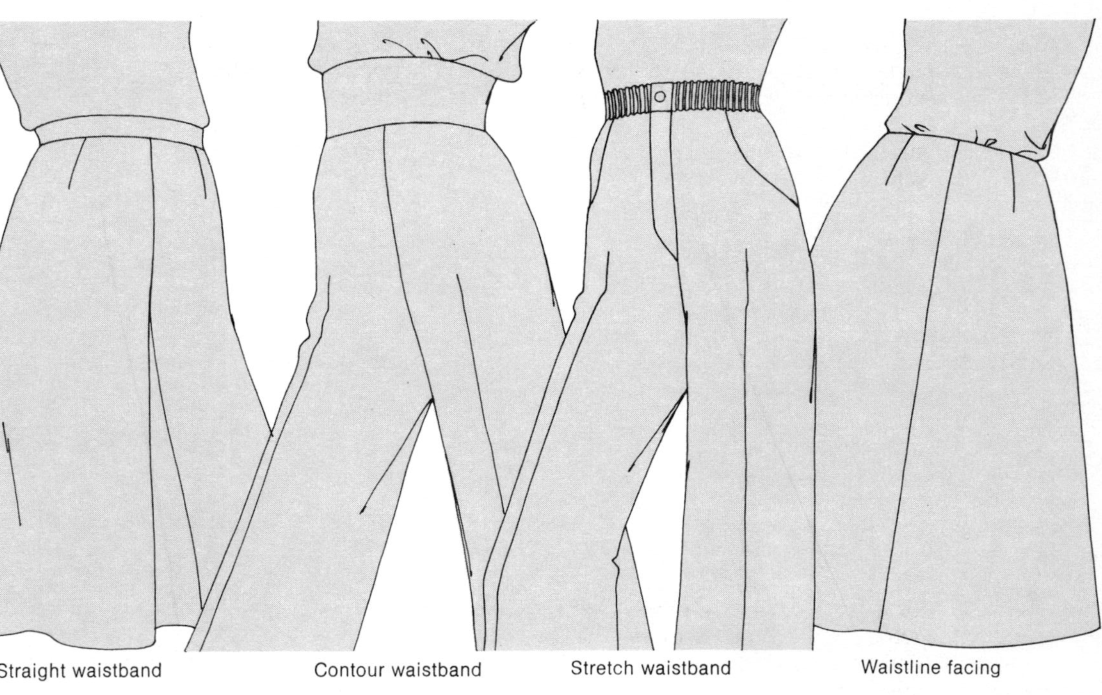

Straight waistband — Contour waistband — Stretch waistband — Waistline facing

Waistline placement

The waistline finish acts as an anchor for the garment, holding it in the proper position on the body. Exact placement of the waistline seam should be determined with the garment on the body. Try it on after all vertical seams and darts have been stitched and before the zipper is inserted; pin the zipper placket closed. Tie a string snugly enough around the waistline to hold the garment up. Settle the garment around the body so that the seams and darts all lie in the proper positions. Pull the waist seamline above or below the string until the garment rides smoothly over the hips and the darts end at the correct position. When adjusting pants, pull them up until they fit well in the crotch and seat area.

After fitting, measure up ⅝ inch from the new seamline and trim away any excess to create a new seam allowance. Apply machine easestitching on the new seamline, then insert the zipper.

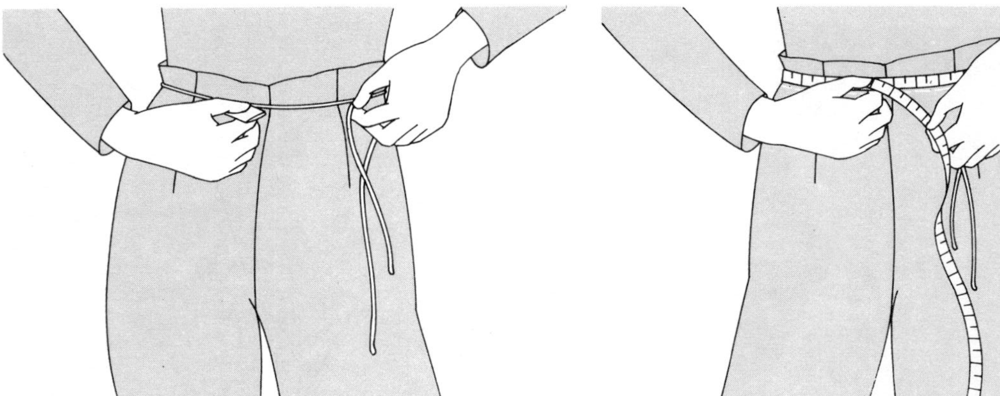

Mark waist seamline location directly beneath the string with pins or chalk after garment has been adjusted so that it fits properly. Seamline may not be level all around the body. Help may be needed for accurate marking.

Measure the waistline circumference while the garment is still on the body and before removing string. Measure with lower edge of tape measure along chalked mark. Use this waistline measurement to determine waistband length.

Cutting the waistband

Before cutting the waistband, decide where the waistband opening will fall and how much extension will be needed on each end of the waistband. The extensions at the ends of the waistband depend on the location of the placket opening on the garment. The ends of the waistband lap right over left when the opening is on the front or left side, and left over right on a center back opening. The overlap end is most often straight and finished flush with the edge of the garment opening. If a special decorative effect is desired, the end may be shaped into a point or a curve, in which case extra length must be allowed. Underlaps have straight ends, and must extend at least 1¼ inches beyond edge of opening to accommodate fasteners.

Patterns will include a piece for the waistband if called for by the design, but it may be easier to cut the waistband without a pattern, especially if the waistline has been altered. The length of the waistband should equal the waistline measurement as determined on the opposite page, plus 1 to 1½ inches for ease, plus two ⅝-inch seam allowances, plus whatever is desired for overlap and underlap. Waistband width is determined by the style of the waistband and how its back is to be finished. A straight waistband should be a maximum of 2 inches wide when finished; contour waistbands may be considerably wider. A straight waistband can be finished with a separate or extended (self) facing; for a self facing, cut the waistband twice the finished width plus seam allowances. When waistband is folded in half, the facing forms the back. Contour waistbands require a separate facing. A fabric facing is cut to the same dimensions as the waistband; grosgrain ribbon (for straight waistbands only) is purchased in the desired finished width.

If the waistband is cut without a pattern, locate and mark the foldline, seamlines, overlap and underlap, center front, center back and side. Waistbands should be cut on the lengthwise grain for greatest stability. If crosswise grain has to be used instead, the waistband must be interfaced.

Finishing. The waistband opening can be fastened with hooks and eyes, a button and buttonhole, or special waistband fasteners that either clamp or sew on. Multiple sets are used except when the fastener is a button; then a snap is added. The inner set of fasteners takes most of the strain; the outer set holds the top edge flat.

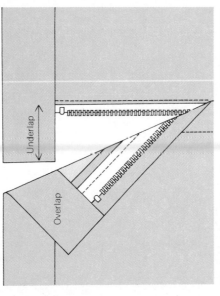

Overlap and underlap allow space for waistband fasteners.

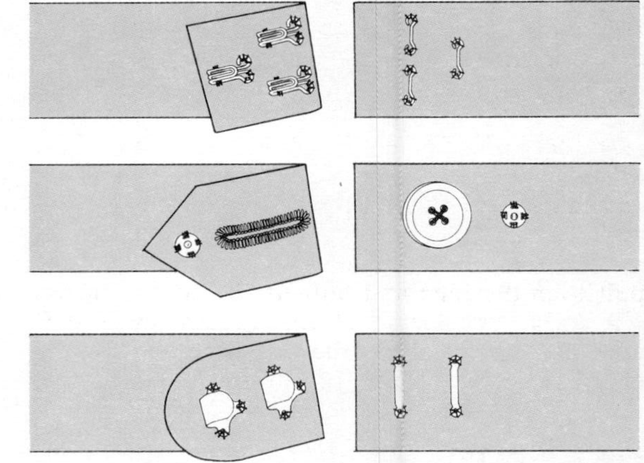

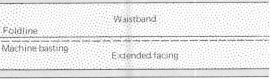

Fastener combinations most often used to close waistband.

Reinforcing the waistband

In order for a waistband to hold its shape and strength throughout the life of the garment, it must be *reinforced with interfacing* or professional waistbanding. (Stretch waistbands, naturally, are exceptions to this.) In addition to reinforcement, an *underlining* may be needed to prevent seams from showing through and to add support to a delicate fabric. A waistband is not lined, but sometimes, to reduce bulk, a lining fabric will be used to make the waistband facing.

The type of interfacing used in a waistband is determined by the garment fabric. It should be sturdy but flexible, crease-resistant, and durable, and it should have the same care properties as the garment fabric. The interfacing that is used in other areas of the garment may be adequate; if it is not, consider using two layers of that interfacing or one layer of a heavier interfacing. If only one layer is needed, it should be attached to the waistband side of the unit (the one that will be outermost in the finished garment). If two layers are required, apply one layer to the waistband and one to the waistband facing. If the waistband has a self facing and the entire unit is interfaced, hold the interfacing to the waistband by machine-basting through both layers slightly below the foldline, on the facing side.

Professional waistbanding can be used in place of regular interfacing. This is a flexible woven synthetic stiffener that has been heat-set in specific widths, ranging from ¾ inch to 2 inches. It should be purchased in the exact width that the finished waistband is to be; it should not be cut down to size, as this will remove the finished edge and expose the sharp cross-yarns, which can scratch the skin. Professional waistbanding is applied differently from regular interfacing; exact instructions follow in this section (see p. 242).

Straight waistband techniques

Interfacing 72-73, 76-79

Grain in fabric 84-85
Slipstitch (uneven) 132

Waistband formed as it is applied

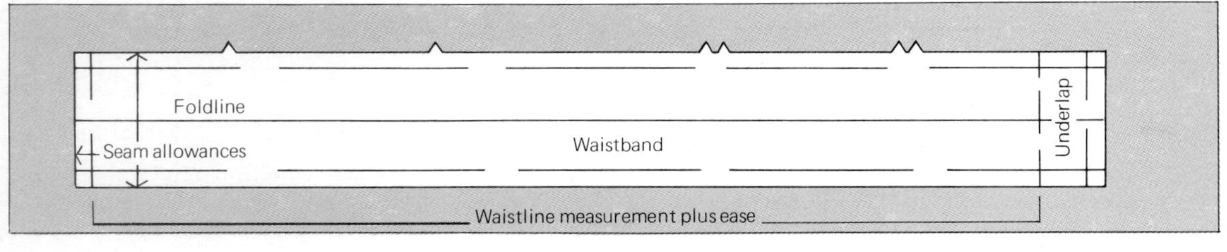

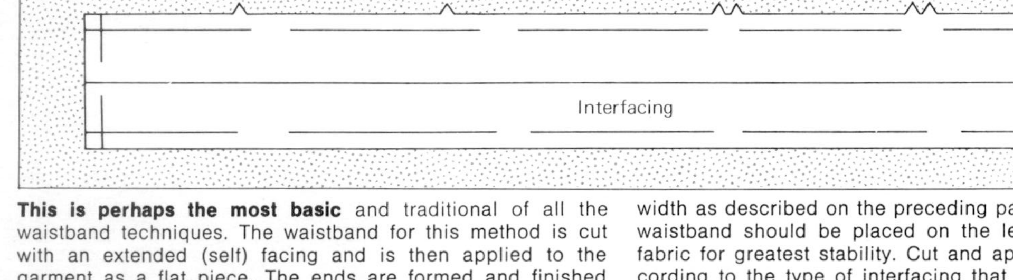

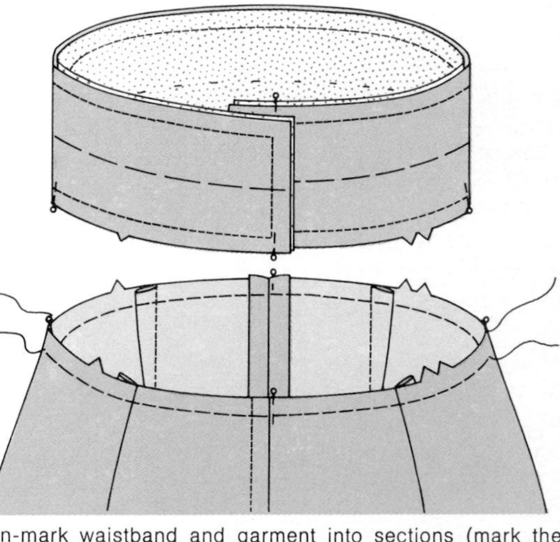

This is perhaps the most basic and traditional of all the waistband techniques. The waistband for this method is cut with an extended (self) facing and is then applied to the garment as a flat piece. The ends are formed and finished while it is being applied to the garment. If the waistband is to be cut without a pattern, determine the correct length and width as described on the preceding pages. The length of the waistband should be placed on the lengthwise grain of the fabric for greatest stability. Cut and apply the interfacing according to the type of interfacing that has been chosen and the number of layers being used. Mark the foldline of the waistband by basting by hand through all thicknesses.

1. Pin-mark waistband and garment into sections (mark the edge of the waistband that will be sewed to the garment). Place a pin at beginning of overlap or seam allowance, another at beginning of underlap. Divide remainder of band into fourths. Pin-mark the garment waistline also into four equal parts, using the zipper opening as the starting point.

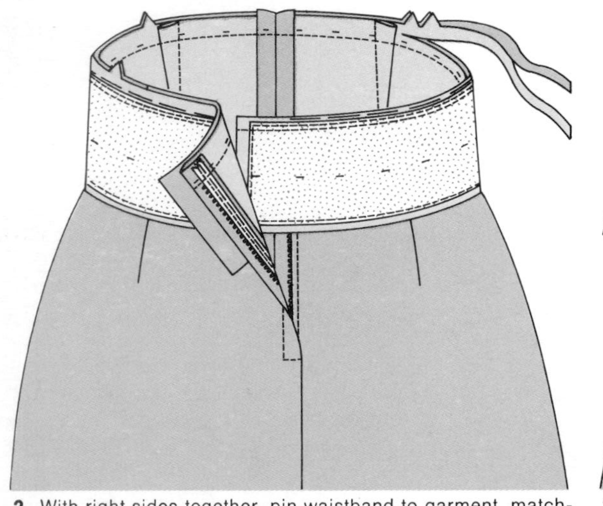

2. With right sides together, pin waistband to garment, matching pin marks and notches. Draw up the ease thread on garment between pins so that the fullness is evenly distributed and the garment lies flat against the waistband. Baste, then stitch, on the seamline. Press seam flat. Grade the seam allowances. Press the waistband and seam up.

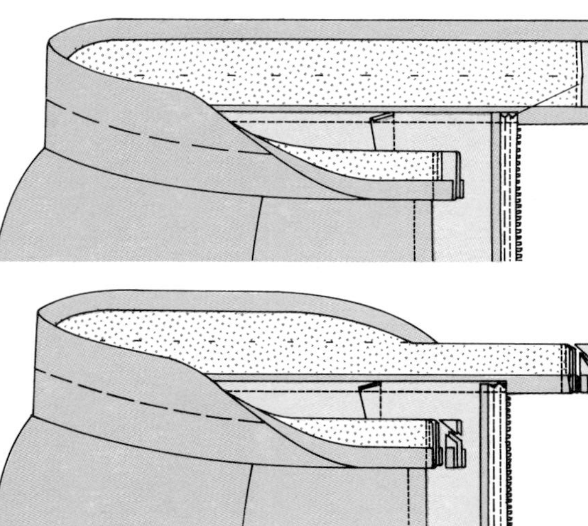

3. Turn the ⅝″ seam allowance on the long unstitched edge of the waistband to the wrong side and press. To finish the ends, fold the waistband along the foldline so that the waistband is wrong side out, with right sides together. Pin at each end and stitch on the ⅝″ seamline. Trim both seams and corners and turn waistband right side out.

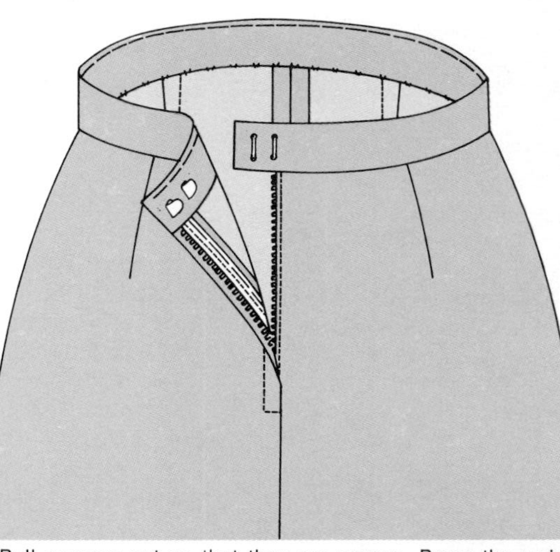

4. Pull corners out so that they are square. Press the waistband facing to the inside of the garment along the foldline, keeping the turned-under seam allowance intact. Pin turned-under seam allowance to garment. Slipstitch folded edge to the seamline, making certain that no stitches show through to the outside. Attach suitable fasteners to ends of waistband.

Backstitch, tying thread ends 137
Cornered seams 146
Reducing seam bulk 147
Seams with fullness 154

Waistband made before application

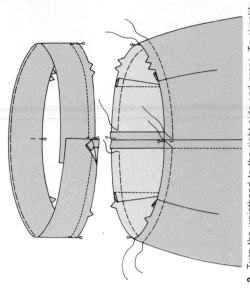

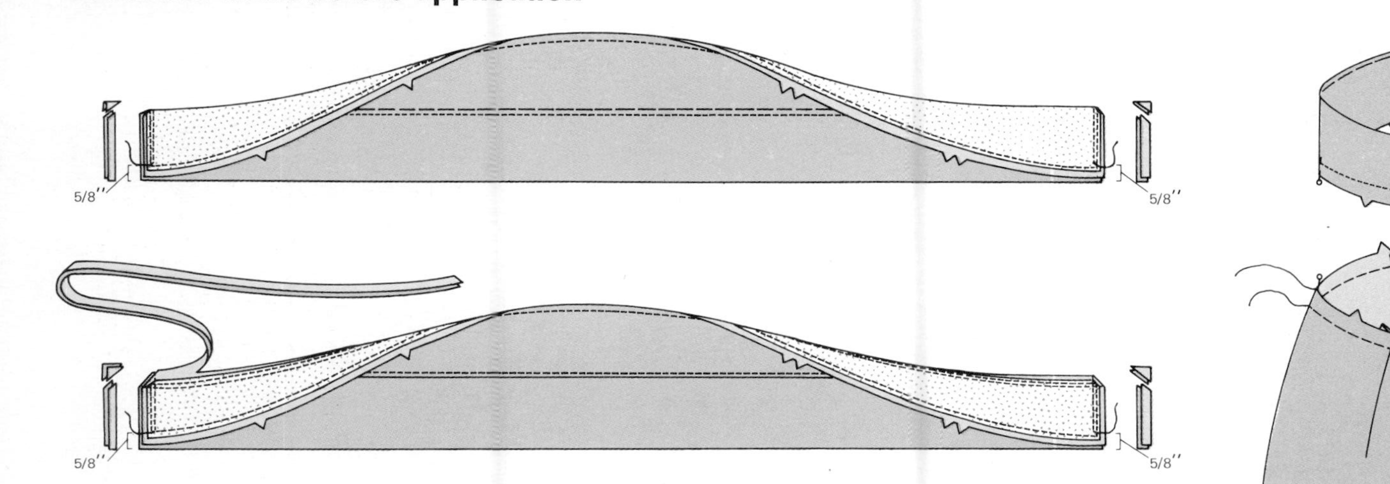

1. This waistband may be cut with an **extended facing,** as in the method opposite, or with a **separate facing.** Apply interfacing according to type and the number of layers being used, making sure it is attached to the side that will be outermost in the finished garment. To construct the waistband with an extended facing, fold the waistband in half lengthwise, right sides together, and stitch across each end from the fold to within ⅝″ of the opposite edge. Secure the stitching. If the band has a separate facing, place right sides of facing and waistband together and stitch across ends and top. Stop and secure stitching ⅝″ from lower edge on ends. Press seams flat, then grade seams and trim corners.

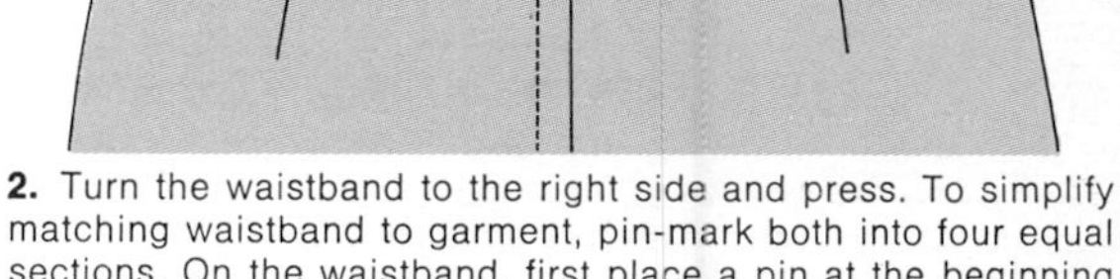

2. Turn the waistband to the right side and press. To simplify matching waistband to garment, pin-mark both into four equal sections. On the waistband, first place a pin at the beginning of the underlap, then divide remainder of band into fourths. Pin-mark the garment seamline evenly into fourths as well, starting at the actual opening of the zipper.

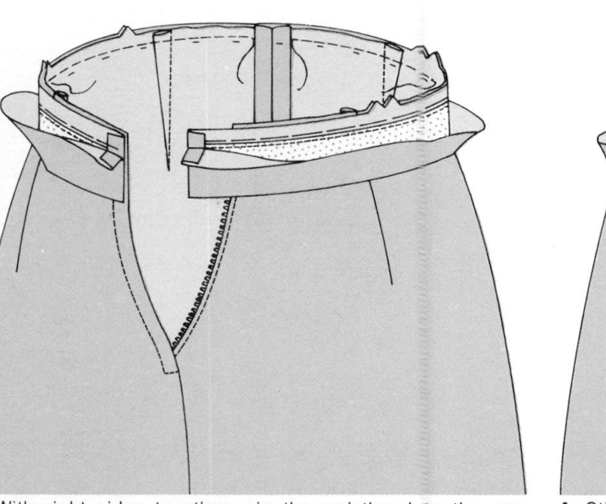

3. With right sides together, pin the waistband to the garment edge. Carefully match all notches and pin marks, making sure that the finished edge of the waistband overlap is flush with the edge of the zipper closing. Pull up the ease thread and adjust fullness evenly between pins so the skirt lies flat against the waistband. Baste along seamline.

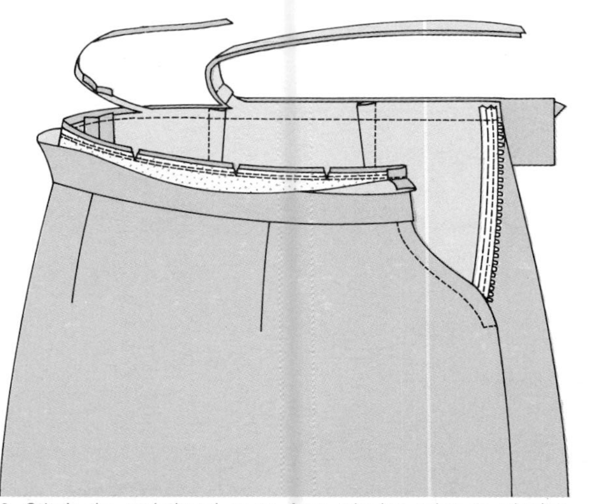

4. Stitch the waistband seam from placket edge to placket edge. Be careful that no tucks are formed in the garment ease and caught in the stitching. Press the seam as stitched, then grade the seam allowances. Clip the seam allowances so they will lie flat when encased in the waistband. Remove any basting that might show from the right side.

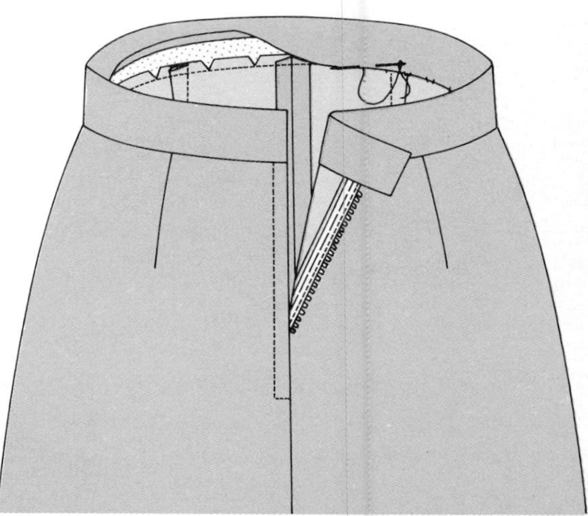

5. Turn the waistband right side out. Press along foldline and ends. Turn under ⅝″ along the unstitched edge and pin to the garment. Slipstitch the fold of the seam allowance to the garment around the waist seamline and underlap. Sew carefully so that no stitches are visible on the right side of the garment. Attach suitable fasteners to ends of waistband.

Straight waistband techniques

Applying professional waistbanding

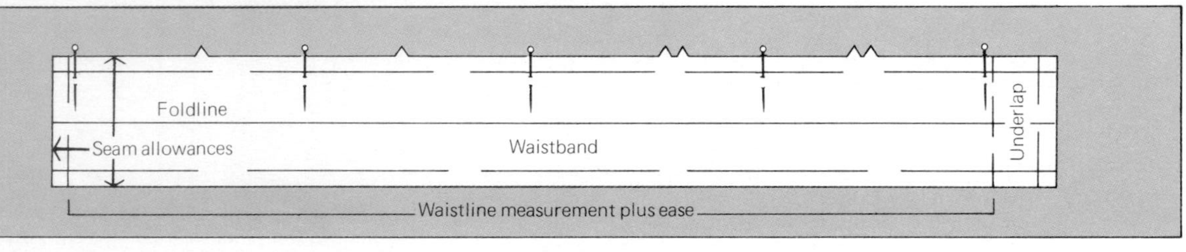

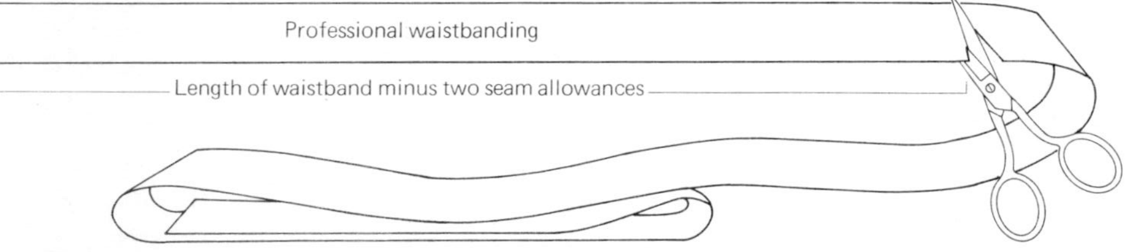

The waistband used for this technique is the straight waistband with self facing. Cut the waistband twice the width of the professional waistbanding plus two seam allowances. The length of the waistband equals the body waist measurement, plus ease allowance, plus two seam allowances, and at least 1¼″ for underlap (allow extra length for an overlap).

1. Pin-mark the area between underlap and overlap or seam allowance into fourths. Cut waistbanding (which has been purchased in the exact width the finished waistband is to be) the length of the waistband minus two seam allowances; extend waistbanding through underlap and overlap but not into seams at ends. (See Cutting the waistband, p. 239).

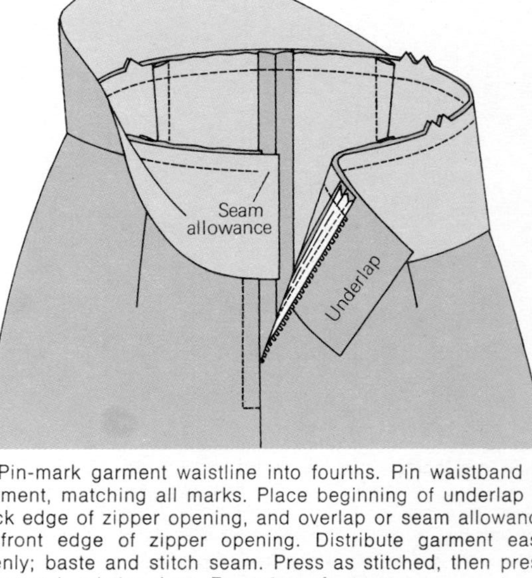

2. Pin-mark garment waistline into fourths. Pin waistband to garment, matching all marks. Place beginning of underlap to back edge of zipper opening, and overlap or seam allowance to front edge of zipper opening. Distribute garment ease evenly; baste and stitch seam. Press as stitched, then press seam and waistband up. **Do not grade seam.**

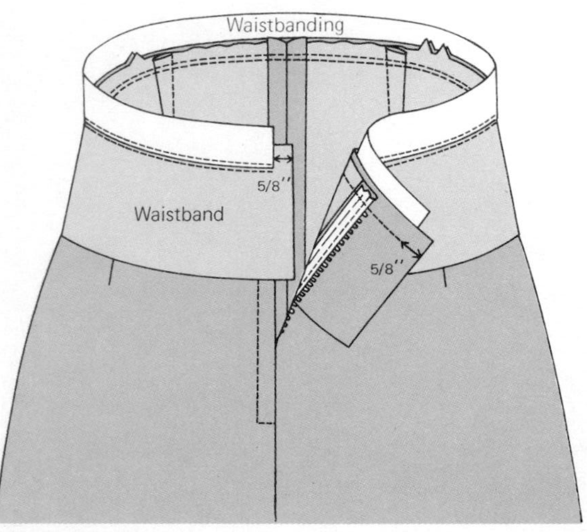

3. With waistband down over garment, lap the waistbanding over seam allowances. Place so that the width of the waistbanding is away from the garment, one edge is aligned exactly to the seamline, and the ends are ⅝″ away from the ends of the waistband. Sew along edge of banding, through both seam allowances. Grade now if desired.

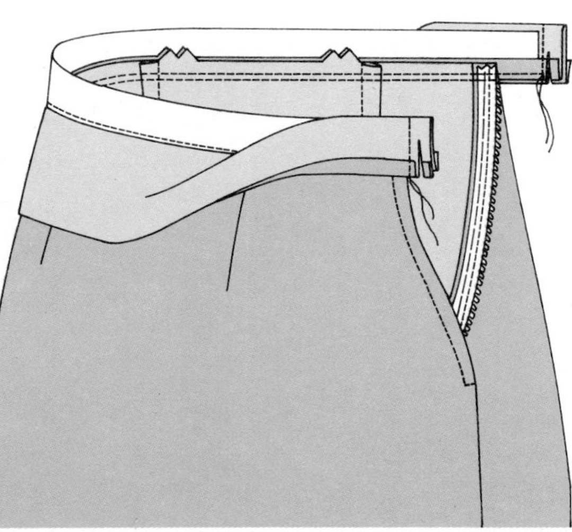

4. To form the ends of waistband, fold band along center foldline so that right sides are together. Pin once at each end to hold the fold in place. Stitch along each end of waistband as close as possible to the waistbanding without actually stitching through it. Trim seams and corners. Turn waistband right side out, over banding.

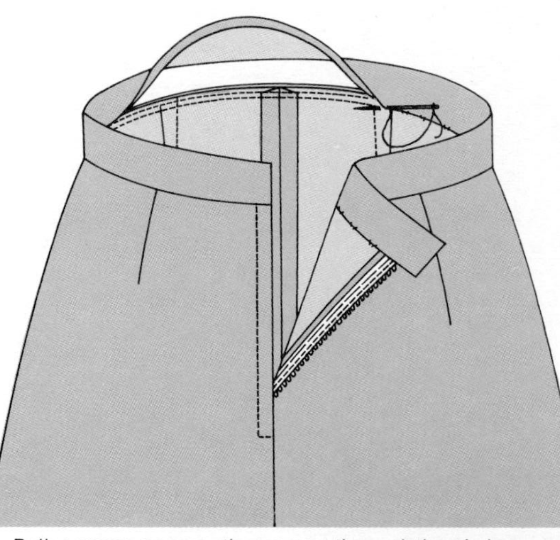

5. Pull corners square, then press the waistband down over the banding. Turn under the ⅝″ seam allowance along the unstitched edge and press in place. Pin the folded edge to the waistband; slipstitch this fold to the waistband seam or just above it. Stitching should not show from the right side. Finish the ends by attaching fasteners.

Grain in fabric 84-85
Hand stitches 129, 136
Reducing seam bulk 147
Zipper underlays 329

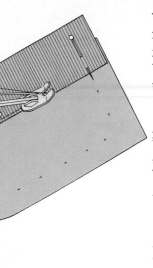

Constructing a ribbon-faced waistband

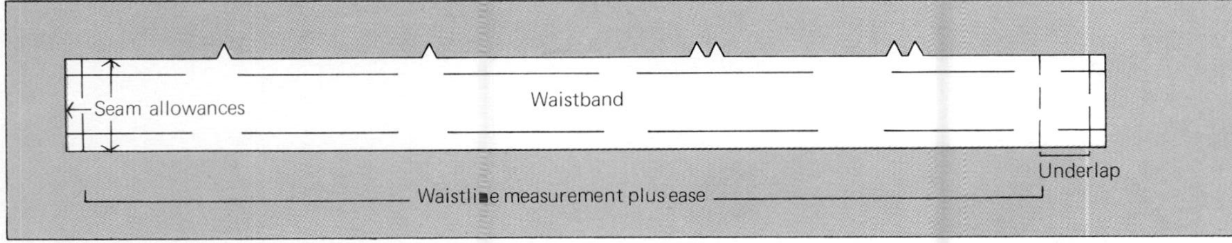

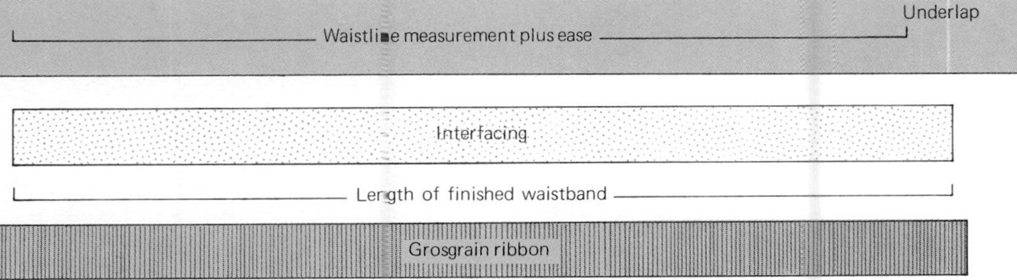

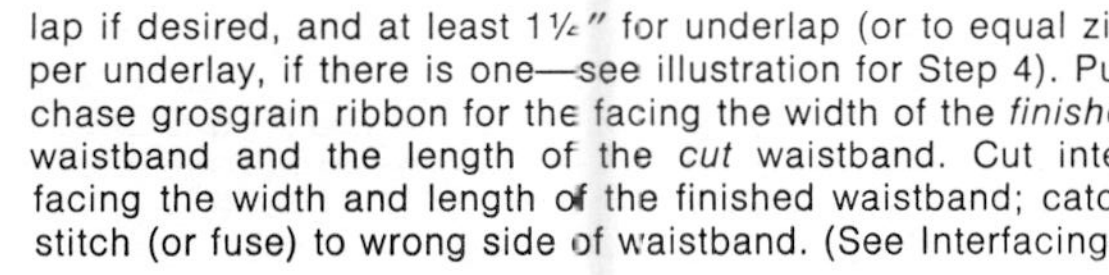

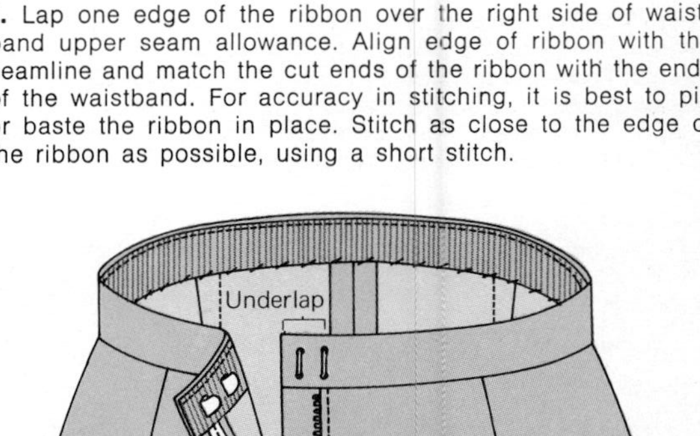

A ribbon facing on a waistband reduces bulk without sacrificing stability, making it a practical choice for nubby or heavy fabrics. Cut the waistband on the lengthwise grain of the fabric. The width should equal that of the finished waistband plus two seam allowances. The length should total the waist measurement, plus ease, two seam allowances, overlap if desired, and at least 1¼″ for underlap (or to equal zipper underlay, if there is one—see illustration for Step 4). Purchase grosgrain ribbon for the facing the width of the *finished* waistband and the length of the *cut* waistband. Cut interfacing the width and length of the finished waistband; catchstitch (or fuse) to wrong side of waistband. (See Interfacings.)

1. Lap one edge of the ribbon over the right side of waistband upper seam allowance. Align edge of ribbon with the seamline and match the cut ends of the ribbon with the ends of the waistband. For accuracy in stitching, it is best to pin or baste the ribbon in place. Stitch as close to the edge of the ribbon as possible, using a short stitch.

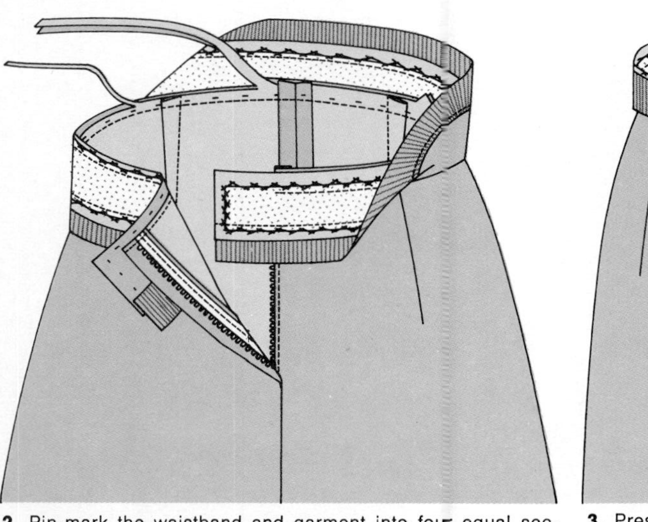

2. Pin-mark the waistband and garment into four equal sections, as described on page 240. Pin waistband to garment, right sides together, matching pin marks and notches. Draw up the ease thread so garment lies flat against waistband; keep ease evenly distributed. Baste and stitch the seam. Press seam as stitched; grade the seam allowances.

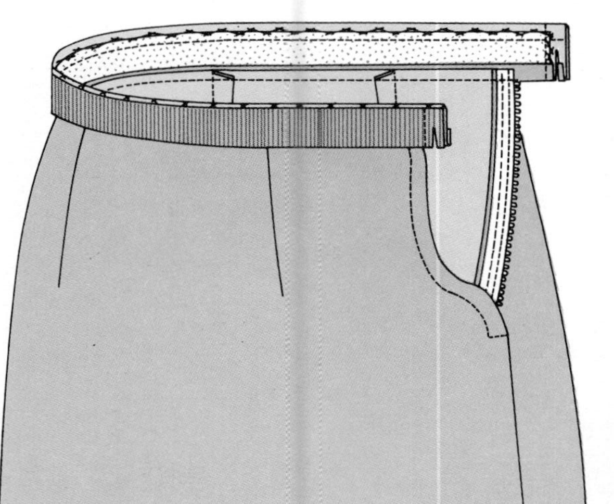

3. Press waistband and seam allowances up. To finish ends, fold right sides of the waistband together along the edge of the ribbon. Pin ends in place and stitch across them on the seamlines. Trim seams and corners; turn waistband to the right side. Press ribbon facing to wrong side along folded edge. Pin free edge of ribbon to waist seam.

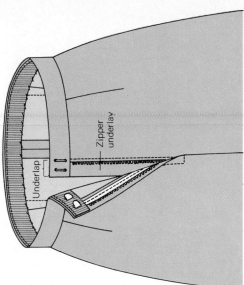

4. Whipstitch free edge of ribbon to waistband seam; attach the fasteners. The zipper underlay illustrated here is used for fine tailored garments, often in conjunction with a ribbon-faced waistband. If this zipper application is used, allow for an underlap equal to the zipper underlay when cutting the waistband, ribbon, and interfacing.

Simplified straight waistbands

Fabric terms 84
Topstitching 143, 152
Reducing seam bulk 147
Seams with fullness 154

Topstitched waistband

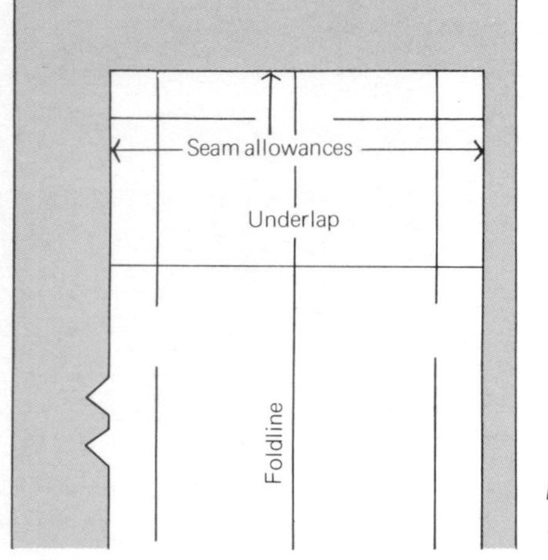

1. This quick and secure waistband is suitable for casual garments. Cut the waistband length to equal the waist measurement, plus ease, seam allowance, underlap, and overlap if desired. Width is twice the finished width plus seam allowances. Apply interfacing (p. 239).

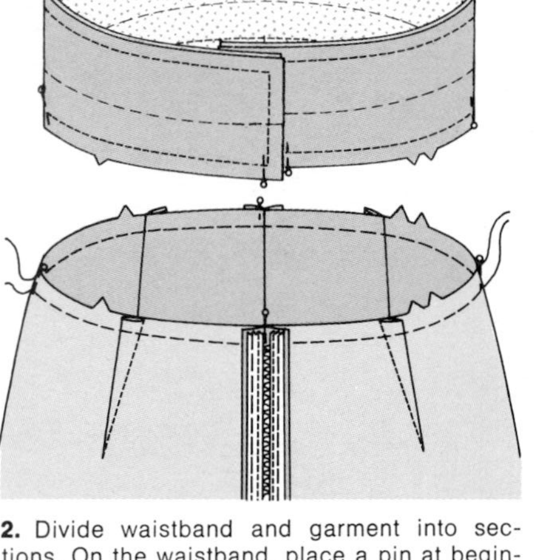

2. Divide waistband and garment into sections. On the waistband, place a pin at beginning of underlap and another pin at overlap or seam allowance; pin-mark space between pins into fourths. Pin-mark the garment waistline into fourths, starting at zipper.

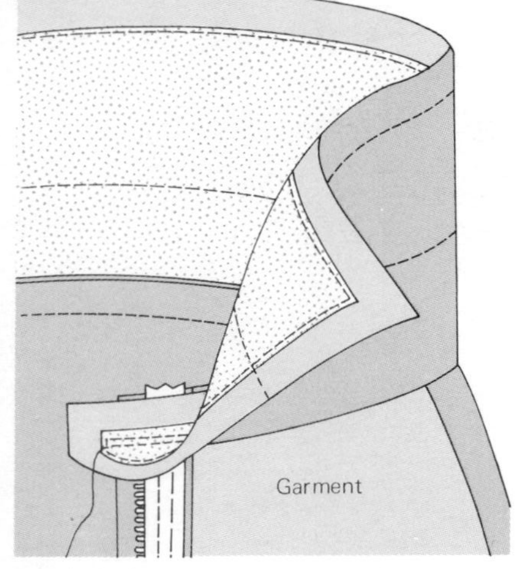

3. Pin the *right* side of the waistband to the *wrong* side of the garment, matching all pin marks and notches. Draw up ease thread and distribute any fullness evenly. Stitch the seam. Press as stitched, then press both seam and waistband up. Grade seam; trim corners.

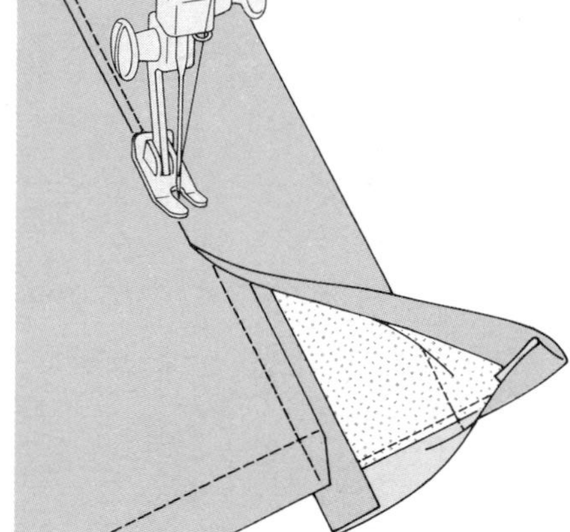

4. Turn under seam allowance on free edge and ends of waistband; press. Turn waistband down to right side on foldline and pin turned-under edge over waistline seam, covering first stitching. Topstitch close to the edge through all thicknesses. Attach fasteners.

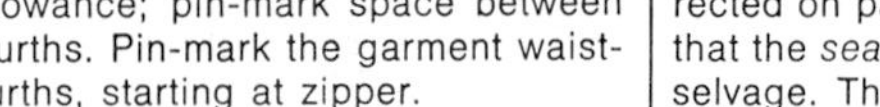

Selvage waistband

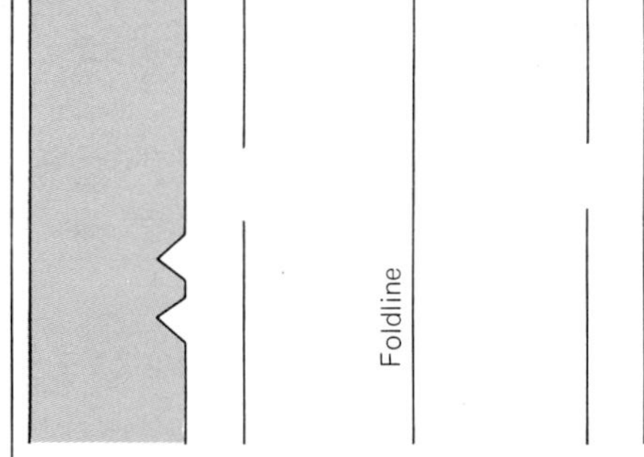

1. Not merely quick, this waistband technique helps to reduce bulk by eliminating a seam allowance. Determine size of waistband as directed on page 238, then cut the waistband so that the *seamline* of one long edge falls on the selvage. This provides one finished edge.

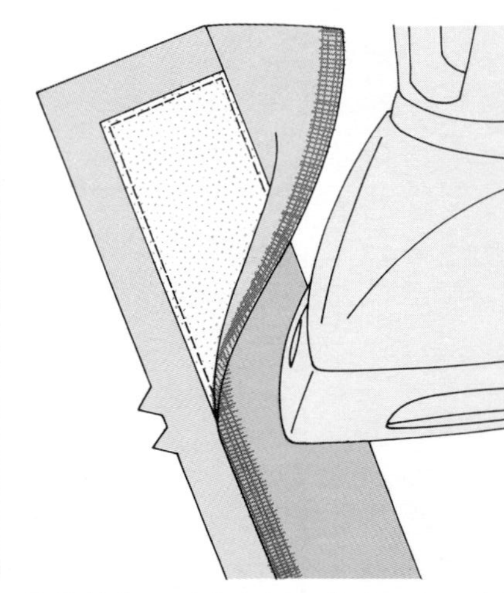

2. Fold the waistband lengthwise along foldline, wrong sides together (the long raw edge should extend ⅝" below the selvage); press. Interface the half of the waistband that has the raw edge. Interfacing should not extend into any seam allowances.

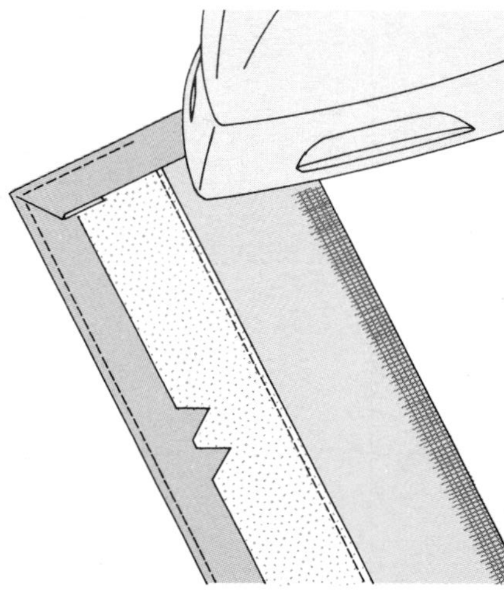

3. Turn the long raw edge and the ends to the wrong side on the seamlines and press. Make certain that pressed-under edge does not extend below selvage edge when waistband is folded in half. Pin-mark waistband and garment into fourths as directed on page 241.

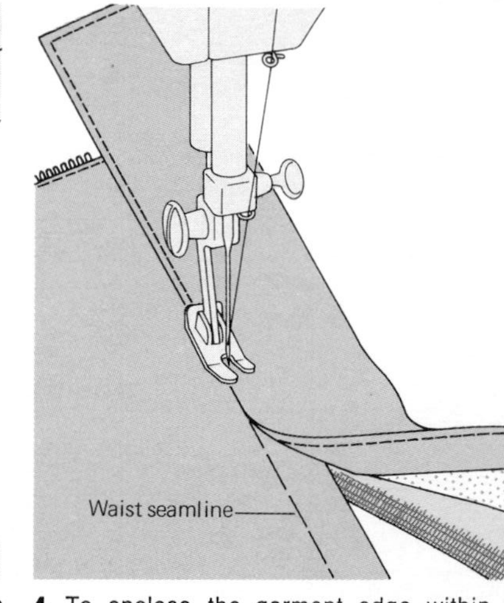

4. To enclose the garment edge within the waistband, place selvage to the inside and fold along waist seamline. Match all pin marks; pin if desired. Topstitch close to fold, from end to end, catching selvage in stitching. Press waistband flat. Attach fasteners.

Contour waistband

Twill tape 16
Interfacing choices 72-73
Hand stitches 125, 132
Machine padstitching 141

Construction and application

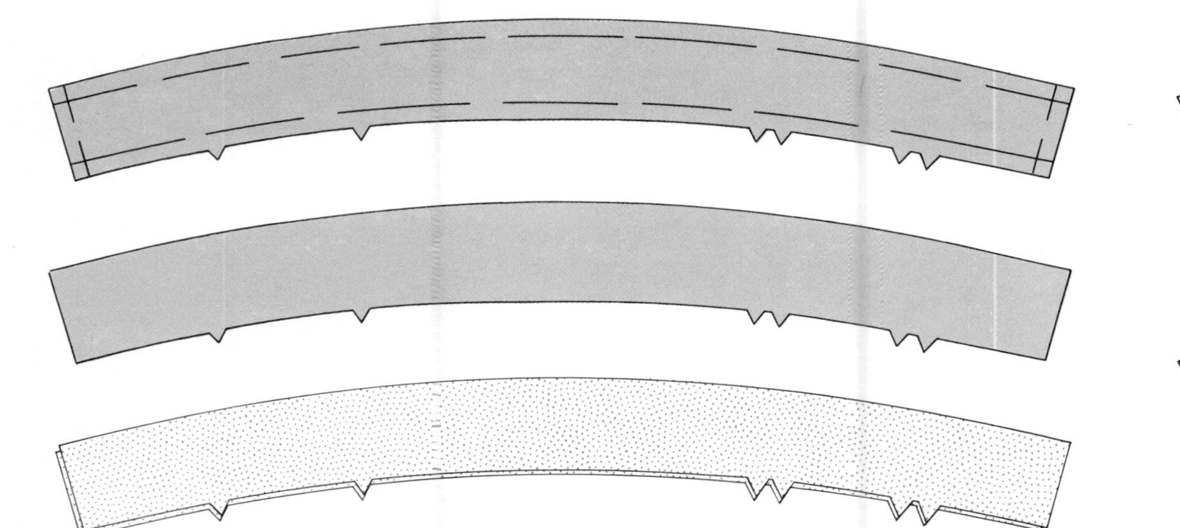

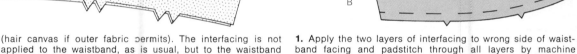

A contour waistband is at least 2″ wide and is formed to fit the body's curves; it is often decoratively shaped along the top edge as well. The width and shape of this waistband requires a separate facing and a double layer of interfacing (hair canvas if outer fabric permits). The interfacing is not applied to the waistband, as is usual, but to the waistband facing. This permits padstitching of the facing, which builds in and holds a permanent shape. (See Padstitching.)

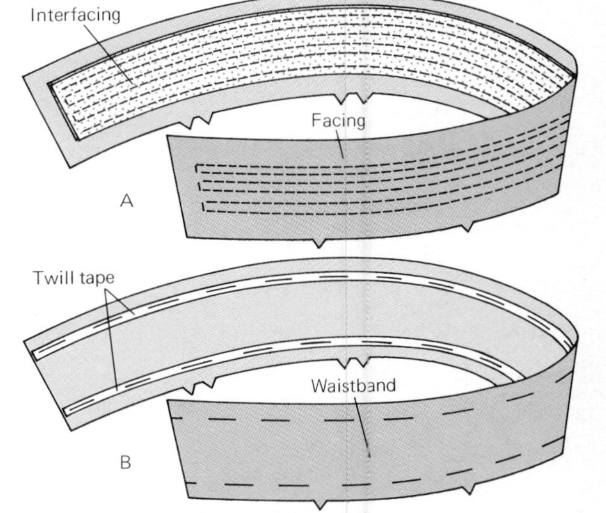

1. Apply the two layers of interfacing to wrong side of waistband facing and padstitch through all layers by machine (A). To prevent stretching of the long edges, baste ¼″ twill tape over seamlines on wrong side of waistband (B).

2. Right sides together, pin and baste waistband to facing along ends and upper edge. Starting and ending ⅝″ from lower edge, stitch as basted, pivoting at corners and stitching through center of twill tape. Press seam flat. Trim and grade seam allowances. Turn the waistband right side out; diagonal-baste around all three finished edges and press.

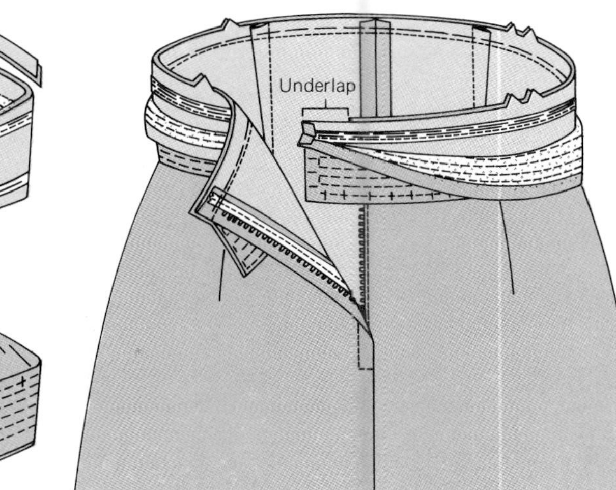

3. Pin-mark waistband and garment waistline into fourths; on waistband, place a pin at beginning of the underlap, then divide remainder of band into fourths. Pin waistband to garment, right sides together, matching all markings and the finished end of waistband to front edge of zipper opening. Adjust ease as needed; baste, then stitch seam.

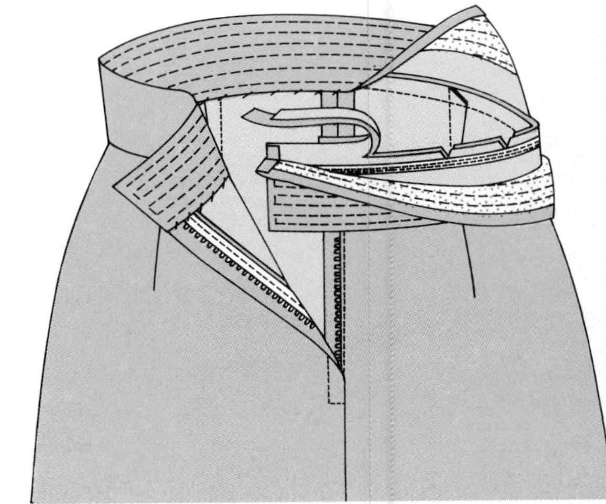

4. Trim and grade the waistline seam; press it and waistband away from garment. Turn under seam allowance on lower edge of the facing and slipstitch the fold to the waistline seam and underlap. Remove all bastings. Press the finished waistband. Apply fasteners; the width of the waistband determines the number of sets and their placement.

Slipstitch (uneven) 132
Maching padstitching 141
Staystitching 144
Fasteners 354, 357

Shaped facing

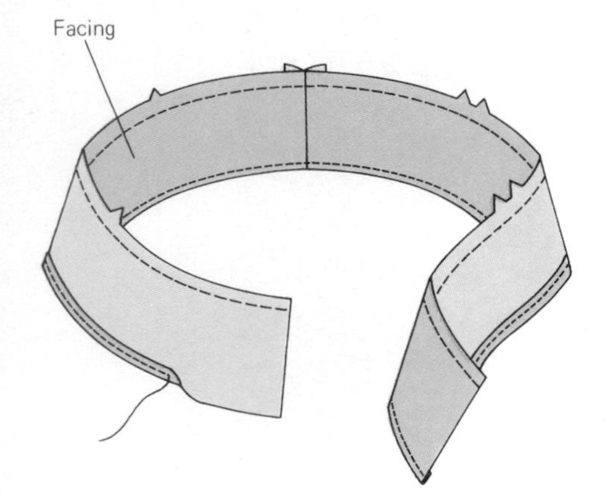

1. Cut facing from garment fabric; if this fabric is heavy, facing may be cut of a sturdy lighter-weight fabric to reduce bulk. Staystitch facing sections ⅛″ inside waist seamline. Stitch sections together, leaving open the seam that corresponds to the placket opening. Apply appropriate seam finish to outer edge of facing. (See Seam finishes.)

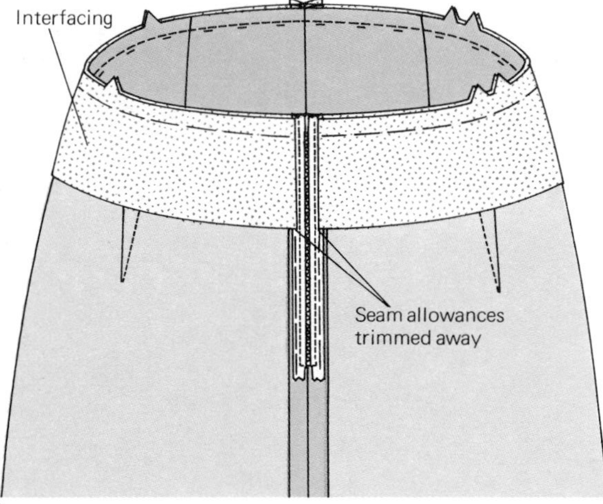

2. Interfacing method depends on garment fabric. **For medium- to lightweight fabrics,** apply one layer of interfacing to garment. Seam interfacing the same as facing; trim away ½″ from outer edge and all of seam allowances at ends. Baste wrong side of interfacing to wrong side of garment, matching markings and positioning ends over zipper tapes.

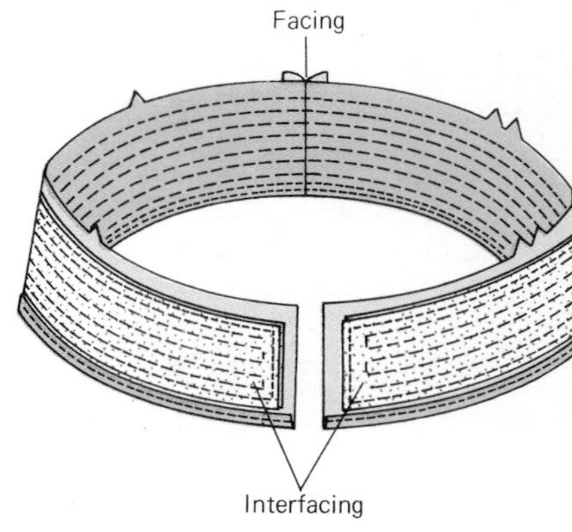
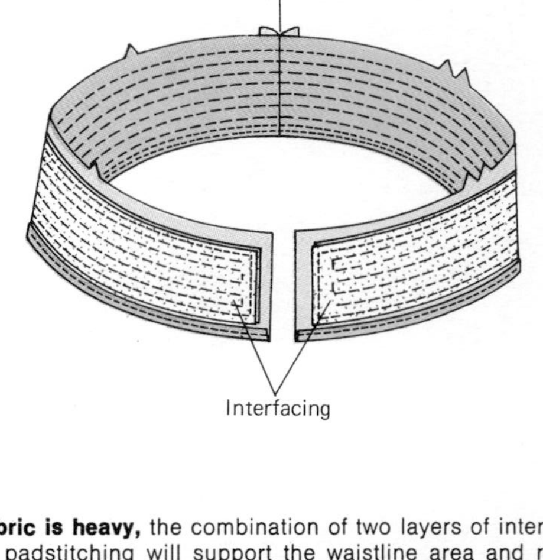

If fabric is heavy, the combination of two layers of interfacing plus padstitching will support the waistline area and reduce wrinkling during wear. Cut the interfacing from facing pattern minus waistline seam allowance; trim lower edge of interfacing to same width as facing. Stitch interfacing seams and apply to wrong side of facing; padstitch. (See Padstitching.)

3. To apply facing of either type, first pin facing to garment, right sides together, matching all seams and notches. Match seam allowances at ends of facing to edges of placket opening. Pin ¼″-wide twill tape over waist seamline; baste through all thicknesses. Stitch seam and press flat. Trim, grade, and clip seam allowances.

4. From the wrong side, with the facing extended away from the garment, press all seam allowances toward the facing. Understitch the seam to keep facing from rolling to the outside of the garment. With facing and seam allowance extended away from garment, stitch from right side close to waist seamline, through facing and seam allowances.

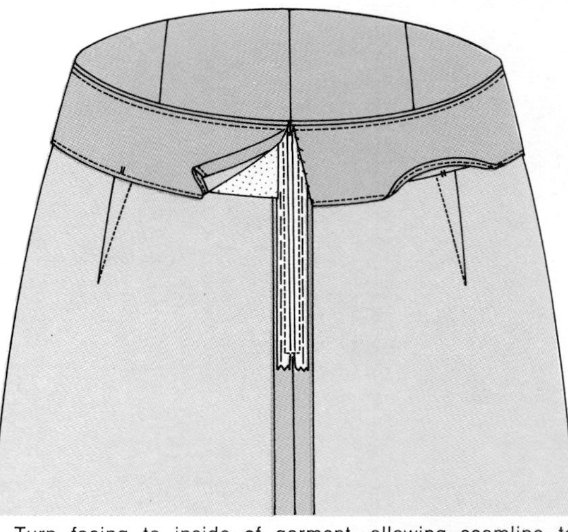

5. Turn facing to inside of garment, allowing seamline to roll inside slightly. Press along waist edge. Tack facing to garment at seams and darts. Turn seam allowances of facing ends to wrong side, making sure facing is turned in such a way that it will not catch in zipper; slipstitch to zipper tape. Attach a hook and eye or hanging snap at top of placket.

Tapes 16
Hand stitches 132, 136
Seam finishes 148-149
Pre-shaping tape 299

Ribbon facing

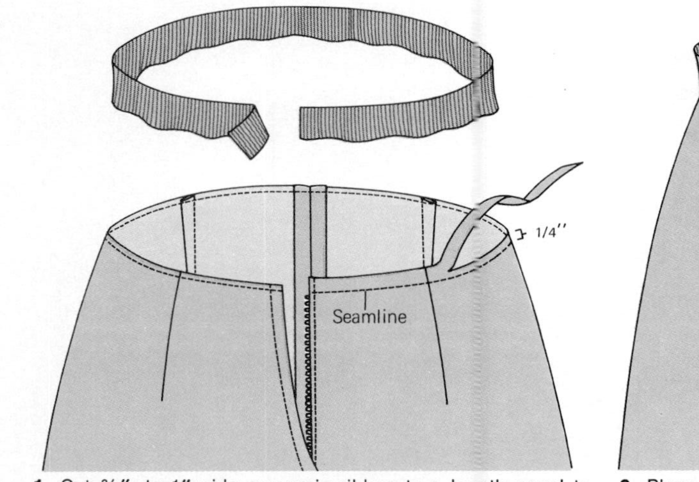

1. Cut ¾″- to 1″-wide grosgrain ribbon to a length equal to the garment waistline measurement plus 1¼″. Shape the ribbon to fit the curve of the garment waistline edge (see How to preshape tape). Staystitch garment waistline on seamline and trim seam allowance to ¼″.

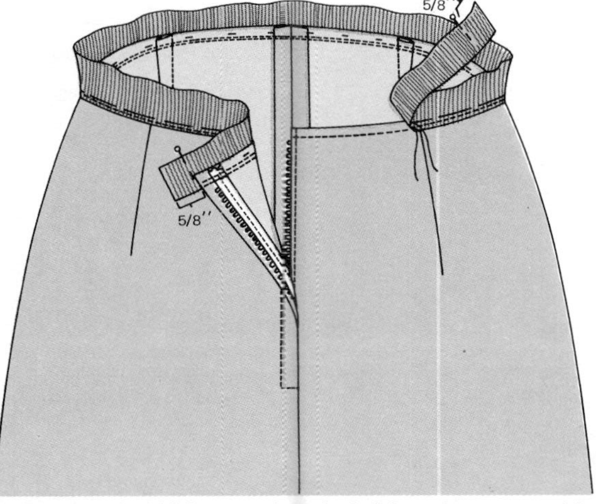

2. Place a pin ⅝″ from each end of ribbon. Lap wrong side of ribbon over right side of garment waistline so that the edge of the *inside* curve of the ribbon is over the staystitched seamline. Match pins at ribbon ends to placket edges. Baste in place. Stitch close to edge of ribbon.

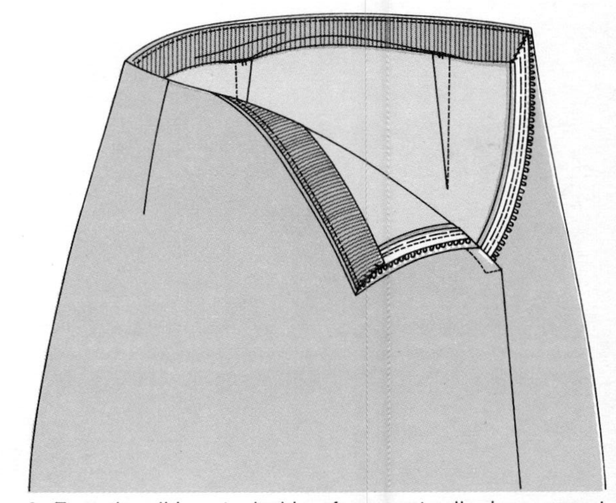

3. Turn the ribbon to inside of garment, allowing garment edge to roll in slightly. Fold under ribbon ends on ⅝″ mark so that they clear zipper, and press entire edge of ribbon. Tack ribbon to garment at all seams and darts; whipstitch ends to zipper tape. Attach fasteners.

Extended facing

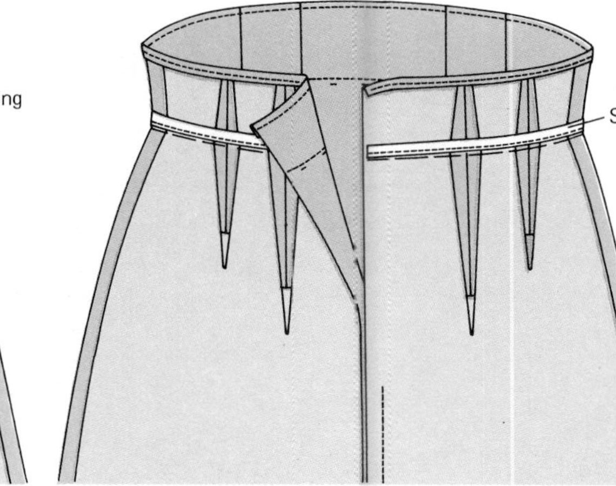

Some patterns are designed with an extended (self) waistline facing. Garment darts extend through the waistline into the facing; pattern foldline marks finished waistline edge.
1. Stitch darts and seams on both the garment and facing. Press the seams open; slash and press open the darts. Finish facing edge as required for fabric. (See Seam finishes.)

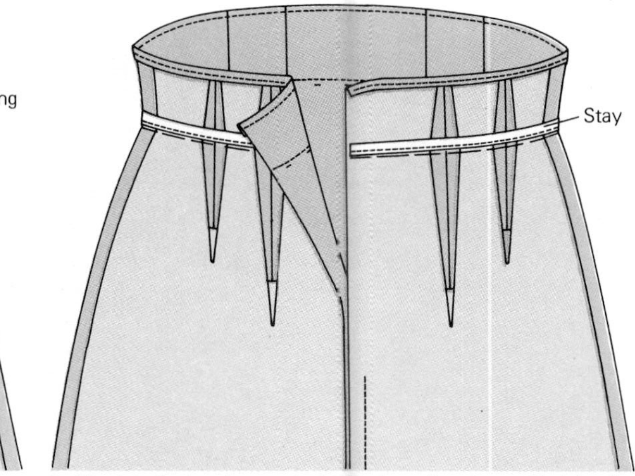

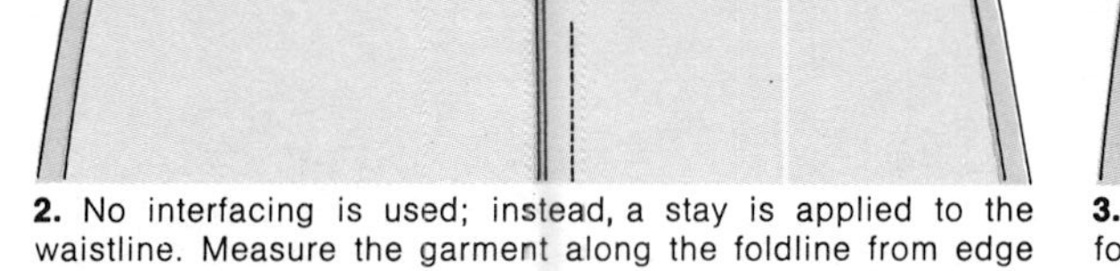

2. No interfacing is used; instead, a stay is applied to the waistline. Measure the garment along the foldline from edge to edge; cut a length of seam tape or twill tape to that measurement. With width of tape on facing, pin the stay along the foldline; have ends of stay even with open edges. Stitch through stay and garment ⅛″ from foldline.

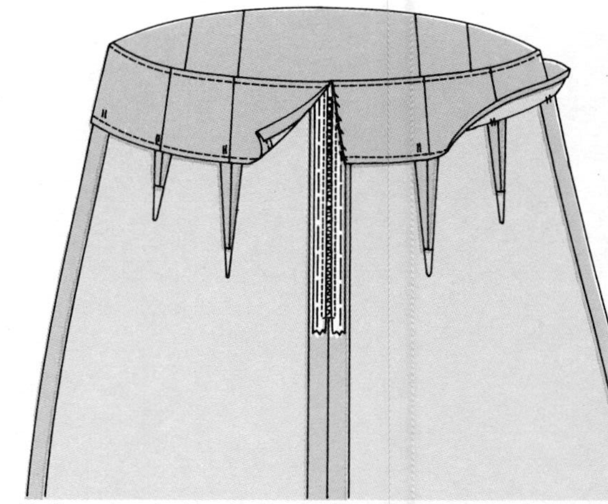

3. Turn the facing to the inside of the garment along the foldline; press. Insert the zipper as recommended by the pattern. Turn in the ends of the facing, being sure to clear the zipper; slipstitch them to the zipper tape. Tack the facing to the garment at all seams and darts. Finish top of closure with hook and eye or hanging snap.

Elastic waistbands

Elastics 17 Zigzag stitching 32-37
Seaming knits 156

Applied elastic (self band)

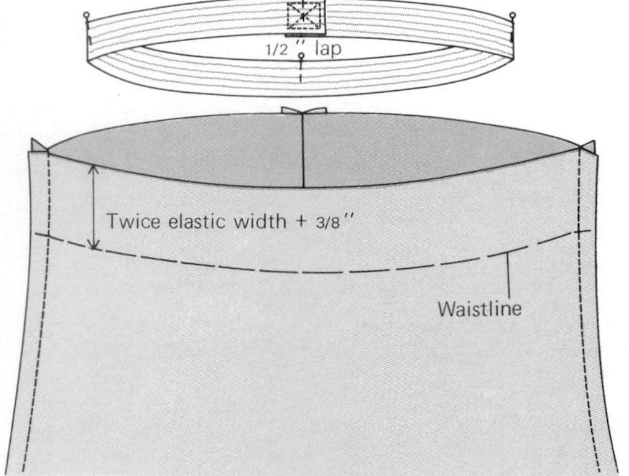

1. This technique can be used only when the garment has not been dart-fitted at waistline. Cut garment with an extension above waistline that is twice the width of the elastic plus ⅜″. Mark waistline with basting. Cut a length of elastic to fit snugly around waist plus ½″. Overlap ends and stitch securely; pin-mark elastic into fourths.

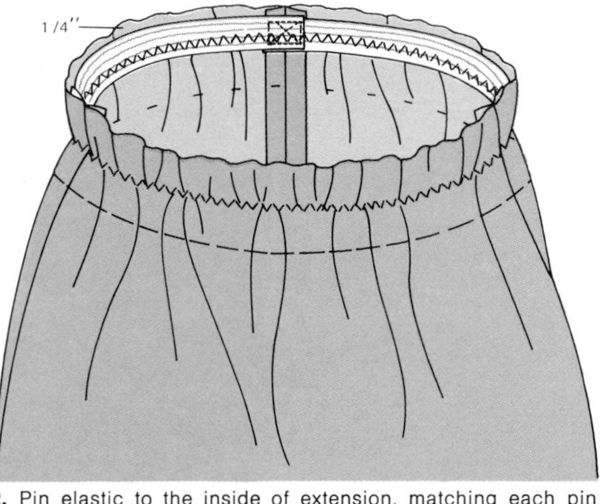

2. Pin elastic to the inside of extension, matching each pin mark to a side seam, center back, or center front. Place top edge of elastic ¼″ down from top edge of the extension. Stitch along the lower edge of the elastic, stretching it between pins as you stitch to fit the fabric. A wide zigzag stitch is best but a short straight stitch may be used.

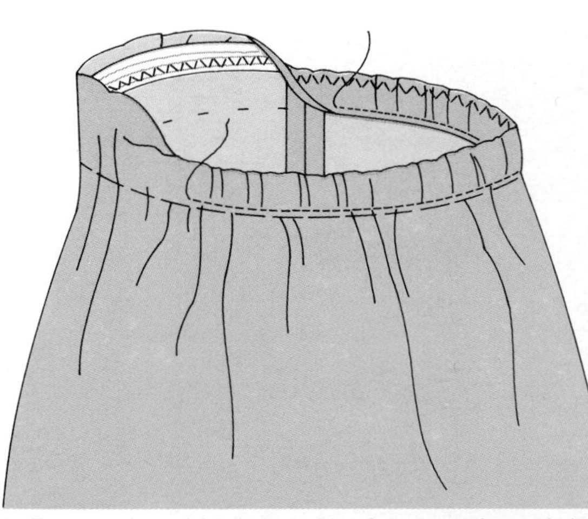

3. Turn elastic and fabric to inside of garment along stitched edge of elastic. The elastic will be completely covered. If fabric does not ravel, raw edge may be left as it is. If fabric ravels, turn under ¼″ on raw edge. Stitch along the waistline marking through the waistband, elastic, and garment, stretching elastic during stitching.

Applied elastic (separate band)

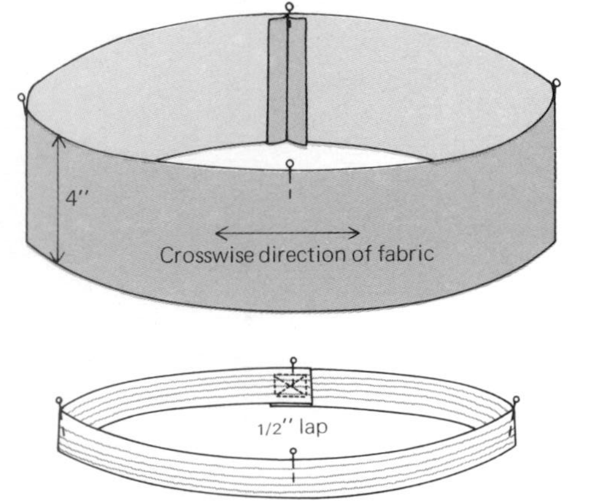

1. This method is suitable only for knits with stretch; waistline may be dart-fitted. Cut waistband on the crosswise grain of the fabric, 4″ wide and the same length as *garment* waist measurement plus seam allowances. Join ends with a ⅝″ seam. Cut 1″-wide elastic to fit *body* waist snugly plus ½″. Overlap ½″ at ends; stitch securely. Pin-mark waistband, elastic, and waistline into fourths.

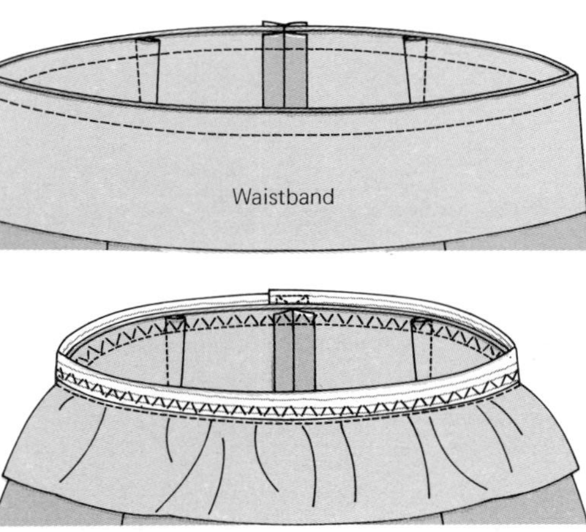

2. Matching pin marks and seams, pin waistband to skirt with right sides together. Stitch a ⅝″ seam, stretching both pieces of fabric as you sew (A). Press seam as stitched. Lap elastic over waistline seam allowance with the bottom edge of the elastic just above first row of stitching. Using a zigzag stitch, sew elastic to seam allowance, stretching it to fit between pins (B) as you stitch.

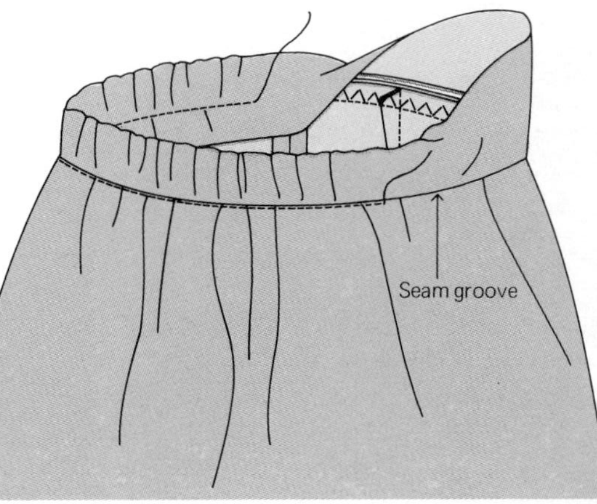

3. Fold waistband over elastic to the inside of garment. Working from the outside, pin the waistband in place, inserting pins just below the seamline so the excess length of the waistband, on the inside, is caught in the pinning. Stitch from right side in the seam groove, stretching elastic so waistband is flat. Trim away excess seam allowance from lower edge of waistband inside garment.

Zigzag stitching 32-37
Staystitching 144

Decorative stretch waistbands

Decorative stretch waistbands are made with specially designed elastic products available in solid colors, plaids or stripes, and prints. Variously woven, braided, or shirred, they come in finished widths from 1 to 2½ inches. Choose a decorative elastic as close as possible to the fabric weight.

The **woven elastics** are called webbings, and their stretchability varies from limited to moderate. Webbings are quite firm and will not roll over during wear. The limited-stretch webbing should be used only when the garment has a placket opening—the stretch is not sufficient to fit over the hips or bust and still fit snugly at the waist. **Braided elastics** have a moderate amount of stretch and can often be used without a placket opening. The **shirred bandings** are basically grosgrain ribbon stitched with elastic thread; their stretch is limited by the amount of shirring, but they are usually stretchy enough to be used without a placket opening.

Edge finishing. On some products, both edges are finished; on others, only one. This determines how the banding is applied. On an unfinished edge, a stitching line will be indicated.

Attaching decorative elastic

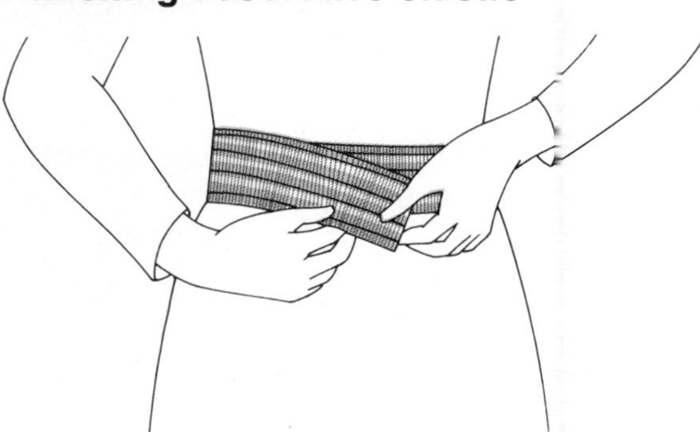

1. Purchase decorative elastic or shirred ribbon in a length to fit around the waistline snugly, allowing an additional 2″ for finishing ends. Width choice depends on the effect desired. To avoid raveling during construction, always cut straight across elastic. As an extra precaution, stitch across cut ends with a straight or zigzag stitch.

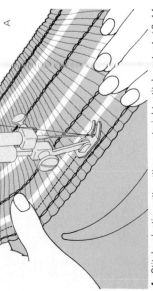

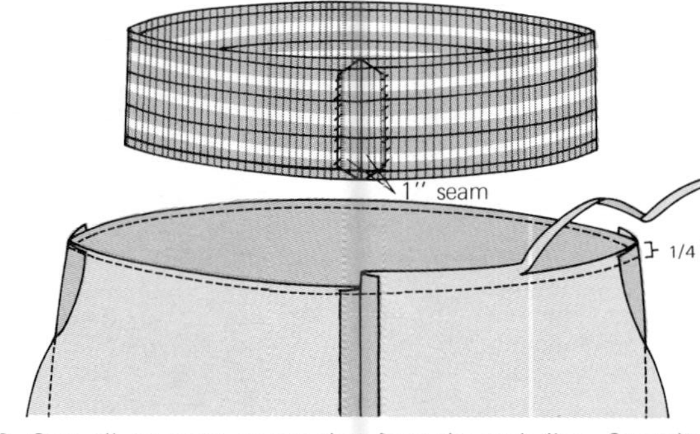

2. Sew all garment seams that form the waistline. Staystitch on garment waistline seam and trim the seam allowance to ¼″. If no closure is being used, seam the ends of the elastic or ribbon by placing right sides together and stitching a 1″ seam. Press open. Turn top edges of seam allowance in diagonally and tack seam allowances to waistband.

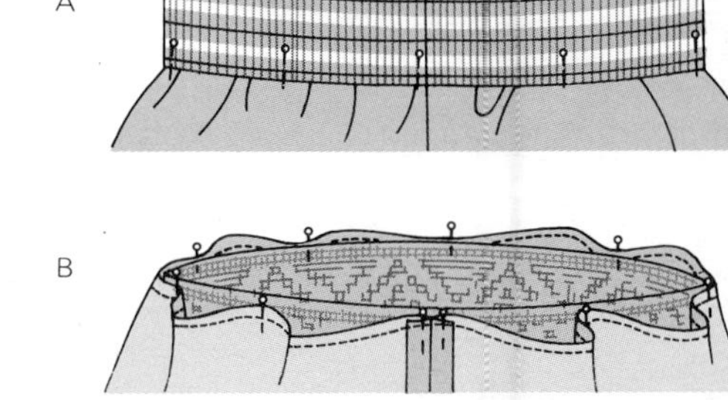

3. Divide garment waistline and elastic or ribbon into four or eight equal parts; pin-mark. If both edges of elastic are finished, lap wrong side of elastic over right side of garment. Place waistband seam at center back and match pins (A). If one edge is unfinished, place elastic inside garment, right sides together, matching pins and stitch lines (B).

A

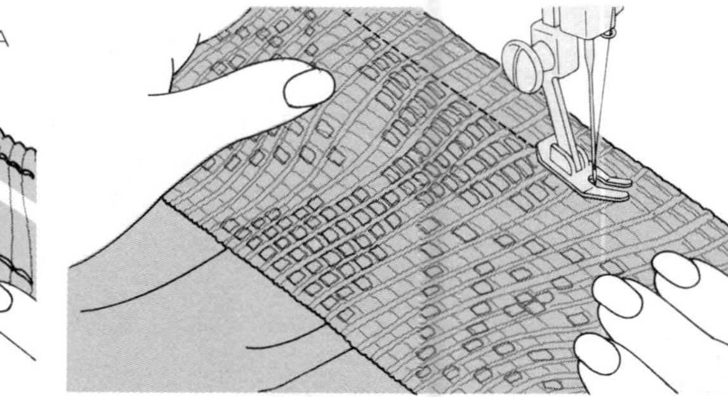

4. Stitch elastic with either a straight stitch set at 12–14 stitches per inch or a zigzag stitch of medium length and width. For a lapped waistline seam (A), stitch just inside the first elastic thread if sewing ribbon, close to the finished edge if elastic webbing is being used. If the elastic has one unfinished edge, sew along indicated stitch line (B). Sew between elastic threads if possible. With one hand behind presser foot and the other in front, carefully stretch elastic between pins as you stitch, to fit the garment. Make certain that stitch line of elastic remains aligned with seamline of skirt. Remove pins as you reach them; do not stitch over them. Overlap stitching at ends. Press seam carefully as it was stitched; test iron temperature first on a scrap to be sure heat you use will not damage elastic.

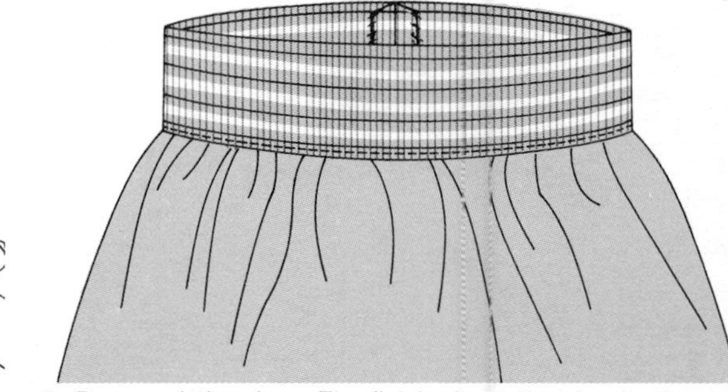

5. Press waistband up. The finished waistband pulls the garment into size by forming soft gathers; the number of gathers depends on size difference between waistline of garment and waistband. If a closure is included in the garment, finish the ends of the elastic by turning them under the desired amount and tacking down. Underlap should extend under overlap enough to allow for fasteners (p. 239).

Belts

Tie belts

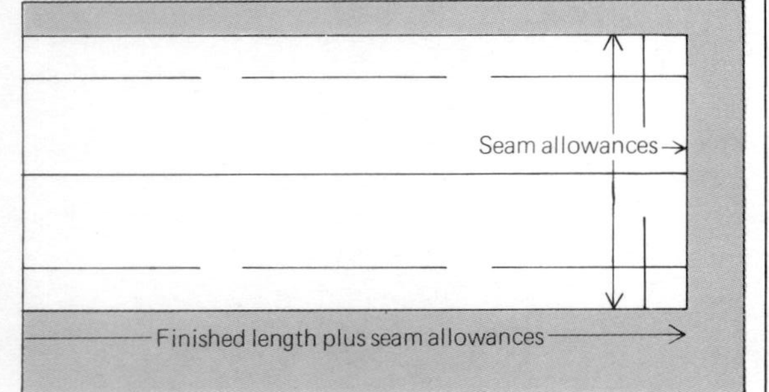

1. Belt may be cut on either the bias or straight grain. Cut it twice the desired finished *width* plus seam allowances, and the necessary *length* plus seam allowances. Length should equal waist circumference plus enough extra to tie ends.

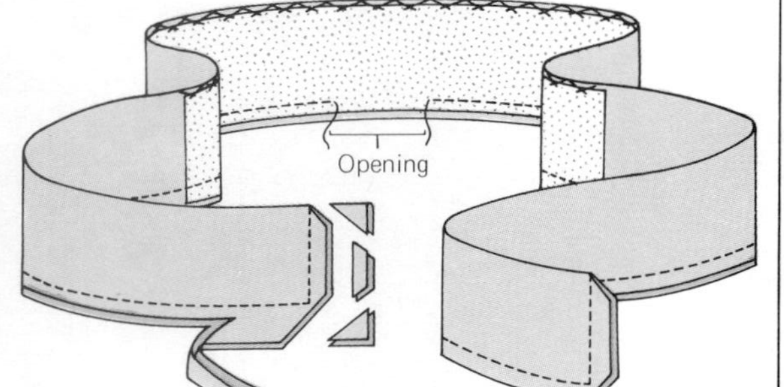

2. If belt is to be interfaced, apply interfacing only to portion that encircles waist. Fold belt in half lengthwise, right sides together. Stitch ends and long edge, leaving an opening for turning. Trim and grade seams and corners.

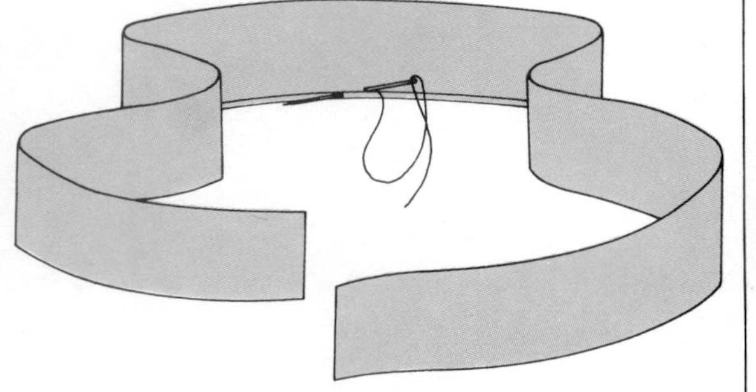

3. Turn belt to the right side through the opening. Pull corners out so that they are square, and press edges carefully. Press in the seam allowances at opening and slipstitch opening closed. Give finished belt a final pressing.

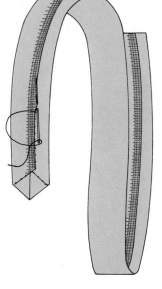

Reinforced belts

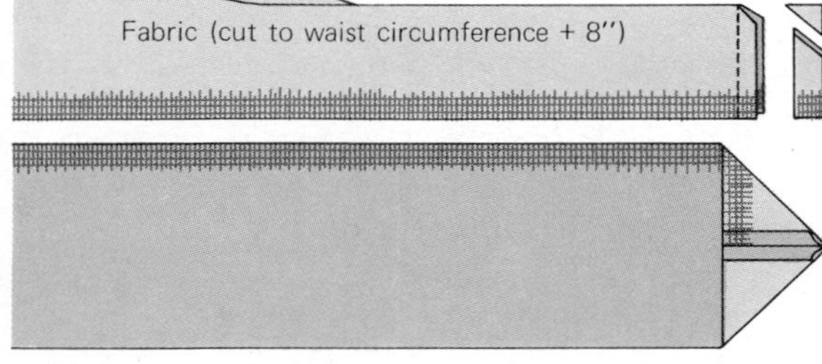

To hand-finish: 1. Cut fabric for belt twice the width of belting plus ½", with one long edge on the selvage. To form a point at one end, fold fabric in half lengthwise and stitch end with ½" seam. Press seam open as illustrated.

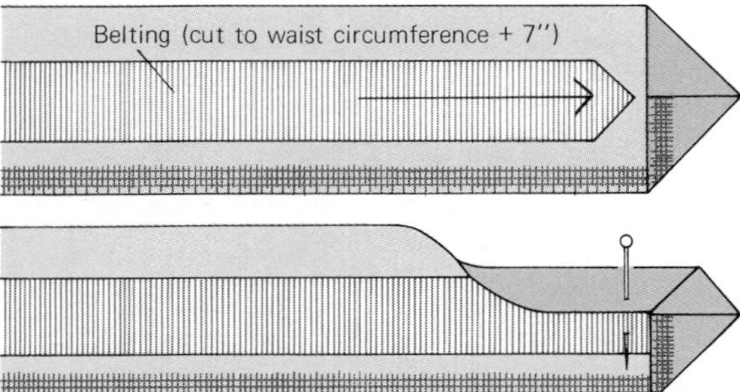

2. Turn finished end right side out. Cut belting so one end has the same point as the fabric. Insert pointed end of the belting into fabric point. Press flat. With belting centered on fabric, pin raw edge of fabric over belting.

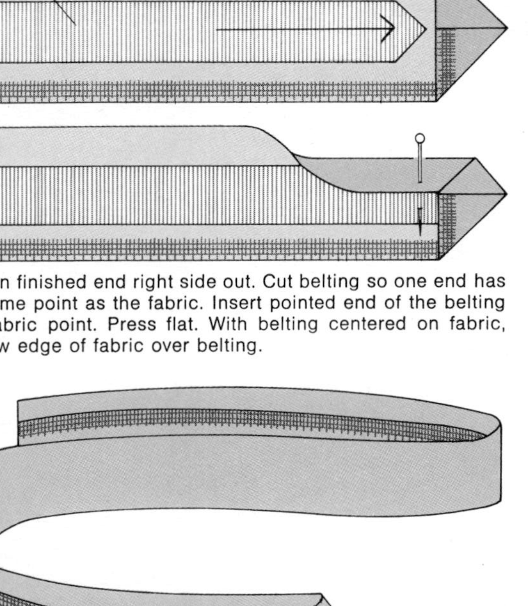

3. Pin selvage edge over raw edge, pulling fabric taut around belting. Slipstitch at point, then along selvage edge. Finish belt by attaching a buckle to unfinished end. If a prong buckle will be used, work eyelets (p. 252).

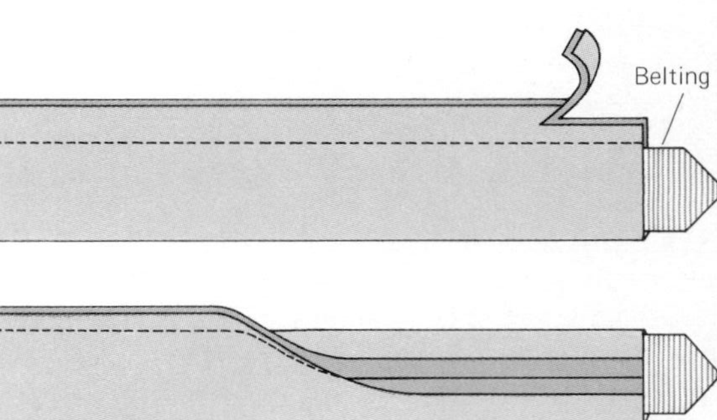

To machine-finish : 1. Cut fabric twice width of belting plus 1¼". Shape one end of belting. Fold fabric over belting, wrong side out. Stitch close to belting, using a zipper foot. Trim seam allowances to ¼"; move seam to center of belting.

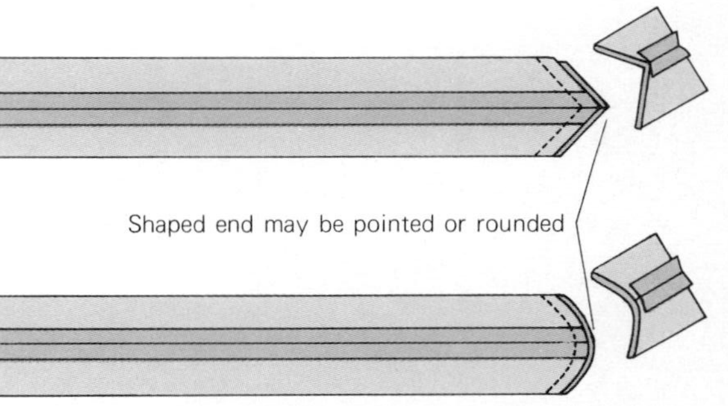

2. Press the seam open with the tip of the iron. Pull shaped end of belting into position inside stitched fabric tube. Carefully stitch close to, but not through the belting. Trim seam. A closely fitted cover for the belting has now been made.

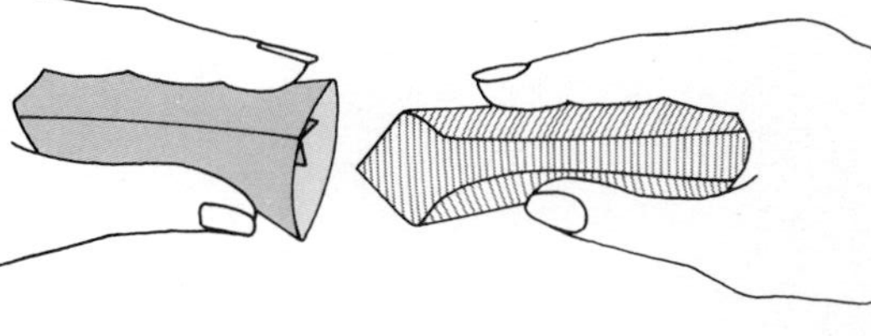

3. Remove the belting and turn the fabric tube right side out. Do not press. Cup belting and slip it into belt, shaped end first. Attach buckle to unfinished end. If a prong buckle will be used, work eyelets in shaped end of belt (p.252).

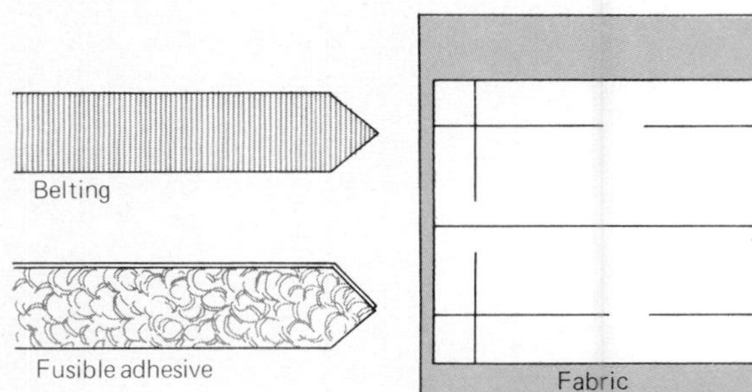

To fuse: 1. Cut belting and two strips of fusible adhesive the length and width that the finished belt is to be. Shape one end of each of the strips into a point. Cut the belt fabric the length and twice the width of the belting.

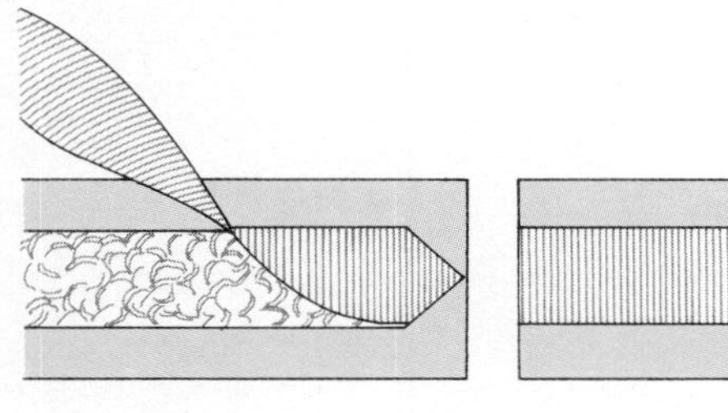

2. Center a strip of adhesive, then the belting, on the wrong side of fabric. Follow manufacturer's directions to fuse layers. Cut a triangular piece of adhesive and place on belting point. Fold fabric over point and fuse point only.

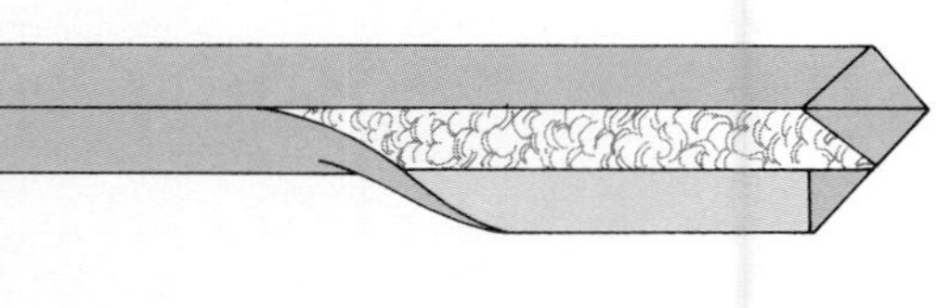

3. Fold long edges of fabric over belting and press. Insert fusible adhesive and cut away any adhesive not covered by fabric at the point. Fuse fabric in place. Attach buckle, work eyelets for a prong buckle (p.252).

Contour belts

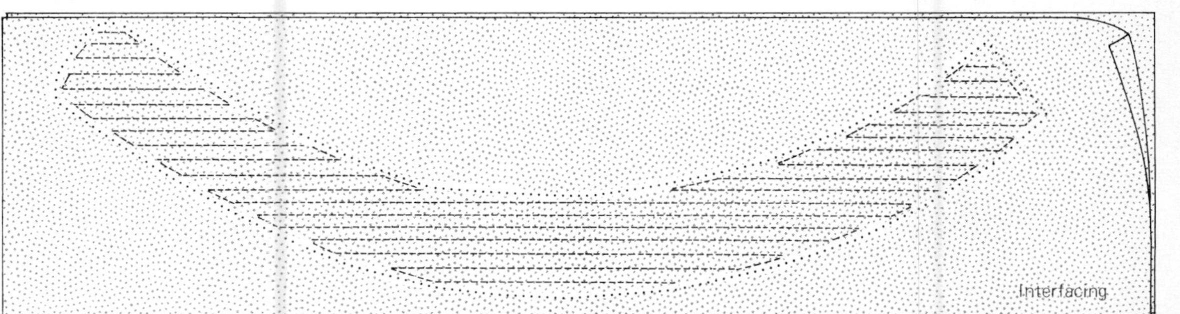

Because a contour belt is shaped to fit the curve of the body, regular straight belting cannot be used for backing. Use two layers of a sturdy interfacing, such as hair canvas (fusible or nonfusible). A separate shaped facing is required.

1. Cut all layers of the belt on the lengthwise grain. If *nonfusible interfacing* is being used, pin the two layers together and trace shape of finished belt onto one. Make rows of machine stitching within outline on lengthwise grain.

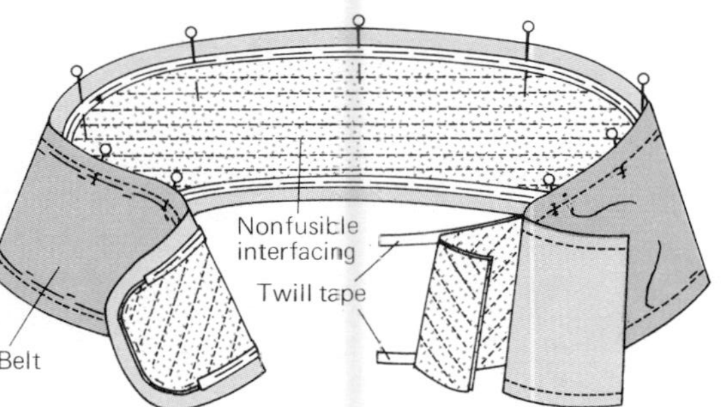

2. Cut the interfacing along the outline. Staystitch the belt along all outer edges. Center the padstitched interfacing on the belt, leaving a ⅝" margin on all sides; baste in place. Center and baste ⅛"-wide twill tape over seamlines.

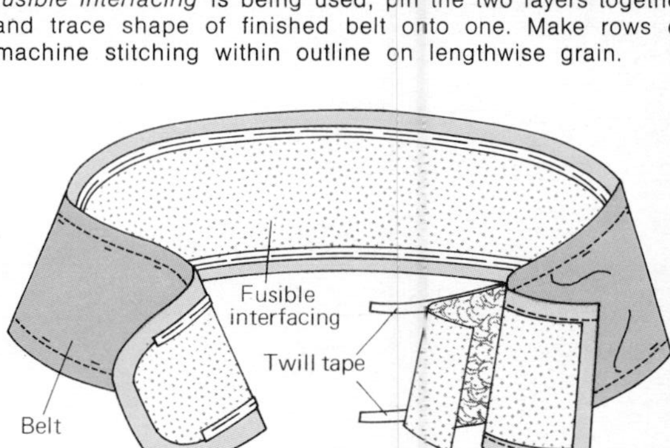

If using fusible interfacing, cut two layers to size and shape of finished belt. Center one layer at a time on the wrong side of the belt, leaving ⅝" on all sides. Fuse in place. Center and baste ⅛"-wide twill tape over seamlines.

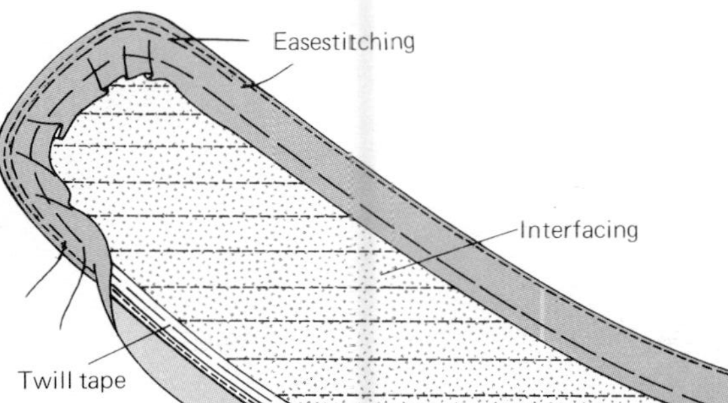

3. Apply a row of easestitching on seamline at curved end of belt. Press seam allowances to wrong side, over interfacing, drawing up easestitching as needed so seam allowances lie flat. Hand-baste to interfacing with long stitches.

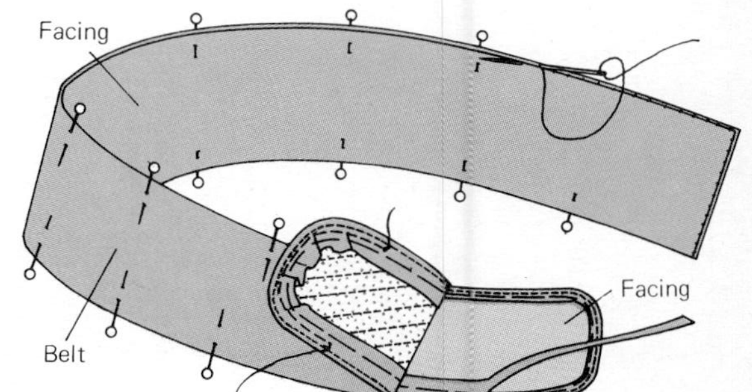

4. Staystitch belt facing and turn all edges in ¾"; baste in place. Trim the seam allowances to ⅜". Pin the facing to the belt and slipstitch into place along all edges. Remove bastings. Attach buckle, work eyelets for a prong buckle (p.252).

Belts

Buckles and eyelets

For any buckle other than one that clasps, try on finished belt and mark center front position on both buckle end and end to be perforated. Cut off buckle end 2 inches from center front mark. Stitch ¼ inch from raw edge, then overcast the edge to prevent raveling of the fabric.

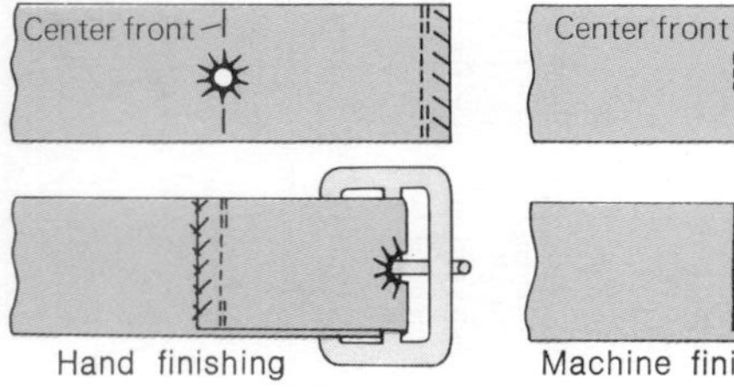

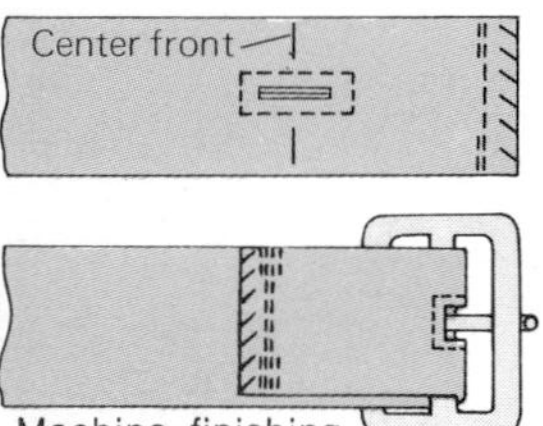

If buckle has a prong, position the prong at the center front mark on straight end of belt. To make an opening for prong, pierce a hole and overcast the edges, or machine-stitch a small rectangle through all layers, then slit between stitches. Slip prong through opening, turn back end of belt and fasten securely with hand or machine stitches.

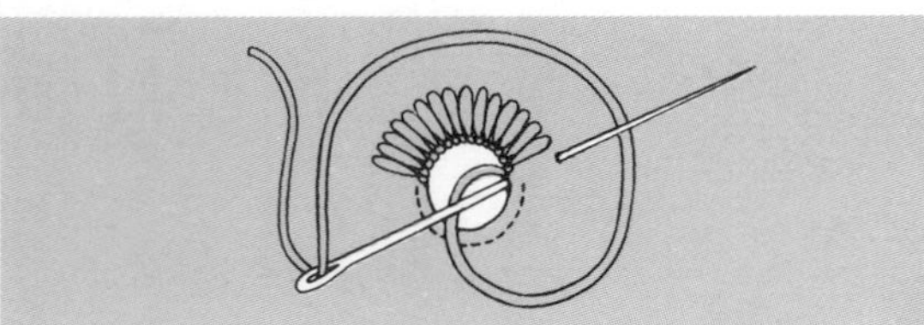

Eyelets can be made three ways: with a special machine attachment, with a tool that punches in metal eyelets, or by hand. To make a hand-worked eyelet, punch a hole with a stiletto, then reinforce opening with small running stitches. Work closely spaced buttonhole stitches over edge of eyelet.

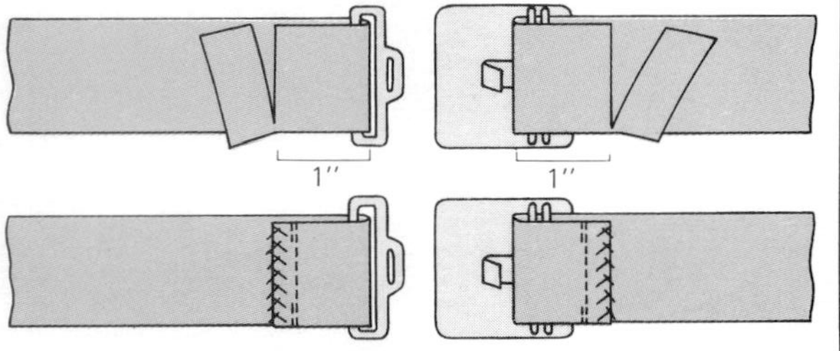

If buckle clasps, slip the ends of the belt through each half of the buckle. Adjust ends until belt fits properly; trim excess at each end to 1″. Stitch ¼″ from each end and overcast. Secure ends to buckle by whipstitching them to back of belt so that no stitching is visible on right side.

Belt carriers

Belt carriers can be made of thread or fabric. Thread carriers, made from a thread chain (see Hand stitches), are nearly invisible and are used primarily on side seams of dresses and coats. Fabric carriers may be very wide or narrow, depending on the style of the garment. They can easily be added to a garment either during construction or afterward. They should be placed around the waistline at strategic points, such as side seams, and 2 to 3 inches on either side of the center front and back. The carriers must be large enough that the belt can slide through easily.

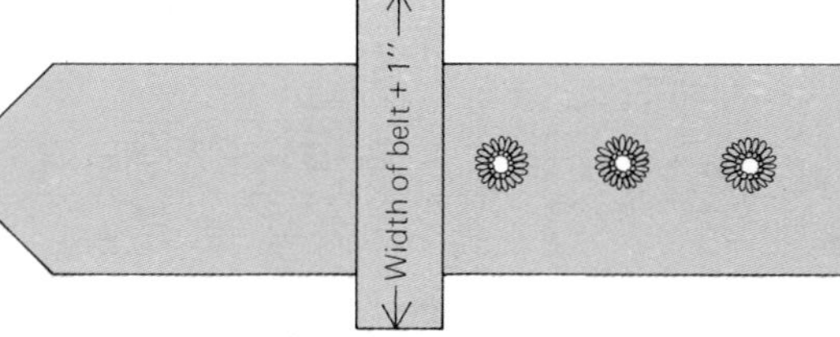

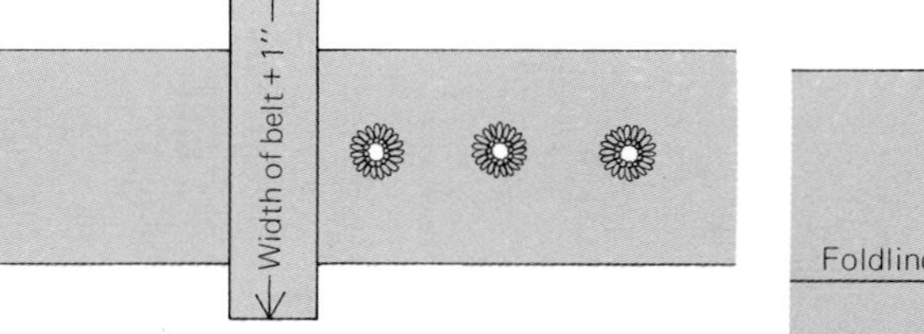

1. The length needed for one carrier is equal to the belt width plus 1″ (allow more for a thick fabric). Prepare total number of carriers needed from a single strip of fabric.

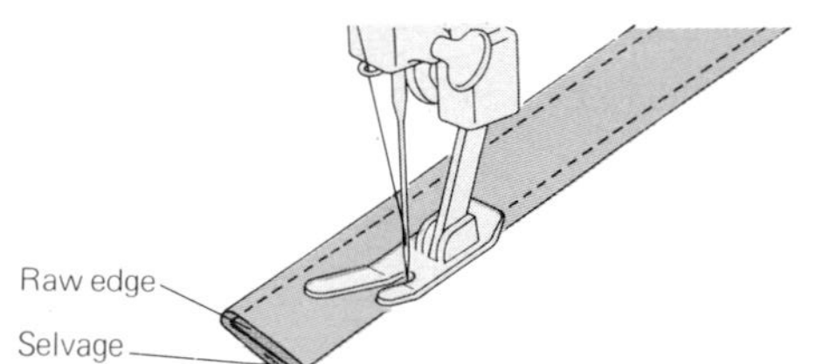

2. Cut strip along selvage, three times desired finished width and total length needed for all carriers. Fold strip to ⅓ original width, raw edge inside. Topstitch both edges.

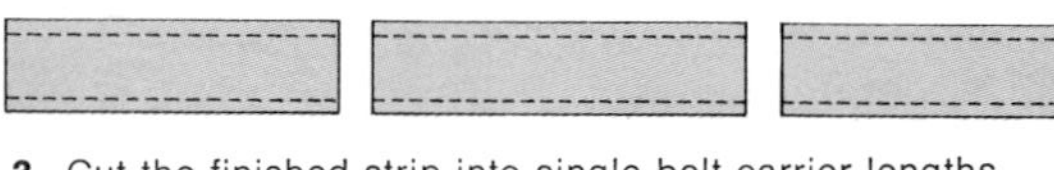

3. Cut the finished strip into single belt carrier lengths.

4. To attach carriers to a garment, fold under ¼″ at each end, and press. Pin carriers in position on garment. To sew by hand, slipstitch raw edges and fold to garment at top and bottom. To sew by machine, stitch across folds at top and bottom. (If a bar tack effect is desired, use a zigzag instead of a straight stitch.)

Foldline

Waistband seamline

To attach carriers to a waistband before it is sewed to garment, position the carriers along the foldline of the waistband. Sew in place as shown on carrier at left, above. Press carrier down and baste free edge to lower edge of waistband so it will be caught in waistline seam.

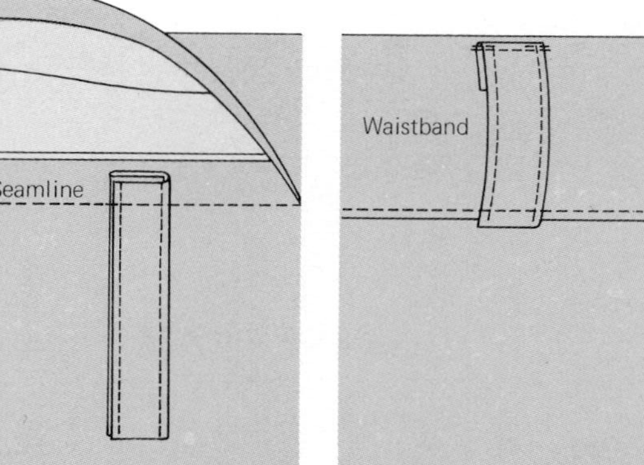

To attach carriers to waistline seam before attaching a waistband, position the carriers on the garment waistline seam as shown on carrier at left, above. This edge of carrier is caught in the stitching of waistline seam. Complete the waistband application. Press carrier up and sew top of carrier to top of waistband, stitching through all layers of waistband.

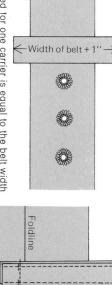

Sleeves & Sleeve Finishes

Sleeves

Pressing 18-19
Sleeve alterations 103-104,115

Basic sleeve types

Today's garments are designed with a wide variety of sleeves, which differ greatly in look and in method of construction. A garment, for example, may have armholes (also referred to as *armscyes*) that are merely finished, producing a **sleeveless** look; or it may have sleeves, either **set-in** or **raglan,** that are separately made and attached to the garment. Still another possibility, **kimono** sleeves, are cut as extensions of the main bodice.

The armscyes on most sleeveless garments are cut to comfortably encircle the arm with upper edge resting at shoulder point. There are variations, however, of the sleeveless look. Garments are sometimes designed with wider-than-usual shoulder widths that drop over the shoulders to create a little cap. Others are styled with narrower shoulder widths that result in a larger and more angled armhole, and something of a halter effect. Whatever an armhole's shape, it is usually finished with a facing unit cut to the same shape, and applied as described on the opposite page. Most patterns use a one-piece armhole facing that is seamed at the underarm; in some, it will be a two-piece facing (front and back) that is seamed together at both shoulder and underarm.

Set-in sleeves are the most widely used type. As the name implies, this sleeve is actually set into the armhole of the garment. Variations of the set-in are numerous: The top edge, or *cap,* can be slightly rounded or fully gathered, the length long or short, the bottom tapered, flared, or gathered. The armscye can also vary, from the standard round armhole to the deeply cut armhole of a dolman sleeve. Most set-in sleeves are designed with a slightly rounded cap; ideally they should fall in a smooth curve from the shoulder edge with no dimpling or puckering. To achieve this, the sleeve cap curvature (which measures slightly more than the corresponding part of the armhole) must be carefully eased into the armscye. For easing method, see page 256.

The raglan sleeve is another type that is attached to the garment. Unlike the set-in sleeve, which is inserted into the armhole, a raglan sleeve is joined to the garment in one continuous seam, which runs diagonally from the front neckline to the underarm and up to the back neckline. For this method, see page 258. The raglan sleeve covers the entire shoulder area. It may be cut from one pattern piece, with shaping achieved by means of a dart along the shoulder line. In some cases, however, raglan sleeves are made from two pattern pieces (front and back), which are shaped as they are seamed together along the shoulder line. Raglan sleeves are comfortable to wear and ideal for hard-to-fit shoulders; the darts or seams are easily alterable to accommodate most figure differences.

The kimono sleeve is one of the easiest types to construct because it is merely an extension of the main bodice. When this sleeve is cut to extend straight out from the neckline, and with a deep "armhole" opening, there is a soft drape under the arm. When it is cut to conform more to the curved shape around the shoulder, and with a shallower armhole opening, the fit becomes closer; arm movement does, however, become more difficult. Such a close fit usually requires a gusset—a small, usually triangular piece of fabric that is inserted into an underarm seam for comfort and ease of movement. Techniques for inserting gussets appear on pages 260–261.

To achieve success with any garment, whether it is sleeveless or made with sleeves, it is wise to observe several principles: (1) Check garment and sleeve fit (see opposite page) and alter the pattern accordingly (see Fitting). (2) Carefully and accurately transfer all sleeve and armhole markings to the fashion fabric. (3) Use proper pressing techniques during construction. (4) Whenever possible, finish the lower edge of the sleeve before attaching it to the garment.

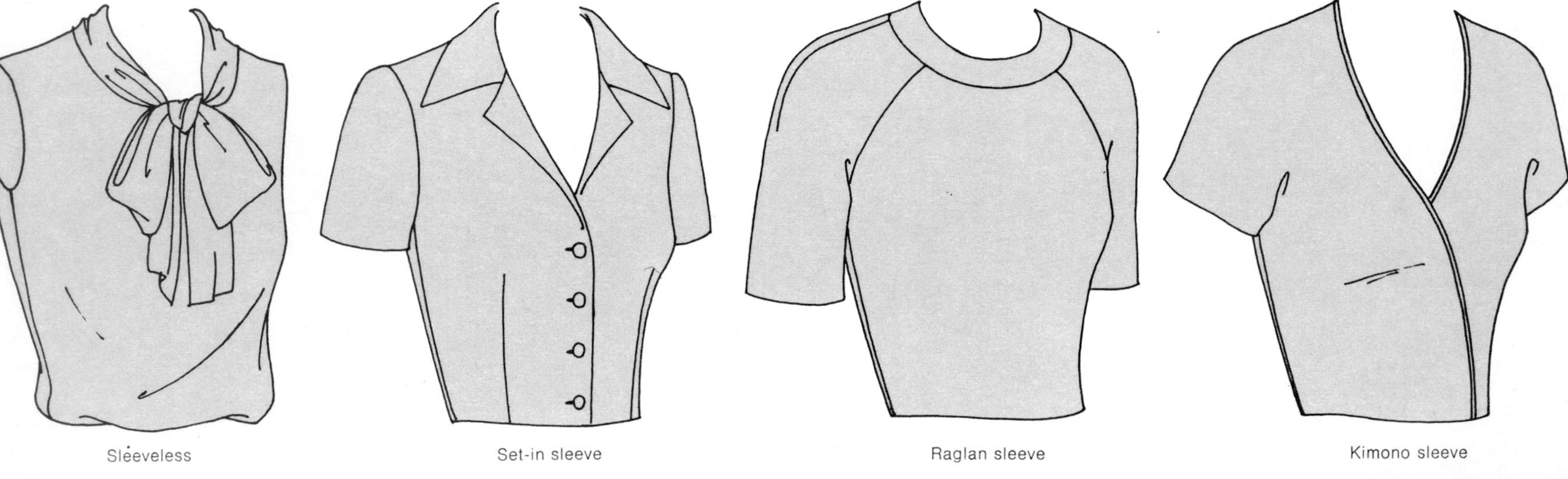

Sleeveless — Set-in sleeve — Raglan sleeve — Kimono sleeve

Hand-stitched tacks 134-136
Reducing bulk 147
Understitching 147

Proper sleeve fit

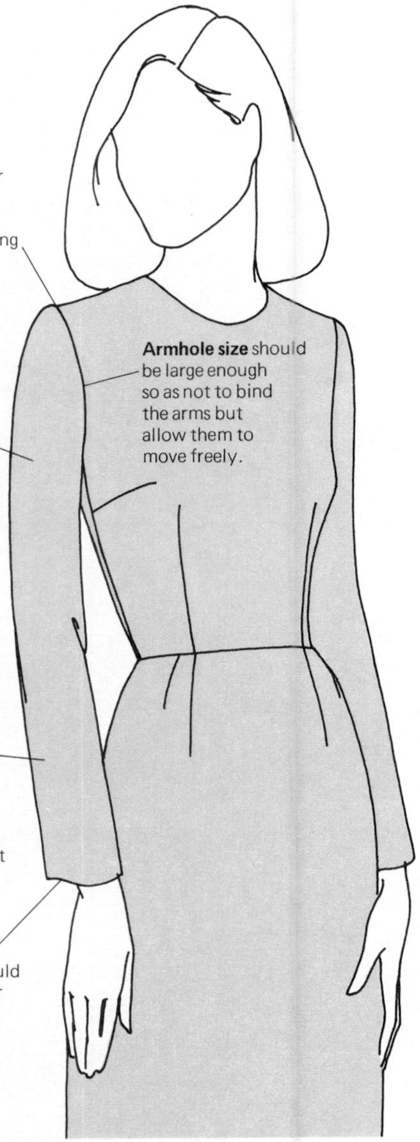

Shoulder line, an important matching point for sleeves, should sit exactly on top of shoulder, dividing front and back portions of body.

Upper arm of sleeve must have sufficient ease around it that sleeve can hang smoothly from shoulder, and arm can move freely.

Lower arm section of sleeve should fit comfortably without being too tight. Darts or easestitching along elbow area can help provide shaping for more comfort and freer arm movement.

Sleeve length should be appropriate for design of garment as well as for individual figure proportions.

Armhole size should be large enough so as not to bind the arms but allow them to move freely.

Sleeveless finish

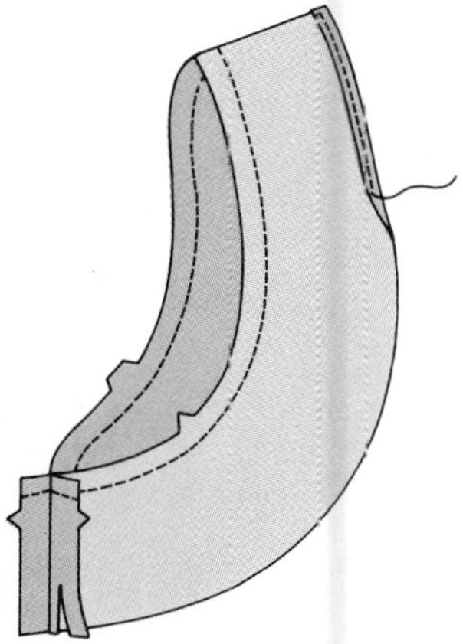

1. Staystitch ⅛" inside seamline of the garment armhole and facing unit. With right sides together, match and seam facing ends together. Press seam flat, then open. Trim seam allowance to half-width. Finish free edges.

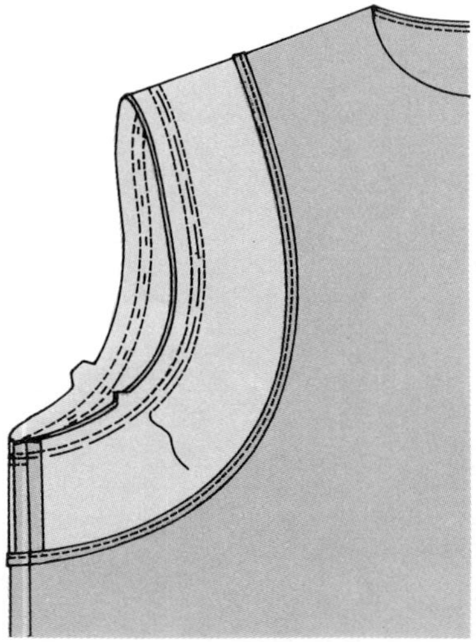

2. With the right sides together, pin and baste facing to garment armhole, matching the underarm seams, notches, and shoulder points. Start at underarm and, with facing side up, stitch the armhole seamline, overlapping a few stitches.

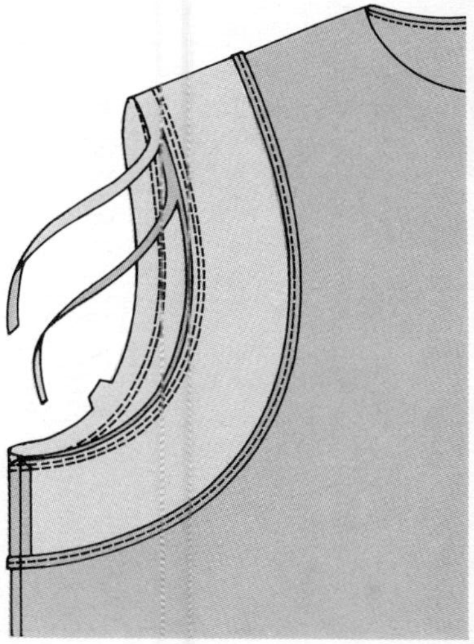

3. Press seam flat to embed stitches. To help reduce bulk around the armhole, trim and grade the seam allowances, making garment seam allowance the widest. Diagonally trim across the underarm seam allowance.

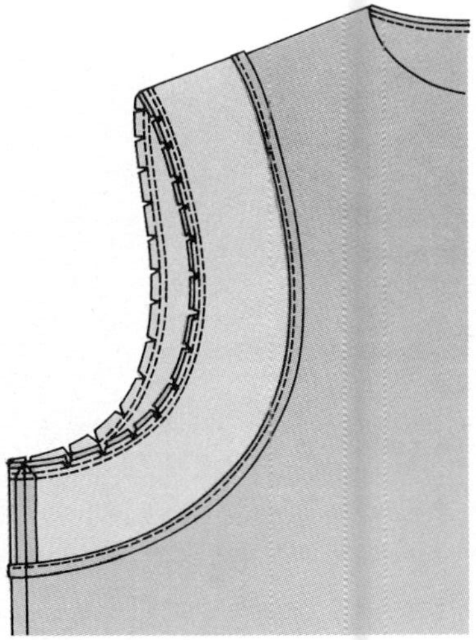

4. Clip into and, if necessary, notch out fullness from seam allowances; this will enable armhole facing to lie flat when it is turned to the inside.

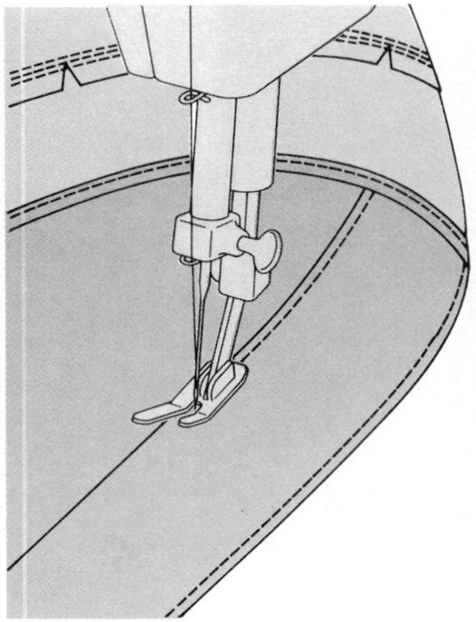

5. Press seam open, then press it toward the facing. Extend facing and seam allowances; from right side, understitch close to seamline.

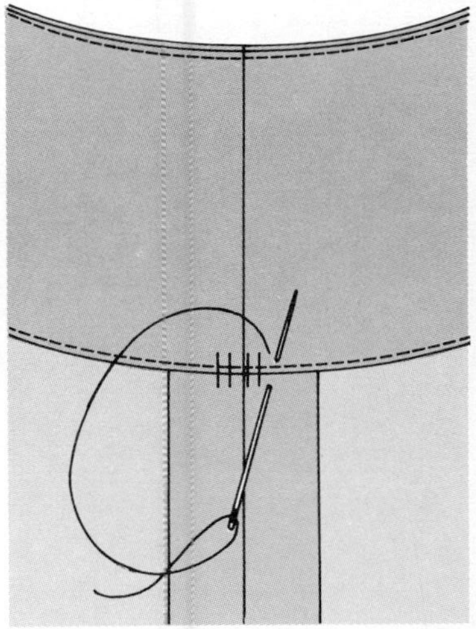

6. Turn facing to inside; roll seamline slightly inside. Align underarm seams, and press. Tack facing to garment seam allowances at underarm and shoulder.

Stitch length for easing 30
Tying thread ends 137
Gathering 178
Tailored sleeve 375

Set-in sleeves

Though set-in sleeves occur in a variety of garments and in many design variations, they are all inserted by a procedure much like the one described at right. Depending on the curve of the sleeve edge, a sleeve cap can be either slightly rounded or full and gathered. If a sleeve is to have

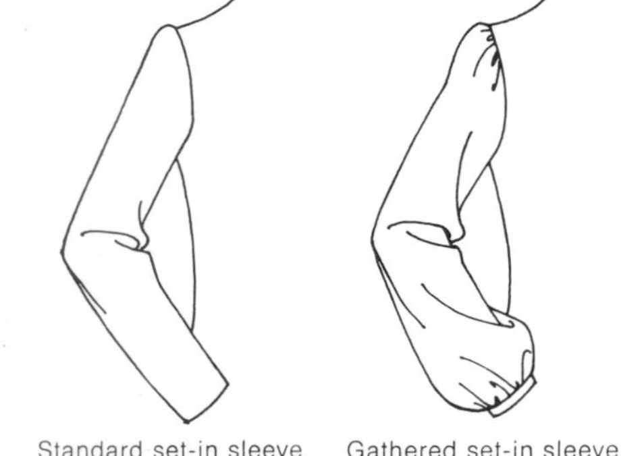

Standard set-in sleeve Gathered set-in sleeve

a nicely rounded cap, it must be carefully manipulated when it is eased into the armscye to avoid puckers and dimples along the seamline. If the sleeve is to have a gathered cap, the shirring must be evenly distributed along the upper curve. The number and form of pattern pieces for set-in

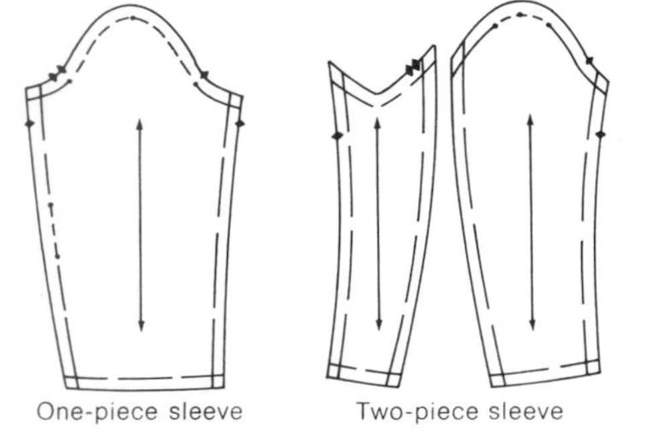

One-piece sleeve Two-piece sleeve

sleeves also varies. The set-in sleeve used most often is cut from a one-piece pattern. Occasionally you will see a two-piece sleeve, usually in tailored garments. Still another available type has a two-piece look but is actually cut as one and the seam positioned at the back of the arm (see Tailoring).

Set-in sleeve method

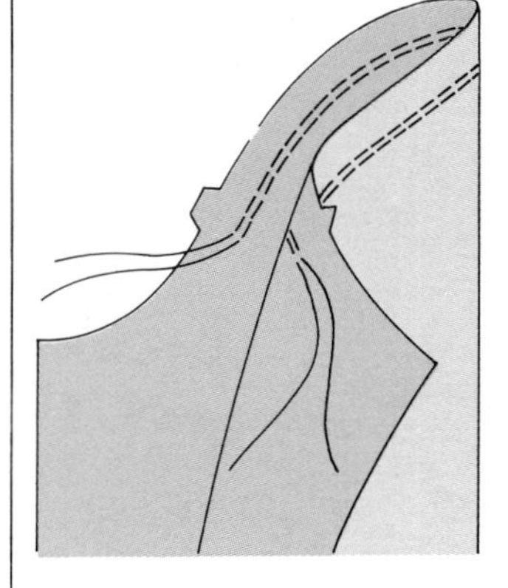

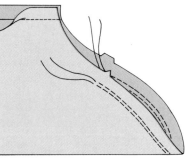

1. The curved edge on most set-in sleeves measures more than the armhole circumference; thus easing along cap is needed to fit the sleeve into the armscye. To provide ease control between sleeve cap notches, place two rows of easestitching within the seam allowance, the first a thread's width from seamline, the second ⅛″ from first.

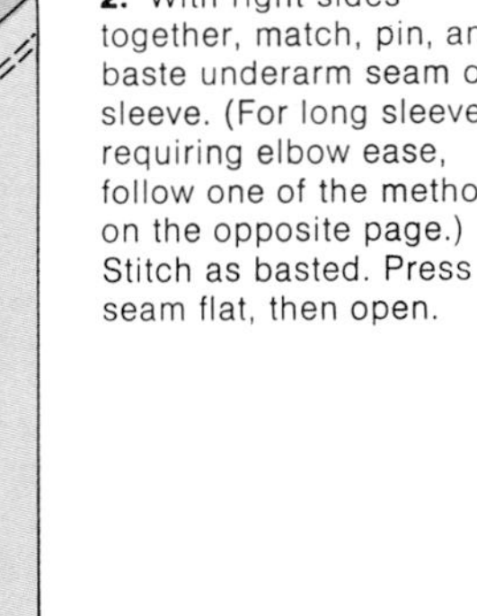

2. With right sides together, match, pin, and baste underarm seam of sleeve. (For long sleeve requiring elbow ease, follow one of the methods on the opposite page.) Stitch as basted. Press seam flat, then open.

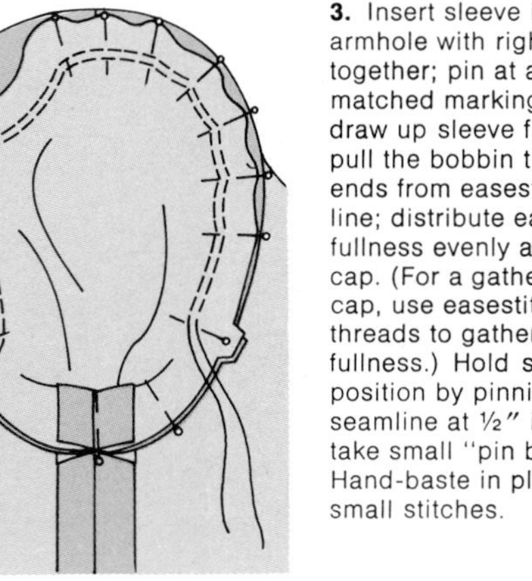

3. Insert sleeve into armhole with right sides together; pin at all matched markings. To draw up sleeve fullness, pull the bobbin thread ends from easestitching line; distribute eased fullness evenly along cap. (For a gathered cap, use easestitching threads to gather excess fullness.) Hold sleeve in position by pinning on seamline at ½″ intervals; take small "pin bites." Hand-baste in place; use small stitches.

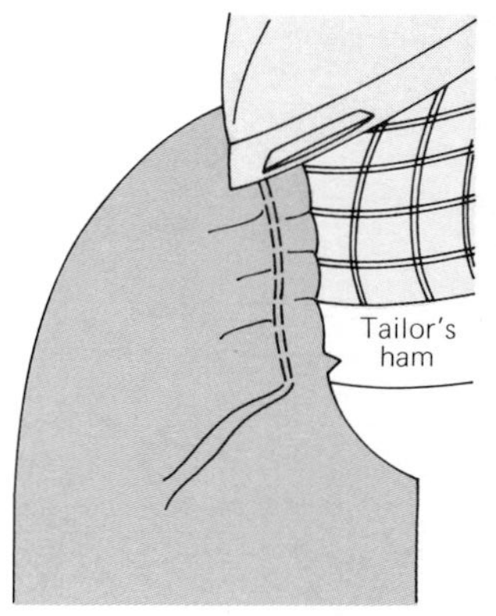

4. Check sleeve from right side; cap should be rounded and smooth. If there are puckers or dimples along seamline, secure easestitching thread ends; remove basted-in sleeve. With right side out, drape sleeve over press mitt or tailor's ham; steam-press along the cap, "shrinking out" as much of the puckering as possible. Re-baste sleeve into armhole.

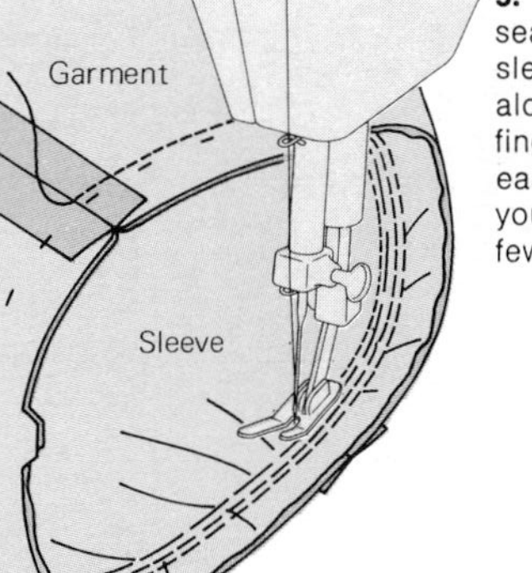

5. Start at underarm seam and, with the sleeve side up, stitch along seamline; use fingers to control eased-in fullness as you stitch. Overlap a few stitches at end.

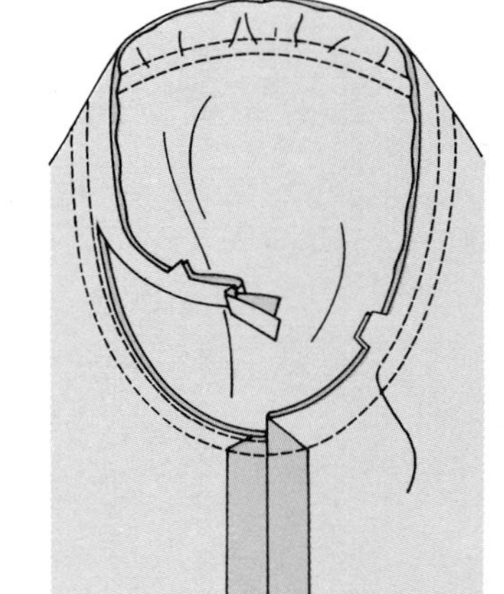

6. Diagonally trim cross-seam allowances at shoulder and underarm. Place another row of stitches (either straight or narrow zigzag) within seam allowance, ¼″ from first row. Trim seam allowances close to second row of stitching. To help maintain rounded cap, turn seam allowances toward the sleeve; *do not press seams.*

Flat-felled seams 150 Seams with fullness 154
Darts 159

Shirt sleeves

One form of the set-in sleeve is attached by the shirt-sleeve method, which permits the sleeve to be sewed into the armhole before garment side and sleeve seams are stitched. Sleeves eligible for this method are less rounded than usual along the shoulder line because the cap is not so steeply curved; there is less difference between the measurement of the armhole and the upper sleeve

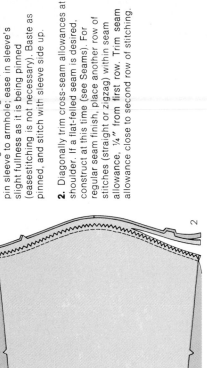

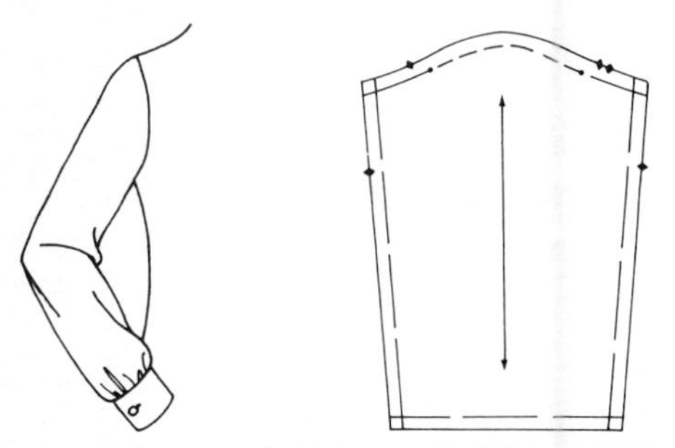

Sleeve cap is less rounded because of shallower curve.

curve, which means easestitching along that curve is usually not necessary. Flat-felled seams are often used in this method; because of the armhole curve, they should be narrow and, contrary to most seam situations, made on the wrong rather than the right side. A popular method for men's shirts, where it originated, the shirt-sleeve technique is also an easy way to handle children's sleeves.

Shirt-sleeve method

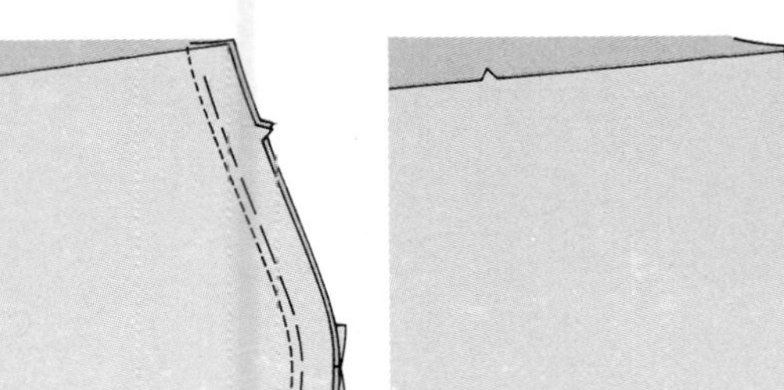

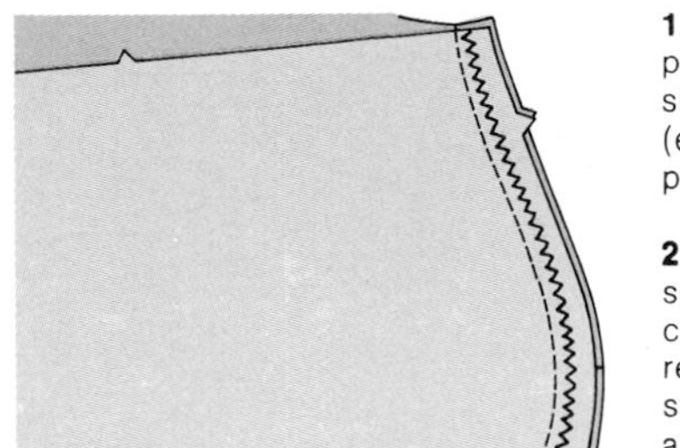

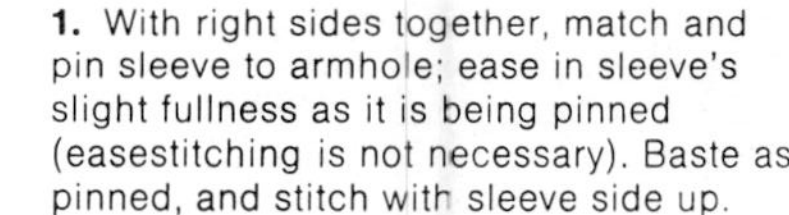

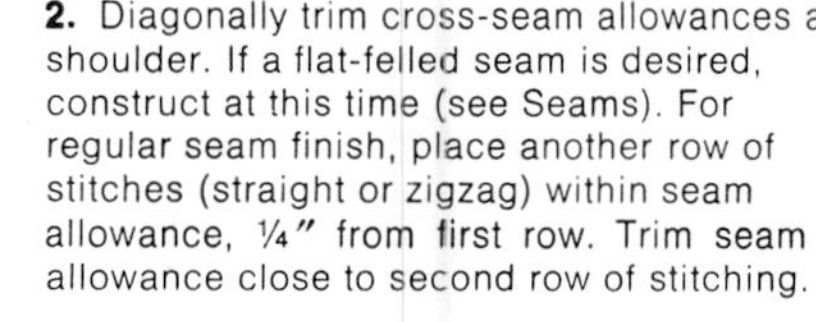

1. With right sides together, match and pin sleeve to armhole; ease in sleeve's slight fullness as it is being pinned (easestitching is not necessary). Baste as pinned, and stitch with sleeve side up.

2. Diagonally trim cross-seam allowances at shoulder. If a flat-felled seam is desired, construct at this time (see Seams). For regular seam finish, place another row of stitches (straight or zigzag) within seam allowance, ¼" from first row. Trim seam allowance close to second row of stitching.

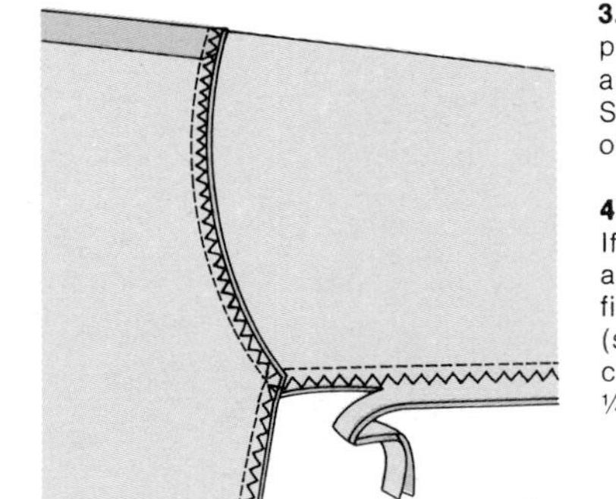

3. With right sides facing, match, pin, and baste underarm seams (turn armhole seam allowances toward sleeve). Stitch in one continuous seam from bottom of garment to bottom of sleeve.

4. Diagonally trim cross-seam allowances. If a flat-felled seam is desired, construct at this time (see Seams). For regular seam finish, place another row of stitches (straight or zigzag) within seam allowance close to second row of stitching ¼" from first row. Trim seam allowance.

Elbow shaping

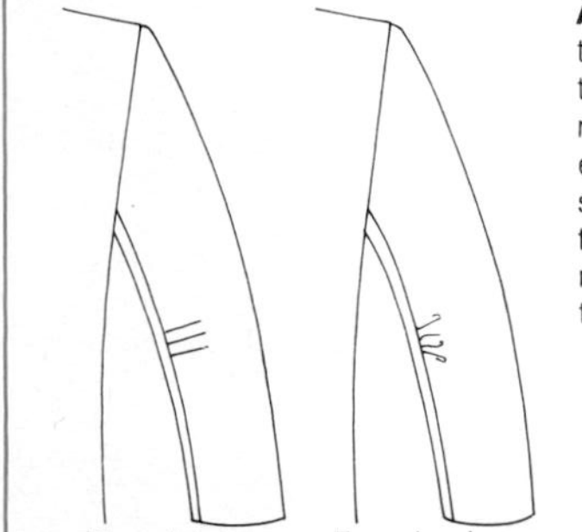

A close-fitting sleeve that extends beyond the elbow usually requires darts or easestitching along the sleeve seam to give the shaping and ease necessary for the elbow to bend comfortably.

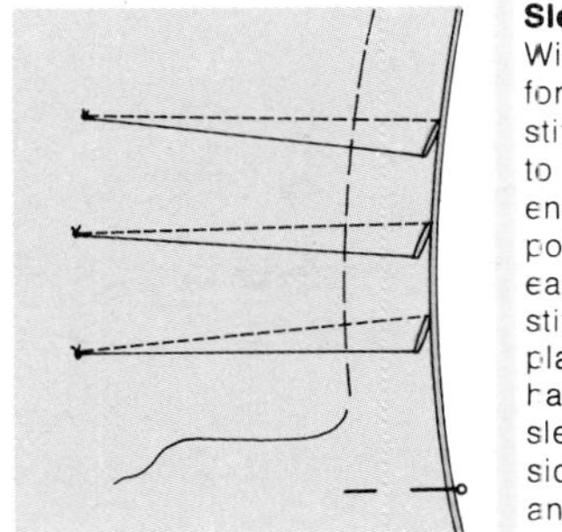

Sleeves with elbow darts: With right sides together, form each elbow dart, stitching from wide end to point; leave 4" thread ends and tie knot at each point (see Darts). Extend each dart and press flat as stitched. With wrong side up, place darts over tailor's ham and press them toward sleeve bottom. With right sides together, match, pin, and baste sleeve seam.

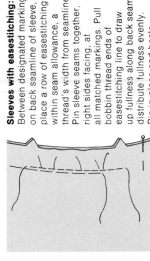

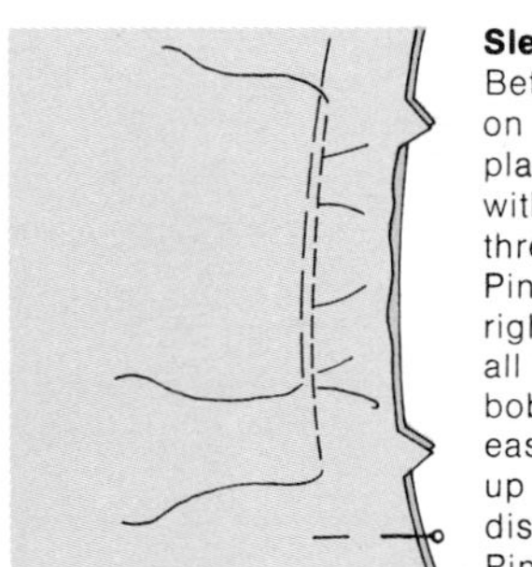

Sleeves with easestitching: Between designated markings on back seamline of sleeve, place a row of easestitching within seam allowance, a thread's width from seamline. Pin sleeve seams together, right sides facing, at all matched markings. Pull bobbin thread ends of easestitching line to draw up fullness along back seam; distribute fullness evenly. Pin in place and baste.

Pressing equipment 18-19
Darts 159

Raglan sleeves

A raglan sleeve is attached to the garment by a seam that runs diagonally down from the front neckline to the underarm, and up to the back neckline. This sleeve covers the entire shoulder and needs some shaping device to make it conform to the shoulder's shape. One device is a dart that ex-

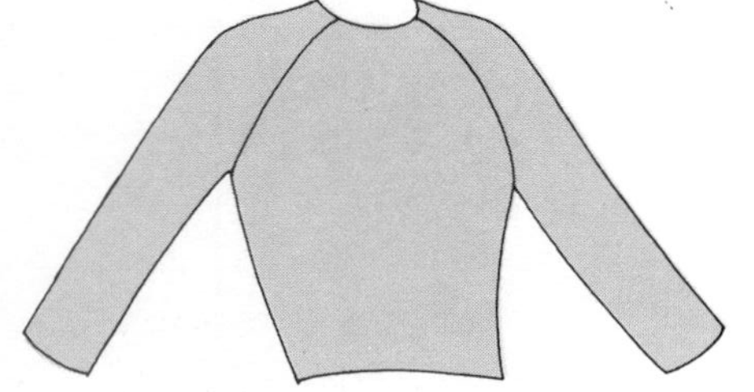

tends from neckline to shoulder edge; here the sleeve pattern is one piece. Another is a shaped seam that runs from the neckline over the shoulder to the sleeve bottom; this sleeve is made from two pieces. Whichever method is used, the deepest part of the curve should fall over the edge of the shoulder without protruding.

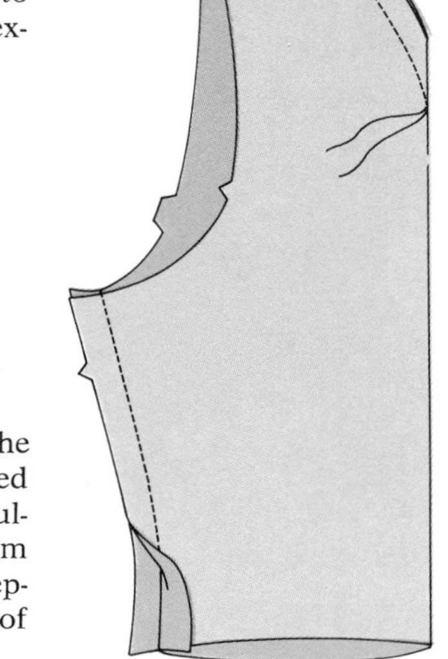

1. With right sides facing, match, pin, and stitch shoulder darts from wide end to point; leave 4″ thread ends. Knot thread ends. Press dart flat. Slash darts if necessary and press open over a tailor's ham. Match, pin, and stitch underarm seams, right sides together. Press flat, then press open.

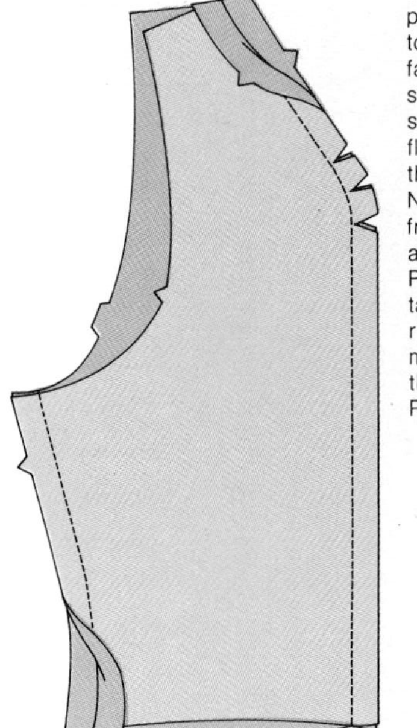

For a two-piece sleeve, place front and back together, right sides facing. Match, pin, and stitch the shoulder seam. Press the seam flat to embed stitches, then finger-press open. Notch out fullness from seam allowance along shoulder curve. Press seam open over a tailor's ham. With right sides together, match, pin, and stitch the underarm seams. Press flat, then open.

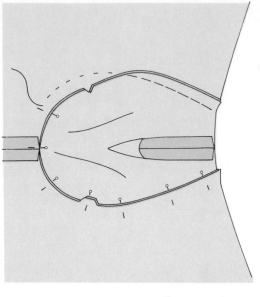

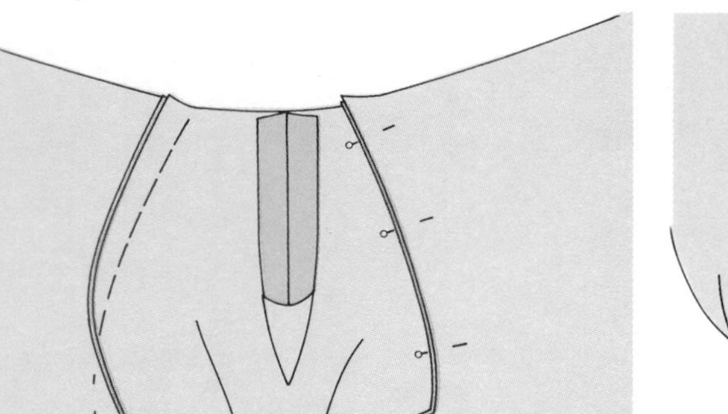

2. Garment side seams should be permanently stitched and pressed open. With right sides together, pin sleeve to armhole, aligning underarm seams, and matching all markings; work with wrong side of sleeve toward you. Baste as pinned.

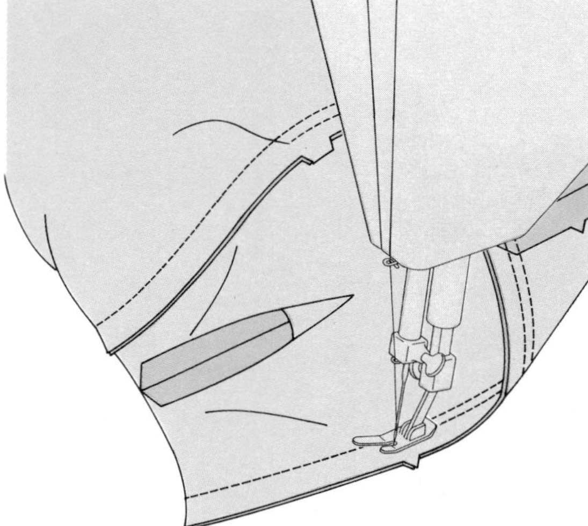

3. With sleeve side up, stitch as basted. Diagonally trim cross-seam allowances at underarm seams. Between front and back notches of underarm curve, place another row of stitching (either straight or zigzag) ¼″ from first row.

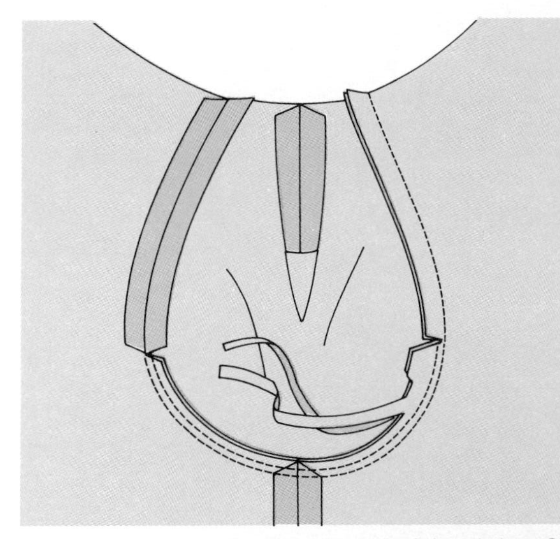

4. Press the seam flat as stitched to embed the stitches. Clip into the seam allowances at the point of each notch. Trim underarm seam allowances close to the second row of stitching. Press seams open above the clips.

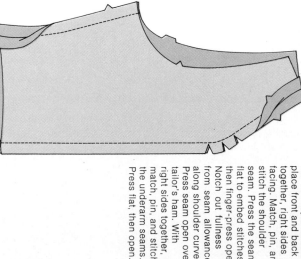

Seam binding, twill tape 16
Pressing equipment 18-19

Kimono sleeves

A kimono sleeve, which is cut as an extension of the main bodice piece, can be either loose or close-fitting, depending on the degree of the sleeve's shoulder slope and underarm curve. If the sleeve fit is very close, a gusset is probably needed for

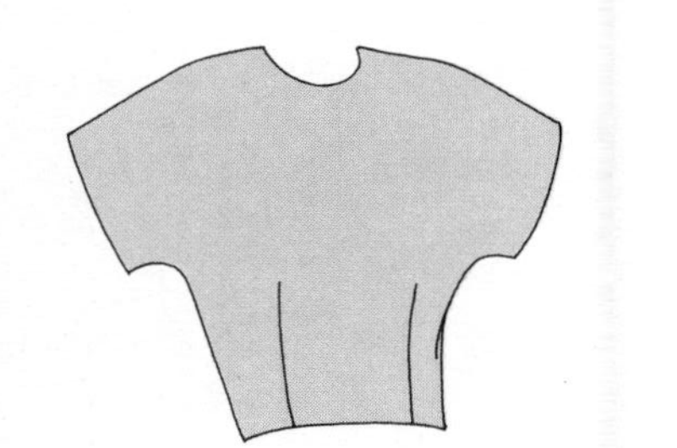

comfort (see pp. 260–261). To construct a kimono sleeve without a gusset, follow one of the methods here, using regular seam binding or ½-inch twill tape for reinforcement under the arm. The first method is easier, but the second is less bulky.

Method 1

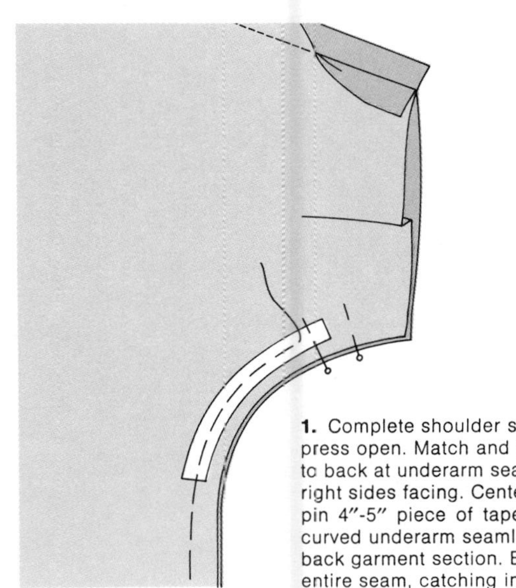

1. Complete shoulder seam; press open. Match and pin front to back at underarm seamline, right sides facing. Center and pin 4″-5″ piece of tape over curved underarm seamline on back garment section. Baste entire seam, catching in tape.

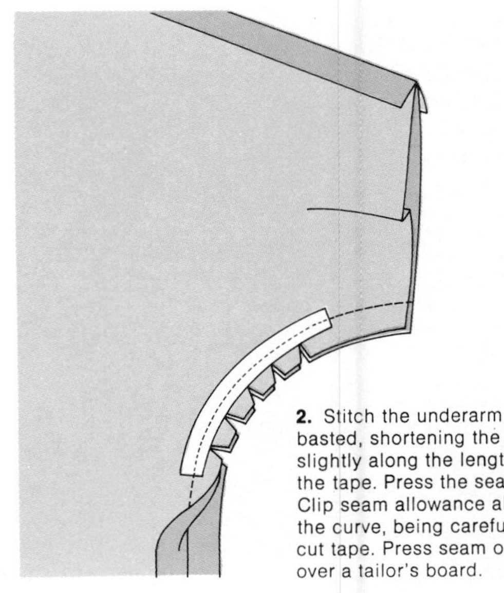

2. Stitch the underarm seam as basted, shortening the stitches slightly along the length of the tape. Press the seam flat. Clip seam allowance along the curve, being careful not to cut tape. Press seam open over a tailor's board.

Method 2

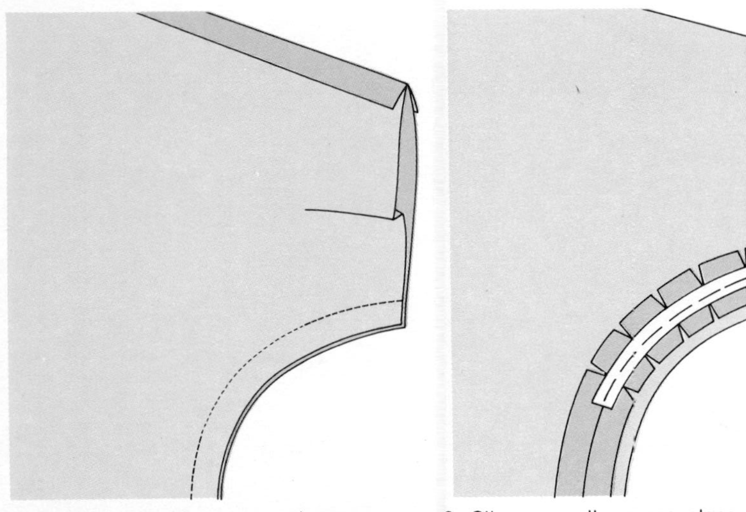

1. Complete shoulder seam and press open. With right sides facing, match, pin, and baste front to back at underarm seamline. Stitch, shortening stitches along curve. Press flat.

2. Clip seam allowances along curve. Press seam open. Center, pin, and baste a 4″-5″ piece of reinforcing tape along curved seamline. Be sure stitches go to right side.

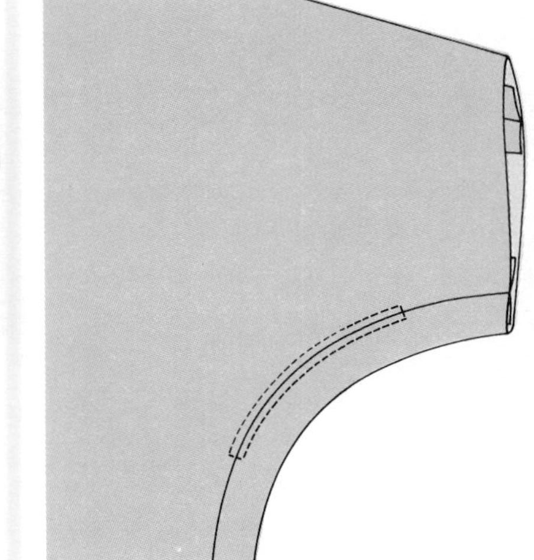

3. From the right side, stitch through all the thicknesses, approximately ⅛″ on each side of basted line. Secure thread ends on wrong side. Remove basting, and press.

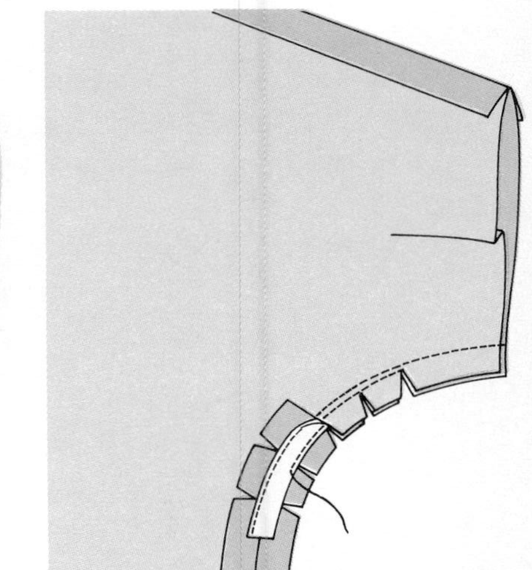

If exposed stitching is not wanted, stitch the tape from wrong side, catching the *tape and seam allowance only* on each side of basted line. Remove basting, and press.

Seam binding 16 Transferring pattern markings 94
Staystitching 144

Gussets

A gusset is a small fabric piece inserted into a slashed opening, usually under the arm of a close-fitting kimono sleeve, to provide ease for a comfortable fit. Although gusset shapes vary, there

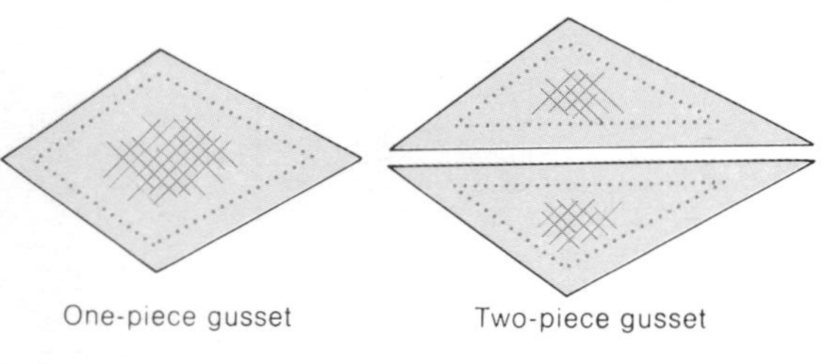

One-piece gusset Two-piece gusset

are basically two gusset types, **one-piece** (usually diamond-shaped) and **two-piece** (usually triangular). The one-piece type is the more difficult to insert because the entire gusset must be sewed into an enclosed slashed opening after underarm and side seams have been stitched. In the two-piece gusset, each piece is separately inserted into a slashed opening on each bodice piece; underarm, both gusset sections, and side seams are then stitched in one seam. Because a two-piece gusset is easier to insert, you may want to convert a one-piece to that type (see next page). Occasionally a gusset will extend into a main garment section; when it does, this is more of a design than a functional feature.

For maximum ease of movement, cut gusset so its length is on the bias. Transfer all pattern markings accurately, especially gusset corners and garment slash points. Reinforce point at marked gusset opening before slashing. For lightweight fabrics or those that ravel, use a bias square or seam binding as described below. A lightweight iron-on interfacing can also be used; fuse it over slash point on garment's wrong side. If fabric is firm, staystitching is sufficient reinforcement.

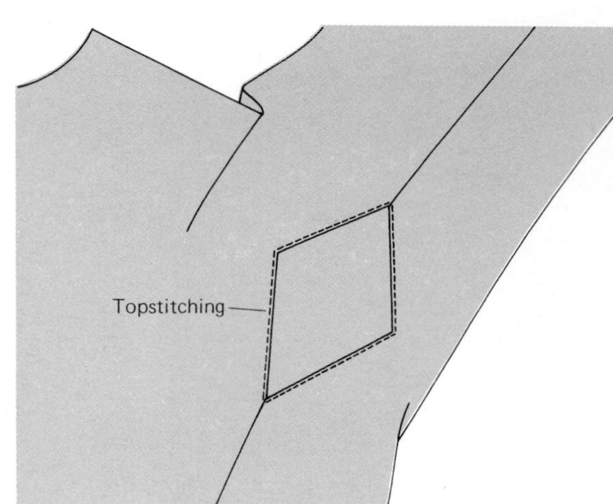

In a well-constructed gusset, all points are precisely related to shape of slashed opening; joining is accurate and smooth. For greater strength, topstitching may be added.

Reinforcing point of slash opening

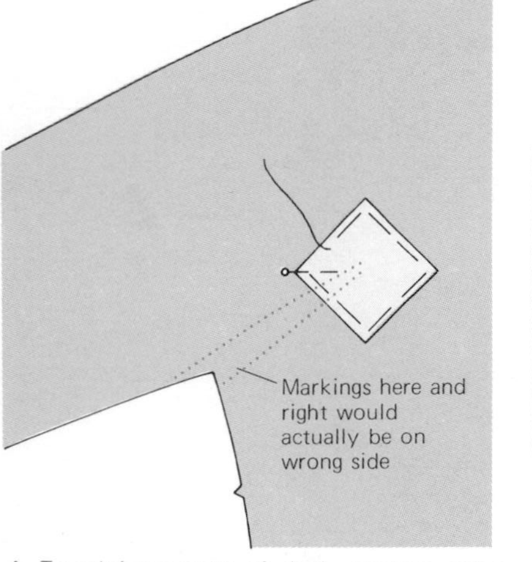

1. To reinforce point of slash opening, cut a 2″ square of bias (self- or underlining fabric). On right side of garment, position the center of the fabric square over the slash point; pin and baste patch in place.

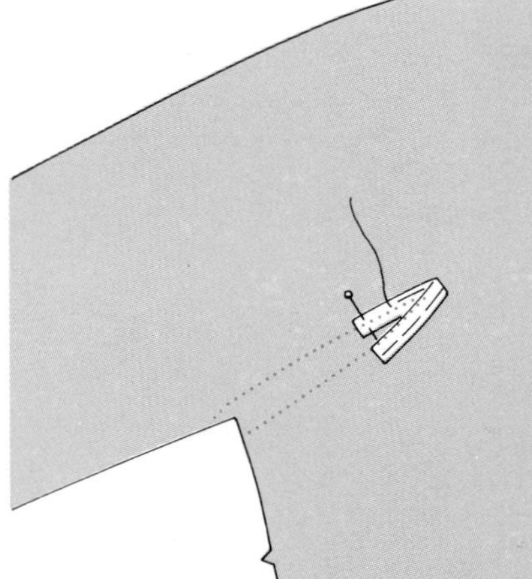

A 4″ piece of regular seam binding can be used in place of bias square; fold tape into a V. Position and pin tape to right side of garment so the V of the tape coincides with the V of the slash point. Baste.

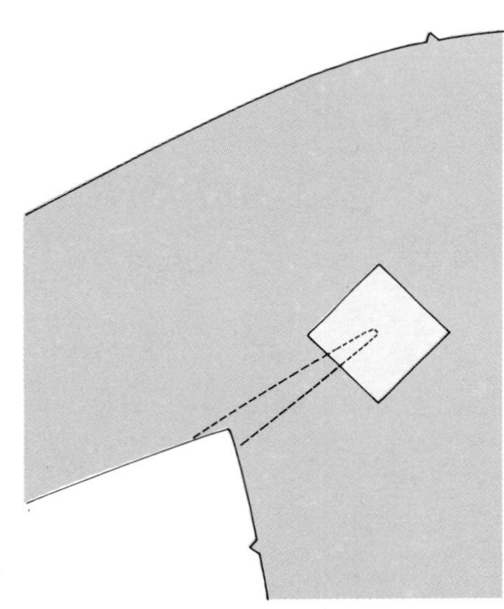

2. Staystitch a thread's width from marked stitching line (shorten stitches around the point). Start at wide end, stitch up one side to point, pivot, take one stitch across point, pivot again, stitch down other side.

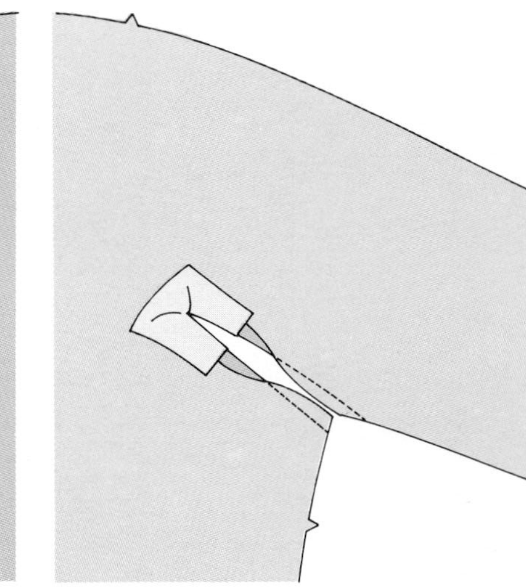

3. Press the staystitched area flat. Then slash through center of opening (between stitching lines) up to reinforced point; cut through fabric square as well. Turn square to wrong side; press lightly so it lies flat.

Securing a seam 137

Inserting a one-piece gusset

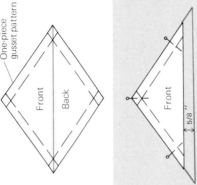

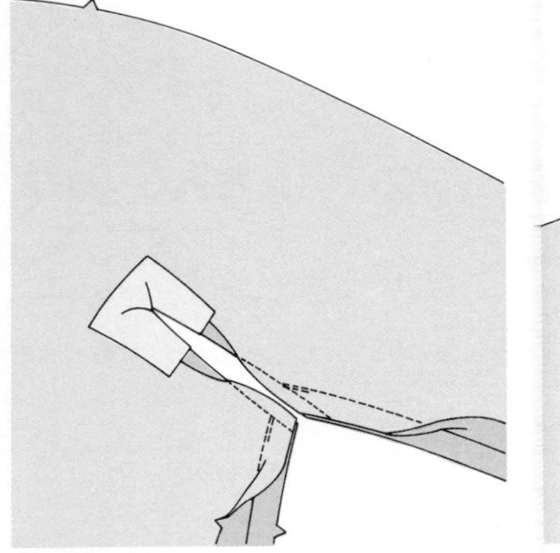

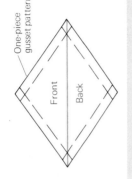

1. With right sides together, match, pin, and baste garment front to back at underarm seams and side seams. Stitch from sleeve bottom to intersecting lines of gusset opening; secure stitches. Stitch from lower edge of bodice to intersecting lines of gusset opening; secure stitches. Press seams flat, then open.

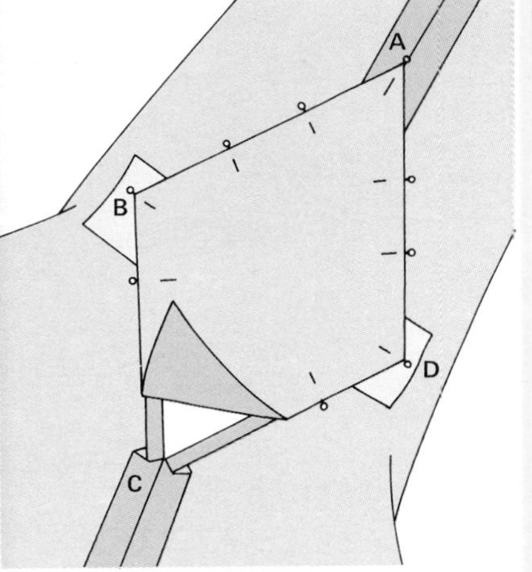

2. Position gusset over slashed opening so marked points of gusset (designated here as A,B,C,D) match corresponding markings of opening. With right sides together, pin the gusset into the slashed opening; match all points accurately and align stitching line of opening to gusset seamline.

A

B

C

3. Baste, but do not remove pins from corners. Garment side up, stitch from point A to B (shorten stitches going around point B); pivot, take one stitch across point, pivot again, and stitch to point C. Leave 4" thread ends at beginning and end. Stitch other side of gusset (C to D to A) the same way.

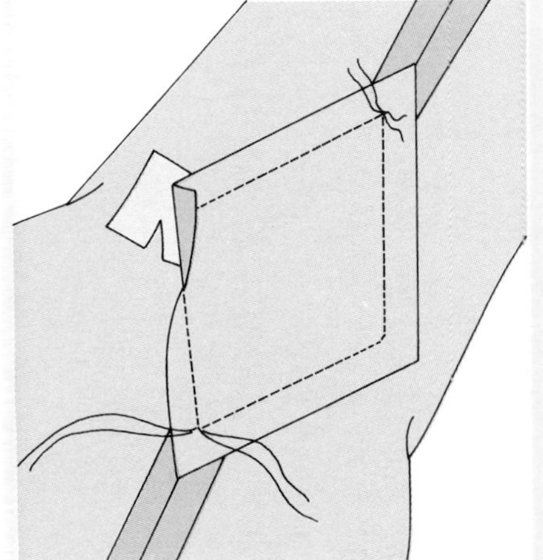

4. Pull all thread ends to wrong side of gusset and knot. Press seams toward garment. Trim extending edges of fabric squares to ⅜"; re-press seams toward garment. If desired, topstitch close to seamline on right side of garment (see preceding page); pull threads to wrong side and knot.

Inserting a two-piece gusset

One-piece gusset pattern

Front

Back

Front

5/8"

1. To convert a one-piece into a two-piece gusset, determine which halves of gusset pattern correspond to front and back bodice pieces; divide with a line; cut in half. Pin triangular pattern pieces to fabric; add ⅝" to cut edge (for underarm seam allowance). Cut out pieces and transfer markings.

A

B

C

2. With right sides together, match and pin gusset to slashed opening of front bodice; align seamlines of opening and gusset. Baste, but do not remove pins from corners. Garment side up, stitch from edge A to B (shorten stitches around B); pivot, take one stitch across point, pivot, stitch to edge C.

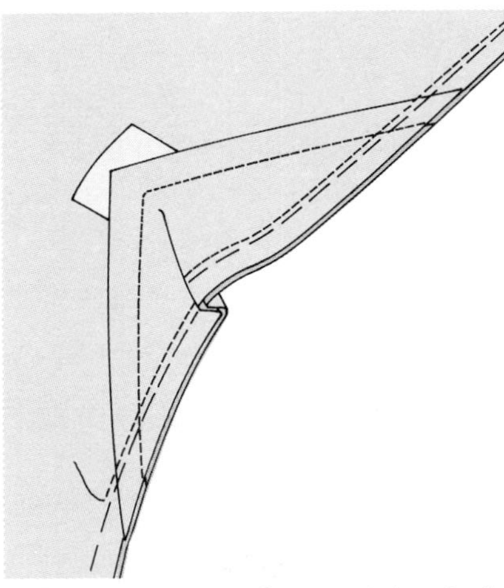

3. Press seams toward garment. Insert other triangular gusset piece into slashed opening of back bodice in same way as for front bodice. With right sides together, pin garment back to front at underarm seam; match intersecting lines of gusset edge and other markings as well. Baste and stitch.

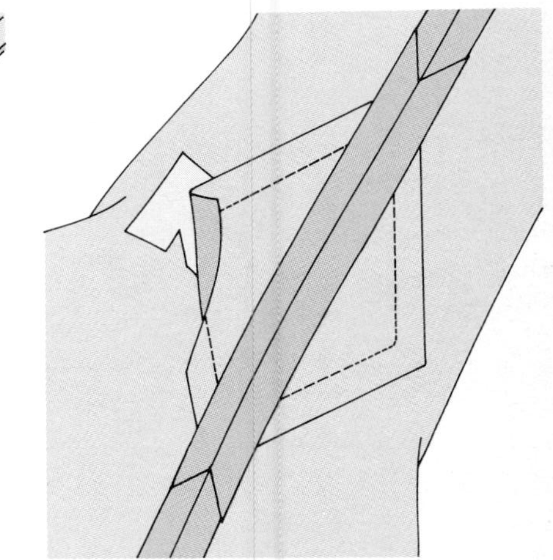

4. Press seam flat to embed stitches, then press seam open. Trim extending edges of fabric squares at gusset points to ⅜"; re-press seams toward garment. If desired, topstitch close to seamline on right side of garment (see illustration on preceding page); pull threads to wrong side and knot.

Sleeve finishes

Pressing 18-19 Diagonal basting 125 Reducing bulk 147 Hem edges 292-293; interfacing hems 295

Types of sleeve finishes

The finishing of a sleeve edge usually depends on the pattern design. It may be a simple **self-hem** or **faced finish** (shaped or bias), or decorative **double binding** made from self or contrasting fabric. The finish is sometimes a design feature, as a **casing** (pp. 264–265) or **cuff** (pp. 266–272) would be. For successful completion of any sleeve, follow these general guidelines: (1) Mark hemline to a length becoming to the wearer; sleeve length helps to determine the total garment silhouette and can easily add to or detract from it. (2) Practice good pressing techniques throughout the finishing process. (3) Reduce bulk wherever possible.

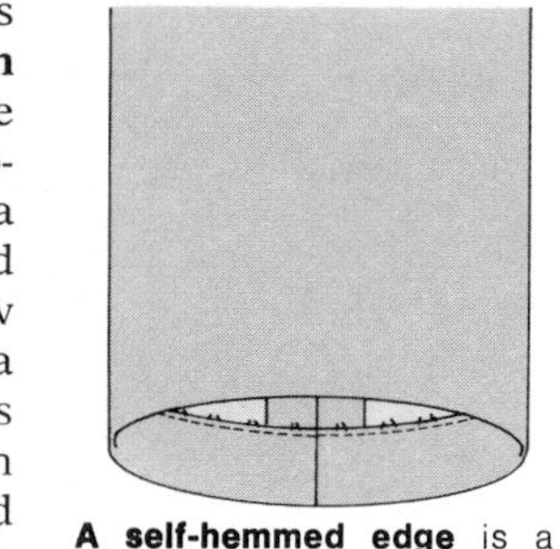

A self-hemmed edge is a simple sleeve finish. A facing can also be used.

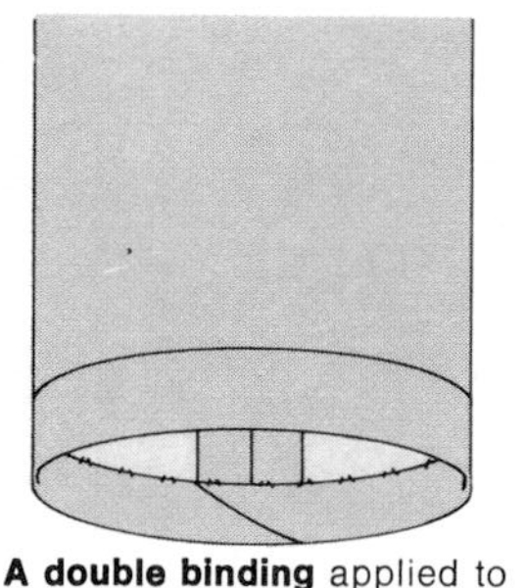

A double binding applied to a sleeve edge gives a decorative finish to the sleeve.

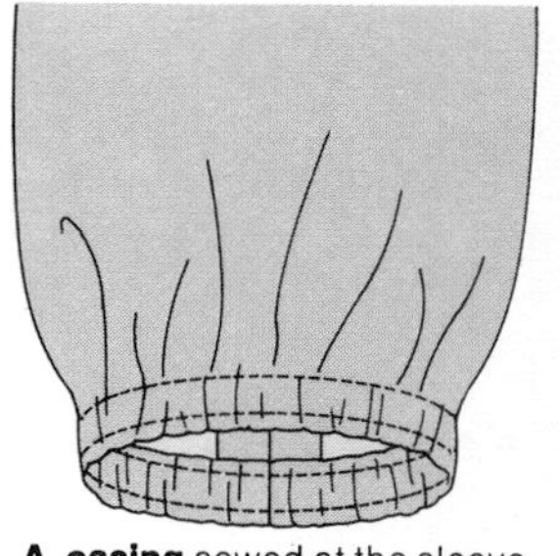

A casing sewed at the sleeve edge can be self-faced or it can be separately applied.

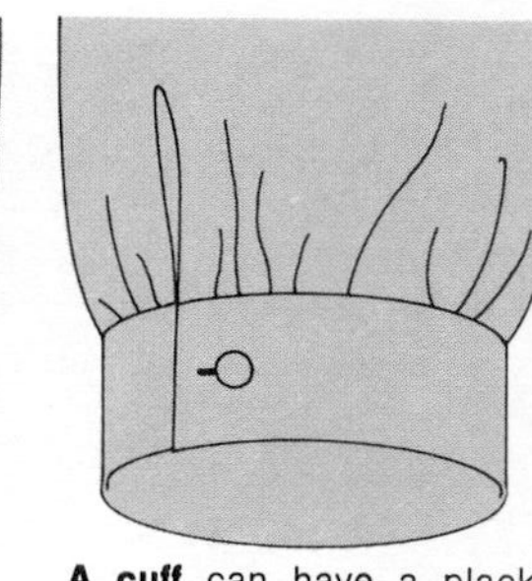

A cuff can have a placket opening or be loose-fitting with no opening.

Self-hem

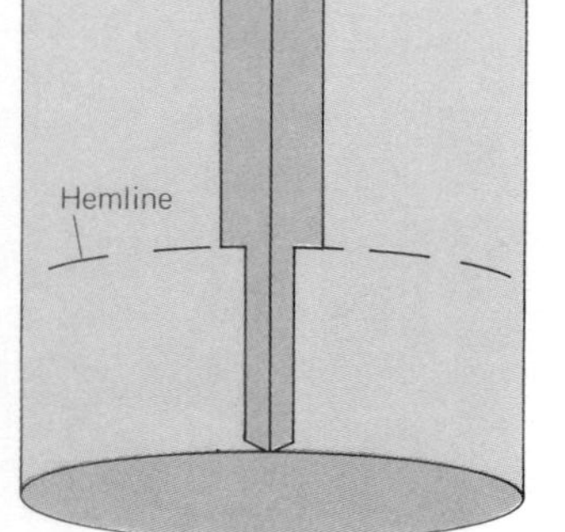

1. Mark sleeve hemline. To reduce bulk at seamline within hem width, trim seam allowance below marked hemline to half width.

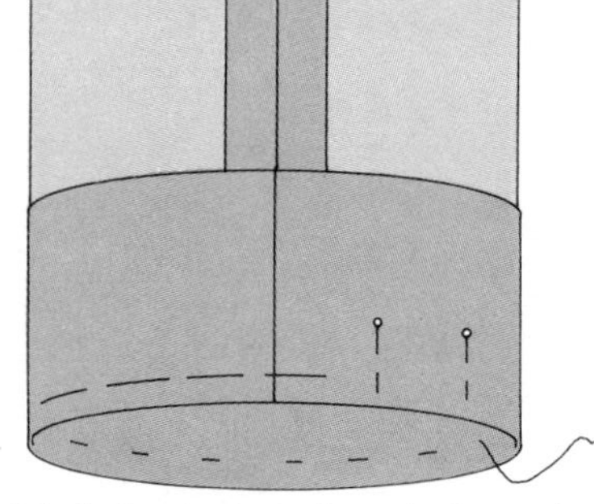

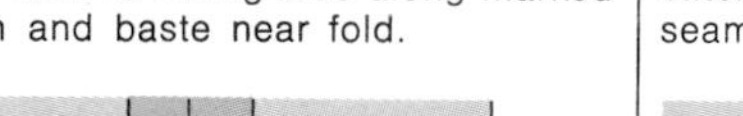

2. If interfacing is desired, apply it now (see Hems). Turn hem to wrong side along marked hemline; pin and baste near fold.

3. To even hem allowance, measure from fold to desired width, and mark that distance around entire hem. Trim along marked line.

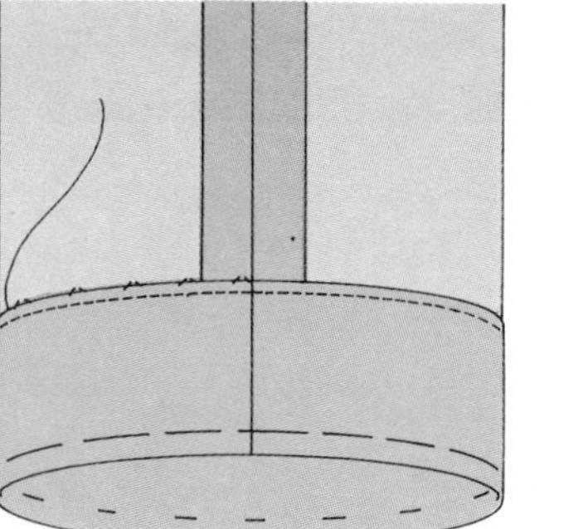

4. Finish raw edges of hem (see Hems). Pin edge to sleeve and secure, using appropriate hand stitch. Remove basting. Press.

Shaped facing

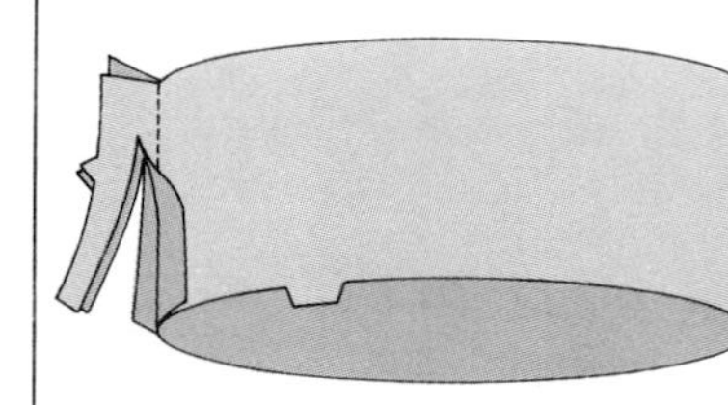

1. With right sides together, match, pin, and stitch facing ends. Press flat, then open. Trim seam allowances to half width.

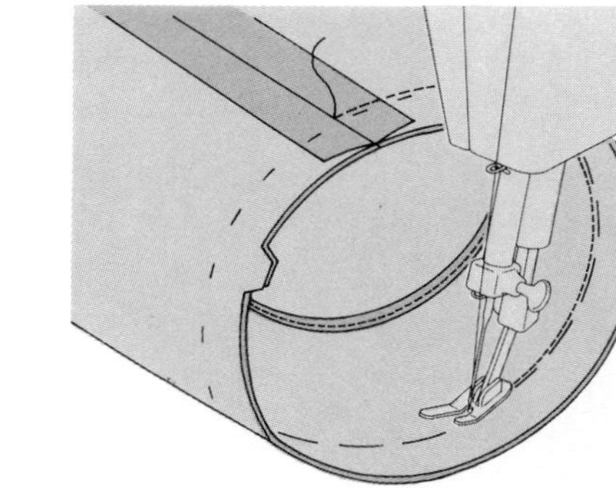

2. Finish unnotched facing edge. With right sides together, match, pin, and baste facing to sleeve edge. Stitch with facing side up.

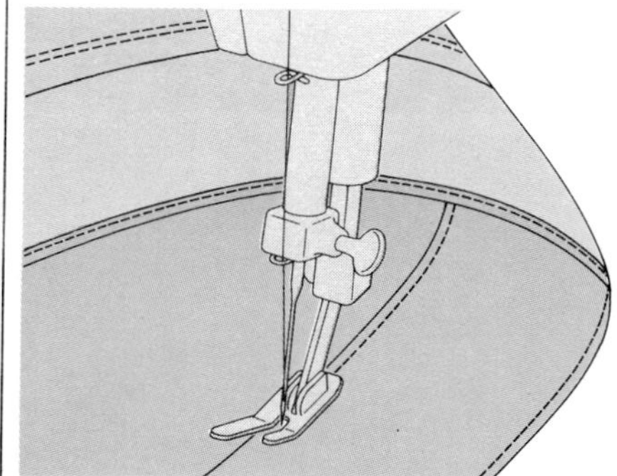

3. Press seam flat. Trim and grade seam allowances; clip if needed. Extend facing and seam allowances; understitch along facing.

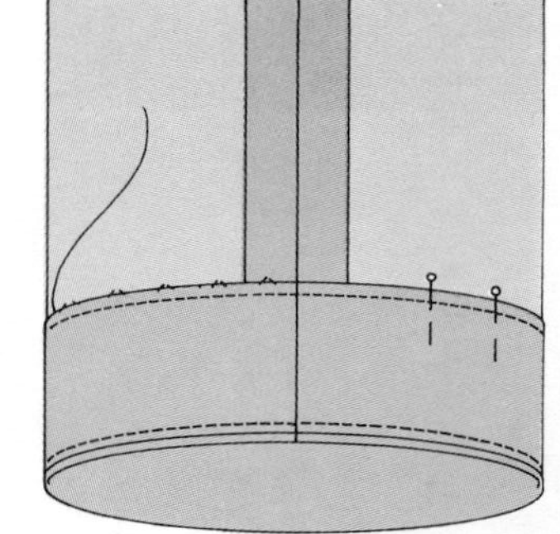

4. Turn the facing to wrong side; roll edges in slightly. Press. Diagonal-baste in place if necessary. Pin edge to sleeve and secure.

Bias tapes 16
Slipstitch 129
Cutting bias strips 298-299

Bias facing

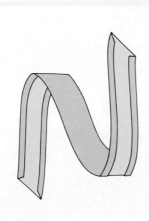

1. Cut a strip of 1½″ bias to sleeve circumference plus 2″. Press under long edges ¼″. If desired, use packaged wide bias tape.

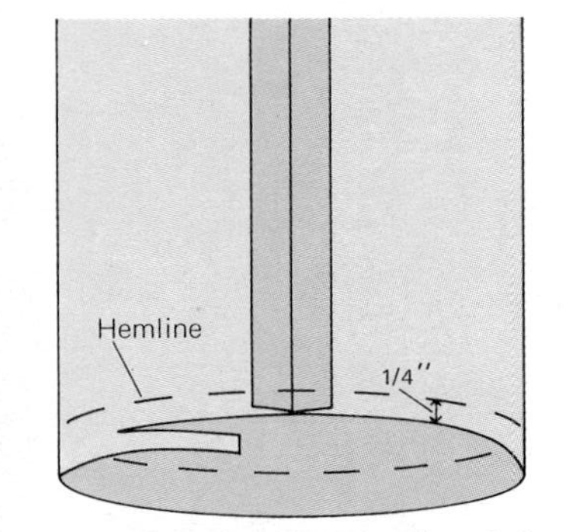

2. Mark hemline along bottom edge of sleeve. To facilitate application of bias facing, trim hem allowance to ¼″ width.

3. Open folded edges and pin facing to sleeve edge, right sides together; pin ends together in diagonal seam (straight grain).

4. Remove facing from sleeve, keeping ends pinned. Stitch ends along straight grain. Trim seam allowances to ¼″ and press open.

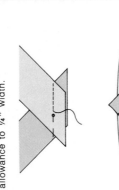

5. Re-pin facing to sleeve, raw edges even. Baste in place; stitch ¼″ from raw edge, using foldline as guide. Press flat.

6. Turn facing to wrong side; roll edges in slightly and press. Pin folded edge of facing to sleeve and slipstitch in place.

Double-fold bias binding

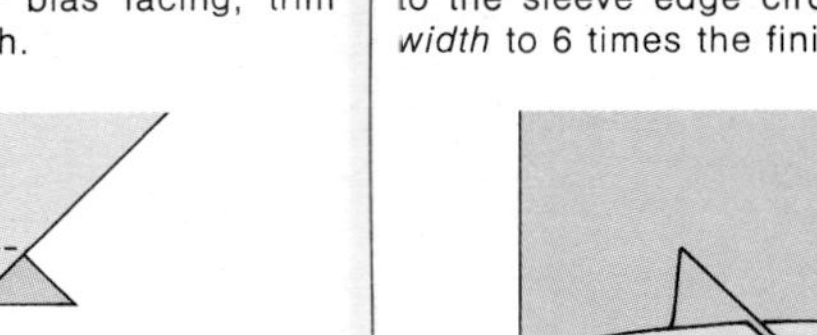

1. Cut a strip of self-fabric bias equal in *length* to the sleeve edge circumference plus 2″, in *width* to 6 times the finished width.

2. Mark sleeve hemline; trim away hem allowance. Mark new seamline a distance from cut edge equal to the finished binding width.

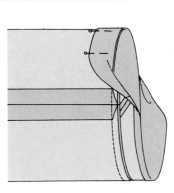

3. With right sides together, pin binding to sleeve, raw edges even. Pin binding ends together in diagonal seam (straight grain).

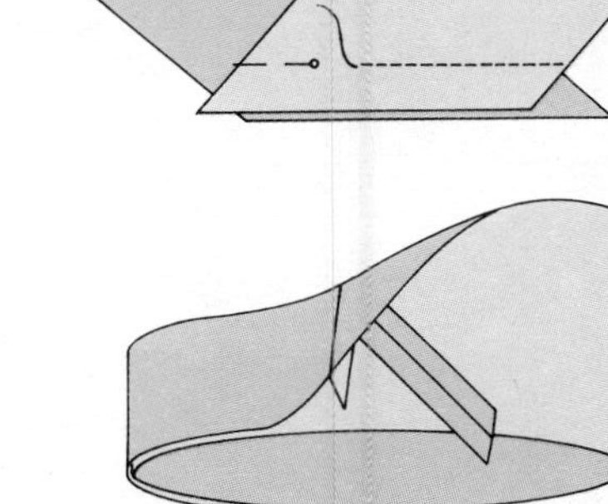

4. Remove binding; keep ends pinned. Stitch. Trim seam allowances to ¼″; press open. Fold binding in half, wrong sides together.

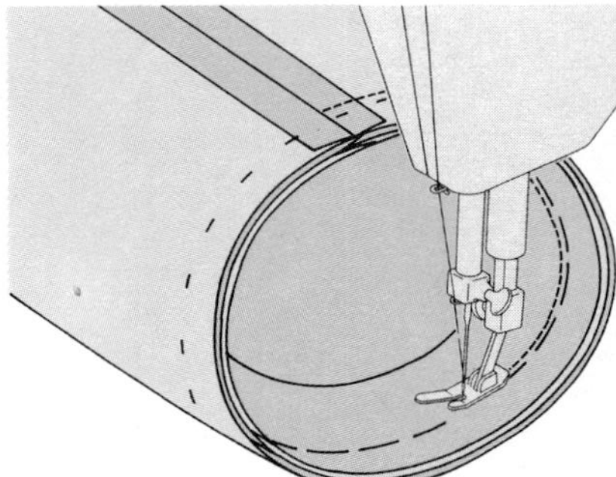

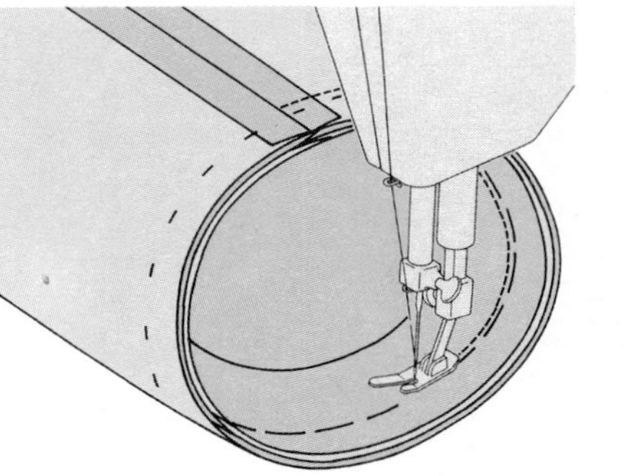

5. Pin binding to right side of sleeve, raw edges even; baste in place along new sleeve seamline. Stitch with binding side up.

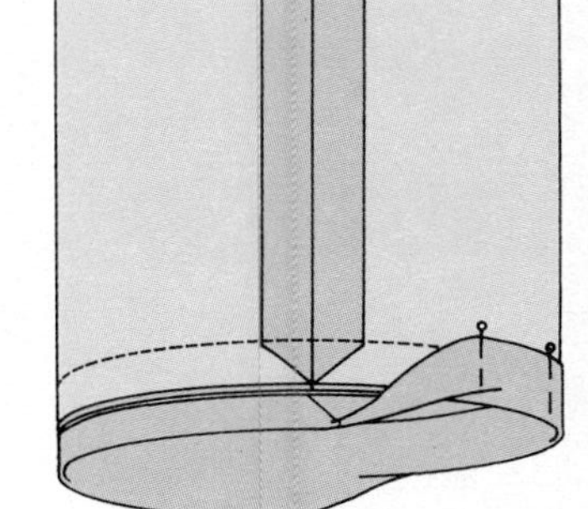

6. Press seam flat. Extend binding up and press; turn to wrong side so fold meets the stitching line. Pin and slipstitch in place.

Sleeve finishes

Hand-sewing aids 12-13 Bias tapes 16 Elastics 17

Casings

A casing is a fabric "tunnel" through which elastic or drawstring can be passed; either will draw up sleeve fullness, creating a puffed effect. Casings are a popular sleeve finish for children's wear, blouses, and sportswear. There are basically two casing types. The first is a **self-faced casing;** in this type the tunnel is created by turning the sleeve edge to the inside. Some self-faced casings are positioned above the sleeve edge so that a gathered flounce, known as a *heading,* will hang below. To construct a self-faced casing (with or without heading), an adequate fabric allowance must be provided below the hemline. The second type of casing is an **applied casing,** actually a separate bias strip that is sewed to the sleeve edge to form the tunnel. The applied type is generally used when there is not enough hem allowance for a self-faced casing or when fabric bulk makes a casing of thinner fabric desirable. Prepackaged bias tapes can be used for this purpose; select the width closest to and slightly wider than the elastic. For both types of casing, it is wise to select a narrow elastic (¼ inch to ½ inch) that is appropriate for tunneling (see Elastics).

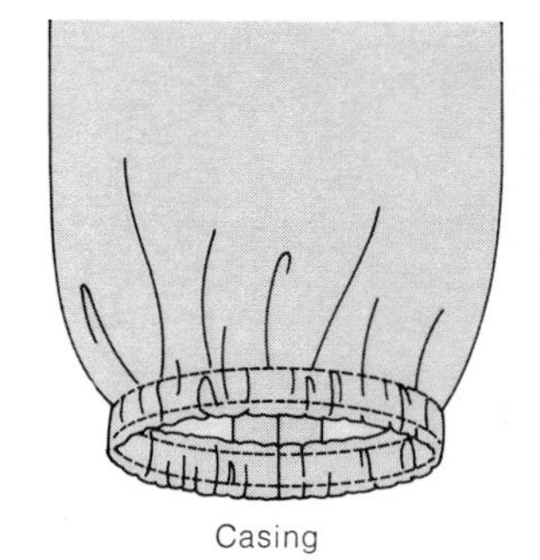
Casing

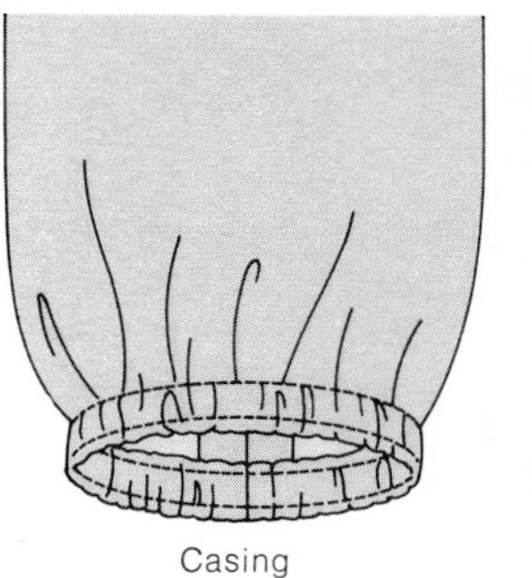
Casing with heading

Self-faced casing

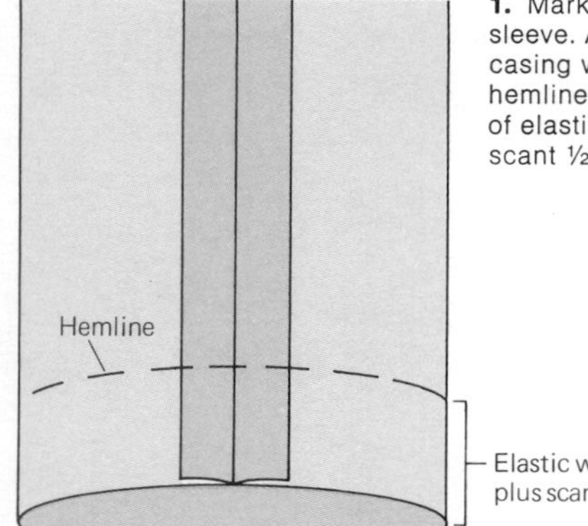

1. Mark hemline on sleeve. Allow enough casing width below hemline to equal width of elastic plus a scant ½".

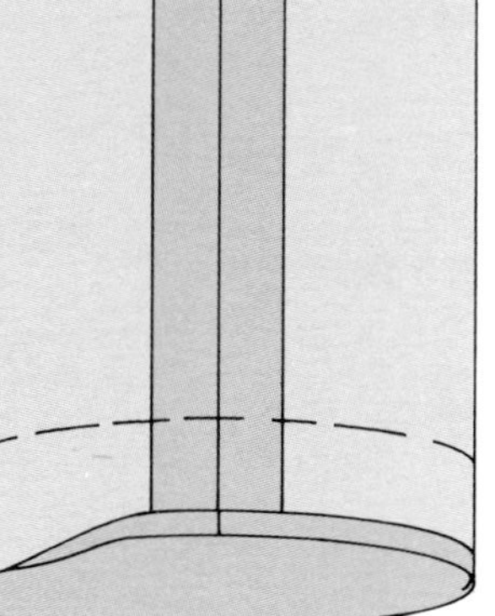
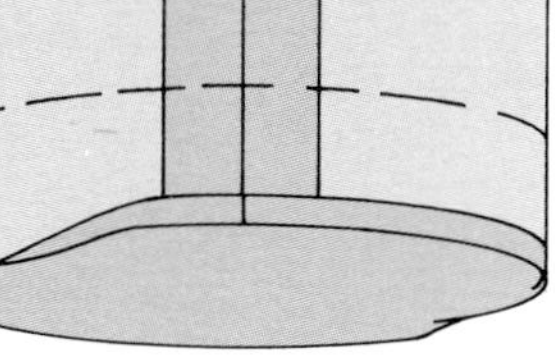

2. Along raw edges of sleeve, turn a scant ¼" to the wrong side and press.

3. Turn casing width to wrong side along marked hemline; pin and baste close to free edge. Stitch along basted line, leaving a small opening at sleeve seamline.

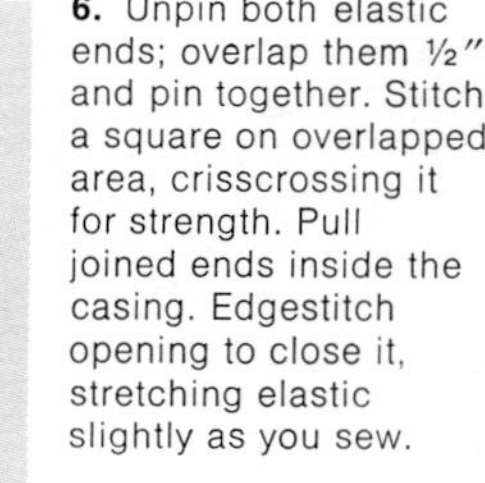

4. Stitch close to fold on lower edge of sleeve, overlapping a few stitches. Fit elastic around arm where the casing will be worn; add ½" and cut elastic.

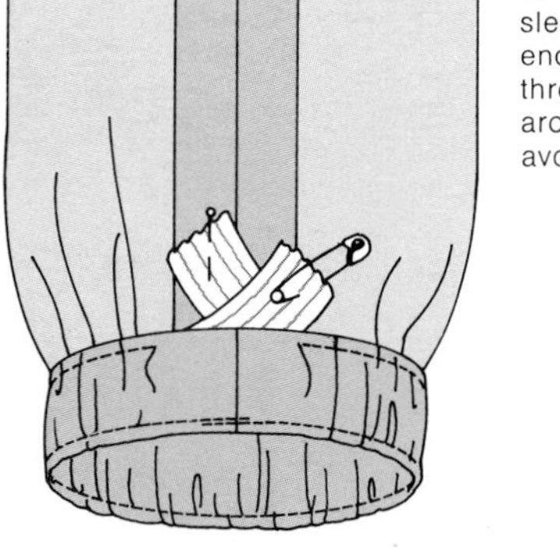

5. Attach a bodkin or safety pin to one end of elastic and insert into casing. Pin other end to sleeve to keep that end from slipping through. Work safety pin around entire casing; avoid twisting elastic.

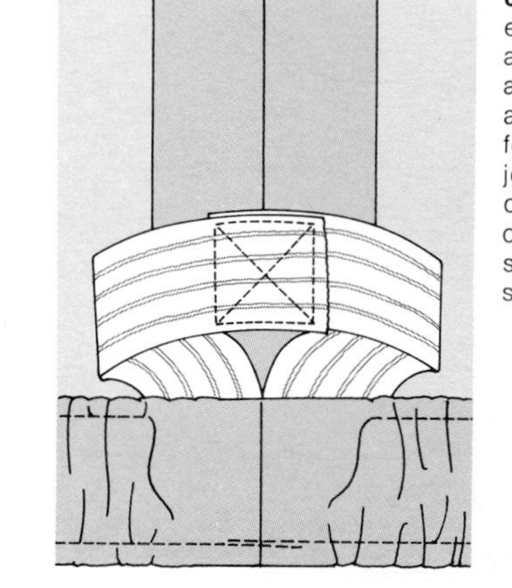

6. Unpin both elastic ends; overlap them ½" and pin together. Stitch a square on overlapped area, crisscrossing it for strength. Pull joined ends inside the casing. Edgestitch opening to close it, stretching elastic slightly as you sew.

Bias tapes 16
Cutting bias strips 298-299

Self-faced casing with heading

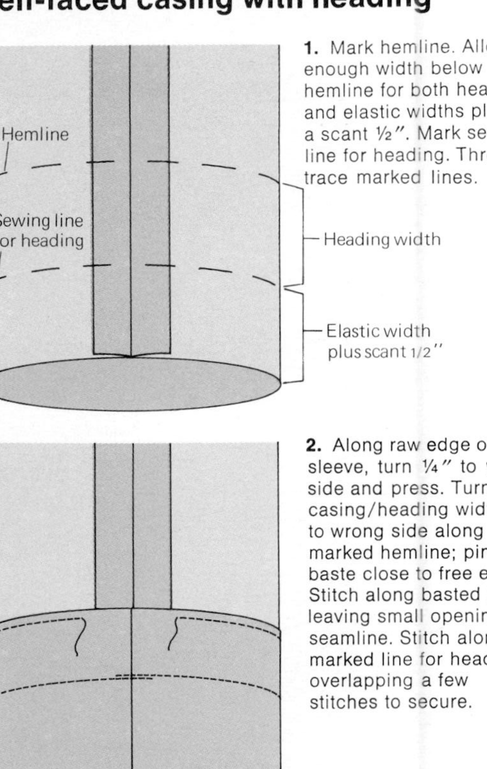

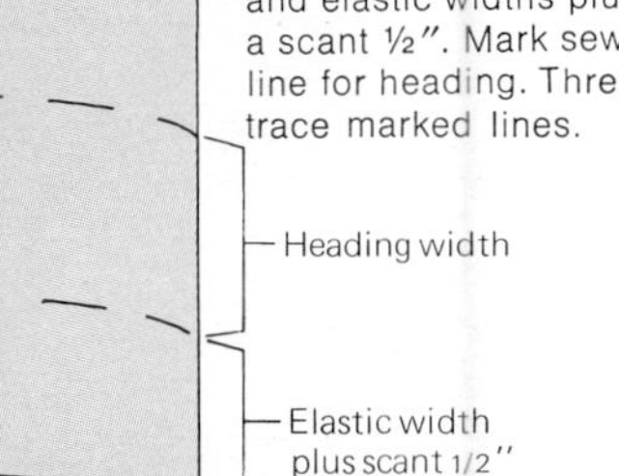

1. Mark hemline. Allow enough width below hemline for both heading and elastic widths plus a scant ½″. Mark sewing line for heading. Thread-trace marked lines.

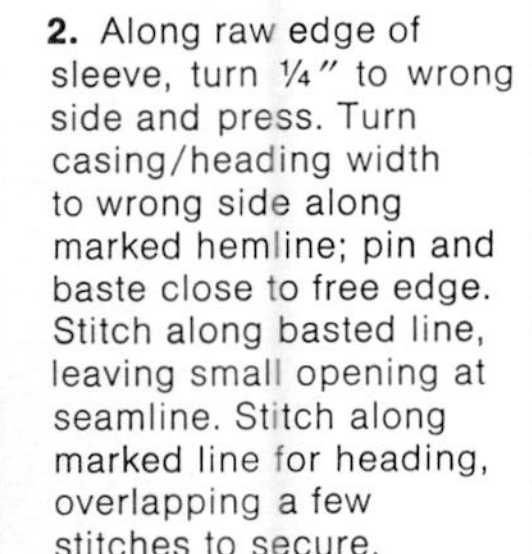

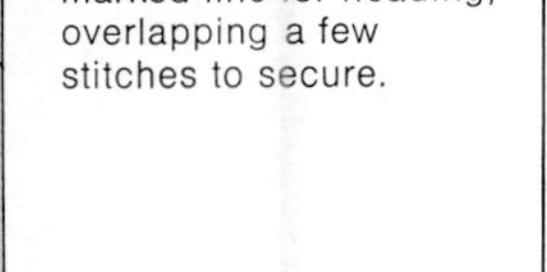

2. Along raw edge of sleeve, turn ¼″ to wrong side and press. Turn casing/heading width to wrong side along marked hemline; pin and baste close to free edge. Stitch along basted line, leaving small opening at seamline. Stitch along marked line for heading, overlapping a few stitches to secure.

3. Fit elastic around arm where the casing will be worn; add ½″ and cut elastic. Insert elastic into casing as described in Steps 5 and 6 on preceding page.

Applied casing

1. To make casing, cut a strip of bias equal in length to the circumference of sleeve edge plus 1″, and equal in width to the elastic width plus ¾″. (If using prepackaged bias, select one slightly wider than the elastic.) Turn under ½″ on both ends of bias strip and stitch across. Press under ¼″ on both long edges.

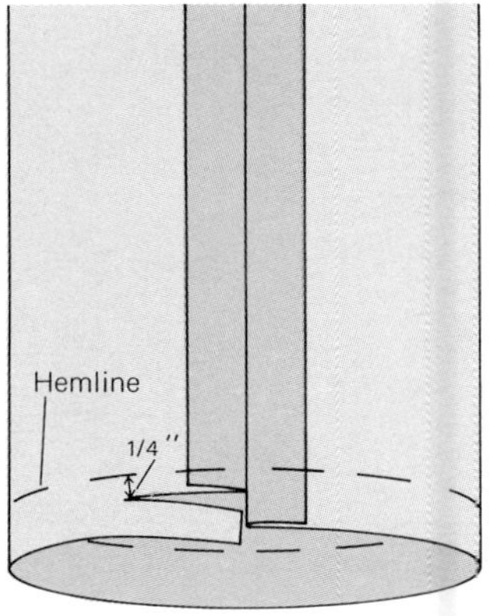

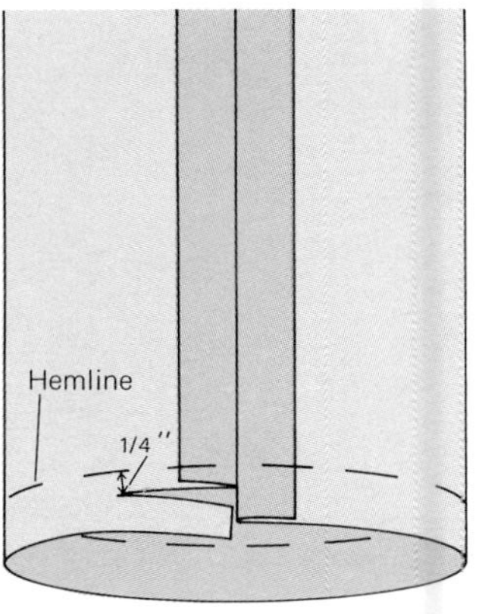

2. Mark hemline on sleeve, and trim the hem allowance to ¼″.

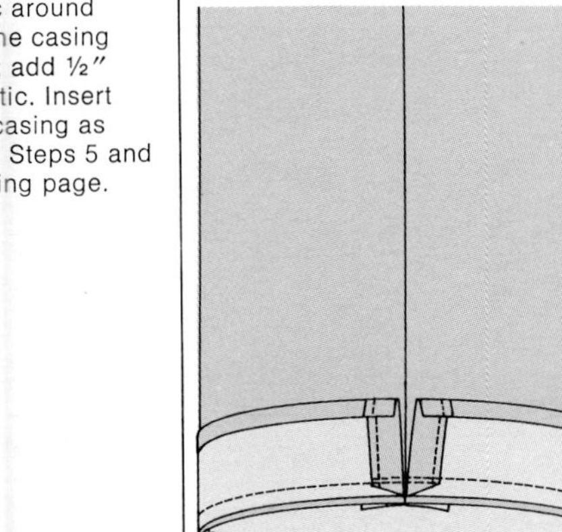

3. Open out one folded edge of casing. Starting at sleeve seam, pin casing to sleeve edge, right sides together and raw edges even; casing ends should meet. Baste and stitch along pressed crease of casing; overlap stitches at ends to reinforce.

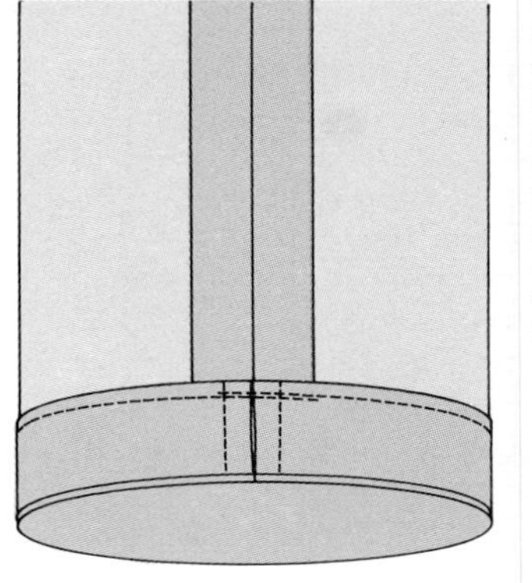

4. Turn casing to wrong side; roll sleeve edge slightly inside. Press. Pin folded inner edge of casing in place and baste; edgestitch along fold, overlapping stitches at end. Fit elastic around arm where casing will be worn; add ½″ and cut elastic.

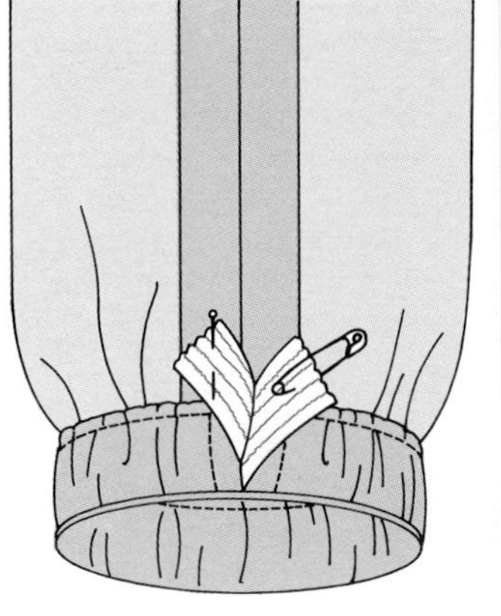

5. Attach a bodkin or safety pin to one end of elastic and insert into casing. Pin other end to sleeve to keep that end from slipping through. Work safety pin around entire casing; avoid twisting elastic.

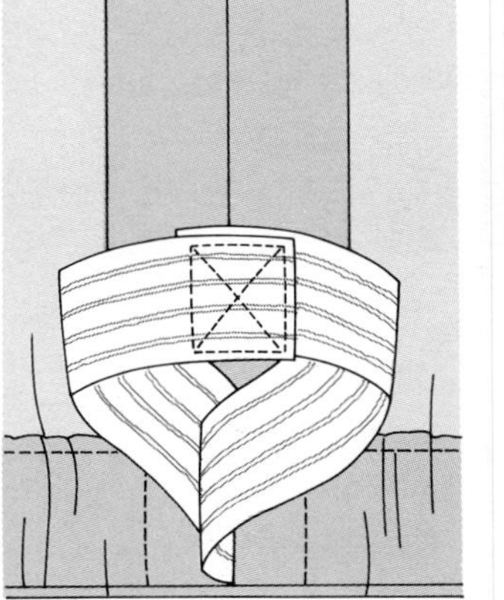

6. Unpin both elastic ends; overlap them ½″ and pin together. Stitch a square on overlapped area, crisscrossing it for strength. Pull joined ends inside the casing. Slipstitch ends of casing together.

Slipstitch (uneven) 132
Seam finishes 148-149

Cuffs with plackets

Cuffs are fabric bands at the bottoms of straight, gathered, or pleated sleeve edges. Although cuff styles vary according to the garment design, any cuff will basically be one of two general types. The first type can be used on both long and short sleeves, and is made large enough around for the hand or arm to slip in and out easily without a cuff-and-placket opening. (For more information about cuffs without plackets, see pp. 270–272.) The second type of cuff is generally attached to a long sleeve and, different from the first type, requires a cuff-and-placket opening fastened snugly around the wrist. Of this cuff type, the three most popular styles are the **lapped cuff, shirt cuff,** and **French cuff.** Each is constructed and applied to the sleeve (see pp. 268–269) after the placket opening is made at the sleeve edge. The three most commonly used plackets are the **faced placket, continuous bound placket,** and **shirt placket.** Note that edges of the faced placket meet at the opening, while edges of the other two plackets lap. The continuous bound placket is finished with a single fabric strip to create a narrow lap; the shirt placket is finished with two separate pieces to create a wider lap.

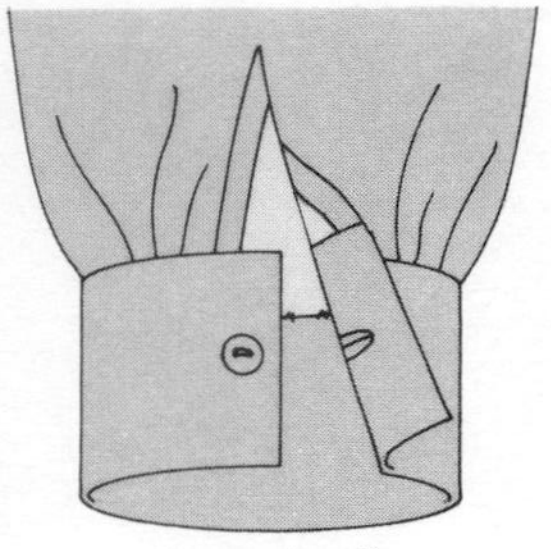

Lapped cuff

The **lapped cuff,** here with a continuous bound placket, has one end projecting from placket edge. The **shirt cuff** is sewed with its ends aligned to the underlap and overlap edges of the shirt placket. The **French cuff,** here with a faced placket, is sewed to the placket edges so cuff ends meet rather than lap; the cuff is cut wide to double back onto itself.

Shirt cuff

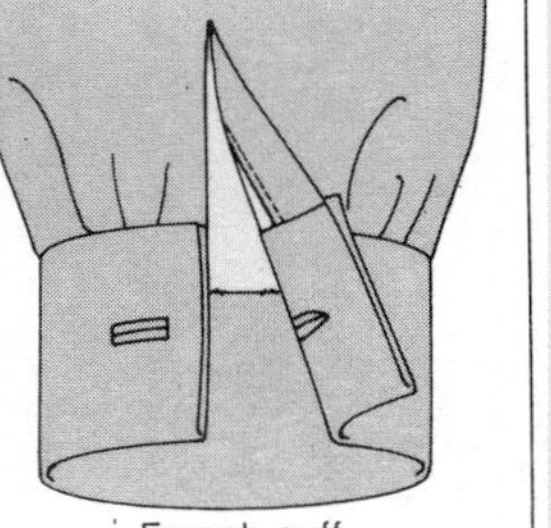

French cuff

Faced plackets

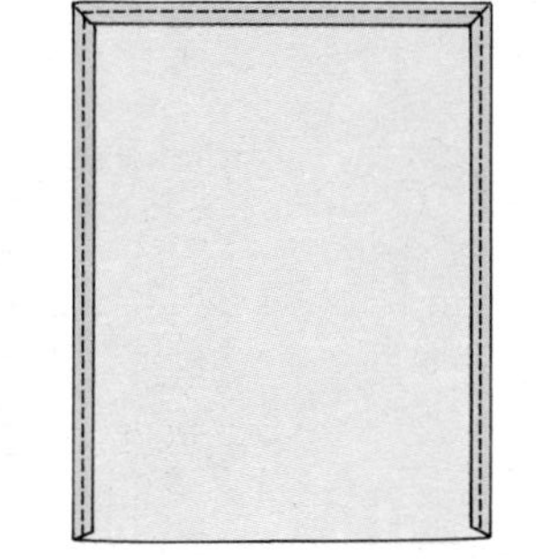

1. Cut a rectangular facing that is 2½″ wide and as long as the length of the slash plus 1″. If garment fabric is heavy, use underlining for facing. Apply a seam finish to the raw edges of the facing except on the bottom edge.

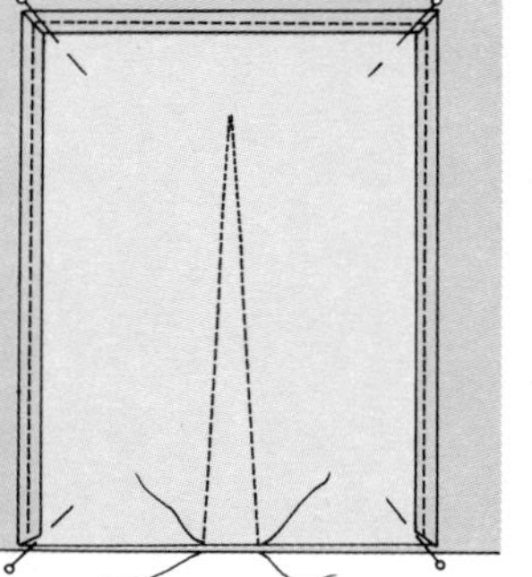

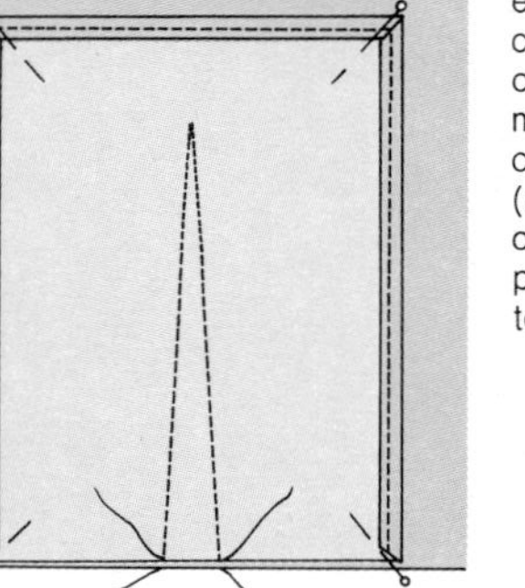

2. Center facing over marked opening, right sides together and raw edges even. Pin at each corner. From wrong side of sleeve, stitch along marked lines: start from one edge, stitch to point (shorten stitches for 1″ on either side of point), pivot, and stitch down to other edge. Press flat.

3. Slash to point; be sure not to clip threads. Press seam open, then toward facing. Turn facing to wrong side of sleeve; roll edges slightly inside. Press. Slipstitch top edge of facing to sleeve.

Continuous bound plackets

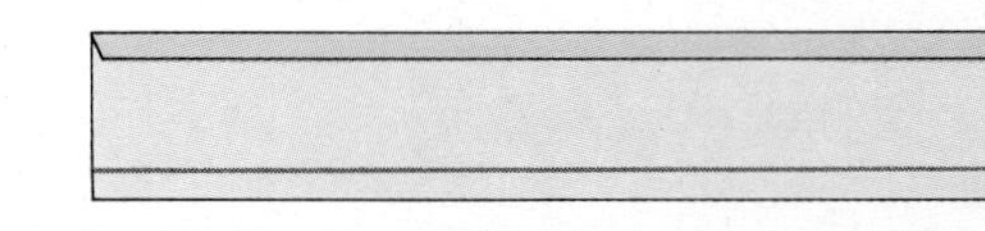

1. Cut binding from self-fabric to measure 1¼″ wide and twice the length of the marked slash. Along one long edge of cut binding, press under ¼″ to wrong side. Mark ¼″ seam allowance along the other long binding edge.

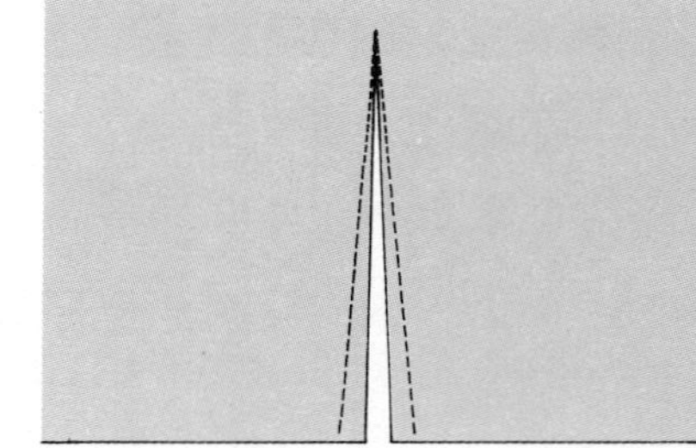

2. Reinforce stitching line of placket opening: Within a thread width of seamline, stitch to point (shorten stitches for 1″ on either side of point), pivot, and stitch down. Press flat. Slash to point; take care not to clip threads.

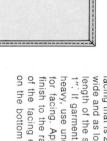

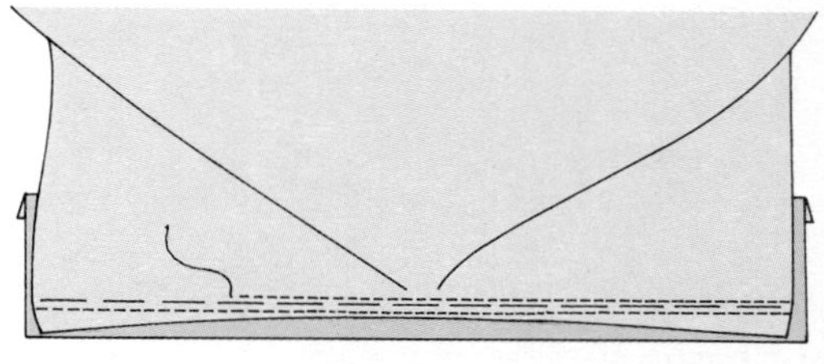

3. Spread slash and pin to unfolded edge of binding, right sides together; align reinforced stitching line to marked ¼″ seamline on binding. Baste, then stitch with sleeve side up. Press seam flat to embed stitches.

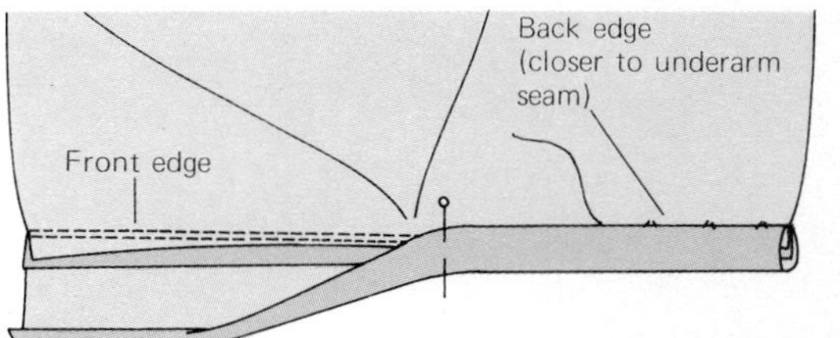

4. Extend binding and fold it to the wrong side, encasing raw edges; folded edge of binding should meet stitching line. Pin in place and secure with slipstitching. Turn front edge of binding to wrong side of sleeve and press.

Shirt plackets

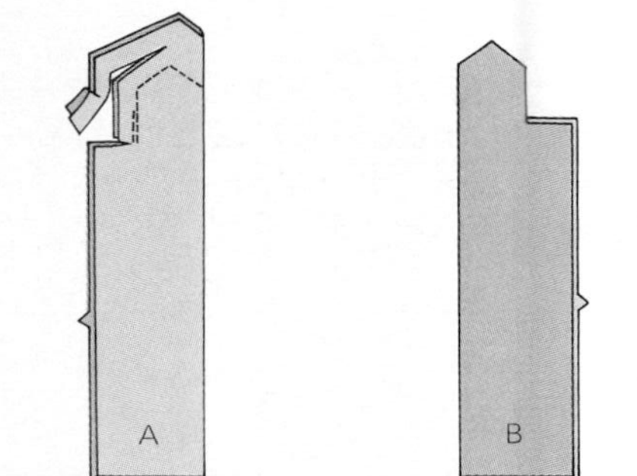
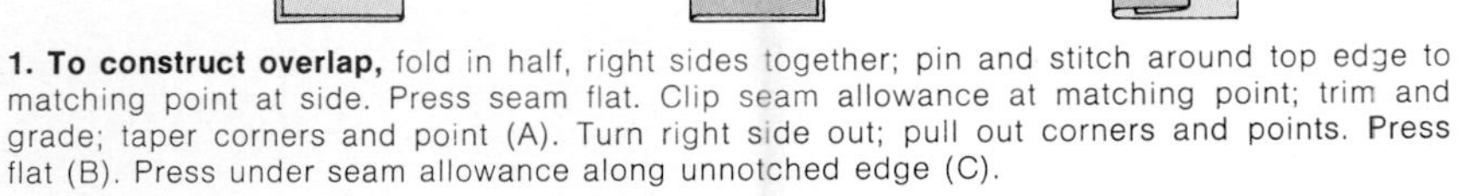

1. To construct overlap, fold in half, right sides together; pin and stitch around top edge to matching point at side. Press seam flat. Clip seam allowance at matching point; trim and grade; taper corners and point (A). Turn right side out; pull out corners and points. Press flat (B). Press under seam allowance along unnotched edge (C).

2. To prepare underlap piece, simply press seam allowance to the wrong side along unnotched edge. Trim this pressed-under seam allowance to about half-width.

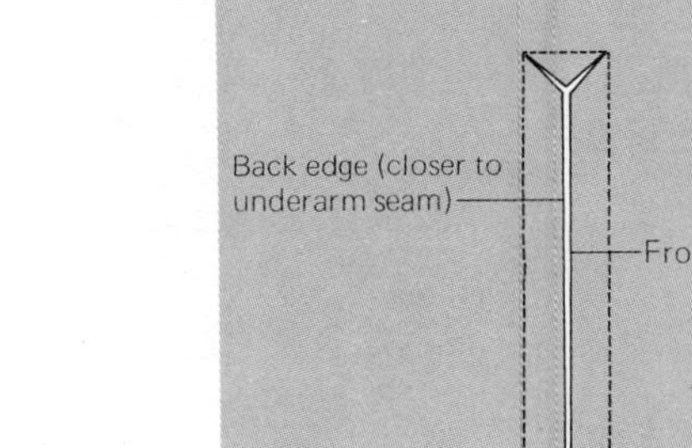

3. Place reinforcing stitches within placket seamline; shorten them at corners. Slash to within ½″ of placket top, then to corners. Determine the front and back edges of opening.

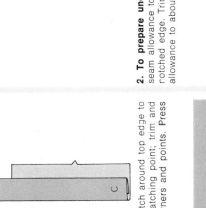

4. With seamlines aligned, pin and stitch right side of underlap raw edge to wrong side of the back placket edge; secure stitches at top corner of placket. Press flat; trim.

5. Press seam allowance toward underlap. Fold underlap to right side; pin its folded edge over stitch line. Edgestitch through all thicknesses; stop at corner; secure stitches.

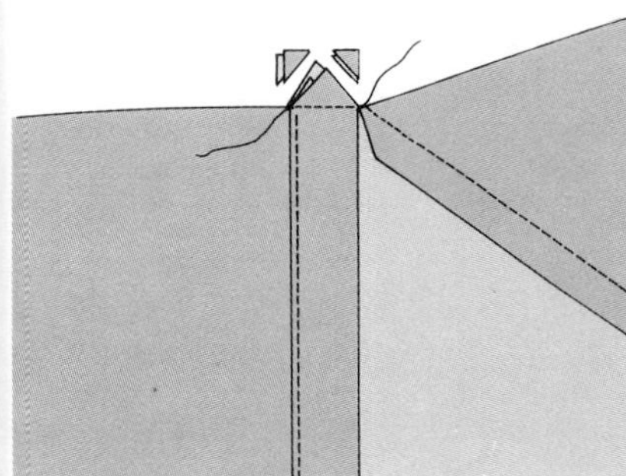

6. At placket top, flip triangular piece up and pin to underlap. Stitch across base of triangle, securing stitches at beginning and end. Taper square corners of underlap.

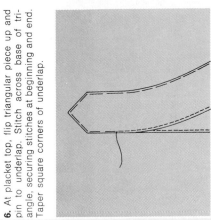

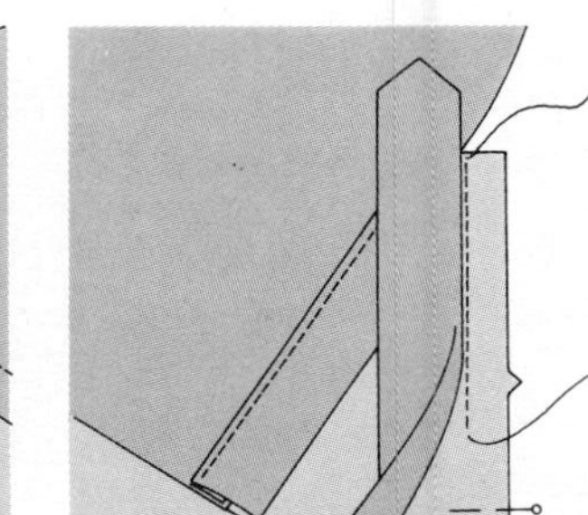

7. Pin right side of overlap's extended edge to wrong side of remaining (front) placket edge; align seamlines, and keep raw edges at bottom even. Stitch; secure stitches at top.

8. Press seam flat. Trim seam allowance to about half-width and press toward overlap. Bring folded edge of overlap to stitching line and pin it in place.

9. Pin the top portion of overlap to sleeve, completely covering the top portion of underlap; pin down as far as placket corner. Baste along all pinned edges.

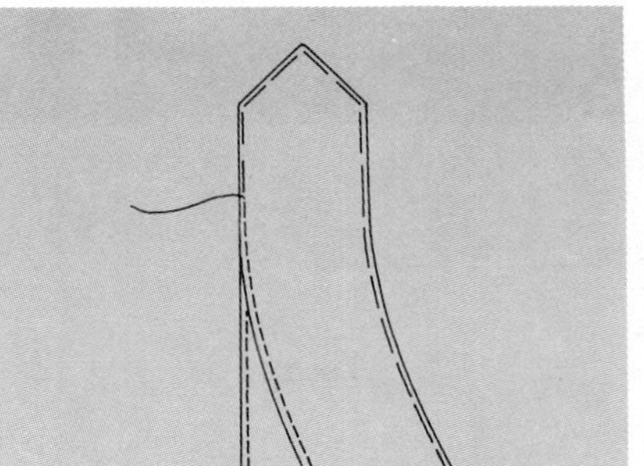
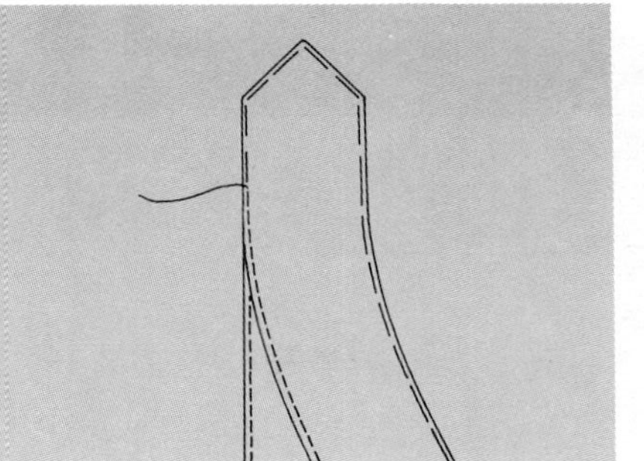
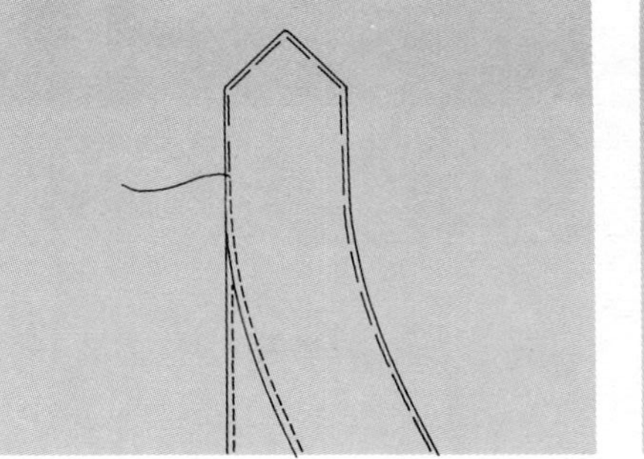

10. Topstitch along unbasted fold of overlap (be sure not to catch any part of underlap in stitching); pull threads to wrong side at stopping point and knot.

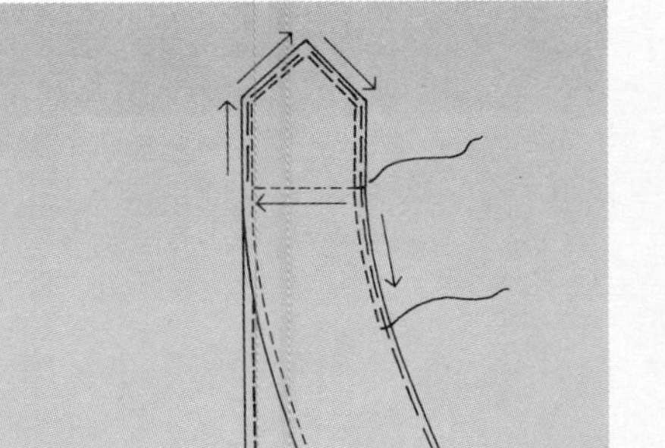

11. Topstitch (through all the thicknesses) across overlap and around basted edges; follow direction of arrows. Secure stitches at beginning. Remove bastings; press.

Sleeve finishes/cuffs

Construction of cuffs with plackets

Cuffs actually consist of a cuff and a facing section, which may be cut all-in-one or as two pieces (see below). Bound buttonholes, if any, should be made before cuff is constructed; worked buttonholes, after cuff is applied to sleeve. Before starting cuff application, complete underarm sleeve seams and prepare pleats or gathers at sleeve edge if called for. Note the placement of cuff end to placket edge. A **lapped cuff** will have one end flush and one end projecting from the placket edges; both ends of the **shirt cuff** and **French cuff** will be flush with placket edges.

One- and two-piece cuff construction

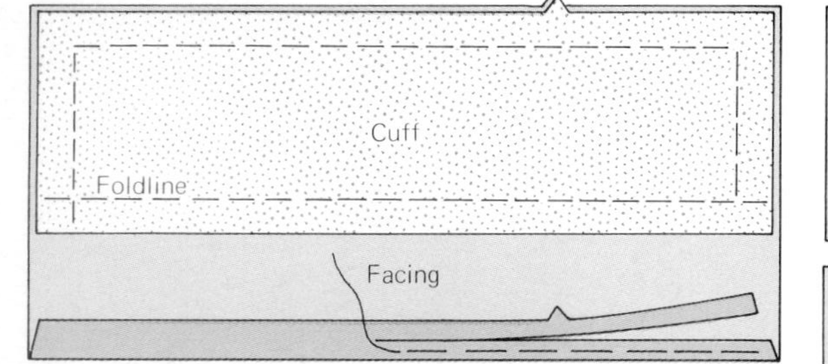

For one-piece cuff, apply interfacing to cuff section. Interfacing can come to foldline or, for a softer fold, extend ½″ beyond it into facing section (see Interfacing). Turn and press seam allowance to wrong side along facing edge and trim to ⅜″; uneven-baste along folded edge.

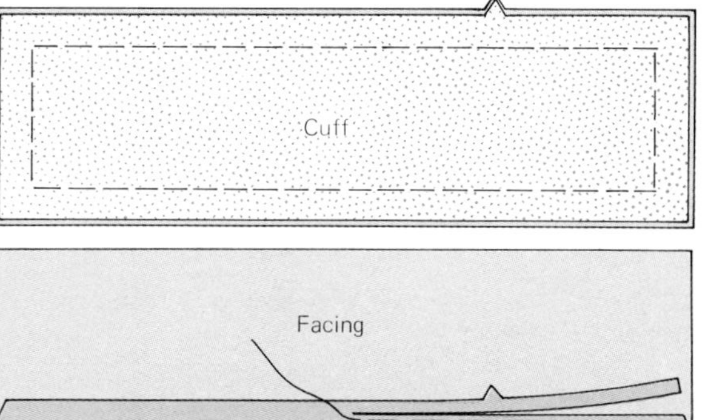

For two-piece cuff, apply interfacing to wrong side of cuff section. Turn, trim, baste notched edge of facing section.

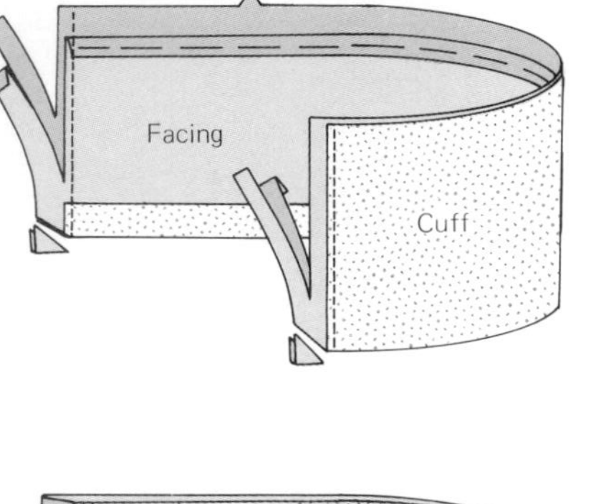

For one-piece cuff, left, fold in half along marked foldline, right sides together, and pin the two ends. **For two-piece cuff,** right, pin cuff to facing, right sides together, leaving notched edge open. Baste either one as pinned, and stitch. Press seam flat. Trim and grade seam allowances; taper corners.

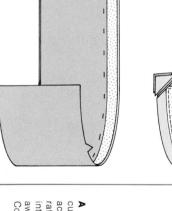

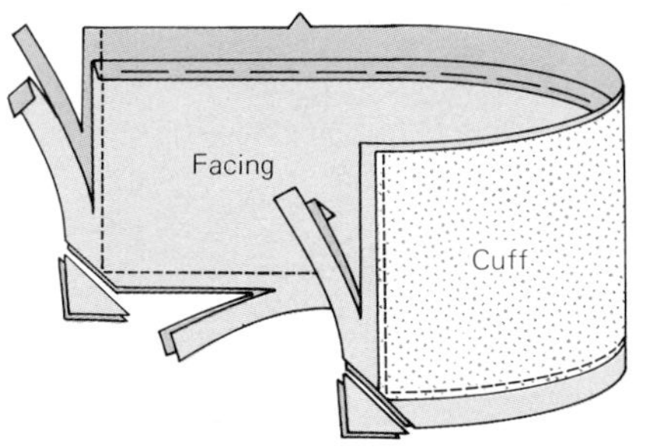
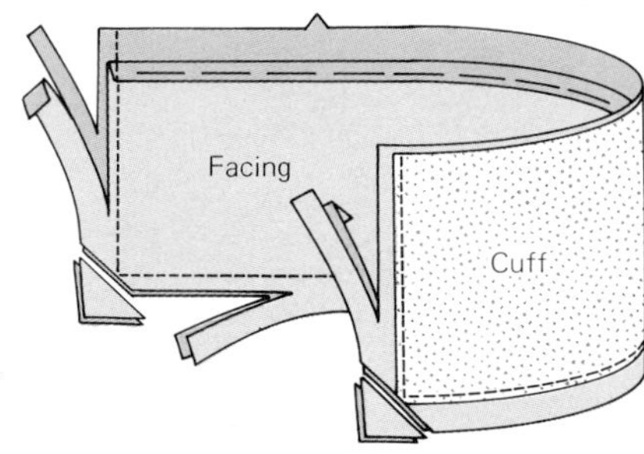

For both one- and two-piece cuffs, press seam allowances open over point presser, then toward facing. Turn cuffs right side out; pull out the corners. Roll facing edges slightly under, and press. If necessary, diagonal-baste around edges of two-piece cuff.

Variations

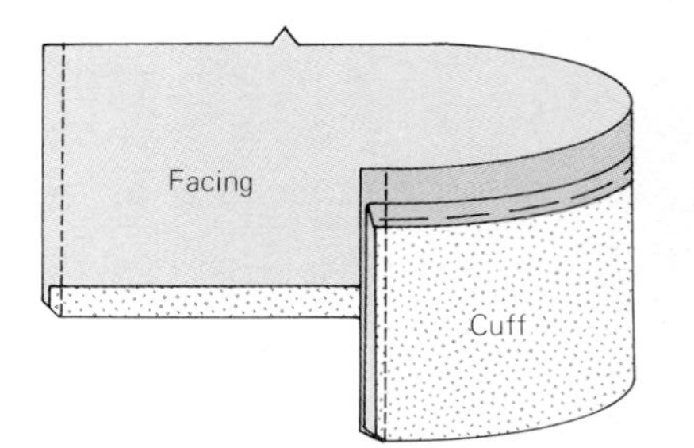

A shirt cuff differs slightly from the cuff constructed at left. Because of the shirt cuff application method (see opposite page), the edge of the *cuff* section rather than the facing section is turned under and basted. Before turning the interfaced cuff edge under, trim away the interfacing seam allowance along that edge. Complete cuff construction as directed.

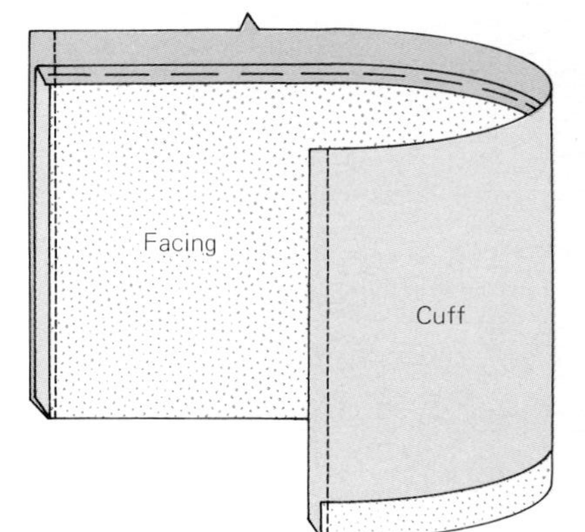

A French cuff is cut double the width of a standard cuff so that it can fold back onto itself. This turnback action exposes the facing, and so the *facing* section, rather than the cuff section (as described at left), is interfaced. Before turning the facing edge under, trim away the interfacing seam allowance along that edge. Complete cuff construction as directed.

Slipstitch (uneven) 132
Seams with fullness 154

Bound buttonholes 330-342
Worked buttonholes 343-348

Lapped cuff application

1. Pin cuff to sleeve at all matched markings, right sides together. Cuff end at back placket edge (edge closer to underarm seam) should project out to create underlap; other end should be flush with remaining placket edge. Pull gathering threads (if any) to ease in fullness of sleeve; distribute gathers evenly while pinning. Baste in place.

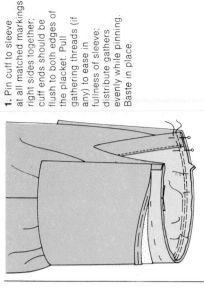

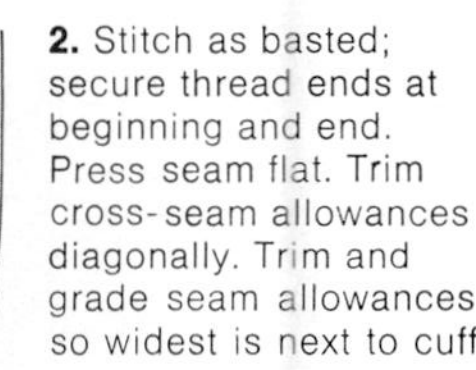

2. Stitch as basted; secure thread ends at beginning and end. Press seam flat. Trim cross-seam allowances diagonally. Trim and grade seam allowances so widest is next to cuff.

3. Pull cuff down; press seam allowances toward cuff. Bring folded edge of facing to stitching line on wrong side of sleeve; pin and slipstitch entire folded edge to sleeve. Remove bastings and press. Complete underside of bound buttonholes or make worked buttonholes. Topstitch if desired.

Shirt cuff application

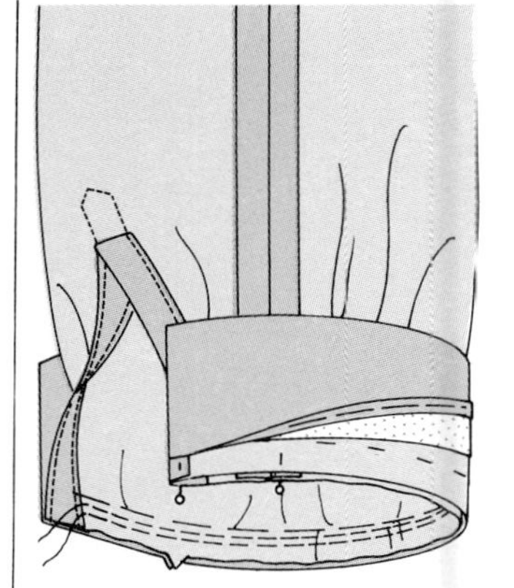

1. Pin right side of cuff facing to wrong side of sleeve at all matched markings. Cuff ends should be flush to the underlap and overlap edges of the shirt placket. Pull gathering threads (if any) to ease in fullness of sleeve; distribute gathers evenly while pinning. Baste in place.

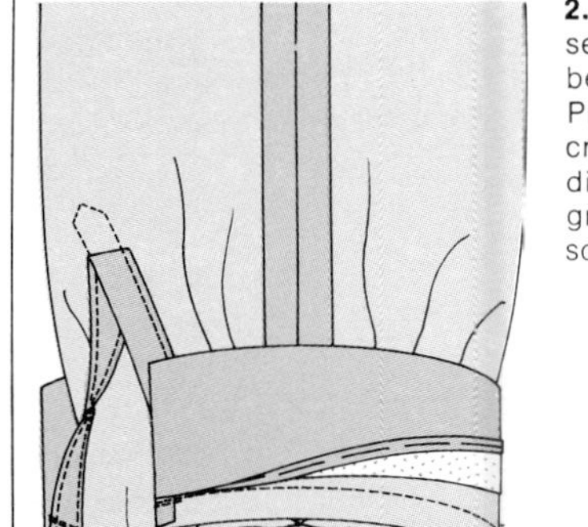

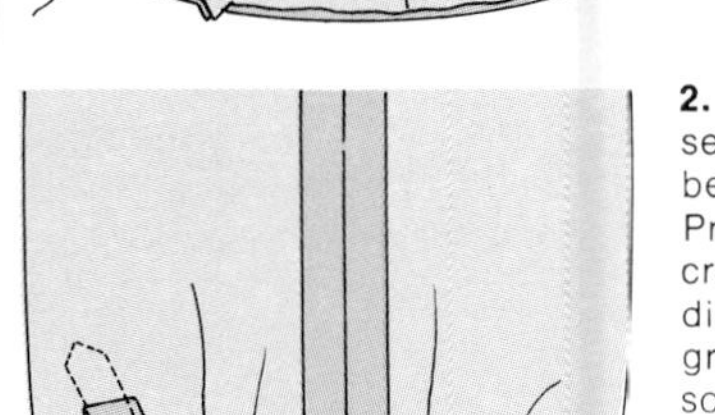

2. Stitch as basted; secure thread ends at beginning and end. Press seam flat. Trim cross-seam allowances diagonally. Trim and grade seam allowances so widest is next to cuff.

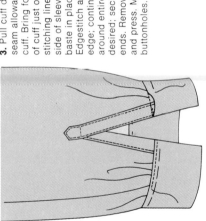

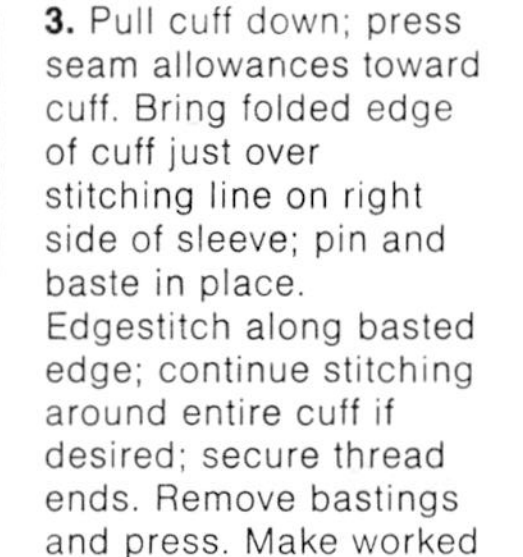

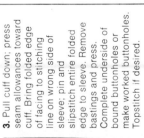

3. Pull cuff down; press seam allowances toward cuff. Bring folded edge of cuff just over stitching line on right side of sleeve; pin and baste in place. Edgestitch along basted edge; continue stitching around entire cuff if desired; secure thread ends. Remove bastings and press. Make worked buttonholes.

French cuff application

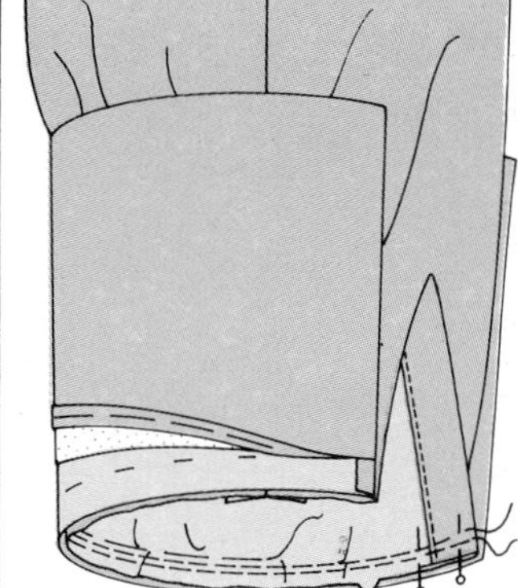

1. Pin cuff to sleeve at all matched markings, right sides together; cuff ends should be flush to both edges of the placket. Pull gathering threads (if any) to ease in fullness of sleeve; distribute gathers evenly while pinning. Baste in place.

2. Stitch as basted; secure thread ends at beginning and end. Press seam flat. Trim cross-seam allowances diagonally. Trim and grade seam allowances so widest is next to cuff.

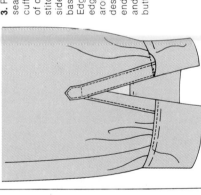

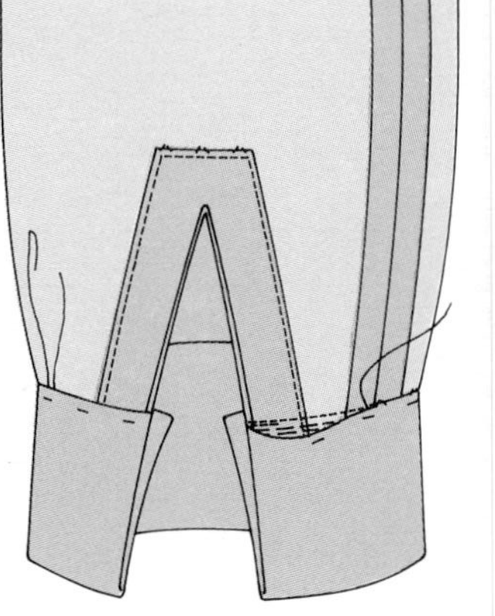

3. Pull cuff down; press seam toward cuff. Bring folded edge of cuff facing to stitching line on wrong side of sleeve; pin and slipstitch folded edge to sleeve. Remove bastings and press. Complete underside of bound buttonholes or make worked buttonholes. Fold cuff in half and press lightly.

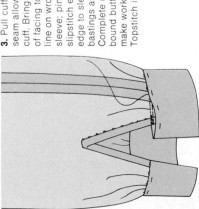

Interfacing 76-79
Slipstitch (uneven) 132
Seams with fullness 154

Cuffs without plackets

Because cuffs without plackets have no openings, they are cut large so the hand or arm can slip easily in and out. There are three basic styles of this cuff type: the **straight band cuff, straight turnback cuff,** and **shaped turnback cuff.** The straight band cuff is made with a separate cuff attached to the sleeve bottom; the straight turnback cuff is made by turning up the deep finished hem of a sleeve. Sometimes, instead of the deep self-hem, a **separate extension piece** is added to the sleeve bottom to form the turnback cuff. The shaped turnback cuff is a separately constructed cuff that is attached to the sleeve with a facing.

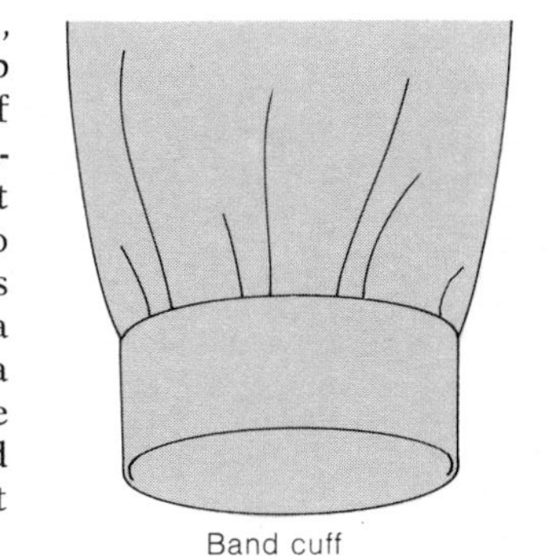
Band cuff

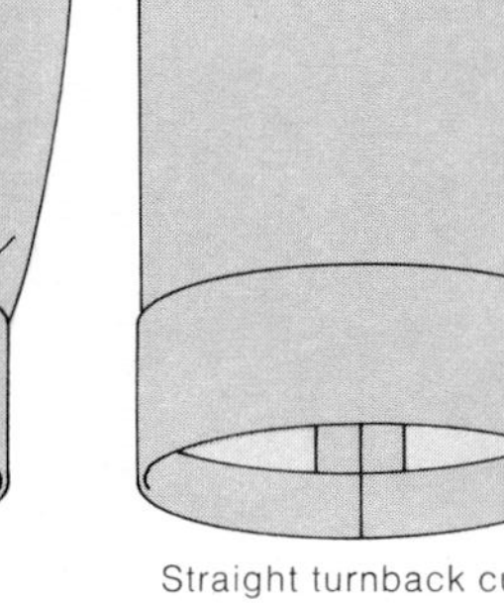
Straight turnback cuff

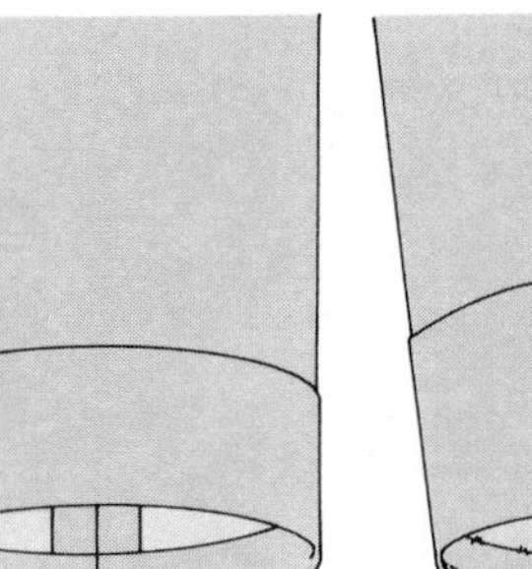
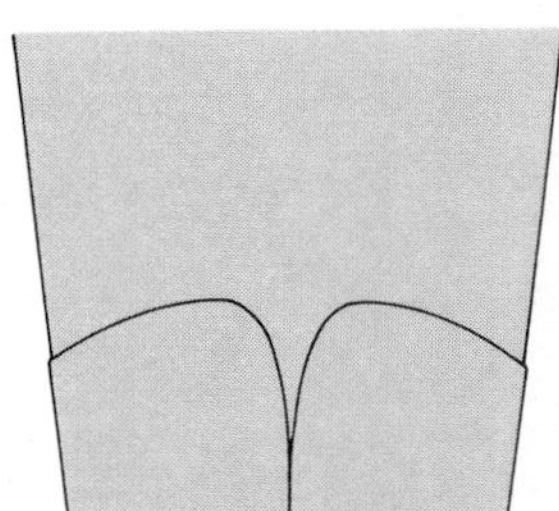
Shaped turnback cuff

Illustrated at left are the three basic styles of cuffs without plackets: the **straight band cuff,** here attached to a full gathered sleeve; the **straight turnback cuff;** and the **shaped turnback cuff** applied with a facing.

Straight band cuff construction and application

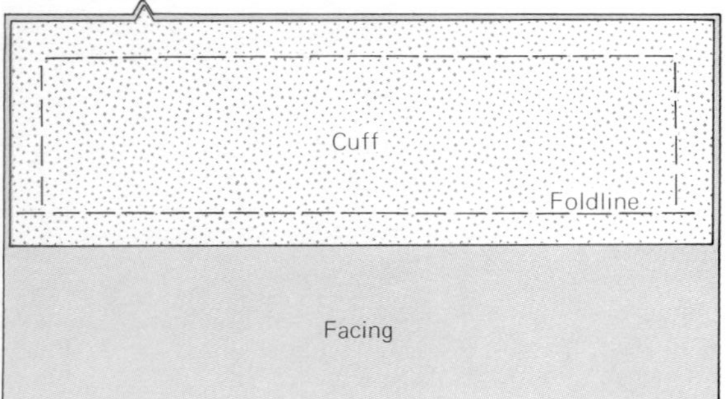

1. To construct cuff, apply interfacing to the wrong side of cuff section. Interfacing can come right to foldline or extend about ½″ into facing section for a softer crease (see Interfacing).

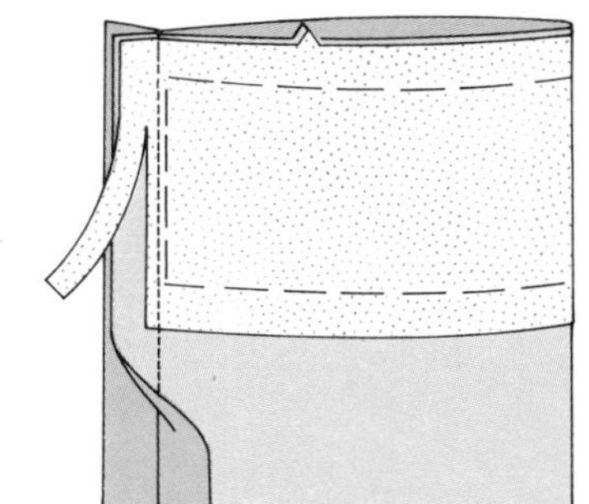

2. With right sides together, match and pin cuff ends together. Stitch and press flat. Trim interfacing seam allowances close to stitching line. Press seam open.

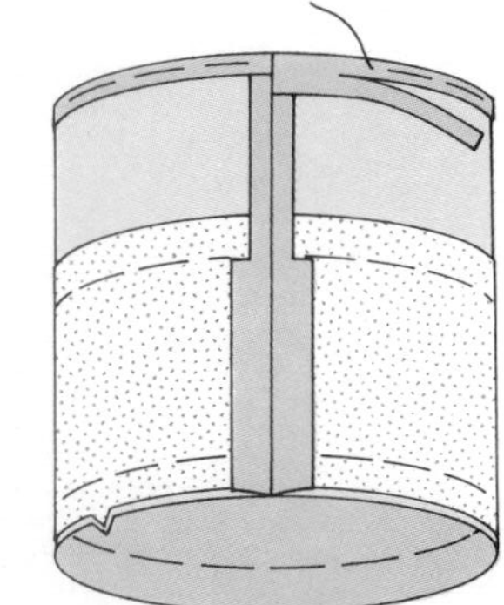

3. Trim seam allowances along the stitched facing section to half-width. Turn and press seam allowance along facing edge to wrong side; trim seam allowance to ⅜″; baste.

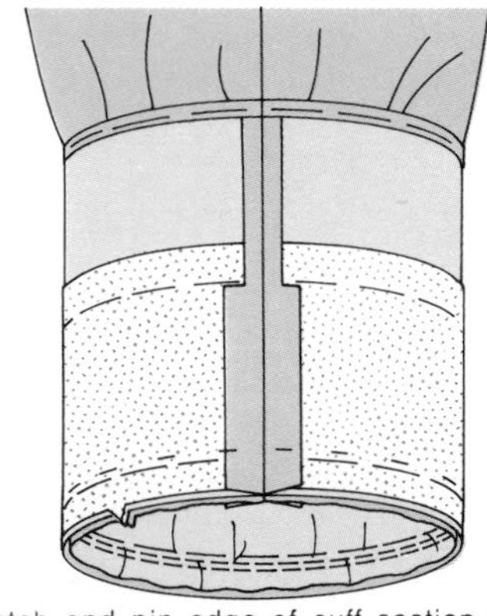

4. Match and pin edge of cuff section to the sleeve edge, right sides together. If sleeve is full, pull gathering threads to ease in fullness. Baste cuff in place.

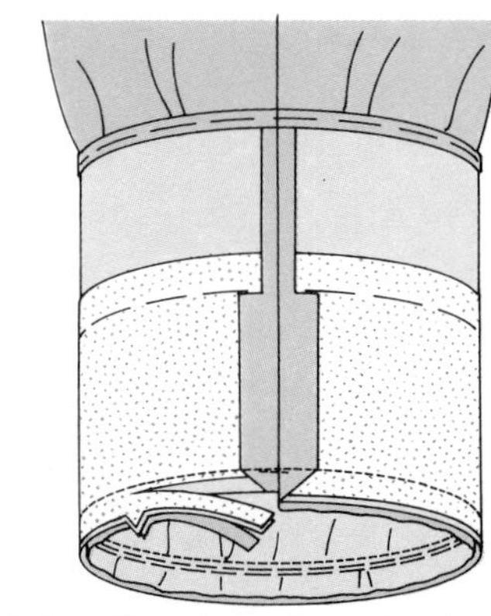

5. Stitch cuff as basted, overlapping a few stitches at the end. Press to embed stitches. Diagonally trim cross seams. Trim and grade so cuff seam allowance is widest.

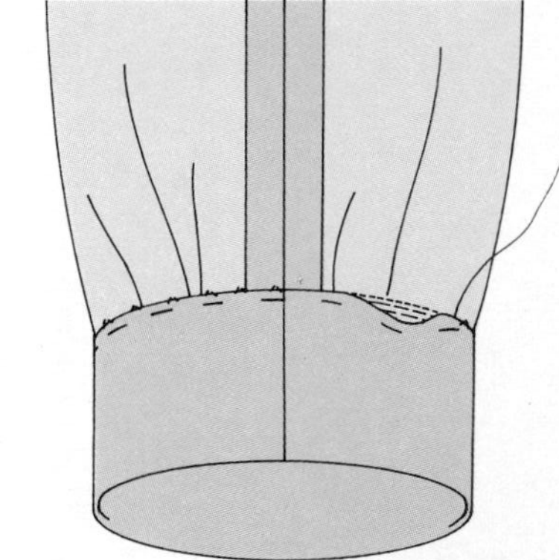

6. Pull cuff down and press seam allowances toward cuff. Fold facing section up to wrong side of sleeve, folded edge meeting stitch line; pin and slipstitch to sleeve. Press.

Interfacing 76-79
Hemming stitches 128-129
Seam finishes 148-149

Straight turnback cuff (self-hem)

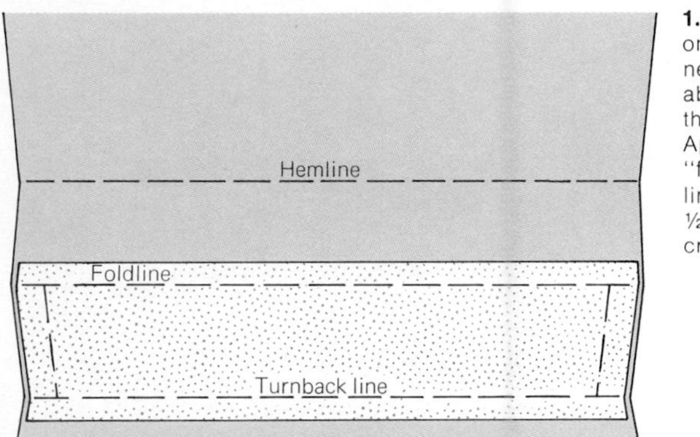

1. Note foldlines for cuff on sleeve bottom. If sleeve needs adjusting, do so above these lines. Mark and thread-trace each line. Apply interfacing between "foldline" and "turnback line"; extend interfacing ½" beyond lines for softer crease (see Interfacing).

2. With right sides together, match, pin, and baste underarm sleeve seam. Stitch. Press seam flat, then open. Trim seam allowance below "foldline" to half-width. Finish edge.

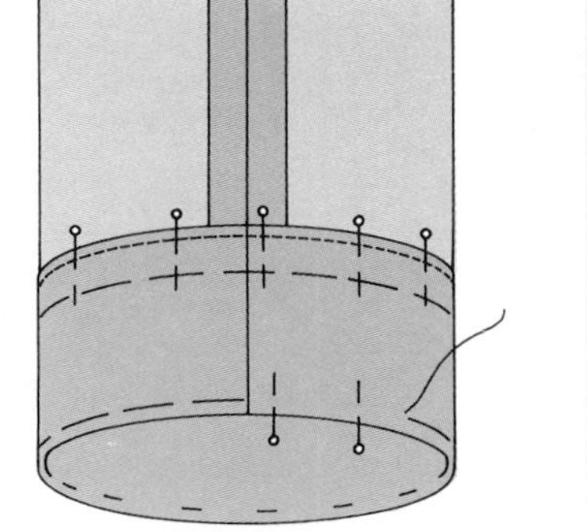

3. Fold sleeve hem to wrong side along "foldline" markings; hold hem in line (do not let it pull) by pinning free edge to sleeve. Pin, then baste close to fold.

4. Remove pins at free edge. Form the cuff by folding sleeve to right side along "turnback line." Pin, then baste through all thicknesses along fold to hold in place.

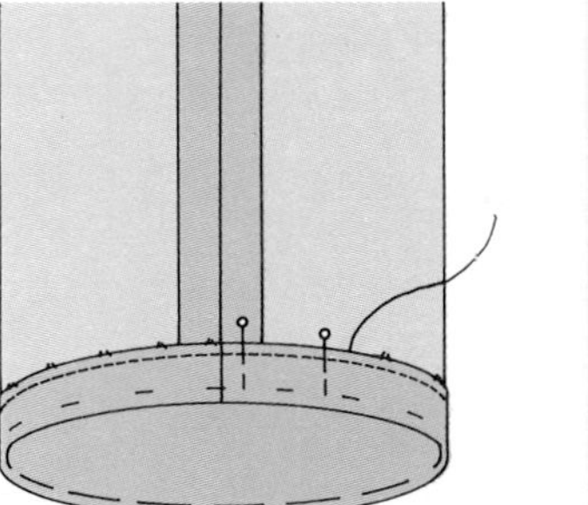

5. Pin hem edge in place on wrong side of sleeve. Secure with an appropriate hemming stitch (see Hemming stitches). Remove all bastings, and press cuff lightly.

Straight turnback cuff (separate extension)

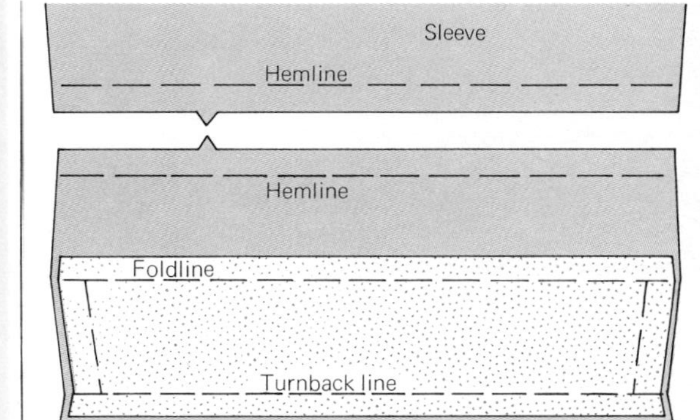

1. Note foldlines for cuff on sleeve extension; mark each line, thread-tracing the "foldline" and "turnback line." If sleeve needs adjusting, do so above the hemline marking on sleeve. Apply interfacing between "foldline" and "turnback line" on extension piece; extend interfacing ½" beyond these lines for softer crease (see Interfacing).

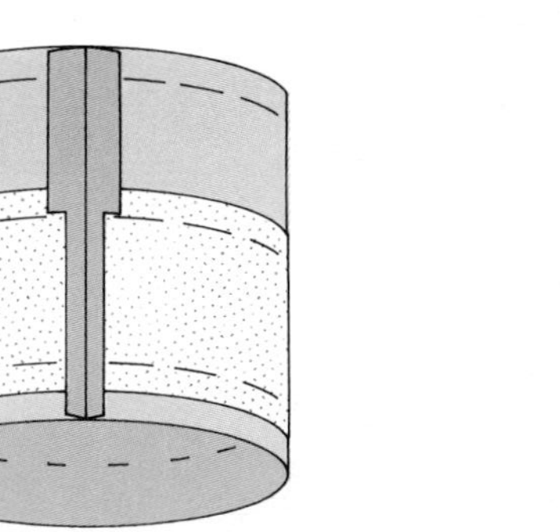

2. Complete sleeve seam. Press open. Right sides together, match, pin, and stitch extension ends. Press flat, then open. Trim seam allowances below "foldline" to half-width.

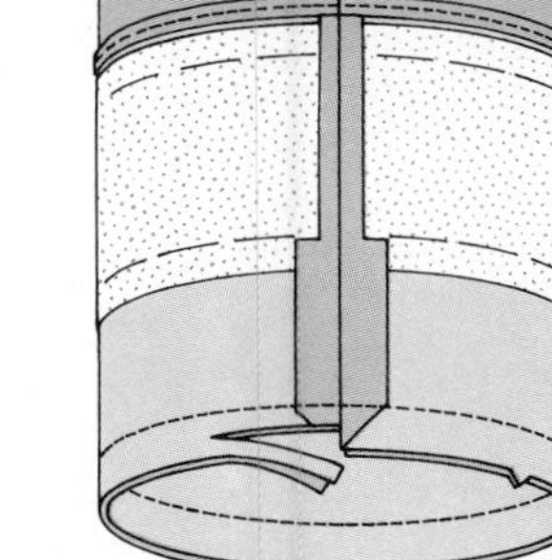

3. Finish unnotched edge of extension. With right sides together, match, pin, and baste extension to sleeve along "hemline"; stitch. Press flat. Trim and grade seam allowances.

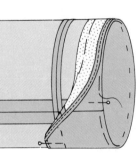

4. Pull extension down; press seam open. Fold extension to wrong side along "foldline." Pin free edge of extension to sleeve to hold in place. Pin, then baste close to fold.

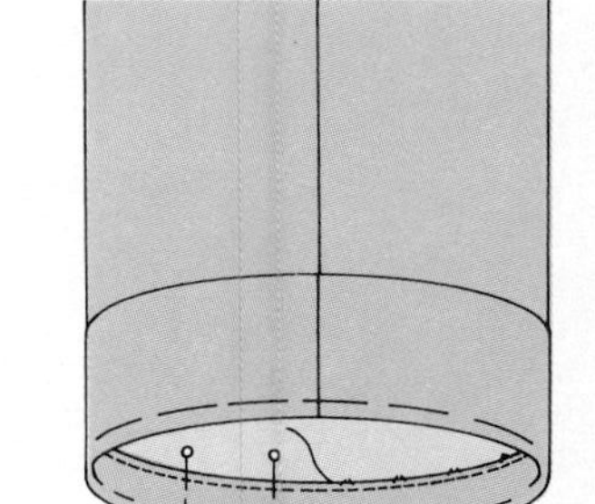

5. Remove pins. To form cuff, fold sleeve to the right side along "turnback line." Pin, then baste through all thicknesses. Pin and secure free edge to sleeve. Remove bastings; press.

Pressing equipment 18-19
Interfacing 76-79
Reducing bulk 147
Seam finishes 148-149

To construct shaped turnback cuff

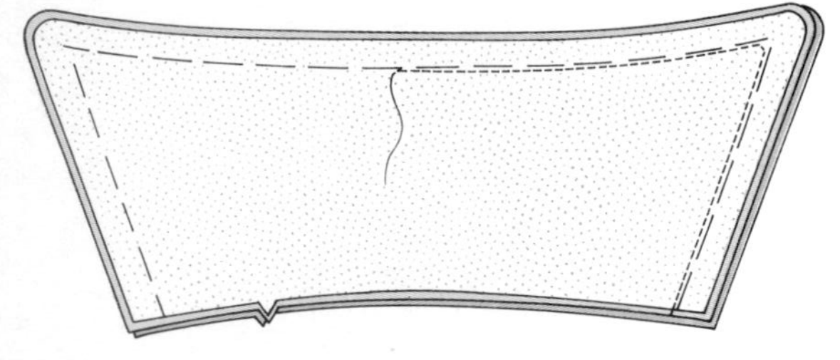

1. Cut and mark cuff and facing sections from pattern. Apply interfacing to wrong side of cuff section. With right sides together, match, pin, and baste cuff to facing; leave the sleeve edge open. Stitch as basted.

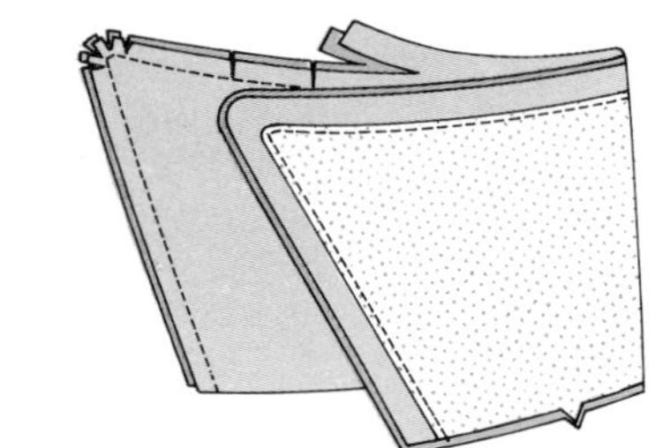

2. Press cuff flat. Trim, then grade seam allowances so widest is next to the cuff section. Clip into or notch out excess fabric from curved seam allowances, as necessary, so seam will lie smooth when cuff is turned.

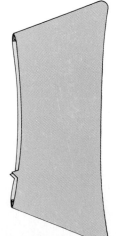

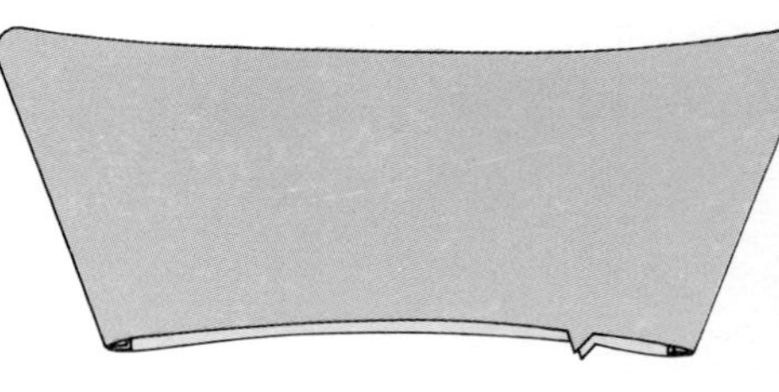

3. Press seams open over a tailor's board, then press seam allowances toward facing section. Turn cuff right side out; roll seams toward facing side. Press, and diagonal-baste if necessary to hold stitched edges in place.

To apply cuff with facing

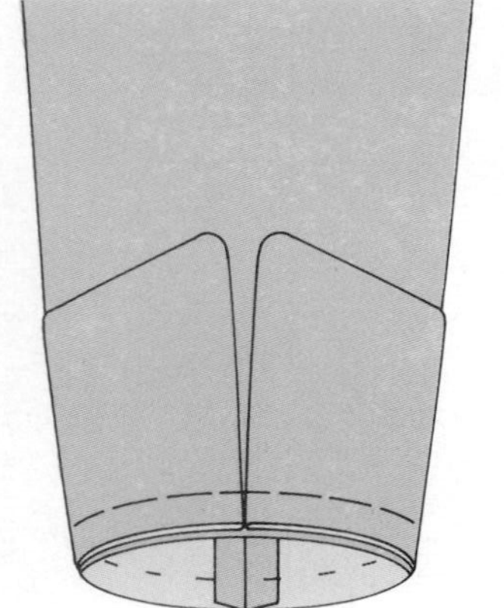

1. Complete underarm sleeve seam; press open. Match and pin the facing side of cuff to the right side of sleeve. Baste in place along seamline.

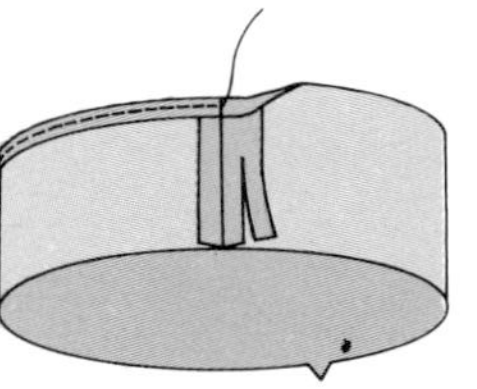

2. With right sides together, pin and stitch ends of sleeve facing. Press seam flat, then open. Trim seam allowances to half-width. Apply seam finish to unnotched edge of facing.

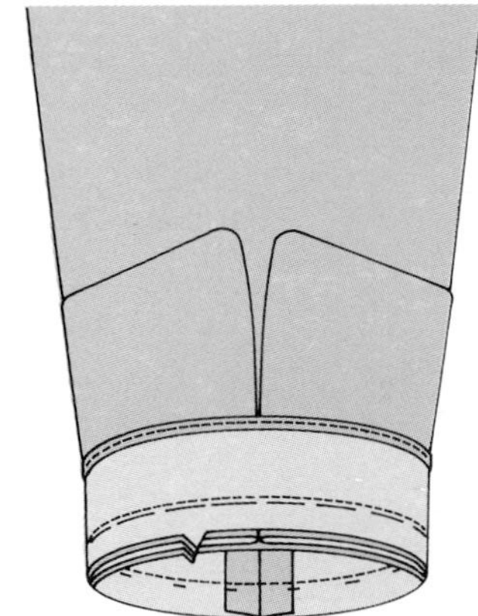

3. Match, pin, and baste sleeve facing to cuff and sleeve. Stitch along seamline. Press to embed stitches.

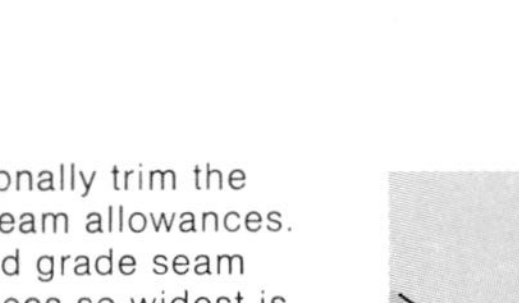

4. Diagonally trim the cross-seam allowances. Trim and grade seam allowances so widest is next to the sleeve.

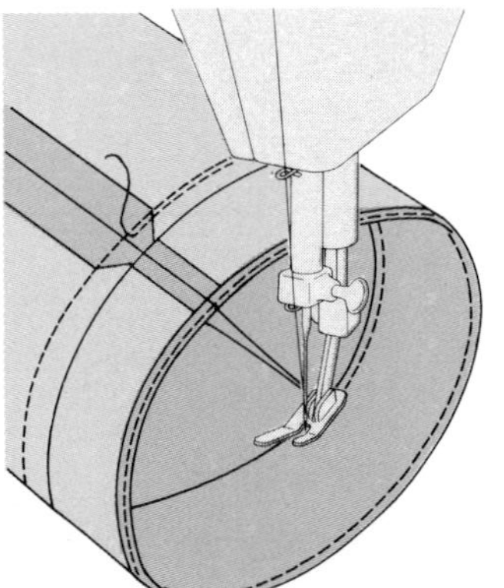

5. Extend the facing and seam allowances and, with right side up, understitch on facing side of seamline. Press seam flat.

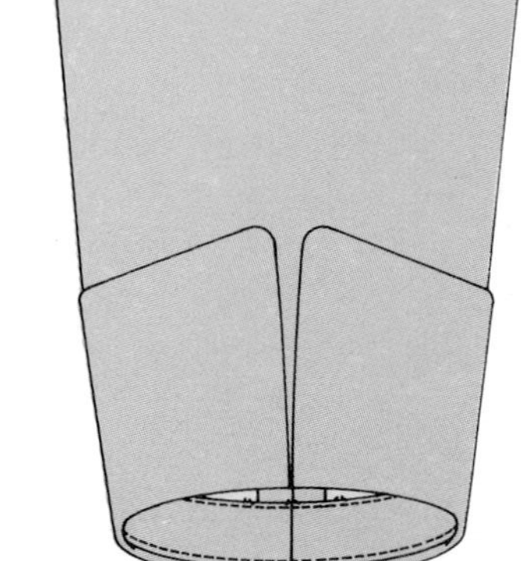
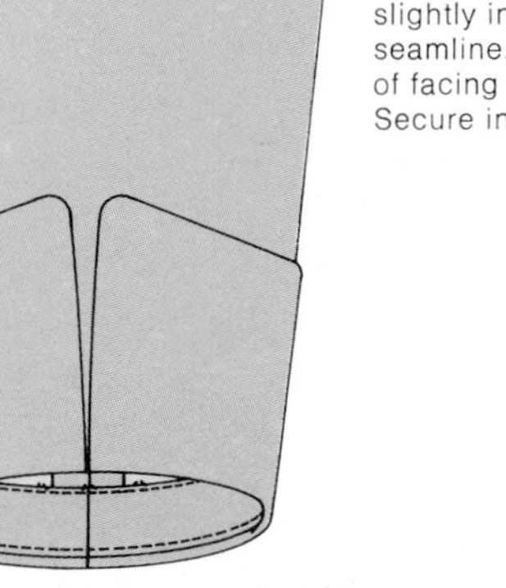

6. Turn facing to the inside, rolling edges slightly inward. Press seamline. Pin free edge of facing to sleeve. Secure in place.

Making & Applying Pockets

Pockets

Interfacing selection and application 72-73, 76-79
Fabric-marking methods 94

Comparison of types

There are two general pocket classifications for women's wear, patch pockets and inside pockets. **Patch pockets** appear on the outside of the garment. They are made from the fashion fabric, can be lined or unlined, and may be attached either by machine or by hand. They can be square, rectangular, pointed, or curved and may be decorated with topstitching, lace or braid trims, or construction details, such as tucks.

Inside pockets are usually made from a lining fabric; they are kept on the inside of the garment, and the opening to the pocket can be either invisible or decorative. There are three types of inside pockets: the **in-seam** pocket, which is sewed to an opening in a seam; the **front-hip** or **frontier** pocket, which is attached to the garment at the waist and side seams; and the **slashed pocket,** which is identified by a slit in the garment, variously finished with the pocket itself, or with a welt, a flap, or a combination of both the welt and the flap.

Placement of the pocket on the garment depends on whether the pocket is functional or strictly decorative. A pocket to be used should be located at a level that is comfortable for the hand to reach. If a pocket is only decorative, as pockets above the waist usually are, it should be placed where it will be most flattering.

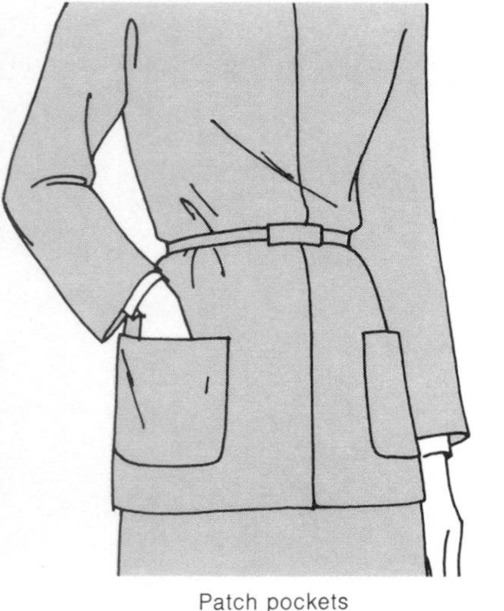

Patch pockets

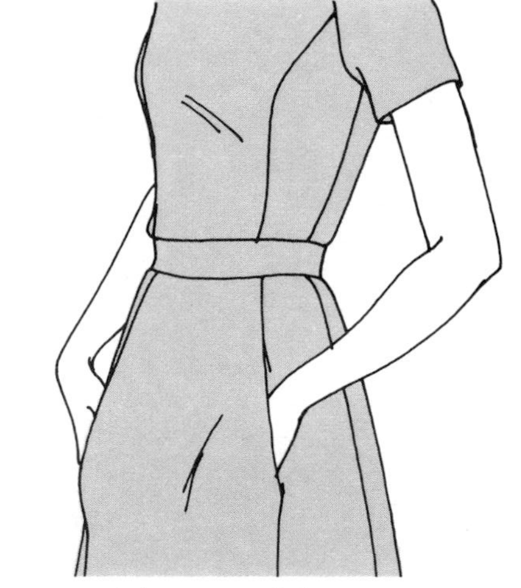

In-seam pockets

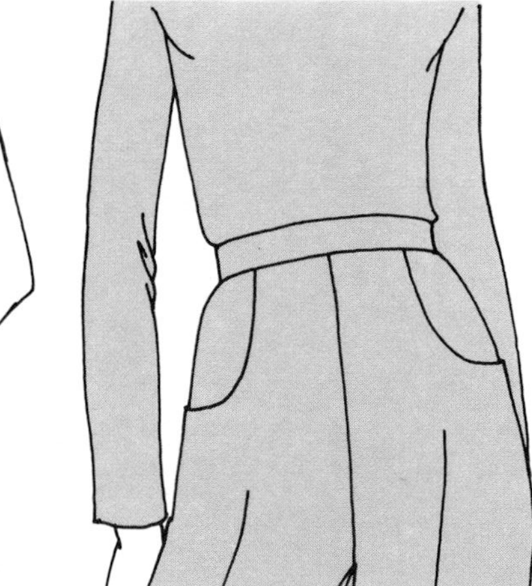

Front-hip or frontier pockets

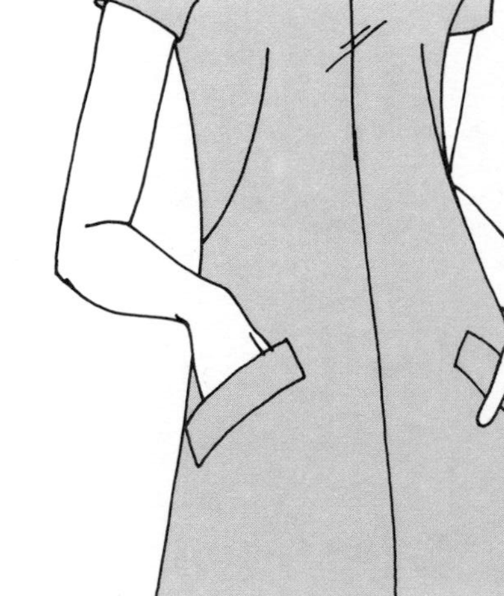

Slashed pockets with welts

Important preliminaries

Pockets are one of the most visible signs of a garment's overall quality and, as such, should be constructed with a close eye to detail. Begin by double-checking the pocket location, particularly if you have made pattern alterations. Transfer pocket location and stitch lines to fabric with careful marking techniques; follow with precise stitching, taking care to neither stop short of nor run beyond the indicated stitch lines. Trim and grade wherever it is possible, and use good pressing techniques at each step.

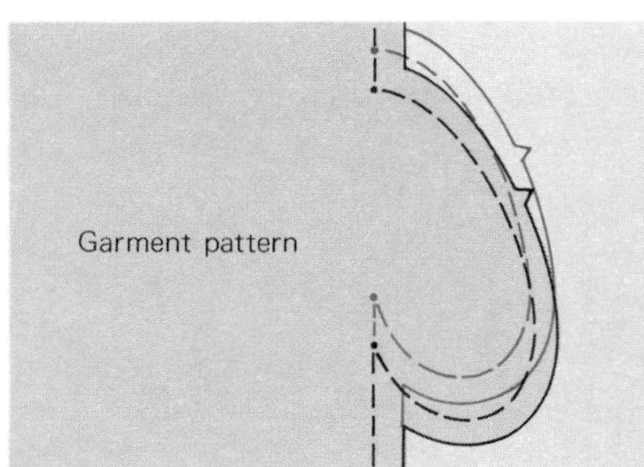

If pocket is re-located to be more flattering or more accessible, be sure to transfer all pocket markings to the new position.

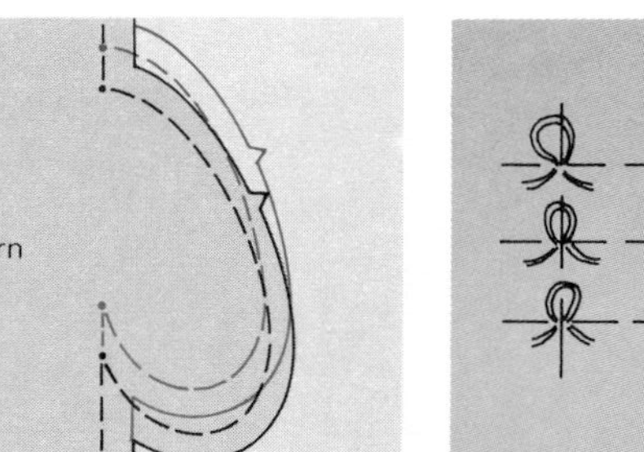

Mark the pocket first with tailor's tacks for positioning, then with thread tracing for all stitching lines.

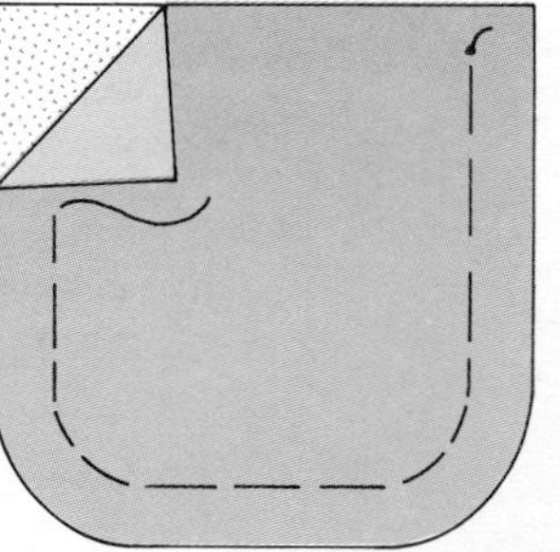

Add interfacing if pocket fabric is lightweight or loosely woven. This adds strength and helps preserve the pocket's shape.

Patch pockets

Uneven basting 124
Slipstitch (uneven) 129

General information

Patch pockets are essentially shaped pieces of fabric that are finished on all sides, then attached to the garment by hand or machine. They may be lined or unlined, and may also be decorated in any of several ways before being attached to the garment. If pockets are to be used in pairs, take care that the finished pockets are the same size and shape; a cardboard template cut to that size is helpful for guiding stitching and pressing. If a plaid, a stripe, or a print is to be matched, the pocket must be cut so this is possible; a striped or plaid pocket may be cut on the opposite grain from the garment or on the bias for added contrast.

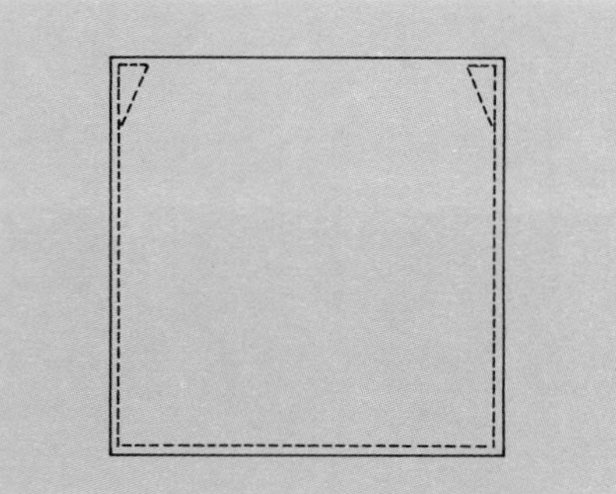

Plain patch pocket, attached with topstitching

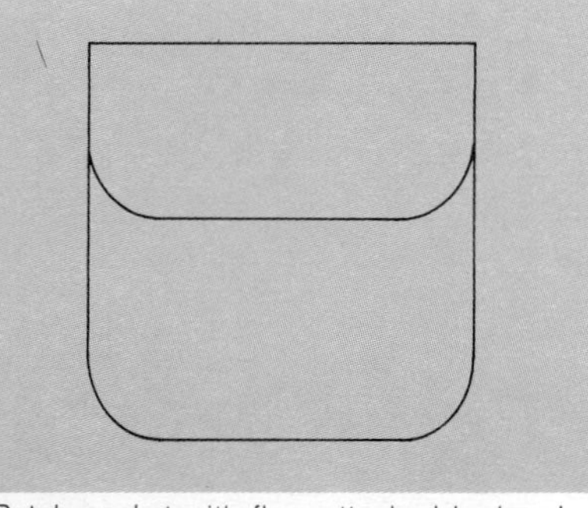

Patch pocket with flap, attached by hand

Unlined patch pockets

Unlined patch pockets are used on casual clothes, such as jeans, shirts, aprons, and the like. Their edges are finished off by turning the facing at the top and the seam allowances at the sides and bottom to the wrong side. If lower corners of pocket are rounded, extra fullness in the seam allowance must be notched out so that there is no overlapping of fabric to cause bulk. If the lower corners are square, they must be mitered.

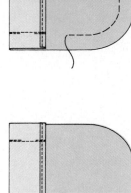

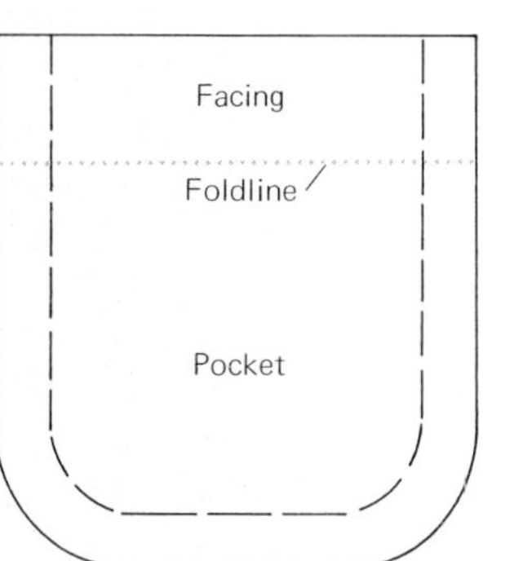

Unlined patch pockets usually have a self-facing at the opening edge, which is turned to the inside during construction.

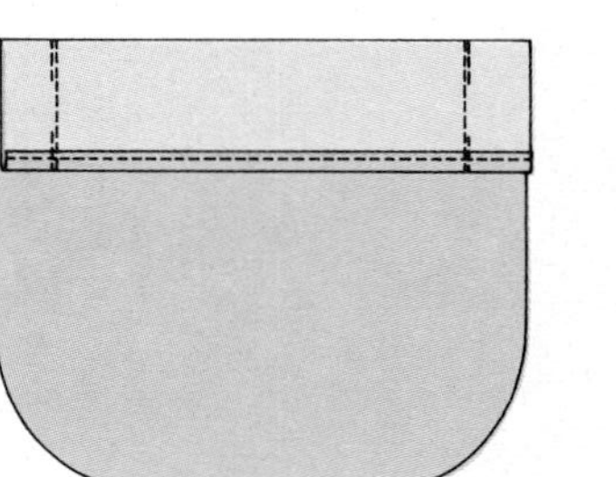

1. Turn under raw edge of pocket facing and edgestitch. Fold facing to the right side along foldline and stitch each side on seamline.

2. If pocket has rounded corners, easestitch at each corner a thread width into the seam allowance from the seamline.

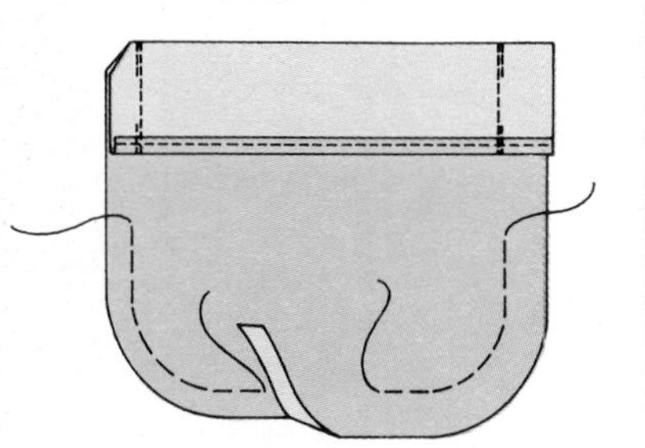

3. Trim entire pocket seam allowance to ⅜" and cut diagonally across each corner at top. Turn facing to wrong side; pull corners out.

4. Press top edge. Pull easestitching at corners to draw in seam allowance and shape pocket curve. Notch out excess fabric.

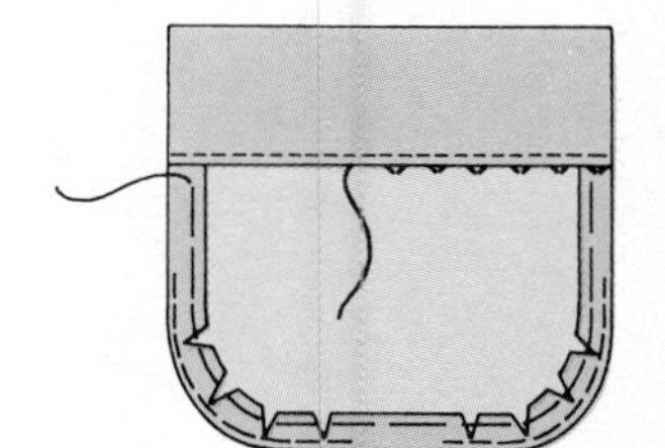
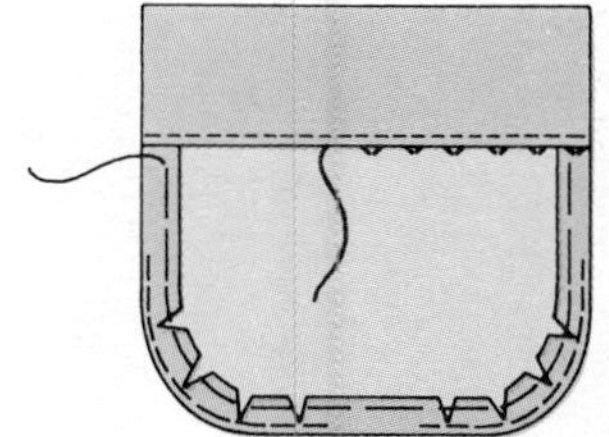

5. Press pocket seam allowances and facing flat. Hand-baste around entire pocket edge and slipstitch facing to pocket.

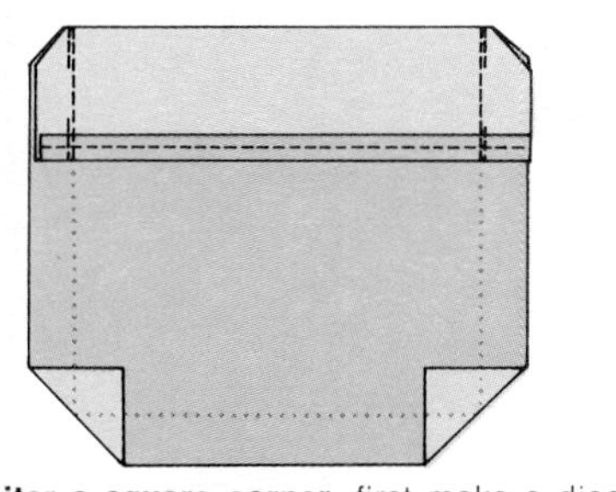

To miter a square corner, first make a diagonal fold to the right side across the junction of the seamlines. Press to crease.

Open the fold and place the *right* sides of the seam allowances together. Stitch on the crease from raw edge to corner. Trim.

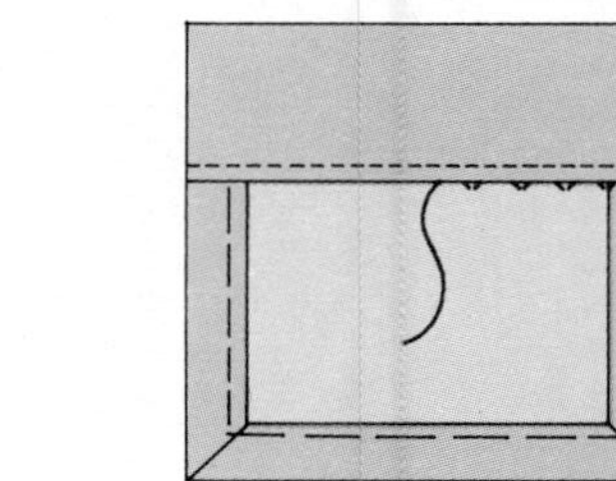

Turn corners and facing to wrong side and press entire pocket flat. Hand-baste around all edges and slipstitch facing to pocket.

Patch pockets

Lined patch pockets

Lining gives patch pockets a neat custom finish. Also, it adds opaqueness to loosely woven or sheer fabrics, which is a great benefit for working pockets that are made of such fabrics. Lining should not be expected to take the place of interfacing, however; it does not support the outer fabric well enough. Quite often you will need to both interface and line a patch pocket. The lining should be color-matched to the outer fabric, and can be of either the garment fabric itself (if it is not too heavy) or a traditional lining fabric. The lining may extend to all edges or, if pocket has a facing, it may go only to the facing.

If a pocket is lined to all edges, use this trick to ensure that no lining shows at the edges. First, cut the lining slightly smaller than the pocket by trimming ⅛ inch from all its cut edges. Center the lining on the pocket so edges correspond, and stitch on the seamline. When the pocket is turned, the lining will pull the finished edge slightly to the wrong side. Press, remembering that the objective is crisp, sharp edges with no lining visible on the right side.

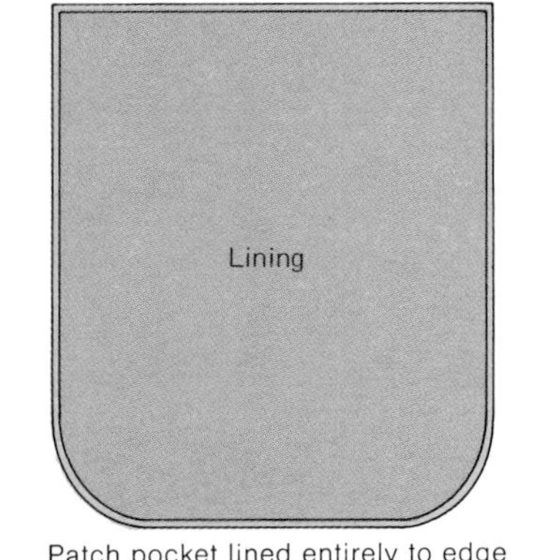

Patch pocket lined entirely to edge

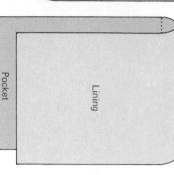

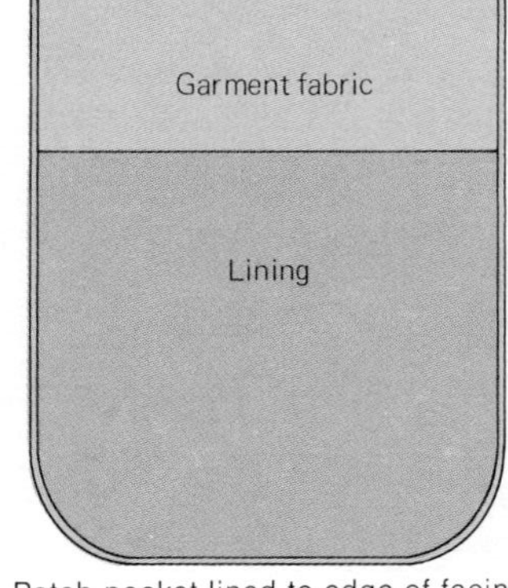

Patch pocket lined to edge of facing

Lining entire pocket

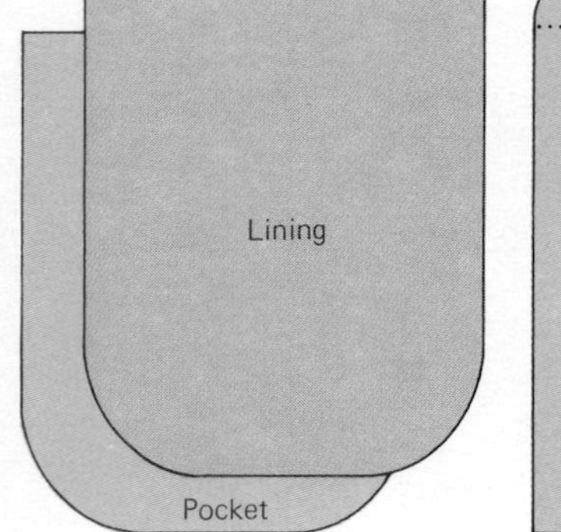

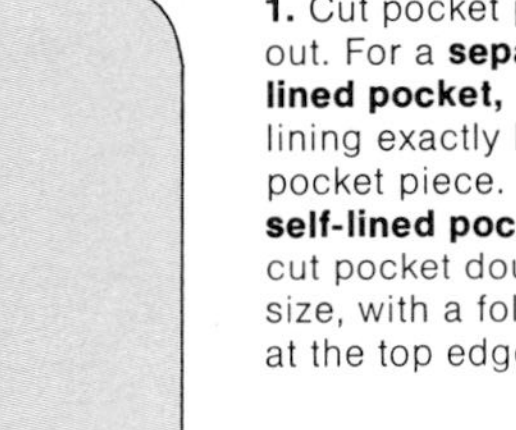

1. Cut pocket pieces out. For a **separately lined pocket,** cut lining exactly like pocket piece. For a **self-lined pocket,** cut pocket double size, with a fold at the top edge.

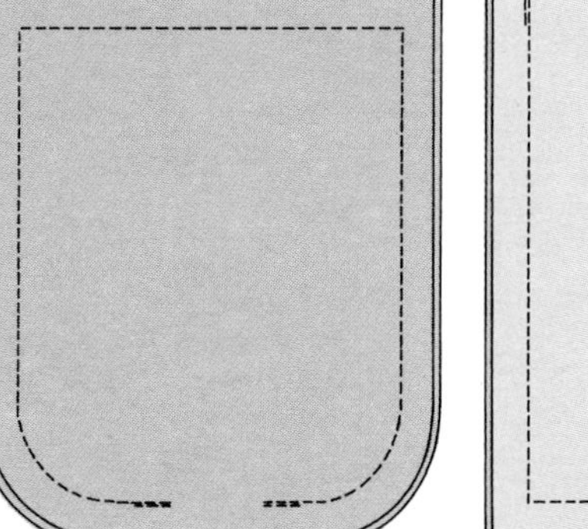

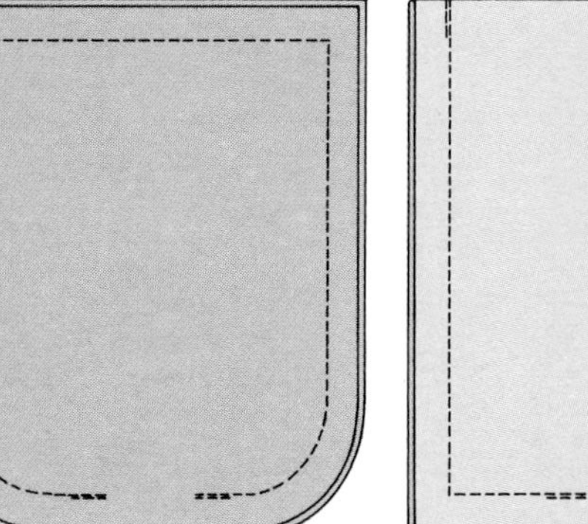

2. For a **separately lined pocket,** place right sides of pocket and lining together and pin along all edges. For a **self-lined pocket,** fold pocket in half, with right sides together, and pin the edges together. Stitch on seamline around raw edges, leaving small portion of bottom edge open. Press flat.

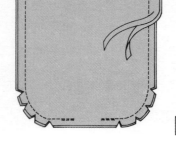

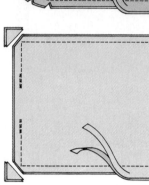

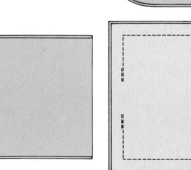

3. Trim and grade seam; taper corners. If pocket is rounded, notch out excess fabric so that when pocket is turned, there is no excess fabric in seam allowances.

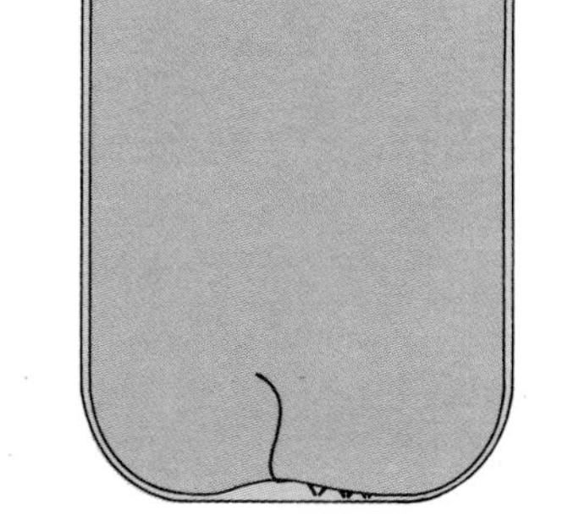

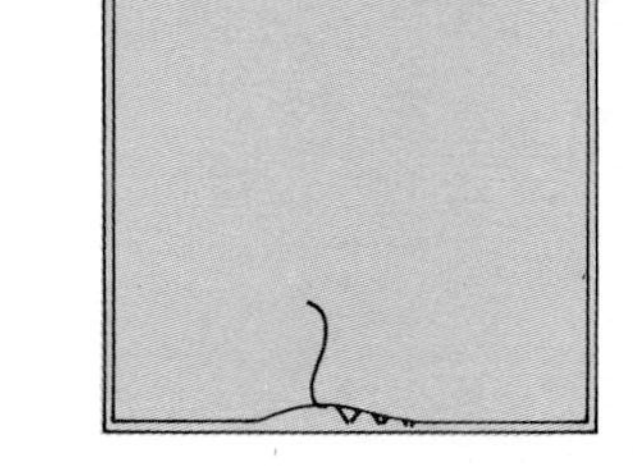

4. Turn pocket to right side, gently pushing it through the open portion in the seam at the bottom edge. Pull out all corners; roll seam to the edge so that it is not visible from the right side. Press. Slipstitch opening at bottom closed.

Separate lining to facing

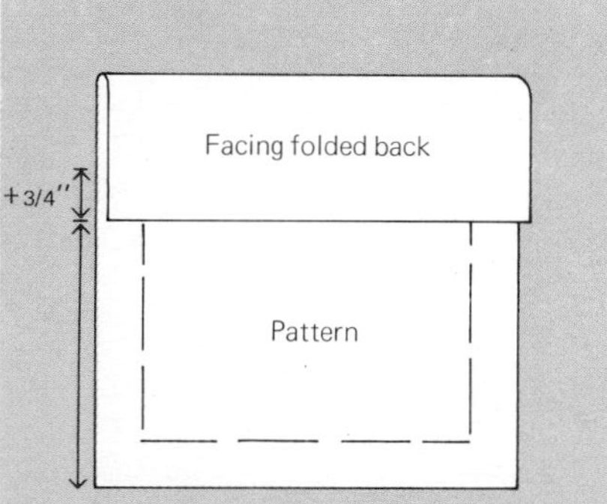

1. Cut lining from the pocket pattern, first folding the facing down out of the way along the foldline. Cut lining from lower edge of pattern to ¾" above the bottom edge of facing.

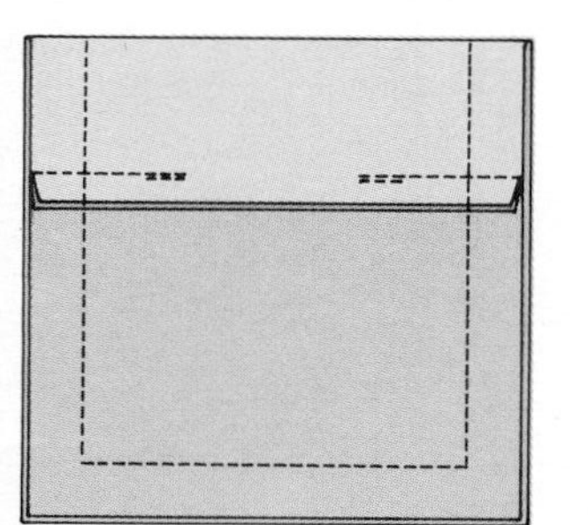

3. With right sides still together, match the bottom and side edges of lining and pocket. Pin, then stitch around the marked seamline. Press flat to embed the stitches.

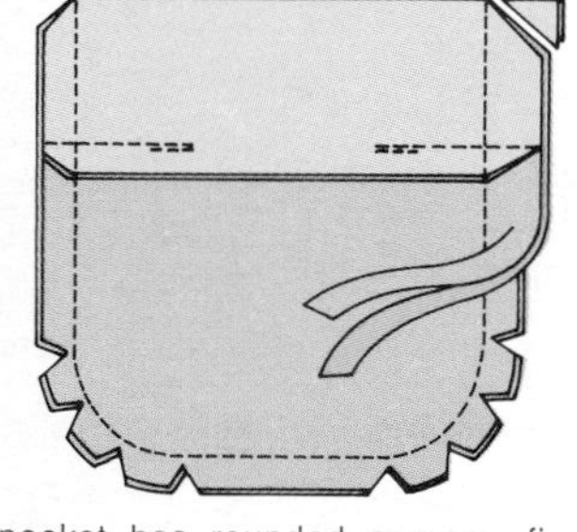

5. If pocket has rounded corners, first trim and grade the seam. Then trim diagonally across corners at top and notch out excess fabric in lower rounded corners.

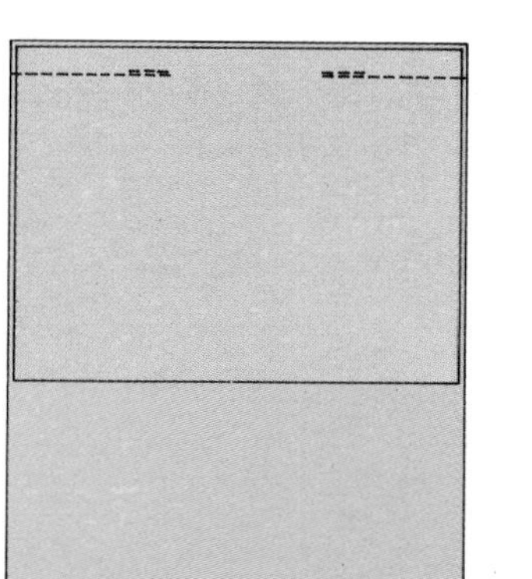

2. Pin top of lining to pocket facing, right sides together. Stitch a ⅜" seam, leaving a small opening in the center of the seam for turning. Press seam toward lining.

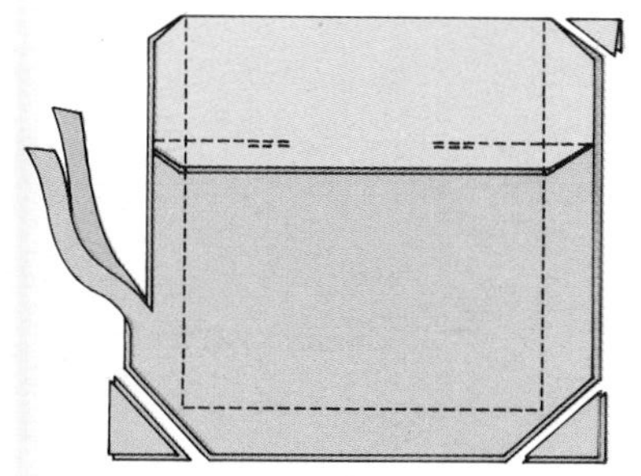

4. Trim and grade seam; trim diagonally across corners at top of pocket and at lower edges so that seam allowances in corners will not be folded back on themselves.

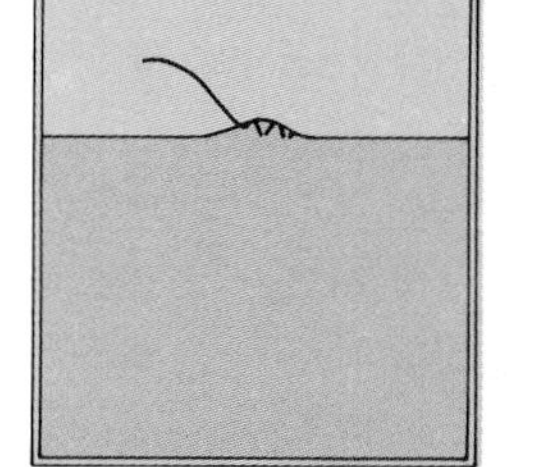

6. Gently turn pocket to right side through opening in facing/lining seam. Press, rolling seam to underside so it will not show on right side. Slipstitch opening closed.

Adding details

Trimming details, such as topstitching, rickrack, lace, or soutache, may be added to pockets during their construction. Topstitching is the most frequent decorative addition. It is most successful when it is done to the pocket before the pocket is applied to the garment (as compared to using the topstitching step as both a decorative measure and a means of attaching the pocket). For better visibility, use a longer stitch length (about 8 stitches per inch) when topstitching.

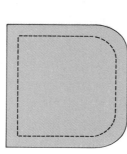

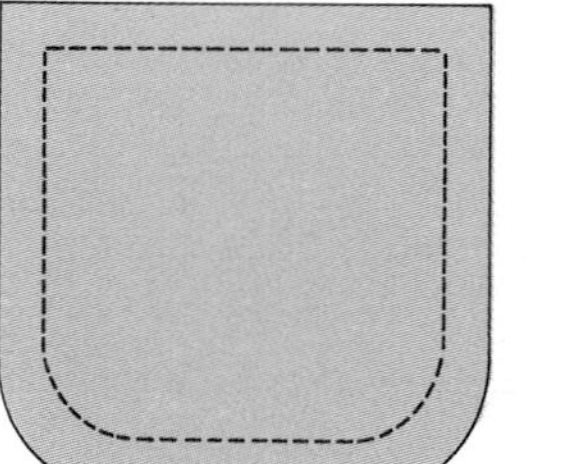

Patch pocket decorated with topstitching

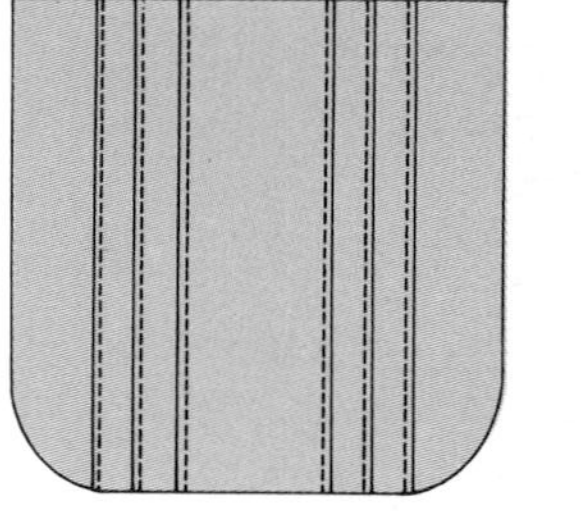

Make tucks before pocket is constructed.

A patch pocket can also be trimmed with buttons and buttonholes, or with appliqués. Studs on jeans and denim skirts contribute decoration along with reinforcement.

Apply any kind of decoration to the pocket before applying it to the garment. Construction details, such as tucks and pleats, should be formed before the pocket is constructed.

Applying pockets

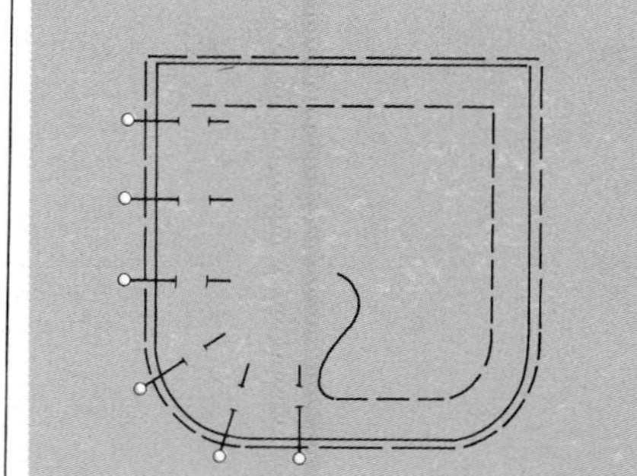

1. Pin and hand-baste finished patch pocket to the right side of the garment, carefully matching it to traced markings.

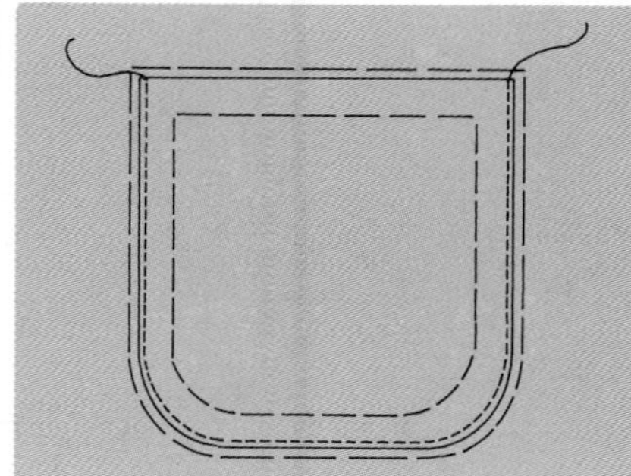

2. To sew pocket on **by machine,** set machine for a regular stitch length; stitch as close as possible to edge of pocket.

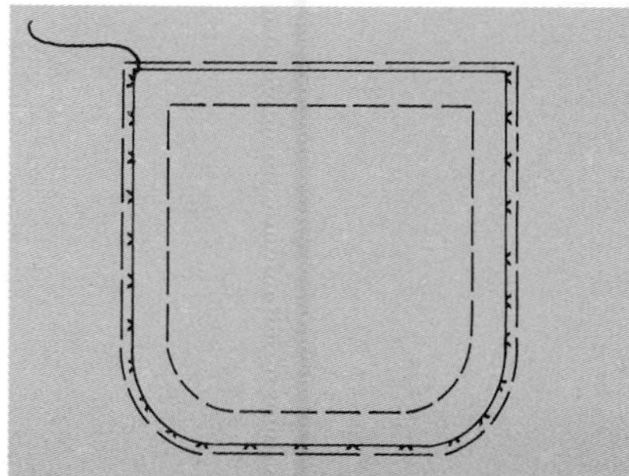

To sew pocket on **by hand,** use an uneven slipstitch. Take care not to pull the stitches too tight, or pocket will pucker.

Zigzag stitching 32-37
Interfacing 72-73, 76-79
Hand bar tack 133; whipstitch 136
Tying thread ends 137

Corner reinforcement

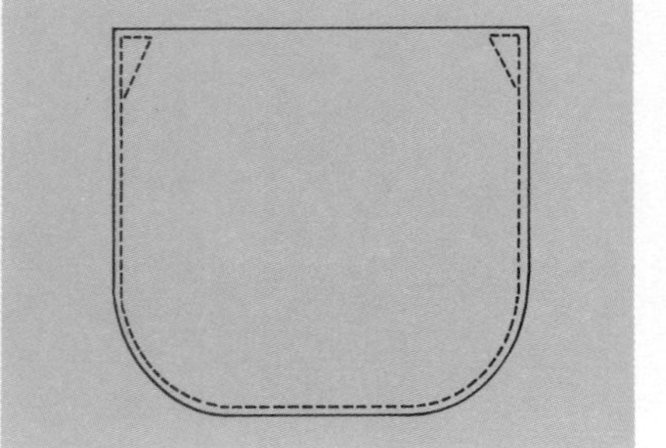

Small, identical triangles stitched at each top corner. This is the pocket reinforcement seen most frequently on shirts.

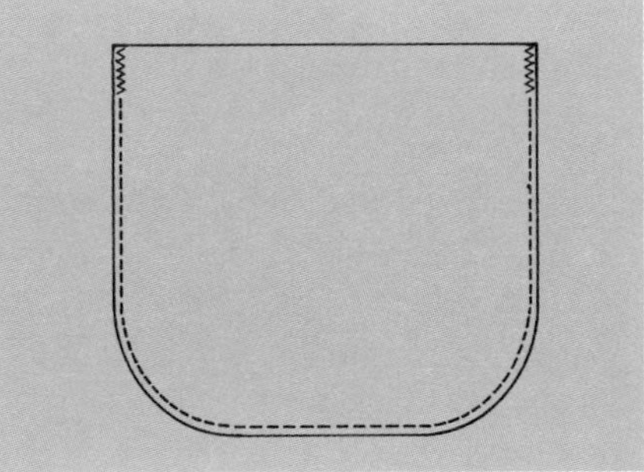

A zigzag stitch about ⅛″ wide and closely spaced, run down ½″ from the top of each side. Good for children's clothes.

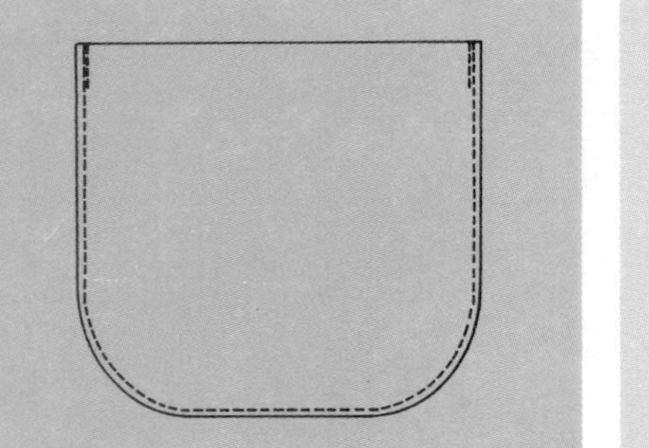

A backstitch for ½″ on each side of the pocket's opening edge, with thread ends tied. This method is often used on blouses.

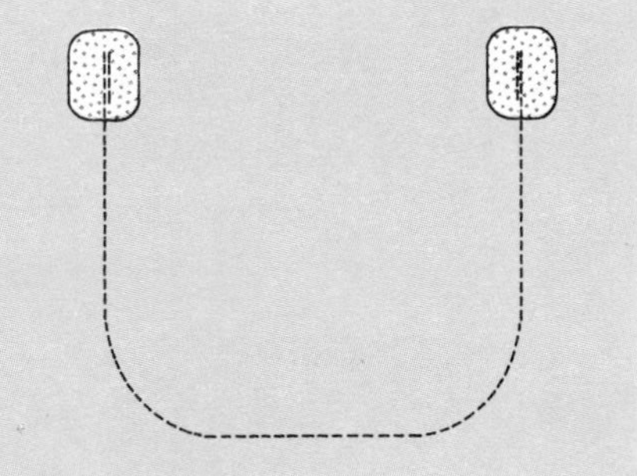

A patch of fabric or fusible interfacing, placed on the wrong side of garment under reinforcement stitching, adds strength.

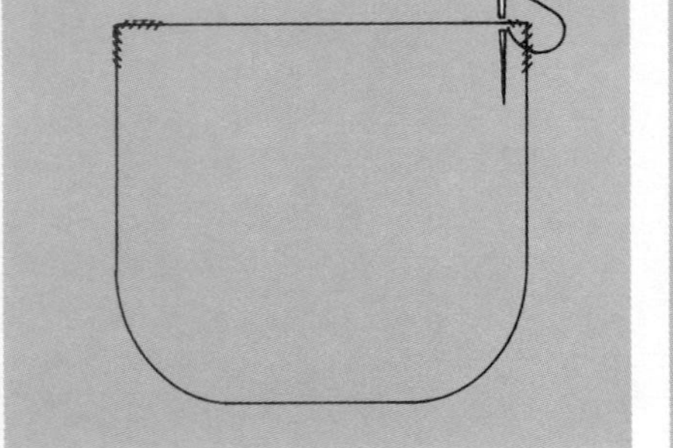

Hand reinforcement may be preferable. One method is to **whipstitch** invisibly for ¼″ on each side of top corners.

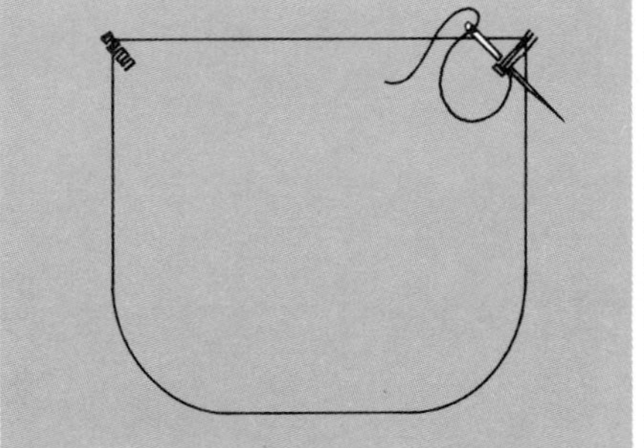

Another hand method is a **bar tack**—¼″-long straight stitches diagonally across corner with blanket stitches worked over them.

Patch pockets with flaps

In addition to such decorative devices as topstitching, patch pockets can be varied by means of flaps. These are finished, sometimes intricately shaped, additions that are free-hanging and located at the top of the pocket. There are two methods for constructing a flap. One is to cut an extra-deep pocket facing, which is turned back over itself to the right side to create a self-flap; the opening of the pocket is above the flap. In the second method, a separate flap is attached to the garment above the opening for the pocket, then pressed down over the opening.

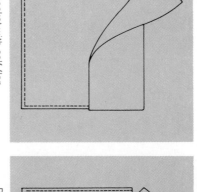

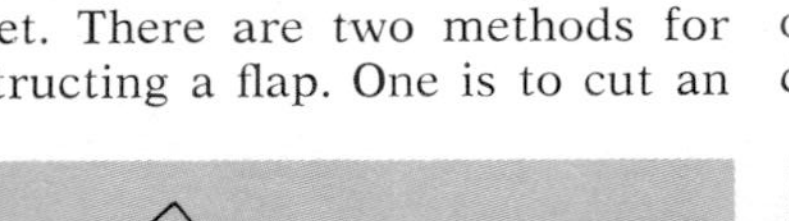

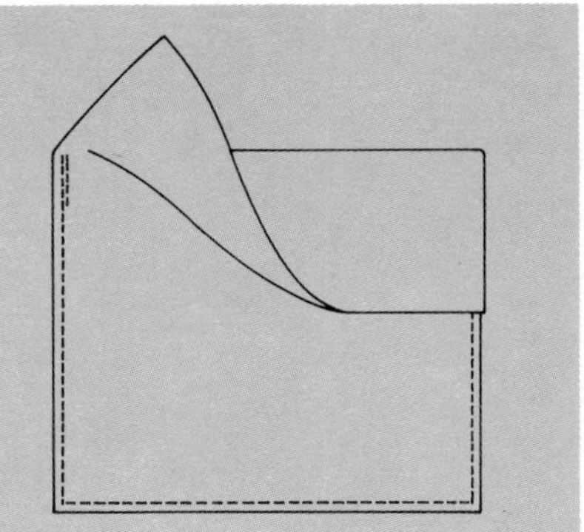

Patch pocket with self-flap

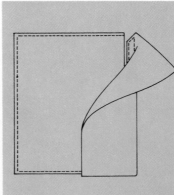

Patch pocket with separate flap

Patch pocket with self-flap

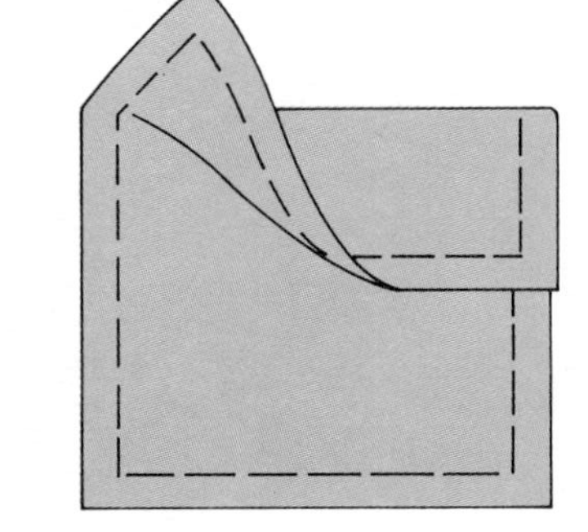

1. Using pattern, cut out the pocket and construct as for any lined or unlined patch pocket with facing. Hand-baste around entire pocket. Fold pocket top down to the right side along line marking depth of flap; press.

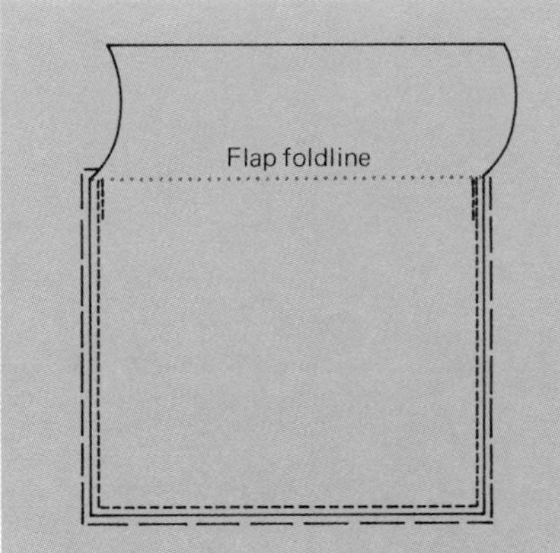

2. Attach pocket to the garment and reinforce corners as for a regular patch pocket, keeping flap up out of the way. Start and end stitching at the flap foldline. Remove all bastings; give pocket a final pressing.

Interfacing 72-73, 76-79
Fabric-marking methods 94
Slipstitch (uneven) 132
Reducing seam bulk 147

Patch pocket with separate flap

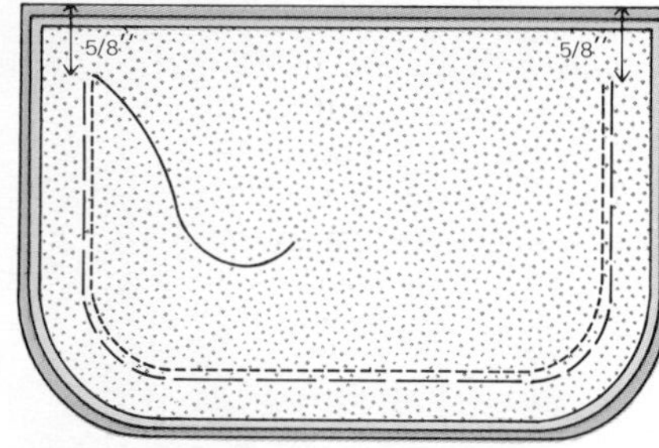

1. To construct flap, cut flap and facing from same pattern; interface flap. Pin flap to facing, right sides together, and stitch on seamline, starting and ending ⅝″ from base of flap. Press to embed stitching.

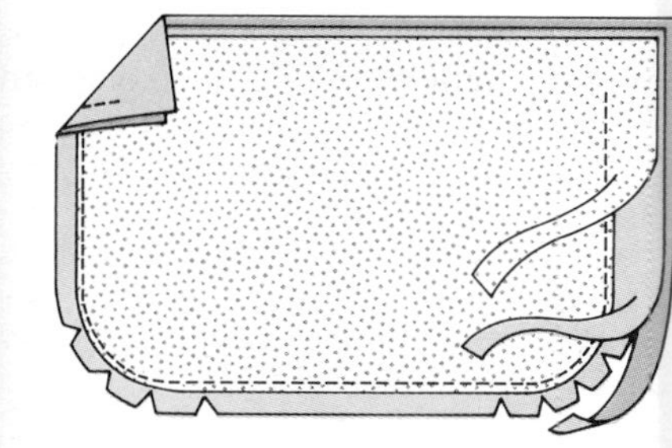

2. Trim and grade the seams; clip or notch curves if the flap has shaped or rounded corners. Interfacing should be trimmed away completely to seamline; the seam allowance of the flap should be left widest.

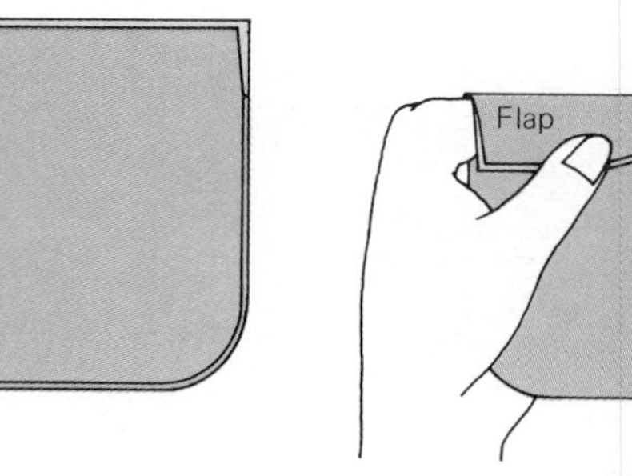

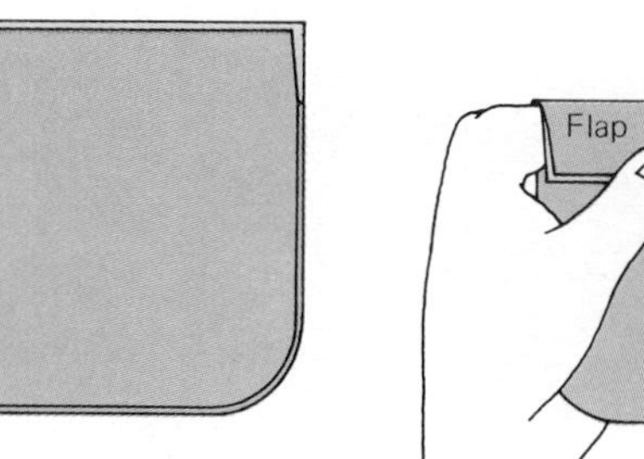

3. Turn flap right side out, easing seamed edge slightly to facing side so that seam will not show on finished flap. **If fabric is bulky,** roll seam allowances at top edge over your finger, with the flap side up, to get additional width from the flap seam allowance. This will help the flap to lie flat and prevent curling on lower edge. Pin, then hand-baste, across the opening a scant ⅝″ away from the raw edges. Carefully press the flap flat.

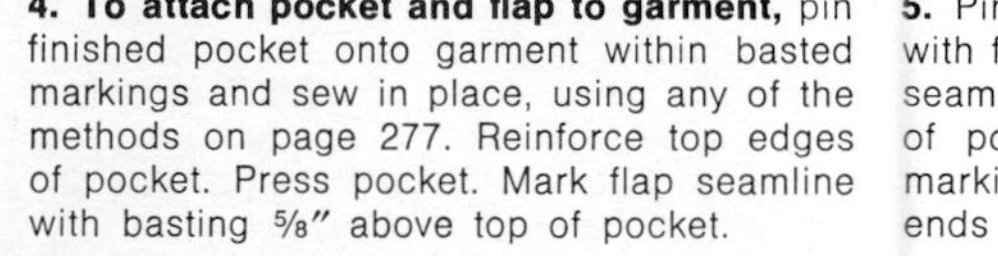

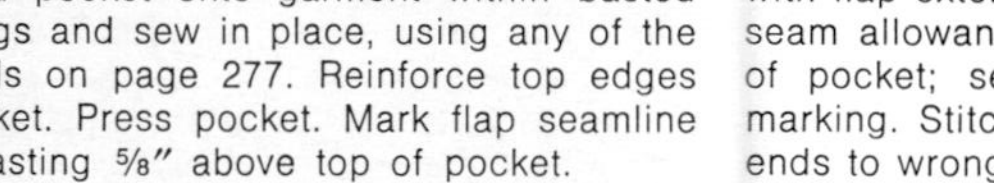

4. To attach pocket and flap to garment, pin finished pocket onto garment within basted markings and sew in place, using any of the methods on page 277. Reinforce top edges of pocket. Press pocket. Mark flap seamline with basting ⅝″ above top of pocket.

5. Pin flap to garment, right sides together, with flap extended away from pocket. Edge of seam allowances should be aligned with top of pocket; seamline of flap should be on marking. Stitch on flap seamline. Pull thread ends to wrong side of garment and tie.

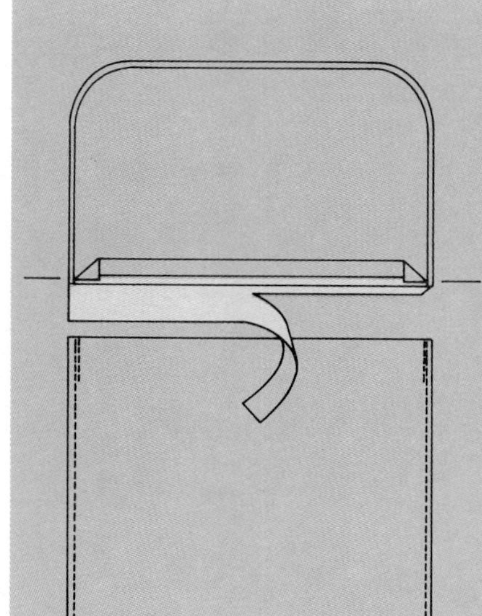

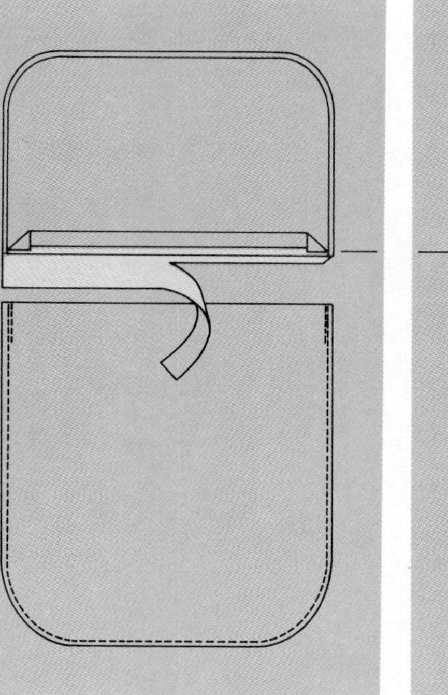

6. With the uppermost seam allowance of the flap held out of the way, carefully trim the lower seam allowance close to stitching. Fold under ¼″ on long edge of upper seam allowance and fold in the ends diagonally to eliminate all raw edges in finished flap.

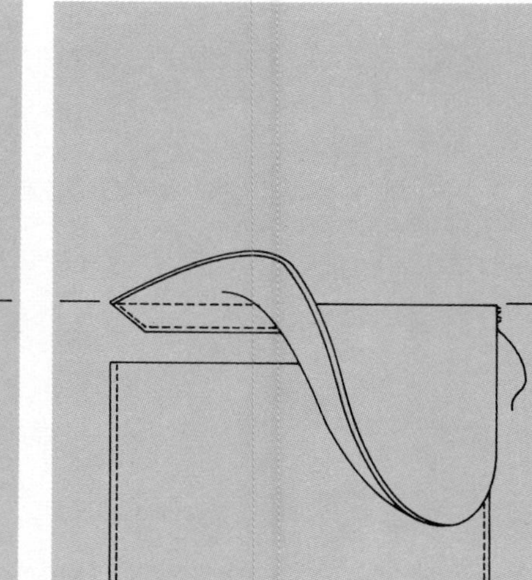

7. Pin upper seam allowance over the trimmed seam allowance and edgestitch around the ends and along the long side. Tie thread ends. Fold flap down over pocket and press. If necessary to hold flap flat, slipstitch the upper corners of the flap to the garment.

Inside pockets

Woven seam tape 16
Lining fabrics 72

In-seam pockets

Although all finished in-seam pockets look the same from the right side of the garment, they may be constructed in three different ways, depending on how the pattern is designed. In the **all-in-one** in-seam pocket, the pocket is part of the garment, so the two are cut as one and there is no seam at the opening of the pocket. The **separate** in-seam pocket is made up of separate pocket and garment pieces that are joined in the seamline to create the pocket. The **extension** in-seam pocket is made up of a separate pocket piece and a garment piece that has a small projection designed to extend into the pocket opening.

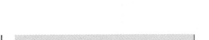

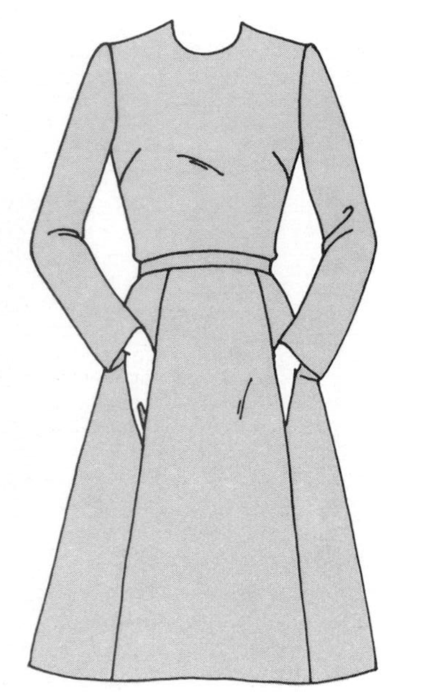

Because inside pockets generally receive a great deal of wear, the seam into which they are set must be reinforced with a stay to prevent stretching. Use a sturdy lining fabric for the pocket to reduce bulk.

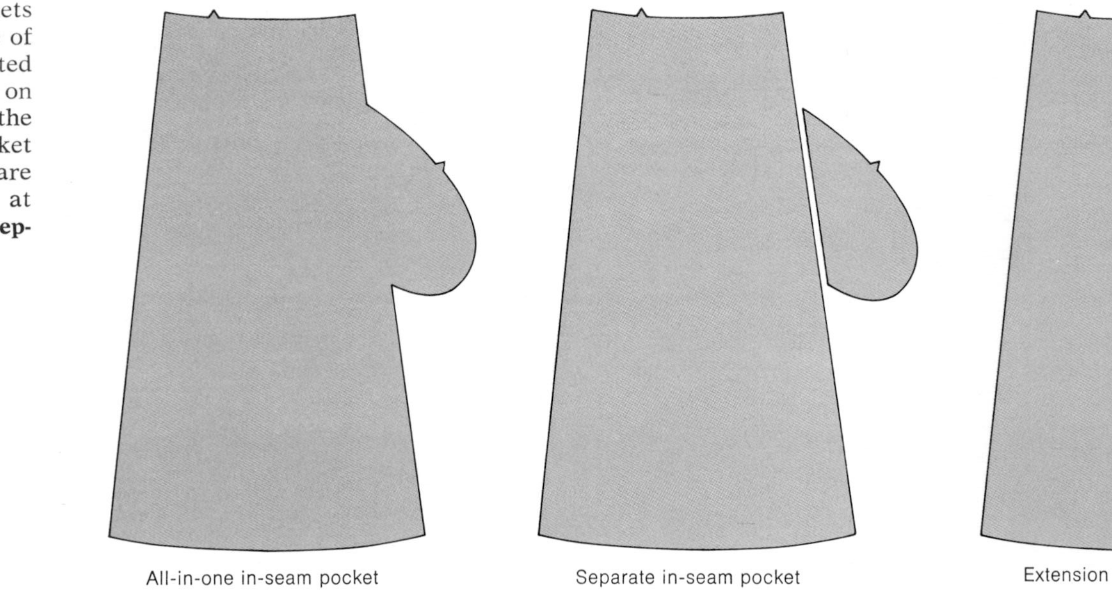

Reinforcing in-seam pockets

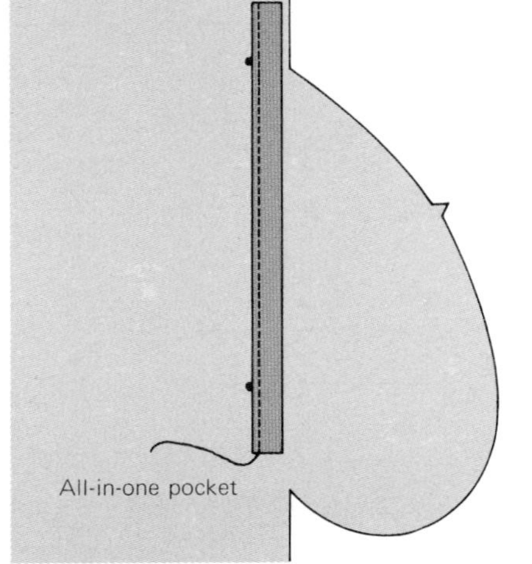

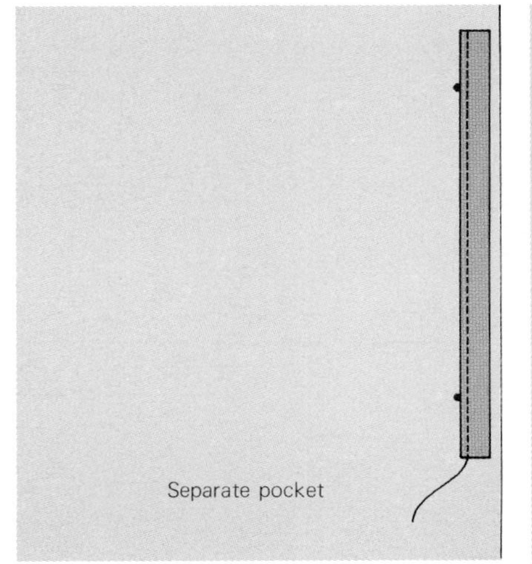

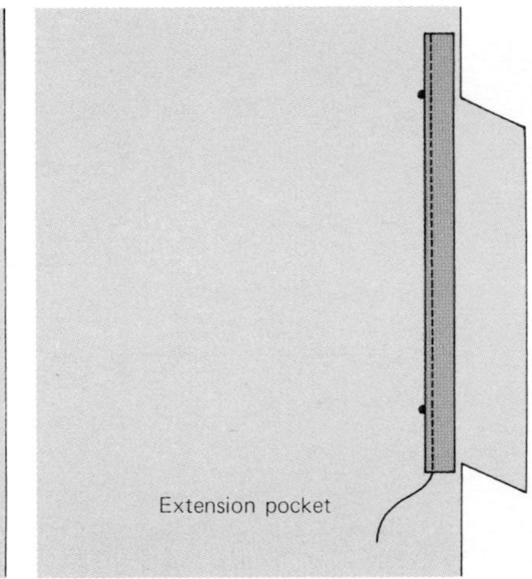

Seamline of front garment section must be reinforced before any in-seam pocket is sewed in, regardless of type. Cut a length of woven seam tape equal to the pocket opening plus 2″. Position tape on the *wrong* side of the pocket seamline, centering it next to the marks for the pocket opening. (Drawings show position for each pocket type.) One edge should be aligned with seamline; the width of the tape should be on the seam allowance or extension of garment. Baste, then stitch tape in place ⅛″ from edge nearest seamline.

All-in-one in-seam pocket

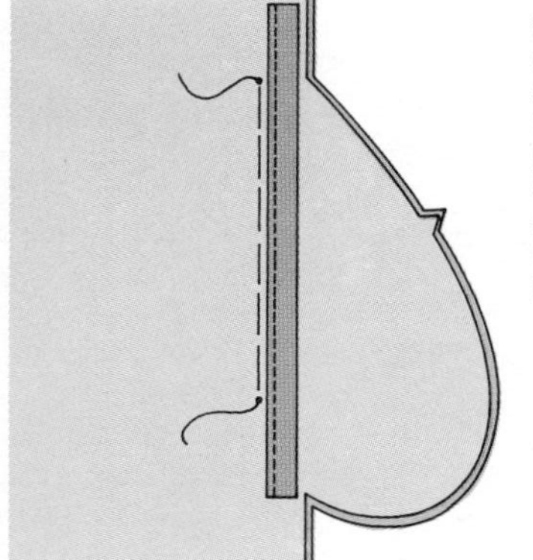

1. Reinforce garment front along pocket opening. With right sides together and markings matched, pin the front and back sections together along pocket opening. Baste by hand along pocket opening.

2. Pin and baste remaining part of seam together. Stitch pocket and seam in one continuous stitching, reinforcing corners of pocket with small stitches. Press flat to embed the stitches. Clip seam allowance of back section of garment at the corners and press open the garment seam allowances above and below the pocket.

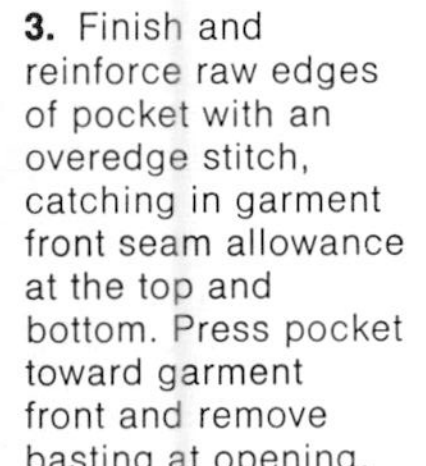

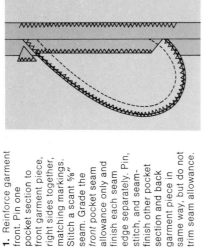

3. Finish and reinforce raw edges of pocket with an overedge stitch, catching in garment front seam allowance at the top and bottom. Press pocket toward garment front and remove basting at opening.

Separate in-seam pocket

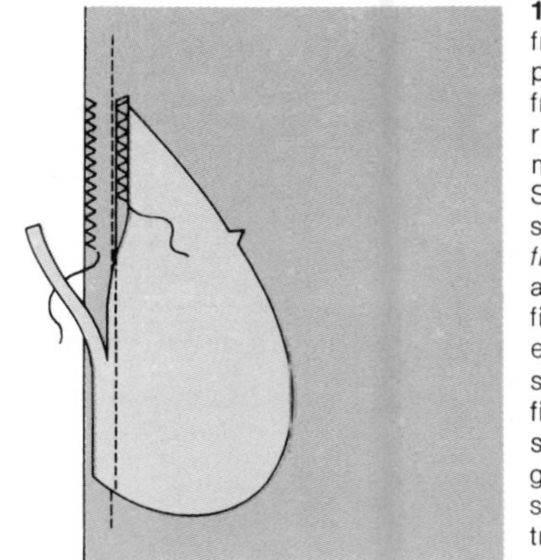

1. Reinforce garment front. Pin one pocket section to front garment piece, right sides together, matching markings. Stitch a scant 5/8″ seam. Grade the *front* pocket seam allowance only and finish each seam edge separately. Pin, stitch, and seam-finish other pocket section and back garment piece in same way, but do not trim seam allowance.

2. With right sides together and pockets extended, match markings and pin front and back sections together along pocket opening; hand-baste across opening. Pin and stitch side seams above and below pocket opening; reinforce with backstitches at pocket markings. Press flat.

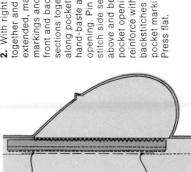

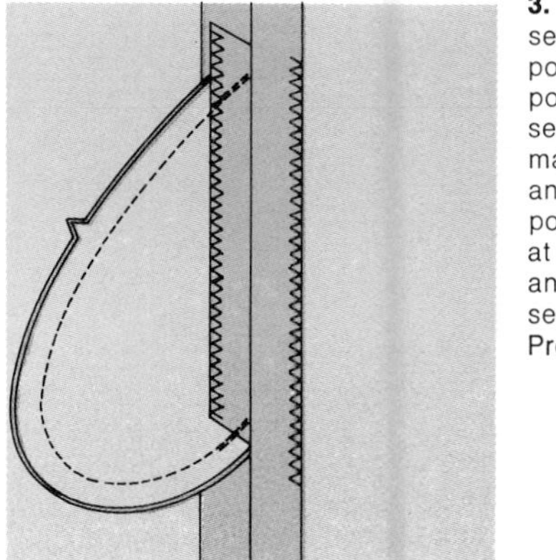

3. Press back pocket seams open and front pocket seams toward pocket. Pin pocket sections together, matching raw edges, and stitch around pocket, backstitching at pocket markings and catching front seam in stitching. Press flat.

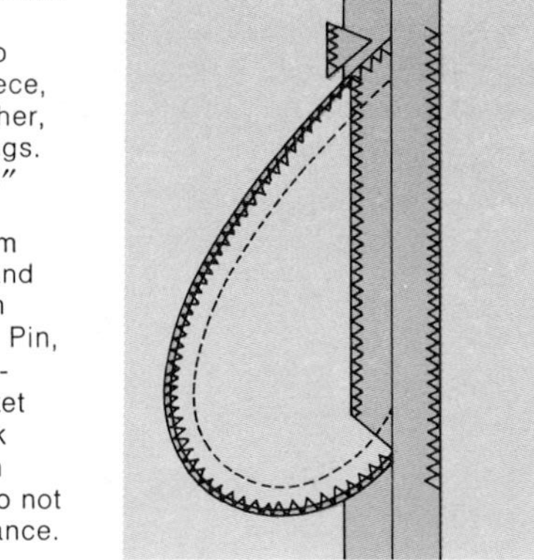

4. Seam-finish edges of pocket together, using the same stitch as on seam allowances. Catch front seam allowance into the seam-finishing at top and bottom of pocket. Press pocket toward garment front and remove basting from opening. Trim off point of pocket at top.

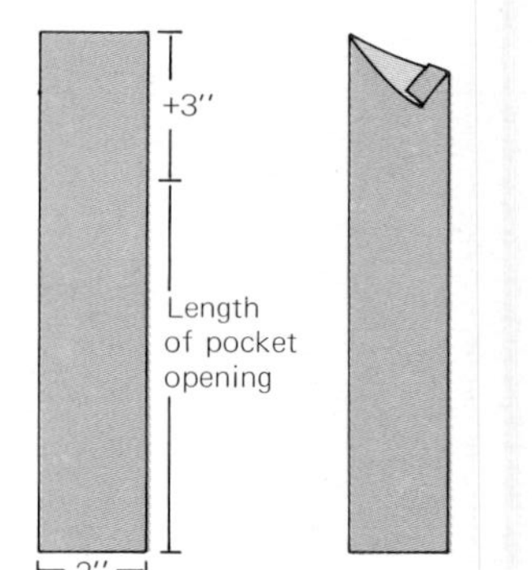

Adding a facing to the opening edge of the pocket will keep any of the pocket fabric from showing if pocket gaps open. **1.** Cut two strips of garment fabric on the straight grain, each measuring 2″ wide by the length of the pocket opening plus 3″. Turn under and press 1/4″ to the wrong side on one long edge of each facing strip.

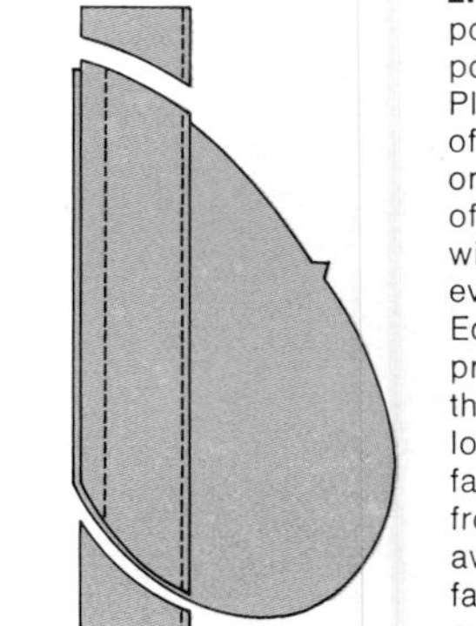

2. Apply facing to pocket before sewing pocket into garment. Place wrong side of each facing on the right side of each pocket piece, with the raw edges even at opening. Edgestitch along pressed-under edge, then stitch other long edge of pocket facing to pocket 1/2″ from raw edge. Trim away excess facing fabric at top and bottom of pocket.

Uneven basting 124
Cornered seams 146
Seam finishes 148-149

Extension in-seam pocket

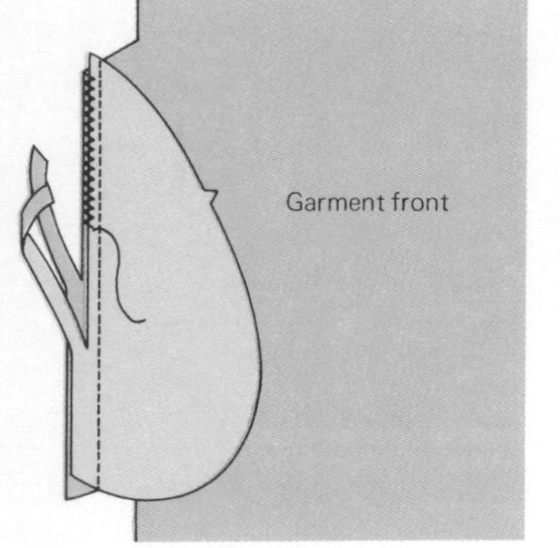

1. Reinforce garment front along pocket opening. Pin and stitch one pocket section to front garment piece, right sides together, matching markings and having raw edges even. Press flat. Trim seam to ¼" and overcast edges together.

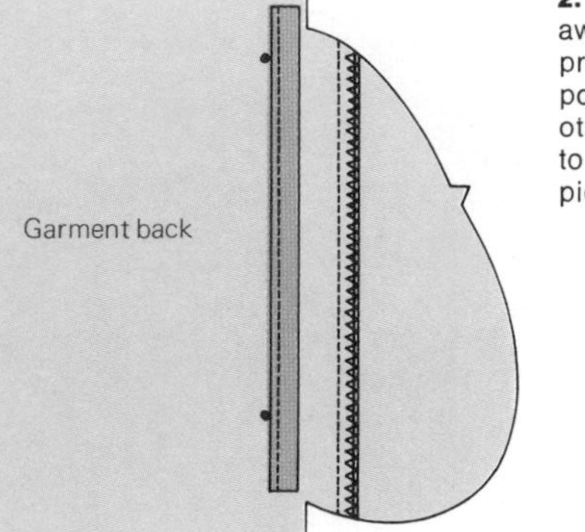

2. With pocket extended away from garment, press seam toward the pocket. Pin and stitch other pocket section to back garment piece as for front.

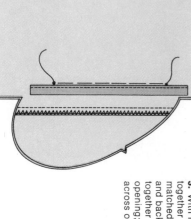

3. With right sides together and all markings matched, pin the front and back sections together along pocket opening; hand-baste across opening.

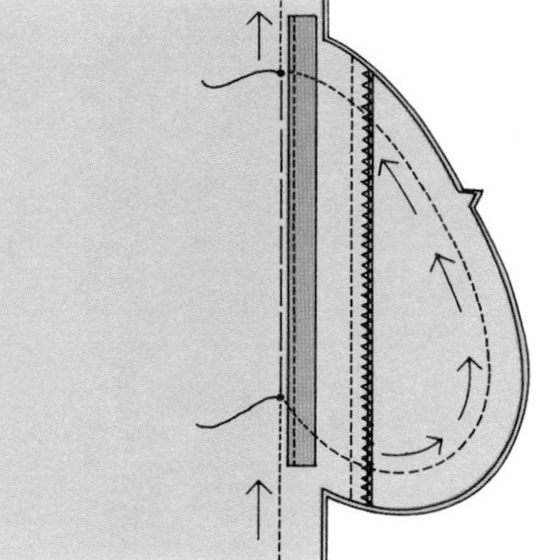

4. Pin and baste remainder of side and pocket seam together and stitch in one continuous seam, reinforcing the corners with small stitches.

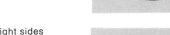

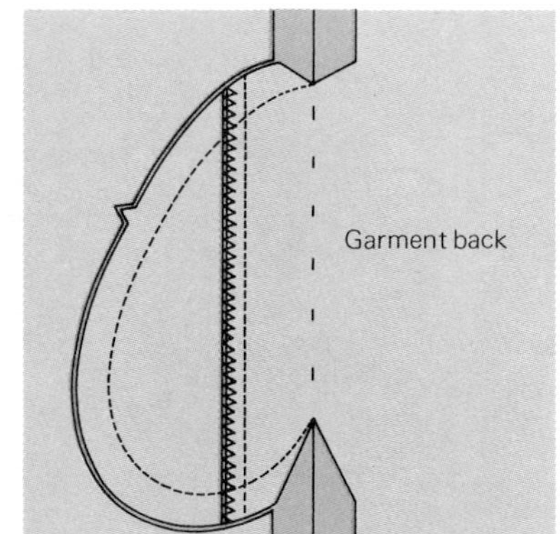

5. Press flat to embed stitches. Clip seam allowance of back garment section to corner and press seam open above and below the pocket.

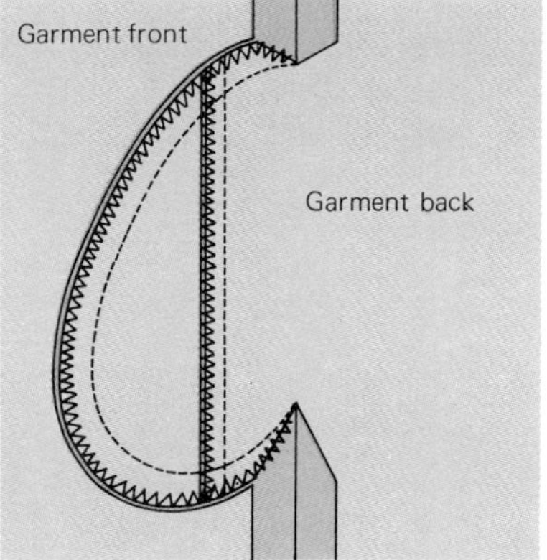

6. Seam-finish edges of pocket together, using the same stitch as on the pocket seam allowance edges. Catch in the garment front seam allowance at the top and bottom. Press pocket toward garment front and remove basting at opening.

Front-hip pockets

Front-hip pockets are attached to the garment at the waist and side seams and must be included in any waist or hip alterations made in the garment. Although these hip pockets can vary greatly in shape and detailing along the opening edge, they are all made up of two pattern pieces, a pocket piece and a facing piece. The shapes of the two are never the same because the facing piece finishes off the pocket opening, while the pocket piece becomes part of the main garment at the waistline. The pocket piece must be cut of fashion fabric, but lining fabric may be used for the facing.

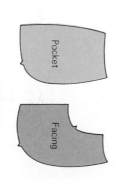

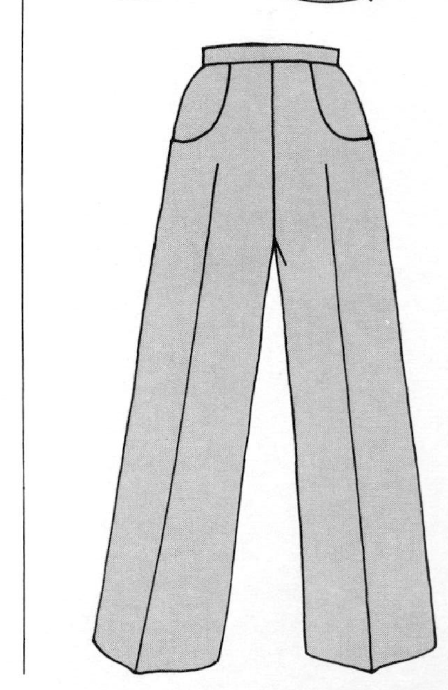

Interfacing selection and application 72-73, 76-79
Understitching, topstitching 143
Reducing seam bulk 147

Construction of front-hip pocket

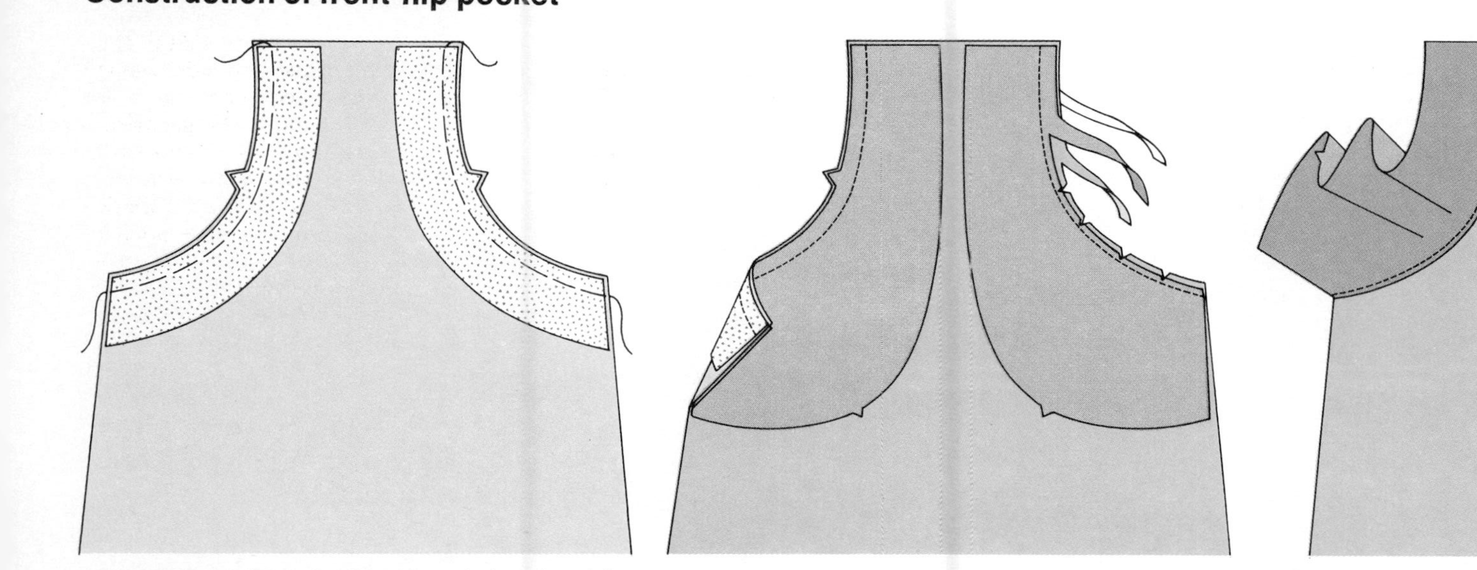

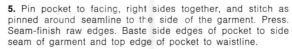

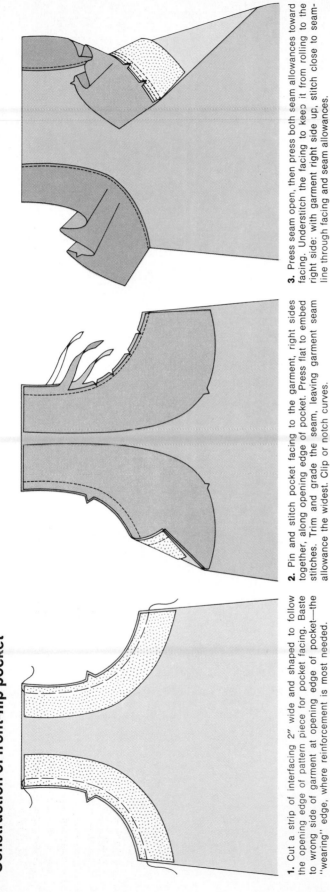

1. Cut a strip of interfacing 2" wide and shaped to follow the opening edge of pattern piece for pocket facing. Baste to wrong side of garment at opening edge of pocket—the "wearing" edge, where reinforcement is most needed.

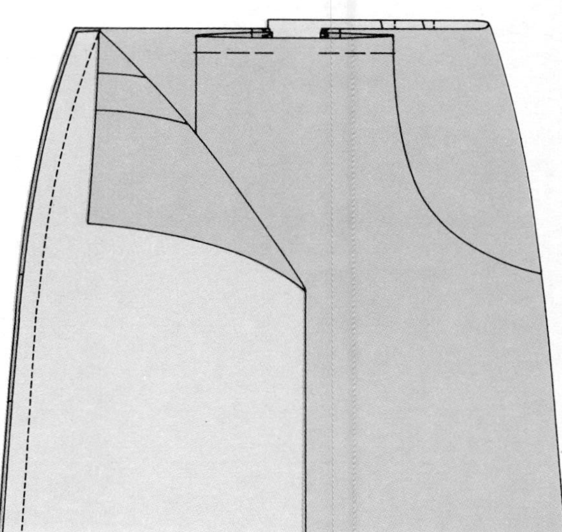

2. Pin and stitch pocket facing to the garment, right sides together, along opening edge of pocket. Press flat to embed stitches. Trim and grade the seam, leaving garment seam allowance the widest. Clip or notch curves.

3. Press seam open, then press both seam allowances toward facing. Understitch the facing to keep it from rolling to the right side: with garment right side up, stitch close to seamline through facing and seam allowances.

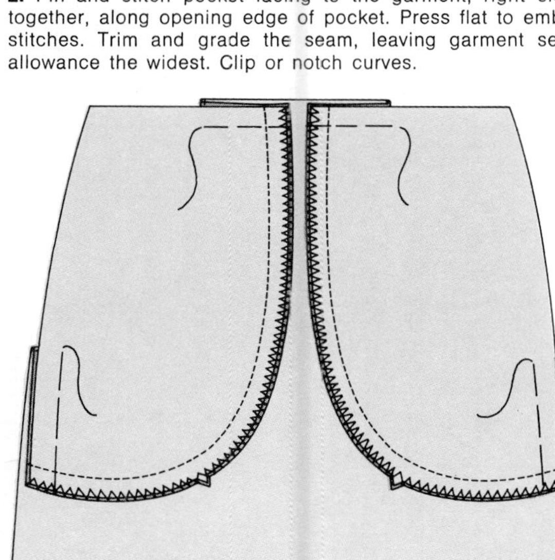

4. Turn facings to inside along seamline and press. Baste around curved edge. If topstitching is desired for a decorative effect, apply it now. (Flaps, if being used, should be made and basted in place before facing is applied.)

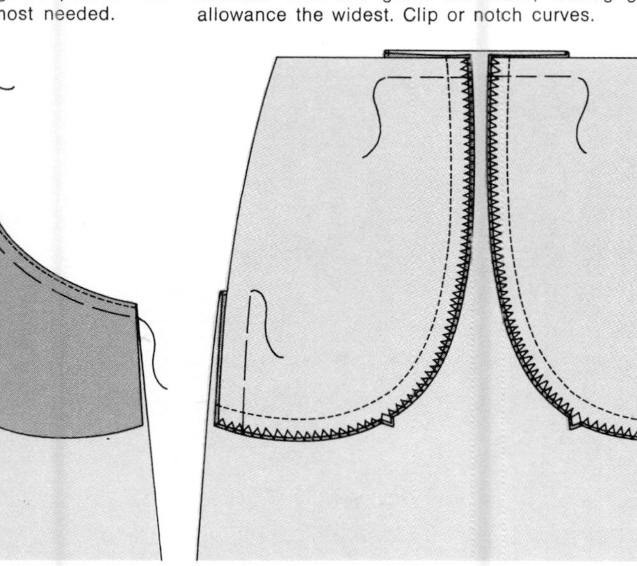

5. Pin pocket to facing, right sides together, and stitch as pinned around seamline to the side of the garment. Press. Seam-finish raw edges. Baste side edges of pocket to side seam of garment and top edge of pocket to waistline.

6. Pin together and stitch side seams of garment, catching in pocket and facing seams. Press seams flat, then open. Treat the upper part of the pocket as part of the waistline seam when applying bodice or waistband.

Inside pockets

Slashed pockets

There are three types of slashed pockets, which differ only in the way the pocket opening is finished. When the pocket acts as a finish, the result is a **bound** pocket, which looks like a large bound buttonhole. A second method is with a **flap,** which covers the pocket after insertion into the upper edge of the slash. Flaps are usually, but not necessarily, rectangular. The third finish, a **welt,** is a rectangular piece, cut separately or as a part of the pocket, that fits over the pocket opening and is sewed into the lower edge of the slash. (A variation is a double welt—one at each edge of the slash.) The three finishes may be used together in almost any combination.

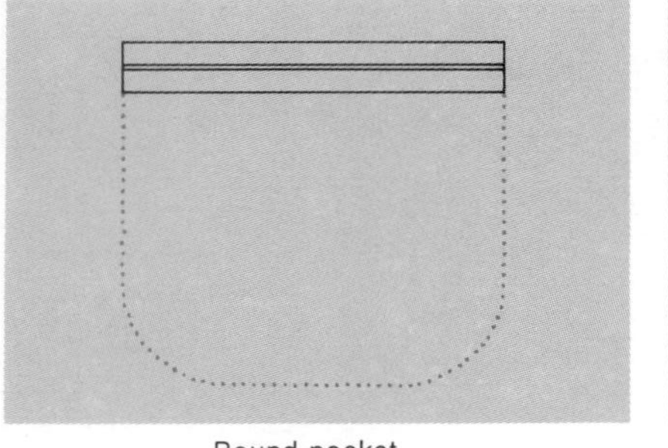

Bound pocket

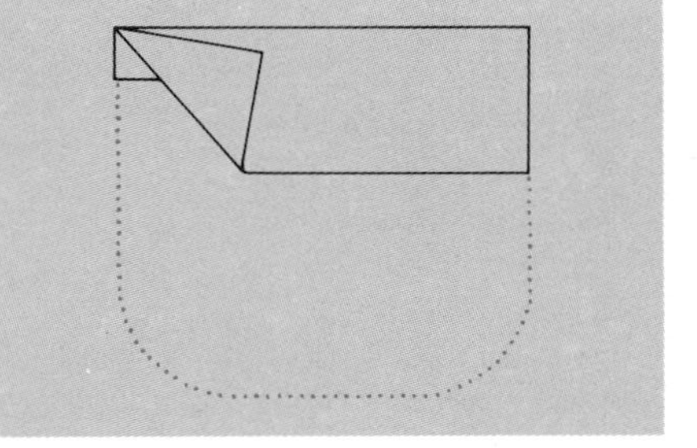

Pocket with flap on top edge

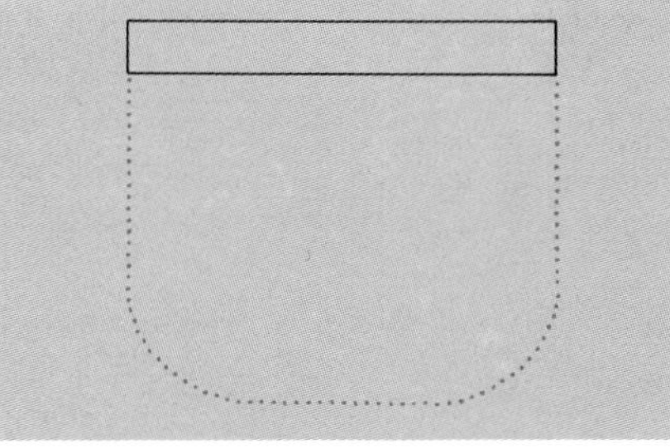

Single welt pocket

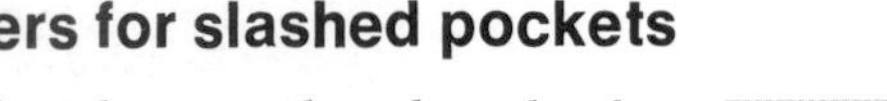

Pointers for slashed pockets

Slashed pockets are thought to be the most difficult of the inside pockets to construct. Actually, they are only a matter of precise marking and exact stitching, combined with very careful cutting. Construction is very much like that of a bound buttonhole, although the finished result is much larger. The pocket back and front are not joined until they have been attached to the opening edge, which is the slash in the garment. The seams of the pocket itself are then formed.

Carefully thread-trace the opening for the pocket on the right side of the garment, using a very small hand stitch. Be sure markings are exactly on grain (unless the pockets are diagonally placed) and that center and stitching lines are exactly parallel. All permanent machine stitching should be done with a very short stitch. Press carefully at each step of construction; a final pressing by itself is not sufficient to set sharp edges.

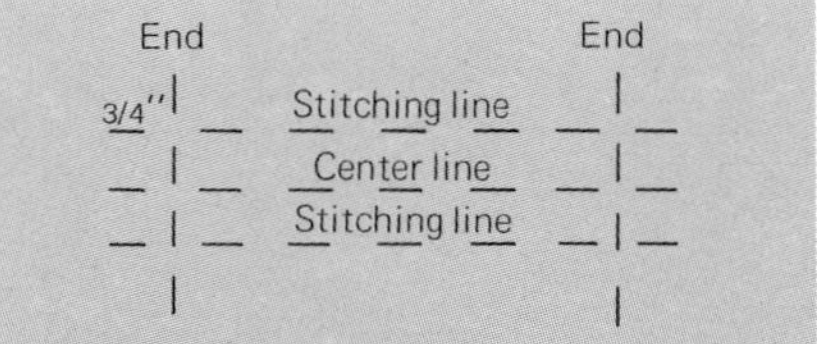

Baste across ends to mark *width* of opening, then through center line and on parallel stitching lines to mark *depth* of opening; extend marks about ¾" beyond the actual limits. Be sure lines are on-grain and parallel.

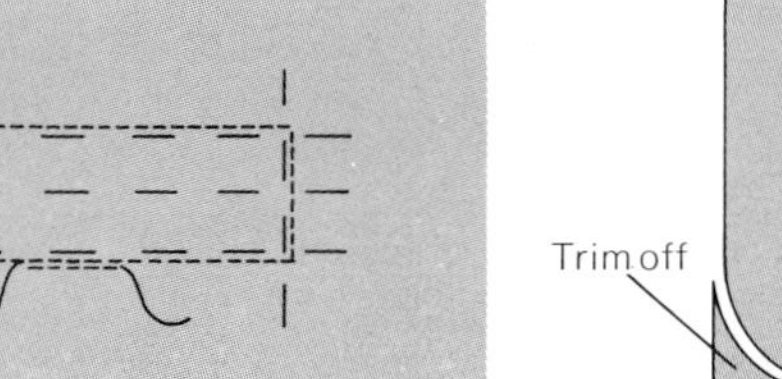

Stitch rectangle precisely for any type of slashed pocket. Begin stitching at center of one side and pivot at corners. Take same number of stitches across each end; overlap stitches at starting point to secure.

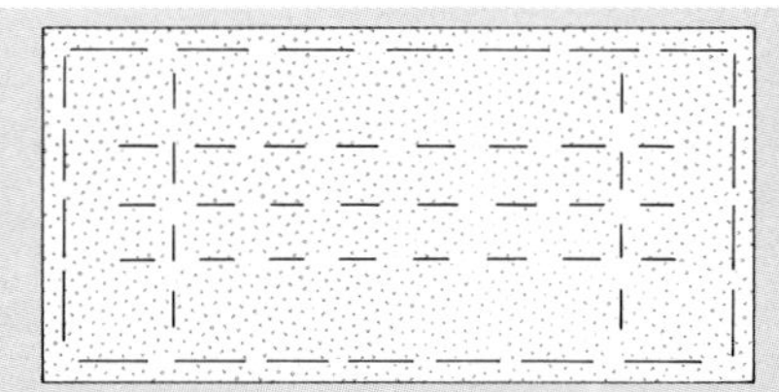

If garment fabric is lightweight or loosely woven, add a stay of lightweight interfacing for stability and crispness. Cut it about 4" long and 2" wider than opening; center it behind pocket opening and baste in place.

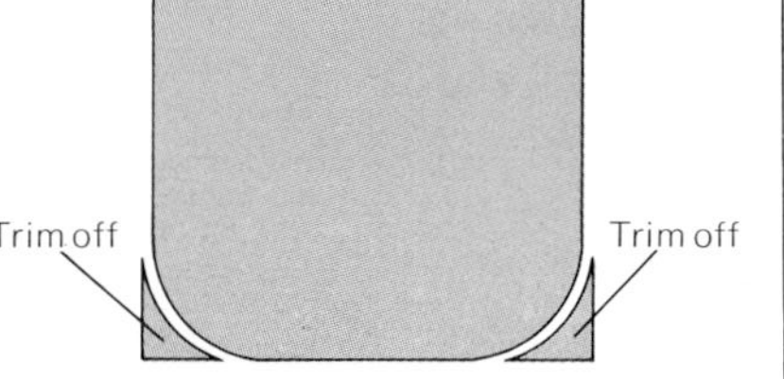

Curve pocket corners if they are square on the pattern, to prevent any lint buildup in the pocket from repeated wearings and washings. Instead of pivoting when stitching the pocket, simply round the corners off.

Bound pockets

Bound pockets are those in which the pocket itself is used to finish off, or bind, the edges of the slash in the garment. From the right side of the garment, the pocket looks like a large bound buttonhole. Although lining fabric is generally recommended for inside pockets, in this pocket type the pocket fabric will show on the outside, so the garment fabric is preferable for the purpose.

When the pocket is completed, arrowhead tacks may be worked at each end for a tailored look (see Hand stitches). Check any pattern you plan to use to be sure that the pocket pieces meet the specifications below. If they do not, alter them to conform.

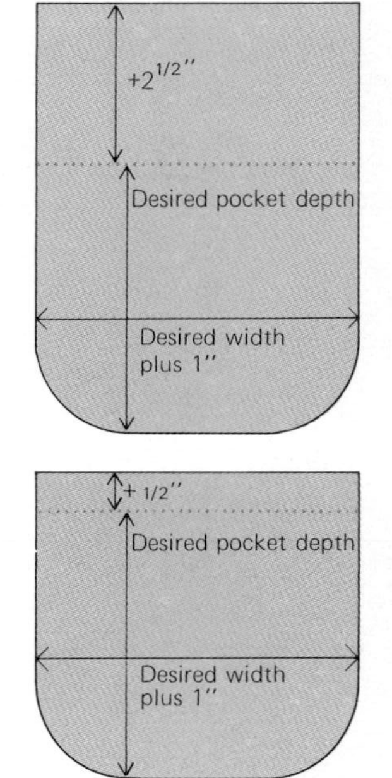

Pieces for bound pocket: This pocket type requires two pocket sections. The first should measure desired pocket depth plus 2½"; the second, pocket depth plus ½". Cutting width of both: desired width plus 1" for side seams.

Constructing bound pockets

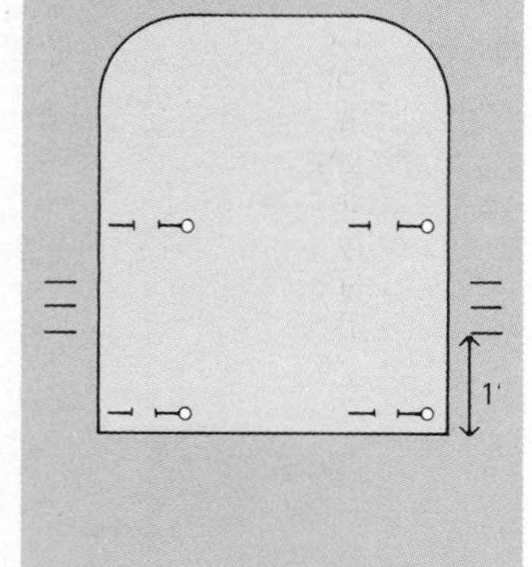

1. With right sides together, pin the long pocket section over pocket markings on garment, with straight (top) edge of pocket 1" below the lower marked stitching line.

2. Turn garment side up for stitching. Following basted markings, stitch a rectangle as shown on preceding page. Slash through all thicknesses between stitching lines; stop ½" before ends and slash diagonally into the four corners.

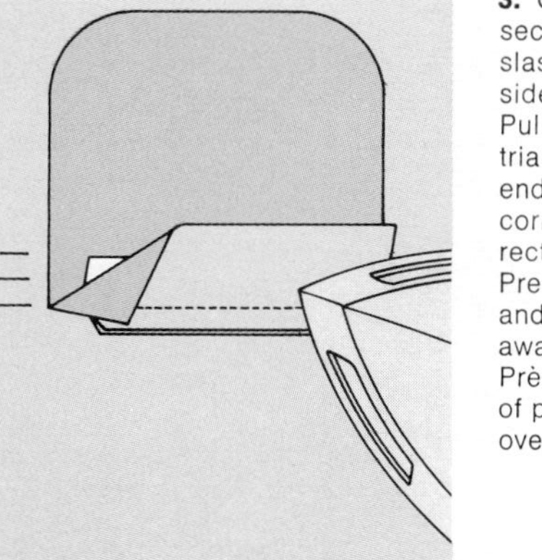

3. Gently push pocket section through slash to the wrong side of the garment. Pull on the small triangles at each end to square the corners of the rectangular opening. Press triangular ends and seam allowances away from the opening. Press straight end of pocket up over the opening.

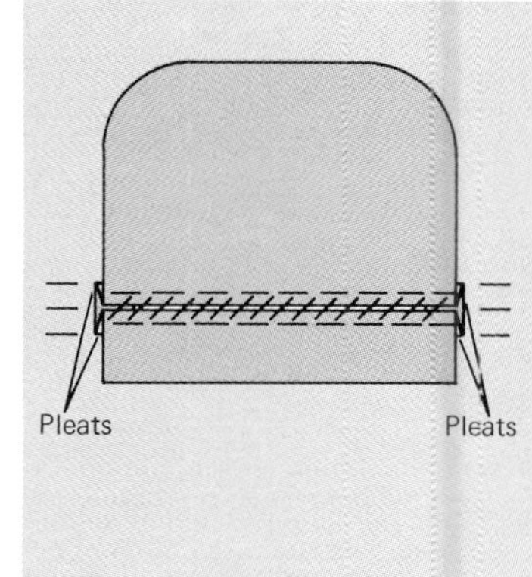

4. Fold pocket to form even pleats that meet in the center of the opening. Check from the right side to make sure that the pleats (or "lips") are equal in depth to one another across the entire width of the pocket. Baste through folded edges and whipstitch lips together. Remove the basted markings from garment.

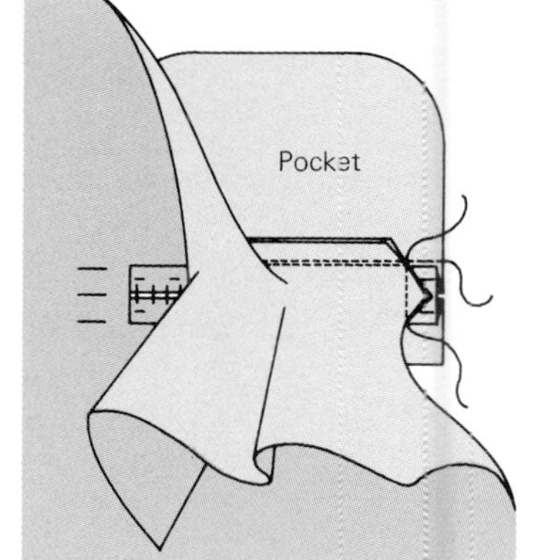

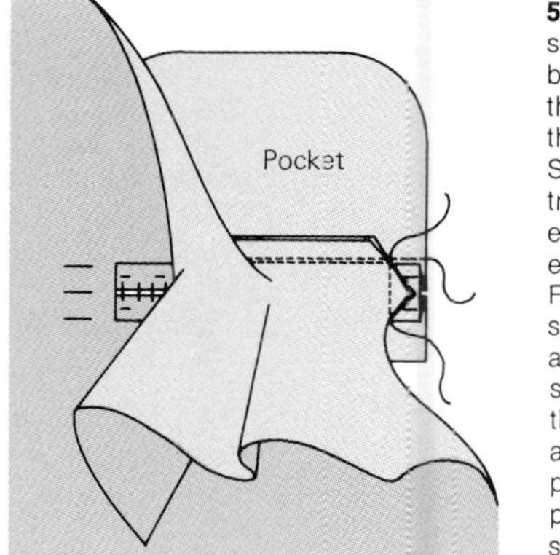

5. Turn garment right side up and flip back garment so that the side edge of the pocket is exposed. Stitch over the triangle and the ends of the lips at each side of pocket. Fold garment down so that top seam allowance of opening shows and stitch through the seam allowances and the pocket, as close as possible to first stitching.

6. Slip remaining pocket section under one sewed to garment and pin along outer edges. Flip garment up so that bottom seam allowance of opening is exposed and stitch through seam allowance and both pocket sections.

7. Turn garment to wrong side. Unpin pocket edges and turn lower pocket section down. Press in place.

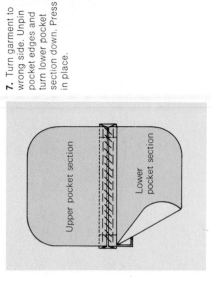

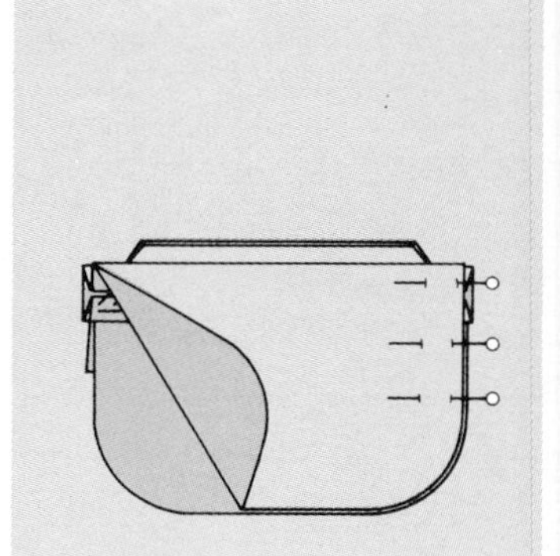
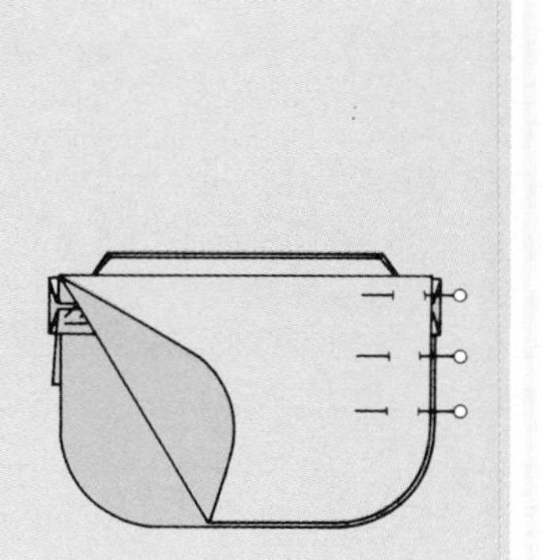

8. Turn upper pocket section down; bottom raw edges of both sections should be even. If they are not, trim them to the same length. Pin sections together.

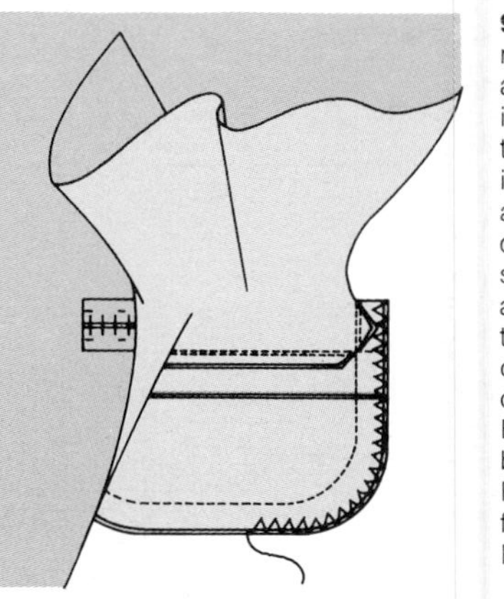

9. Turn garment to right side again and fold garment in such a way that side of pocket is exposed. Stitch around pinned pocket on the seamline, starting at the top and stitching across triangular ends as close as possible to original stitching. Backstitch at beginning and ends. Press flat. Seam-finish outer raw edges. Remove all bastings.

Inside pockets

Interfacing 72-73, 76-79

Flap and separate welt pockets

In these two pockets, either a flap or a welt is completely constructed, then attached to one of the seam allowances of the pocket opening. The **flap** is attached to the top seam allowance, the **welt** to the bottom one. This is the only difference in the construction of the two pockets.

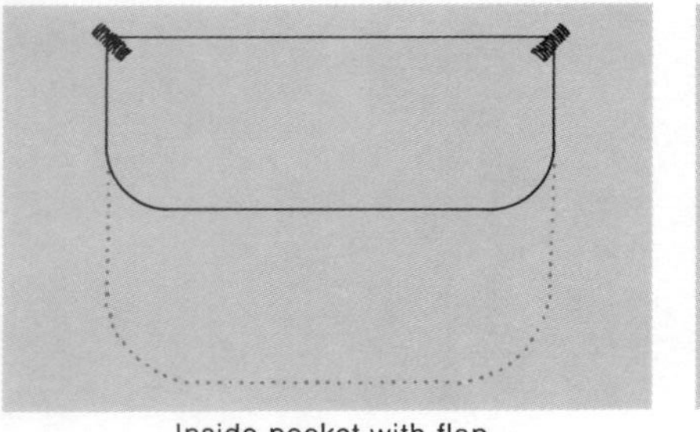

Inside pocket with flap

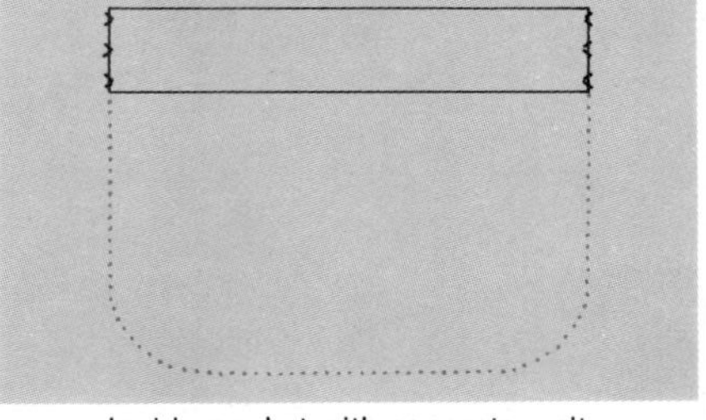

Inside pocket with separate welt

Making the flap or welt

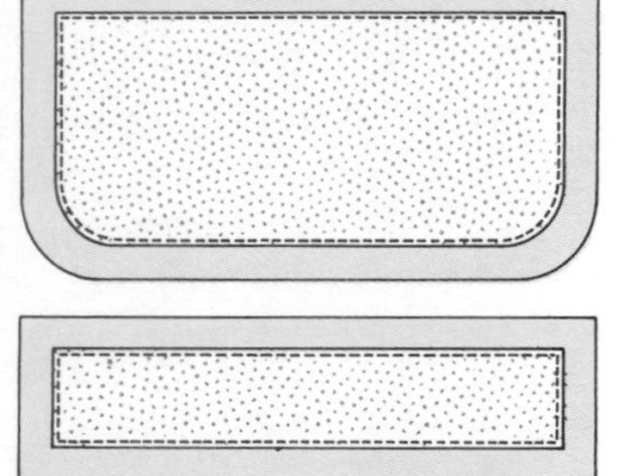

1. Cut welt or flap and its facing from pattern and interface wrong side of welt or flap. Trim interfacing seam allowance.

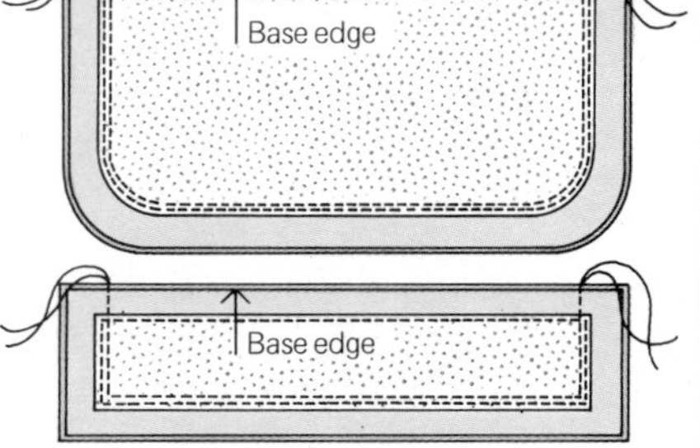

2. Pin welt or flap to facing, right sides together, and stitch around marked seamline, leaving base edge open. Press flat.

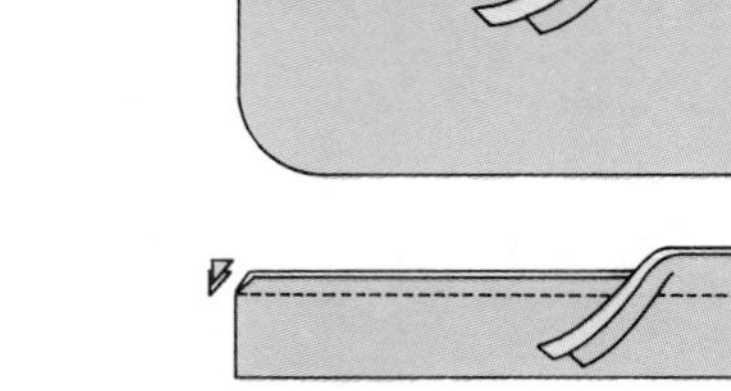

3. Trim and grade seam; clip or notch curves if corners are rounded. Turn and press, easing the facing under slightly.

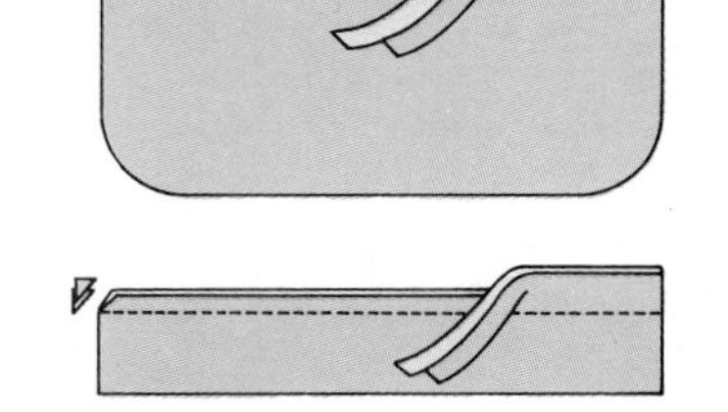

4. Trim base edge to ¼″. Machine-stitch a scant ¼″ from raw edge to hold layers together. Trim across corners diagonally.

Making the pocket

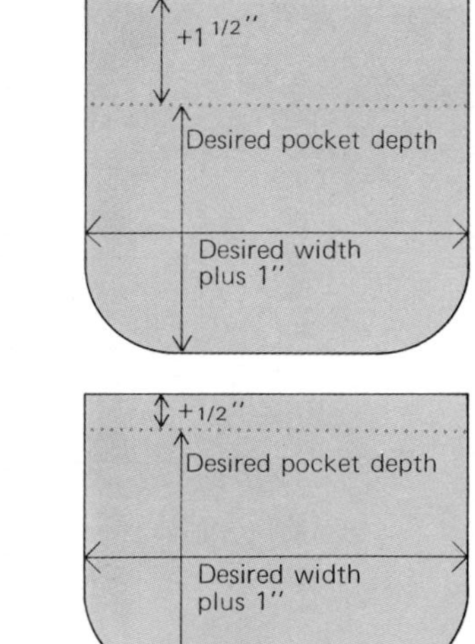

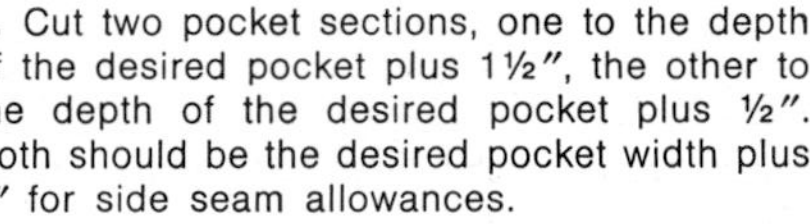

1. Cut two pocket sections, one to the depth of the desired pocket plus 1½″, the other to the depth of the desired pocket plus ½″. Both should be the desired pocket width plus 1″ for side seam allowances.

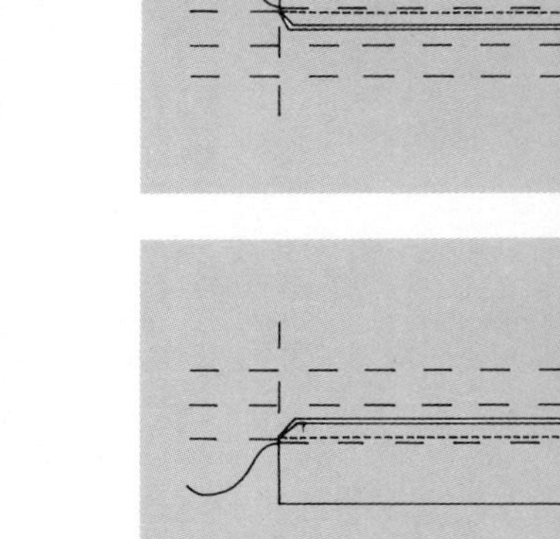

2. Baste right side of welt or flap to right side of garment over pocket markings. If a flap is being used, the seamline of flap should align with **upper** stitch line; if a welt is used, match its seamline to **lower** stitch line.

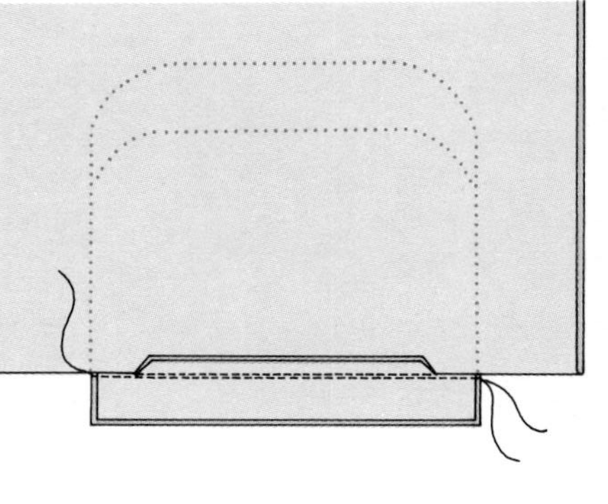

7. With garment right side up, flip up garment to expose pocket edge. Slip remaining pocket section under opening, right side up, matching raw edges of pocket sections; pin. Stitch, as shown, on first stitch line.

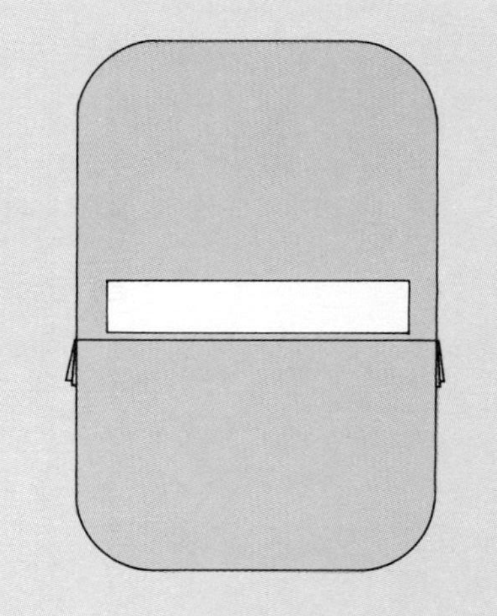

8. Press seam allowance of the opening back away from opening, then turn garment to the wrong side and bring down lower pocket section. Press flat. One edge of pocket is now completely finished.

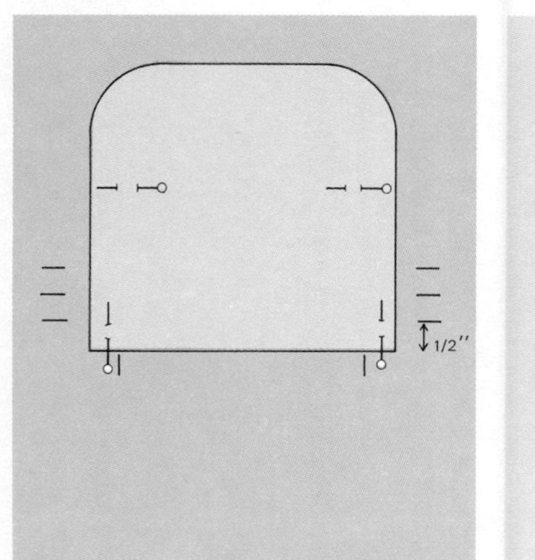

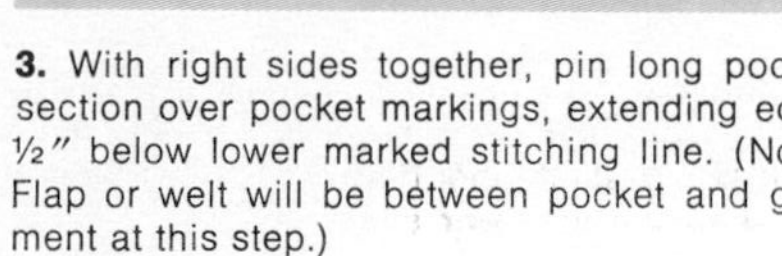

3. With right sides together, pin long pocket section over pocket markings, extending edge ½" below lower marked stitching line. (Note: Flap or welt will be between pocket and garment at this step.)

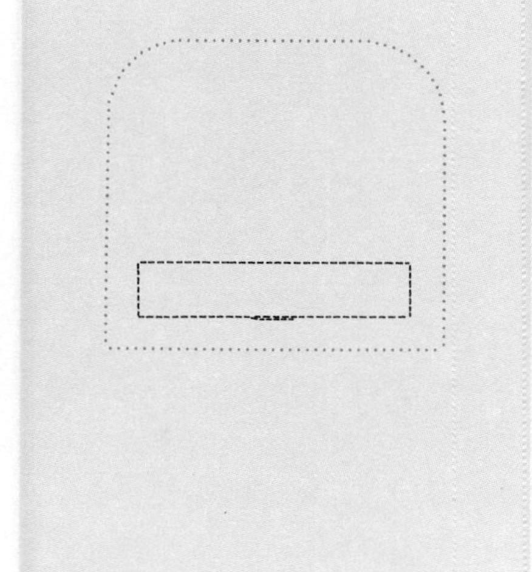

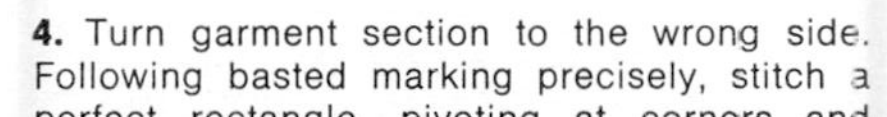

4. Turn garment section to the wrong side. Following basted marking precisely, stitch a perfect rectangle, pivoting at corners and overlapping stitching on one long side. Remove all bastings.

5. Very carefully slash through all the thicknesses at center of rectangle; stop ½" before ends and cut diagonally into the four corners, forming small triangles at each end. Do not cut into stitching.

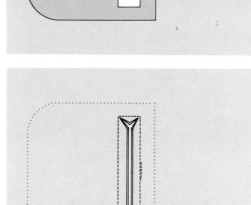

6. Gently push pocket through slash to wrong side. Turn a flap *down* over opening; turn a welt *up.* Pull on small triangles to square corners of opening. Press triangles and seam allowances away from opening.

9. Turn the upper pocket section down over the opening. Bottom raw edge of both pocket sections should be even. If they are not, trim them to the same length. Pin sections together, taking care not to catch garment.

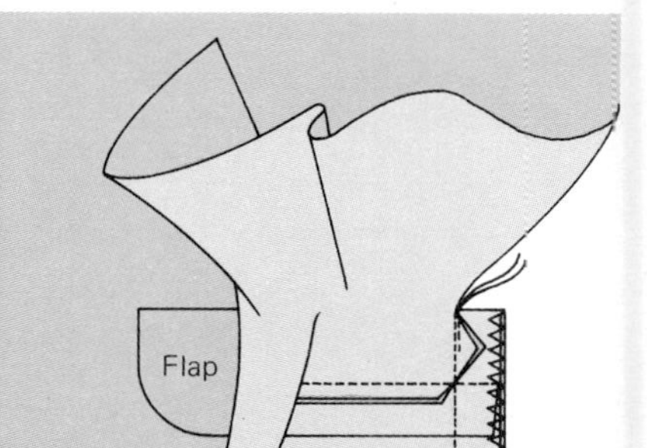

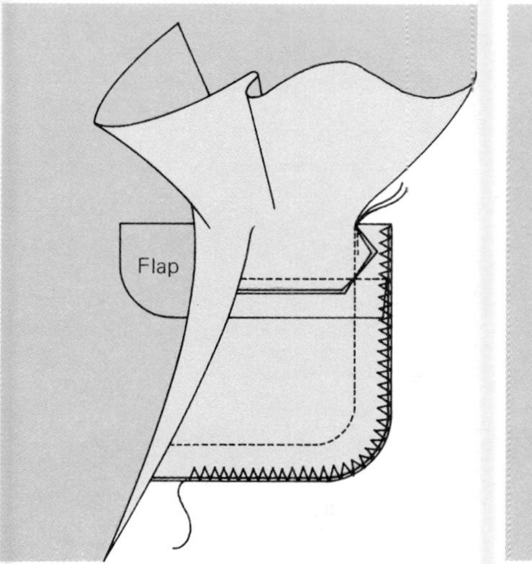

10. Turn garment right side up. A **flap** (see above) should be in a downward position, pocket opening completely covered. A **welt** (above right) will point upward and also cover pocket opening. Flip garment back so pocket is exposed. Stitch around pinned pocket, starting at top. Stitch across triangle ends as close as possible to original stitching; backstitch at beginning and end. Press flat. Seam-finish outer edge of pocket.

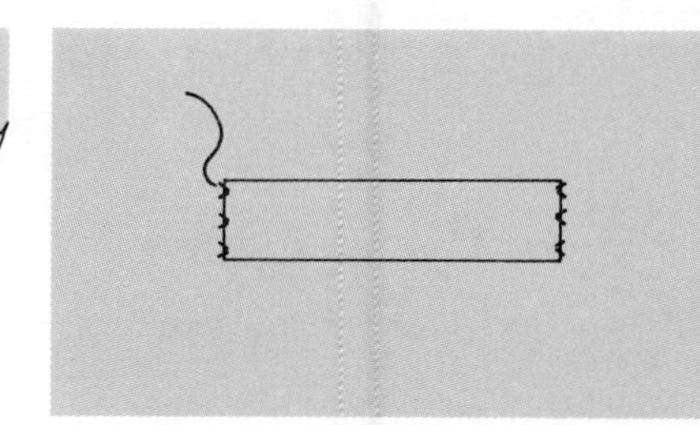

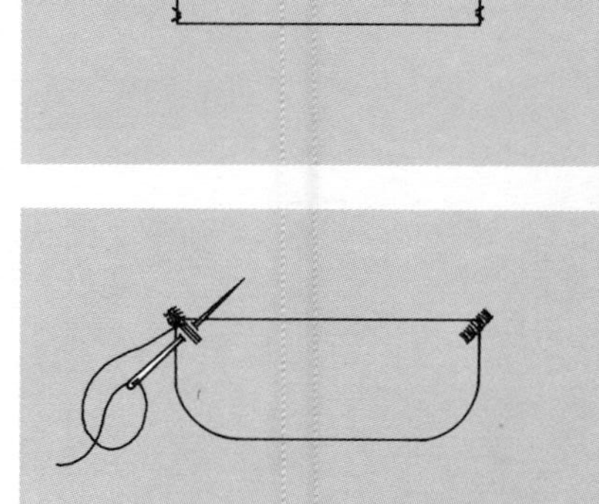

11. To finish off the **welt** pocket (top), slipstitch ends of the welt invisibly to garment. This will hold the welt in an upright position. To finish the **flap,** make a tiny bar tack by hand to hold the flap down.

Inside pockets

Self-welt or stand pocket

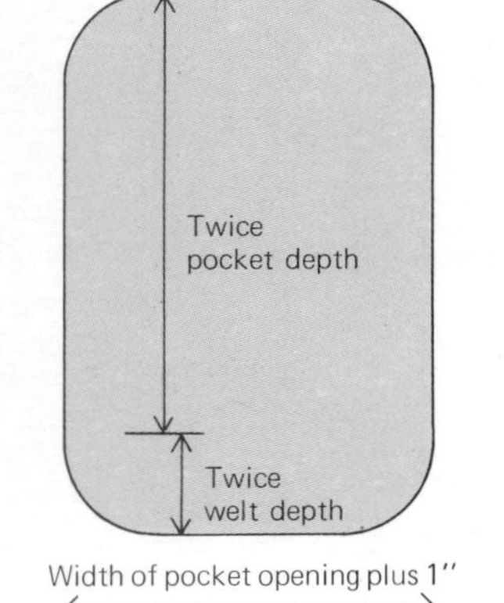

In this method, a welt is formed of pocket fabric during pocket construction.
1. Cut pocket from garment fabric on the lengthwise grain. Pocket length should be twice the desired depth of the finished pocket plus twice the desired depth of the welt; pocket width should equal that of the pocket opening plus 1″ for side seam allowances.

2. Fold pocket in half horizontally and press in a crease at the fold. With right sides together, pin pocket section to the garment, aligning crease with marked lower stitching line.

3. Turn garment to wrong side. Following basted guidelines, stitch around pocket, forming a perfect rectangle (see p.284). Remove basted markings.

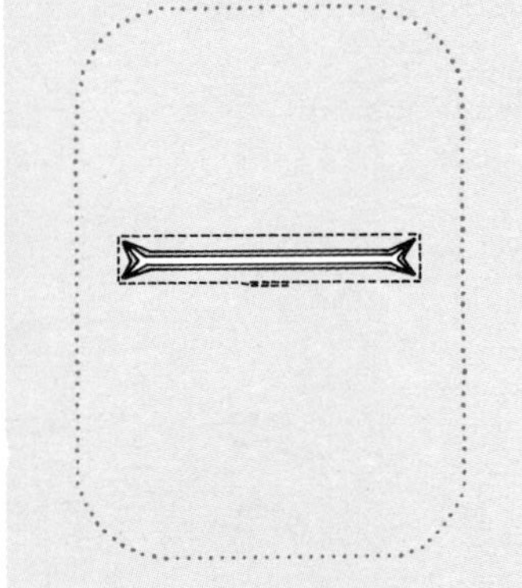

4. Carefully cut through garment and pocket at center of rectangle; stop ½″ before ends and cut diagonally into the four corners, forming a small triangle at each end of opening.

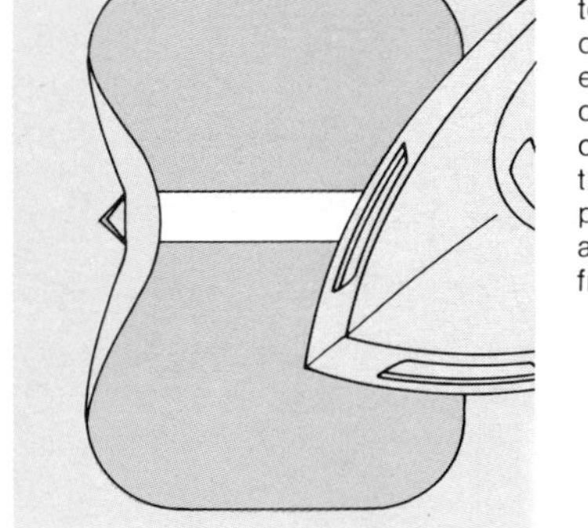

5. Gently push pocket through slash to wrong side. Pull on small triangular ends to square the corners of the opening. Press triangular ends and pocket opening seam allowances away from the opening.

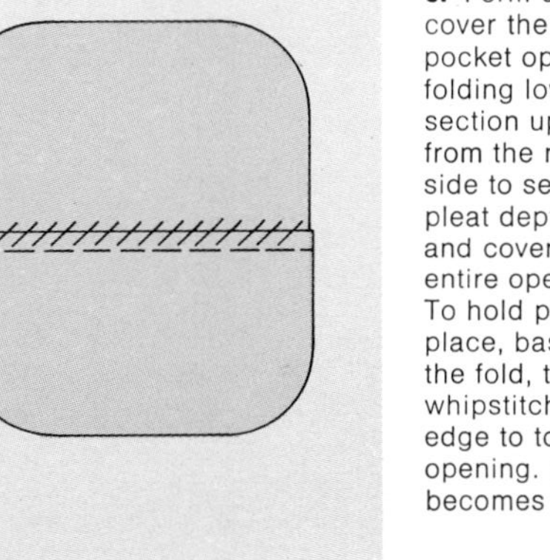

6. Form a pleat to cover the pocket opening by folding lower pocket section up. Check from the right side to see that pleat depth is even and covers the entire opening. To hold pleat in place, baste through the fold, then whipstitch folded edge to top of opening. (Pleat becomes the welt.)

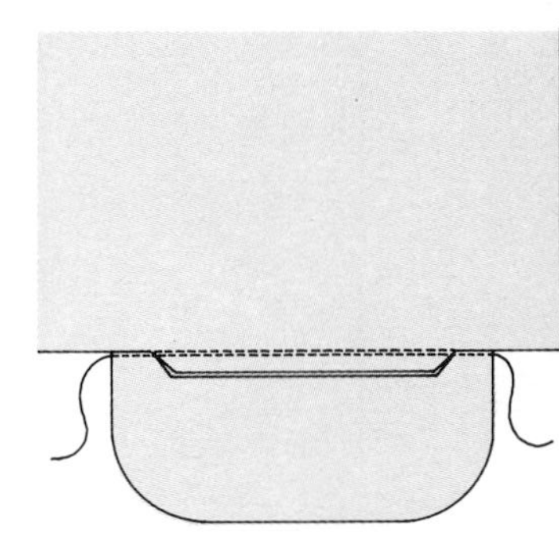

7. Turn garment right side up. Flip up bottom portion of garment to expose lower seam allowances of opening. Stitch through seam allowances and pocket.

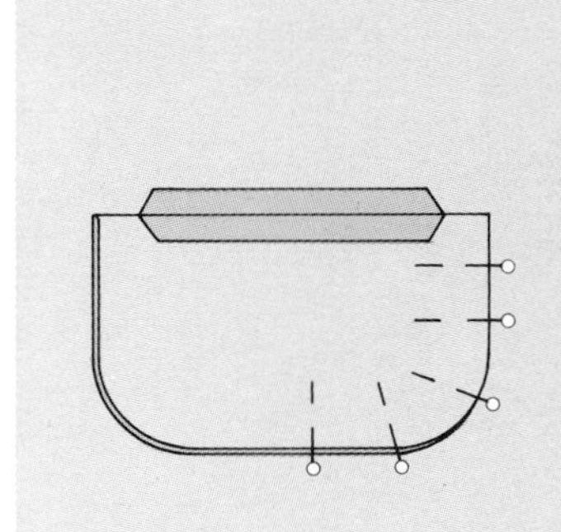

8. Turn garment back to wrong side and fold upper portion of pocket down over bottom section. Right sides of pocket should be together and the edges should be even. Pin around pocket. Press open the seam allowance at the top.

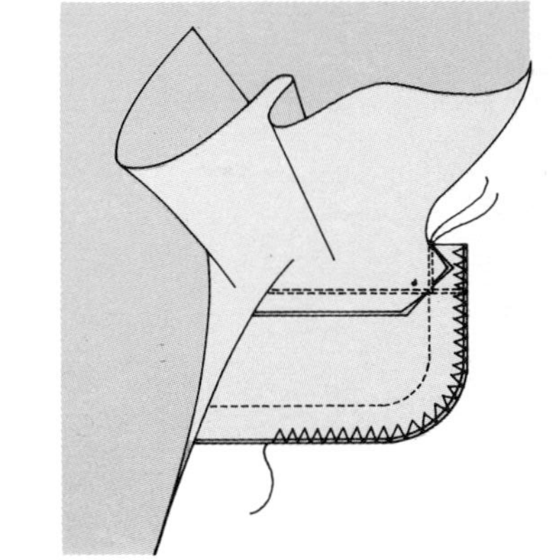

9. Turn garment right side up again and flip it out of the way to expose the pocket. Stitch around the pinned pocket, starting at the top and stitching across triangular ends as close as possible to original stitching; backstitch at beginning and end. Press flat. Seam-finish outer raw edges of pocket. Remove all bastings.

Hems & Other Edge Finishes

Hems and other edge finishes

Skirt markers 8
Hemming pleated garments 172-173

General information

A hem is a finish for any bottom edge of a garment. There are three basic forms—**turned-up edge** (the most common), **faced edge,** and **enclosed edge.** Though all are dealt with here as hem treatments, any might be used for other edges as well.

Selection of a hemming method depends largely on garment style and fabric. Whatever the choice, certain criteria should always be met: (1) The garment should hang evenly and gracefully; (2) there should be no lumpiness in the hem allowance; (3) unless meant to be decorative, finished hems should be totally inconspicuous.

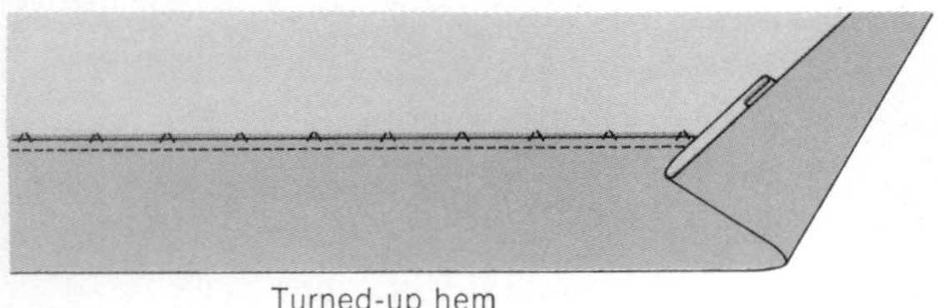

Turned-up hem

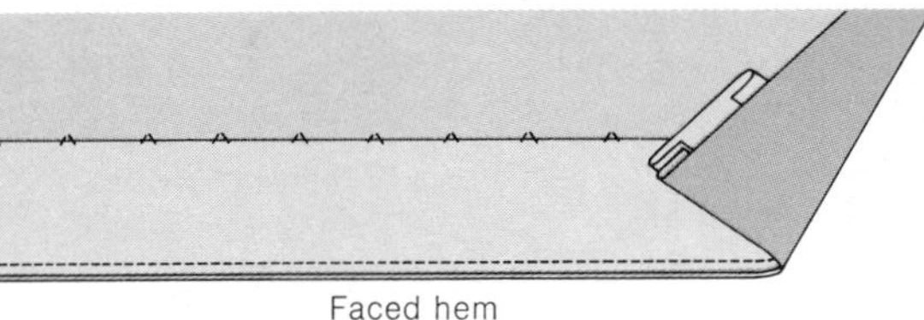

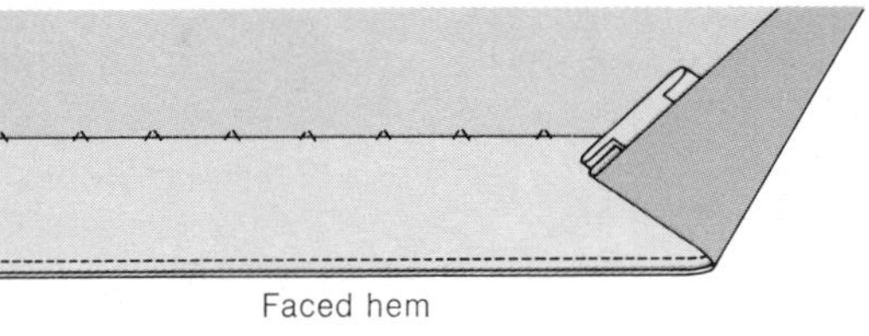

Faced hem

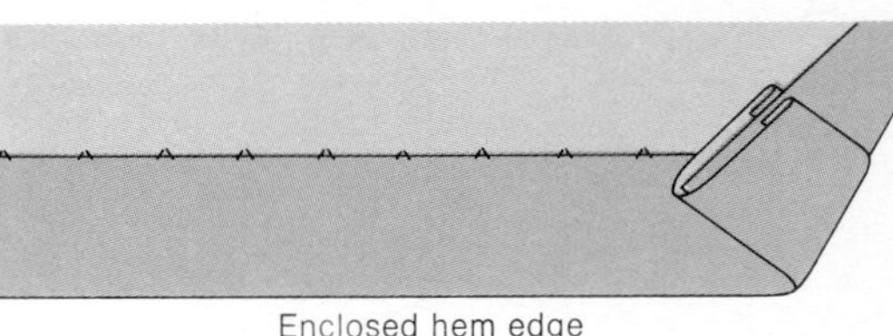

Enclosed hem edge

Marking the hemline

The first step, common to all hem finishes, is marking the hemline. Except for certain pleated styles, marking is done after garment construction has been completed. Though a garment's finished length is largely determined by the pattern style and current fashion, it should be modified if a different length will be more flattering to the wearer. It is wise to check the hemline location before cutting the pattern, in case a change is required.

Basically, there are two ways to mark a hem—on a flat surface or on the wearer. The first is suitable for a hem on the hipline or above, the second for any length below the hip. If someone is marking a garment for you, it is best to wear the undergarments and shoes you will wear with it, and to stand in one place while your helper moves around you to mark. Before marking a bias or circular garment, allow it to hang for 24 hours.

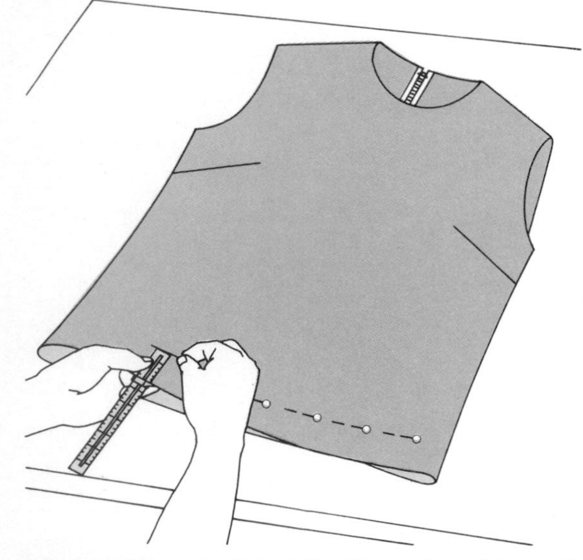

Before marking a hemline at the hip or above (also pants legs), check the pattern to see how much hem allowance has been provided. Measure and turn up this amount, pinning fabric from right side. Try on garment; adjust length if necessary. Remove garment; measure and mark the hemline.

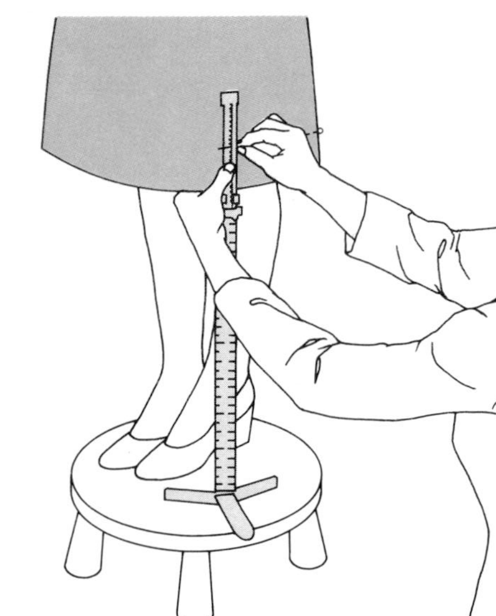

To mark a hemline below the hips, put garment on over appropriate undergarments; wear shoes and belt that go with it. Stand on a low stool, while a helper moves around you with a marker (pin marker as shown, yardstick, or suitable substitute), placing pins or marks every 2″.

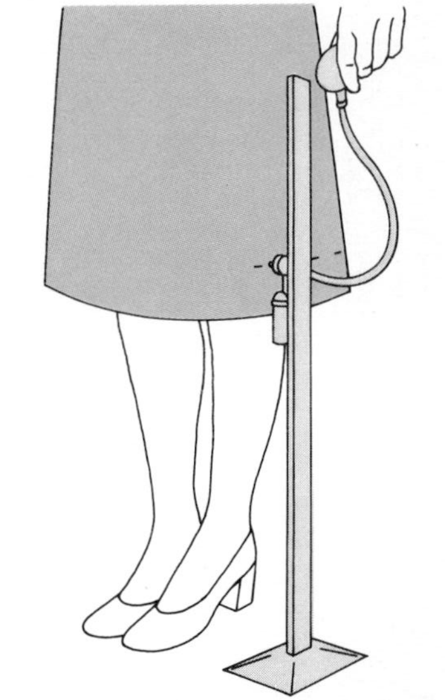

To mark a hemline without help, use a marker of the chalk type shown here. Test it on a scrap beforehand; the chalk cannot be removed from some fabrics. Standing straight, with feet together, move the marker around you, marking every 2″. Try to avoid changing posture as you work.

Turned-up hems

Measuring devices 8
What pattern markings mean 57

Turning up the hem edge

In a turned-up hem, a certain width of fabric, the *hem allowance,* is folded inside the garment, then secured by hand, machine, or fusing. This is the hem type usually provided for in pattern designs, with the amount of turn-up indicated on the pattern by a line or written instructions. It is wise to check this allowance before cutting out the garment, should a change be desirable.

The hem's shape, straight or curved, generally determines how much should be turned up. As a rule, the straighter the edge, the deeper the hem allowance; the more it curves, the shallower the allowance. Exceptions are sheer fabrics, in which a very deep or a narrow rolled hem (p. 314) may be preferable, also soft knits, where a narrow turn-up will minimize sagging (p. 294 and p. 314).

Hem up to 3"

Hem 1 1/2" to 2"

Hem allowance varies according to garment shape. Up to 3" is usually allowed for a straight garment, 1½" to 2" for a flared one. Fabric weight should also be considered.

A hemline may look distorted if the hem curve is too extreme for, or does not align with, the fabric design. A slight adjustment may be necessary, for a better effect.

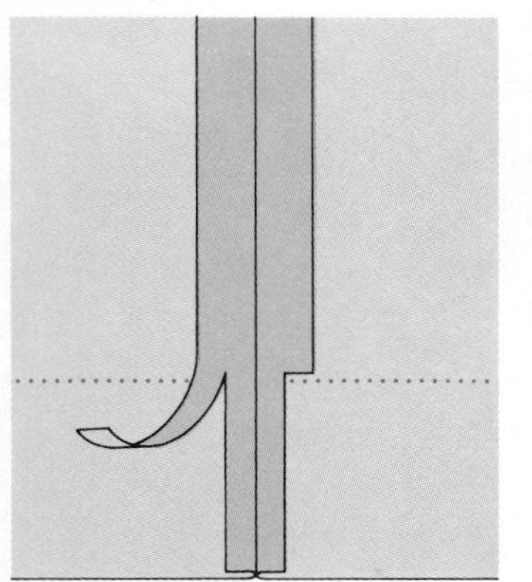

1. Before turning up the hem, reduce bulk within the hem allowance by trimming seam allowances to half their original widths. This will make the hem smoother at the seamlines.

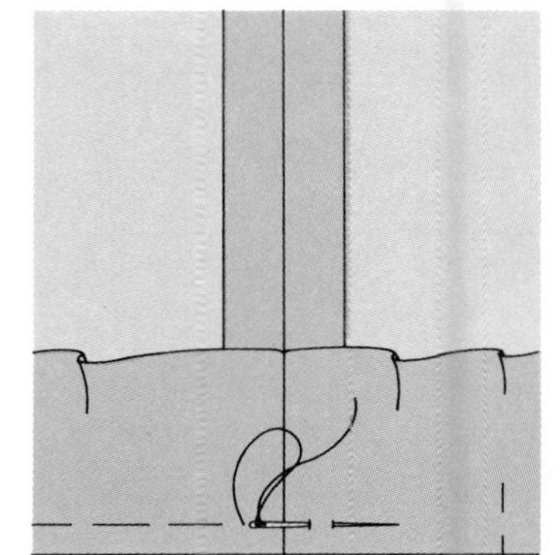

2. With wrong side facing you, fold hem on the marked line, placing pins at right angles to the fold about every 2". (If a mark should be greatly out of line with the others, ignore it, and align the fold with the marks on either side.) Try on garment; make adjustments if necessary. After removing the garment, baste close to the folded edge.

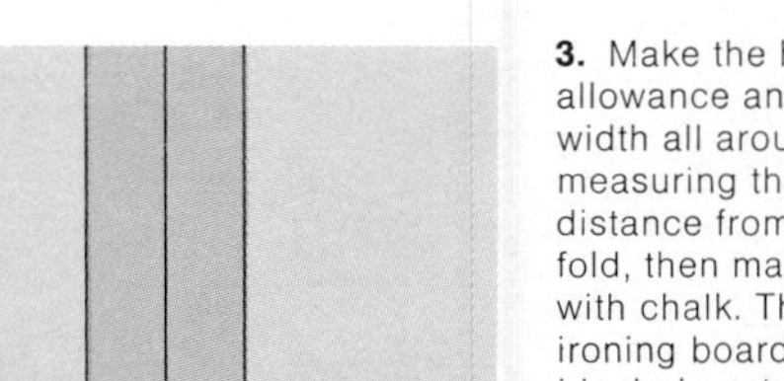

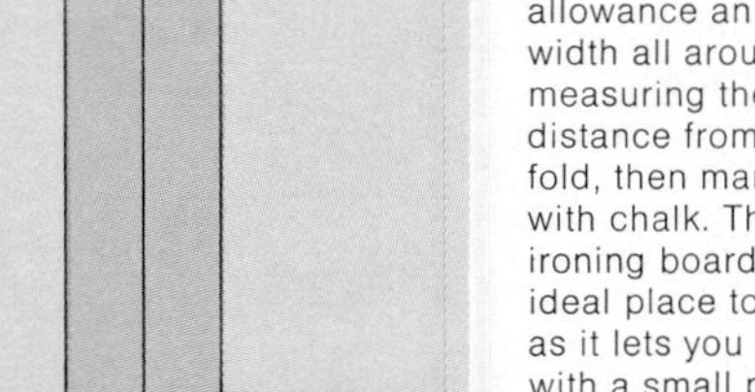

3. Make the hem allowance an even width all around by measuring the desired distance from the fold, then marking with chalk. The ironing board is an ideal place to work, as it lets you deal with a small part of the hem at a time. A sewing gauge is the easiest measuring device to use.

4. Trim excess hem allowance along the marks. At this stage, you can see whether or not the hem edge lies smoothly against the garment. If there are ripples, the fullness should be controlled by easing, a step that is usually necessary with gored skirts and other flared styles.

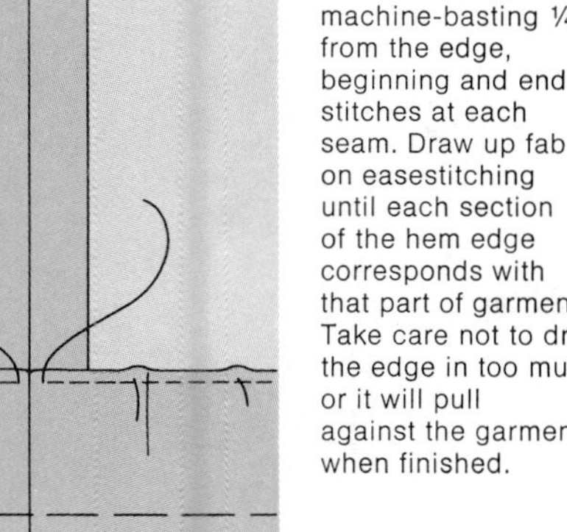

5. Ease the hem by machine-basting ¼" from the edge, beginning and ending stitches at each seam. Draw up fabric on easestitching until each section of the hem edge corresponds with that part of garment. Take care not to draw the edge in too much, or it will pull against the garment when finished.

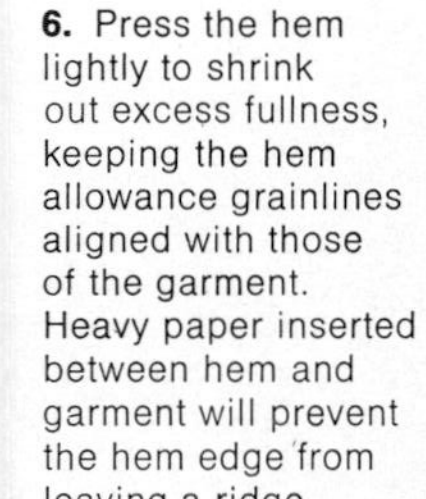

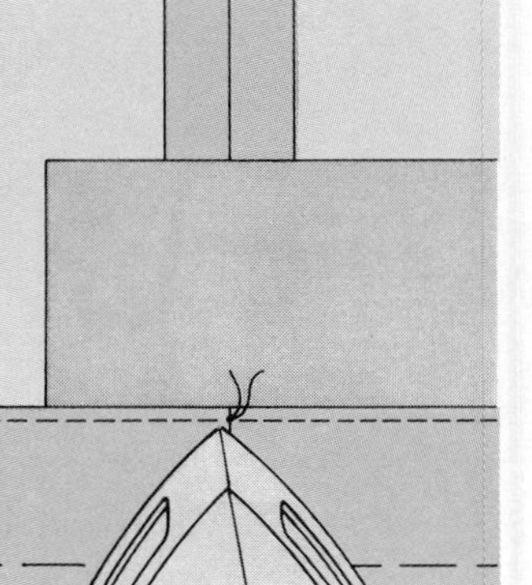

6. Press the hem lightly to shrink out excess fullness, keeping the hem allowance grainlines aligned with those of the garment. Heavy paper inserted between hem and garment will prevent the hem edge from leaving a ridge.

Turned-up hems

Zigzag stitching 32-33, 140, 148
Hand sewing techniques 122
Hand stitches: hemming 128-129; overcast 130; uneven slipstitch 132

Sewing hems by hand

Before a hem is secured by hand, the raw edge should be neatly finished. The finish chosen depends first on fabric characteristics and garment style, second on personal preference. The edge can be left uncovered on fabric that does not ravel, also where a lining will cover the hem; use a covered edge for fabric that ravels a great deal, and in those situations where a more finished look is wanted.

There are two basic hand-hemming methods—*flat,* where stitches pass over the hem edge to the garment, and *blind,* where stitches are taken inside, between hem and garment. Blind hems are best for heavier fabrics and knits because the hem edge is not pressed into the garment. (See Hand stitches for techniques.)

Uncovered hem edges

A turned-and-stitched edge is suitable for all lightweight fabrics, especially crisp sheers; an excellent, durable finish for washable garments.

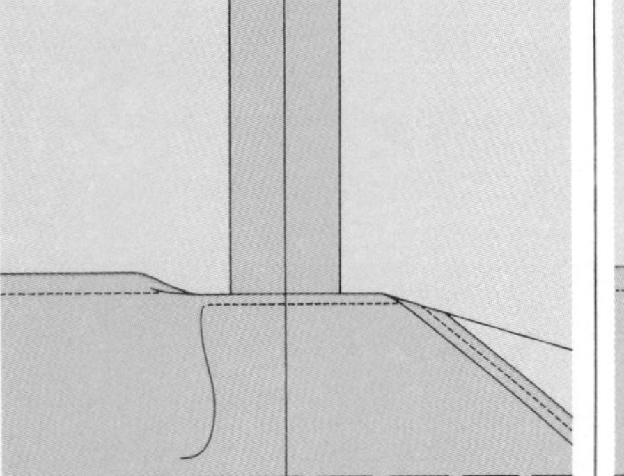
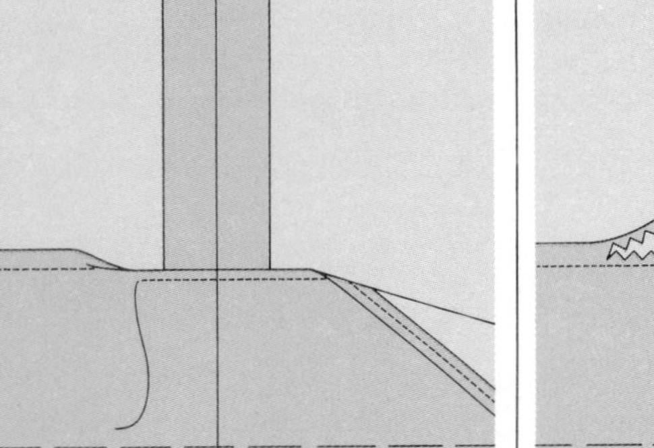

Turn the hem edge under ¼″ and press. (If using an easestitch, turn the edge along the stitching line.) Topstitch ⅛″ from fold.

Secure hem with vertical hemming stitches (shown) or use uneven slipstitches, spacing the stitches ⅜″ apart. Do not pull thread taut.

A stitched-and-pinked edge is a quick hem finish for fabrics that ravel little or not at all; it is a particularly good choice for knits.

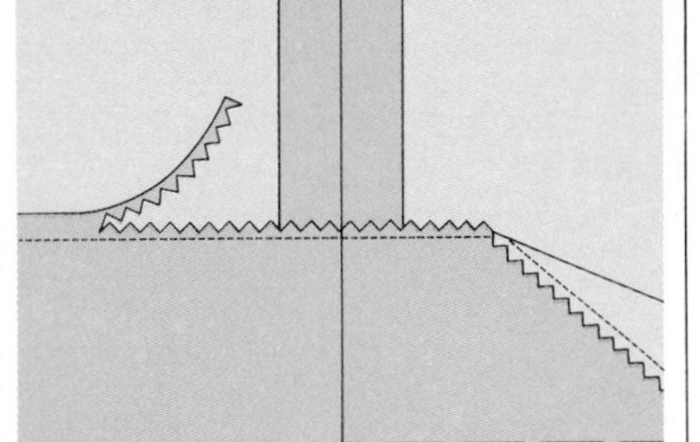

Stitch ¼″ from the hem edge, using regular stitching or easestitching (see p. 291) as required. Trim the edge with pinking shears.

Turn hem edge back ¼″; secure with a blind-hemming stitch, as shown, or with the blind catchstitch (for a heavy fabric).

A stitched-and-overcast edge, though slower than pinking, can be used on medium-weight and heavy fabrics that ravel; often used on coats and suits.

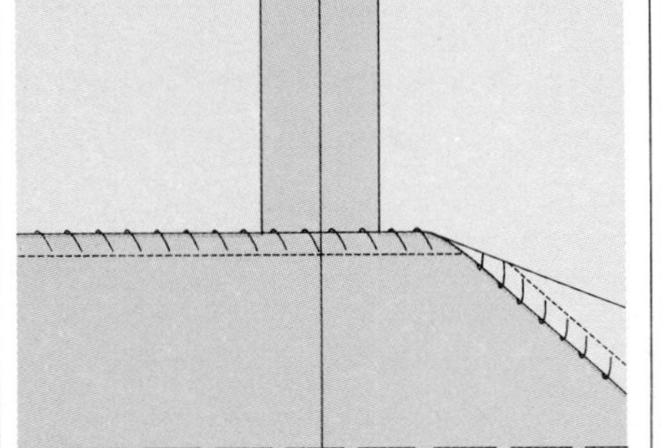
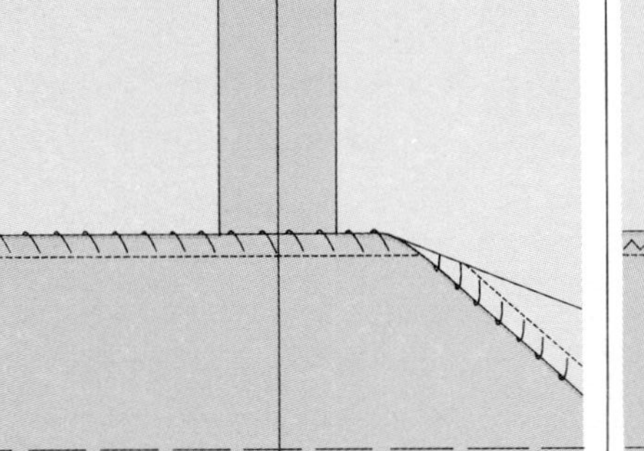

Stitch ¼″ from hem edge, using regular stitch or easestitch as needed. Overcast edge, spacing stitches evenly. Use stitching as guide.

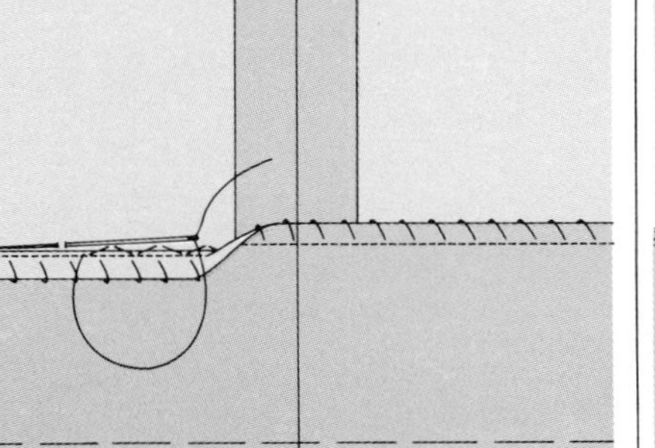

Turn hem edge back ¼″; secure with a blind-hemming stitch, as shown, or the blind catchstitch (for a heavy fabric).

A zigzagged edge is a fast and relatively neat finish usable for any fabric that ravels; also for knits, taking care not to stretch the edge.

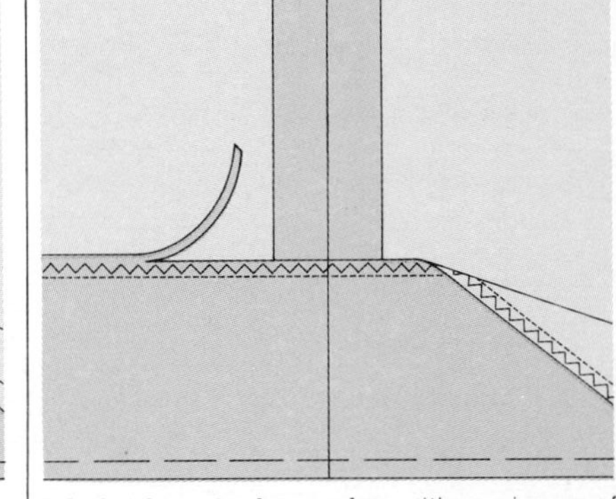

Stitch close to hem edge with a zigzag of medium width and length. If necessary, easestitch just below zigzag. Trim excess fabric.

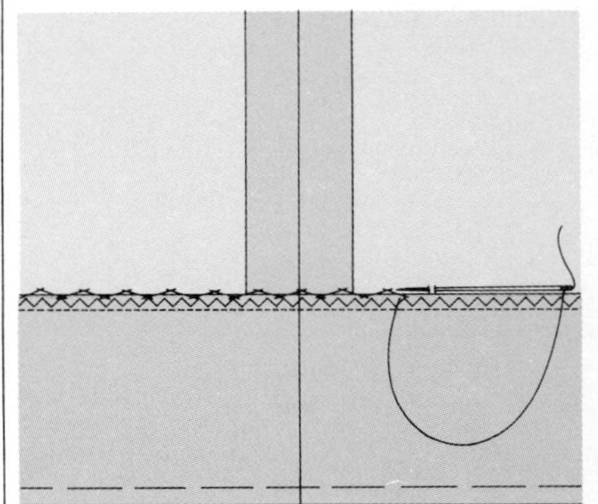

Secure hem with catchstitch if material is lightweight or tends to curl. For heavier fabric, use a blind-hemming stitch.

Tapes used in construction 16
Underlining fabrics 72-73
Cutting bias strips 298-299

Covered hem edges

Seam binding provides a clean finish for fabric that ravels. Use the woven-edge type for a straight-edge hem, a stretch lace for a curved shape and for knit or other stretch fabric.

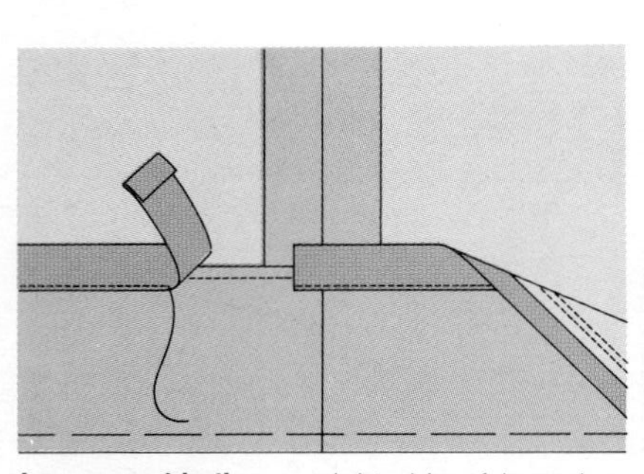

Lay seam binding on right side of hem, lapping it ¼″ over the edge. Edgestitch, overlapping ends at a seam, as shown.

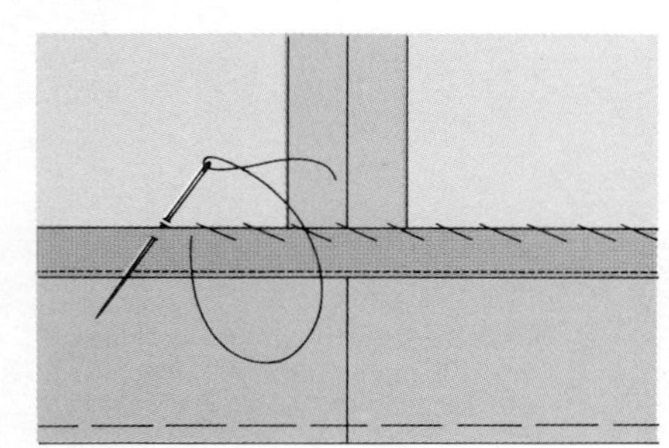

For **light-to medium-weight fabric,** secure hem with one of the flat hemming stitches—slant (shown), vertical, or catchstitch.

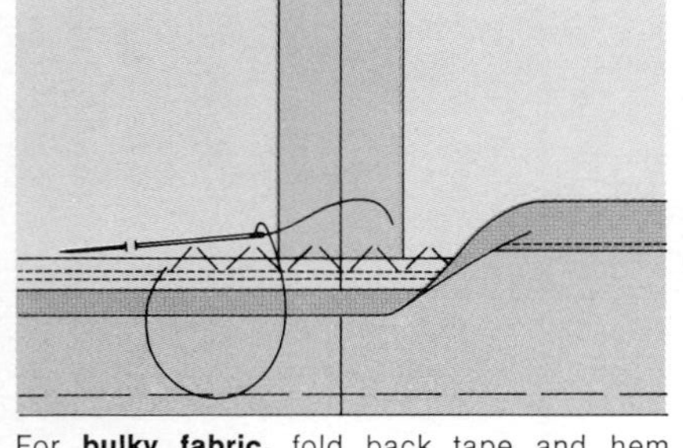

For **bulky fabric,** fold back tape and hem edge; blindstitch, as shown, catching the stitches through the hem edge only.

Bias tape is a neat hem finish for garments with a flared shape—the bias adjusts to curves. Use the ½-inch width, in matching color, if available, otherwise a neutral shade.

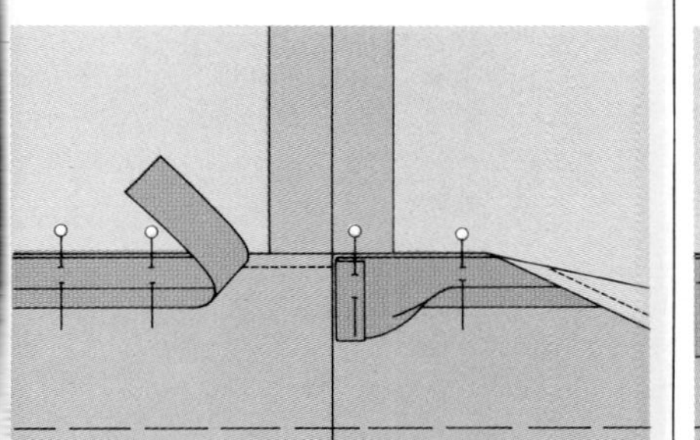

Open one fold of tape; place crease just below easestitching on right side of hem. Fold end back ¼″; align with a seam; pin.

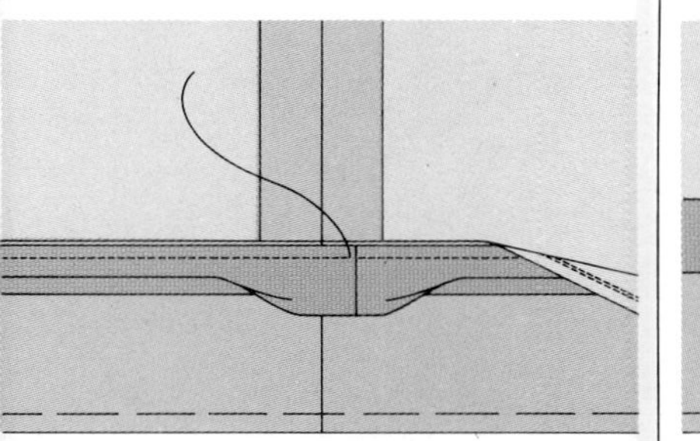

Stitch to within 3″ of starting point. Trim tape to lap ¼″ beyond fold of starting end; stitch the rest of the way across.

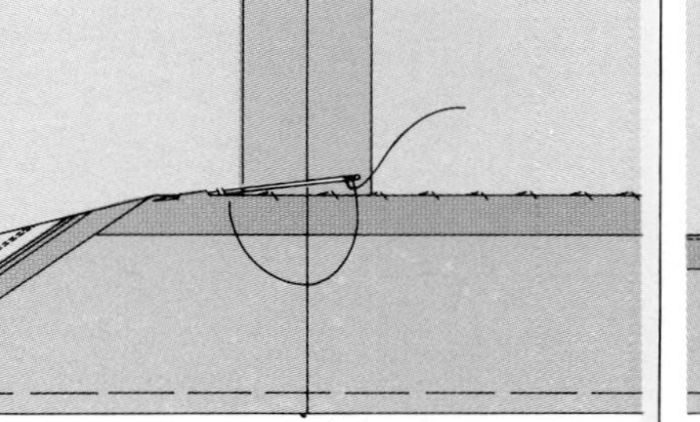

Secure hem edge with uneven slipstitches, as shown, or use either vertical or slant hemming stitches to secure it.

Hong Kong finish is suitable for any garment style or fabric, but especially good for heavy or bulky fabrics; recommended also for velvet or satin, using net in place of a bias strip.

Cut 1″ bias of underlining fabric, or use packaged ½″ width. Stitch to the hem, ¼″ from edge, lapping ends as for bias tape.

Wrap bias over the raw edge and press. From the right side, stitch in the groove formed by the first row of stitching.

Secure the hem with the blind-hemming stitch, or use blind catchstitch. Be careful not to pull thread too tight.

Double-stitched hem

This technique is recommended for very wide hems, also for heavy fabrics, as it gives better support. The edge is left uncovered as a rule, but a Hong Kong finish is also appropriate.

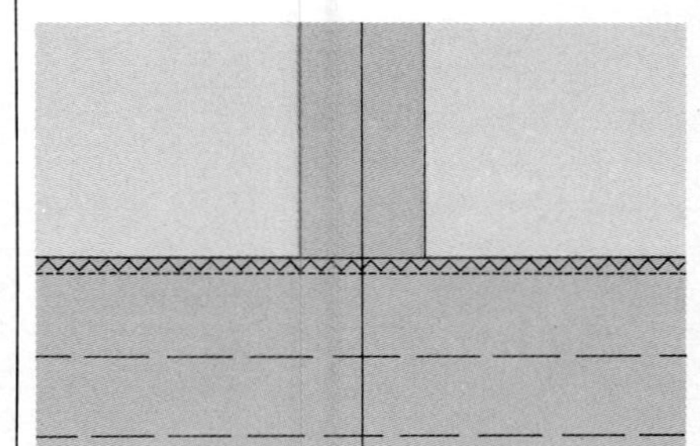

After finishing the hem edge, place a row of basting stitches halfway between the edge and the fold at the hemline.

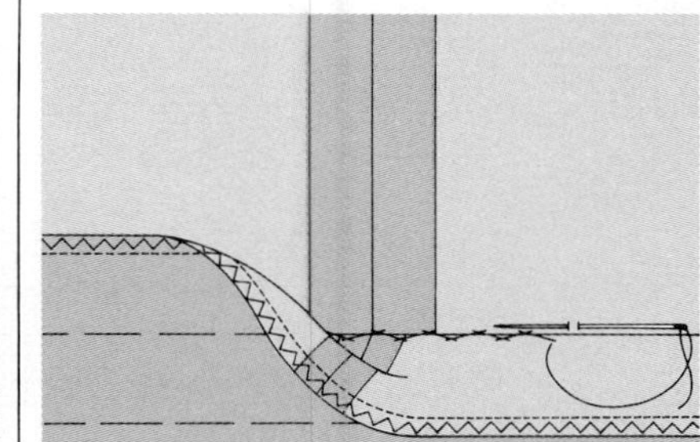

Fold the hem back along this basting and secure the fold with the blind catchstitch, spacing the stitches ⅜″ apart.

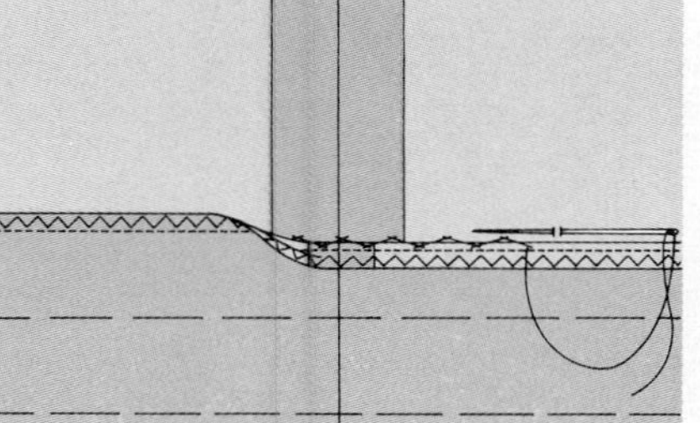

Turn the upper half of the hem up again, and secure the edge with a blind catchstitch. Do not pull the thread too tight.

Turned-up hems

Sewing a hem by machine

The major assets of machine hems are speed and extra sturdiness. They can also provide a decorative touch, and are especially appropriate if topstitching is part of the design.

Machine stitches are more casual on a hem than hand stitches, so careful consideration should be given to their suitability for the garment. Of the several methods, the blindstitched hem is the least conspicuous (about every sixth stitch catches the right side). On the garment, however, the stitch is usually $\frac{1}{16}$ to $\frac{1}{8}$ inch long, and should be used only where such stitches would not be too unsightly.

Take special care with all machine-stitched hems to keep stitching an even distance from the hemline (see Topstitching seams for suggestions).

Types of machine-stitched hems

Blind hemming by machine is a sturdy yet fairly inconspicuous finish; used mainly for children's clothing, very full skirts, and household decor.

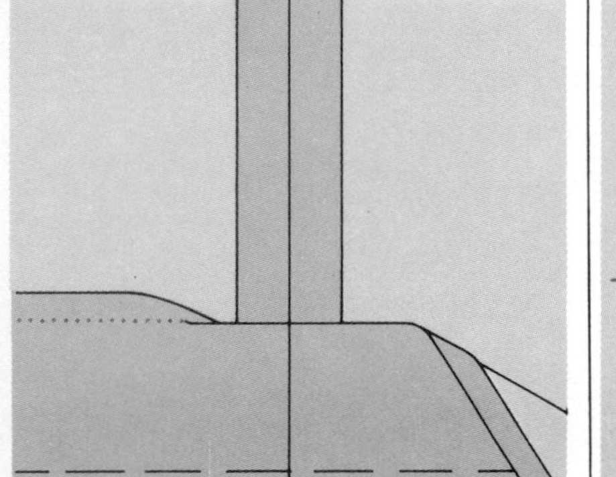

Mark, fold, and baste hemline. Make the hem allowance even; turn edge under ⅜"; press. Adjust machine for blind-hemming stitch.

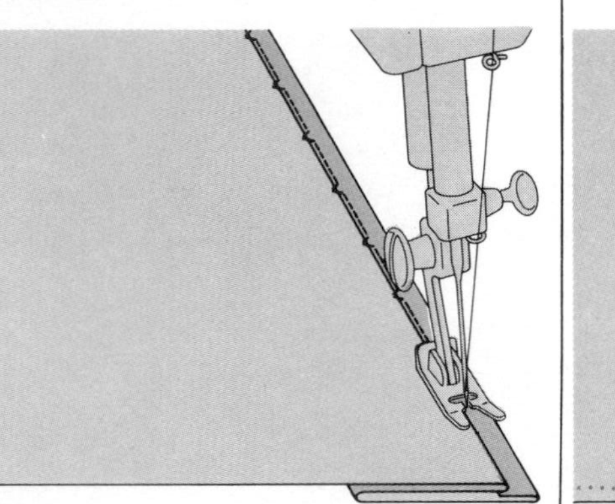

Lay hem allowance face down; fold garment back to reveal the hem edge. Stitch, catching only the garment in the zigzag stitch.

A narrow machine-stitched hem is suitable where neither a deep nor an inconspicuous hem is required; best for blouses, shirts, and dress linings.

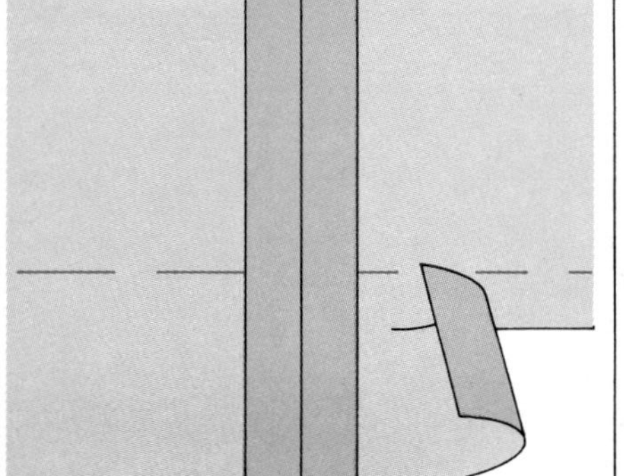

Mark the hemline. Trim hem allowance to ½". Turn edge under ¼" and press. Turn the edge again and press along the hemline.

Stitch along the hem edge. Take care to keep the hem and garment grainlines aligned; if edge is allowed to slant, hem will ripple.

A topstitched hem is essentially a decorative finish, particularly appropriate where topstitching is used elsewhere in garment construction.

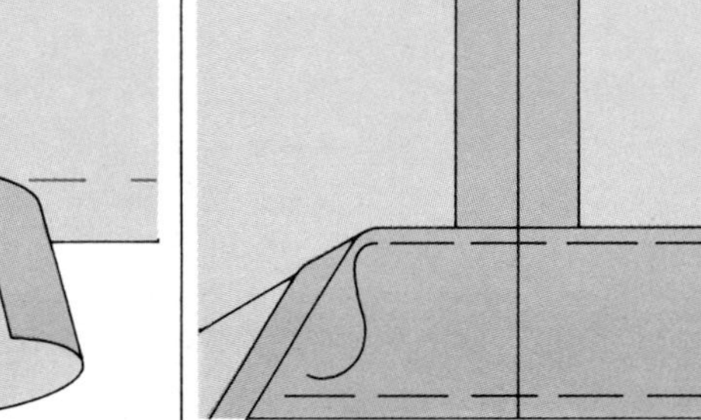

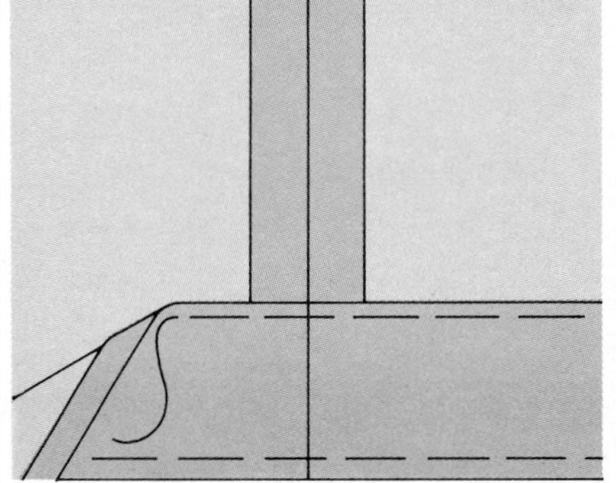

Mark, fold, and baste hemline. Adjust hem allowance to desired width. Fold hem edge under ⅜". Baste to garment along fold.

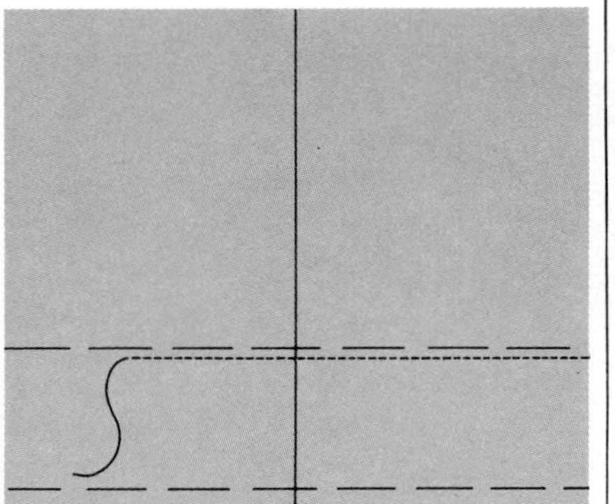

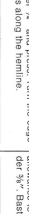

Topstitch from the right side, using a straight stitch or, if desired, a zigzag or another of the decorative stitch patterns.

A narrow topstitched hem is fine for knits, especially soft ones, which may sag with a hand finish; suitable for any fabric that does not ravel.

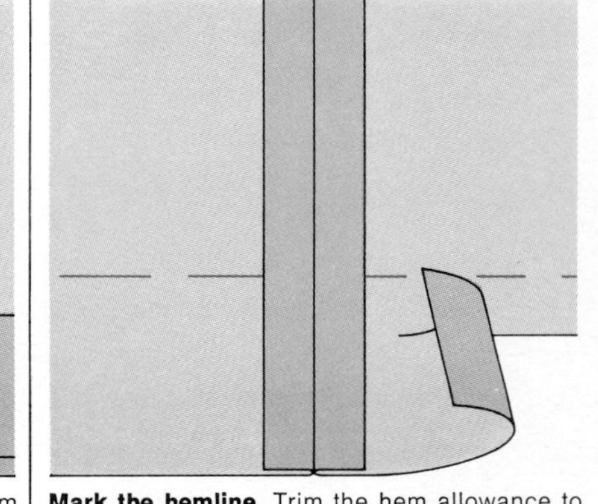

Mark the hemline. Trim the hem allowance to ⅝". Turn the hem up on the hemline and press. Baste ½" from the edge.

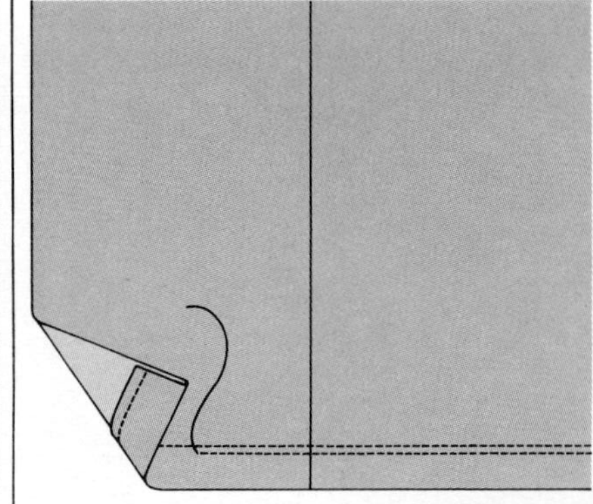

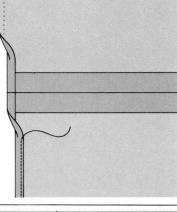

Topstitch, ½" from fold. Stitch a second row ⅛" below the first one (or use a twin needle to stitch both rows at once).

Fusing webs 17
Underlying fabrics 72-73
Hand sewing techniques 122
Hand hemming stitches 128-129

Fusing a hem

A fast and inconspicuous way to secure a hem is to bond it with fusible web (a sheer nonwoven material that melts with application of heat and moisture). This web is available in packaged precut strips, suitable for most hem jobs, also in larger sheets from which you can cut strips.

A hem can be fused on any fabric that can be steam-pressed, but pressing time varies with different fabrics, so a test is essential. Check on a scrap to see if the bond is secure and the appearance satisfactory.

If properly done, the fusing lasts through normal washing and dry-cleaning procedures. Removal is possible, but messy, so adjust your hem carefully before application. The following additional precautions are necessary: (1) avoid stretching a fusible during application; (2) do not let it touch the iron; (3) do not glide the iron over the fabric.

1. Slip a 3/4″ strip of fusing web between hem allowance and garment, placing top edge of strip just below hem edge; pin.

2. With iron at steam setting, heat-baste the hem in place by pressing between pins with the tip of the iron. Remove pins.

3. Cover hem with damp press cloth. Press a section at a time, holding iron on cloth until dry. Let fabric cool before handling.

To fuse heavy fabric, use a 2″ strip of fusing web to support the extra weight. This may take extra pressing time, especially at seams.

Interfacing a hem

Interfacing adds body and support to a hem, and can also serve as a cushion to keep the edge from being pressed sharply against the garment.

Hem interfacing is cut on the bias (see pp. 298–299 for the method) from underlining fabric, or from light- or medium-weight interfacing, whichever best suits the garment fabric.

The interfacing technique illustrated below is used in a lined, tailored garment, usually one of medium-weight or heavy fabric. It can be accommodated to lightweight fabric by cutting the interfacing to fit just to the hemline. In either case, the lining will cover the part of the interfacing above the hem edge.

To interface the hem in an unlined garment, cut the interfacing to extend just 1 inch above and below the hemline. This produces a softly rolled or padded effect, especially suitable for velvet or satin garments.

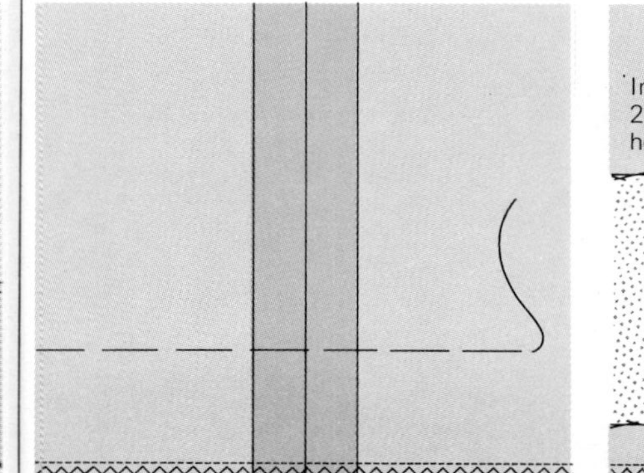

1. Baste hemline with contrasting thread. Make the hem allowance even; finish the edge. Lay garment with wrong side toward you.

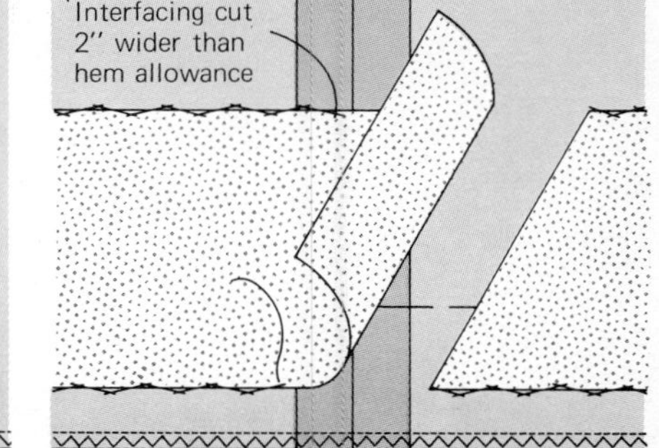

2. Pin interfacing in place with lower edge extending 1″ below the hemline. Catchstitch both edges. Overlap ends where they meet.

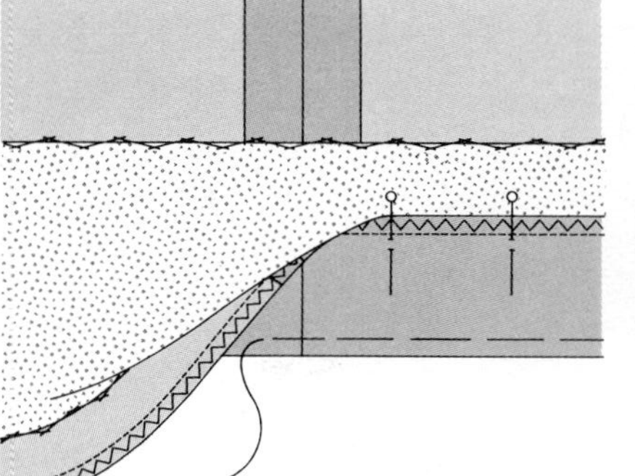
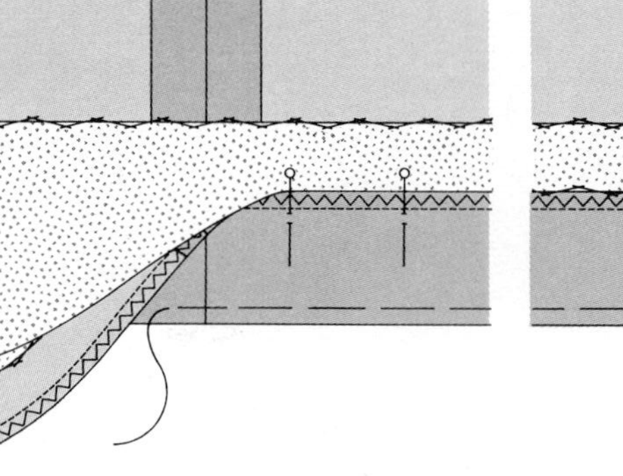

3. Turn hem up along basted line and pin, then baste close to the fold. (Interfacing will extend above the hem edge about 1″.)

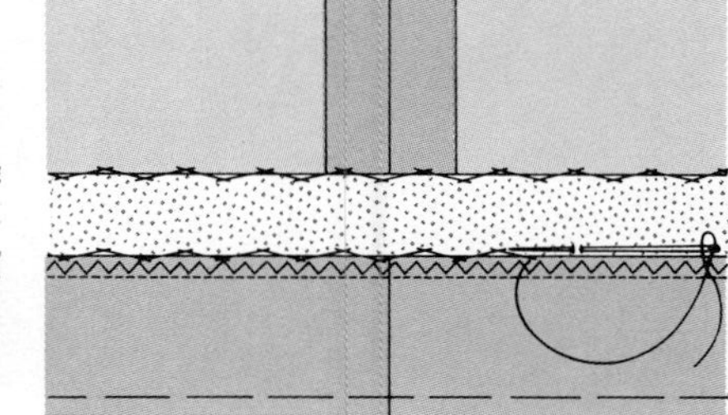

4. Secure hem edge with a flat catchstitch, as shown, taking the stitch that is above the hem edge through interfacing only.

Pressing equipment 18-19
Hand sewing techniques 122
Hand hemming stitches 128-129
Whipstitch 136

Hemming a faced opening

There are two ways to finish the hem edge of a faced opening. One is to hem the facing itself, then fold and secure it inside the garment. This is appropriate for all light- to medium-weight fabrics, and permits later lengthening of the hem. In the second method, the hem allowance is trimmed at the facing and the part of the garment that is covered by it. The bottom of the facing is then sewed to the garment by hand or machine. This technique is suitable for any fabric, but

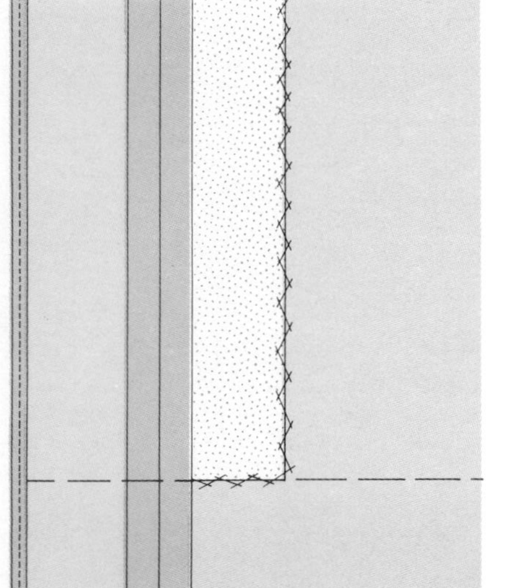

is especially good for a heavy one because it eliminates so much bulk. It does not, however, permit the hem to be lengthened.

Whichever method is used, the lower edge of the completed facing should be smooth and flat. One way to achieve this is to trim the interfacing at the hemline and catchstitch it in place, as shown above. Another is to flatten the edge with a clapper (see Pressing equipment).

Method 1

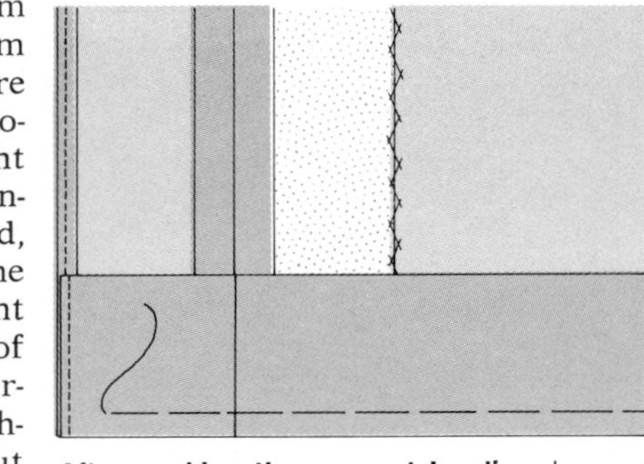

After marking the garment hemline, be sure the faced edges are the same length. Press facing seam open; fold and baste hemline.

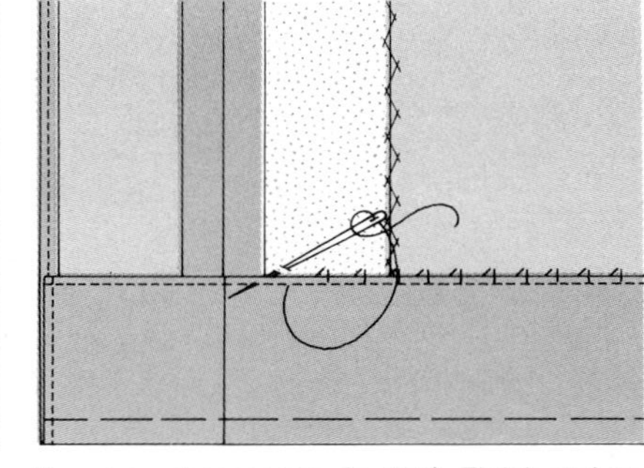

Ease hem if necessary (p. 291). Finish and secure hem edge in appropriate way (see pp. 292-293), hemming to the edge of the facing.

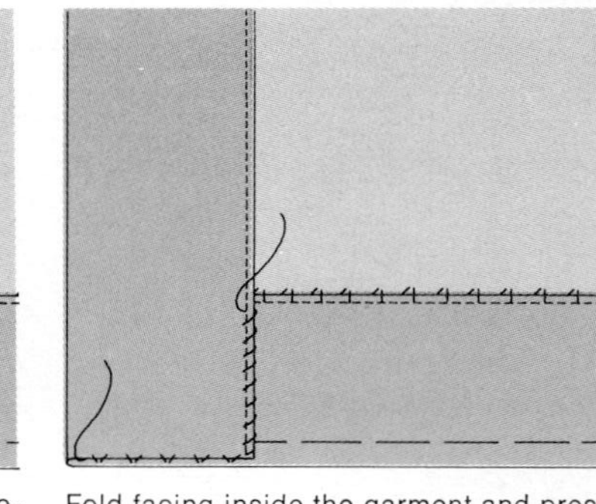

Fold facing inside the garment and press. Slipstitch bottom edge of facing to hemline. Whipstitch free edge of facing to hem.

Method 2

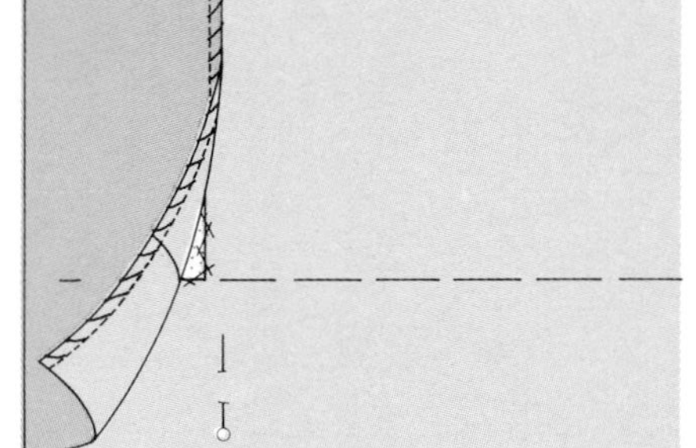

1. Mark hemline with thread tracing; be sure the faced edges are the same length. On the hem allowance, pin-mark where facing ends.

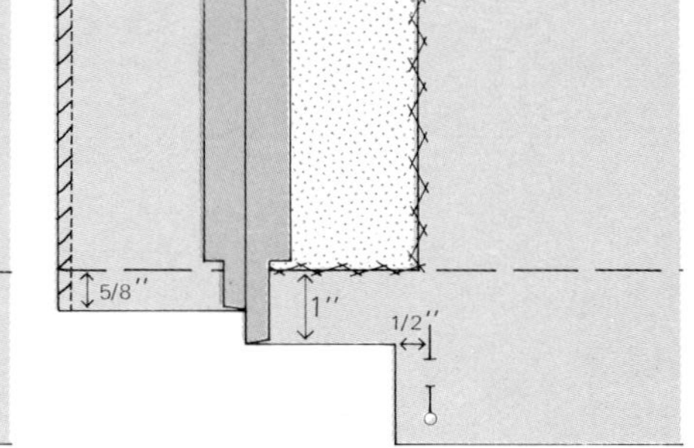

2. Open out facing; trim hem allowance of facing to ⅝", of garment to 1", ending ½" from pin. Trim seam allowances as shown.

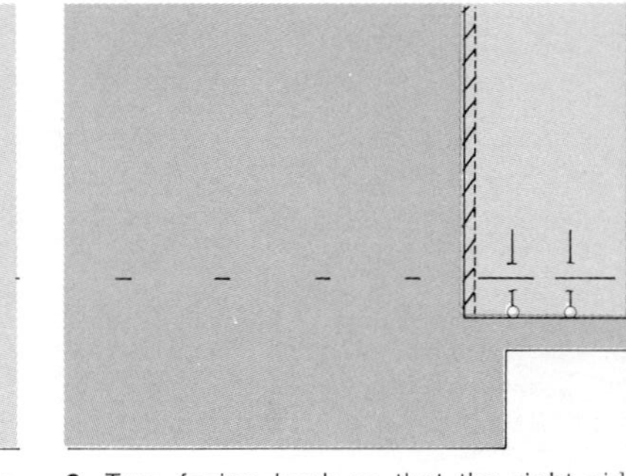

3. Turn facing back so that the right side is toward the garment. Pin and baste the bottom edge, aligning traced hemlines.

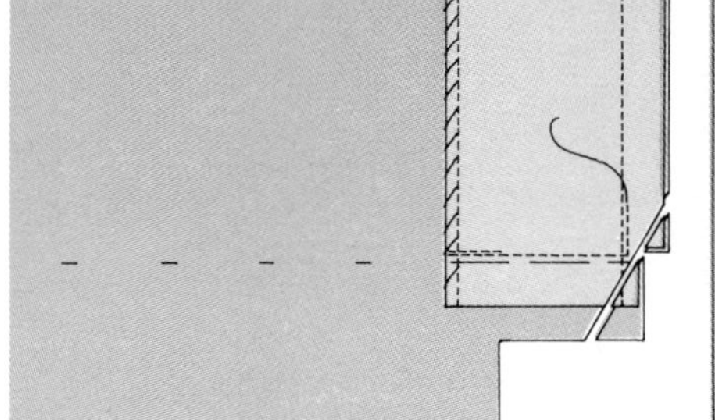

4. Stitch from inner edge of facing to seam at garment edge; pivot, and stitch up seam for 1". Trim corners diagonally.

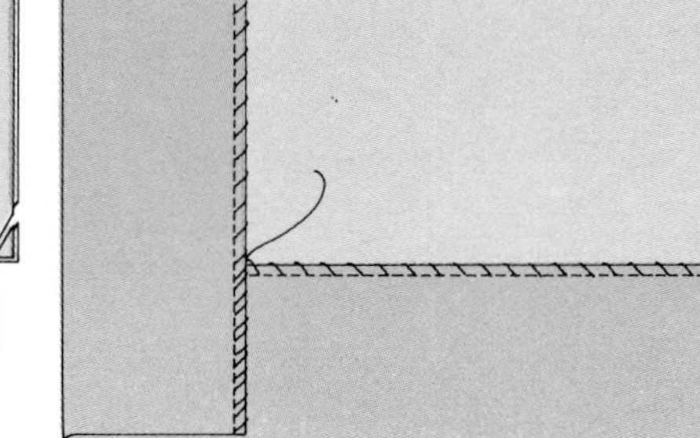

5. Turn facing inside garment; whipstitch inner facing edge to hem allowance. Secure hem with appropriate stitch (pp. 292–293).

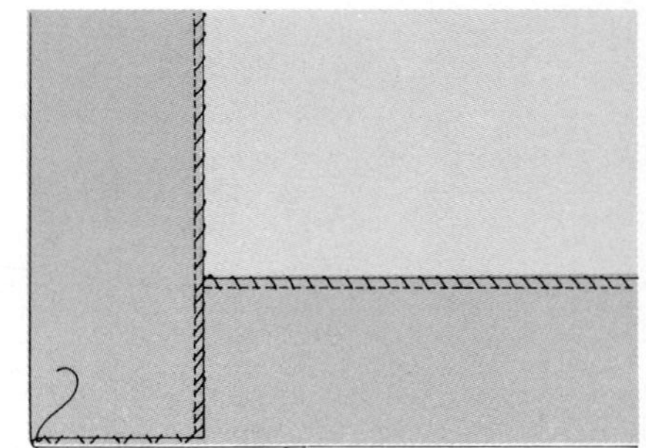

If preferred, omit the stitching in Step 4, and slipstitch the lower edge. On a very heavy fabric, this edge can be left open.

Hemming a lining

There are two ways to handle a lining hem: (1) Sew it to the garment, providing a fold for easy movement; (2) hem the lining separately, securing it to the garment with French tacks. The first is appropriate for a jacket or vest, also a sleeve lining; the second, for a garment that extends below the hips, as a skirt, dress, or coat.

Before a lining is hemmed, the garment hem should be finished and the lining sewed in place except for 6 inches at lower edge (see Underlying fabrics). To adjust lining length, put garment on wrong side out and have someone pin lining to the garment all around, about 6 inches above the hemline. If there is no one to help, drape garment on a dress form or the ironing board and smooth the lining carefully, pinning it first at the seams, then at intervals in between.

When the lining is anchored, trim excess fabric. For an attached hem, trim lining to ⅝ inch below garment hemline; for free-hanging style, the amount left should equal the lining hem allowance minus 1 inch (for a 2-inch hem, lining would be trimmed to 1 inch below garment).

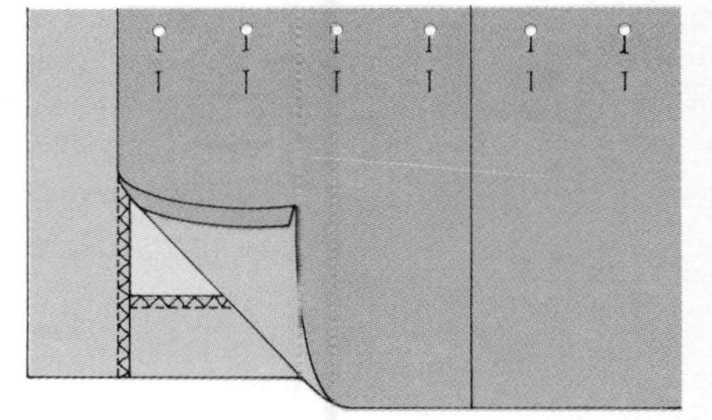

Hem of lining attached to garment

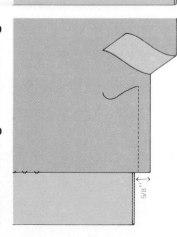

Trim lining to ⅝" below finished garment edge. If hem must be eased, place a row of easestitching ½" from the hem edge.

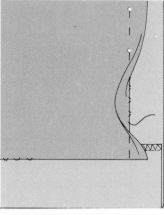

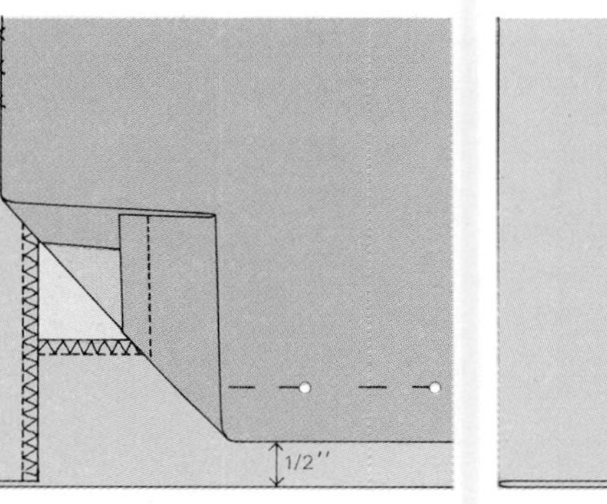

Turn lining under 1⅛", so that fold is ½" from garment edge. Pin lining to garment, placing pins ½" above and parallel to fold.

Fold lining back along the pinned line and slipstitch it to the garment hem, taking care to catch underlayer of lining only.

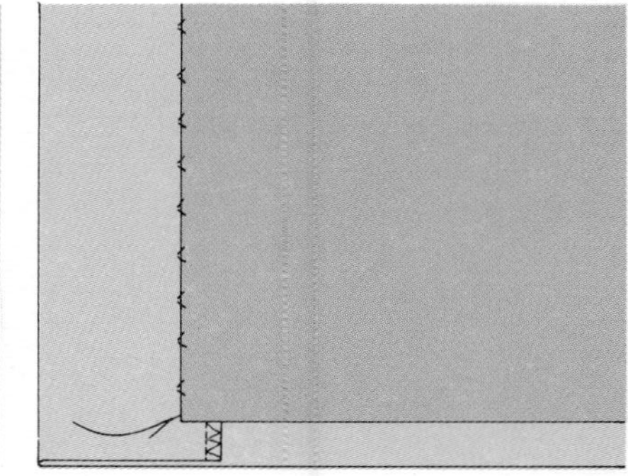

Remove pins and press lining fold lightly. If garment has a faced opening, slipstitch remaining lining edges to the facing.

Hem of free-hanging lining

Turn under the lining so that the fold is 1" from garment hemline; baste close to the fold. Make the hem allowance an even width.

Ease the hem edge if necessary (see p. 291) finish and secure the hem by an appropriate method (see pp. 292–293 for the choices).

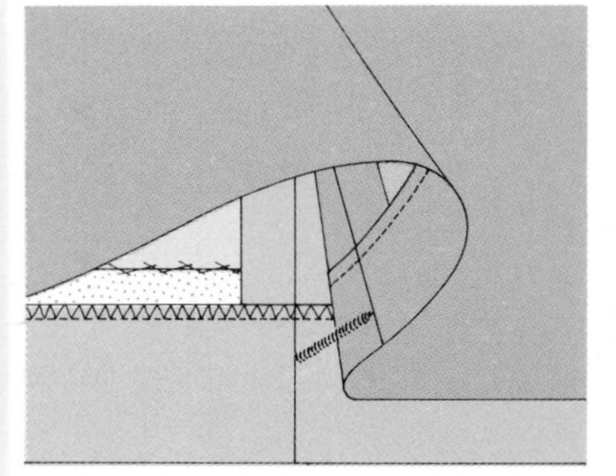
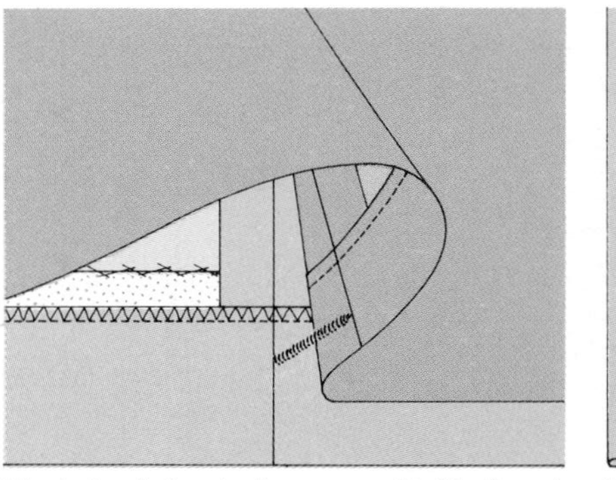

Attach the lining to the garment with French tacks, 1" long, placing one at each seam (see Hand stitches for details of the method).

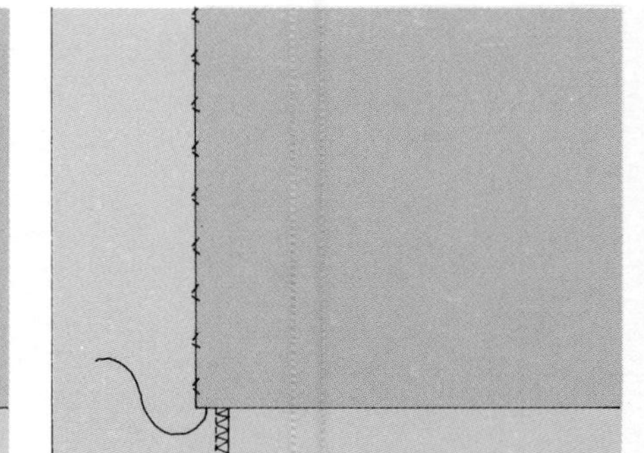

If garment has a faced opening, slipstitch remaining lining edge to the facing. Lining is now secured, yet moves freely.

Faced hems

Ready-made hem facings 16
Fabric grainlines 84
Hand sewing techniques 122
Hand hemming stitches 128-129

The basic uses of hem facings

In a faced hem, most of the hem allowance is eliminated; a band of lightweight fabric is then stitched to the hem and turned inside so it does not show. There are two basic facing forms—**shaped** (cut with grainlines and shape conforming to the hem) and **bias** (cut as a bias strip, then shaped to fit). Two-inch wide stretch lace is an alternative to bias.

A shaped facing is applied, as a rule, where a hem shape is unusual, as in the wrap skirt, right. Its use is limited to a hem with minimal flare. A bias (or lace) facing is ideal for a widely flared hem, especially when the garment itself is cut on the bias. It is recommended in place of a turned-up hem when (1) there is not enough hem allowance to turn up; (2) fabric is exceptionally bulky; (3) a skirt is circular in style.

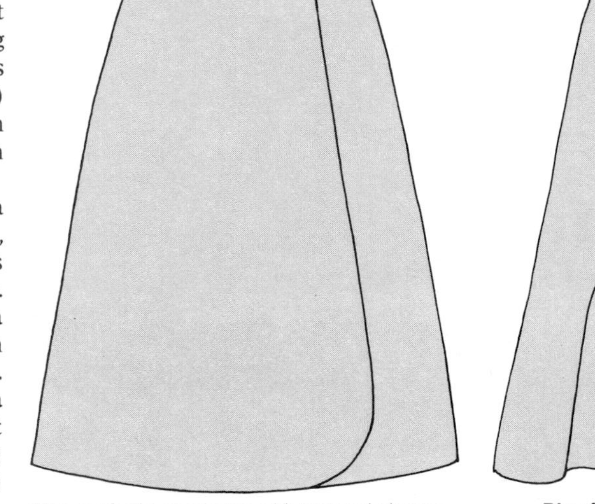

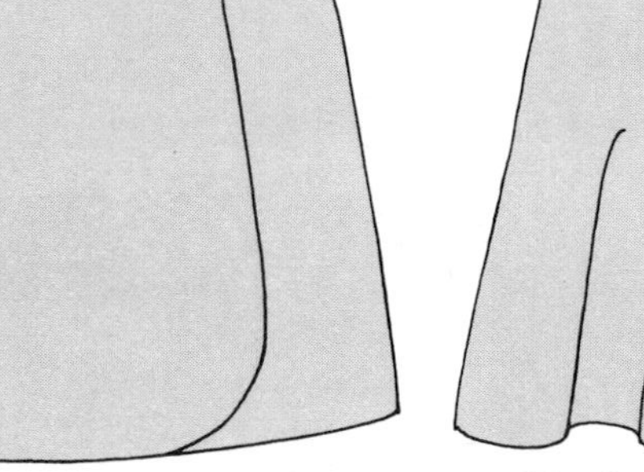

Shaped facing for hems with unusual shapes.

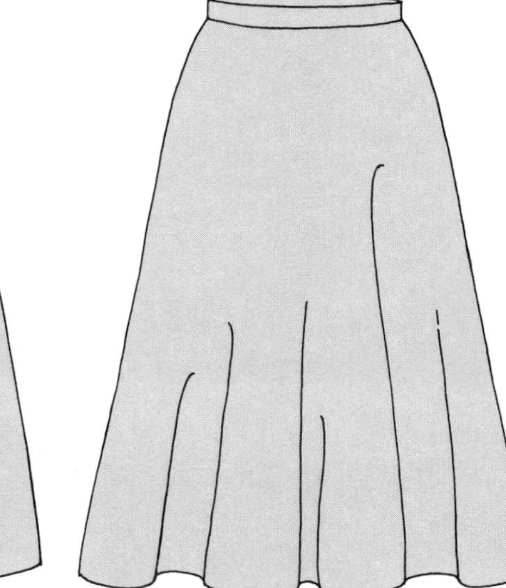

Bias facing for widely flared skirts.

Shaped hem facing

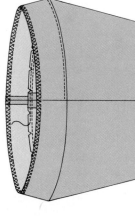

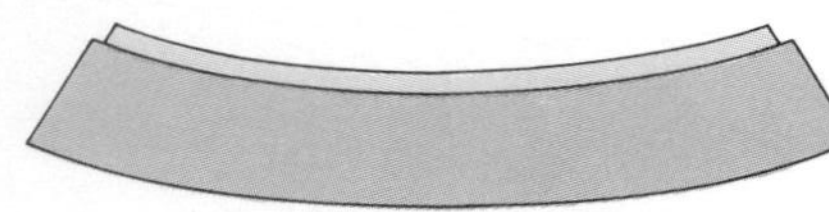

1. Cut facings to fit the hem. If there are no patterns, make your own, tracing the hemline from garment pieces. Cut them 2½" wide.

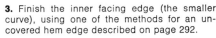

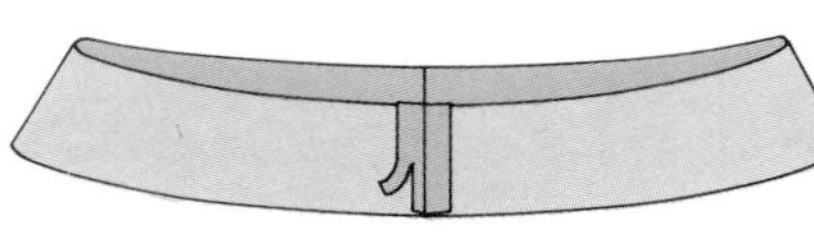

2. Join the facing sections and press the seams open. Trim the seam allowances to half their original width.

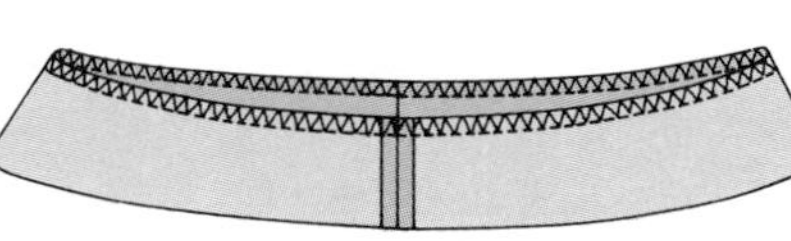

3. Finish the inner facing edge (the smaller curve), using one of the methods for an uncovered hem edge described on page 292.

4. Before attaching facing, mark hemline and trim hem allowance to ⅝". Right sides together, stitch facing to garment with ½" seam. Trim, grade, and notch seam allowances.

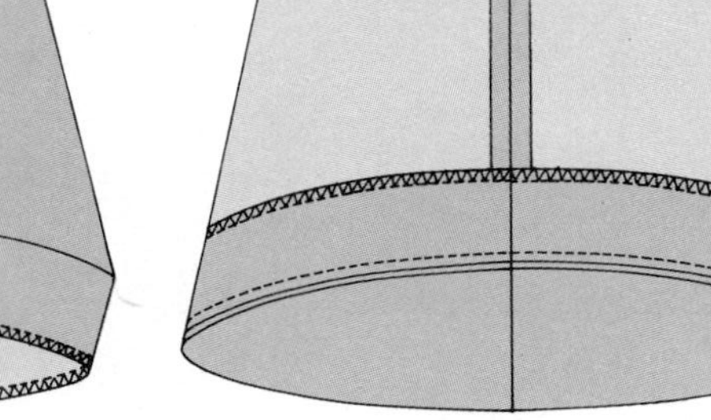

5. Press the seams open, then toward the facing. With the facing pulled out flat, stitch the facing close to the seam edge, through all of the seam allowances.

6. Turn facing inside the garment and press the hemline (seam should be ⅛" from fold). Secure free edge of facing to garment with an appropriate hem stitch (see p. 292).

Cutting bias strips

Bias strips are bands of fabric cut on the true bias (that is, any diagonal at a 45-degree angle to the lengthwise or crosswise grain). They have many uses, ranging from hem facings (directions on opposite page) to piping and covered cording (p. 300), bandings and bindings (pp. 301–303), neckline facings, casings, and ruffles.

When more than one strip is required, joining is done on the straight grain, either individually (two to four sections), or continuously (several strips at once). Both methods are shown on the opposite page. When bias is attached to a garment, the final seam is sometimes joined on the bias and aligned with a garment seam for a neat effect (see Enclosed edges, pp. 301–303, for examples).

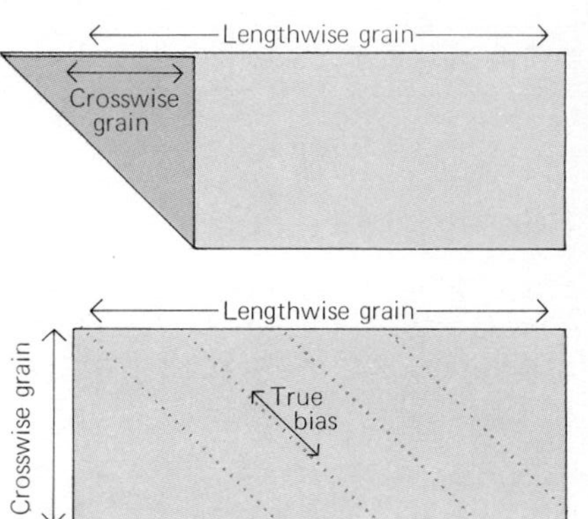

To cut the needed pieces, first locate the true bias by folding fabric diagonally so that a straight edge on the crosswise grain is parallel to the lengthwise grain (selvage). Press fabric along the diagonal fold; open it out and, using the crease as a guide, mark parallel lines, spacing them the width of one strip.

Purchased bias can be used if width, color, and fabric are suitable.

Lengthwise grain 84

Clipping seams 147
Grosgrain ribbon waistband facing 243

Joining bias strips

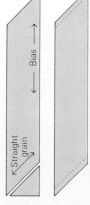

To join bias strips individually, first cut on the marked lines; make sure all ends are on the straight grain. Mark ¼″ seam allowances.

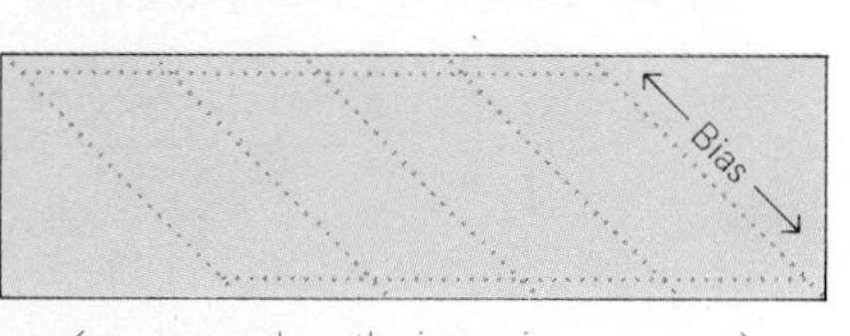

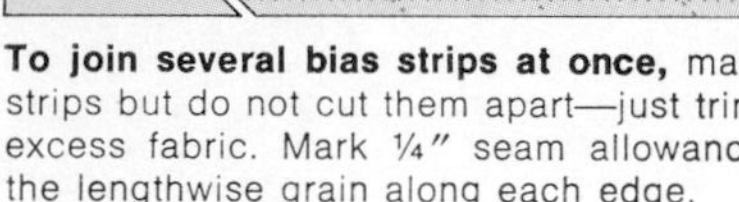

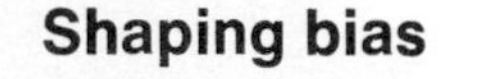

To join several bias strips at once, mark all strips but do not cut them apart—just trim the excess fabric. Mark ¼″ seam allowance on the lengthwise grain along each edge.

Right sides together, pin two strips with seamlines matching. Strips should form a V exactly as shown, with seam ends aligned.

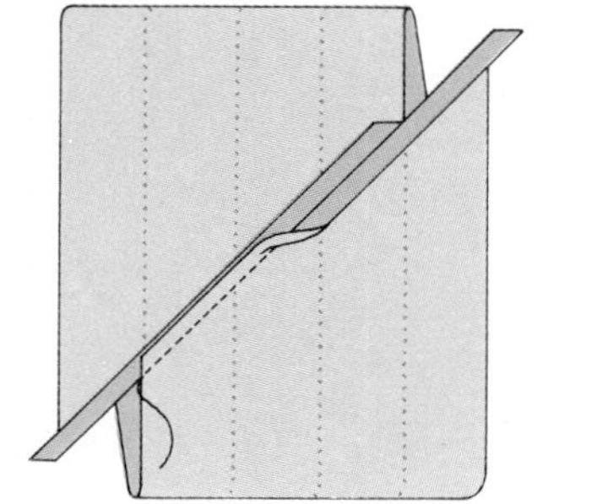

Fold fabric into a tube, right sides together; align the seams, and the marks, having one strip width extending beyond the edge on each side. Stitch; press seam open.

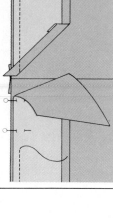

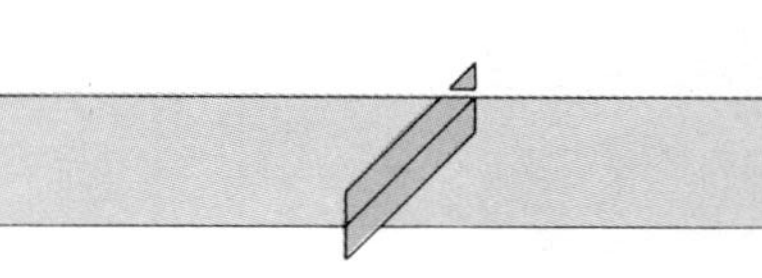

Stitch; press seam open. Trim protruding corners of seam allowances to align with edge of strip. Join as many strips as needed.

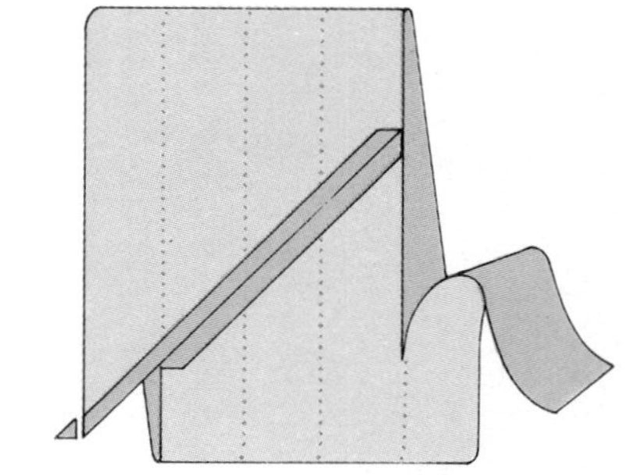

Beginning at one end, cut along the marked line, cutting continuously until you reach the edge of the strip at the opposite end. Trim protruding corners at each end.

Shaping bias

When bias is to be stitched to a curved edge, application will be easier and the finished edge smoother if you shape it first to conform to the curve. Do the shaping with a steam iron, shrinking in fullness along one edge while stretching the opposite edge.

The shaping method shown at the right is mainly for hem facings, whether your own bias or a packaged variety. This technique can be used also to shape grosgrain ribbon for waistband facing, but is less effective because grosgrain has little stretch.

Before applying shaped bias, determine how its edges should relate to the garment curves. With a hem facing, for instance, the stretched edge would be stitched to the hemline.

To shape bias, set the iron for steam; using the tip of the iron to hold bias in position on one edge, stretch and mold the opposite edge into a curve. After each section is shaped, press it gently to set the curve. When bias is to be used for a banding or binding, fold strip in half before shaping it.

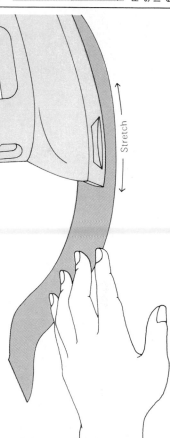

Stretch

Bias hem facing

Cut bias 2½″ wide and long enough to span hem edge plus 3″. Join and shape strips if necessary. Press under ¼″ along each edge. Trim all but ½″ of garment hem allowance.

Open out one folded edge of bias; fold the end back ¼″. Beginning at a garment seam, pin bias to hem, right sides together and raw edges aligned. Stitch along the creaseline to within 3″ of starting point.

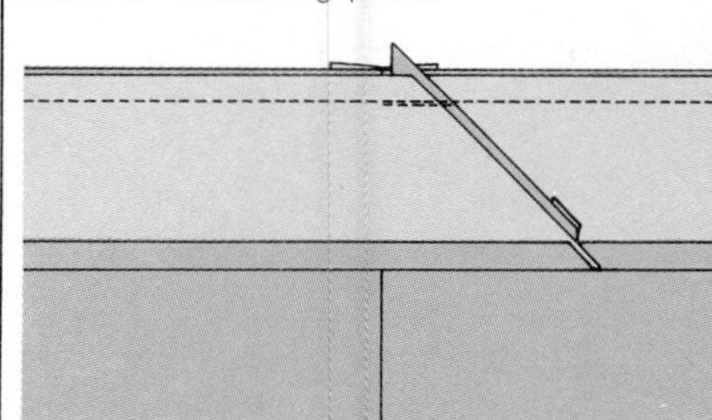

Trim excess facing to align with edge of starting end. Lap this end over the first one; stitch the rest of the way across.

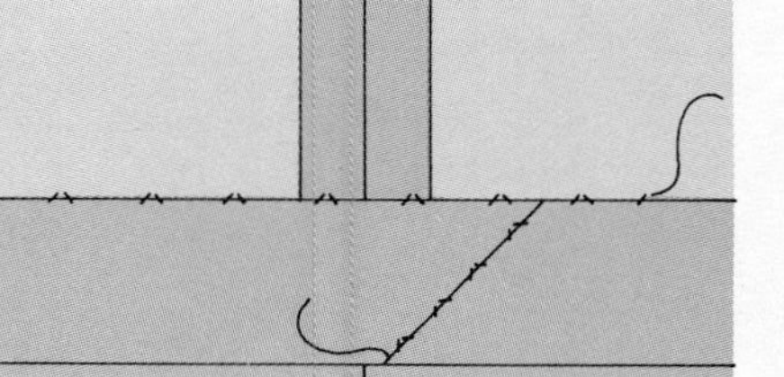

Press the seam open, clipping where necessary. Fold bias inside garment along the hemline; press. Secure bias to garment; finish the ends with a slipstitch.

Decorative hem finishes

Cable cord 16
Zipper foot 38
Hand hemming stitches 128-129
Understitching 147

Faced hem with decorative insert

One way to accent a hemline is with a decorative insert. Many ready-made trims will serve this purpose, lace and ruffled eyelet being just two examples. Each such trim has a plain or unfinished edge meant to be caught between facing and hem edge.

Two of the more popular insert trims are **piping** and **cording,** both made with bias strips, folded and stitched (see below). Piping is flat; cording is filled with a length of cable cord. Though either can be purchased, ready-made piping and cording come in a limited range of fabrics, widths, and colors, so it may be necessary or preferable to make your own.

Any inserted edging adds body and often some stiffness to a hem, causing it to stand away from the figure. Before proceeding, consider how this will affect your garment style.

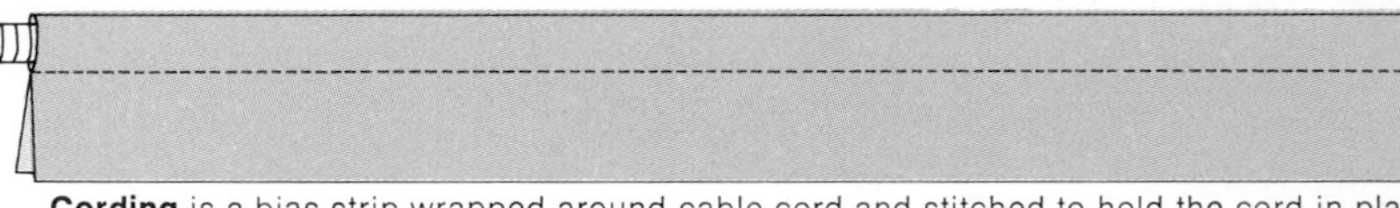

Piping is a bias strip folded wrong sides together, then stitched to form a flat welt.

Cording is a bias strip wrapped around cable cord and stitched to hold the cord in place.

How to make piping and cording

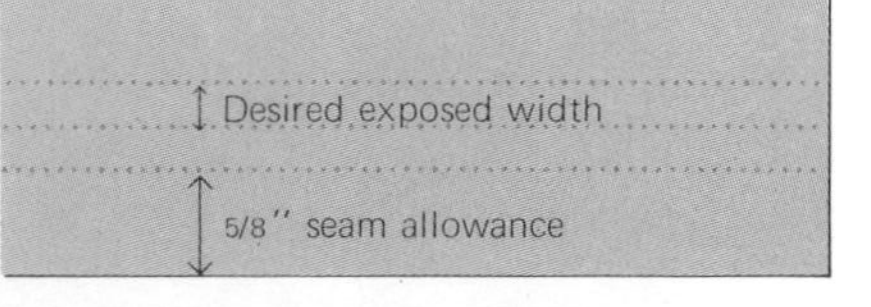

To make piping, cut bias twice the exposed width plus 1¼" for seam allowances. Fold strip in half lengthwise, wrong sides together; stitch ½" from raw edges.

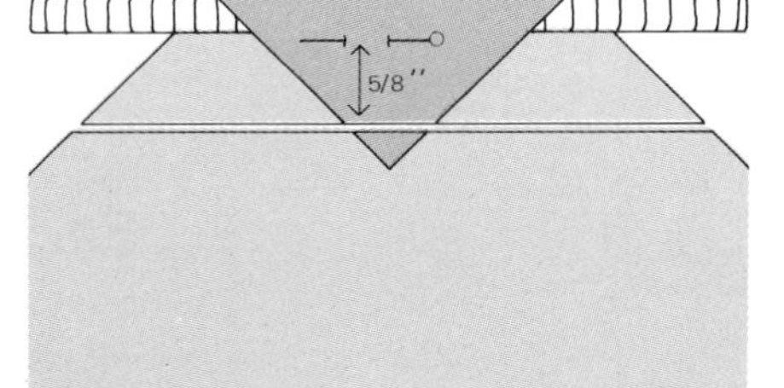

To make cording, first select a cable cord thickness; fold a corner of fabric (or tissue paper) over it and pin, encasing cord snugly; measure ⅝" out from pin and cut.

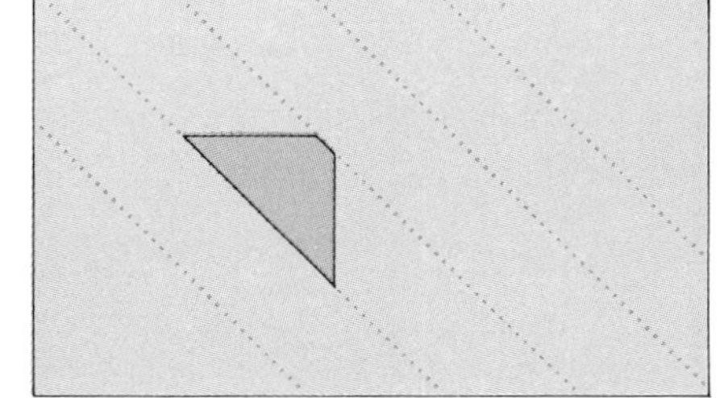

Use the measured piece as a pattern for marking the width of the bias strips. Join cut strips individually or continuously (see pp. 298–299 for cutting and joining bias).

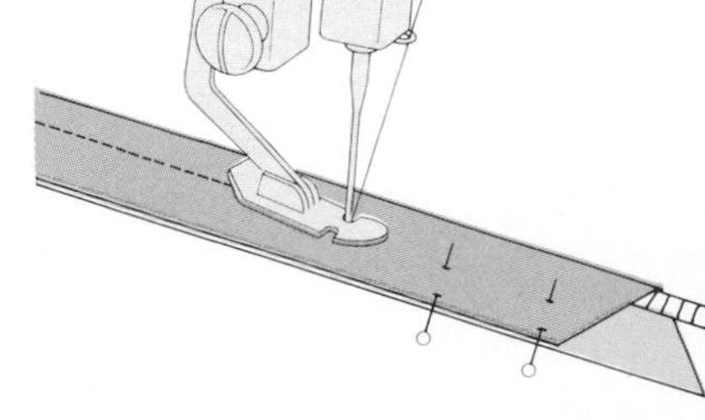

Wrap bias around cord with right side of fabric out, seam edges even; pin. With zipper foot to left of needle, stitch close to cord, but do not crowd stitching against it.

Applying piping or cording to a hemline

Application of piping or cording is done in two stages. It is stitched first to the garment, then to the facing, with each successive line of stitching placed closer to the trim. When completed, no stitching should show on the right side. Any trim to be inserted can be applied in the same way.

Before proceeding, hemline should be marked and the hem allowance trimmed to ⅝ inch. If the exposed portion of the trim is more than ¼ inch wide, adjust the hemline to allow for the amount that will show. For example, if trim is 1 inch wide after insertion, raise hemline 1 inch.

Baste piping to right side of hem, aligning piping seam and hemline. With zipper foot to right of needle, stitch left of piping stitches.

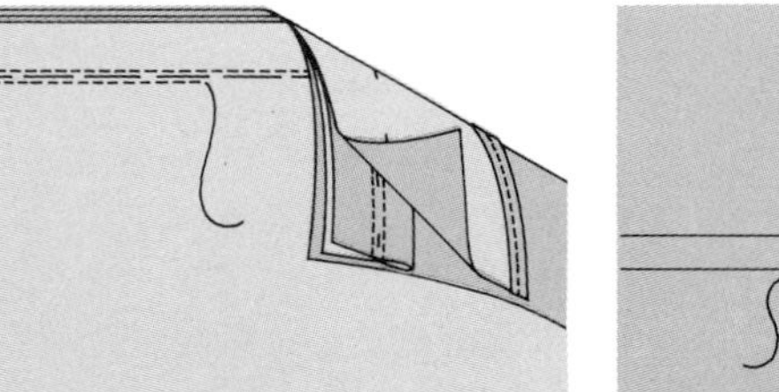

Baste facing to hem with right sides together, raw edges even. Stitch on the hem, crowding stitches between piping and first stitching.

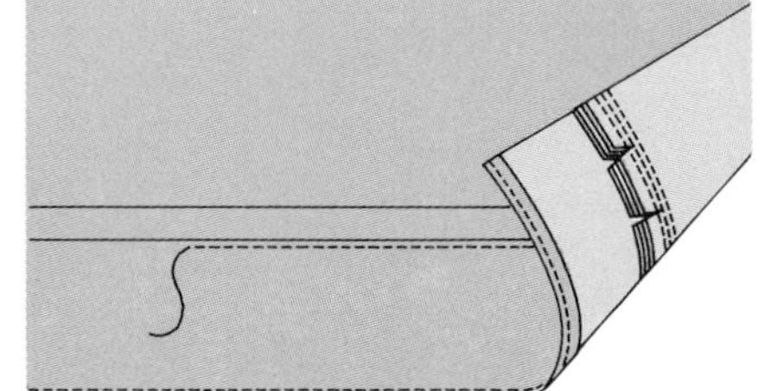

Trim, grade, and notch seam allowances. Press seams open, then toward facing. Understitch the facing, using a zipper foot.

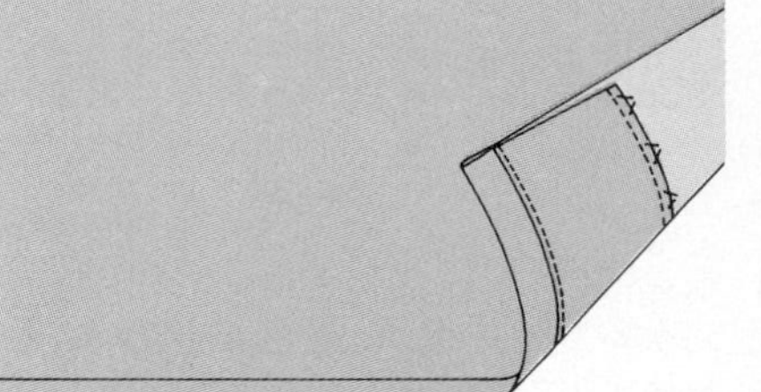

Press facing inside garment so that piping falls at the hem edge; secure facing with appropriate hemming stitch (see p. 292).

Shaped neckline band 206
Slipstitch 132

Enclosing a hem edge

For an enclosed hem edge, all of the hem allowance is eliminated and the raw edge encased by either a **banding** or a **binding.** Preparation and application of these two finishes are similar but, when completed, banding becomes an extension of the hem and binding wraps around it (see comparison below). The decision as to which should be used depends on garment style and fabric. A banding would be the choice if a garment needs lengthening (a child's dress, for example) or when a wide edging is desired. A binding is used most often for reversible styles and for garments made from sheer fabrics.

When preparing your own banding

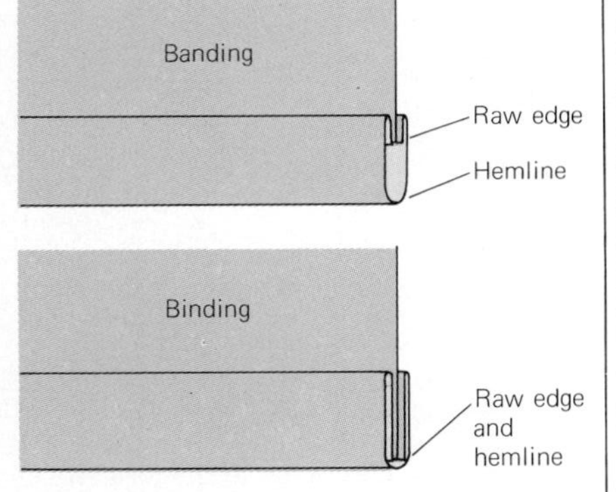

or binding, cut it on the fabric grain with the greatest stretch—bias for a woven, crosswise grain for a knit. The natural flexibility of these grains makes application smoother, especially on a curved edge. Bias strips are usually joined on the straight grain, but the method is different for banding and binding. For these uses, the ends of the strip are squared off and joined on the bias, and the juncture aligned with a garment seam for a trim look. Take special care not to stretch the fabric in joining.

Banding

Banding is an extension of a garment edge. It can be cut the same shape as the edge (see Necklines) or on the bias, the usual approach for a hem because it is ideal for adding length.

To prepare the hem for banding, mark the hemline at the desired length. Measure up from the hemline a distance equal to finished banding width; mark a new line and trim all but ¼ inch of fabric below it. (Omit second line to lengthen the garment.)

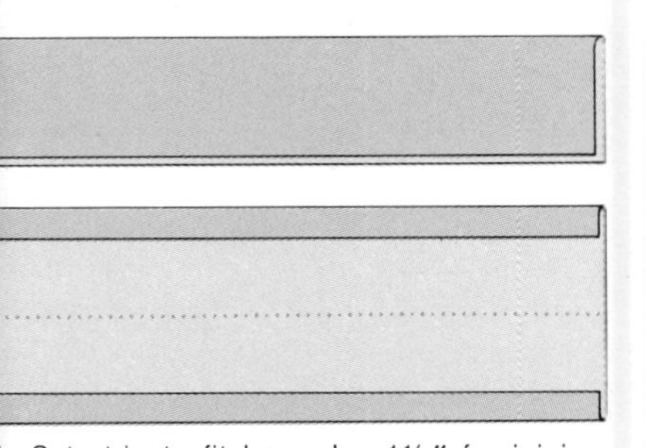

1. Cut strip to fit hem plus 1¼″ for joining. Press it in half lengthwise, wrong sides together. Open strip; press edges under ¼″.

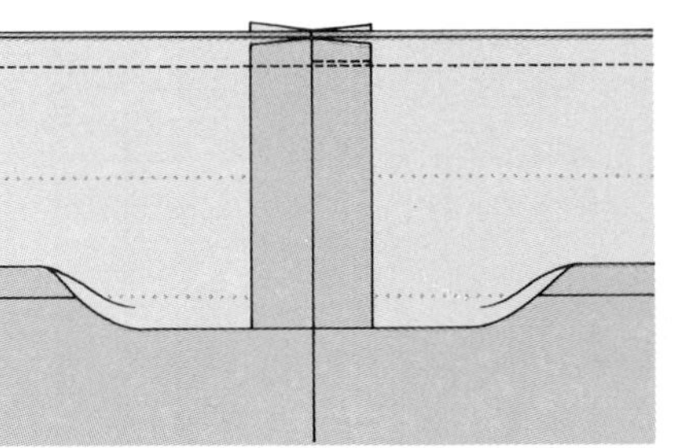

2. Open out folds; stitch ends and press seam open. Right sides together and seams aligned, stitch band to garment ¼″ from edge.

3. Press seam allowances toward the banding. Fold banding in half. If the banding is **woven,** bring folded edge to meet the seamline; pin.

If the banding is a **knit,** open out the raw edge and finger-press it flat. Baste in place with the raw edge extending ¼″ beyond the seamline.

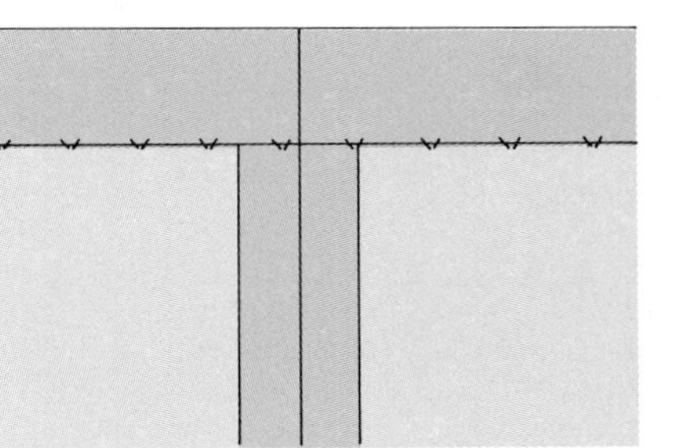

4. Finish woven banding by slipstitching the folded edge to the seamline. Stitches should not show on the right side of garment.

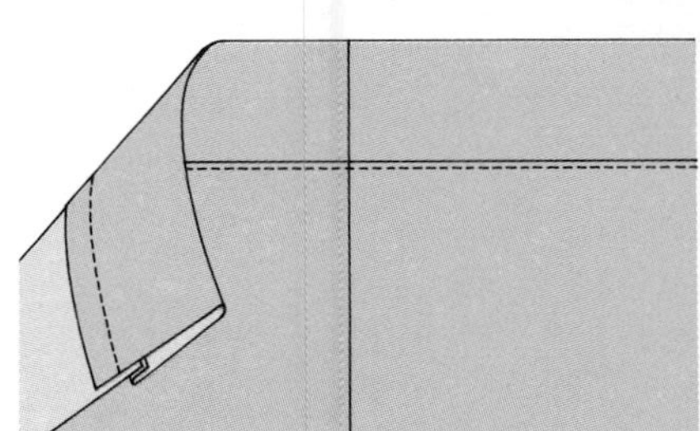

Finish a knit banding by stitching from the right side in the seam groove. Leave inside edge as is, or trim with pinking shears.

Quick application method for knit banding

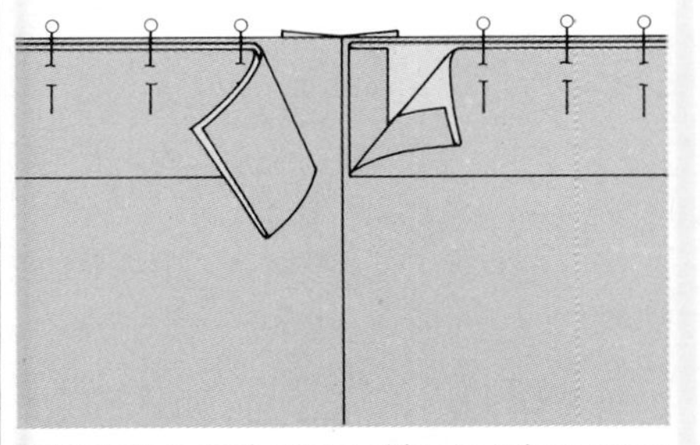

Fold strip in half, wrong sides together; press Fold one end under ½″. Pin band to garment raw edges even, folded end at seam.

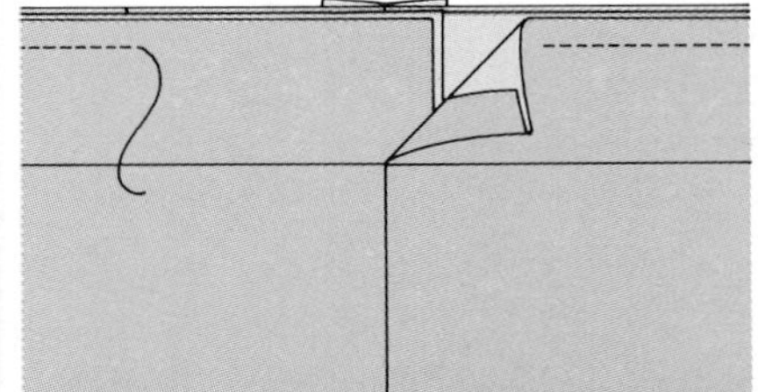

Stitch ¼″ from edge; begin 1″ from folded end and stop 3″ from starting point. Slip end between folds; lap ½″. Continue stitching.

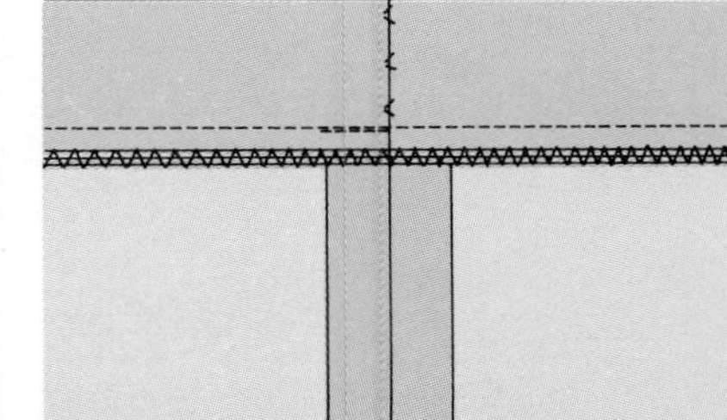

Zigzag edges together. Press band away from garment, seam allowances toward garment. Slipstitch ends of band where they overlap.

Hems with enclosed edges

Tapes and trimmings 16
Slipstitch 132

Binding

Binding is a strip of fabric that encases a hem or other garment edge. It is a neat and practical finish for the hem of a reversible garment, and can also be an attractive trim, especially in a contrasting color or texture.

The strip used for binding can be woven fabric cut on the bias, or knit cut on the crosswise grain. It might also be a folded braid, bias tape, or grosgrain ribbon (the most difficult to apply), all available by the yard or in packaged lengths.

There are two basic binding types, **single** and **double.** Single binding is suitable for any fabric; double binding is most appropriate for sheers.

To prepare the hem for binding, mark the hemline, then trim away all hem allowance (binding fold should be against hem edge when it is completed). Cut strips with seam allowances same width as finished binding. Completed width should be narrow.

A single binding can be applied in two stages (as shown on this page) or in a single operation (on the opposite page). The latter depends for success on careful pressing to make one side slightly wider than the other.

Single binding can be applied to any fabric.

Double binding is most appropriate for sheers.

Preparation of a single binding

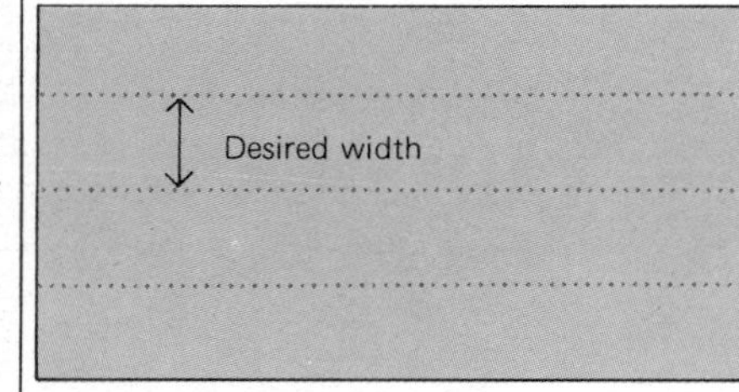

Cut bias strips four times the finished *width* of the binding, and the *length* of the edge to be bound plus 2″ for ease and joining.

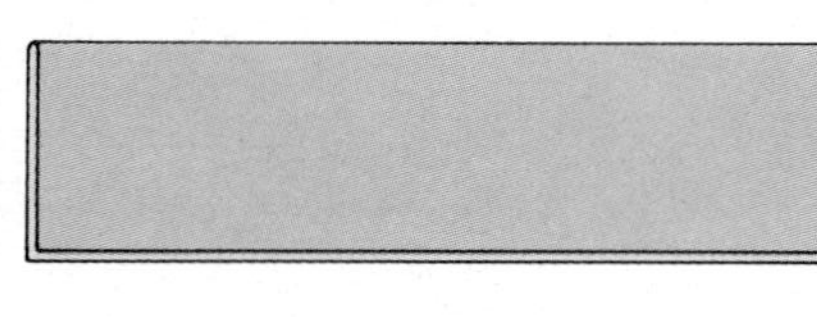
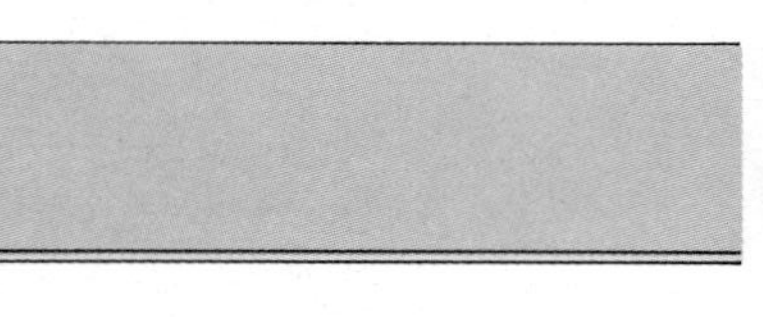

Fold the strip in half lengthwise, with wrong sides together. Press it lightly, taking care not to stretch the fabric.

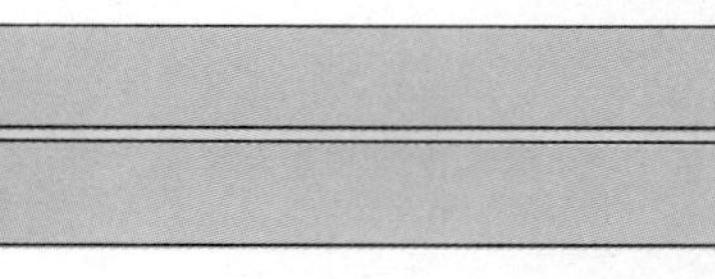

Open out binding and fold edges to meet at the center crease; press. Shape the binding if necessary (see p. 299 for method).

Applying a single binding

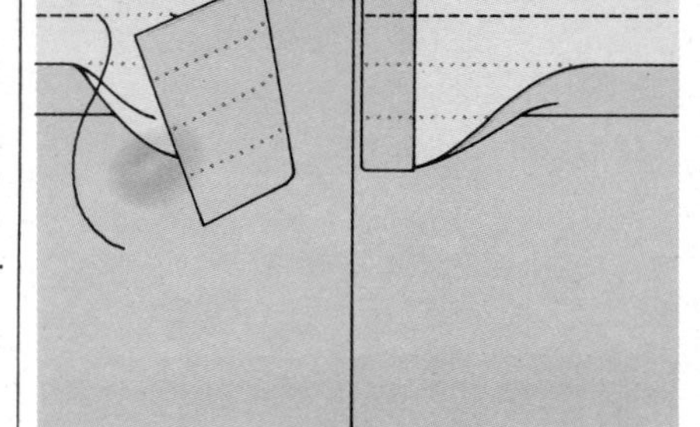

1. Open out one fold of binding; pin it to the hem edge, right sides together and raw edges aligned. Turn back the starting end ½″ and align the fold with a garment seam; stitch to within 3″ of the starting point.

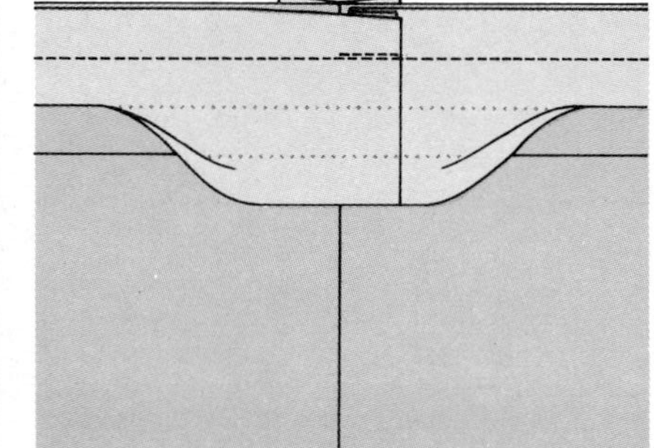
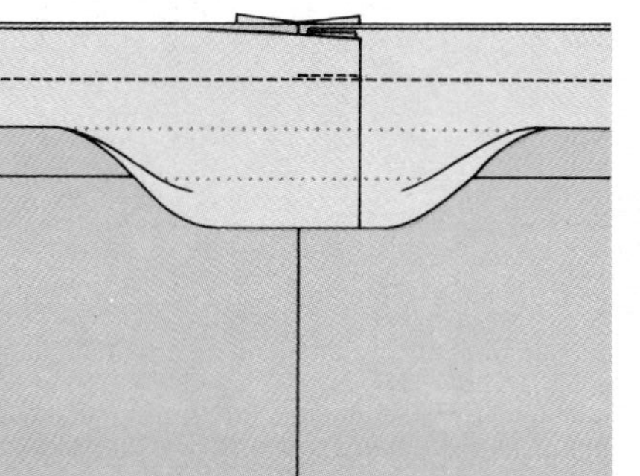

2. Trim away excess binding at this end so that it laps ½″ beyond the fold of the starting end. Lap the second end over the first one and stitch the rest of the way across, through all of the thicknesses.

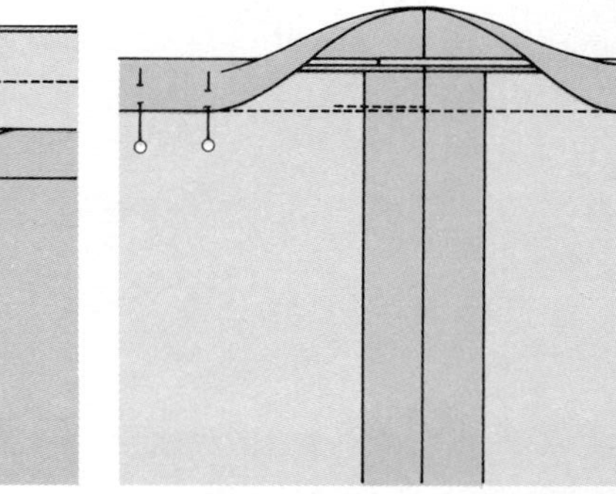

3. Press seam allowances toward the binding. Fold binding in half on the pressed line. If the binding fabric is **woven,** bring the turned-under edge to meet the seamline; pin in place, taking care not to stretch the fabric.

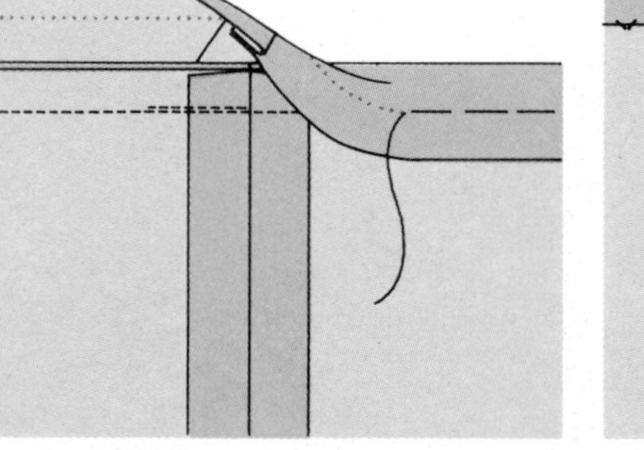

If binding is a **knit,** open the raw edge and finger-press it flat. Baste in place, matching the binding crease and garment seamline.

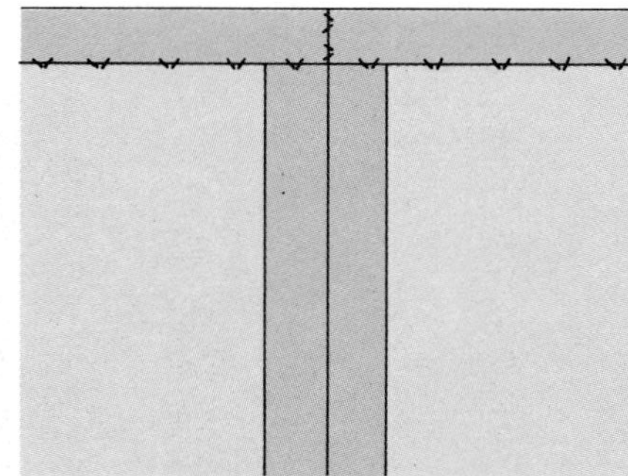

4. Finish woven binding by slipstitching the folded edge to the seamline. Slipstitch the binding ends where they overlap.

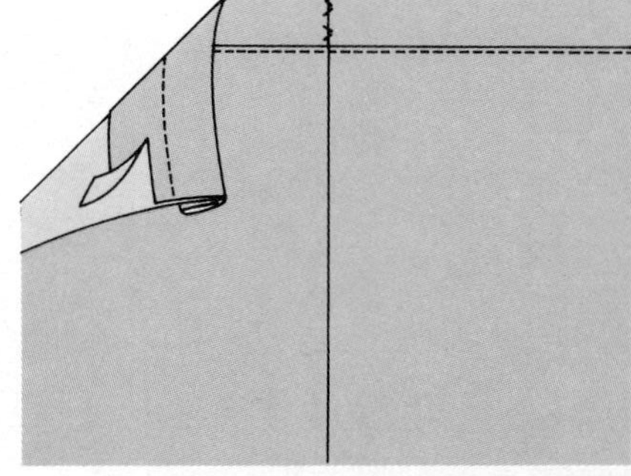

To finish a knit binding, stitch on right side in the seam groove. Slipstitch binding ends. Trim excess binding inside garment.

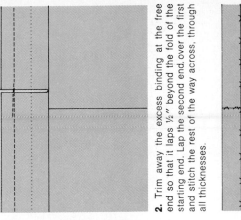

Preparing single binding for topstitching

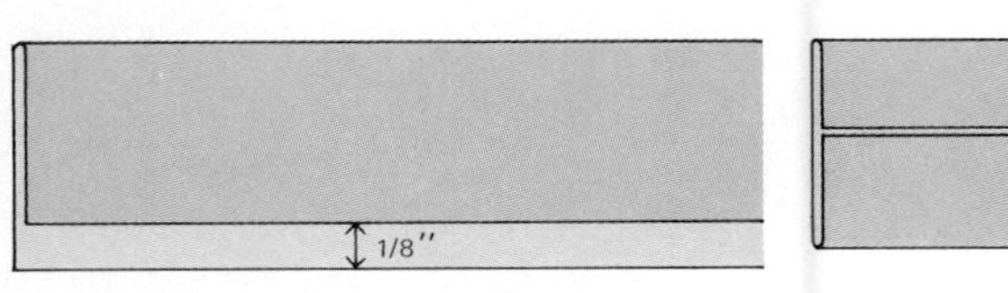

Fold bias strip lengthwise, a little off center, so that one side is 1/8" wider than the other; press strip lightly.

Open out strip and fold cut edges to meet at pressed crease; press folds lightly. Shape if necessary (see p. 299 for method).

Topstitch application of single binding

1. With garment right side up, wrap binding over the hem edge with wider side beneath. Pin binding, positioning the starting edge to extend ½" beyond a garment seam. Stitch to within 3" of the starting point.

2. Trim away the excess binding at the free end so that it laps the starting end by 1". Fold the second end under ½" and lap it over the first one, aligning the second fold with the garment seam.

3. Tuck all edges in neatly, then continue stitching, ending at the garment seam (do not reverse stitch at end). Remove pins.

4. Pull threads to the wrong side and tie a knot. Slipstitch the folded edge where binding overlaps. Press binding lightly.

Preparing a double binding

Cut binding strip six times desired width, and the length of edge to be bound plus 2". (Seam allowances equal finished width.)

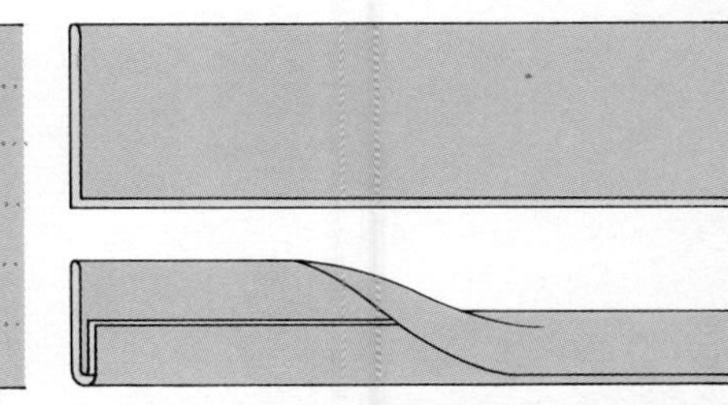

Fold strip in half lengthwise, wrong sides together; press. Fold the halved strip in thirds; press. Shape if necessary (p. 299).

Applying a double binding

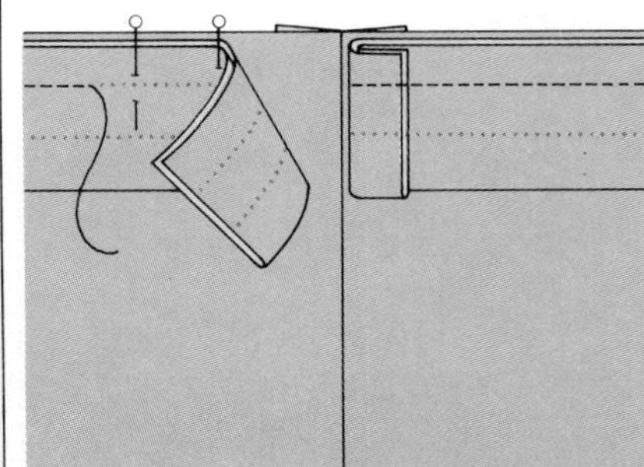

1. Lay binding on right side of hem with raw edges aligned. Turn back the starting end ½" and align the fold with a garment seam; pin. Stitch, in binding crease nearest the edge, to within 3" of the starting point.

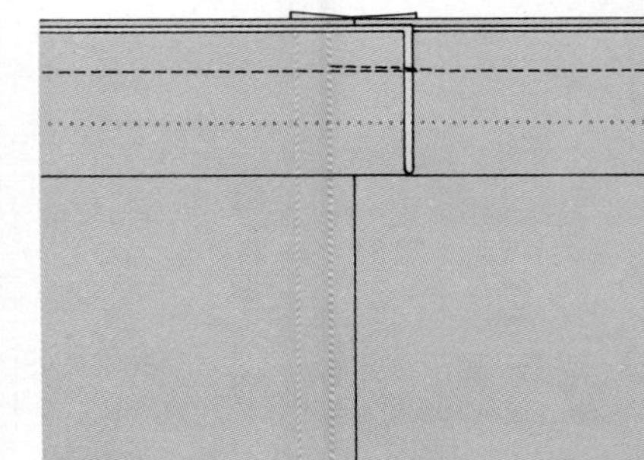

2. Trim away the excess binding at the free end so that it laps ½" beyond the fold of the starting end. Lap the second end over the first and stitch the rest of the way across, through all thicknesses.

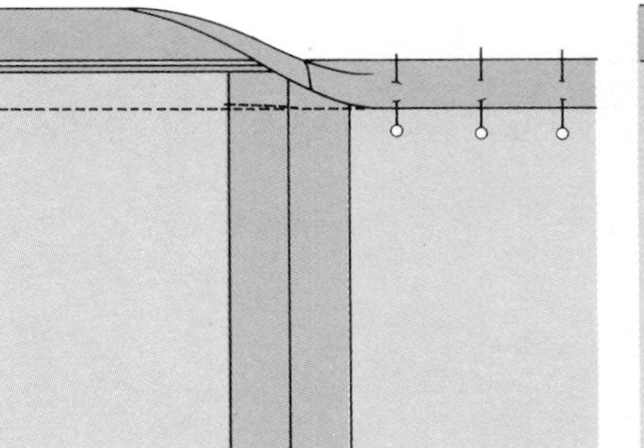
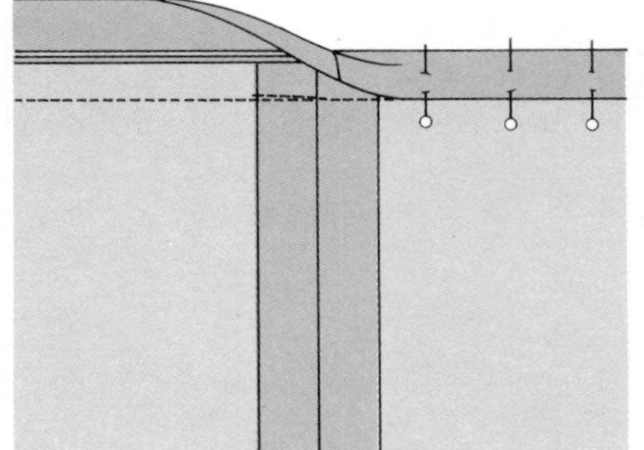

3. Turn binding inside the garment, bringing the long folded edge just to the stitching line. The folded end will be on top.

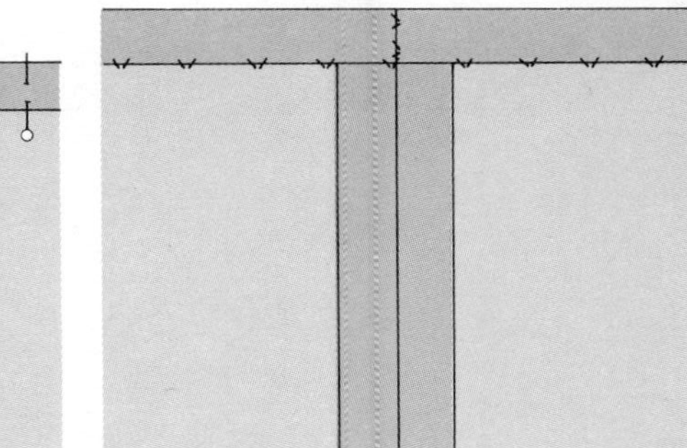

4. Slipstitch binding to seamline, taking care that stitches do not show on right side. Slipstitch binding ends where they overlap.

Finishing corners

Tying thread ends 137

Mitering

Corners that occur at garment edges can be satisfactorily finished in any hem style (turned-up, faced, bound, etc.) by means of a technique called **mitering**—the diagonal joining of two edges at the corner. The join may be stitched or just folded in place. The key to successful mitering is accurate pressing of folds at the corner, with the mitered piece always at a right angle to the corner's sides. These pressed lines sometimes act as stitching guides for the miter.

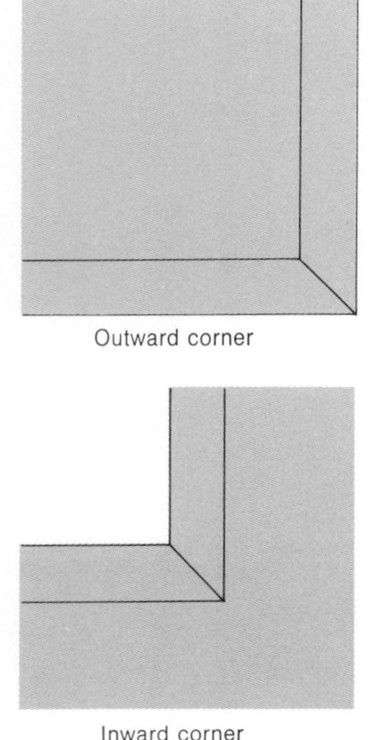

Outward corner

Inward corner

Corners divide basically into two types, **outward** and **inward** (see illustrations above); mitering techniques will differ for each. If the mitered piece (e.g., binding) *goes around* the corner, it is an outward corner; if the piece *lies within* the corner, it is an inward corner.

Mitering turned-up hems

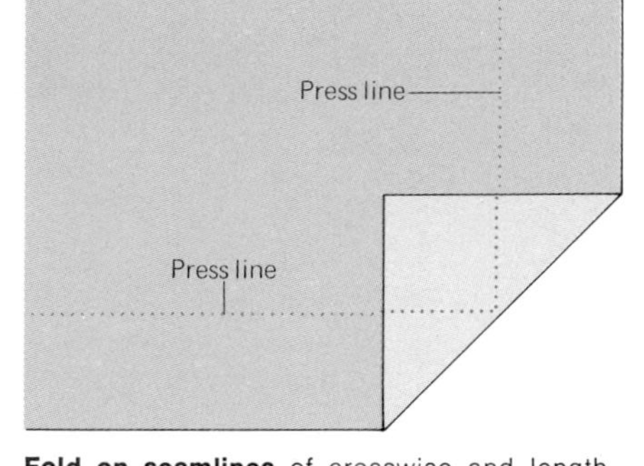

Fold on seamlines of crosswise and lengthwise edges; press. Open out edges. Fold corner up, aligning creased lines; press.

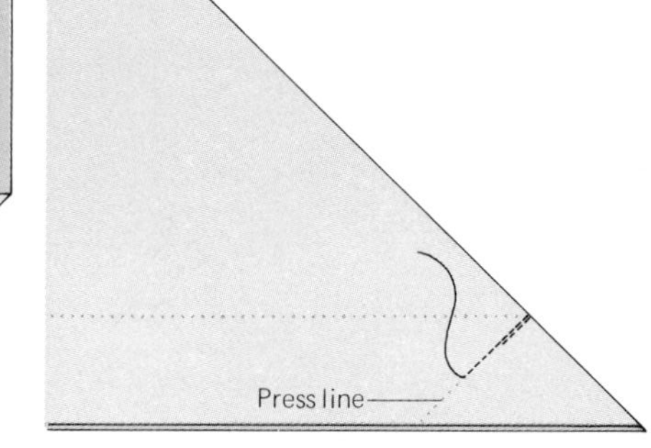

Open out corner. Fold garment diagonally (on bias), right sides together and raw edges even. Stitch on diagonal press line.

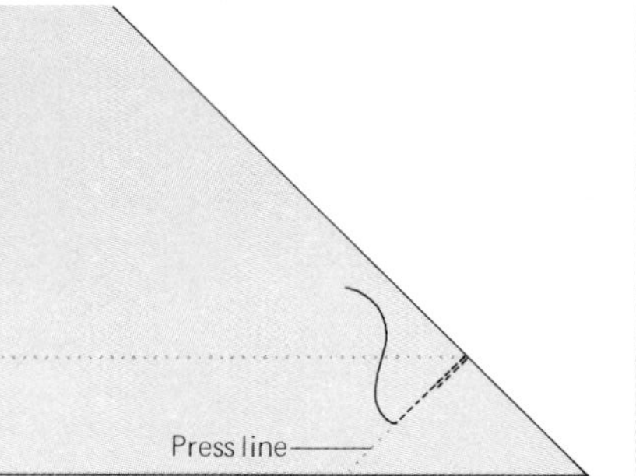

Trim point, leaving ¼″ seam allowance. Taper seam allowance at corner; press seam open. Turn corner right side out; press.

Mitering a flat trim

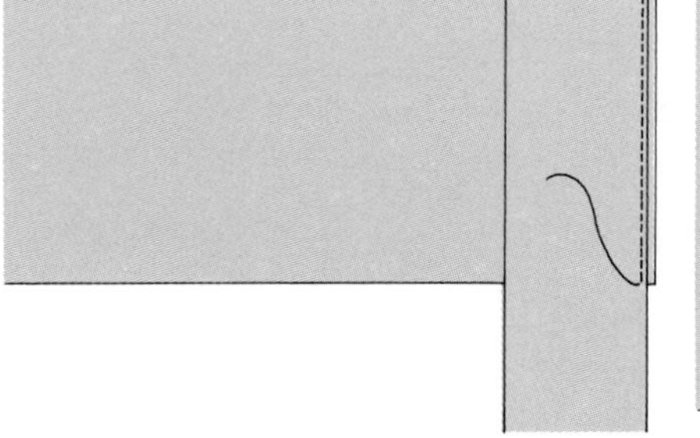

1. Pin the trim to finished edge of garment. Stitch along outer edge of trim; stop at corner; pull threads to wrong side and knot.

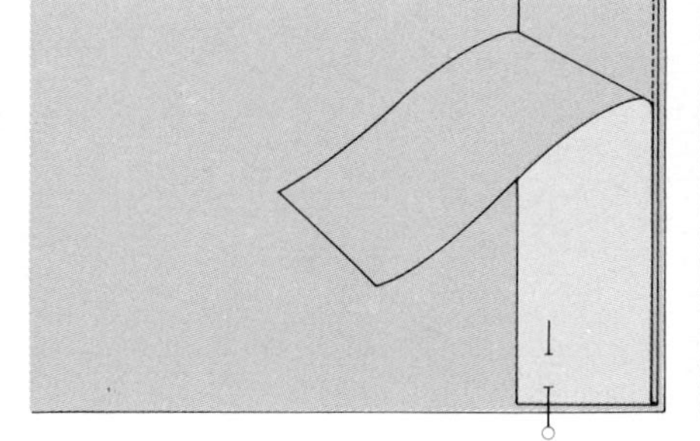

2. Fold trim straight back on itself so that fold of trim aligns with lower garment edge; pin at fold to hold in place.

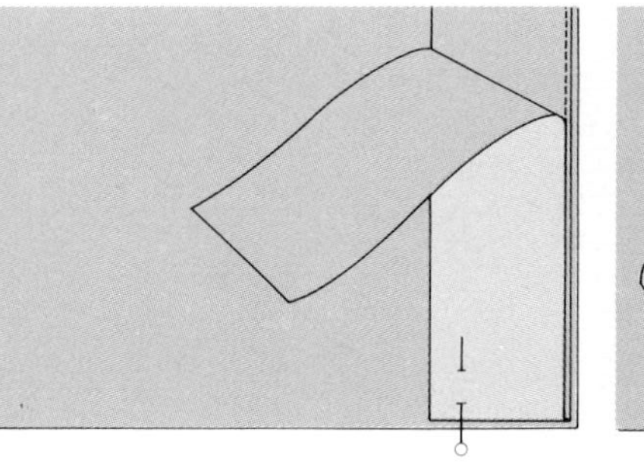

3. Fold trim down, creasing a diagonal fold at corner and aligning outer edge of trim with lower edge of garment. Press diagonal.

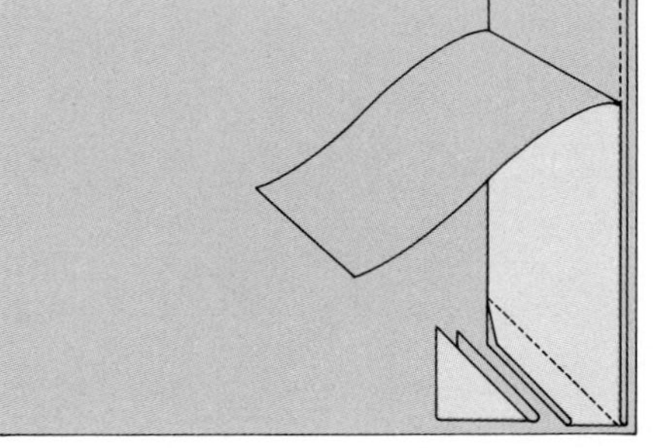

4. Lift up trim at corner and stitch on diagonal press line through all thicknesses. Trim the corner to reduce bulk.

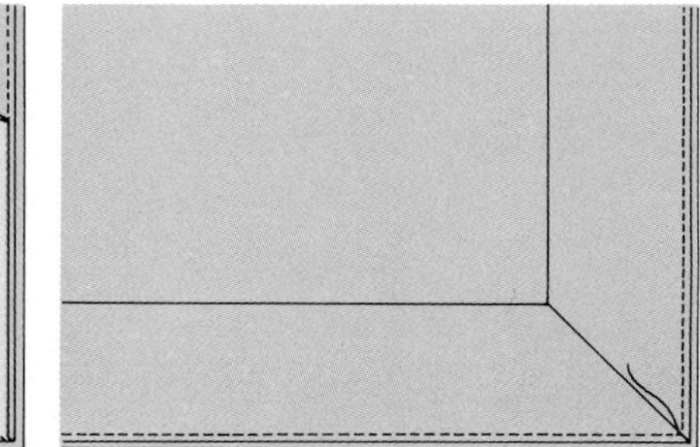

5. Fold trim back, aligning its lower edge with garment edge. Starting in last stitch at corner, stitch along outer edge of trim.

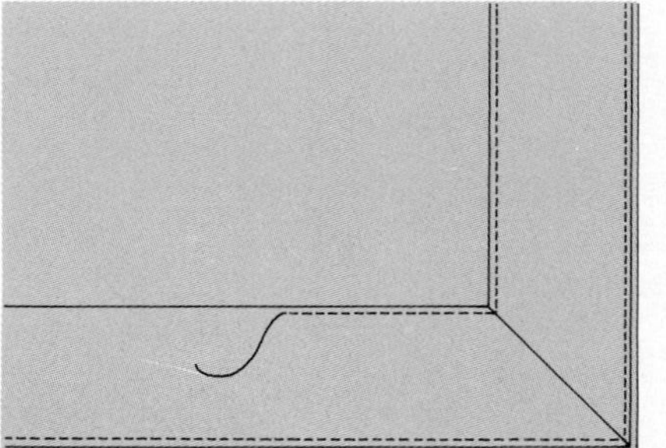

6. Pull threads at corner to wrong side and knot. Then stitch along inner edge of trim. Press entire trim and garment.

Mitering a bias facing

When applying a bias facing to a garment edge with corners, care must be taken to get the facing to turn inside and lie flat at each corner. Before starting, trim the seam allowances to ¼ inch along the edge to be faced. A prepackaged bias facing can be used,

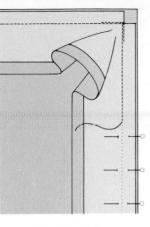

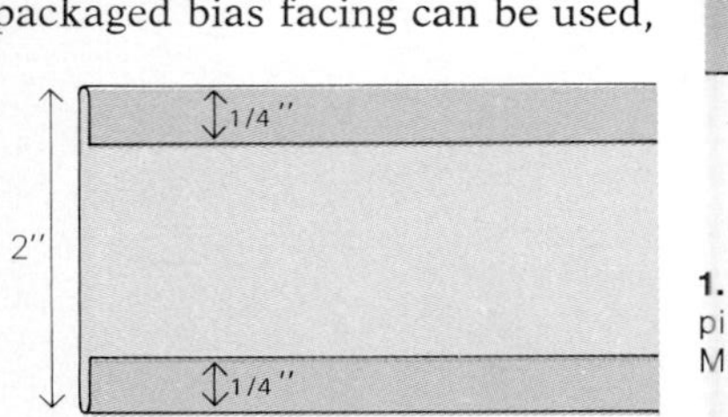

or facing can be cut from a lightweight underlining as shown above. Cut a bias strip (see pp. 298–299) 2½ inches wide, and press both long edges ¼ inch to the wrong side. Follow the instructions at the right for mitering at an outward corner. To miter an inward corner, follow the steps illustrated below; basically this technique enables you to change a straight bias piece into a shaped facing. Trim carefully during construction to help eliminate bulk.

Mitering a bias facing (outward corner)

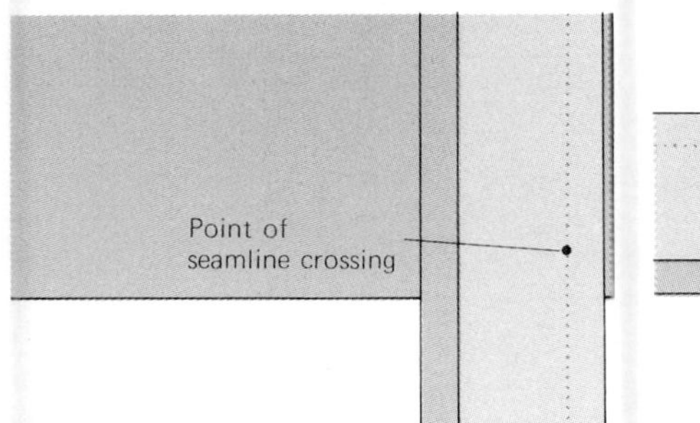

1. Open out one folded edge of bias facing; pin to garment edge, right sides together. Mark facing at point of seamline crossing.

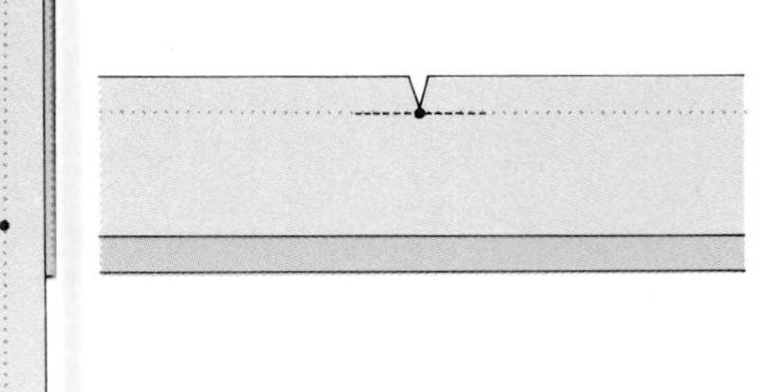

2. Place a short row of stitches within foldline in area of marked point. Clip seam allowance to point; avoid cutting threads.

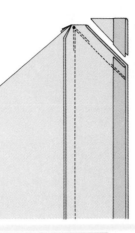

3. Pin facing to garment as before; at the slash point, bring facing around corner. Stitch along foldline, pivoting at corner.

4. Trim off seam allowances at the corner. Carefully fold the facing so it is at right angles to itself. Press lightly.

5. Fold garment, right sides together, so facing edges are even. Stitch on diagonal press line. Trim off point; leave ¼" seam allowance.

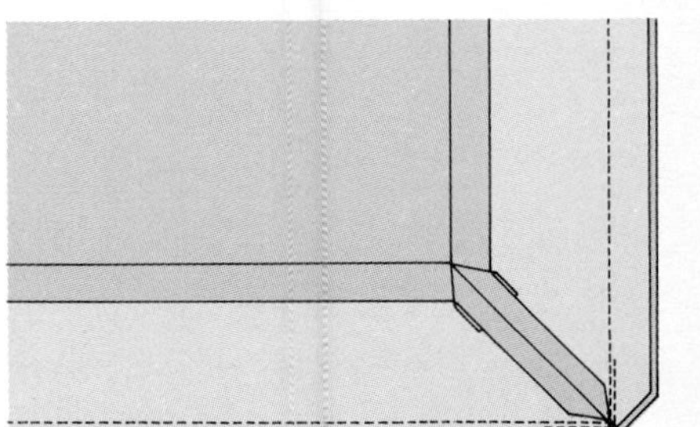

6. Clip seam allowance at corner; press mitered seam open. Press open seam allowances at edges; turn facing to wrong side; press.

Mitering a bias facing (inward corner)

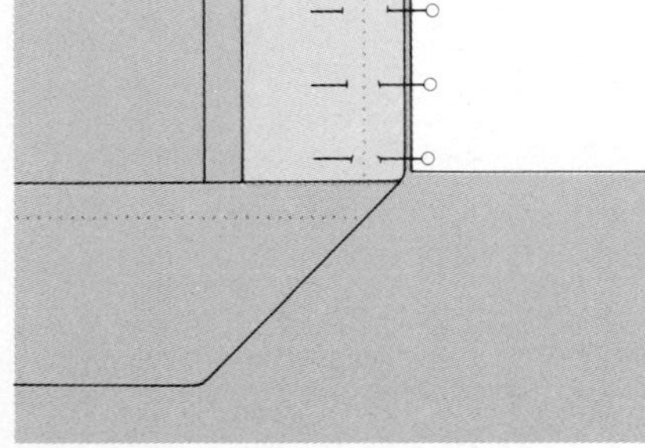

Open one folded edge of bias facing; pin to garment edge, right sides together. Diagonally fold facing at corner edge; press.

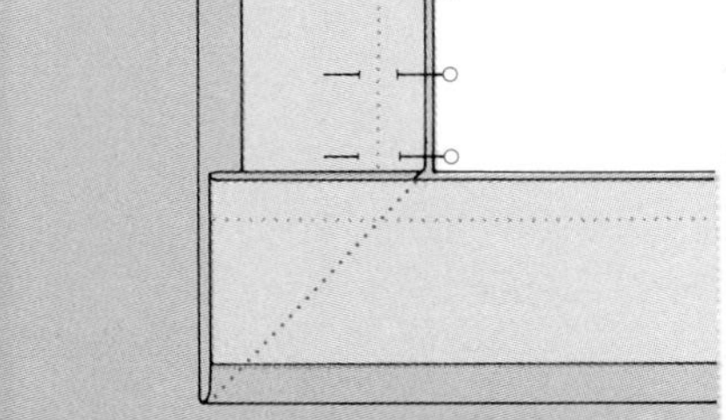

Fold facing straight back toward the corner, aligning fold with the outer edge of facing; press lightly. Remove facing.

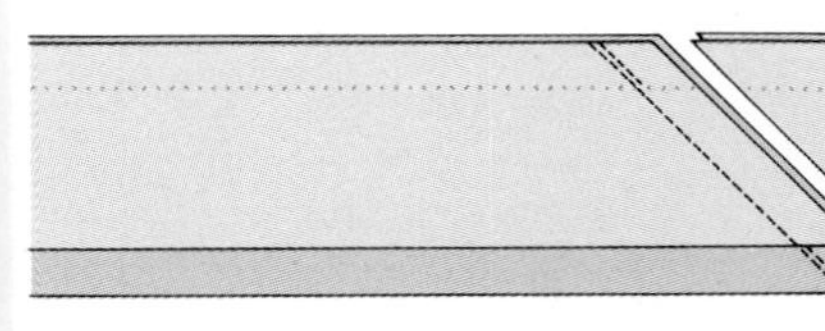

Fold facing along press line, right sides together. Stitch on the diagonal press line. Trim corner point, leaving ¼" seam allowance.

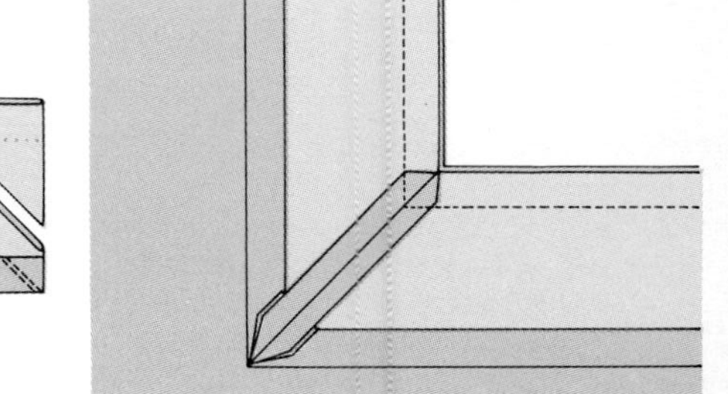

Clip seam allowance at point; press open. Treat mitered facing as a shaped facing and apply to garment (see Neckline facing).

Finishing corners

Mitering banding (outward corner)

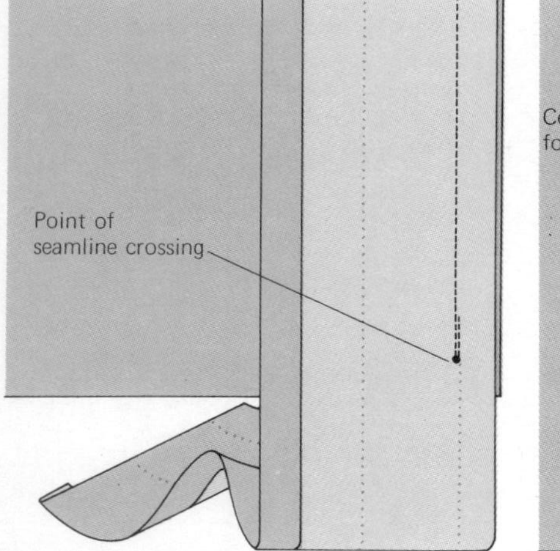

Prepare banding as described on page 301. Open out one folded edge. With right sides together, pin banding to garment edge; stitch along the banding foldline; stop and secure stitches at seamline crossing.

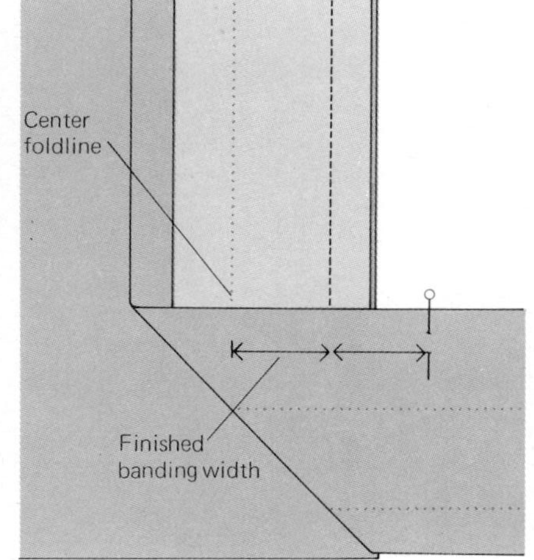

Diagonally fold banding away from garment; press lightly. From the center foldline of the banding, measure a distance equal to twice the width of the finished banding, and mark that point with a pin.

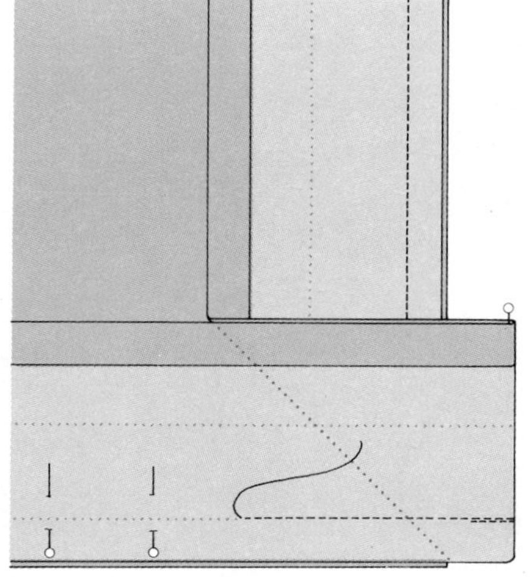

Fold the banding straight back from the pin mark, and pin banding edge to the adjoining garment edge. Stitch along the banding foldline, securing stitches at the beginning. Then press the seam flat.

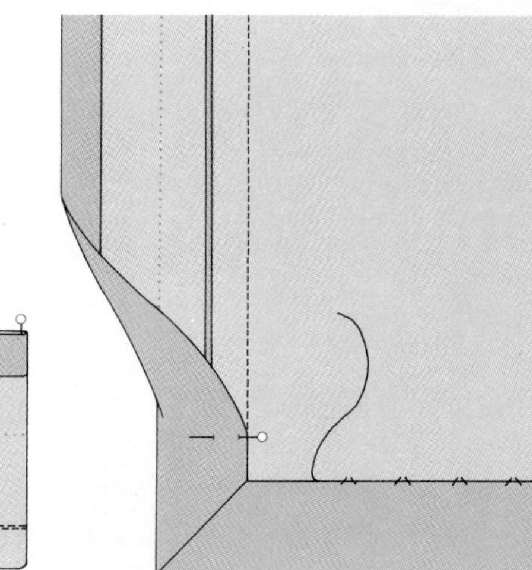

Form a neat miter on right side of garment; fold banding over edges to wrong side and form miter on that side. Bring folded edge of banding to stitching line; pin and slipstitch banding edge and mitered fold in place.

Mitering banding (inward corner)

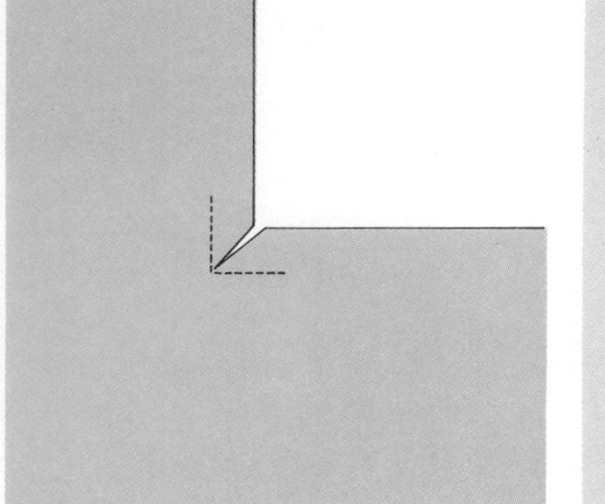

Reinforce inner garment corner with small stitches: Stitch within a thread's width of the seamline for 1″ on either side of the corner. Clip into the corner, being careful not to cut threads of reinforcement stitches.

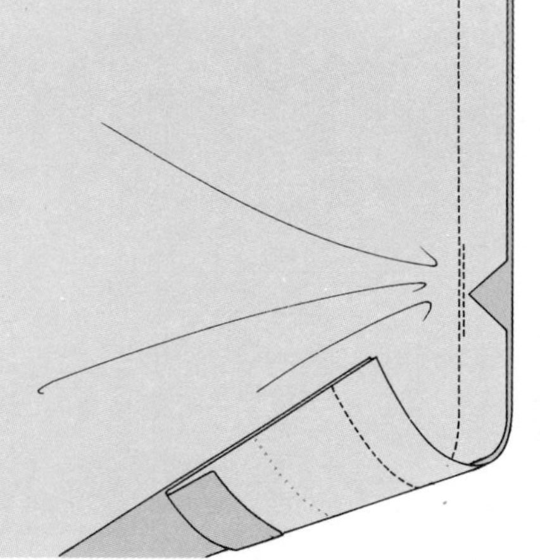

Prepare banding (see p. 301). Open out one folded edge. Spread the slashed corner and pin edge to banding, right sides together; keep banding foldline aligned with garment seamline. Stitch from the garment side.

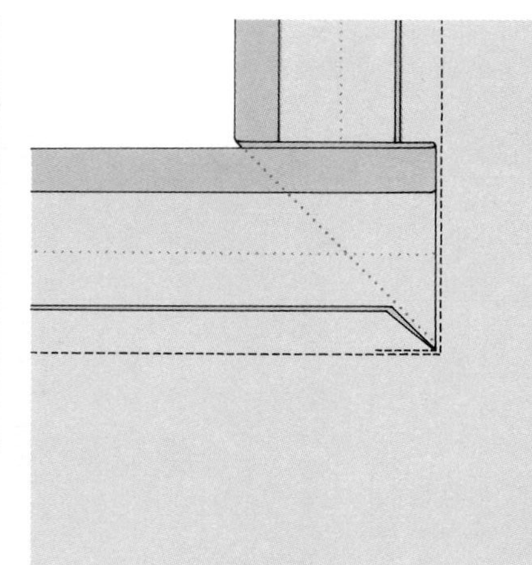

Carefully fold banding to form miter on the right side. Illustration above shows folds from the wrong side; note straight fold of mitered banding is placed between edges of clip. Keep edges at right angles to one another.

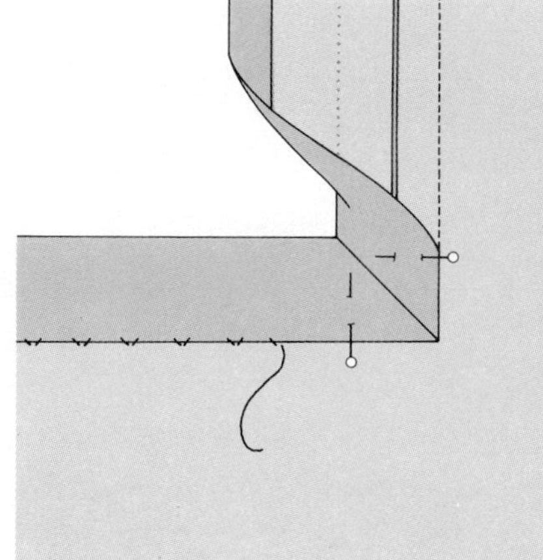

Turn banding down over seam allowances, forming miter on the wrong side; folded edge of banding should come to the stitching line. Pin and slipstitch the banding edge and mitered fold in place.

Mitering knit banding (outward corner)

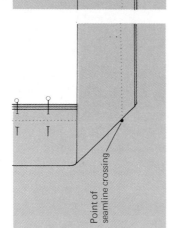

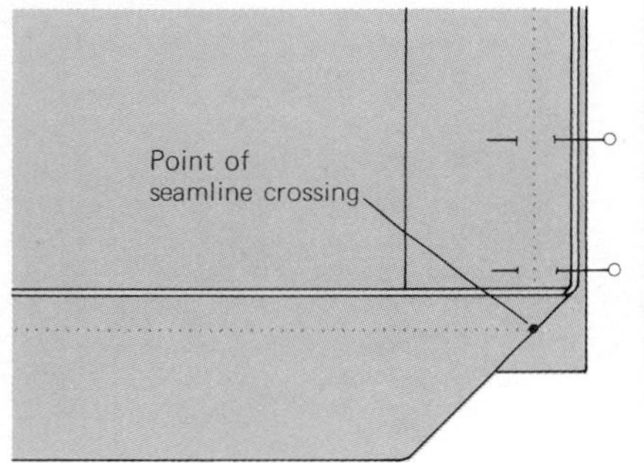

1. Prepare banding (see p. 301). Open folded edges, then fold banding along center foldline. Pin to garment; stop at seamline crossing; fold banding diagonally toward garment.

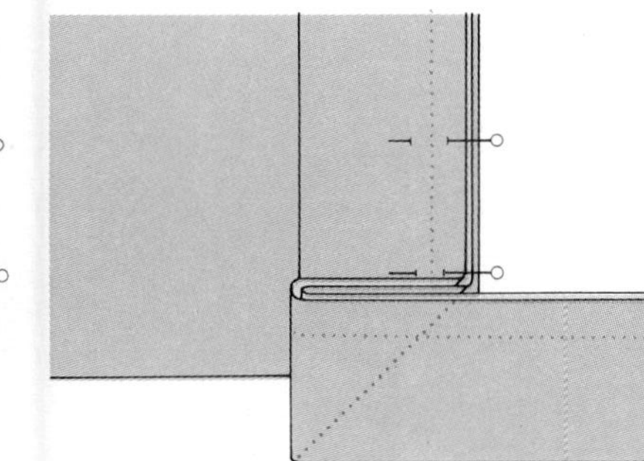

2. Fold the banding straight back toward the corner so that the fold is aligned with the banding edge; press lightly. Remove banding, and open it out completely.

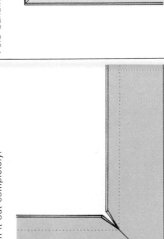

3. Fold the banding along the horizontal press line, right sides facing. Stitch along the press lines that form a "pyramid"; start and stop ¼" from edges; secure stitches.

4. Trim excess at corners, leaving a ¼" seam allowance on each side; clip to point. Press seam allowances open, and turn mitered banding right side out. Press.

5. Pin banding onto garment as before, bringing banding around corner. Stitch along banding foldline; shorten stitches around corner. Trim off garment seam allowance at corner.

6. Place another row of stitches (either zigzag or straight) within the seam allowance. Press flat, then press banding away from garment. Whipstitch corners together.

Mitering knit banding (inward corner)

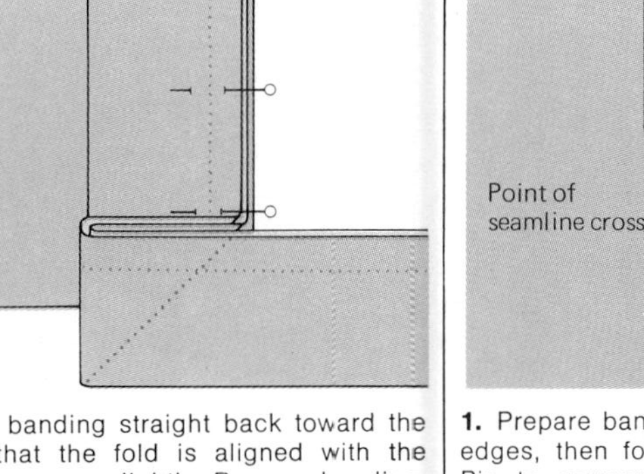

1. Prepare banding (see p. 301). Open folded edges, then fold banding on center foldline. Pin to garment; stop at seamline crossing. Fold banding diagonally away from corner.

2. Fold banding straight back toward the garment so that the fold is aligned with the raw edge of the banding; press lightly. Remove banding, and open it out completely.

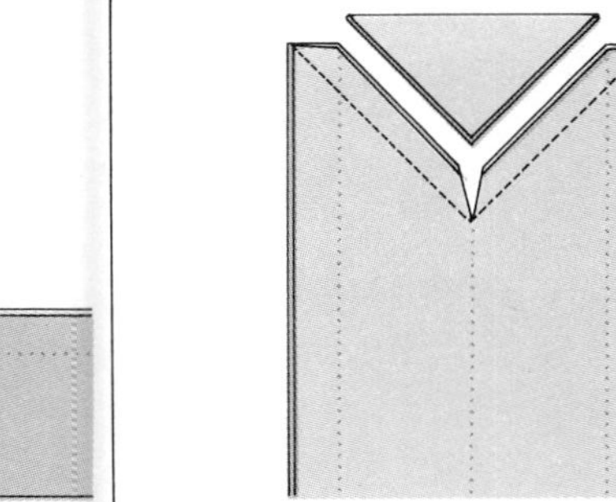

3. Fold banding along horizontal press line, right sides facing. Stitch press lines that form "inverted pyramid." Trim triangular piece; leave ¼" seam allowances; clip; press open.

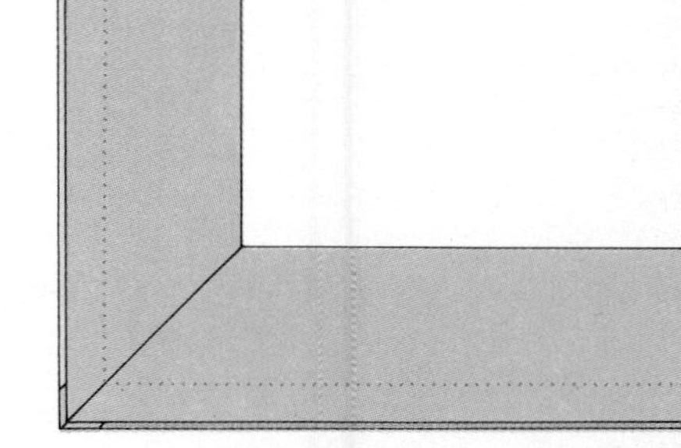

4. Turn banding right side out. Press. Reinforce inner garment corner with small stitches: Stitch within a thread's width of seamline for 1" on either side of corner.

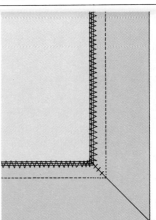

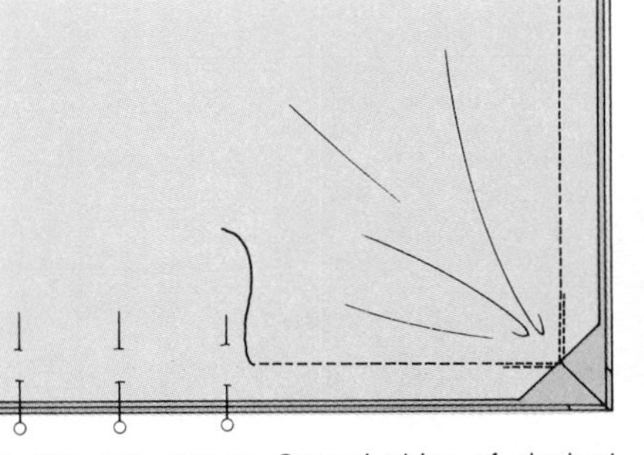

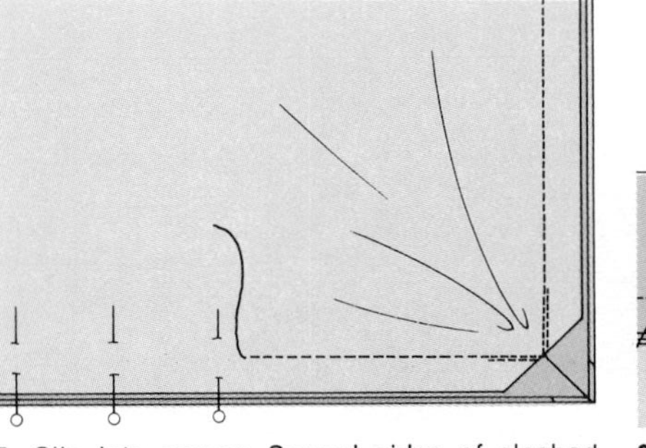

5. Clip into corner. Spread sides of slashed corner, and pin banding to right side of garment, foldline and seamline aligned. Stitch from garment side, pivoting at corner.

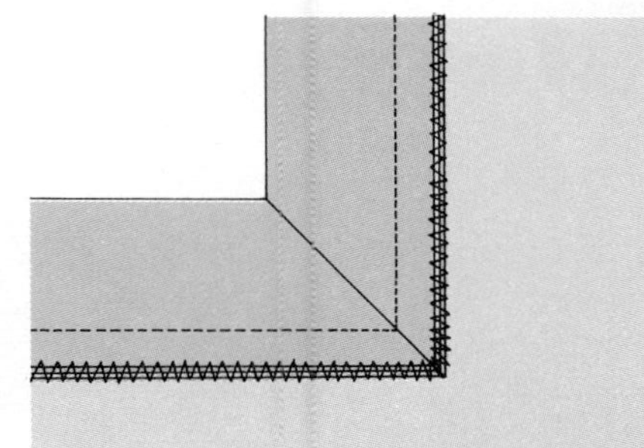

6. Place another row of stitches (either zigzag or straight) within the seam allowance. Press flat to embed stitches. Press banding away from the garment.

Finishing corners

Slipstitch (uneven) 132

Mitering bindings

Methods of constructing and applying single and double bindings are dealt with earlier in this chapter (see pp. 302–303). Though these methods differ according to the type of binding, mitering techniques for both single and double binding are similar for outward and for inward corners. The illustrations below show a single binding being mitered; note that one folded edge is opened before application begins. When mitering a double binding, keep the binding folded in half, and proceed as directed below. Techniques for mitering a topstitched binding are on the opposite page.

Mitering single or double binding (outward corner)

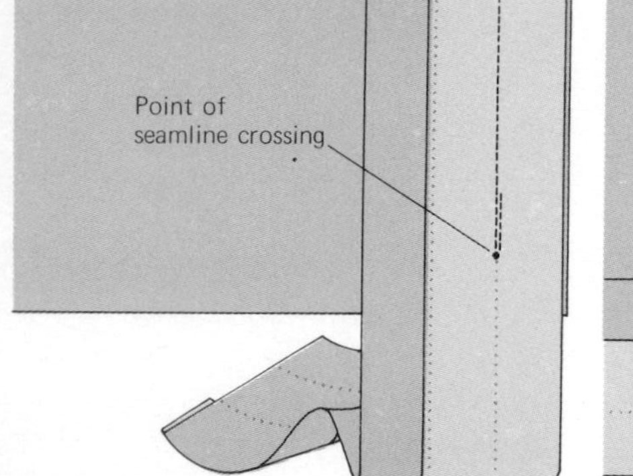

Prepare the single or double binding (see pp. 302–303). With right sides together, pin binding to garment, aligning foldline and seamline. Stitch along the binding foldline; stop and secure stitches at seamline crossing.

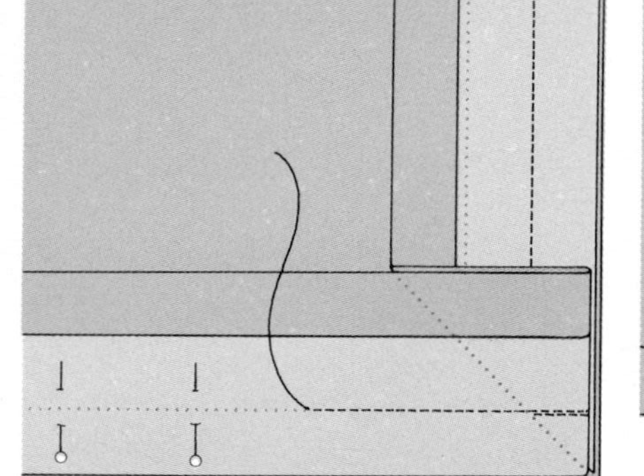

Diagonally fold binding away from garment; press. Fold banding straight back toward garment so fold is aligned with binding edge. Stitch along the binding foldline, securing stitches at the beginning.

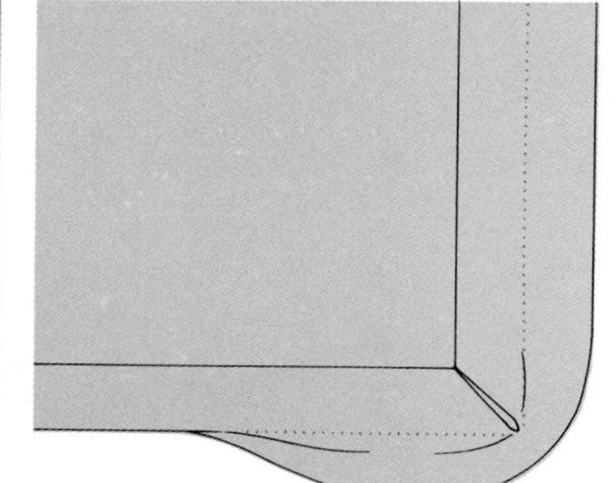

Press the seam flat to embed stitches. Fold the binding over raw edges to the wrong side; at the same time, carefully form a neat miter on the right side of garment. Keep the mitered corner squared.

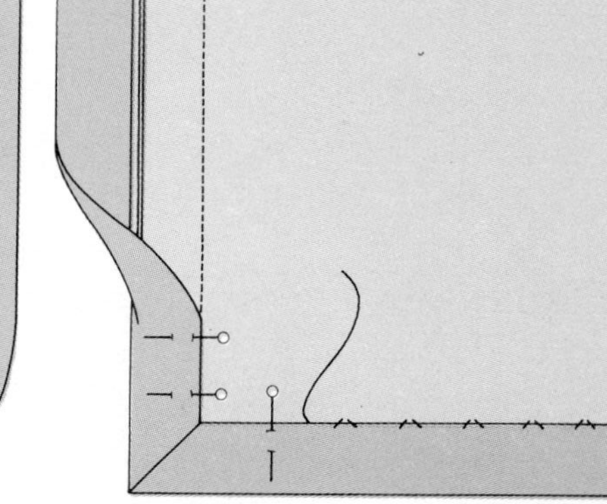

Form a miter on the wrong side as well; bring the folded edges of the binding to the stitching line; pin and slipstitch the edge of the binding and the fold of the miter in place. Press the entire binding.

Mitering single or double binding (inward corner)

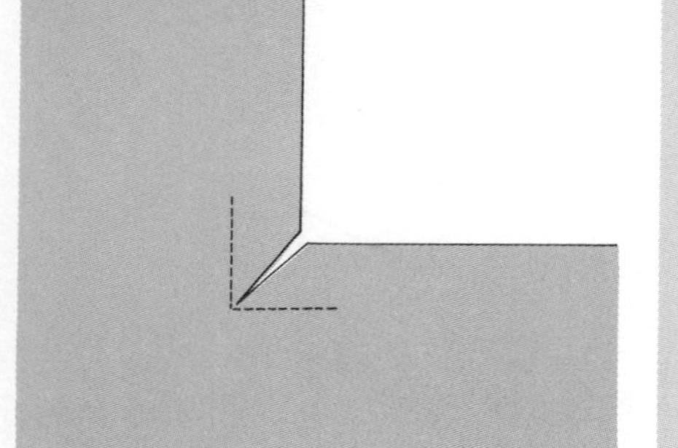

Reinforce the inner garment corner with small stitches: Stitch within a thread's width of the seamline for 1″ on either side of the corner. Clip into the corner, being careful not to cut the threads.

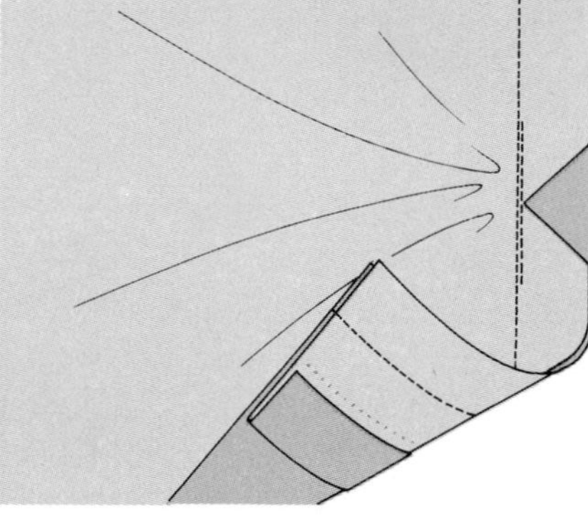

Prepare the single or double binding (see pp. 302–303). Spread the slashed corner, and pin edge to binding, right sides together; keep binding foldline aligned with garment seamline. Stitch from the garment side.

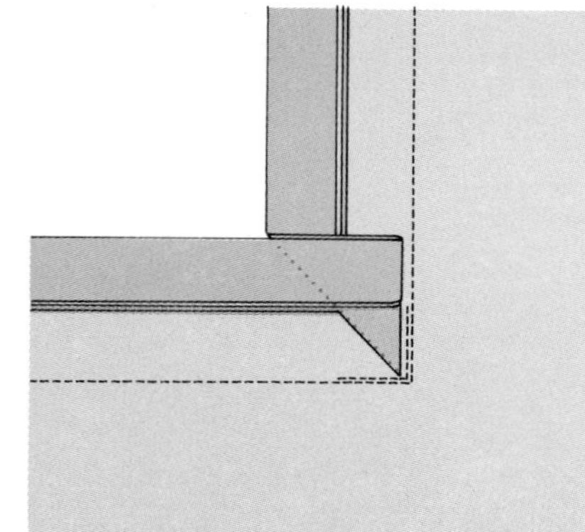

Carefully fold binding to form miter on right side. Illustration above shows folds from wrong side; note straight fold of mitered binding is placed between edges of clip. Keep edges at right angles to one another.

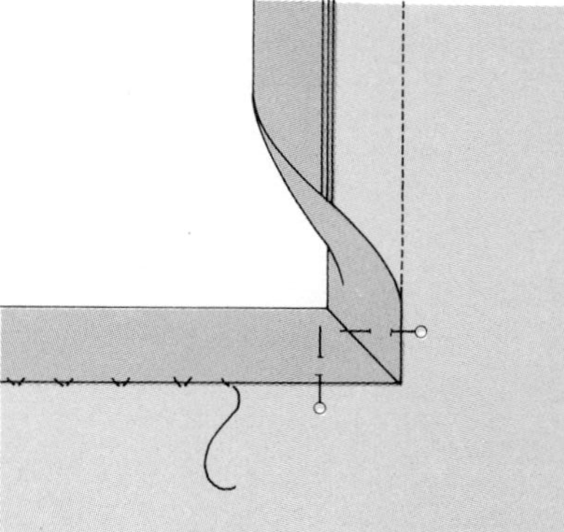

Turn binding down over seam allowances, forming a miter on the wrong side; folded edge of binding should come to the stitching line. Pin and slipstitch the binding edge and mitered fold in place.

Mitering topstitched binding (outward corner)

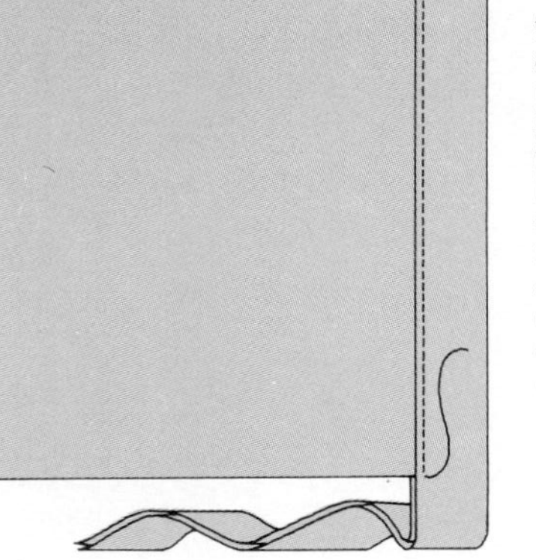

1. Prepare binding for topstitching application (see p. 303) or use prepackaged double-fold binding. Insert one garment edge into fold of binding; pin and stitch along inner edge of binding; stop at the bottom of the garment edge.

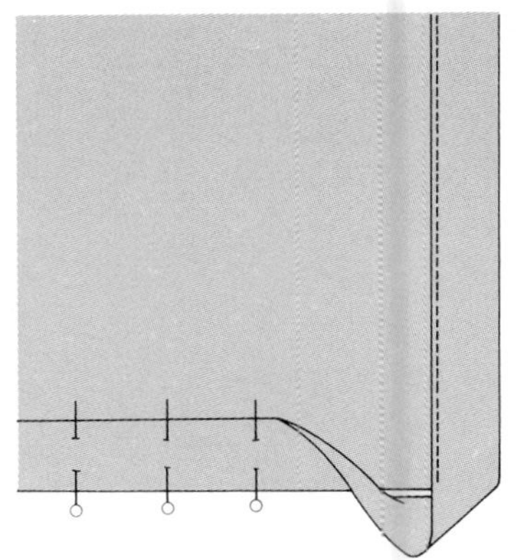

2. Bring binding around the corner, encasing bottom raw edge of garment; pin in place, forming miter around corner.

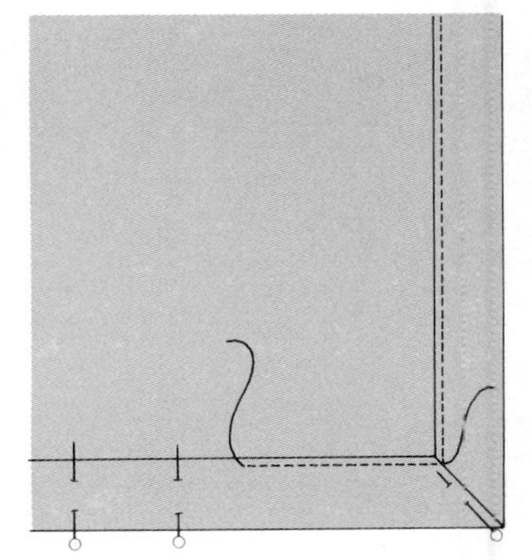

3. Pin mitered fold in place. Resume stitching at last stitch in inner corner. Pull threads through at starting point and knot. Slipstitch mitered fold if necessary.

Mitering topstitched binding (inward corner)

1. Reinforce the inner garment corner with small stitches: Stitch within a thread's width of the seamline for 1" on either side of the corner. Clip into the corner, being careful not to cut threads.

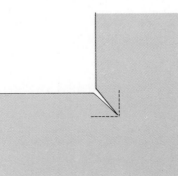

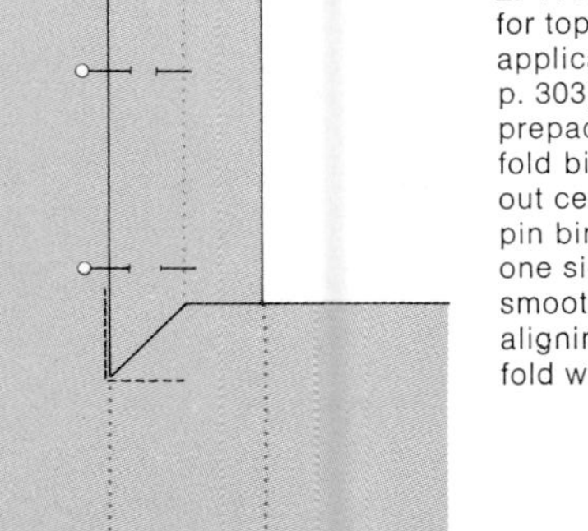

2. Prepare binding for topstitching application (see p. 303) or use prepackaged double-fold binding. Open out center fold and pin binding to one side of corner, smooth side out, aligning center fold with raw edge.

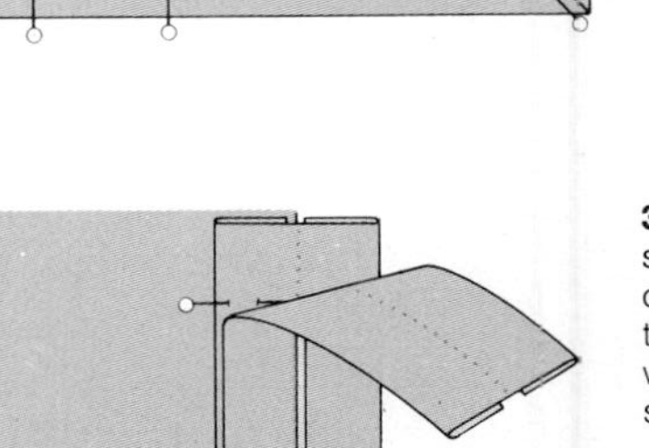

3. Fold the binding straight back on itself so that the fold is aligned with the garment's stitching line.

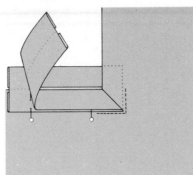

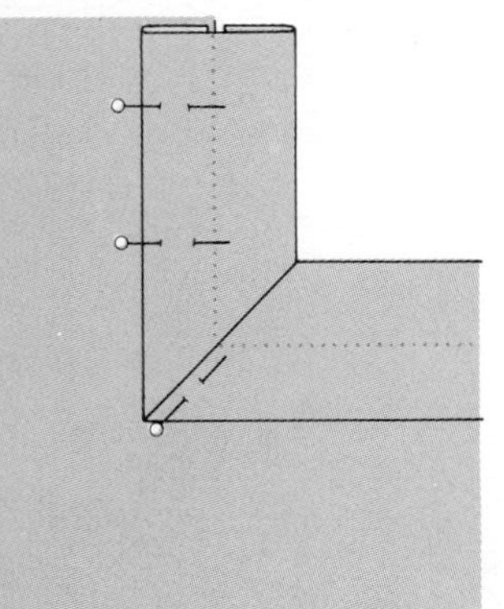
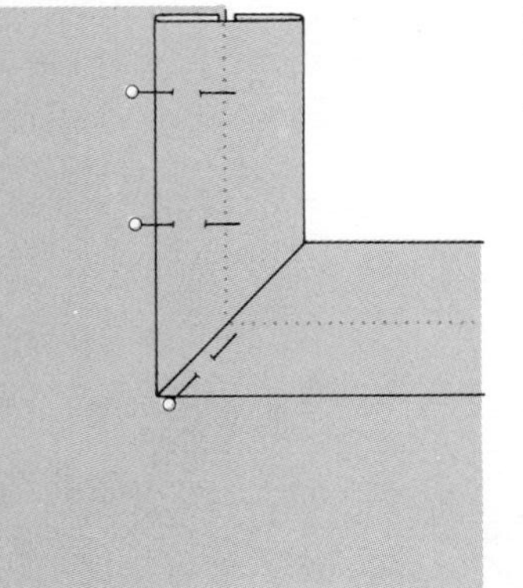

4. Then fold binding diagonally; press lightly. Pin diagonal fold to hold it in place.

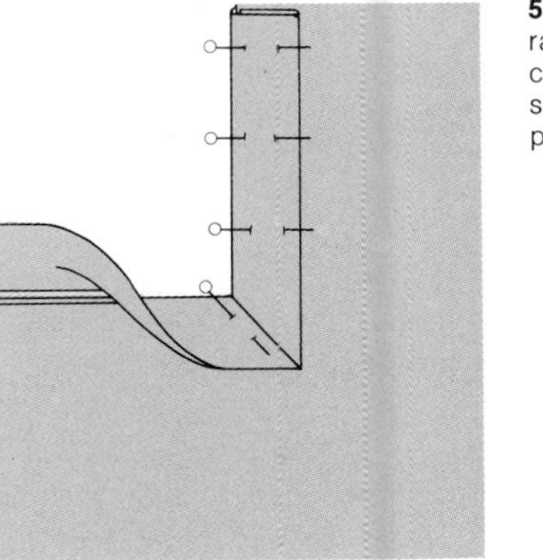

5. Fold binding over raw edge, mitering corner on the wrong side of the garment; pin in place.

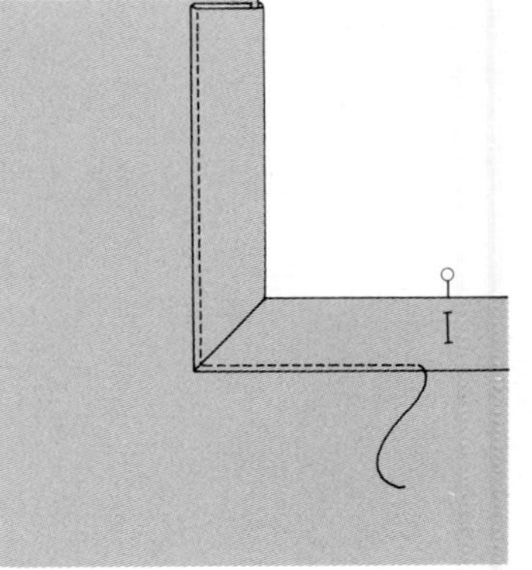

6. From the right side, stitch along binding edge through all thicknesses. Slipstitch mitered fold in place if necessary.

Special hemming situations

Pattern alterations 100-110, 116-117
French tack 134

Examples of problem hems

Special techniques are required on some garments to achieve a satisfactory hem finish. Sometimes the garment itself creates the need. An even, smooth hem on pants cuffs, for example (see right), demands careful handling of the lines that form the cuff and hem. A long evening gown may need help to hold its hemline flare; horsehair braid added to the hem fortifies it (see opposite page).

Hems in standard garments may need special handling because of unusual fabric characteristics, mainly texture or structure. Pages 312–314 suggest techniques for such problem fabrics: lace, fake fur, leather, velvet, stretchy knits, and sheers.

Another category of fabrics can be treated normally except for small special considerations at the hemline. For example, permanent press and tightly woven fabrics are both difficult to ease. When a garment made of such hard-to-ease fabrics has a shaped hem, the hem allowance should be kept narrow; it will be far easier to control the excess fullness. Brocade and fabrics like it can quickly become worn-looking; as a preventive measure, use a light touch when pressing the hem fold. Some such fabrics may even waterspot; this can be avoided by pressing with a dry iron set low. To retain the reversibility in garments of double-faced fabrics, hems can be either banded or bound (see pp. 301–303).

Adding cuffs to an uncuffed pattern

To make cuffed pants using a favorite pants pattern not designed for cuffs, alter the pattern as follows:

1. Make all pattern alterations that occur in the waist-to-hip area (the waist, crotch, etc.).
2. Determine finished pants length from the waistline; have a friend measure you along the side, or take the side seam measurement from another pair of pants that fits well.
3. Measure this same distance down from the waistline marking on pattern pieces and mark them.
4. Decide on the cuff depth; double this measurement and add it to the pattern (if necessary, tape tissue paper to bottom for added length).
5. To this amount, add another 1¼ inches for a hem allowance.
6. Mark and identify each line.
7. Cut out pants; thread-trace hem, fold, and turn-up lines.
8. Construct and hem the cuff as directed above right.

Waistline
Finished length of pants
Hemline
Foldline
Turn-up line

Hemming pants cuffs

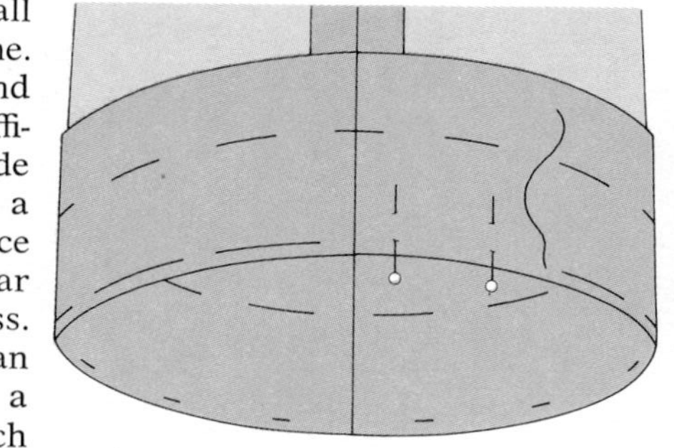

1. Complete pants construction. Press seams open. Turn hem allowance to wrong side along foldline; pin, then baste close to fold.

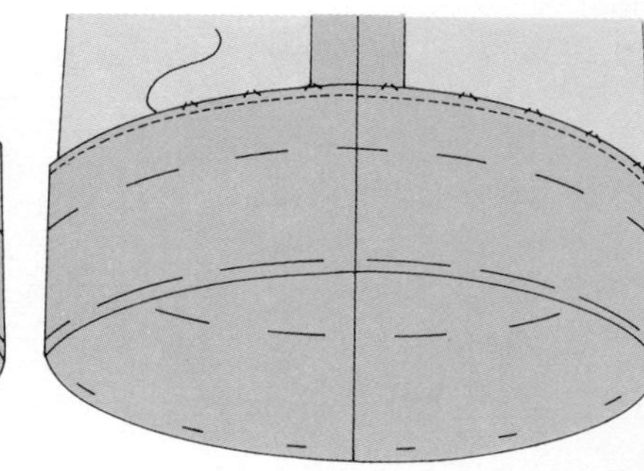

2. Finish raw edge, and secure to pants leg; if desired, machine-stitch in place (stitching will not show when cuff is turned).

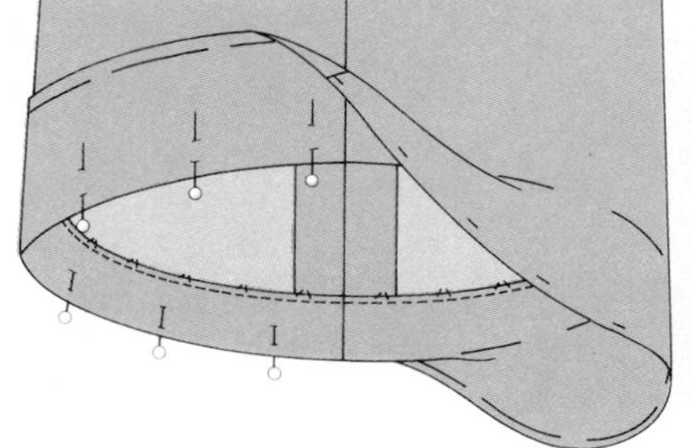

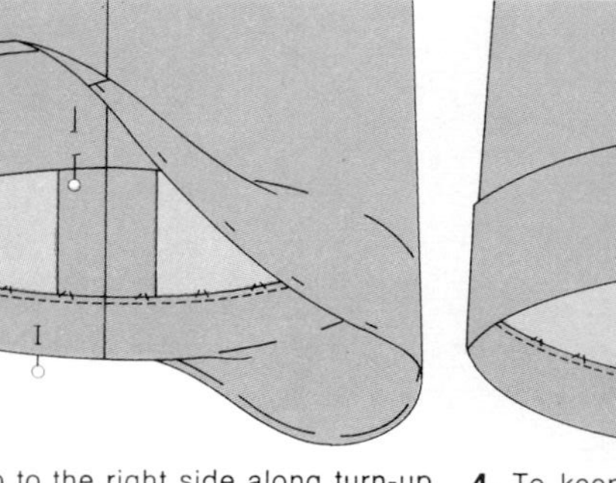

3. Turn cuff up to the right side along turn-up line; pin in place. Baste close to fold, through all thicknesses. Press gently.

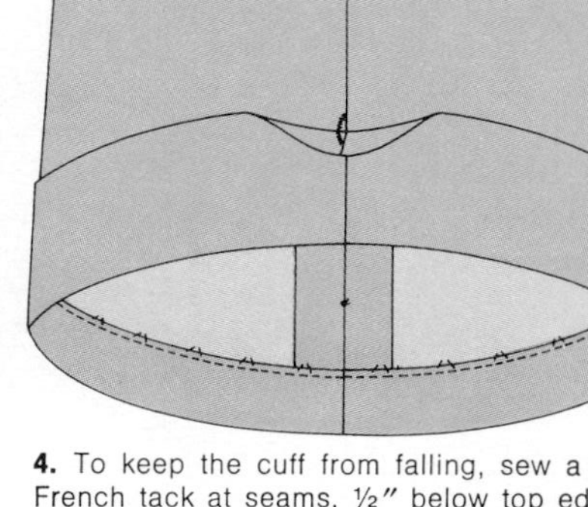

4. To keep the cuff from falling, sew a short French tack at seams, ½″ below top edge of cuff. Remove all bastings, and press.

Adding cuffs to shaped pants

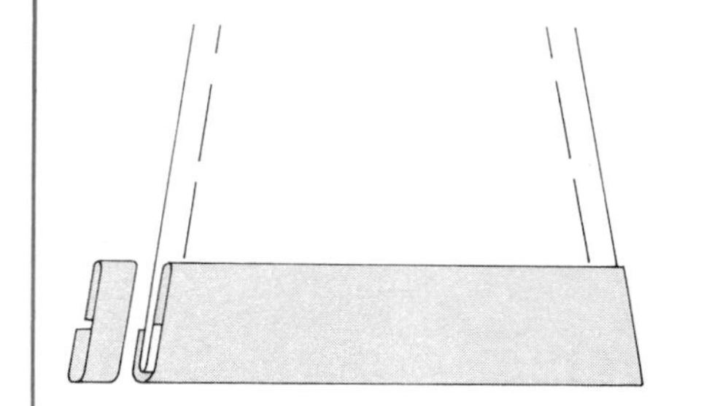

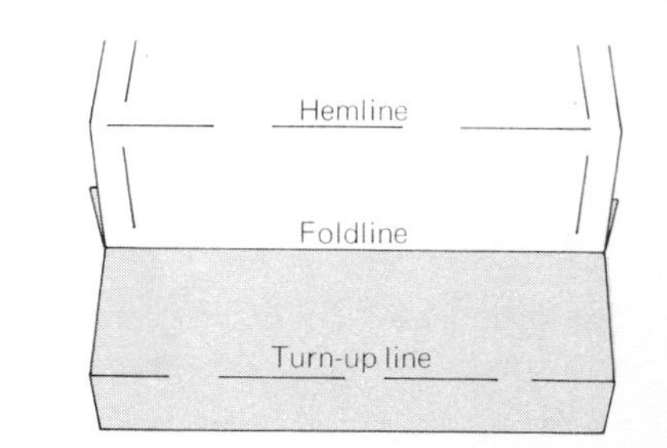

To add cuffs to a shaped pants pattern, add length to pattern as explained at left; fold pattern according to the line indications; make cutting edges at bottom continuous with those above. Open out pattern piece; use to cut and mark pants.

Single cross-stitch tack 134
Whipstitch 136

Hemming with horsehair braid

Horsehair braid is a loosely woven braid made from transparent strands of nylon thread. It is usually sewed to the hemline of dressy garments, such as evening gowns, designed to flare at the bottom edge. By stiffening the edge, the braid enables the skirt to hold the desired shape.

Horsehair braid comes, as a rule, in ½ and 1 inch widths, the narrower of the two used most often on lightweight and the wider on mediumweight fabrics. Shaping of wider braids can be facilitated by easestitching along one edge. Before applying the braid, steam-press it to remove any folds or creases; do not stretch the braid in handling. The application procedure is similar for both widths of the braid (see below).

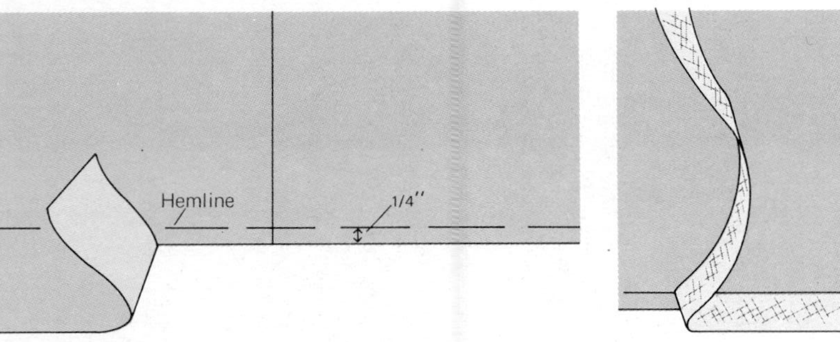

1. Mark the hemline at the bottom of the skirt. Trim the hem allowance below the marked hemline to ¼″.

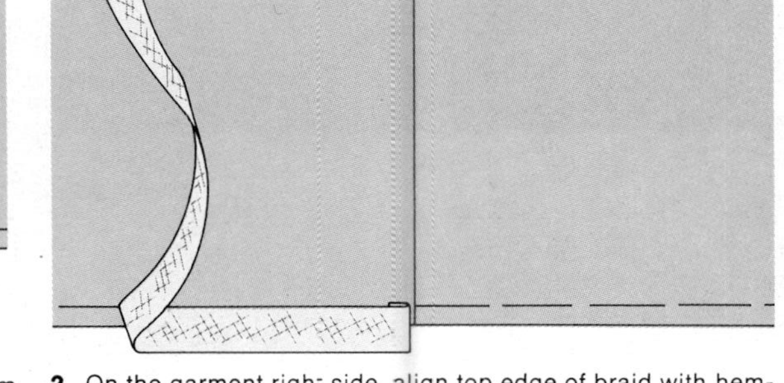

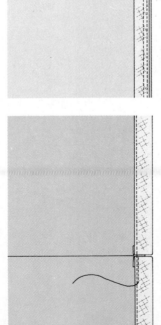

2. On the garment right side, align top edge of braid with hemline; start at back or side seam; fold under starting end.

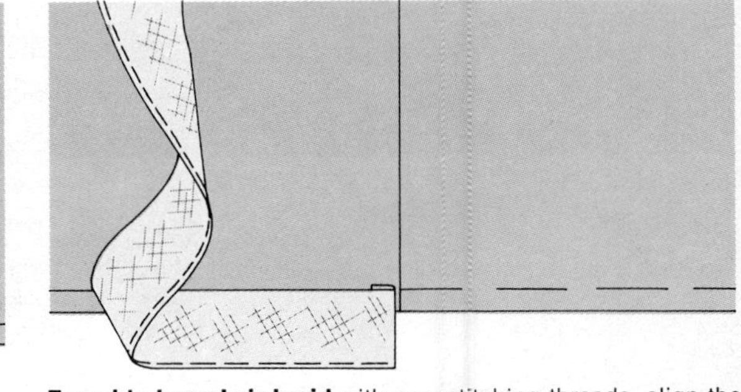

For wide horsehair braid with easestitching threads, align the unstitched edge of the braid with the hemline.

3. Edgestitch braid all the way around garment hem; fold under finishing end of braid to abut the starting end

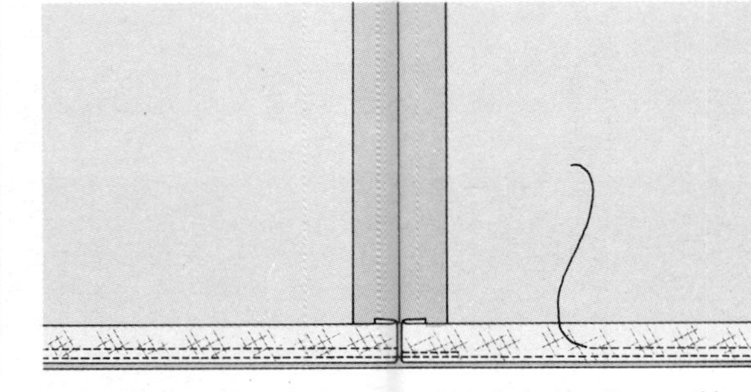

4. Fold hem and braid to wrong side along hemline marking. Edgestitch along folded edge through all thicknesses.

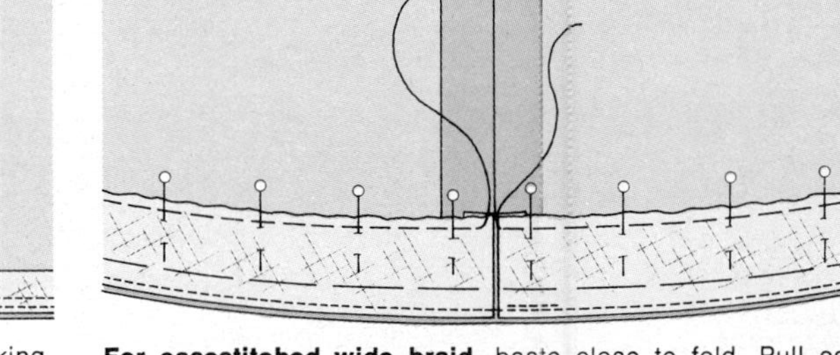

For easestitched wide braid, baste close to fold. Pull ease threads if necessary to draw up fullness; press and pin.

5. Secure the free edge of horsehair braid to the garment by tacking it to the seams only.

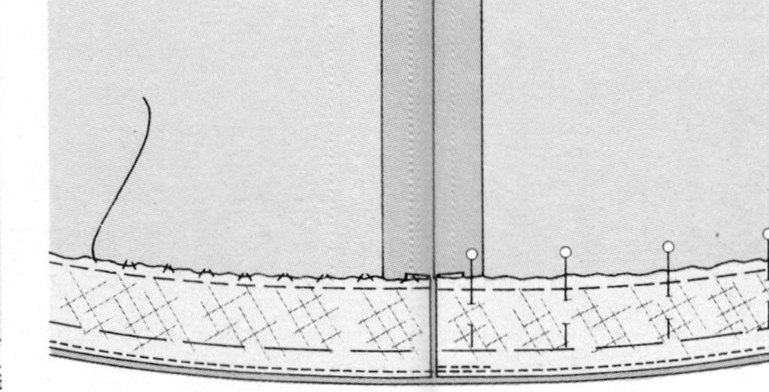

For wide horsehair braid that has been easestitched, slipstitch the entire free edge to the garment.

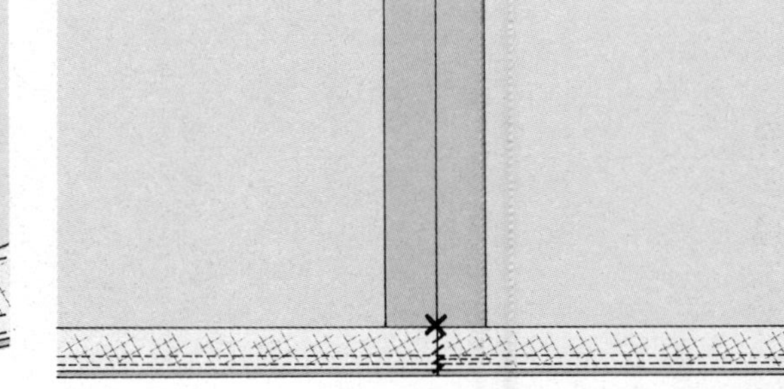

6. Whipstitch the abutted braid ends together. Remove any bastings. Press entire hem carefully.

Special hemming situations

Lace 70, deep pile 71
Flat catchstitch 129
Slipstitch (uneven) 129
Whipstitch 136

Hemming laces

Lace fabrics range from lightweight to heavy, and are made in a variety of patterns with straight or scalloped edges. The hemming method depends upon the lace. Laces that are backed can be finished by one of the turned-up hem methods discussed on pages 292–293; hems for heavy laces can be faced. For lightweight laces, a rolled hem (p. 314) or a horsehair braid finish (p. 311) is recommended; an alternative is a lace trim appliquéd to the hemline for a decorative finish (see below). If the lace is already scalloped, the finished edge can be used as the hemline (see below).

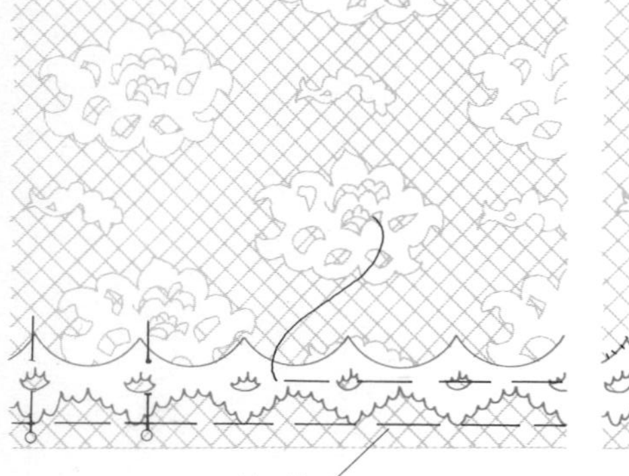

To appliqué a lace trim to the edge, mark hemline. Place trim on right side of garment, aligning lower edge with garment hemline. Pin, then baste through center of trim.

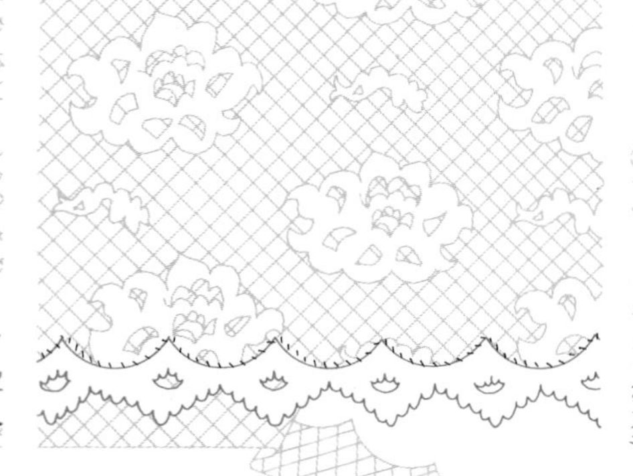

Stitch trim to garment by the appliqué method (whipstitch along inner edge of trim's motif, or use a narrow machine zigzag). Cut away hem allowance underneath the lace trim.

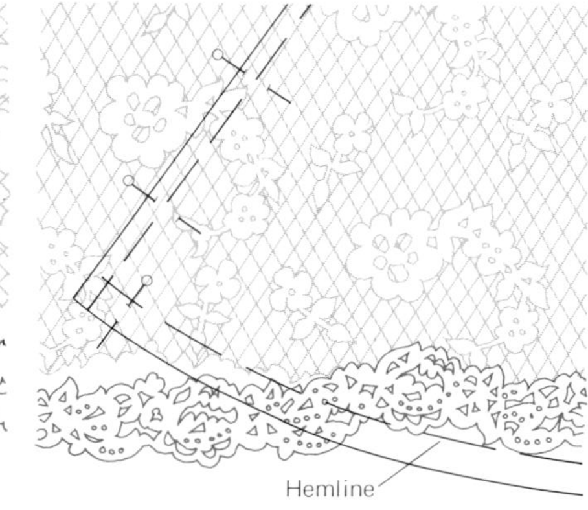

To use scalloped edge as hem, pin pattern to fabric; align hemline with bottom edge of scallop motif. Cut above scallop to separate part of motif that falls below hemline curve.

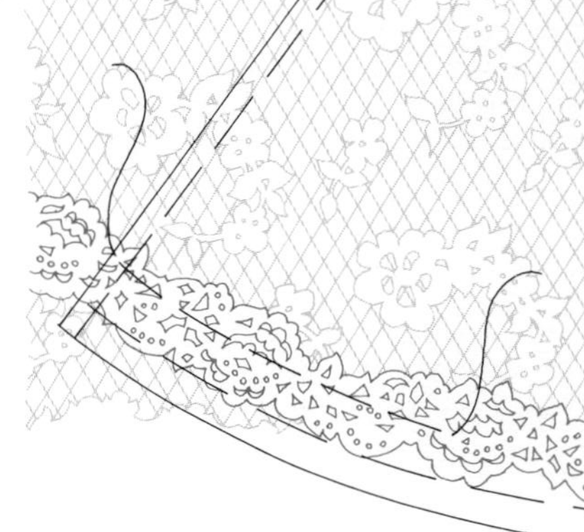

Re-position separated portion of scallop to follow hemline curve; pin and baste. Cut out garment. Secure re-positioned part of scallop with whipstitching or machine zigzag.

Hemming fake furs

The problem associated with hems in fake fur is usually caused by the bulk and weight of the fur's long hairs. When a fake fur has short hairs, as many do, it can be handled like a medium-weight fabric. A turned-up hem is the finish to use; the raw edge is covered with seam binding and the hem secured with double stitching (p. 293). Garments of exceptionally heavy or dense fake fur require a bias facing, either the packaged type or one made from lining fabric (p. 299). The facing method for such fake furs (see below) is similar to the standard facing technique.

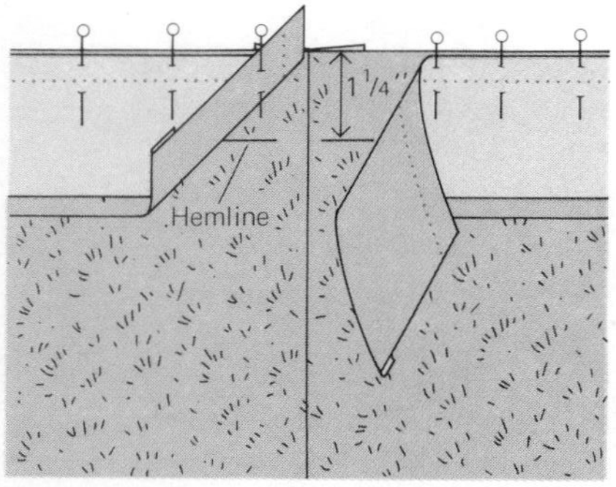

Mark hemline. Trim hem allowance to 1¼″. Open one folded edge of facing; fold end back ¼″. Starting at garment seam, pin facing to hem, right sides together and raw edges even.

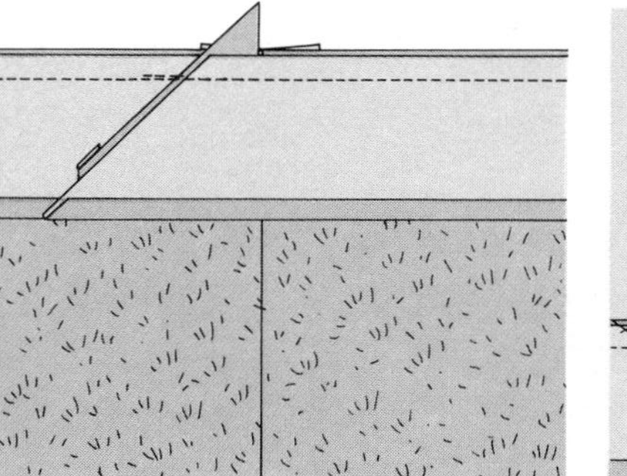

Stitch on crease of fold to within 3″ of the starting point, removing pins as you go. Cut excess facing to overlap the first end, and continue stitching across. Press flat.

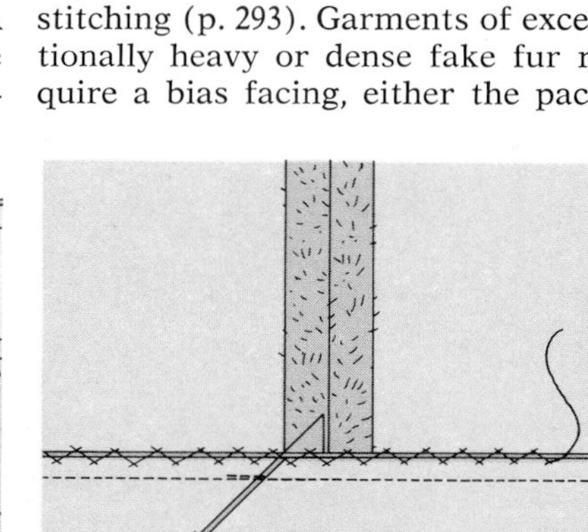

Turn hem up to wrong side along marked hemline on garment; pin and baste through hem fold to hold in place. Catchstitch raw edges of fur fabric and facing to the garment.

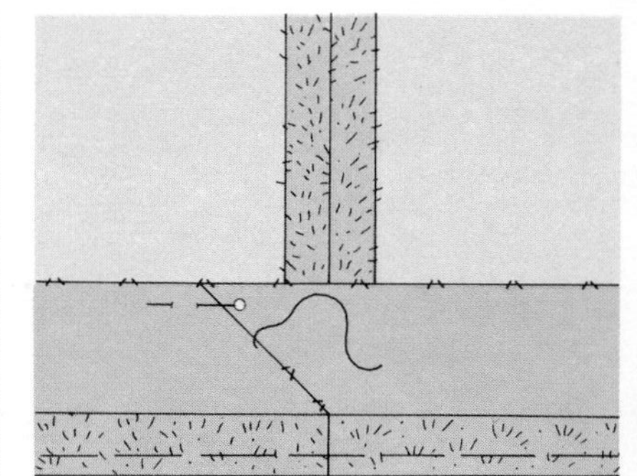

Press facing up, and pin to back of fur fabric; secure. Slipstitch lapped ends in place. Remove all bastings; if necessary, steam-press gently, using a press cloth.

Marking chalk 9
Wedge-point machine needle 12
Self-stick sewing tape 12
Leather, velvet 71

Hemming leathers

Certain precautions must be taken in hemming leather and some leather-like fabrics because they tend to retain surface pin marks and to tear easily. Avoid pins entirely by using chalk to mark the hemline, and paper clips to hold the hem in place. To solve the tearing problem, hems can be either topstitched or glued. **Topstitching** is the easier of the two techniques; a wedge-shaped needle and a fairly long stitch are best for this job. The alternative procedure, **gluing**, must be done with meticulous care. For the adhesive, use rubber cement. Apply a thin coat over the appropriate area; take care not to use too much. To help reduce hem bulk, trim the seam allowance below the hemline to half-width. If the leather is very firm and heavy, you can just mark and trim off the hem allowance.

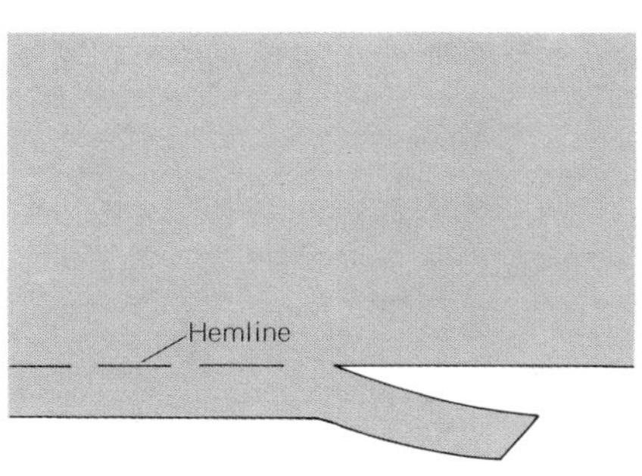

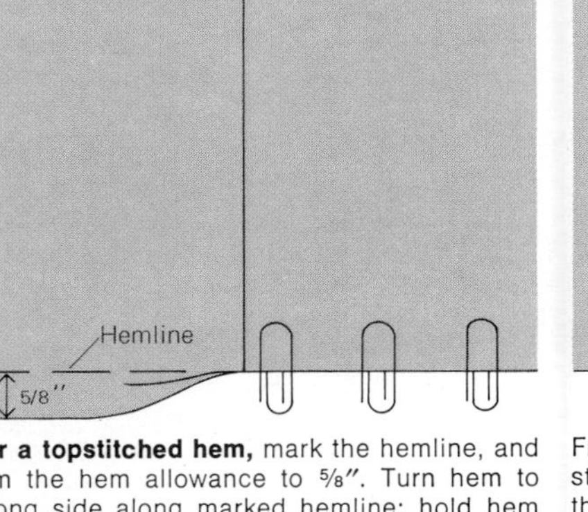

For a topstitched hem, mark the hemline, and trim the hem allowance to ⅝". Turn hem to wrong side along marked hemline; hold hem in place with paper clips.

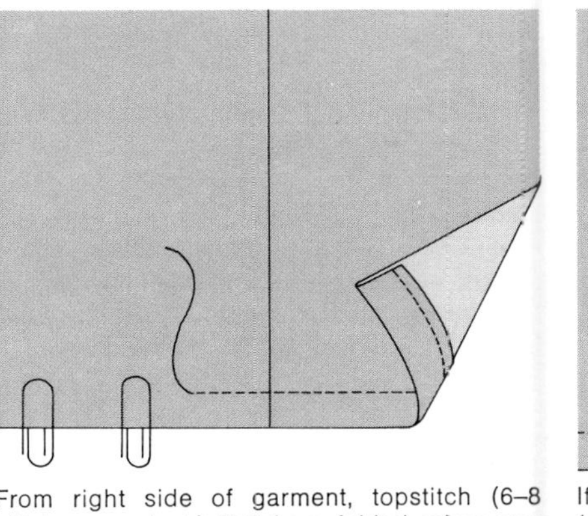

From right side of garment, topstitch (6–8 stitches per inch) ½" from folded edge; use the sewing machine gauge or a self-stick sewing tape for easy, accurate guidance.

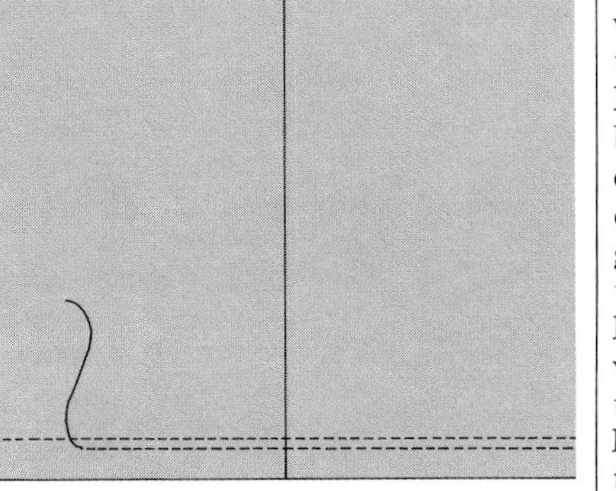

If desired, place another row of topstitching ⅛" below the first row. With a press cloth beneath the iron, press the hem with the iron set at low temperature.

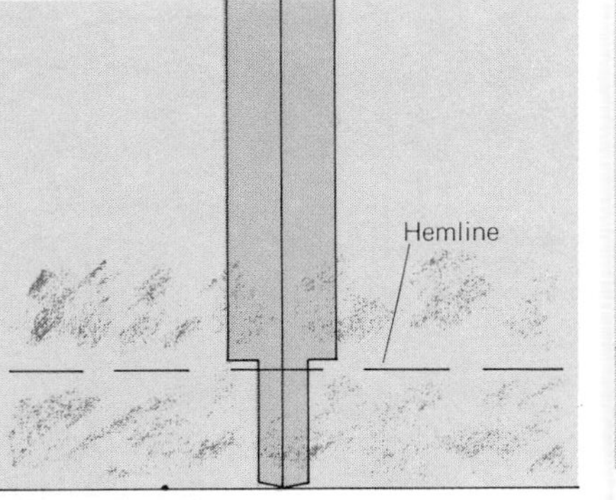

For a glued hem, mark hemline; trim hem allowance to 2" or less. Spread rubber cement over wrong side of hem and garment area hem will cover, also under seam allowances.

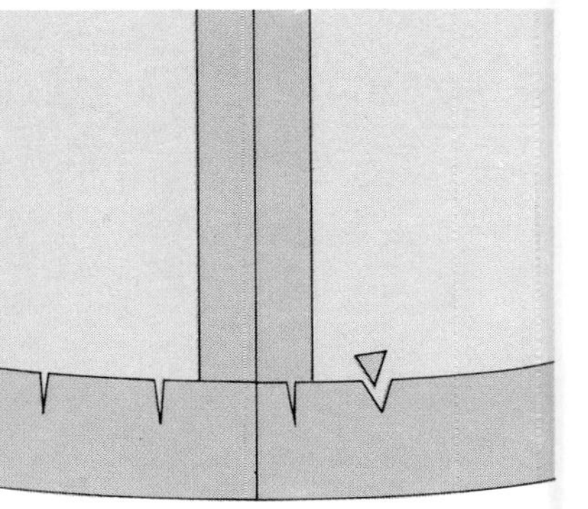

Turn hem up and finger-press, working from center toward side seams. If hem is curved, snip small wedges from the full areas of the hem and bring their cut edges together.

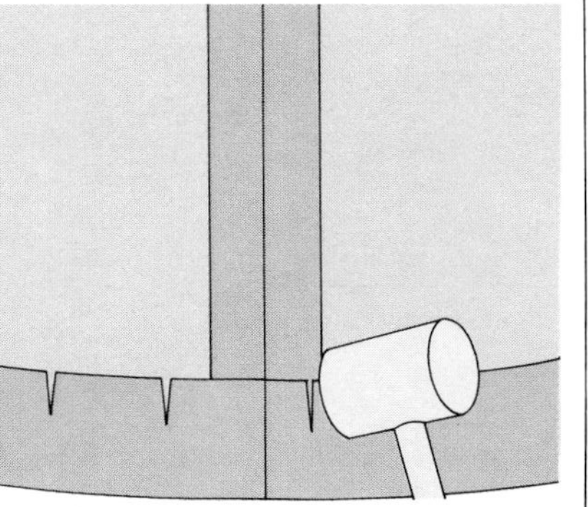

When entire hem is complete, gently pound the glued portion of the hem from the inside with a mallet. Let the glue dry completely before handling the garment again.

Hemming velvets

Velvet is a plush and elegant fabric that belongs in the general category of pile fabrics; the pile creates a definite "up" and "down" nap that must be carefully considered when a garment is cut. Because velvets have a tendency to mar easily, hems on velvet demand special care and techniques. Of course, such pile fabrics as corduroy and velveteen also have naps, but they are less susceptible to marring and can, for the most part, be handled like any ordinary medium-weight fabric. A recommended hem treatment for velvets is the Hong Kong finish (p. 293) with, as shown below, a strip of nylon net used to encase the raw edge. Often a soft roll is desired at the bottom edge of a velvet garment; to obtain this soft roll and to keep the shape of the hemline, the hem is interfaced (see p. 295). If the velvet garment has a circular skirt, the finish can also be a hand-rolled hem (p. 314). A good general precaution with velvet is the use of silk thread to hand stitch any hem. Keep a light touch in pressing, and always use a needle board.

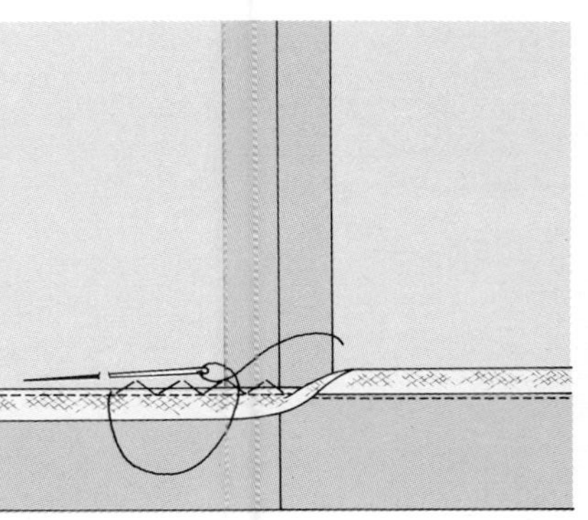

Hong Kong hem: Follow the directions on page 293, using a strip of nylon net to cover the raw edge of the velvet; loosely blindstitch edge in place, tacking securely every 4" to 5".

Special hemming situations

Zigzag stitching 32-33
Machine blindstitch 34
Narrow hemmer foot 38

Hemming stretchy knits

The extreme stretchiness of soft and stretchy knits, such as jersey and lingerie tricot, makes hemming troublesome and results often far from satisfactory. Along the edge of a turned-up hem, for example, it can cause unsightly sagging and rippling. Fusing (p. 295) can relieve this to some extent. Better alternatives are a narrow **topstitched** hem (p. 294) or a **rolled** hem, as shown at the right. Other possibilities are such decorative finishes as a **shell-stitched edge** or a **lettuce edge** (see below).

Shell-stitched edge

The shell-stitched edge is a popular finish for lingerie and nightgowns. To achieve this multiple scalloped effect, use the blindstitch on your machine (see Machine stitching); the zigzag stitches reach over the folded edge of the garment to create tiny scallops. Consult your machine instruction book for settings, and make a test swatch before starting.

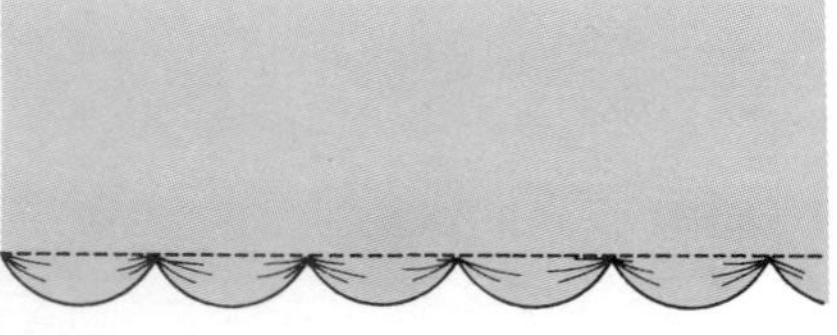

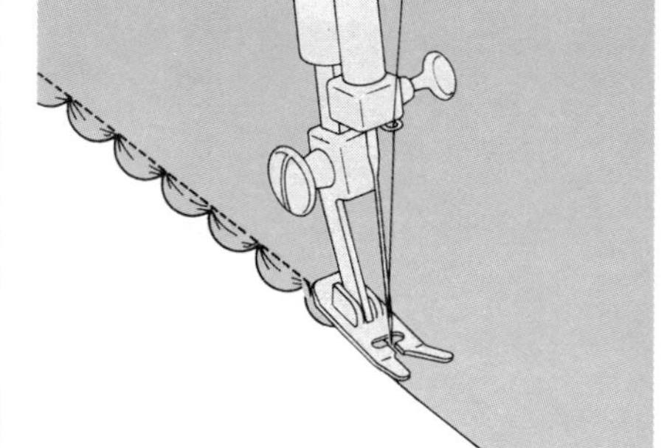

Mark hemline; trim hem allowance to ⅜″; press to wrong side. Stitch on right side, a scant ¼″ from fold. Zigzag stitches go left, so bulk of garment is to right of presser foot.

Lettuce edge

A lettuce edge is a decorative finish that takes advantage of the knit's stretchiness. To get the frilly effect, stretch the fabric while stitching the garment edge with a medium-width zigzag; the more that the fabric is stretched, the smaller and more numerous the ripples become. Some knits develop runs if stretched near the cut edge, so test a swatch first.

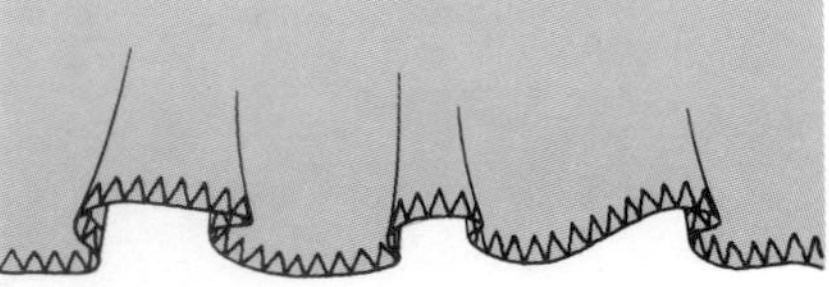

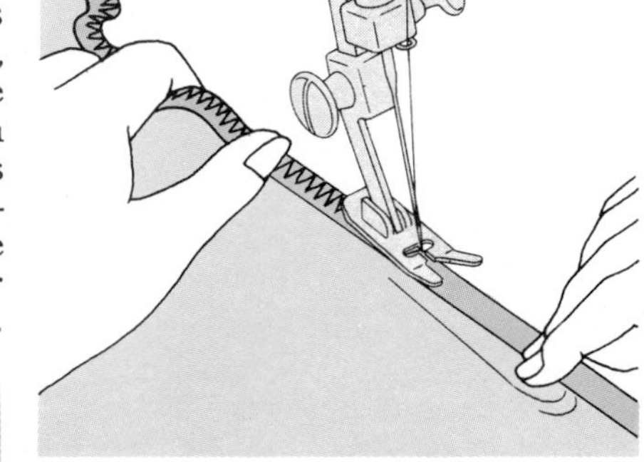

Mark hemline; trim hem allowance to ⅜″; press to wrong side. With wrong side up, grasp fabric firmly with both hands and stretch it as you zigzag along the fold. Trim excess.

Hemming sheer fabrics

Garments made of sheer fabrics can be finished with a simple turned-up hem. If the hem edge is cut straight and the sheer is crisp (e.g., voile), the hem can be very deep, a popular effect in children's wear. Garments of soft sheers (e.g., chiffon) tend to stretch at the bottom; hems of these are better rolled than turned up. Rolled hems can be made by hand, or by machine with the aid of the hemmer foot (see below). Although a machine-rolled hem is faster, one that is hand-rolled has a more elegant look.

Hand-rolled hem

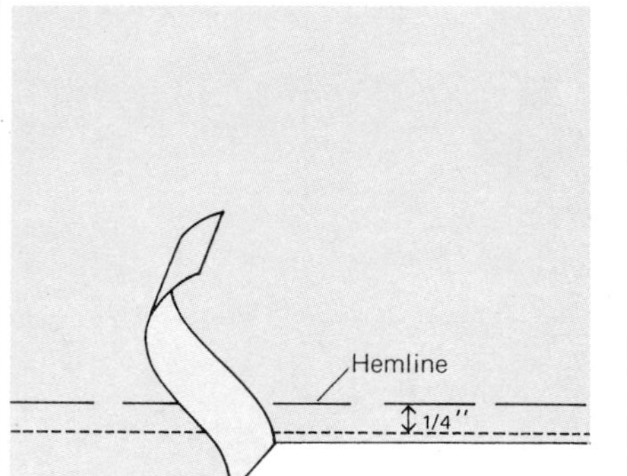

Mark hemline; machine-stitch ¼″ below marked hemline. Trim off hem allowance ⅛″ below stitching. Fold hem to wrong side, turning just far enough that the stitch line shows.

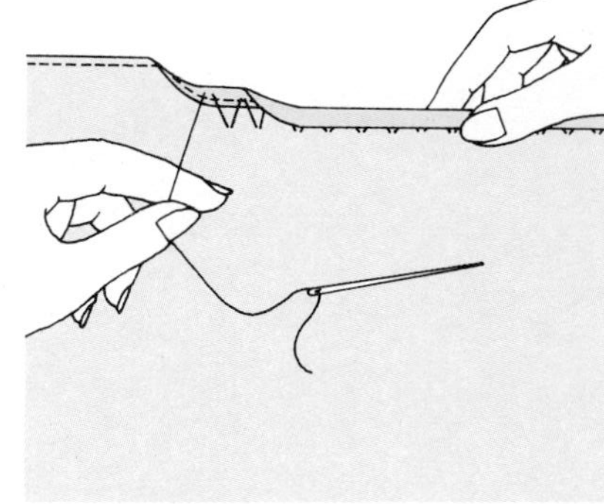

Working right to left, take a small stitch through fold; then, ⅛″ below and beyond that stitch, catch a few threads of garment. Pull thread to roll hem to wrong side.

Machine-rolled hem

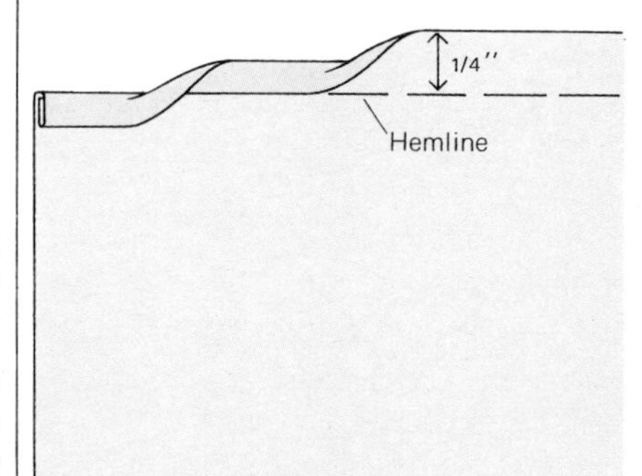

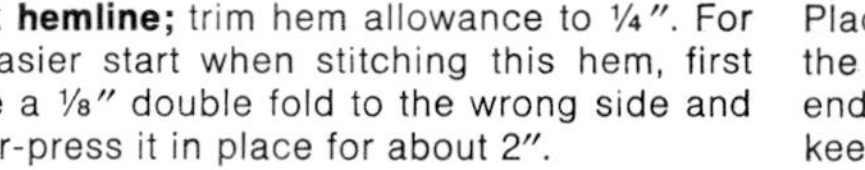

Mark hemline; trim hem allowance to ¼″. For an easier start when stitching this hem, first make a ⅛″ double fold to the wrong side and finger-press it in place for about 2″.

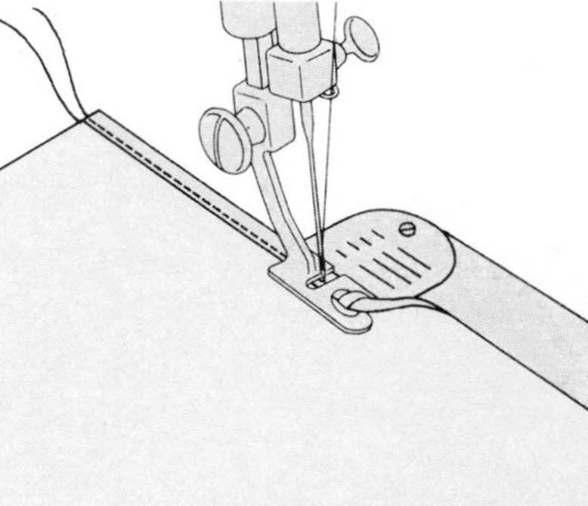

Place the finger-pressed starting edge under the hemmer foot attachment, hold the thread ends back, and start stitching. Use hands to keep garment feeding evenly.

Handbook of Closures

Zippers

Buttonholes

Fabric closures

Attaching buttons

Making buttons

Hooks and eyes

Snaps

Tape fasteners

Zippers

Basic types

Basically, zippers are of three types: **conventional, separating,** and **invisible.** Conventional zippers are closed at one end and sewed into a seam that is closed to the zipper placket. Separating zippers are open at both ends and are sewed into a seam that will open completely. The invisible zipper is constructed so as to disappear into a seam; like conventional zippers, it has one closed end.

All zippers consist of either a *chain* of metal or plastic teeth or a synthetic *coil* joined to fabric tapes. Coils are essentially tightly twisted spirals of polyester or nylon. Chains and coils are made in many weights and sizes, heavier ones being stronger. Since metal and coil zippers are about equal in strength and performance, the choice is largely a matter of personal preference. Coil zippers are lighter in weight, and usually more flexible, than chain zippers. Unlike metal, they will not rust, and they are available in more colors. Metal zippers are less affected by heat and they come in heavy-duty forms (see Zipper chart).

Zipper tapes are woven, generally of all cotton (usual with chain zippers) or a blend of cotton and polyester. Some tapes for coil zippers are stabilized nylon or polyester knit. In most zipper brands, a sewing guideline is woven into the tapes to direct stitching. Zippers are opened and closed by means of a slider, with a handlelike tab that moves it up and down the coil or chain. Top and bottom stops keep the slider from running off the zipper.

If fabric or thread jams a coil zipper, fold the zipper crosswise and separate the coil. Close the coil by moving the slider to the bottom stop, then returning it to the top.

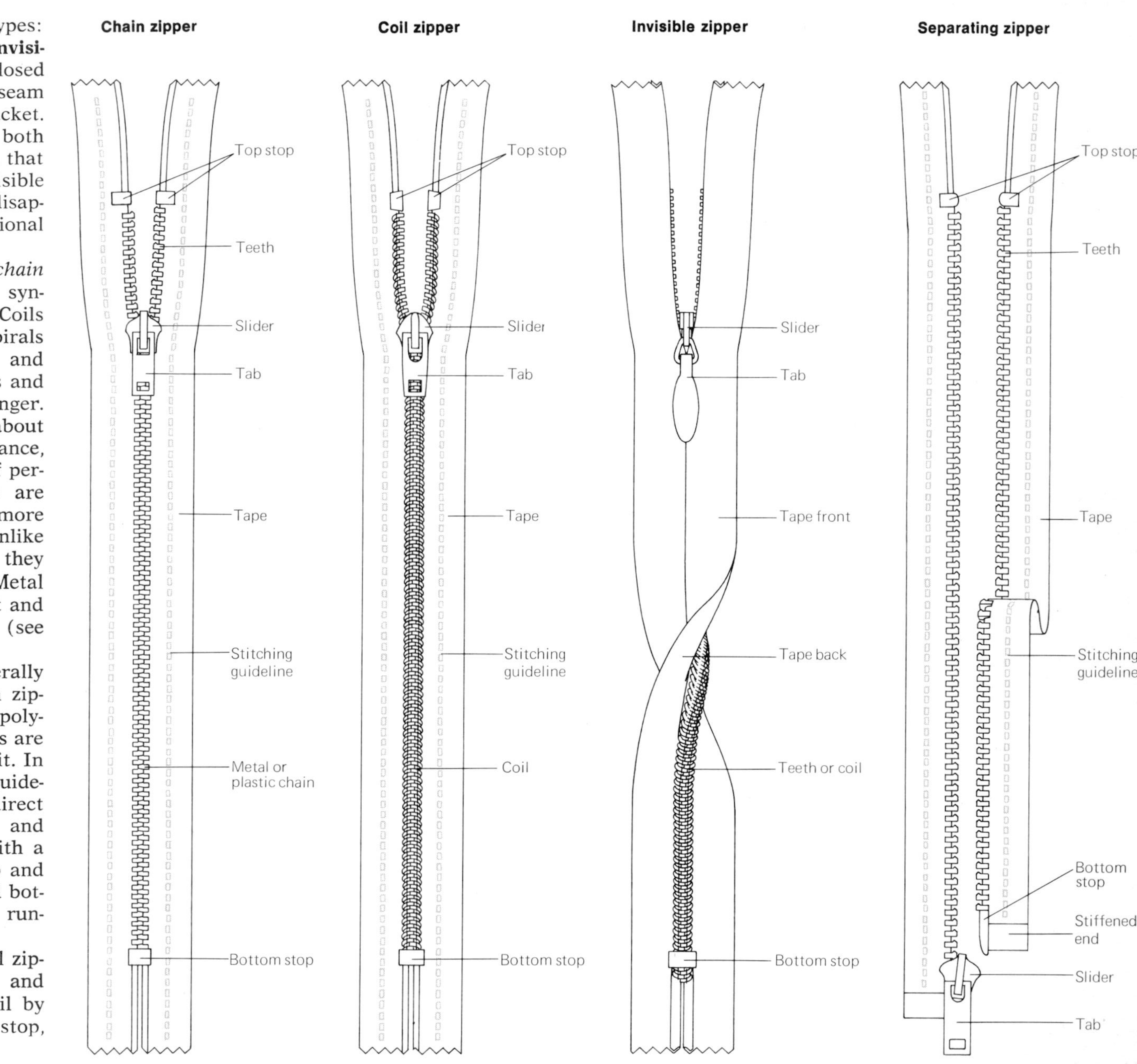

Seam binding 16
Whipstitch 136
Staystitching 144
Seam finishes 148-149

Basic applications

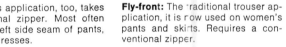

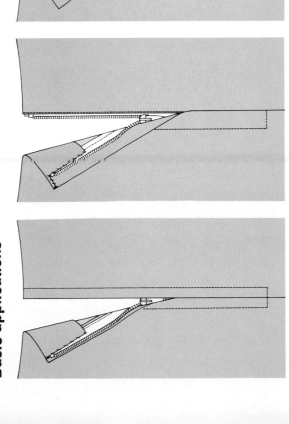

Centered: Application involving a conventional zipper. Used at center front or back of garment, at edges of sleeves, in home decorating.

Lapped: This application, too, takes a conventional zipper. Most often used at the left side seam of pants, skirts, and dresses.

Fly-front: The traditional trouser application, it is now used on women's pants and skirts. Requires a conventional zipper.

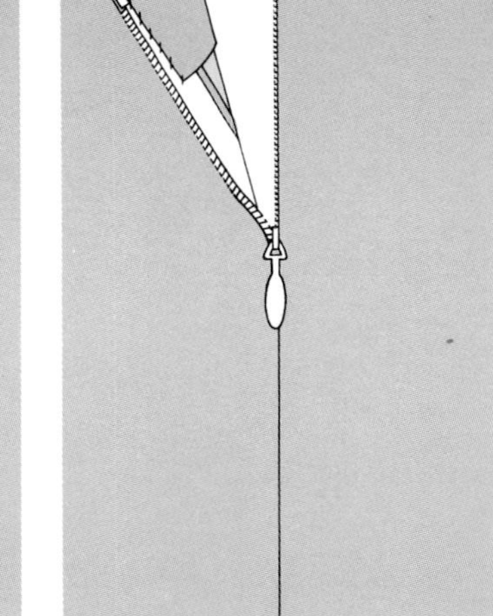

Invisible: Possible only with the special invisible zipper, this application can substitute for either a lapped or centered application.

Separating: The separating zipper may be sewed in with either a centered or lapped application. Usable on jackets, vests, or skirts.

Installation tips

Before any zipper is sewed into a garment, the placket seam should be **seam-finished** and then, in most cases, basted and pressed open. **Staystitch** any curved or bias placket seamlines ¼″ from the cut edge to prevent possible stretching. **Preshrink the zipper** to avoid puckering after laundering. Immerse zipper in hot tap water for a few minutes, roll in a towel to absorb excess moisture, then allow to air-dry. If you expect a great deal of shrinkage from the fabric, preshrink the zipper twice.

Use of a **zipper adhesive** eliminates basting and pinning, and is excellent for fabrics that show needle and pin punctures. It is basically a double-faced tape; for use, see information accompanying the product.

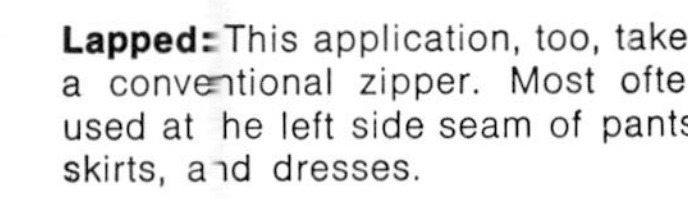

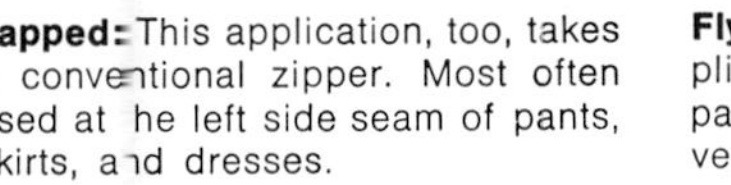

Enlarging seam allowances: This is necessary if they are less than ⅝″ wide. Edgestitch woven seam binding to edge of seam allowances only.

Reduce bulk in cross-seam allowances at, for example, yokes and waistlines. Trim seam allowances slightly past zipper seamline as shown, and press open.

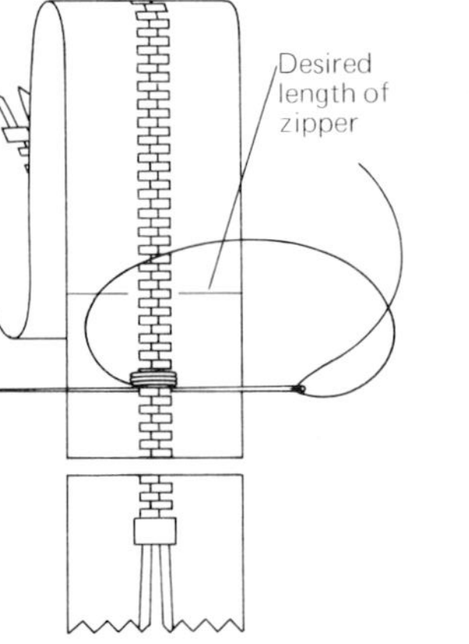

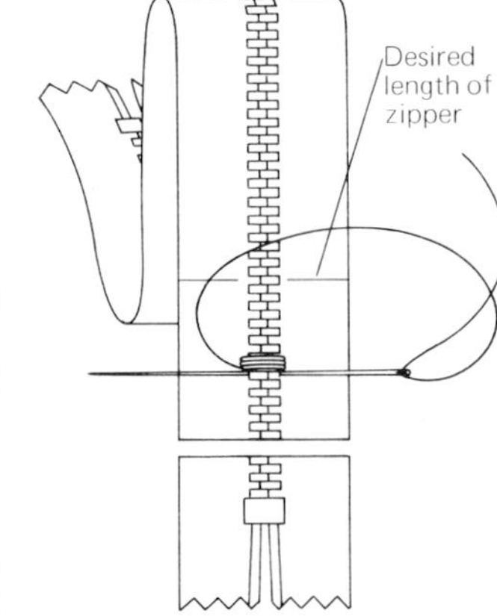

To shorten a zipper, whipstitch several times over coil or chain as shown, 1″ below desired new length, then cut off the excess zipper and tapes.

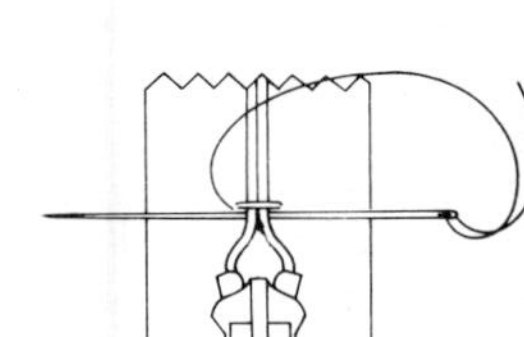

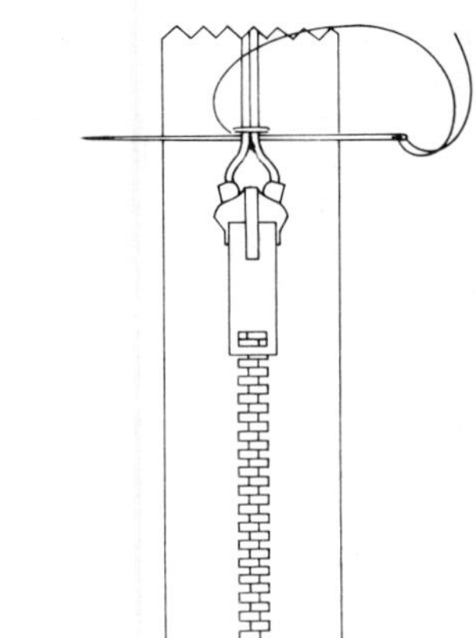

For dress placket use, a zipper must be closed above the top stop. Whipstitch the edges of the tapes together ¼″ above top stop, or attach a straight-eye fastener.

Centered zipper

Machine attachments 38-39
Hand basting 124, machine 137
Tying thread ends 137
Seam finishes 148-149

Basic application

The method for applying a centered zipper is the same regardless of the garment type; the only variable is in the placement of the zipper below the top edge of the garment. Where it is placed depends on how this edge will be finished. If a facing is to be used, you should place the top stop of the zipper ½ *inch below* the seamline of the garment. This allows extra space for turning down the facing and for attaching a hook and eye. If the finish does not require that seam allowances be turned down, as with a waistband or standing collar, place the top stop *just below* the seamline (a scant ¼ inch).

All work is done on the *inside* of the garment except for topstitching. **Work from bottom to top** of placket, in both preliminary basting and topstitching. Keep the zipper closed, except in Step 3, and slider tab up.

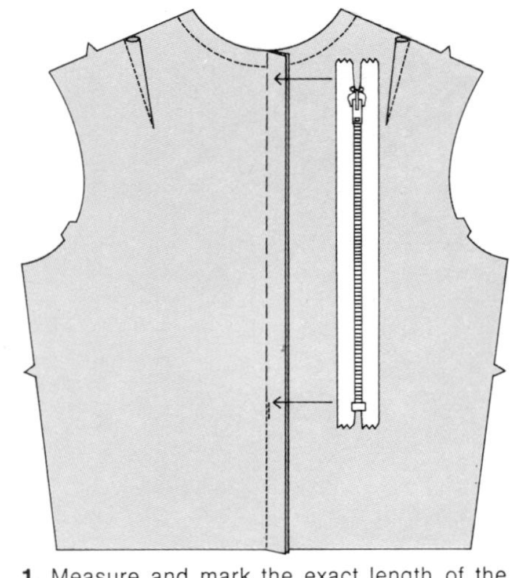

1. Measure and mark the exact length of the placket opening, using the zipper as a guide. Close the seam with machine stitching: stitch up to the mark for bottom of zipper with a regular stitch length, backstitch, then change to machine basting for placket seam.

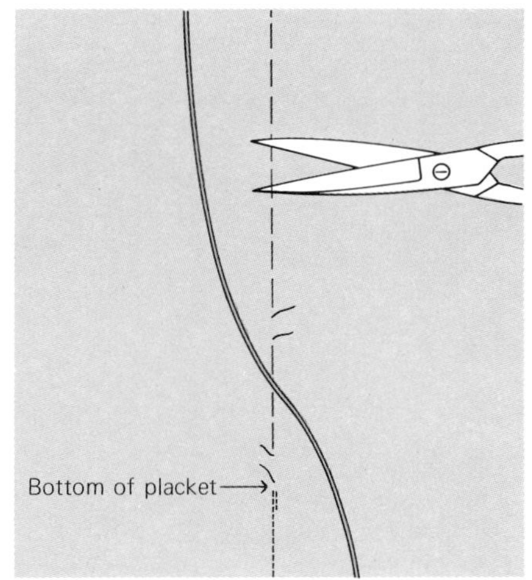

2. Clip both of the machine basting threads at the bottom of the placket; then clip only the bobbin thread at 1" intervals—this will make removal of basting easier. Press the seam open and, if necessary, seam-finish the edges with a finish suitable to fabric.

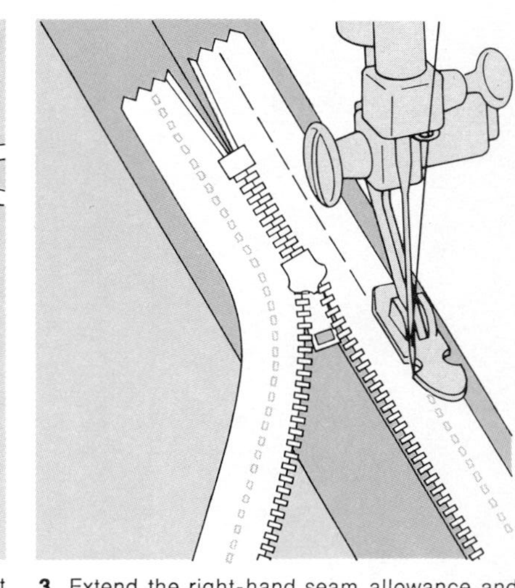

3. Extend the right-hand seam allowance and place zipper face down, with the top stop at mark and the edge of the opened coil or chain along the seamline; pin in place. Using a zipper foot, machine-baste along stitching guideline on zipper tape.

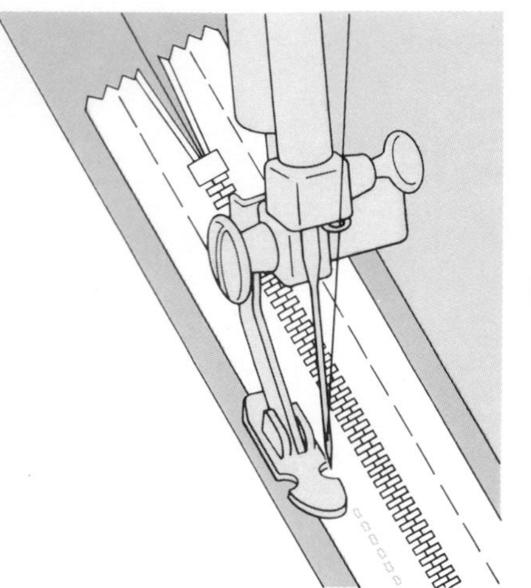

4. Close the zipper and keep the pull tab up. Extend the remaining seam allowance. Position the zipper foot to the left of the needle and machine-baste the unstitched zipper tape, from bottom to top, to the seam allowance, following the guideline on the tape.

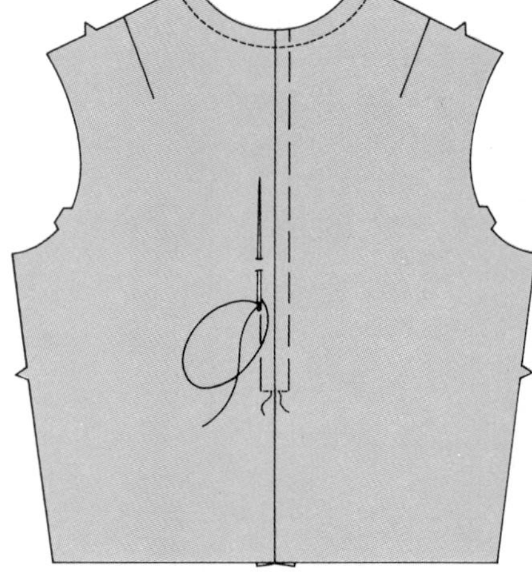

5. Turn garment right side up and spread it as flat as possible. Starting at the center seam, hand-baste across bottom and up one side, ¼" from the seamline, catching garment, seam allowance, and zipper tape in basting. Repeat for the other side.

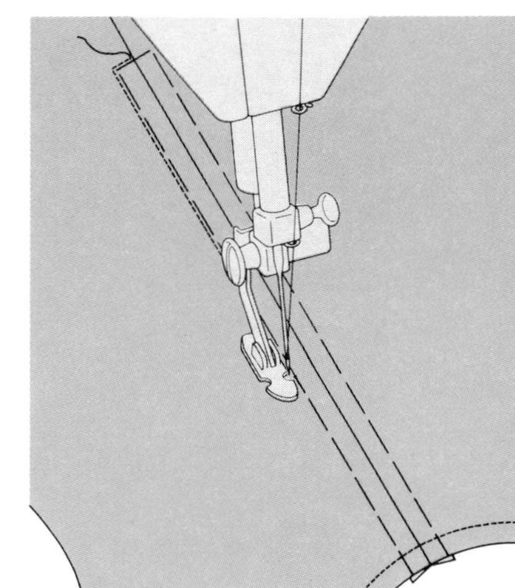

6. Change to a regular stitch length. Begin at the bottom of the placket, just outside the basting, and topstitch through all three layers—garment, seam allowance, and tape. Take 2 or 3 stitches across bottom of placket, pivot, and stitch to top.

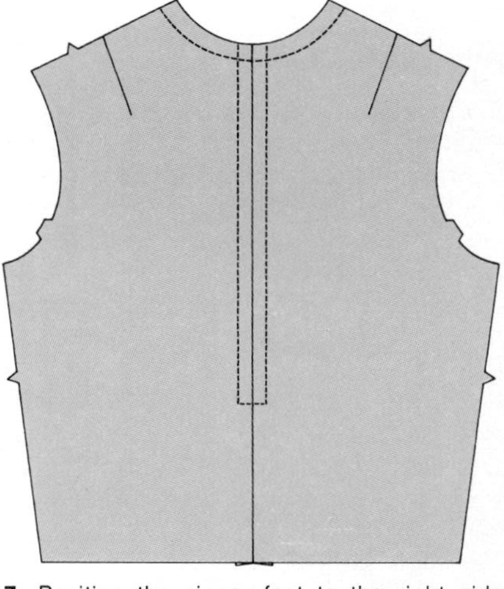

7. Position the zipper foot to the right side of the needle and topstitch the remaining side in the same way, taking the same number of stitches across bottom of placket. Pull thread ends to wrong side and tie. Remove hand bastings and open the placket.

Various finishing techniques

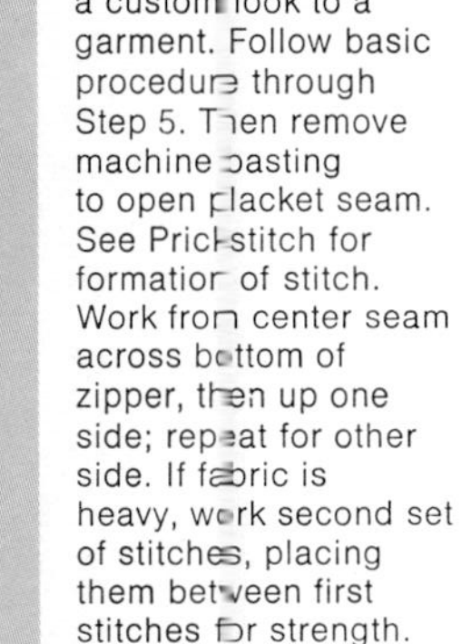

Hand-finishing gives a custom look to a garment. Follow basic procedure through Step 5. Then remove machine basting to open placket seam. See Prickstitch for formation of stitch. Work from center seam across bottom of zipper, then up one side; repeat for other side. If fabric is heavy, work second set of stitches, placing them between first stitches for strength.

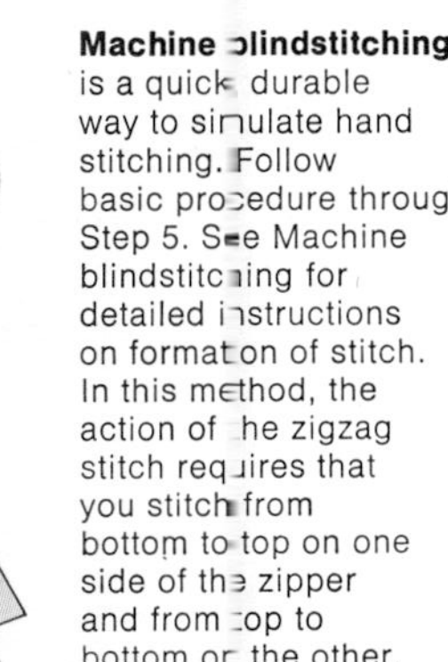

Machine blindstitching is a quick durable way to simulate hand stitching. Follow basic procedure through Step 5. See Machine blindstitching for detailed instructions on formation of stitch. In this method, the action of the zigzag stitch requires that you stitch from bottom to top on one side of the zipper and from top to bottom on the other.

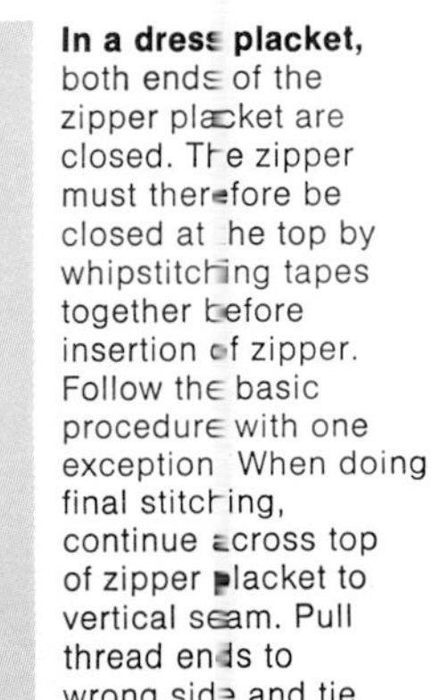
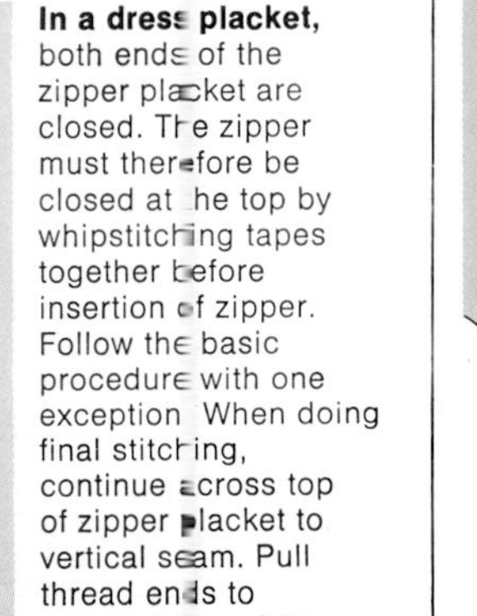
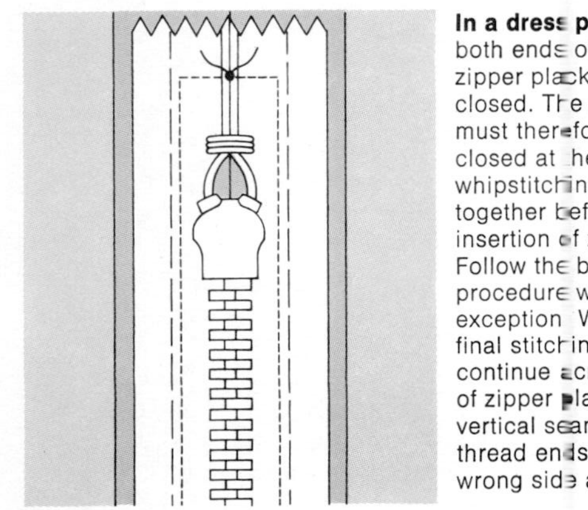

In a dress placket, both ends of the zipper placket are closed. The zipper must therefore be closed at the top by whipstitching tapes together before insertion of zipper. Follow the basic procedure with one exception. When doing final stitching, continue across top of zipper placket to vertical seam. Pull thread ends to wrong side and tie.

Separating zipper (centered application)

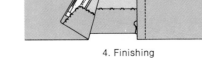

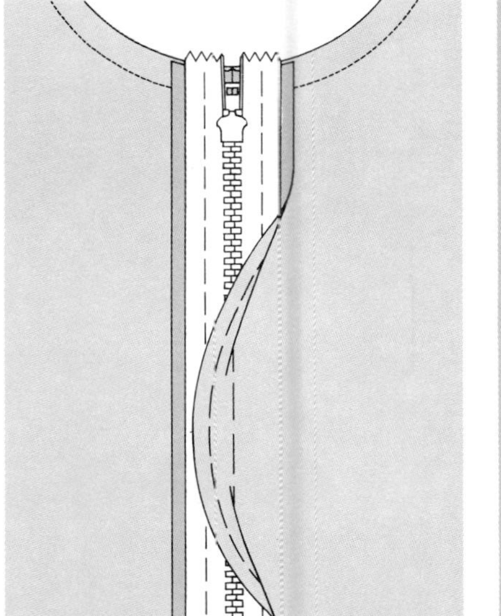

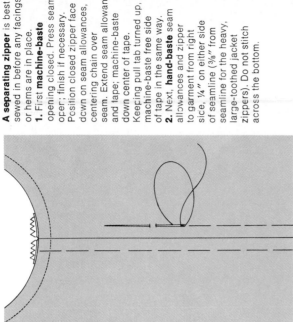

1. Machine basting

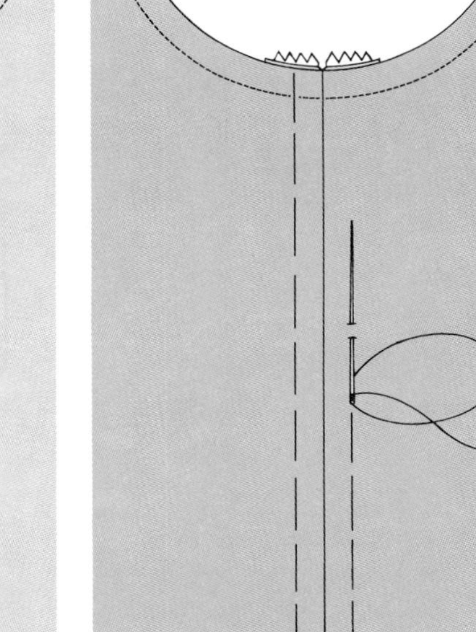
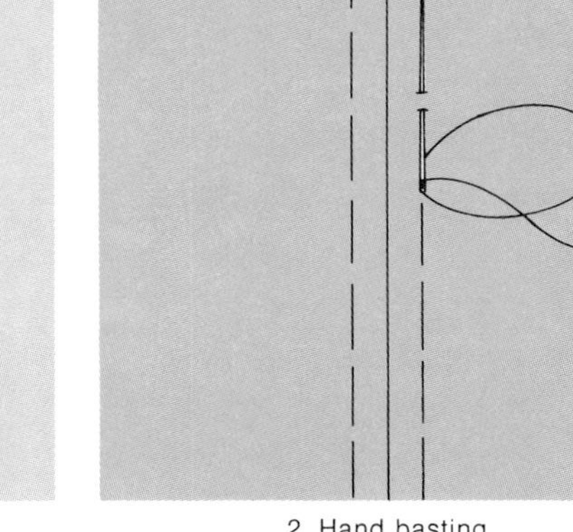

2. Hand basting

A separating zipper is best sewed in before any facings or hems are in place.
1. First **machine-baste** opening closed. Press seam open; finish if necessary. Position closed zipper face down on seam allowances, centering chain over seam. Extend seam allowance and tape; machine-baste down center of tape. Keeping pull tab turned up, machine-baste free side of tape in the same way.
2. Next, **hand-baste** seam allowances and zipper to garment from right side, ¼″ on either side of seamline (⅜″ from seamline for the heavy, large-toothed jacket zippers). Do not stitch across the bottom.

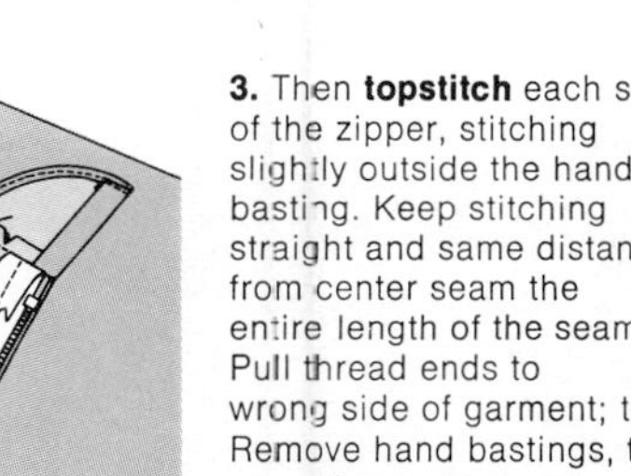
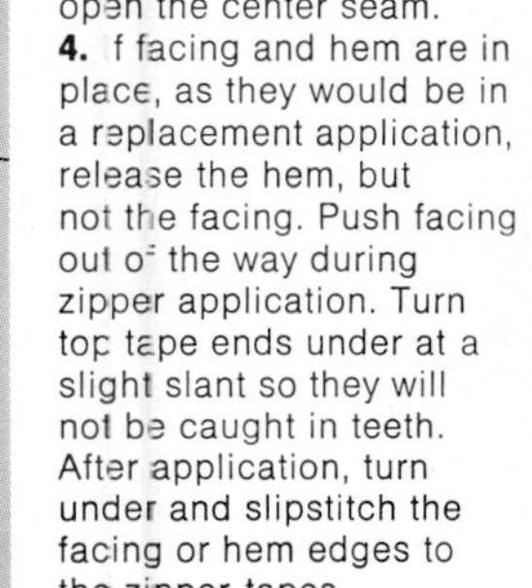

3. Topstitching

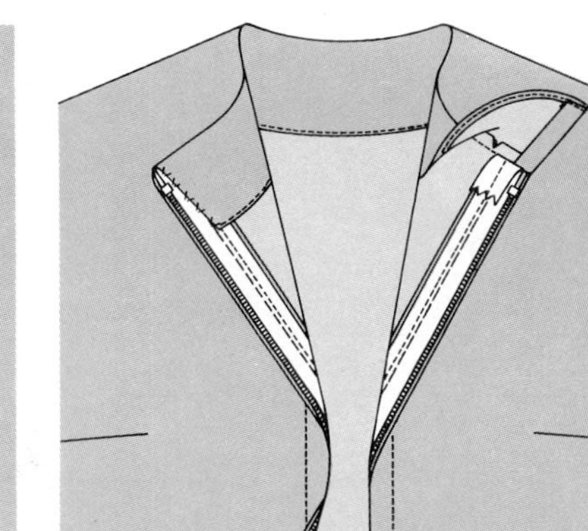
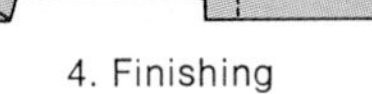

4. Finishing

3. Then **topstitch** each side of the zipper, stitching slightly outside the hand basting. Keep stitching straight and same distance from center seam the entire length of the seam. Pull thread ends to wrong side of garment; tie. Remove hand bastings, then open the center seam.
4. If facing and hem are in place, as they would be in a replacement application, release the hem, but not the facing. Push facing out of the way during zipper application. Turn top tape ends under at a slight slant so they will not be caught in teeth. After application, turn under and slipstitch the facing or hem edges to the zipper tapes.

Exposed zipper

Machine attachments 38-39

Uneven basting 124
Slip basting 125

Basic application

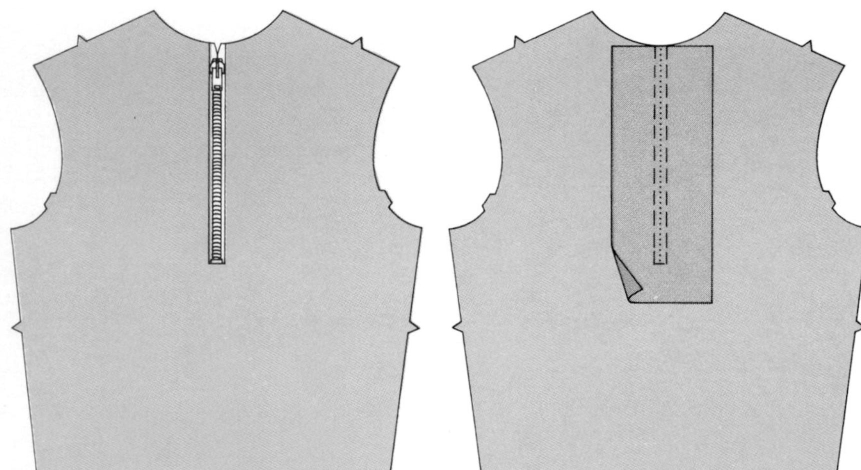

The exposed zipper can only be applied where there is no seam. Although it can be used on woven fabrics, it is most often seen on sweater knits. Before installation of the zipper, a stay is sewed to the placket area, which prevents sagging and stretching.

1. Cut a stay 3″ wide and 2″ longer than the zipper from lightweight, firmly woven lining fabric. Mark opening down center of garment and stay to equal the length of zipper coil or chain plus ⅝″. Right sides together, match markings and baste stay to garment.

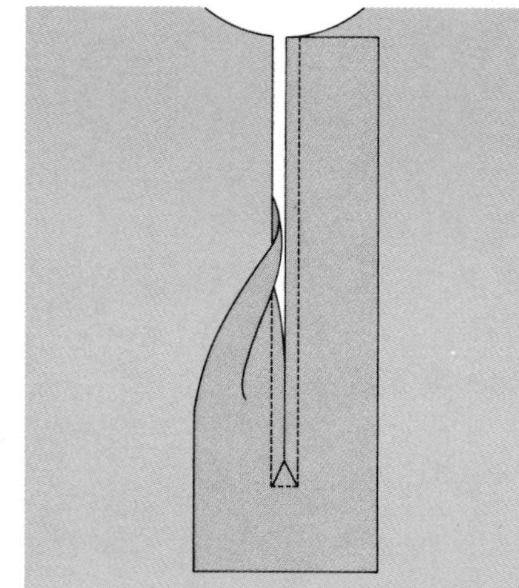

2. The opening for the zipper should be wide enough to expose only the zipper coil or chain. Stitch ⅛″ on each side of the center line and across bottom at end of center marking. Remove bastings. Slash down center line to within ½″ of bottom; cut into corners.

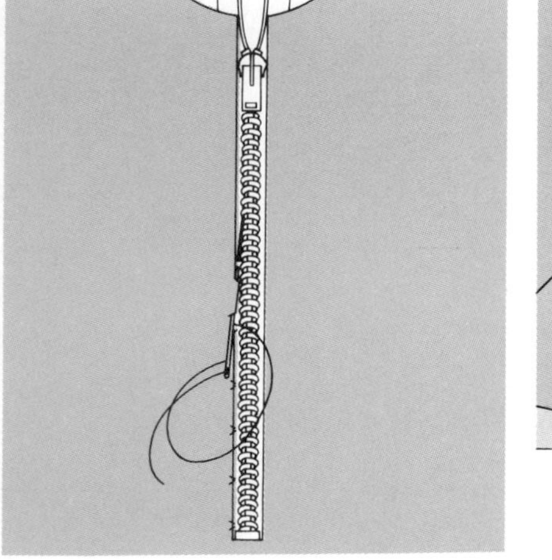

3. Turn stay to inside and press, making sure that none of the stay shows on right side of garment. Center zipper under opening with bottom stop of zipper at bottom end of opening. Slip-baste zipper to garment along the folds on each side and at bottom of zipper.

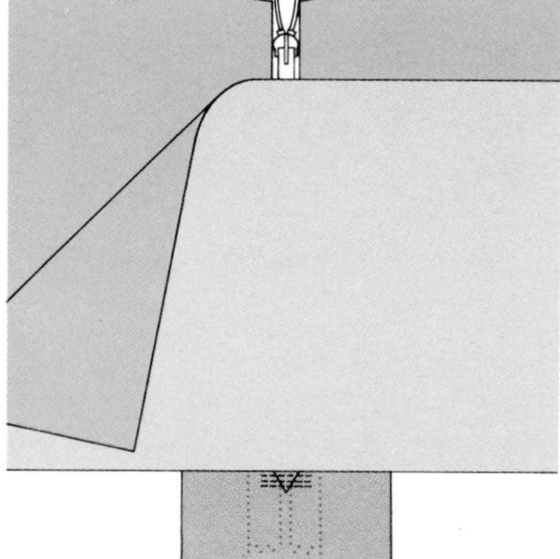

4. Lift the bottom part of the garment to expose the ends of the zipper tape and the triangle of garment and stay fabric at the bottom of the opening. Using a zipper foot, stitch across the base of the triangle to secure it to zipper tapes and stay.

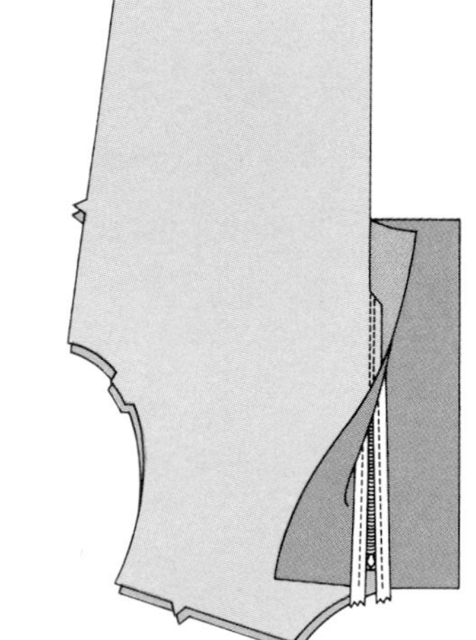

5. Fold back one side of the garment until the original stitching line is visible. Working from bottom to top, stitch the garment to the zipper tape along this stitching line. Repeat for the other side of the zipper. Remove the slip bastings that held zipper in position.

Enclosed exposed zipper

Appearance of finished zipper

Stay basted on all sides

If both ends of the zipper opening are closed, as with a pocket or a pillow cover, follow the basic procedure opposite, with these exceptions:
Cut the stay 3″ wide and 4″ longer than opening. Center stay over mark for opening. Stitch across both ends when stitching stay onto fabric.

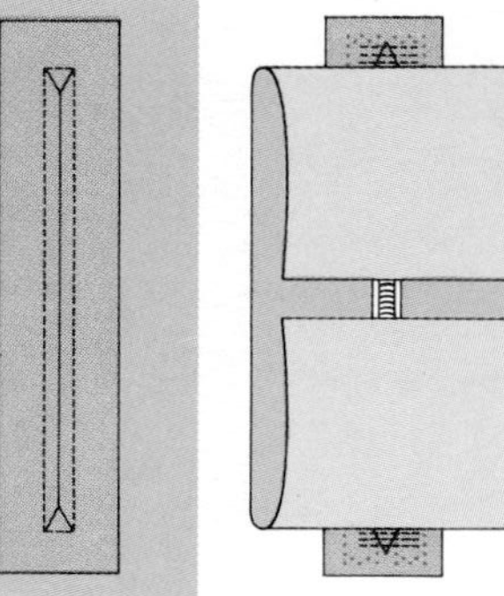

Corners slashed after stitching

How triangular ends are secured

Slash after stitching as in Step 2, but cut into corners at both ends.
Close the zipper tapes above top stop with a bar tack. Baste the zipper into finished opening as in Step 3, basting top as well as bottom.
Stitch triangles at both top and bottom (see Step 4) to zipper tape.

Machine attachments 38-39
Uneven basting 124
Neckline finishes 192-211

Decorative exposed zipper

1. Length of opening equals length of zipper coil or chain (plus 5/8″ if facing has not been applied). Mark opening down center of garment. Stitch around opening 1/8″ from center mark on both sides and across bottom.

2. Cut carefully along center line to within 1/2″ of bottom, then cut diagonally into each corner. This will form a 1/8″ seam allowance on each of the long sides of the opening and a small triangle at the bottom.

3. Turn the 1/8″ seam allowance on the long sides to right side of garment. Baste seam allowances in place and press opening flat. When application is completed, seam allowances will be covered by the decorative trim.

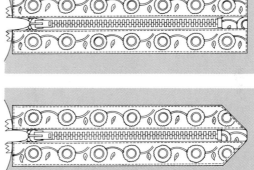

4. Center the zipper under the opening with the bottom stop at bottom end of opening and top stop at finished edge (5/8″ from upper edge if facing has not been applied). Using a zipper foot, edgestitch zipper from garment side through all thicknesses.

5. Trim should be at least 1/4″ wide to cover seam allowances. Position the trim around the zipper; miter trim to make a square or pointed end, as you prefer. Try, if possible, to match the design horizontally across zipper. Baste trim in place by hand.

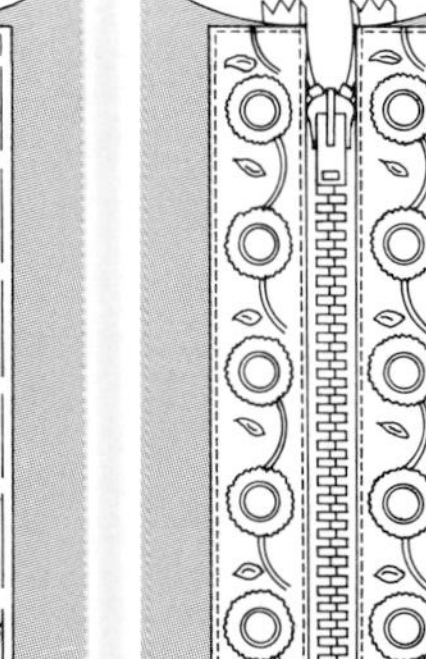

6. Using the zipper foot, topstitch the trim to the zipper, first next to coil or chain, then on outer edge. (If the trim contrasts in color with the garment, choose thread and zipper colors to match the trim.) If facing is not already in place, apply it now.

Mitering trim

For mitering purposes, trim should be twice the length of the zipper tape plus whatever extra is required to match a design. Some additional length is also needed for finishing the ends: **twice** the width of the trim for a pointed end; **four times** the width of the trim for a square end.

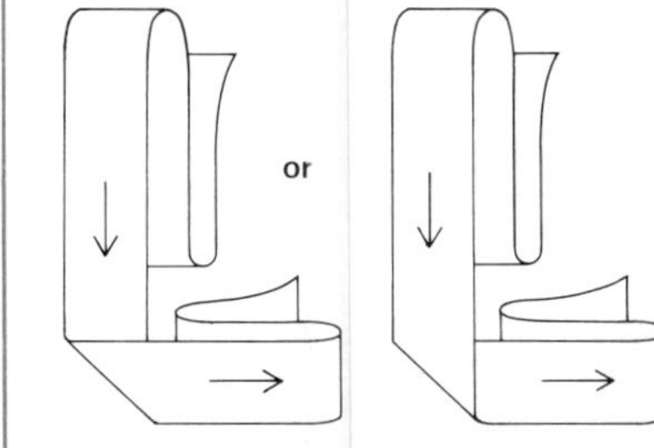

For a point, first fold the trim straight across itself, making a 45° angle.

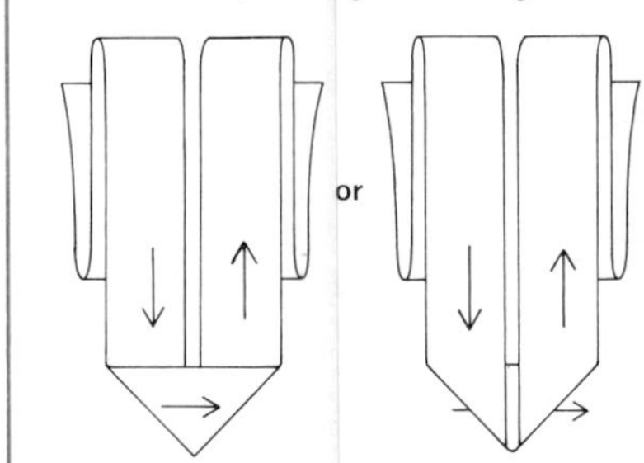

Then fold again, forming an opposite 45° angle, to complete the miter.

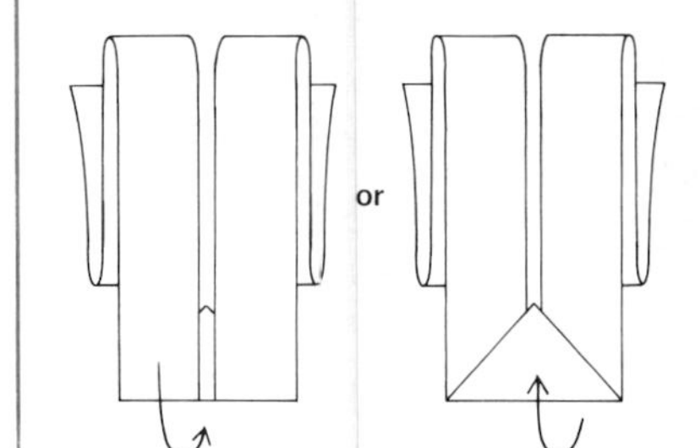

For a square end, complete steps for triangular miter; then fold point either under or back onto trim.

Lapped zipper

Machine attachments 38-39
Hand basting 124, machine 137
Whipstitch 136
Tying thread ends 137

Basic application

A lapped zipper is applied the same way regardless of garment type; the only variable is in the placement of the zipper in relation to the garment edge. If there will be a facing finish, place the top stop *½ inch below* the seamline. If the garment will have a waistband or standing collar, place the top stop *just below* the seamline. Do all work on inside of garment, except topstitching; keep zipper closed throughout application. **Work from bottom to top** on all steps; this will ensure that the lap goes in the proper direction on the garment.

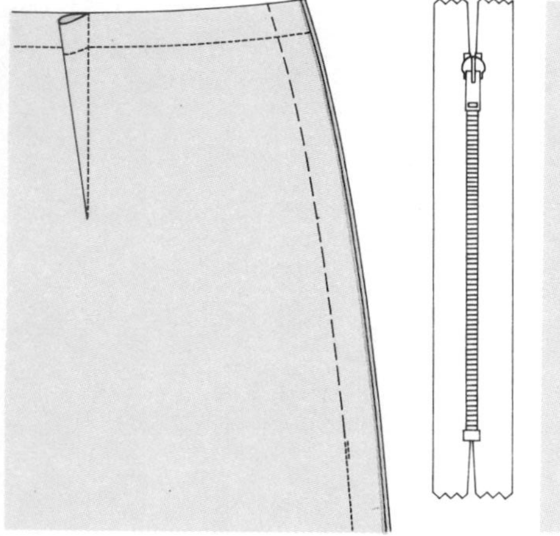

1. Mark the exact length of the placket opening, using the zipper as a guide. Stitch seam up to bottom of zipper placket with a regular stitch length, backstitch, then change to machine basting for placket. Clip basting thread at intervals. Press seam open; seam-finish.

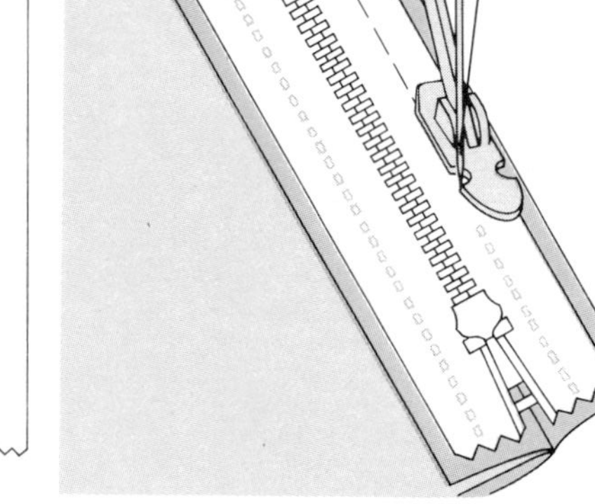

2. To position the zipper, extend the right-hand seam allowance and place zipper on it face down, with top stop at mark and edge of coil along the seamline; pin in place. Using a zipper foot, positioned to right of needle, machine-baste on stitching guideline.

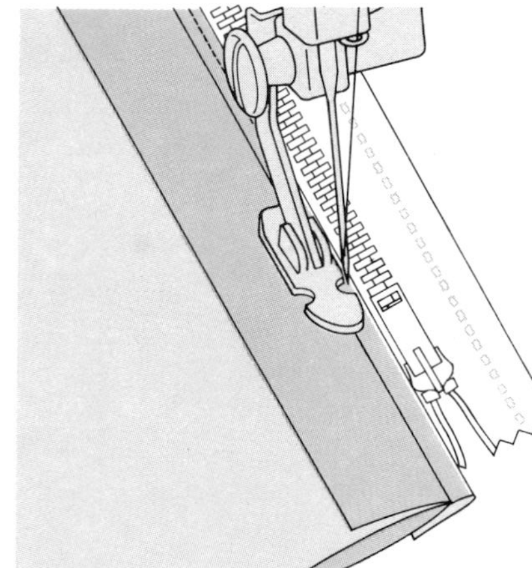

3. Position zipper foot to the left of the needle. Turn the zipper face up, forming a fold in the seam allowance. Bring the fold close to, but not over, the zipper coil or chain; pin if necessary. Stitch along edge of fold through all thicknesses.

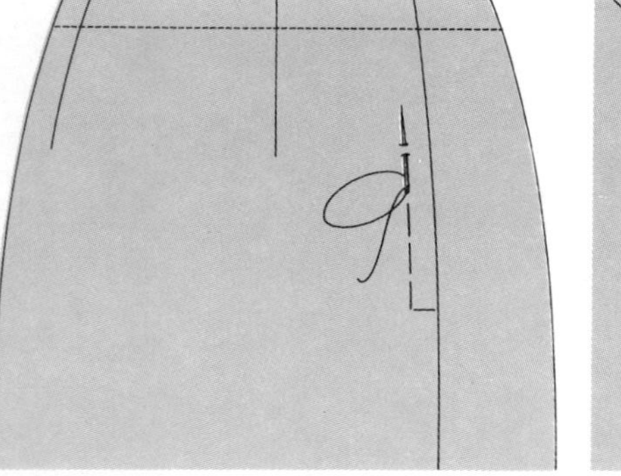

4. Turn garment to right side; spread fabric as flat as possible over unstitched zipper tape. Hand-baste across bottom of zipper, then up along the side, ⅜" to ½" from seamline. This should place basting close to stitching guideline on zipper tape.

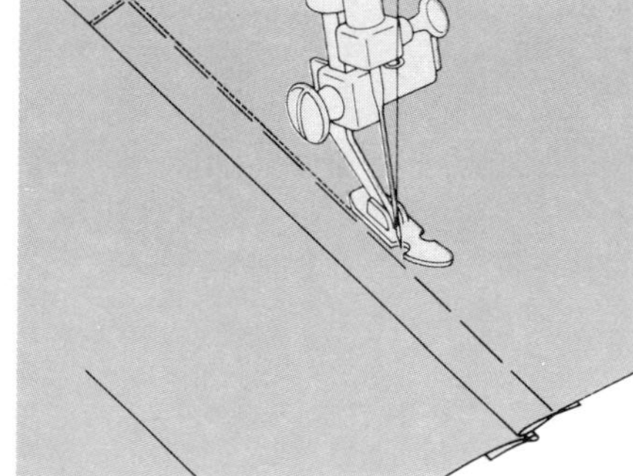

5. Position zipper foot to the right of the needle. Topstitch close to the basting across the bottom of the zipper and up along the side, pivoting at the corner. Take care not to stitch over the basting. Bring thread ends to underside and tie. Remove hand bastings.

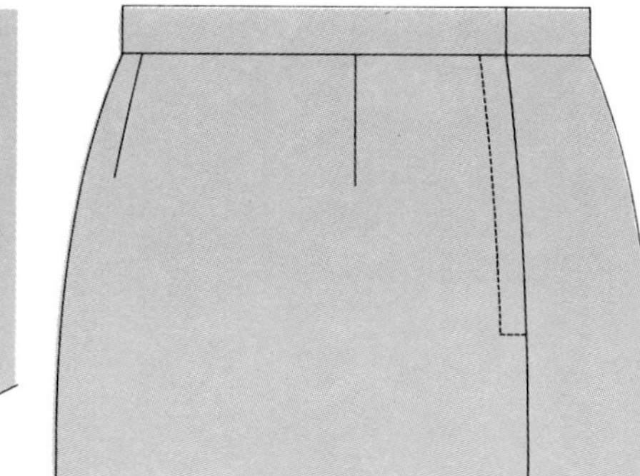

6. Open the zipper placket by removing the machine bastings in the placket seam. Tweezers are helpful for getting out any stubborn thread ends. Finish top edge of garment with appropriate finish—facing, collar, or waistband—as pattern directs.

Dress application

Before beginning the basic application, whipstitch zipper tapes together above top stop. The length of the placket should be equal to the distance from bottom stop to whipstitches.

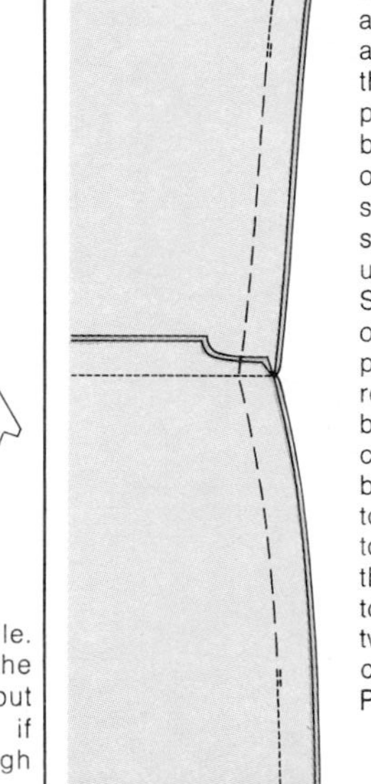

If placket intersects a cross seam, such as a waistline, make sure the seam is matched perfectly before basting the placket opening. Trim cross-seam allowances as shown to reduce unnecessary bulk. Stitch from bottom of seam to bottom of placket using a regular stitch length, backstitch, then change to machine basting and stitch to top of placket. At top of placket, return the stitch length to normal, backstitch two stitches, and complete the seam. Press seam open.

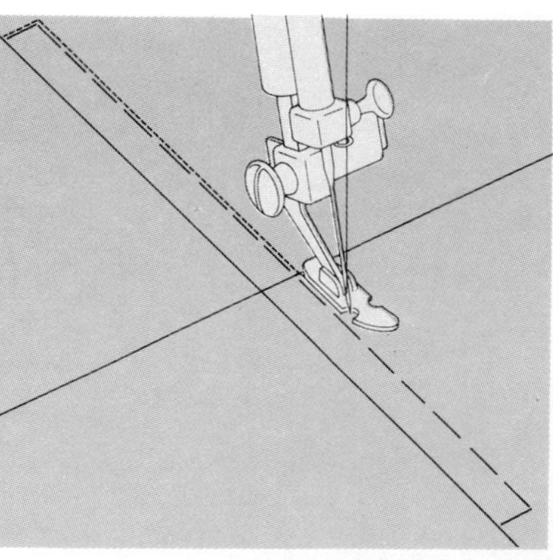

Start and stop topstitching at the vertical seam. Stitch from seam across bottom of zipper, up along the side, then back across top. Pull thread ends to wrong side and tie.

Various finishing techniques

Hand-finishing is a sign of careful craftsmanship. Follow basic instructions to Step 5. See Prickstitch for formation of the hand stitch. Work from bottom to top of zipper. For extra strength, turn garment to inside and machine-stitch edge of front *seam allowance* to zipper tape.

Machine blindstitching gives the appearance of hand finishing, but is more durable.
1. Allow ⅞" seam allowances when cutting out garment. Follow instructions for basic application through Step 3. Baste free zipper tape to remaining seam allowance through center of tape.

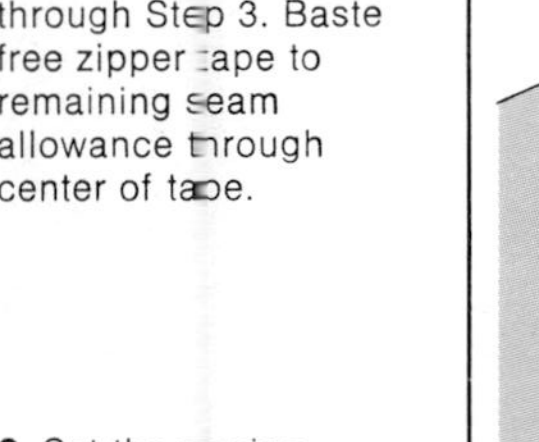

2. Set the sewing machine for a short, narrow blindstitch. Keep foot to right of needle. Fold back garment on basting line and, with bottom of placket away from you, position zipper tape over machine feed. With zipper foot on seam allowance, blindstitch full length of placket, closely following fold. Prickstitch by hand across bottom. Remove bastings.

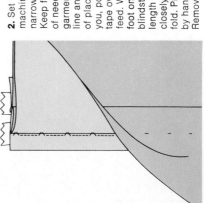

Separating zipper (lapped application)

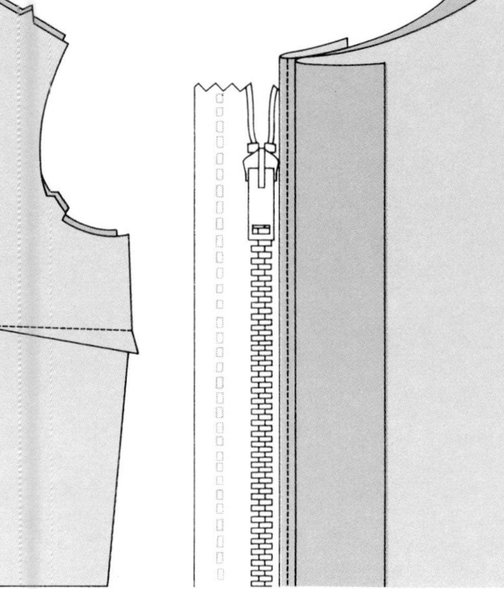

1. Positioning zipper

2. Stitching first seam allowance

A separating zipper should be sewed in before facings or hems are in place.
1. Machine-baste placket seam closed. Press open and seam-finish if necessary. **Position closed zipper** face down on seam allowances, with zipper teeth centered over the seam and bottom stop at bottom of opening. Keeping tab turned up, machine-baste right-hand tape to seam allowance from bottom to top.
2. Turn the zipper face up, forming a fold in the seam allowance. Bring the fold close to, but not over the zipper coil or teeth; pin if necessary. Change to a zipper foot, positioned to the left of the needle. **Stitch along edge** of fold through all thicknesses.

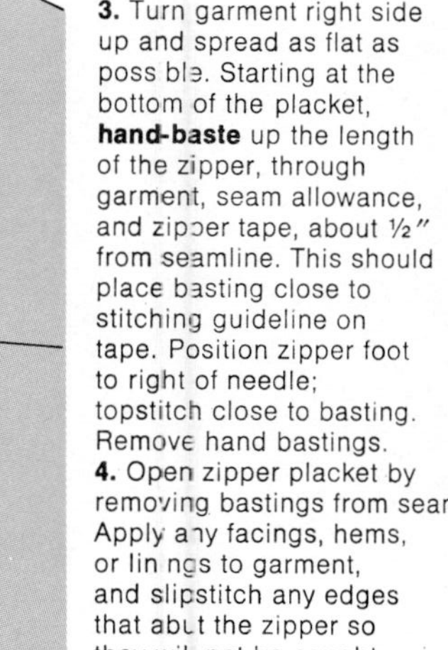

3. Hand basting before topstitching

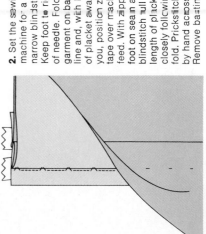

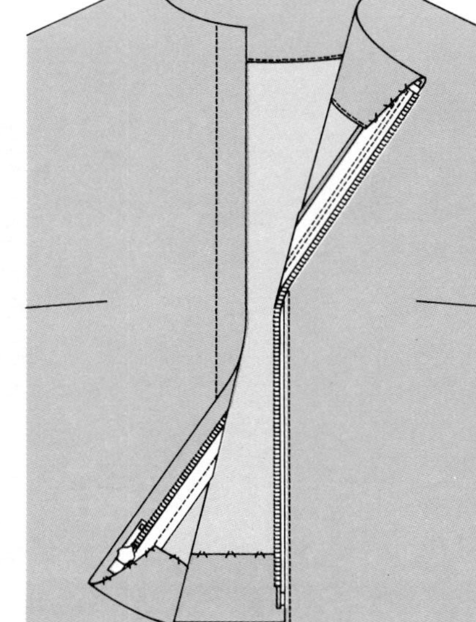

4. Finishing

3. Turn garment right side up and spread as flat as possible. Starting at the bottom of the placket, **hand-baste** up the length of the zipper, through garment, seam allowance, and zipper tape, about ½" from seamline. This should place basting close to stitching guideline on tape. Position zipper foot to right of needle; topstitch close to basting. Remove hand bastings.
4. Open zipper placket by removing bastings from seam. Apply any facings, hems, or linings to garment, and slipstitch any edges that abut the zipper so they will not be caught in zipper teeth during wear.

Fly-front zipper

Chart of zipper types 14
Uneven basting 124
Reducing seam bulk 147
Men's trouser zipper 396-397

Application

The fly-front zipper is the traditional zipper application for men's trousers. It is often used on women's sport clothes as well, however, because it provides such a neat and durable closing. The placket has a definite lap direction: in women's clothes it laps right over left as shown here; in men's garments it laps left over right (see Sewing for men).

A special trouser zipper is often recommended for use with this application. If a trouser zipper is not suitable because of its weight, or the limited color range, a neck or skirt zipper can be used. No matter what type of zipper is used, it will probably require shortening; fly-front plackets are not as long as most other zipper plackets. See instructions at right.

It is best to buy a pattern designed with a fly-front closing—it will supply all the necessary pattern pieces.

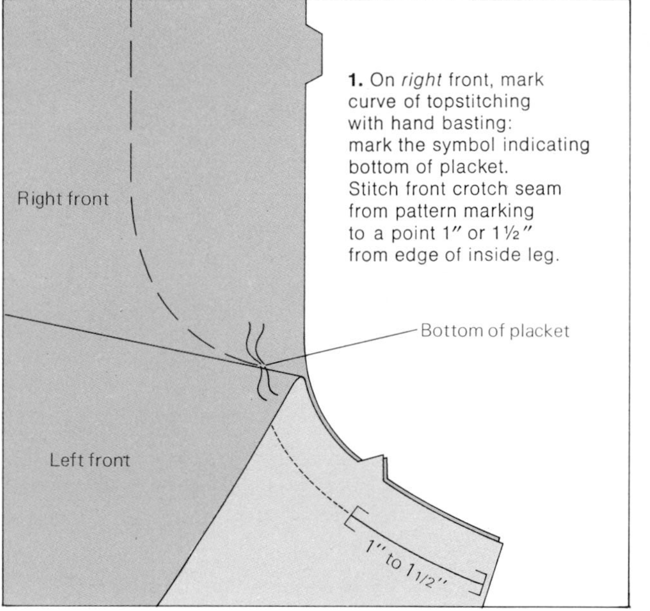

1. On *right* front, mark curve of topstitching with hand basting: mark the symbol indicating bottom of placket. Stitch front crotch seam from pattern marking to a point 1" or 1½" from edge of inside leg.

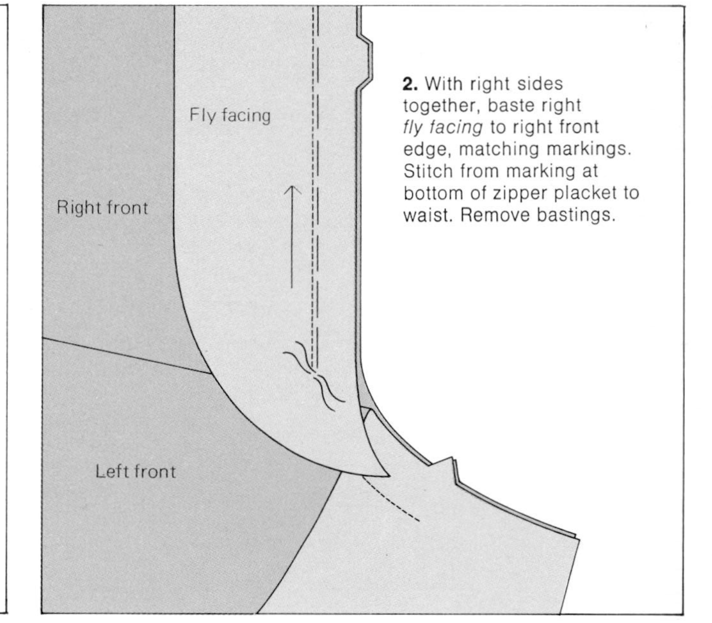

2. With right sides together, baste right *fly facing* to right front edge, matching markings. Stitch from marking at bottom of zipper placket to waist. Remove bastings.

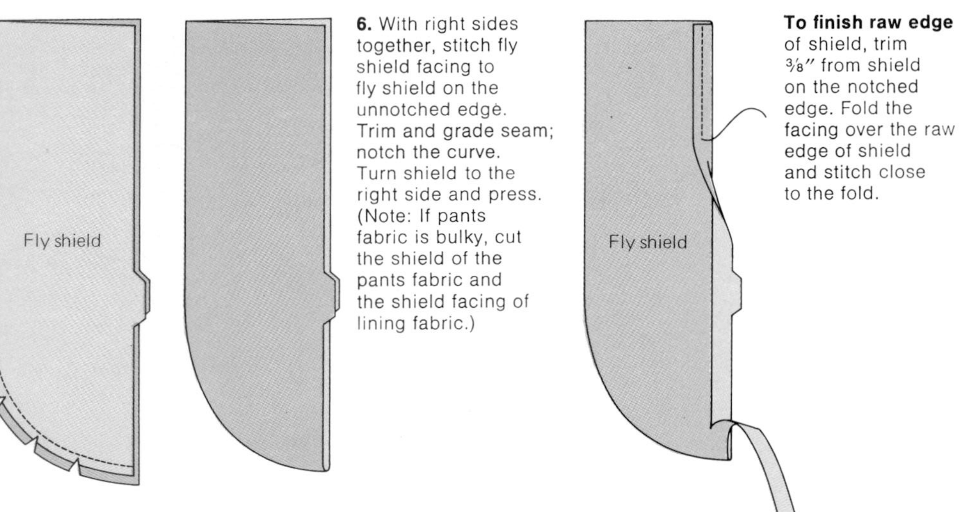

6. With right sides together, stitch fly shield facing to fly shield on the unnotched edge. Trim and grade seam; notch the curve. Turn shield to the right side and press. (Note: If pants fabric is bulky, cut the shield of the pants fabric and the shield facing of lining fabric.)

To finish raw edge of shield, trim ⅜" from shield on the notched edge. Fold the facing over the raw edge of shield and stitch close to the fold.

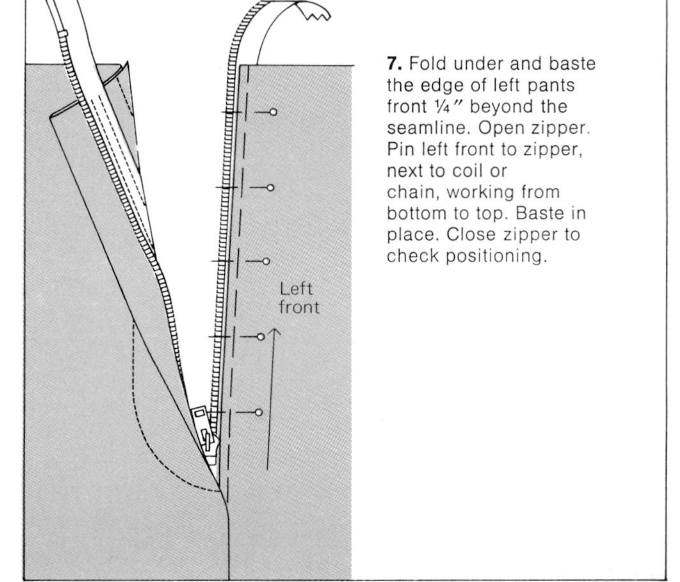

7. Fold under and baste the edge of left pants front ¼" beyond the seamline. Open zipper. Pin left front to zipper, next to coil or chain, working from bottom to top. Baste in place. Close zipper to check positioning.

Machine attachments 38-39
Hand bar tacks 133
Machine bar tacks 142

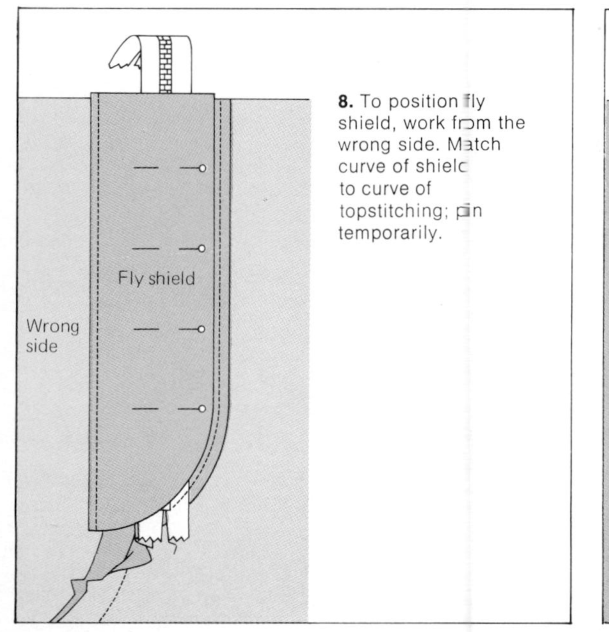

3. Trim and grade the seam allowances; open out the facing and press it and the seam allowances away from the garment.

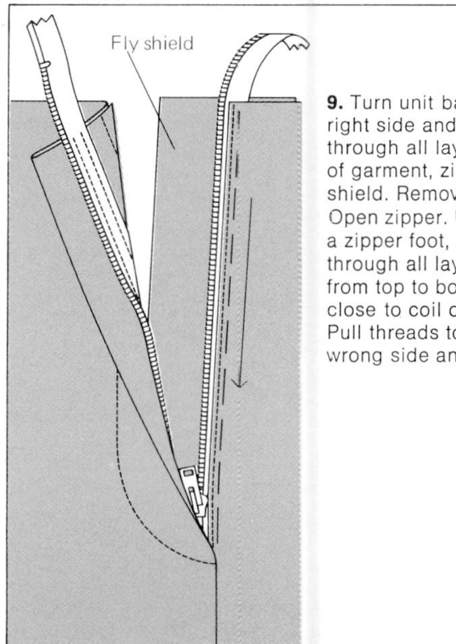

4. Position closed zipper face down on *right* side of facing. The *left* edge of zipper tape should lie along facing seam and *bottom stop* should be ¾" from raw edge of facing. Top of zipper may extend beyond upper edge of facing. Baste zipper in place, turning up bottom of left zipper tape even with bottom stop. Baste left zipper tape to facing from bottom to top. On right zipper tape, stitch close to chain or coil, using zipper foot and regular stitch length. Stitch a second time, close to edge of tape.

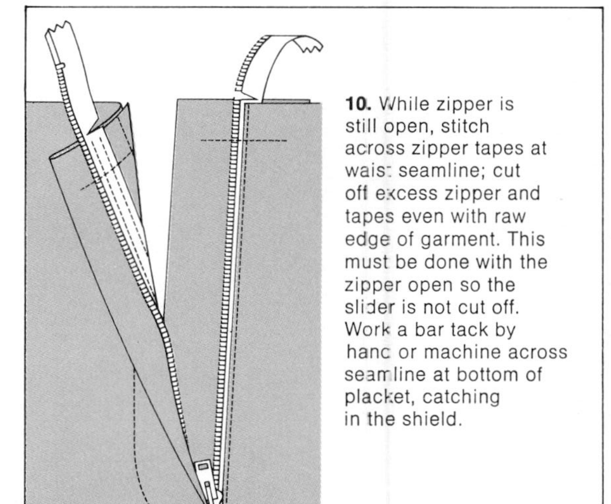

5. Turn facing to the inside on seamline. Press. On outside of garment, baste fly facing to front, following original basted markings. Then topstitch from bottom to top along basted markings, being careful not to catch left zipper tape in stitching. Pull threads to wrong side and tie. Remove all basting threads.

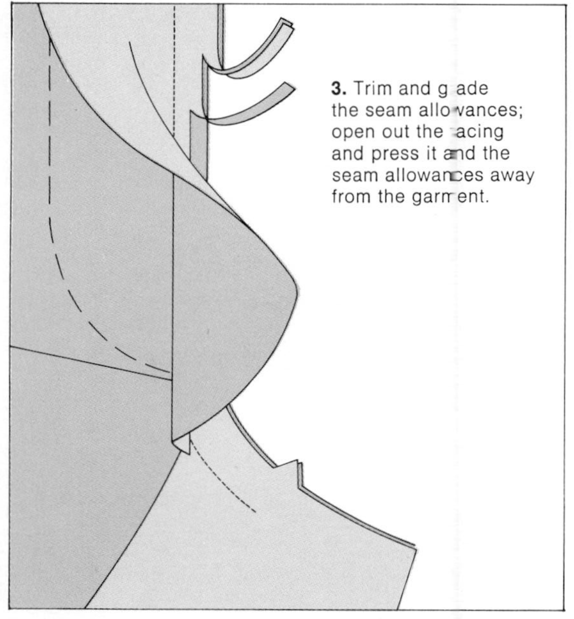

8. To position fly shield, work from the wrong side. Match curve of shield to curve of topstitching; pin temporarily.

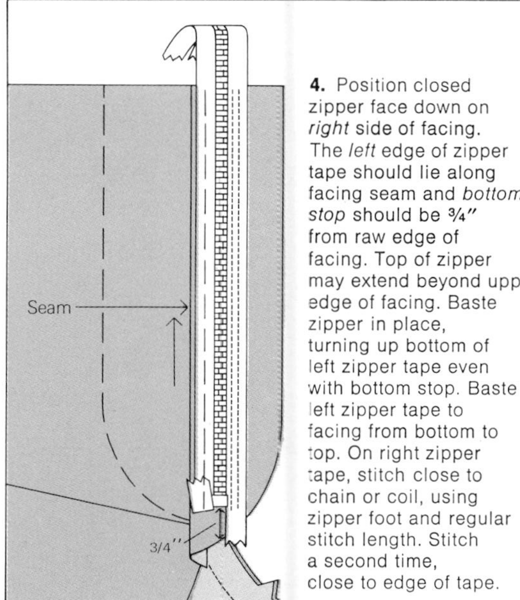

9. Turn unit back to right side and baste through all layers of garment, zipper, and shield. Remove pins. Open zipper. Using a zipper foot, stitch through all layers from top to bottom, close to coil or chain. Pull threads to the wrong side and tie.

10. While zipper is still open, stitch across zipper tapes at waist seamline; cut off excess zipper and tapes even with raw edge of garment. This must be done with the zipper open so the slider is not cut off. Work a bar tack by hand or machine across seamline at bottom of placket, catching in the shield.

Bar tack

Invisible zipper

Chart of zipper types 14
Tying thread ends 137
Seam finishes 148-149

General information

The invisible zipper is different from a conventional zipper in both appearance and installation. When this zipper is closed, all that shows on the garment is a plain seam and tiny pull tab. Invisible zippers are applied to an open seam, to seam allowances only—there is no stitching on the outside of the garment. They can be used wherever conventional zippers are.

Manufacturers supply a special zipper foot to sew in this zipper. It is impossible to apply a synthetic coil invisible zipper without one, although a metal invisible zipper can be applied with a regular zipper foot.

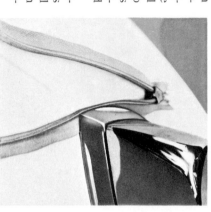

Press synthetic coil invisible zippers from wrong side with the zipper open so that the tapes are smooth and the coils stand away from tapes. Zipper will then feed smoothly through grooves in the foot. Do not close the zipper until both sides have been stitched in place.

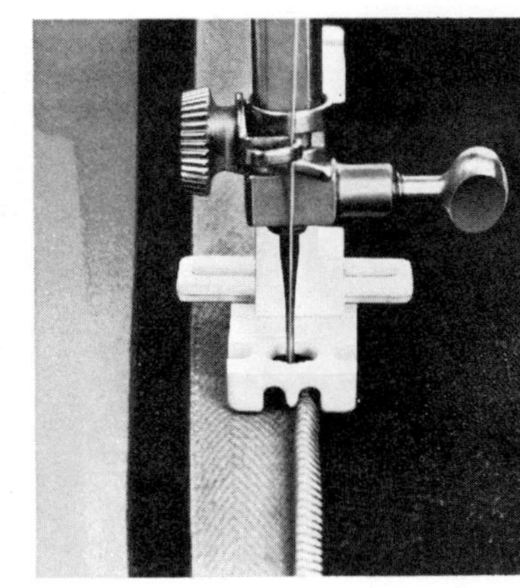

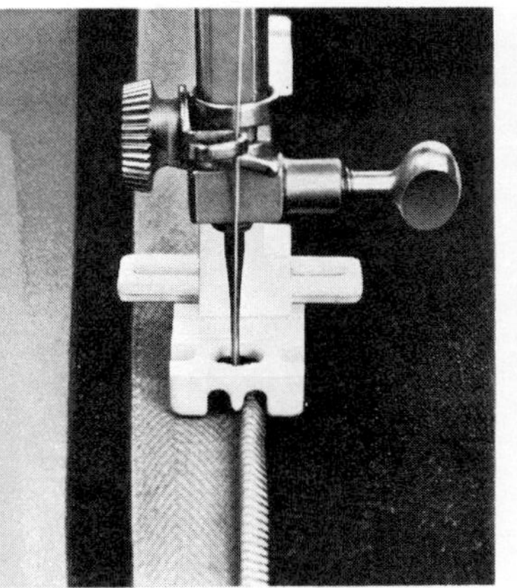

A special foot for invisible zippers is designed with grooves that hold the coil or chain upright and out of the way so needle can stitch right alongside chain or coil. Be sure to get the foot made for the brand of zipper you buy. Also, the feet for metal and coil zippers are not meant to be interchangeable.

Basic procedure

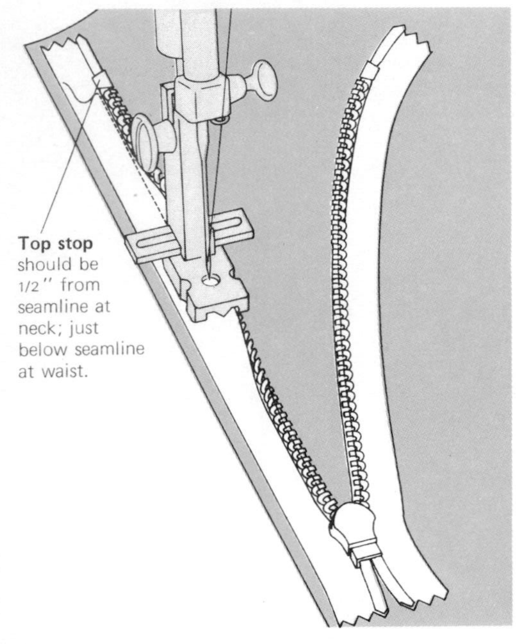

Top stop should be 1/2" from seamline at neck; just below seamline at waist.

1. Seam-finish garment edges, if needed. Place open zipper, face down, on the right side of garment—coil along seamline, top stop at appropriate mark. Pin if necessary. Fit right-hand groove of the foot over coil. Stitch to slider; backstitch; tie thread ends at top.

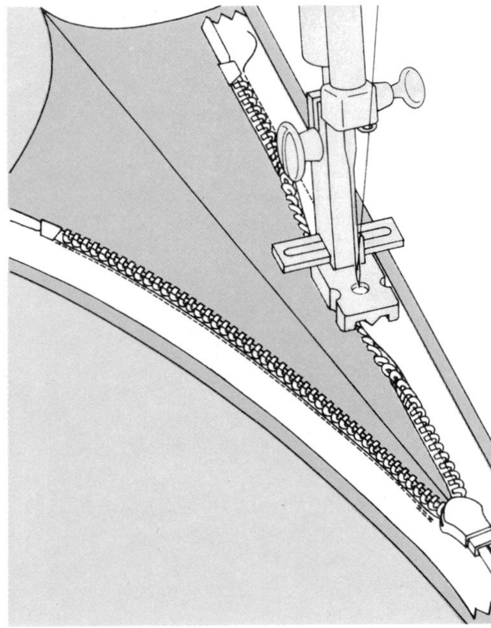

2. Pin the unstitched tape, face down, to right side of other garment piece. Width of zipper tape should be on garment seam allowance. Position top stop at appropriate mark and coil along seamline. Fit left-hand groove of foot over coil. Stitch as in Step 1.

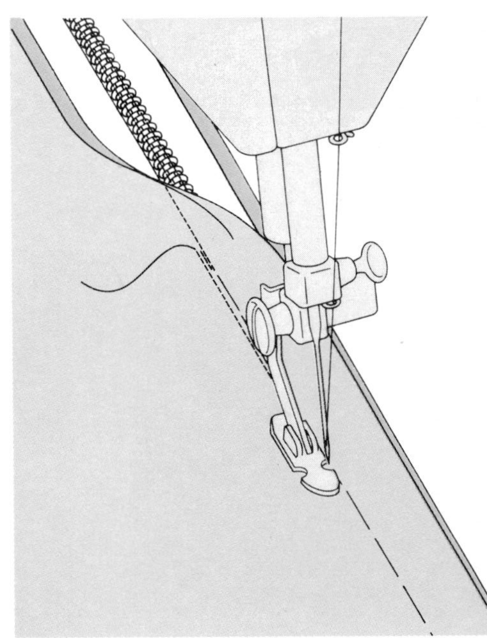

3. Close zipper. Attach regular zipper foot and position to left of needle. Pin and baste seam below zipper. Lower needle into fabric at end of stitching, slightly above and to the left of the last stitch. Stitch seam to lower edge. Tie thread ends.

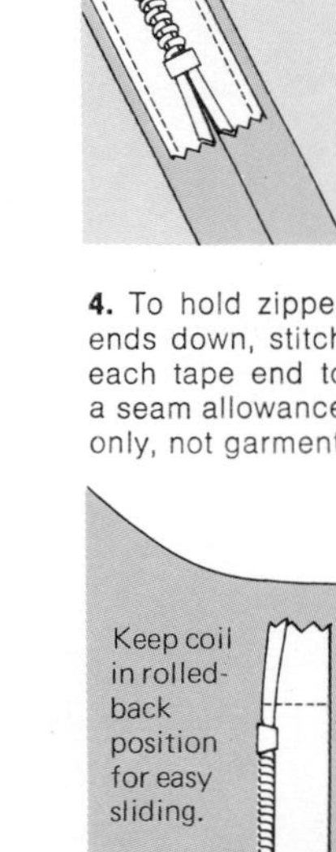

Keep coil in rolled-back position for easy sliding.

4. To hold zipper ends down, stitch each tape end to a seam allowance only, not garment.

5. Open up zipper; stitch across tops of tapes with the coil held upright as shown.

Optional steps; alternative method

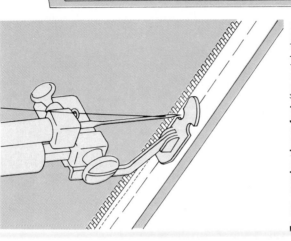

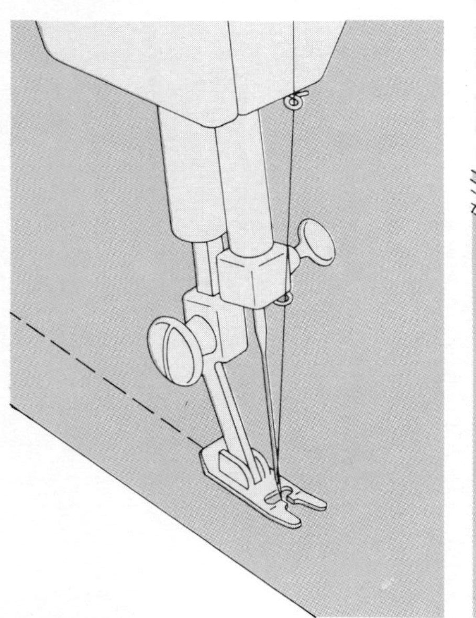

Basted guideline: To help in positioning the zipper, hand- or machine-baste a seam guideline on both garment pieces. Place coil exactly on this line, and use it for matching the seamlines below zipper.

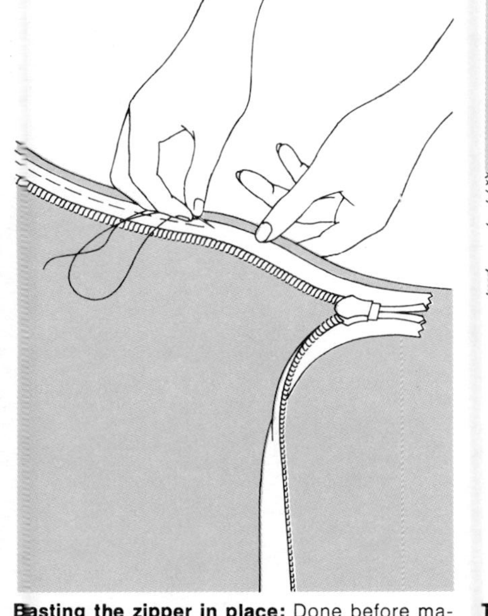

Basting the zipper in place: Done before machine stitching, basting is especially helpful when applying an invisible zipper with a regular zipper foot. Baste, then stitch, one tape at a time from top to bottom.

To use regular zipper foot (for metal zipper only): Baste first tape in place; with foot to left of needle, stitch close to teeth. Move foot to right of needle and repeat for other side. Finish as in Steps 3, 4, 5, left.

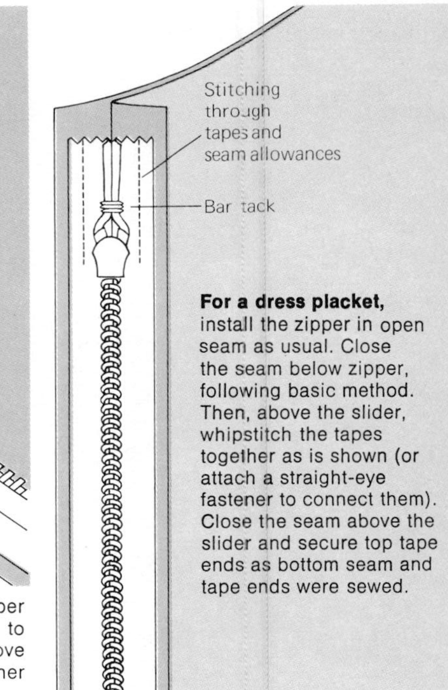

For a dress placket, install the zipper in open seam as usual. Close the seam below zipper, following basic method. Then, above the slider, whipstitch the tapes together as is shown (or attach a straight-eye fastener to connect them). Close the seam above the slider and secure top tape ends as bottom seam and tape ends were sewed.

Special tips

To reduce puckering: Puckering may occur when sewing fabrics with a permanent press finish and some sheers. To avoid this, hold fabric and zipper firmly behind and in front of zipper foot and keep them taut as they pass under the needle. Let feed dog move fabric; do not pull it.

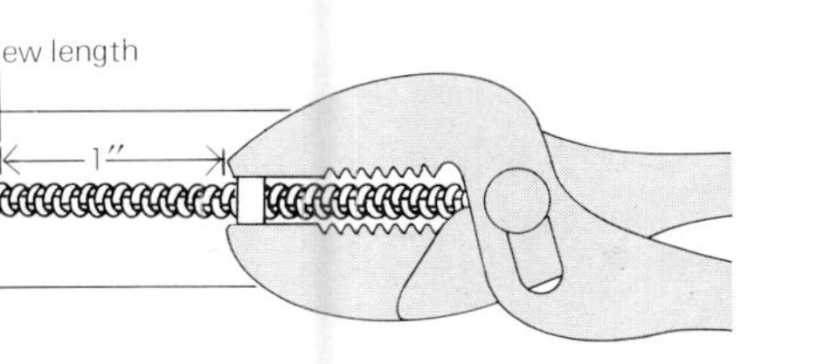

To shorten zipper, measure and mark new length on tape. Make new bottom stop by whipstitching several times over chain about 1″ below mark. (Zipper shown above has an adjustable bottom stop, which can be clamped in place with pliers.) Cut off zipper ½″ below new bottom stop and insert as usual.

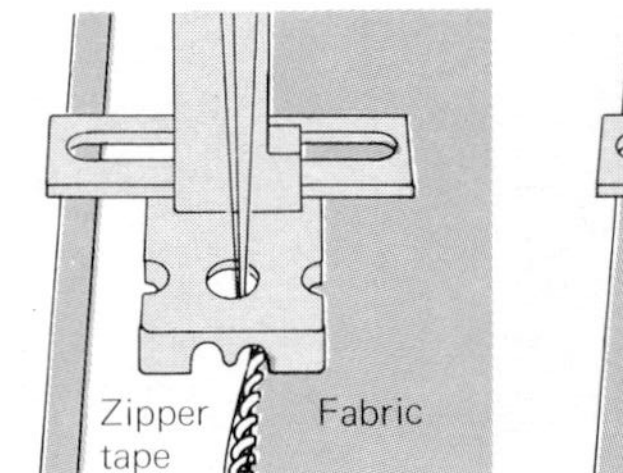
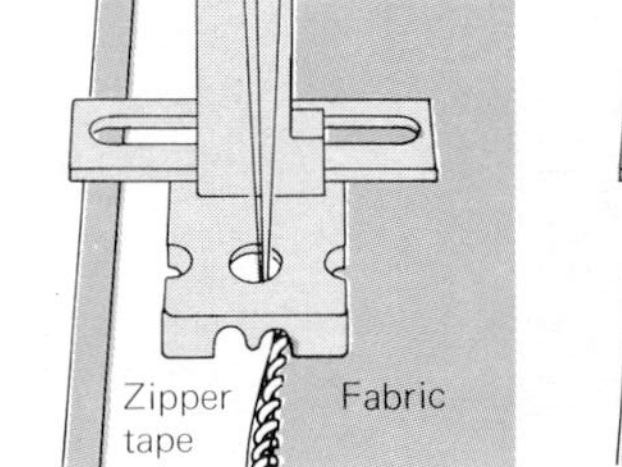

Adjusting for different fabrics: For average-weight fabrics, the needle should stay in center of needle hole on the invisible zipper foot. It may be advisable, however, to move the foot so needle is off-center—*closer* to coil for lightweight fabrics (left, above), *farther away* for heavy fabrics (right, above).

Seam and pattern matching (invisible zipper)

The situations below may occur in the installation of an invisible zipper. The extra matching steps are necessary because this zipper is applied to an *open* seam. When zippers are applied to a closed seam, as is usually the case, matching is easily taken care of when the seam is basted before zipper installation. The method for matching diagonals can also be used to match garment seams, or to match a large print motif, such as a floral. The fabric must, of course, be cut so that it is possible to match the stripe, plaid, or design.

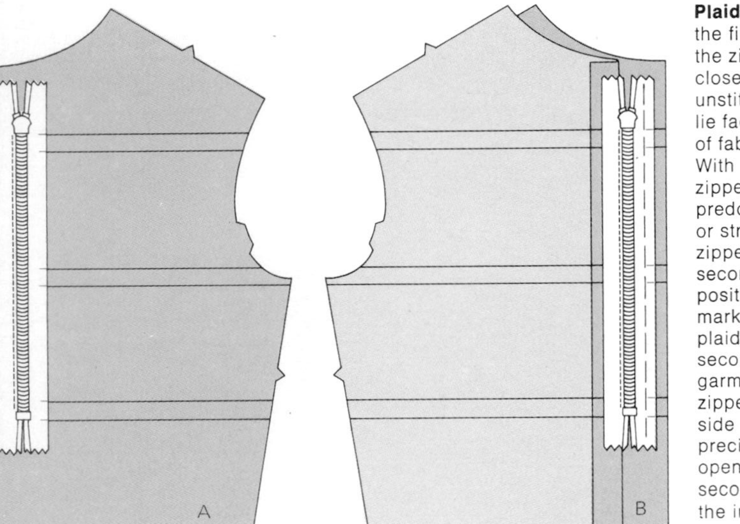

Plaids or stripes: Sew the first side of the zipper in place, then close the zipper. Let unstitched side of zipper lie face down on outside of fabric (drawing A). With a pencil, mark the zipper tape at each predominant cross bar or stripe. Open the zipper and baste the second zipper tape in position, matching the marks on the tape to the plaid or stripe on the second side of the garment (B). Close the zipper and check on right side of garment for a precise match. If correct, open zipper and stitch second side; complete the installation.

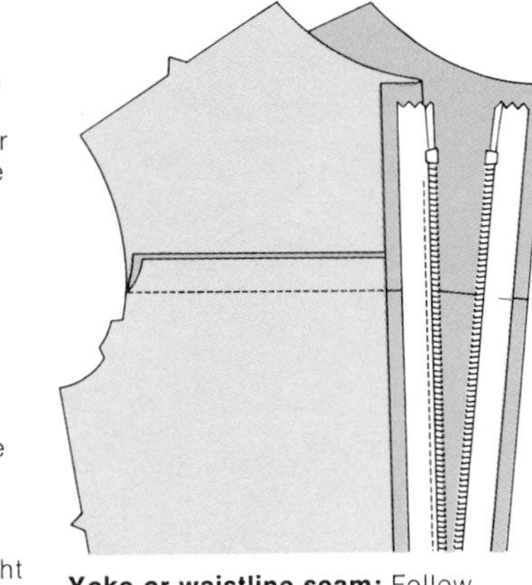

Yoke or waistline seam: Follow procedure at left for matching plaids or stripes, first trimming the cross-seam allowances to eliminate bulk.

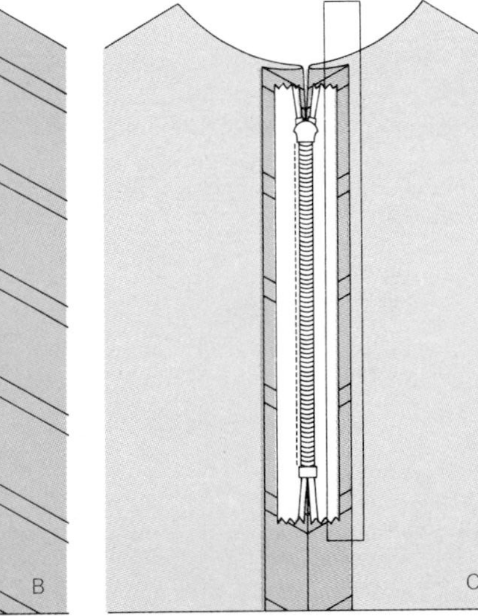

To match diagonals or large designs, stitch the first side of the zipper in place, then fold back fabric so that right side of zipper and fabric are both visible (A). Fold back seam allowance of unstitched side. Match second side to first side, taping in place temporarily (B). Turn fabric to wrong side and tape unstitched side of zipper tape to fabric seam allowance (drawing C). Remove tape from face side of fabric. Open zipper; stitch the taped side of zipper; finish application.

Knits, leather, fake fur

Knits: Stabilize a zipper opening in a moderately stretchy knit by staystitching ½ inch from cut edges (see Staystitching for knits). If fabric is very stretchy, stabilize zipper area on both seams with woven seam binding. Stitch it to the wrong side, over the seam allowance, with the stitching ½ inch from cut edge.

Leather, suede, and vinyl: A centered application is recommended. The zipper placket seam cannot be basted closed because punctures from the needle would remain. To close the placket temporarily for installation of zipper, turn back the seam allowances on the seamline and glue them down to wrong side of garment. Then, on outside of garment, hold the placket edges together with a transparent tape. Use a zipper adhesive (see product instructions) to position zipper face down on seam allowances. Stitch on *inside* of garment from bottom to top, taking the same number of stitches across bottom of zipper on each side of seam. Pull thread ends to wrong side; tie.

High-pile fake fur: Use grosgrain ribbon to form a smooth, flat facing between zipper and fur fabric. First, clip pile from placket seam allowances. Edgestitch 1-inch-wide grosgrain ribbon, cut 1 inch longer than zipper, to right side of both seam allowances, aligning edge of ribbon with seamline. Trim the fabric seam allowances underneath the ribbon to ¼ inch. Place opened zipper face down on ribbon with bottom stop at end of opening and chain or coil even with seamline; baste and stitch. Repeat for other side. Turn the ribbon and zipper inside garment along seamline. Hand-backstitch zipper tape and ribbon to fur fabric *backing* only. Catchstitch ribbon edge to backing.

Zippers in pleated skirts

The primary considerations in sewing a zipper into a pleated skirt are that the zipper be as inconspicuous as possible, and that it not interfere with the fold or hang of the pleats. In order for both to be accomplished, the positioning of the zipper seam must be considered when the pattern is laid out on the fabric. If the pleats are box or inverted, try to position the zipper seam down the center of the pleat *underfold;* then install the zipper with either the centered or invisible method. If the garment is side-pleated, try to position the seam where the pleat *backfold* will fall; then insert the zipper by means of the special lapped application that is shown and described at right. (See Pleats for definition of terms.)

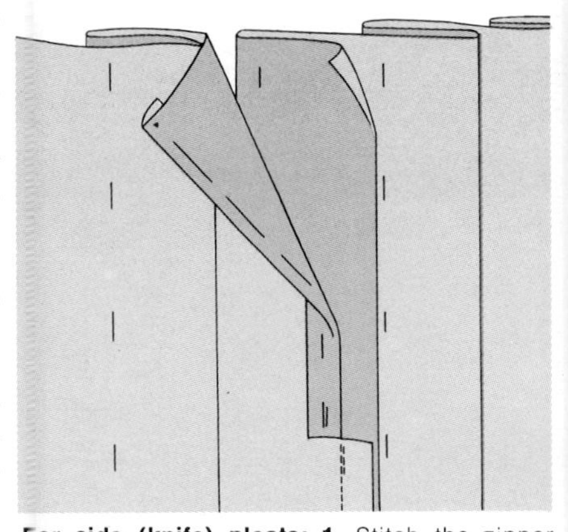

For side (knife) pleats: 1. Stitch the zipper seam at the pleat backfold after pleats have been formed. Leave the top part open for the zipper. Clip into the left seam allowance; turn it to the wrong side of the garment and baste in place, as shown.

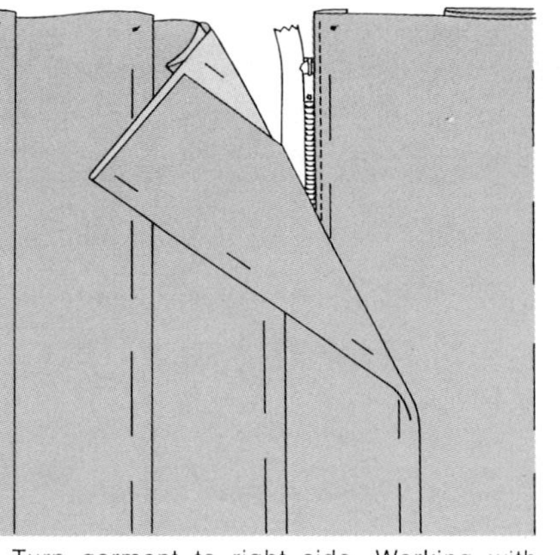

2. Turn garment to right side. Working with the open part of the seam, position closed zipper under basted seam allowance with the folded edge close to the teeth and top stop just below top seamline. Baste. Then, using a zipper foot, stitch close to fold.

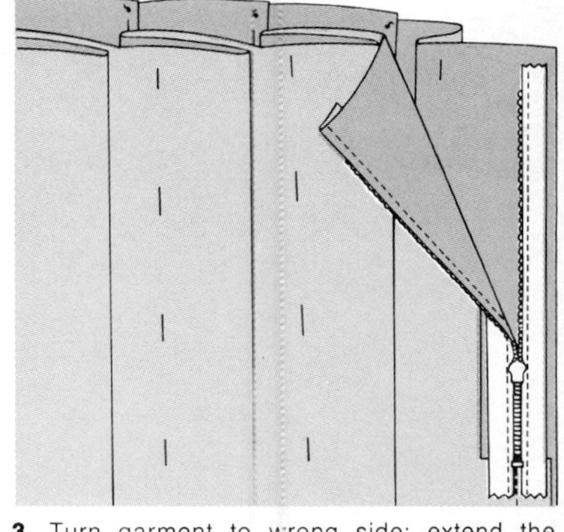

3. Turn garment to wrong side; extend the unclipped (right-hand) seam allowance. Place unstitched half of zipper face down on seam allowance with teeth ⅛" beyond seamline. Pin and baste. Open zipper and stitch to seam allowance only, not to top fold of pleat.

Post-application procedures

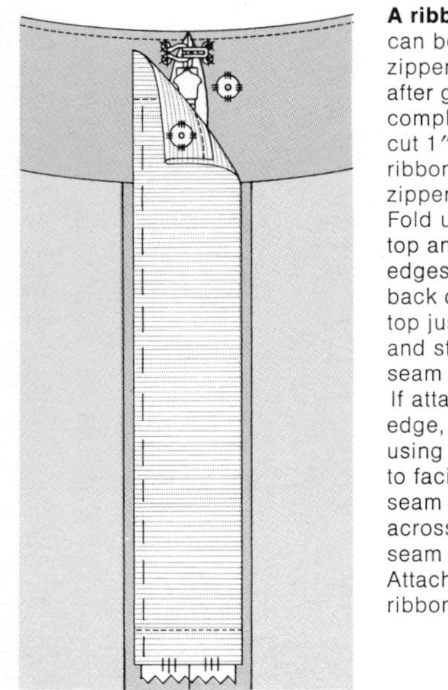

A ribbon underlay can be added to any zipper application after garment is completed. To make it, cut 1"-wide grosgrain ribbon 1" longer than zipper chain or coil. Fold under and finish top and bottom edges. Center over back of zipper, with top just above slider, and stitch to left seam allowance only. If attaching at a neck edge, hand-stitch, using a running stitch, to facing and then to seam allowance. Tack across bottom to both seam allowances. Attach snap at top of ribbon as shown.

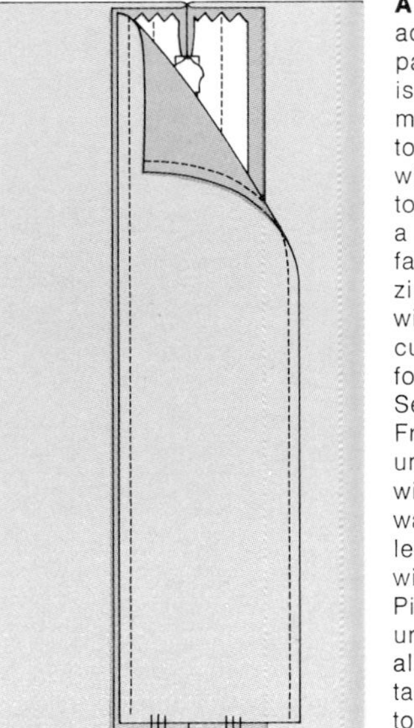

A fabric underlay is added to a skirt or pants before waistband is applied. (Waistband must be cut long enough to extend across entire width of underlay at top.) For underlay, cut a strip from garment fabric the length of the zipper tape and 2½" wide. (For a self-facing, cut fabric 5" wide and fold in half lengthwise.) Seam-finish raw edges. From wrong side, place underlay over zipper with top edge meeting waistline edge and lengthwise edge even with the left seam edge. Pin, then stitch underlay to seam allowance only. Hand-tack across bottom to both seam allowances.

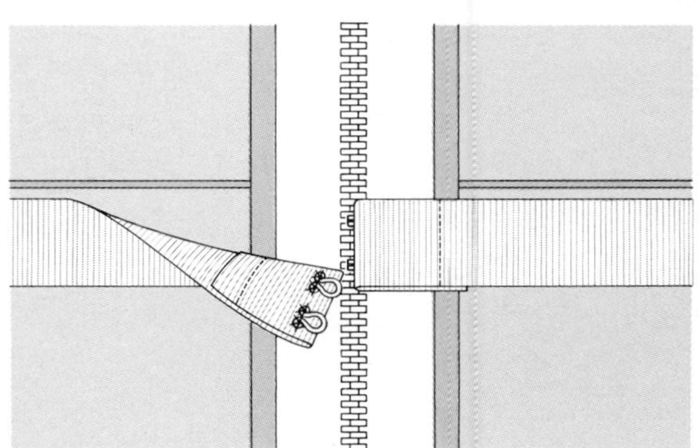

A waistline stay relieves strain on a zipper and makes it easier to close. To make the stay, cut a length of grosgrain ribbon equal to the measurement of the garment at waistline plus 2". Finish the ends by folding them back 1", then turning raw edges under ¼" and machine-stitching in place. Sew hooks and round eyes to ends. Position ribbon at waistline with ends at either side of zipper. Leaving 2" free at each end for easy fastening, tack stay to allowance of waistline seam if there is one; to seams and darts if there is not.

Buttonholes

Description of types

All of the many buttonhole methods are variations of two basic types, worked and bound. The method you choose for a garment will depend on the design of that garment, the fabric, and your particular level of sewing ability.

Bound buttonholes are made by stitching strips or patches of fabric to the buttonhole location in any of several ways. The garment fabric is then cut as specified, and the strips or patches are turned to the wrong side, thus "binding" the edges of the opening. Bound buttonholes are particularly suited to tailored garments, but are not recommended for sheer or delicate fabrics where the patch might show through or add bulk.

Machine-worked buttonholes consist of two parallel rows of zigzag stitches, and two ends finished either with a fan arrangement of stitches or with the bar tacks shown below (which it is depends on the specific sewing machine or attachment). A machine-worked buttonhole is opened only after stitching is completed. These buttonholes are used on sportswear, washable garments, children's clothes, and men's jackets. They are not recommended for fragile fabrics because zigzag stitching could damage the fabric.

Hand-worked buttonholes are made by finishing a cut in the fabric with hand buttonhole stitches. They are used on men's jackets and women's tailored garments, and on fabrics too sheer for bound buttonholes or too fragile for machine stitching.

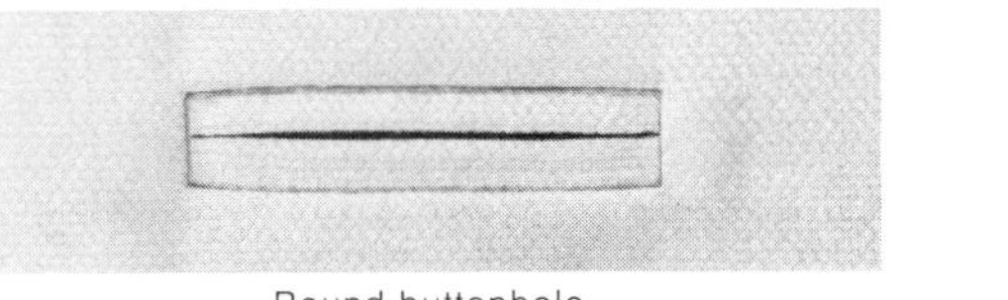

Bound buttonhole

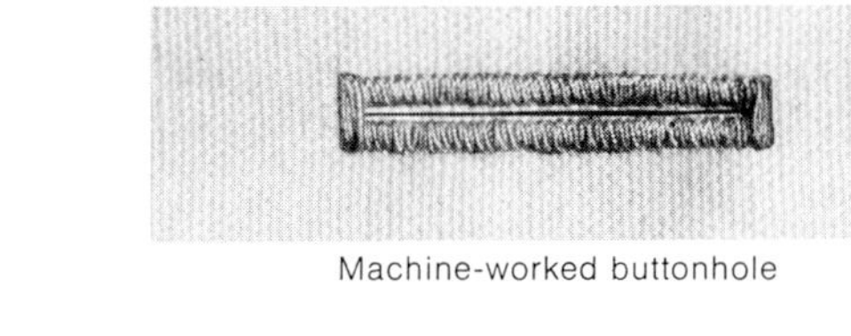

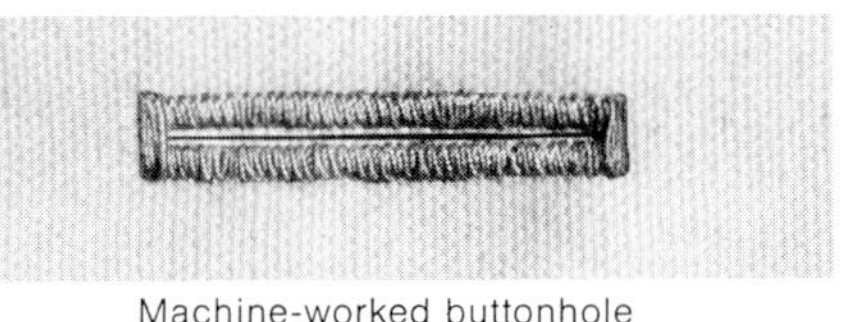

Machine-worked buttonhole

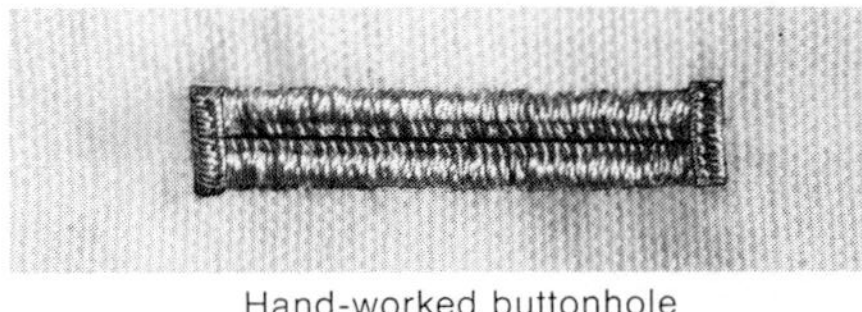

Hand-worked buttonhole

Determining and testing buttonhole length

It is important to make your buttonholes exactly the right length, so that they allow the button to pass through easily, yet hold the garment securely closed. The **length of the buttonhole opening** should equal the diameter of the button plus its height. On a bound buttonhole, this measurement will be the total length of the buttonhole from end to end; on a worked buttonhole, however, because of the finishing that is involved at each end, the space allowed for must be ⅛ inch greater than the actual opening.

To check buttonhole length, make a slash in a scrap of the garment fabric equal to the length desired for the buttonhole opening. If the button slips through easily, buttonhole length is correct. **Test the buttonhole method** on a scrap of fabric before working on the actual garment; be certain to include all the layers of fabric, such as interfacing and underlining, that will be present in the finished garment. Also, go through all construction steps when testing the technique.

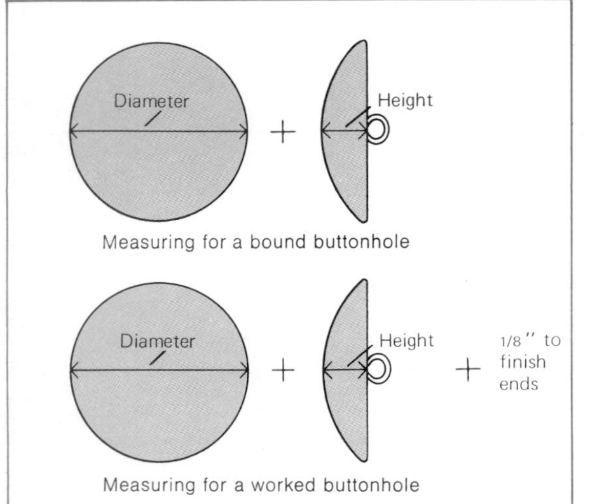

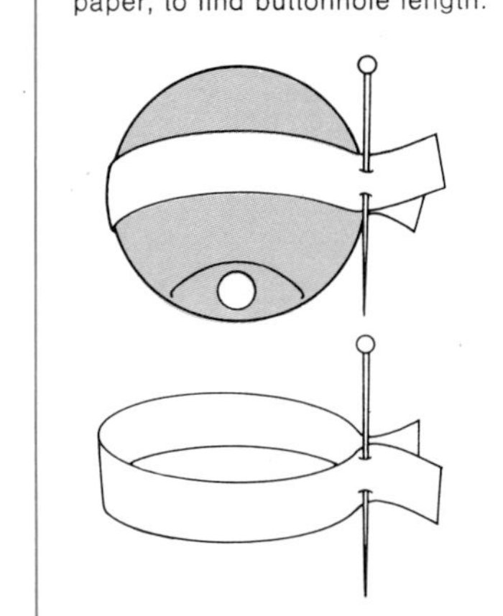

Pin a strip of paper around a ball button, then measure the paper, to find buttonhole length.

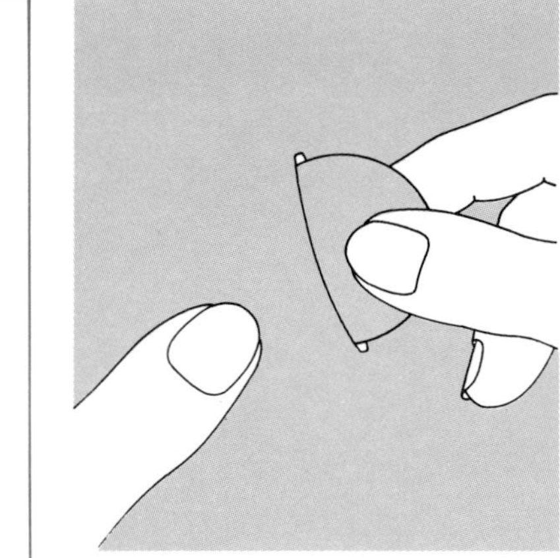

Test the proposed buttonhole length by slipping the button through a slash cut in a scrap of the garment fabric.

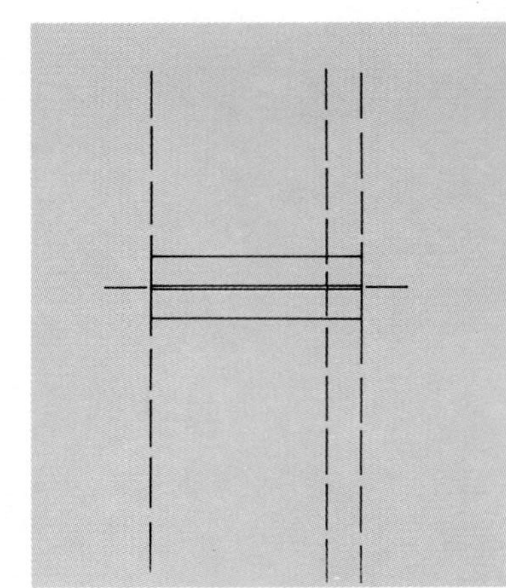

Make a practice buttonhole to test the technique, using all layers of fabric that will be in the final garment.

Fabric-marking methods 94
Basic pattern alterations 103-105

Positioning buttonholes

Buttonholes in women's garments are placed on the right-hand side of a garment that closes in the front; if a garment closes in the back, the buttonholes go on the left-hand side.

Buttonholes must be positioned on the garment in relation to the button placement line, which, in turn, is located according to the center line of the garment. The button placement line must be marked on each half of the garment so that the center lines of the garment will match when the garment is closed.

The three key placement points for buttonholes are at the neck, the fullest part of the bust, and the waist. Additional buttonholes are evenly spaced between these points. The lowest buttonhole must always be above the bulk of the hem.

Horizontal buttonholes are the most secure, therefore used on most garments. When buttoned, the pull of the closure is absorbed by the end of the buttonhole, with very little distortion. These buttonholes are placed to extend 1/8″ beyond the button placement line.

Vertical buttonholes are often used with a narrow placket, such as a shirt band, or when there are many small buttons involved in closing the garment. They are placed directly on the button placement line, and the top of the buttonhole is 1/8″ above the mark for center of button.

Markings for horizontal buttonholes: Marking A is the button placement line of the garment; B and C mark the ends of the buttonhole (B is 1/8″ from button placement line); D marks the center of the buttonhole. These markings should all be transferred to the garment before the construction begins.

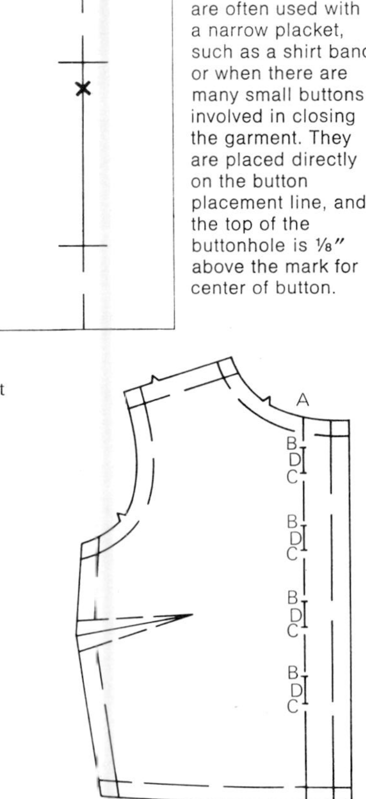

On double-breasted garments, the two rows of buttons must be equidistant from the center line of the garment. If buttons are to be 3″ from the center line, locate the B line of the left-hand row of buttonholes 2 7/8″ from center and the B line of the right-hand row 3 1/8″ from center line. Mark remaining lines.

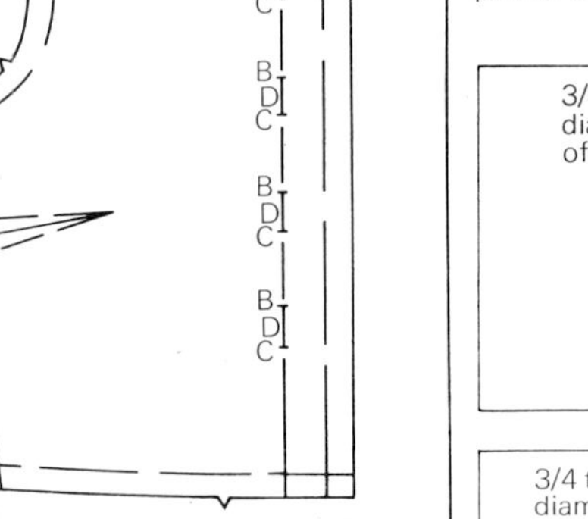

The markings for vertical buttonholes are placed directly on the button position line A. The D lines should be marked first, on top of the A line to prevent confusion between buttonholes and spaces. The B and C lines mark the ends of the buttonhole, with the B line placed 1/8″ above the mark for the button center.

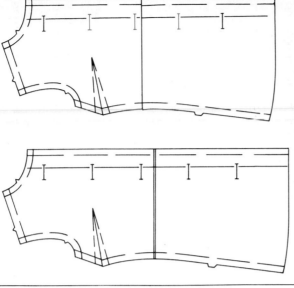

Making changes

If a pattern with a button closing is altered lengthwise, the buttonholes must be re-spaced on the pattern itself after the alteration is complete. Shown above is the procedure for a shortened pattern; when one is lengthened, it is reversed. In either case, a buttonhole may have to be added or subtracted for the sake of design. Remember the three key positioning points when re-spacing.

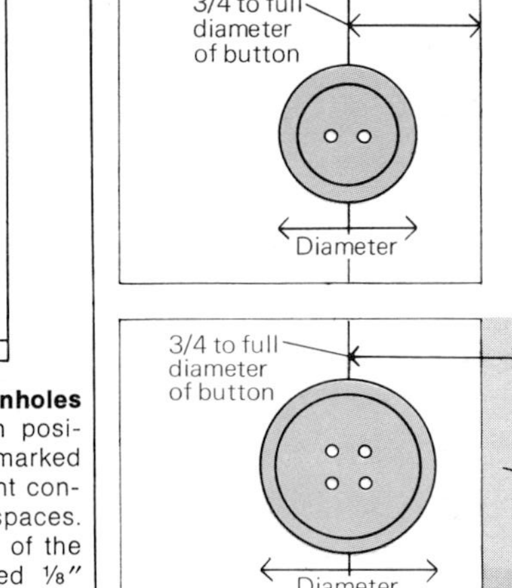

If button size is changed from pattern specification, the space between button position line and finished edge of garment must be changed accordingly. This space must always measure from three-fourths to the full diameter of the button.

Bound buttonholes

Interfacing selection and application 72-73, 76-79
Underlining 72-75
Grain in fabric 84-85

Basic information

A well-made bound buttonhole is flat, and the inner fabric edges, or "lips," are set into a rectangle that has perfectly square corners and is no wider than ¼ inch. (The exception to the ¼ inch width is made when a fabric is very bulky. A slightly wider rectangle may look better.) Each of the buttonhole lips should be no wider than ⅛ inch, and they must meet exactly in the center of the buttonhole. In most cases, the lips will be cut on the straight grain of the fabric, but the bias grain can be an attractive contrast if a plaid or stripe is being used. Cut one continuous strip of fabric for all the buttonhole lips, and make all of them at one time. When constructing the buttonholes, **complete the same step on all buttonholes** before proceeding to the next step. This is much likelier to produce a look of uniformity than if

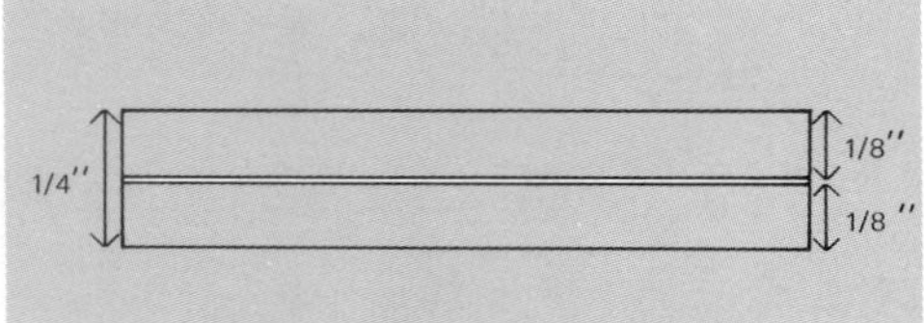

If total buttonhole is ¼", lips should be ⅛" wide.

the buttonholes are finished one at a time.

If possible, use silk thread for all bastings in the bound buttonholes; it is least likely to mar the fabric. Machine-baste all markings unless the fabric shows stitch marks. When doing the permanent stitching, use a short stitch (20 per inch) to add strength and to help achieve sharper corners. Do not backstitch; backstitching can inadvertently get off the stitching line. Instead, pull thread

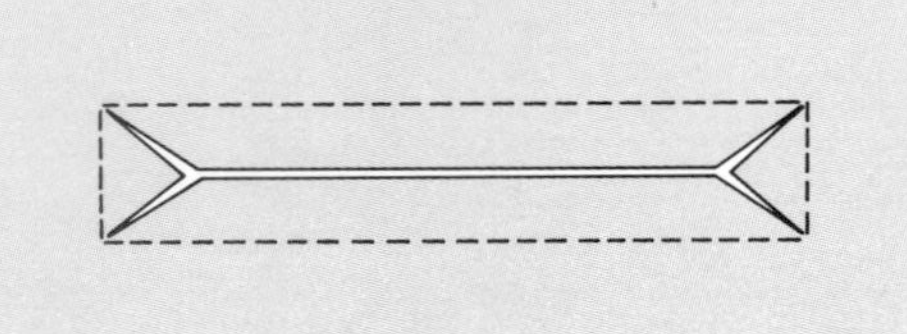

Opening cut first in center, then into corners.

ends to the wrong side and tie them securely.

At some point in the construction of the buttonhole, a rectangular-shaped opening must be cut through the garment. Before cutting, make sure

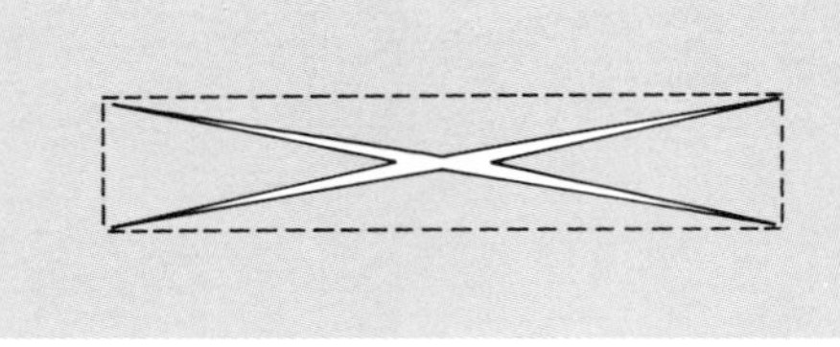

Opening cut straight into corners from center.

that all stitching for the buttonhole is in precisely the right place and that all rows are straight and parallel to one another. It is extremely difficult to correct stitching once the slash has been made. There are two different ways of cutting a buttonhole. One is to cut in the center to within ¼ inch of each end, then diagonally into each of the four corners. This produces the small triangles at each end that are eventually stitched to the buttonhole patch or lips. The other way of cutting, suggested for fabrics that ravel easily, is to cut directly into the corners from the center of the buttonhole area.

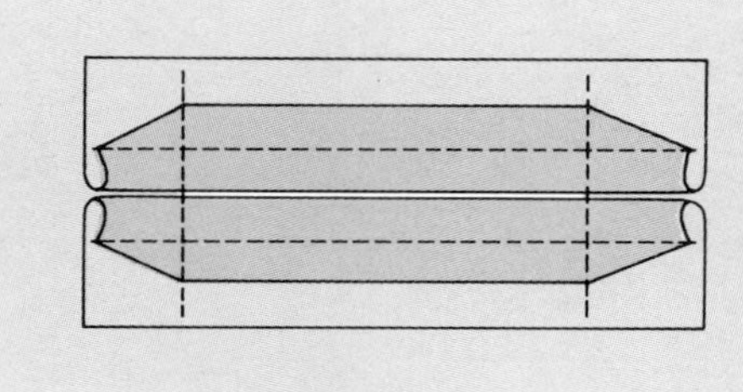

Reduce bulk by grading edges of lips.

The triangular ends produced by this method are much larger and easier to work with. In either case, take care to cut exactly to, but not through, the stitching lines.

The edges of the patches or strips must be graded to reduce bulk when the buttonhole is finished. The layer of fabric nearest the outside (or next to the garment) is left widest. Successive layers should be trimmed ⅛ inch narrower.

Support fabrics in the buttonhole area must be treated very carefully. If the garment is underlined, work the buttonholes through the underlining. If the garment is not underlined, a strip of support fabric may be added underneath the buttonhole area only. Cut a strip of lightweight underlining or interfacing fabric (an iron-on fabric may be used) 1 inch wider and 1 inch longer than the buttonhole area. Center it over the area and baste in place before beginning any construction, including marking, on the buttonholes.

Bound buttonholes should never be worked

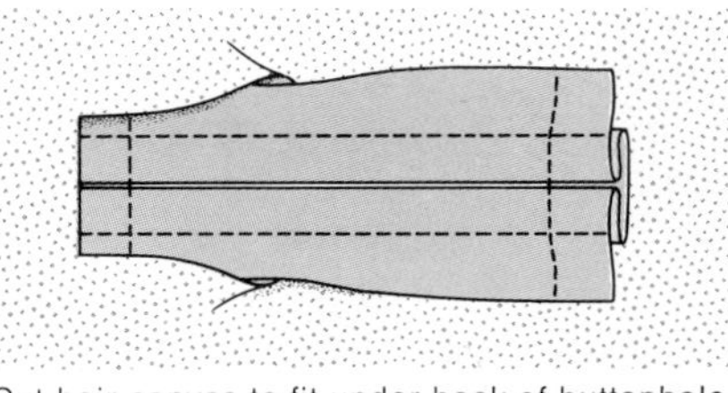

Cut hair canvas to fit under back of buttonhole.

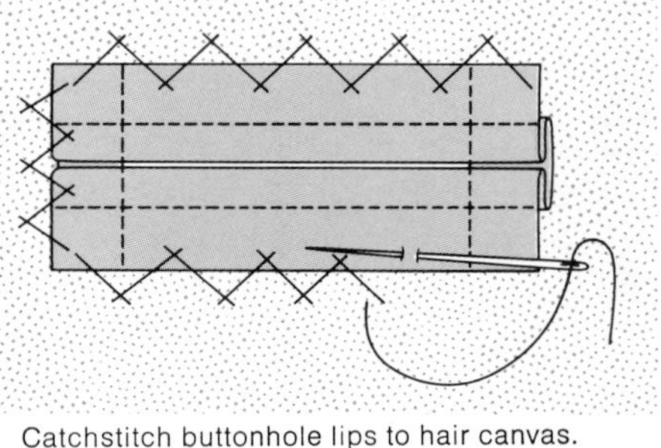

Catchstitch buttonhole lips to hair canvas.

through hair canvas interfacing because of the difficulty in pressing and because of the excess bulk. Instead, work the buttonholes in the garment, then cut openings in the hair canvas the same size as the buttonhole rectangles and in the exact same position as the buttonholes. The interfacing should fit up close to the buttonhole stitching. Pull the back of the buttonhole through the opening, then catchstitch the outer edges of the buttonhole patch or strip to the interfacing.

Cable cord 16
Machine accessories 38
Hand basting 124-125
Cutting bias strips 298-299

Corded method

In this method, corded bias strips are used for the buttonhole lips. The cord produces soft, rounded edges instead of crisp ones, making this method particularly suitable for spongy fabrics that do not hold a sharp crease well, such as textured knits.

The strip for each lip should be 1½ inches wide by the length of the buttonhole plus 1 inch. Save time by cutting and sewing the lips for both sides of all buttonholes at one time. Use a cable cord not over ⅛ inch in diameter, considering also the thickness of the fabric so that the lips have body but not too much bulk.

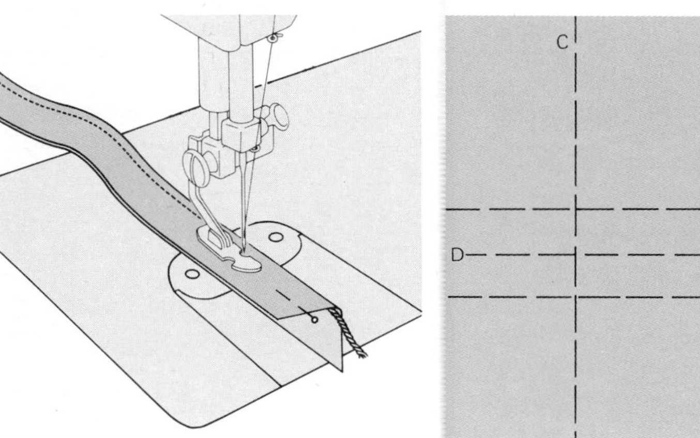

1. Fold bias piece, right side out, around the cable cord and pin the edges together to hold the cord in place. Stitch close to the cord, using a zipper foot. Cut into individual strips for buttonholes, each strip 1″ longer than width of buttonholes.

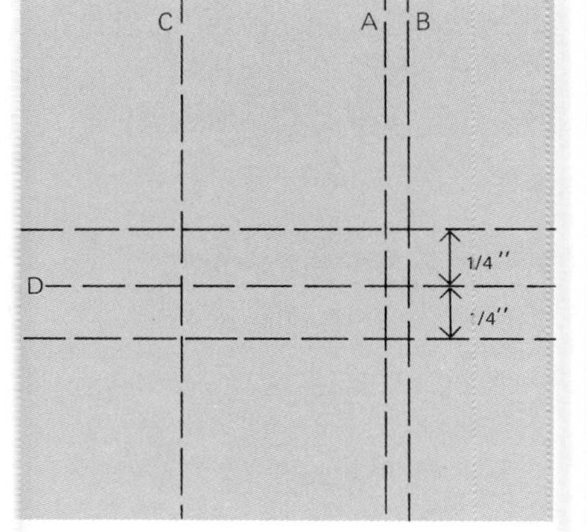

2. Baste-mark the four positioning lines on garment as described on page 331. Baste additional marking lines ¼″ above and below the buttonhole positioning line. If the fabric is very heavy, baste these lines 5/16″ from the buttonhole positioning line.

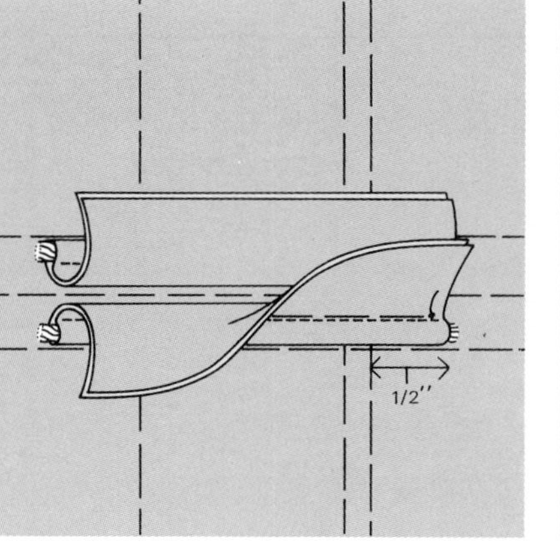

3. Center strips over markings on right side of garment so ends extend ½″ beyond lines for ends of buttonhole. Corded edges should lie along the outer ¼″ markings, with excess fabric of strips toward center of buttonhole. Baste each strip in place by hand.

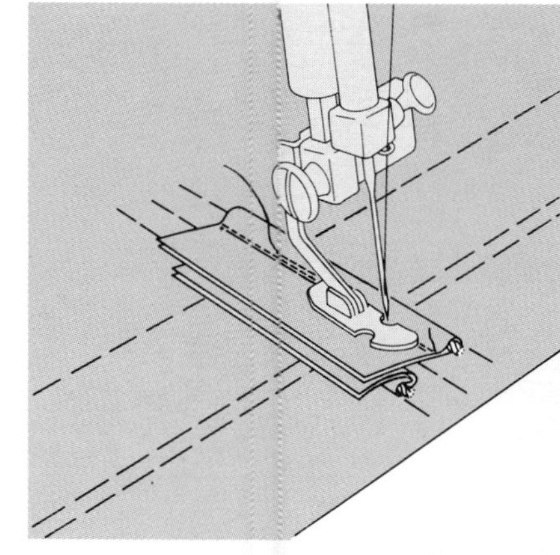

4. Attach zipper foot to machine. Lower needle through strip and garment precisely on the mark for end of buttonhole and just to the inside of the existing stitching. Stitch with a 20 stitch length, stopping at mark for other end. Repeat for remaining side.

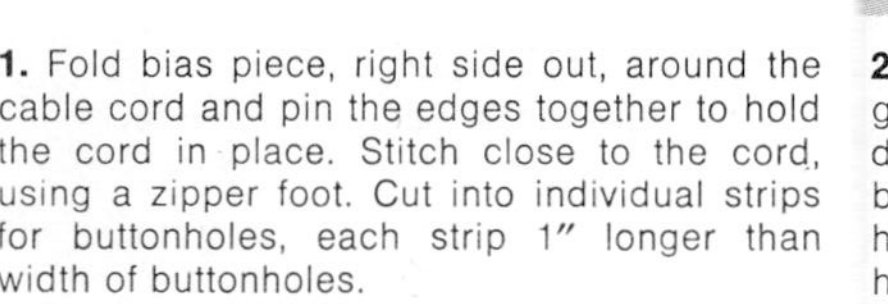

5. Bring thread ends to the wrong side of the garment and tie. Cut along the center line of the buttonhole to within ¼″ of each end, then cut diagonally into each corner. Or, cut directly from center into each corner. Take care not to cut through stitching.

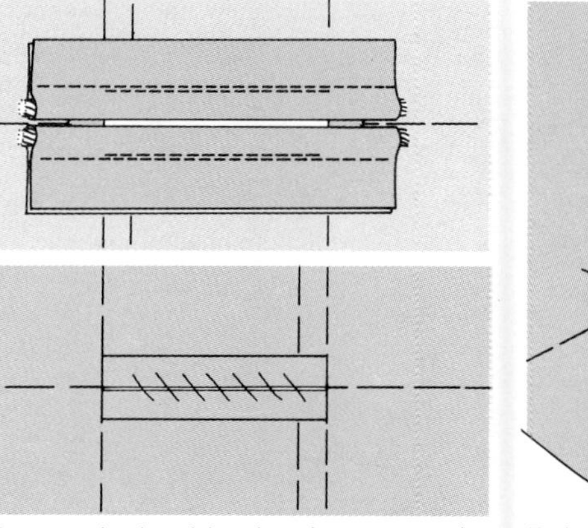
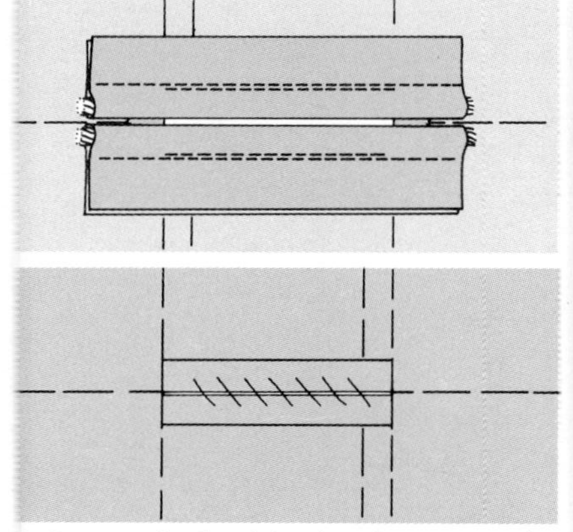

6. Remove the hand basting that was used to hold the strip to the garment. Turn the strips through to the wrong side and pull the triangular ends into place. Press as directed on page 339. From the right side of the garment, diagonal-baste lip edges together.

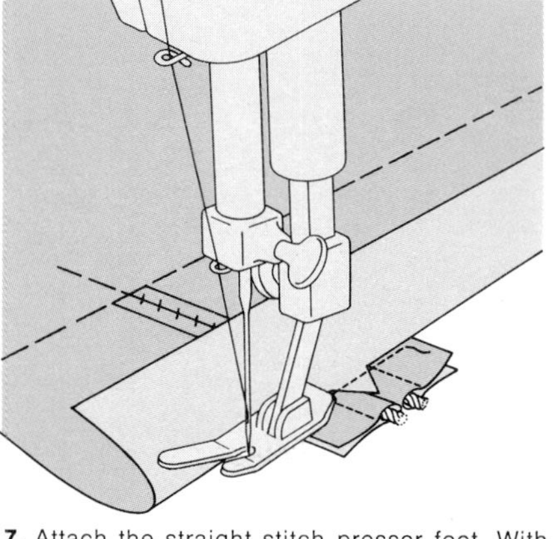

7. Attach the straight stitch presser foot. With the garment right side up, fold back enough of the garment to expose one triangular end. Stitch back and forth across triangle several times to secure it to ends of strips. Repeat for other end of buttonhole.

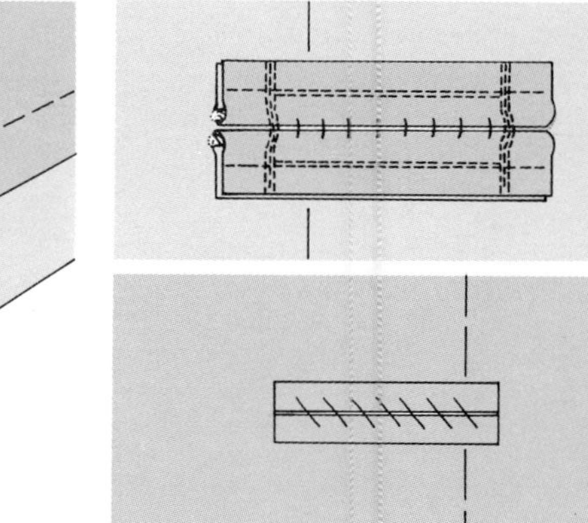

8. Remove all the basted markings except center front markings. Trim the strips to within ¼″ of the buttonhole stitching lines. Press the entire area. The diagonal basting stitches holding the lips together should stay in until the garment is completed.

Bound buttonholes

Grain in fabric 84-85
Hand basting 124-125

Patch method

The patch method involves making a rectangular opening the size of the buttonhole, with a patch of garment fabric as the facing. The patch facing is then folded so as to create the buttonhole lips. This method is a good choice for buttonholes in fabrics that are light to medium in weight, do not ravel, but do retain a crease readily. For each buttonhole, cut a patch of fabric 2 inches wide and 1 inch longer than the buttonhole. To mark the center of the patch, fold it in half lengthwise and finger-press the fold. Straight grain is preferred for the patch, although bias may be used.

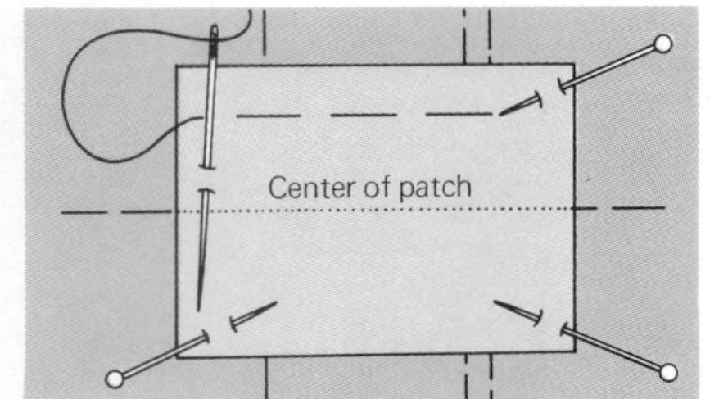

1. With right sides together, center patch over buttonhole markings, placing the crease of the patch along the buttonhole position line. Baste in place over markings.

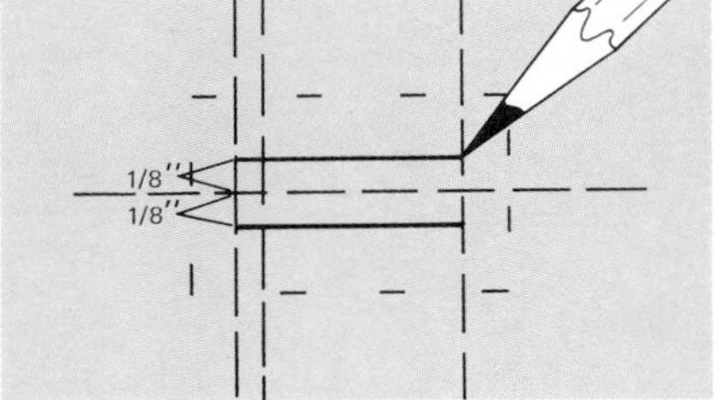

2. On wrong side of garment, mark lines ⅛" above and below the buttonhole positioning lines. On heavy fabric, mark these lines $^{3}/_{16}$" to ⅜" away from the positioning lines.

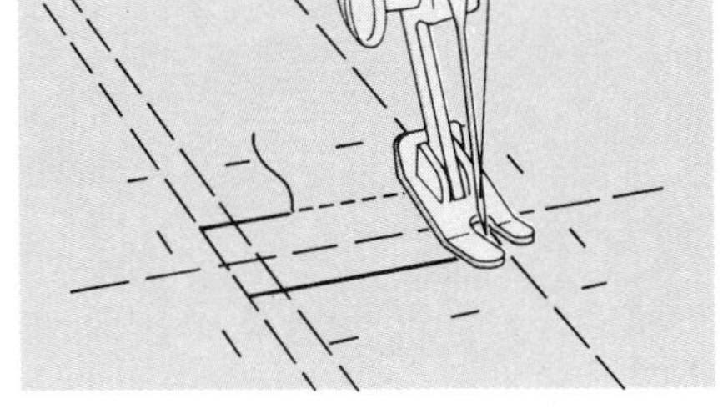

3. Using a 20 stitch length, stitch around the "box" made by the pencil markings and the buttonhole length markings. Begin on one of the long sides and pivot at the corners.

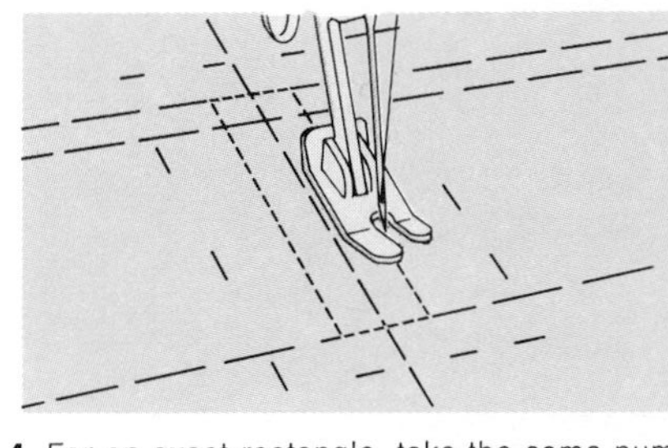

4. For an exact rectangle, take the same number of stitches (5 or 6) across each of the short sides. Overlap several stitches at the end. Remove hand bastings and press.

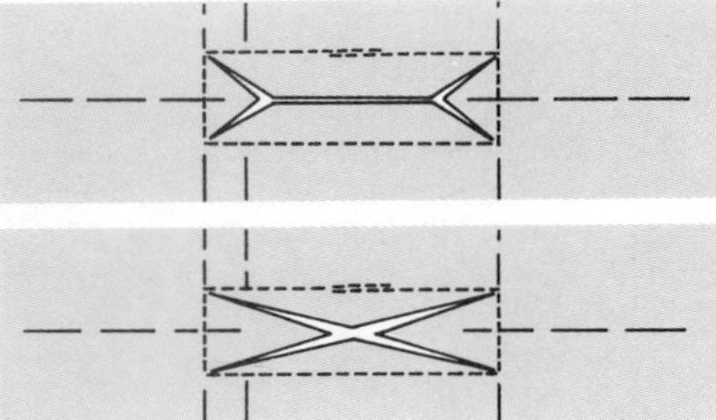

5. Cut through patch and garment along center to within ¼" of the ends, then diagonally to corners. Or cut directly into the corners from the center. Do not cut stitching.

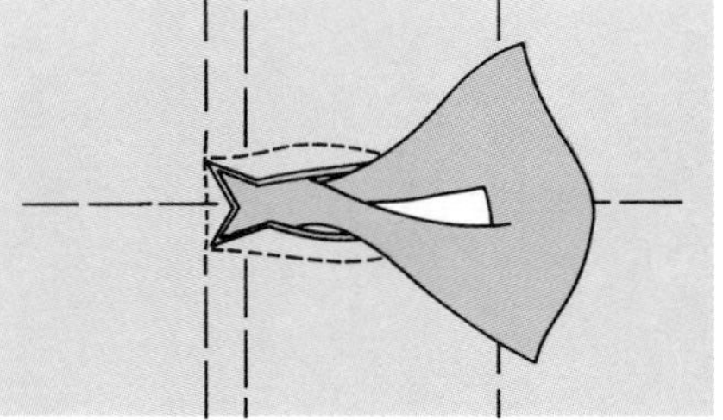

6. Gently turn patch through opening to wrong side of garment. A properly stitched opening will be a perfect rectangle. Pull on the ends to square the corners.

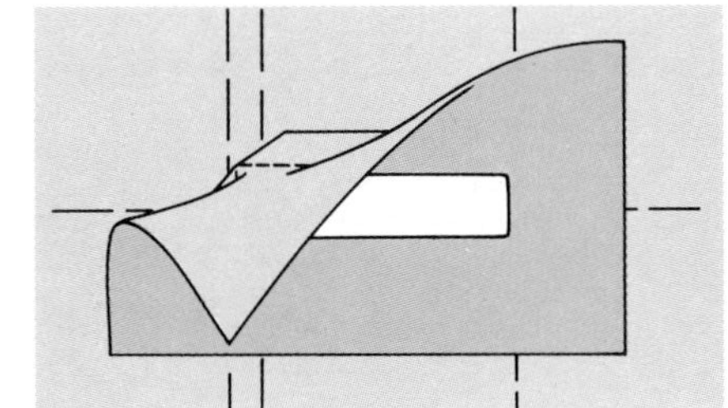

7. Roll edges of opening between your fingers until the seam is precisely on the edge of the opening. Press carefully so that none of the patch shows on the right side.

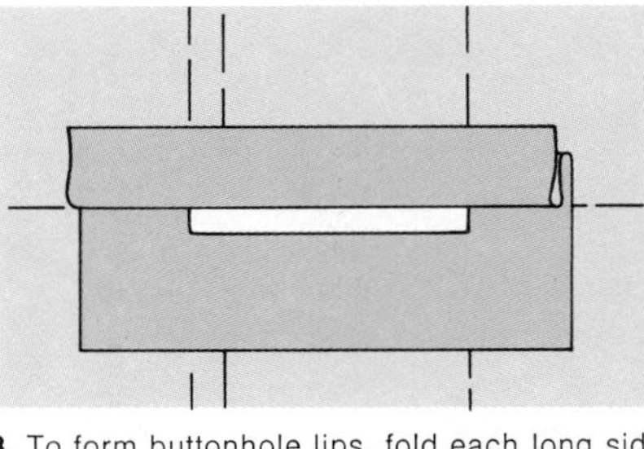

8. To form buttonhole lips, fold each long side of the patch over the opening so that the folds meet exactly in the center. For accuracy, fold along a true grain line.

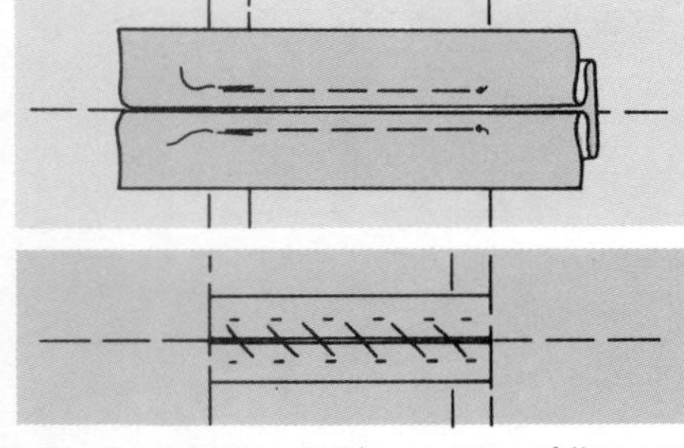

9. From right side, check accuracy of lips and manipulate them until exactly right. Baste along the center of each lip to hold the fold in place. Then diagonal-baste the lips together at their fold lines and press.

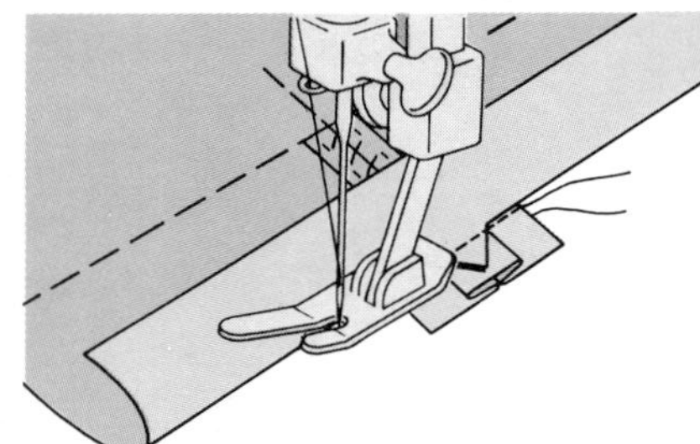

10. Place garment right side up on the machine. Flip back enough of the garment to expose one of the triangular ends, then stitch back and forth across both it and the patch. Repeat at the other end.

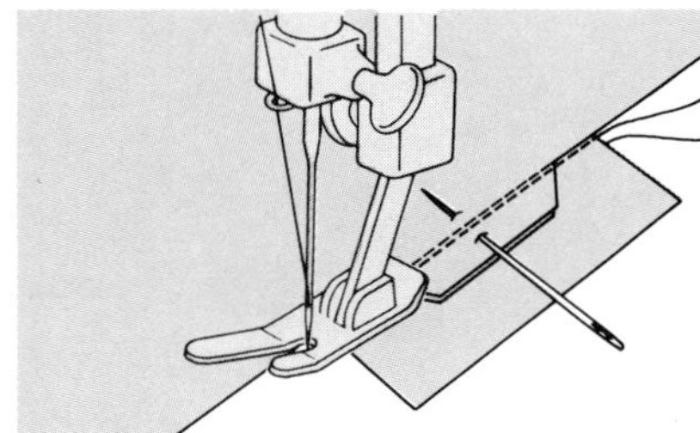

11. With the garment still right side up, turn it back to expose one of the horizontal seam allowances. Stitch through the seam allowance and the patch, just slightly inside the original stitching line. Repeat on other seam.

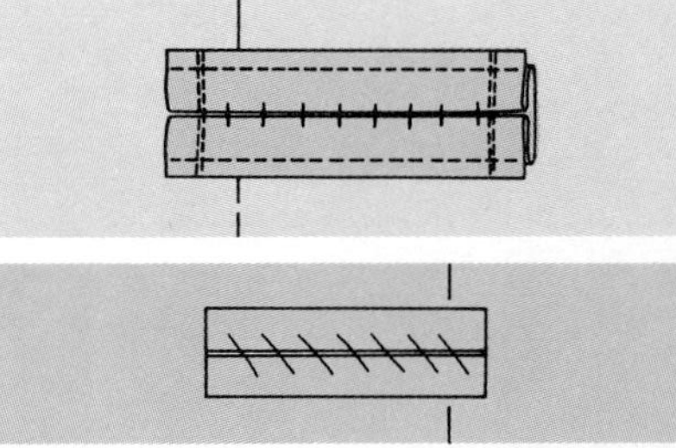

12. Tie thread ends. Remove all markings and bastings except center front line. The diagonal basting holding the lips together should remain in place until the buttons are added. Trim patch to within ¼" of machine stitching.

Grain in fabric 84-85
Diagonal basting 125
Slipstitch (uneven) 132
Machine basting 137

Simplified patch method

This buttonhole method is an ideal choice for a beginner because both the positioning and the formation of the lips are done in one easy step. Also, there is an easy way to check that the lips and stitching lines are properly located before the buttonhole is cut, which virtually assures success. Because this method relies on machine-basted markings, it cannot be used on fabrics that are easily marred by a machine needle. Cut a patch of fabric for each buttonhole that is 2 inches wide and 1 inch longer than the buttonhole, on either the bias or the straight grain.

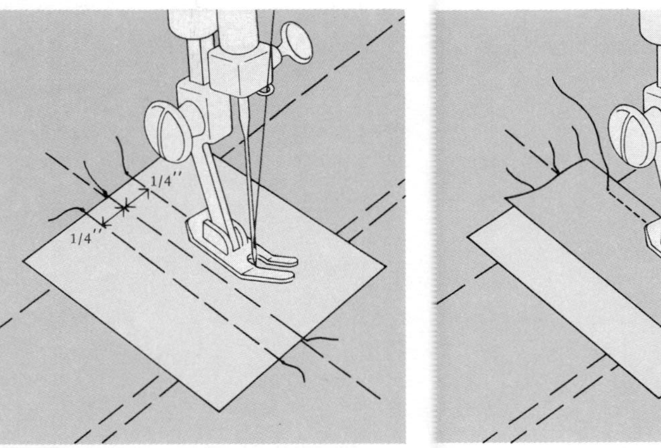

1. Placing right sides together, center the patch over the buttonhole markings on the garment. Machine-baste through center of patch along the buttonhole position line, then exactly ¼″ above and below this line.

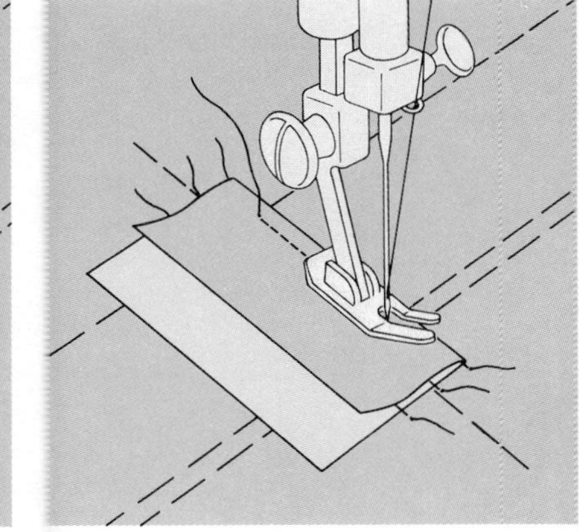

2. Fold one long edge of patch toward center on the ¼″ basted line and finger-press it in place. Using a 20 stitch length, sew precisely ⅛″ from fold, beginning and ending exactly on buttonhole length markings.

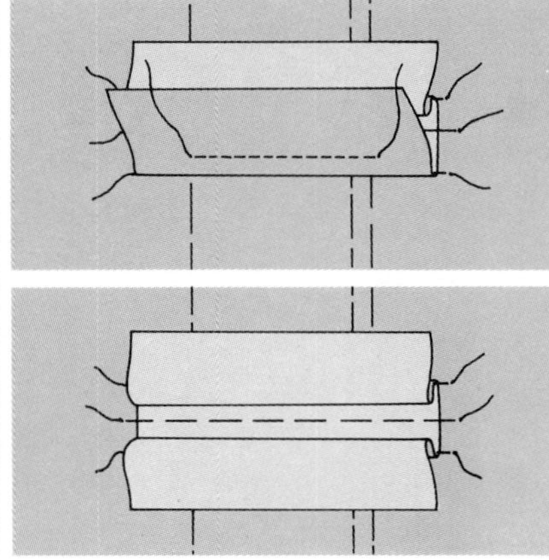

3. Fold other edge of patch toward center on ¼″ basted line. Finger-press it in place and stitch as above. The lips have now been formed and stitched in place. Press edges of lips away from center line of buttonhole.

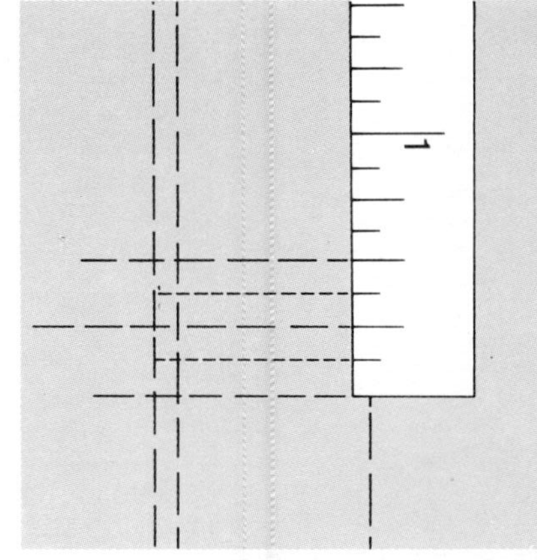

4. Five rows of stitching are now visible on wrong side of garment. Use a ruler to check that all five are precisely ⅛″ apart along their entire length. Re-stitch if necessary; tie thread ends. Remove machine basting.

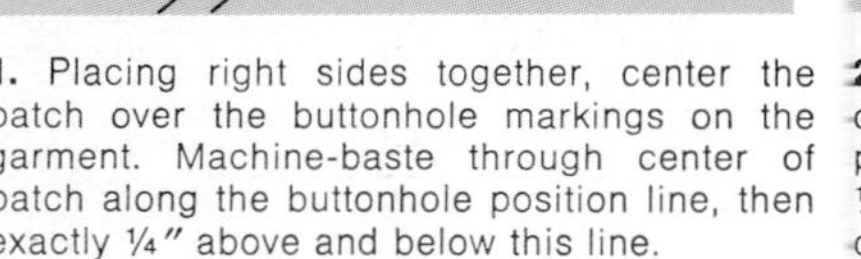

5. From wrong side, cut along center line to within ¼″ of ends. Then cut diagonally into corners. Or cut directly into corners from center. From the right side, cut through ends of patch so there are two strips.

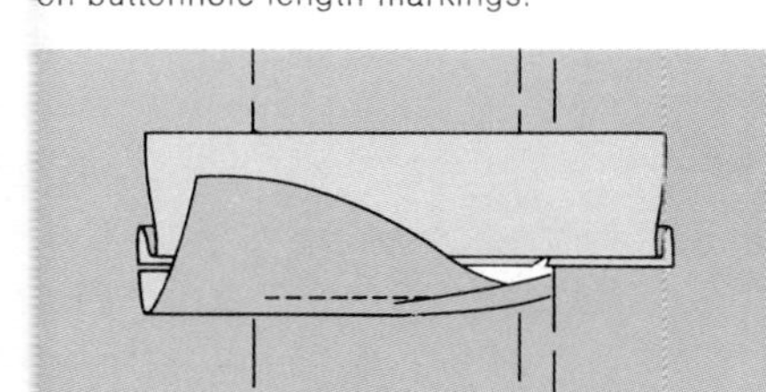
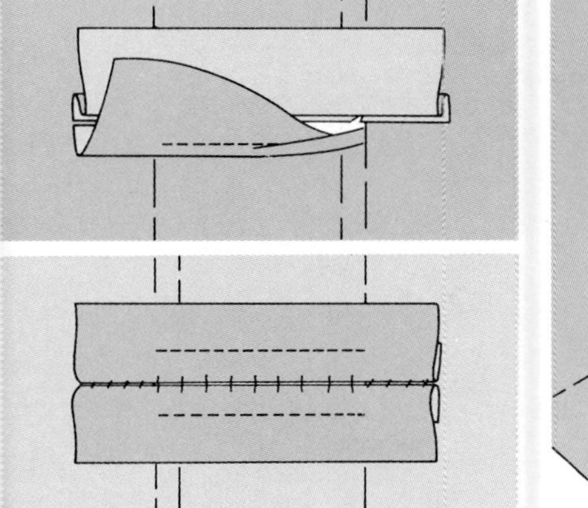

6. Carefully push the lips through the opening to the wrong side and press. Diagonal-baste them together. From wrong side, slipstitch the ends of the lip strips together on the fold lines, beyond buttonhole area.

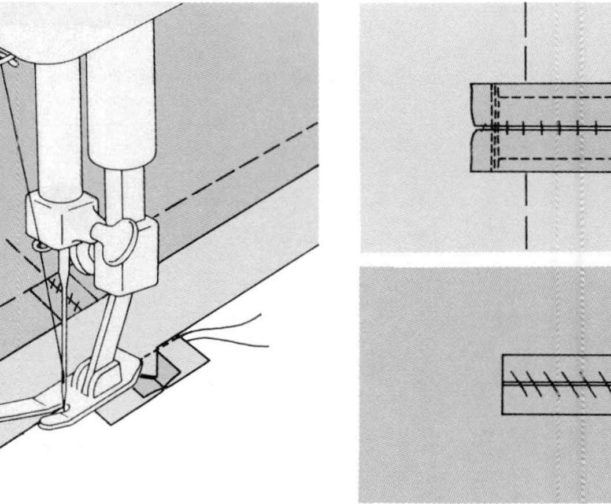

7. Place garment on the machine, right side up. Fold back just enough of the fabric to expose one tiny triangular end of buttonhole. Stitch back and forth across this end, attaching it to strips. Repeat at other end.

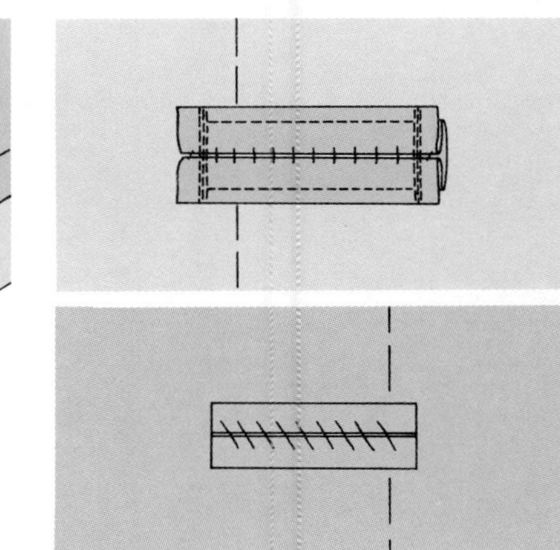

8. Remove all markings except center front line and press. Trim ends and sides of strips to within ¼″ of stitching lines. The diagonal basting holding lips together should stay in until garment is finished.

Bound buttonholes

Tapestry needle 11; loop turner 13
Cable cord 16
Hand basting 124-125
Tying thread ends 137

One-piece folded method

This buttonhole method is recommended for light- to medium-weight fabrics that crease easily and do not ravel. Like regular patch buttonholes, it involves a patch of fabric, but it differs from them in that the lips are formed before the patch is attached to the garment. In addition to assuring uniform lip widths, this method eliminates almost all bulk from the buttonhole area.

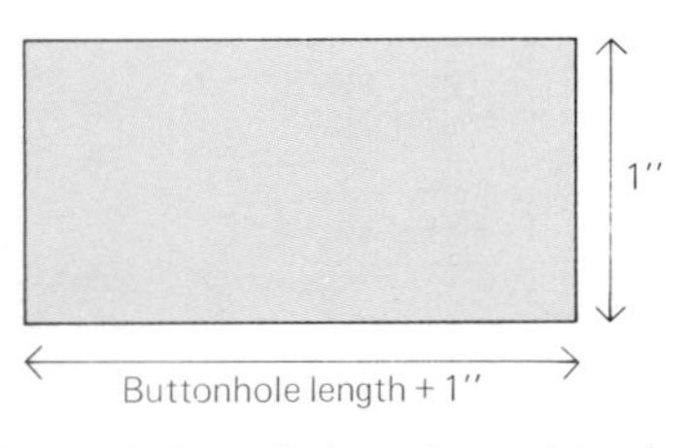

1. For each buttonhole, cut a patch of garment fabric 1″ wide and 1″ longer than the buttonhole. For best results, cut the patch on the straight grain.

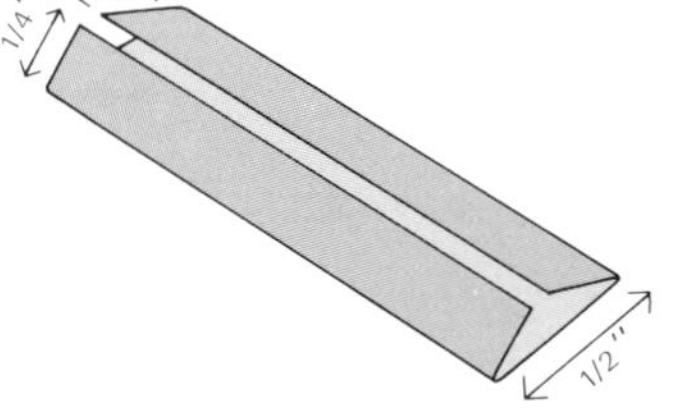

2. With wrong sides together, fold long edges so they touch. Baste through center of each fold and press. Patch is now ½″ wide; open side has two ¼″ sections.

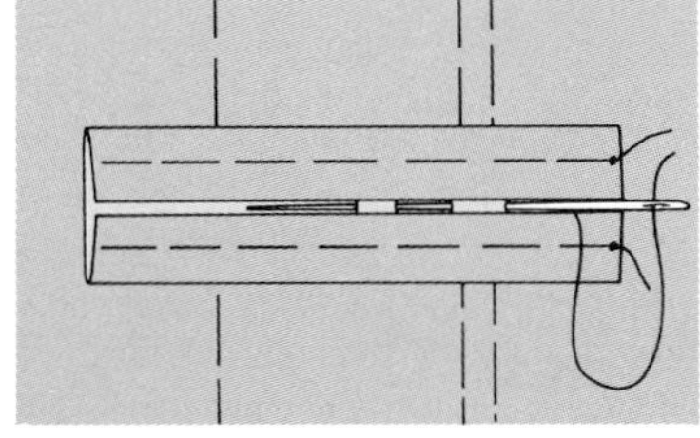

3. Center the patch, open side up, on the right side of the garment directly over the buttonhole markings. Baste the patch in place through the center.

4. Selecting a 20 stitch length, stitch through exact center of each half of the patch, starting and stopping exactly on markings for end of buttonhole.

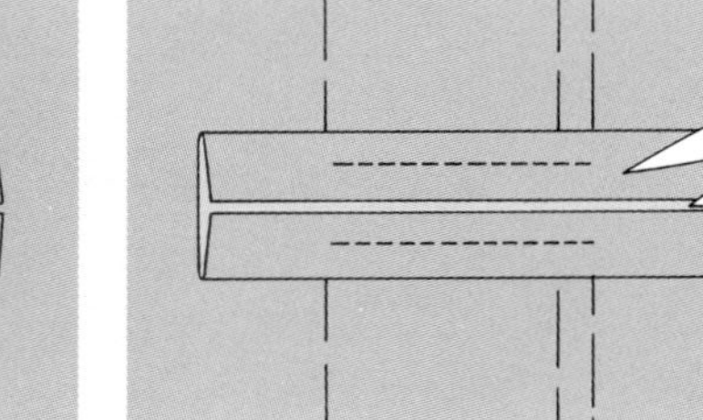

5. Pull thread ends to the wrong side of the garment and tie. Remove basting threads; press. Cut through the center of the patch to form two strips.

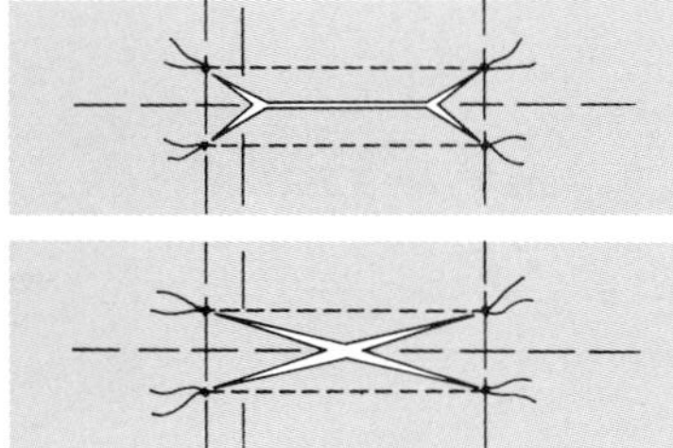

6. Turn to wrong side to cut into corners. Cut along center line and then into corners. Or cut directly into corners from center. Stop short of stitching.

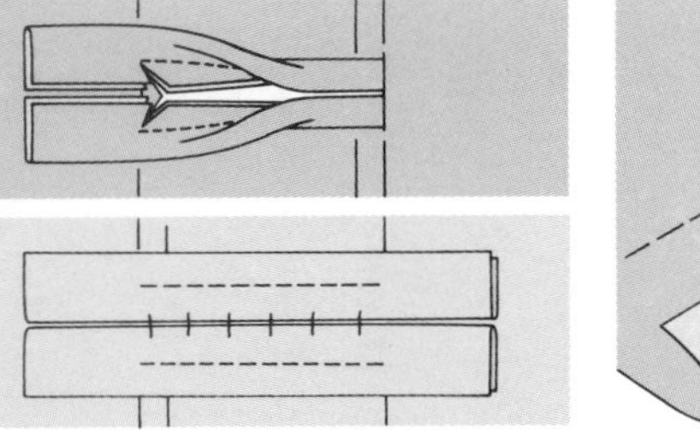

7. Carefully push the buttonhole strips through the opening to the wrong side. Pull on the ends of the strips to square off the corners of the rectangle. Baste the lips together diagonally from the right side of the garment. Press.

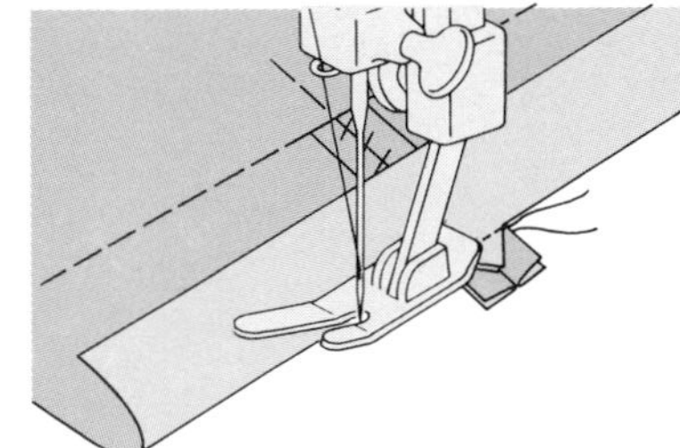

8. Place the garment right side up on the machine. Fold back enough fabric to expose one of the triangular buttonhole ends. Stitch back and forth across this triangle to secure it to the strips. Repeat at the other end.

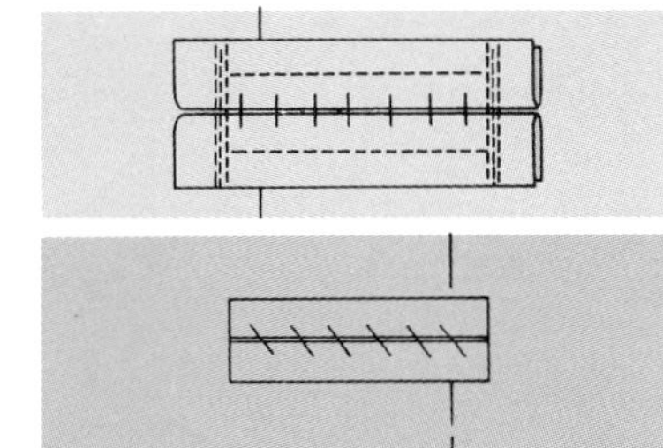

9. Remove all markings except center front line. Trim the edges of the buttonhole strips to within ¼″ of the ends of the buttonhole. Press. The diagonal basting should remain in place until the garment is completed.

One-piece tucked method

This method is the same as the one at the left, except that the lips are stitched before the patch is sewed to the garment. For each buttonhole, cut a patch (bias or straight) 1½ inches wide and 1 inch

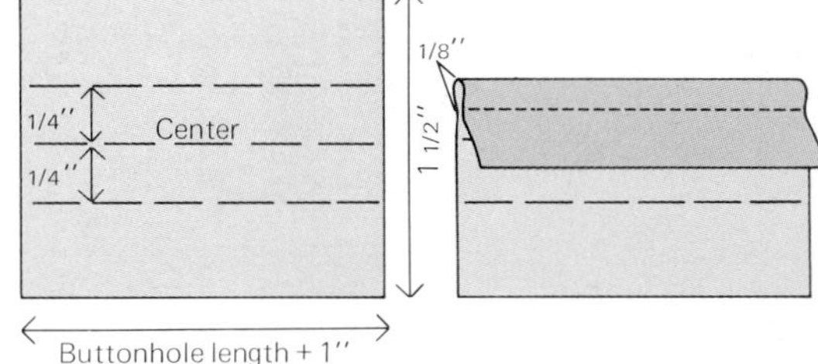

longer than the buttonhole. Mark the lengthwise center of the patch, then mark lines ¼ inch above and below the center. Fold the patch, wrong sides together, on the ¼ inch lines. Press, then stitch ⅛ inch from the folds. Proceed with Step 3, left.

Cording bound buttonholes

If the lips of a buttonhole seem limp and somewhat thin in relation to the rest of the garment, both problems can be remedied by drawing yarn or soft cord into the lips. This extra step is taken after the lips have been formed, but **before** the tri-

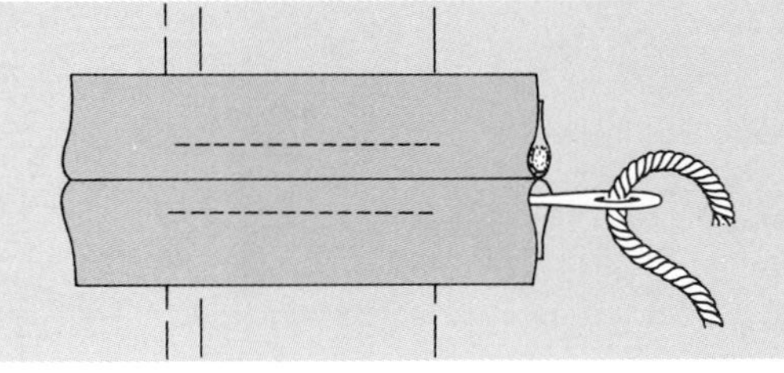

angular ends of the buttonholes are stitched. Also, the only buttonhole methods adaptable to this are the simplified patch and the one-piece folded and tucked methods. Choose a yarn or soft cord in a diameter that will just nicely plump the lips. If the garment fabric is washable, choose an acrylic yarn. Use a loop turner or a blunt-pointed (tapestry) needle to pull the yarn through the lips. Cut the yarn even with the ends of the patch strips, then stitch across the ends.

Lining fabrics 72-73 Uneven basting 124
Reducing seam bulk 147

Two-piece piped method

In this procedure, a completely faced "window" is made in the garment, then the buttonhole lips are constructed and sewed in behind the "window." An advantage of the method is that the corners of the buttonhole, sometimes a troublesome area, can be made perfectly square before the lips are sewed in. It is an excellent choice for fabrics that tend to ravel, because the raw edges of the garment are finished off early in construction. The lips in the finished buttonhole are slightly wider than in other buttonhole techniques, which makes it an excellent choice for heavy, bulky fabrics.

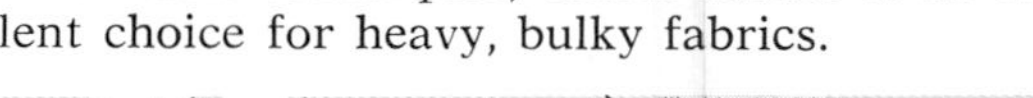

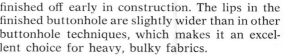

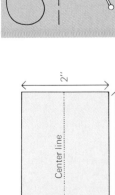

1. Cut a facing for the "window," 2" wide and 1" longer than buttonhole, from a sheer, lightweight fabric, color-matched to the garment fabric. Finger-press center crease.

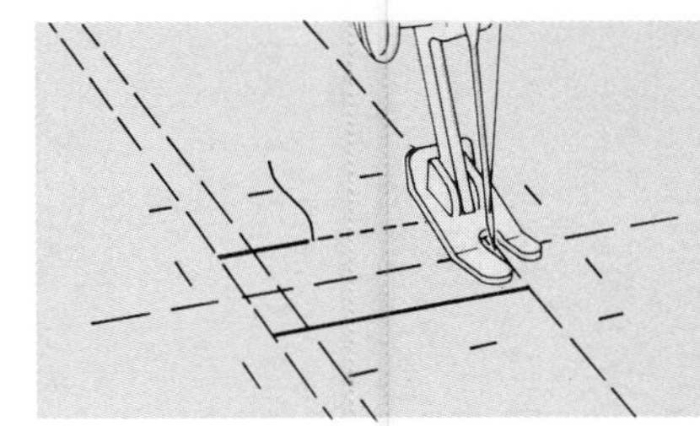

2. Center the sheer patch over the buttonhole markings on the right side of the garment. Carefully pin at each of the corners, then hand-baste in place.

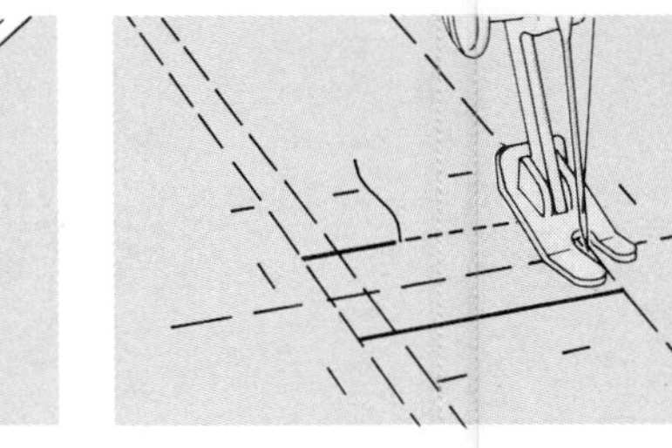

3. On garment wrong side, pencil-mark lines, above and below buttonhole positioning line, setting off a span of 3/16" to 1/4". These and buttonhole end lines together form rectangle.

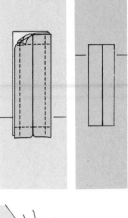

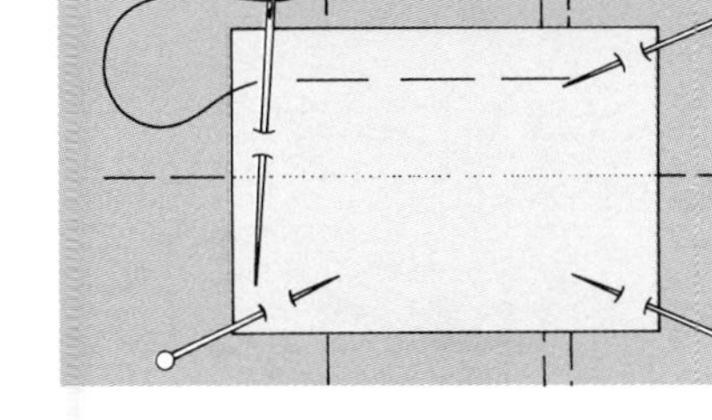

4. Using a 20 stitch length, stitch around the rectangle. For best results, start at the center of one long side, pivot at the corner, and stitch across the end.

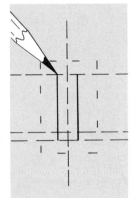

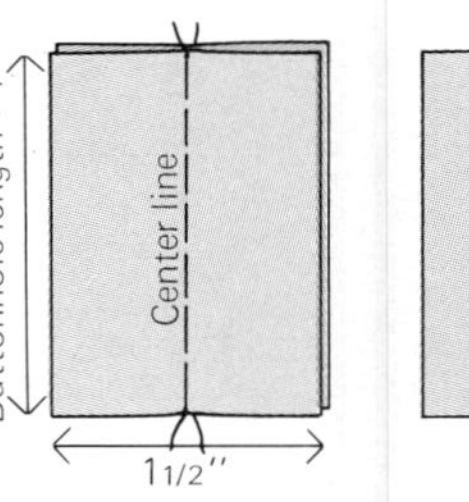

5. Continue stitching, pivoting at corners and making sure that the same number of stitches are taken across each end. Overlap about four stitches at the starting point.

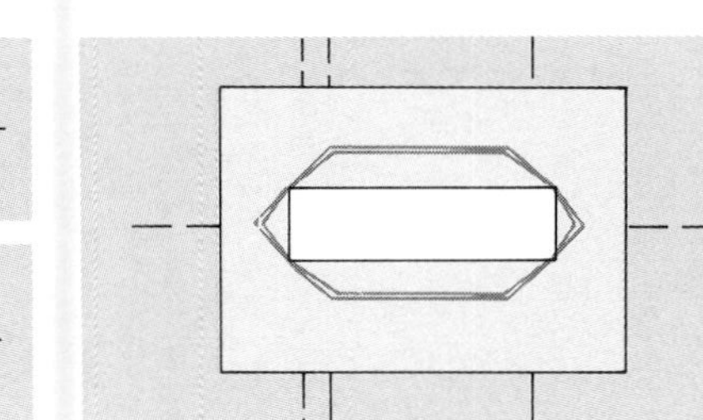

6. Next cut into corners. Cut through center of rectangle to within 1/4" of each end, then into corners. Or cut directly into corners from center. Do not cut through stitching.

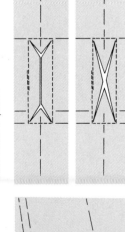

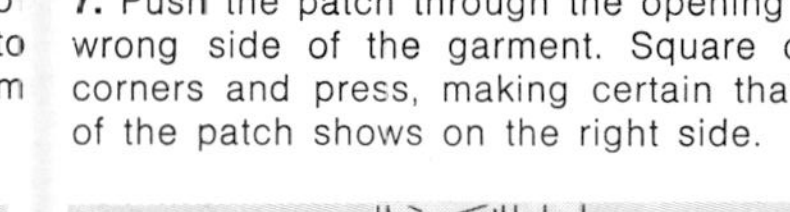

7. Push the patch through the opening to the wrong side of the garment. Square off the corners and press, making certain that none of the patch shows on the right side.

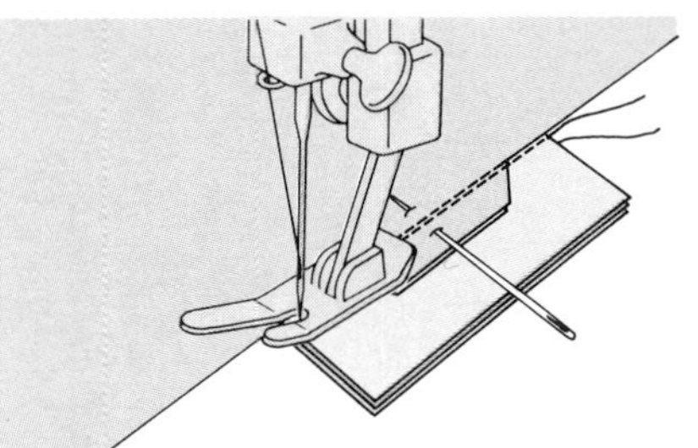

8. For lips, cut two fabric strips 1 1/2" wide and 1" longer than buttonhole. Right sides together, machine-baste strips through center. Open out on basting; press flat.

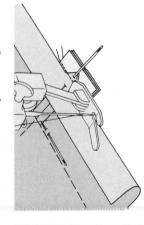

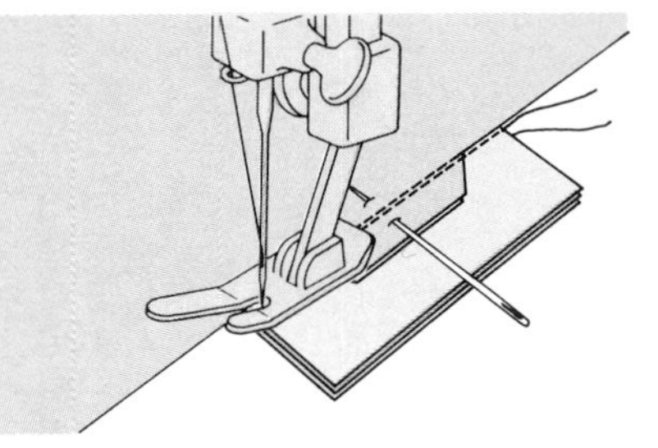

9. With the garment right side up, position the lips underneath the "window" so that the joining of the lips is aligned with the center of the buttonhole opening. Use fine needles instead of pins to hold lips in place so presser foot can get next to the ends.

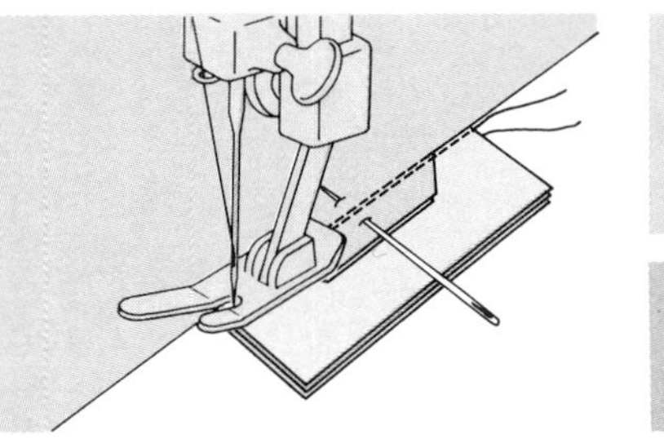

10. With garment right side up, fold back fabric on buttonhole end marking. The triangular end, and the ends of the sheer patch and the lips, will be exposed. Use a needle to pin triangle to other layers. Stitch triangle back and forth exactly on end of buttonhole.

11. After both buttonhole ends are stitched, sew top and bottom to buttonhole lips. Use a needle to hold seam allowances of opening to the lips, and stitch through all layers as close as possible to the first stitching; take care to keep stitching straight.

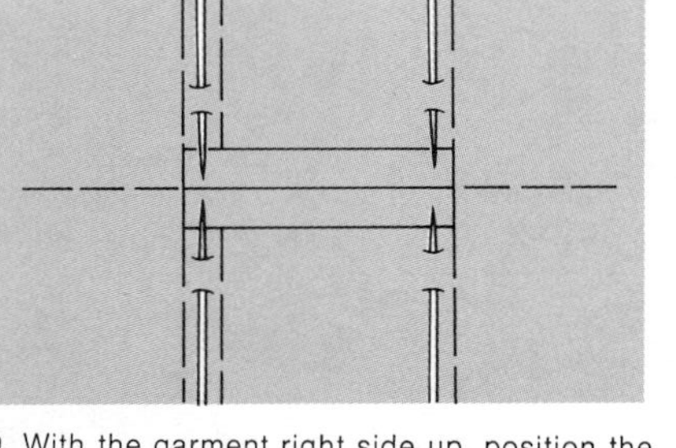

12. Trim and grade excess width of lips and patch so the layer nearest the garment is 3/8" and the top layer 1/4" from the stitching. Remove all markings except center front line and press. Leave machine basting in center of lips until garment is complete.

Bound buttonholes

Fabric-marking methods 94
Even basting 124
Slipstitch (uneven) 132
Tying thread ends 137

In-seam method

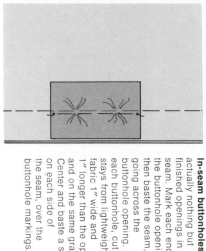

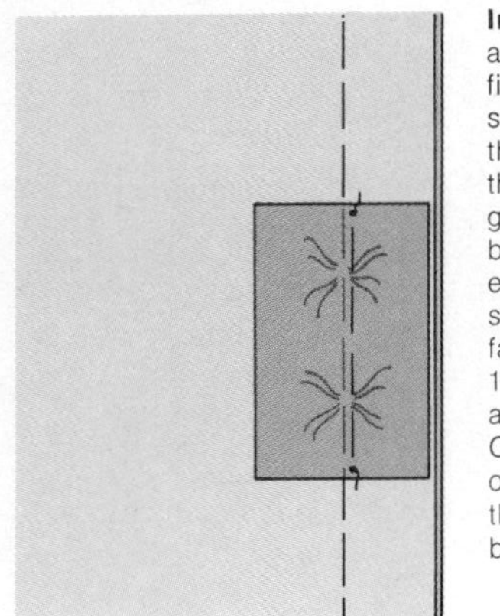

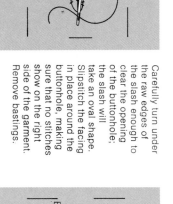

In-seam buttonholes are actually nothing but finished openings in a seam. Mark each end of the buttonhole opening, then baste the seam, going across the buttonhole opening. For each buttonhole, cut two stays from lightweight fabric 1″ wide and 1″ longer than the opening, and on the same grain. Center and baste a stay on each side of the seam, over the buttonhole markings.

Stitch the garment seam, interrupting the stitching at the buttonhole markings. Leave long thread ends at each end of the buttonhole. Pull thread ends to one side of the garment and tie them together.

Press seam open and trim stay so it is slightly narrower than the seam allowances. If the buttonhole is in a horizontal seam that also runs through the facing, remember to leave a similar space in the facing. Make the opening in the facing the same way as the buttonhole, eliminating the stays. Then slipstitch facing and garment together.

Facing finishes

After bound buttonholes have been constructed, the interfacing is attached (see p. 332) and the garment facing is ultimately sewed into the garment. The areas in the facing that lie behind the buttonholes must then be opened, finished off, and attached so that the buttonhole is ready for use.

There are three principal methods for finishing a facing. Which you choose depends mainly on the type of garment fabric, but also on the amount of time you want to spend. The **oval method** is a quick

Oval method

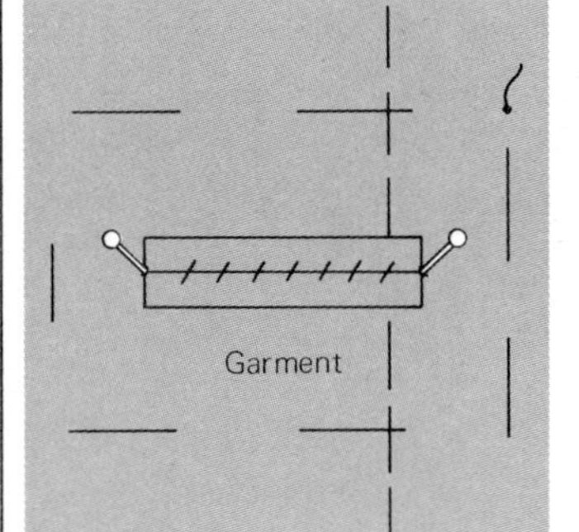

Position facing in garment exactly as it will be worn. Baste around each buttonhole through all the garment layers to hold the facing in place. Insert a straight pin from the right side through the facing at each end of the buttonhole.

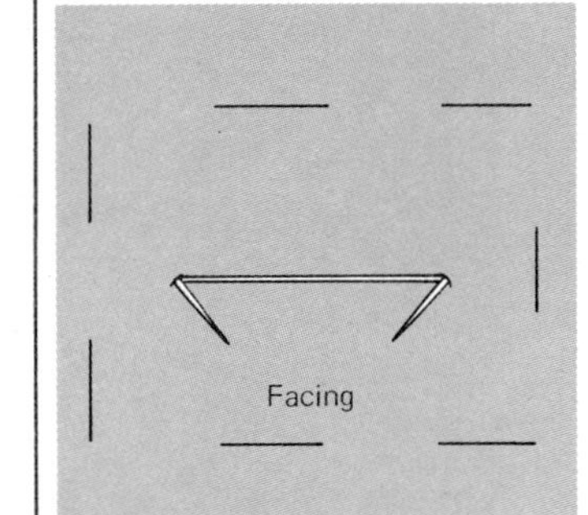

Working from the facing side, cut the facing between the two pins. This slash must not be longer than the buttonhole, and it should be on the straight grain if possible. Remove pins.

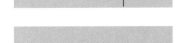

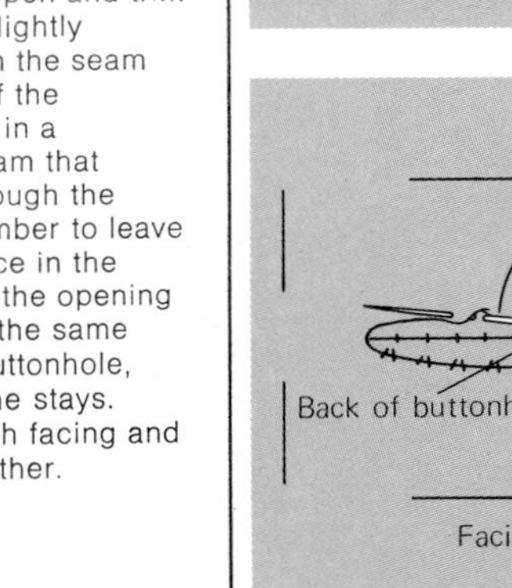

Carefully turn under the raw edges of the slash enough to clear the opening of the buttonhole; the slash will take an oval shape. Slipstitch the facing in place around the buttonhole, making sure that no stitches show on the right side of the garment. Remove bastings.

Rectangle method

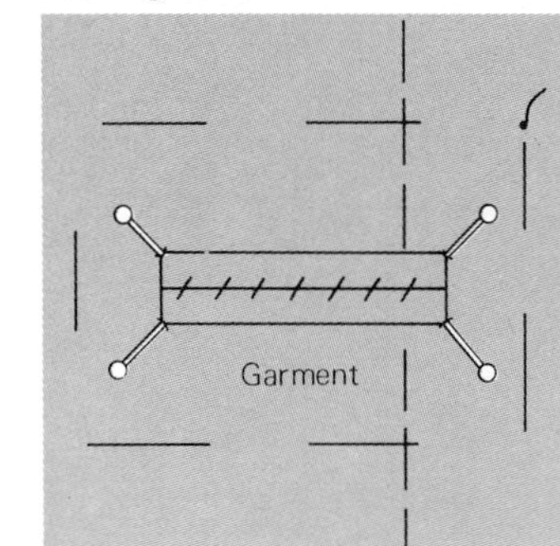

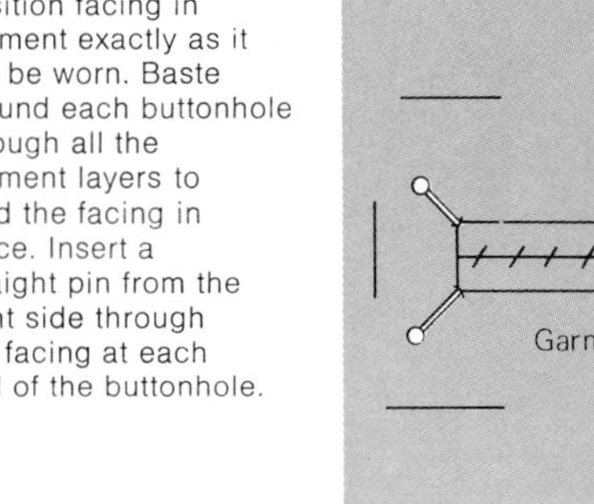

Position facing in garment exactly as it will be worn. From the right side, baste around each buttonhole through all garment layers. Insert a straight pin from the right side through the facing at each of the four corners of the buttonhole.

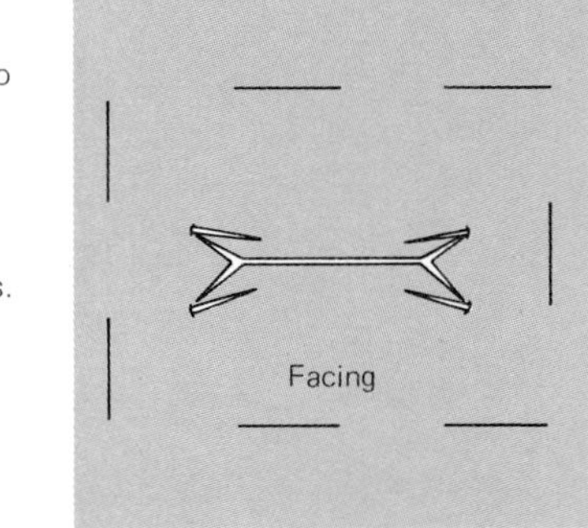

Working from the facing side, cut along the center of this pin-outlined area to within ¼″ of each end. Then cut diagonally to each of the four pins. Remove pins.

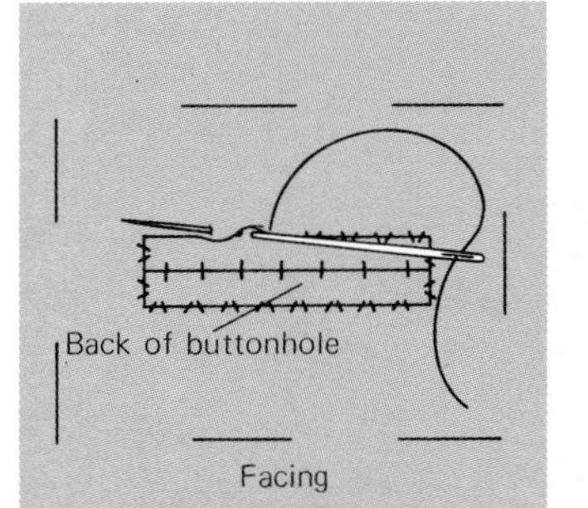

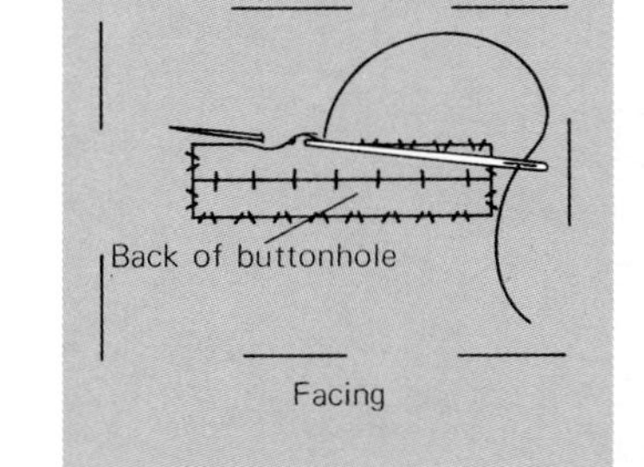

Turn under the raw edges so that the fold is even with the stitching on all four sides of the buttonhole. The slash will take a rectangular shape. Slipstitch the facing in place to the back of the buttonhole.

Pressing equipment 18-19
Thread tracing 94
Uneven basting 124

and easy finish, good for fabrics that ravel easily because little handling is involved. The **rectangle method** is similar to the oval method, except that the shape is more exacting, and requires more manipulation. For this reason, it is recommended only for tightly woven fabrics that will not ravel easily. The **windowpane method** can be used for all types of fabric. It is the neatest of all the facing finishes, but requires more time in the execution than either of the other methods.

Windowpane method

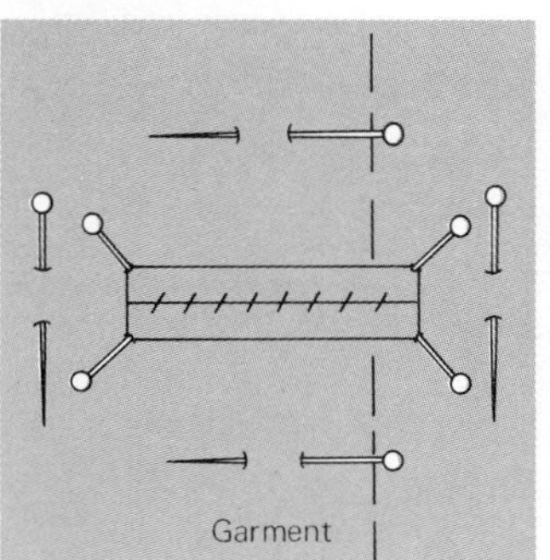

1. Position facing in garment exactly as it will be worn. From the right side, pin the garment to the facing around the buttonhole. Insert a straight pin from the right side through the facing at each of the four corners of the buttonhole.

2. Turn the garment to the facing side and insert four more pins at the corners. Then remove the pins originally inserted from the right side. Facing and garment can then be opened out and the facing will still be pin-marked.

3. Remove the pins that hold the garment and facing together and carefully lift the facing away from the garment. Thread-trace the rectangular outline of the buttonhole on the facing, using the pin markings as a guide. Remove pins when outline is completed.

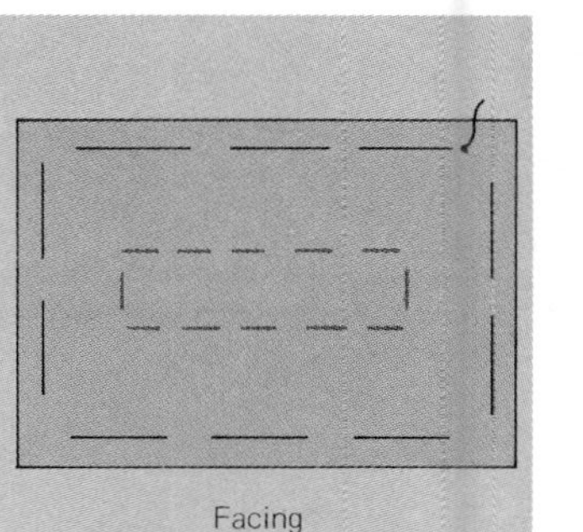

4. Using a lightweight fabric color-matched to the garment, cut a patch 2" wide and 1" longer than the buttonhole. Center the patch over the basted outline of the buttonhole and baste in place.

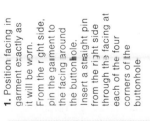

5. From the wrong side of the facing, stitch the patch in place along the basted outline of the buttonhole. Cut, turn, and press the patch to the wrong side as described for the two-piece piped method, Steps 4, 5, 6, 7, page 337.

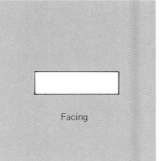

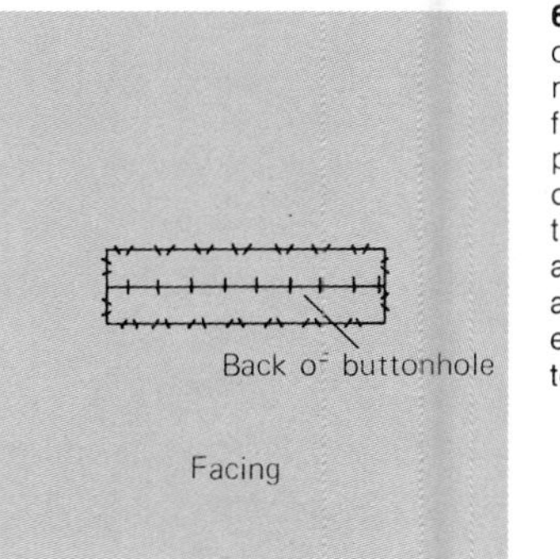

6. When all windowpane openings have been made, replace the facing in its permanent position on the garment. Pin the openings in place at the buttonholes and slipstitch the edges of the opening to the buttonhole.

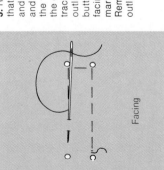

Pressing during construction

Pressing during construction is essential to a well-made bound buttonhole. To avoid imprints or shine on the right side, place strips of brown paper between the patch or strips and the garment, and use a soft press cloth between the garment and the ironing board. Choose the proper temperature setting and amount of moisture for the particular fabric. Press carefully at each of the following stages: (1) after initial stitching of patch or strips to garment; (2) when the patch or strips have been pulled to the wrong side (press triangular ends with the tip of the iron and the top and bottom seams with the side); (3) after basting lips together; (4) when the edges of the patch or strip have been trimmed and/or graded; (5) after facing has been completely attached.

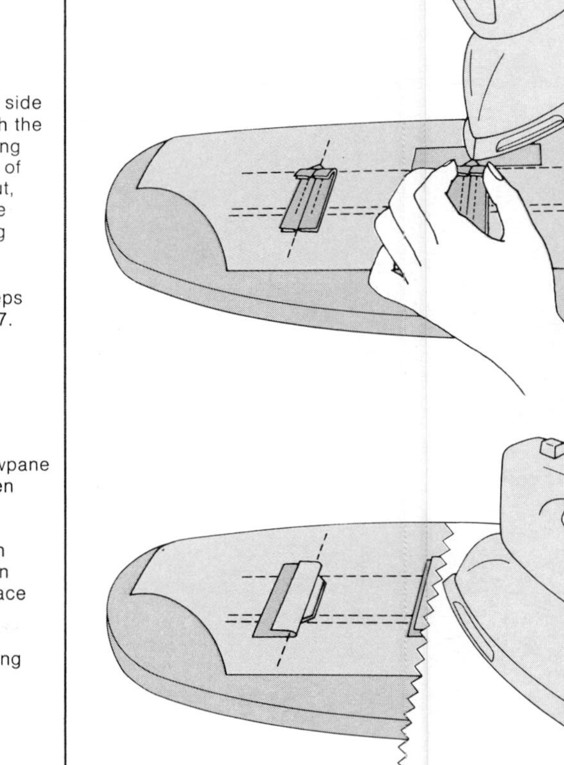

Buttonholes for fur, leather, and similar materials

Real and fake fur, leathers, and vinyls cannot accept regular bound buttonhole techniques, for several reasons. One is that usually they cannot be marked on the right side, either because marking would damage the face of the material, as in leathers, or that the markings would not show, as in deep pile furs. Other considerations are the bulk inherent in some of these materials, and the fact that self-material often cannot be used for the lips. The end result of these special limitations is that bound buttonholes in these fabrics quite often do not look like regular bound buttonholes, and are not made in the same way.

To mark for buttonholes in leather, fur, and similar materials, use chalk, pencil, or a felt tip pen on the back side of the material. Some leathers and vinyls can be marked with a tracing wheel. If a deep pile fur must be marked on the right side, use T-pins or extra-long glass-headed pins. Cut these materials with a sharp razor blade, using a metal ruler as a guide if needed.

A false buttonhole, for real or fake leathers

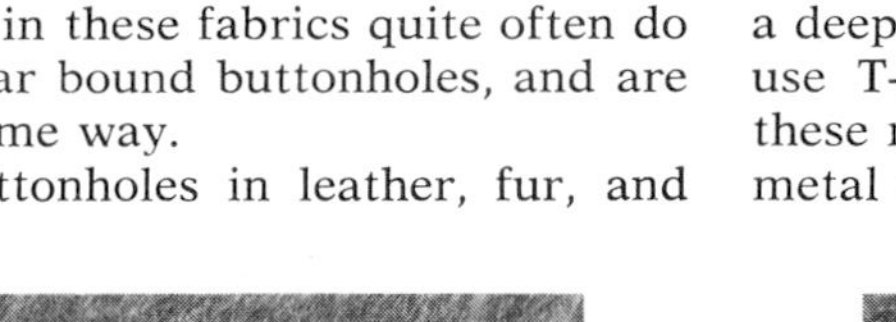

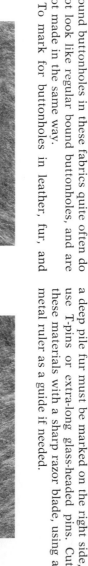

A buttonhole for fur made with grosgrain lips

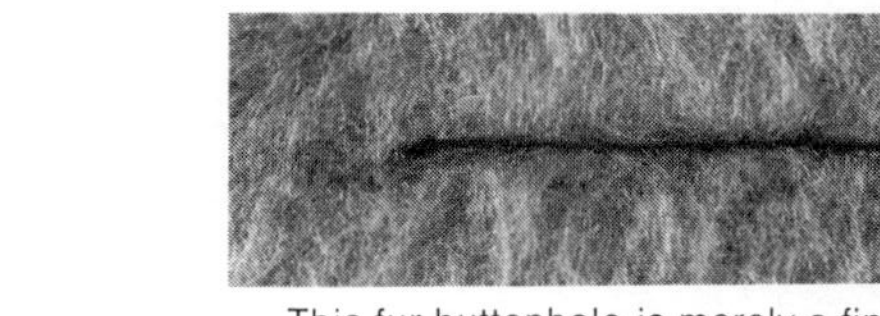

This fur buttonhole is merely a finished slit.

False buttonholes for real and fake leathers

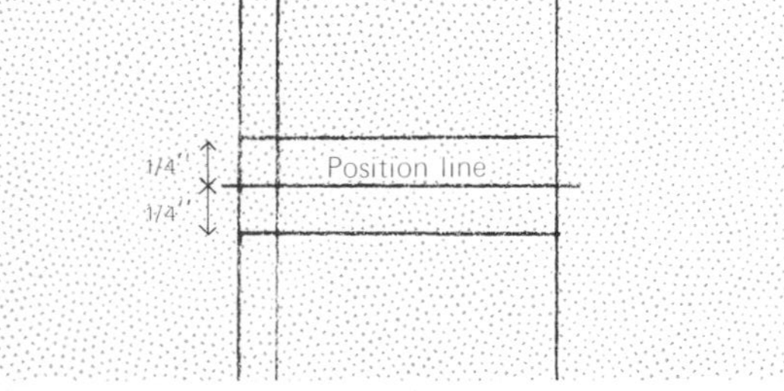

This is not a bound buttonhole in the true sense; it is actually two rectangles stitched to look like a buttonhole, with a slit in the center. **1.** Apply a suitable interfacing and pencil-mark buttonhole (see p. 331). Draw additional lines ¼" or ⅜" above and below buttonhole position line.

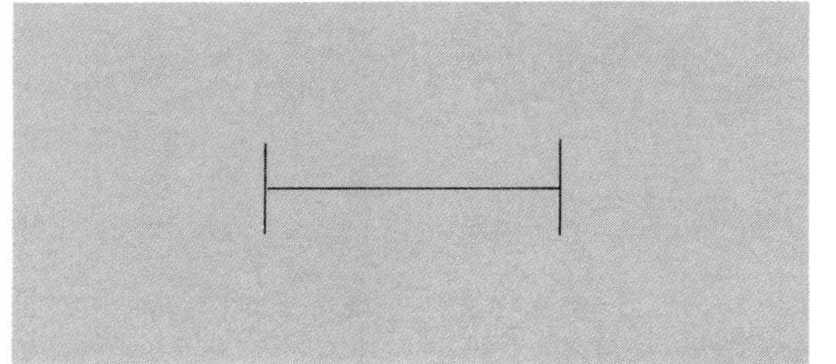

2. Transferring of markings to right side of fabric must be done carefully to avoid puncture marks from needles and pins that would show in the finished garment. Basted markings must be placed so needle punctures will be hidden in final stitching. This is done with three hand stitches, in this way: Using the pencil markings on the wrong side as a guide, take one basting stitch across each end and a third, longer stitch along the center of the buttonhole. Leave long thread ends on all stitches. This makes only six puncture marks, which will be covered by machine stitches.

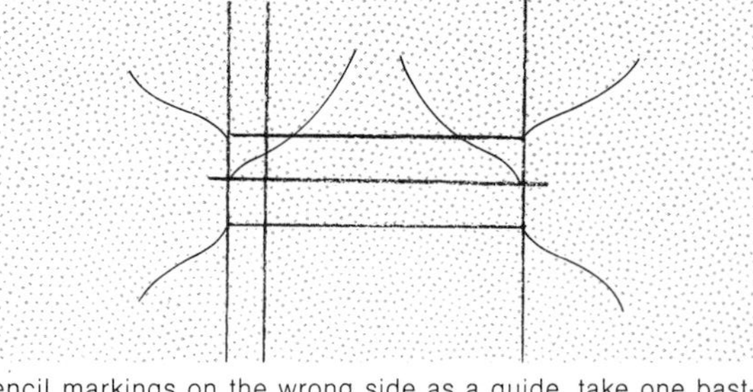

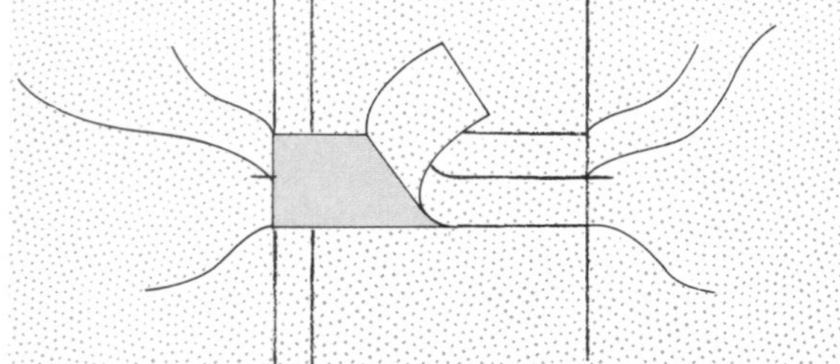

3. Remove the interfacing from within the rectangular buttonhole area carefully so as not to disturb the three long basting threads. To do this, trim out interfacing along the pencil marks for buttonhole sides and ends. To remove a fusible interfacing, slit with a razor blade on markings, then apply a warm iron to the area to soften the adhesive.

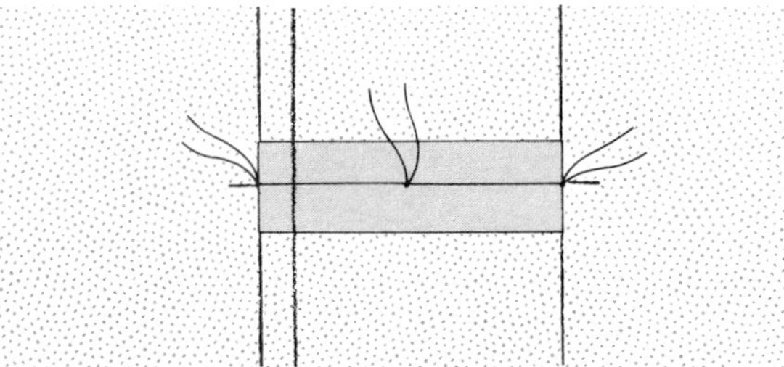

4. Now tie the thread ends together so that the thread markings on the right side of the garment are straight, taut, and secure. Before continuing with the buttonholes, apply the garment facing. Turn the facing to its permanent position, and anchor it securely, with either leather glue or topstitching, before stitching buttonholes.

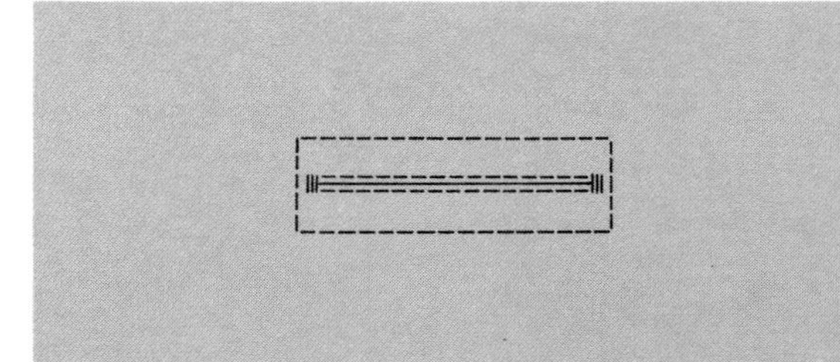

5. Stitch buttonhole from right side of garment as shown above. Stitch outer rectangle first, then one side of center to within one stitch of end. Pivot on the needle and take one stitch forward, then one back; repeat for a total of five stitches. Stitch other side and end. Tie all thread ends. Cut buttonhole between center stitches. Remove basting.

Interfacing selection
and application 72-73, 76-79
Tying thread ends 137

Strip method for real and fake leathers

This is a true bound buttonhole, made in a way much like the strip method for fabric, except that several stitching steps are eliminated to avoid weakening the leather with excess needle punctures. Vinyls and leathers vary greatly in thickness and suppleness, which affects the width of the lips in the finished buttonhole. The thicker the material, the wider the lips. Use the guide, right, to select the correct width, then make a test buttonhole. The length of each strip should be 1 inch greater than the length of the buttonhole to provide a ½-inch extension on each end.

Buttonhole width	Lip width	Strip width
¼″	⅛″	½″
⅜″	3/16″	¾″
½″	¼″	1″

If garment facing is leather, use Step 6 to finish back of buttonhole; for fabric see pages 338–339.

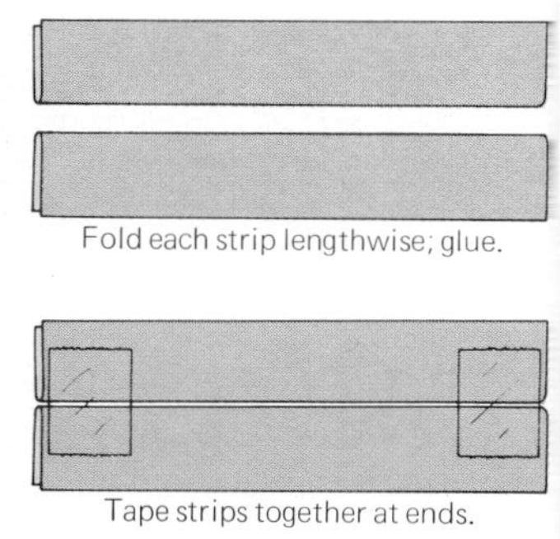

Fold each strip lengthwise; glue.
Tape strips together at ends.

1. Cut two strips for each buttonhole in the recommended width for the size buttonhole you are making. Fold strips in half lengthwise, apply leather glue or rubber cement to wrong side, and allow to dry, weighted if necessary. Abut folded edges and tape together ½″ from ends.

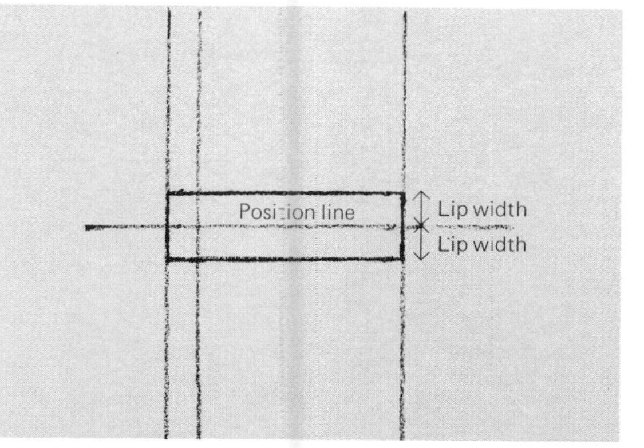

2. Mark the ends and the buttonhole position (center) line on the back of the fabric with chalk or a felt tip pen (see p. 331). Mark additional lines above and below the center line, making them the same distance from the center line as the recommended lip width.

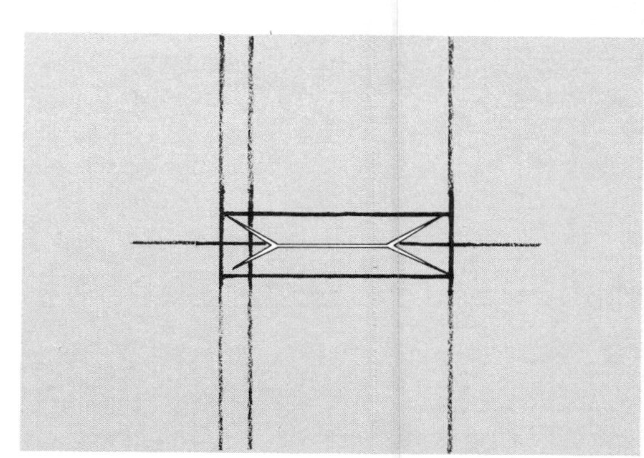

3. Draw additional lines into the corners from a point on the center line ½″ from each end. Cut along the center of the buttonhole to within ½″ of the ends, then cut diagonally into each of the four corners, following the marked lines. Use a razor blade and metal ruler for a clean cut.

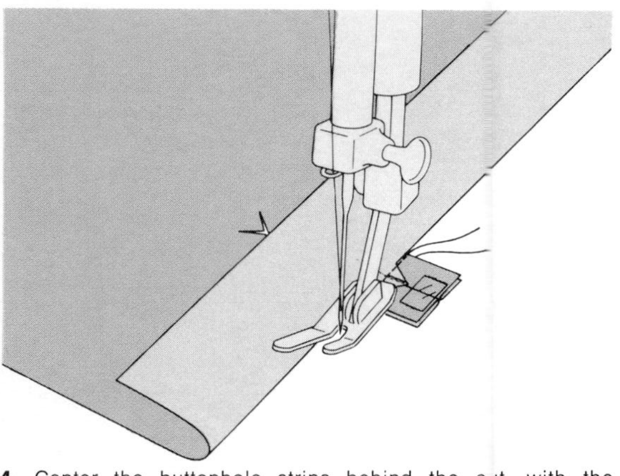

4. Center the buttonhole strips behind the cut, with the abutted edges of the lips exactly in the center of the buttonhole. With right side up, fold garment back to expose the end of the buttonhole. Turn out the little triangle so it is on top of the strips and stitch exactly on the drawn line at the base of the triangle. Repeat at the other end.

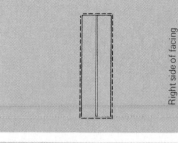

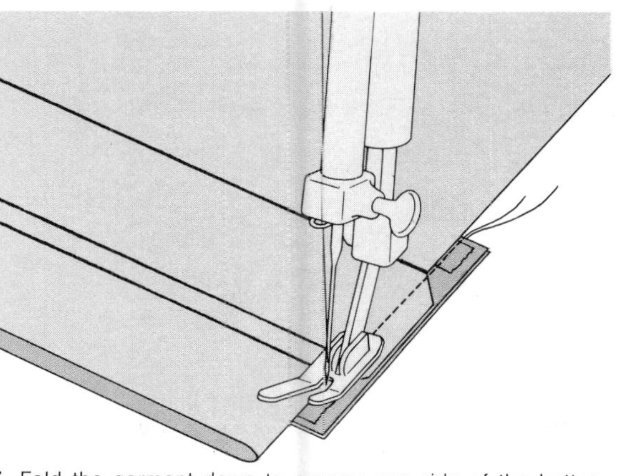

5. Fold the garment down to expose one side of the buttonhole. Match the edge of the seam allowance of the slash to the edge of the buttonhole strips and stitch exactly on the marked line of the base of the seam allowance. Repeat on the other side of the buttonhole. Tie all thread ends; do not backstitch. Remove tape from strips.

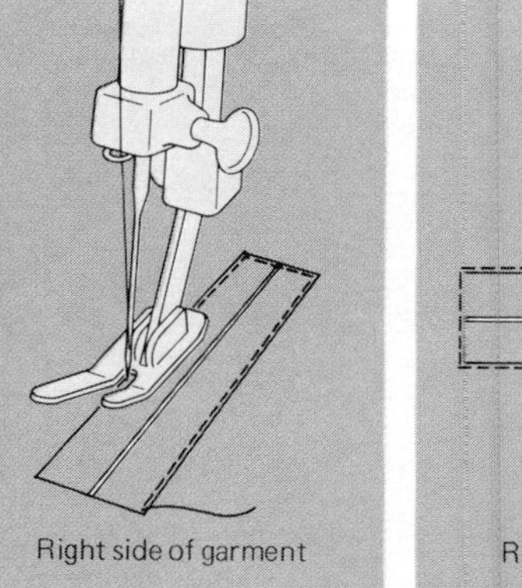

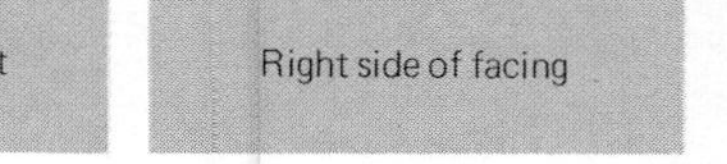

6. Apply interfacing, trimming it out of buttonhole area (see p. 332). Sew facing to garment. To finish the facing, stitch the lips to facing from the right side of the garment by sewing in the seam crevices that form the buttonhole rectangle. Tie all thread ends. Trim away the facing inside the stitching lines to open the buttonhole.

Leather needles 11, twill tape 16
Backstitch 123, catchstitch 129

Overhand stitch 130, running stitch 131
Slipstitch 132, whipstitch 136

Taped method for real and fake furs

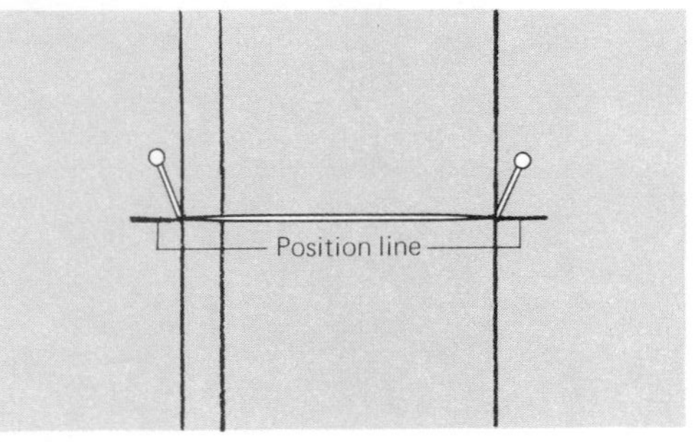

This easy buttonhole method for fur can also be used as a facing finish for the strip method described at right.

1. Using a pen or pencil, mark the buttonhole length and position lines on the wrong side of the material. Place a pin at mark for each end and cut between pins on buttonhole position line. Use a single-edge razor blade so only the leather back, not the fur, is cut.

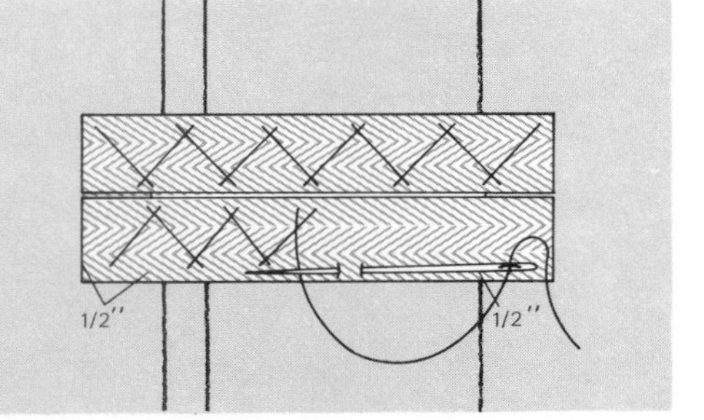

2. Cut four strips of ½" twill tape for each buttonhole, each piece 1" longer than the buttonhole. On the wrong side, center a strip of tape along one edge of slash, aligning edge of tape exactly to edge of slash. Catchstitch tape to skin. If a regular needle will not penetrate the skin, use a special wedge-shaped leather needle. Repeat on other edge.

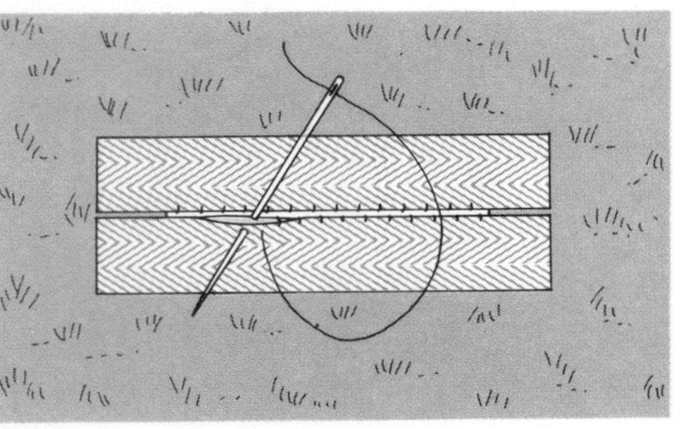

3. The remaining two pieces of twill tape are stitched on from the right side. Center them at slit in the same way as explained above. Sew edges of tape to buttonhole edges with a small overhand stitch. Push fur away from slit to ensure that it is not caught in stitching.

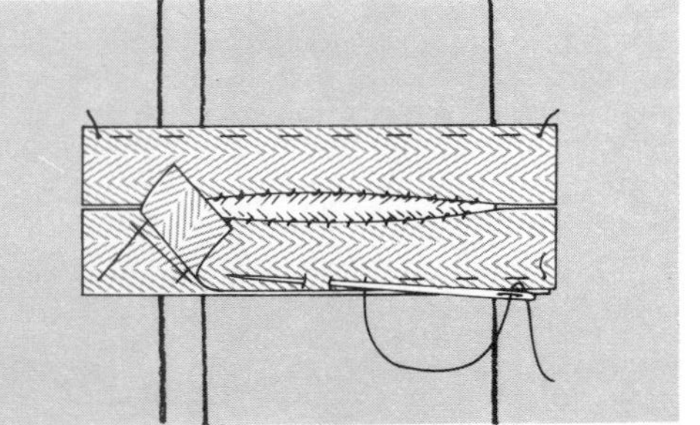

4. Turn both pieces of tape to the inside. Using a running stitch, secure these pieces to the corresponding catchstitched tapes. This method may also be used for a facing finish. (An alternative facing finish involves simply slashing a marked opening in the facing and whipstitching edges of slash to the back of the buttonhole.)

Strip method for real and fake furs

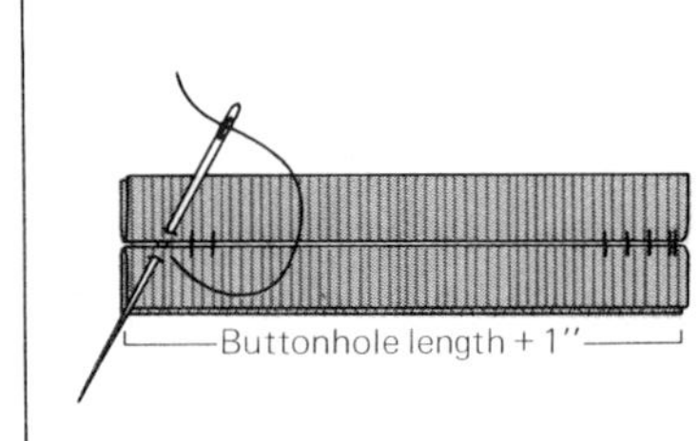
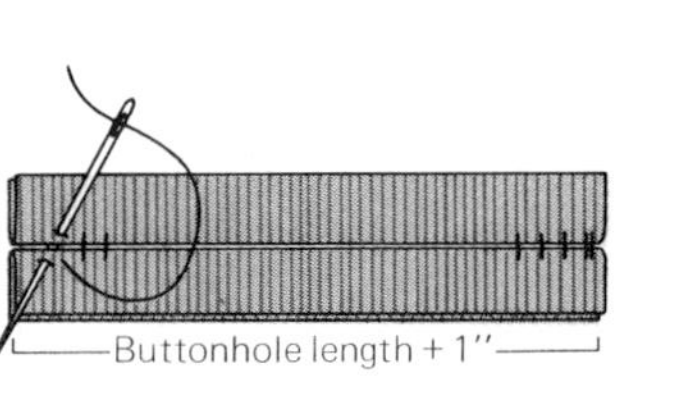

1. Mark buttonholes (see p. 331), drawing additional lines ⅛" above and below the center line to extend beyond length lines. Cut two strips of ⅝" grosgrain ribbon, color-matched to the fur, 1" longer than the buttonhole. To form lips, fold pieces of ribbon in half and press. Tack strips together for ½" at ends.

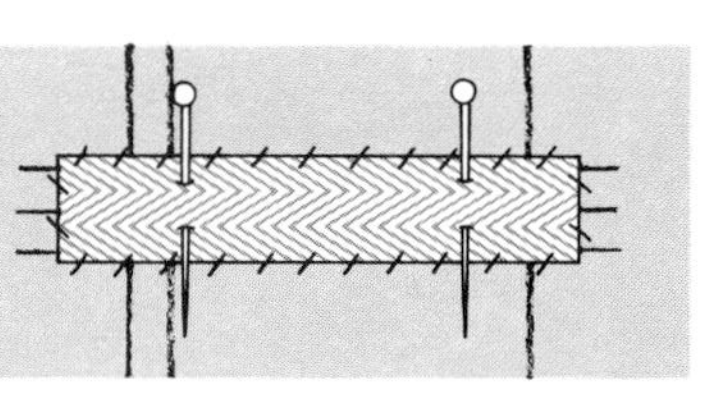

2. A stay of twill tape will keep material from stretching. Cut a strip of ½" twill tape, 1" longer than the buttonhole, and center it over the buttonhole marking. Whipstitch the tape edges to the garment, using a wedge-shaped needle if needed. Place straight pins ½" from each end of buttonhole to guide slashing.

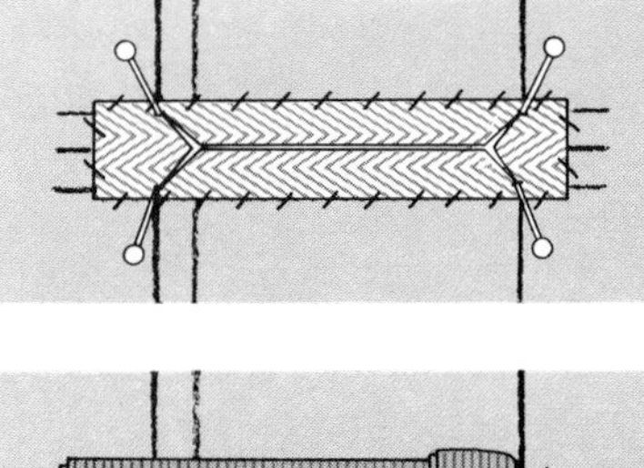

3. Slash through tape and fur between the pins, using a single-edge razor blade. Now place a pin in each of the four corners of the buttonhole—exactly where the ⅛" lines above and below center cross the buttonhole length lines. Slash diagonally into each corner.

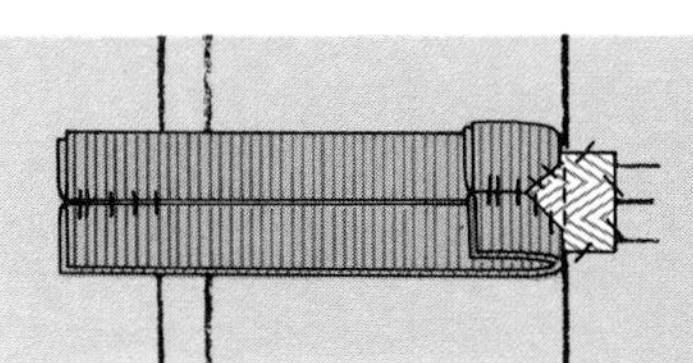

4. Carefully cut hair away from the buttonhole seam allowances formed by the slashing. Center the ribbon lips at the slash so the opening in lips exactly matches the slit in the fur. Whipstitch edges of the little triangle at each end to the ribbon lips. Hand-backstitch across base of triangle.

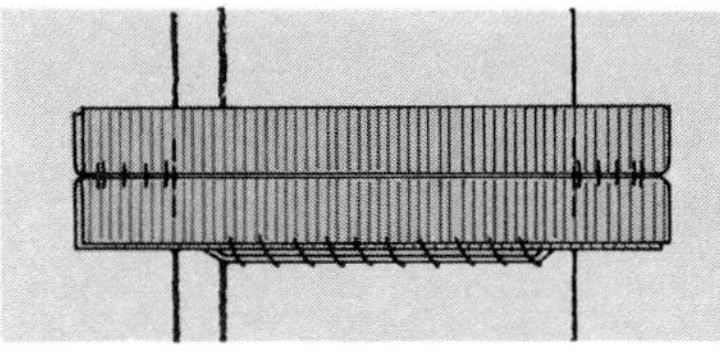

5. Match the edge of one seam allowance of slash to outside edge of the ribbon lip so that the sheared area lies against the ribbon. Whipstitch these edges together for the entire length of the buttonhole. Repeat on other seam allowances.

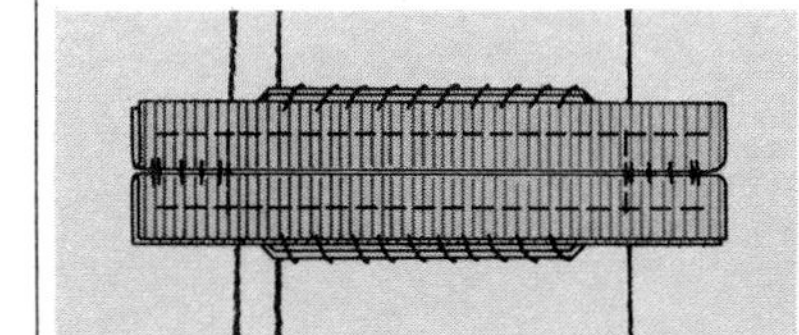

6. Stitch along each side of the opening, ⅛" from the edge. Use a short machine stitch or a hand backstitch. To finish garment facing behind buttonhole, use the taped method at the left and slipstitch facing opening to back of buttonhole.

Worked buttonholes

The two types

A worked buttonhole is a slit in the fabric finished with either hand or machine stitches. It has two sides equal in length to the buttonhole opening, and two ends finished either with a fan-shaped arrangement of stitches (see center photo, below left) or with bar tacks (at immediate right). A worked buttonhole is stitched through all fabric layers, after interfacing and facing are in place; all fabrics should be color-matched to avoid the possibility of color contrast at the cut edge. A hand-worked buttonhole is slit first, then stitched; a machine-worked buttonhole is stitched and then slit.

Worked buttonholes are marked as described on page 331. For a worked buttonhole, the measurements for the actual buttonhole opening and for the stitched buttonhole are different. The finished length of a worked buttonhole will equal the opening plus an extra ⅛ inch for the stitches that are used to finish each end (see p. 330).

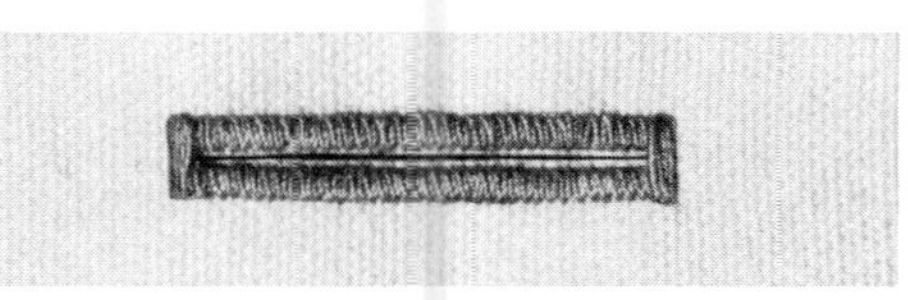

Machine-worked buttonhole with bar-tacked ends

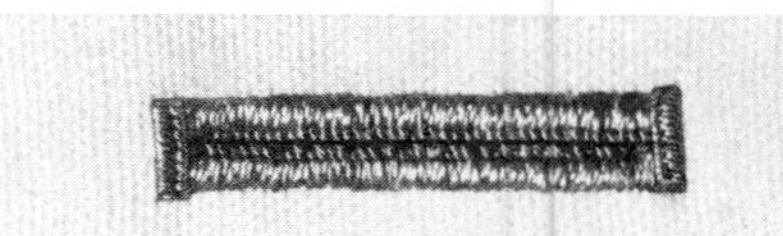

Hand-worked buttonhole with bar-tacked ends

Machine-worked buttonholes

There are three different ways to make a machine-worked buttonhole. The first method involves turning the fabric by hand for each side and end, and using zigzag stitches of different widths; it is called a **manual machine method.** The second way is with **built-in buttonhole stitches** that come with the machine; by means of a few movements of a lever or turns of a dial, a buttonhole with finished ends (bar-tacked or rounded) is stitched. There is no need to turn the fabric by hand.

These two methods require that the machine have a built-in zigzag stitch capability. The third method makes use of a **special attachment** that clamps onto the needle bar and presser foot of the machine; attachments of this sort are available for both straight stitch and zigzag machines. They are especially valuable for straight stitch machines, since a buttonhole cannot be made with a straight stitch alone. Although the results produced by a straight stitch attachment are similar to those of attachments used on zigzag machines, the method is quite different. In the straight-stitch situation, the attachment grips the fabric firmly and, as the machine stitches forward, simultaneously jogs the fabric from side to side and moves it in the buttonhole shape. Together, these three movements produce a buttonhole that looks very much like those made with a zigzag stitch. The attachment for the zigzag machine moves the fabric in the buttonhole shape, while the machine does the zigzag stitching. Attachments will vary from machine to machine, but in most cases the size and shape of the buttonhole is determined either by a cam or by a button placed in the attachment. Buttonhole size is limited by the capability of the attachment. With the other two methods, the buttonhole can be any size you wish.

The choice of method determines the shape of the buttonhole. Buttonhole shapes are variously *rectangular,* with straight bar tacks at each end; *oval,* with two rounded ends; or *keyhole,* which is basically an oval but has an eyelet at one end. The manual machine method always results in rectangular buttonholes; buttonholes produced by built-in buttonhole stitches may be either rectangular or oval; attachments may make any of the three shapes, depending on the cams that come with the attachment. There is very little difference in the end-use applications of rectangular and oval buttonholes. The keyhole, however, is used mainly on tailored clothing and menswear. It stays closed better than the other two shapes because there is a ready-made space for the button shank to rest without distorting the buttonhole.

Always test machine-worked buttonholes, through all fabric layers involved, before beginning buttonhole work on the garment. Machine-worked buttonholes should be stitched with the same needle and thread as are used for other construction.

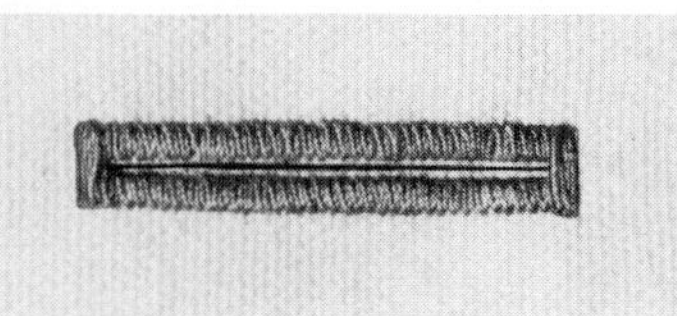

Rectangular buttonhole made with two widths of zigzag stitches, with fabric turned by hand.

Oval buttonhole can be made with either built-in stitches or a special attachment.

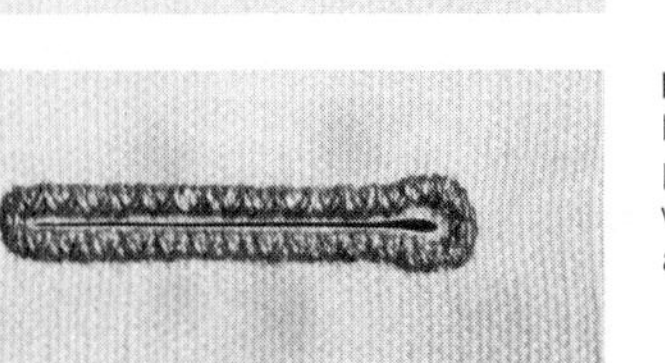

Keyhole buttonhole is possible only with a special attachment.

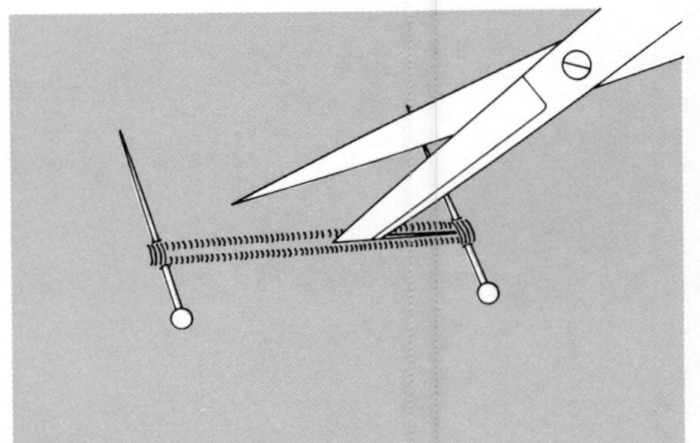

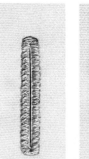

Machine-worked buttonholes are opened only after stitching is completed. Cut slowly and carefully with a small, sharp scissors to avoid snipping accidentally through stitches. To prevent cutting through the ends, place straight pins at each end of the buttonhole opening, then cut down the center on the buttonhole position line to the pins.

Machine-worked buttonholes

Zigzag stitching 32-33
Machine accessories 38-39

Manual (hand-guided) method

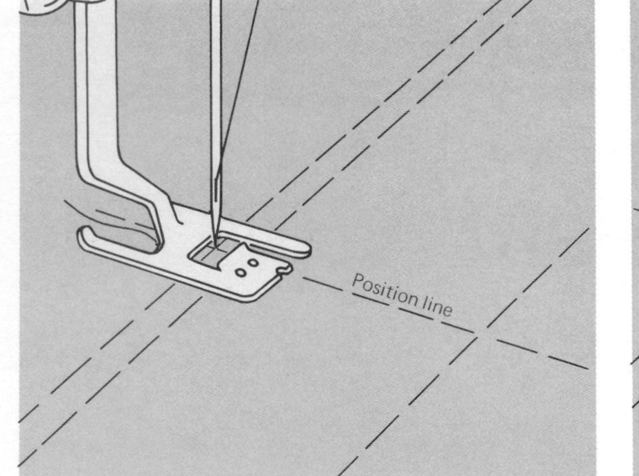

1. Attach the zigzag throat plate and the appropriate foot for your machine. Set needle position at "left," stitch *length* on "fine," and stitch *width* on "medium." Working on right side of garment, center the buttonhole position line under the foot. Position the needle in the fabric, at one end of buttonhole, on the left side of the position line.

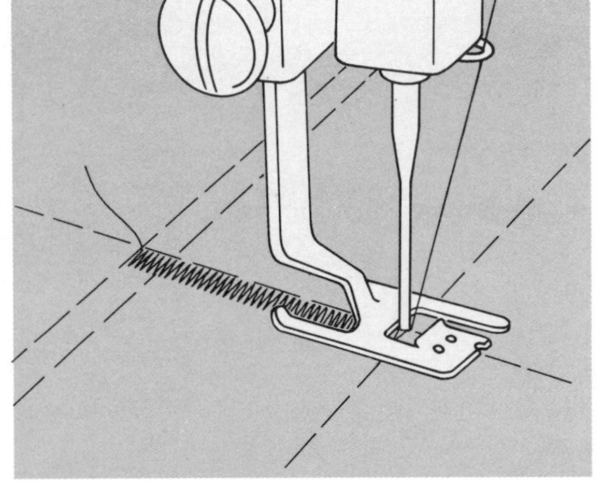

2. Lower the foot and stitch slowly to the opposite end of the buttonhole. End this stitching with the needle in the fabric *next to* the buttonhole position line. This method has the best results when great care is taken to leave the needle in the right spot for pivoting. Such care insures accuracy, since the needle is never positioned by hand.

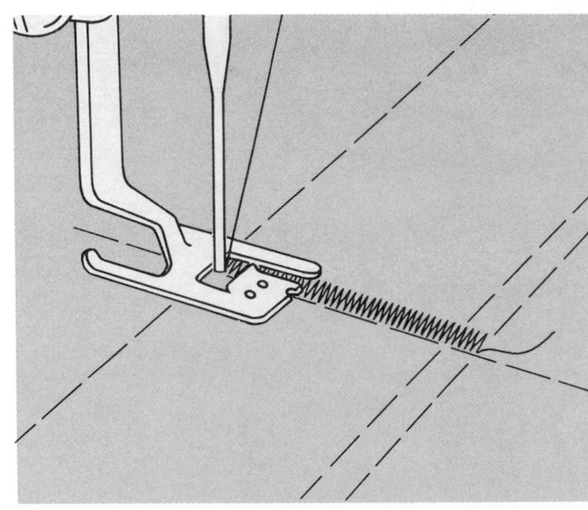

3. Raise the foot and pivot the fabric on the needle to turn the garment 180° (complete turn). Buttonhole position line will be centered under the foot, and the garment positioned for stitching one of the bar tacks and the other side of the buttonhole. Lower the foot and take one stitch to bring needle to outer edge of buttonhole. Lift needle.

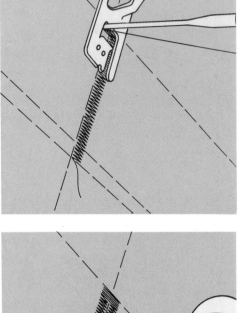

4. For the first bar tack, set the stitch width selector at the *widest* setting. Take 6 stitches, ending with the needle at the *outside* edge of the buttonhole. You will notice that one half of the bar tack is stitched over the initial row of buttonhole stitches. The other half leads directly into the second row of buttonhole stitches.

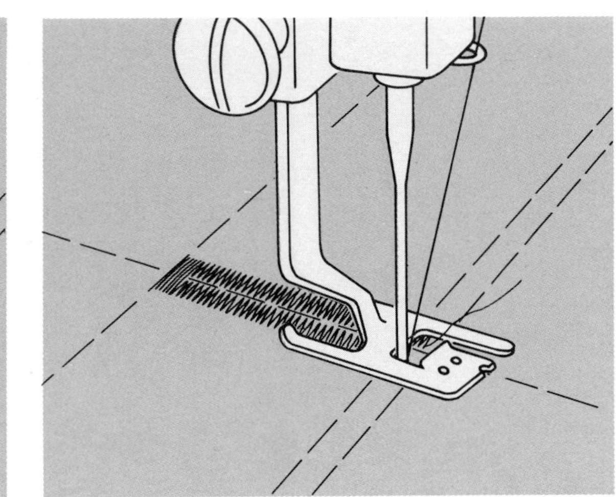

5. Lift the needle just out of the fabric at the outside edge of the buttonhole, and re-set the stitch width to medium. Stitch the second side of the buttonhole to within $\frac{1}{16}''$ of the actual end of the buttonhole, ending this row of stitching with the needle again at the outside edge. The last $\frac{1}{16}''$ will be part of the second bar tack.

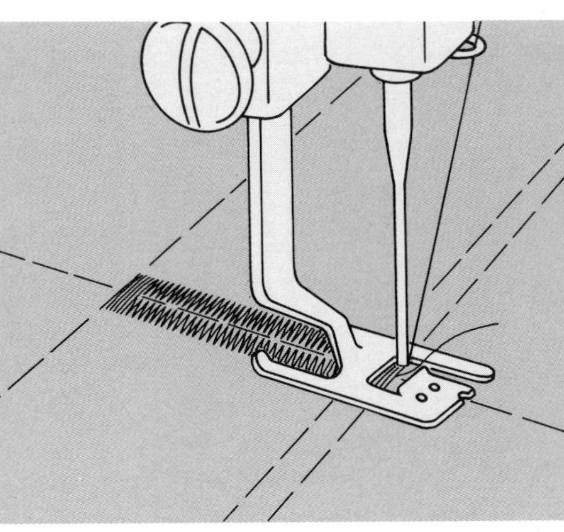

6. With needle up, change to the wide stitch width. Take 6 stitches for the other bar tack. To secure stitching, set the stitch width selector at "0" width for straight stitching and take 3 stitches. Draw threads to the underside and tie. Place a straight pin in front of each bar tack and cut the buttonhole open. Remove pins and markings.

Zigzag stitching 32-33
Machine accessories 38-39

Buttonholes from built-in capabilities

Many sewing machines of comparatively recent design have built-in mechanisms that stitch machine-worked buttonholes automatically. There is no need to pivot, change needle position, or turn the fabric when a machine has these built-in capabilities. By manipulating a single control, each step of the buttonhole is automatically positioned and stitched. Half of the buttonhole is stitched forward, the other half is stitched backward.

Before stitching is begun, all buttonhole position and length marks must be made (see p. 331). The markings are then located under the presser foot as directed by the machine booklet. Depending upon the machine, the buttonhole is stitched in two, four, or five steps as described at the left. The instructions will vary according to the number of steps; directions in the machine booklet must be followed carefully. Also check the booklet to see whether there is a presser foot designed expressly for stitching buttonholes.

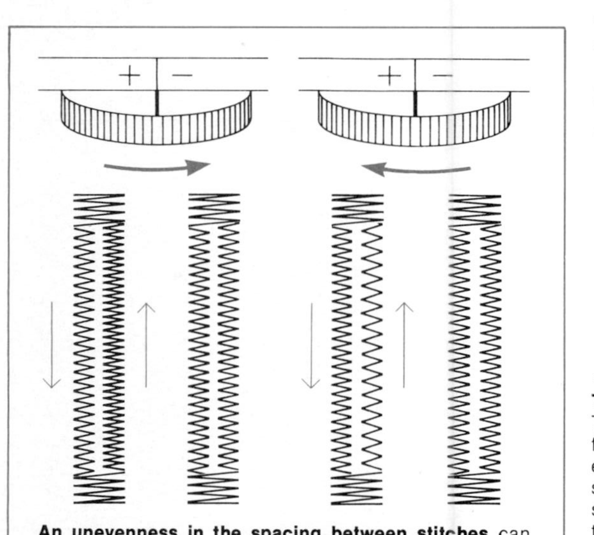

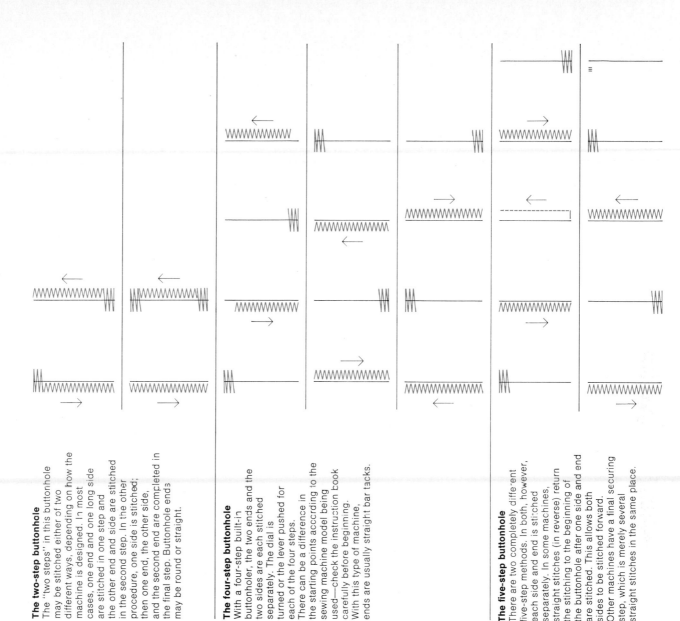

An unevenness in the spacing between stitches can occur when a machine sews in reverse, causing sides of buttonhole to look mismatched. There is a special mechanism to control this tendency; consult your machine booklet for instructions in its use. As a rule, if reverse stitches are too close together, the mechanism is turned to a minus setting; if they are too far apart, toward a plus setting.

The two-step buttonhole
The "two steps" in this buttonhole may be stitched either of two different ways, depending on how the machine is designed. In most cases, one end and one long side are stitched in one step and the other end and side are stitched in the second step. In the other procedure, one side is stitched; then one end, the other side, and the second end are completed in the final step. Buttonhole ends may be round or straight.

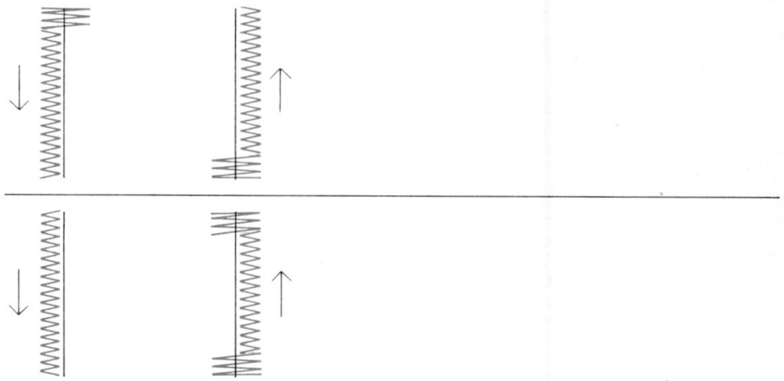

The four-step buttonhole
With a four-step built-in buttonholer, the two ends and the two sides are each stitched separately. The dial is turned or the lever pushed for each of the four steps.
There can be a difference in the starting points according to the sewing machine model being used—check the instruction book carefully before beginning.
With this type of machine, ends are usually straight bar tacks.

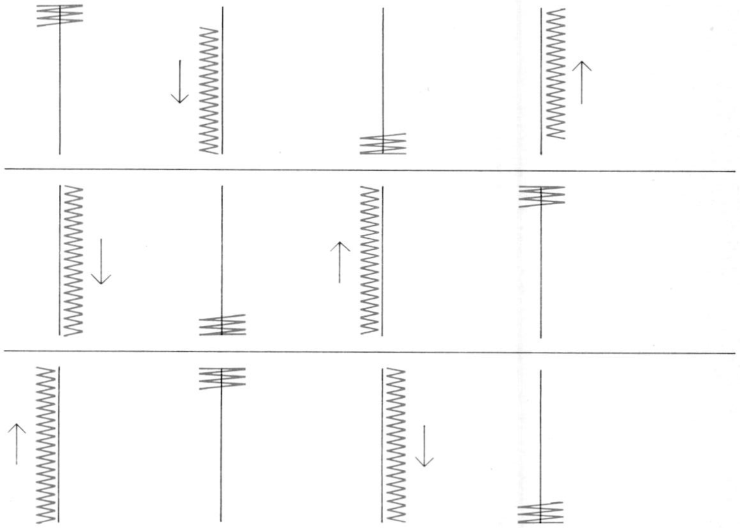

The five-step buttonhole
There are two completely different five-step methods. In both, however, each side and end is stitched separately. In some machines, straight stitches (in reverse) return the stitching to the beginning of the buttonhole after one side and end are stitched. This allows both sides to be stitched forward.
Other machines have a final securing step, which is merely several straight stitches in the same place.

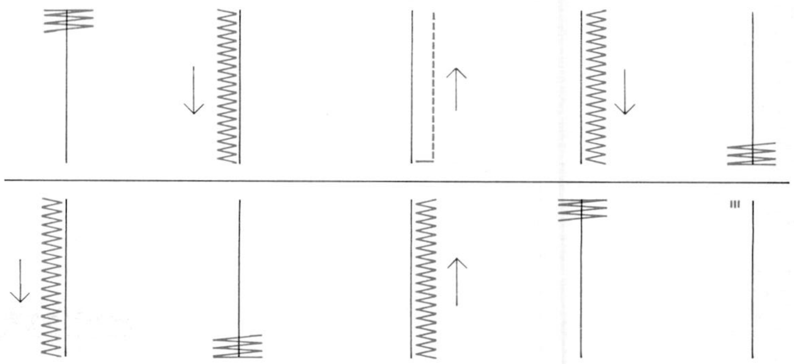

Machine-worked buttonholes

Buttonhole attachments

A buttonhole attachment is a special accessory that is attached to a machine at needle bar and presser foot. It is used in conjunction with a special feed cover plate and comes with a variety of templates or cams for different buttonhole lengths and styles, including those with eyelets. These attachments are available for both straight stitch and zigzag sewing machines. Make sure the one you use is the right type for your machine.

Although it is possible to make neat buttonholes with just a zigzag machine, an attachment does the guiding of the fabric for you and eliminates the need to turn the fabric by hand.

Such an attachment on a straight stitch machine increases its capability; straight stitches alone cannot make a worked buttonhole. The buttonhole produced by an attachment on a straight stitch machine looks like one sewed on a zigzag model. It accomplishes this by gripping the fabric firmly and moving it back and forth under the needle, while also producing the buttonhole shape.

Read the instructions that accompany the attachment carefully, since each attachment is different. Always test any buttonhole through all the fabric thicknesses that will be in that area of the garment. The look of the buttonhole may be improved by stitching around it twice.

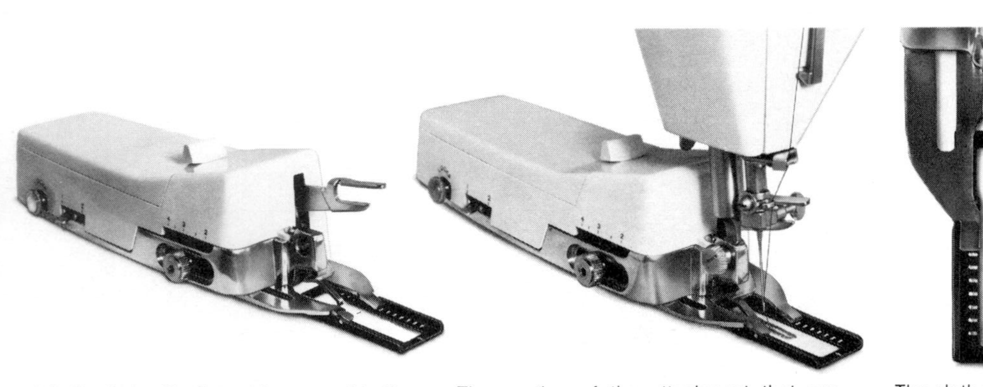

A buttonhole attachment is secured to the sewing machine at the presser foot area and also with a fork arm on the needle clamp. It is equipped with dials with which to control the stitch width and the starting position of the template.

The section of the attachment that surrounds the stitching area is called the *cloth clamp*. The under side of this clamp has a textured surface that grips the fabric firmly so it will not shift while the buttonhole is being stitched.

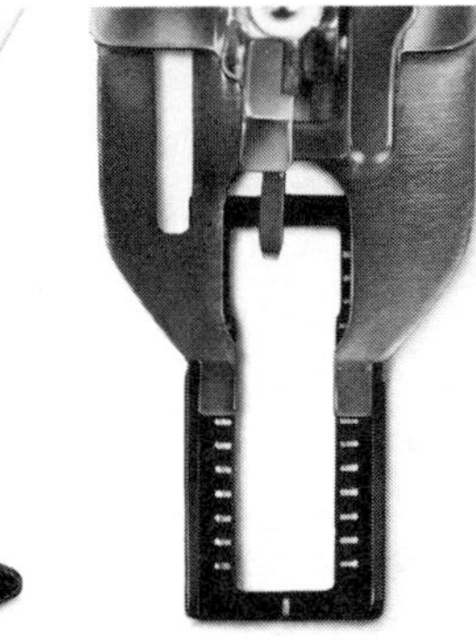

The cloth clamp, shown in close-up above, has many horizontal markings, used to position template at buttonhole markings on fabric.

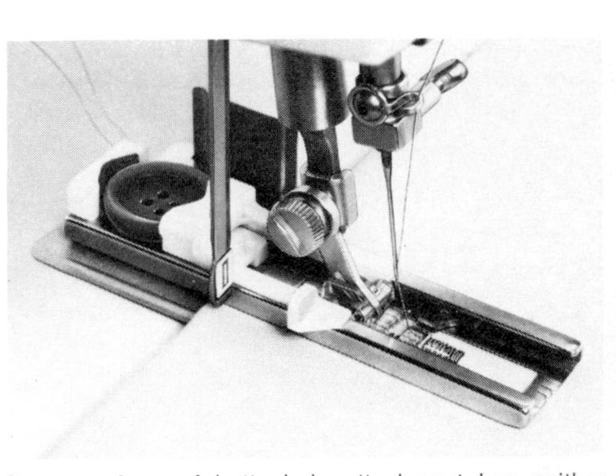

A newer type of buttonhole attachment has neither cams, fork arm, nor feed cover plate. It is limited in length selections, and makes only rectangular buttonholes. The button chosen for the garment, inserted at the back of this attachment, guides the stitching of a buttonhole of the correct length.

Cording machine buttonholes

Corded machine buttonholes are made by stitching with a special cording foot over a filler cord. The filler may be embroidery or crochet thread, or a double strand of ordinary sewing thread. How the cord is inserted will depend on the type of buttonhole the machine produces, and the precise cording foot used. The cord is either looped around a "toe" located in the front or at the back of the cording foot, or threaded through an eyelet in the cording foot. Consult your machine booklet for instructions. When stitching is completed, the looped end of the cord is pulled under one end of the buttonhole. At the other end, loose ends are tied, trimmed, and hidden under the bar tack.

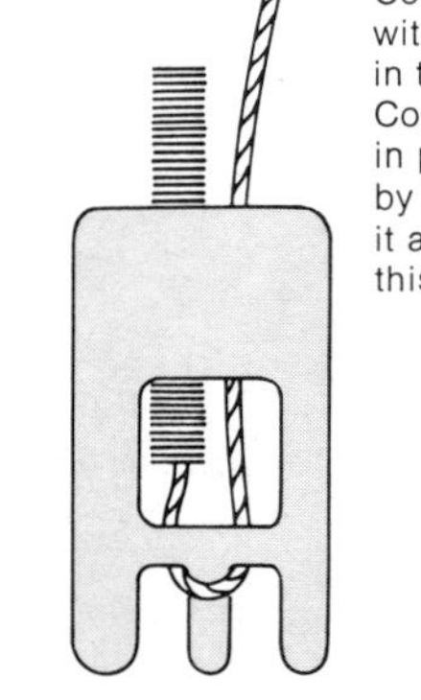

Cording foot with toe in the front. Cord is held in place by looping it around this toe.

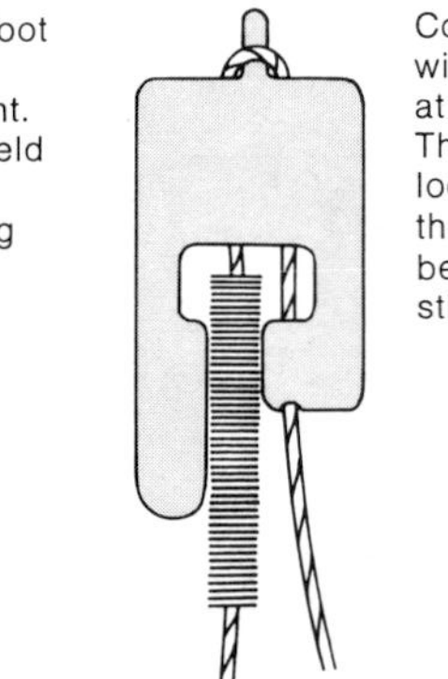

Cording foot with toe at the back. The cord is looped over the toe before stitching.

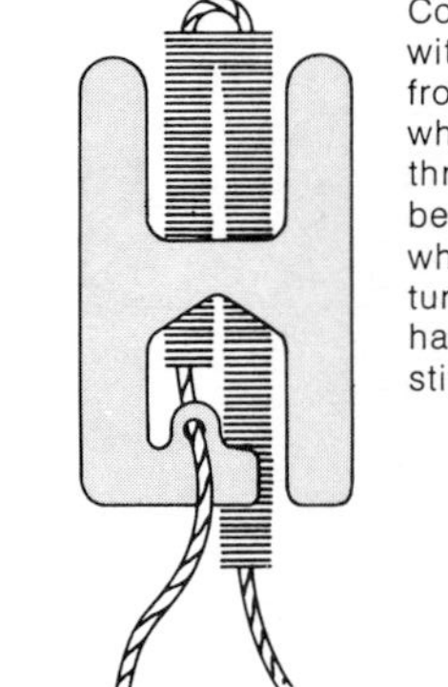

Cording foot with eyelet in front through which cord is threaded. Can be used only when fabric is turned by hand during stitching.

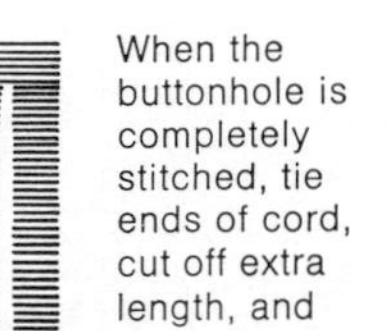

When the buttonhole is completely stitched, tie ends of cord, cut off extra length, and hide the knot under bar tack.

Hand-worked buttonholes

Thread chart 10 General hand-sewing suggestions 122 Bar tack 133

Basic information

Hand-worked buttonholes are made by cutting a slit in the fabric equal in length to the buttonhole opening, then stitching over the edges with a combination of buttonhole and blanket stitches.

Horizontal buttonholes usually have a fan arrangement of stitches at the end where the button will rest, and a straight bar tack at the other; a fan accommodates a button shank better. The tailored form of a horizontal buttonhole, the keyhole buttonhole, has an eyelet at the fanned end.

Vertical buttonholes are made like horizontals, except that both ends are finished in the same shape, either fanned or bar-tacked.

Test the buttonhole through all layers of fabric that will be in the finished garment. Stitch with a single strand of buttonhole twist or regular sewing thread. (If you prefer a double strand of the regular thread, take great care to pull up both strands uniformly with each stitch.) Stitch depth can be from $\frac{1}{16}$ to $\frac{1}{8}$ inch, depending on the fabric type and the size of the buttonhole. A deeper stitch is used on loosely woven fabrics and large buttonholes. The stitch depth must be taken into consideration when determining the buttonhole length, because it affects the ends as well as the edges. Note that the markings for the ends of the buttonholes are a stitch depth away at each end from the actual end of the cut opening.

Keep the stitches closely spaced and uniform when working buttonholes; do not pull them too tight. Fasten the stitching on the wrong side by running the thread under a few completed stitches. Remove markings only after all buttonholes are completed. To start a new thread, come up through the last purl, and continue stitching.

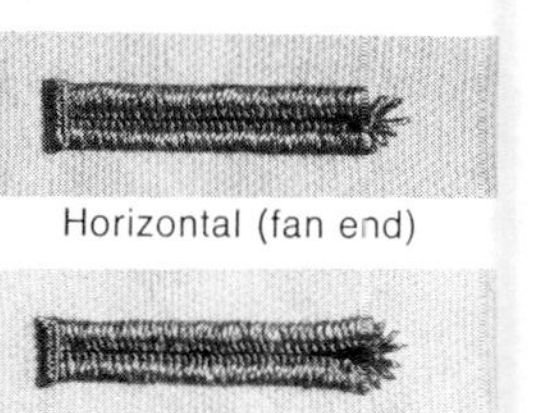

Horizontal (fan end)

Horizontal (keyhole)

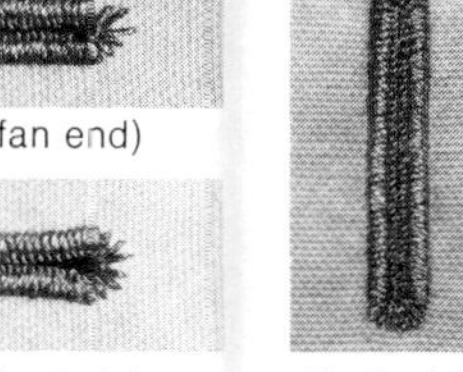

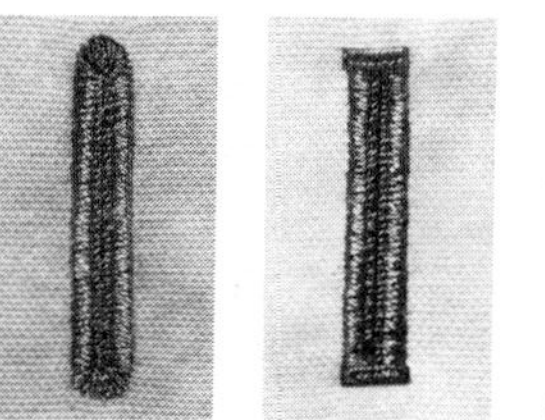

Vertical (fan and bar-tack)

Standard hand-worked buttonholes

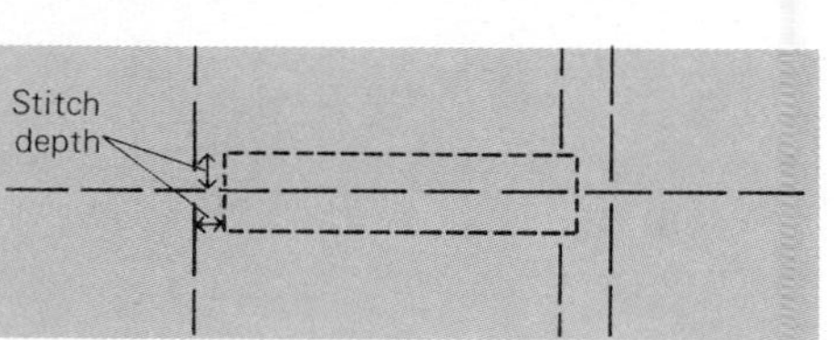

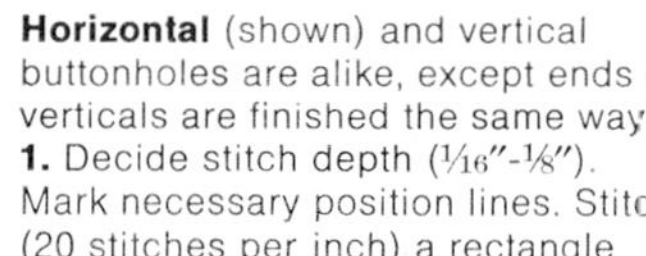

Horizontal (shown) and vertical buttonholes are alike, except ends of verticals are finished the same way.
1. Decide stitch depth ($\frac{1}{16}$"-$\frac{1}{8}$"). Mark necessary position lines. Stitch (20 stitches per inch) a rectangle that is the stitch depth away from the center line and end markings.

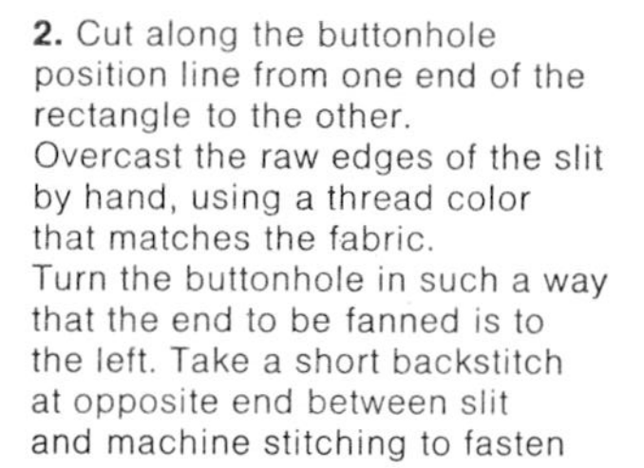

2. Cut along the buttonhole position line from one end of the rectangle to the other. Overcast the raw edges of the slit by hand, using a thread color that matches the fabric. Turn the buttonhole in such a way that the end to be fanned is to the left. Take a short backstitch at opposite end between slit and machine stitching to fasten thread for hand stitching.

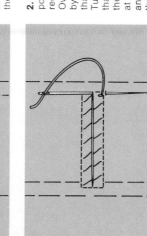

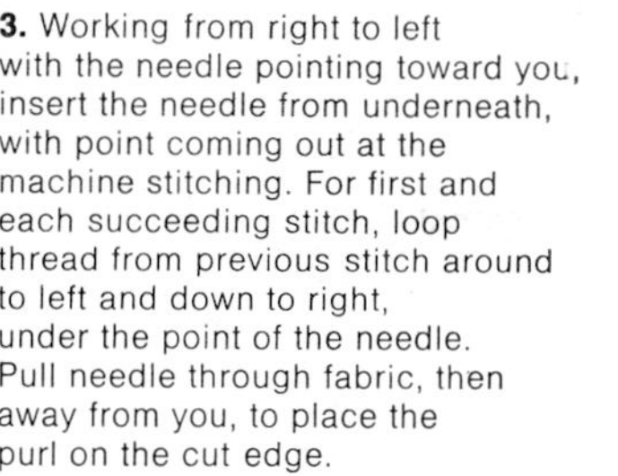

3. Working from right to left with the needle pointing toward you, insert the needle from underneath, with point coming out at the machine stitching. For first and each succeeding stitch, loop thread from previous stitch around to left and down to right, under the point of the needle. Pull needle through fabric, then away from you, to place the purl on the cut edge.

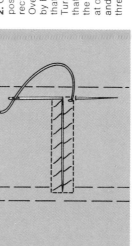

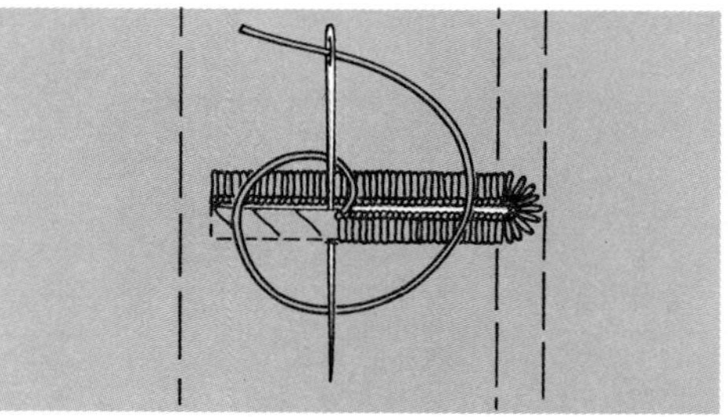

4. Take successive stitches very close together, continuing until that entire side is covered. Then fan the stitches around the end, turning the buttonhole as you work. Take 5 to 7 stitches around the fan, keeping them an even depth. When fan end is completely stitched, continue along the second side.

5. Stitch along second side until other end of the opening is reached. Then insert the needle down into the purl of the first stitch to wrong side of buttonhole; bring needle out just below the last stitch, at outer edge of buttonhole. Take several long stitches close together across the width of the two rows of buttonhole stitches to form the base for the bar tack.

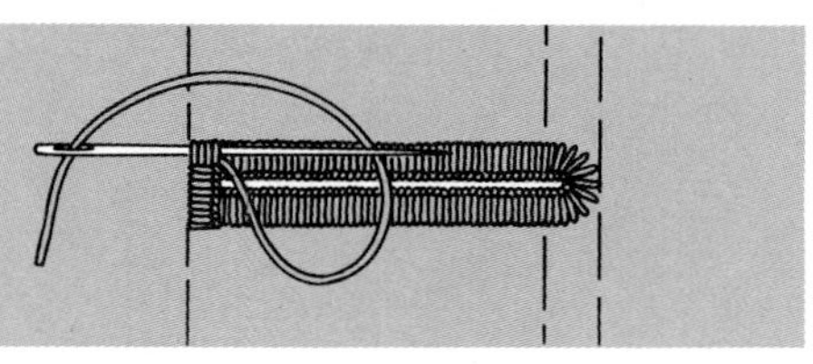

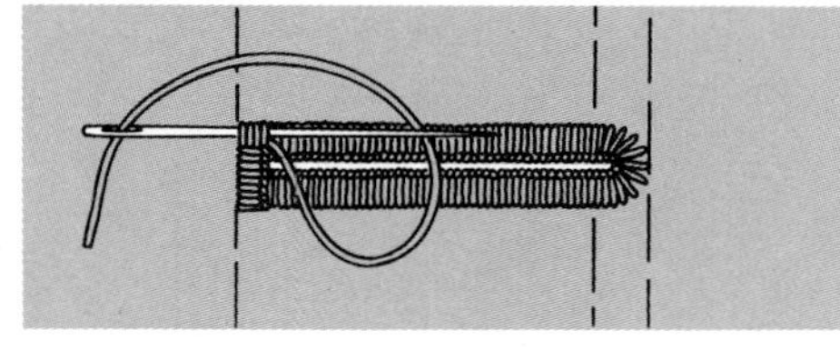

6. Working with point of needle toward buttonhole and beginning at one end of the bar tack, insert needle into fabric under long stitches. Keep thread from previous stitch under needle point; draw up stitch. Continue, completely covering long stitches. Secure on wrong side.

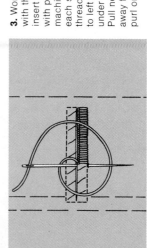

Hand-worked buttonholes

Thread chart 10
Awl 13
Blanket stitch 125
Overcast stitch 130

Keyhole buttonholes

The tailored worked buttonhole, or keyhole buttonhole, is similar to the horizontal hand-worked buttonhole on the preceding page. The difference is an eyelet, or enlarged "resting place" for the button shank, at one end instead of the usual fan arrangement of stitches. By providing more room for the shank, the eyelet ensures that the buttonhole will not be distorted when the garment is buttoned. This makes the tailored buttonhole the best choice for men's jackets and other finely tailored garments. Remember, on a man's coat or jacket, that the buttonholes are placed on the opposite side from the side used for women's garments.

Use a single strand of buttonhole twist or heavy-duty thread for buttonhole stitches. For a professional touch, it is suggested that a tailored worked buttonhole be corded. The filler can be heavy-duty thread, buttonhole twist, or fine string.

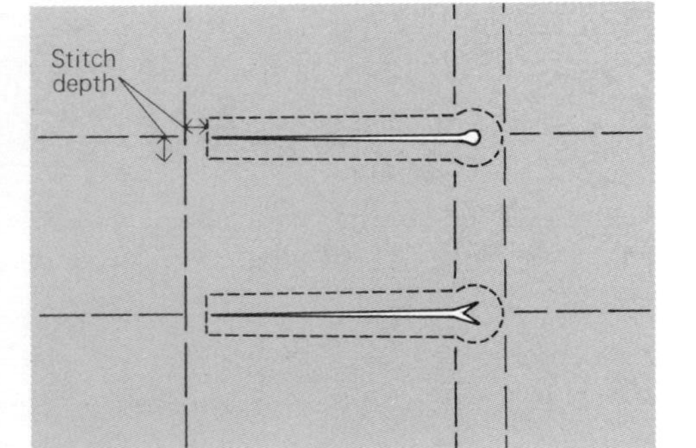

1. Machine-stitch at 20 stitches per inch around the buttonhole the stitch depth away from the buttonhole position line and ends. There are two ways to open the buttonhole and eyelet: Use an awl to punch the eyelet hole, then cut along the position line to within 1/8" of the other end; or cut along position line to within 1/8" of keyhole end of opening, then cut two tiny diagonal slashes to machine stitches.

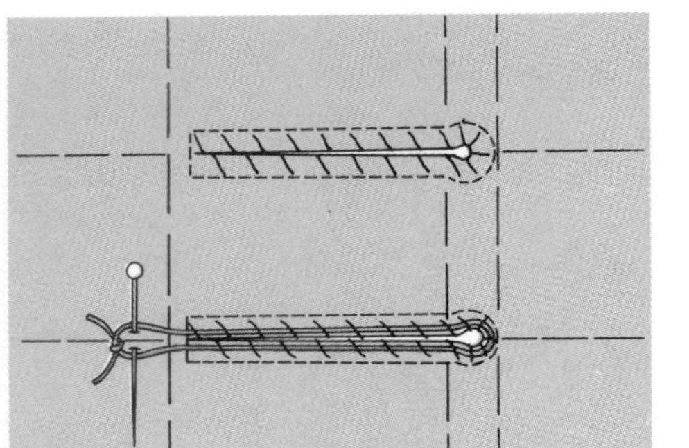

2. Overcast the edges of the slash by hand. If the buttonhole is to be corded, cut a length of cord and knot it to fit loosely around the buttonhole. Place the cord around the buttonhole so that the knot is at the end that will be bar-tacked; secure with pins. Overcast as above, enclosing the cord in the stitching.

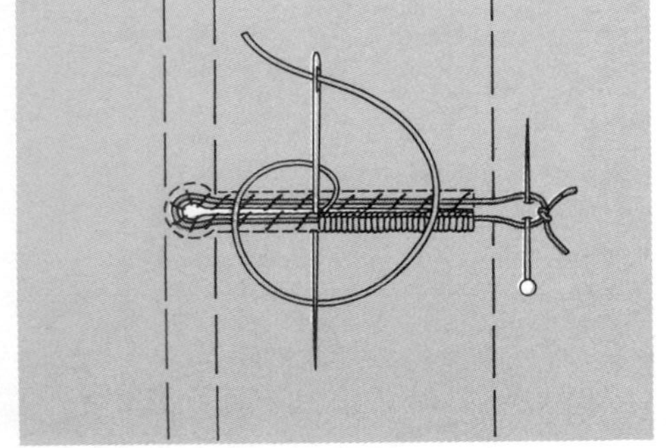

3. Work the buttonhole stitches with the keyhole opening at the left when work begins. Use the machine stitching as a guide for stitch depth. For each stitch, be sure thread from the needle eye goes around and under needle point. To form a purl on the edge, draw the needle straight up. Place stitches close together so that the edge is covered with purls.

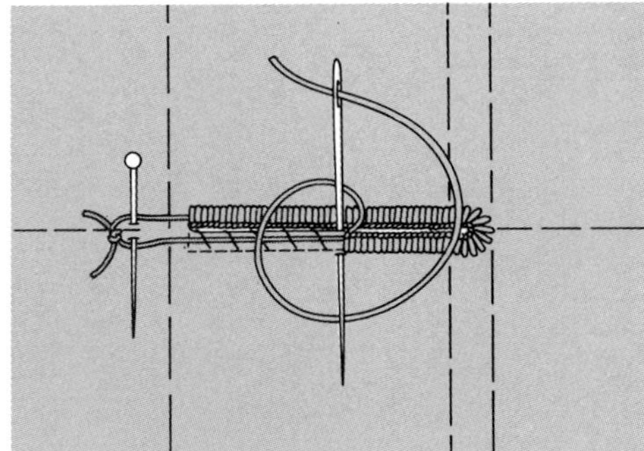

4. Continue the buttonhole stitches around the keyhole, keeping the purls close together along the edge. To form a smooth line, the stitches may have to be fanned slightly apart around the curve. Turn the buttonhole as work progresses and cover cut edge completely with buttonhole stitches.

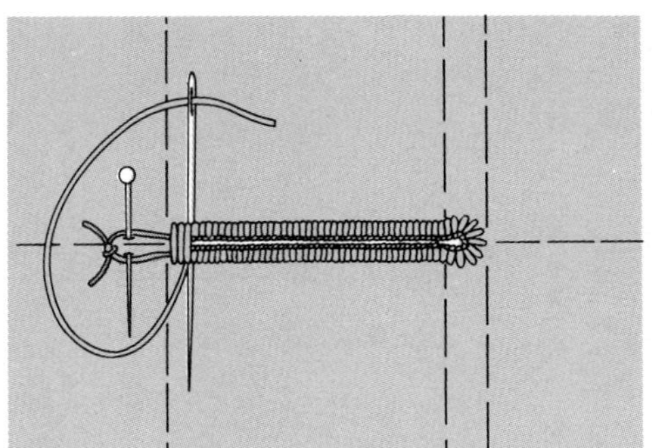

5. To make a bar tack at the unfinished end, take several long stitches across the end to equal the combined width of the rows of buttonhole stitches. Work blanket stitches across these long stitches, catching in fabric underneath, and keeping thread from previous stitch under the point of the needle with each new stitch.

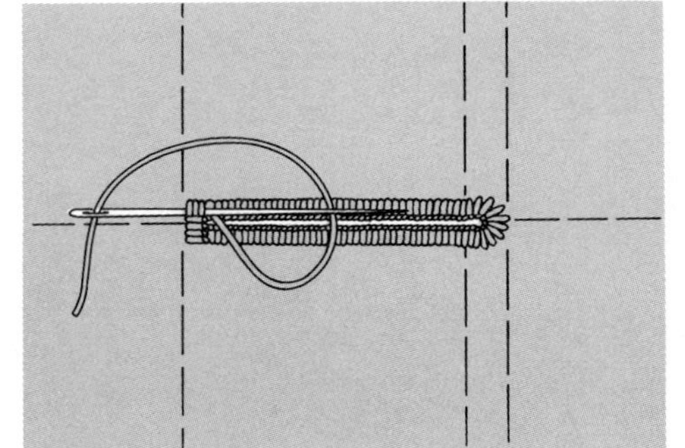

6. Cover long stitches completely with blanket stitches. When finished, fasten the thread on the underside. Pull slightly on the tied ends of the cording so the buttonhole looks smooth and taut. Tie a new knot if necessary. Cut off excess cord and tuck knot into bar tack.

Fabric closures

Cable cord 16
Slipstitch (uneven) 132
Whipstitch 136
Cutting bias strips 298-299

Button loops

Button loops can often be substituted for buttonholes, provided loops are compatible with the overall styling of the garment. They are particularly useful for fabrics such as lace, where handling should be kept to a minimum. Although any type of button can be used, ball buttons fit best.

Button loops may be set into the seam at the opening edge of the garment, or they may be part of an intricate, decorative shape called a frog, which is sewed in place on the outside of the finished garment. Frogs are most frequently used in pairs, with one frog containing the button loop and the frog opposite sewed under the button, which is usually the Chinese ball type.

Because loops go at the edge of the garment, the pattern may need some slight adjustment before the fabric is cut. First, cut the side of the garment to which the buttons will be sewed according to the pattern. Then mark the center line of the side to which the loops will be sewed, add ⅝ inch for a seam allowance, and draw a new cutting line at this spot. Adjust the facing in the same way. (This adjustment eliminates any overlap.)

Always make a test loop to see how the fabric works into tubing, and to determine the proper size for the loop. Sew a button onto a scrap of fabric to be sure that the loop will slip easily but also fit snugly over the button, which it must if it is to hold the garment edges securely closed. Also check the diameter of the tubing to see whether it is suitable to the button size.

Frog closure

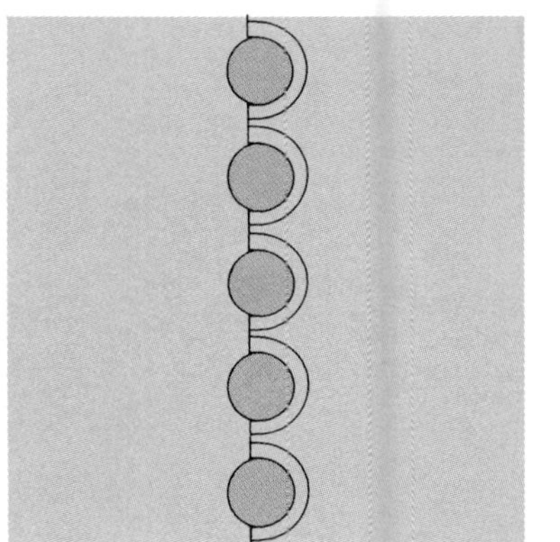

Button loop closure

How to make tubing

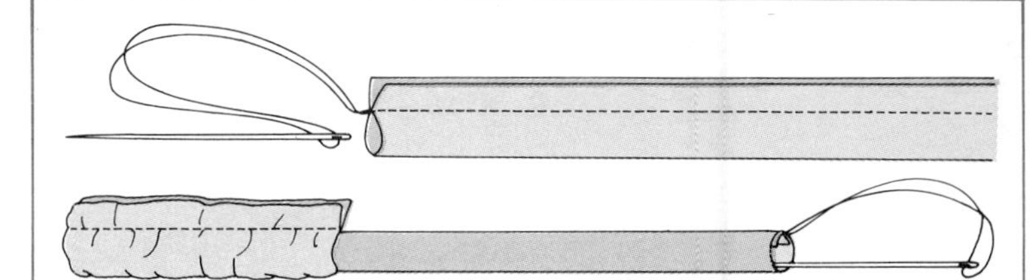

Self-filled tubing: Cut true bias strips 1⅛″ wide; fold in half lengthwise, right sides together. Stitch ¼″ from fold, stretching bias slightly; do not trim seam allowances. Thread a bodkin or large needle with several inches of heavy-duty thread. Fasten thread at seam at one end of tubing, then insert needle, eye first, into tube and work it through to other end. Gradually turn all the tubing to the right side. This can be accomplished by pulling on thread and feeding seam allowances into tube.

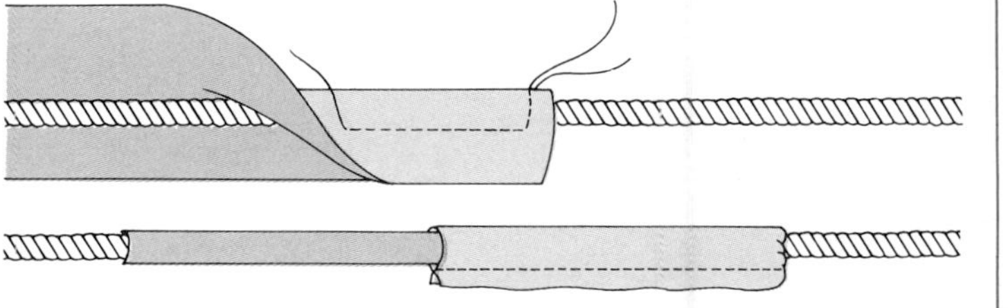

Corded tubing: Cut a length of bias equal in width to the diameter of cord being used plus 1″. Cut cord twice as long as bias. Fold the fabric around one half of the length of the cord, right sides together. Using a zipper foot, stitch across end of bias that is at center of cording, then stitch down long edge close to cord, stretching bias slightly. Trim seam allowances. To turn right side out, simply draw enclosed cord out of tube; free end will go into tube automatically. Trim off excess cord, including stitched end.

How to make frogs

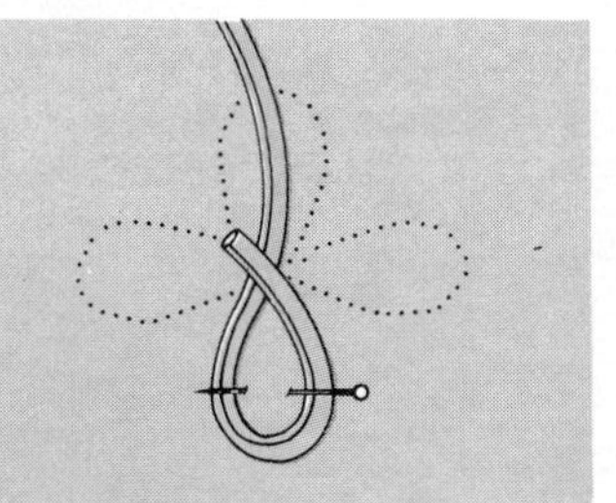

Draw the design for frog on paper. Place end of tubing at center of the design, leaving a ¼″ end.

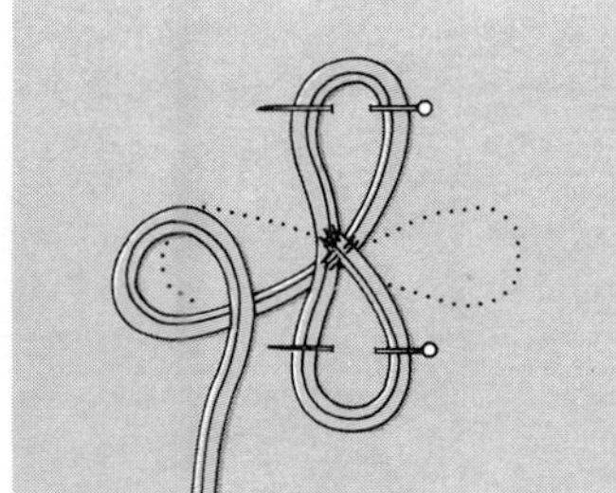

Pin tubing to paper, following design and keeping seam up. Conceal first end on wrong side of frog.

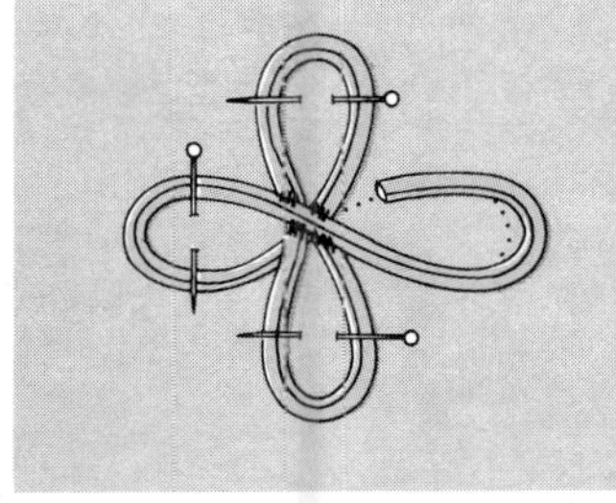

Whipstitch crossings securely, making sure that stitches and ends do not show on right side.

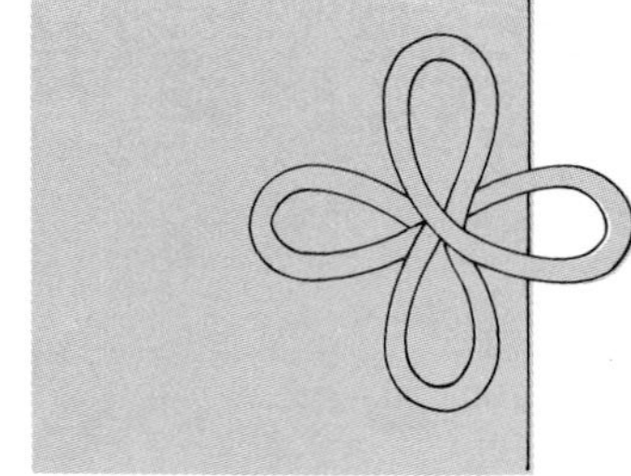

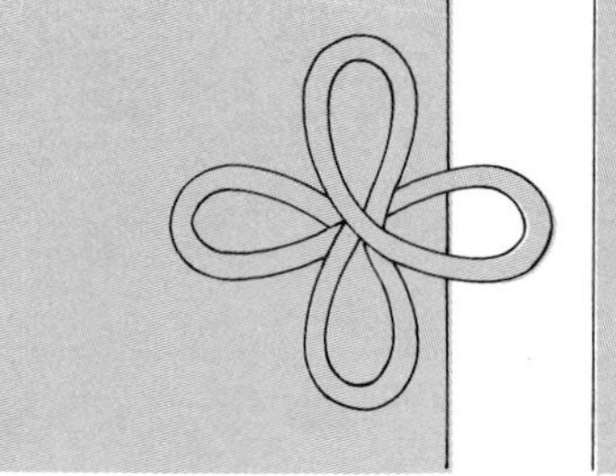

Remove frog from paper and place it face up on garment with button loop extending over the edge. Then

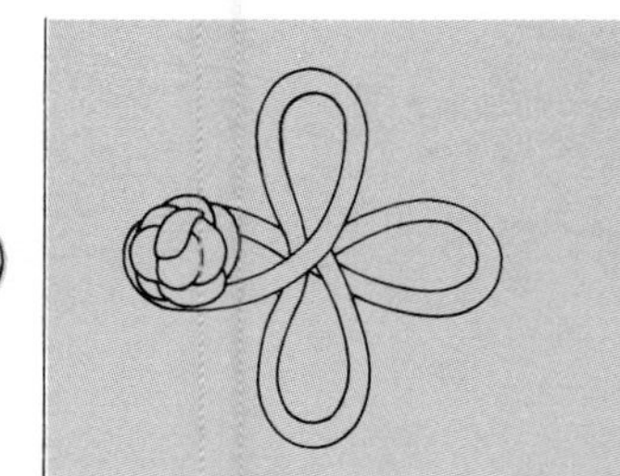

slipstitch to garment from underside. Make another frog for button and attach at button position.

Feed-related machine accessories 39
Understitching 147
Positioning buttonholes 331

How to make button loops

Button loops are used on cuffs of sleeves, as well as at the front or back of blouses and dresses as the main garment closing. Button loops with pearl buttons are the traditional closure for brides' dresses. Though loops are most often made of self-fabric tubing, soutache braid can be used instead.

If you are substituting button loops for some other type of closure, be certain to adjust your pattern as instructed on the preceding page. In addition to adjusting the pattern, you will need to make a diagram to establish the spacing and size of the button loops. This is explained in detail in the step-by-step instructions.

When making your paper diagram, you must decide whether the button loops will be applied individually or in a continuous row. The choice depends on fabric weight and desired spacing. Use single loops when the buttons are large, or if the loops are to be spaced some distance apart. Continuous loops are advisable when buttons are small. The smaller the button, the closer together they should be to close the garment effectively.

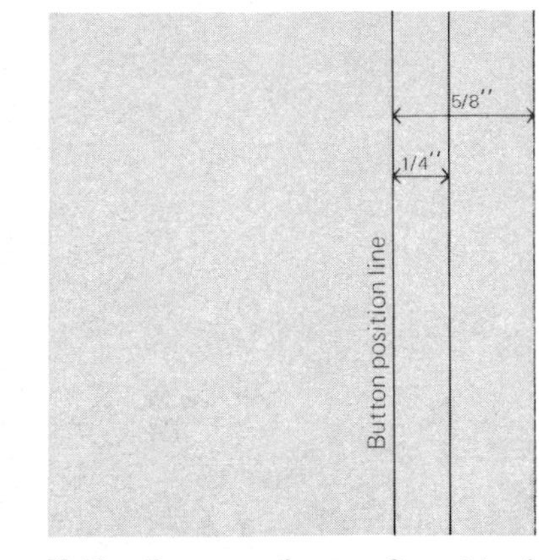

Making the paper diagram: On a strip of paper, draw a line ⅝″ from the edge to represent the button position line (the line on which the buttons will be sewed). Draw a second line ¼″ from the first, into the seam allowance. This is where the ends of each loop should be placed for either application.

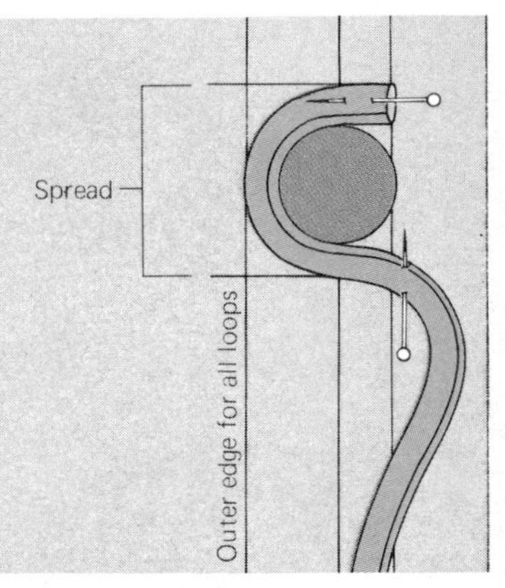

Place the exact center of the button on position line and lay the tubing around it, with seam side up. Pin the end of the tubing at the ¼″ line, then pin again below the button where tubing meets the ¼″ line. Mark at edge of tubing above and below the button; this is the *spread* (top-to-bottom spacing). Mark outer edge.

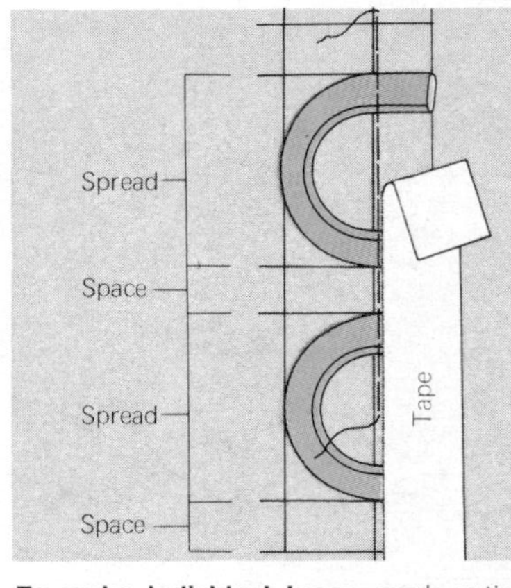

To make individual loops, mark entire length of placket, indicating spread of each loop and space between loops. Place tubing on guide and mark it at both places where it crosses ¼″ line to determine tubing length needed for each loop. Position loops on guide; tape in place. Machine-baste.

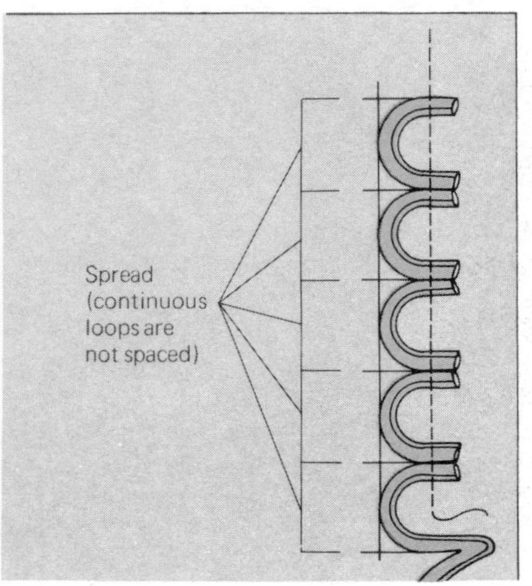

For continuous loops, determine loop size as with individual loops; prepare a paper guide marked with seamline and lines for loop formation. (Omit the spaces between the loops.) Place tubing on paper guide, turning it at ¼″ marks in seam allowance. Trim or clip at turns so the loops lie flat and close together. Tape loops in place, then machine-baste.

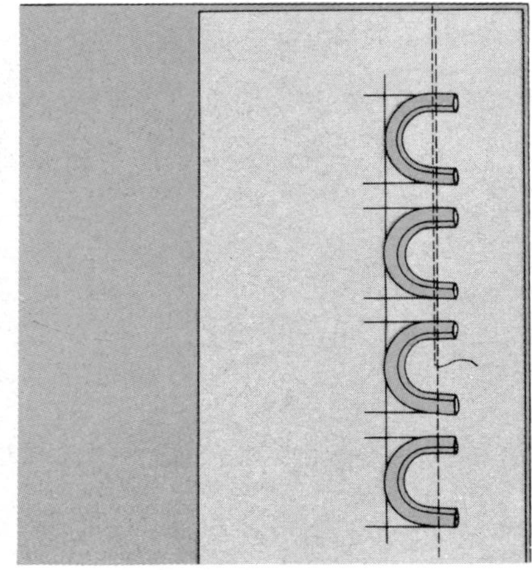

To attach loops of either type to garment, pin paper guide to appropriate side of garment on right side of fabric, matching ⅝″ line to seamline of garment. Remove tape and machine-baste next to first machine-basted line. Stitch carefully, making certain that the machine goes over the tubing without skipping. Then carefully tear the paper away.

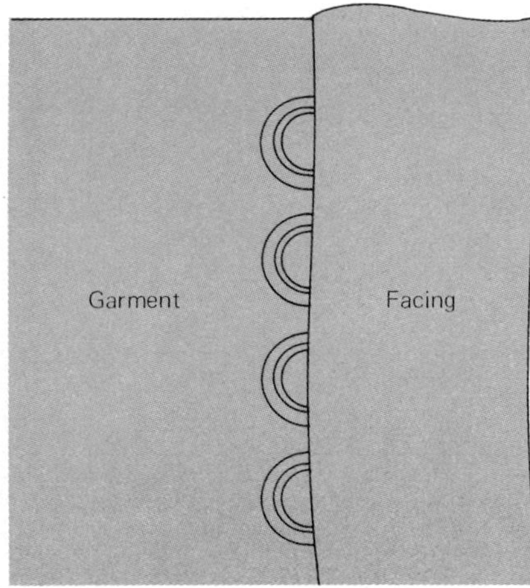

Pin and baste facing to garment, right sides together. Loops will be between facing and garment. Then, from garment side (so you can use the previous stitching as a guide), stitch on the seamline. This will conceal previous rows of basting. If your sewing machine has a "top feed" assist, it is helpful to use it. Grade seam allowances; turn facing to inside.

Trim and grade seam allowances. Fold the facing to the inside along seamline. Understitch, then press. Loops will extend beyond the garment edge. Lap this side of garment over opposite side, carefully matching *finished* edge to the button position line on the button side. Mark button locations, then sew buttons to garment at the correct positions.

Attaching buttons

Thread chart 10
Beeswax 13
Buttons 15
Positioning buttonholes 331

Button placement

Button position should be marked when the garment is nearly completed and after the buttonholes or button loops are made. Although button position line should be marked at the beginning of construction and button location can be tentatively marked, the location should be finally determined when buttonholes are finished. Lap buttonhole side of garment over button side as garment will be worn, matching center front or center back lines; pin securely between buttonholes.

For *horizontal* buttonholes, place a pin through buttonhole opening, ⅛ inch from the end that is nearest the finished garment edge, into fabric beneath. For *vertical* buttonholes, button should be positioned ⅛ inch below the top of the buttonhole opening. Carefully lift buttonhole over pin and refasten the pin securely at the proper location. Center button at pin mark, directly on center line, and sew in place according to the type of button you are using. Be especially careful in double-breasted garments that layers are completely smooth and flat before positioning pins.

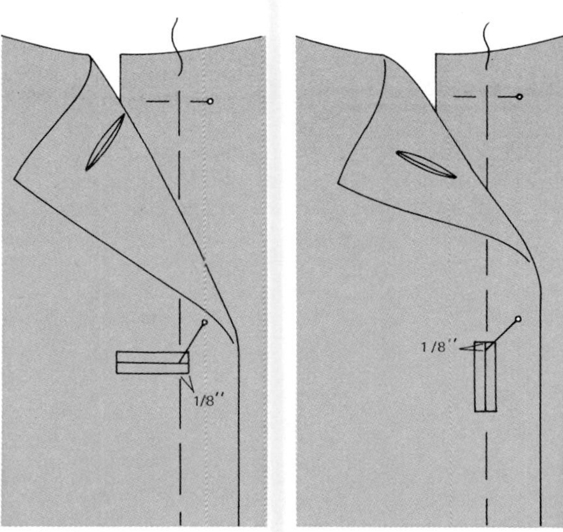

To establish button position, first lap garment sections with buttonholes on top and match up center lines. Push a pin through buttonhole ⅛" from end to locate place for button.

Thread/needle choices

Buttons can be attached with any of several thread types, depending on the weight of the fabric. With **fine fabrics,** use silk thread, size A, or a general-purpose sewing thread compatible with the fiber content of the fabric. For **light- to medium-weight fabrics,** use silk buttonhole twist, size D, or a general-purpose thread compatible with the fiber content of the fabric. For all **heavy fabrics,** use silk buttonhole twist, size D, or heavy-duty thread, or button and carpet thread. Thread should match the button in color unless a contrast is wanted for its effect with sew-through buttons.

A single strand of thread is generally the best; double thread has a greater tendency to knot. Waxing with beeswax will strengthen thread and smooth its "glide" through the fabric (especially recommended for silk twist). To wax thread, pass it across beeswax through slots in the container.

Your needle should be long enough to reach easily through the several thicknesses of button and fabric, but the diameter should not be greater than the holes in the button.

Shank buttons

There are two basic types of buttons, shank buttons and sew-through buttons. Shank buttons are those that have a little "neck," or shank, with a hole in it, on the lower side. The shank allows the button to rest on top of the buttonhole instead of crowding to the inside and distorting the buttonhole. The shank button is especially recommended for closures in heavy and bulky fabrics. If garment fabric is very bulky, as in a coat, it may be necessary to make an additional shank of thread below the regular shank to allow enough space for the buttonhole to fit under the button.

To sew a shank button onto fabric that is not very thick, take enough small stitches through fabric and shank to make the button secure. Position the button so that threads are parallel to the opening edge and the shank aligns with the buttonhole. This will keep the shank from spreading the buttonhole open. Fasten the thread between garment and facing with several stitches. Buttons used only as decoration are also sewed this way.

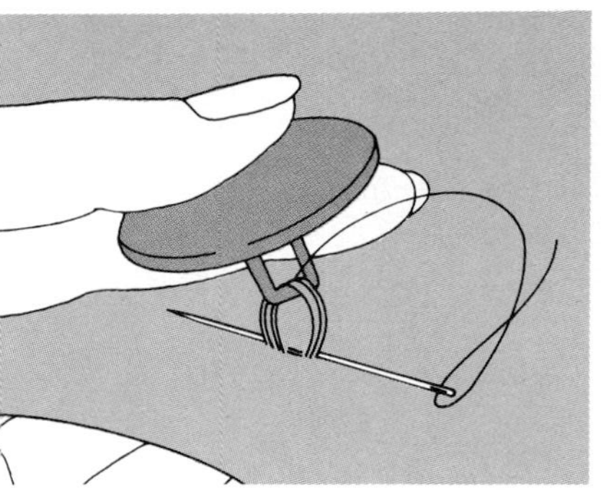
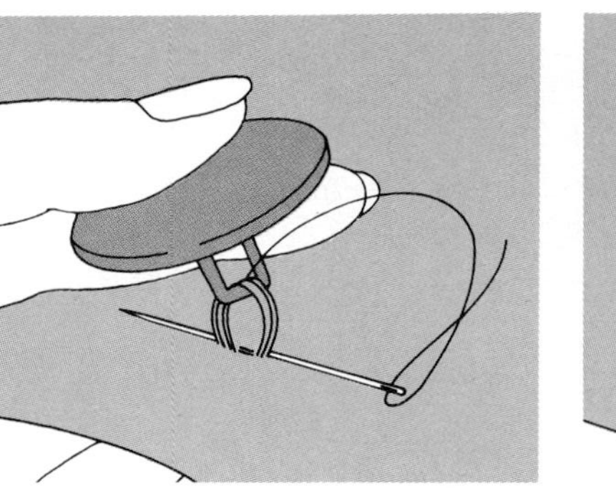

To make an additional thread shank, first take a few stitches where button is to be placed on the garment's right side. Holding forefinger between button and garment (this keeps the two apart until the button is secure), bring thread several times through shank and back into fabric. On last stitch, bring thread through button only, then wind thread tightly around stitches to form thread shank. Fasten securely on underside.

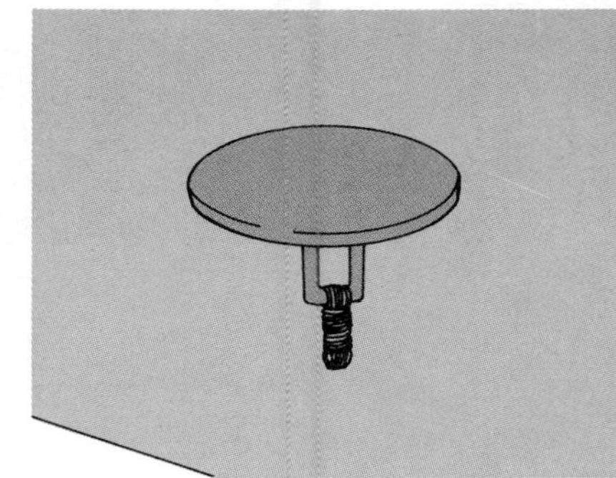

Attaching buttons

Buttons 15 Machine attachments 38
Eyelets 252

Sew-through buttons

A sew-through button has either two or four holes through which the button is sewed to the garment. When sewed flat, this button can be used as a closure only for very thin, lightweight fabrics, or as a decorative button. If a thread shank is added, the button can be used to close heavy or bulky fabrics as well. The shank permits the closure to fasten smoothly and will keep the fabric from pulling unevenly around the buttons. The shank length should equal the garment thickness at the buttonhole plus ⅛ inch for movement.

Buttons with four holes can be sewed on in a number of interesting ways. Use thread in a color that contrasts with the button and treat the four holes as a grid for different arrangements of stitches. The thread can be worked through the holes to form a cross, a square, a feather or leaf shape, or two parallel lines.

If the holes are large enough, a button can be attached with narrow ribbon, braid, or cord. (This may require an eyelet to be worked in the garment.) Run the ribbon or braid through the holes in the button and tie it in a secure knot on the wrong side of the garment or on top of the button.

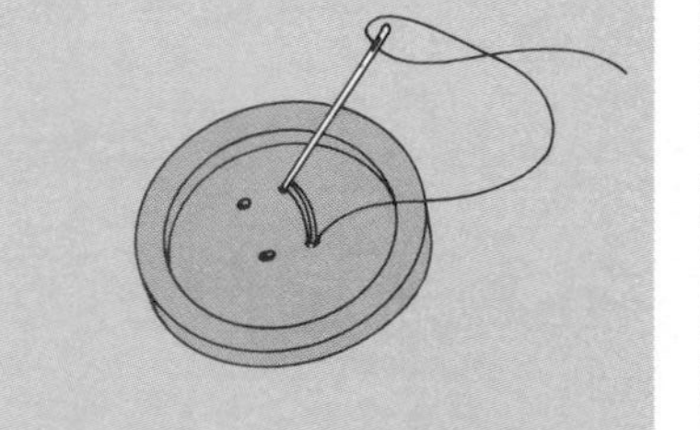

To sew button flat to a garment, take several small stitches at mark for the button location, then center button over marking and sew in place through holes in button. Fasten stitches on wrong side or between garment and facing.

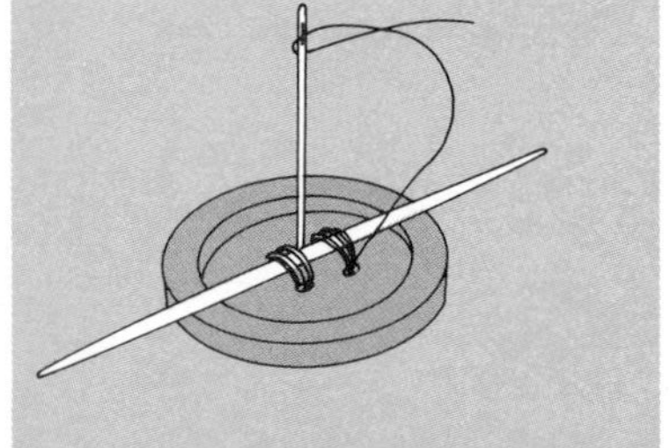

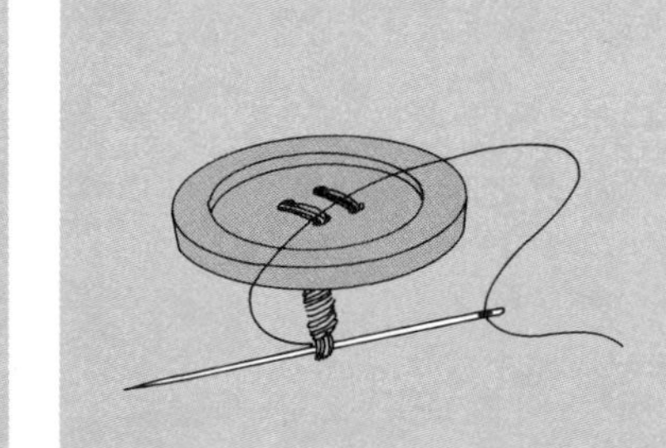

To make a thread shank, secure thread at button mark, then bring needle up through one hole in button. Lay a pin, toothpick, or matchstick across top of button. Take needle down through second hole (and up through third, then down through fourth, if a 4-hole button); make about six stitches. Remove pin or stick, lift button away from fabric so stitches are taut, and wind thread firmly around stitches to make shank. Backstitch into shank to secure.

Another thread shank method

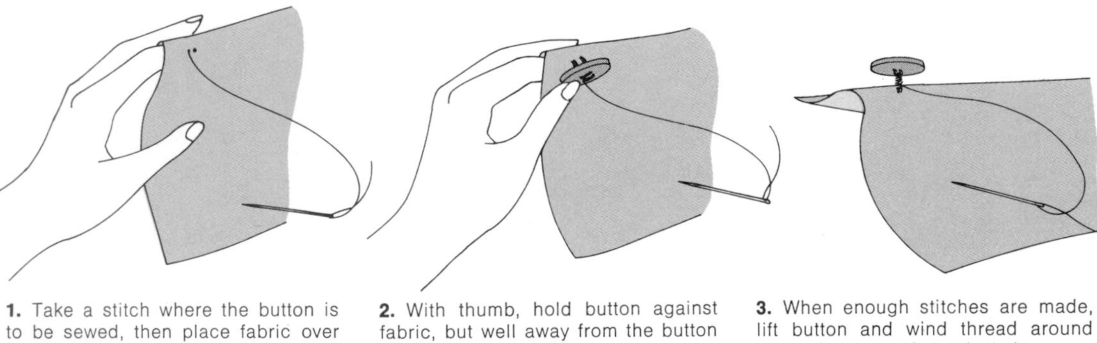

1. Take a stitch where the button is to be sewed, then place fabric over index finger of left hand.

2. With thumb, hold button against fabric, but well away from the button mark, and sew on button.

3. When enough stitches are made, lift button and wind thread around them. Secure with backstitches.

Sewing on buttons by machine

A zigzag sewing machine can be used to sew on sew-through buttons. Check machine booklet for exact instructions. A four-hole button may have to be sewed with two separate stitchings.

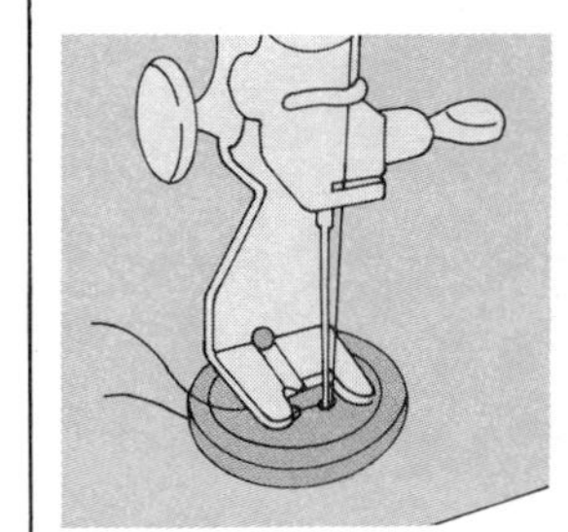

A special button foot is included in many machine accessory boxes. It holds the button in place while the needle stitches from side to side. Stitch width must equal the space between the holes in the button. Some experimentation will be necessary with each new style of button.

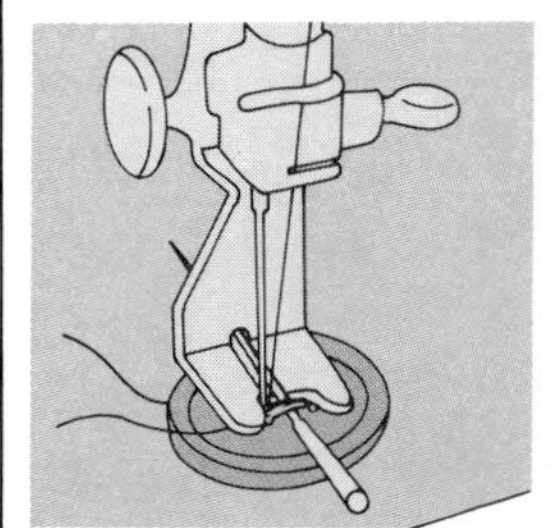

If a shank is desired with a machine-sewed button, a machine needle is pushed into a special groove in the foot; the stitches then pass over the shaft of this needle. The length of the shank is determined by the thickness of the shaft of the needle under the stitching. The thicker the shaft, the longer the shank.

Reinforcing buttons

Reinforcing buttons are useful at points of great strain and on garments of heavy materials. By taking the stress that would otherwise be on the fabric, they keep top buttons from tearing it.

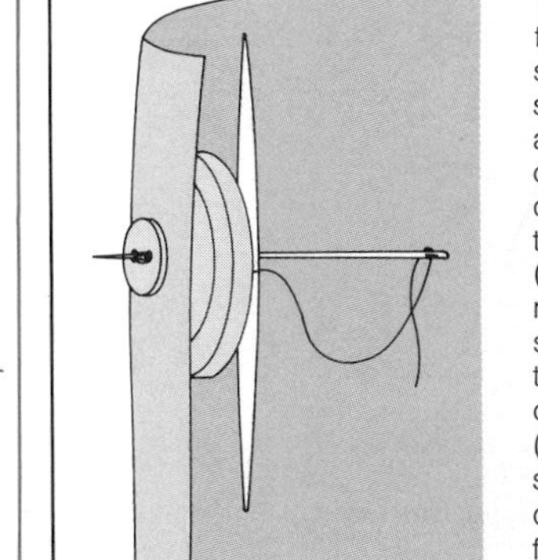

To add a reinforcing button, follow steps for attaching a sew-through button with a shank, additionally placing a small flat button on inside of garment directly under outer button. Sew as usual through all sets of holes (buttons should have same number of holes). On last stitch, bring needle through hole of top button only and complete shank. (If fabric is delicate, substitute a doubled square of fabric or seam binding for the small button.)

Making buttons

Thread chart 10
Buttons 15

Hand backstitch 123
Running stitch 131

Fabric buttons

Fabric buttons made to match the garment are the answer when suitable ready-made buttons cannot be found. Full instructions come with each of the many kits available for making covered fabric buttons. Covered buttons can also be made using plastic or bone rings, sold at notions counters.

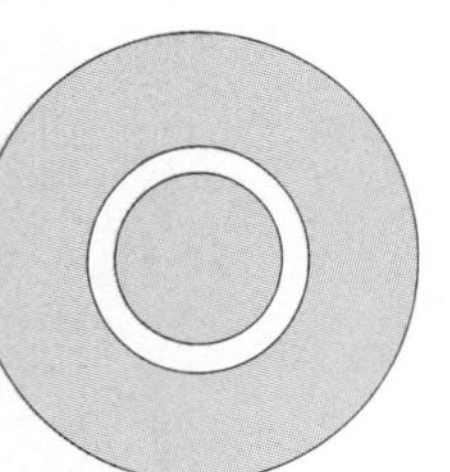

1. Select a ring of the diameter required for the finished button. Cut a circle of fabric slightly less than twice the diameter of ring.

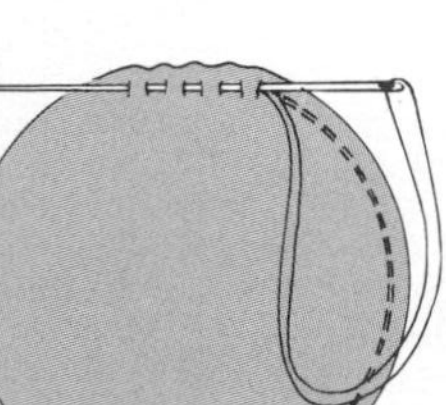

2. Using a double thread, sew around fabric circle with a small running stitch, placing stitches close to the edge. Leave thread and needle attached to fabric at the end of stitching.

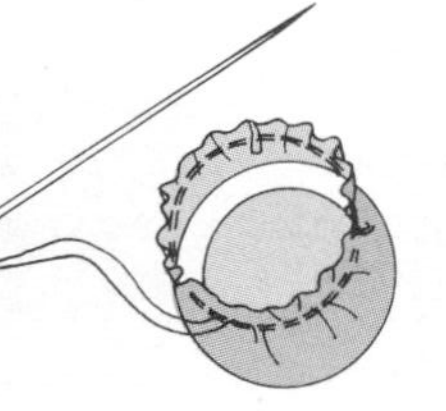

3. Place the ring in the center of fabric circle. Gather fabric around the ring by pulling on the needle and thread until the hand stitches bring the cut edges of fabric together.

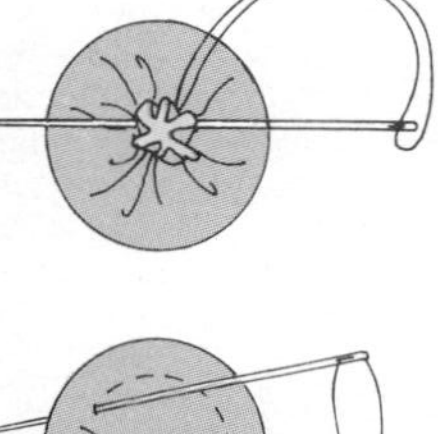

4. Secure gathered-up fabric around ring by pulling up hand stitches tightly. Fasten with several short backstitches.

5. Decorate button by taking small backstitches around and close to ring, through both fabric layers. Use buttonhole twist. Attach button to garment with a thread shank.

Leather buttons

Leather buttons can be made at home using commercial cover-your-own kits. The easiest forms to cover are those with prongs all around the inside of the rim. Almost any type of leather, even fairly thick ones, can be used. This is a practical place to use small scraps and remnants.

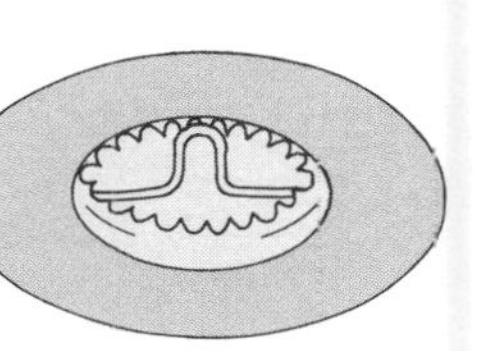

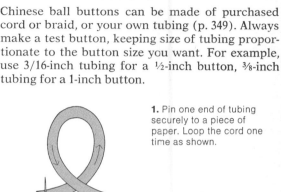

1. Use pattern in kit to cut a circle of leather for each button.

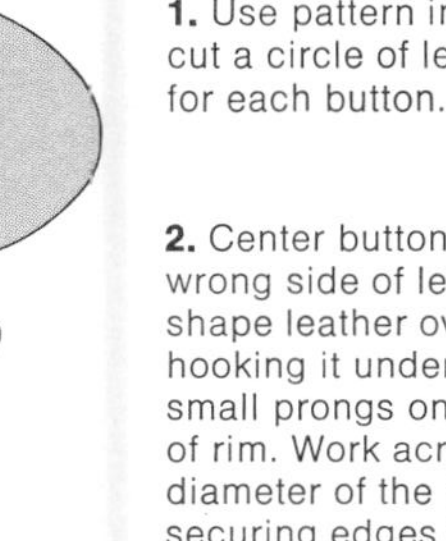

2. Center button front on wrong side of leather; shape leather over button, hooking it underneath small prongs on inside of rim. Work across the diameter of the button, securing edges that are opposite one another.

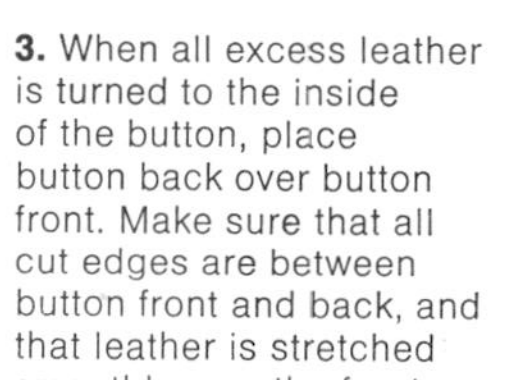

3. When all excess leather is turned to the inside of the button, place button back over button front. Make sure that all cut edges are between button front and back, and that leather is stretched smoothly over the front.

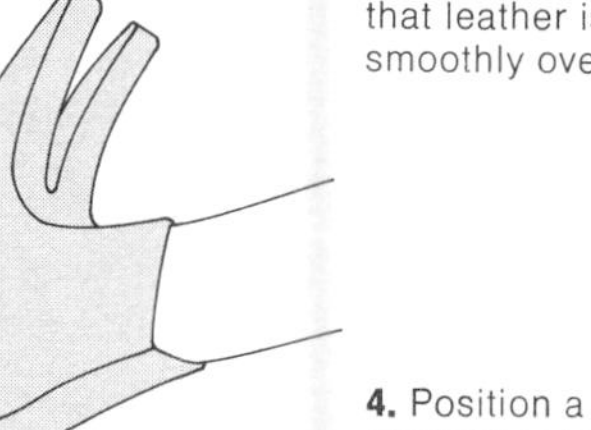

4. Position a thread spool over the button back, with shank of button in hollow center of spool. Rap the spool sharply with a hammer to force button back into place. This will flatten the button, and should lock the back permanently in place. If back is not secure, rap it again, using spool and hammer as before.

Chinese ball buttons

Chinese ball buttons can be made of purchased cord or braid, or your own tubing (p. 349). Always make a test button, keeping size of tubing proportionate to the button size you want. For example, use 3/16-inch tubing for a ½-inch button, ⅜-inch tubing for a 1-inch button.

1. Pin one end of tubing securely to a piece of paper. Loop the cord one time as shown.

2. Loop a second time over first loop, then go under end. Keep seam of tubing down at all times as you work.

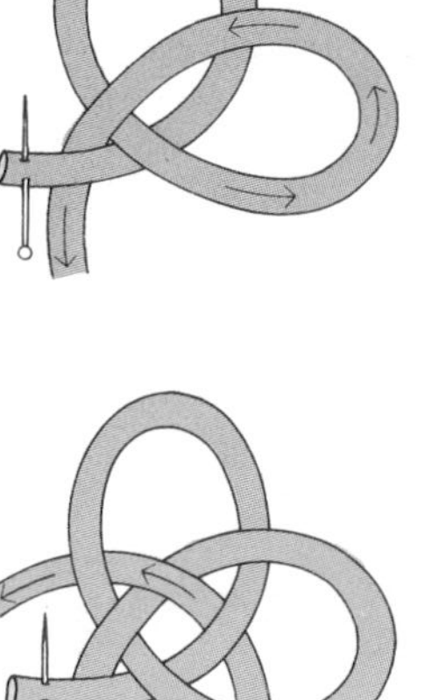

3. Loop a third time, weaving through previous two loops. Take care tubing does not become twisted at any point in either looping or weaving.

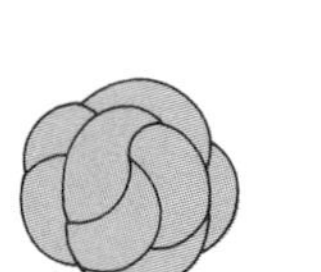

4. Gradually tighten up on loops, easing them into a ball shape. Trim the ends of the tubing and sew them flat to the underside of the button.

Hooks and eyes

Hooks and eyes 15 Blanket stitch 125 Whipstitch 136

Types and uses

Hooks and eyes are small but comparatively strong fasteners. Though they are most often applied at single points of a garment opening, such as a waistband or neckline, they can also be used to fasten an entire opening.

There are several types of hooks and eyes, each designed to serve a particular purpose. General-purpose hooks and eyes are the smallest of all the types and are used primarily as supplemental fasteners; a familiar example is the hook and eye at the top of a zipper placket. This type ranges in size from fine (0) to heavy (3); finishes are either black or nickel. Special-purpose hooks and eyes are larger and heavier, and so can withstand more strain than those of the general-purpose type. Included in this group are plain and covered hooks and eyes for use on coats and jackets. The covered ones are advisable where a less conspicuous application is desired. The covered fasteners can be bought ready-made, or standard hooks and eyes can be covered with blanket stitches as shown and explained below, right. Another special-purpose type is the waistband hook and eye, different in form from all the other types, but also made with either a black or nickel finish.

Two eye shapes are made for most hook types, the purpose being to accommodate both lapped and abutted garment openings. The *straight eye* is intended for use on lapped edges; the *round eye* for those that are abutted. An exception is the special-purpose hook and eye designed for waistband use. The eye in this case is always straight, because the fastener will be used only on a lapped edge.

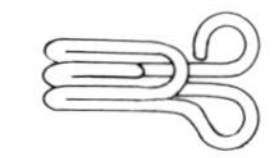
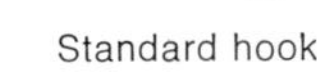
Standard hook

Straight eye

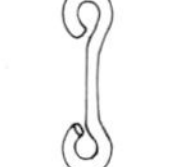
Round eye

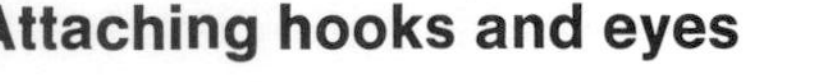

Attaching hooks and eyes

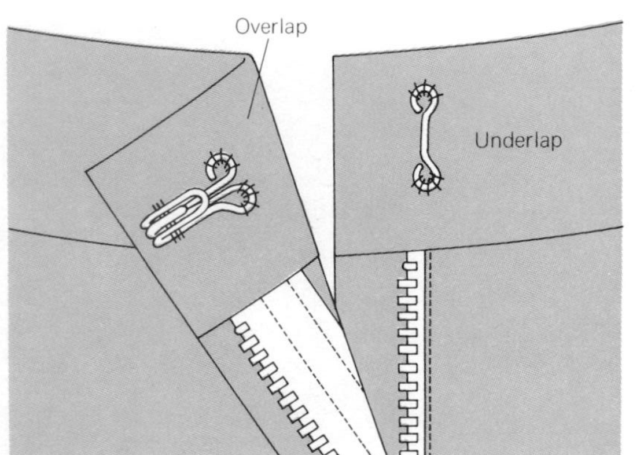

With lapped edges, the hook is sewed on the inside of the garment, the eye on the outside. Place *hook* on the underside of overlap, about ⅛" from the edge. Whipstitch over each hole. Pass needle and thread through fabric to end of hook; whipstitch around end to hold it flat against garment.
Mark on the outside of underlap where the end of the hook falls—this is the position for the eye. Hold *straight eye* in place and whipstitch over one hole. Pass needle and thread through fabric to other hole and whipstitch.

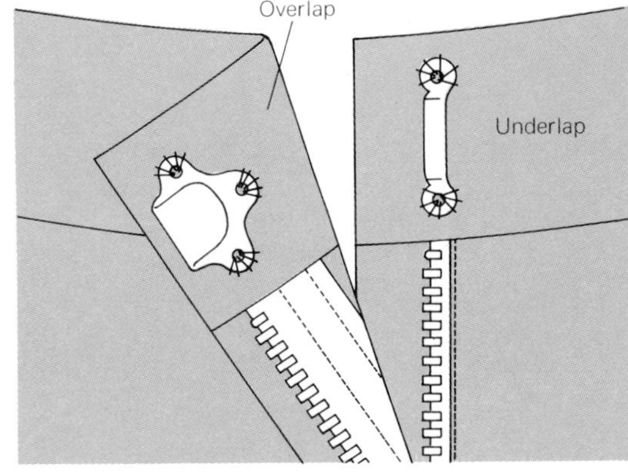

For use on waistbands of skirts or pants, special hook and eye sets are available. They are strong and flat, and designed so the hook cannot easily slide off the eye. They can be used only for lapped edges. Position and sew on the hook and eye as for a lapped application of a standard hook and eye (end of hook need not be secured).

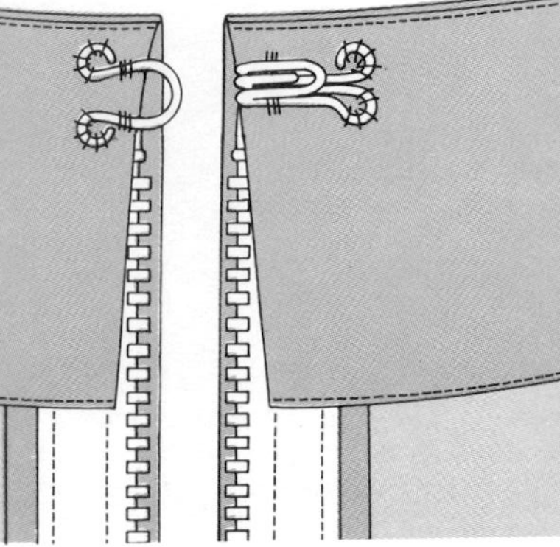

With abutted edges, both the hook and the eye are sewed to the inside of the garment. Position *hook* 1/16" from one of the edges. Whipstitch over both holes. Pass needle and thread through fabric to end of hook; whipstitch over end to hold it flat against garment. Position *round eye* on other edge so that loop extends slightly beyond edge. Whipstitch over both holes. Then pass needle and thread through fabric toward edge and whipstitch both sides of loop to garment.

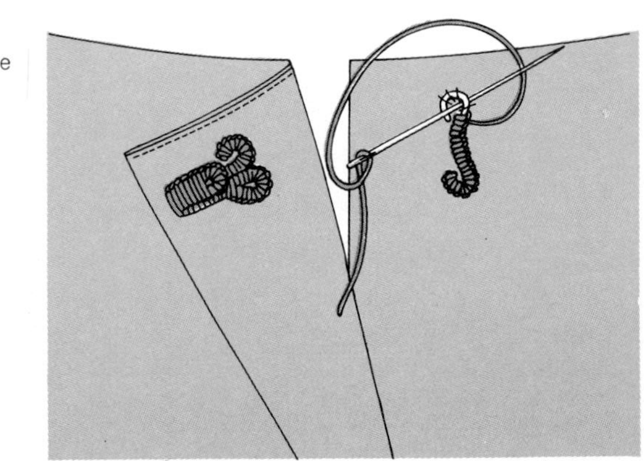

Covered hooks and eyes are used as a fine finishing touch. They can be purchased ready-made but you can cover your own as follows:
Sew a large hook and eye to the garment, by the lapped or the abutted method, whichever is appropriate. Then, using a single strand of silk twist that matches the fabric, cover both hook and eye with closely spaced blanket stitches. Do not catch the fabric between the holes of the eye. Secure the stitches.

Thread eyes

Essentially, a thread eye is a substitute for the metal eye. A thread eye is not as strong, however, as a metal eye and so should not be used at places where there is much strain. There are two ways to form a thread eye: (1) the **blanket stitch method** (the stronger of the two) and (2) the **thread chain method.** For both, use a single strand of heavy-

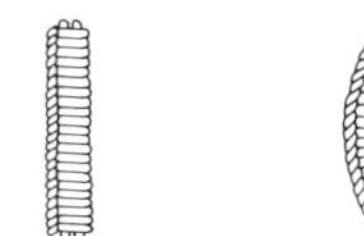

Straight eye   Round eye or loop

duty thread or buttonhole twist color-matched to the fabric. A *straight eye* should be as long as the space between its two placement marks; a *round eye* should be longer than the space between marks, actual length depending on the end use.

These two methods can also be used for forming button loops and belt carriers. For a button loop, the length should be equal to the combined total of button diameter and thickness. A straight belt carrier should be as long as the belt is wide, plus ¼ to ½ inch for ease.

Blanket stitch method

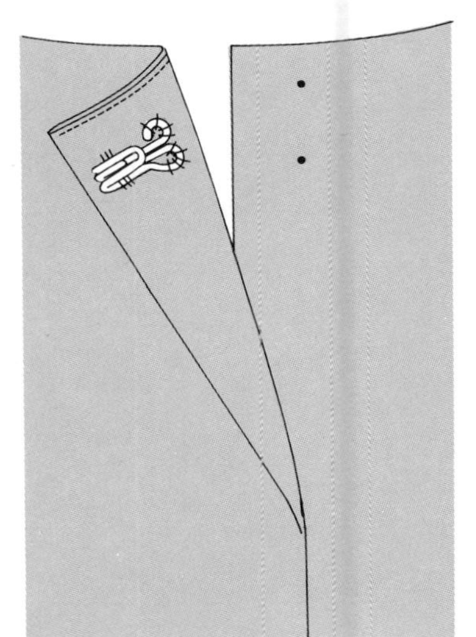

Sew hook to one edge of the garment by either the lapped or abutted method (see opposite page) as required. Close the placket and mark beginning and end positions for eye on other edge.

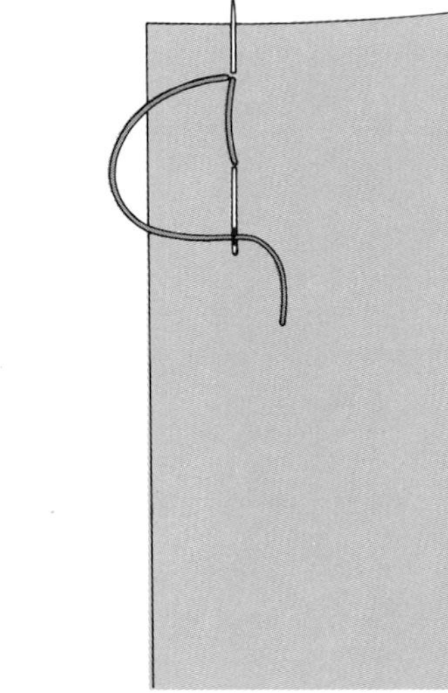

Insert needle into fabric at one mark and bring it up at other mark. Take 2 or 3 more stitches in the same way; secure. (If the eye is round, let the thread curve into the intended size.)

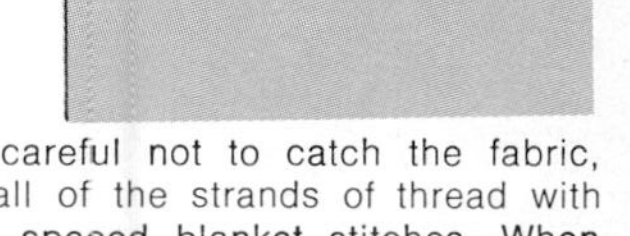

Being careful not to catch the fabric, cover all of the strands of thread with closely spaced blanket stitches. When finished, bring needle and thread to the underside and secure stitching.

Thread chain method

Mark on garment where thread chain will begin and end. Bring needle and thread up through one mark; take a small stitch over this mark, leaving a 4" to 5" loop.

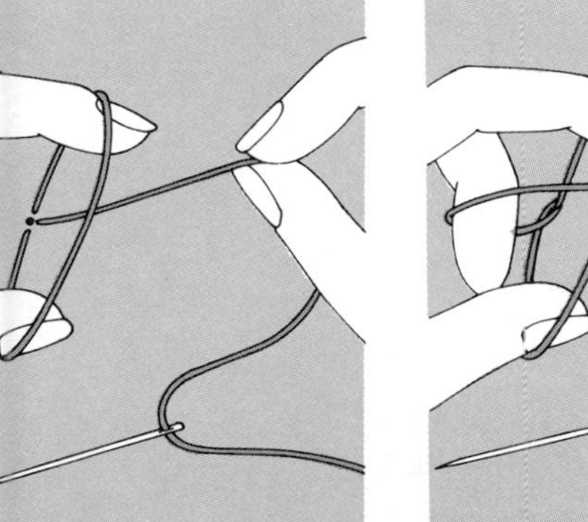

As shown above, hold the loop open with the thumb and index finger of the left hand; hold supply thread taut with the thumb and index finger of the right hand.

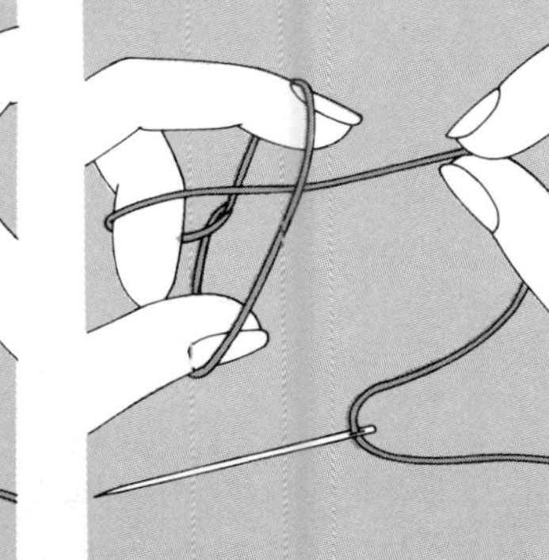

Bring second finger of left hand through loop to grasp the supply thread. Pull supply thread through loop; let loop slide off finger and be drawn down to fabric.

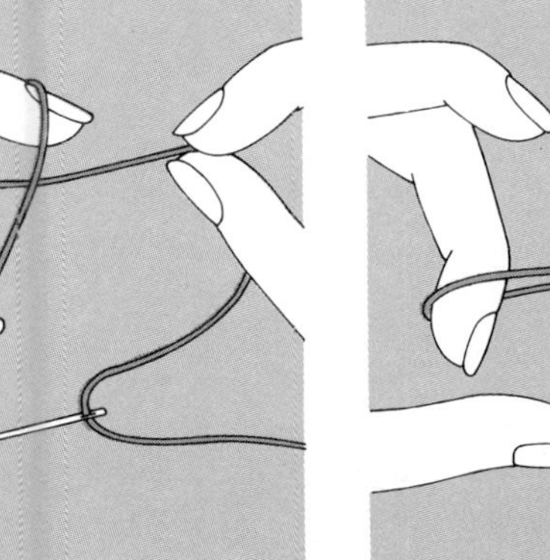

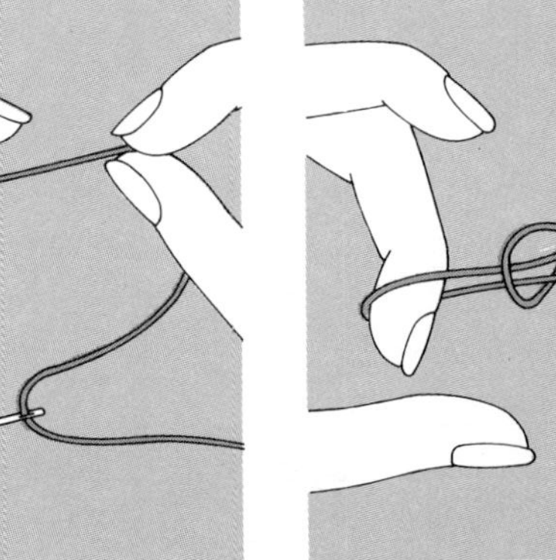

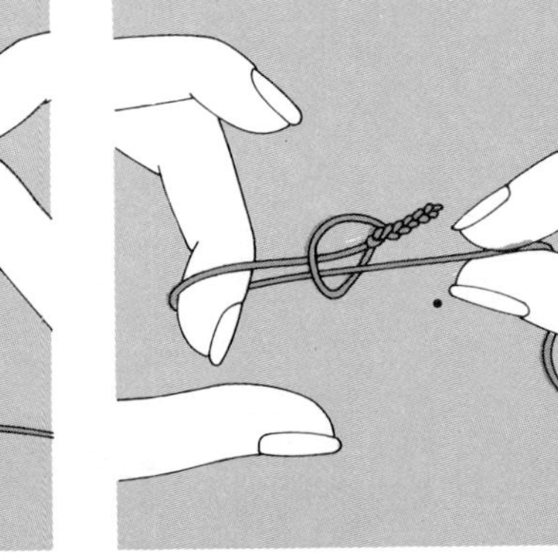

Repeat Steps 2 and 3 until chain is desired length. For straight eye, marked space and chain length are equal; for a loop, chain is longer than space between marks.

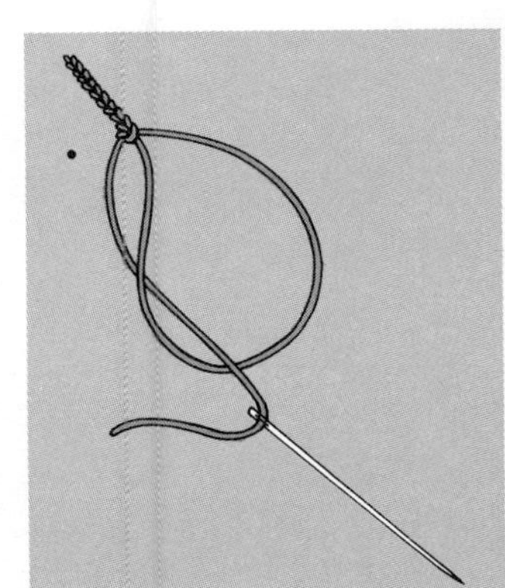

To secure the last loop of chain, pass needle and thread through final loop and pull taut. Fasten the free end of the chain to the garment at the second (end) mark.

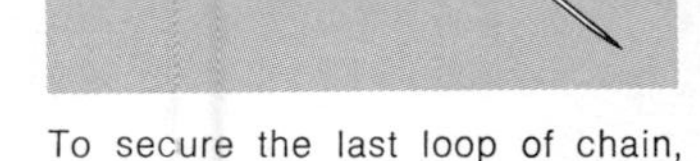

Hooks and eyes

Awl 13
Hooks and eyes 15
Seams in pile fabrics 157
Eyelets 252

Hooks and eyes on fur garments

Large, covered hooks and eyes are sometimes used as fasteners for fur garments. Because of the difficulty of hand-sewing through furs, a special lapped method has been developed for attaching hooks and eyes (see below). The hooks are inserted into the seamline of the overlapping edge, and the ends of the eyes passed through punctures to the underside of the opposite edge. (If the garment edges are abutted, both hooks and eyes can be inserted into the seamlines.)

To facilitate the sewing of hooks and eyes, it is recommended that the garment opening be underlined or interfaced. The seamlines should not be machine-understitched; they can be hand-understitched after hooks and eyes are attached.

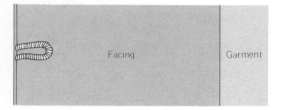

Attaching the hooks

Hooks in fur garments extend out from the seamline of the overlapping garment edge. Before stitching this seam, mark on the seamline the position of each hook. In stitching this seam, leave a ¼" opening at each mark. Then proceed as follows.

1. Working from the wrong side of the garment, open out the facing. With curve of hook toward the facing, insert hook through a ¼" opening and allow curve of hook to wrap around to the right side of the facing.

2. Pass a 3" length of ¼" twill tape under the stem of the hook. Cross the tape ends, then pull on them to bring the stem of the hook to the garment. Pin tape ends to garment and whipstitch in place. Be sure that the hand stitches do not show on the finished side of the garment.

3. Repeat Steps 1 and 2 for each hook. Then secure the facing to the twill tape, using small, close whipstitches.

Attaching the eyes

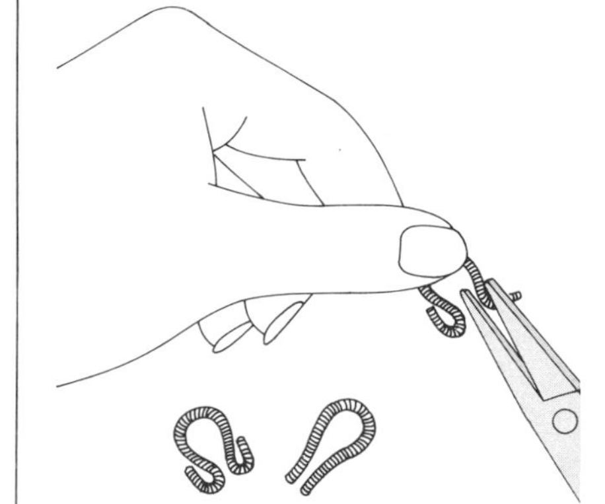

1. Using a long-nose pliers, straighten the ends of each eye. This prepares the ends so they can be passed through to the inside of the garment and then sewed in place.

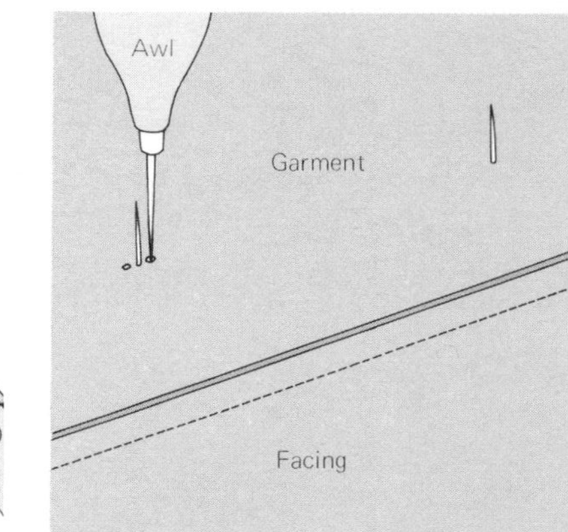

2. Pin-mark position for each eye on the underlap. From garment inside, pierce garment ¼" to each side of each pin. If necessary, hand-finish holes (make eyelets).

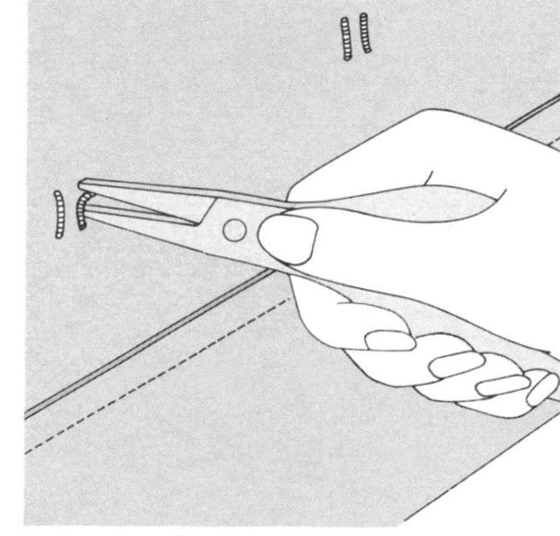

3. Insert ends of each eye into holes until just enough of the eye remains on garment right side for the hook to catch. Using the long-nose pliers, re-shape ends of each eye to form open loops.

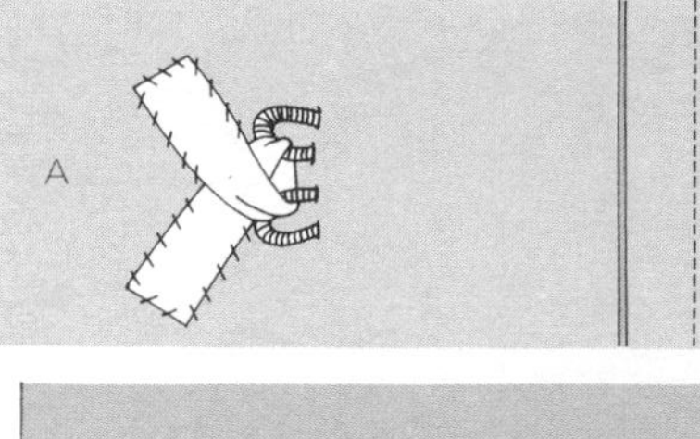

4. Pass a 3" length of ¼" twill tape under the stem of the eye and cross the ends. Pin the tape to the garment and whipstitch in place (A), being sure the stitches do not show on the finished side (B).

Snaps

Snaps 15 Running stitch 131 Whipstitch 136

Basic types and application

Snaps, another kind of small fastener, have less holding power than hooks and eyes. Each snap has two parts—a *ball* half and a *socket* half. General-purpose snaps range in size from fine (4/0) to heavy (4); finishes are either nickel or black (clear nylon snaps are also available). Other snap types are covered snaps and no-sew snaps. Covered snaps can be bought ready-made or you can cover your own. They are intended for use on garments, such as jackets, where it is desirable that the snaps not be apparent when the garment is worn open. No-sew snaps are strong fasteners that are not sewed to the garment, but cleated into the fabric (see package instructions).

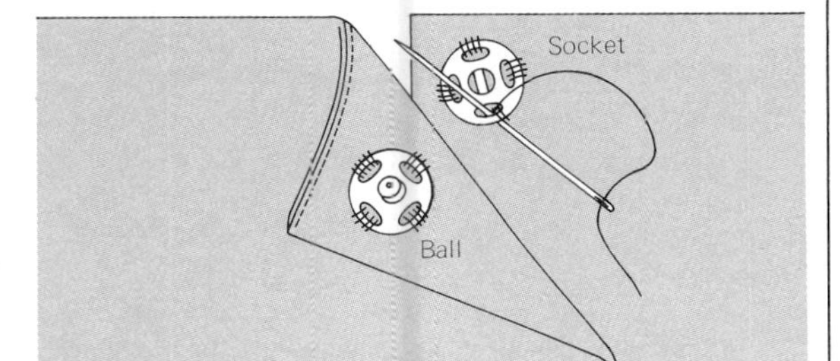

To attach a snap, position ball half on underside of overlap far enough in from edge so it will not show; whipstitch over each hole. Position socket half on right side of underlap to align with ball; whipstitch over each hole.

Special uses and applications

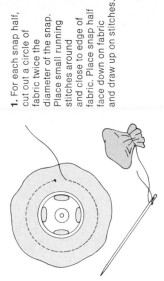

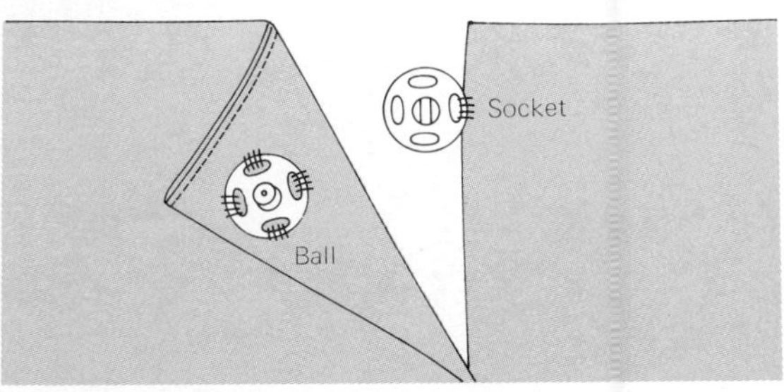

An extended snap is used on garment edges that abut. Attach ball half of snap to underside of one garment edge. Position socket half at the other garment edge; whipstitch over only one of the holes to secure socket to edge.

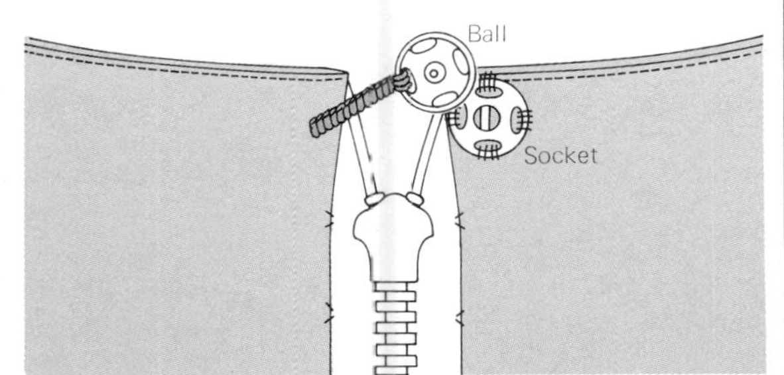

A hanging snap can also be used for garment edges that abut. Attach socket half to underside of one garment edge. To attach the socket half to the other edge, adapt the blanket stitch method for forming a thread eye (p. 355).

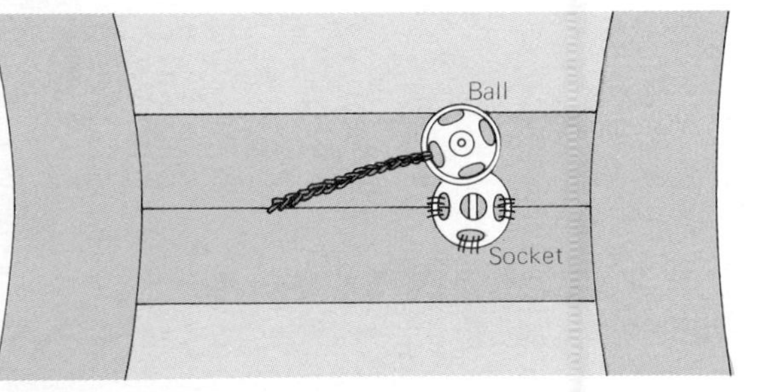

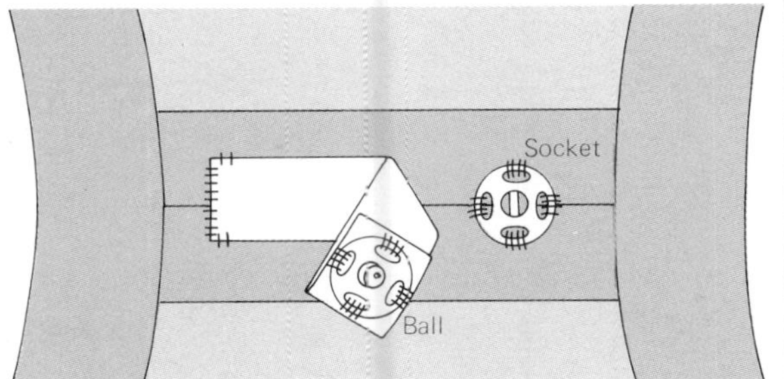

Lingerie strap guards are attached to the underside of a shoulder seam. Sew socket half of snap to seam, ¾″ from center of shoulder, toward neck edge. For a *thread chain guard* (above), start chain in garment about 1½″ from snap socket. Form a 1½″ chain (p. 355). Take a few whipstitches over one hole of ball half of snap; pass needle and thread through chain and fasten in garment. For a *tape guard* (above), use a 2¼″ length of tape. Turn under one end ¼″; whipstitch to garment 1½″ from snap socket. Turn under free end of tape ½″ and sew ball half to underside.

Covering snaps

Fabric-covered snaps can be purchased ready-made or you can cover your own. If making your own, use large snaps and cover them with a lightweight fabric that is color-matched to the garment fabric. Follow covering instructions below, then attach the snap to the garment. To keep fabric from fraying, lightly coat the raw edges with clear nail polish before sewing snap to garment.

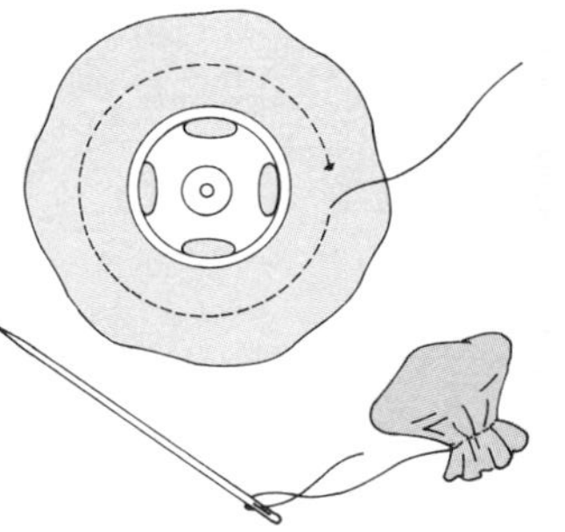

1. For each snap half, cut out a circle of fabric twice the diameter of the snap. Place small running stitches around and close to edge of fabric. Place snap half face down on fabric and draw up on stitches.

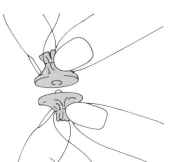

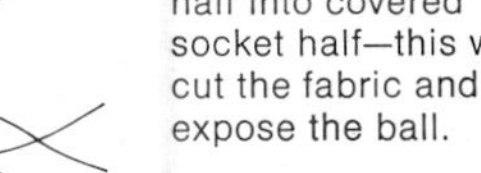

2. Push covered ball half into covered socket half—this will cut the fabric and expose the ball.

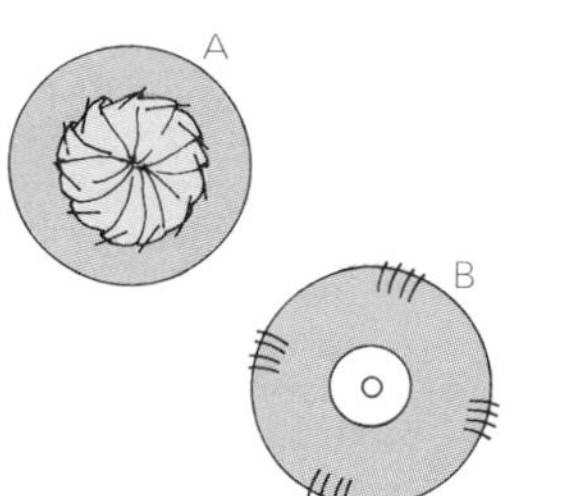

3. Pull snap apart. Draw stitches up tightly and secure. Trim excess fabric on the underside; whipstitch over edges if necessary (A). Attach snap to garment (B).

Tape fasteners

Types and uses

Tape fasteners are made in three types, **snap, hook and eye,** and **nylon.** Tapes are practical fasteners for pillow and slipcovers, for infants' and children's clothing, and for such items as bassinet skirts because they permit easy removal for laundering. Since uses and applications differ so widely, it is difficult to specify exact rules about extra fabric allowances for finishing edges. If a pattern calls for a tape fastener, as those for infants' clothes sometimes do, these allowances will be given. When you must determine for yourself how to cut fabric pieces, as with slipcovers, the fabric allowances become your decision. You must allow, for example, a double seam allowance for the underlap in a lapped application. Top and bottom edges are usually caught into cross seams and need no further finishing. Never let the metal parts of any fastener extend into such seams.

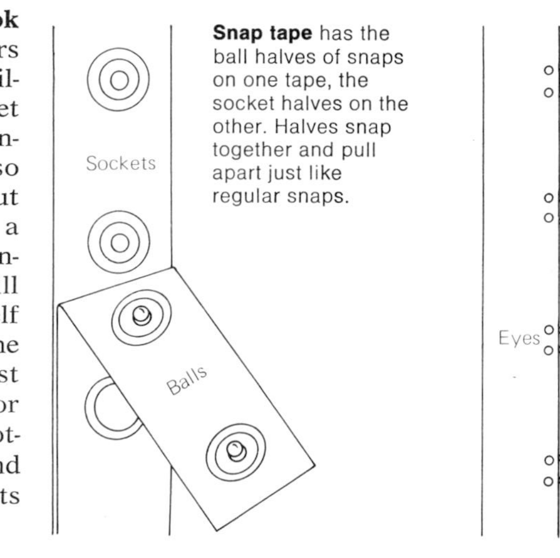

Snap tape has the ball halves of snaps on one tape, the socket halves on the other. Halves snap together and pull apart just like regular snaps.

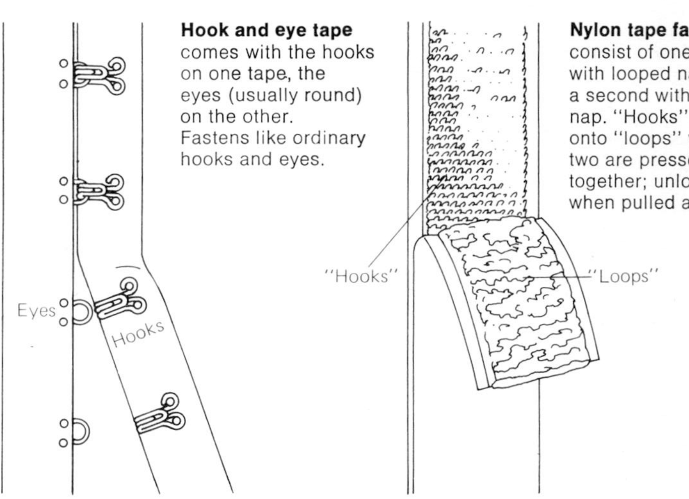

Hook and eye tape comes with the hooks on one tape, the eyes (usually round) on the other. Fastens like ordinary hooks and eyes.

Nylon tape fasteners consist of one tape with looped nap, a second with hooked nap. "Hooks" lock onto "loops" when the two are pressed together; unlock when pulled apart.

Applying tape fasteners

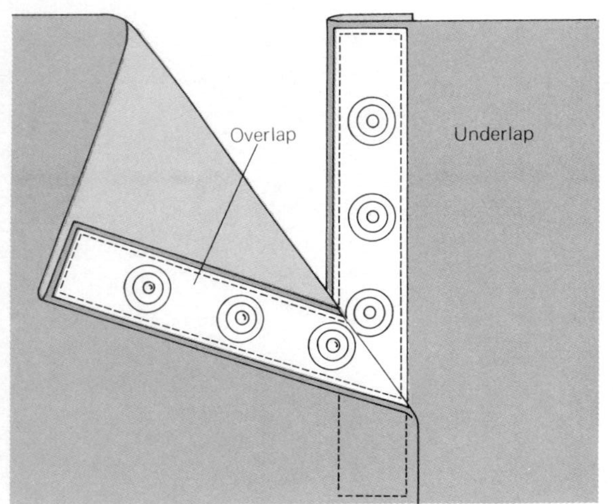

Snap tape requires a lapped application because of the way the ball half must enter the socket half. Both garment edges should be wider than the tapes; for greater strength, cut a double-width seam allowance for the underlap. Position socket tape on underlap and stitch around all edges through all layers. Place ball tape on underside of overlap, align ball halves with sockets, and stitch around all edges through all layers. For a less obvious application, stitch ball tape to underlayer of overlap, fold edge under, and stitch along free edge through all layers.

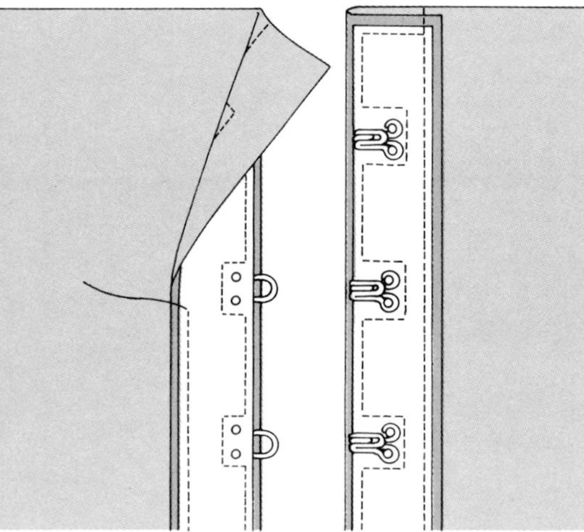

Hook and eye tape calls for a centered application because hooks and eyes must abut to be fastened. As with snap tape, both garment edges should be wider than the tapes. To apply, position hook tape on the underlayer of one edge, with hooks along fold. Stitch through both layers around each hook. Fold edge and stitch through all layers along the free edge (be sure needle does not hit hooks). Stitch eye half to the opposite edge in the same way, aligning eyes with hooks and positioning eyes just beyond fold. Again, take care that needle does not hit eyes.

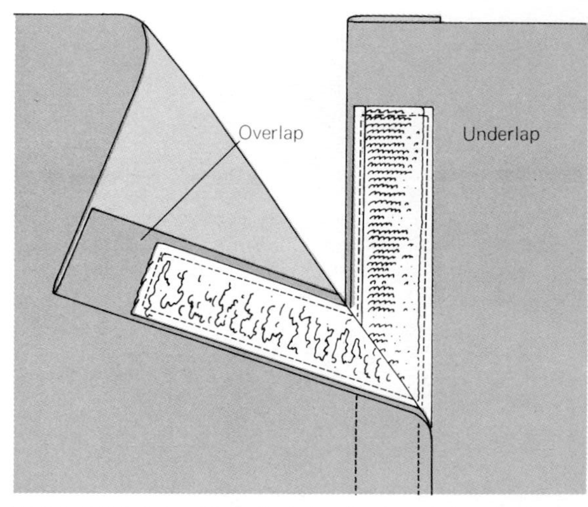

Nylon tapes must be lapped for the two halves to fasten. Because the hooks and loops lock on contact, application to an open seam is best; this lets them stay separate during application. Garment edges should be wider than tapes; for extra strength, cut a double-width seam allowance for the underlap. Position hook tape on underlap; stitch around all edges through all layers. Align and position loop tape on overlap; stitch around all edges through all layers. For a less obvious application, stitch loop tape to underlayer of overlap, fold edge under, and stitch along free edge.

Techniques of Tailoring

Tailoring basics

Pressing 18-19 Design considerations in fashion sewing 50-53 Buying fabric 67-69 Underlying fabrics 72-83

Introduction

To many, the word "tailoring" immediately suggests a sewing impossibility that is meant only for the "experts." Though this may be a common impression, it is a false one. Tailoring is just a refinement of standard sewing procedures, aimed at building *permanent* shape into the garment.

Tailoring does require more than the usual amount of detail work. For example, the lapels

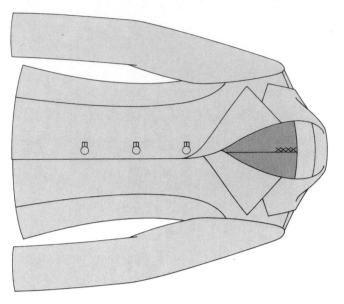

and under collar of the garment are padstitched to help mold and shape them; additional sewing notions, such as twill tape, sleeve headings, and shoulder pads, are used in construction to help define and mold the garment lines; the need to permanently set certain garment areas calls for unusually frequent steam pressing. Patience is essential when tailoring, since each step must be carefully completed before going on to the next.

The jacket illustrated above will be used as a demonstration model for the step-by-step procedures in this chapter. Before starting, be sure you understand the special considerations at the right.

Advance considerations

A successful tailored garment begins long before a stitch is sewed—with an understanding of pressing procedures and purposes, of fabric choices and the reasons for them, and of the special fitting requirements of tailored styles.

PRESSING EQUIPMENT

An ironing board and a steam iron are, of course, standard equipment; in addition to these, a tailor's ham is needed to provide the desired rounded surfaces for pressing shaped areas. Although a sleeve board and tailor's board are not absolutely necessary, they can be very useful when tailoring. Other valuable pressing aids include the seam roll, press mitt, and dressmaker clapper. Consult the pages on Pressing for the proper use of each equipment piece. When pressing the right side of the fabric, always use a press cloth to prevent fabric shine. To produce additional steam, use a dampened cloth, but allow that pressed area to dry before handling it. Avoid pressing seams so flat that their edges mark through to the right side.

PATTERN SELECTION

When selecting a pattern for your tailored garment, choose a design that is becoming to you (see Pattern selection/style), and try to avoid styles you have never worn before. You will be investing many hours of work in your tailored garment, and you want to be sure that the style suits you. If possible, select a pattern designed for tailoring; that way, all the necessary pattern pieces, such as separate under collar and lining, will be available.

SELECTION OF GARMENT FABRIC

After having chosen your pattern, select a fabric that is appropriate for the style. You may want to consult your pattern envelope for fabric recommendations. Keep in mind that worsted wools and wool blends shape and mold well when pressed, and are thus excellent choices for tailoring. Other fabrics suitable for tailoring include firmly woven linens and tweeds, double knits and heavy silks. Limp fabrics cannot generally be molded or shaped and are thus poor choices. When purchasing fabric, be aware of fabric nap, if any (print or pile), and buy yardage accordingly.

SELECTION OF UNDERLYING FABRICS

To give the tailored garment adequate body, and to maintain its shape, the garment fabric must be used in combination with various underlying fabrics. These fabrics include **underlining, interfacing,** and **lining;** interlining is sometimes used for additional warmth (see Interlining). Each of these underlying fabrics must be carefully selected so that when they are combined, the garment will look natural and not be unduly stiff.

Underlining, the second fabric layer in your garment, is attached to the wrong side of the garment fabric before the garment units are connected. The underlining helps to maintain the shape of the garment as well as supplying additional strength and durability. Although most underlinings are lightweight, they can still vary in fiber content and in the type of finish (soft, medium, or crisp). Select the one that is most complementary to the garment fabric, and is similar in color; also consider its care compatibility.

Interfacing is the third layer of fabric in the tailored garment; it provides extra support and shape in designated areas such as collar, lapels, upper back, and hemline. Interfacings are available in different weights, fiber contents, forms (woven and nonwoven), and degrees of crispness. For tailoring, a woven hair canvas is generally recommended since it has the ability to shape well. Select a hair canvas that is of a suitable weight for your garment, and is of good quality (usually with a high goat hair content and a balanced weave of even-sized warp and weft yarns).

Lining, the last fabric layer to be attached, conceals the inner construction of the garment to give a clean finish on the inside. Because the lining lies next to the skin, a smooth, silky fabric is usually recommended for this purpose. Linings are available in many different fiber contents and in a range of weights from light (e.g., China silk) to heavy (e.g., taffeta). Choose a lining that is of a proper weight and is compatible, in care requirements, with the other fabrics; it should also be sturdy enough to withstand normal garment wear. Because the lining is usually visible, its color should either match or be coordinated with the garment fabric.

PATTERN ALTERATIONS
As in all construction situations, the pattern for a tailored garment must be altered to size, as necessary, before the fabrics are cut; flat pattern alterations are critical, as major changes are difficult to make after a garment is cut and sewed. For more specific information, turn to the section on Pattern alterations. When comparing pattern and figure measurements, remember that the minimum ease required in a tailored jacket is slightly more than in a standard dress, and the minimum ease in a coat is slightly more than in a jacket; take into consideration, further, the designed-in fullness of your particular garment style. If you are in serious doubt as to the fit of your garment, take the time to make up a test garment, and then transfer all of the alterations made on that garment onto the flat pattern.

Patterns for interfacing

Pattern pieces for interfacing vary from pattern to pattern. Some provide only a partial front and back interfacing; others may supply pattern pieces with seam allowances already trimmed; still others specify use of the same pattern piece for cutting both facing and interfacing. To give support and shape across the chest area and upper back of the tailored garment, full front and back interfacing pieces are recommended. If your pattern does not contain such interfacing pieces, make up your own from the main pattern pieces. Follow the directions below after basic pattern alterations have been made, then transfer all markings to the new pattern. For a knit, use a two-piece interfacing across the back (see p. 369).

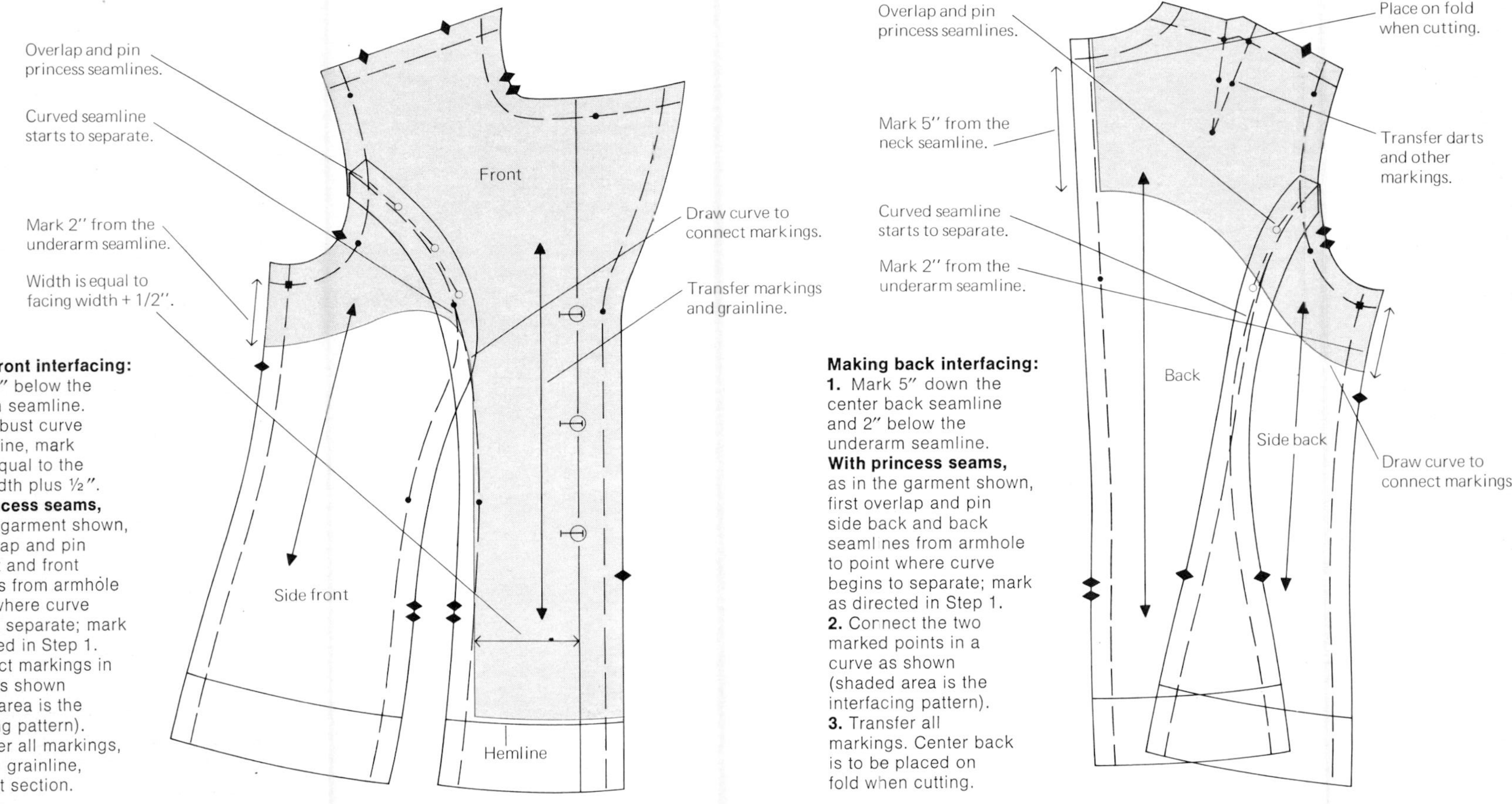
Overlap and pin
princess seamlines.
Curved seamline
starts to separate.
Mark 2" from the
underarm seamline.
Width is equal to
facing width + 1/2".
Front
Side front
Hemline
Draw curve to
connect markings.
Transfer markings
and grainline.
Overlap and pin
princess seamlines.
Mark 5" from the
neck seamline.
Curved seamline
starts to separate.
Mark 2" from the
underarm seamline.
Back
Side back
Place on fold
when cutting.
Transfer darts
and other
markings.
Draw curve to
connect markings

Making front interfacing:
1. Mark 2" below the underarm seamline. Between bust curve and hemline, mark a width equal to the facing width plus ½".
With princess seams, as in the garment shown, first overlap and pin side front and front seamlines from armhole to point where curve begins to separate; mark as directed in Step 1.
2. Connect markings in a curve as shown (shaded area is the interfacing pattern).
3. Transfer all markings, including grainline, from front section.

Making back interfacing:
1. Mark 5" down the center back seamline and 2" below the underarm seamline.
With princess seams, as in the garment shown, first overlap and pin side back and back seaml nes from armhole to point where curve begins to separate; mark as directed in Step 1.
2. Cor nect the two marked points in a curve as shown (shaded area is the interfacing pattern).
3. Transfer all markings. Center back is to be placed on fold when cutting.

Tailoring preliminaries

Treating underlining and garment fabric as one layer 74

Preparing and cutting fabric 84-93
Fabric-marking methods 94

Cutting

Before the garment is cut out, prepare the fabric as described in the Cutting section, straightening and re-aligning the fabric ends, and preshrinking the garment and underlining fabrics if necessary. If you are using wool, you can preshrink by an alternative method—careful steam pressing of the dampened fabric. Work on small sections at a time and keep the grainlines straight as you press.

Lay the pattern pieces out according to the pattern instructions. As a precautionary measure, leave 1-inch seam allowances on all side seams as you cut (see illustration); do the same when cutting out the underlining. Cut out the interfacing pieces and lining pieces (see p. 376).

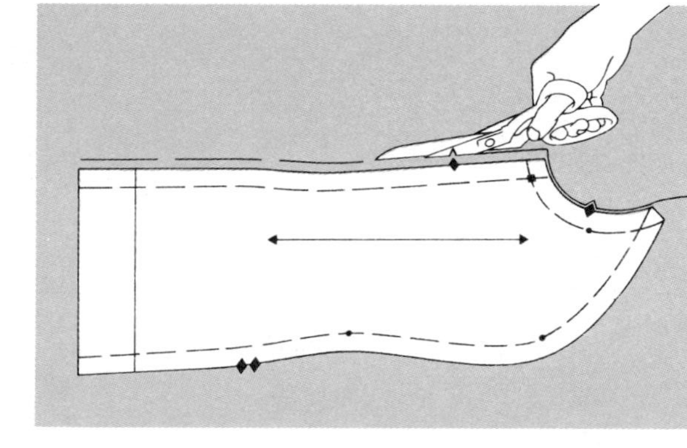

Marking

Markings for all garment pieces must be carefully transferred to each fabric layer. The recommended method of marking, and the markings most likely to be transferred to garment fabric, underlining, and interfacing, are shown below. Note that the marking methods most often used in tailoring include tailor tacks and thread tracings as well as tracing paper and wheel (see Marking methods).

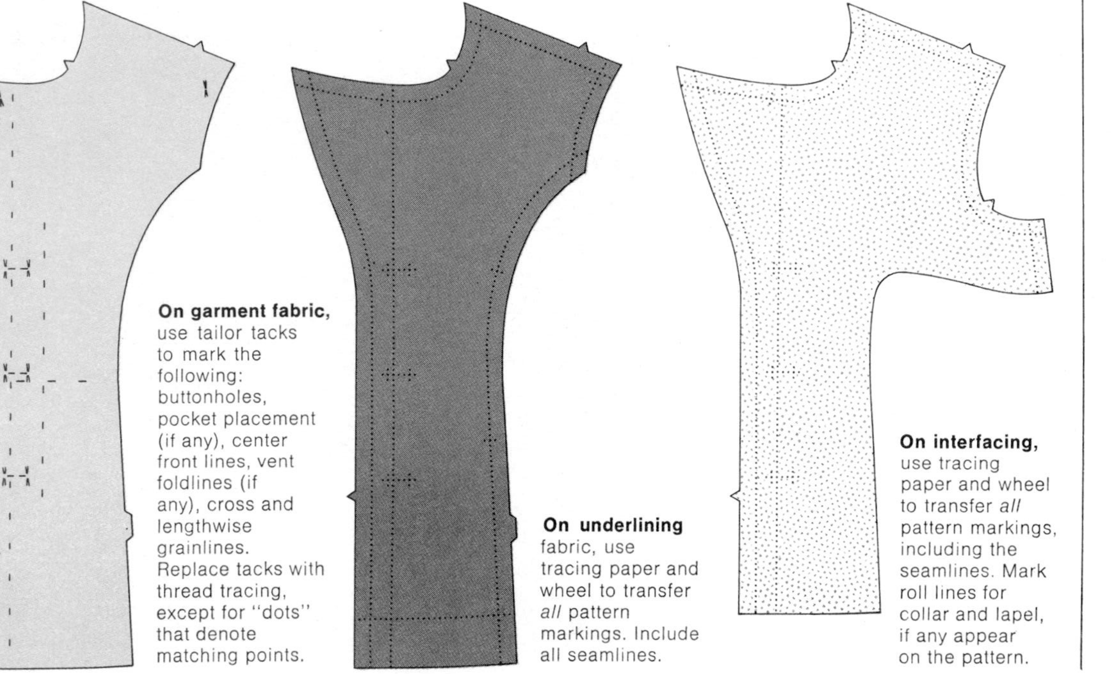

On garment fabric, use tailor tacks to mark the following: buttonholes, pocket placement (if any), center front lines, vent foldlines (if any), cross and lengthwise grainlines. Replace tacks with thread tracing, except for "dots" that denote matching points.

On underlining fabric, use tracing paper and wheel to transfer *all* pattern markings. Include all seamlines.

On interfacing, use tracing paper and wheel to transfer *all* pattern markings, including the seamlines. Mark roll lines for collar and lapel, if any appear on the pattern.

Basting underlining to fabric

After garment and underlining fabric pieces have been marked, the two layers of fabric are then basted together (see below) so they can be handled as one (see Underlinings). Note that, for easier comprehension, the diagonal basting threads have been eliminated in drawings that follow.

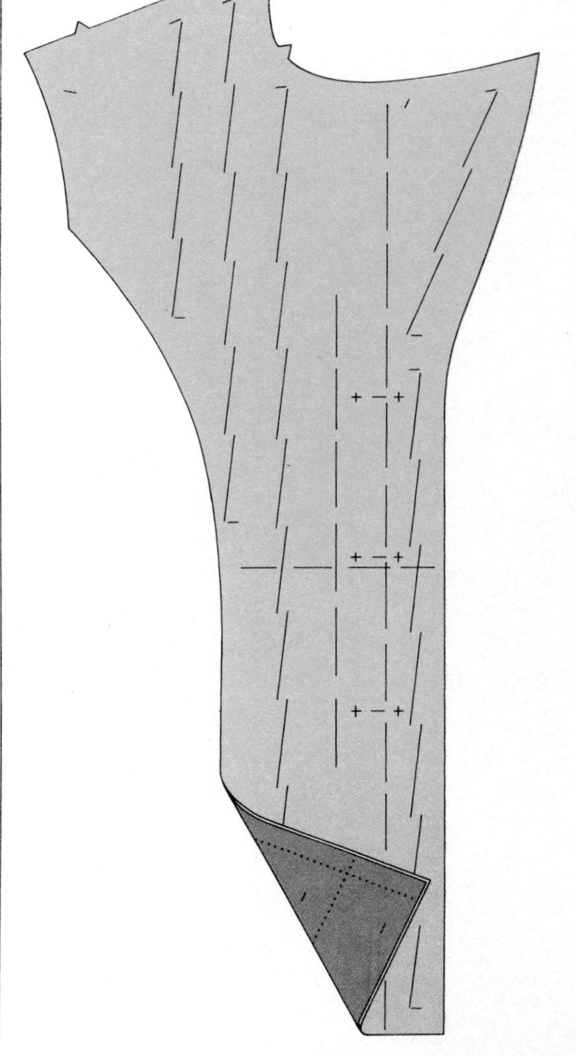

Finger-pressing 18
Test garment 120
Even and uneven basting 124
Staystitching 144

Preparation for first fitting

Proper fit is all-important to the look of your tailored garment; to obtain this fit, your garment will go through not one but a number of fittings along the way. The first fitting is probably the most important one. It is at this point that the general fit of the garment is checked and the roll lines on the collar and lapels are established. To prepare for this fitting, all darts and internal seams are first basted; if possible, the clipping of any seam allowance should be avoided until the seam is permanently stitched. The interfacings are basted in place, and the main sections then basted together. Before starting this preparation, be sure to staystitch the necklines of each garment section (see Staystitching). If a test garment has already been made and fitted, this first fitting is usually not necessary; you can simply proceed with construction after making needed alterations.

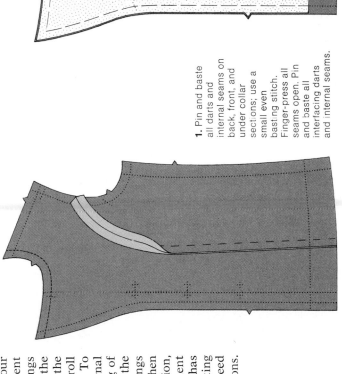

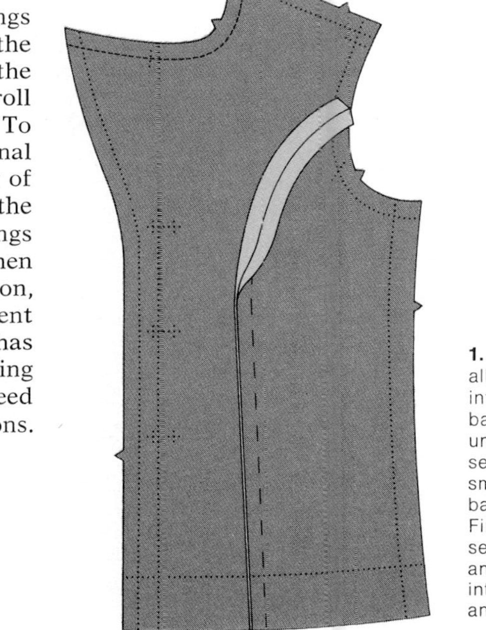

1. Pin and baste all darts and internal seams on back, front, and under collar sections; use a small even basting stitch. Finger-press all seams open. Pin and baste all interfacing darts and internal seams.

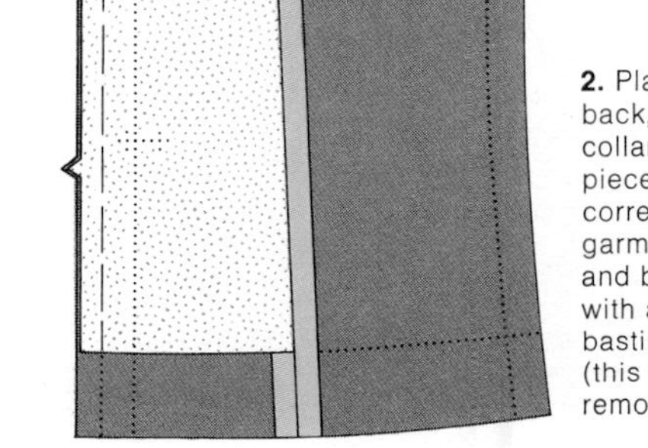

2. Place front, back, and under collar interfacing pieces onto corresponding garment pieces, and baste in place with an uneven basting stitch (this will be removed later).

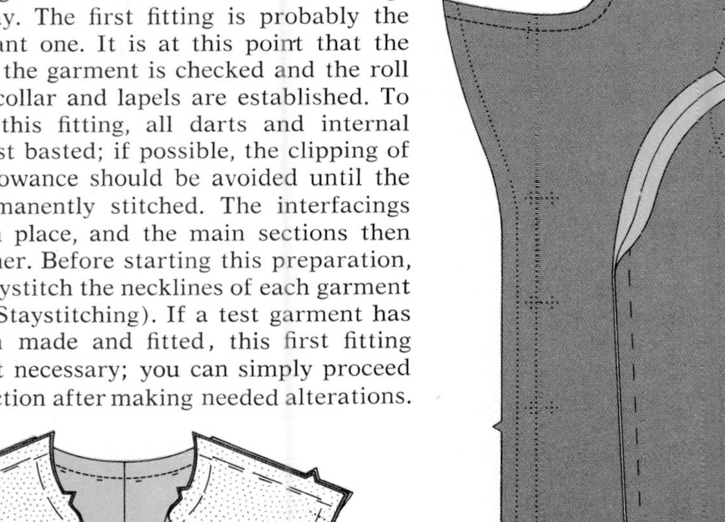

3. With right sides together, pin and baste front sections to back at shoulder and side seams; use a short even basting stitch. Finger-press seams open.

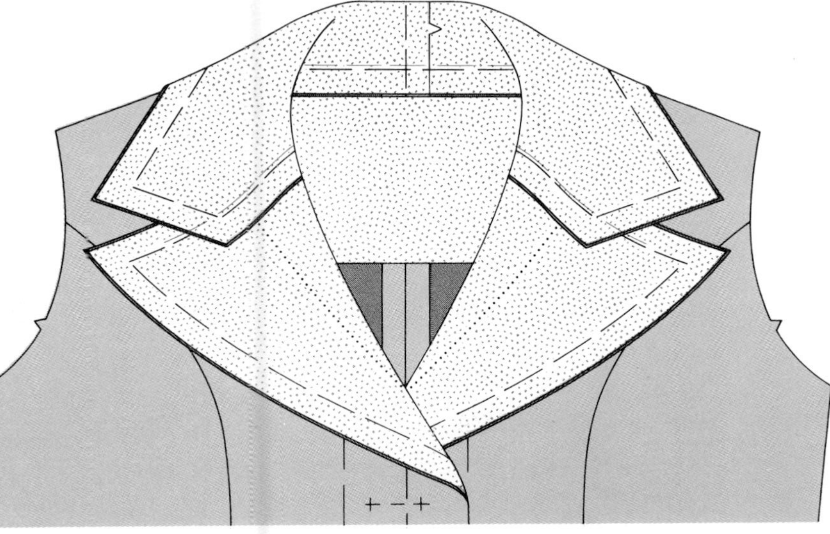

4. Lap right side of under collar over wrong side of garment neckline, matching markings and aligning seamlines; pin in place, starting from center back and working toward center front. Baste on seamline through all thicknesses.

First fitting

Most of the necessary adjustments should be noted during the first fitting of the garment shell; the garment seams at that stage are only basted together, and alterations can be easily made. To get an accurate fit, the garment shell should ideally be worn by the person for whom it is intended, with another person checking for fitting details. If the completed garment is to be worn with another piece of clothing, such as a blouse, it should also be worn during the fitting. If fitting on the real model is not possible, the next best choice is a dress form in the proper size. When neither of these two models is available, a heavy, rounded suit hanger will suffice.

Place the garment shell on the model, and adjust the garment so the shoulder seams are lying squarely on the shoulder line. If shoulder pads are to be used, position them under the garment. Align the center lines on each front section and pin the front opening together. Roll back the lapels and the under collar so that they are lying smoothly. Pin the hemline up so the length and proportion of the garment can be checked.

Examine the fit of the garment carefully: Is there ample ease around the bust, waist, and hip areas? Are the darts or princess seams properly positioned over the bust? Are the lengthwise and crosswise grains straight? Are such details as buttonholes, pockets, flaps, etc., marked at flattering positions? Now check the roll of the lapel and collar: Is the collar stand at a comfortable height? Does the fall of the under collar cover the neck seamline? If the lapel/collar fit is satisfactory in these respects, pin-mark the roll lines on both under collar and lapels.

Checklist for first fitting (below and at right).

Shoulder seam squarely on shoulder line.

Princess seams or darts in proper position over bust.

Center front lines aligned.

Such details as pockets marked at flattering positions.

Hem pinned up.

Buttonholes positioned properly.

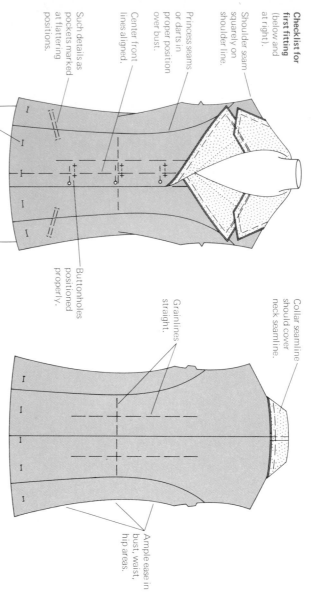

Collar seamline should cover neck seamline.

Grainlines straight.

Ample ease in bust, waist, hip areas.

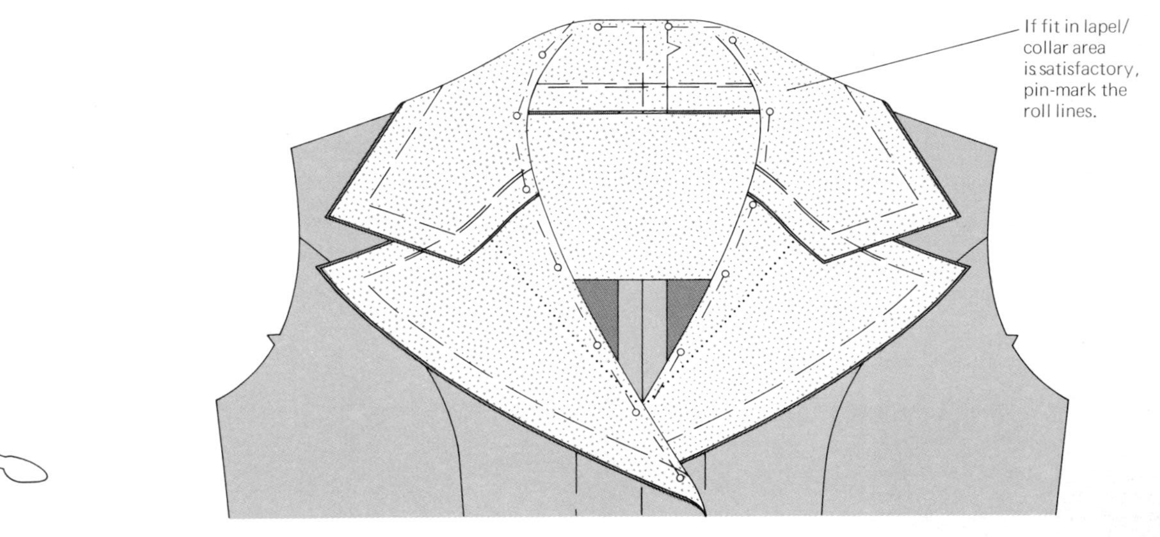
If fit in lapel/
collar area
is satisfactory,
pin-mark the
roll lines.

Tailoring/construction

Pressing equipment 18-19
Princess seams, darts 158-161
Pockets 274-288
Bound buttonholes 330-342

Construction procedure

When the garment shell has been fitted, remove the bastings and separate the main sections. Remove the interfacing pieces as well and thread-trace the pinned roll line markings onto them. If alterations are needed, make all the necessary changes on the garment and interfacing units; when these have been completed, the permanent construction of the tailored garment can begin.

To start construction, complete all internal seams within the main garment sections (see below), and all darts as well. To eliminate bulk from each dart, slash through its center to within ½ to 1 inch of its point, and press dart open over a tailor's ham. To keep the dart flat, catchstitch its raw edges to the underlining (see right).

The interfacings are then applied to the garment while the front and back sections are still unattached. The lapels and under collar are carefully padstitched, and preshrunk ¼-inch twill tape is applied to designated seams on the front sections to help prevent stretching and to define lapel lines. After the main sections are joined, the under collar is stitched to the assembled unit, and the upper collar/facing unit attached.

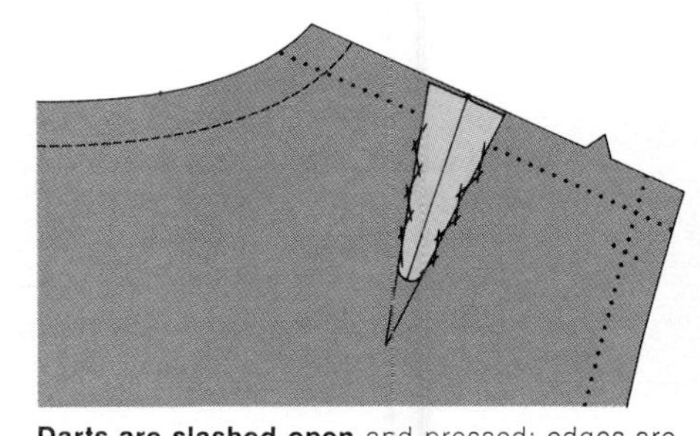

Darts are slashed open and pressed; edges are then catchstitched flat.

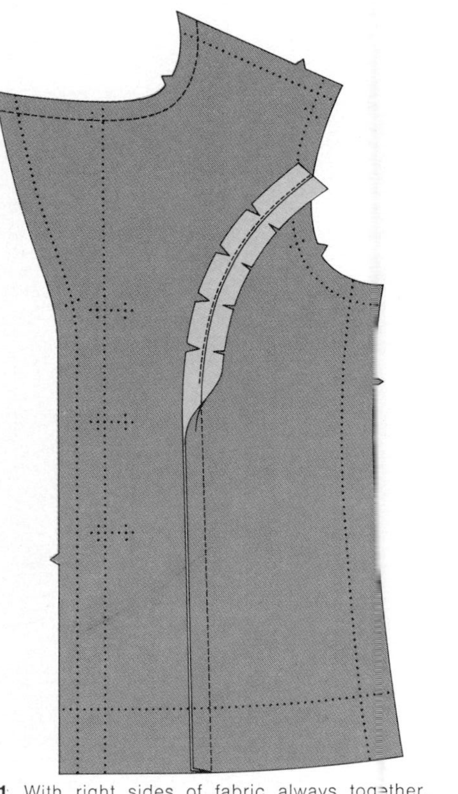

1. With right sides of fabric always together, match, pin, and stitch all the internal seams and darts on both the front and back sections. (Clip and notch princess seams if the garment has them.) Press each seam flat, then press it open over a tailor's ham.

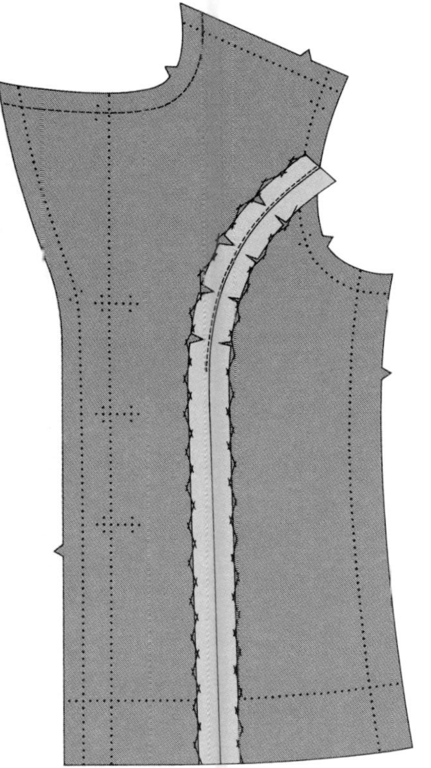

2. Finish darts as described at the top of the page. To ensure that internal seams lie flat, catchstitch their seam allowances to the underlining; take care that the stitches do not catch the garment fabric below. Re-press each dart and seam over a tailor's ham.

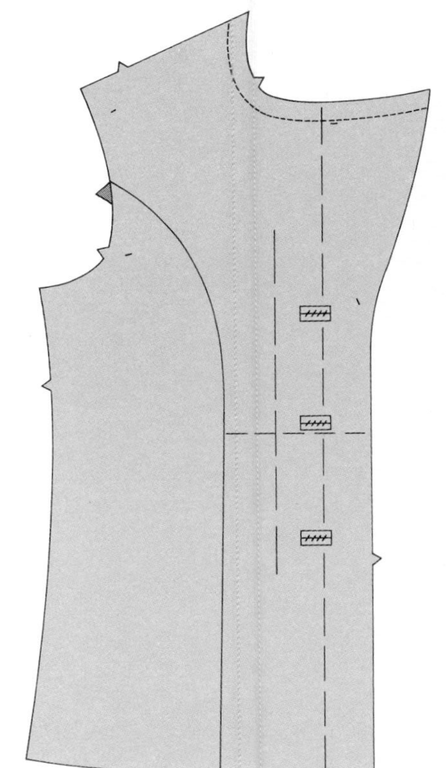

3. At this point in the process, make all bound buttonholes on the garment front, following the appropriate instructions in the Buttonhole section. At this same stage, construct pockets, if the garment is to have them, following instructions in the section on Pockets.

Catchstitch (flat) 129
Padding stitches (chevron and parallel) 131
Darts in interfacing 162

Applying front interfacing

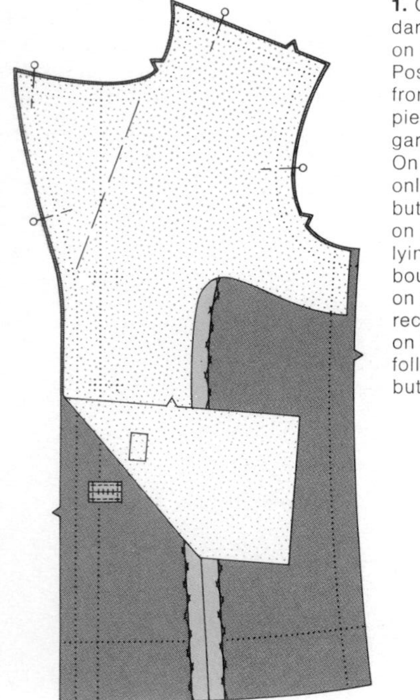

1. Construct all darts that appear on front interfacings. Position and pin front interfacing pieces onto front garment sections. On right front section only, check whether buttonhole markings on interfacing are lying exactly over bound buttonholes on garment; cut out rectangular openings on the interfacing, following the buttonhole markings.

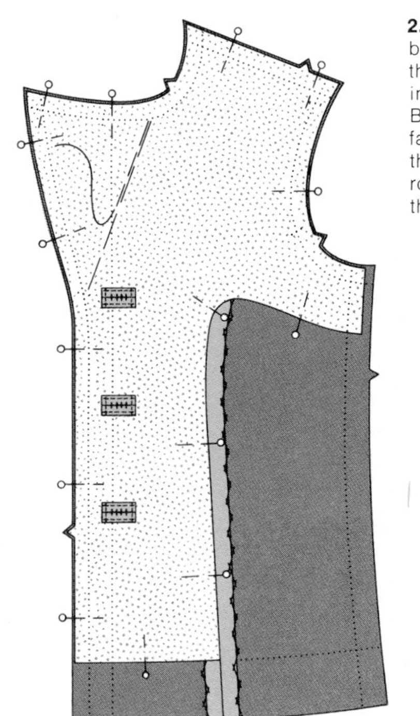

2. Pull raw edges of bound buttonholes through cut openings in interfacing. Baste through all fabric layers along the thread-traced roll line. Remove the thread tracing.

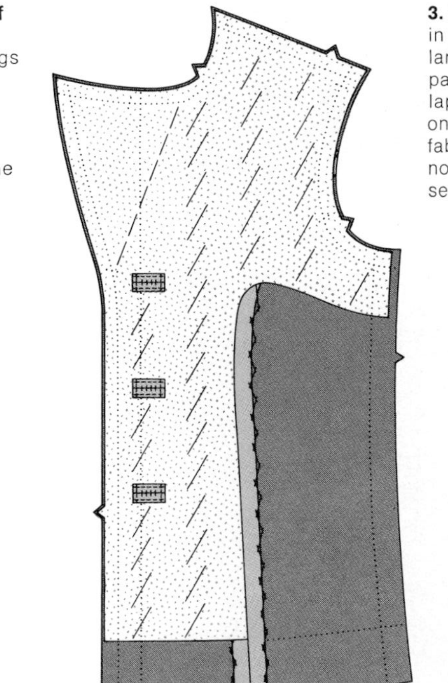

3. Hold interfacing in place, using a large parallel padstitch outside the lapel area; catch only the underlining fabric below, and do not stitch into any seam allowances.

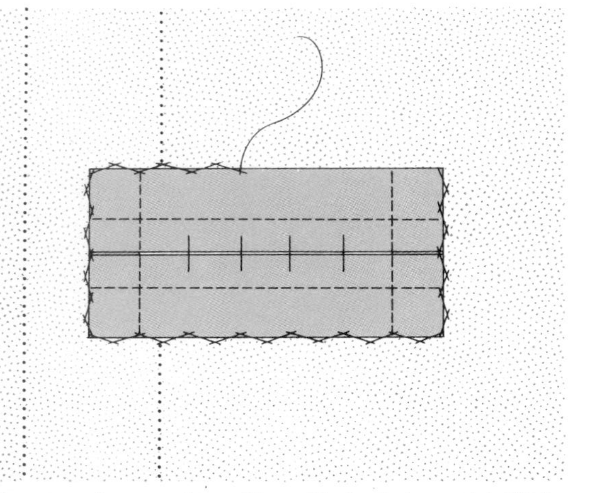

4. To secure the raw edges of bound buttonholes, catchstitch them to the interfacing.

5. Fill in lapel area with short chevron padstitching; catch only a yarn or two of the garment fabric below. Start at the roll line and shape the lapel, rolling it over your hand as shown; do not padstitch into any of the seam allowances.

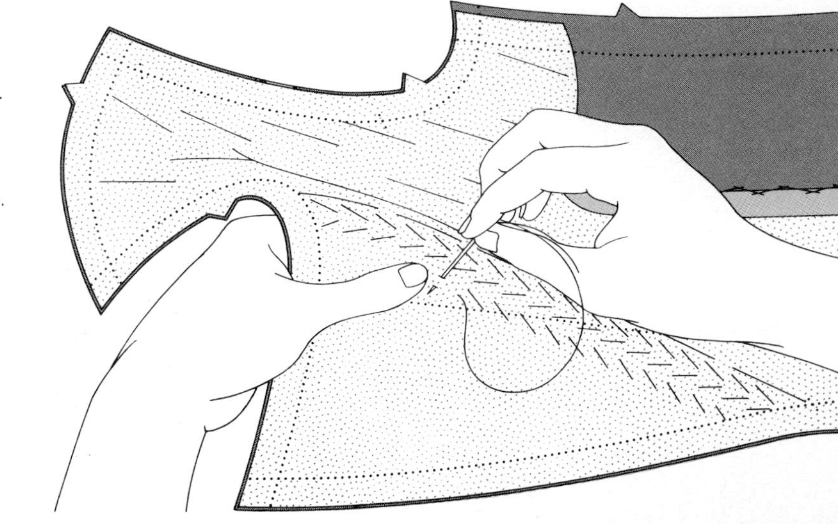

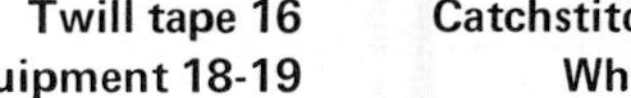

Twill tape 16
Pressing equipment 18-19
Catchstitch (flat) 129
Whipstitch 136

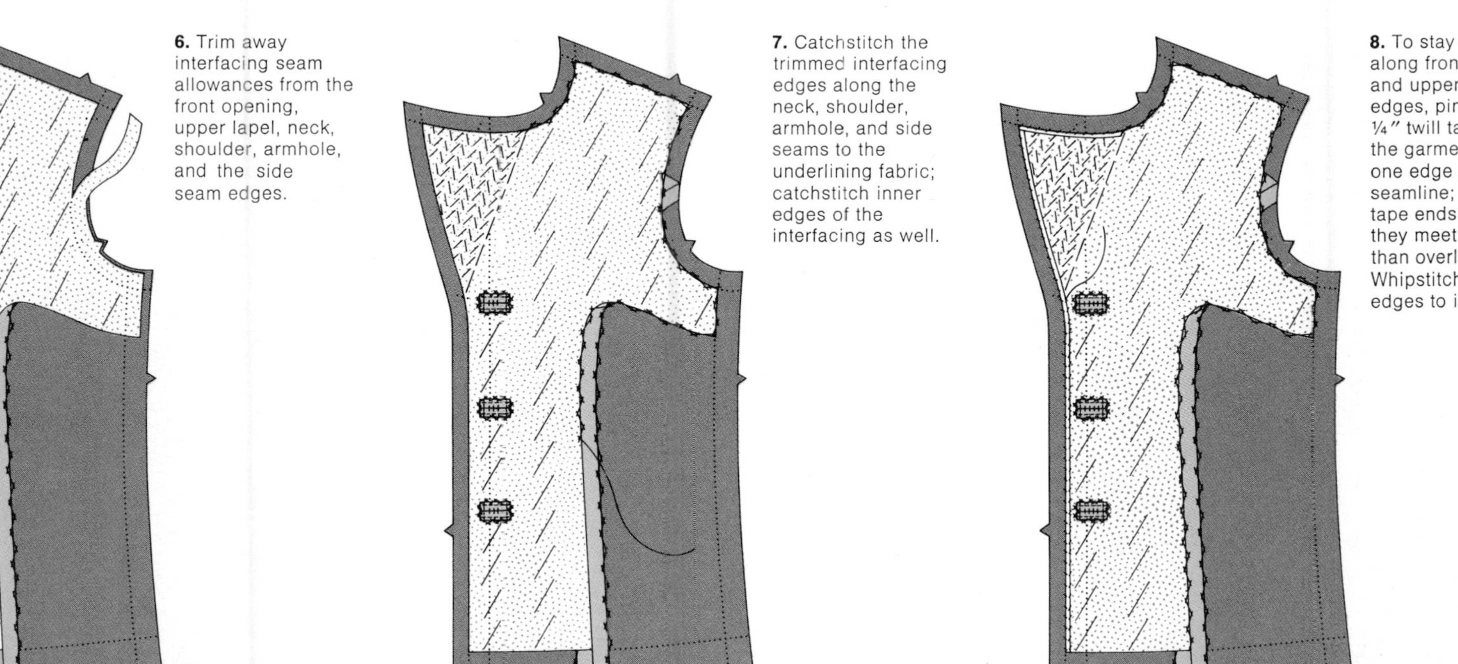

6. Trim away interfacing seam allowances from the front opening, upper lapel, neck, shoulder, armhole, and the side seam edges.

7. Catchstitch the trimmed interfacing edges along the neck, shoulder, armhole, and side seams to the underlining fabric; catchstitch inner edges of the interfacing as well.

8. To stay seamlines along front opening and upper lapel edges, pin preshrunk ¼" twill tape onto the garment with one edge against the seamline; cut the tape ends so that they meet rather than overlap. Whipstitch both tape edges to interfacing.

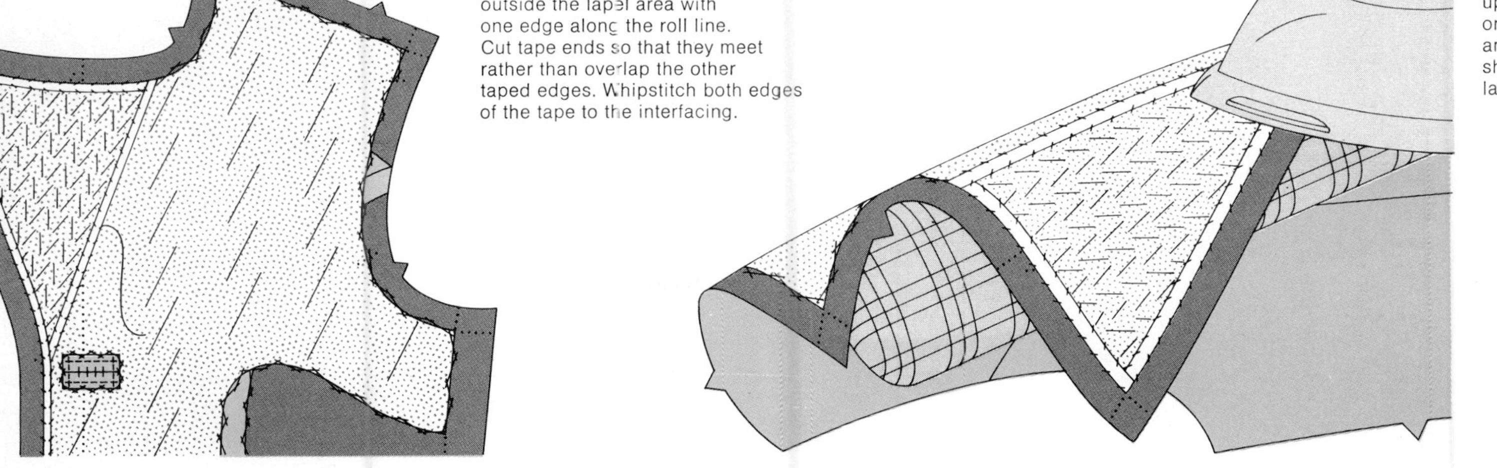

9. To stay the lapel roll line, pin the twill tape onto the garment, outside the lapel area with one edge along the roll line. Cut tape ends so that they meet rather than overlap the other taped edges. Whipstitch both edges of the tape to the interfacing.

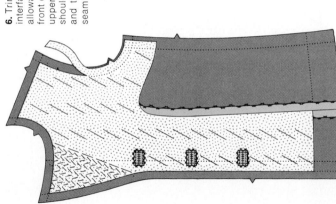

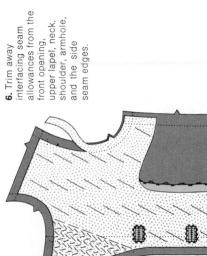

10. Position the lapel, wrong side up, over a seam roll or tailor's ham, and steam-press to shape and set the lapel roll.

Tailoring/interfacing

Darts in interfacing 76, 162
Catchstitch (flat) 129
Padding stitch (parallel) 131

Applying back interfacing

The back interfacing provides the necessary support for the upper back and underarm of the tailored garment. Application of the back interfacing can be done by either of two methods. The first utilizes a one-piece interfacing (see p. 361 for instructions on making its pattern), and is the method most often used, especially if the tailoring fabric is woven. Unlike the front interfacing, the one-piece back interfacing does not require fine padstitching; only long parallel padstitches are necessary to hold the interfacing in place (see below). The second application method uses a two-piece interfacing that is ideal when tailoring with a knit fabric; the two separate interfacing pieces are not secured with long padstitches, and so are free to give with the movement of the knit fabric. (See the opposite page for cutting instruction and method of application.)

Darts in the back interfacing, like those in the front, are handled in a special way so that much of their bulk is eliminated. The lapped method, illustrated at right, is one way to treat darts in interfacing. Directions for this and other methods are given in the section on Interfacing.

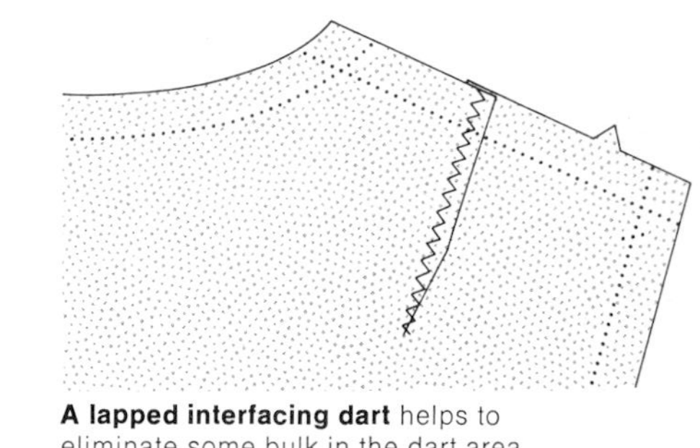

A lapped interfacing dart helps to eliminate some bulk in the dart area.

One-piece method

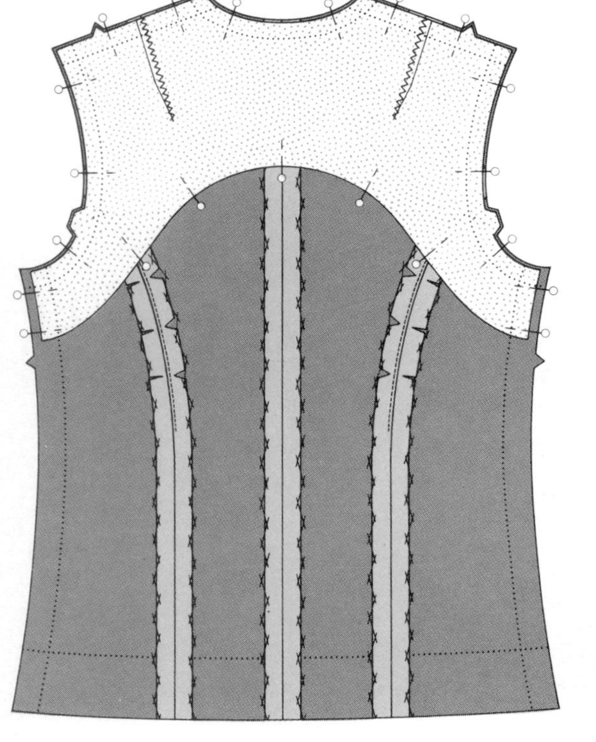

1. Construct all darts that occur on the interfacing unit. Position the interfacing on the wrong side of the garment, matching all of the markings. Pin around the edges.

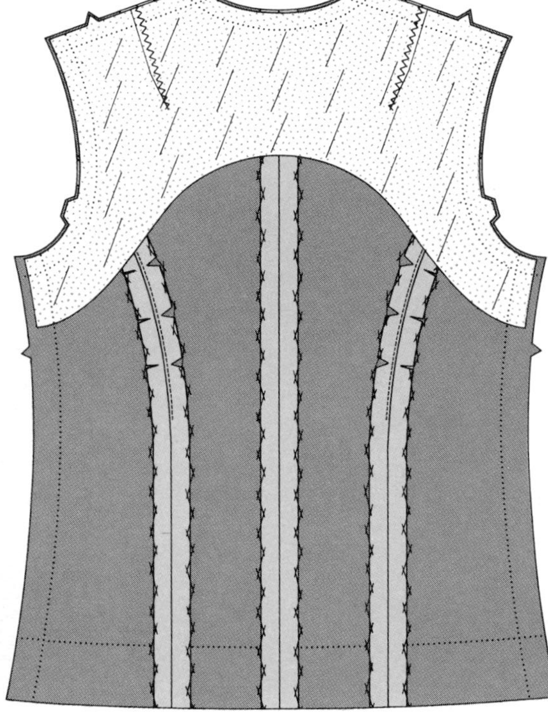

2. Secure the interfacing to the garment, using long parallel padstitches (see Hand stitches); catch only the underlining below, and do not padstitch into any seam allowances.

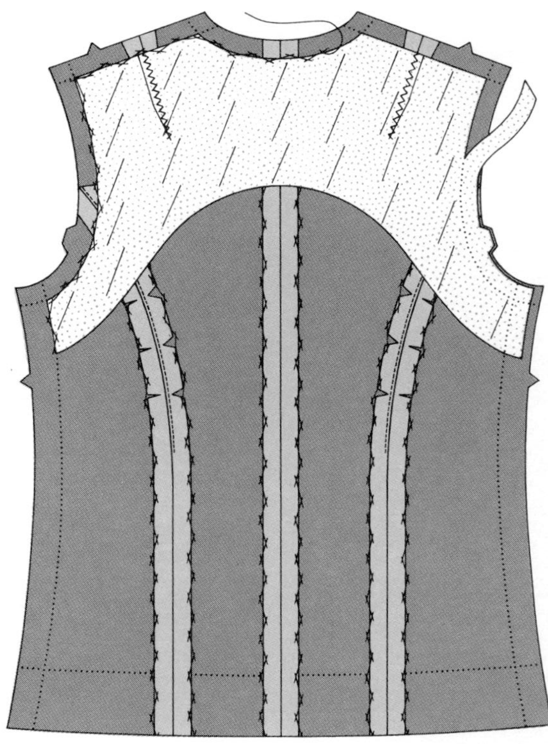

3. Trim away all of the interfacing seam allowances along the neck, shoulder, armhole, and side seam edges. Catchstitch the cut edges to the garment seam allowances.

Uneven basting 124
Catchstitch (flat) 129

Two-piece method

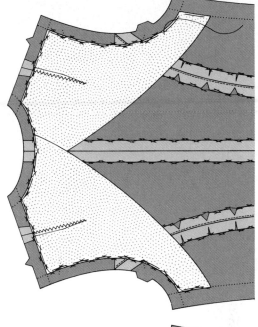

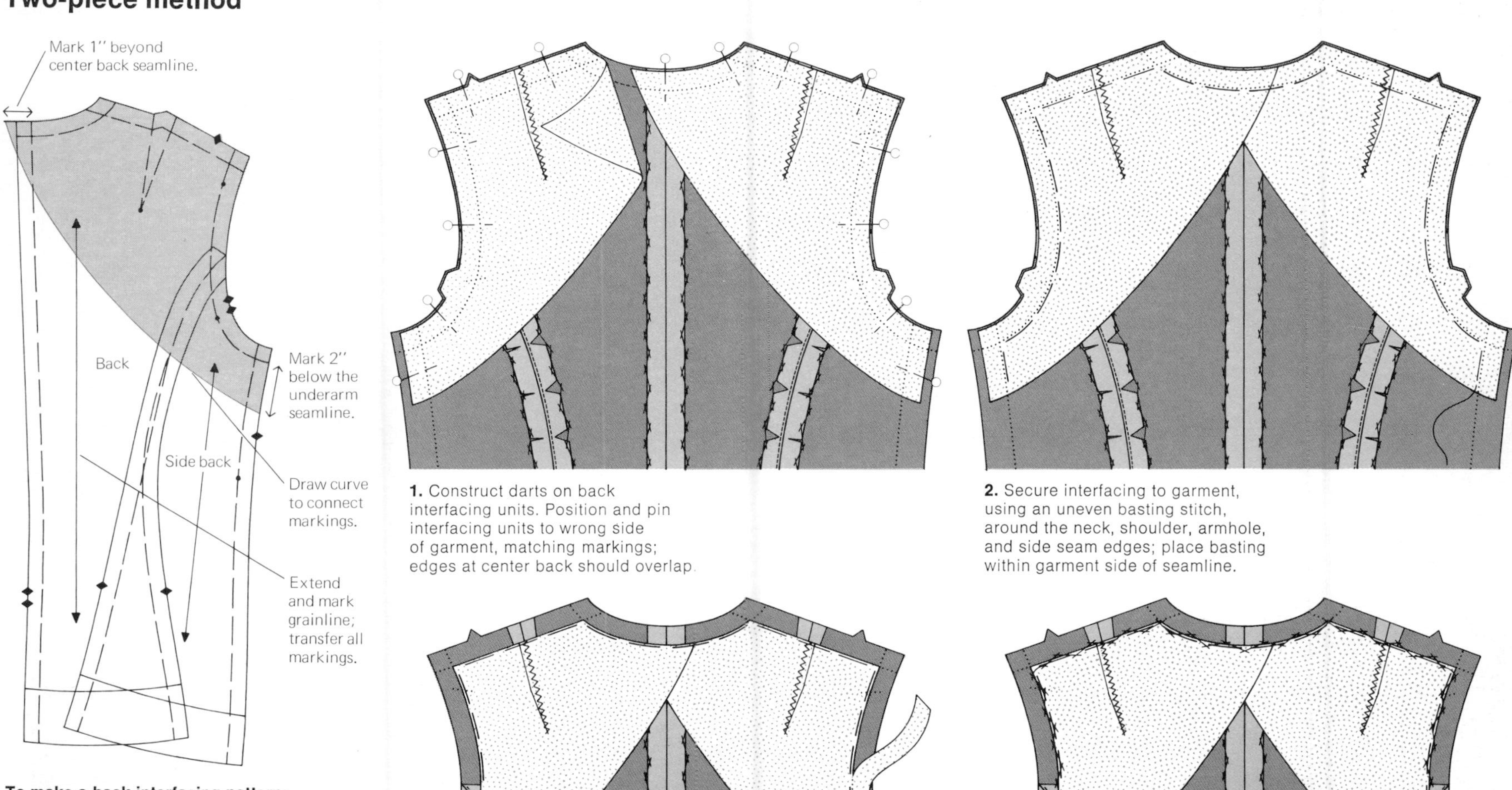
Mark 1" beyond center back seamline.
Back
Side back
Mark 2" below the underarm seamline.
Draw curve to connect markings.
Extend and mark grainline; transfer all markings.

To make a back interfacing pattern:
1. Mark 1" beyond the center back seam on pattern.
2. Mark 2" below underarm seamline.
3. Draw a curve connecting the two points (shaded area is interfacing).
If garment has princess seams, as shown, first overlap and pin side back and back seamlines from armhole to point where curve begins to separate; mark as directed.
4. Transfer all markings. Extend and mark the grainline.

1. Construct darts on back interfacing units. Position and pin interfacing units to wrong side of garment, matching markings; edges at center back should overlap.

2. Secure interfacing to garment, using an uneven basting stitch, around the neck, shoulder, armhole, and side seam edges; place basting within garment side of seamline.

3. Trim away all interfacing seam allowances along the neck, shoulder, armhole, and side seam edges; do not pull or shift the interfacing while working.

4. Catchstitch trimmed edges to garment seam allowances; remove the bastings. The back interfacing is now secured in place, but is still allowed some give across the back.

Abutted and lapped seams 76

Catchstitch (flat) 129
Padding stitch: hand 131, machine 141

Applying interfacing to under collar

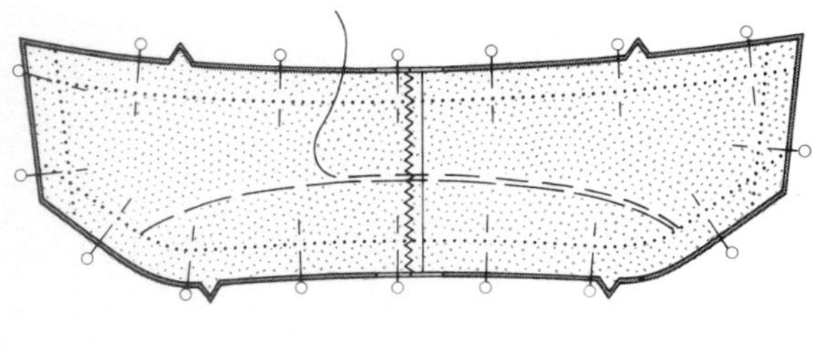

1. Complete under collar seam; press open. Thread-trace roll line on interfacing units. Join interfacing units with an abutted or lapped seam. Pin interfacing to wrong side of under collar; baste the two together along the roll line.

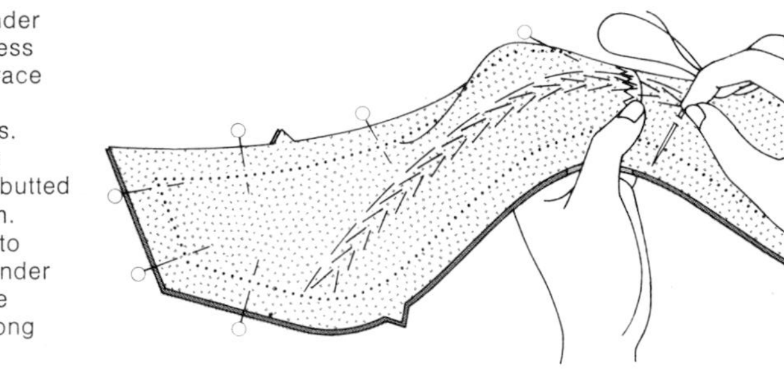

2. Remove thread tracing. Fill in the *stand* area with short chevron padstitching; catch only a yarn or two of garment fabric below. Start at roll line and shape under collar over your hand as shown; do not padstitch into any seam allowances.

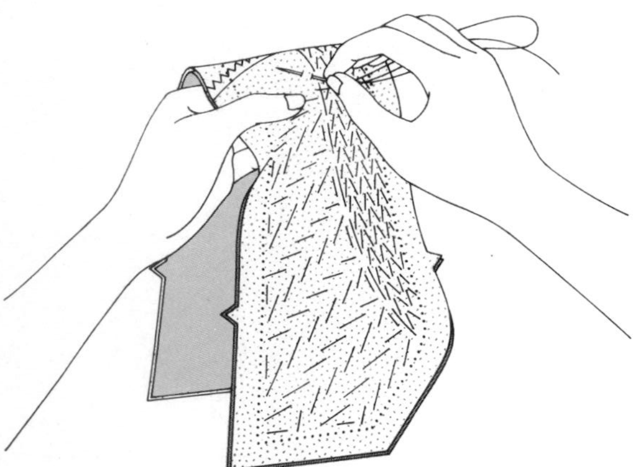

3. Using a slightly longer chevron padstitch, fill in *fall* area of under collar, following the grainline of the interfacing; shape the under collar over your hand as shown, and do not padstitch into any seam allowances.

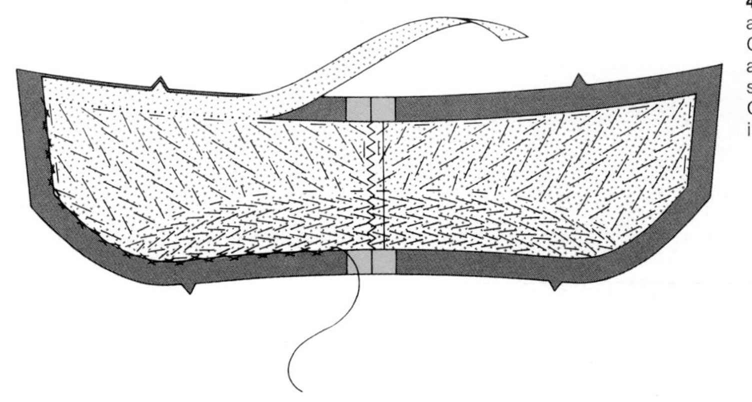

4. Remove basting along roll line. Carefully trim away all interfacing seam allowances. Catchstitch trimmed interfacing edges.

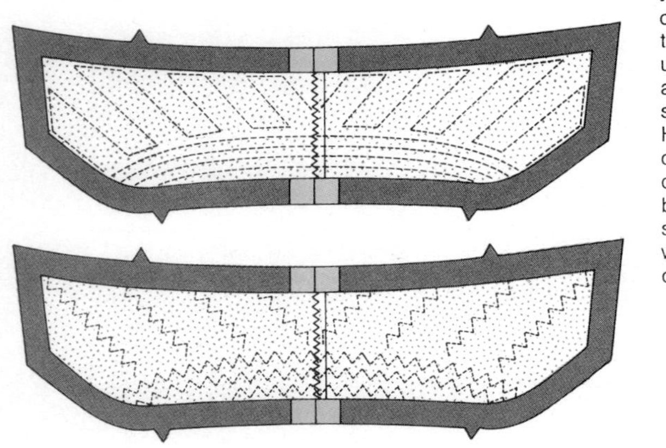

Padstitching can be done by machine to save time, using a straight or a zigzag stitch as shown (see Stitches). However, the shaping quality of an under collar padstitched by machine is not as satisfactory as when padstitching is done by hand.

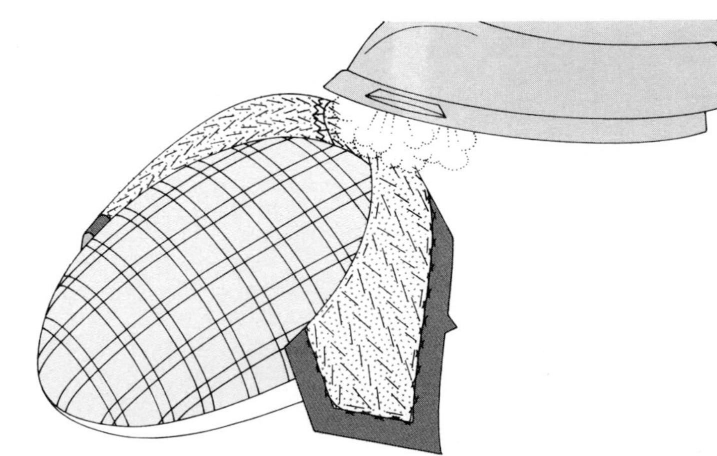

5. Pin under collar to tailor's ham as shown, and steam-press along roll to set its shape. If under collar is not to be used immediately, do not store it away flat; instead, maintain its shape by pinning the under collar over a rolled-up towel.

Tailoring/assembling garment

Pressing equipment 18-19
Catchstitch (flat) 129
Staystitching 144
Reducing seam bulk 147
Seam finishes 148-149

Attaching under collar to garment

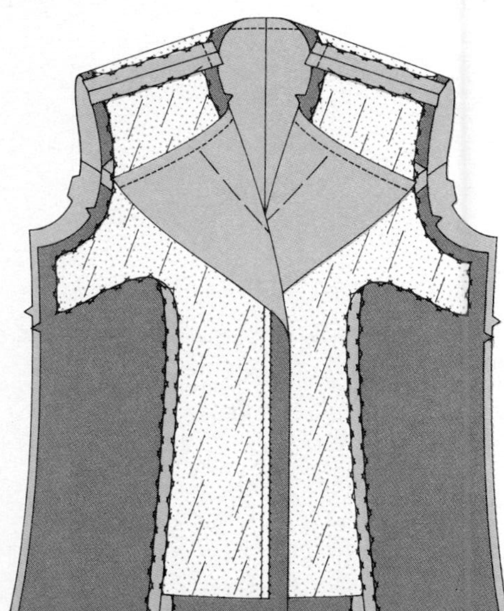

1. Before the under collar can be attached, the front and back garment sections must be stitched together: With right sides facing, match, pin, and stitch back to front sections at shoulder seamlines. Press seams flat, then open. Catchstitch seam allowances to the interfacing below. Side seams have been left unstitched to facilitate subsequent steps in collar construction.

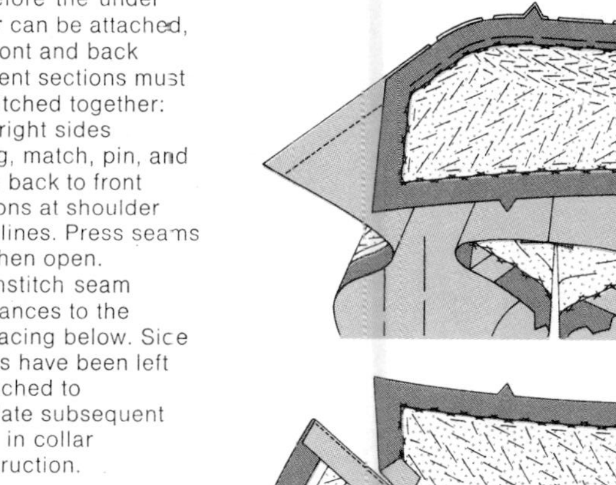

2. With right sides together, match and pin under collar to garment along neck seamline; clip garment seam allowance if necessary for collar to fit smoothly. Baste and stitch with garment side up, securing stitches at both ends of seamline crossing. Press seam flat.

3. Trim stitched seam allowances to ⅜"; diagonally trim cross seams. Finger-press seam open; clip garment seam allowance and notch the under collar seam allowance as necessary until they both lie flat. Press seam open over tailor's ham.

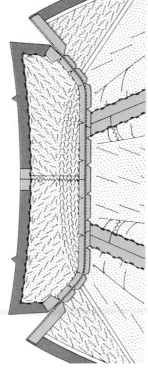

Attaching upper collar to facing

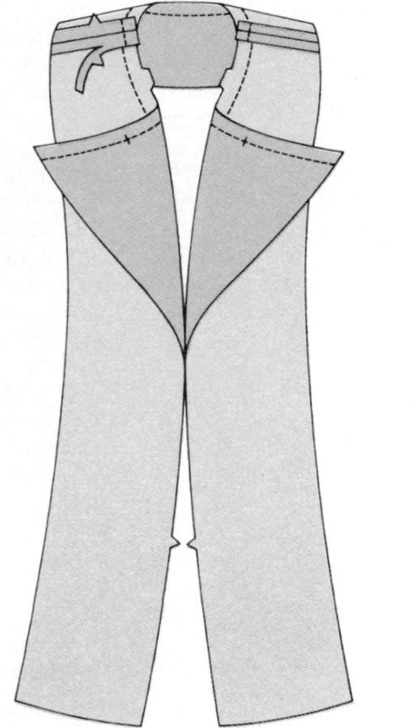

1. Staystitch neck seamlines on front and back facing units. With right sides together, match and pin front and back facings together along shoulder seamlines. Press seams flat, then open. Trim seam allowances to half width. If fabric tends to ravel easily, apply a seam finish to outer edges of the facing.

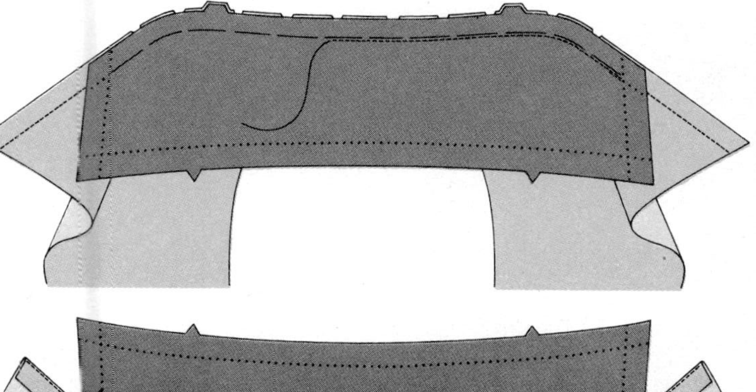

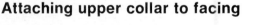

2. With right sides together, match and pin upper collar to facing along neck seamline; clip facing seam allowance if necessary for collar to fit smoothly. Baste and stitch with facing side up, securing stitches at both ends of seamline crossing. Press the seam flat.

3. Trim stitched seam allowances. Diagonally trim cross-seam allowances. Finger-press seam open; clip facing seam allowance and notch upper collar seam allowance as necessary until they both lie flat. Press the seam open over a tailor's ham.

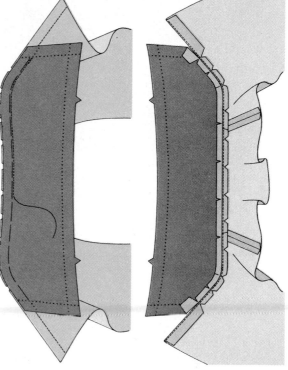

Blunting corners 146

Attaching upper collar unit to under collar and garment

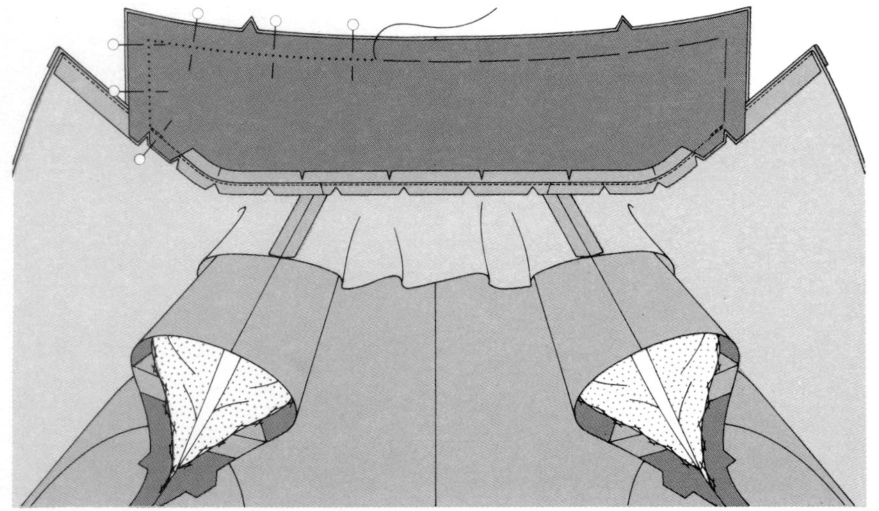

1. With right sides together, accurately match and pin upper collar to under collar; if necessary, ease in upper collar to fit. Baste in place; at the seamline junction of collar and lapel, turn down neckline seam allowances on upper and under collars so that they are not caught in the stitching.

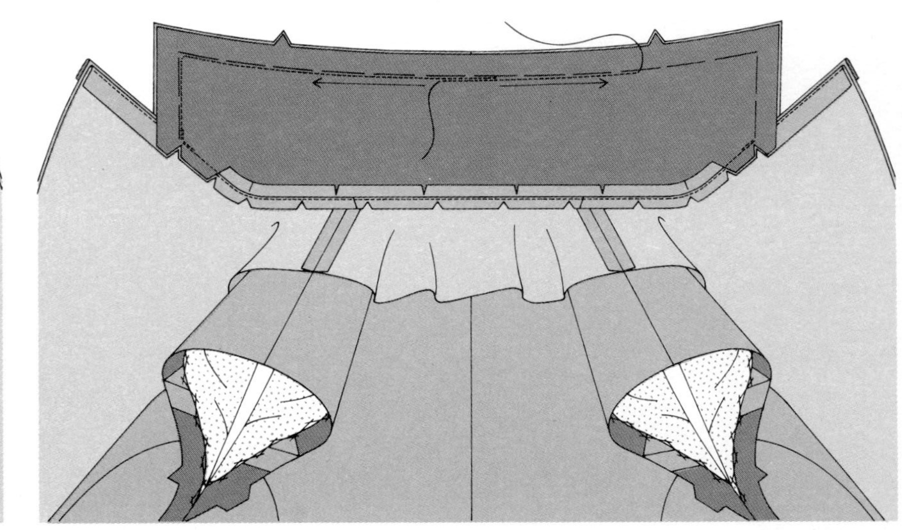

2. Stitch as basted, starting at center of collar: Stitch around collar, reinforcing stitches at corners and stitching across corners to blunt them (see Seams); secure stitches at junction of collar and lapel. Stitch remaining half of collars together in the same way; overlap a few stitches at the beginning. Press seam flat.

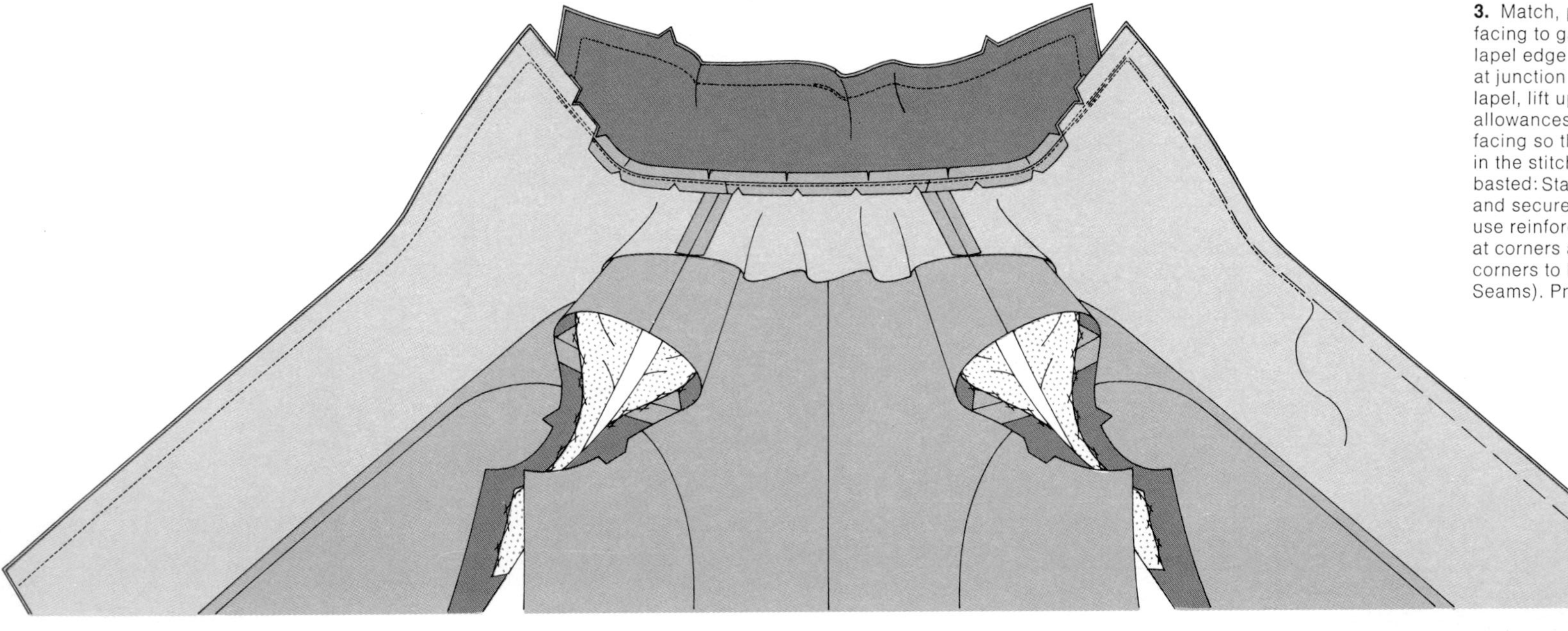

3. Match, pin, and baste front facing to garment along upper lapel edge and front opening; at junction of collar and lapel, lift up neckline seam allowances on garment and facing so they are not caught in the stitching. Stitch as basted: Start at upper edges and secure beginning stitches; use reinforcement stitches at corners and stitch across corners to blunt them (see Seams). Press seam flat.

Pressing equipment 18-19
Pickstitch (for hand understitching) 124
Diagonal basting 125
Catchstitch (flat) 129
Reducing bulk 147

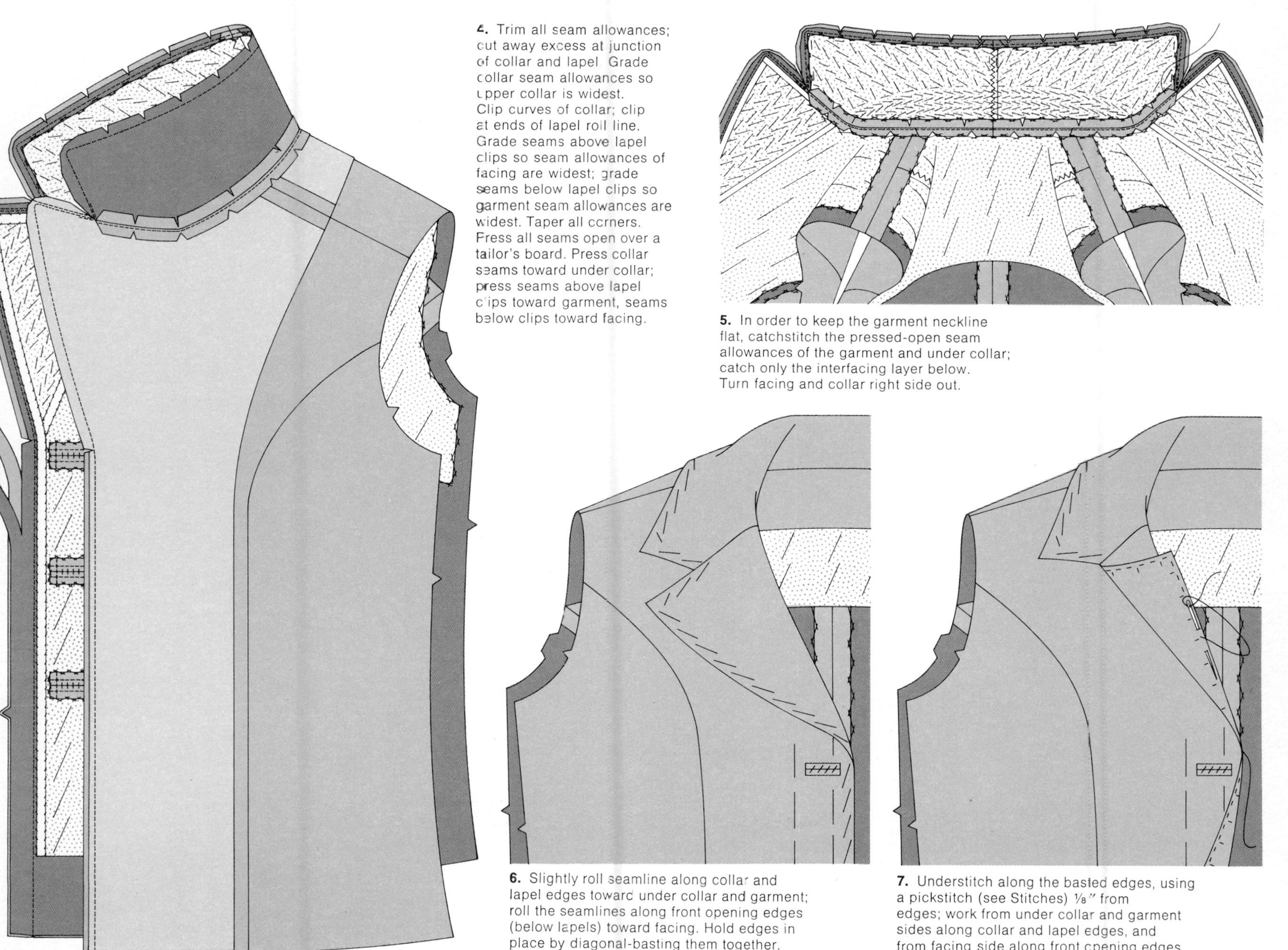

4. Trim all seam allowances; cut away excess at junction of collar and lapel. Grade collar seam allowances so upper collar is widest. Clip curves of collar; clip at ends of lapel roll line. Grade seams above lapel clips so seam allowances of facing are widest; grade seams below lapel clips so garment seam allowances are widest. Taper all corners. Press all seams open over a tailor's board. Press collar seams toward under collar; press seams above lapel clips toward garment, seams below clips toward facing.

5. In order to keep the garment neckline flat, catchstitch the pressed-open seam allowances of the garment and under collar; catch only the interfacing layer below. Turn facing and collar right side out.

6. Slightly roll seamline along collar and lapel edges toward under collar and garment; roll the seamlines along front opening edges (below lapels) toward facing. Hold edges in place by diagonal-basting them together.

7. Understitch along the basted edges, using a pickstitch (see Stitches) ⅛" from edges; work from under collar and garment sides along collar and lapel edges, and from facing side along front opening edges.

Plain-stitch tack 135
Finishing bound buttonholes 338-339

Completion of collar and lapel

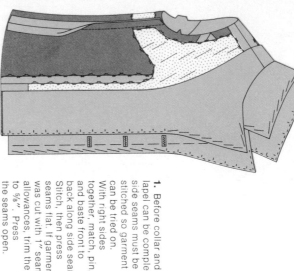

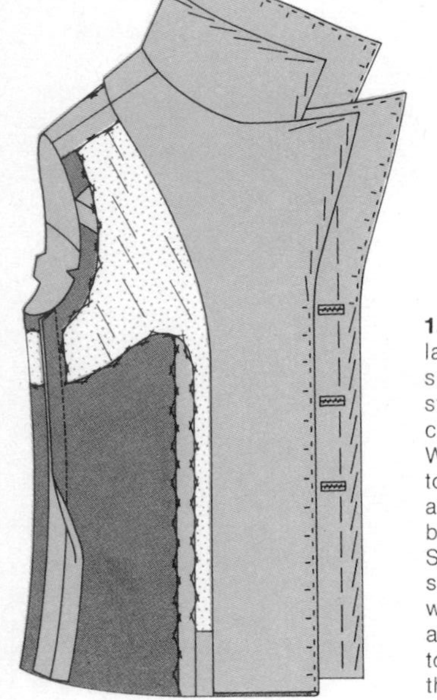

1. Before collar and lapel can be completed, side seams must be stitched so garment can be tried on. With right sides together, match, pin, and baste front to back along side seams. Stitch, then press seams flat. If garment was cut with 1″ seam allowances, trim them to ⅝″. Press the seams open.

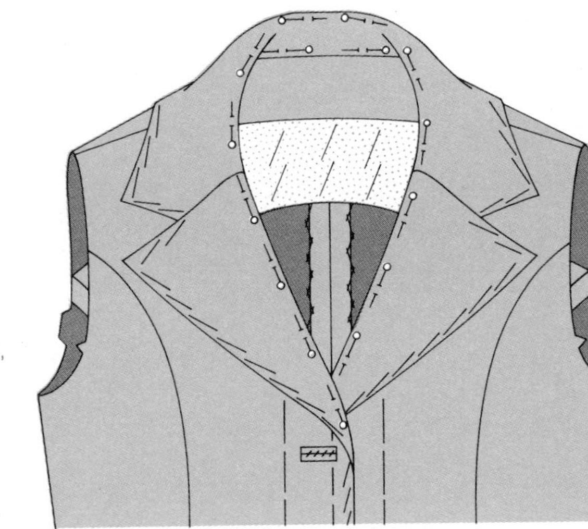

2. Place garment on model. Roll back collar and lapels, and allow them to fall smoothly into place. Hold them in position by pinning along the roll lines and just above back neck seamline. Remove garment.

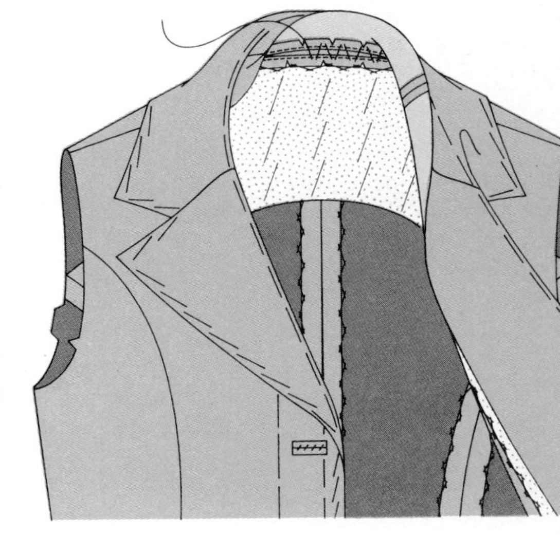

3. Baste along the pinned roll lines of collar and lapels. Lift up back neck facing and, using plain-stitch tacks, stitch facing and garment neck seamlines together as they have fallen in the pinning.

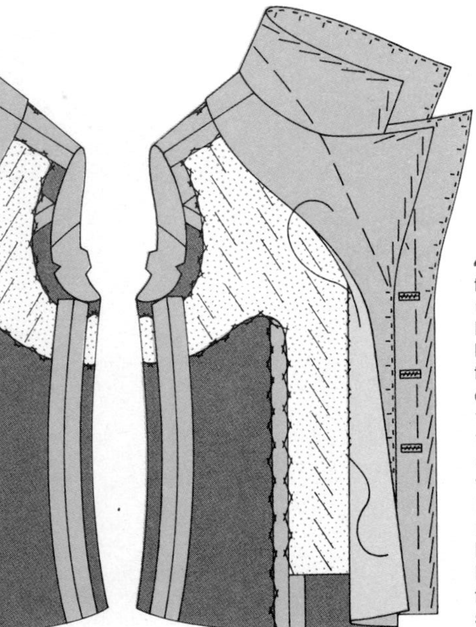

4. On buttonhole side of front opening, complete underside of bound buttonholes as shown at far left (see Buttonholes); to hold facing in place on opposite side of garment front, turn facing back 2″ from finished edge, and secure facing to interfacing with plain-stitch tacks between first and last button markings (see left). If last button and buttonhole are less than a double hem width from hemline, take these steps after hem is completed.

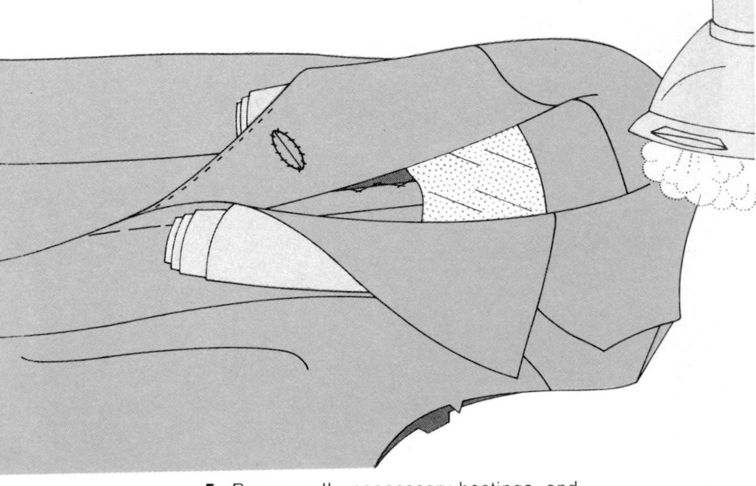

5. Remove all unnecessary bastings, and press front openings of garment. Place a rolled-up towel under collar and lapels for support, then pass a steaming iron over the garment, holding it close enough for the steam to set the roll of collar and lapels.

Sleeves

Because sleeve procedures in a tailored garment are similar to those used in standard garments, it is recommended that the Sleeve chapter be reviewed before tailored sleeve construction is undertaken. One difference, called for by the more structured character of tailored garments, is extra shape-building steps. A **sleeve heading,** for example, usually made from a rectangular piece of lamb's wool, is sewed to the sleeve's upper seamline to support and smooth out the sleeve cap. A **shoulder pad** can be added to help define the shoulder line and compensate for figure faults.

Set-in sleeves in tailored garments are usually shaped according to one of three basic pattern types: (1) standard one-piece sleeve with an underarm seam; (2) two-piece sleeve with seams along the front and back of the arm; and (3) a variation on the one-piece sleeve in which the seam is at the back of the arm (see below). Most tailored sleeves are of the second and third types because their seam positions give a better fit.

As an optional step, to sharpen line definition around the sleeve, the armhole can be taped. This is done before the sleeve is inserted, by pinning and basting twill tape over the armhole seamline, easing the garment in slightly as you do. Because taping causes armhole fit to be closer, it is not recommended for coats.

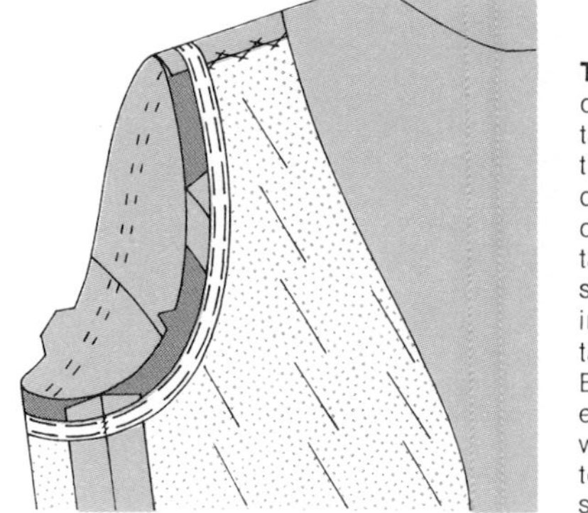
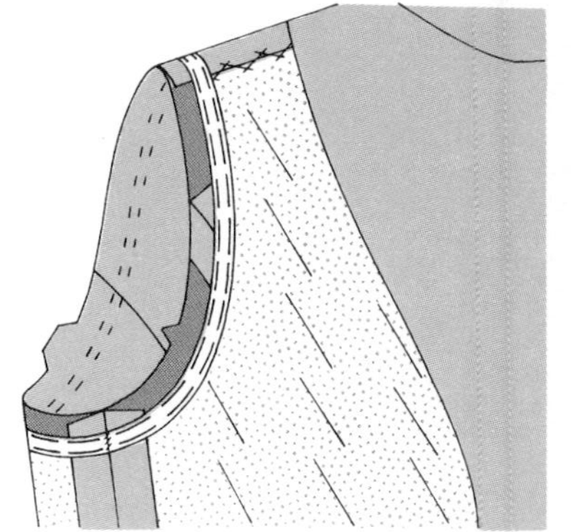

To tape armhole, cut ¼″ twill tape ½″ shorter than armhole circumference; center and pin tape over seamline; ease in garment so tape ends meet. Baste along both edges of tape; whipstitch ends together. Insert sleeve as shown.

1. If sleeve is designed with elbow ease, complete the darts or place a row of easestitching within designated markings on the seamline, as pattern requires.

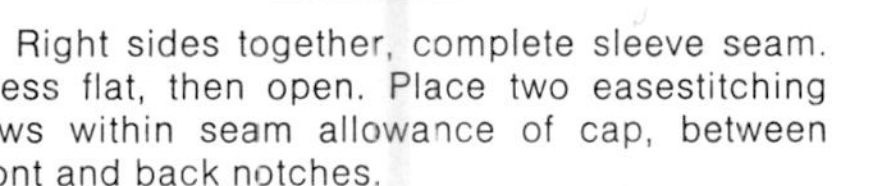

2. Right sides together, complete sleeve seam. Press flat, then open. Place two easestitching rows within seam allowance of cap, between front and back notches.

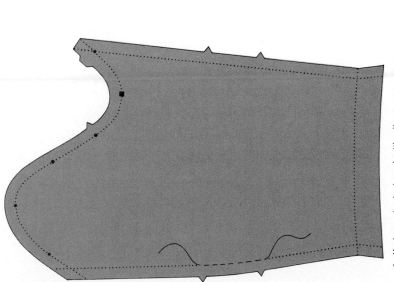

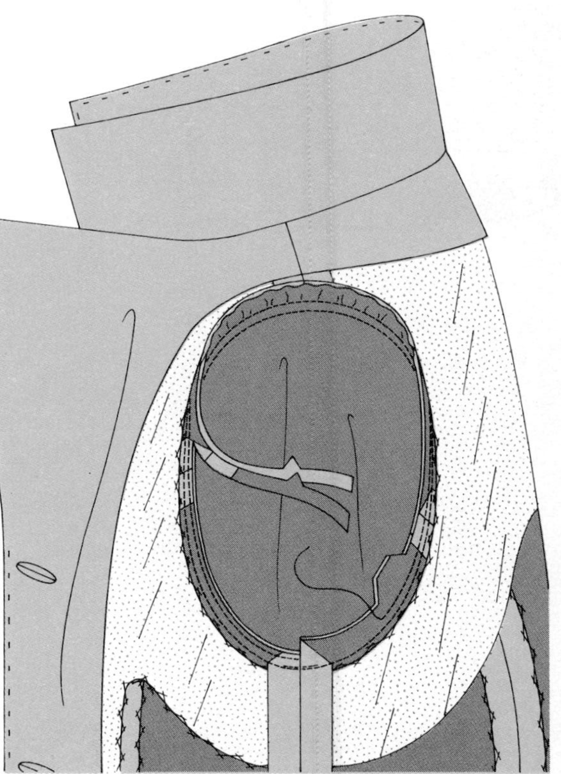

3. Pin and baste sleeve into armhole. If sleeve fit is satisfactory, stitch it in permanently. Finish seam allowance with a second row of stitching, then trim close to second stitching line.

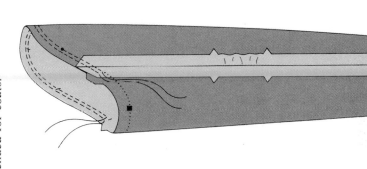

Running stitch 131
Whipstitch 136

Sleeve heading

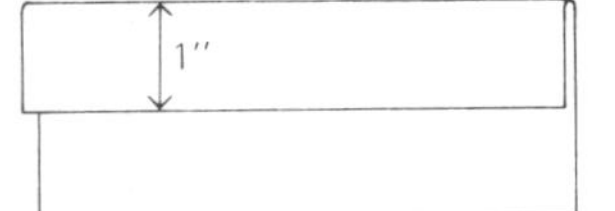

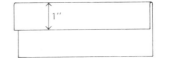

Sleeve headings can be purchased or made. To make sleeve heading, cut a 3" x 5" piece of lamb's wool, flannel, or polyester fleece; make a 1" fold on long side.

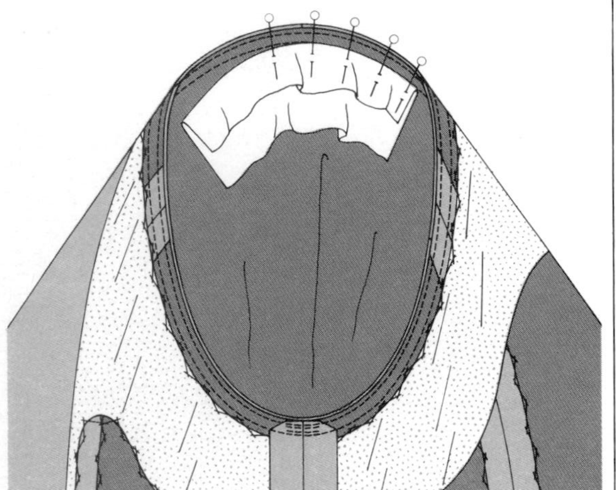

Center and pin heading to wrong side of sleeve cap with fold against seamline, wider half of heading against sleeve.

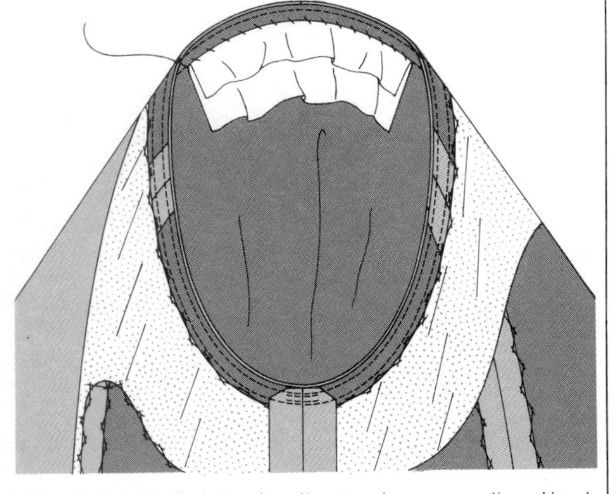

Whipstitch fold of sleeve heading to sleeve seamline. Heading now supports and rounds out sleeve cap.

Shoulder pads

Shoulder pads are sometimes needed in a tailored garment to help maintain the shoulder line. They are also useful for disguising such figure faults as rounded shoulders and uneven shoulder heights. Thicknesses of shoulder pads can vary, depending on their precise purpose; select one that does the job without distorting the natural shape of the garment. Shoulder pads such as the one shown below can be purchased in various shapes, or pads can be made for a more exact fit. To make a shoulder pad pattern, overlap shoulder seams on the front and back pattern pieces; pin any darts or seams that extend into the shoulder seam or armhole. Draw shape of pad as shown at upper right: Connect armhole curve between front and back notches, gradually extending curve ⅜ inch out at shoulder line. Draw shoulder curve with its top edge 1 inch from the neckline. Use pattern to cut out graduated layers of polyester fleece. Stitch layers together and insert shoulder pads.

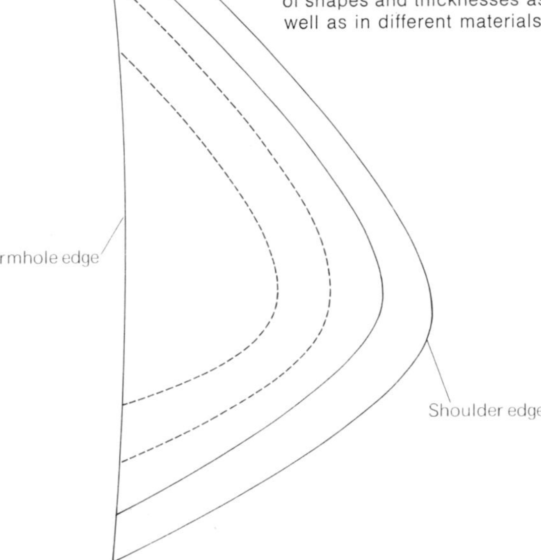

A purchased shoulder pad of the type shown here is sometimes called a *shoulder shape*. They come in a variety of shapes and thicknesses as well as in different materials.

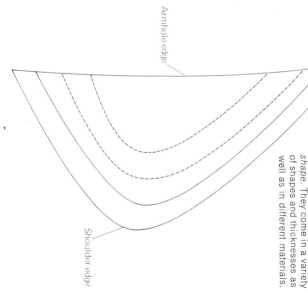

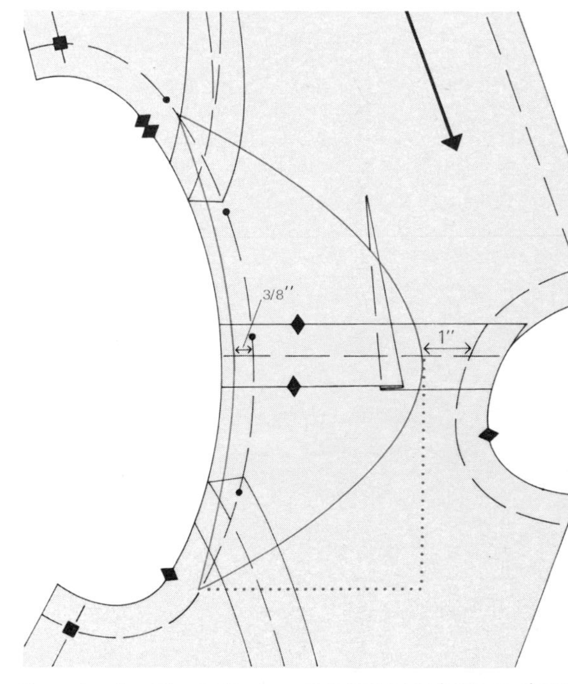

To make shoulder pads, draw shoulder pad shape as shown. For a hollow-chested person, square off the front portion of the pad, as indicated by the dotted lines.

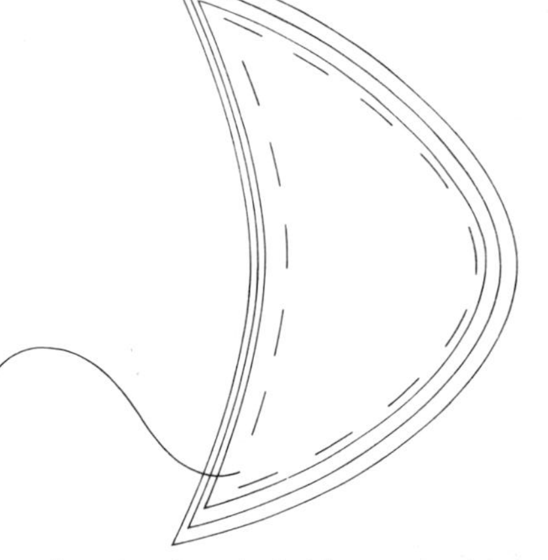

For each pad, cut graduated layers of polyester fleece; hold layers together with long running stitches.

Catchstitch (flat) 129 Single cross-stitch tack 134 Interfaced hems 295

Inserting shoulder pad

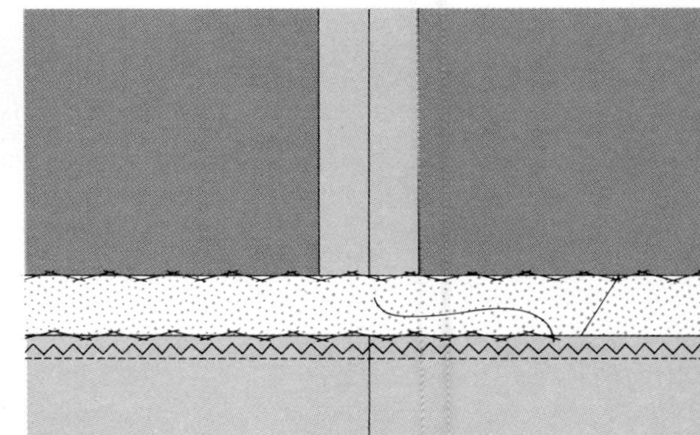

Place garment on model; insert pad and adjust its position as shown, with top edge extending ⅜" from armhole seamline. Pin pad in place along shoulder line, and remove garment.

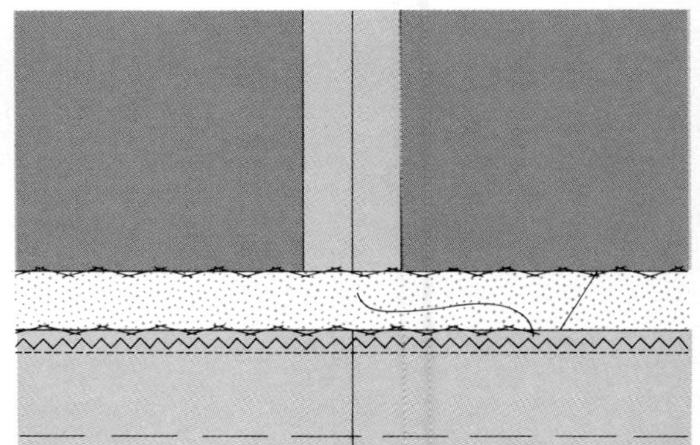

Turn garment wrong side out; stitch edge of pad to armhole seam allowance with a running stitch. Flip up facing, and tack shoulder end of pad to shoulder seam allowances.

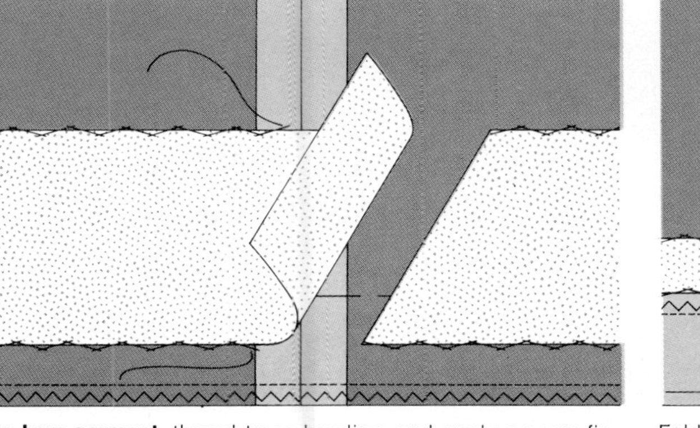

To complete shoulder pad application, bring facing down, then pin and catchstitch the upper portion of the front facing to the top layer of the shoulder pad.

Hemming tailored garments

As a rule, the hem of a tailored garment is interfaced to give body to the area and to help maintain the hem's shape along the lower edge. The interfacing in the completed hem usually extends past the finished edge; this distributes the bulk and has the effect of "grading" the two layers. The interfacing is generally positioned so it goes over the hemline, producing a softly rounded crease; in a man's tailored jacket, however, the interfacing stops at the hemline so that the crease at the bottom edge will be sharp. Detailed instructions on how to interface a hem are given in the chapter on Hems. When the hem is completed, all bastings are removed from the garment. Before attaching the lining, have the entire garment professionally steam-pressed to permanently set all seams.

To hem garment, thread-trace hemline, and apply a seam finish to the raw edge. Catchstitch interfacing to underlining.

Fold hem up along hemline marking and baste along the folded edge. Catchstitch free edge of hem to interfacing.

Pressing equipment 18-19
Cross-stitch tacks 134
Staystitching 144
Darts 159

Lining

Lining is the last fabric layer to be added to the tailored garment. It should fit smoothly within the garment, providing a neat, clean inside finish. As a rule, the lining is constructed from a smooth fabric that complements the outer fabric layer (see p. 360). Any alterations in the garment should also be made in the lining. To ensure sufficient ease for body movement without strain on lining seams, there is usually a vertical pleat down the back of the lining, and a fold at the bottom of the sleeve and at the garment hem. If your pattern does not supply lining pieces, these can easily be made up from the main garment patterns. Instructions for preparing front and back lining sections are given at the right; the sleeve lining can be cut from the sleeve pattern piece. In tailoring, the lining is generally hand-sewed to the garment; it should be handled carefully to avoid stretching. Press lightly to protect lining from getting a worn look. For additional warmth, an interlining may be installed (see p. 382).

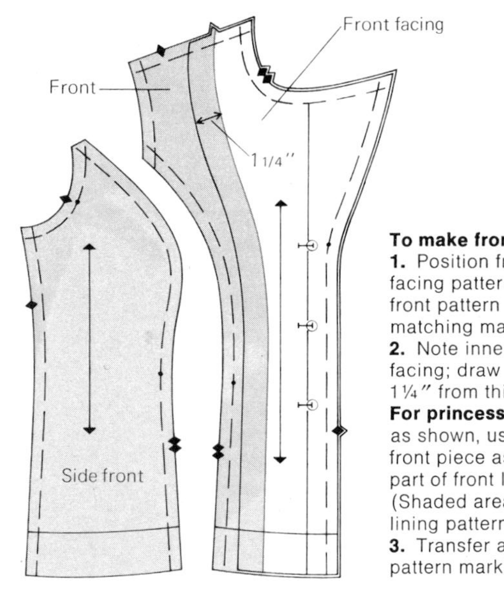

To make front lining:
1. Position front facing pattern *under* front pattern piece, matching markings.
2. Note inner edge of facing; draw new line 1¼" from this edge.
For princess seams, as shown, use side front piece as is for part of front lining. (Shaded areas are lining patterns.)
3. Transfer all pattern markings.

Back facing
1 1/4"
1"
Back
Side back

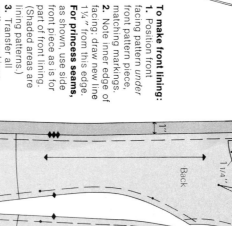

To make back lining:
1. Tape a strip of tissue paper to pattern's back edge.
2. Position back facing *under* back pattern piece.
3. Mark 1" beyond pattern's center back edge (not seamline) to allow for pleat.
If garment does not have a center back seam, mark 1" beyond center back foldline.
4. Note inner edge of facing; draw new line 1¼" from this edge.
For princess seams, as shown, use side back piece as is for part of back lining. (Shaded areas are the lining pieces.)
5. Transfer all pattern markings.

Joining main lining pieces

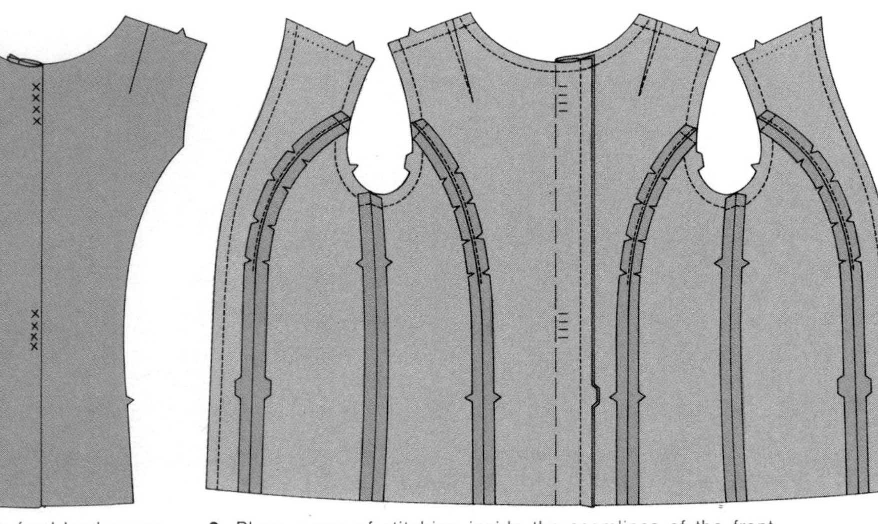

1. Stitch darts (and back seam, if any). Baste up the back pleat; press to one side; tack through all layers with cross stitches below neckline and at waistline.

2. Place a row of stitching inside the seamlines of the front opening, back shoulder, neck and armhole edges (staystitching can serve for this stitching line). Complete internal seams and side seams. Press seams flat, then open; clip and notch the seam allowances as necessary.

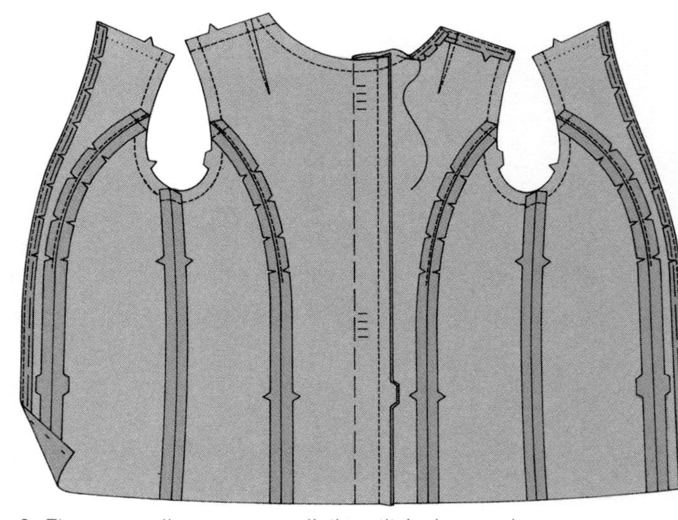

3. The seam allowances on all the stitched raw edges, except for the armhole edges, should be turned and pressed to the wrong side; clip and notch the seam allowances as necessary so that they lie flat. Baste the turned edges in place.

Running stitch 131
Slipstitch (uneven) 132

Attaching lining to garment

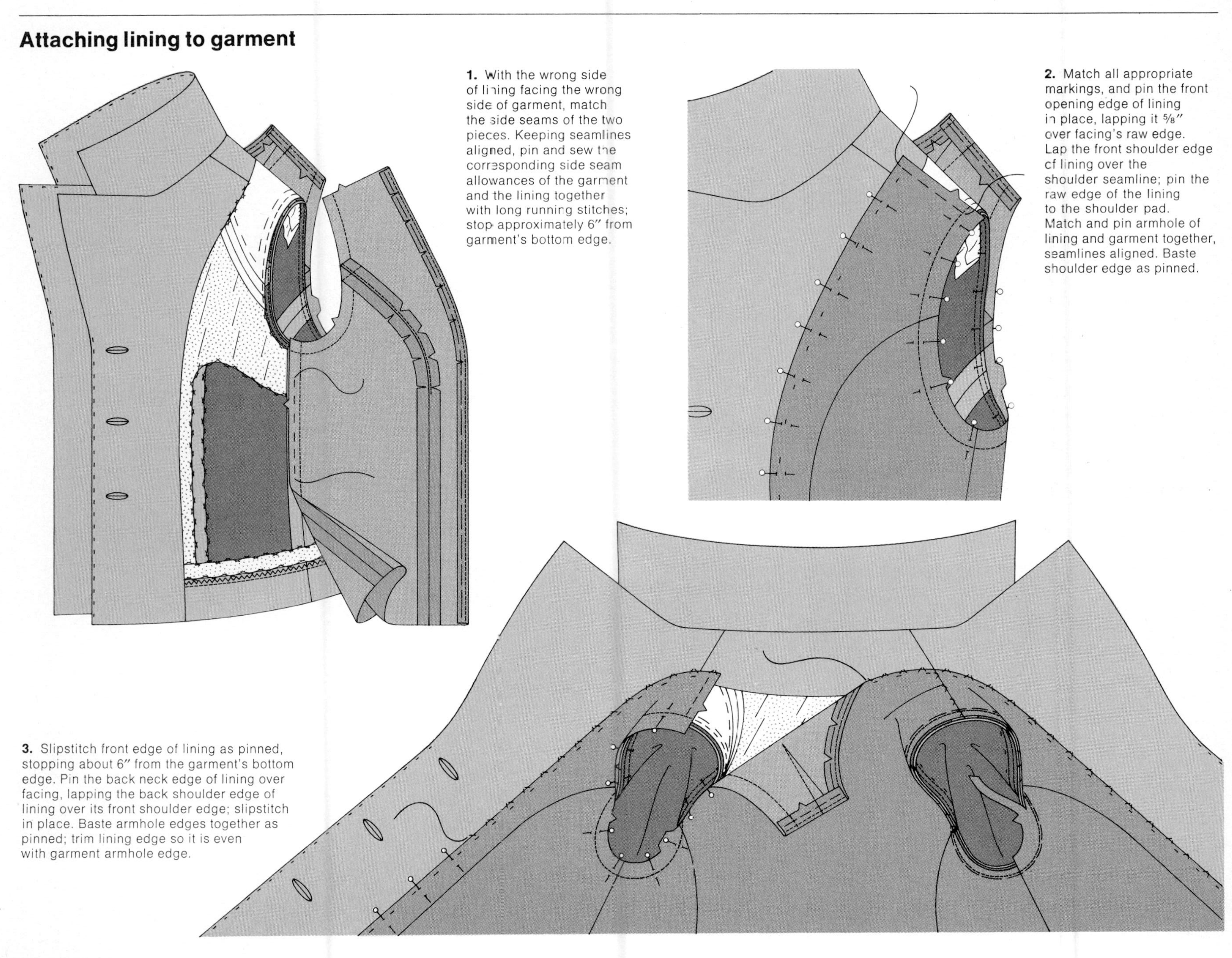

1. With the wrong side of lining facing the wrong side of garment, match the side seams of the two pieces. Keeping seamlines aligned, pin and sew the corresponding side seam allowances of the garment and the lining together with long running stitches; stop approximately 6″ from garment's bottom edge.

2. Match all appropriate markings, and pin the front opening edge of lining in place, lapping it ⅝″ over facing's raw edge. Lap the front shoulder edge of lining over the shoulder seamline; pin the raw edge of the lining to the shoulder pad. Match and pin armhole of lining and garment together, seamlines aligned. Baste shoulder edge as pinned.

3. Slipstitch front edge of lining as pinned, stopping about 6″ from the garment's bottom edge. Pin the back neck edge of lining over facing, lapping the back shoulder edge of lining over its front shoulder edge; slipstitch in place. Baste armhole edges together as pinned; trim lining edge so it is even with garment armhole edge.

Stitch length for easing 30
Running stitch 131
Staystitching 144

Sleeve lining

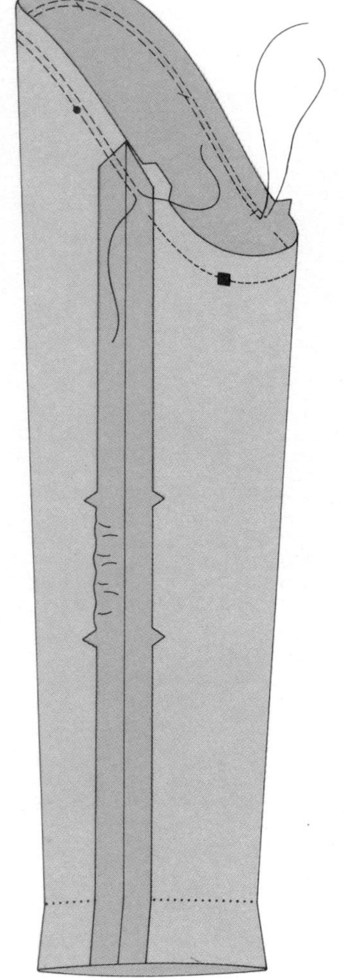

1. With right sides facing, complete sleeve seam; press open. Place two rows of easestitching within seam allowance of cap, between front and back notches. Staystitch sleeve underarm between same two notches.

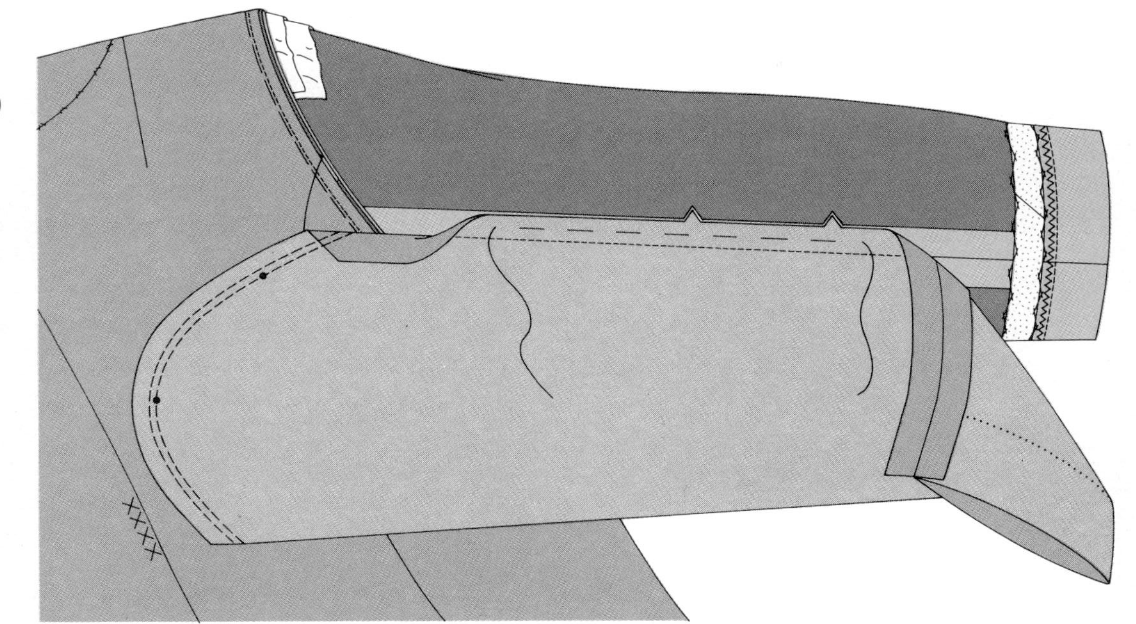

2. Turn both garment and sleeve lining wrong side out. Match and pin corresponding sleeves of lining and garment together along seam allowances. Hold the seam allowances together with a long running stitch, stopping about 4" from bottom edge of garment sleeve.

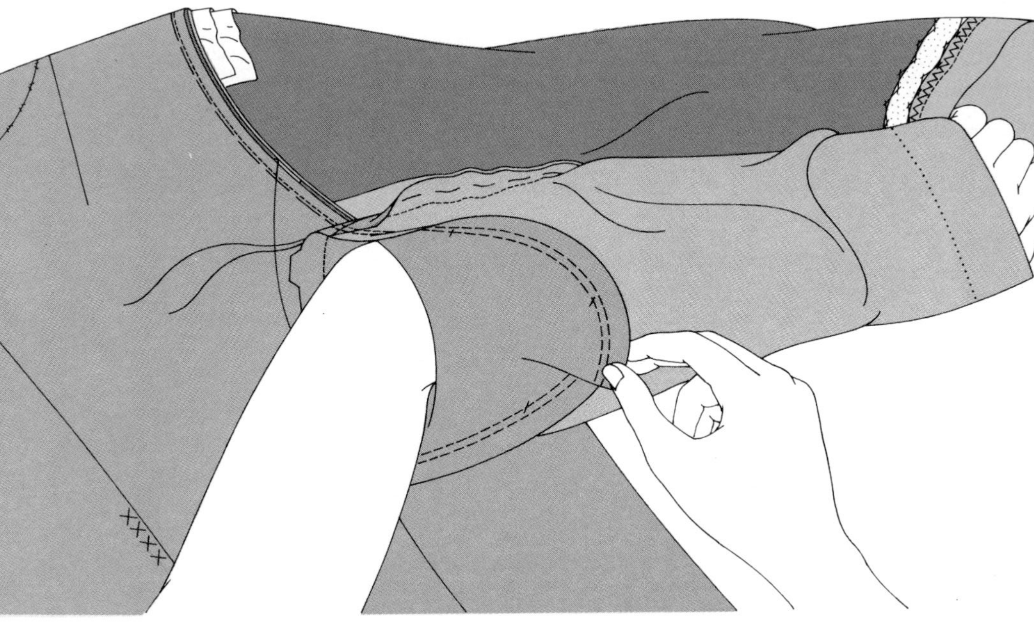

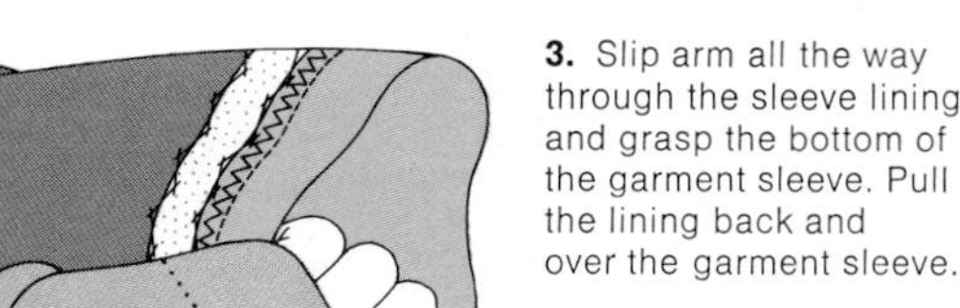

3. Slip arm all the way through the sleeve lining, and grasp the bottom of the garment sleeve. Pull the lining back and over the garment sleeve.

Slipstitch (uneven) 132
Hemming a lining 297

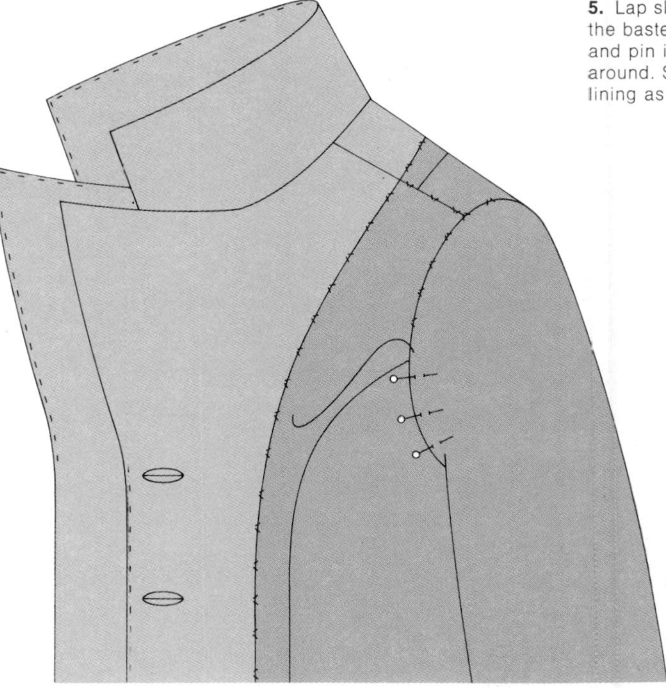

4. Pull sleeve lining up and over entire garment sleeve. Draw up the easestitching threads so cap of sleeve lining fits around the armhole. Turn under seam allowance of sleeve lining, clipping the underarm curve as necessary.

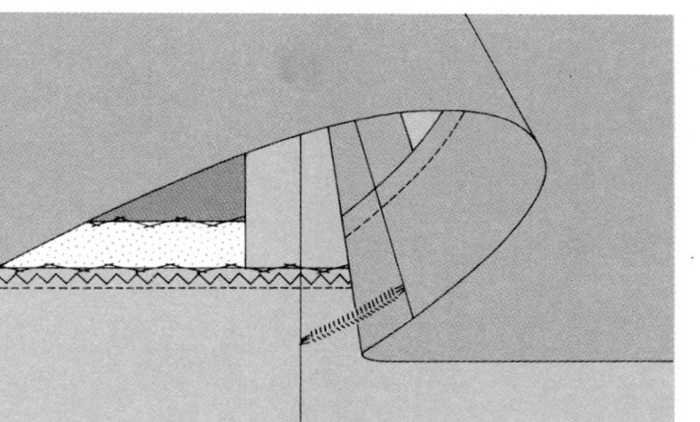

5. Lap sleeve lining over the basted armhole line, and pin in place all around. Slipstitch sleeve lining as pinned.

Hemming methods for linings

The lining hem can be completed by one of two methods. The first is used most often at the bottom edges of jackets and sleeves; in this procedure, the lining is attached to the garment hem and a fold created for greater wearing ease. The second method is used principally at the bottom edge of coats; here the lining is separately hemmed and secured to the garment with French tacks. Refer to the chapter on Hems for detailed directions for both methods. Before beginning either method, place the garment wrong side out on a model, and pin lining to garment 6 inches above hemline.

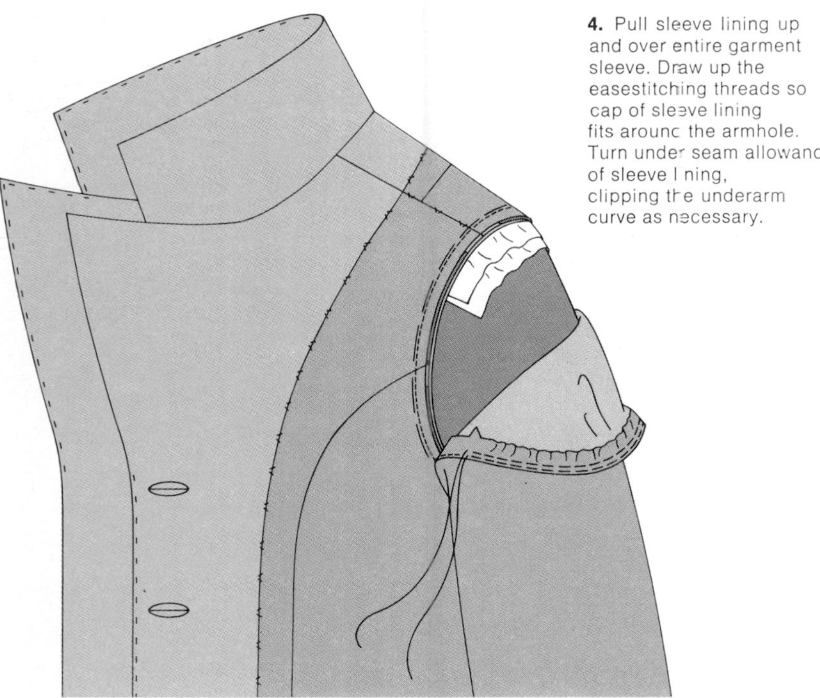

An attached lining is completely secured to the garment hem, with a small fold at the bottom to provide additional wearing ease within the lining. Attached hems are most often used at the bottom edges of tailored jackets and sleeves.

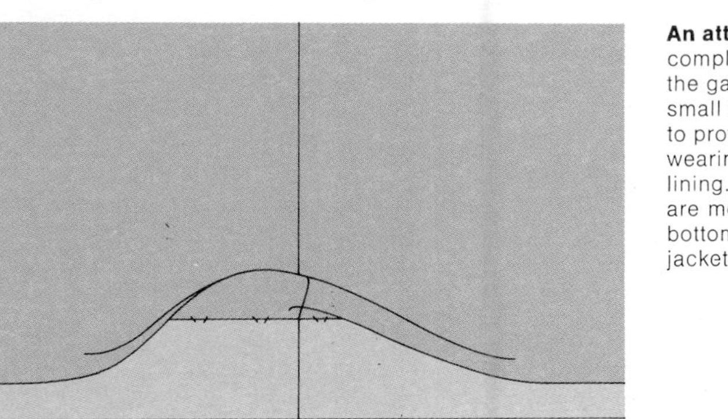

A free-hanging lining is hemmed separately from the garment, then secured to the garment at each seam with French tacks. Free-hanging linings are most often used at the bottom of tailored coats.

Tailoring/special techniques

Interlining 83 Whipstitch 136 Staystitching 144 Darts 159 Fasteners 351-357

Interlining

If additional warmth is desired in a tailored garment, another layer of fabric known as an interlining can be applied between the lining and the constructed garment. Popular fabrics for this purpose include lamb's wool, polyester fleece, and flannel. Because the interlining contributes extra bulk, more wearing ease must be allowed when adjusting the garment and lining patterns. The interlining is usually cut from the lining pattern, but without a back pleat. In working with interlining, each section is basted to its corresponding lining section and both are then handled as one layer. To help reduce bulk, the interlining is cut off at the hemline and excess seam allowances are trimmed away wherever possible.

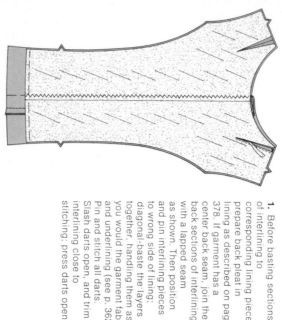

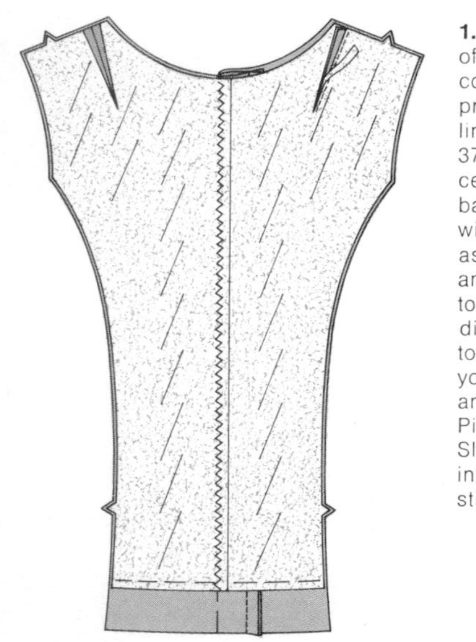

1. Before basting sections of interlining to corresponding lining pieces, prepare back pleat in lining as described on page 378. If garment has a center back seam, join the back sections of interlining with a lapped seam as shown. Then position and pin interlining pieces to wrong side of lining; diagonal-baste the layers together, handling them as you would the garment fabric and underlining (see p. 362). Pin and stitch all darts. Slash darts open, and trim interlining close to stitching; press darts open.

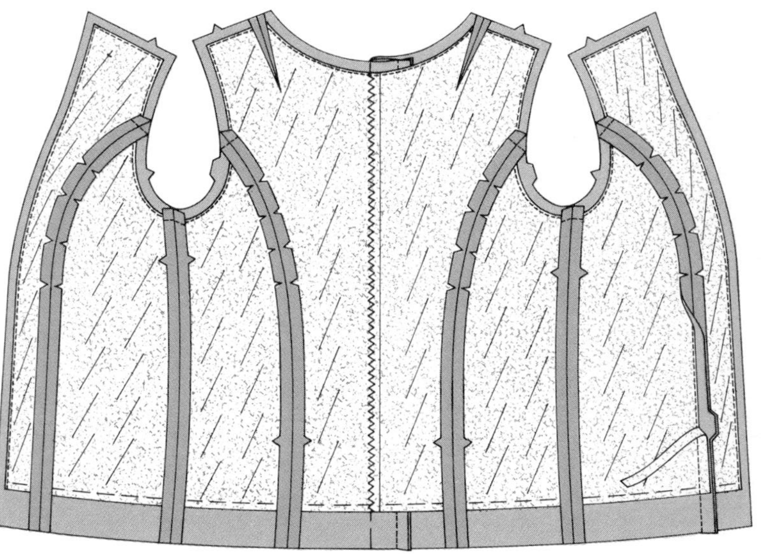

2. Baste around each interlined lining piece to keep the raw edges of the two layers from shifting. Then place a row of stitching inside the seamlines of the front opening, front and back shoulders, neck and armhole edges; trim interlining seam allowances close to the stitching. With right sides together, complete all internal seams within front and back sections. Then join front to back along side seams. Press each seam flat; trim interlining seam allowances close to stitching line, and press seams open. Remove basting. Proceed with lining construction (see p. 378).

Professional touches

Certain finishing touches, none of them difficult to manage, can give your tailored garment a professional look. Buttons, for example, can be important accessories if they are carefully coordinated with the garment. If snaps are used to hold the garment closed, buy or make the covered kind; they will be less conspicuous. When sewing such visible items to the garment, position them properly and sew them on neatly and securely.

Weights at the hemline, either the chain or drapery type, will help to maintain the hang of the garment. Chain weights are sewed under the lining hem fold, and are used most often in tailored jackets. Drapery weights are placed in small "pockets," which are sewed to seams and openings before the garment is hemmed; they work best in tailored coats. Be sure any weight you select will hold the garment in place without distorting its line.

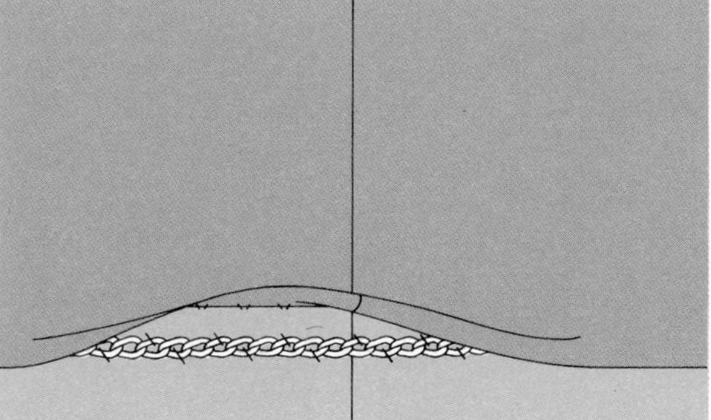

Chain weights are placed under the fold of the hem lining. They can be used either around the entire garment or along sections of it. To install, position the chain flat against the garment hem and secure it in place with a whipstitch every 2" on each side of the chain.

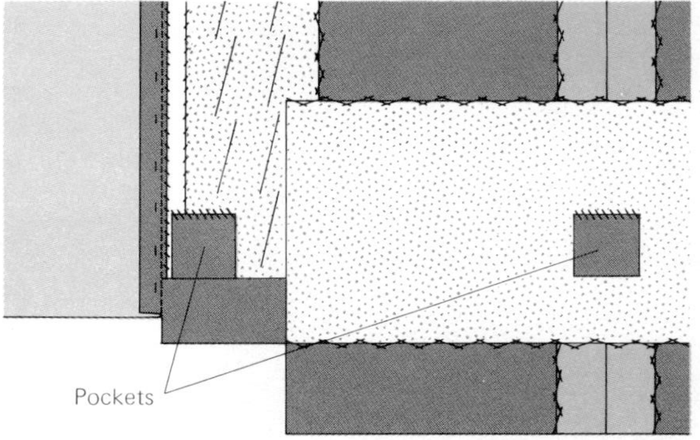

Drapery weights are first put in fabric "pockets," which are then sewed to the garment. To make pockets, cut rectangles of fabric. Fold each in half; seam two sides; turn. Drop in the weight and stitch the pocket across the top. Whipstitch pockets to seams and front openings.

Sewing for Men & Children

Sewing for men and boys

Introduction

When sewing is done for men and children, some of the goals and certain techniques differ from those for women's garments. It is the intent of this chapter to deal with those aspects that vary from the usual. To make clear how these variations fit into the customary procedure, a step-by-step checklist has been provided for each of several garment types. These lists are not intended to take the place of your pattern direction sheet, but to supplement it, and to guide you in locating techniques that are to be found elsewhere in the book. Page numbers are listed alongside each step.

In the construction of a man's garment, the principal goal is clothes with individual styling plus good fit. Since most men prefer results that resemble ready-to-wear or custom tailoring, the procedures for men's garments are adapted from manufacturers' and tailors' methods. Many of these techniques are complex, particularly those for a tailored jacket. It is advisable to have a basic knowledge of sewing and some experience before undertaking such intricate projects.

In sewing for children, two primary aims are durability and allowance for growth. Speedy completion of the garment is also important. Hints and techniques in the children's section, which begins on page 404, are based on these criteria.

Selecting pattern size

Pattern sizes for men and boys are grouped in three categories, each of them related to body build. A comparison of body types is shown at the right. (For Toddlers' and Little boys', see p. 404.) To determine the correct size, first take and record measurements on a chart like one on the opposite page. Compare the starred measurements with those in the size charts below. Select a **jacket or coat** size according to chest measurement, a **shirt** by the neckband size, **trousers** according to waist measurement. If measurements fall between two sizes, buy the larger size for a husky build, the smaller size for one that is slender. When pattern types are grouped, jacket or shirt plus trousers, for instance, choose the size by the chest measurement and adjust the trousers, if necessary.

Size range charts

BOYS'					**TEEN-BOYS'**			
Size	**7**	**8**	**10**	**12**	**14**	**16**	**18**	**20**
Chest	26	27	28	30	32	33½	35	36½
Waist	23	24	25	26	27	28	29	30
Hip (seat)	27	28	29½	31	32½	34	35½	37
Neckband	11¾	12	12½	13	13½	14	14½	15
Height	48	50	54	58	61	64	66	68

MEN'S								
Size	**34**	**36**	**38**	**40**	**42**	**44**	**46**	**48**
Chest	34	36	38	40	42	44	46	48
Waist	28	30	32	34	36	39	42	44
Hip (seat)	35	37	39	41	43	45	47	49
Neckband	14	14½	15	15½	16	16½	17	17½
Shirt sleeve	32	32	33	33	34	34	35	35

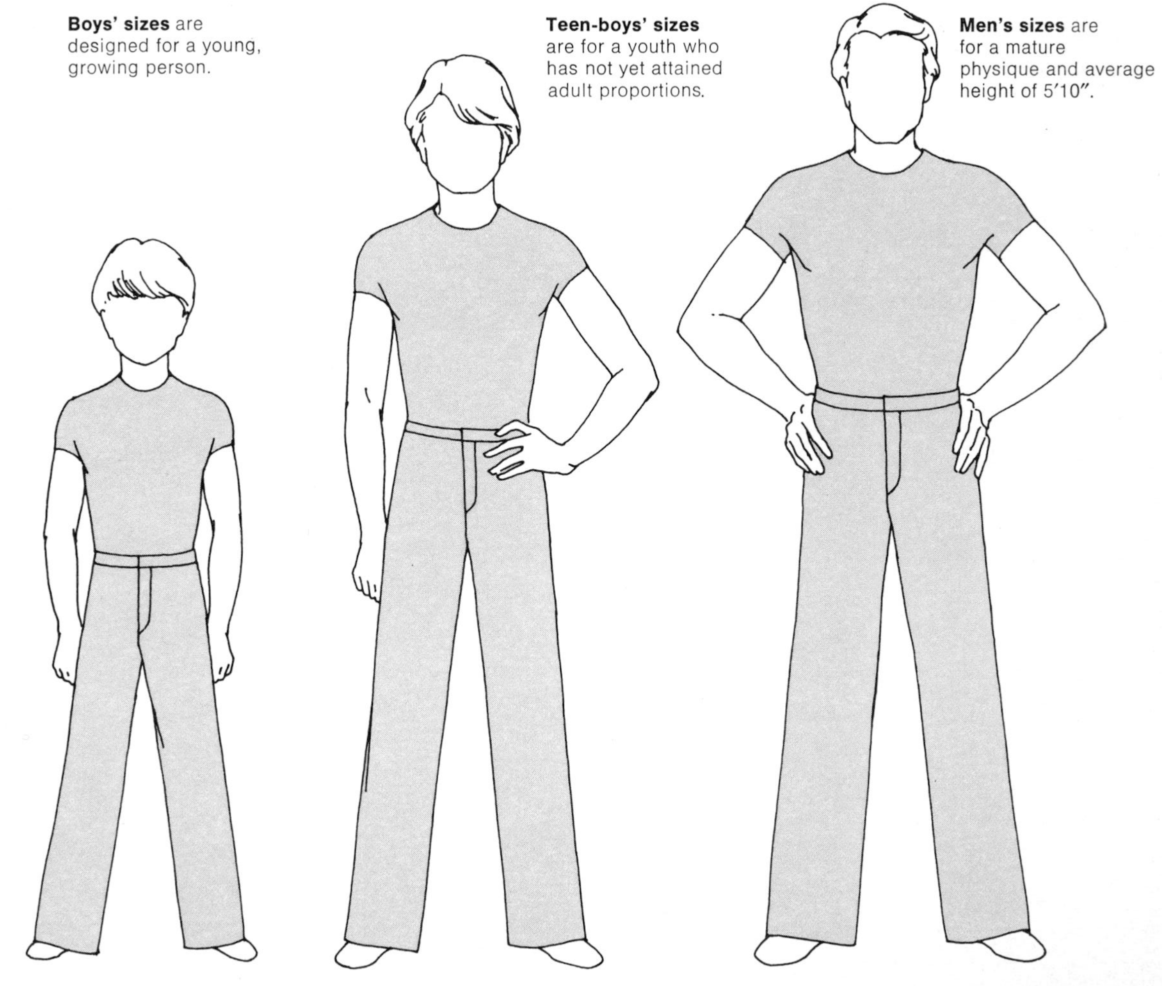

Boys' sizes are designed for a young, growing person.

Teen-boys' sizes are for a youth who has not yet attained adult proportions.

Men's sizes are for a mature physique and average height of 5'10".

How to take measurements

Directions for taking two sets of measurements are given below; for convenience, all can be taken at one time. Those in the **first group** (marked with asterisks) are used primarily for choosing a pattern size (see opposite page). They might also indicate the need for pattern adjustments. If the "difference" column shows a variance of ½ inch or more, the pattern needs to be adjusted by that difference (see Fitting section for methods).

Measurements in the **second group** (no asterisks) are useful for achieving good fit. These can be compared to actual pattern dimensions to see if the pattern needs adjusting in these areas.

The best way to take measurements is over an undershirt and lightweight trousers—no belt. Use a flexible tape measure, and pull it snug, but not too tight. When measuring *waist, outseam,* and *inseam,* trousers should be adjusted to the preferred wearing position. The *crotch depth* can be measured by the method that is given on page 405, or it can be calculated instead by subtracting the inseam from the outseam measurement.

Measurements for growing boys should be checked often to keep pace with growth spurts. Arms and legs can grow longer without an accompanying change in girth. If this happens, a lengthening of the present size may be all that is needed.

Measurement chart

MEASUREMENT	YOURS	PATTERN	DIFFERENCE
Height*			
Chest*			
Waist*			
Hip (seat)*			
Neckband*			
Shirt sleeve*			
Shoulder			
Arm length			
Trouser outseam			
Trouser inseam			
Crotch depth			

FOR PATTERN SIZE:

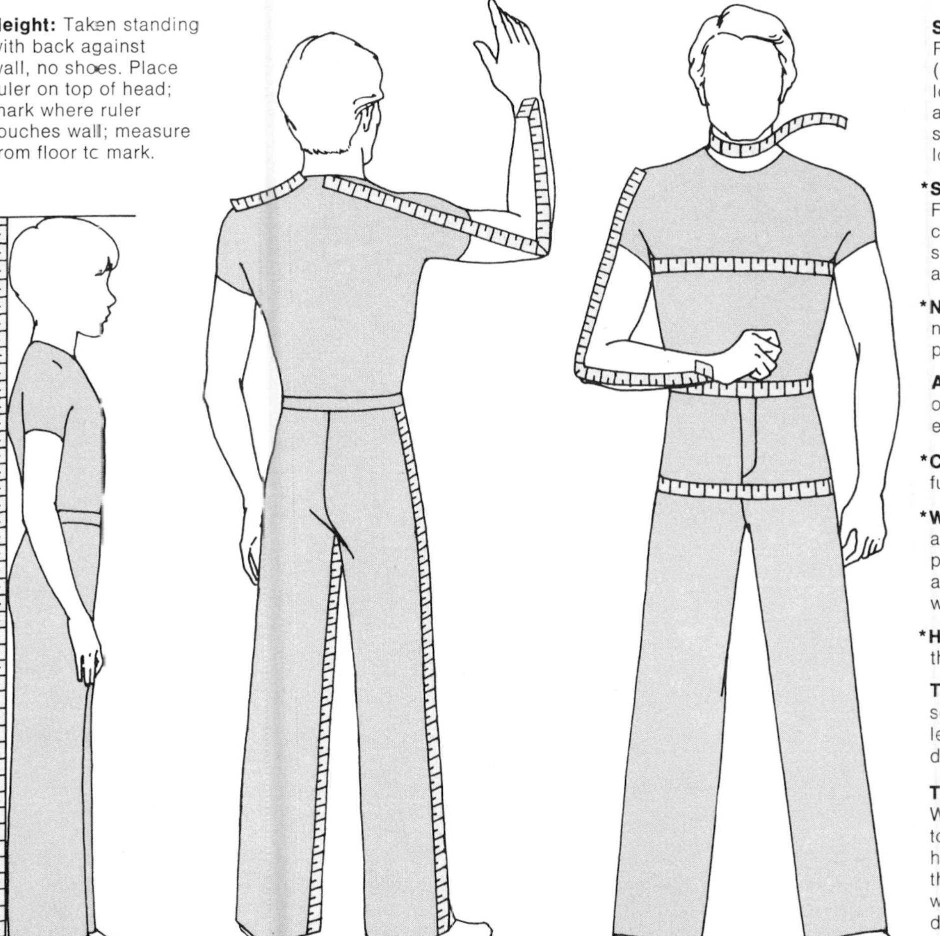

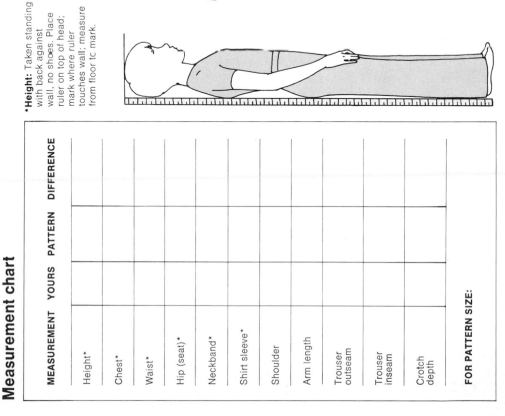

***Height:** Taken standing with back against wall, no shoes. Place ruler on top of head; mark where ruler touches wall; measure from floor to mark.

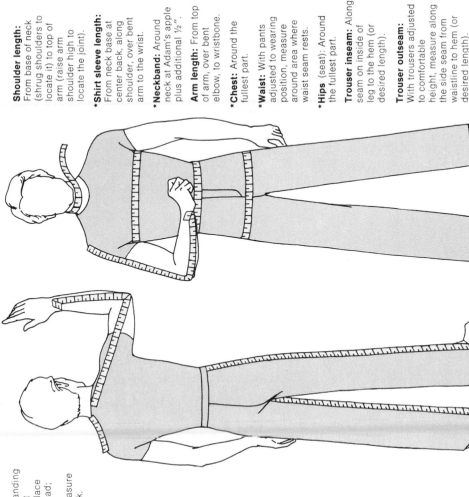

Shoulder length: From base of neck (shrug shoulders to locate it) to top of arm (raise arm shoulder high to locate the joint).

***Shirt sleeve length:** From neck base at center back, along shoulder, over bent arm to the wrist.

***Neckband:** Around neck at Adam's apple plus additional ½".

Arm length: From top of arm, over bent elbow, to wristbone.

***Chest:** Around the fullest part.

***Waist:** With pants adjusted to wearing position, measure around area where waist seam rests.

***Hips** (seat): Around the fullest part.

Trouser inseam: Along seam on inside of leg to the hem (or desired length).

Trouser outseam: With trousers adjusted to comfortable height, measure along the side seam from waistline to hem (or desired length).

Pattern alterations 102-104, 106-109

Making and fitting a trial garment 120, 364
Tailoring 360-382

Making a jacket

There are two basic approaches to tailoring a man's jacket, one traditional, the other modern. The first produces a jacket that is molded and crisp, qualities that have for many years been characteristic of men's styles. The second results in a less structured look, suitable for today's casual trend in dressing. Both require basic knowledge of sewing and precise handling of details.

The **traditional method** encompasses all techniques explained in the Tailoring chapter, with these few differences: (1) Underlining is omitted; (2) more shape is built into the jacket with additional layers of interfacing (see discussion and handling of chest piece, below and opposite); (3) the collar is structured almost entirely by hand (see p. 389); (4) the sleeve is pressed differently (p. 389); (5) an inside pocket is added to the front.

Fabrics most suitable for traditional tailoring are wools and wool blends, which shape easily. A type with medium thickness and moderate sponginess, such as flannel, is particularly good. Menswear worsteds and gabardines are the most durable, but their close weave and hard surface makes them more difficult to handle. Interfacing should always be a wool and hair combination.

Traditional findings, such as twill tape, chest pieces, shoulder pads, and sleeve headings, can be bought at tailors' suppliers and notions counters.

In **modern tailoring**, fusing and machine stitching are substituted for hand techniques. This approach is not only speedier, but in many ways sturdier. Such construction will even withstand machine washing. Applicable to any fabric type, modern methods are especially suited to washable ones such as cotton or synthetic double knit.

In both tailoring methods, the lining options are three—full, half, or none. The choice is partly a matter of preference, but style and fabric also have a bearing. Where a lining is used, the back neck facing, found in women's jackets, is omitted.

Whatever the construction method, preliminary steps should include careful checking of measurements (see p. 385), careful appraisal of proportions (see below), and adjustments, if necessary.

Before proceeding, go through the Tailoring chapter, then note the variations that begin here and continue through page 390. You can use the checklist at the right as a general guide to procedure and for locating techniques; follow your pattern's directions for specific design features.

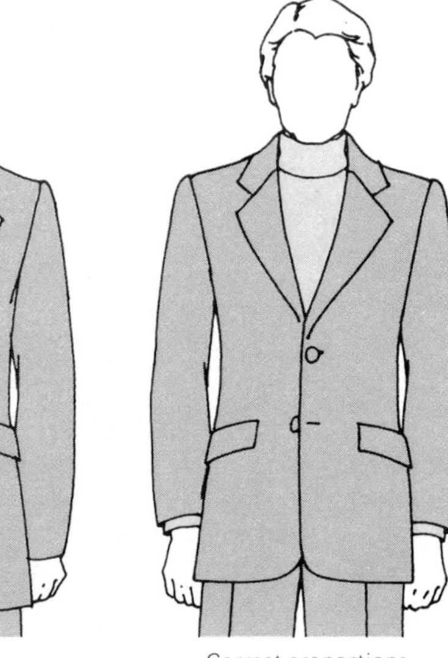

Too short — Too long — Correct proportions

A well-fitted jacket should be long enough to cover the seat, ending where legs and buttocks join; sleeves should just touch the wristbone, allowing the edge of the shirt cuff to show. Lapel length and pocket placements should be in proportion with the wearer's build. If your pattern's proportions need adjusting, you may wish to make a trial garment in heavy muslin (see Fitting chapter for the method).

Checklist/jacket procedure

Cut out jacket shell, 84-93, 362; interfacing 361

Transfer pattern markings 94, 362

Check garment fit 363-364

Stitch darts and internal seams of main garment sections 365

Apply front interfacing: padstitched method 366-367; fused method 388

Construct front pockets 275-279, 284-288

Attach chest pieces 386-387

Apply back interfacing: woven fabric 368; knit fabric 369

Join jacket fronts and back 371

Construct inside pocket 390

Attach facings and collar sections: traditional method 389; modern method 371-374

Set in sleeves 256, 375

Press armhole seams 389

Insert sleeve headings and shoulder pads 376-377, 389

Hem jacket 295, 377

Cut, construct, and attach lining: full lining/traditional 379; full lining/modern 80; half lining 390; sleeve lining 380

Make buttonholes 343-348

Attach buttons 351-352

The jacket chest piece

A chest piece is used to round out the hollow in the front of a man's shoulder. It consists of several layers of specially shaped interfacing, caught loosely together, and attached to the front interfacing. The exact number and shaping of pieces can be varied to accommodate individual styling or physique, but a typical chest piece has four layers like the ones shown opposite. For a boy's jacket, also for an unlined style, the chest piece is usually omitted because it would add too much bulk.

Ready-made chest pieces are available, made with four layers (one of felt) fused together. One size fits any jacket up to size 44. These are especially suitable for washable garments.

Padding stitches 131, 366

Constructing a chest piece

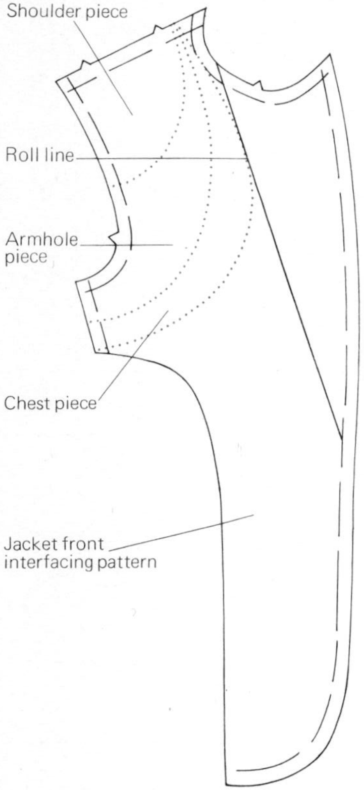

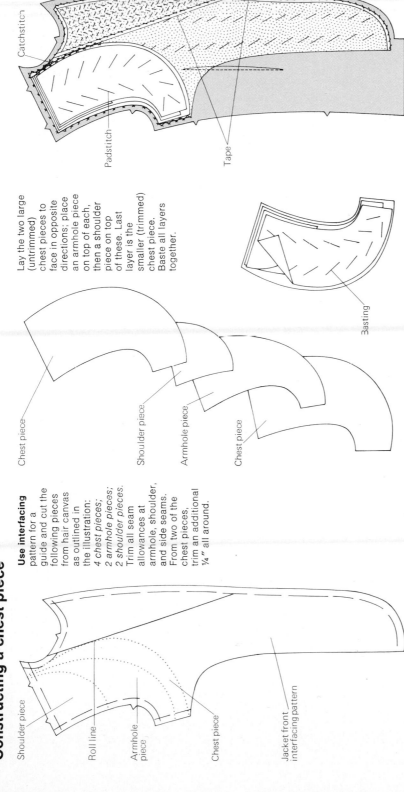

Shoulder piece
Roll line
Armhole piece
Chest piece
Jacket front interfacing pattern

Use interfacing pattern for a guide and cut the following pieces from hair canvas as outlined in the illustration: *4 chest pieces; 2 armhole pieces; 2 shoulder pieces.* Trim all seam allowances at armhole, shoulder, and side seams. From two of the chest pieces, trim an additional ¼″ all around.

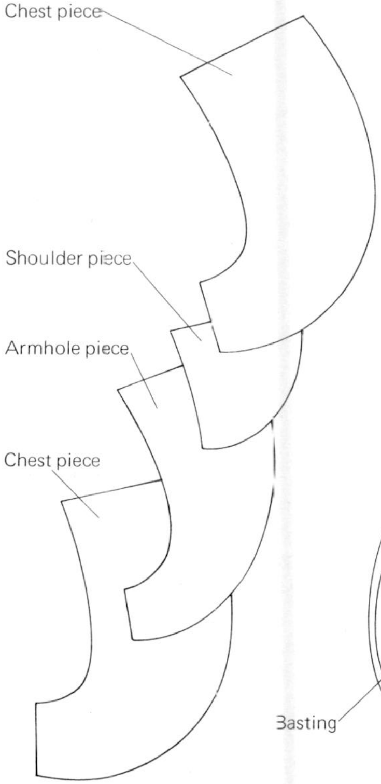

Chest piece
Shoulder piece
Armhole piece
Chest piece

Lay the two large (untrimmed) chest pieces to face in opposite directions; place an armhole piece on top of each, then a shoulder piece on top of these. Last layer is the smaller (trimmed) chest piece. Baste all layers together.

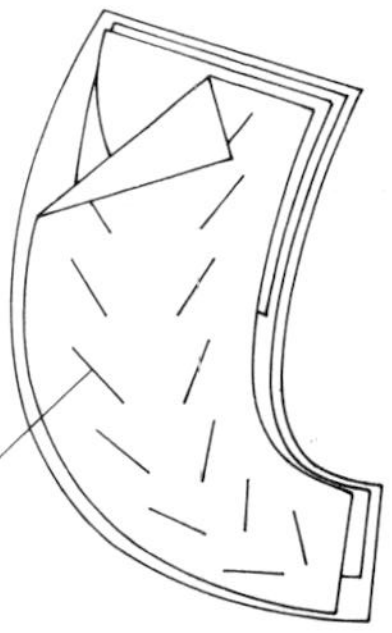

Basting

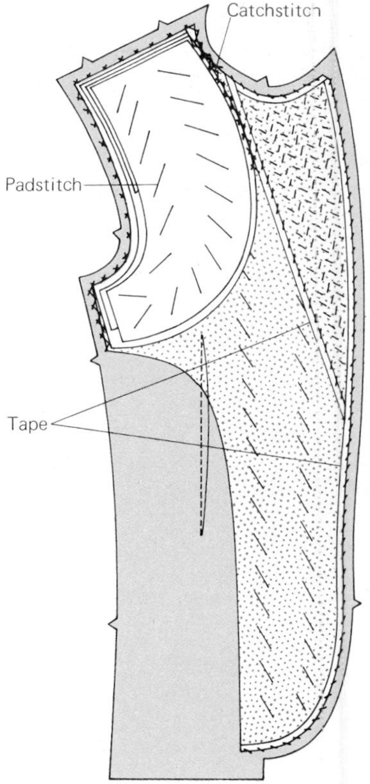

Catchstitch
Padstitch
Tape

Position chest piece on jacket front, with smaller chest-piece layer on top, armhole and shoulder edges aligned with jacket seams. Use long padstitches to hold chest piece in position, catching stitches through the front interfacing only. Catchstitch the upper part of the curved edge (next to roll line) to jacket interfacing. Remove basting.

Attaching a commercial chest piece

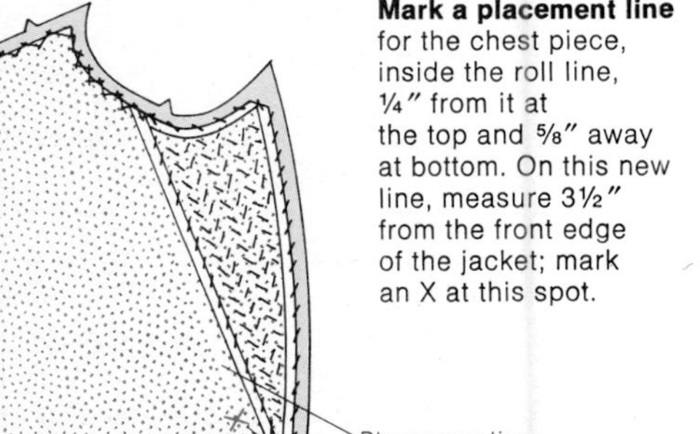

Mark a placement line for the chest piece, inside the roll line, ¼″ from it at the top and ⅝″ away at bottom. On this new line, measure 3½″ from the front edge of the jacket; mark an X at this spot.

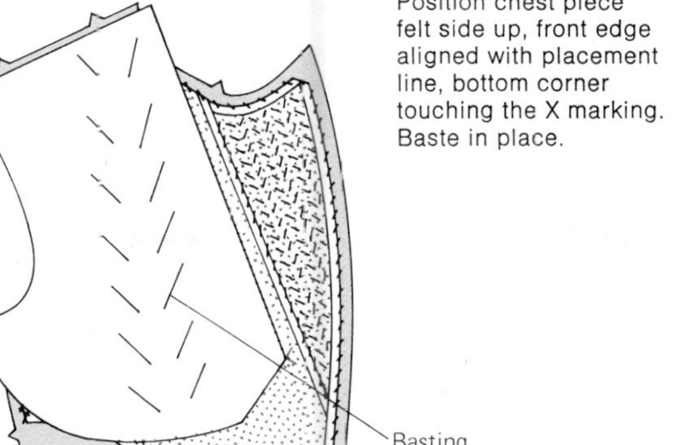

Position chest piece felt side up, front edge aligned with placement line, bottom corner touching the X marking. Baste in place.

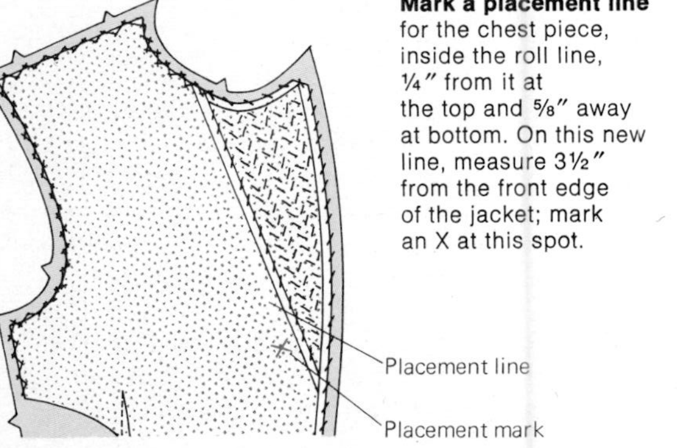

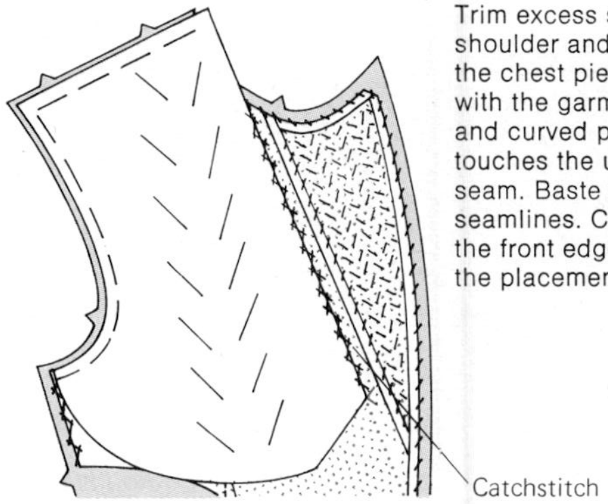

Trim excess so that shoulder and armhole of the chest piece align with the garment edges, and curved part just touches the underarm seam. Baste on the seamlines. Catchstitch the front edge to the placement line.

Attaching jacket collar and facing 371-374

Modern tailoring method/fused interfacing

For a jacket tailored the modern way, interfacing with fusible backing is used. It adds firmness but relatively little shape to jacket front and collar; is omitted entirely from the jacket back. For adequate support, the best type is a lightweight woven canvas. It is applied before pattern markings are transferred; collar and front facing are later completed by the method described in Tailoring.

Fusible interfacing is suitable wherever padding stitches would be impractical—on a knit, for example, or a firmly woven cotton or synthetic. It is particularly recommended for a washable jacket.

A chest piece is optional with fused interfacing. If you choose to add one, use a commercially prepared type (see p. 387 for the application).

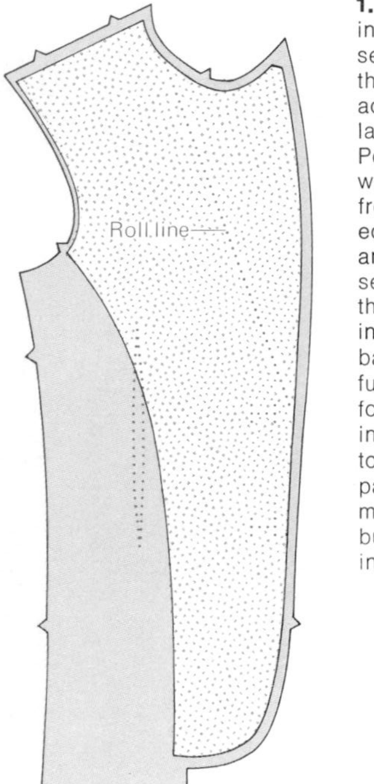

1. Cut out jacket front interfacing; trim away all seam allowances except at the armhole, and an additional ¼″ across the lapel point (to reduce bulk). Position interfacing on wrong side of jacket so that front, neck, and shoulder edges align with seamlines and armhole aligns with seam edge. Using the tip of the iron, touch interfacing in several places to heat-baste (anchor) it, then fuse the entire section, following the manufacturer's instructions. Allow fabric to dry. Then, with tracing paper, transfer the pattern markings for roll line, buttonholes, and dart to interfacing and jacket front.

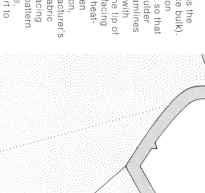

2. Cut a triangle of interfacing to fit the lapel point between seam allowances, as shown; trim ¼″ from the point, as in Step 1. Fuse the triangle on top of the first layer. This additional bit of padding improves the roll of the lapel by weighting the lapel point so it will lie flat against the jacket.

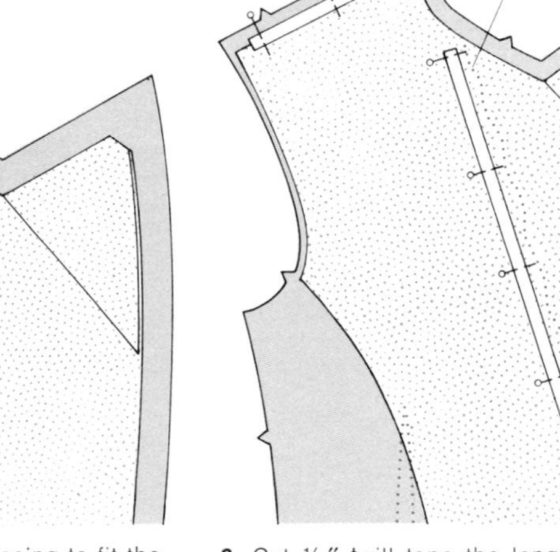

3. Cut ¼″ twill tape the length of the shoulder seam less 1¼″; center it over the seamline between neck and armhole seams; pin in place. Cut twill tape the length of the lapel roll line less ½″. Pin tape ¼″ from roll line, stretching tape to fit. This will cause slight rippling, which should be evenly distributed.

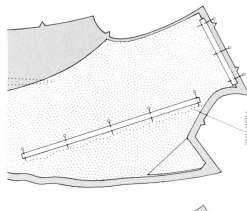

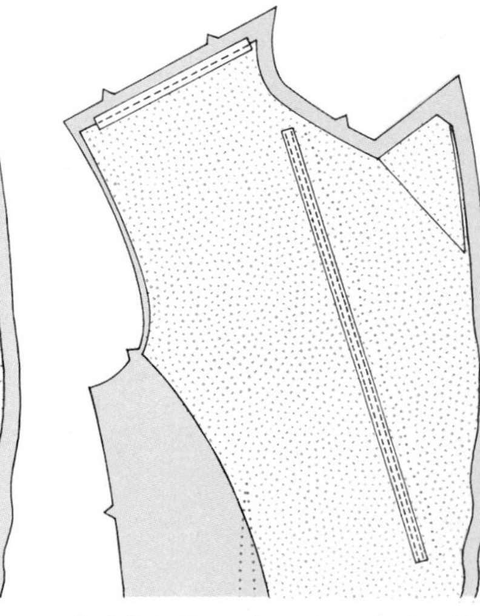

4. Stitch through center of shoulder seam tape. Stitch along each edge of the lapel tape, stretching tape as you stitch. (If preferred, small catchstitches can be substituted for machine stitching.) This slight easing along the roll line is important because it forces the lapel to roll outward.

Fusing interfacing to the jacket collar

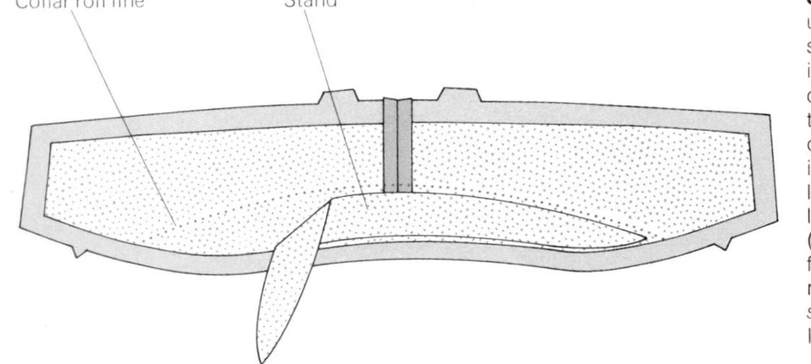

Cut interfacing for under collar; trim off seam allowances. Fuse interfacing to under collar sections, within the seamlines. Stitch center back seam; press it open. Mark the roll line. Cut a second layer of interfacing (on a bias fold) to fit from roll line to neck seam (called the *stand*). Fuse second layer to under collar.

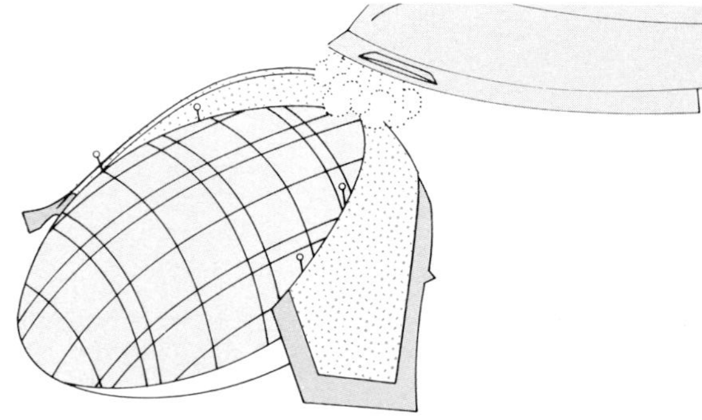

Fold the under collar on the roll line. Shape it over a tailor's ham so that the roll curves as it would if fitted around a neck; place one or two pins at each end to anchor it. Hold a steaming iron above the collar, allowing the steam to penetrate. Do not remove collar from the ham until it is dry.

Hand stitches: padding stitch 131; running stitch 131; slipstitch 132
Jacket sleeves 375
Shoulder pads, sleeve headings 376-377

Traditional method for jacket collar

When a man's jacket is traditionally tailored, the collar is structured almost entirely by hand. This technique permits careful control of the edges to achieve the flat, sharp look that is part of the tradition. For this effort to be successful, the under collar fabric must be lightweight and firmly woven. If your jacket fabric does not fit this description, buy a different, more suitable type for the under collar. (It should blend with, but need not match, the jacket.) A tailor would use French melton for this purpose, and trim away the seam allowances, whipstitching raw edges to neckline and upper collar. Because French melton is not easy to obtain, the method we show is an adaptation, with seam allowances folded under. Pay careful attention to the padstitch instructions on the under collar; they affect the way the collar lies.

Before the collar is attached, the front lining and facing sections should be joined and the inside pocket completed (see p. 390 for pocket method). Stitch the front facings to the jacket fronts from the top of the lapel to the end of the bottom curve. Grade and clip seam allowances; trim lapel corners diagonally. Turn facings to the inside and press so the seams are slightly to the inside along the front edge, slightly to the underside of the lapel. Clip the neck seam allowance to the staystitching.

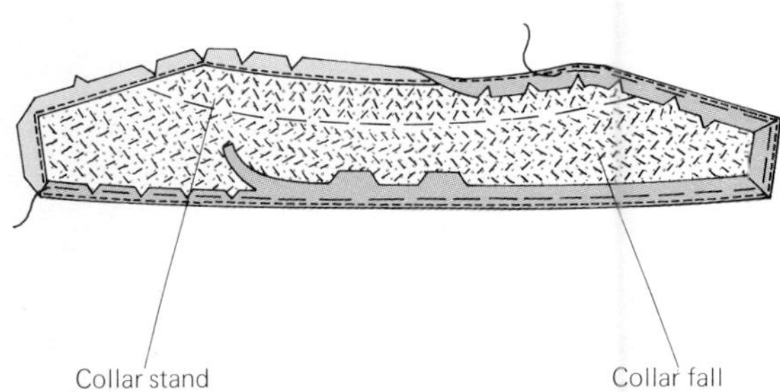

To prepare under collar, cut and assemble fabric and interfacing as pattern directs; staystitch seams. Fill in *stand* with short chevron padstitches, working perpendicular to neck seam; fill in *fall* with longer chevron padstitches, working parallel to top. Trim corners diagonally; trim seam allowances to ⅜"; press under; clip as needed. Shape on tailor's ham.

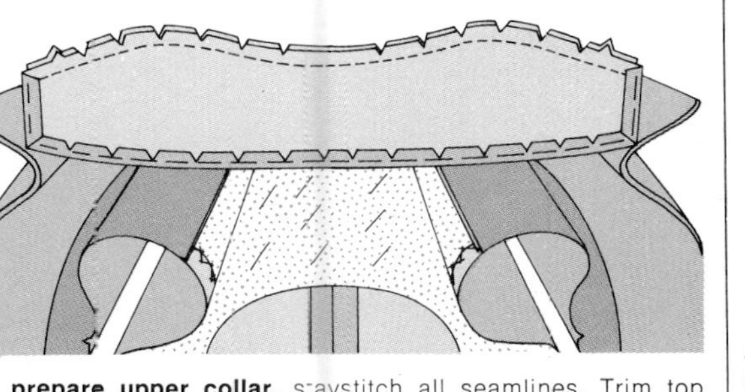

To prepare upper collar, staystitch all seamlines. Trim top and side seam allowances to ⅜" and press under, clipping as needed; baste. With right side of collar facing wrong side of jacket, stitch upper collar to neckline (do not catch facing), aligning ends of collar with inner corners of lapels. Clip to the stitching about every 1" along the neck seamline.

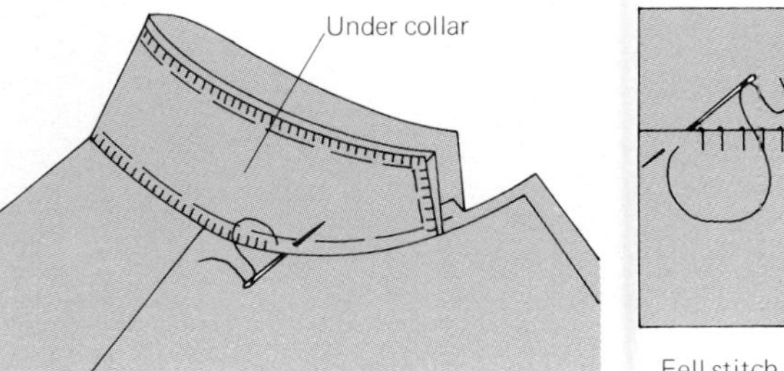

To join upper and under collars, baste them, wrong sides together, with all seam allowances enclosed and under collar edges slightly inside upper collar edges. Sew with small, closely spaced fell stitches (see insert).

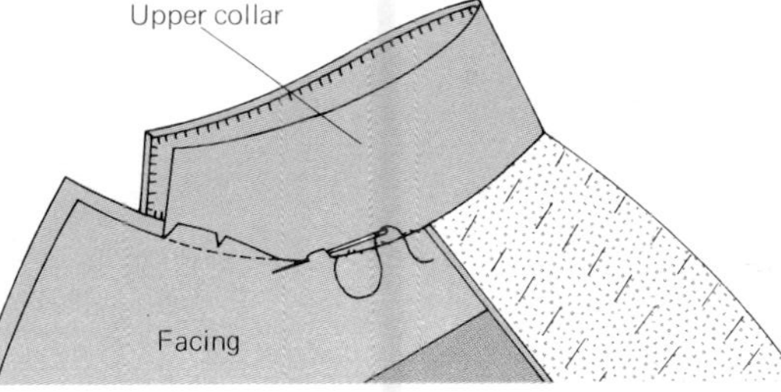

To finish neck edge of facing, fold under and press the seam allowance along the staystitching line. With tiny, closely spaced stitches, slipstitch facing to upper collar along seam where upper collar is joined to jacket.

The jacket sleeve

Techniques for fitting and setting in a man's jacket sleeve are the same as for a woman's (see Tailoring), with one basic difference—the sleeve cap seam is pressed open, giving the shoulder and sleeve area a flatter, squarer look, and permitting the sleeve to shape properly over a shoulder pad.

Men's shoulder pads and sleeve headings are like women's, but larger. It is best to purchase these. The pad is positioned with one-third in the jacket front, two-thirds in back. Sleeve heading is the same length as the shoulder pad, and is positioned the same way (see below).

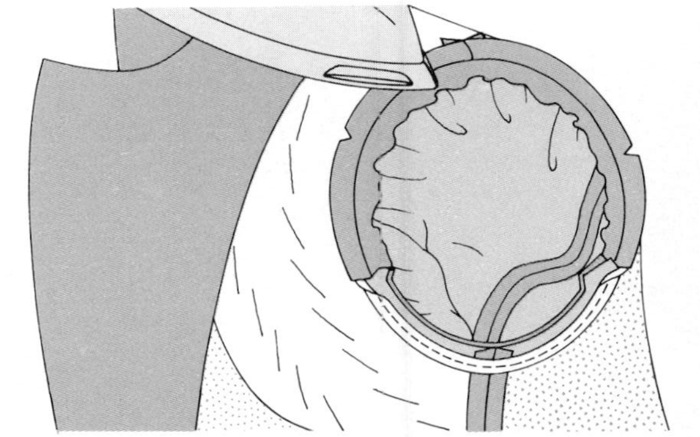

After setting in the sleeve, clip to the stitching at each jacket armhole notch. Place armhole over a tailor's ham, wrong side out. Using the tip of the iron and light pressure, press open the sleeve cap seam between notches.

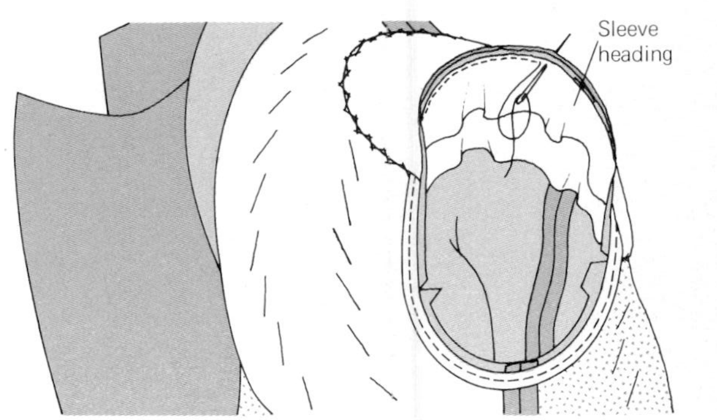

Position shoulder pad with edge extending ⅜" into sleeve; baste. Insert and baste sleeve heading; align fold with cut edge of pad. Check the fit. Sew all layers to the sleeve seam allowance with small running stitches.

Jacket lining: machine application 80; hand application 378-381

Fabric-marking methods 94
Hems 290-297

The inside jacket pocket

For convenience, a man's jacket has a pocket inside the right front or, if preferred, both fronts. In a lined jacket with narrow lapel, the pocket fits entirely on the lining. In a lined jacket with wide lapel, it fits mostly on the lining, but a small portion extends into the front facing (see below). In an unlined jacket, the pocket goes on the facing, which is cut extra wide. In these last two instances, the pocket must be completed before the facing is sewed to the jacket (see p. 389).

Preparation: (1) Turn up and finish the hem on the front lining. Join the front lining to the jacket front facing; press seam allowances toward the lining. **(2)** With thread tracing, mark pocket placement on right side of the lining and facing. (If pattern does not provide for this pocket, mark a line perpendicular to the underarm seam, 1″ below the bottom of the armhole. The opening should be 5¼″ long, with ¾″ of the total extending into the facing.) **(3)** For the pocket, cut a rectangle of lining fabric, 6¾″ wide by 13½″ long. On the wrong side, mark the pocket opening 7″ down from top and ¾″ from each side. Mark a stitching line ¼″ to each side of opening and across the ends.

Partially lined jacket

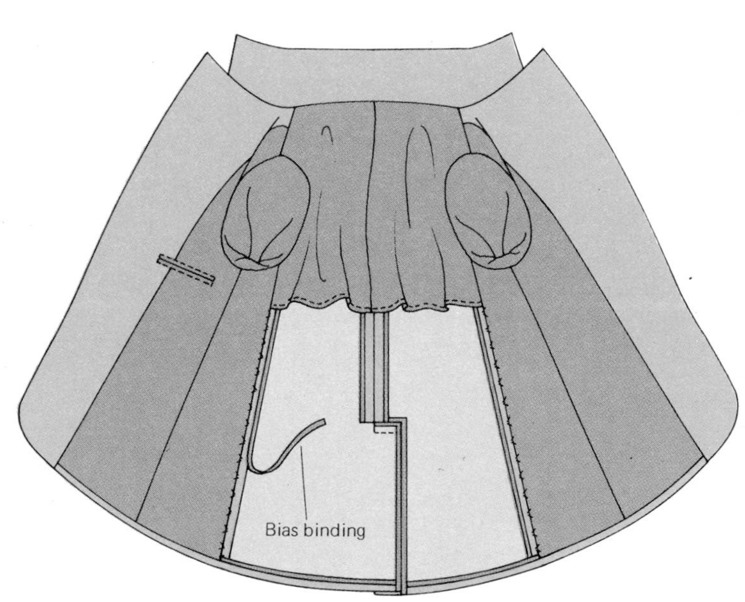

A partially lined jacket is often preferred to one with a full lining for coolness and lighter weight. The construction and application are basically the same as for a full lining, with the following exceptions:

The back lining section is cut to extend just 3″ below the armhole at the underarm seams. Its lower edge is narrowly hemmed with either a machine stitch or slipstitch.

The exposed part of the jacket back is neatly finished by (1) cutting hem and vent interfacings ¼″ less than the finished widths so that they will not show; and (2) binding the exposed seam and vent edges with either bias tape or bias strips cut from the lining fabric.

The front lining side seams are finished by slipstitching them to the front underarm seam allowances.

Constructing the inside jacket pocket

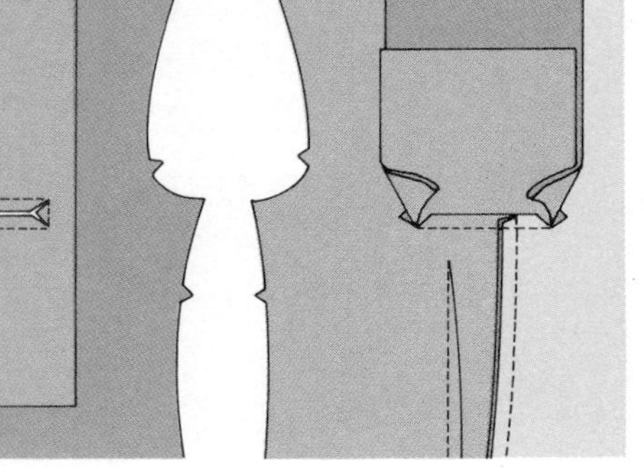

Baste pocket to right side of lining, matching markings. Stitch around opening, using a 15 stitch length. Slash center of opening, through both thicknesses, to within ½″ of each end; clip diagonally to the corners.

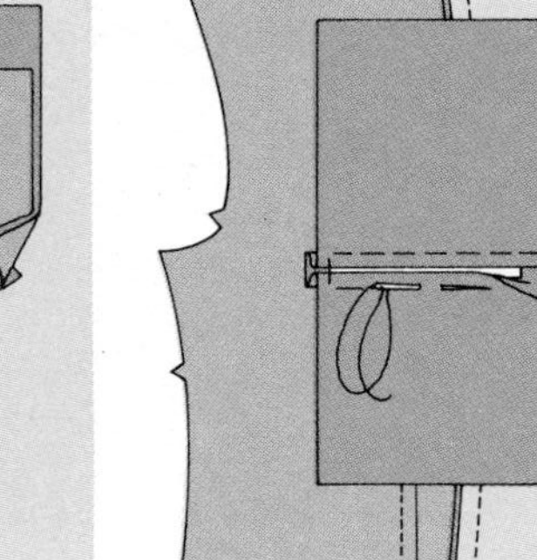

Slip pocket through the opening to the wrong side. Press the seams open on the long slashed edges, then press them flat (toward the opening). Press the V-shaped corners away from the opening.

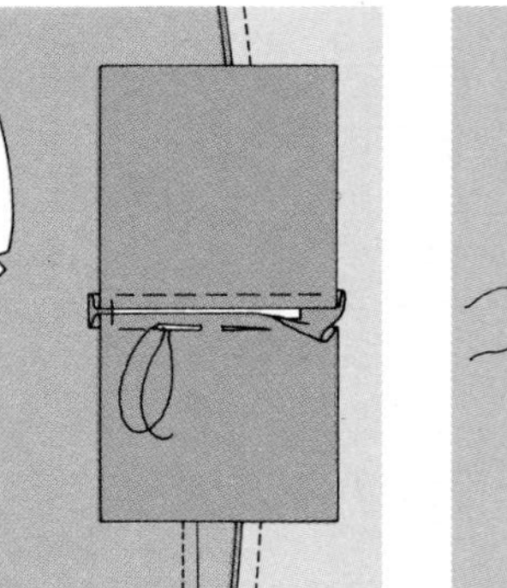

Form welts by folding each half of the pocket back over the stitching, having the two folds meet in the center of the opening. Press folds lightly. Baste around the opening, using silk thread, to hold the welts in place.

From the right side, stitch each welt in the groove formed by the seam. Before proceeding with this step, make sure that the seam is flat; if necessary, press the seam lightly with just the tip of the iron.

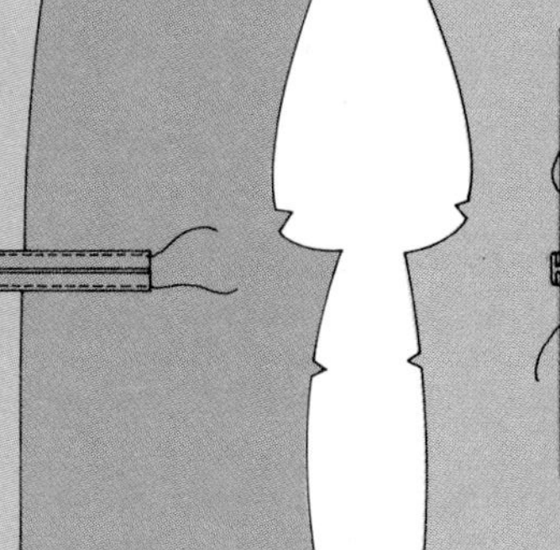

With the right side still facing you, fold back the lining to expose the V-shaped corner. Stitch across end of the V and welts, on top of original stitching. Repeat for other end. Turn garment to wrong side.

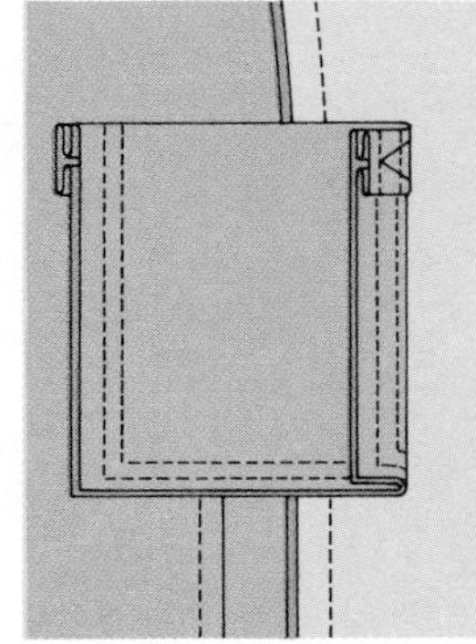

Fold the two halves of the pocket together, edges meeting; stitch around three sides, ⅝″ from the edge. Stitch a second time, ¼″ from the first stitching, in the seam allowance; trim close to the second stitching.

Making trousers

The construction of men's trousers involves a few techniques and some terminology (see Glossary of terms below) that are not encountered elsewhere. Directions for special techniques begin here and continue through page 401. For other methods that apply to trouser construction, see pages listed in the Checklist for procedure, below right.

A good fit is essential to well-made trousers. The best and easiest way to achieve it is by adjusting the pattern dimensions to those of a pair that fits well. (The chart, right, indicates which measurements should be compared.) If you do not have such a well-fitted pair, take the appropriate body measurements, as directed on page 385, and compare these with the pattern's. If lengthwise adjustments are needed, consult the Fitting chapter. Adjustments, up to 2 inches, in waist or hip circumference can usually be made at the center back seam. If you re-style the leg, be careful to make equal adjustments on both inseam and outseam so the crease line position will not be changed.

Glossary of terms

Bar tack: A reinforcement tack used at points of strain. Bar tacks can be made by hand (refer to Hand stitches for method) or by machine (see Machine facsimiles of hand stitches).
Inseam: The seam on the inside of the leg.
Outlet: Extra fabric allowance in trousers, which is usually added to the center back seam and the top of the front inseam.
Outseam: The seam that falls along the outside of the leg (the side seam).
Overtacking: Three or four hand stitches in the same spot; used to hold two areas together.
Pin-tack: Several machine stitches in the same stitch, made by lifting the presser foot slightly so the fabric does not feed; used to reinforce machine stitching where the usual backstitching would be unsightly.
Pocketing: A tightly woven, lightweight fabric of cotton or cotton-synthetic blend; used for inside pockets, the zipper fly stay and shield lining, also waistband facing in men's trousers.
Stay: A piece of fabric (usually pocketing) used to reinforce an area and prevent stretching.

Trouser measurement chart

PLACE TO MEASURE	TROUSERS	PATTERN	DIFFERENCE
Waist (at the seamline)			
Crotch front (from waist to inseam)			
Crotch back (from waist to inseam)			
Hips (7″ below waist)			
Thighs (3″ below crotch seam)			
Outseam (waist to hemline)			
Inseam (crotch to hemline)			
Circumference of leg at knee*			
Circumference of leg at hem*			

*These measurements are needed only where an exact duplication of the trouser style is desired.

Checklist/trouser procedure

Check pattern measurements 391

Adjust pattern: crotch seam 110; crotch allowance 392; center back seam allowance 392

Cut out and mark: trousers 84-94; crotch stays 392

Establish crease lines 392

Stitch back darts 159

Construct back pockets: patch 275-279; inside 393

Construct front pockets: patch 275-279; front-hip 282-283; in-seam 394

Stitch outseams: plain 145; with in-seam pocket 394

Apply zipper: boys' fly 324; men's fly 396-397

Stitch inseams 145

Attach waistbands 398-401

Construct change pocket 395

Anchor pocket tops 399

Stitch crotch seam 399

Finish waistband facings 398-401

Construct belt carriers 401

Attach trouser hooks 354

Hem trousers: turned-up hem 290-295; cuffed 310

Pockets: patch 275-279; front-hip 283; flap 286-287; separate welt 286-287

Cutting additions for trousers

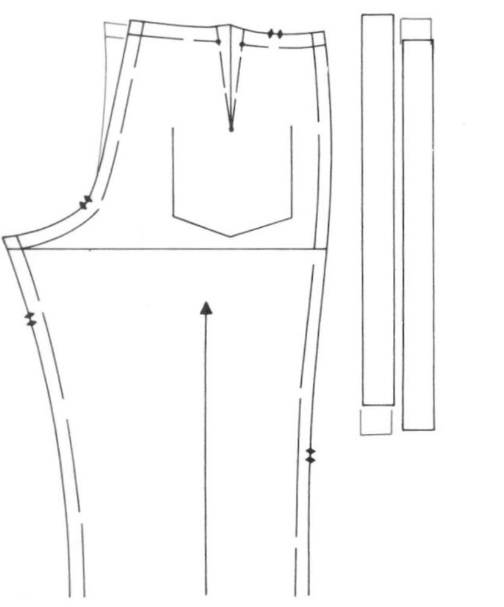

Extra back waist allowance is usually provided at the center back seam of men's trousers. This makes adjustments possible in the waist and upper hip areas where they are most often needed in case of a weight gain. If your pattern does not have this provision, add it yourself before cutting out the trousers: Draw a line, starting 1" from the cutting line at the waist and tapering to the existing cutting line at the seat. Add the same amount (1") to the waistband pieces.

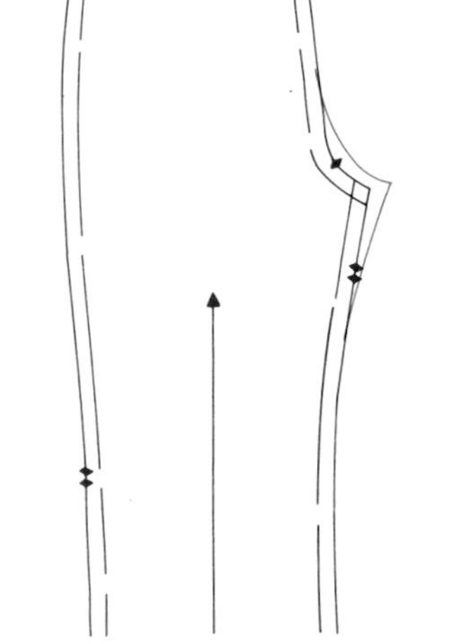

Extra crotch allowance should be added to the trouser left front (or the right, if a man prefers) so they will fit comfortably. Do this by drawing an addition on the pattern piece at the center front seam and the inseam, as is shown. The addition is ¾" at the crotch, and tapers to existing cutting lines at the waist, and at a point 5" below crotch on the inseam. Cut both trouser sections from the altered pattern piece, then trim the opposite side back to the original cutting line.

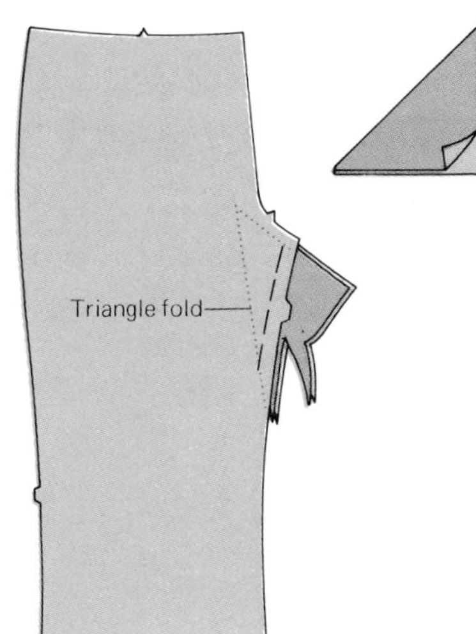

The addition of crotch stays gives extra life and durability to trousers by limiting the possibility of stretching or ripping in this area. To add stays, cut two 6" squares of pocketing; fold each square diagonally to form a triangle. Position one triangle on the wrong side of each trouser front, with the fold extending 2¼" from the inseam edge at the crotch, and tapering to meet the inseam edge about 6" below the crotch. Baste. Trim raw edges of the stay to match the seam edges.

Establishing the crease line

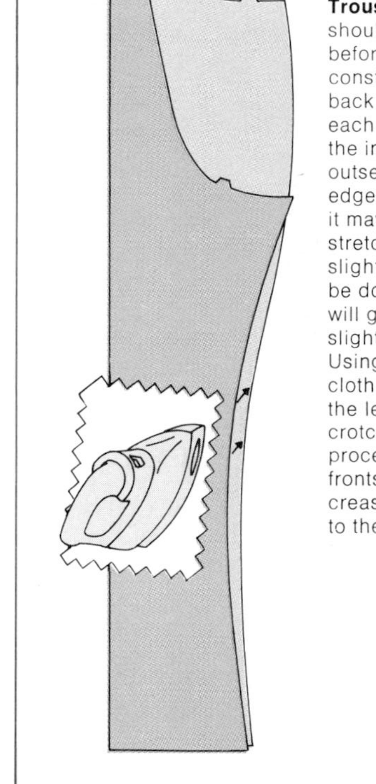

Trouser crease lines should be established before proceeding with the construction. Begin with back sections, folding each in half and aligning the inseam with the outseam. (To bring seam edges together at the top, it may be necessary to stretch the crotch area slightly upward. This can be done gently, and will give the crotch a slightly better curve.) Using a dampened press cloth, press the crease from the leg edge to 3" above crotch level. Repeat the procedure for trouser fronts, pressing the creases from the leg edge to the waistline.

Trouser pockets

Several different pocket styles are used for men's trousers. Three types of inside pockets—a *back-hip* pocket, a *front in-seam* style, and a *change* pocket—are dealt with in this section. Directions for other types, such as front-hip and patch pockets, are described in the chapter on Pockets.

Men's trouser pockets are rarely just decorative. To satisfactorily serve their many purposes, they should be smooth and sturdy, with opening edges neatly finished and reinforced. For smoothness, an inside type is usually made of pocketing (see Glossary, p. 391), cut so that it extends, and is later attached, to the waistline; the pocket sections are joined with a French seam. Constructed in this way, the pocket is strong and well supported to better withstand the downward thrust frequently exerted on it. For good appearance, opening edges are faced with trouser fabric; the opening ends are bar-tacked for reinforcement.

For ease in handling, most trouser pockets are attached before the trouser sections are joined—back pockets first, then the front ones. One exception is the change pocket, which is added after the waistband is attached, but before the waistband facing is anchored inside.

Instructions for the back-hip pocket (opposite page) and the change pocket (p. 395) include explanations of how to cut the needed pieces and mark the placement. If you wish, you can add these pockets to trousers not designed to include them.

The pocket tab

The back left pocket often has a tab closure to protect the man's wallet. The way to construct it is explained below. Its insertion in a double-welt pocket is illustrated on the opposite page.

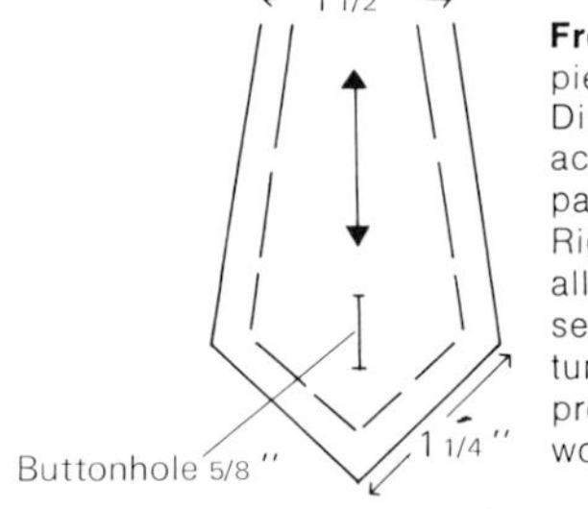

From trouser fabric, cut two pieces shaped as illustrated. Dimensions are 3" long; 1½" across top; 2" across widest part; 1¼" each side of V. Right sides together, stitch all but the top with a ¼" seam. Trim corners diagonally; turn unit right side out; press. Make hand- or machine-worked buttonhole, ⅝" long.

Back-hip pocket

A typical back-hip pocket has edges finished with trouser fabric; the inside is cut from pocketing and extends to the waistline. Instructions are given here for a double-welt style. If you prefer a single-welt or a flap style, cut the pocket sections as specified below, then follow directions in the chapter on Pockets for finishing the edges.

Instructions below include a tab for securing the opening. An alternative is a hand-worked buttonhole, centered vertically ½″ below pocket opening.

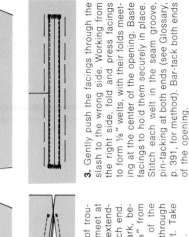

Preparation: (1) Stitch the back trouser darts, if any; slash them to within ½″ of the points; press the darts open. **(2)** With thread tracing, mark pocket placement. (If your pattern gives no placement indication, place the pocket 3½″ below waist, or at the bottom of dart. Opening begins 1½″ from the outseam, is 5½″ long, and aligns with the cross grain.) **(3)** From pocketing, cut two rectangles, each 11″ by 7″ (cut twice as many if you are constructing two pockets). **(4)** From trouser fabric, cut three rectangles (six for two pockets), each 6¼″ by 1½″. Two of these will be used for facings (welts) to bind the pocket edges; the third, for an underlay that fits behind the pocket opening.

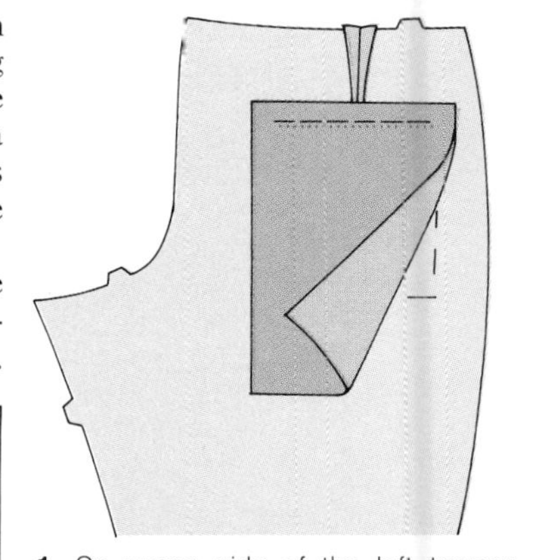

1. On wrong side of the left trouser back, position one pocket section so that the top edge extends 1″ above the placement mark, the sides ¾″ beyond each end. Baste it to the trousers just above the mark. (This is called the inside pocket; the other section, added later, is called the outside pocket.) If you are making two pockets, repeat procedure for right trouser back.

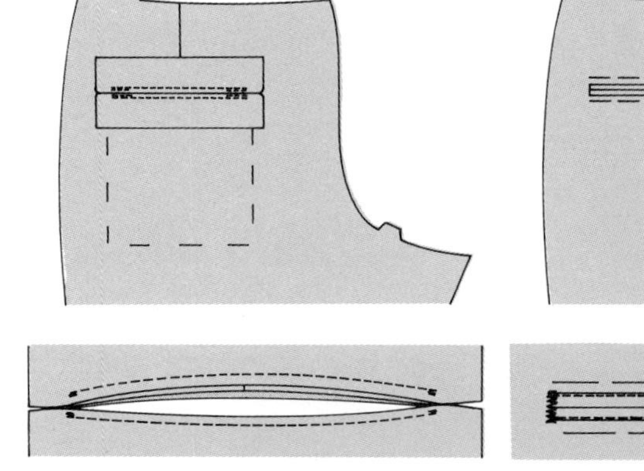

2. Baste facings to right side of trousers, having lengthwise edges meet at the placement mark, and ends extending ⅜″ beyond the mark at each end. Stitch facings ⅛″ from the mark, beginning and ending stitches ⅜″ from each end. Starting at center of the mark, cut to each end, slashing through the trousers and inside pocket. Take care not to cut beyond stitches.

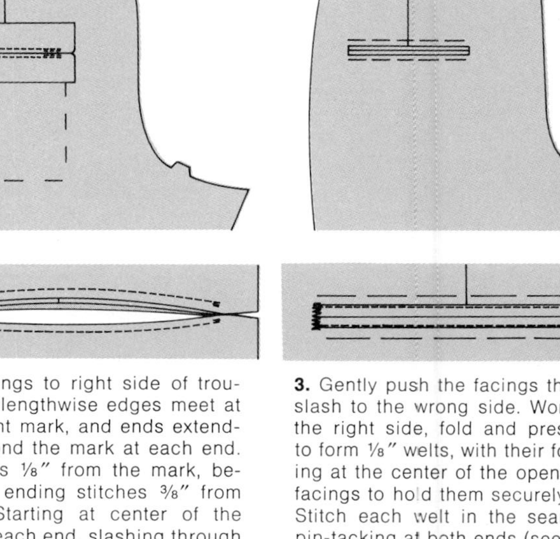

3. Gently push the facings through the slash to the wrong side. Working from the right side, fold and press facings to form ⅛″ welts, with their folds meeting at the center of the opening. Baste facings to hold them securely in place. Stitch each welt in the seam groove, pin-tacking at both ends (see Glossary, p. 391, for method). Bar-tack both ends of the opening.

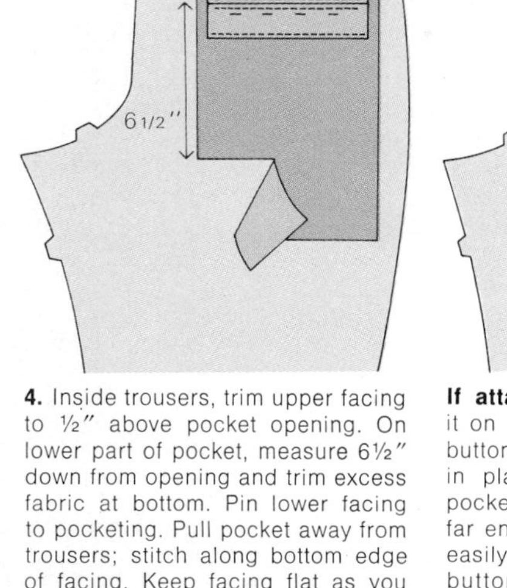

4. Inside trousers, trim upper facing to ½″ above pocket opening. On lower part of pocket, measure 6½″ down from opening and trim excess fabric at bottom. Pin lower facing to pocketing. Pull pocket away from trousers; stitch along bottom edge of facing. Keep facing flat as you stitch; do not let it slide toward pocket opening.

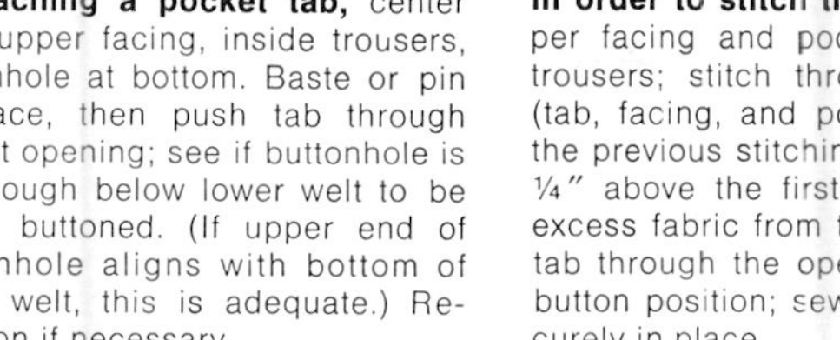

If attaching a pocket tab, center it on upper facing, inside trousers, buttonhole at bottom. Baste or pin in place, then push tab through pocket opening; see if buttonhole is far enough below lower welt to be easily buttoned. (If upper end of buttonhole aligns with bottom of lower welt, this is adequate.) Reposition if necessary.

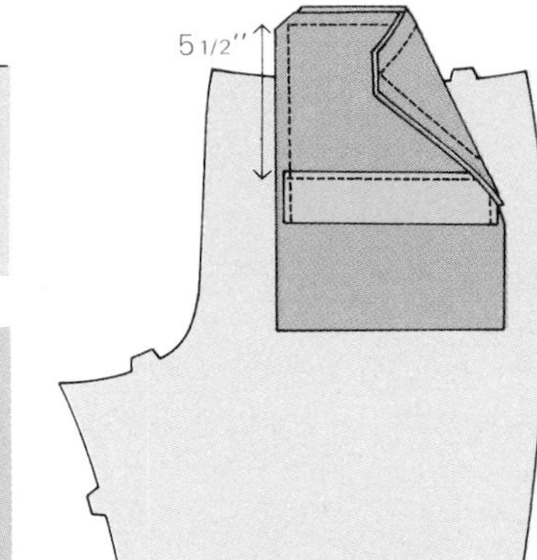

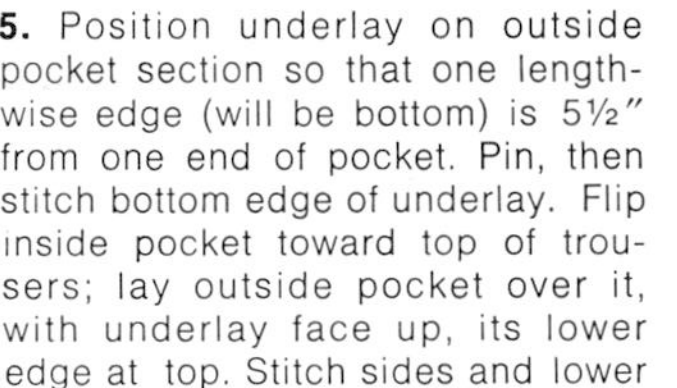

In order to stitch the tab, pull upper facing and pocket away from trousers; stitch through all layers (tab, facing, and pocket), close to the previous stitching. Stitch again, ¼″ above the first stitching. Trim excess fabric from top of tab. Push tab through the opening; mark the button position; sew the button securely in place.

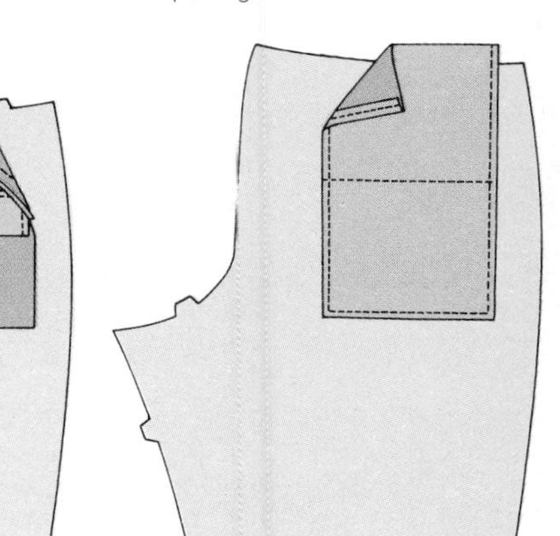

5. Position underlay on outside pocket section so that one lengthwise edge (will be bottom) is 5½″ from one end of pocket. Pin, then stitch bottom edge of underlay. Flip inside pocket toward top of trousers; lay outside pocket over it, with underlay face up, its lower edge at top. Stitch sides and lower edges with ¼″ seam.

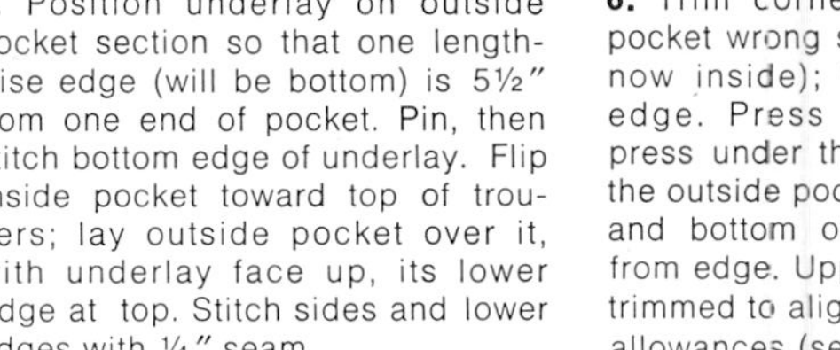

6. Trim corners diagonally; turn pocket wrong side out (underlay is now inside); work seams out to edge. Press seam edges, then press under the top side edges of the outside pocket ¼″. Stitch sides and bottom of pocket again, ⅛″ from edge. Upper edge will later be trimmed to align with the waist seam allowances (see p. 399).

Pockets: patch 275-279; front-hip 283

Trouser in-seam pocket

A front in-seam pocket is found most often in trousers of a traditional or tailored style. The inside sections are cut from pocketing, and the pocket opening (which is sewed to the outseam) is faced with the trouser fabric.

Construction of this pocket is begun after the back-hip pockets are completed and before the trouser outseam is stitched. Instructions include the addition of a back stay, which serves to both reinforce and finish the back inside edge of the pocket. Ends of the opening are reinforced with bar tacks.

This particular pocket fits well only in trousers with a certain cut. It should not be attempted unless the pattern style is designed to incorporate it. If your pattern has front-hip or patch pockets, see the chapter on Pockets for directions.

Preparation: (1) From pocketing fabric, cut four pocket sections, carefully indicating the opening edge with notches. **(2)** From the cross grain of pocketing, cut two pocket stays, each 1½″ wide and the length of the pocket opening plus 1¼″. **(3)** From the lengthwise grain of the trouser fabric, cut four pocket facings, each 2¼″ wide and the length of the pocket opening plus 1¼″. Cut notches on all of the facings to indicate pocket openings. (If your trouser pattern provides separate pieces for the cutting of pocket facings, use the pattern pieces instead.)

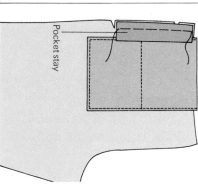

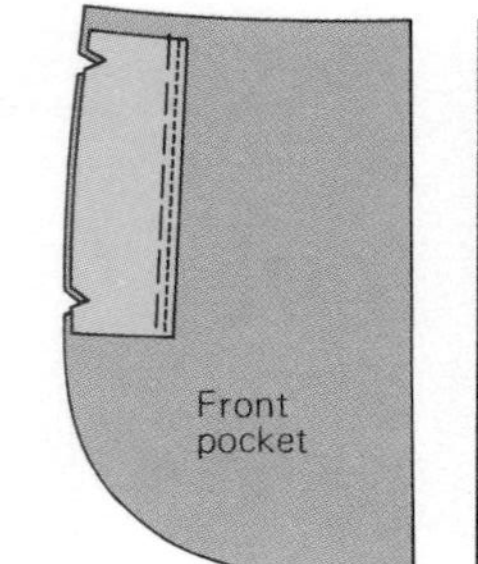

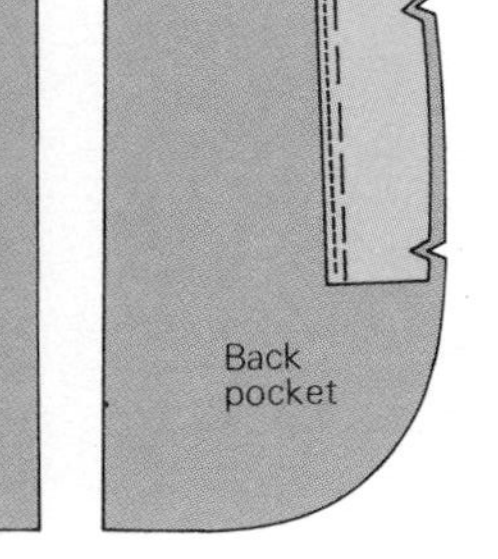

Lay front and back pocket sections, right side up, as shown. Baste a facing to each section, positioning the front pocket facing along the edge and the back pocket facing ⅜″ from the edge, matching notches carefully. Stitch along each inside facing edge. Repeat the procedure for the second pocket, reversing the pocket positions, so that the back pocket is on the left, the front pocket on the right.

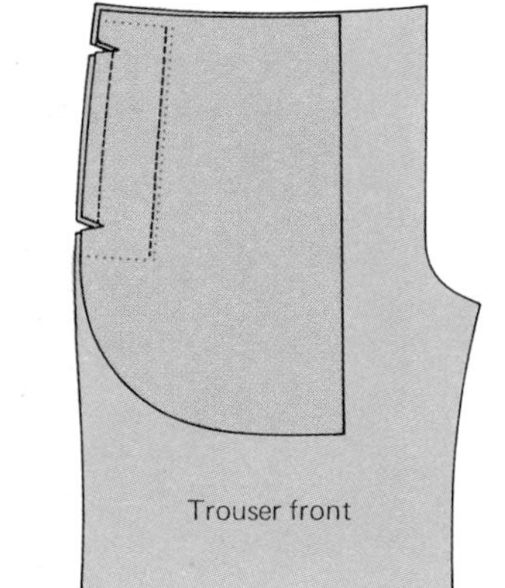

1. With right sides together, stitch the front pocket to the trouser front, between notches, ½″ *from the edge.* At each end of the stitch line, clip to the stitches and ⅛″ beyond (the clip should be ⅝″ deep).

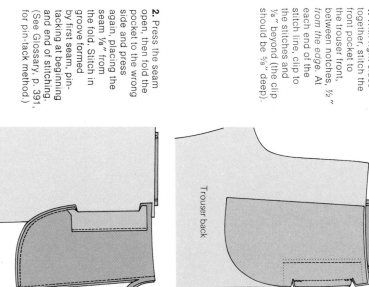

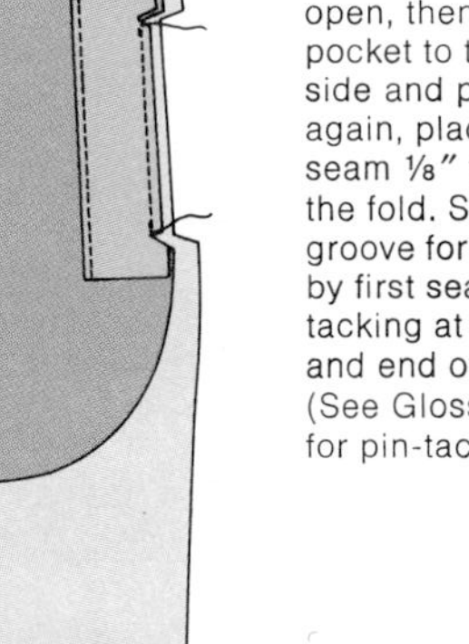

2. Press the seam open, then fold the pocket to the wrong side and press again, placing the seam ⅛″ from the fold. Stitch in groove formed by first seam, pin-tacking at beginning and end of stitching. (See Glossary, p. 391, for pin-tack method.)

Pocket stay

3. Baste the pocket stay to the wrong side of the trouser back, aligning the bottom of the stay with the lower end of the pocket opening.

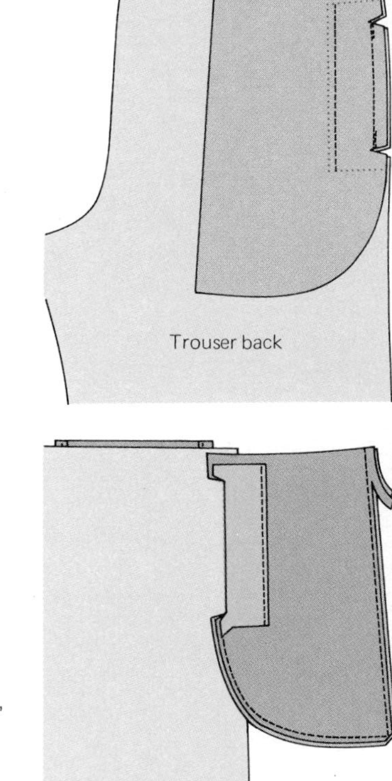

4. With right sides together, stitch the back pocket to the trouser back, between notches, ⅝″ from the edge. Clip to the stitches at each end.

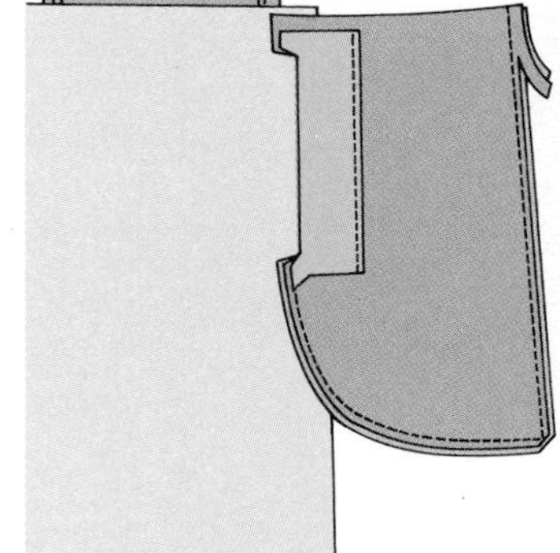

5. Pull the two sides of the pocket away from the trousers. Wrong sides together, stitch pockets with ¼″ seam, from the top edge to the lower notch for the pocket opening. Trim seam allowances to ⅛″. Trim the corners diagonally.

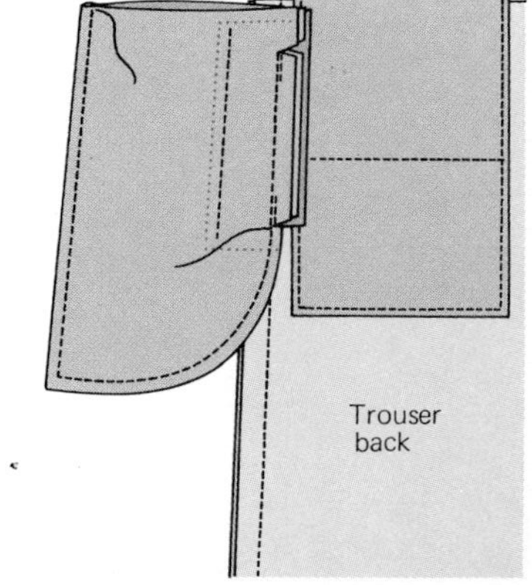

6. Press the pocket seam open. Turn the pocket wrong side out, work the seam out to the edge, then press again. Stitch the pocket a second time, ¼″ from the edge. Next, stitch front and back of trousers together along the outseam, above and below the pocket opening; reinforce with backstitches at each notch.

Bar tack: hand-stitched 133;
machine-stitched 142

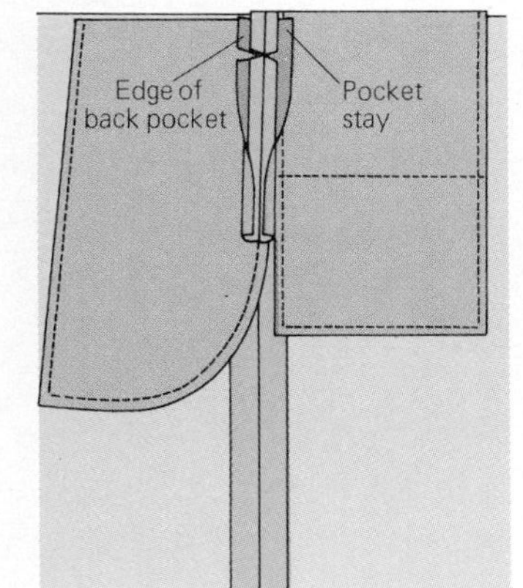

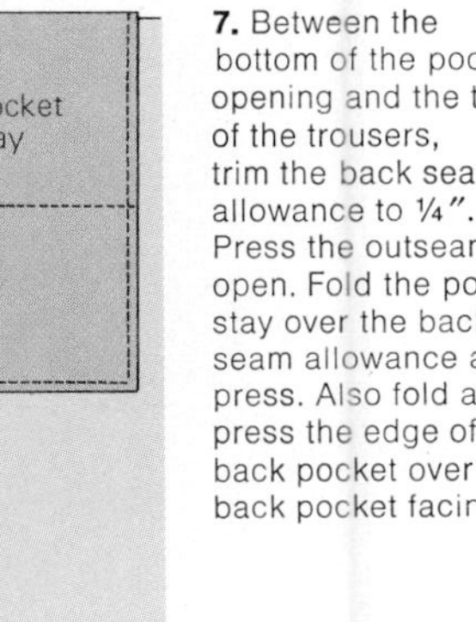

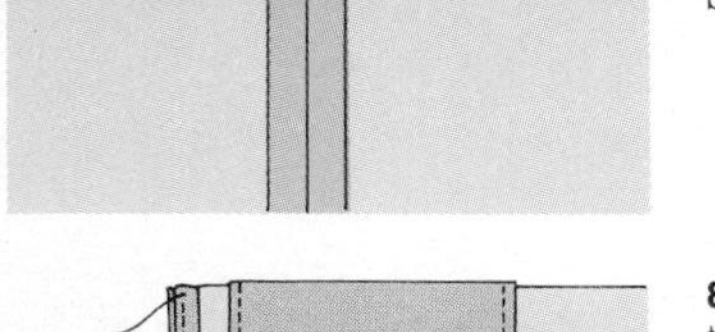

7. Between the bottom of the pocket opening and the top of the trousers, trim the back seam allowance to ¼". Press the outseam open. Fold the pocket stay over the back seam allowance and press. Also fold and press the edge of the back pocket over the back pocket facing.

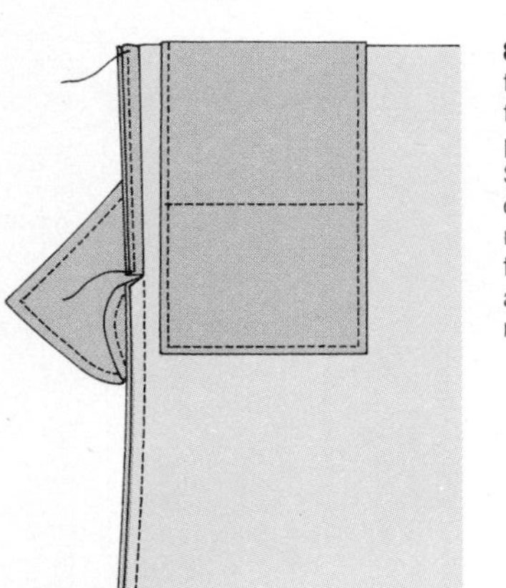

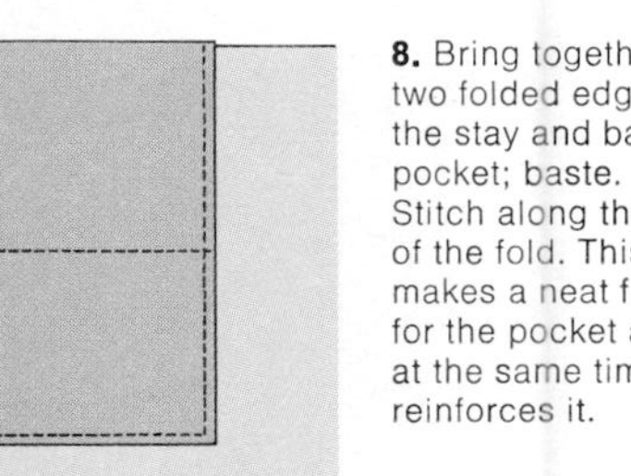

8. Bring together the two folded edges of the stay and back pocket; baste. Stitch along the edge of the fold. This makes a neat finish for the pocket and, at the same time, reinforces it.

9. On the right side of the trousers, pull the front edge of the pocket toward the outseam. Bar-tack the ends of the pocket opening, either by hand or machine, taking one stitch beyond the outseam.

Change pocket

The change pocket, sometimes called a watch or a ticket pocket, is an in-seam type, inserted just under the waistband on the right trouser front; its opening is in the waist seam. An optional addition to any trouser style, the change pocket is constructed after the waistband is attached, but before the waistband facing is completed.

Preparation: (1) Trim seam allowances to ⅜" on trouser waist and waistband. **(2)** On the right front waist seam, mark pocket position with first edge ¾" from outseam. (Opposite end of pocket will be 4¾" from the outseam.) **(3)** From pocketing, cut two 4" squares. **(4)** From trouser fabric, cut a facing 2" by 3½".

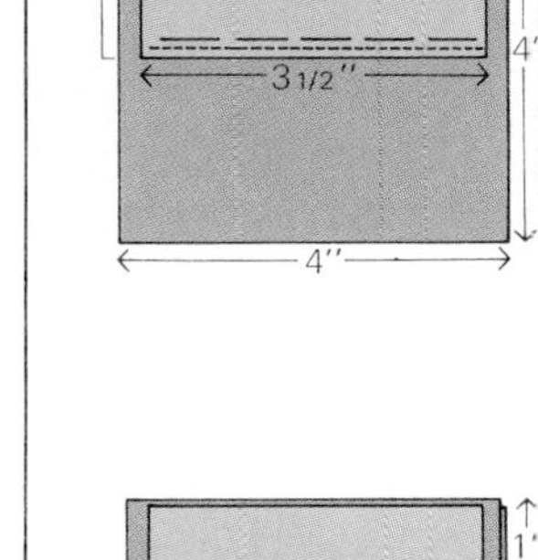

1. With right sides up, baste the facing to one pocket section with the top edges aligned, as shown. Stitch the lower edge of the facing.

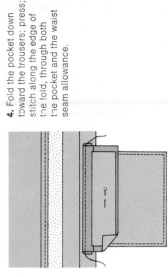

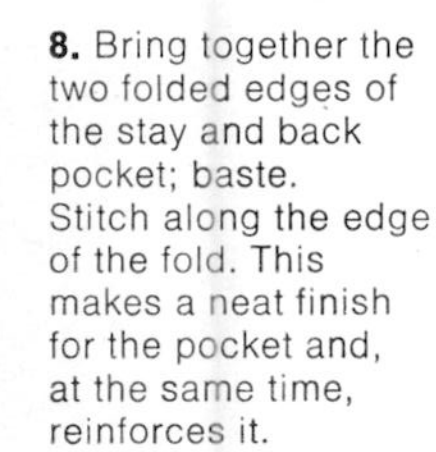

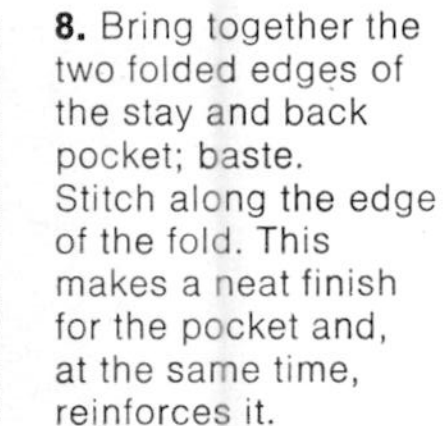

2. Wrong sides together, stitch the two pocket sections with a ¼" seam, beginning and ending the stitching 1" from the top on each side; clip to the stitching. Trim corners diagonally; trim sides to ⅛". Press seams open.

3. Turn pocket wrong side out; work seams out to edge; press. Stitch again, ⅛" from the edge. Fold back and pin the faced side out of the way. Place the unfaced side against the trouser waist (faced side underneath), aligning sides with pocket placement marks, top edge with edge of trouser waist seam. Stitch, ¼" from the edge, through pocket and waist seam allowance.

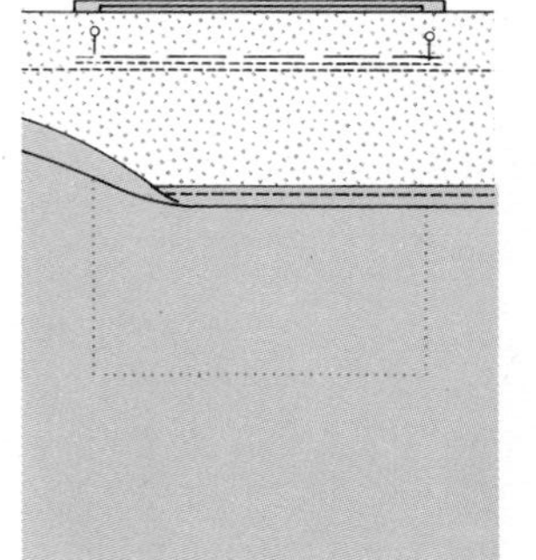

4. Fold the pocket down toward the trousers; press; stitch along the edge of the fold, through both the pocket and the waist seam allowance.

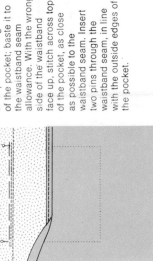

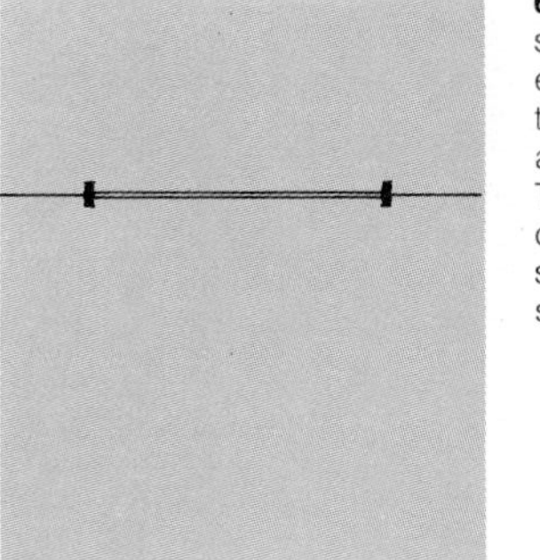

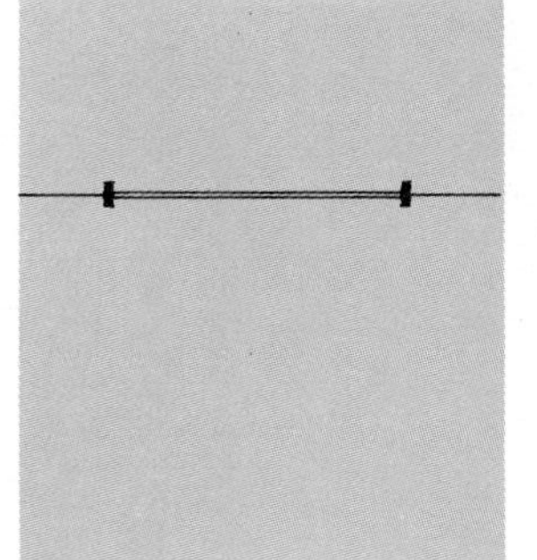

5. Unpin the facing side of the pocket; baste it to the waistband seam allowance. With the wrong side of the waistband face up, stitch across top of the pocket, as close as possible to the waistband seam. Insert two pins through the waistband seam, in line with the outside edges of the pocket.

6. From the trouser right side, make a bar tack at each pin mark, extending the tack ⅛" above and below the waist seam. To open the pocket, carefully remove the stitches from the waist seam, between the tacks.

Zipper types 14 Fly-front zipper 324-325 Pin-tack 391

Trouser zipper

A man's trouser zipper is applied in a fly closing that laps from left to right, the fly completed before the crotch seam is stitched. The method shown here is adapted from one used by many tailors and trouser manufacturers. To follow these directions, you will need to cut a fly facing, shield, and shield lining, using your trouser pattern for a guide, and substitute these pieces for the ones included in the typical pattern. The dimensions are suitable for all men's sizes up to 44.

A trouser zipper is recommended for use with this application. If this type is not available, or not suitable for your fabric, an 11-inch skirt or neck zipper can be substituted. The zipper will be cut to the length of the fly opening when the application is complete. Besides a zipper, you will need ½ yard of pocketing for fly stay and shield lining (see cutting instructions, right).

For the fly front in boys' trousers, the method in the Zipper section is more suitable than the one here. Be sure, however, in using that technique, to reverse the opening from right to left.

Cutting fly facing and shield

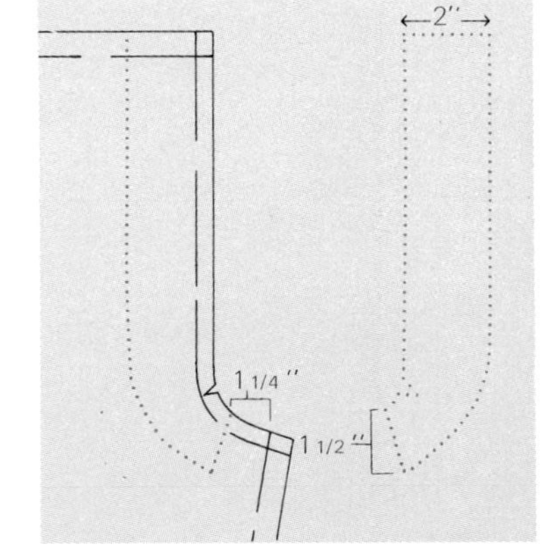

Before cutting fly facing and shield, trim the center front seam to ⅜" on both trousers and trouser pattern; cut a notch on the front seam allowance, 1¾" from the inseam. On the trouser pattern, draw a guide for the facings—2" wide at the top and 1½" wide at the bottom, ending 1¼" from the inseam. Trace the facing guide twice to the wrong side of trouser fabric (see first drawing). Mark one tracing left (L), the other right (R); cut them out. The left facing is usually interfaced with pocketing, cut on the bias, using facing as pattern (above). This is called the *fly stay* because it reinforces and also supports the fly.

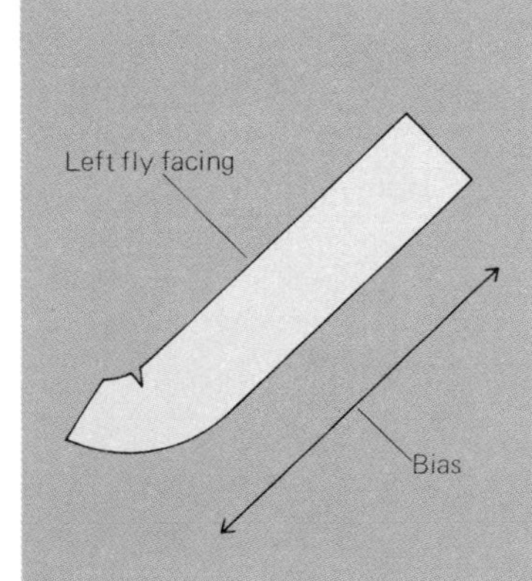

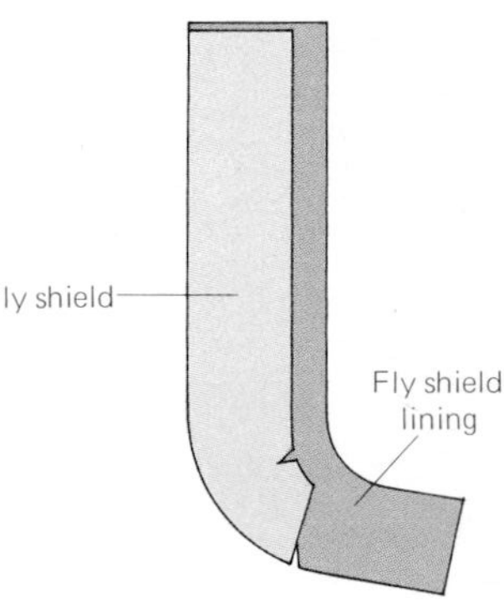

The right facing becomes an extension of the trousers called a *fly shield*. From the cross grain of pocketing fabric, using the facing as a guide, cut a fly shield lining, making it 3" longer at the bottom and ¾" wider along the inside (notched) edge. Clip into the lining ⅛" at the bottom end of the shield.

Stitching the left fly front

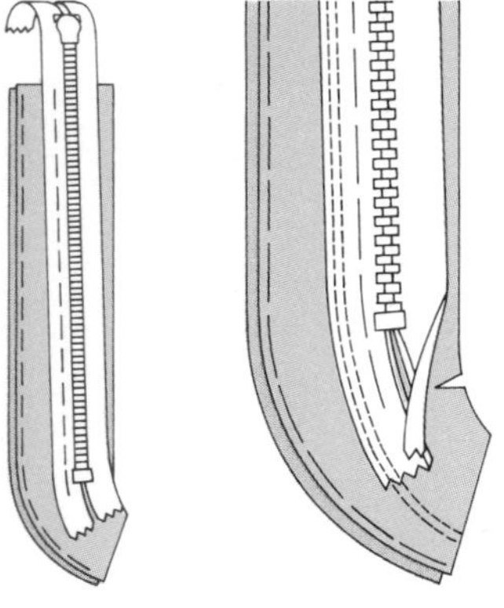

Baste the stay to the wrong side of the left facing. Place closed zipper on the facing, face down, with bottom stop ½" above the notch. Baste the zipper so that right edge of tape aligns with the facing edge at the bottom and is ¼" away at the top. Stitch zipper tape along left edge, then again ⅛" from edge.

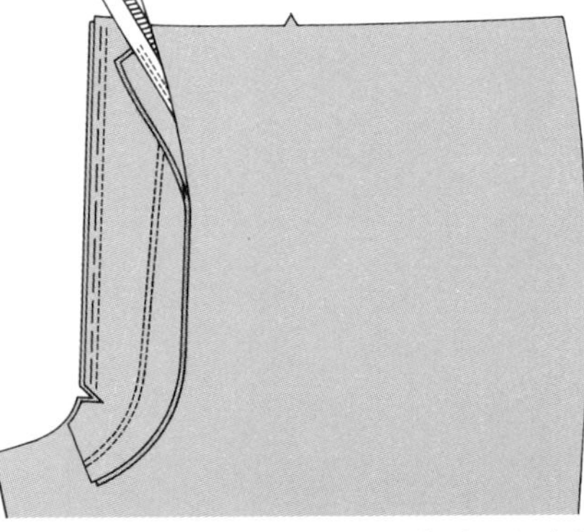

With right sides together, baste facing to left trouser front, taking care not to catch zipper. (Fold zipper back and, if necessary, pin to hold it out of the way.) Stitch facing from notch to waist edge, taking ¼" seam. Carefully cut the notch to ⅜", so that it extends ⅛" beyond the stitch line.

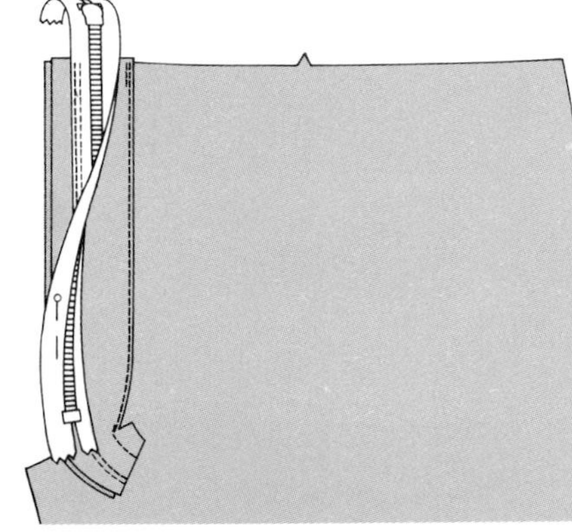

Pull the facing out and away from trousers, and press seam allowances toward it. If necessary, notch seam allowances on the curve so that the facing lies flat. From right side, stitch through the facing and all seam allowances, close to the seam. End the stitching and reinforce with a pin-tack at the notch.

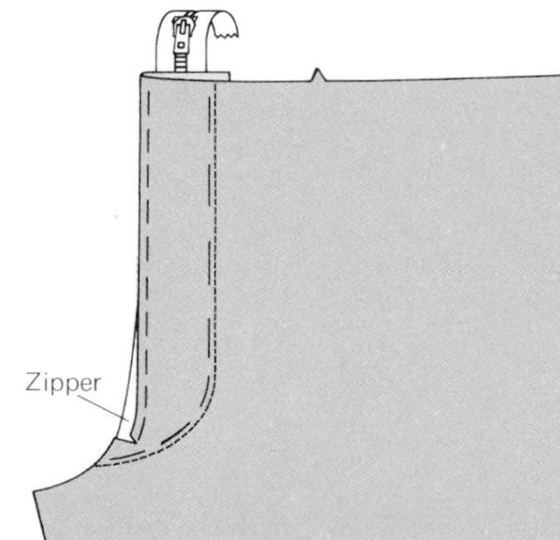

Fold the facing inside the trousers, placing the seam ⅛" from the fold. Baste close to the seam to hold facing in position. From the right side, baste a guideline 1½" from the fold, tapering the line to ½" opposite notch and extending it to trouser edge ¾" below the notch. Topstitch close to basting.

Stitching the right fly (shield)

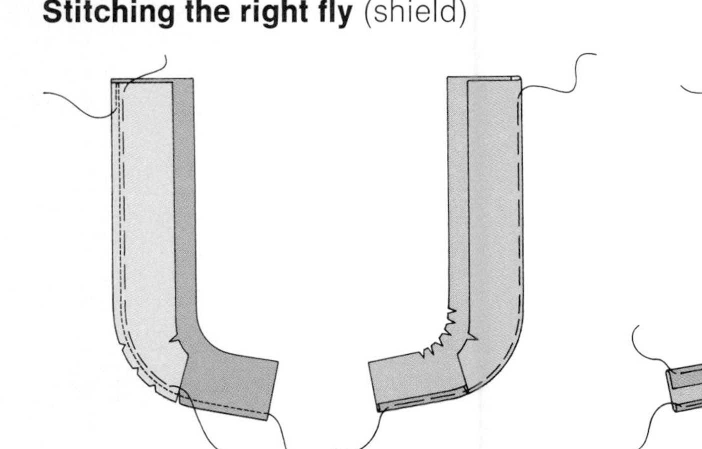

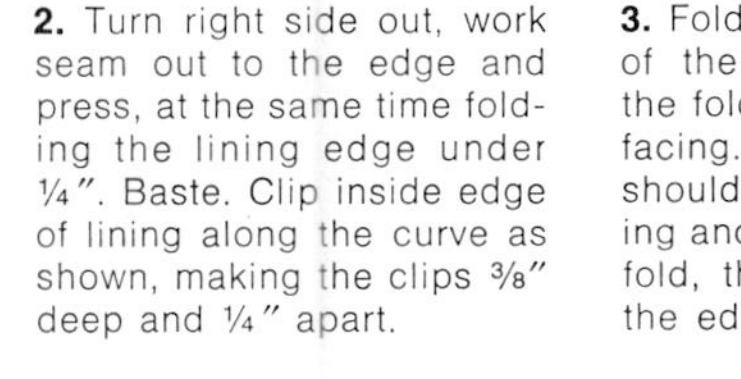

1. With right sides together, baste right fly facing and lining along the outside edge. Stitch with ¼″ seam, beginning at the top of the facing and ending at bottom edge of lining. Notch curve. Press seam open.

2. Turn right side out, work seam out to the edge and press, at the same time folding the lining edge under ¼″. Baste. Clip inside edge of lining along the curve as shown, making the clips ⅜″ deep and ¼″ apart.

3. Fold under the front edge of the lining ¾″, aligning the fold with the edge of the facing. (The seam allowance should lie between the facing and the lining.) Press the fold, then baste it close to the edge.

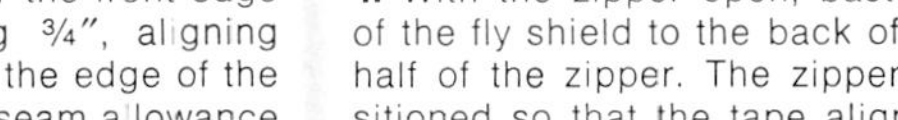

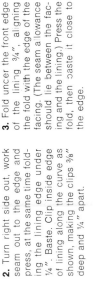

4. With the zipper open, baste the right side of the fly shield to the back of the unattached half of the zipper. The zipper should be positioned so that the tape aligns with the facing edge, and the bottom stop is ½″ above the notch. Stitch through zipper and shield, ¼″ from the edge. Do not catch the shield lining in the stitching.

5. Close the zipper. With right sides together, baste shield and zipper to the right trouser front from notch to waist edge. (Do not catch the shield lining in the basting.) Stitch through all layers, from notch to waist, placing stitches just to the left of the previous stitch line. Clip the notch to the stitching.

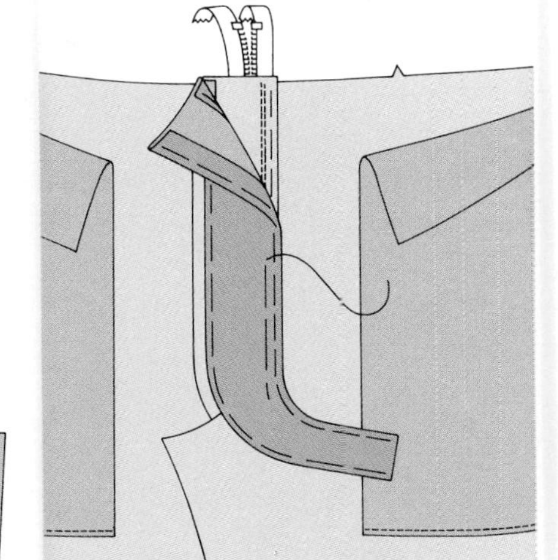

6. Open the zipper. Inside the trousers, press shield lining flat. Baste close to the fold, through all layers—shield, trousers, and zipper. The upper lining should completely cover the back of the shield. The lower lining is left free, and will be finished when trousers are completed (see Final steps, right).

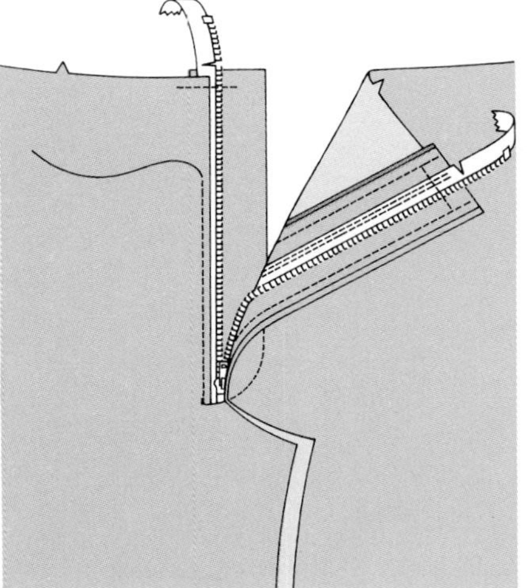

7. From right side of trousers, stitch close to the left fly seam, pin-tacking at the notch, keeping the zipper tape and fly shield flat as you stitch. On each side of the zipper, stitch across the top of the tape, ½″ from the edge of the trousers. Trim the tops of the zipper even with the trouser edge.

Final zipper steps

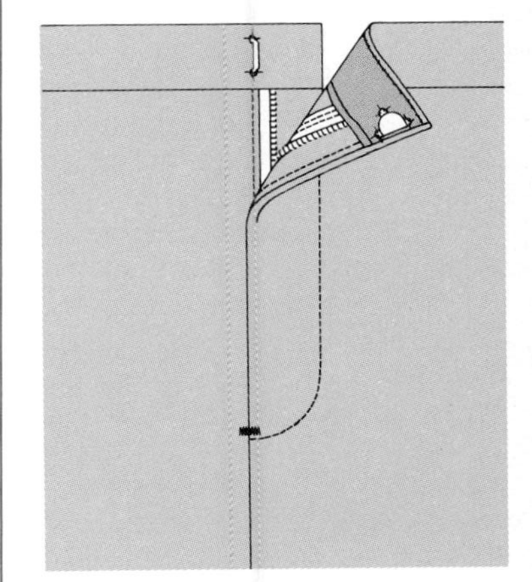

After waistband and crotch seam have been stitched, pull the bottom of the left fly slightly to the right so fly shield seam is covered. Bar-tack by hand or machine, extending the tack one or two stitches into the right front.

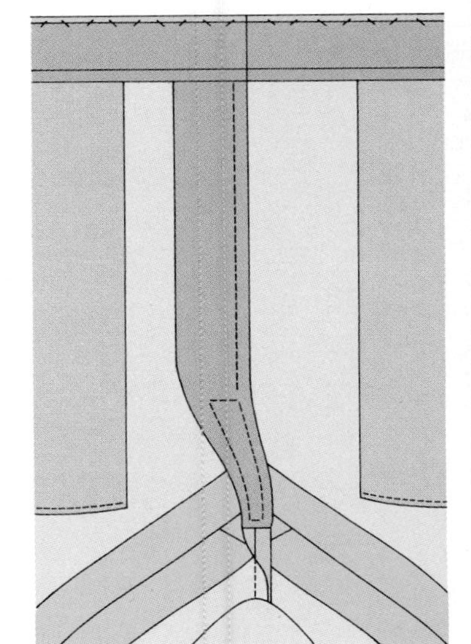

Inside the trousers, sew the lower end of the fly lining to crotch seam allowances with tiny backstitches.

Waistband stiffenings 17
Grain in fabric 84-85
Catchstitch (blind) 129
Grading seam allowances 147

Trouser waistbands

The methods for constructing a waistband for men's trousers vary according to the pattern, the fabric, and the waistband material. The following, however, are common to all methods.

The waistband is cut of garment fabric in two sections, one for the right side of the body and one for the left. Each section is sewed to the corresponding trousers half, then the back seam of garment and waistband are sewed in one step. This makes any future waist alterations easier. (The top 1 inch to 1¼ inches of the back seam may be left open in a "V" for greater comfort.)

The left waistband must be cut longer than the right so that it equals fly facing and whatever extension is allowed for waistband fasteners.

The facing for the waistband is rarely of the garment fabric; instead, a firmly woven, lightweight fabric, such as pocketing, is used. The reinforcement is often a special stiffener, similar to buckram, instead of regular interfacing.

The waistband seam holds the front and back pocket tops securely in place.

Follow our instructions carefully; the cutting of the pieces and the point at which the waistband is applied may differ from the pattern's specifications. Leave crotch seam unstitched until directed to join waistband sections at center back.

Waistband with professional waistbanding

There are several products available for supporting a trouser waistband. Professional waistbanding is a flexible woven synthetic product that has been heat-set to precise widths from ¾ inch to 2 inches. Purchase it in the exact width desired for the finished waistband. Do not cut it to make it narrower; this will remove the finished edge and expose sharp cross-yarns that could penetrate fabric and scratch skin. (Note: Technique using this product is shown with a left front extension.)

Cutting: Cut the *left waistband* in a length to fit from the raw edge of the back seam to the finished edge at the front plus 3". Cut the *right waistband* to fit from the edge of the back seam to the finished edge of the fly shield plus ⅝". The width should equal the width of the professional waistbanding plus 1½". Cut *facing sections* the same length but 2" wider than the waistbanding, placing them on the true bias of the pocketing. Cut *waistbanding* to equal the length of the waistband sections minus ⅝".

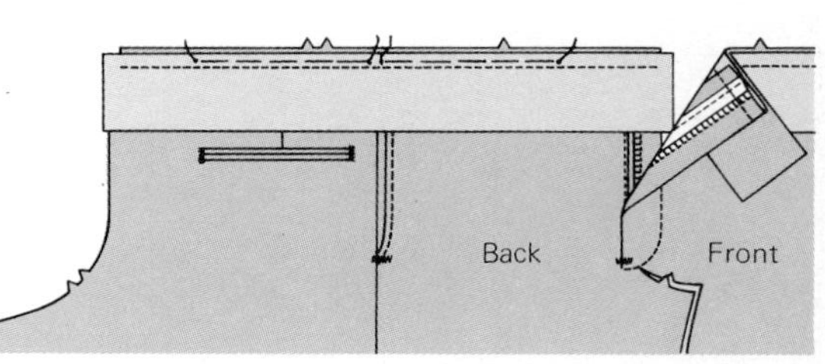

1. Right sides together, stitch waistband sections to garment sections. Baste pockets to waist seam.

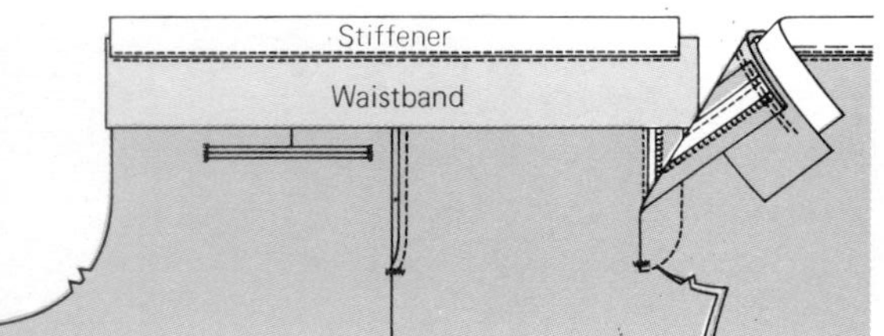

2. Lap the waistbanding over waistband seam allowances, aligning long edge with the stitching on seamline. End of waistbanding should be ⅝" from front edge of each section. Stitch close to edge through all layers.

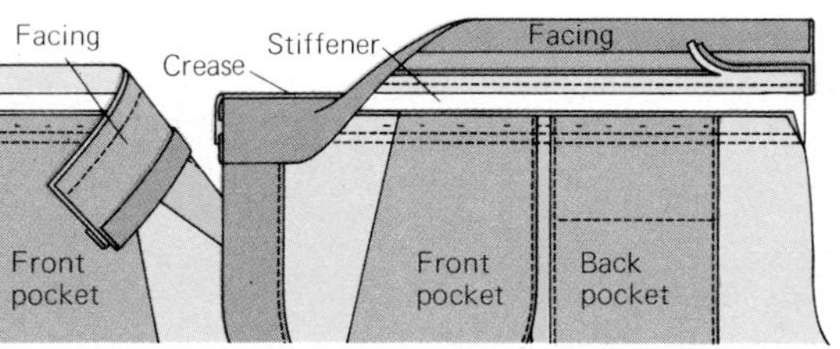

3. Stitch facings to waistbands with a ⅝" seam, right sides together. Grade seam allowances; press toward facing. Turn free edge of facing under 1"; press. Fold facing down; press a crease where waistband touches stiffener.

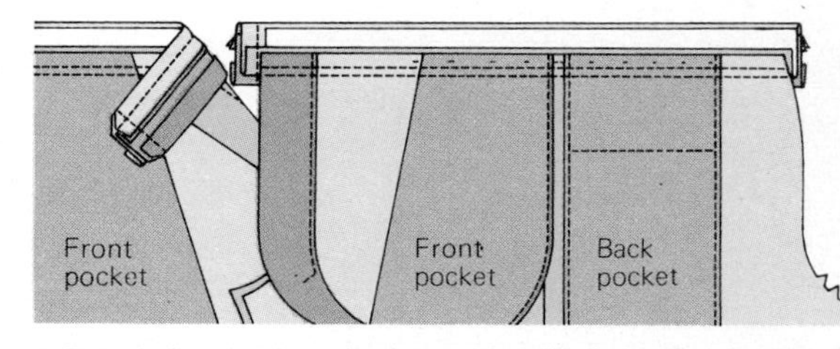

4. Turn facing back to the right side. Match inside of pressed crease to the top edge of the stiffener. Stitch across the front ends on each section. Trim seam and clip across corners diagonally, as shown.

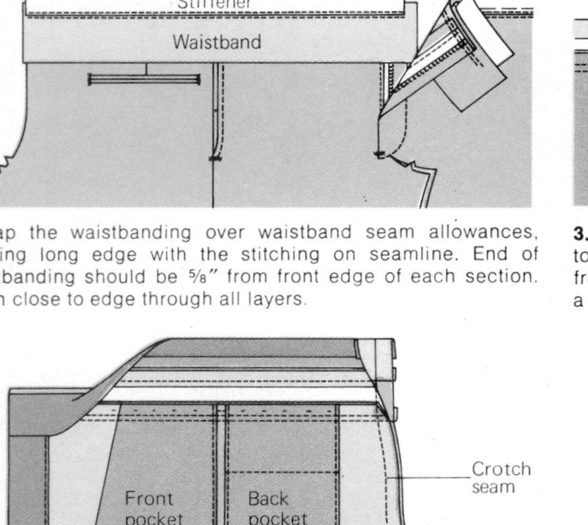

5. To sew center back seam and waistband, lift facing up; pin seam, matching cross seams. Stitch; press open; fold facing to inside of waistband. (For a V-shaped opening at top of waistband, see Step 6, opposite page.)

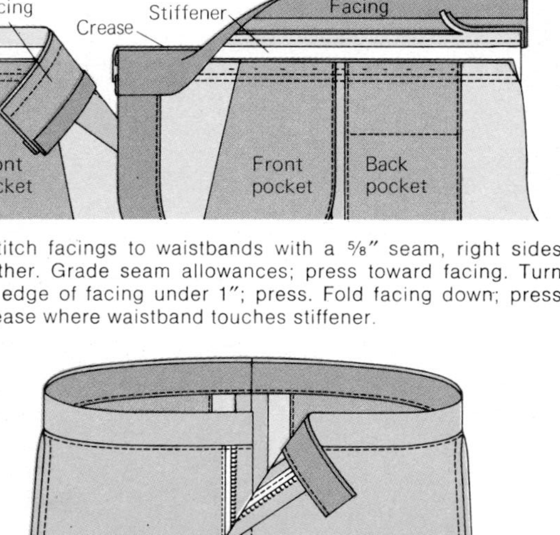

6. Press facing into position on inside of garment, keeping seam allowances of waistline seam toward top of waistband. Baste facing to trousers along waistline seam. From right side, stitch in seam groove, through the facing.

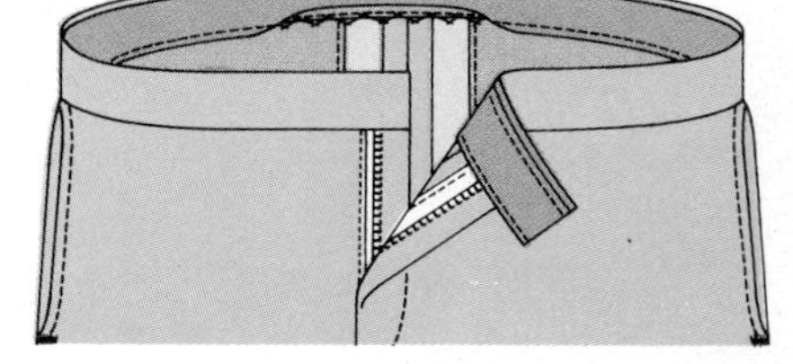

An alternative method: Machine-stitch ⅜" from lower edge of facing to hold fold in place. Secure facing to waist seam with a blind catchstitch, using machine stitches as a guide for placement of catchstitches on facing.

Interfacing selection 72
Grain in fabric 84-85
Slipstitch (even) 132
Trouser zipper 396-397

Tailored waistband

This smooth, flat, flexible waistband, made with hand-finishing, is the one used by professional tailors in the trousers of fine suits. The stiffener should be more flexible than for other methods. Professional tailors use buckram, sold by the yard and in pre-cut strips in specialty stores. Be sure the strips are cut on the bias, not the straight grain. If buckram is not available, you can substitute a very heavy hair canvas, only in a nonfusible.

Instructions are given here for a finished waistband width of 1¾ inches; this method works best when the finished waistband width is kept under 2 inches. The zipper should be in the trousers, but the crotch seam should still be open, when construction is begun. Cut the waistband sections, on the lengthwise grain, from garment fabric.

Cutting: *Waistband sections* should be cut to length equal to waist seamline from edge to edge of each half plus ⅝″. Width is 2¾″. *Facings and finishing strips* are cut the same length as waistband sections, from cross grain of pocketing. Facings are 2½″ wide, finishing strips 1½″ wide. *Buckram:* Same size as waistband; cut on the bias grain.

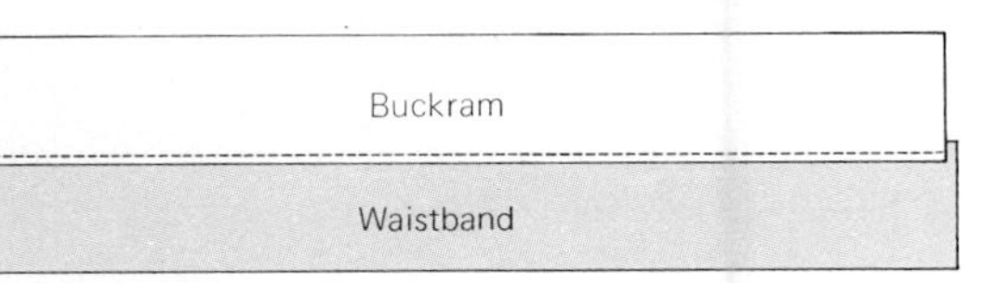

1. Lap one long edge of the buckram or hair canvas ¼″ over the **wrong** side of the waistband section. Stitch through center of lapped edges. When folded, this is the top edge.

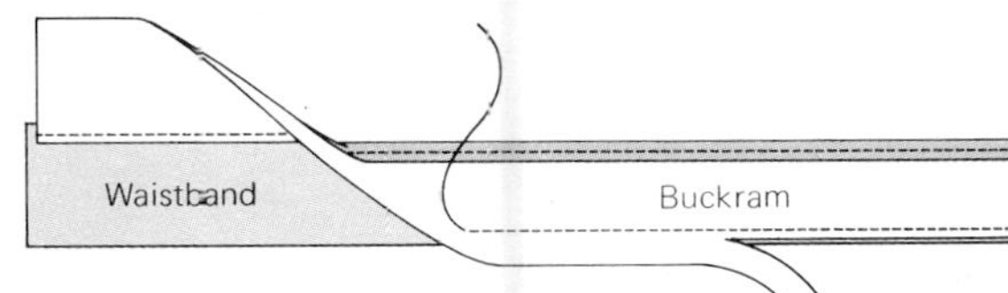

2. Turn buckram to wrong side of waistband; ¼″ of waistband fabric is now at top edge of buckram. At lower edge, trim buckram even with fabric; stitch the two together.

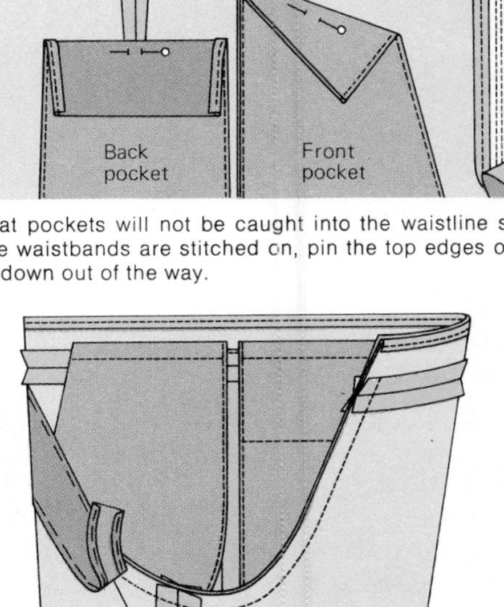

3. So that pockets will not be caught into the waistline seam when the waistbands are stitched on, pin the top edges of the pockets down out of the way.

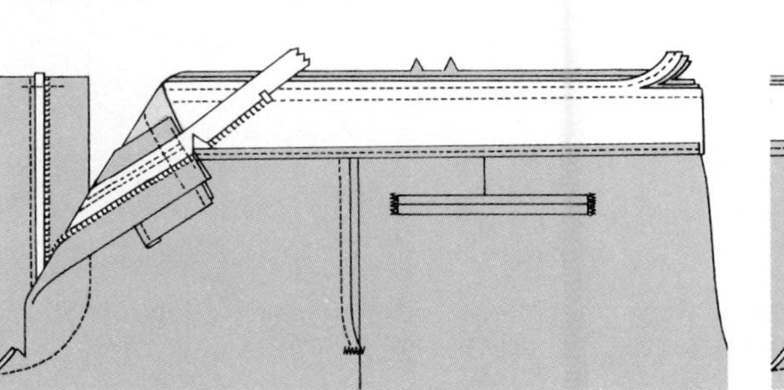

4. Working with the waistband side up, pin left waistband to left trouser half. Front edge of waistband should extend ⅝″ beyond finished edge of trousers. Stitch, then trim seam allowances to ⅜″. Repeat for right side.

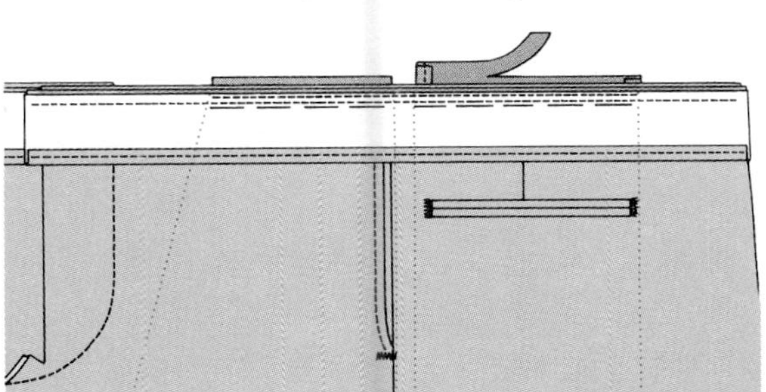

5. To secure pockets to waistline seam, first adjust them so they lie flat. Baste top edges to waist seamline. Waistband up, stitch through center of waistband seam allowance, catching pockets. Trim pockets to ¼″ above seam allowance.

6. Sew crotch seam with one leg inside the other, right sides of fabric together. Stitch, beginning at bottom of zipper and ending 1¼″ from top edge of waistband (for the comfort "V"), stretching seat area slightly as you stitch.

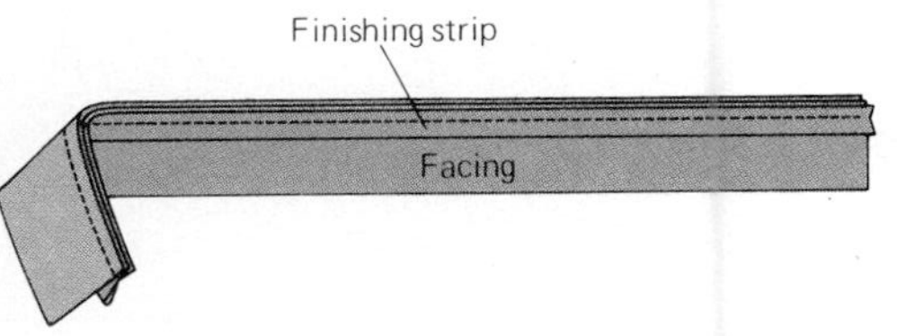

7. Fold facing finishing strips in half lengthwise. With right sides together, stitch them to one long edge of each of the facings, taking a ¼″ seam. Press seam flat to embed the stitches, but do not press strips away from facing.

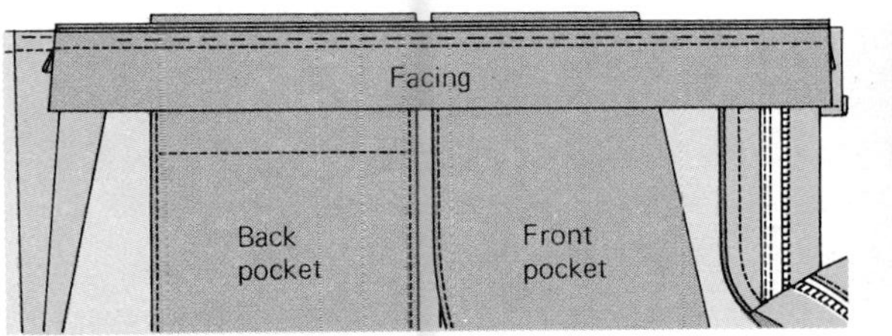

8. With finishing strip between wrong side of pants and facing, hand-sew facing seam allowance to seam allowance of waistband, using a running stitch. Facing will cover center back seam. Leave facing loose at back seam and zipper.

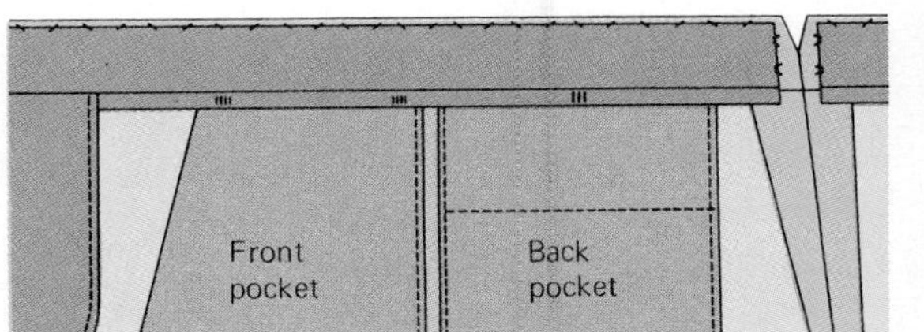

9. Press under remaining edges of facing ⅜″ all around, and slipstitch to waistband edges at tops and ends. Overtack facing finishing strips to pockets at each side on front pockets, at center on back pockets (see p. 391).

Waistband with men's waistbanding

This technique employs a specially designed product called men's waistbanding with extremely durable results. It is a combination of waistband stiffener and facing, the stiffener a sturdy buckram-type material, the facing a firmly woven fabric similar to pocketing. Facing and stiffener are joined at the lower edge; the top is left open for sewing to the waistband. In the method that follows, the ends of the waistbanding are machine-stitched to waistband seam allowances at center back and front for maximum durability. The waistbanding is secured all around the waist seam.

Cutting: *Waistband sections* should be cut to length equal to the waist seamline of each half from edge to edge plus ⅝″; to a width 1¼″ wider than the facing part of the waistbanding. *Waistbanding:* Same length as waistband sections.

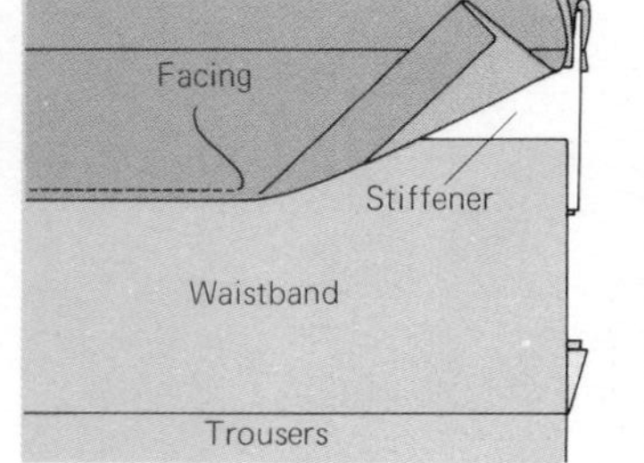

1. Right sides together, stitch waistband section to trouser section with a ⅝″ seam. Press under free edge of facing part of waistbanding ½″. Place waistband top between facing and stiffener so it overlaps stiffener ⅝″. Stitch close to facing fold through all thicknesses.

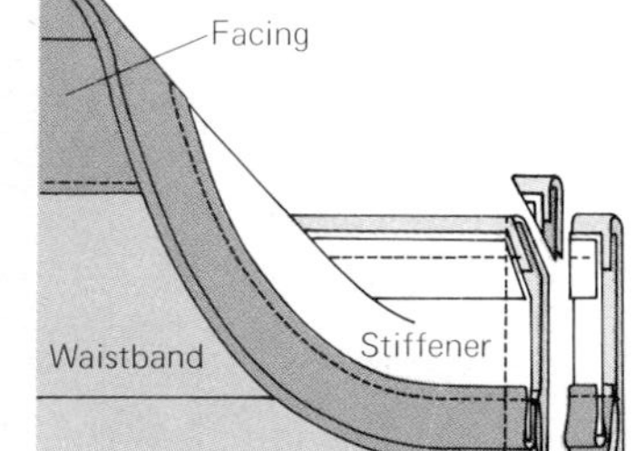

2. Repeat for other half of waistband. Finish front edge of each section by turning waistband so right sides are together, and stitching across ends with a ⅝″ seam. Trim and grade seam; clip corner diagonally. Turn band right side out, press; press a crease at top edge.

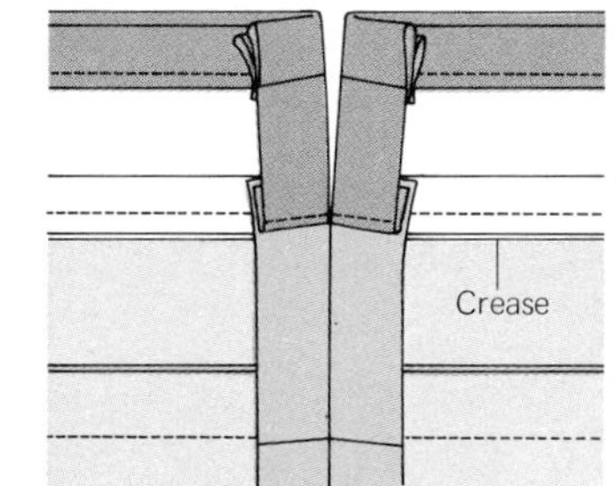

3. To form center back seam, first open out waistbanding so it will not be caught in seam. Stitch entire seam from crease at top of waistband (or from 1″ below for a comfort "V") to zipper in the front. Press *seam* open, seam *allowances* back on unstitched waistbanding.

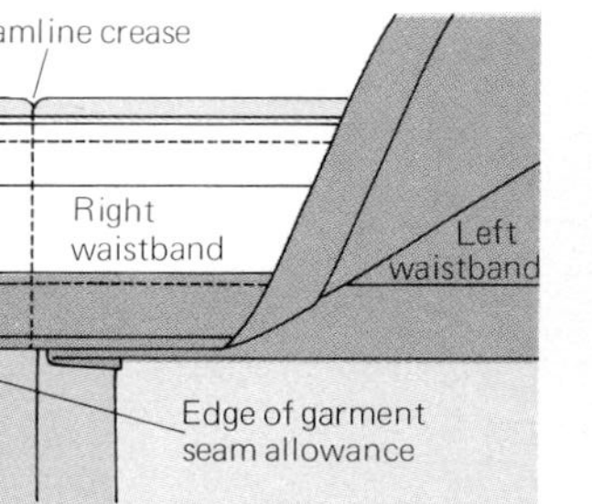

4. To finish back edges, fold the waistband so right sides are together. Work on half of garment at a time. Open out center back seam allowance; match its edge to edge of waistbanding. Stitch in pressed seam allowance crease of waistbanding the width of waistband.

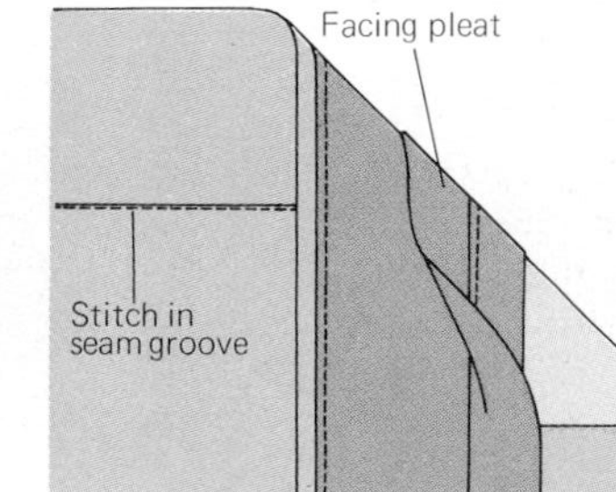

5. Turn waistband right side out. To finish waistband, stitch in the seam groove from right side of garment, lifting facing pleat out of the way and stitching only through the pleat in the stiffener. Or tack stiffener pleat to the pockets and seam allowances all around.

Waistband with elastic

This waistband method can be used only with knit fabrics. It is ideal for them because it takes advantage of the fabric's stretchability, and at the same time gives the waistband a sturdy support that will not roll over. The elastic used, a woven spandex designed especially for men's trousers, serves as both facing and interfacing. It is sold by the yard in 1½- and 2½-inch widths; the elastic width determines that of the finished waistband. You should purchase enough elastic to fit both waistband sections. Usually, the waist measurement plus 8 inches is sufficient. The left waistband is cut with an extension to allow for finishing the front edge with garment fabric.

Cutting: *Waistband sections* should be cut to length equal to the waist seamline of each half, plus an extra amount equal to the zipper fly facing on the left half and an additional ⅝″ on the right. Width is that of the elastic plus 1¼″. *Elastic:* Length equal to waistbands minus zipper facing on left.

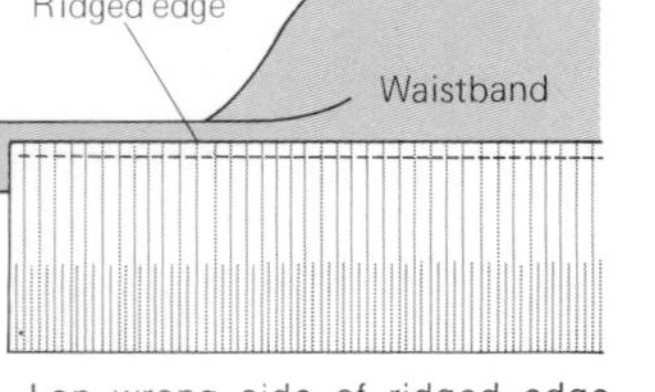

1. Lap wrong side of ridged edge of elastic ¼″ over right side of one long edge of waistband. On left half, match end of elastic to beginning of extension. Stitch.

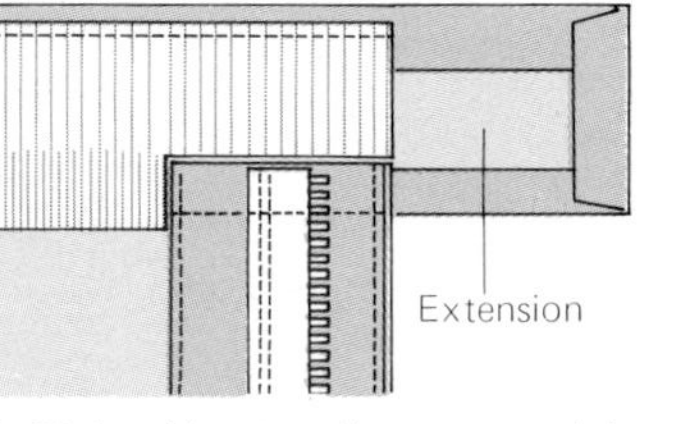

2. Right sides together, sew waistband to trousers; trim seam allowances to ⅜″. Fold elastic and ¼″ of waistband to wrong side. On left side, trim out elastic over zipper.

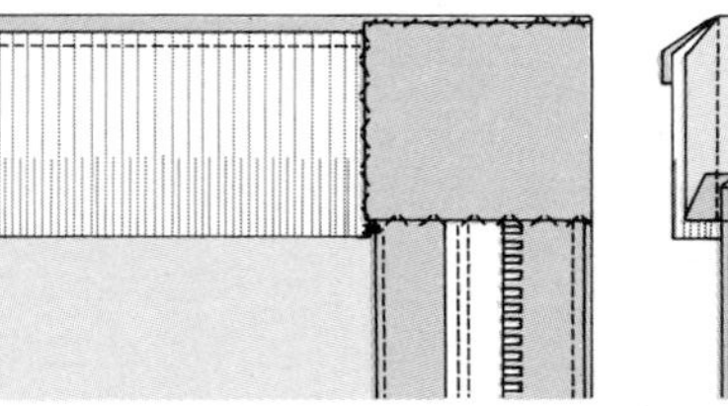
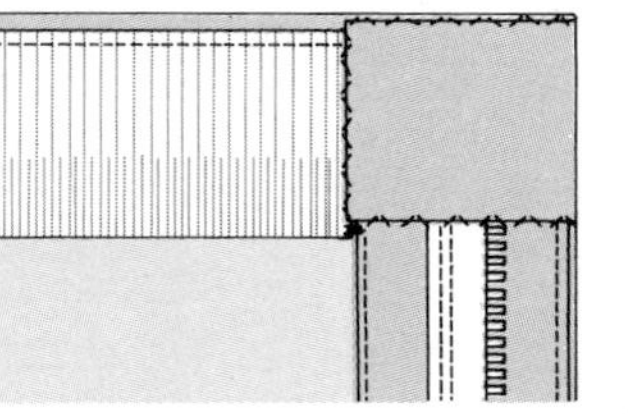

3. Fold the extension to inside of waistband; turn under seam allowances all around and slipstitch in place. Whipstitch cut end of elastic to zipper facing.

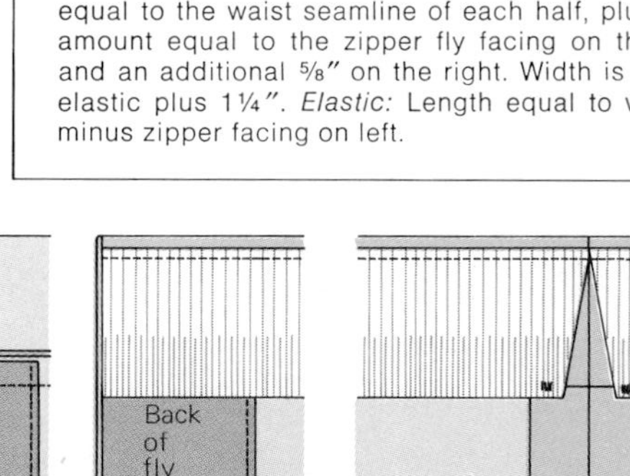

4. To finish right-hand side, fold waistband, right sides together. Stitch across end, aligning stitching with edge of trouser front. Trim seam and turn waistband right side out.

5. Stitch center back seam, leaving elastic open. Turn waistband to inside; turn ends of elastic in on a diagonal, and tack each securely to center back seam allowances.

Fusible interfacings and their application 79
Slipstitch (uneven) 132

Waistband with iron-on interfacing

In this method, the width of the waistband is not limited by the width of the stiffener; the interfacing may be cut to any desired width. Select a sturdy hair canvas iron-on interfacing. The construction method is the same as for the tailored waistband, page 399, beginning with Step 3.

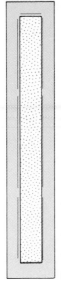

Cutting. *Waistband sections, facings, and finishing strips:* Cut these the same as for a tailored waistband, page 399, in the chosen width. *Interfacing* should be cut to the *finished* size of the waistband; trim away all seam allowances.

Match edges of interfacing to seamlines of wrong side of waistband. Fuse in place; proceed with technique.

Belt carriers

Belt carriers appear on most men's trousers, the exception being those made with an elastic waistband. There are usually seven such carriers, evenly spaced around the waistline seam, with one carrier located at center back. If the waist is very large, more carriers should be added.

Carriers vary in width and length to suit trouser style and belt width. In general, the wider or heavier the belt, the wider the loops should be to support the weight. The total length of a carrier should equal the belt width plus 1 inch to allow the belt to slip through easily.

There are three ways to make belt carriers. The first method is quick and easy, and the selvage need not be used if the fabric is a firmly constructed knit. The second method is preferred for fine, tailored trousers in any fabric. The third is an alternative suitable for very crisp, firmly woven, lightweight fabrics only.

Preparation of belt carriers

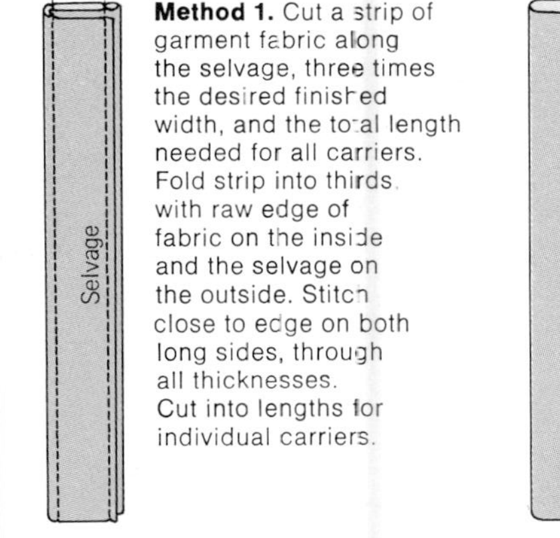

Method 1. Cut a strip of garment fabric along the selvage, three times the desired finished width, and the total length needed for all carriers. Fold strip into thirds with raw edge of fabric on the inside and the selvage on the outside. Stitch close to edge on both long sides, through all thicknesses. Cut into lengths for individual carriers.

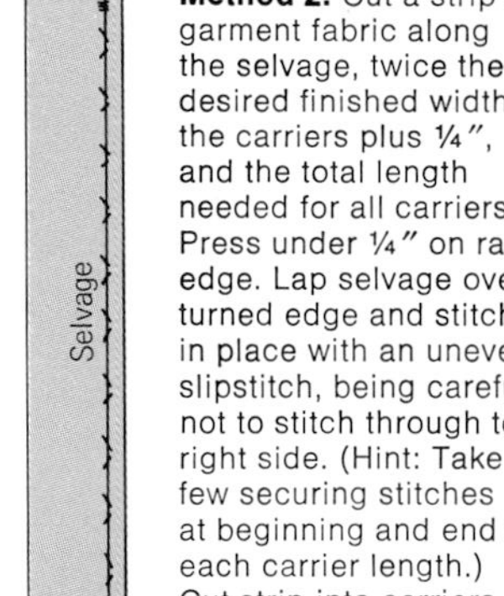

Method 2. Cut a strip of garment fabric along the selvage, twice the desired finished width of the carriers plus ¼″, and the total length needed for all carriers. Press under ¼″ on raw edge. Lap selvage over turned edge and stitch in place with an uneven slipstitch, being careful not to stitch through to right side. (Hint: Take a few securing stitches at beginning and end of each carrier length.) Cut strip into carriers.

Method 3. If strips cannot be placed on the selvage, cut a strip of fabric twice the desired width of the finished carrier plus ½″, in a length sufficient for all carriers. Press under ¼″ on both long edges. Fold strip in half lengthwise, carefully matching the folded edges. Press. Topstitch close to both edges. Cut strip into the individual lengths needed for each carrier.

Marking location of carriers: Locate a carrier at center back, one at each side seam, and halfway between each side seam and centers front and back. Baste a mark ¼″ below top edge of waistband and ¼″ below waistline seam (or lower, if the belt is wider than the waistband).

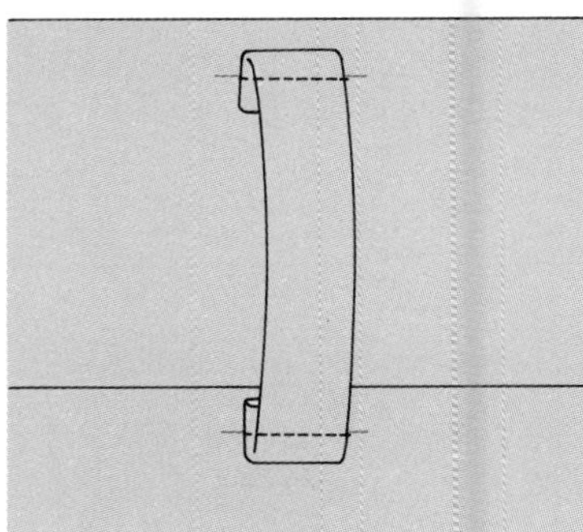

To attach carriers (except at center back), fold each end under ¼″; press. Place one fold ⅛″ above top waistband mark, the other fold ⅛″ below lower mark. Machine-stitch in place.

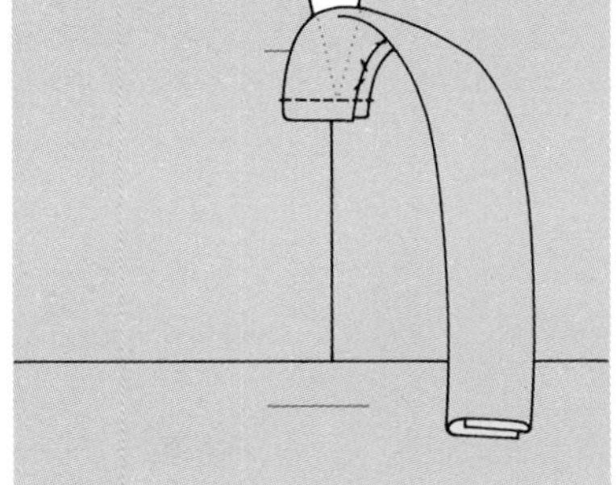

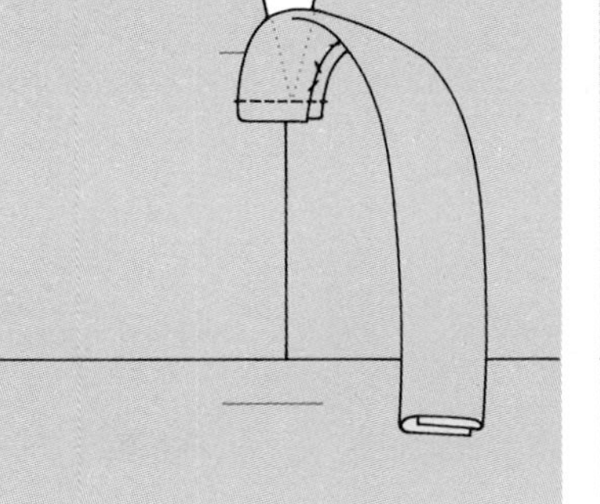

To attach center back carrier where there is a V-shaped opening at the top of waistband, place one end of the carrier wrong side up just below the end of the "V". Stitch across the width of carrier at the bottom of the V-shaped opening, as shown. Bring the carrier down over the waistband, fold the other end under ¼″, and sew in place below waistline seam. Press.

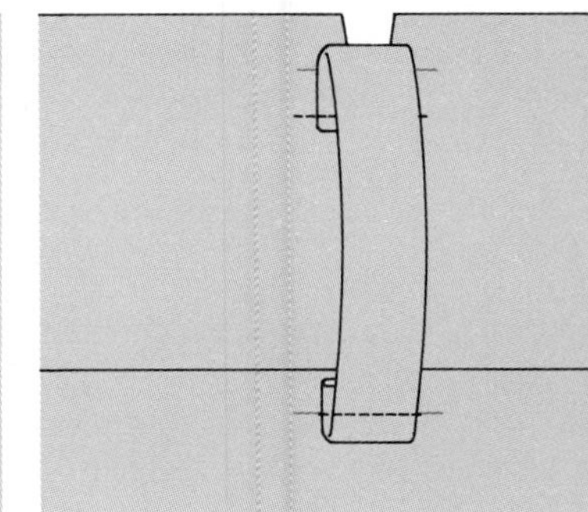

Hand basting 124
Trimming and grading seams 147
Flat-felled seams 150

Making a shirt

Although a man's shirt may seem a masterpiece of precision, it requires little more than regular sewing techniques, very carefully executed.

Listed at the far right are the steps, in order, for constructing a shirt. The numbers after each step are the pages on which an explanation of that technique can be found. Because styles vary, not all steps will apply to every shirt.

The traditional seam choice for men's shirts is the flat-felled seam, preferred because it gives a uniformly clean finish. The fell, or overlap, is usually on the inside of the shirt, the exact opposite of most other applications, in which the flat-felled seam is formed on the right side. The result is one visible row of stitching (rather than two) on the right side of the garment. This and the other recommended techniques ensure that there are no exposed raw edges anywhere in the shirt.

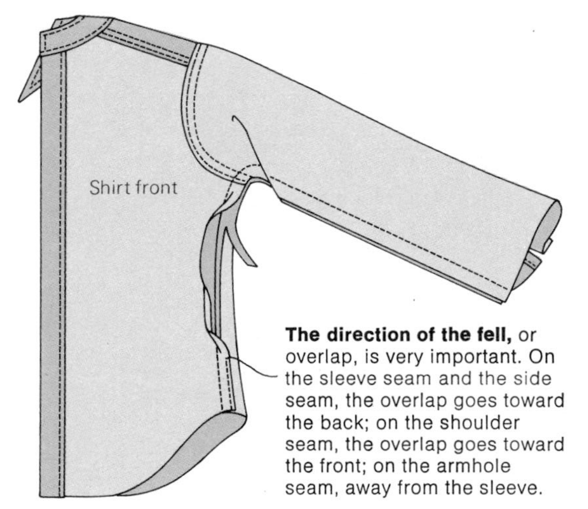

The direction of the fell, or overlap, is very important. On the sleeve seam and the side seam, the overlap goes toward the back; on the shoulder seam, the overlap goes toward the front; on the armhole seam, away from the sleeve.

Checklist/shirt procedure

Adjust pattern fit 101-104, 106-109

Lay out pattern, cut out shirt 84-93

Transfer pattern markings 94

Attach pockets and shirt tabs 275, 277

Attach yoke 402-403

Construct collar: insert collar stays 403; attach interfacing 403; join collar sections 227; attach to band 227; attach band to neckline 228

Construct sleeve plackets 267

Set in the sleeves 257

Stitch underarm seams of sleeves and shirt 257

Construct and attach cuffs 268-269

Hem shirt 294

Make buttonholes 343-347

Attach buttons 351-352

Classic shirt yoke

The classic shirt yoke is fully lined so that all seams are enclosed. In the first of these two techniques, the yoke is topstitched in place along the front seam; it may also be topstitched at the back seam, if you like. The second method uses machine sewing throughout, but no topstitching. It is not difficult, but demands care in positioning for the stitching of front shoulder seams. Make fitting pleat at center back before starting either yoke.

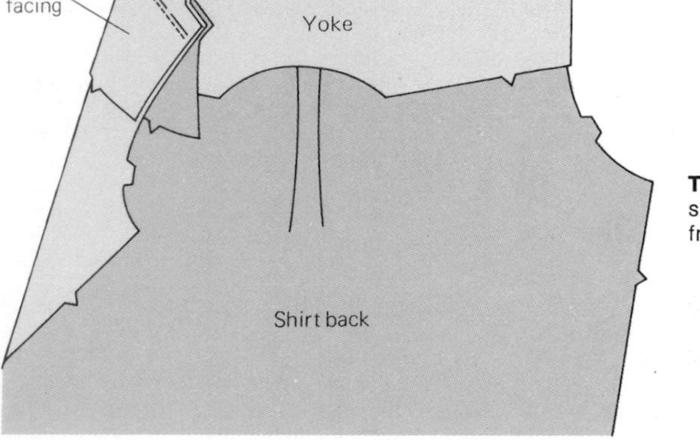

Step 1, both methods: Right sides together, baste the yoke to the shirt back. Baste the right side of the yoke facing to the wrong side of the shirt back. Stitch a ⅝" seam, sewing through all three layers. Grade seam allowances, leaving yoke seam allowance the widest. Press yoke and facing up, away from shirt, into yoke's permanent position.

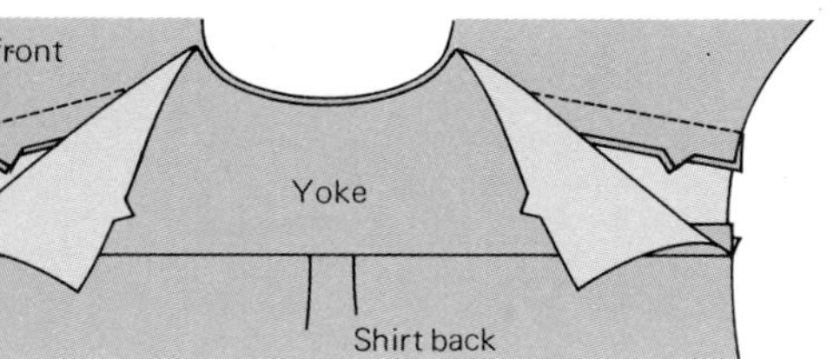

Topstitched method: Topstitch yoke seam if desired (not shown). Baste right side of yoke facing to wrong side of front shoulder seams. Stitch; press seam toward facing. Trim

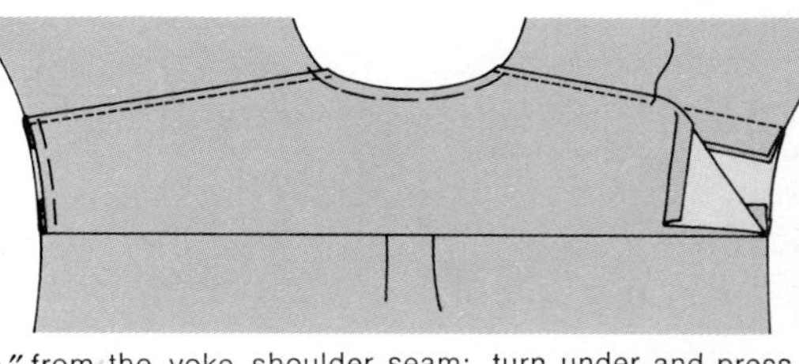

¼" from the yoke shoulder seam; turn under and press the remaining ⅜". Match folded edge to yoke facing seamline; topstitch. Baste neck and shoulder edges together.

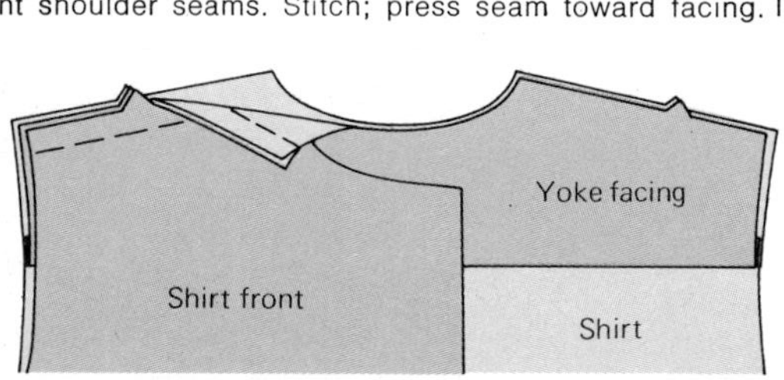

Couture method: Do not topstitch yoke seamline. Baste right side of yoke facing to wrong side of shirt fronts at shoulder seam. Right sides together, match shoulder seams of yoke

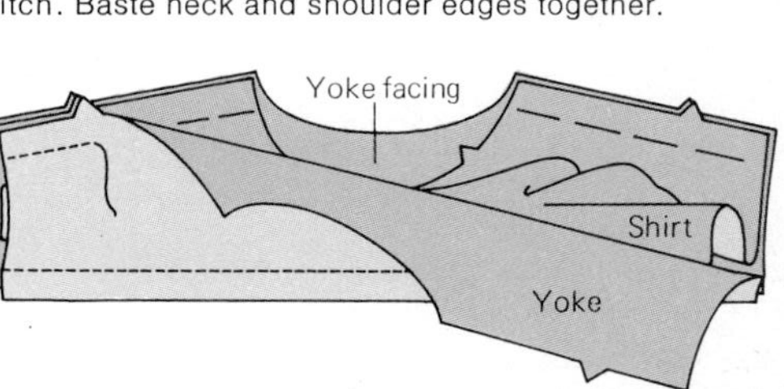

and shirt front. (Shirt will be between yoke and yoke facing.) Stitch through yoke, shirt front, and yoke facing. Turn shirt to right side and press.

Western shirt yoke

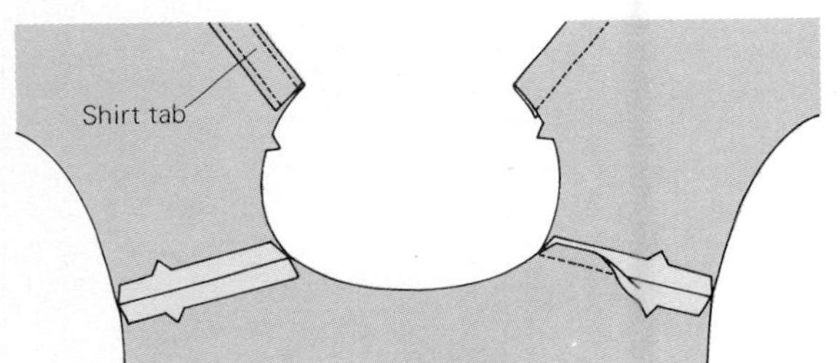

The western-style shirt yoke is basically a big appliqué sewed on over the shoulder area of the shirt. Unlike the traditional yoke, it is not an integral part of the shirt.
1. With wrong sides together, stitch the shoulder seams of the shirt and press them open.

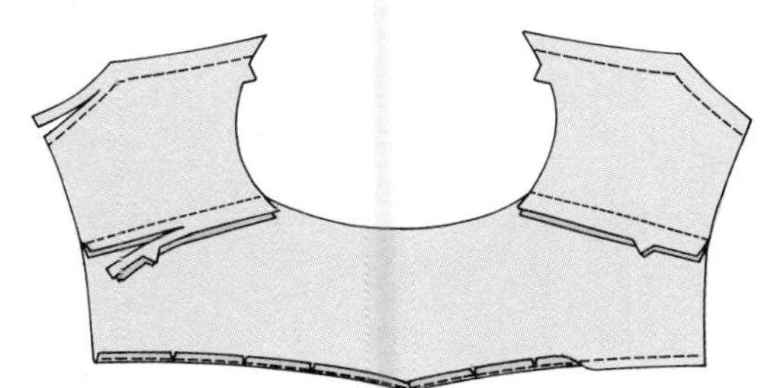

2. Right sides together, stitch yoke sections together at shoulder. Trim and grade, making front seam allowance the widest; press toward back. Stitch on seamline of pointed edges; trim seam allowances to ¼″. Press under, rolling stitching slightly to underside; clip as needed.

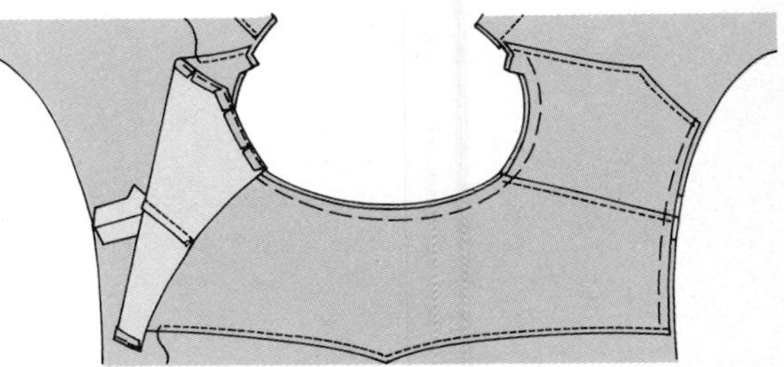

3. Pin yoke to right side of shirt as shown, matching markings and shoulder seams and carefully aligning edges of neck and armholes; baste yoke in place. Topstitch yoke along shoulder seams, then along folded seam allowances on front and back. Baste neck and armhole edges together.

Shirt collar stay

Collar stays are plastic strips with one pointed end that are used to support the front of a collar and prevent the collar point from curling upward. Stays are an optional detail, but you must decide before beginning collar construction if you will use them. Choose stays that are just long enough to reach diagonally from the collar roll to the finished collar point (this would be to the topstitching on most collars). Collar stays can usually be found in notions departments, or you can use the stays from another shirt, provided they are the correct length.

Note: Fusible interfacing cannot be used in a stayed collar, because the pocket for the stay is formed between interfacing and under collar.

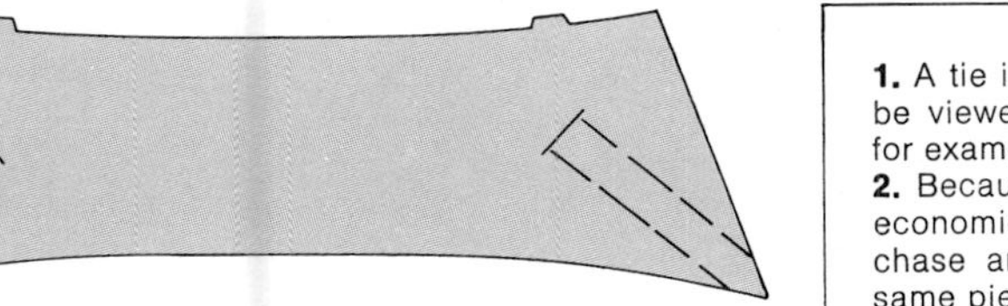

1. On the right side of the under collar, center a stay diagonally between the collar edges at each corner, with the point ⅝″ from the corner. (Place it ⅜″ from the corner if there is to be no topstitching.) Lightly, with a lead pencil, mark each side of the stay. Then mark straight across the end, making mark slightly longer than the width of the stay. Using a ruler, draw parallel lines from the end mark to the collar point.

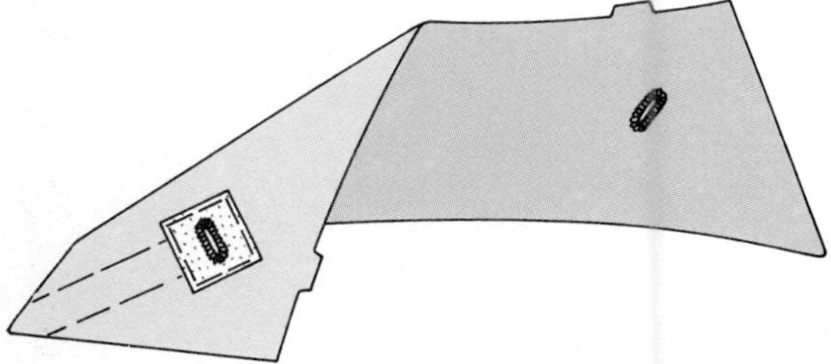

2. The mark at the end of the stay is for a buttonhole. Baste or fuse a small square of interfacing on wrong side of under collar under the buttonhole mark. Make machine- or hand-worked buttonholes on right side exactly at mark on under collar. Carefully open buttonholes.

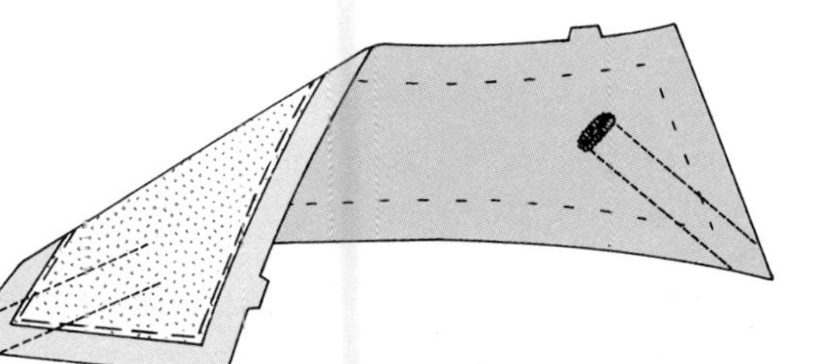

3. Baste interfacing to the wrong side of the under collar. Stitch along the parallel lines so that a pocket is formed for the stay. Complete collar construction. Slip stay into pocket. The end should protrude about ¼″ from the buttonhole to permit easy removal for laundering.

Tips on making men's ties

1. A tie is cut on the bias, so any fabric choice should be viewed from this angle before purchase. A stripe, for example, will become a diagonal.
2. Because a tie is cut from the bias grain, it is more economical (because it avoids wasted fabric) to purchase an extra ⅛ yard and make two ties from the same piece of fabric.
3. There are two types of interfacing especially for ties: one is made of wool (or a wool and rayon blend) and can be dry-cleaned only; the other is made of synthetic fibers and is washable. If you must use another type of interfacing, choose one with a high loft, or use two layers of a type that is of medium weight and softness.
4. When any tie is being worn the bottom tip should reach to the top of the belt. After determining the proper length for the tie, compare it with that of the pattern, adding or subtracting length as needed at the center seam. Remember to alter the interfacings by the same amount.
5. For easier control in hand-stitching and pressing, cut cardboard pieces to the finished shape of each end of the tie, and place them inside the tie until stitching and pressing are completed.
6. The finished edges of the tie should be rolled, not flattened; do not put the full weight of the iron on the tie while pressing. Use a lightweight press cloth and, holding the iron just above it, allow steam to penetrate for a few seconds.
7. To keep the narrow end in place when the tie is worn, sew a loop of ribbon or fabric to the underside of the wide end about 6 inches from the point. Make a loop equal to the width of the narrow end plus ⅜″. Turn the ends of the loop under ¼″ and slipstitch each in place.

Sewing for children

Introduction

There is probably no sewing activity so immediately satisfying as sewing for children. You get quick results, for one thing, because the garments have smaller dimensions. Also, more shortcuts can be taken in techniques. Children's garments should be constructed to survive vigorous activity and endless washings. Other special considerations include providing room for sudden growth spurts, and planning garments that are easy to put on.

Size range charts

BABIES

Age	**Newborn (1-3 months)**	**6 months**
Weight	7-13 lbs.	13-18 lbs.
Height	17″-24″	24″-26½″

TODDLERS'

Size	**½**	**1**	**2**	**3**	**4**
Breast or chest	19	20	21	22	23
Waist	19	19½	20	20½	21
Approximate heights	28″	31″	34″	37″	40″
Finished dress length	14″	15″	16″	17″	18″

CHILDREN'S

Size	**1**	**2**	**3**	**4**	**5**	**6**	**6X**
Breast or chest	20	21	22	23	24	25	25½
Waist	19½	20	20½	21	21½	22	22½
Hip				24	25	26	26½
Back waist length	8¼	8½	9	9½	10	10½	10¾
Approximate heights	31″	34″	37″	40″	43″	46″	48″
Finished dress length	17″	18″	19″	20″	22″	24″	25″

GIRLS'

Size	**7**	**8**	**10**	**12**	**14**
Breast	26	27	28½	30	32
Waist	23	23½	24½	25½	26½
Hip	27	28	30	32	34
Back waist length	11½	12	12¾	13½	14¼
Approximate heights	50″	52″	56″	58½″	61″

CHUBBIE

Size	**8½c**	**10½c**	**12½c**	**14½c**
Breast	30	31½	33	34½
Waist	28	29	30	31
Hip	33	34½	36	37½
Back waist length	12½	13¼	14	14¾
Approximate heights	52″	56″	58½″	61″

Selecting pattern type and size

Patterns for children's clothes are grouped into several types, intended to reflect in their styling the size and physical development of the average child at certain ages. For purposes of identification, the pattern groupings are named to correspond with the different stages in a child's growth. You should not assume, however, that just because your child is a toddler, he or she will automatically fit into the toddler size range. A child who is not yet walking may be larger than the largest set of measurements in the toddler range. To make an accurate size selection, you must measure your child and compare his or her individual measurements with those listed for each pattern type to see which type and what size most closely approximates the child's own measurements. The object is to choose a pattern type and size that fits with as few alterations as possible.

The captioned figures below represent the groupings of pattern types for children's wear. (For boys, see p. 384.) To make an accurate choice, measure your child and compare body measurements with those listed in the chart at left to determine which pattern type and size is suitable.

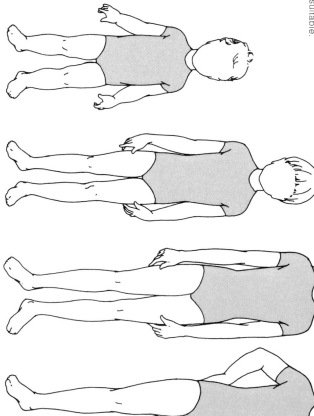

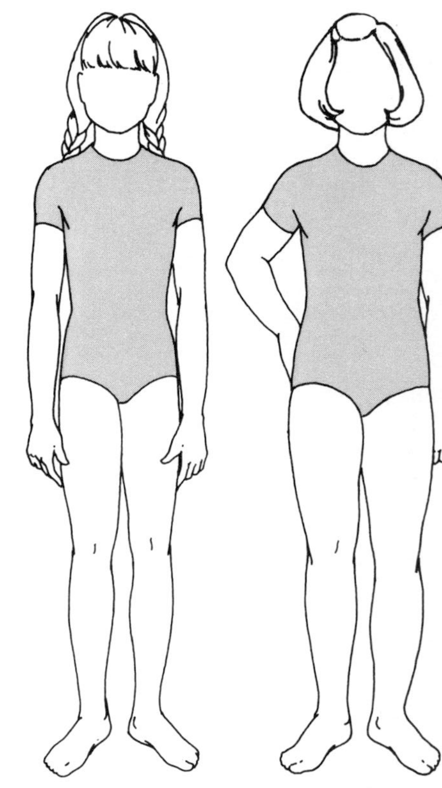

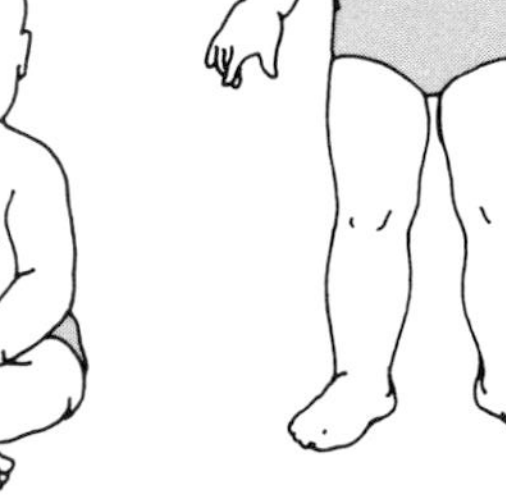

Babies patterns are for infants who do not yet walk. There is a diaper allowance, and styles are usually suitable for both boys and girls.

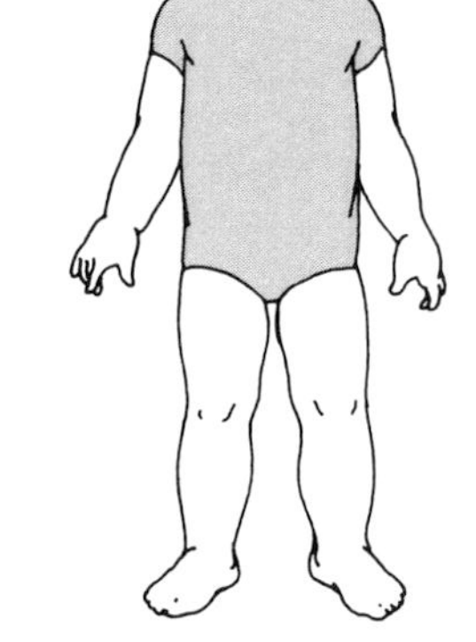

Toddlers' sizes are for the stage of development between a baby and a child. A diaper allowance is included, and styles often suit both boys and girls.

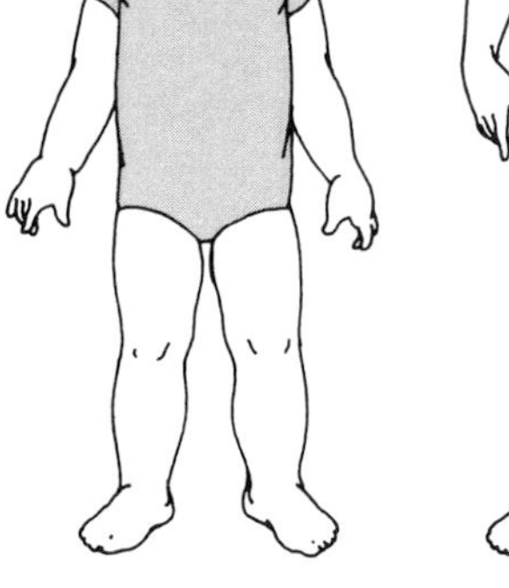

Children's sizes have the same breast and waist measurements as Toddlers' but are meant for a taller child, so shoulder, arm, and dress lengths are longer.

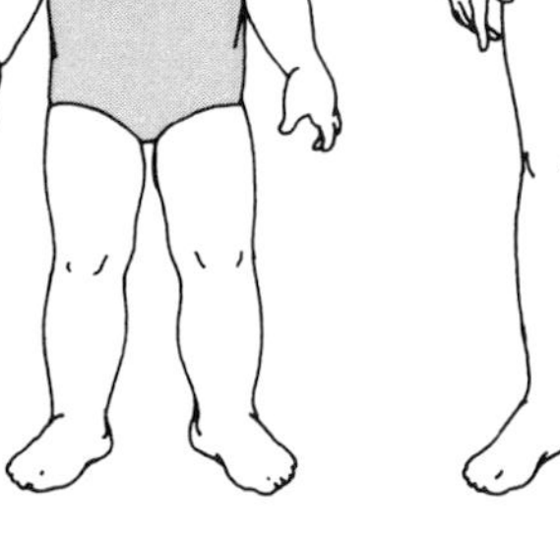

Girls' sizes are for the figure that has not yet begun to mature. Sizes are comparable to those for boys (see p. 384) but the height is greater for girls.

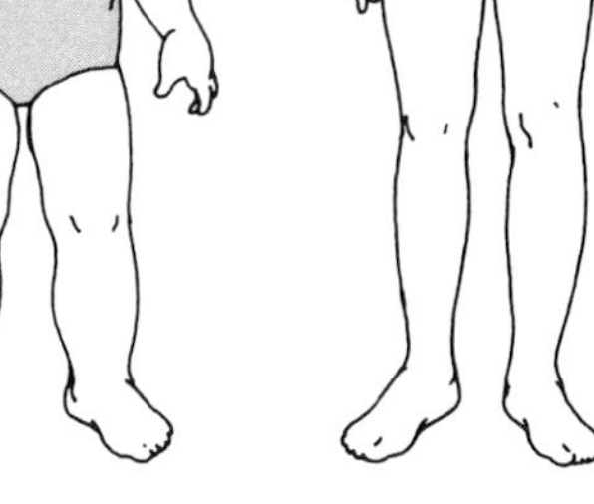

Chubbie sizes are for the growing girl whose weight is above average for her age and height. The height range is approximately the same as for Girls'.

Taking measurements

Two sets of measurements must be taken for children's clothes. One set is used to select the correct pattern size (and to help with alterations); the other is used only for the alterations that may be needed to make the pattern fit better.

In using the two sets of measurements, it is important to remember that the first set is compared to the measurements on the *back of the pattern envelope*, the second set to measurements of the *actual pattern pieces*. In comparing the second set, you need to know how much you should add for ease; on the first set, ease will be taken care of when differences, if any, between the body and the measurement on the pattern envelope are reconciled. This reconciliation is accomplished through basic pattern alterations. Another way to check measurements is to compare the pattern's with those of a garment that fits the child well.

Measure the child over undergarments only. Use a tape measure that will not stretch. Remember to check a child's measurements often; they can change quite rapidly. Also, height can sometimes increase with no change in circumference. If a child's measurements fall between sizes, it is generally wiser to go with the larger size. Record measurements on your chart in pencil, to allow for frequent re-recordings as changes occur.

Measurement chart

Measurements for pattern selection

MEASUREMENT	CHILD	PATTERN ENVELOPE	DIFFERENCE
Weight (for babies)			
Height			
Breast			
Waist			
Hips			
Back waist length			
Finished dress length			

Measurements for pattern alterations only

MEASUREMENT	CHILD	PATTERN PIECE	EASE	DIFFERENCE
Arm length			None*	
Shoulder length			None	
Crotch depth			Up to ½″	
Pants inseam			Up to ½″	
Pants outseam			None	

*For fitted sleeve; add extra length for full sleeve.

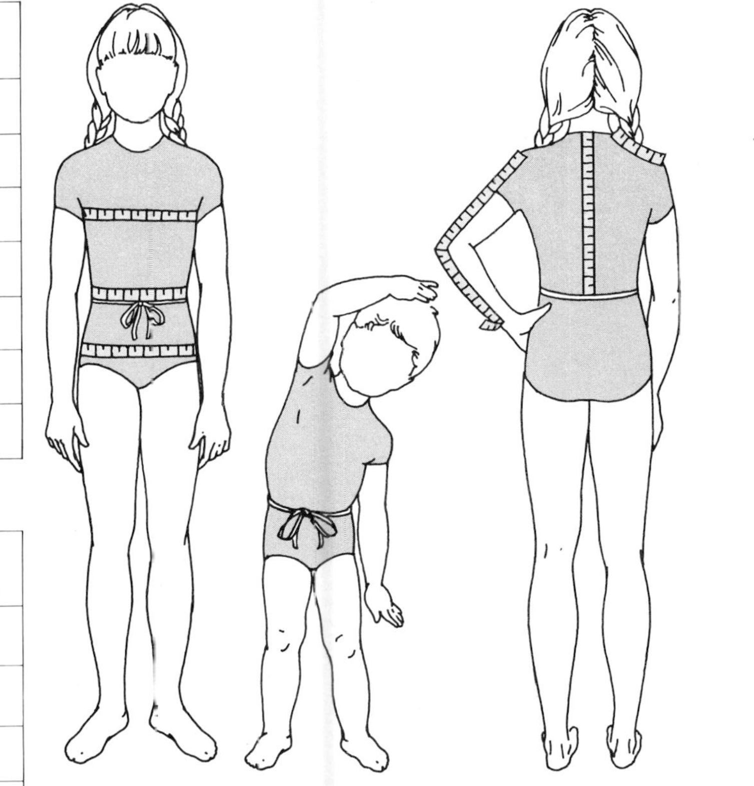

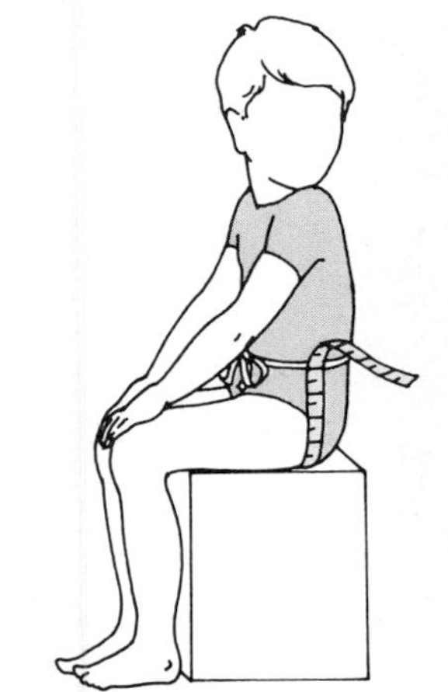

Breast: Under arms over fullest part of chest in front, just under the shoulder blades in back.
Waist: Around natural indentation (tie string around middle and have child bend sideways; the string will settle at the waistline).
Hips: Around fullest part of buttocks.

Back waist length: Prominent bone at base of neck to waist.
Shoulder length: Base of neck (have child shrug shoulders to locate it) to prominent bone at outer shoulder.
Arm length: From top of arm, over bent elbow, to wrist.

Height: Have child stand with back against wall, no shoes. Place ruler on top of head; mark where ruler touches; measure from floor to mark.

Crotch depth: With child seated on a firm chair, feet flat on floor, measure from waist to chair seat. Or measure a pair of pants that fits the child well and subtract the inseam from the outseam.

Sewing for children

Pattern alterations 103,106
Machine basting 137; chainstitch 139
Tucks 164
Applied casings 235-237

Special sewing hints

1. For speed, modifications of mass production techniques can be applied. The basic idea is to group similar tasks, doing as much of one as is practical before changing to another. For example, you might cut out several garments at once; complete as much stitching as possible (even on unrelated units) before pressing; press a number of areas before returning to the machine; set hand work aside for a time when you will be sitting still anyway—when you are watching television, for instance.

2. To quickly finish hems of sleeves, skirts, and pants, substitute fusing web for hand stitches.

3. For durability, substitute machine for hand stitches wherever it is practical and not unsightly to do so. (To tack down facings, for example.)

4. For extra strength, stitch areas of strain, such as armholes, twice.

5. For ease in handling really small garments, attach the sleeves before closing the underarm seam.

6. For ease of care, choose fabrics that are washable; also check the care requirements of white or pastel colors. Though cottons and synthetic blends are usually the first choices for children's garments, washable wools are candidates too.

7. To please the child, pick bright colors and lively prints. Be careful, though, to keep patterns in scale with the child's size. Too large a design can be overwhelming.

8. For convenience, always provide a pocket or two, even if the pattern does not include them. Children like places to keep small possessions.

9. For safety, sew reflective tape strips to outer garments—jackets, coats, caps, and so on. This material is available at notions counters in precut packaged quantities. It can be seen by motorists when children are outdoors during twilight hours and after dark, when visibility is not good.

10. To personalize a hand-me-down, particularly one from an older sister or brother, add a special appliqué, pocket, or monogram. Also, consider changing the garment style somewhat: could a former jumper become a tunic top for the new owner?

Providing room to grow

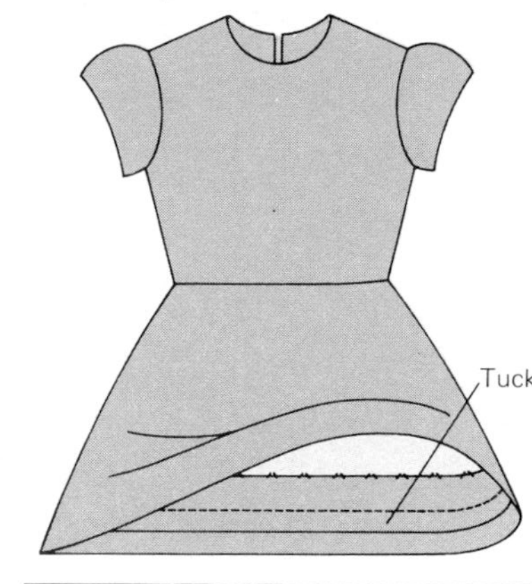

Three ways are described on this page to build some provision for sudden growth spurts into children's garments. The adjoining page tells how to add life to outgrown or worn garments.

A hem tuck introduces extra fabric into a skirt or dress hem without adding too much extra bulk. Illustration at the left shows how the finished garment looks from the right side.

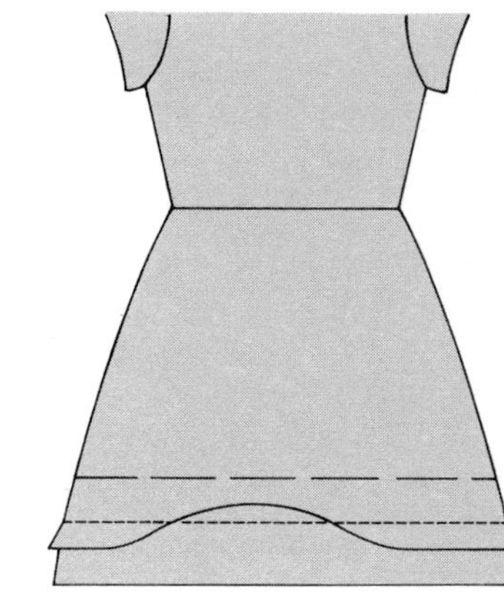

To make a hem tuck, add 1" to 4" of extra hem allowance when cutting garment. Mark hemline, then make the tuck within hem allowance, far enough above the hem edge that it will not show. Sew tuck with the most easily removed stitch on your machine. Complete the hem; press tuck toward hemline. To lengthen garment, release the tuck stitching and either re-stitch a narrower tuck or use all of the tuck allowance.

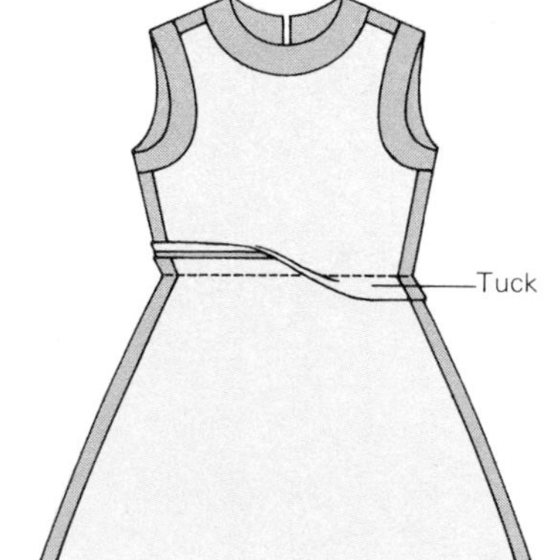

A bodice tuck is a way of providing extra length in the waist-to-shoulder area. This tuck is made before the zipper is inserted; to release the tuck, zipper stitching must be taken out to the bottom of the placket. The extra length that the released tuck adds to the center back seam will make the zipper space too long. To remedy this, sew up a part of the seam at placket bottom equal to tuck depth. Re-stitch zipper.

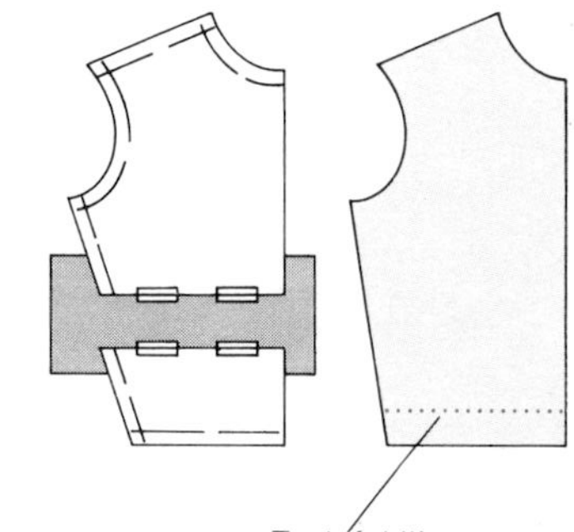

To make a bodice tuck, add 1½" to bodice length; cut out garment. On the wrong side of each bodice section, mark a tuck foldline ¾" above waist seam. Stitch bodice to skirt, then fold along tuck foldline and press. With skirt up, baste through waist seam and folded bodice. Machine-stitch just below waist seamline, using most easily removed stitch. Press tuck and seam allowances toward bodice.

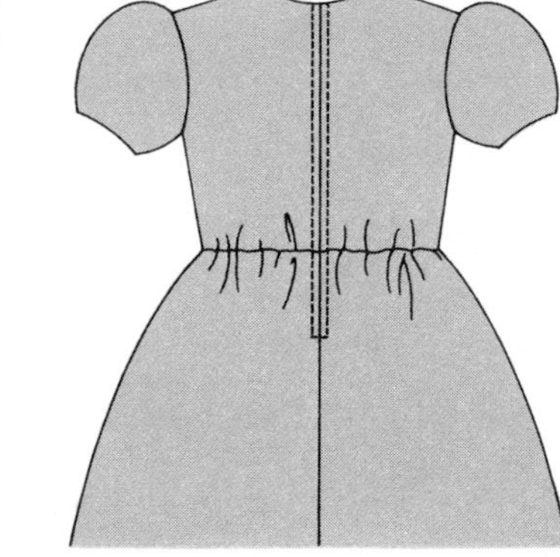

An expandable waistline can be made for any garment by adding extra fabric to the waistline, then controlling the fit with elastic. This is particularly suited to children's wear because it makes movement less constricted as well as allowing for growth. The elastic is generally put only in the back waist seam. Omit any darts in the back bodice or skirt.

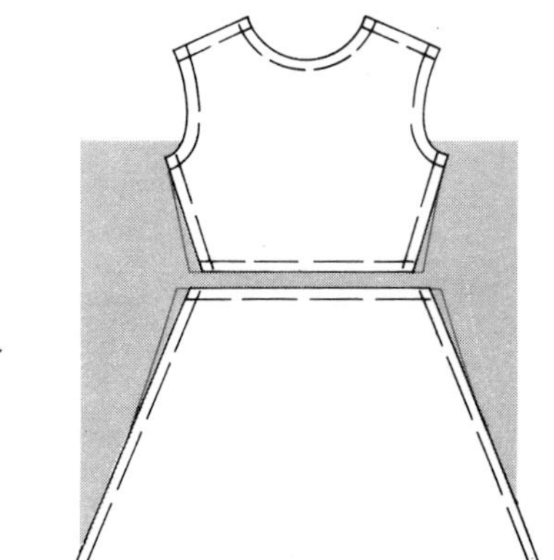

To make such a waistline, first add ½" to the side seams at waist, front and back, on bodice and skirt. Taper to original cutting line at hip and chest. Construct garment as usual; it will be about 2" too big in the waist. Sew a casing of bias tape to the back waist seam allowances; insert a length of narrow elastic (this will pull in the waistline); secure elastic ends at center back and side seams.

Extending garment life

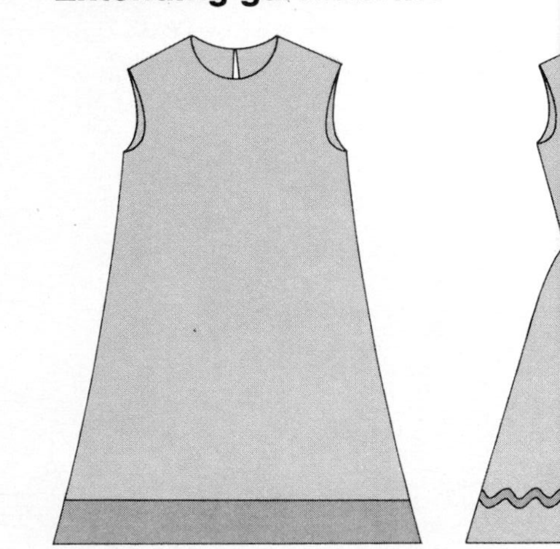

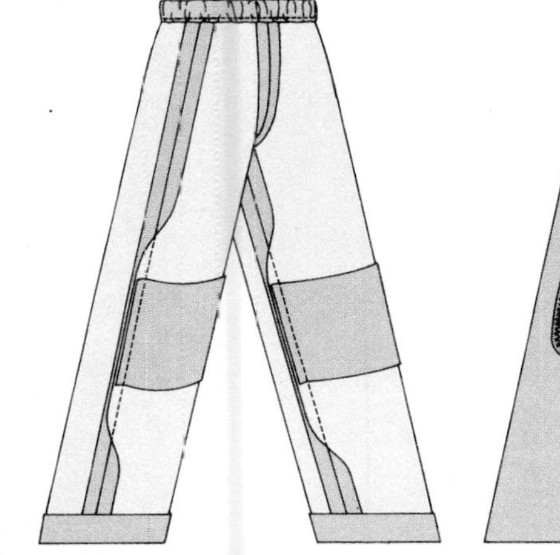

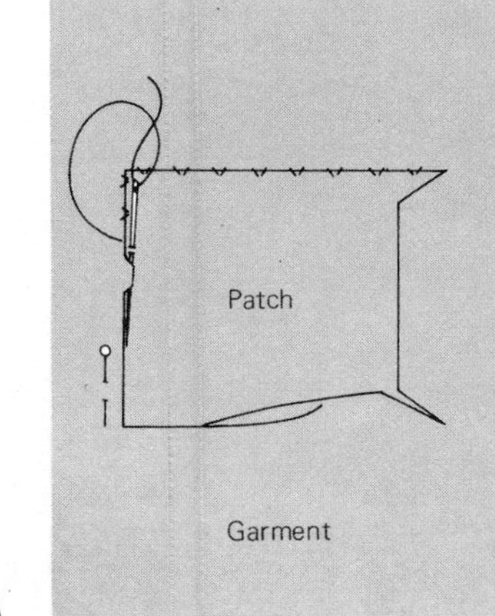

To lengthen a garment with little or no extra hem allowance, you can add a band of fabric. It could be a matching or contrasting plain fabric, or a harmonizing print. (See Hem finishes for methods of adding bands.) This same technique will work equally well for lengthening sleeves at the lower edges.

To conceal a worn line—it may be from fading, or from stitch marks where a hem or a tuck has been let out—sew a trim over it. Among the possibilities: rickrack, soutache braid, embroidered ribbon, bias tape, a bias band of garment fabric. Try a sash to conceal any such lines at the waist.

To make pants knees last longer, a number of things can be done.
1. Fuse a patch to the inside of the pants, at the knees. Use iron-on interfacing or lightweight fabric with an underlayer of fusing web. Cut the patch as wide as the pants; stitch it to the seam allowances at inseam and outseam.

2. Fuse a patch to the outside of the pants over the knee area; use iron-on patches, or scraps of fabric bonded with fusing web. After fusing, stitch around the outside edges of the patch with a decorative machine or hand stitch. This method is good for patching knees that already have holes in them.

3. Insert a patch into a worn or torn knee by first cutting away the damaged area, then sewing new fabric in its place. Cut the worn spot into a square; clip ¼" into each corner; press edges under ¼" all around. Place patch under hole, matching grain or design; slipstitch folded edges to patch.

Making garments easy to put on and take off

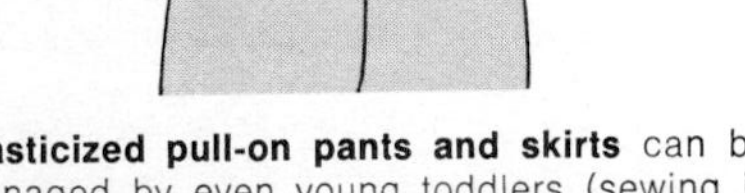

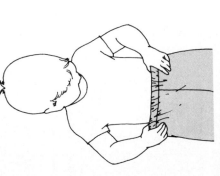

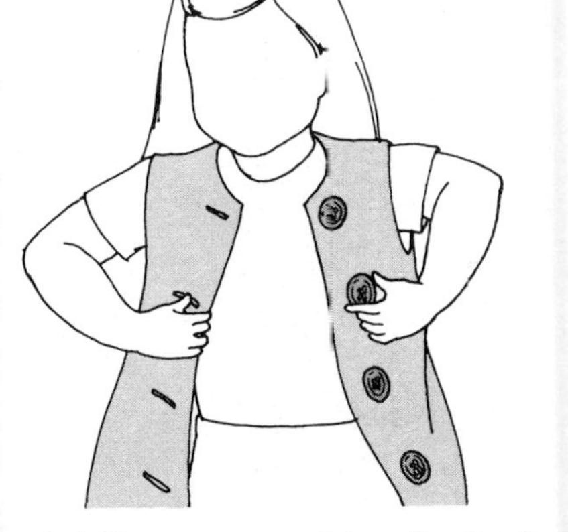

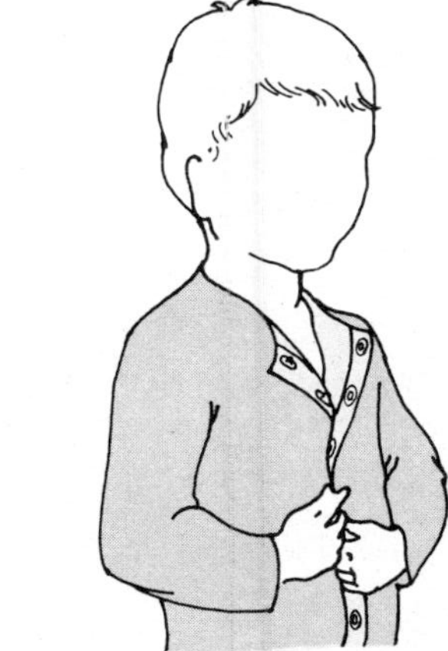

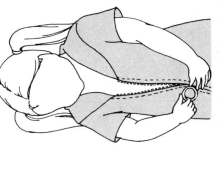

Elasticized pull-on pants and skirts can be managed by even young toddlers (sewing is easy, too). If garment front and back are different, mark back with ribbon or tape.

Large buttons are a great incentive for do-it-yourself dressing, because they don't take much dexterity and are easy for little fingers to grasp. Sew buttons very securely.

A zipper with a large pull is best for first attempts at zipping up. Buy a decorative zipper with a fancy pull, or add a ring to any type. Install zipper in garment front.

No-sew snaps are the easiest type for small fingers to cope with, and they have good holding power. Use single snaps for spot closings and snap tape for longer plackets.

Slipstitch 132
Seams 147-149
Collars 214-215
Cutting bias strips 298-299

Necklines

For necklines on children's garments, special finishes are recommended. Some are advised because they are easier to handle with the tiny neck seams and neck openings. A **bias finish** is simpler to work with than a tiny facing. A **combination facing** incorporates what would be three small neck and armhole facings into one facing of manageable size. It must be applied while the center back seam is still open or the garment cannot be turned right side out. Some finishes are preferred just for their charm and appropriateness—**scallops,** for example, at the necklines of little girls' clothes.

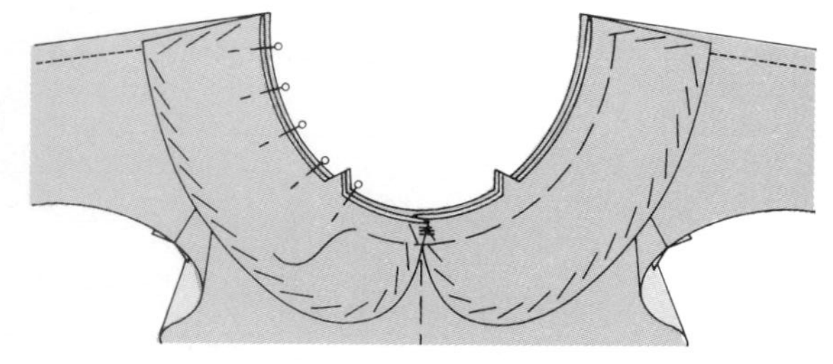

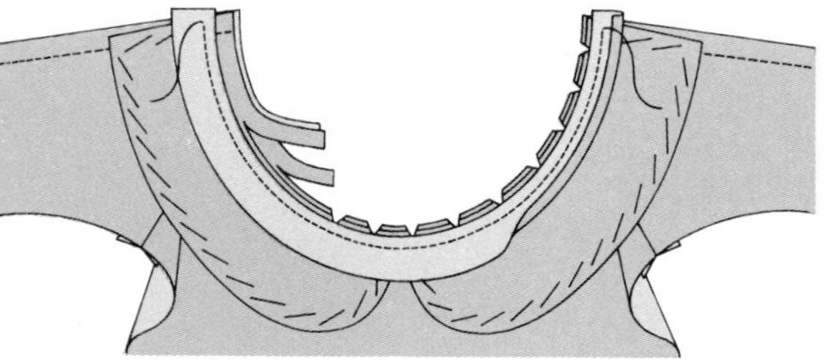

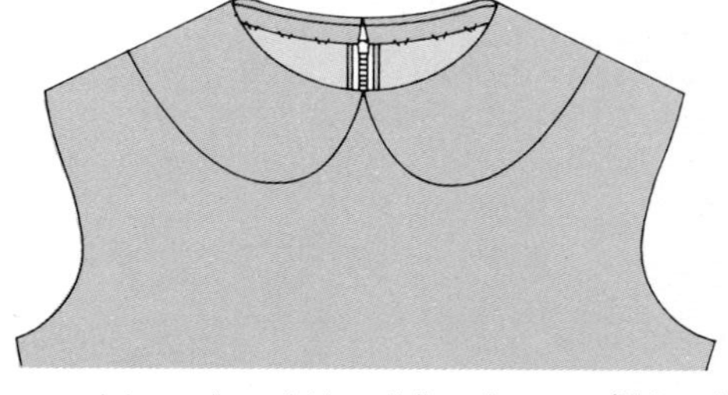

A bias finish for a neckline with collar is much easier to work with than a shaped facing on very small sizes. Construct collar and baste it to garment neckline. Cut a strip of ½″ bias tape to fit neckline seam (or a true bias strip, 1″ wide, from collar fabric). Baste to the neck seam, using ¼″ seam allowance. Stitch neckline; trim, grade, and clip seam allowances. Turn under remaining edge of bias ¼″ and press. (This edge in purchased tape is already pressed.) Slipstitch the bias to the inside of the garment at neckline seam.

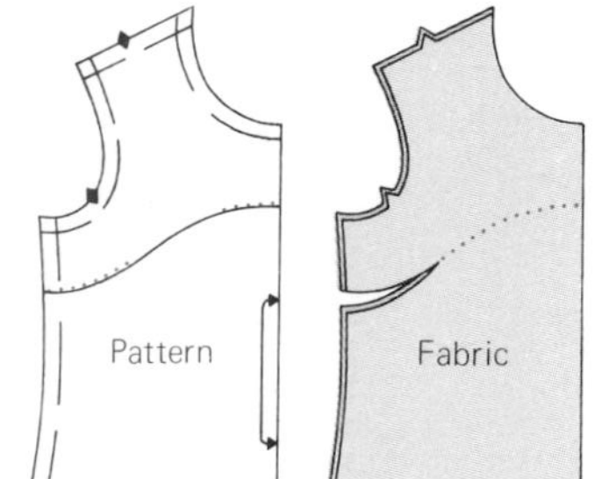

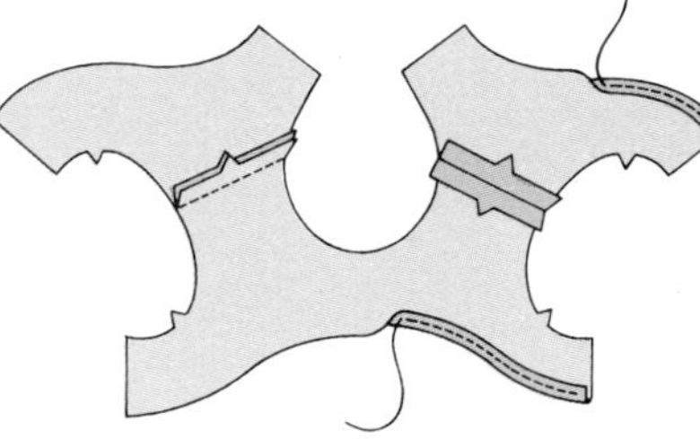

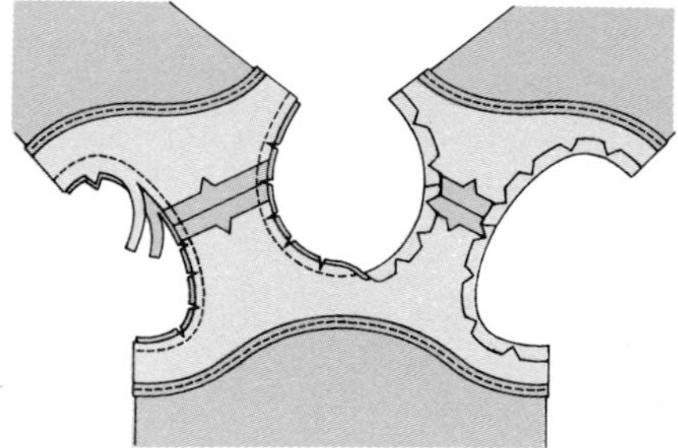

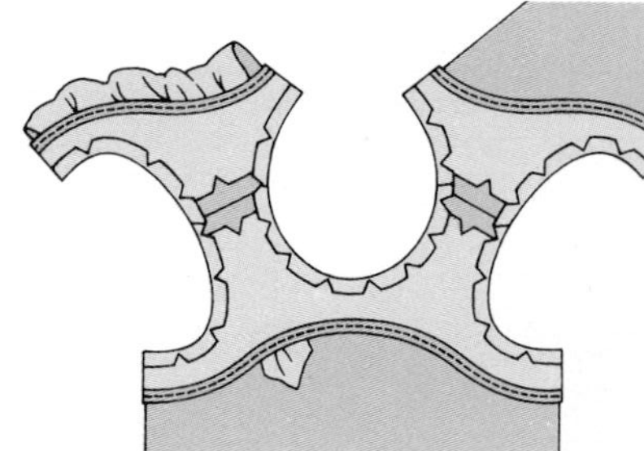

Combination facings are cut from patterns for garment front and back. Measure and mark several points 3″ below neck edge and armhole; connect marks with curved lines. Lay pattern on fabric and transfer the curved lines with tracing paper. Cut out neck, shoulder, and armhole edges; remove pattern and cut curved lines. Stitch and press garment darts and shoulder seams. Stitch and press facing shoulder seams. Seam-finish lower edges in a way that suits fabric. Right sides together, stitch facing to garment at neckline and armholes. Trim, grade, and clip seam allowances. Press seams toward facing. Turn garment right side out by pulling backs of garment through shoulders to front. Lift facings away from garment and stitch side seams of garment and facings in one continuous seam; press open. Tack facings to seam allowances at underarm and to zipper at center back.

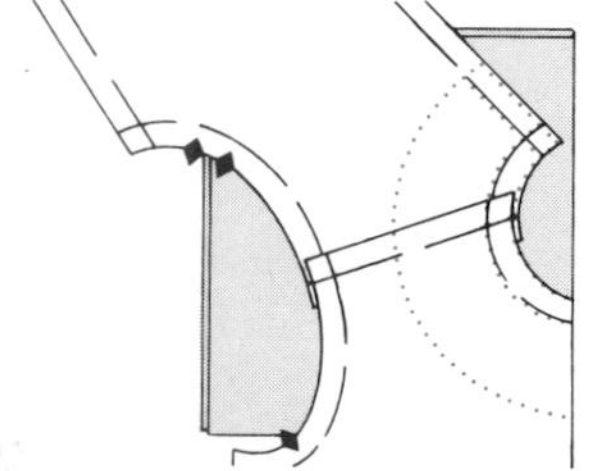

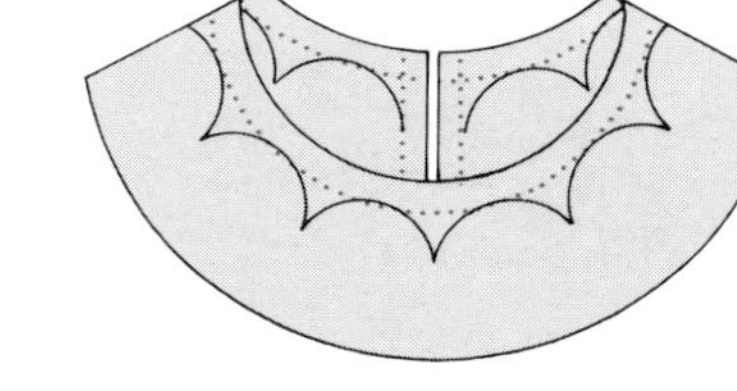

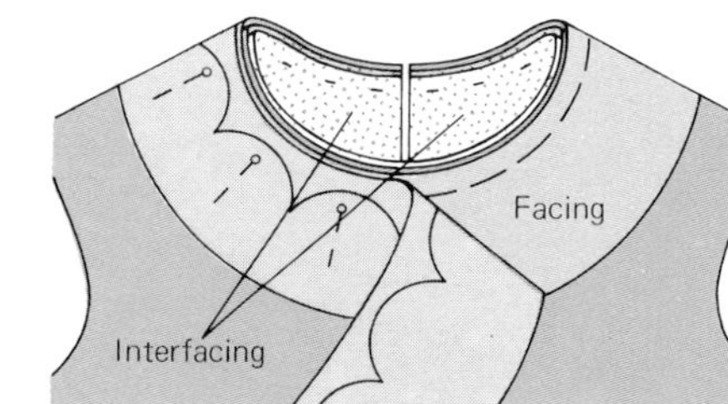

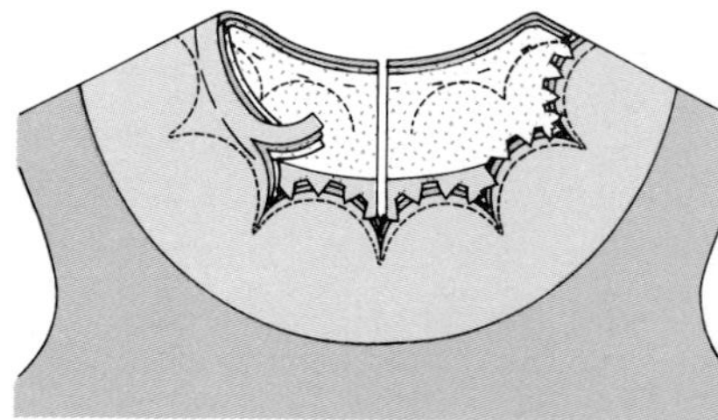

Scalloped edges begin with a paper pattern. Pin front and back pattern pieces together, overlapping and aligning the shoulder seams. Trace the neck seamline onto tissue paper. Figure the size and number of scallops that will fit along the seamline, keeping scallop size proportionate to the garment. Height of scallop should be about one-third its width at base. Draw scallops with curves at seamline, centering pattern at front so finished edges are at center back. Baste interfacing to wrong side of garment at neck edge. Right sides together, baste neck facing to garment; pin tissue pattern on right side of garment over facing with scallop edges at seamline. Stitch through tissue and all fabric layers, using small (15 per inch) stitches. Carefully remove tissue. Trim, grade, and notch curves; clip to stitch line at each point. Turn all scallops right side out and press carefully for smooth curves.

Fusible interfacing selection and application 72, 76, 79
French tack 134; whipstitch 136

Making a child's coat

A child's coat can be a real money-saver. It is doubly worth the time and money if you invest in a durable fabric so that the coat can be handed on to another child. To make the coat adaptable for both boys and girls, buttonholes can be worked on both sides (see below, right).

Because there is relatively little shaping in a child's coat, there is no need for the time-consuming hand padstitching and other traditional methods of shaping a tailored garment and hemming the bottom edge and sleeves. Interfacing can be done with fusibles. A machine method for attaching the lining is not only quicker, but actually stands up better to active wear. Special techniques are discussed on this page; see the checklist at the right for techniques covered elsewhere.

Choose fusible products according to the fabric weight and the function the fusible is to perform. For light- to medium-weight coat fabric, use iron-on interfacing in an all-purpose weight; for a heavy coat fabric, an iron-on hair canvas. Trim away all seam allowances and across corners of interfacing before fusing. Use a fusing web for hems on sleeves and at the coat's lower edge. Before fusing, however, consider whether you might later wish to alter the length; it is best to fuse hems only when you do not expect to change them. Fusing directions here are general; for specifics, see information accompanying the product.

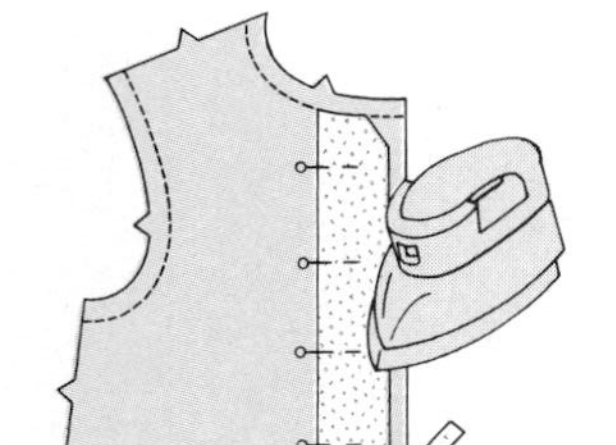

Heat-baste interfacing in place with the tip of the iron. Take care not to press over pins. Remove all pins, then lay a dampened press cloth over the whole interfacing section and press with an iron set for wool. The iron should be held in place for at least ten seconds. It is important to allow each piece to dry thoroughly before handling it—the garment piece will retain the shape in which it dries.

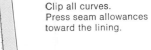

Checklist/child's coat procedure

Adjust pattern fit 101-109
Lay out pattern, cut out coat 84-93
Cut out lining 378
Transfer pattern markings 94
Attach interfacing 409
Stitch side, shoulder, and under collar seams 144-146
Attach under collar, upper collar, and facings 371-373
Set in sleeves 375
Fuse hem and sleeve hems 409; tack facings 374
Make lining 378; attach lining 409
Make buttonholes 343-348, attach buttons 351-352

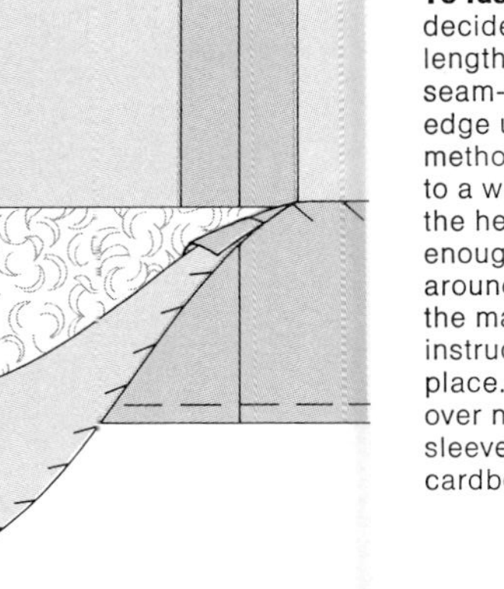

To fuse a hem, first decide the garment length and hem depth; seam-finish the fabric edge using an appropriate method. Cut fusing web to a width ½" less than the hem depth and long enough to go completely around the hem. Following the manufacturer's instructions, fuse hem in place. Press sleeves over narrow end of sleeve board or a sturdy cardboard tube.

Dual buttonholes—that is, separate sets worked on both the left and right sides of the garment—can greatly lengthen the garment's life. Open buttonholes only on the side where they are needed, and sew buttons right over the unopened ones. If the coat is handed on to a child of the opposite sex, the closed set can be opened and the other set closed with tiny whipstitches. Buttons can then be re-attached over the newly closed set.

Lining the coat

This machine method for lining a coat is excellent for children's wear because it is so secure; can also be used for adult garments where extra sturdiness is required. At the lining stage, all construction on the coat should be completed, including hems and tacking in place of front facings.

Do all lining construction by machine, including setting in of sleeves and formation of center back pleat. Press all seams open. Fuse the lining hem into place, after measuring and adjusting it to hang 1 inch above the coat hemline.

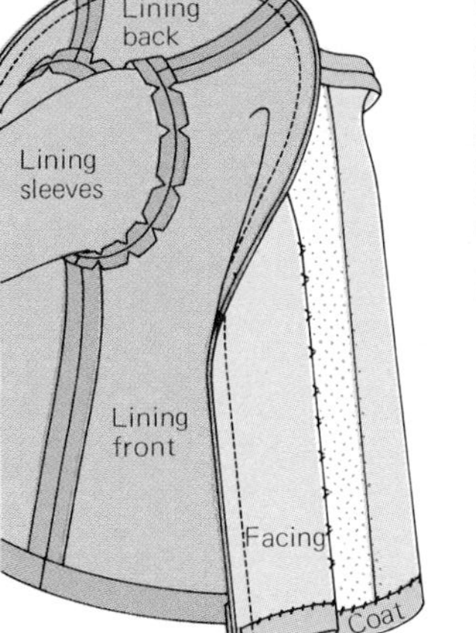

Pin lining to coat facings with right sides together, beginning at the hem on one front and ending at the opposite front hemline. Match shoulder seams and center back. Stitch with a ⅝" seam. Clip all curves. Press seam allowances toward the lining.

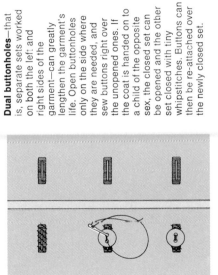

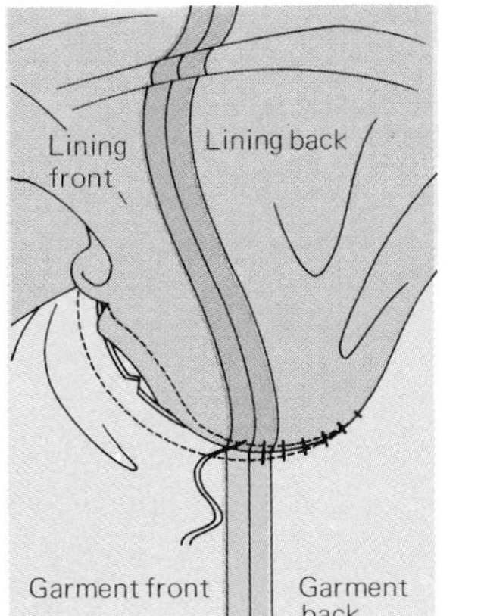

The lining is tacked to the coat at the underarm armhole seams to keep the lining in place. Lift the lining up at side seams so that underarm area of armhole seams is exposed. Match the seamlines of lining and coat at underarm; make sure seam allowances are all going toward sleeve. With a double thread, whipstitch lining seamline to coat seamline. Use French tacks between lining and coat hems at side seams. Whipstitch front facings to coat hem.

Sewing for children

Hand stitches 123, 125-126, 131, 136
Seams 145-146
Gathering 178-179
Fold-down casings 234
Hems 295
Sewing on buttons 351-352

Encouraging children to sew

The chances are very good that when a child sees you working at your sewing machine, especially if you are making something for him or her, the youngster will show an interest in learning to sew. The way you treat the first spark of interest can make all the difference in the child's future attitude toward sewing. Nurture this beginning curiosity by answering questions as patiently as possible, and initiating sewing projects that the child can complete with a sense of achievement.

What projects a child can do will depend on the diligence and physical abilities he or she brings to them. Some children will spend more time with their sewing, and do more of it, so their capabilities will develop faster than those of children whose attention tends to wander. Also, some youngsters will be able to cut out intricate shapes, while others of the same age will be doing well to manage simple hand stitches.

Just when to start a young person using the sewing machine depends on the individual child's coordination and desire, but around nine years old is usually a good time. For younger children, there are toy machines you may want to consider. One model makes a lockstitch and has a guard to keep fingers from getting caught under the needle. It can be operated by means of a hand crank, or with batteries. Another model joins seams with a special gluing process instead of a stitch.

Stitches and projects for different age groups

AGE	STITCHES TO LEARN	SUITABLE MATERIALS	SUGGESTED PROJECTS
2-3	None	Spools, fabric scraps, zippers, bits of trim	Free play Make a collage
4-5	Simple embroidery, such as cross stitch, outline Sewing buttons	Sewing cards: large needlepoint canvas, blunt needle, yarn Medium to large buttons Large needle Yarn	Embroidered pictures Sew buttons on a toy or favorite garment
6-7	Basic hand stitches, such as whipstitch, running stitch, backstitch Toy sewing machine	Felt Cotton fabrics that are not too tightly woven	Pocket animals Eyeglass case Doll clothes Bib Babushka Drawstring bag
8-9	Advanced embroidery stitches, such as chainstitch, blanket stitch, buttonhole stitch Begin use of standard sewing machine, plain straight seams	Linen Cotton Terry cloth (woven)	Pillow cover Potholder Tote bag
10-12	Progress with sewing machine techniques —curved seams, gathers, casings or hems	Cottons and cotton blends	Simple-to-sew pattern, such as skirt, pull-on pants, smock

Sample projects

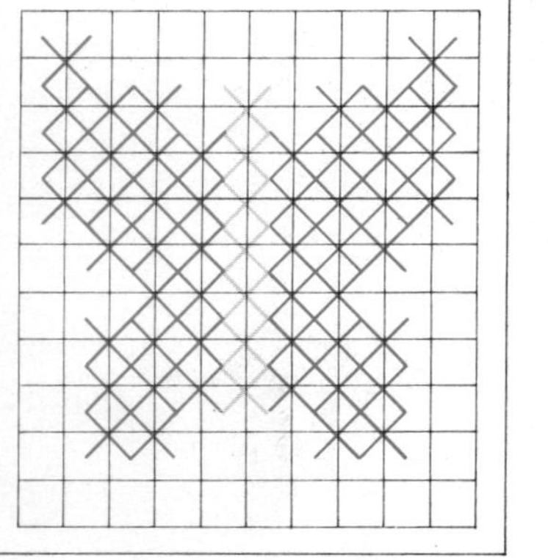

Sewing cards are made with the needlepoint canvas that has the fewest holes per inch (often called "quickpoint" canvas). Bind raw edges of canvas with masking tape. Using colored marking pens, draw a simple stitch pattern on the canvas. The child stitches over markings with blunt needle and yarn.

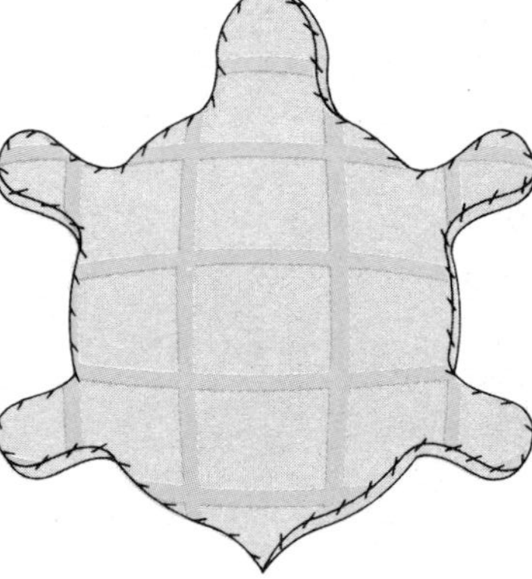

Pocket animals are made by cutting a bottom and top of a simple, familiar animal shape. The child sews the top and bottom pieces together (wrong sides of fabric together), leaving a small opening for stuffing. Good stitches for young hands: the whipstitch and the blanket stitch. After stuffing, sew up the opening.

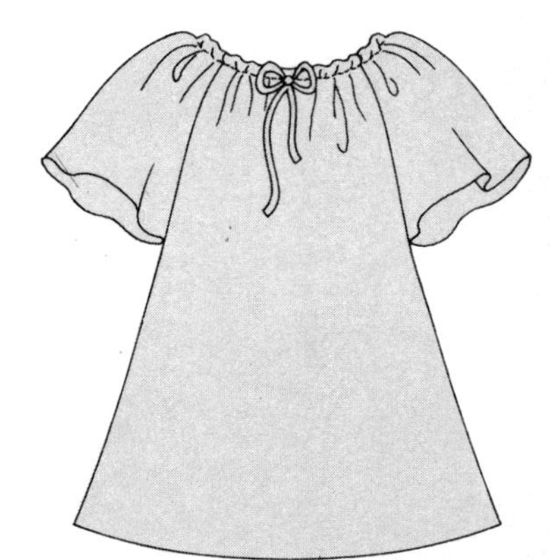

A simple garment is a good first project at the sewing machine. It should have few pattern pieces, no set-in sleeves, and casings instead of shaped facings or waistbands. Teach the child to use fusing web for hems; hand-stitch control is not likely to be good enough for a really invisible hem.

Sewing for the Home

Sewing for the home

Sewing tools and supplies 8-16
Sewing machine and attachments 26-39
Fabrics 58-71
Seams 145-153

Advance considerations

In this chapter, you will find various methods for making major home decorating items—slipcovers, pillow covers, bedspreads, curtains, and draperies. Sewing for the home calls for the same basic skills as dressmaking does, but they are often differently applied. For example, the "pattern" for cutting out slipcover fabric may be the upholstered chair or sofa being covered. With curtains and draperies, it will be just a set of key measurements.

In most home projects, you must remember to add your own seam and hem allowances. Some techniques normally done by hand are here better done by machine, for example, hems in slipcovers, curtains, and draperies. The machine not only does such jobs faster, but the results are more durable. Large quantities of fabric must often be handled, and the working area should be modified or enlarged to accommodate the extra bulk. It is also helpful to arrange things so that the sewing machine, the work area, and the project being worked on are close to each other.

CHOOSING FABRICS

Certain fabrics are made especially for sewing for the home. Generally classified as "decorator fabrics," they are usually at least 48 inches wide and often are treated to resist wrinkles, stains, or fading. Fabrics basically meant for use in clothing, if they share these same qualities, are just as appropriate. Choosing the correct fabric for any project means relating the fabric's weight and weave to the day-to-day wear the fabric will get, the construction methods that will be used, and the final appearance you want from it.

Fabric for a slipcover, for instance, should be closely woven and heavy enough to hold its shape. If the fabric is also treated to resist wrinkles and stains, it will be practical as well as durable. The fabric's design is also a factor. Slipcover fabric might well be cut into pieces of many sizes, causing the design to look very different in use than it did as uncut yardage. The best way to picture the effect is to test-drape a large swatch of fabric over the areas to be covered.

Test curtain or drapery fabric by holding it up to the window to see how its design and texture look when they are backlit. Sheers, semisheers, and open weaves will filter the light gently. If you want to block the light, choose an opaque fabric or consider adding a lining to make the fabric more opaque at the window. Drape the fabric in folds as you test to check its character in the intended use. Fabrics for curtains and draperies should also be resistant to sun fading.

Bedspreads, curtains, and draperies are most effective constructed with a minimum of seams. The best choice, to provide a large, unbroken expanse of fabric, is a fabric with a generous width. Wide fabrics are the most economical, as a rule, for any major home sewing project.

Consider also how the color, design, and texture of fabric will blend with the rest of the room. This becomes very important when the item being made is massive or will span a large area. Be sure, too, that the fabric suits the mood of the room. It will help, in shopping for new fabric, to carry samples of fabrics already in the room. You can often get a sample by carefully trimming a scrap from a seam allowance or hem. If this cannot be managed, ask for a swatch of the fabric you are considering, and test it at home before making a final purchase. Such testing is a good precaution in any case because the light in the store may well be different from that in your room.

Finally, is the fabric's cost in proportion to the value you put on the project? A fabric must be right for its purpose, and durable enough to justify the time you spend sewing. But you may want more from bedroom than from kitchen curtains, for example, and be willing to invest more in them.

EQUIPMENT AND SUPPLIES

In addition to your basic equipment, you should consider other tools that might come in handy when sewing for the home. For example, you can cut upholstery fabrics better and more comfortably with heavy-duty shears. When fitting a slipcover to a chair, use long (1¼-inch) pins or T-pins—both long types with large heads, which makes it easier to pin heavy fabrics together or pin fabric to upholstery. A carpenter's folding rule is ideal for long, straight, above-the-floor measurements for curtains and draperies. For curves, use a flexible rule or tape measure.

There are also supplies designed specially for home decorating—some to be stronger, others to streamline construction or to give a quality finish to your project. Examples of such special items are heavy-duty zippers for use in slipcovers; pillow forms for making covered pillows; metal weights that, when sewed to the bottom of draperies, will make them hang properly; pleater tapes and hooks for easy construction and automatic pleating of both curtains and draperies.

SEWING

You will undoubtedly use your sewing machine more often than usual when sewing for your home, because so much traditional hand work is done by machine—hemming, for example. To use your machine to its fullest, investigate feet and attachments available for it that can save you time. These are just a few useful examples. A zipper foot is indispensable for inserting a zipper or forming corded seams. The narrow hemmer foot enables you to stitch a narrow rolled hem fast and efficiently with neat results. An adjustable seam gauge or a quilter guide-bar is helpful if you are stitching a wider-than-normal seam allowance. The gathering foot and the ruffler attachment make quick work of gathering long lengths of fabric. The binder attachment lets you stitch a binding to a raw edge in one operation, without pinning. A roller foot or other "top feed" assist attachment can help to make difficult fabrics feed evenly.

The appropriate seaming method can vary, depending on your fabric and the project you are engaged in. For most situations, a plain seam is all that is required; it can be seam-finished if necessary. If the fabric is a sheer, say a voile for kitchen curtains, a French seam is recommended. A flat-felled seam is valued mainly as a sturdy seam for heavy fabrics, but it also gives an attractive informal look to fabrics of other weights. It is best confined to straight seams.

For any sewing, choose the proper needle, thread, and stitch length for the fabric. Test and adjust tension before starting, and whenever the items being sewed have changed. Be sure to use a proper foot pressure, especially when matching motifs at seams or stitching extra-long fabric lengths.

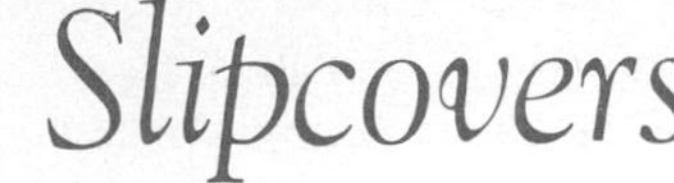

Slipcovers

General introduction

A slipcover is a practical and economical way to restore a worn piece of furniture or to give it a new look. If the slipcover is to be a replacement for an old cover, an easy way to cut the new one is to take the original apart and use the resulting pieces, first, for a trial layout to determine the yardage needed, and then as patterns for cutting the new slipcover.

If you are starting fresh, fabric requirements are ascertained by measuring the piece of furniture (see below), then adding yardage for any specific requirements of the fabric, for the slipcover's skirt, and for making cording for the seams if necessary (see next page). The fabric is pinned directly to the furniture to develop the sections that make up the slipcover. An advantage of this method is that it allows for the fitting of any irregularities in the furniture's shape.

In a third cutting method for a slipcover, you first make a trial slipcover in muslin, then use the muslin pieces as a pattern.

In choosing a fabric, the basic requirements are that it be sturdy, resistant to soil, and easily cleaned. Generally, a medium-weight fabric is better than a heavy one because it is easier to handle where several layers must be joined, and adds less bulk when layered over upholstery. To check your fabric choice for color and design, take home a large swatch (minimum of ¼ yard or one design motif) and drape it over the furniture. Some stores will lend you a sample; if your store will not, a swatch could prove a good investment by preventing a costly mistake.

In addition to the fabric, you will need thread and machine needles suitable to it, and heavy-duty slipcover zippers for both the slipcover and cushions (see p. 417 for length requirements). If the slipcover will not have a skirt, get either snap or nylon tape, or tacks, to secure the slipcover to the frame. Other findings that you might need are cable cord for the cording, seam or twill tape to reinforce occasional seams, and T-pins. T-pins are better than regular straight pins because they are heavier and longer, and their tops are easier to hold for this kind of pinning.

Taking measurements for yardage

A basic estimate of the yardage needed for a slipcover can be arrived at by measuring the piece of furniture to be covered. There are three key measurements to take, as shown and explained at the right; the tape direction corresponds to the lengthwise fabric grain. Extra yardage will be needed for matching or special placement of a fabric, for making cording, and for a gathered or pleated skirt (p. 414). Add these extra amounts to the basic measurement to get the total yardage required. Record all measurements on a chart similar to the one below. If you need or want to convert the inch measurements to yards, divide each figure by 36.

Measurements for total yardage	inches	yards
Measurement A ____ x ____ sections		
Measurement B ____ x 2 (both arms)		
Measurement C ____ x ____ cushions		
Allowance for special fabric needs		
Allowance for covering cord		
Allowance for skirt		
Total		

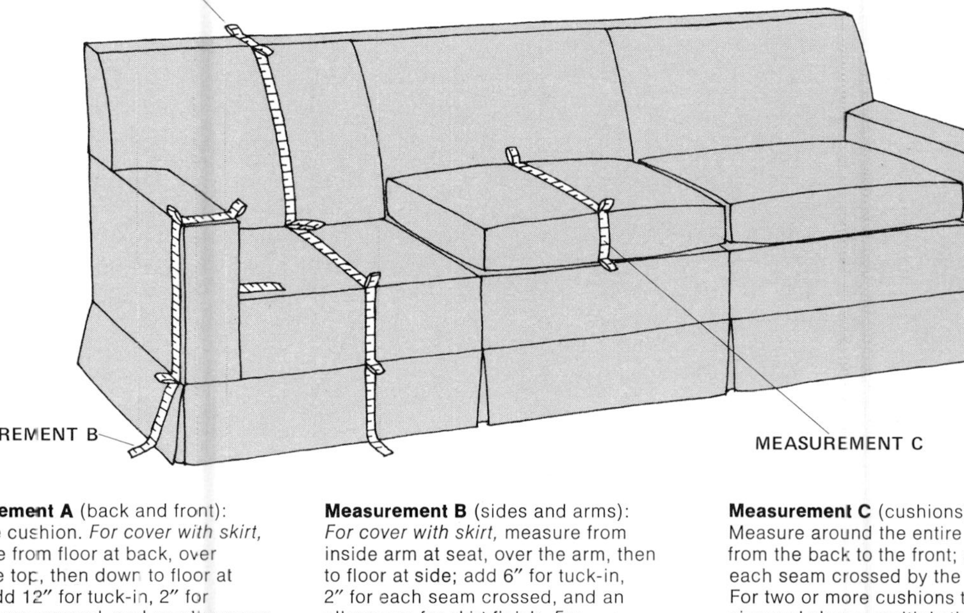

Measurement A (back and front): Remove cushion. *For cover with skirt,* measure from floor at back, over furniture top, then down to floor at front; add 12″ for tuck-in, 2″ for each seam crossed, and an allowance for skirt finish. *For cover without skirt,* measure just to bottom edges of furniture; add 11″ for facings. For a wide piece (sofa), multiply length by number of fabric widths needed.

Measurement B (sides and arms): *For cover with skirt,* measure from inside arm at seat, over the arm, then to floor at side; add 6″ for tuck-in, 2″ for each seam crossed, and an allowance for skirt finish. *For cover without skirt,* measure just to the bottom edge of furniture and add 5½″ for facing. Double either of these measurements to arrive at total length needed for both arms.

Measurement C (cushions): Measure around the entire cushion from the back to the front; add 2″ for each seam crossed by the tape measure. For two or more cushions the same size and shape, multiply this total by the number of cushions that need to be covered. For cushions of varying sizes, measure each cushion separately, then add all of these measurements together.

Matching and positioning special fabrics 68-69
Pleats 166-169, 172, 176-177

Special yardage considerations

Basic yardage needs are estimated by measuring the furniture to be covered (see the preceding page). Some adjustments may be needed in this basic estimate because of the construction, design, or width of the fabric, as well as for variations in slipcover style. The following should be considered before any fabric is actually purchased.

The width of many upholstery and slipcovering fabrics is 48 inches, which is usually sufficient for each lengthwise section of a chair or sofa. If the fabric is narrower, more than one fabric length might be needed for each section; if the fabric is very wide, less than the full width of a fabric length might suffice. If a section should take less than a full fabric width, the excess may be usable on the front of an arm, as a boxing strip, and so on. Before buying your fabric and while measuring your furniture, carefully appraise both fabric and furniture to see if less yardage will do. Be careful, though, not to skimp.

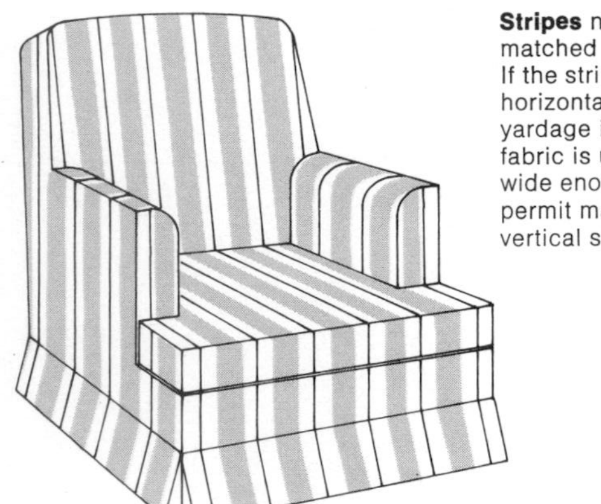

Stripes need to be matched at seams. If the stripe is horizontal, extra yardage is needed; fabric is usually wide enough to permit matching of vertical stripes.

Motifs on fabrics should be placed at strategic points on the various sections of the slipcover. Such positioning will require extra yardage.

Extra yardage will be needed when the fabric has a large motif that must be centered strategically on the slipcover, or a horizontally striped design that must be matched at the seamlines. The supplementary amount is usually the length of one extra motif for each section of the slipcover.

If the seams of the slipcover are to be corded, extra fabric is required to cover the cord. For an average-sized chair, allow 1 yard; for a large chair, 1½ yards; for a sofa, 2 yards. The cord requirement can be calculated by measuring the seams of the upholstery. If you want to cover the cording in a fabric other than the slipcover fabric, this yardage is of course a separate quantity.

Skirt yardage depends on the style of the skirt and the method chosen for finishing its lower edge (see pp. 418-419). Skirts can be plain, pleated, or gathered. Two measurements are necessary to estimate the yardage: (1) total skirt length and (2) total skirt width. **Total skirt length** is the finished skirt length (distance from floor to seamline where the skirt is joined to the slipcover), plus a 1-inch top seam allowance, plus an allowance for finishing the lower edge. **Total skirt width** is the finished skirt width (equal to the measurement of the skirt's top seamline), plus allowances for pleats or gathers, plus 1-inch seam allowances for finishing ends and joining fabric lengths. To arrive at the approximate number of fabric lengths that are needed to produce the total skirt width, divide the width of the fabric that is being used into the total skirt width.

The illustrations at the right show a range of typical furniture types that lend themselves to slipcovering; the adjoining captions give the approximate yardages that would be needed to slipcover each one. These measurements are intended to give you an idea of yardage differences from one type of furniture to another. They are not intended to replace actual measurement of the piece of furniture you are slipcovering.

Approximate yardages

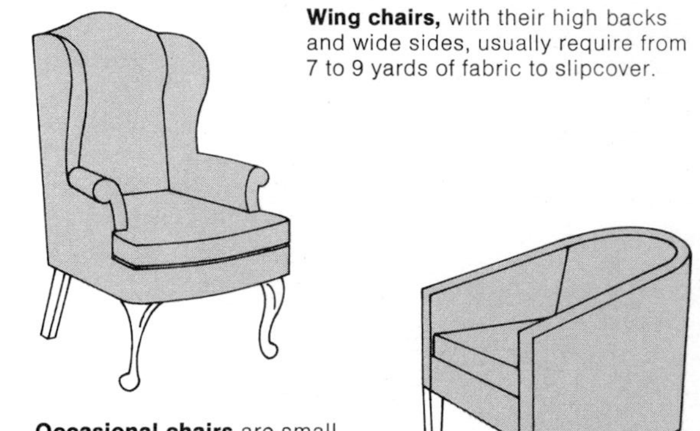

Wing chairs, with their high backs and wide sides, usually require from 7 to 9 yards of fabric to slipcover.

Occasional chairs are small chairs with yardage needs usually from 4½ to 6 yards.

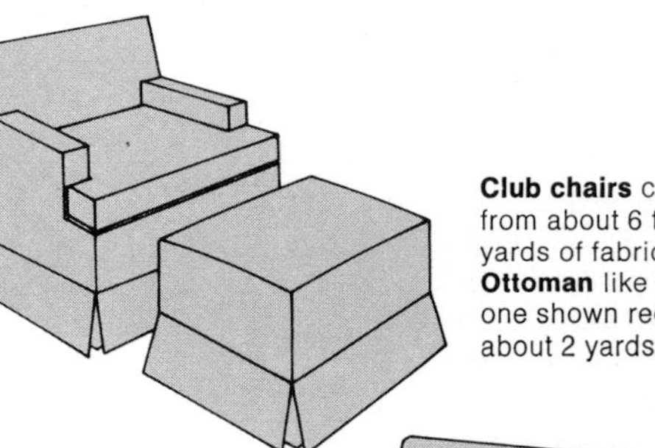

Club chairs can take from about 6 to 7½ yards of fabric. **Ottoman** like the one shown requires about 2 yards.

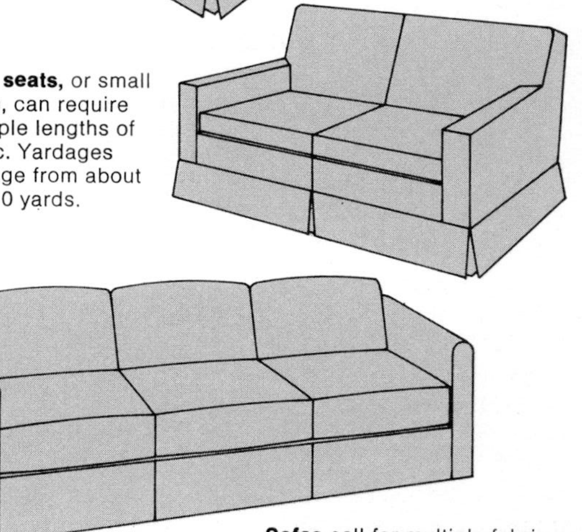

Love seats, or small sofas, can require multiple lengths of fabric. Yardages average from about 8 to 10 yards.

Sofas call for multiple fabric lengths. Yardage requirements are about 11 to 14 yards.

Fitting and cutting slipcovers/the unit method

An accurate way to make a slipcover is to use the piece of furniture being covered as a guide, fitting and cutting each section to correspond to the seams of the furniture's upholstery. With this method, the fabric is pinned to the furniture with its right side out. This permits precise placement of the fabric's motifs, matching of fabric at seamlines, and accurate fitting of any of the furniture's irregularities.

Although some slipcovers will have more seams and sections than others, most can be divided into units, and the units cut, fitted, and sewed in the following order: (1) **top and inside back,** (2) **seat platform and apron,** (3) **arms,** (4) **outside back,** (5) **cushion,** and (6) **skirt.**

The general procedure is to pin the fabric to the center of a section, then smooth it toward each side, then upward and downward, keeping the grainlines straight and pinning to the furniture as you progress. Lengthwise grain should run from top to bottom of each vertical section, from back to front of horizontal sections (cushions). Cut out the section, allowing 1-inch seam allowances on all edges, and tuck-ins (extra fabric) where necessary. Tuck-ins are needed at points where movement occurs when furniture is sat upon—where back and arms meet at the seat platform, for example, or where wing and back meet in a wing chair.

If fabric is plain and of a solid color, you can mark and remove each section after its fitting. It is better, however, to pin the entire slipcover before removing any part of it, especially when the fabric requires careful placement of a motif or matching at the seamlines. Where two or more sections must be cut identically, such as the top and bottom of a cushion, you can cut one and then unpin it to use as a pattern for cutting the other. When the other piece is cut, pin-fit all of the sections to check their fit.

When the fabric has a motif, center it on the front, back, and each side of the arms, a bit more than halfway up from the center point. Center a motif on each side of a cushion so it can be reversible. With directional fabrics (naps, one-way prints), be sure to place fabric consistently on all sections—from top to floor of vertical sections, from back to front on horizontal sections.

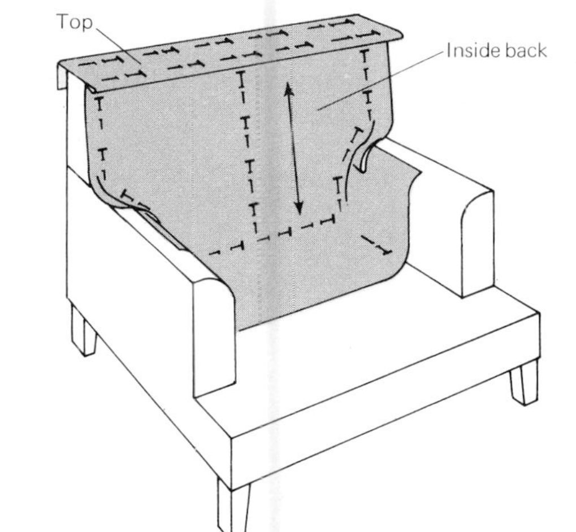

Top and inside back: With right side out and lengthwise grain running vertically, drape fabric over top and back. (Center design if necessary.) Pin in place down center. Then, working from the center out, smooth fabric until it is taut, and pin at sides. Leaving a 2″ fold between back and top, pin fabric across top; pin along seamline.

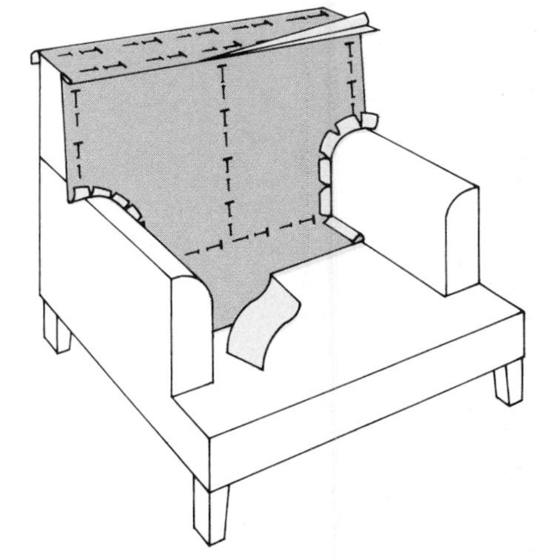

Leaving 1″ seam allowances, trim the back of the top, the sides, and the arms (if tuck-ins are necessary between back and arms, allow an extra 3″ of fabric). Clip and notch seam allowances where this is necessary for fabric to fit. Trim at seat, allowing 6″ for tuck-in. Cut fabric along fold between top and inside back.

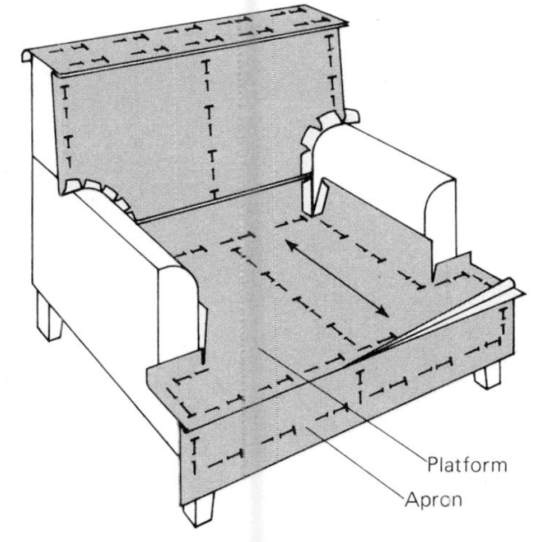

Seat platform and apron: Allowing 6″ to extend up the back, position fabric on seat as was done for inside back. Leaving a 2″ fold between seat and apron, pin fabric to apron. At back and arms, trim fabric, allowing 6″ for tuck-ins. Trim other edges, except bottom, to 1″ seam allowances (2″ at bottom). Cut along fold at seat and apron.

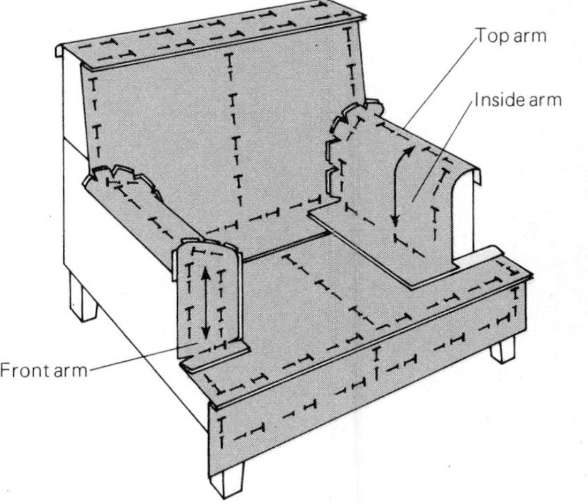

Arms: Positioning lengthwise grain vertically, center and pin fabric to top of arm, then down inside of arm. Trim all edges that do not need tuck-ins to 1″ seam allowances (at seat, allow 6″ for tuck-in; if tuck-in is needed at back of arm, allow 3″). Position and pin fabric to front of arm; trim to 1″ seam allowances. *(Continued next page)*

Darts 159
Gathering 178-179

Fitting and cutting slipcovers/the unit method

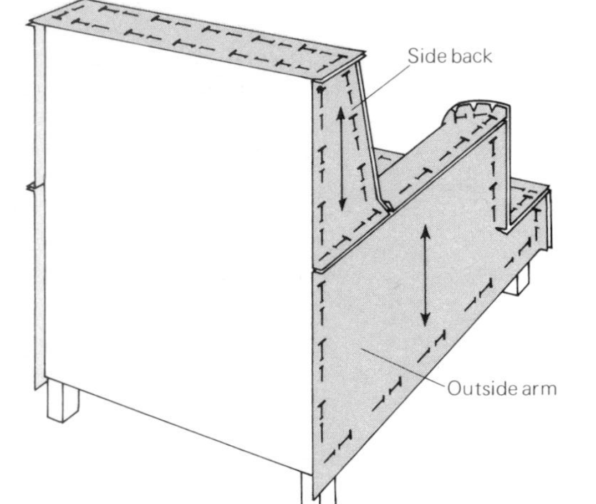

Outside arm and side back: Depending on upholstery seams, these may be cut as one piece, or as two (shown). With the lengthwise grain vertical, drape fabric down arm, then up side back (if two pieces, allow an extra 2″ between). Center as needed; pin. Trim edges, allowing 1″ for seams (2″ at bottom). If necessary, cut along fold between sections.

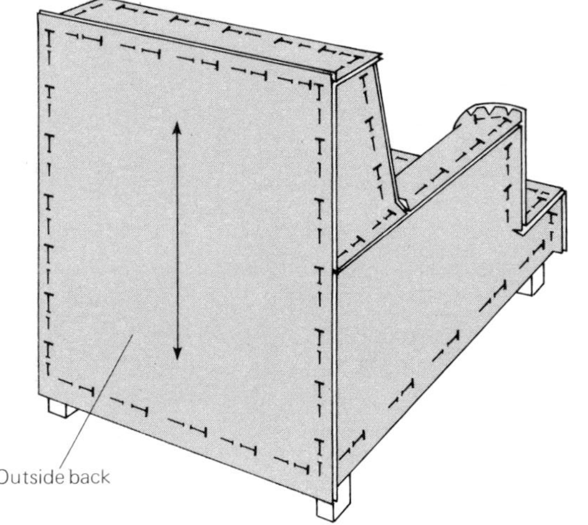

Outside back: With the lengthwise grain vertical, drape the fabric down the back. Center the fabric and pin it down the center. Working from the center, smooth the fabric toward the sides and top and bottom edges, pinning as you progress. Trim the top and side edges, providing for 1″ seam allowances; trim bottom edge, leaving a 2″ seam allowance.

Cushion: Placing lengthwise grain as shown, center and pin fabric on cushion top (match motif with rest of slipcover). Cut, leaving 1″ seam allowances. Cut an identical piece for cushion bottom; pin in place. Cut and fit boxing pieces; allow for two placket seam allowances at center of piece to contain zipper. Trim edges to 1″ seam allowances.

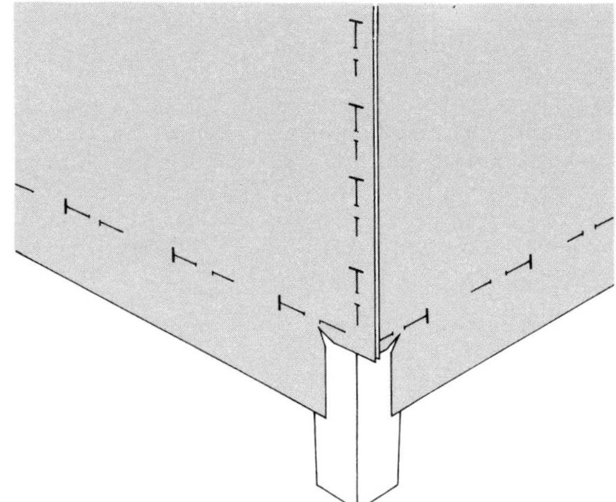

At each leg: After checking to see that all sides of the slipcover fit and are pulled taut, re-pin the entire bottom edge of the slipcover. At each leg, trim away fabric, leaving ½″ seam allowances and forming a three-sided edge as shown. Clip diagonally into corners of top seam allowance, being careful not to clip beyond seamline.

Special shaping techniques

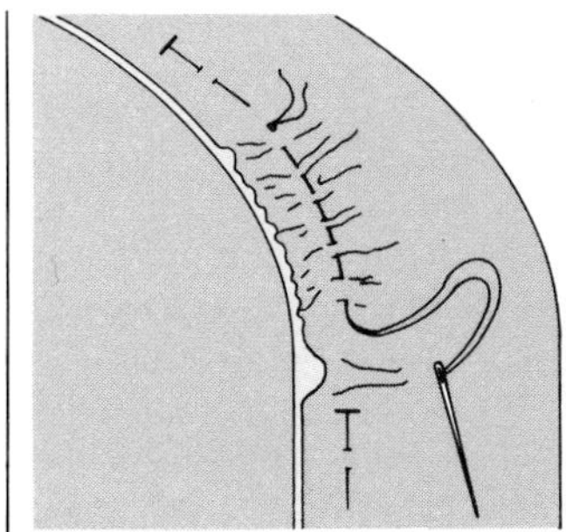

Gathering is one way to control fullness at a curve. Pin both layers of fabric along seamline up to curved area. Then, using a double thread, place hand-gathering stitches along seamline of edge to be gathered. Draw up on fabric to fit other fabric edge; secure gathers.

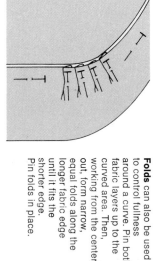

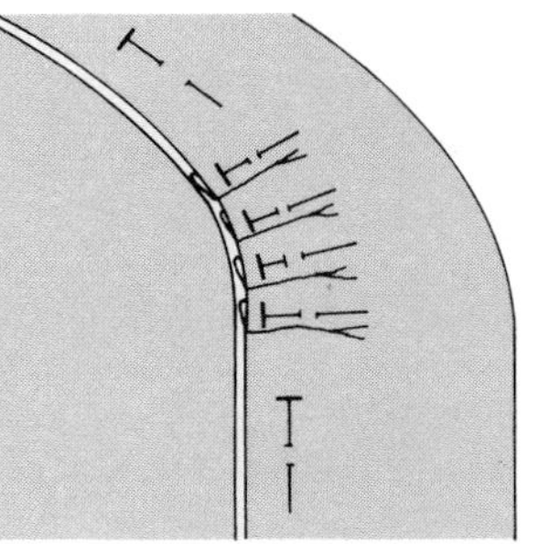

Folds can also be used to control fullness around a curve. Pin both fabric layers up to the curved area. Then, working from the center out, form narrow, equal folds along the longer fabric edge until it fits the shorter edge. Pin folds in place.

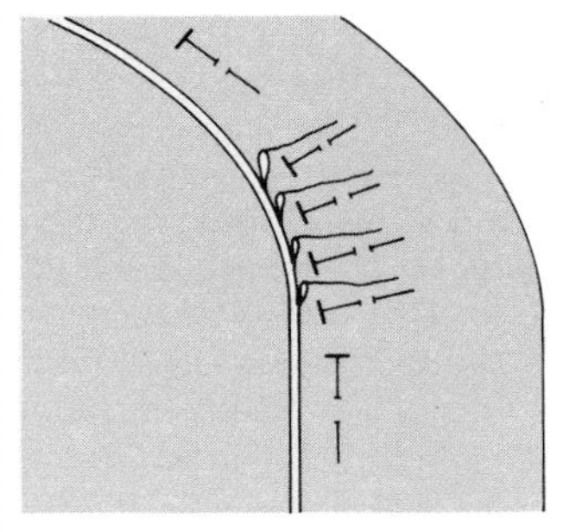

Darts are another method of controlling fullness at curved edges. Pin fabric layers together up to the curved area. Then, working from the center out, form narrow, equal darts in the longer fabric edge to fit it to the shorter edge. Pin darts in place.

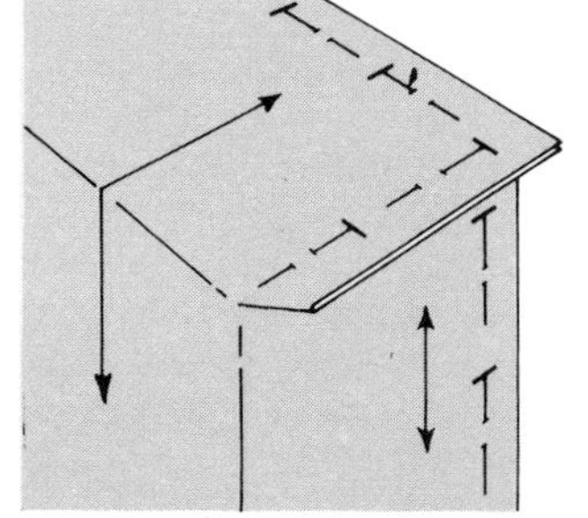

A miter can be formed to shape a continuous piece of fabric around a corner. With lengthwise grain placed as shown, pin fabric to sections on both sides of corner. Then pin the fabric along the corner. Trim excess fabric to the 1″ seam allowances.

Needle/thread/stitch length selection 27
Seams 144-149, 153, 155
Making cording 298-300
Centered zipper application 318

Preparing to sew

After the slipcover has been satisfactorily fitted and pinned, mark the seamlines (see the adjoining drawing and explanation). It may also be useful to label each section by writing its name and location on a piece of paper or tape and placing the label on the top seam allowance. Arrange the work area so that the furniture being worked on is reasonably near the sewing machine. To support the quantity of fabric you will be handling, it is helpful to have a large table at the machine. If your machine is a portable, set it on the table; if the machine is in a cabinet, move the table to the side or back of the machine as necessary.

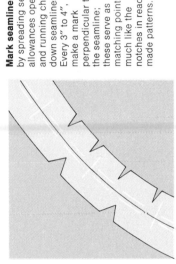

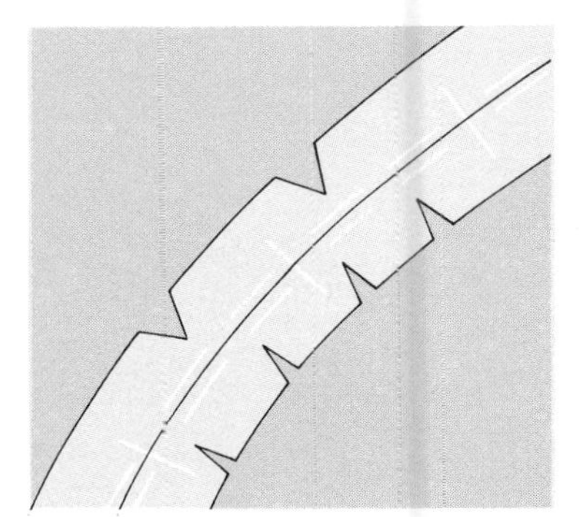

Mark seamlines by spreading seam allowances open and running chalk down seamlines. Every 3″ to 4″, make a mark perpendicular to the seamline; these serve as matching points, much like the notches in ready-made patterns.

Sewing the slipcover

The most accurate way to sew slipcovers is to handle one unit at a time. Remove a unit from the furniture and unpin the pieces. Lay them out flat and trim the seam allowances even. Stitch the unit together and put it back in place to be sure that it fits the furniture and the adjoining units. Then remove, stitch, and check the next unit.

Where possible, it is best to use corded seams. They are stronger than plain seams and better define a slipcover's edges. To construct the required quantity of cording (welting), cut continuous bias strips, then cover the cord. For all stitching, use a needle, thread, and stitch length suitable to the fabric. Shorten the stitch length around curves and corners. It is best to apply the cording to the half of the seam that needs control and staystitch the other seamline. For instance, apply the welting to larger rather than smaller sections; cord the gathered seamline rather than the ungathered one. As the cording is being applied, clip and notch its seam allowances as necessary so it will fit around curves and corners. Where ends of cording meet, treat them as explained below. In constructing a corded seam, use a zipper foot, and place successive rows of stitching between the preceding row and the seamline (in effect, bringing each row closer to the seamline). Form plain seams where seams will not be corded—joining boxing pieces, for example. Trim, grade, clip, or notch seam allowances where necessary; press all seams open; seam-finish as needed. Leave the placket seam of the slipcover open for the zipper. The zipper of a cushion cover should be inserted in a part of the boxing before the boxing unit is formed. For reinforcement, tape the seams at the ends of any zipper placket.

When cording ends meet, start stitching ½″ from end. At the other end, trim *cord* to meet first cord, *fabric* to ½″.

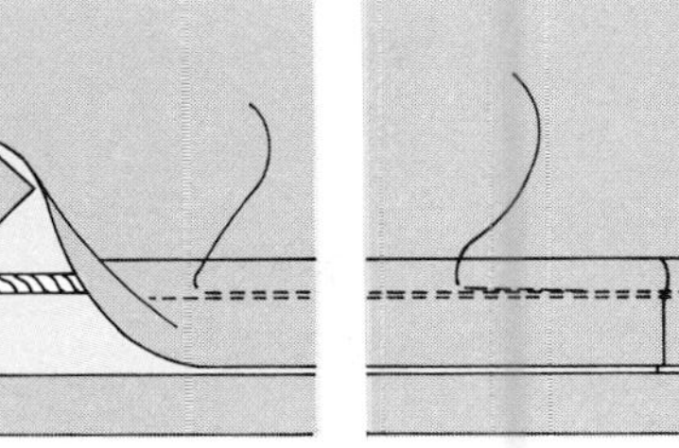

Fold the trimmed fabric edge under ¼″. Wrap the fold around the starting end of cording, letting cord ends meet.

Stitch across both ends to ½″ beyond the point where stitching was started. If necessary, backstitch to reinforce.

Applying zippers

On a chair cover, the zipper is usually applied to a side back seam; on a sofa cover, to one or both side back seams. If the sofa will stand against a wall, the zipper can be installed in one or two of the lengthwise seams between slipcover sections. A zipper should span at least three-fourths of the seam and should not extend into the skirt. The zipper for a cushion cover should be at the back of the boxing unit, and should be long enough to go across the back and around at least one corner.

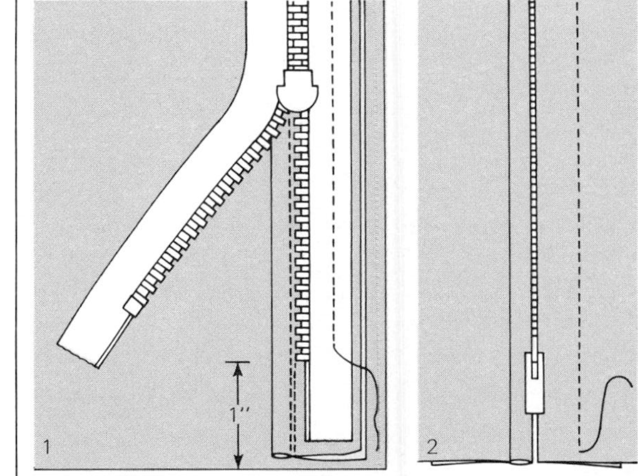

Zipper at slipcover back: (1) Open zipper. With face down and top stop 1″ above bottom seamline, place teeth along stitching that holds cording. Stitch. (2) Turn back corded edge; close zipper. Turn under and abut other placket edge to cording; stitch other zipper half to this edge.

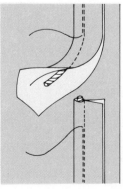

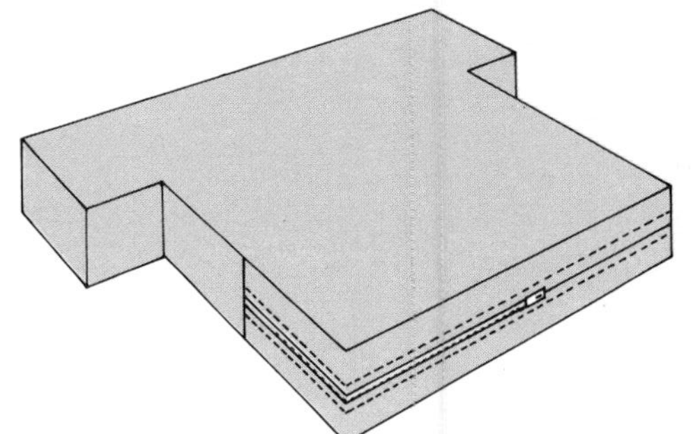

Zipper in cushion cover is usually applied by the centered method to a part of the boxing. Entire boxing unit is then formed and attached to cover pieces (see p. 422).

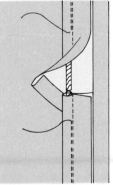

Finishing bottom slipcover edge

When the slipcover is completely sewed, try it on the furniture to check the fit and to mark the bottom seamline. For a facing, mark the seamline along the bottom edge of the furniture; for a skirt, an equal distance from the floor on all sides.

To construct and apply a **facing,** see the opposite page. If the finish is a **skirt,** first cut enough fabric lengths to produce the finished width (see below and p. 414). Whether these are joined immediately or later depends on the skirt style. For a *gathered skirt,* join the lengths first, finish the skirt's lower edge, then apply gathering stitches to the top seamline. Pin and gather the skirt to fit the slipcover; pin the cording to the skirt. Remove the skirt and stitch the cording; remove the slipcover and attach its skirt.

For a *pleated skirt,* work first with unjoined strips so you can place the joining seams at the backs of pleats. Pin the strips to the slipcover, forming and marking the pleats and the joining seams as you go. Remove the marked strips and open them out flat. Join the lengths and finish lower edge of skirt. Re-pin skirt to slipcover, repleat, and pin cording to skirt. Remove skirt to stitch cording; remove slipcover to attach skirt.

Before facing or skirt is constructed and applied, mark seamline at lower edge of slipcover: for facing, at bottom of furniture; for skirt, an even distance from floor.

Calculating total skirt widths

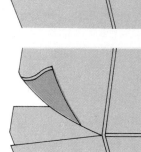

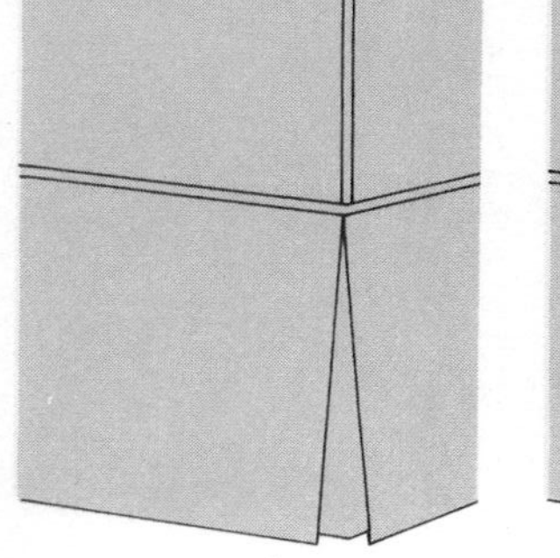

Single pleats: Allow for finished skirt width, plus joining seams and twice the depth of each pleat. Position pleats at the corners and at lengthwise seams of slipcover.

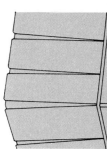

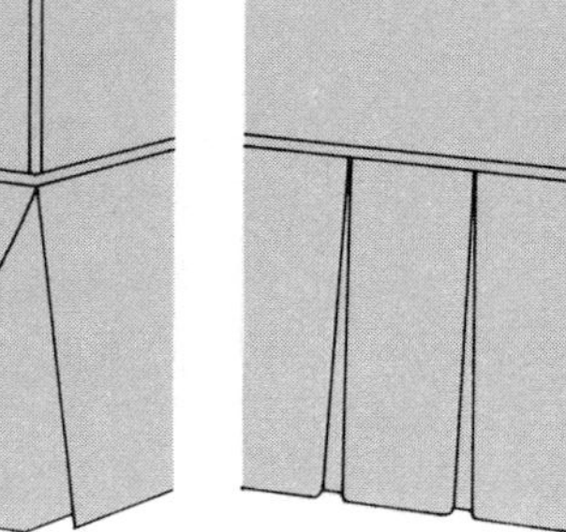

Separate underlay pleats: Finished skirt width, plus joining-seam allowances, the depth of each pleat, seam allowances at all pleat ends for a lined finish.

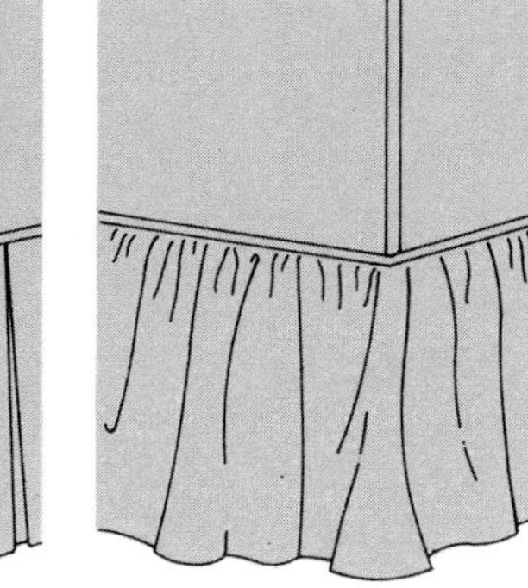

Continuous pleats: Three times the finished skirt width, plus joining-seam allowances. Place a pleat at each corner and at center front and back, then form pleats in between.

Gathers: This type of skirt calls for twice the finished skirt width, plus joining-seam allowances. Fullness should be evenly distributed around the entire skirt.

Finishing lower edge of skirt

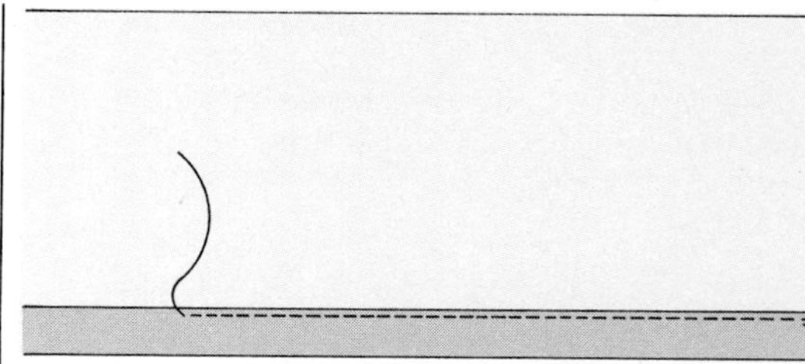

A machine-stitched hem can be the finish for skirt's lower edge. Start with 1½″ hem; for methods, see Hemming.

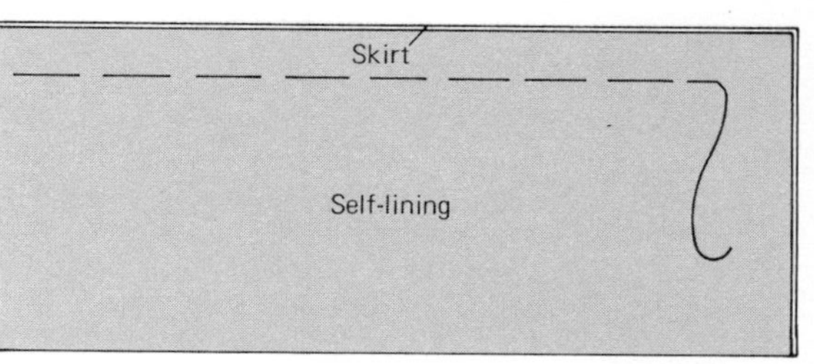

For self-lined skirt, cut skirt twice the finished length, plus two seam allowances. Fold at hemline; baste at top.

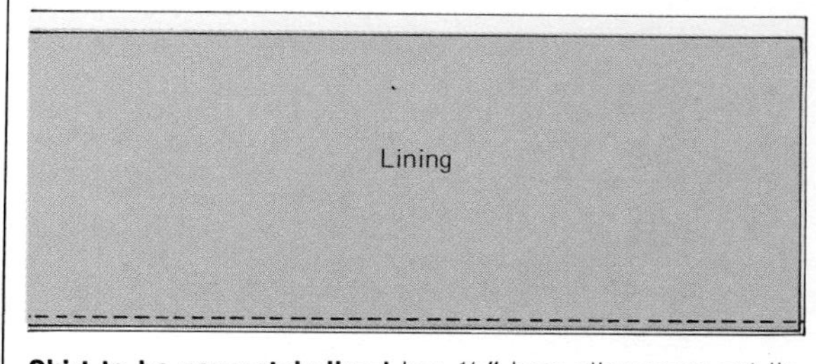

Skirt to be separately lined has ¼″ hem allowance; cut lining ¼″ shorter than skirt. Right sides together, sew lining to skirt at lower edge. Trim seam; press toward lining.

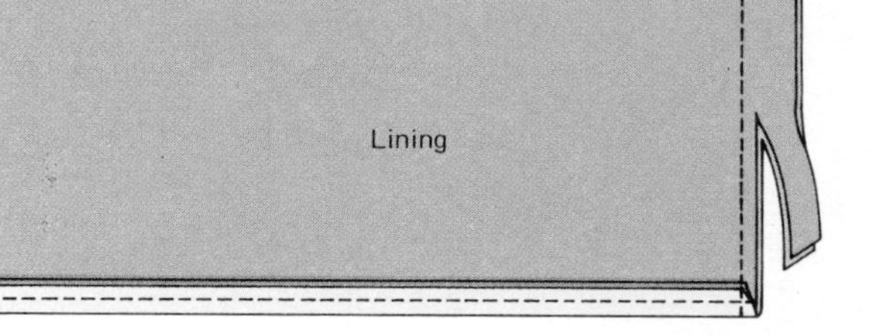

To seam the free ends, fold in half, right sides together, and align top edges; stitch, trim, and press seams. Turn skirt right side out; align and baste top edges.

Skirt closures

The lapped edges that occur with pleated skirts can be held closed with snaps. When applying the skirt, leave the underlap of the pleat free beyond the placket and finish its top edge. The overlap can be sewed to the slipcover. Sew snaps to back of pleat.

The abutted edges that occur with gathered skirts can be fastened with hooks and round eyes. When applying skirt, be sure to turn back placket seam allowances so the placket edges will meet; if necessary, turn under or seam-finish placket seam allowances.

Skirtless (faced) finish

When seamline has been marked at bottom of furniture, pin the cording in place along markings (See p. 416 for an explanation of cutting around the legs.) Sew cording to slipcover.

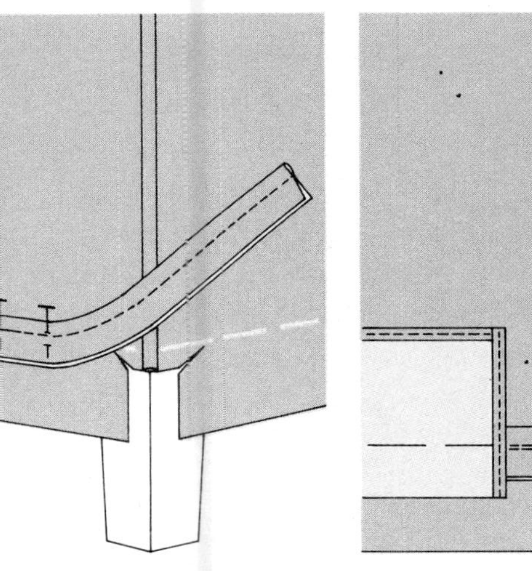

For each side of slipcover, cut a facing that will be, with outer edges finished, the length of the side from leg to leg, and 3" wide. Finish edges; apply facing to slipcover.

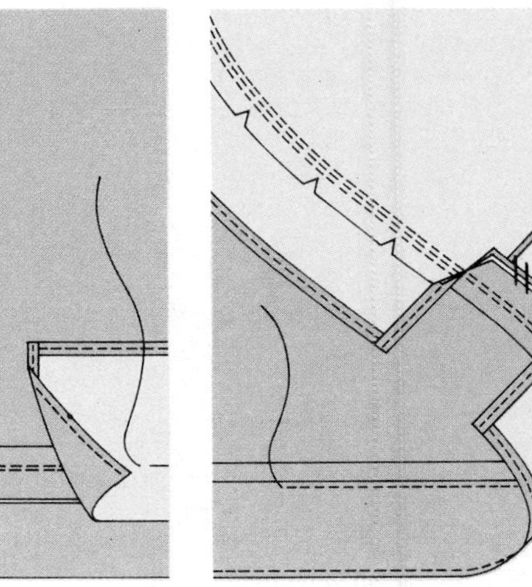

Clip into seam allowances at each end of facings. Trim, grade, and notch seam allowances; understitch the seamlines. Turn unfaced parts of seams to inside; whipstitch in place.

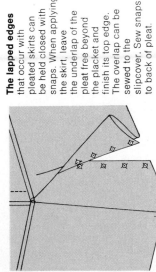

Securing bottom edge of slipcover

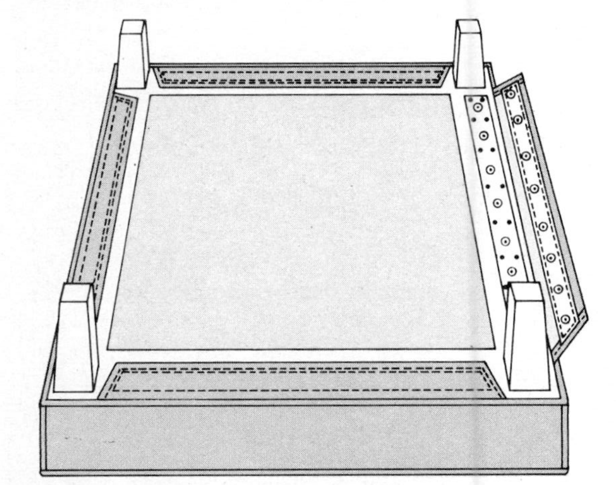

A skirtless finish can be held in place with snap or nylon tape. Sew one half of the fastener to the wrong side of the facings; align and tack the other half to the frame.

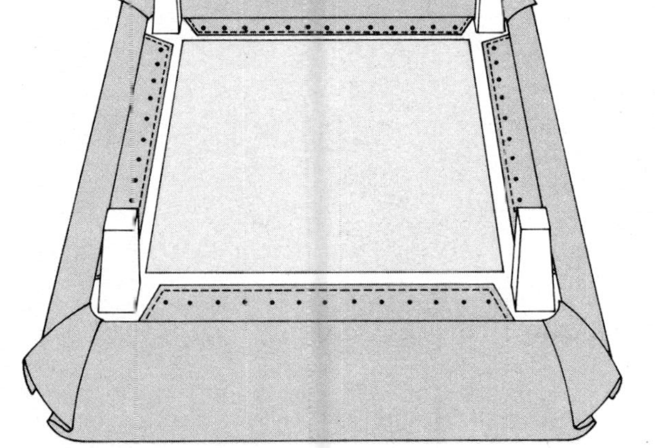

Skirt can be secured to the frame by tacking slipcover and skirt seam allowances to it. Another way is to add a facing to seam of slipcover and skirt and tack facing to frame.

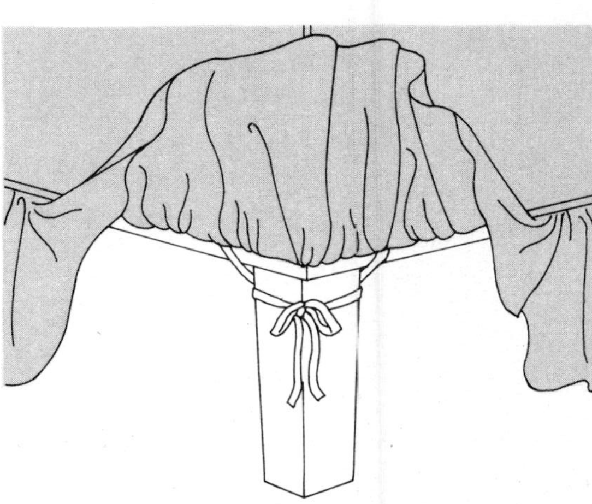

Tapes tied at each leg are another way of holding a skirted slipcover in place. Simply insert 12" lengths of twill tape at sides of legs as skirt is being stitched to cover.

Pillows

Slipstitch 132

Corded seams 153
Making cording 298-300

Types of pillows

Though pillows vary greatly in size and shape, there are basically only two types, knife-edge and box-edge. A **knife-edge pillow** is one that is thickest at the center and tapers off to the edges, so that there is very little side depth. A **box-edge pillow** is uniform in thickness from center to edges, and so has a side depth that must be covered with a boxing strip. The bolster, to the surprise of many, is actually a type of box-edge pillow. Typical shapes for any of these pillows are rectangular and circular; one bolster form is wedge-shaped.

The forms for pillows can be preshaped (cut foam shapes and polyester-filled covers are examples), or you can buy or make a shaped fabric cover and fill it with batting. To arrive at the basic measurements of the fabric pieces for the pillow cover, measure the pillow form (see below); allow for a seam at each edge. If a placket will fall at one of the seams already allowed for in the basic measurements, no additional allowances are necessary. If a placket opening will be within a section,e.g.,in a part of the boxing strip, extra allowances are needed; these are explained as they occur on the next few pages.

When a pillow shape is intricate, it is best to make a pattern for cutting the fabric sections. When fabric is expensive or fragile, a muslin test cover is advisable; it can serve later as an inner cover for the pillow. If the pillow is to be trimmed, apply the trimmings before constructing the cover. Some trims, such as ruffles, can be added to the outside seams so as to extend out from the edges and increase the cover's size. This is often done with pillow shams.

Basic measurements

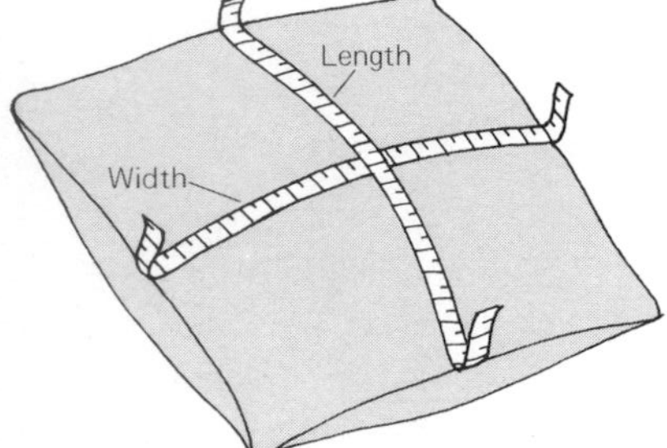

Knife-edge form: If *rectangular*, measure the length and width; if *circular*, measure diameter. Add seam allowances to all edges.

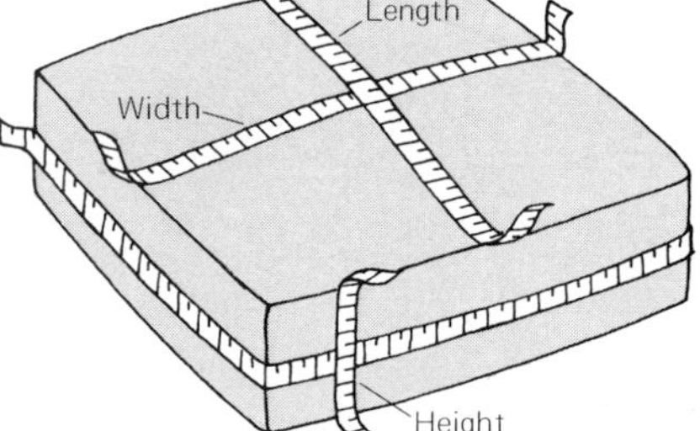

Rectangular box-edge form: Measure length, width, height, then around form for length of boxing. Add seam allowances to edges.

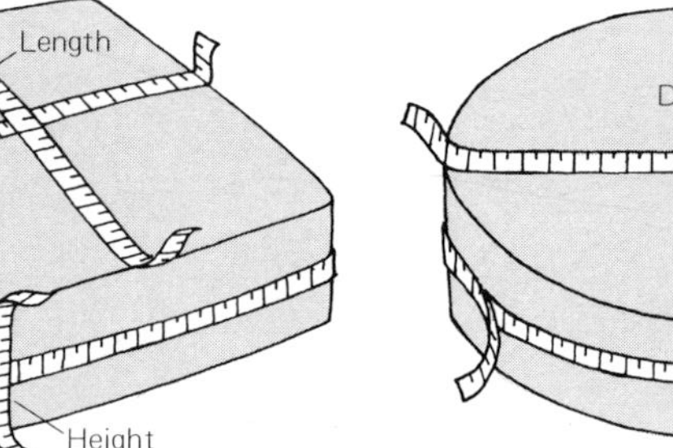

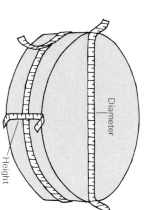

Circular box-edge form: Measure diameter and height, then around form for length of boxing. Add seam allowances to all edges.

Circular bolster form: Measure diameter of ends, width of bolster, then around bolster. Add seam allowances to all edges.

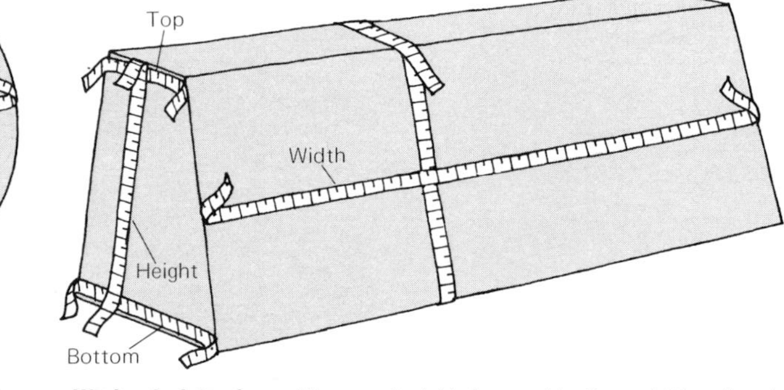

Wedge bolster form: Measure height, top and bottom widths of ends, width of bolster, around bolster. Add seam allowances to edges.

Knife-edge pillow covers

The cover for a basic knife-edge pillow consists of a top and a bottom section. To allow for insertion of the form, an opening must be provided in one of the cover's seams. The opening can be closed with hand slipstitches but a zipper inserted in the seam makes it easier to remove the cover and put it back on. The instructions at the right are for inserting a zipper into a seam of a rectangular cover. It is easier, in a circular cover, to insert the zipper across the center of the bottom. This requires creating a placket seam. Allow for it by cutting two semicircles with an extra seam allowance along their straight edges. Insert the zipper, then sew the bottom to the top.

If cording will be used in the seams, prepare a suitable quantity of covered cord. Use a zipper foot to apply cording and to stitch the seams.

Tufting a knife-edge pillow, besides adding a decorative touch, keeps the cover and form from shifting. It is done after the form is inserted into the cover. Once a pillow is tufted, the cover is rarely, if ever, removed, and so a zippered opening is not needed. Tufting can be done with thread only, or with thread and buttons.

Pillow shams are relatively loose-fitting knife-edge covers, popular as decorative daytime covers for bed pillows. To be most attractive, a sham should cover the full width of a single bed or half the width of a double bed. Extra size is added to the body of the sham by means of trims or borders that extend out from the cover portion. The placket for a sham is placed along the center of the bottom; it should be finished before the top and bottom sections are joined. Be sure to allow for the placket when cutting out the bottom section.

Thread 10, hand needles 11
Ruffles 184-186
Hems 294
Zipper applications 318-319, 322

Constructing a knife-edge pillow cover

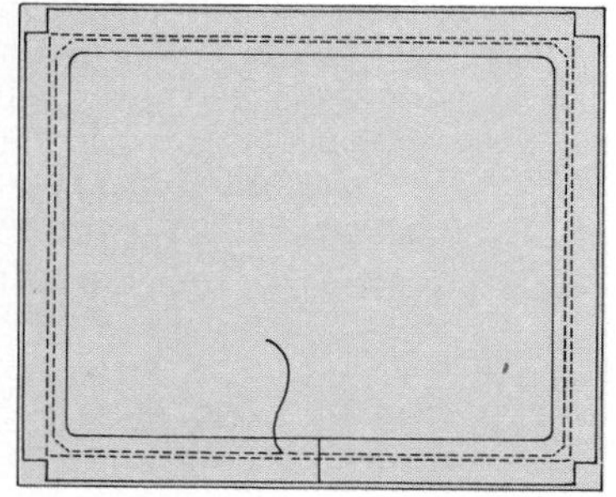

1. Baste cording to right side of cover top, along the seamline (to join cording ends, see p. 417). Clip into cording seam allowances at corners. Stitch the cording in place, stitching across corners to blunt them.

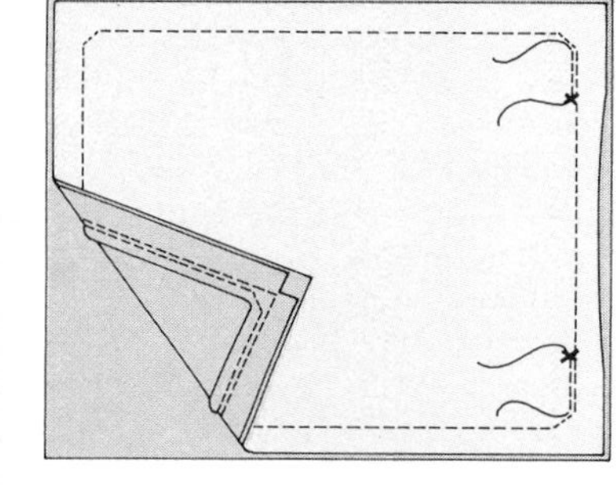

2. On wrong side of cover top, mark top and bottom of placket opening. With right sides together, stitch cover top to cover bottom above and below placket. Start at each marking and stitch to each corner's seamline.

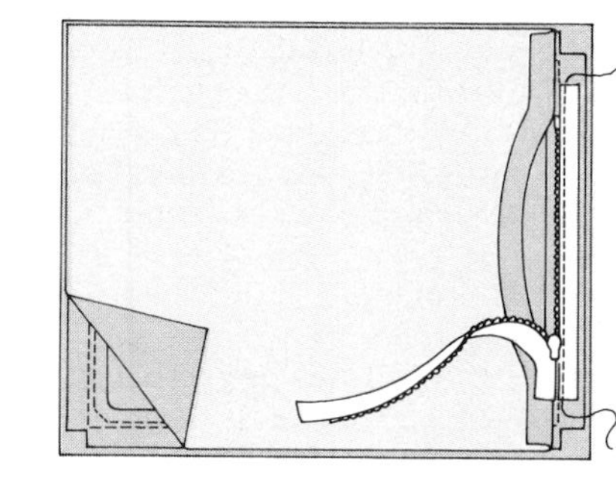

3. Extend placket seam allowance of top section. Open zipper and place half of it face down on seam allowance, with teeth along cording and top and bottom stops at top and bottom of opening. Stitch in place.

4. Close zipper; form bar tack across tapes at top. Spread open the cover sections and placket seam. From right side, baste, then stitch the free zipper tape to bottom of cover; stitch across ends and along the side of the zipper. Remove bastings; open zipper.

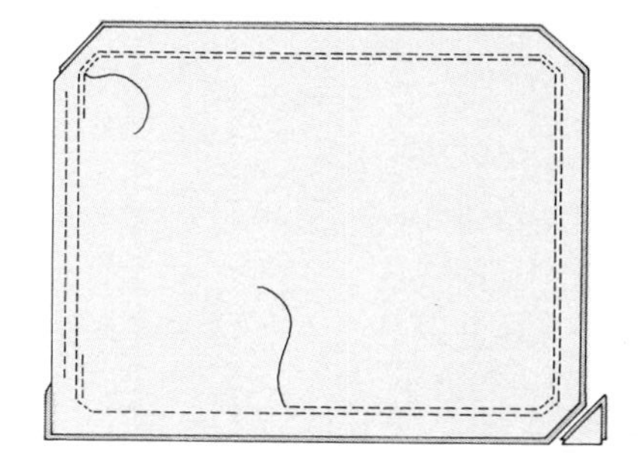

5. Right sides together, stitch cover top to the bottom (begin and end at the placket seam). Sew across corners to blunt them; trim seams.

Tufting pillows

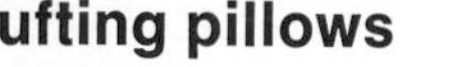

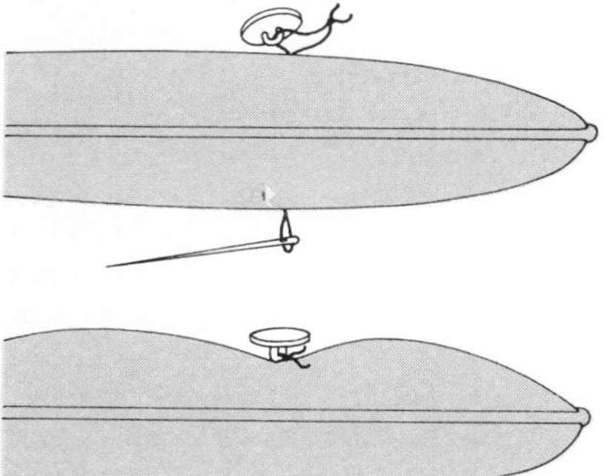

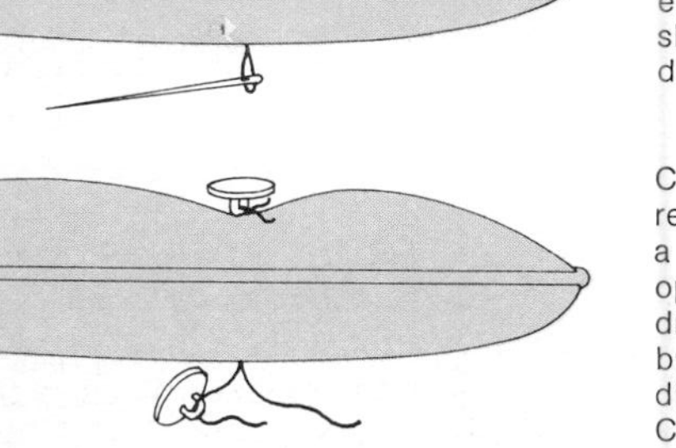

To tuft with buttons, thread a long needle with a double strand of strong thread. Tie thread ends to button shank. Push needle down through pillow.

Clip the thread to remove needle. Tie a second button opposite the first; draw up knot and button tightly to dimple the pillow. Clip thread ends.

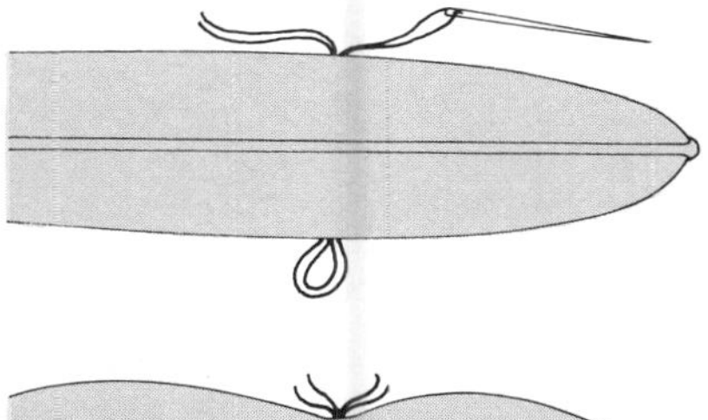

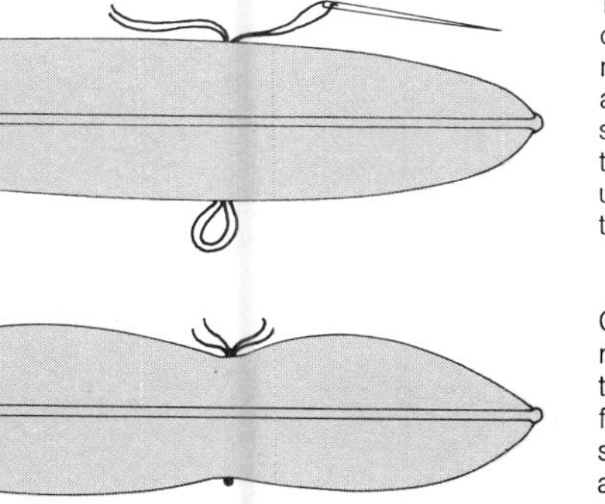

To tuft with thread only, push a long needle, threaded with a double strand of strong thread, down through pillow, then up, coming out next to starting point.

Clip thread to remove needle. Tie the thread ends, forcing knot down so it presses into and dimples the pillow. Clip, leaving some thread ends.

Pillow shams

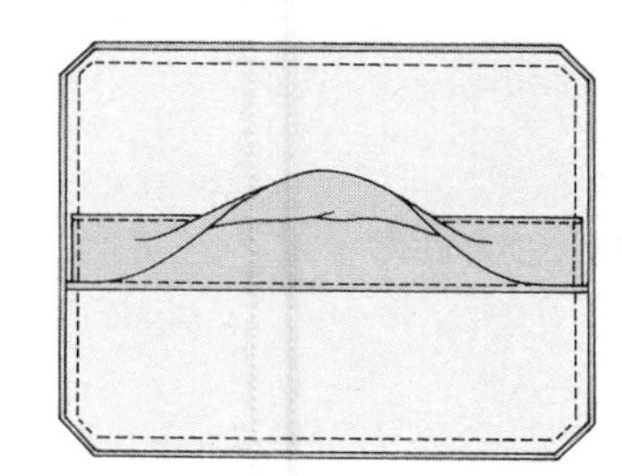

Pillow sham is a loose-fitting knife-edge cover unique for its placket opening, which is placed along center of sham bottom. Placket is finished before top and bottom are joined; usually takes the form shown—1½" wide overlapping hemmed edges. See other forms below.

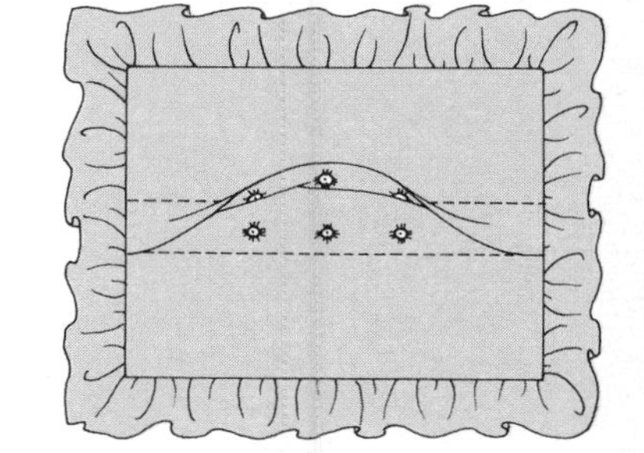

Ruffle, attached to the sham top before top is sewed to bottom, increases sham size. Here snaps secure placket's overlapping edges.

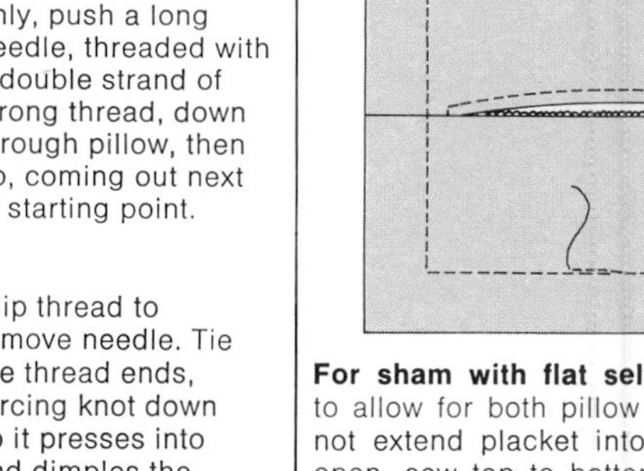

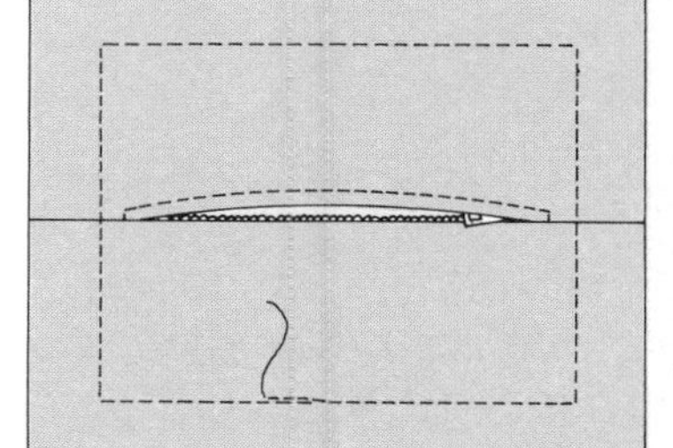

For sham with flat self-border, cut sections to allow for both pillow and border width. Do not extend placket into border. With placket open, sew top to bottom; turn right side out; topstitch on line between pillow and border. Placket here has lapped zipper closing.

Staystitching 144
Seams 144, 146-147, 153
Making cording 298-300
Zipper applications 318, 326

Box-edge pillow covers

A box-edge pillow cover consists of top and bottom sections, plus a boxing strip to cover the sides. A zipper is usually inserted into a part of the boxing strip, and applied before the strip is sewed to the pillow top and bottom. If cording will be used in the seams, prepare the necessary quantity of covered cord before constructing the pillow. A boxed effect can be achieved on a rectangular cover without a separate boxing strip. For this method, both top and bottom sections must be cut to include half the pillow depth along each edge.

Rectangular box-edge cover

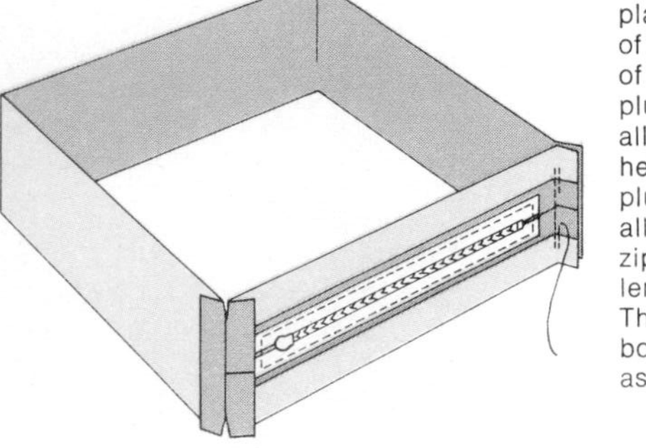

1. To provide for a placket, cut one part of boxing the length of the pillow side plus two seam allowances, by the height of the pillow plus four seam allowances. Insert zipper along the lengthwise center. Then seam the boxing strip unit as shown at left.

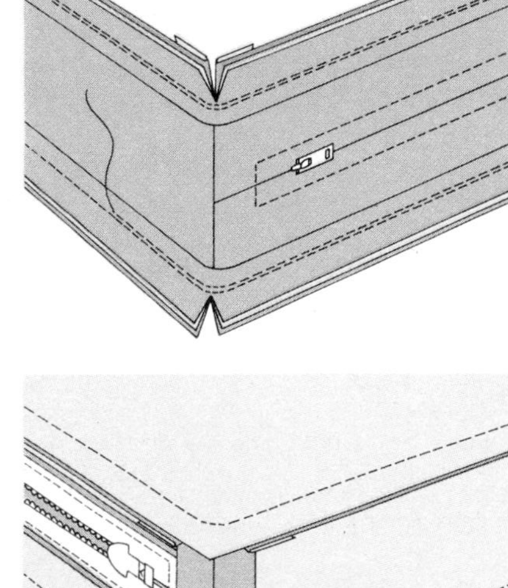

2. If cording the pillow, sew cording to top and bottom seamlines of boxing. Position cording to right side of boxing with raw edges of cording toward raw edges of boxing. Join cording ends as on page 417; clip into seam allowances at the corners.

3. With right sides together and the boxing side up, stitch bottom section to the bottom seamline of the boxing. Stitch just inside stitching that holds cording to boxing. Spread the boxing seam allowances open at the corners; stitch across the corners to blunt them.

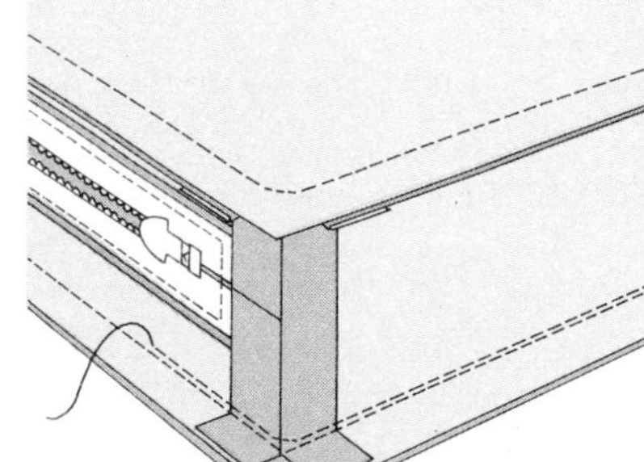

4. Open zipper. With right sides together and the boxing side up, sew top section to the top seamline of boxing, using techniques in Step 3. Trim seams if necessary. Turn cover to right side through zipper opening; push out on fabric at corners.

Boxed effect without boxing strip

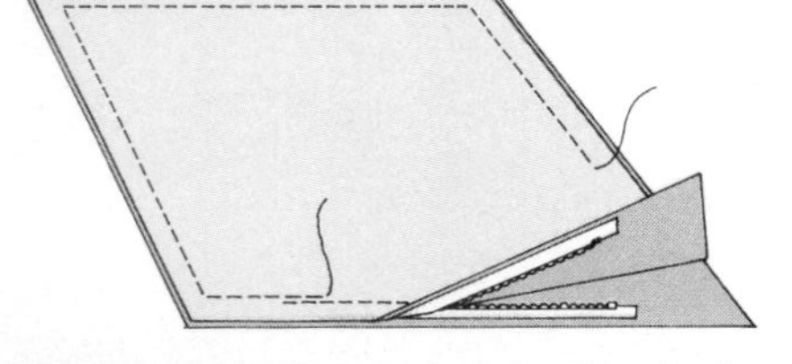

Cut top and bottom to include side depth. Apply invisible zipper to one seam; open. Sew top to bottom from one placket end to other.

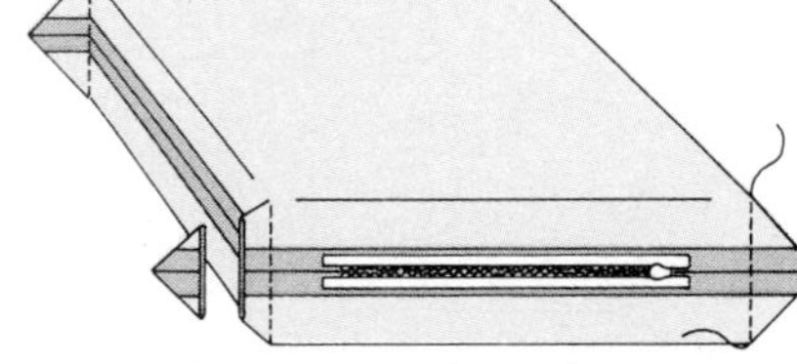

Fold cover at corners to align cross seams; stitch across as shown, and trim. Length of stitch line should be equal to height of pillow.

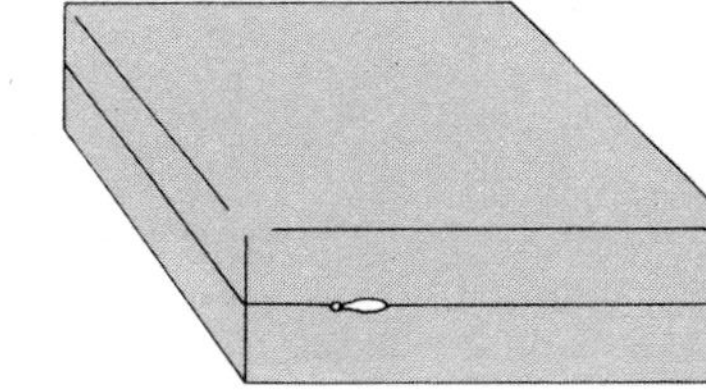

Turn the cover to the right side through the zipper opening. Push out on the seamlines to shape the corners and their edges.

Circular box-edge cover

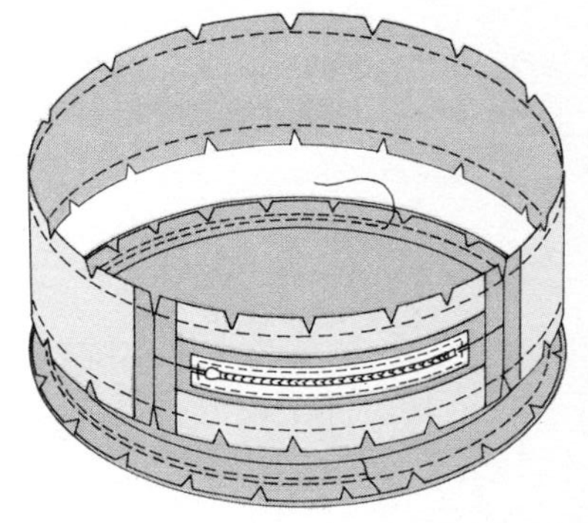

1. Allow for and insert the zipper into about one-fourth of the boxing (Step 1, left). Staystitch and clip both edges of boxing. Stitch cording as shown to top and bottom pieces.

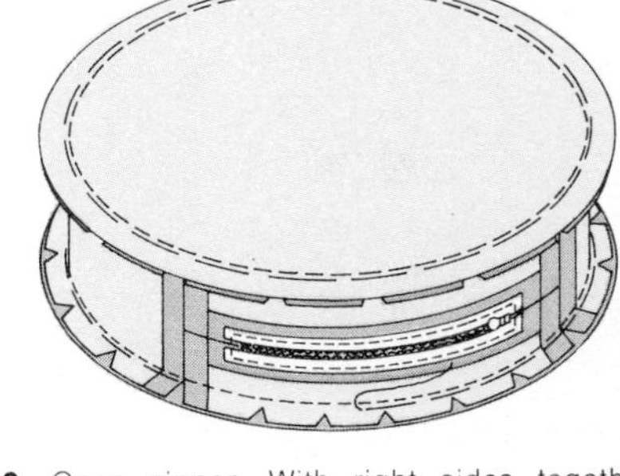

2. Open zipper. With right sides together, baste top section to the top seamline of the boxing; baste bottom section to the bottom seamline of the boxing.

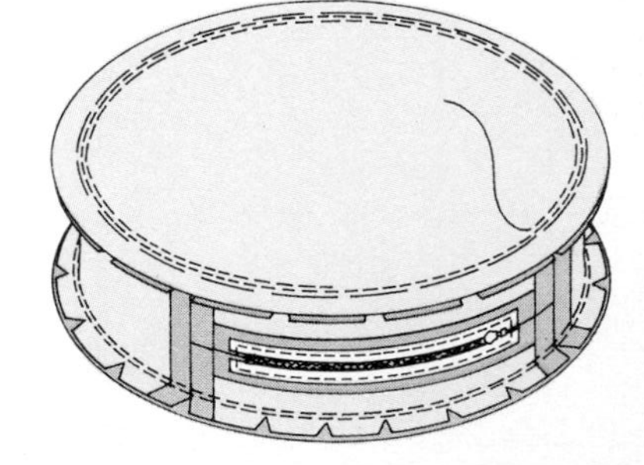

3. With boxing side up, stitch top and bottom to the boxing. Trim seams if necessary. Turn cover to right side through zipper opening. Push out on seamlines to shape edges.

Bolster covers

A bolster is a type of box-edge pillow in which the boxing strip area has become the largest part, actually the body of the pillow, and the top and bottom merely the pillow ends. The two most typical bolster shapes are round and wedge. Since both are relatively complicated to cover, it is best to make a pattern for cutting the fabric pieces. As shown below, the closures occur in joining seams and thus need no special provision. In a **round-bolster** cover, the zipper is inserted into the seam that joins the ends of the body piece. In a **wedge-bolster** cover, the placket opening spans that joining seam and the bottom seam of both end pieces as well. Snap tape is the easiest closure to apply and is used in the example.

Cover for round bolster

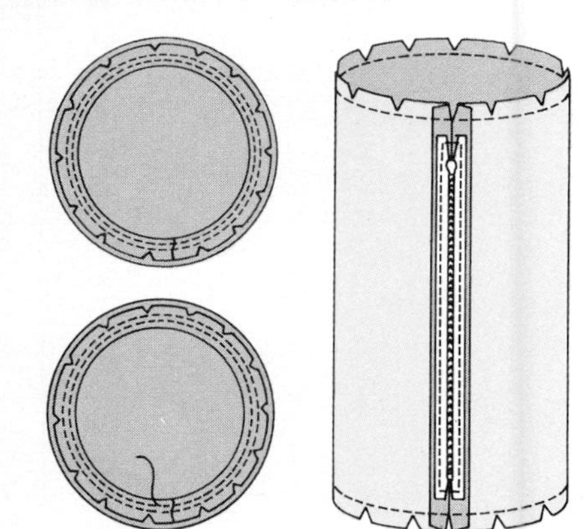

Stitch cording to right side of each bolster end piece; clip into seam allowances of cording so it will curve. Insert zipper in seam that will join ends of body piece; staystitch and clip into seam allowances of both edges of body.

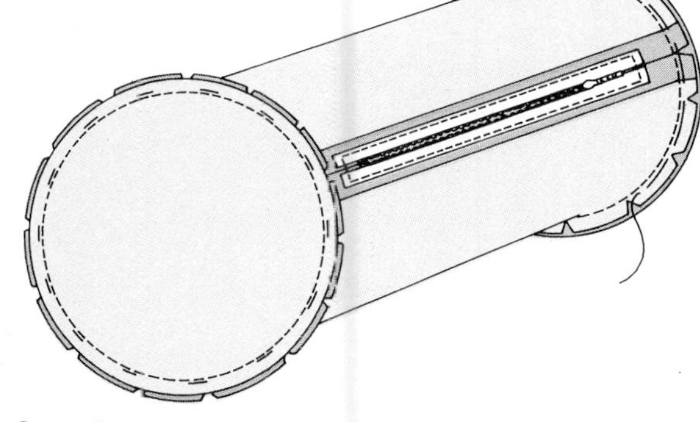

Open the zipper. With right sides together, baste an end piece to one edge of the body; spread the clipped seam allowances of the body so seamlines can be matched. Baste the other end piece to the other edge in the same way.

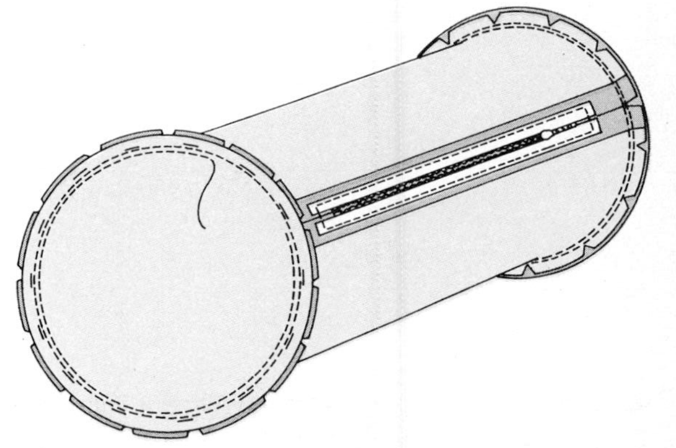

With body part of cover nearest the needle, stitch both of the end pieces to the body. Remove bastings; trim seams if necessary. Turn cover to the right side through the zipper opening. Push out on seamlines to curve the edges.

Cover for wedge bolster

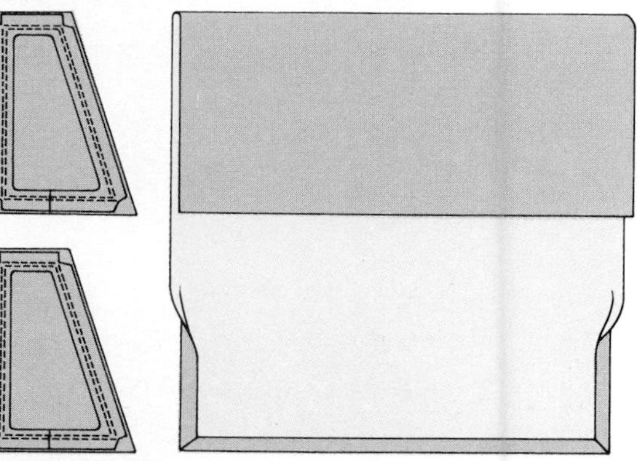

Stitch cording to right side of both ends; clip seam allowances of cording so it will go around corners. At one end of the body piece, fold in and miter the corner seam allowances (this prepares edge for snap tape, far right).

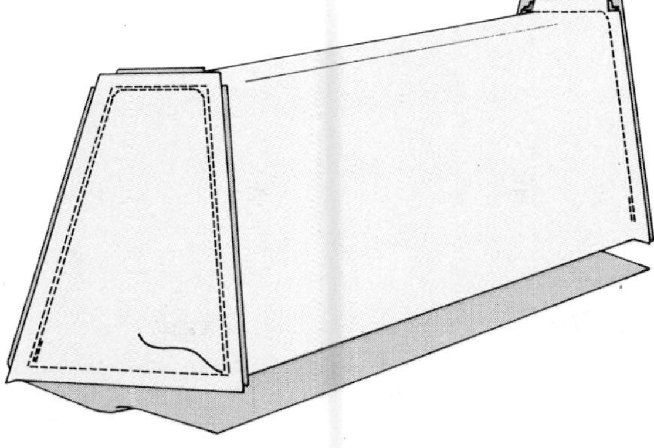

Right sides together, stitch both end pieces to body piece, starting and ending stitching at bottom seamline. Clip into seam allowances of body pieces at top corners; stitch across corners to blunt them. Turn cover right side out.

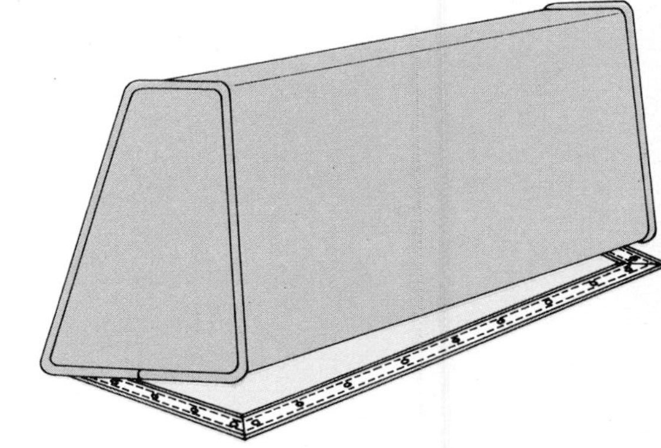

Sew ball half of snap tape to upper seam allowance of open seam; miter tape at corners (keep snaps free of miters). Position socket half on lower seam, aligning sockets and balls; miter at corners; topstitch through all layers.

Bedspreads

Introduction

Basically, there are three bedspread styles—*throw, flounced,* and *tailored.* The first is simply a flat piece that drapes over the bed. The second two have fitted drops (sides) that may be gathered, pleated, or straight.

Whatever the style, a spread is made with a full fabric width in the center and seams an equal distance from the center. Unless covered by lining, seam allowances should be neatly finished, preferably self-enclosed or bound, but they can be zigzag-stitched. Because of the many yards involved, machine-finished hems are practical.

Any fabric will do for a spread, but generally, the more body it has, the better. Lining is optional, but a soft or sheer fabric will probably need one. If a bed is to be used for lounging, the spread fabric should be sturdy and easy to clean.

If there is nap (or one-way design), it should run the same way on all throw sections. The effect is most pleasing on a fitted spread if the nap runs down from top to floor, but this may require some piecing. The alternative is to run the nap around the sides *in one direction only.*

Any of the basic styles can be adapted for a *coverlet*—a short spread that ends 3 inches below the mattress. Extra care should be taken in finishing a coverlet edge because it is more visible than one that hangs to the floor. Lining and/or cording would be appropriate here.

A coverlet is usually combined with a *dust cover*—a fitted top piece with a straight, pleated, or gathered skirt—that conceals the box springs and legs. For economy, the top can be muslin or other inexpensive fabric.

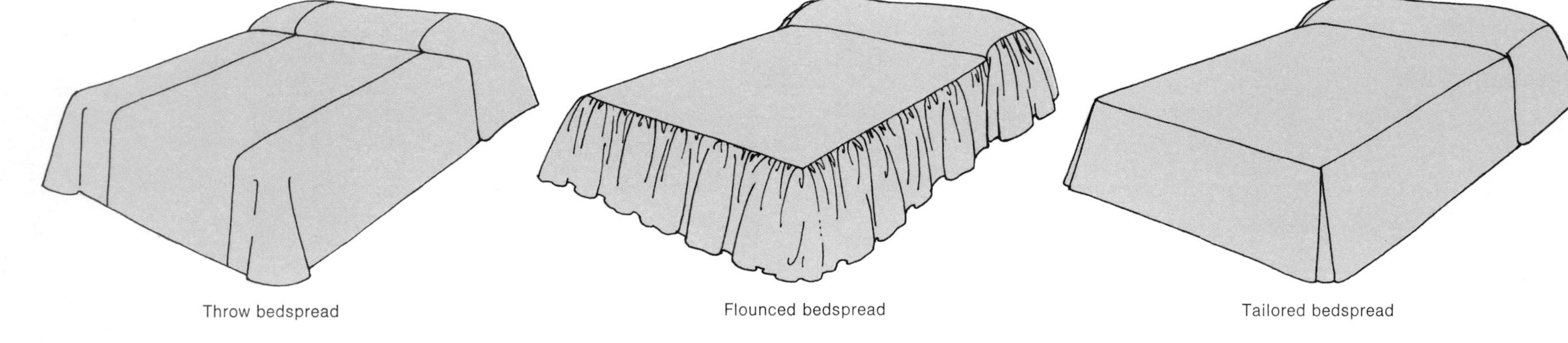

Throw bedspread

Flounced bedspread

Tailored bedspread

Estimating yardage for a spread

To estimate yardage, decide on the style, then take appropriate measurements as explained at the right. To them, add ½ inch for seam allowances (see Flounced spread for exceptions) and 2 inches for hems, including hem for head end. In general, the fabric required depends on fabric width in relation to bed width and height. A throw for a bed 54 inches wide by 20 inches high, for example, would require an overall width of 100 inches. You would need two bed lengths (top length plus foot drop) of *54-inch* fabric, or three lengths of *36- or 45-inch;* another yard to cover cable cord; and an extra motif for each length, if fabric must be matched.

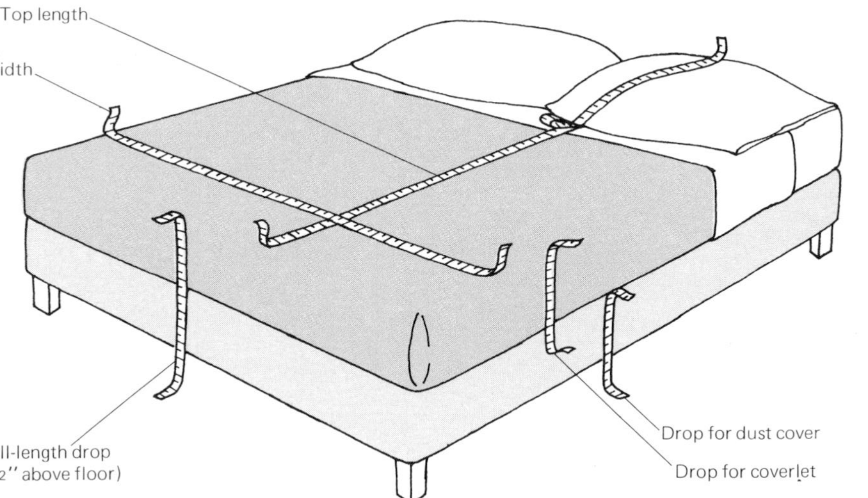

To measure the bed, first make it up with sheets and blankets, also pillows, if the spread is to cover them. Use a flexible tape measure; where it does not reach the full distance being measured, pin at the place where the tape ends, and continue measuring from the pin.
Top length: Measure from the head to the foot, allowing 14" for pillow tuck-in.
Top width: From edge to edge.
Drop for full spread: From the edge of the top to ½" from the floor.
Drop for coverlet: From the top edge to 3" below the top mattress.
Drop for dust cover: From the top edge of the box spring to ½" from the floor.
Top for dust cover: Length and width of the box spring.

Zigzagged seam finish 148
Bias-bound seam finish 149
Self-enclosed seams 150
Applying cording to hemline 300

Throw style

A **throw bedspread** is made of three panels that form a flat rectangle, long and wide enough to cover the entire bed. The center panel is the width of the top or less, and long enough to include foot drop and pillow tuck-in. Side sections extend from center panel to floor on each side; corners at the foot end are often rounded so they do not touch the floor. Any bulky or heavy fabric, especially a quilted one, is a good choice for a throw, being less inclined to wrinkle or to become rumpled.

Basic procedure is to join the sections, then hem all around. Unless a throw is lined, self-enclosed seams are most suitable. Two types, *flat-felled* and *French,* are shown below. For two others, *mock French* and *self-bound,* consult the Seams chapter.

For more emphasis on seams, welting or a flat trim can be added. If welting is used, finish seams with a zigzag stitch or bias binding. If a flat trim is added, it is simplest to topstitch the trim over seam allowances on the right side (see below).

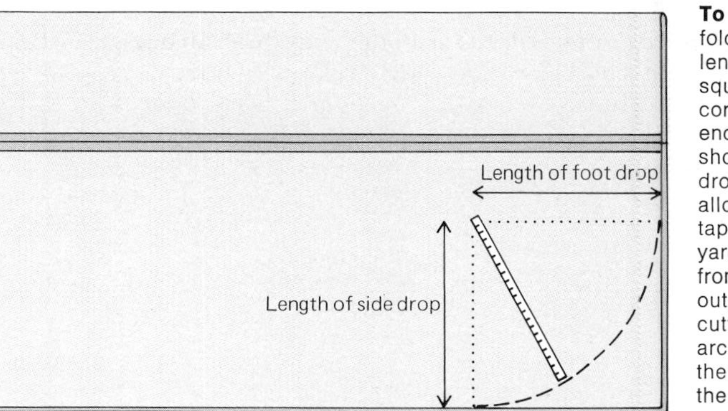

To round off corners, fold spread in half lengthwise; mark a square on the outer corner at the foot end. Sides of square should equal the drop depth plus hem allowance. Using a tape measure or yardstick, measure from the inner corner out, marking a cutting line in an arc. Cut one corner, then mark and cut the second one.

Recommended seams

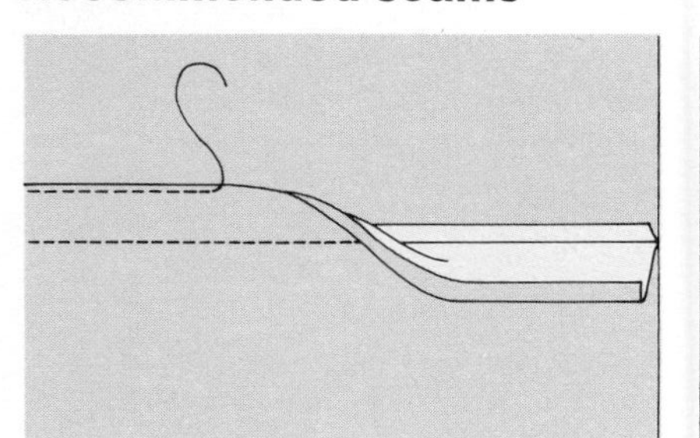

For a flat-felled seam, stitch on seamline, wrong sides together. Trim one seam allowance to ⅛". Fold under ⅛" of second allowance; fold second over first and topstitch.

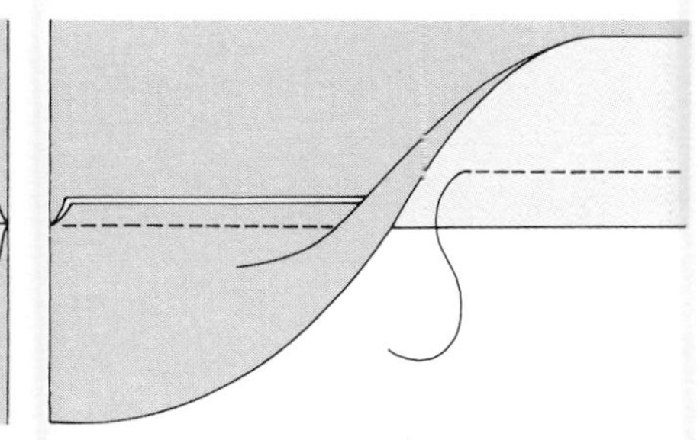

For a French seam, stitch ¼" from seamline, wrong sides together. Trim seam allowances to ⅛". Fold fabric right sides together, stitched line on fold; stitch ¼" from fold.

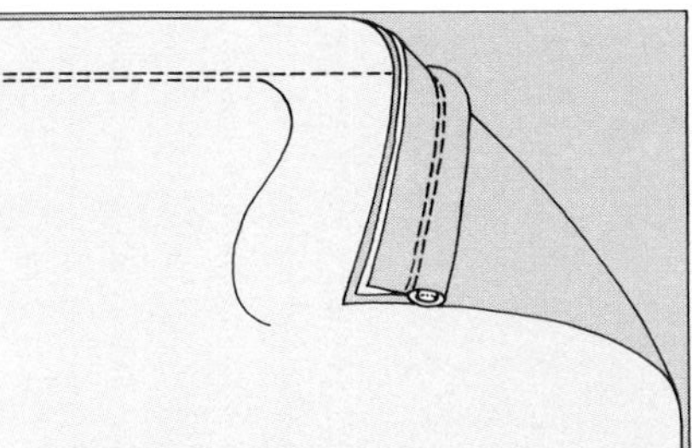

For a corded seam, stitch cording to right side of one seam allowance, crowding stitches between cording and stitches that hold it. Stitch seam, placing this row closer to cording.

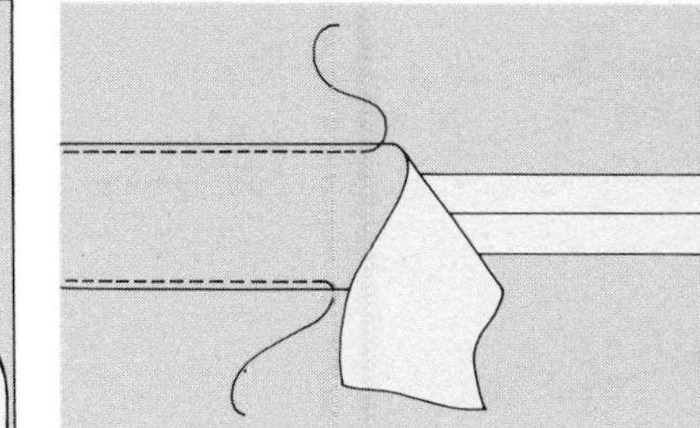

For a seam with trim, stitch on the seamline, wrong sides together. Press seams open; trim seam allowances, if necessary. Topstitch the trim over the seam.

Suggested edge finishes

For topstitched hem, turn up hem allowance; fold hem edge under ⅜"; baste hem. Topstitch from right side, close to basting.

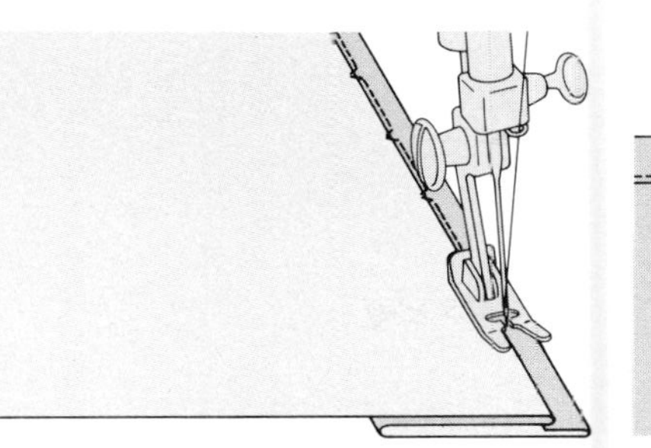

For blindstitched hem, turn up hem allowance; fold edge under ⅜". Blindstitch as shown, catching only the spread with zigzags.

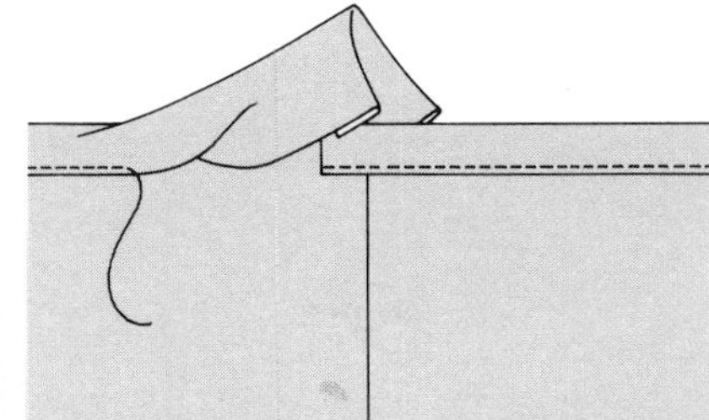

For topstitched binding, wrap binding over hem edge, wider side underneath. Edgestitch as shown, catching both sides of binding.

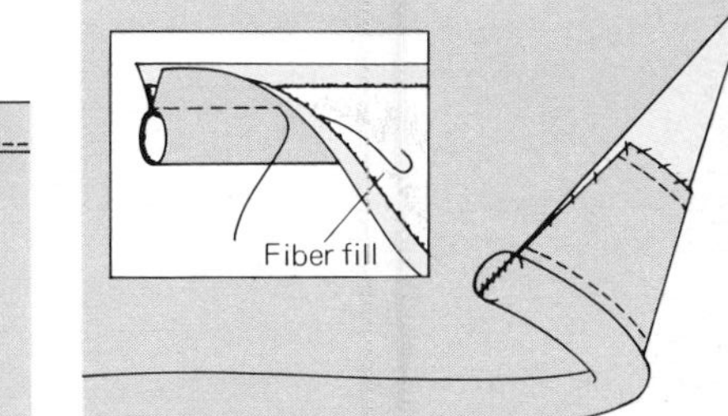

For a padded edging, cover a strip of fiber fill with bias (see inset); attach filled bias in the same way as cording (see Hems).

Gathering foot 38 Zigzagged seam finish 148
Corded seams 153

Fitted spread with flounce

A **flounced bedspread** has a fitted top and sides that are gathered or pleated all around. Medium- or lightweight fabric is best for this style.

The top is cut the length and width of the bed, plus seam allowances, and a hem allowance for the head end. If fabric must be pieced, use a full width for the center panel and a split width (or portion) for each side. The top will fit better if you blunt corners at the foot end (take a few stitches diagonally when joining top to drops). Corners can also be rounded, using the mattress for a pattern.

The drop is cut in several sections, joined with French seams (see p. 425) or interlocking fell seams (p. 431). Allow twice the length to be covered for a gathered drop, three times this length for pleats. Sections are usually cut from fabric width (so lengthwise grain goes from top to floor). For a fuller look, or special effect (stripes run horizontally, for example), sections can be cut lengthwise.

A ruffled flounce can be made with or without a heading. For style with no heading, cut top with 1-inch seam allowances; flounce with ¾-inch allowances at top edge, 2 inches for bottom hem. For a headed ruffle, allow 2-inch seams at the top, ¾ inch for top of ruffle, 2 inches for a hem.

The general procedure is to join flounce sections, hem bottom and free edges, then gather and join flounce to top. Before gathering, divide drop into 10 to 12 equal parts; mark with notches. Do the same with top. Align notches when joining.

Cording, if desired, can be added to a style with no heading; attach it to the flounce before stitching flounce to top. Instead of self-binding (near right), zigzag seam edges or line the top (opposite page).

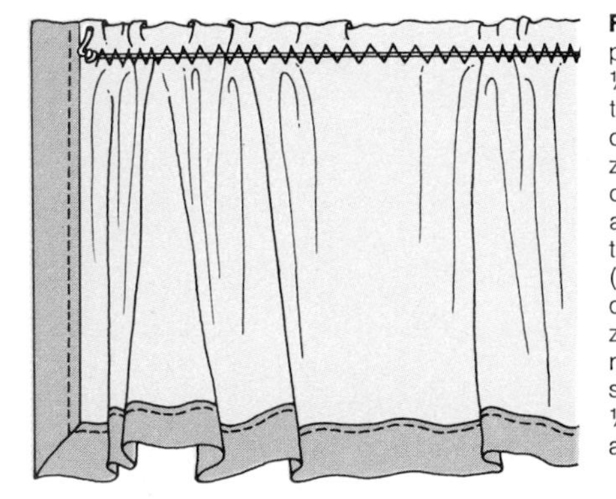

For a plain flounce, place a thin cord ½″ from top edge on the wrong side; stitch over it with widest zigzag. Pull the cord to form gathers, adjusting flounce to fit top section. (If your machine does not have a zigzag, make two rows of straight-stitch gathering, ¼″ apart, or use a gathering foot.)

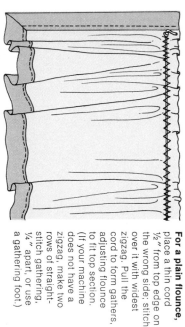

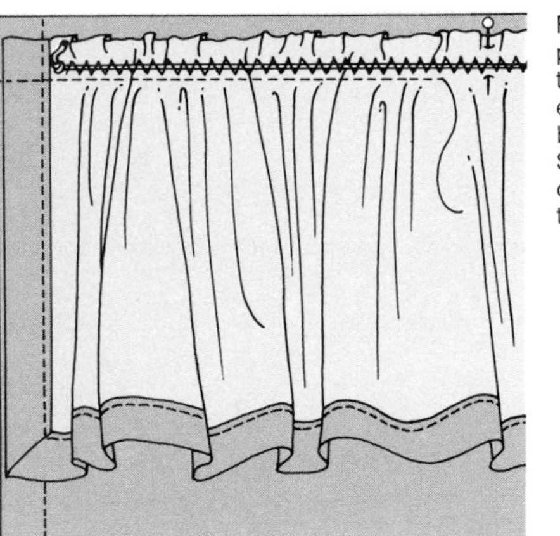

Right sides together, pin flounce to the top section, with edge of flounce ¼″ below edge of top. Stitch just below the cord, or 1″ from the top edge.

Trim flounce seam allowance to ¼″. Fold under the edge of untrimmed seam allowance ⅛″, then fold again, aligning fold with seamline and enclosing the edge of the flounce; press. Stitch folded edge through seam allowances only.

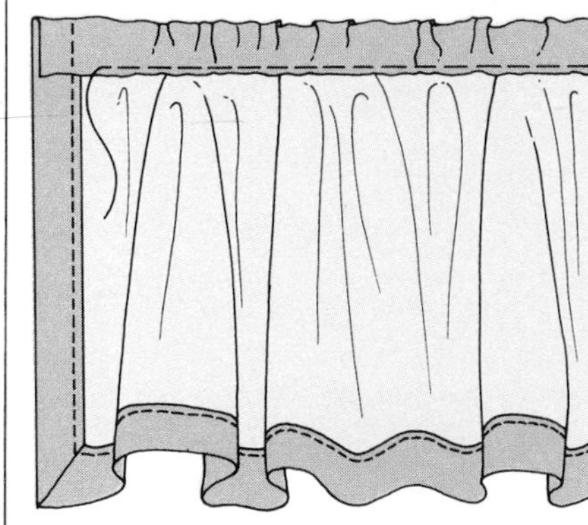

For headed flounce, fold and press the top edge 1″ to the wrong side. Place one row of straight-stitch gathering ⅛″ from the raw edge (or use a gathering foot). Do not gather over the hem at the end. Draw up gathers to fit the top of the spread.

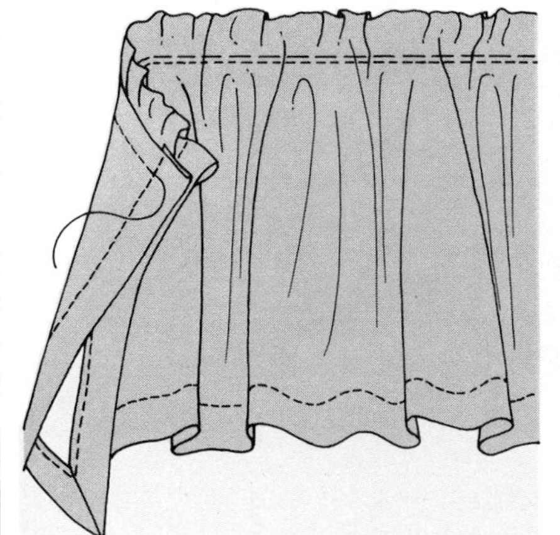

Wrong sides together, pin flounce to the top section, extending flounce ½″ beyond the edge of the top. Stitch ⅛″ below the gathering line. (This distance might be a little more than ⅛″, but should not be less, or the raw edge of the flounce will not be covered.)

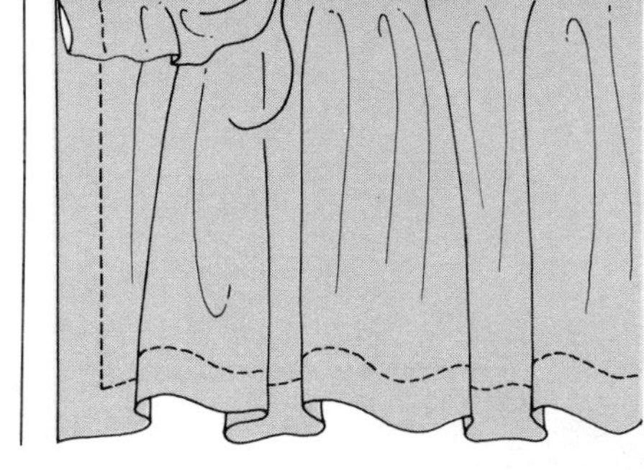

Trim seam allowance on the top section to ⅛″. Fold flounce to right side of the top, and stitch in place ⅛″ above the gathering stitches. All seam allowances are now enclosed.

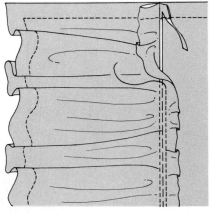

Fitted spread with tailored sides

A **tailored bedspread** has a fitted top and straight sides. The top is the same as for a flounced spread (see opposite page). The drops, where they meet at corners, can be (1) stitched together; (2) pleated; (3) hemmed, with an underlay backing; or (4) hemmed, with no underlay.

Stitched corners produce a snug fit, and a trim look if the fabric is heavy or the spread is lined.

Inverted pleats permit a more flexible fit; work best with light- or medium-weight fabric. Sections should be cut so seams will be at the edge of a backfold, allowing 10 inches for each side of pleat (5 inches folded).

Hemmed edges with an underlay resemble pleats, but are better with bulky fabric. Cut each drop section to fit the top, plus 2 inches for hems. Cut underlays 12 inches wide (omit them if bed has corner posts).

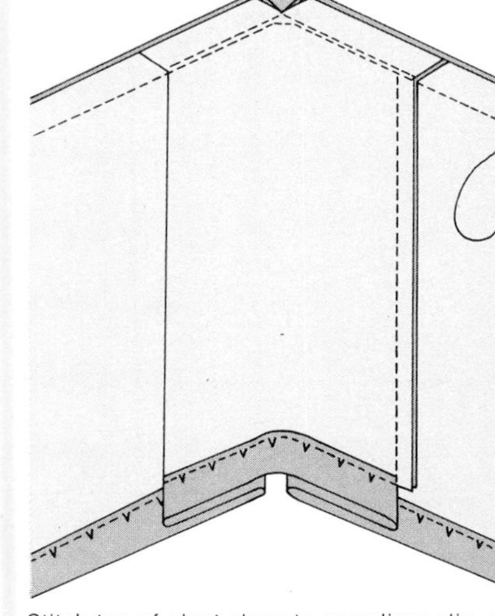

For drop with corner pleats, join sections with ½" seams, having each seam fall at the backfold of a pleat. Finish hem at the bottom, clipping seams above the hem edge.

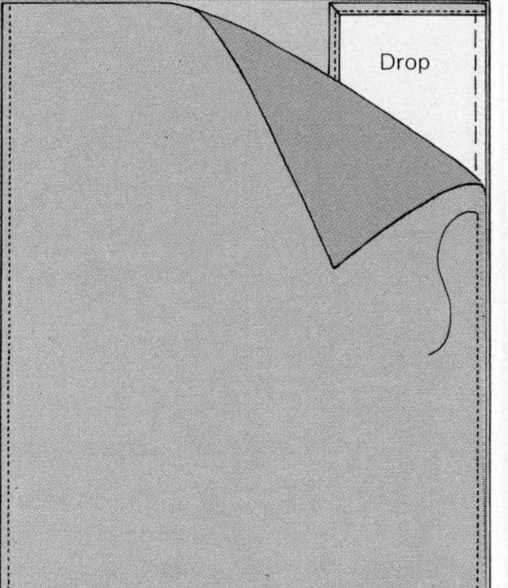

Stitch top of pleat close to seamline; clip center back to stitching. Right sides together, pin sides to top, aligning pleat folds with corners and spreading back of pleat; stitch.

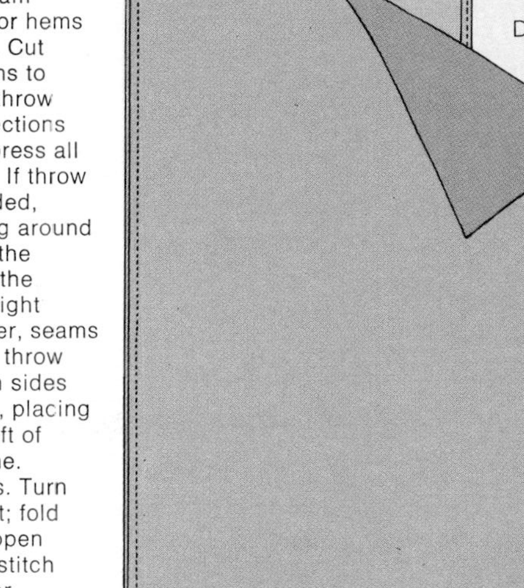

For corner with underlay, hem side and bottom edges of drop sections and underlays. Stitch top of underlay behind opening; clip to stitching at center. Join sides to top.

Lining a bedspread

A bedspread lining can serve several purposes at once. It can add body, enclose seam allowances, take the place of a hem, even, if desired, make the spread reversible. A lining also adds durability when fabric is loosely woven, or has loose floats on the back (brocade, for example).

Lining fabric should be compatible with the spread in care requirements, and at least as wide, so that seams will correspond. A bed sheet might be used, eliminating lining seams.

A throw style is lined from edge to edge. In flounced or tailored styles, usually only the top is lined, though tailored drops might be lined if more body is needed. Directions for lining a fitted top are given at the far right. See the Classic bedroom project for a way to line side sections.

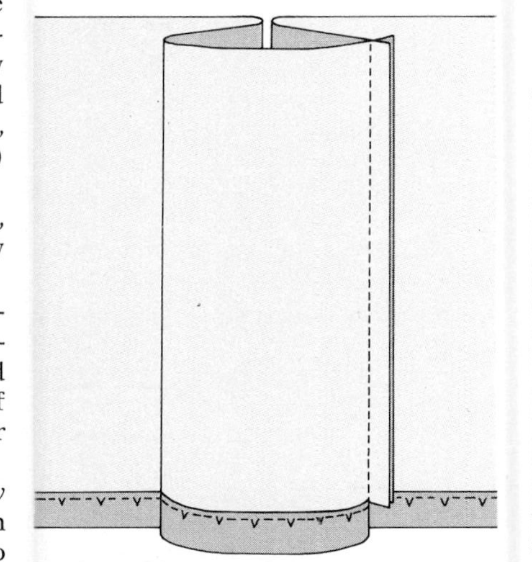

To line a throw, substitute seam allowances for hems on all edges. Cut lining sections to match. Join throw and lining sections separately; press all seams open. If throw is being corded, stitch cording around the edge on the right side of the throw. With right sides together, seams aligned, and throw on top, stitch sides and foot end, placing stitches to left of first stitch line. Notch curves. Turn right side out; fold in edges of open (head) end; stitch folds together.

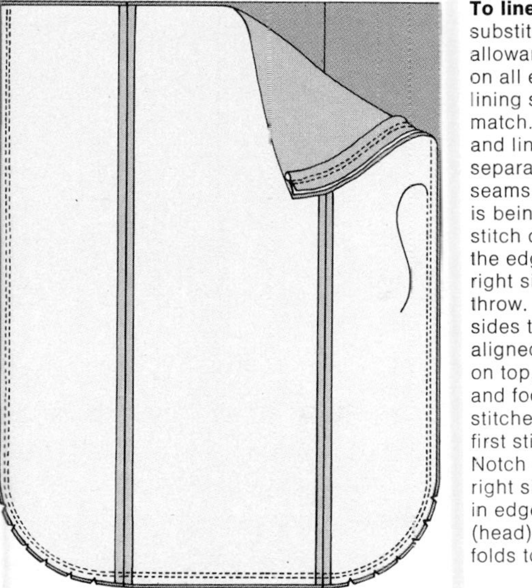

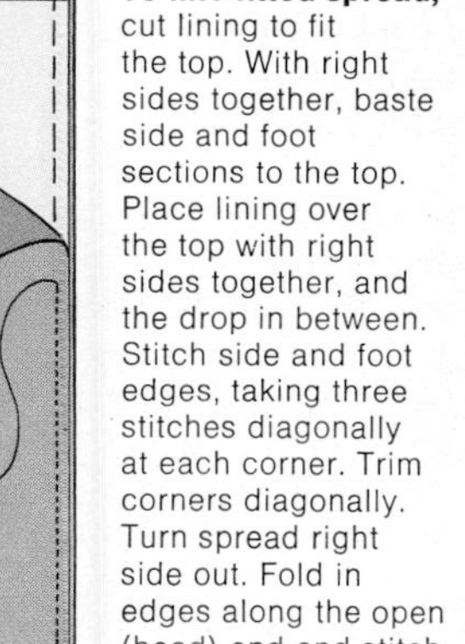

To line fitted spread, cut lining to fit the top. With right sides together, baste side and foot sections to the top. Place lining over the top with right sides together, and the drop in between. Stitch side and foot edges, taking three stitches diagonally at each corner. Trim corners diagonally. Turn spread right side out. Fold in edges along the open (head) end and stitch folds together.

Curtains and draperies

Re-aligning grain 85

Introduction

Curtains and draperies are sewing projects even a novice can undertake. Success depends less on sewing skill than it does on careful measuring and thoughtful relating of style and fabric.

Procedure is basically the same for all window treatments in this section. When you have decided on a style, install the hardware and measure the window area to determine yardage needs (p. 430). Then buy the fabric and proceed with construction according to the requirements of your plan.

Before buying any fabric, appraise its impact on the room. If possible, borrow a large sample from the store, or purchase ½ yard. See how it looks at the window; light behind a fabric can change its look considerably. Check whether the fabric is resistant to sun fading and deterioration and to wrinkles, and what sort of cleaning it will require.

When you shop for rods, mounting fixtures, and accessories, look for types that will support the fabric, as well as create the effect you want. The illustrations, opposite, show the basic varieties; those below show a typical use for each type.

Before you cut or sew, be sure the work area is adequate—two tables side by side for cutting if you do not have one large one; a table next to the machine to support fabric weight during stitching.

Prepare fabric first by straightening ends and pressing out wrinkles. It is best, before cutting each panel, to draw out a crosswise thread and cut on the line that is left (see p. 431 for special considerations in cutting fabric to be matched). Re-align grain, if necessary (see Cutting).

The order of construction, generally, is to sew sides first, heading next, and then hems. Final steps often include weighting of hems and setting of pleats (see p. 435).

Choosing the style

To decide on a window treatment, you must consider far more than mere looks. First, there is **the view.** Do you want to conceal it or frame it? Will an uncovered window create a privacy problem? What about **sunlight?** Should it be controlled? Does the **window type** limit your choice (a French window, for example, that opens in)? Might the look be improved by rods set above or to the sides of the frame? Finally, there is the **room itself.** Will the style harmonize with it? Do you want your window treatment to blend in or stand out?

Window coverings classify into these basic types:

Glass curtains. Made of sheer or semisheer fabric; not lined. The heading is a casing that slips directly over the rod. A *panel* curtain has top casing and bottom hem, and is sometimes embellished with embroidery or flocking. *Casement* style has casings at both top and bottom. *Ruffled* variation (also called priscilla) has ruffles at sides and bottom, is often tied back to the window frame.

Café curtains. Made with any fabric type and heading style; can be lined or not. Cafés cover only a part of the window lengthwise; can provide privacy at one level and light (if desired) at another; are best in informal settings. With overlapping tiers, upper tier covers heading of one below.

Draperies. Made with any fabric type, but generally heavier weights; can be lined or not; heading is usually pleated. Depending on fabric choice and construction, draperies can be decorative, provide privacy, darken a room, insulate against cold. *Panel* draperies cover only the sides of a window area; *draw* draperies span the entire width.

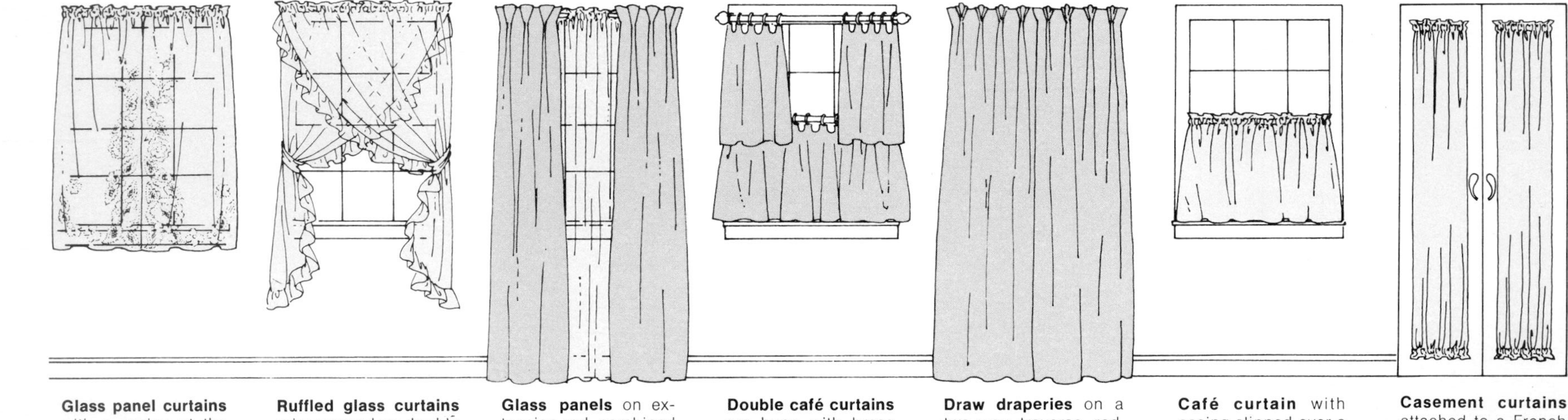

Glass panel curtains with a casing at the top, slipped over a flat curtain rod.

Ruffled glass curtains crisscrossed on double flat rods and tied back to window frame.

Glass panels on extension rod, combined with **panel draperies** on a swinging rod.

Double café curtains are hung with brass rings on the traditional café rod.

Draw draperies on a two-way traverse rod, with traditional pleating at the top.

Café curtain with casing slipped over a tension-rod, mounted in the window frame.

Casement curtains attached to a French door with sash rods at top and bottom.

Rods and fixtures

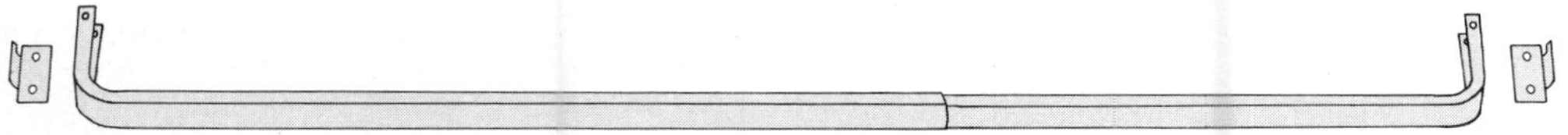

Flat curtain rod, used mainly for stationary curtains; comes in standard and heavy-duty weights, adjustable length.

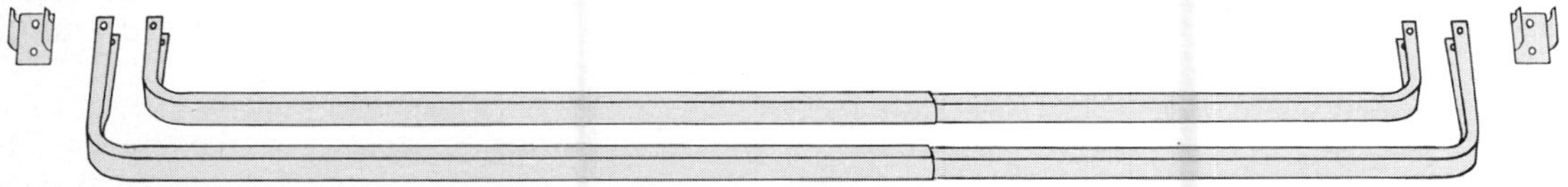

Double flat rods have different return depths; used for multiple curtain layers, such as crisscross style.

Curved flat rod serves the same purpose as flat rod above; fits a curved window frame.

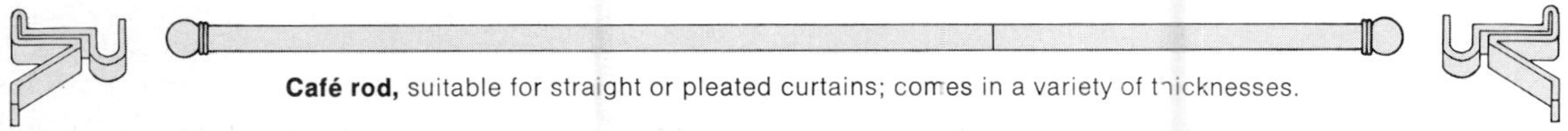

Café rod, suitable for straight or pleated curtains; comes in a variety of thicknesses.

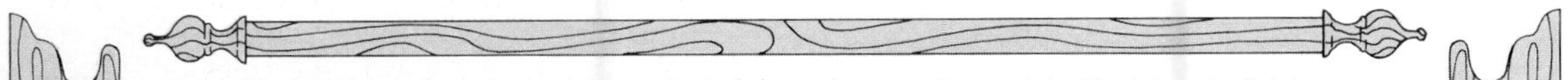

Decorative rod supports plain or pleated draperies; wood or metal with elaborate finials.

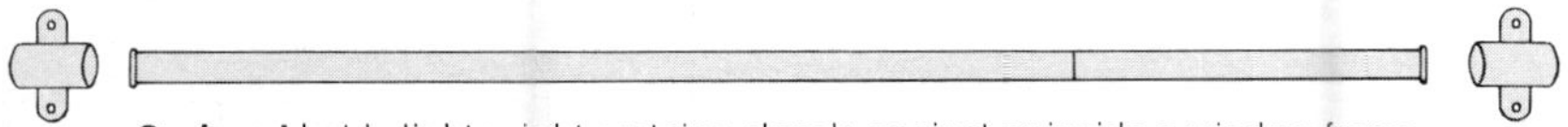

Sash rod holds lightweight curtains closely against or inside a window frame.

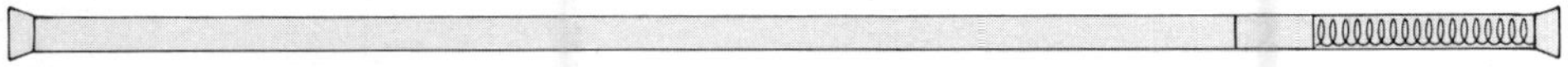

Tension rod holds lightweight curtain inside window frame by means of tension spring; no fixture needed.

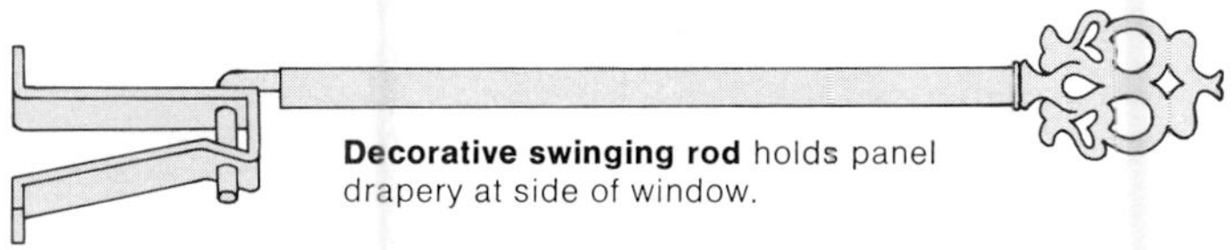

Decorative swinging rod holds panel drapery at side of window.

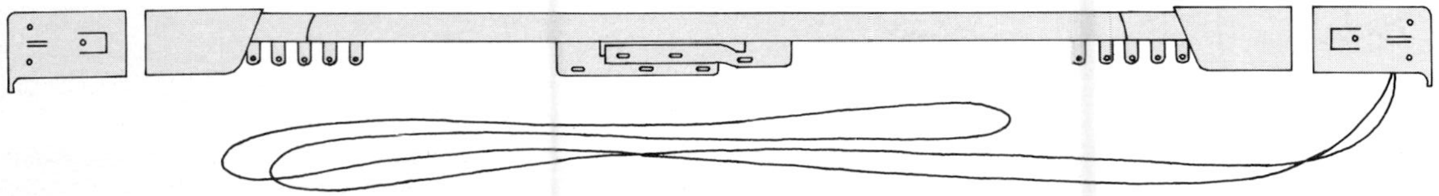

Traverse rod holds draperies to be opened and closed; availabile in one- or two-way draw, also a curved shape.

Accessories

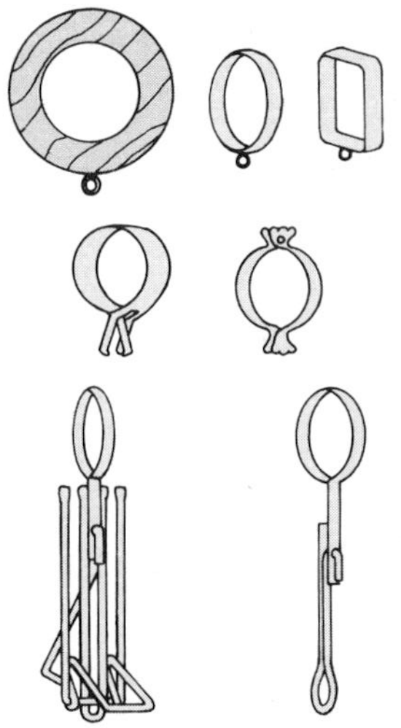

Rings with eyes must be sewed to curtain or drapery; come in variety of shapes and sizes to suit different rod styles.

Clip-on rings are quickly attached and easily removed for laundering; used mainly for café curtains; three-pronged style holds together a simple pleat (see p.433).

A ring-and-hook combination is used with a heading of pleater or scallop tape.

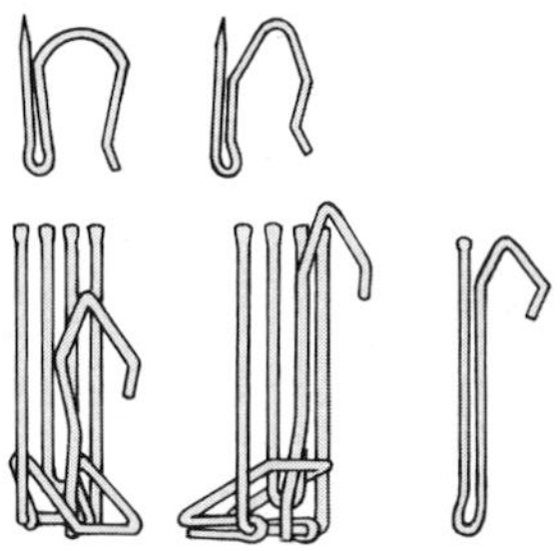

Pin-on hooks hold draperies pleated with plain stiffener; rounded shape is for flat rod, V-shape for traverse.

Pleater-tape hooks slip into pleater pockets; types for regular or ceiling traverse, to hold pleats or ends.

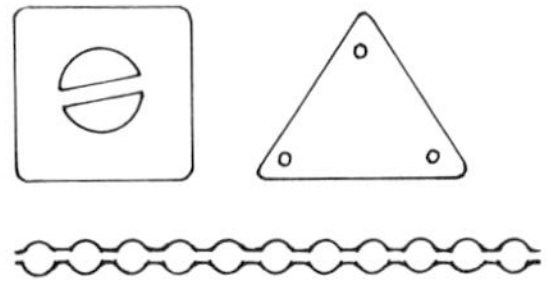

Weights improve hang of draperies or curtains; individual weights are tacked to corners; chain type is inserted in the hem fold.

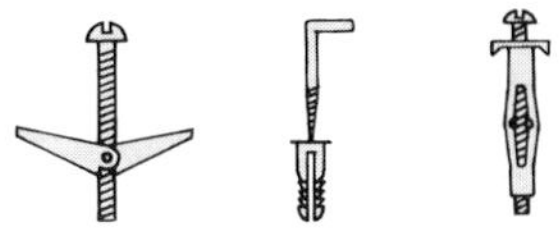

Anchors (toggle, screw, molly) hold bolts or screws securely to support drapery weight.

Curtains and draperies

Estimating yardage

Two measurements are basic for estimating curtain or drapery yardage, finished length and finished width. Install all hardware before measuring; fabric is sewed to fit the supporting device rather than the window. For most accurate results, use a steel tape or folding ruler. If more than one window is being covered, measure each one, even if they all appear to be the same. General measuring procedure is given here. See illustrations below for the specifics of measuring for various styles.

Finished length: Measure from top of rod to place where hem will fall; standard choices are *sash, sill,* bottom of *apron,* or *floor* (see right). For a floor-length style, substract ½ inch to clear the floor, more if there is baseboard heating.

Finished width: Measure the entire span of the rod. If it projects from the wall or frame, include the *return* (distance from fixture to bend in rod). On a traverse rod, measure each half separately from end of slider *(overlap)* to the fixture.

To assure adequate fullness, double the finished width figure; triple it for sheers or other lightweight fabrics. (To achieve the necessary fullness, you may have to join one or more fabric widths—see opposite page.) To this doubled or tripled width, add side hem and/or seam allowances; divide the total by the width of your fabric. If necessary, adjust the figure to the nearest whole number. The result is the *number of panels* required.

To determine the *length* that each panel should be cut, add hem and heading allowances to the finished length measurement. These will vary with the window treatment; for specifics, consult directions for the type you plan to use. In general, it is better to be generous than too exact; some length is always taken up by the fullness. If you plan to include a shrinkage tuck (see p. 432), allow extra fabric for this. If the heading will extend above or fall below the top of the rod (see below), further adjustment in length must be made.

To estimate the yardage requirement, multiply the *total length* for each panel times the *number of panels* needed for each window. (If your measurements are in inches, divide by 36 to convert to yards.) When fabric design must be matched, add one extra motif for each length required.

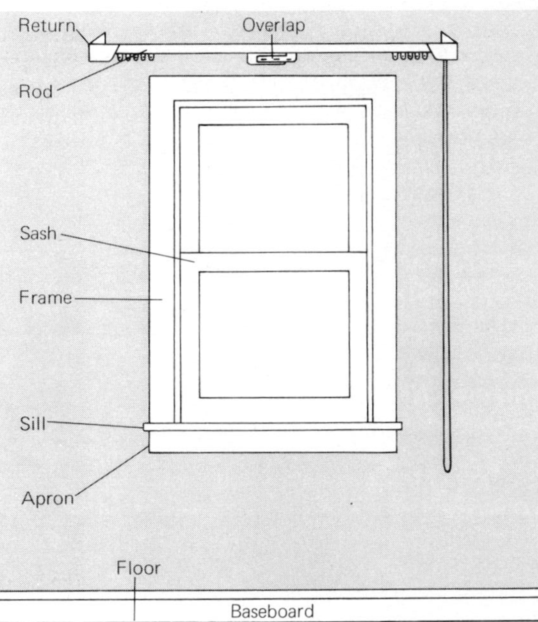

Representative measuring situations

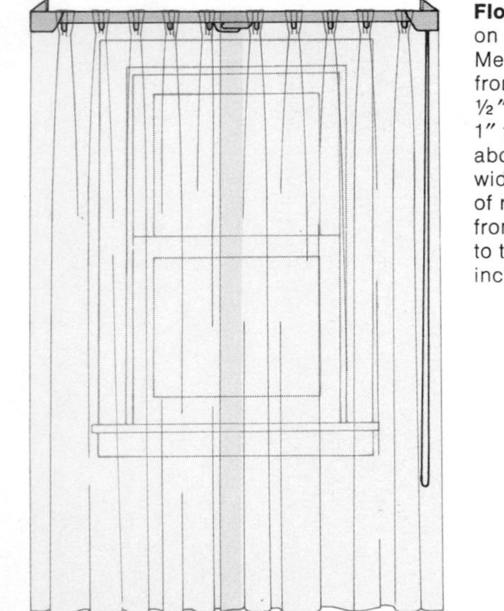

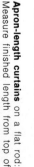

Floor-length draperies on a traverse rod: Measure finished length from top of rod to ½" above the floor; add 1" for heading extension above the rod. For width, measure each half of rod separately, from end of slider to the mounting fixture, including the return.

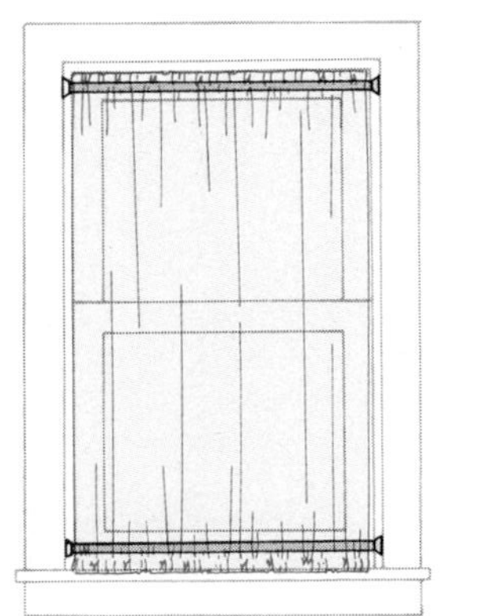
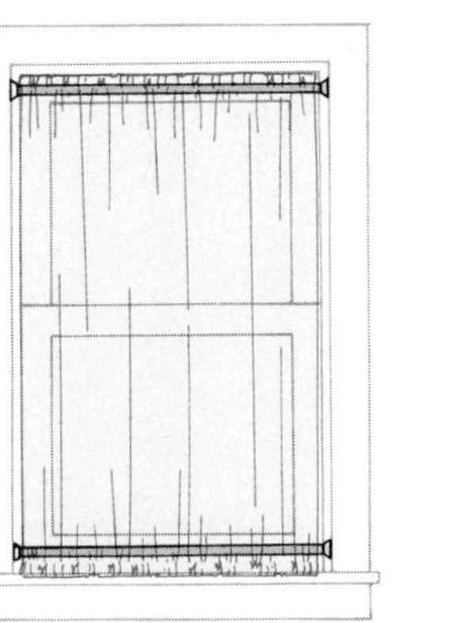

Casement curtains on tension rods: Measure length from top of upper rod to bottom of lower one; add ½" for heading extension at each end. Measure width across inside of frame.

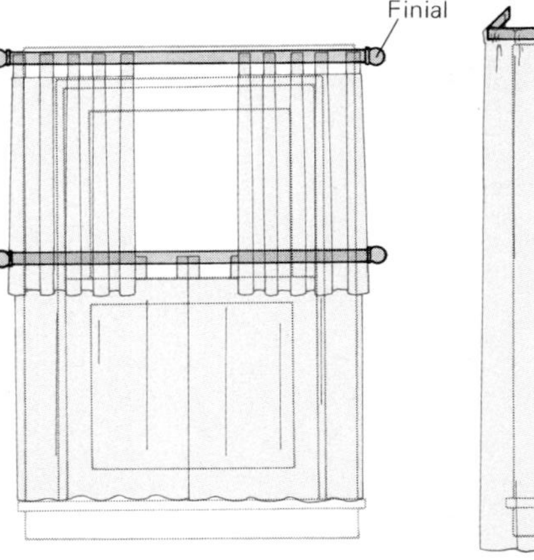

Double café curtains on café rods: Measure upper tier from top of rod to bottom of lower rod; measure lower tier from top of rod to sill. Measure width between finials.

Apron-length curtains on a flat rod: Measure finished length from top of rod to bottom of apron. Measure finished width between the mounting fixtures, including the return.

Adjusting stitch length 30
Machine blind-hemming stitch 138
French and mock French seams 150
Fused hems 295

Matching techniques

When a fabric requires matching, the design should flow without interruption from heading to hem and from side to side. Treatment of the design must be duplicated exactly for each window in the room. Always relate motif placement to finished edges. If the fabric has a vertical repeat, be sure to allow for the overlap, if any. See below for matching and placement of horizontal motifs.

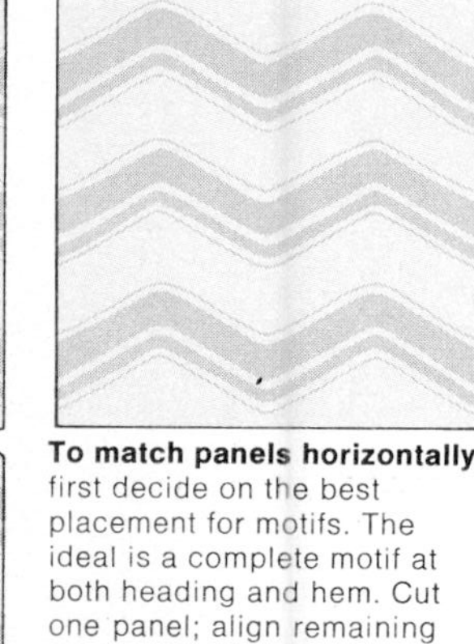

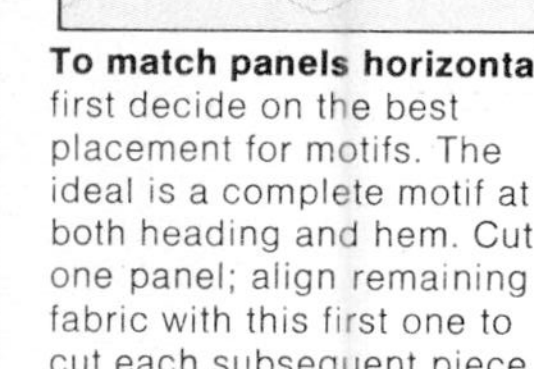

To match panels horizontally, first decide on the best placement for motifs. The ideal is a complete motif at both heading and hem. Cut one panel; align remaining fabric with this first one to cut each subsequent piece.

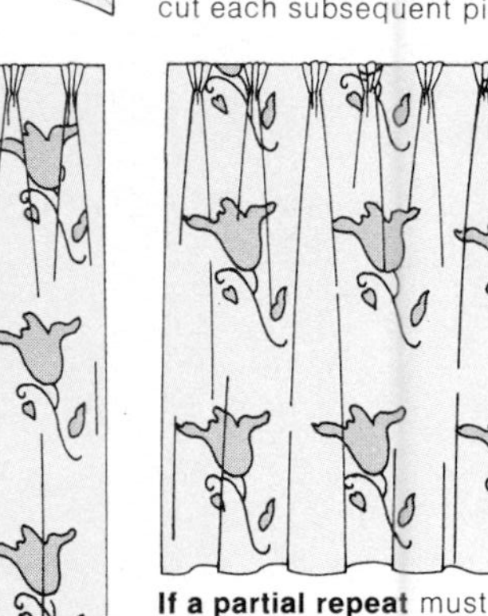

If a partial repeat must be used at one edge, place it at the hem for a floor-length treatment, at the heading for a shorter length. Use a full motif at the opposite end. Such placement makes the cut-off less noticeable.

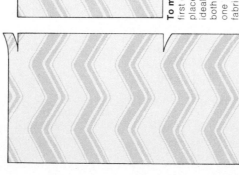

Joining panels

A simple and neat way to join curtain sections is with the interlocking fell seam, illustrated below. In this technique, one edge is pressed and then machine-hemmed over another. An interlocking seam can also be made using a hemmer foot, which will fold the extending edge while you stitch. For better control of fabric that must be matched, use a French or mock French seam.

For interlocking fell seam, lay sections with right sides together, and top piece ¼" from edge of piece beneath (a bit more than ¼" for heavy fabric).

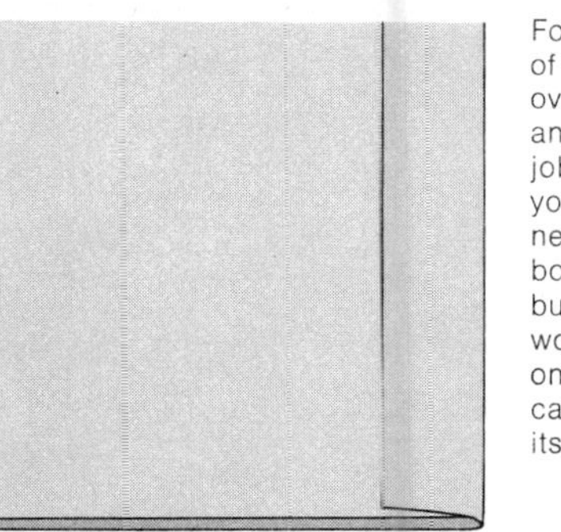

Fold extended edge of under layer over the top one, and press. This job is easier if you set a table next to the ironing board to support bulk of fabric. Or work directly on a large table, carefully protecting its surface.

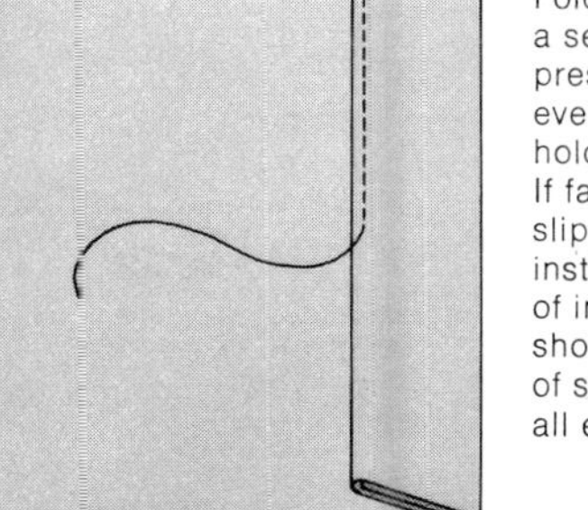

Fold both layers a second time and press again. Pin every 4" or 5" to hold layers in place. If fabric is very slippery, baste instead. Stitch edge of inside fold, as shown. This one line of stitching holds all edges enclosed.

Side hems

Side hems for unlined panels are made before the heading or bottom hem (except for a covered heading, p. 432). Machine techniques and fusing are recommended. Side hems can be single, as below, or double (p. 435); standard finished width is 1 inch. A finishing alternative (for sheers only) is to use the selvage, provided it does not pull. Also, a ruffle can be added (p. 435).

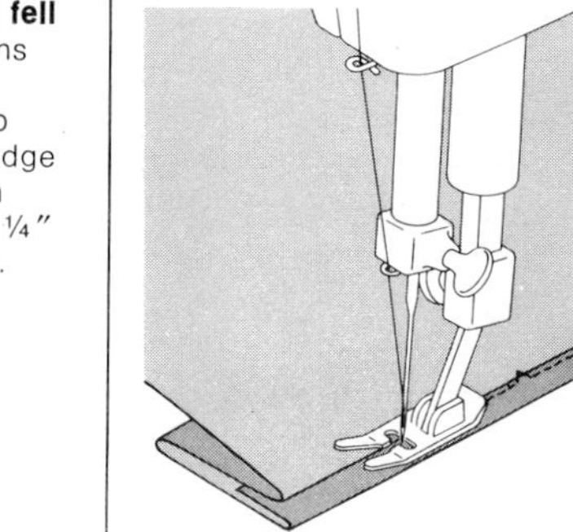

For blindstitched hem, turn and press hem allowance; press the hem edge under at least ⅜". Adjust your machine for blind-hemming stitch. Fold back curtain or drapery portion to reveal hem edge. Stitch, catching only the curtain in the zigzag stitch.

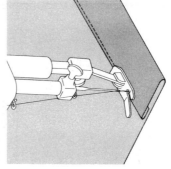

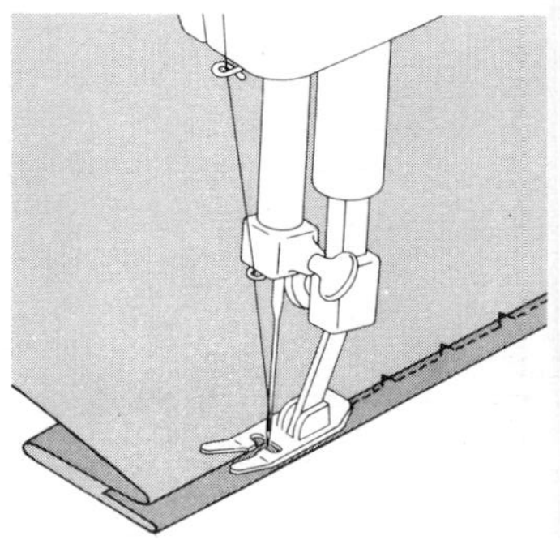

For straight-stitched hem, turn and press the hem allowance; press the hem edge under at least ¼". Adjust machine for 8 to 10 stitch length. Stitch along the hem edge, taking care to keep grainlines of hem and curtain aligned.

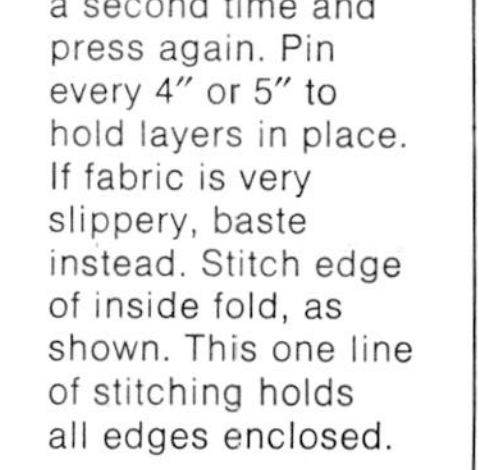

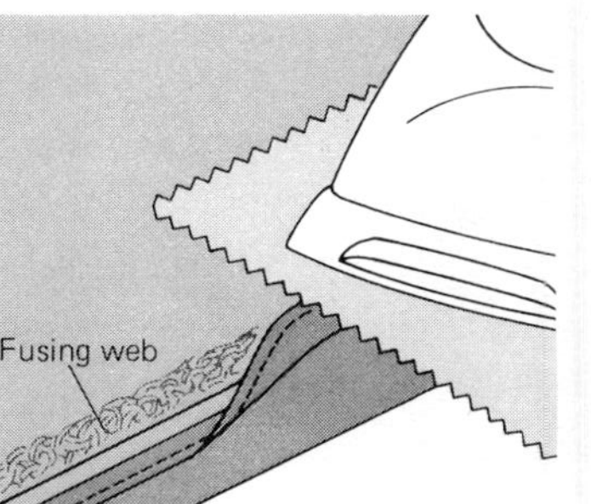

For a fused hem, turn and press the hem allowance; press the hem edge under at least ¼"; stitch close to fold. Slip fusing web between hem and curtain. Set iron for steam and heat-baste, then fuse, covering hem with damp press cloth (see Hems for more details).

Casings

The fullness of a glass curtain is generally controlled with a casing. This is a hem that slips over the curtain rod, forcing the fabric to gather in soft folds. The casing can be plain or have a heading that extends above the rod (see right).

Fabric allowance for a plain casing should equal the diameter of the rod, plus ½ inch for turning under the edge, and some ease allowance so the fabric will slip easily over the rod. Ease should be ¼ to ½ inch, depending on fabric thickness. (You can pin the fabric over the rod to determine the right amount.) If you want a heading, add twice the desired depth to the above measurements. To provide a shrinkage tuck (if you want to avoid preshrinking washable fabric), add 2 more inches.

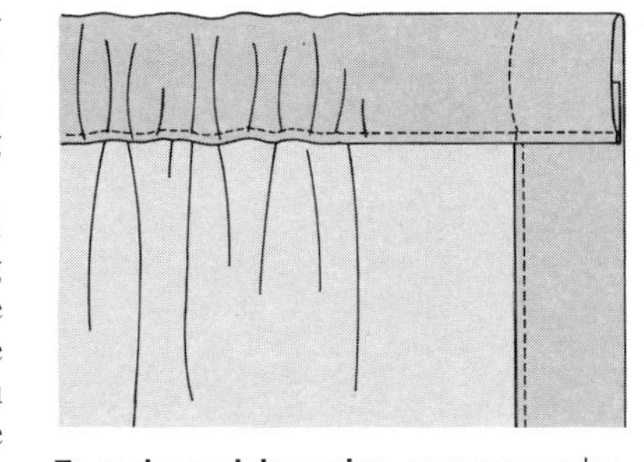

To make a plain casing, press raw edge under ½″, then turn down a casing equal in depth to the diameter of the rod, plus the suitable ease allowance. Stitch in place on pressed edge.

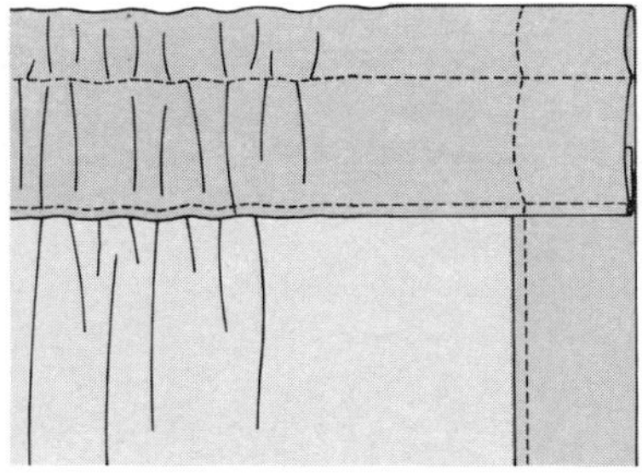

To stitch casing with heading, decide casing width as above, adding in half of the total heading allowance. Turn raw edge under ½″, press, and stitch. Stitch again at the heading depth.

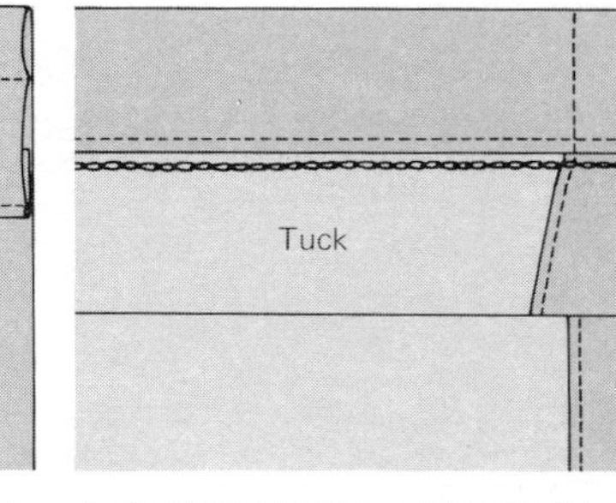

A shrinkage tuck is added on the wrong side, just below the casing. Sewed with the machine stitch that is easiest to remove, it can be let out if the curtain should shrink in laundering.

Preparing the heading for pleats

A pleated heading is used for most drapery styles, and sometimes for café curtains as well. It can be made with plain stiffener, on which pleats must be measured and sewed; or with pleater tape, into which hooks are inserted to form the pleats.

Plain stiffener (backing) permits greater flexibility in depth, spacing, and style of pleats. Materials suitable for backing are firm, nonwoven interfacing, or buckram (for a stiffer result). To attach plain backing, you can use either of the methods below. Backing in the first method is covered completely, so that the heading is finished, but somewhat bulky. In the second, it is left exposed. In both cases, the heading depth is usually 4 inches, but might be less for a short panel.

With *pleater tape,* only one pleat style is possible (see opposite). The procedure is quick, however, and the heading flattens out for cleaning or laundering. Before attaching pleater tape, you must calculate the number and spacing of pleats, adjusting drapery width to fit the tape, if necessary. Use Method 2, below, to apply it.

Prepare drapery for pleated heading as follows:

Method 1: Allow 4½ inches for the heading; fold and press this allowance to the wrong side. Cut stiffening 4 inches wide and long enough to fit the hemmed drapery width. Do not hem the sides.

Method 2: Allow ½ inch for heading. Cut stiffening to fit the hemmed drapery width plus 1 inch. Turn under and finish the side hems (see p. 431).

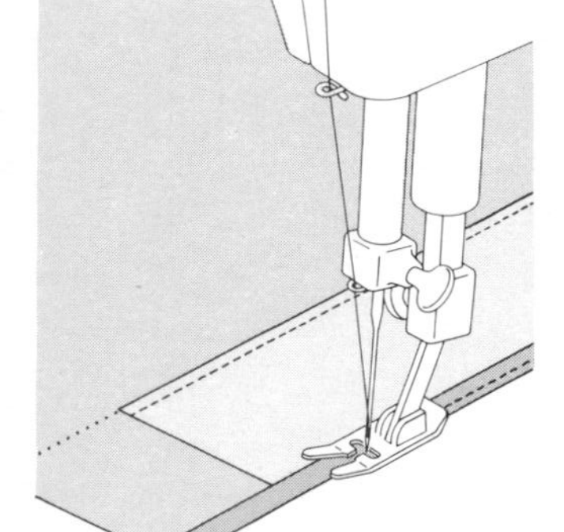

Method 1: Open out heading; align lower edge of stiffener with the crease; stitch ¼″ from this edge. Fold and press top edge of fabric over stiffener; stitch as shown.

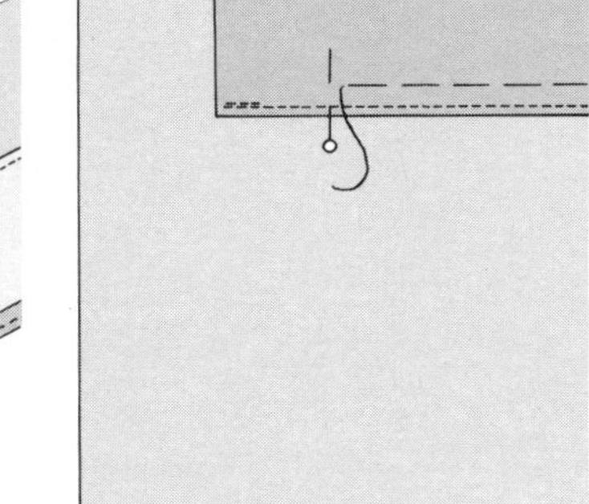

Re-fold heading to the wrong side. Pin, then baste. Trim hem allowances from the heading, cutting it to within ½″ of top fold, then cutting diagonally to the fold.

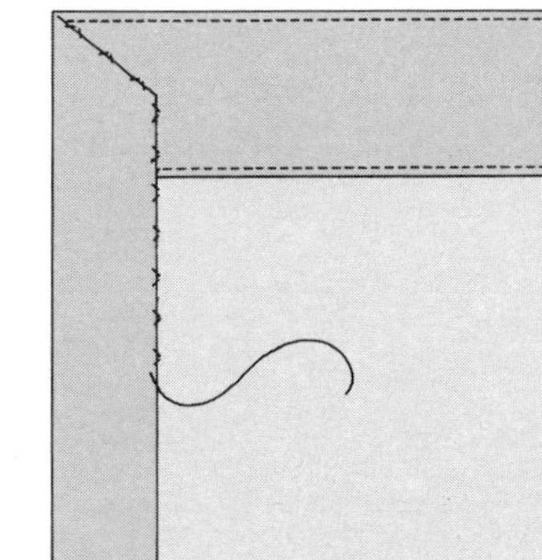

Fold and press the side hems in place, turning in the top corner diagonally to form a miter. Finish with a slipstitch, or a machine stitch, if preferred. Remove basting.

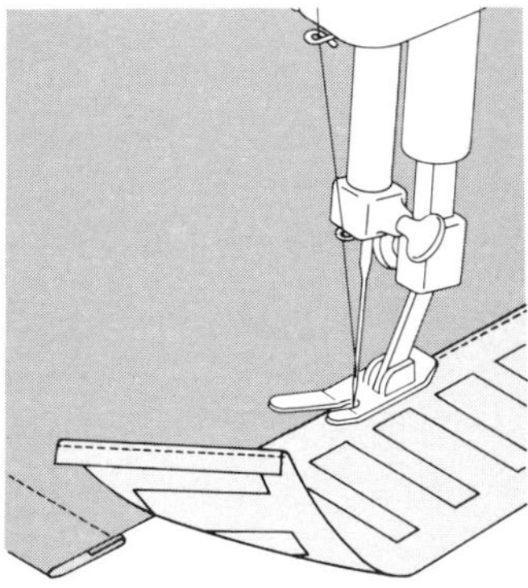

Method 2: Turn stiffener ends under ½″; stitch fold. Lay it over right side of fabric, lapping edges ½″. Stitch on edge. (For pleater tape, stitch on woven guideline.)

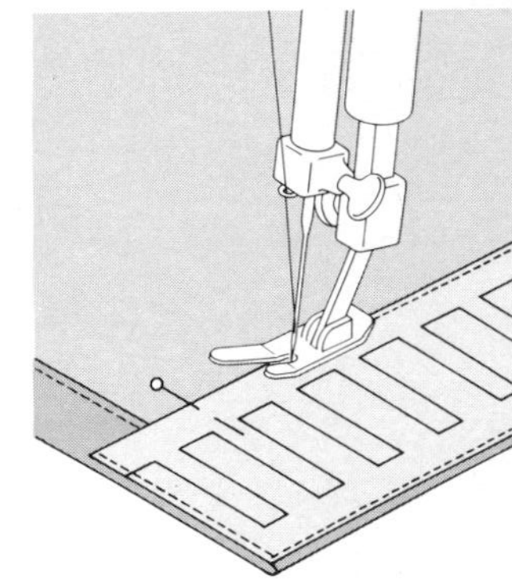

Fold and press the stiffener to the wrong side of fabric, making sure that none of it shows on the right side; pin in place; stitch ¼″ from the lower edge.

Gathering by hand 131, 179

How to space the pleats

To determine the depth and spacing of pleats, first measure and pin-mark the returns and overlaps on the right side of each panel. If there are none, mark off a 2-inch space at both ends. Subtract the combined widths of these unpleated areas from the finished width (as measured on p. 430), and divide the adjusted figure by the number of panels to be pleated. This is the *finished width* that the pleated portion of each panel should be.

To establish how much fabric should be taken up by pleats, measure between your two pin marks and subtract the *finished width* from this amount. To calculate the number of pleats, divide this figure by the amount allotted for each one (see below). Result should be an *uneven* number.

Make the first two pleats at each end and the third pleat midway between these two, then space the remaining pleats in between.

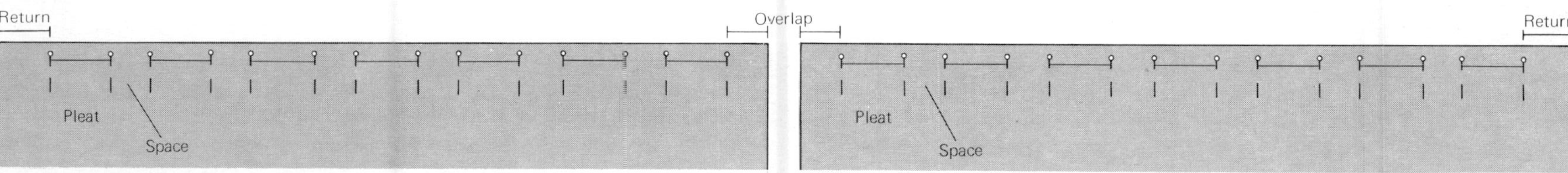

Panels marked with returns and overlaps are made to fit the right and left sides of a window and will not be interchangeable. Space the pleats evenly between the overlap and the return.

Forming the pleats

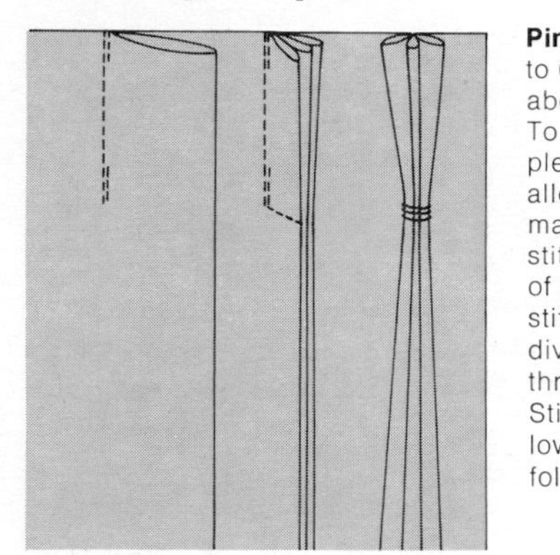

Pinch pleats: Allow 5″ to 6″ for each pleat, about 4″ in between. To make the basic pleat, fold the pleat allowance in half, matching pin marks; stitch from top of heading to end of stiffener. Next, divide the pleat into three parts; press. Stitch across the lower end, or tack folds by hand.

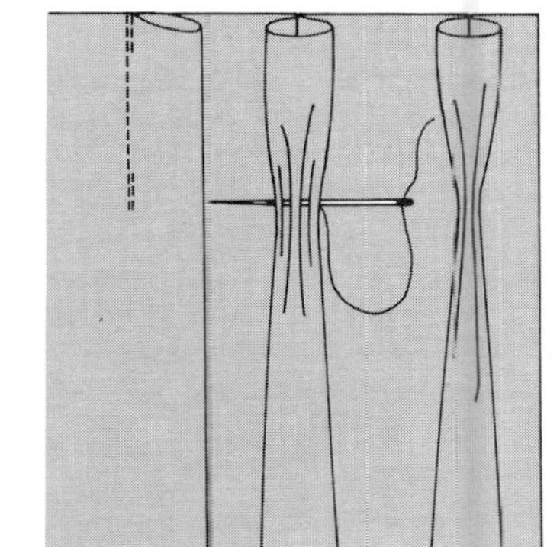

French pleats: Allow 5″ to 6″ for each pleat, 4″ in between. Make a basic pleat and divide it in thirds, but do not press the folds. Using heavy-duty thread or buttonhole twist, gather pleat by hand across the bottom of the heading, drawing thread tightly. For heavy fabric, sew through the pleat more than once.

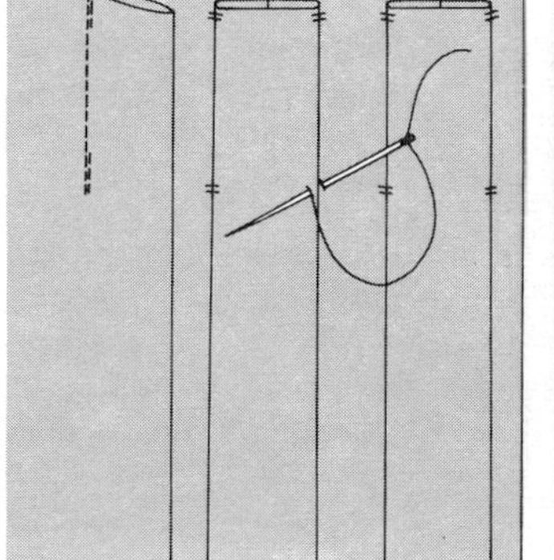

Box pleats: Allow 4″ for each pleat, about 4″ in between. Make the basic pleat as directed for pinch pleats; then press the pleat allowance flat to make two folds each the same distance from the stitching. Tack the folds by hand at top and bottom of heading.

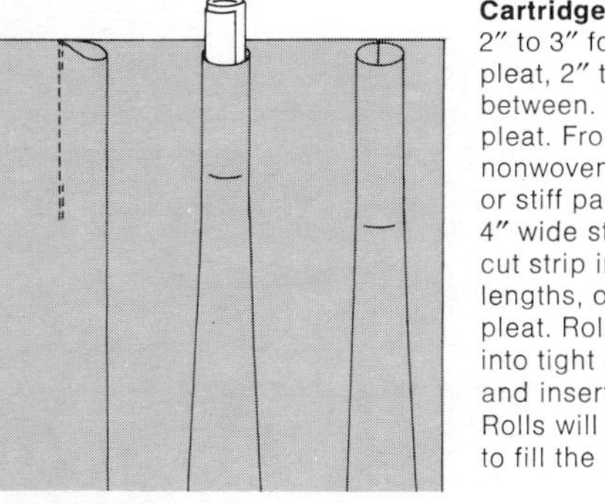

Cartridge pleats: Allow 2″ to 3″ for each pleat, 2″ to 3″ in between. Sew a basic pleat. From buckram, nonwoven interfacing, or stiff paper, cut a 4″ wide strip, then cut strip into 3″ lengths, one for each pleat. Roll stiffener into tight cylinders and insert into pleats. Rolls will expand to fill the pleats.

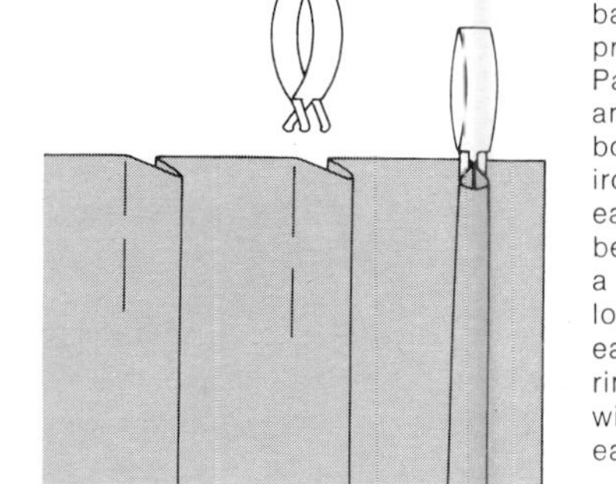
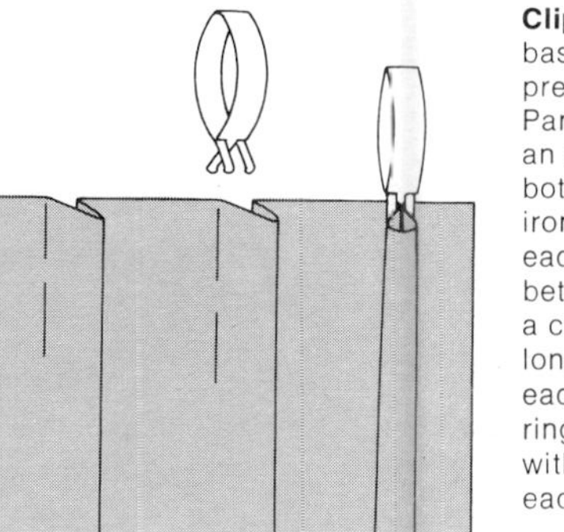

Clip-on rings hold a basic pleat that is pressed, not stitched. Panels remain flat, an advantage in both laundering and ironing. Allow 2″ for each pleat, 3″ in between. Press a crease, 4″ to 6″ long, at the center of each pleat. Clip the rings to pleats, with a prong holding each side, as shown.

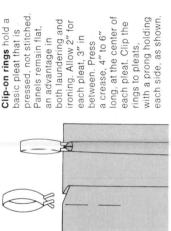

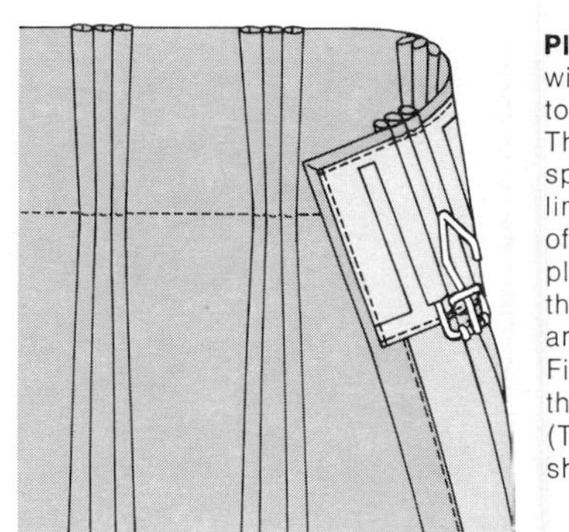

Pleater hooks are used with pleater tape to form pinch pleats. The pleat depths and spaces between are limited by the spacing of pockets. To form a pleat, insert each of the four prongs into an adjacent pocket. Finger-press the folds that are formed. (These cannot be sharply creased.)

Curtain and drapery headings

Slipstitch 132 Grading and clipping seam allowances 147
Making belt carriers 252, 401

Scallops

A graceful top finish for café curtains, scallops can be used on a plain or a pleated heading. There should be an *uneven* number on each panel, with at least ½ inch or a pleat width between them. To make your own pattern, cut a strip of paper the width of the hemmed curtain. Across the top, mark scallop widths and spaces between them, centering the first scallop. Make the scallops half as deep as they are wide, using a compass, scallop ruler, or plate to draw them. When cutting the curtains, allow for a self-facing at the top equal to the scallop depth plus 2½ inches. Cut stiffening (from nonwoven interfacing) the length and depth of the facing less ½ inch. The rod will be visible so choose one to complement your fabric.

To prepare the heading, turn the facing edge under ½" and press. Fold facing allowance to the right side. Baste stiffener to the curtain top on the wrong side. Pin pattern over stiffener and carefully trace the scallops. Remove pattern.

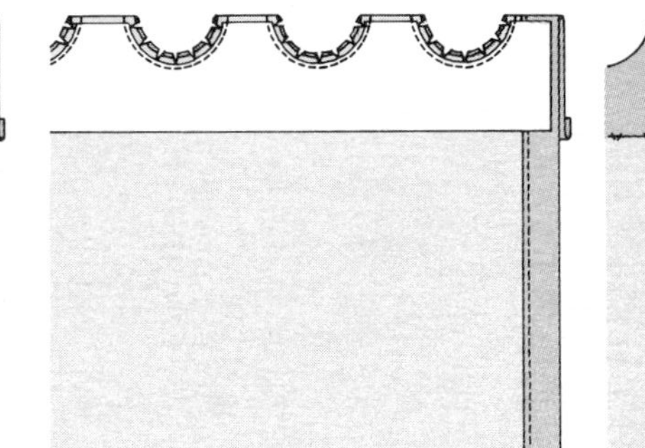

Stitch around scallops on the traced lines. Trim the stiffener close to the stitching. Grade seam allowances within each scallop. Clip the curves.

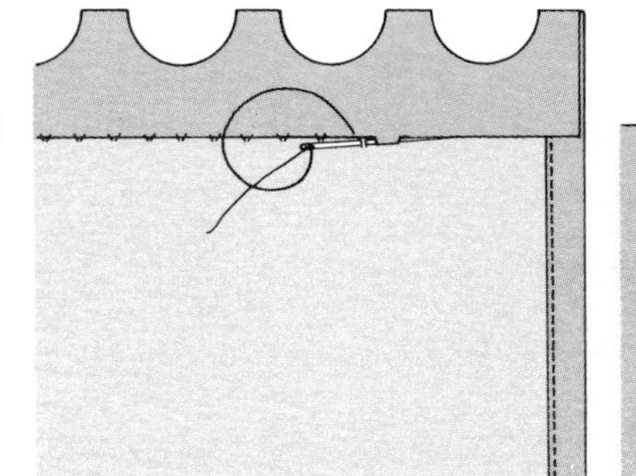

Turn the facing to the wrong side, over the stiffener. Slipstitch the facing to the curtain along the folded edge, and at the side hems. Machine-stitch, if preferred.

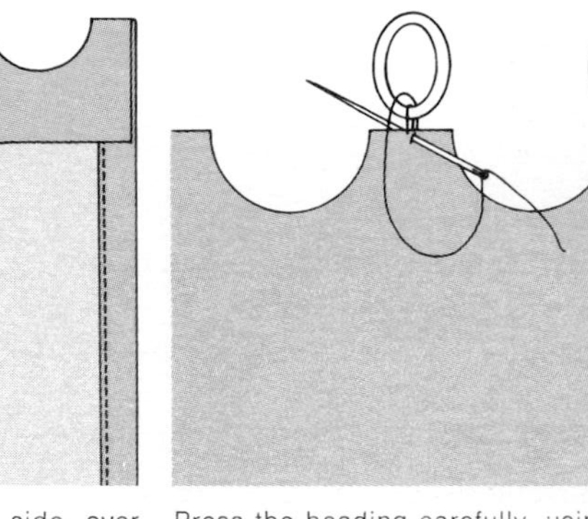

Press the heading carefully, using a pin, if necessary, to pull out corners at the top of each scallop. Attach rings (clip-on or sew-on) between the scallops.

Loops

A looped heading can give special interest to an otherwise plain window treatment. The loops should be long enough to slip easily over the rod. The number and spacing of the loops depends to some extent on their width, but there should be enough to support the curtain adequately.

When planning panel length, be sure to figure the finished loop length into the total; also, allow ½ inch for a top seam. Fabric loops can be prepared by one of the methods for making a belt carrier. Braid loops require no preparation, unless you want to sew two lengths back to back.

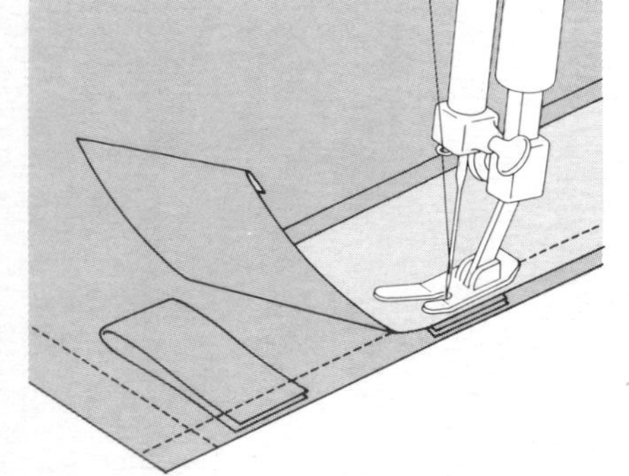

Fabric loops. Prepare loops. Fold and baste to right side of curtain, raw edges aligned. Stitch ¼" from the edge. Apply a facing over the loops, stitching ⅜" from edge.

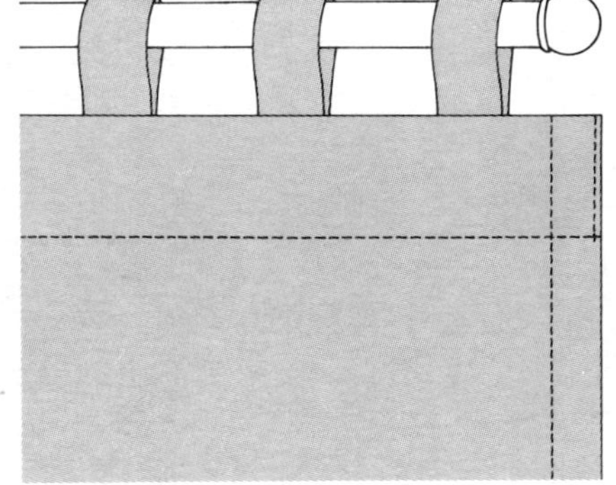

Press facing to wrong side. Machine-stitch side and lower edges of facing to curtain or, if preferred, slipstitch them. Slip curtain over a café or decorative rod.

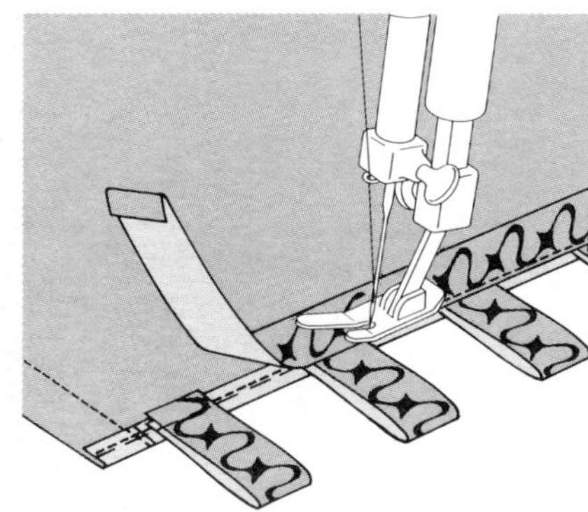

Braid or ribbon loops. Cut the loops. Press top of curtain ½" to right side. Baste loops over folded edge, as shown. Stitch them ¼" from the fold. Cut a length of braid to the width of the curtain plus 1"; fold the ends under ½". Position top edge close to fabric fold and stitch, then stitch ends and lower edge. All loop ends will be neatly enclosed.

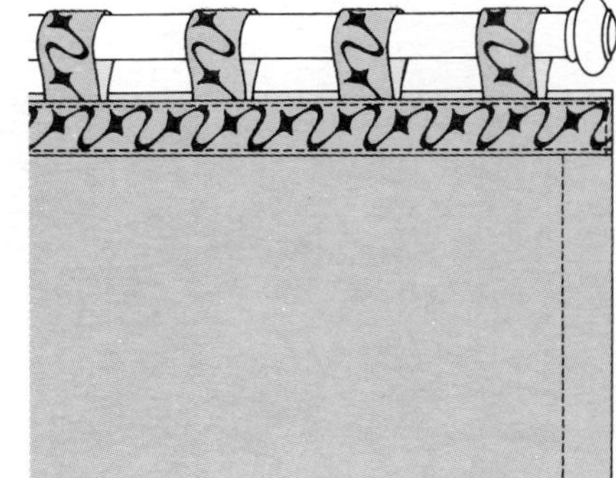

Hems

Hemming techniques: hand 128-129, 292; machine 294
Making a ruffle with heading 184-185
Narrow machine-stitched hem 294

Allowances and methods

To assure accuracy in the finished length of curtains or draperies, fold and baste hem allowances, hang panels a few days, then adjust if necessary. A hem at the sill should just clear; one at the floor should clear by ½ inch; combined curtains and draperies should be the same length. If using weights, pin or tack them in place to test the effect.

Average hem allowances are 2 inches for curtains, 3 to 6 inches for draperies, depending on length. While a single hem is adequate for medium-weight or heavy fabric, a double hem is recommended for sheers, and will improve the hang of any fabric. Of various ways to finish hems, machine methods and fusing are most practical but many people prefer hand-finished draperies.

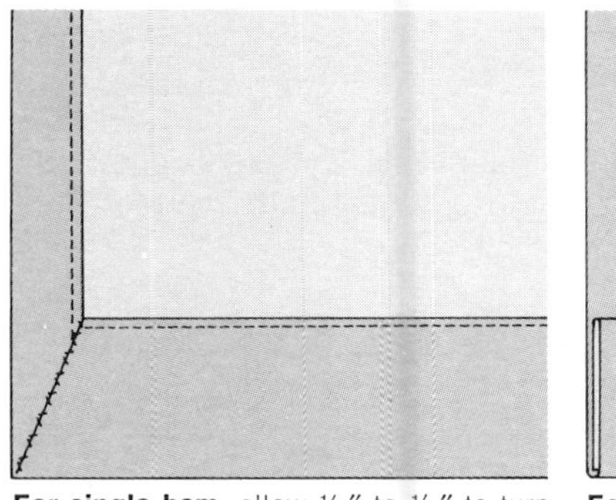

For single hem, allow ¼″ to ½″ to turn under at edge. At each corner, turn edge in diagonally to form a miter.

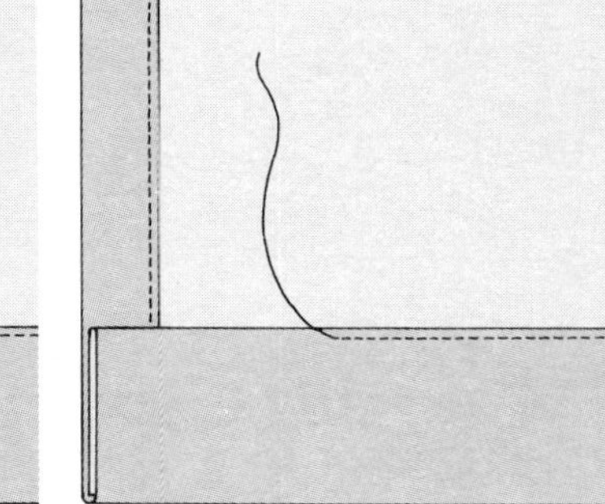

For double hem, allow turn-under equal to hem depth. Keeps edge from showing through sheers, and adds weight.

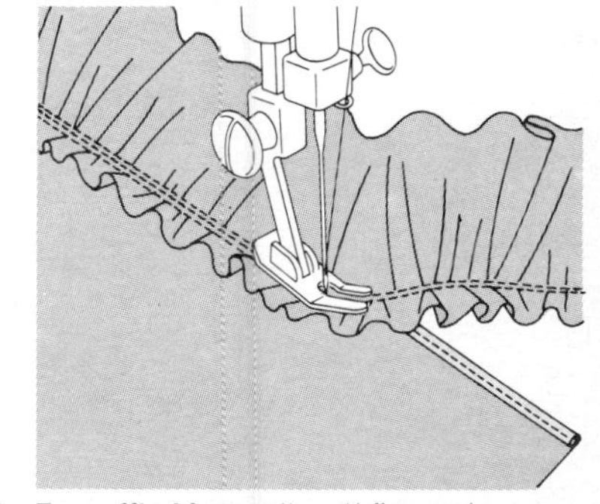

For ruffled hem, allow ½″ to make a narrow machine-stitched hem, folded to right side. Topstitch ruffle over hem.

Weighting and anchoring hems

Curtains and draperies hang better when hems are weighted or anchored. Individual weights are used for heavier fabrics. They are attached at corners and at bottoms of seams to prevent drawing. Chain types are run through the hems of sheer and other lightweight panels to encourage even hanging and minimize billowing. Cup hooks can also be used to hold side hems straight and stationary.

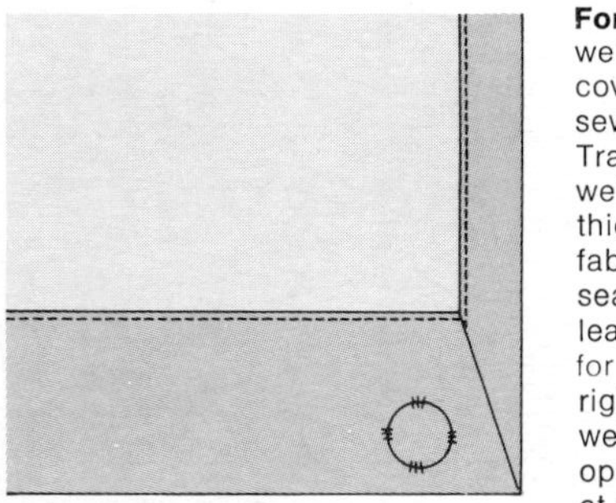

For unlined curtains, weights should be covered before sewing to the hem. Trace shape of weight onto a double thickness of curtain fabric; add ¼″ for seaming. Stitch, leaving an opening for turning. Turn right side out, slip weight in, and close opening. Sew to hem at corners and seams.

For lined draperies, cover the weight with lining fabric as described above for unlined panels. Sew the weight to the drapery hem, high enough so that lining hangs over it. If preferred, the weight can be sewed on, with no covering, as you would a button.

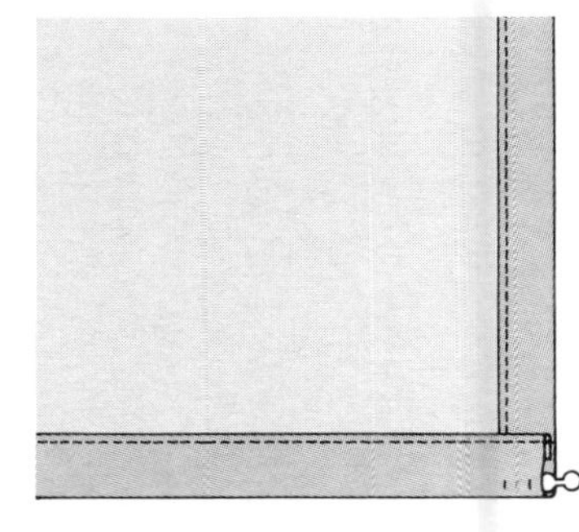

For sheer curtains, the best choice is a covered chain weight. It should be purchased in a length to equal the width of the curtain. Slip weight through the hem, then tack in place with a few stitches at side hems and at any seams.

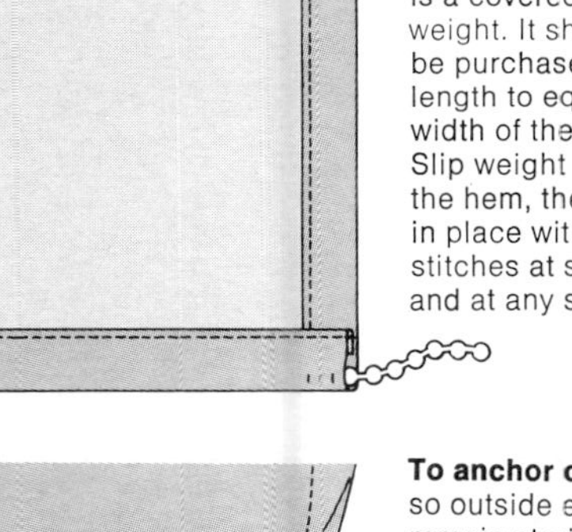

To anchor curtains so outside edges will remain straight and taut, use small plastic rings and cup hooks. Sew rings to bottom hem of curtains at outer edge, then screw cup hooks into the wall behind the rings. Hooks should point down to hold most securely. Place ring in hook.

Setting pleats

To hang gracefully, pleat folds may need setting: When draperies are hung, arrange the folds carefully. Pin them in position at the bottom, or tie them loosely with soft cord or tape, using T-pins to support tape, if necessary. Leave them in place for a few days.

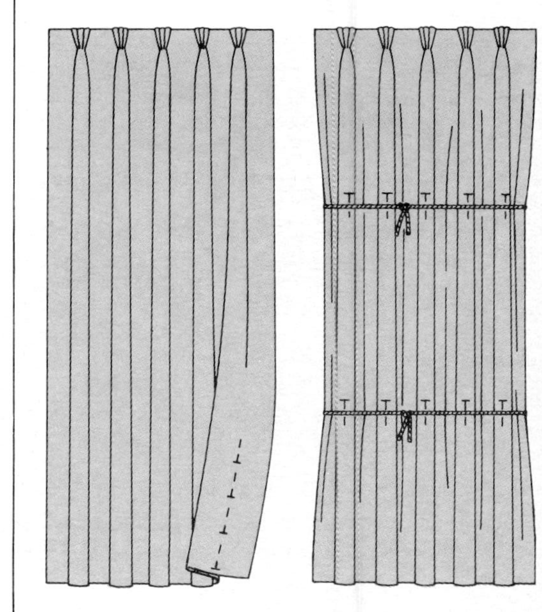

Hemming techniques: hand 128-129, 292; machine 294

Slipstitch 132
French tack 134

Making a lining

Lining gives a more finished look to draperies or café curtains and, at the same time, adds opaqueness, protects fabric from fading, and helps insulate against cold or heat. Lining fabric is usually an opaque cotton, such as sateen or muslin, in white or off-white. Specially treated fabrics are also available for extra insulation.

When cutting panels to be lined, allow 5 inches for self-facings at sides, 3½ inches for a bottom hem, and ½ inch for the top seam. Cut the lining 5 inches narrower than the drapery at the sides, 3½ inches shorter at the bottom. The hem allowances here are for short curtains. For floor-length panels, allow more depth—at least 5 to 6 inches for the drapery panels, and about 3 inches for the lining.

The basic procedure is to hem the lining, then stitch it to each side of the drapery panel (when drapery is turned right side out, it will have a 2-inch self-facing on each side). Next, prepare the heading, then form the pleats as directed on page 433. Finish the lower edges as specified below.

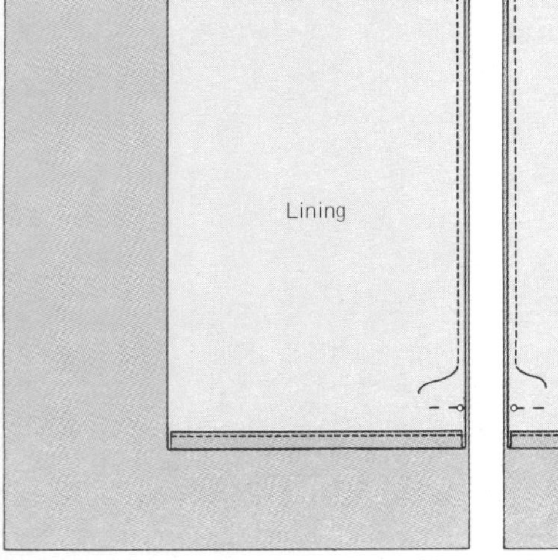

1. Make a 1" hem at lining bottom. Place lining on drapery, right sides together, top and right edges aligned. Stitch ½" seam from top to 2" above lining hem.

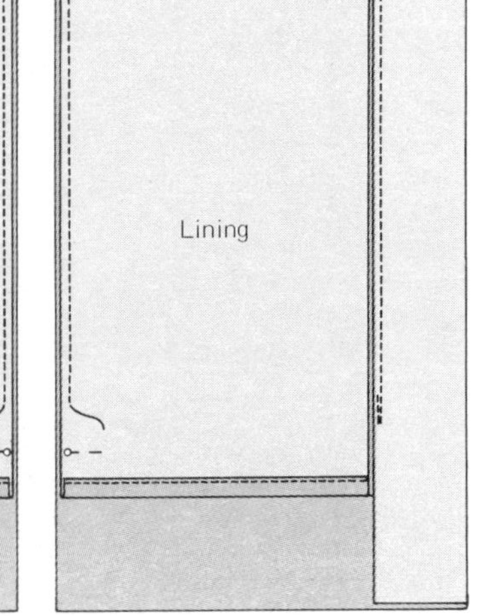

2. Pull lining over to left side, aligning edge with that of drapery. Stitch ½" seam, starting at top, ending 2" above lining hem.

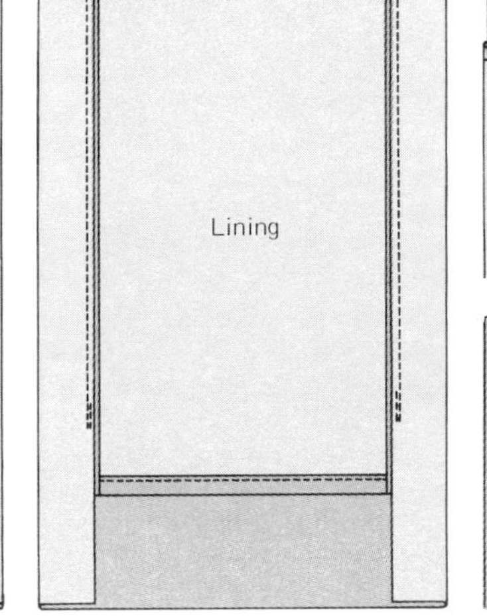

3. Center lining on the drapery; press seams toward the lining. Stitch across top of lining and drapery, ½" from the edge.

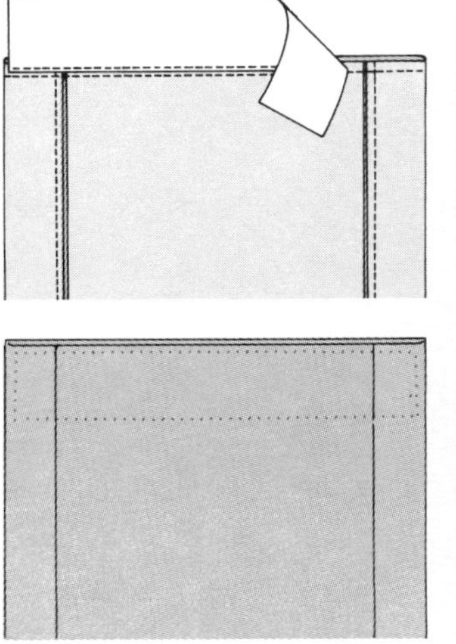

For covered heading, align edge of stiffener with top seam, as shown; stitch the edge. Turn panel right side out. Press sides.

For pleater tape heading, do not stitch top in Step 3. Turn drapery right side out; baste top edges. Sew tape as in Method 2, p. 432.

Finishing lower edges of lined draperies

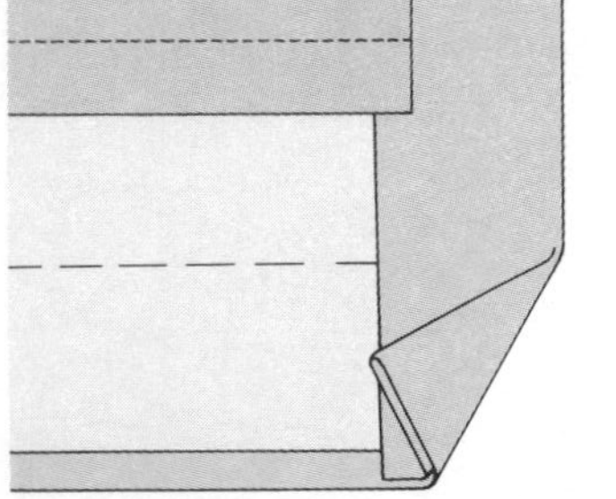

To hand-finish lower edges, fold and press hem edge under ½"; turn corner in diagonally. (For bulky fabric, trim excess from corner.)

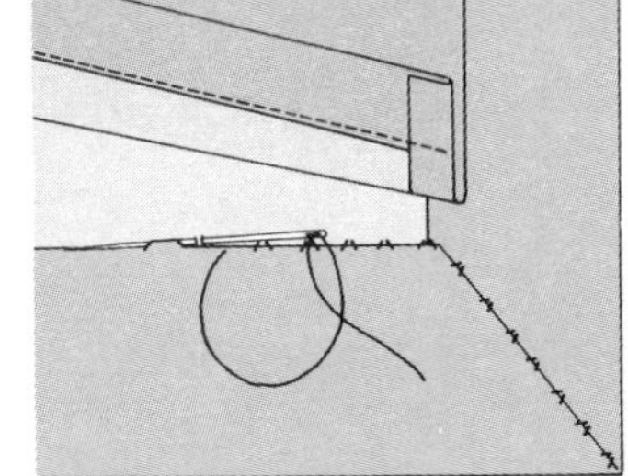

Turn up hem; slipstich in place. If a different hand or machine finish is preferred, consult the Hems chapter for suitable method.

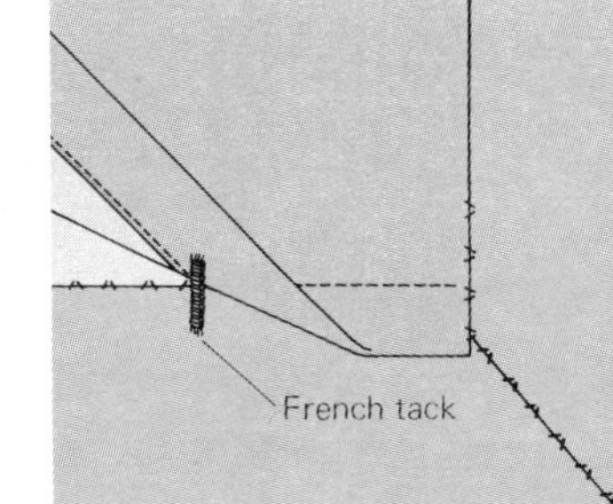

Slipstitch remainder of lining to the facing and hem. Anchor lining to drapery hem every 10 inches to keep the layers aligned.

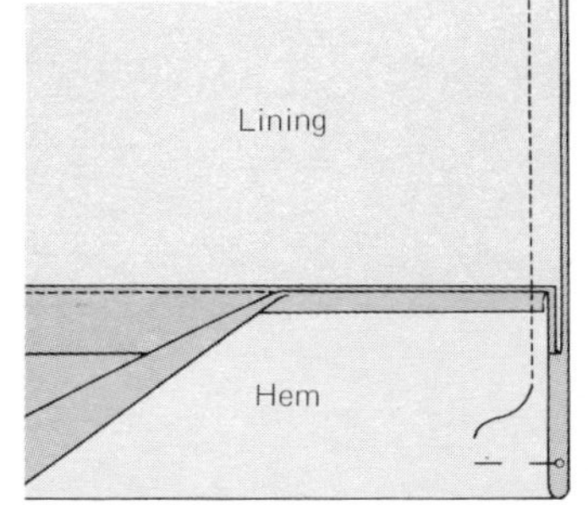

To machine-finish lower side edges, have panel wrong side out, as in Step 3, above. Fold right side of hem over drapery and lining; pin.

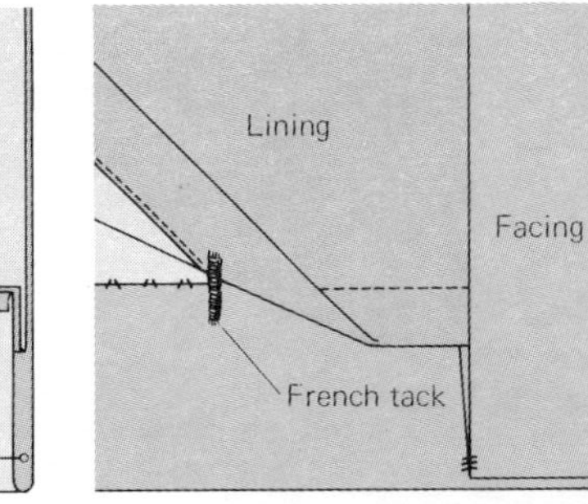

Stitch side seam down to hem fold. Turn drapery right side out. Slipstitch hem. Tack bottom end of facing to hem. French-tack the lining.

Projects to sew for your home

For carefree living: Foam "furniture" / room dividers / magazine holder

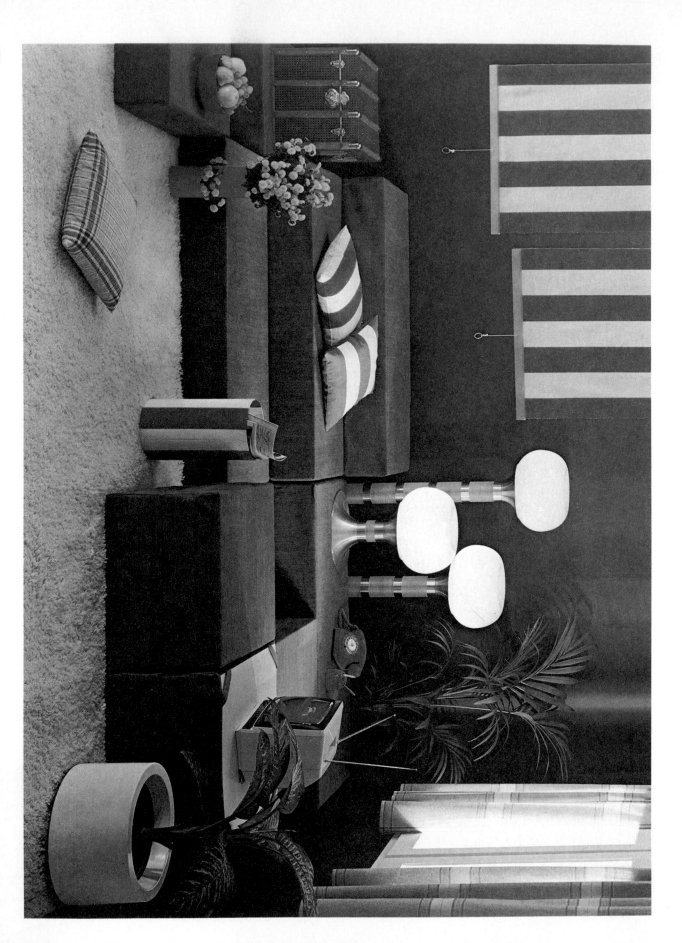

This modern, versatile furniture system is perfectly suited to today's informal life styles. (It is inexpensive and easy to care for, too, which should please the keeper of the house and the budget.) The oversize foam blocks, covered here in casual denim, can be rearranged quickly and easily to suit changing moods or needs. A seat converts in seconds to a handy table with the addition of a square of plastic laminate, held in place by four slim straps. Patch pockets, in a variety of sizes, can be added at the sides of the seats to hold books, magazines, anything you want close by.

The **covers** are simple and quick to sew; zippers make them removable for laundering. Shown here is a combination of several cushions and mattress-size seats. You may decide to make more or fewer. The instructions provide for this, giving fabric quantities required for individual units.

Boldly striped **room dividers** are original and easy to make. Just staple a length of reversible fabric onto a spring shade roller, attach the bottom strips and pullcord, and suspend from brackets in the ceiling. Pull the shades down to screen off a dining area (as is shown on page 446), or perhaps a work/study corner. Raise them to use the entire room again.

The same striping is repeated on the **magazine holder**, actually a wastebasket covered with fabric.

Curtains have a plain heading and large rings that slip over a rod. (For curtain instructions, see pp. 428-436.) They are made of sheer fabric, which has special advantages here, letting in natural light and offsetting heavier fabrics used elsewhere in the room.

Toss pillows not only add comfort, but are a smart way to use up fabric scraps, in this case perhaps left over from the room dividers or curtains. For an appliqué idea, coordinated to this scheme, see page 449. Basic instructions for covering toss pillows begin on page 420.

For the color scheme, we have chosen blue denim with predominantly red and white accents. Other possibilities are shown at the right. To cover the foam blocks, a practical alternative might be corduroy, denim in another of its many colors, or sailcloth — all suitably heavy, durable, and washable. Look at other upholstery fabrics as well. You may find a nubbed tweed in natural off-white more to your taste. Or consider a backed vinyl, which can be sponged clean. If the cushions are plain, accent colors and patterns can be just about anything you like. But before you buy, do look through your scrap bag!

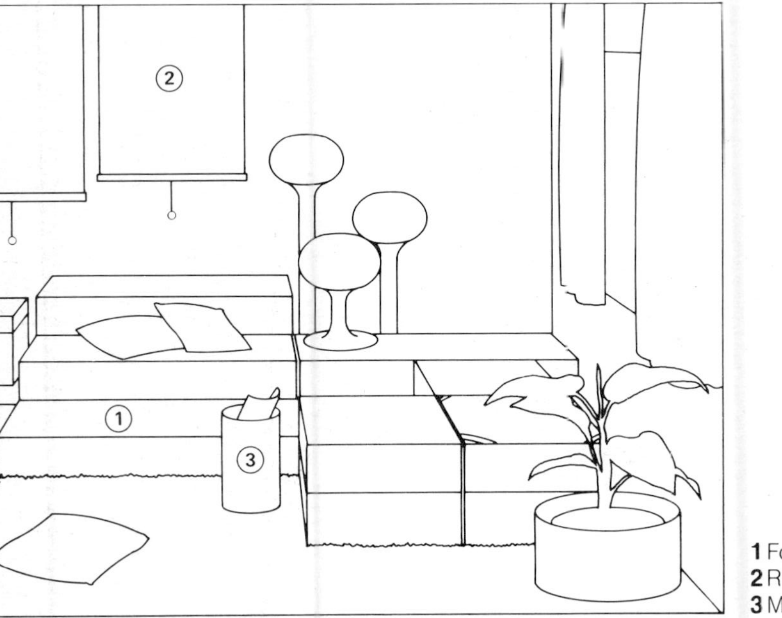

1 Foam "furniture" 440
2 Room dividers 444
3 Magazine holder 445

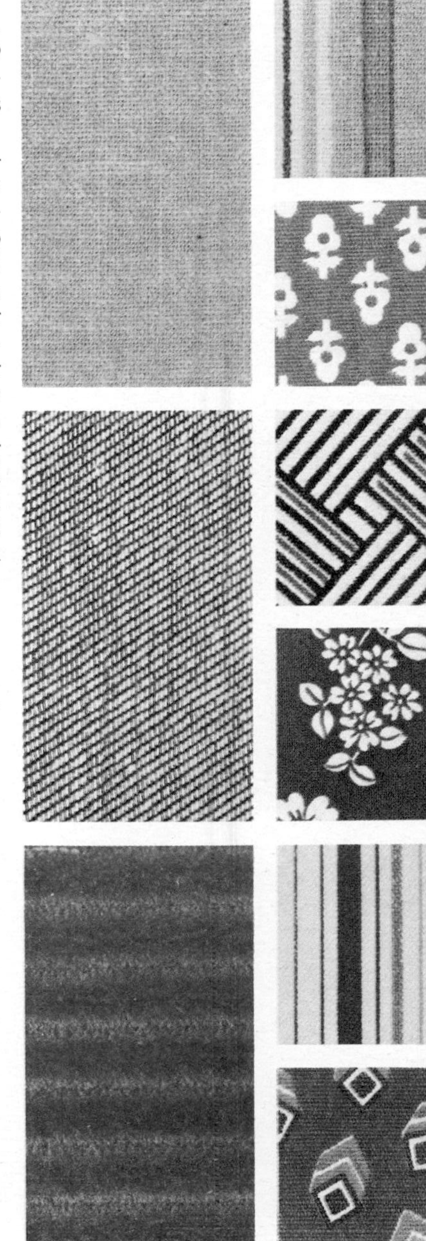

Foam "furniture"

These mattresses and cushions can be arranged in a variety of combinations to suit changing needs. They not only provide comfortable seating, but the cushions can be turned into tables just by adding a strap across each corner and inserting plastic laminate under the straps. Also, patch pockets can be added to either the mattresses or the cushions.

Materials are given for one mattress and one cushion so you can make any number you wish. Covers are zippered for easy removal.

MATERIALS NEEDED

For a cushion:

One 28 x 24 x 8-inch piece of dense foam *or* two 28 x 24 x 4-inch foam pieces glued together
2¼ yards of 44/45-inch fabric
One 24-inch zipper

For a mattress:

One 55 x 24 x 8-inch piece of dense foam *or* two 55 x 24 x 4-inch foam pieces glued together
3⅔ yards of 44/45-inch fabric
Two 24-inch zippers
Appropriate thread

GLUING FOAM

If you are using 4-inch-thick foam pieces, glue two layers together to form an 8-inch thickness of foam for each mattress or cushion. Apply rubber cement or special foam adhesive to both surfaces and, making sure the layers are properly aligned, press them together. Careful positioning of the two layers is important because once they are pressed together, they may be difficult to separate. Remeasure the foam piece before cutting the fabric for its cover.

CUTTING

If foam blocks are the same size as those shown here, use the given dimensions when cutting the fabric pieces. If blocks are not the same size, substitute the correct measurements for those given. Remember to cut a top and a bottom piece for each block of foam.

The cushion. Cut a rectangle for the top and sides, measuring 45¼ inches long x 41¼ inches wide. Cut another rectangle for the bottom, 29¼ inches long x 25¼ inches wide.

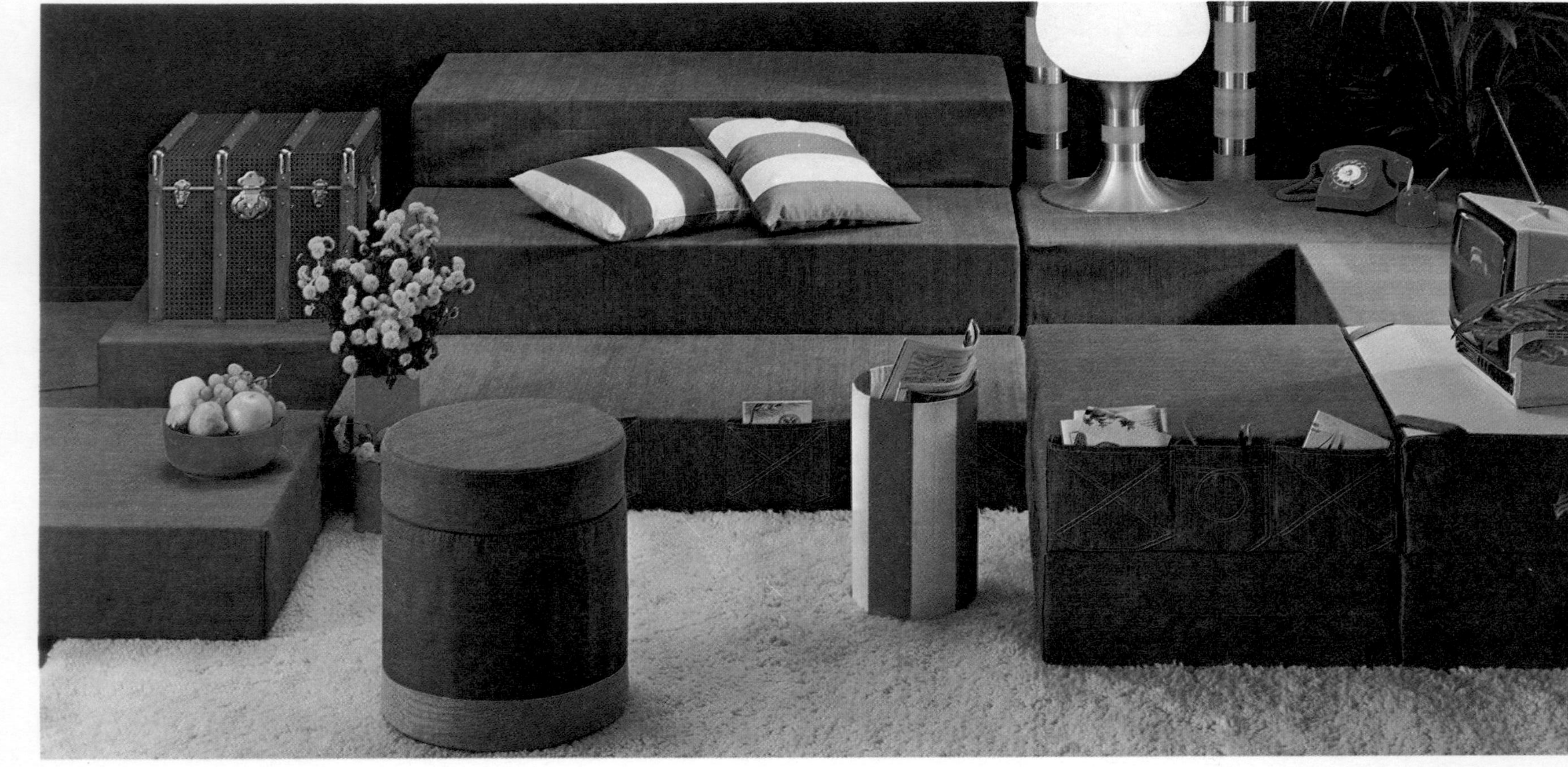

If your foam piece is a different size than the one used here, calculate the size of the two rectangles as follows: The length of the rectangle for the top and sides must equal the length of the foam, plus twice the side depth of the foam, plus two ⅝-inch seam allowances; its width should be equal to the width of the foam, plus twice the side depth of the foam, plus two ⅝-inch seam allowances. Cut a rectangle for the bottom to measure the length and width of the foam, plus a ⅝-inch seam allowance on all of the edges.

On the larger rectangle, make a row of hand-basting 8⅝ inches in from each edge. These bastings separate the top and side areas and mark the stitching lines for forming a miter at each of the corners.

The mattress. Cut one rectangle for top and sides, measuring 72¼ inches long x 41¼ inches wide. Cut another for bottom, measuring 56¼ inches long x 25¼ inches wide.

If your foam piece is a different size than the one used here, calculate the size of the two rectangles as follows: The length of the top and side rectangle should equal the length of foam, plus twice the side depth of the the foam, plus two ⅝-inch seam allowances. The width of the top rectangle should equal the width of the foam, plus twice the side depth of the foam, plus two ⅝-inch seam allowances. The rectangle for the bottom should measure the length and width of the foam, plus a ⅝-inch seam allowance on all edges.

On the larger rectangle, make a row of hand-basting 8⅝ inches in from each edge. These bastings mark the division between the top and side areas of the rectangle and also the stitching lines for forming a miter at each corner of the rectangle.

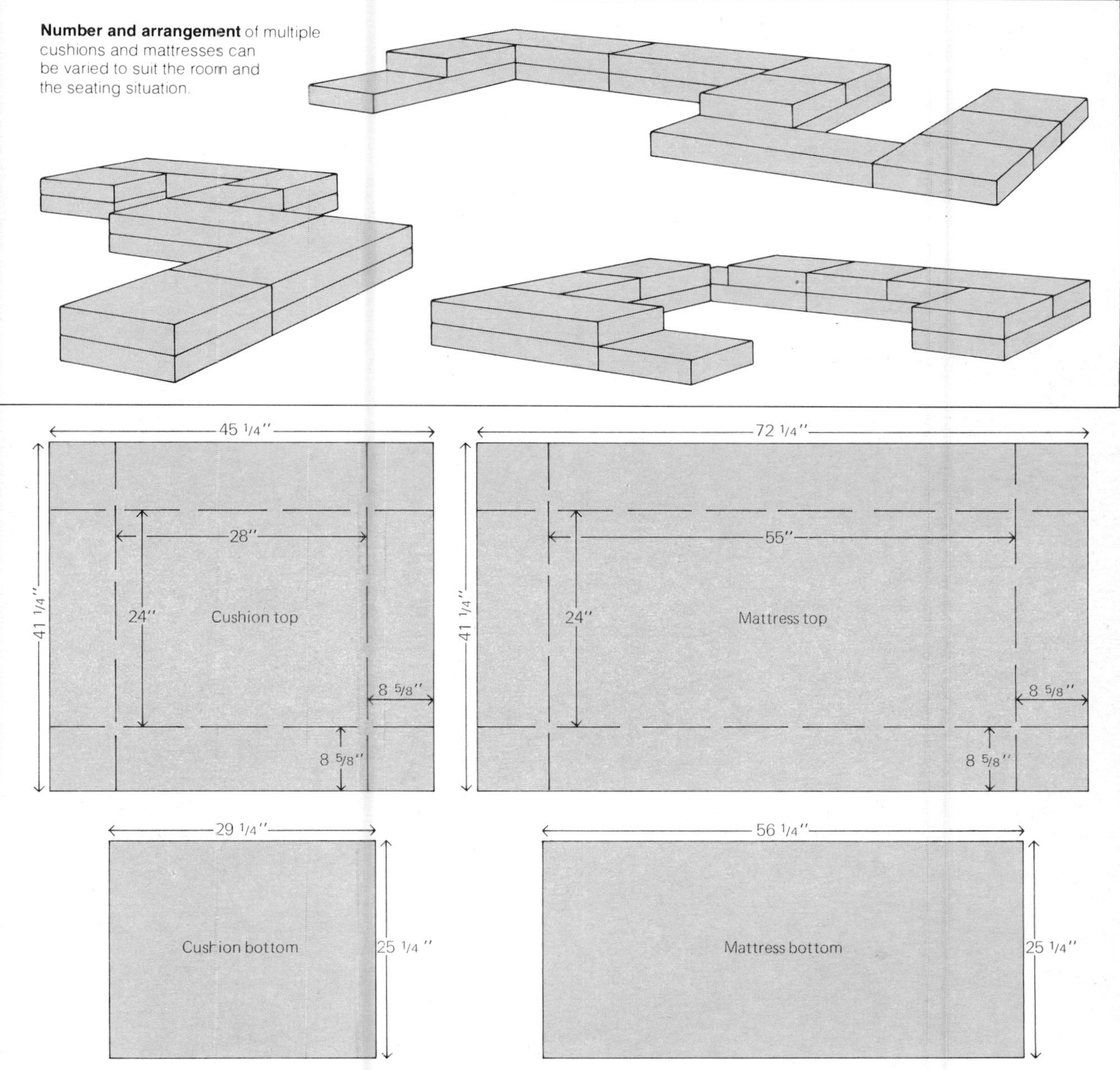

Number and arrangement of multiple cushions and mattresses can be varied to suit the room and the seating situation.

Cut out a top and a bottom rectangle for each cushion or mattress cover. Rectangle for cover's top must be large enough to span side depth of foam block.

Foam "furniture"

Centered zipper application 318-319

SEWING
If you plan to add pockets, they must be constructed and applied before the mattress or cushion cover is sewed. Directions for cutting and stitching the pockets are on page 443.

The cushion. With their right sides facing, form a placket seam between the top and bottom rectangles along one of the longer edges. Start and stop the stitching at the cross seamlines. Press seam flat, then open.

With the seam and both rectangles spread open, insert a zipper into this seam, using the centered method. For extra reinforcement form a bar tack across the tapes at top of zipper.

Keeping the bottom rectangle free of the stitching, miter the four corners of the top rectangle. Miter each corner as follows: Diagonally fold the top rectangle to match the two mitering stitching lines. Stitch from point to the cross seamline; secure thread ends. Trim seam allowances, then press the seam open.

Open the zipper. With right sides together, match and stitch top rectangle to bottom rectangle along the remaining three seamlines. Start and stop the stitching at the placket seamline; spread seam allowances open at corners. Press seams open.

Turn cover right side out through the zippered opening. Push out on the corners to shape the cover. Insert foam into cover; close zipper.

The mattress. Seam the top and bottom rectangles together along one of the longer sides, as for the cushion cover. Insert the two zippers into this seam, using the centered method and having the top ends of the zipper meet at the middle of the seam. Do not form bar tacks across tapes.

Proceed with construction, following the instructions for the cushion cover above and at the right.

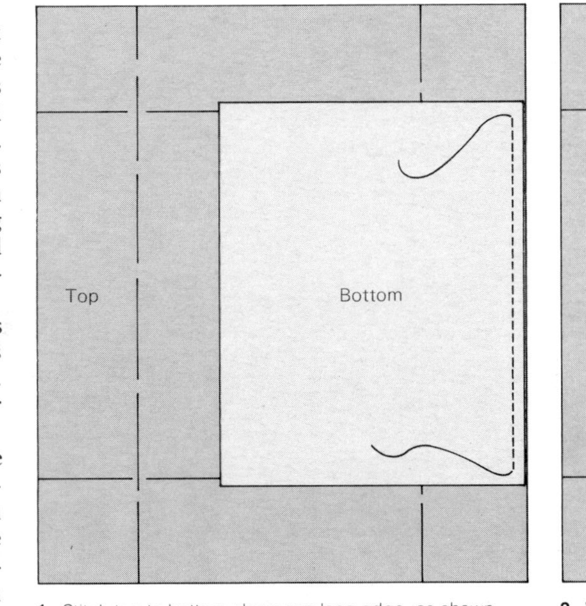

1. Stitch top to bottom along one long edge, as shown.

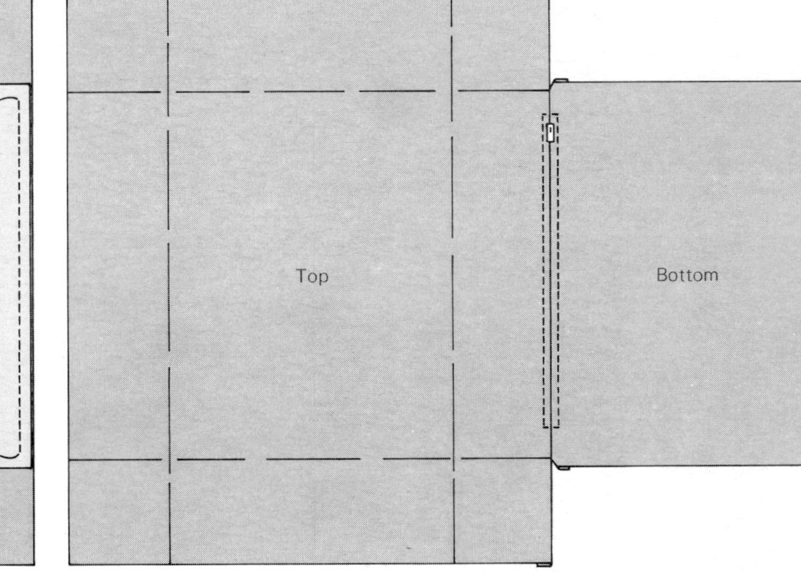

2. With seam and rectangles spread open, insert the zipper, using the centered method.

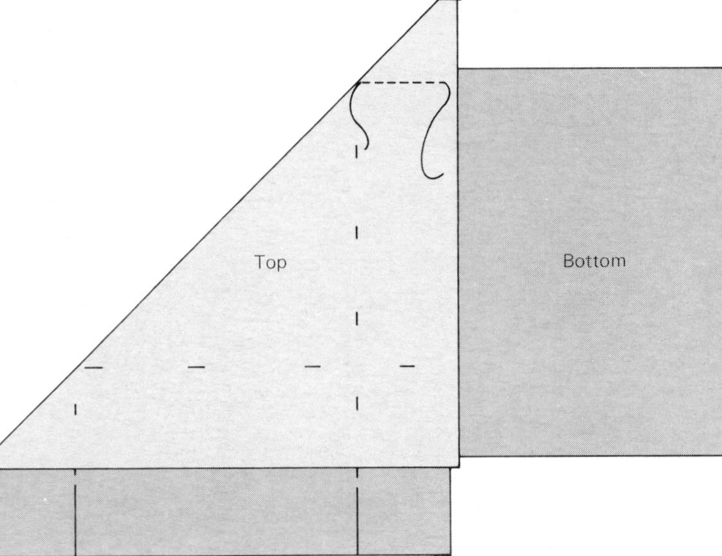

3. Keeping bottom rectangle free of the stitching, miter corners of top rectangle.

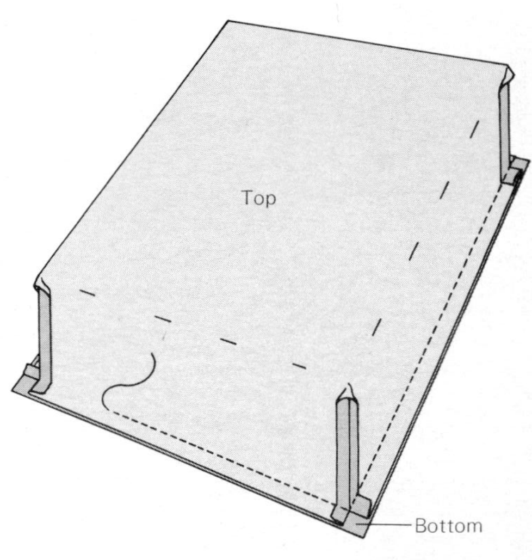

4. Stitch top rectangle to bottom along remaining seamlines.

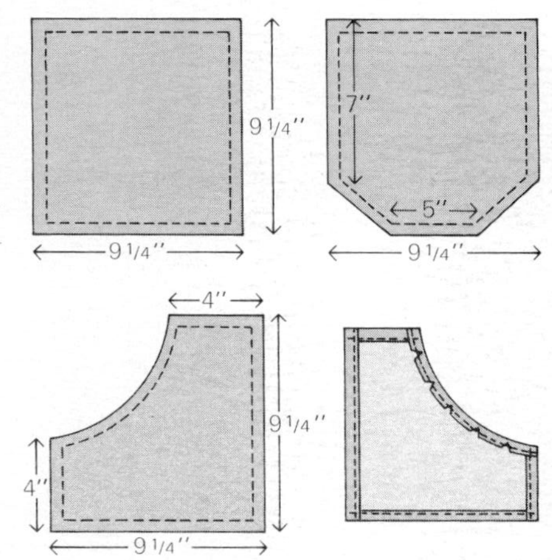

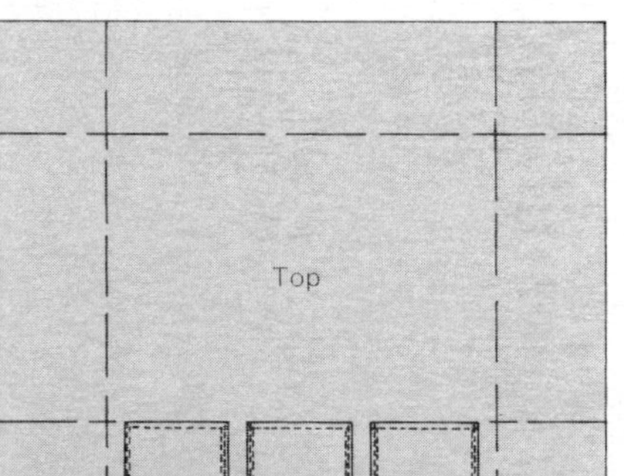

Pockets can vary in shape; are sewed to cover top.

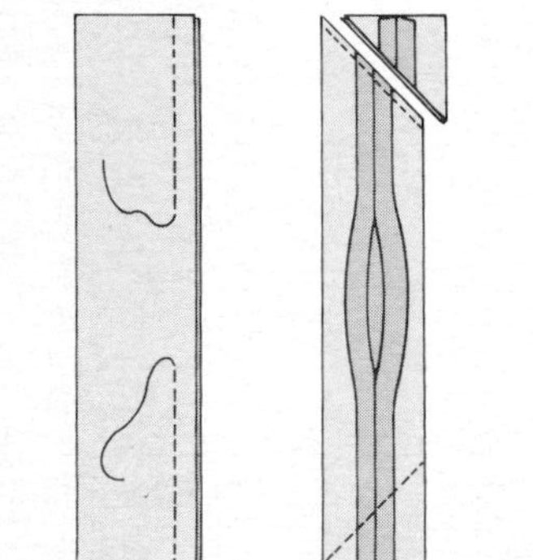

Straps are trimmed at an angle before application.

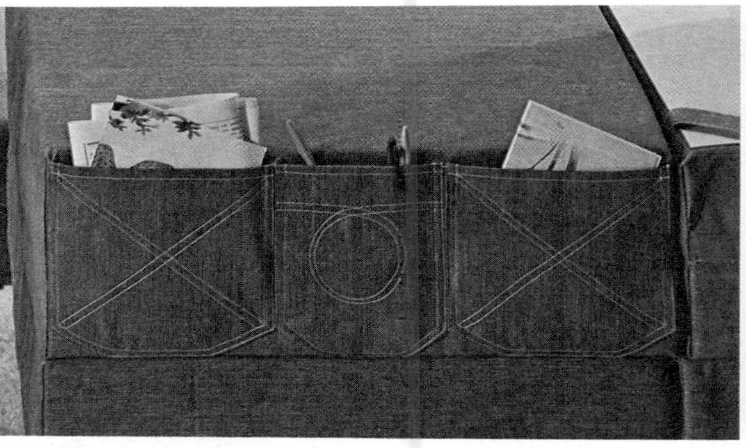

Pockets can be decoratively stitched as shown, or in any pleasing pattern.

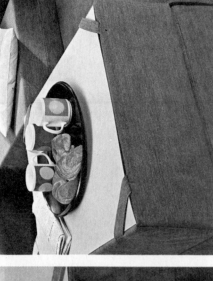

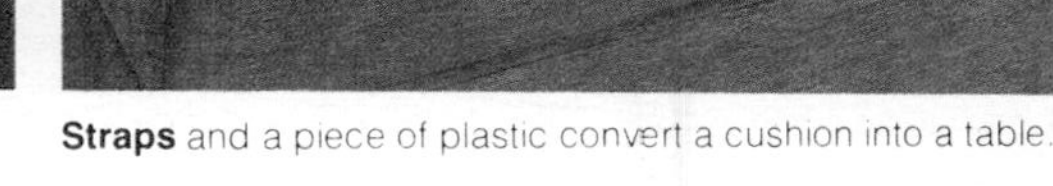

Straps and a piece of plastic convert a cushion into a table.

MATERIALS FOR POCKETS
One 9¼-inch square of fabric for each pocket
Appropriate thread

CUTTING POCKETS
For each pocket, start with a square of fabric that is equal in size to the side depth of the cushion or mattress, plus a seam allowance on all edges. For example, if the side depth is 8 inches, cut a 9¼-inch square for each pocket. The shape of the pocket can vary — it can be square, pointed at the bottom, or curved along the top edge. Decide how many pockets are needed and what shape each will be, then cut them out.

SEWING POCKETS
Staystitch each pocket piece ½ inch from each edge. Turn the edges to the wrong side, clipping and notching the fabric if necessary; press edges flat. From right side, topstitch along all edges. At this time, do any other decorative topstitching, such as rows stitched diagonally across pocket.

APPLYING POCKETS
Pockets can be added to a cushion or a mattress cover. They can be applied to any of the side areas of the top rectangle except the side that will contain the zipper (see p. 442).

With the top rectangle flat and its right side up, position and baste each pocket to the side area. Topstitch or hand-slipstitch each pocket in place; be sure to reinforce stitching at both top edges of each pocket.

Continue to construct cushion or mattress cover, following the directions on page 442.

MATERIALS FOR TABLE TOP
One 27 x 23-inch piece of firm, smooth plastic (piece should be slightly smaller than cushion top)
4 x 9-inch fabric piece for each strap (four needed for each set)
Appropriate thread

CUTTING STRAPS TO HOLD PLASTIC
For each set of straps (four to a set), cut out four rectangles, each measuring 4 inches x 9 inches.

SEWING STRAPS
Fold strap in half lengthwise with right sides together. Stitch along the lengthwise edge, taking a ¼-inch seam and leaving a 2-inch opening at the center of the seam. Press the seam open, moving it to the center of the strap and carefully pressing the seam allowances of the unstitched part of the seam as well.

With seam side up, position a strap across corner of cushion, allowing ¼ inch of the strap to extend beyond both edges of the cover. Across each end of the strap, mark a line at an angle that is flush with the edge of the cushion. Stitch along the marked lines; trim. Turn the strap right side out through the seam opening; pull out corners. Slipstitch the opening closed. Press the strap well, then topstitch along all of the edges. Repeat the same procedure for each of the straps in the set.

Position each strap across a corner, with the ends of the strap at the sides of the corner; whipstitch in place. Slip plastic under straps.

Room dividers

Grain in fabrics 84-85

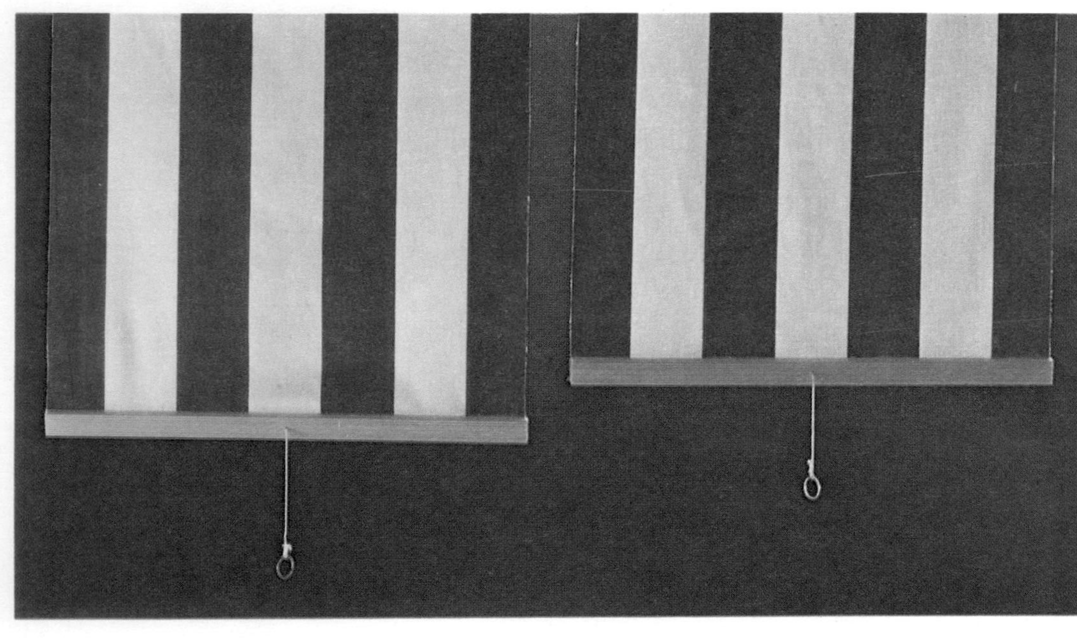

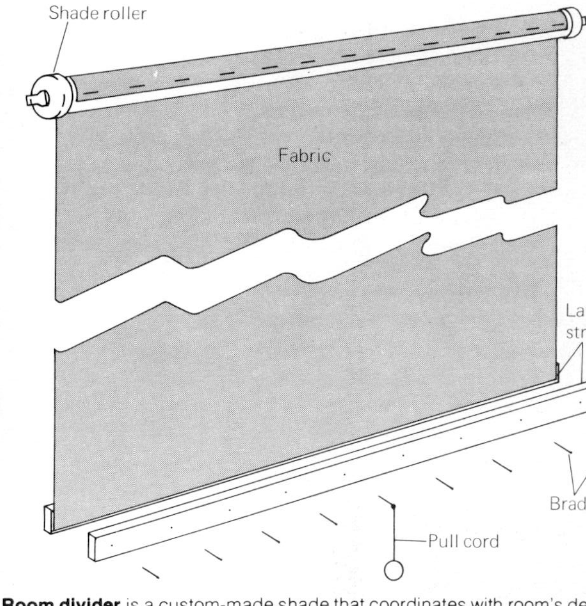

Room divider is a custom-made shade that coordinates with room's decor.

These room dividers take very little time to make. Make two or more of them, depending on the width of the roller and the amount of space that needs to be divided.

The best fabric choice is one that is medium-weight and closely woven, with a smooth surface. It should be (or be made) reversible, since both sides will be visible. The wooden strips used to finish the bottom can be bought at a lumberyard.

MATERIALS NEEDED

For each divider:

1 shade roller
Fabric for divider: The best choice is a reversible fabric, but two lengths of regular fabric, fused together, can work the same way. In either case, fabric length should equal the distance from floor to ceiling, plus 15 inches. Reversible fabric should be ½ inch narrower than the roller; other fabric should be 2 inches wider.
Two ¼-inch thick wood lattice strips, each ½ inch narrower than the roller
Glue
½-inch brads
1 pull cord and tack
Heavy-duty staples
1 set roller shade brackets
Fusible web (if nonreversible fabric)

CUTTING

If the fabric is reversible, cut one length for each divider. If the fabric is not a reversible type, cut two lengths of the fabric and a piece of fusible web long enough to bond the two layers together. Cut the fabric on the straight grain; if it is off grain, the shade will not pull down or roll up satisfactorily.

PREPARING NONREVERSIBLE FABRIC

For best results, arrange a working surface at least as large as the fabric. Protect it with a blanket or several sheets. Press the fabric to remove any wrinkles.

To fuse together the two lengths of fabric, lay out one fabric length wrong side up, and position fusible web on top. Smooth out these two layers. Then place the other length of fabric, with its wrong side down, onto the fusible web. Smooth out the layers. Following the instructions that accompany the fusible web, first partially fuse (heat-baste) the layers together, then fuse the fabrics permanently. Fuse from the center out to the edges, being careful to smooth out any bubbles or wrinkles. Let the bonded fabrics cool before further handling. Re-measure and compare the widths of the roller and the fused fabrics. Mark trimming points on each side of the fabric that will make the fabrics ½ inch narrower than the roller. Using a ruler, draw a trimming line along each edge of the fabric; be sure the lines are absolutely straight and parallel. Trim excess fabric. Because fabrics are fused, there should be no need for seam-finishing the cut edges.

CONSTRUCTION

Spread glue on one side of both lattice strips. With glued side toward fabric, position a strip on either side of bottom edge; align carefully and press into place. Let glue dry. Every 3 to 4 inches, drive a brad through fabric and strips. Tack a pull cord to one strip. Center top edge of fabric to roller and staple in place. Fasten shade brackets to ceiling; suspend divider from them.

Magazine holder

Cover a cylinder with the same fabric that you used to make the room dividers, and you will have a coordinated magazine holder, umbrella stand, or container for your needlework. This cylinder is a metal wastebasket that measures 16 inches high by 9 inches in diameter, but many other types and sizes could be used. For real economy, consider recycling a commercial container.

MATERIALS NEEDED

For a 16 x 9-inch cylinder:

1 yard of 44/45-inch fabric
Glue
Adhesive tape
Appropriate thread

CUTTING

Measure the height of the cylinder, then measure the circumference and the diameter of its base.

Cut a rectangle as long as twice the height of the cylinder, plus 1¼ inches; and as wide as the circumference of the cylinder's base, plus 1¼ inches. (For the 16 by 9-inch cylinder, the rectangle measures 33¼ inches long by 29½ inches wide.) On wrong side of fabric, mark a foldine along the crosswise center.

Cut out a circle with a diameter equal to the diameter of the base of the cylinder, plus 1¼ inches. (For the 9-inch base, the cut circle measures 10¼ inches in diameter.)

SEWING

Staystitch ½ inch from the top and bottom edges of the rectangle. With right sides together, fold rectangle in half lengthwise. After matching the edges on the long side, baste, then stitch them together, using a ⅝-inch seam allowance. Press seam flat, then open.

Clip into the staystitching along the bottom edge of tube. With right sides together, baste, then stitch circular base to clipped edge. Trim seam; press toward body of cover.

Insert cover into cylinder with the wrong side of the cover toward the inside of the cylinder. Push base of cover down to fit the base of the cylinder. Smooth cover to the inside of the cylinder. At top of cylinder, match foldline of cover to edge of cylinder; fold remaining half of cover down over the outside. Smooth out any wrinkles and make sure that the cover is not twisted; be sure the seamline runs straight up and down. Turn cylinder upside down and spread glue around edge of base. Fold bottom edge of cover over bottom edge of cylinder and push fabric onto glued part of base. Allow glue and fabric to dry. Notch out the excess fabric, being careful not to trim beyond the staystitching. To neaten edge and prevent fabric from working loose, tape fabric edge to base.

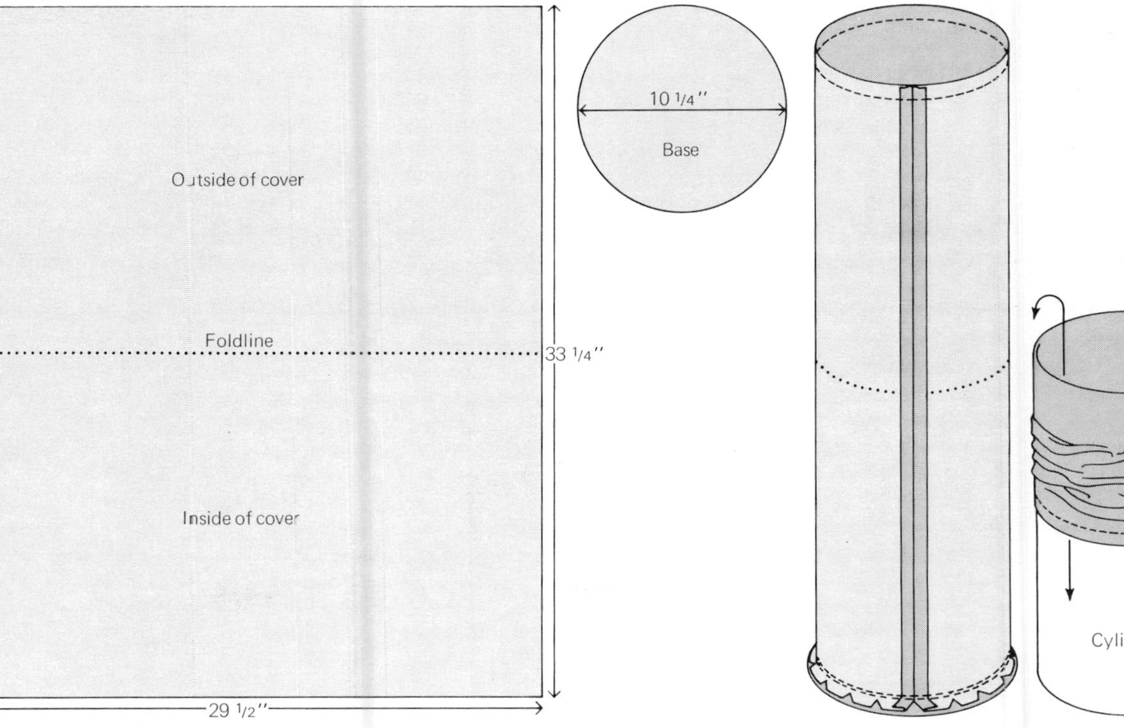

Cover pieces are a large rectangle and a circle. Rectangle is seamed to form a tube; circle is sewed to tube. Cover is then slipped over cylinder.

For casual dining: Foam pads / pillows / hassock / place mats / napkins

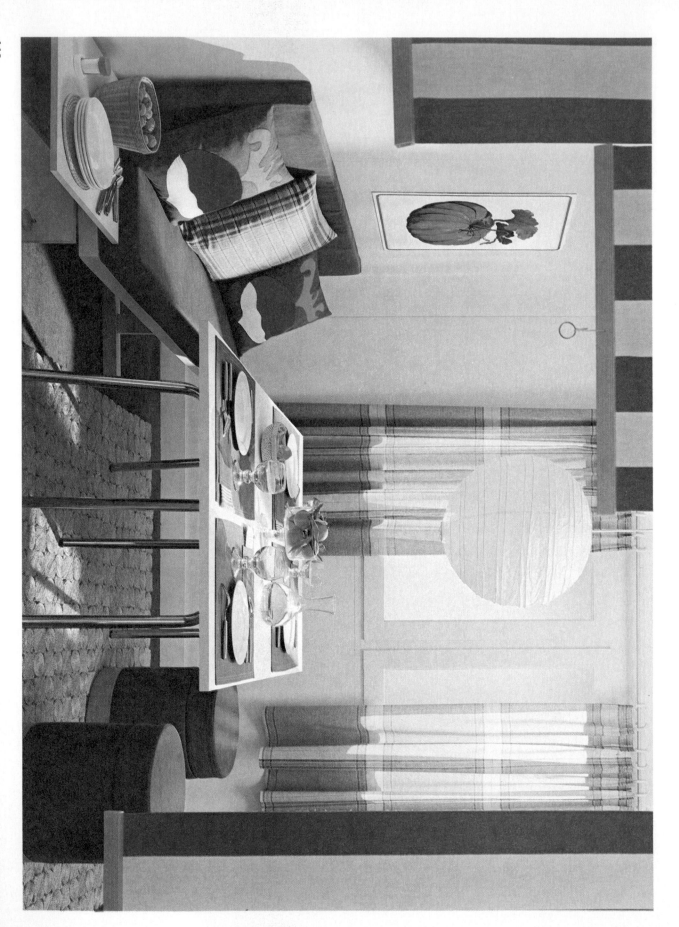

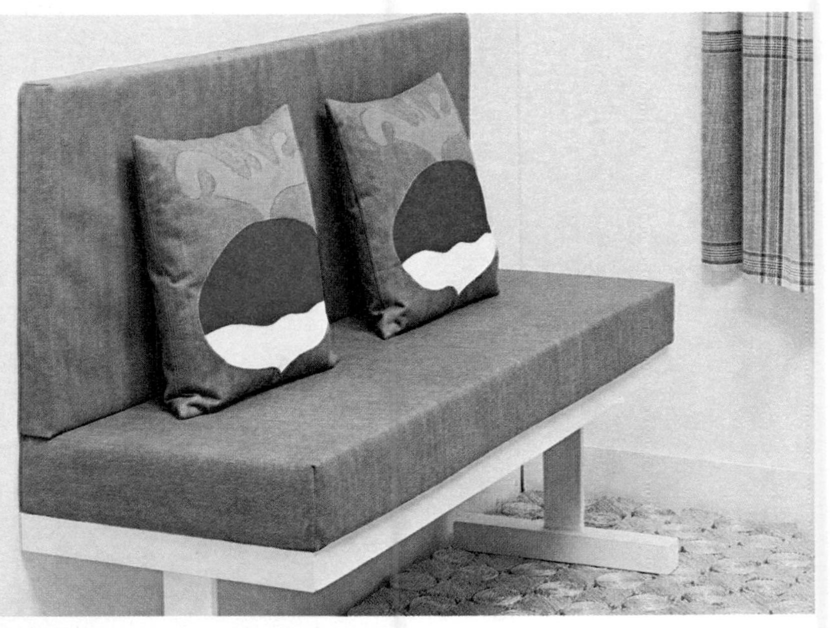

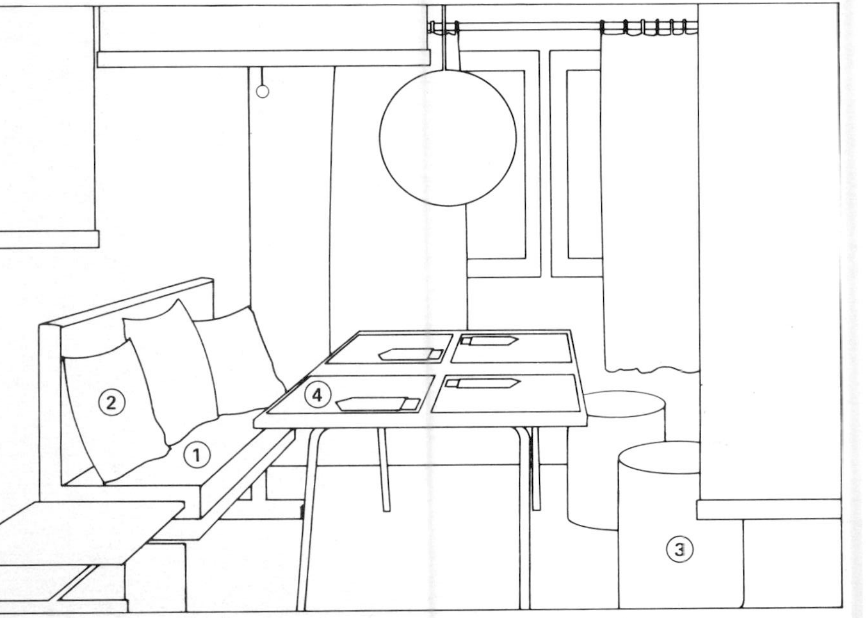

1 Foam pads 448
2 Pillows 449
3 Hassock 450
4 Place mats and napkins 451

This cheerful dining area, done in the color scheme of the room on page 438, is a prime example of what can be achieved with imaginative use of fabric and minimum sewing skill.

The ideas for the decor originated in France, as did the room's dominant fabric, denim being a serge first produced in Nimes. The French phrase *de Nimes* (from Nimes) is pronounced, allowing for its "French accent," almost exactly the same way.

No special sewing skill is called for by these versatile furnishings — just reasonable care in following directions. The **foam seat pads**, like the foam units on page 438, are covered with durable denim, zippered for easy removal. Shown here on a bench, they could also top a low chest, contributing storage space to the area along with seating convenience.

The **radish appliqué pillows** add comfort and color. Though they need not be confined to the dining area, they do look right at home here. The appliqués are simple to make, using scraps of washable fabrics in bold colors and a machine satin stitch. If you prefer, you can create a motif of your own—carrots or mushrooms, lemons or strawberries—and follow our instructions only for method.

The **hassocks**, constructed in two sections, can be moved around easily, and used in various ways according to the need of the moment. The bottom section is a cylinder covered in denim with a contrasting band stitched all around the base. It can serve as a hassock or all-purpose table, as the occasion requires. Add the matching foam pillow on top, and it converts instantly to extra seating. Covers unzip for easy removal at laundering time.

Place mat styling is reminiscent of blue jeans and every bit as sensible, especially for family dining. A patch pocket in the upper right corner holds a napkin. Both mats and pockets, like blue jeans, are finished with topstitching to hold them firm.

The **napkins** are simply hemmed rectangles, charming in a gingham or polka dot fabric. If you would rather buy than make them, use a bandanna or other large handkerchief.

Suggestions for other fabrics and colors appear on page 439, opposite the living/family room featuring foam "furniture" in the same blue-jean blue. Consider only fabrics that you know will wash well, and make sure fabric is preshrunk before you start to cut. When you are deciding on contrasts, remember that texture is a possibility along with color and pattern. You could, for example, cover the bench and hassocks in wide-wale corduroy and make place mats and perhaps pillows of linen or canvas.

Foam pads

Centered zipper application 318

The denim-covered foam cushions, illustrated on page 447, are meant to rest on a bench or chest placed up against a wall. Zippered for easy removal, the covers are constructed in the same way as the cushions and mattresses in the living area.

MATERIALS NEEDED:

One 52 x 18 x 4-inch foam block for the seat cushion
One 52 x 18 x 2-inch foam block for the back cushion
6¼ yards of 44/45-inch fabric
Four 24-inch zippers
Appropriate thread

CUTTING

For the top and side part of the *seat cover*, cut a rectangle 61¼ inches long x 27¼ inches wide. For the top and side part of the *back cover*, cut a rectangle 57¼ inches long x 23¼ inches wide. For the bottoms of both the seat and back covers, cut two rectangles, each 53¼ inches long x 19¼ inches wide. If your foam blocks are a different size than the ones called for here, cut top pieces the length and width of the foam, plus the depth of the foam and a seam allowance on each edge; cut bottom pieces the length and width of the foam plus a seam allowance on each edge.

On the seat top rectangle, stitch a row of hand-basting 4⅝ inches from each edge; on the back top rectangle, place basting rows 2⅝ inches from each edge. Bastings mark the division between top and side areas of the cover as well as the stitching lines for a miter at each corner.

SEWING

For either the seat or back covers, proceed as follows: With right sides facing, form a placket seam between top and bottom rectangles along one long edge. Start and stop stitching at the cross seamlines. With seam and both rectangles spread open, insert two 24-inch zippers into this seam. Use the centered method of application and have the top ends of the zippers meeting at center of seam.

Keeping the bottom rectangle free of the stitching, miter the four corners of the top rectangle as follows: Fold the top rectangle diagonally to match top mitering stitching lines. Stitch from point to cross seamline; secure stitching. Trim the seam allowances; press seam open.

Open the zippers. With right sides together, match and stitch top rectangle to bottom along the three remaining seamlines. Start and stop stitching at placket seam; spread seam allowances at the corners.

Turn cover right side out through zippered opening; push out on corners. Insert foam and close zippers.

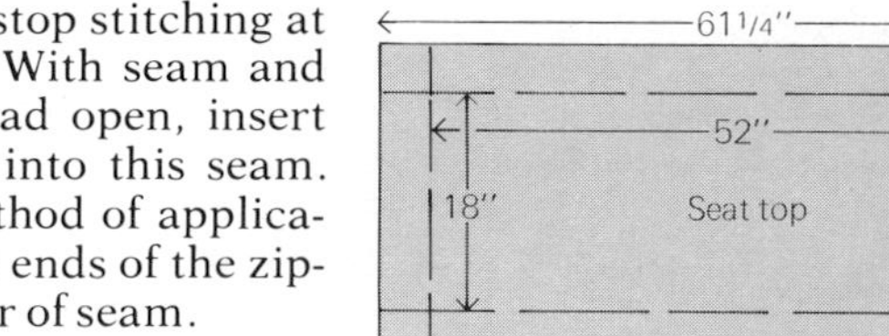

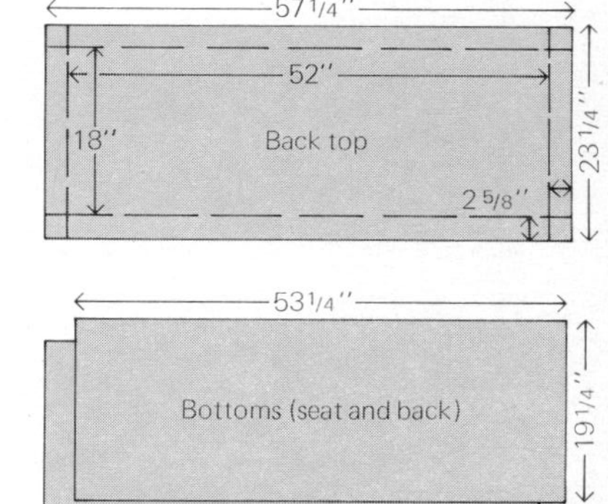

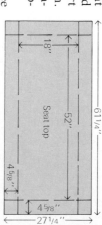

Cut a top and bottom piece for each cushion cover.

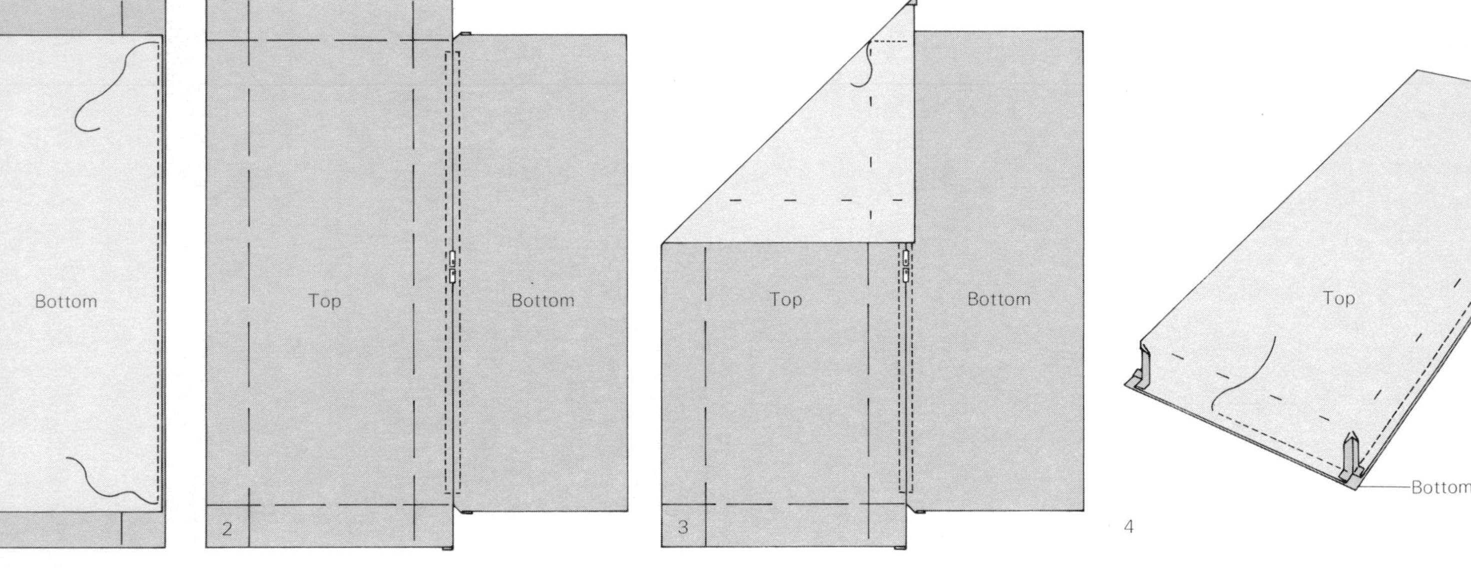

To construct cover, sew top and bottom rectangles together along one long edge (1); apply zippers to this seam (2). Miter the four corners of top rectangle (3). Sew top to bottom along remaining seamlines (4).

Pillows

Satin stitching 30, 32-35
Knife-edge pillow covers 420-421

Bold radish appliqués make these pillows right at home in a dining area. The colors coordinate well with the denim seat and back cushions, but you might want to select others — or even design your own appliqué.

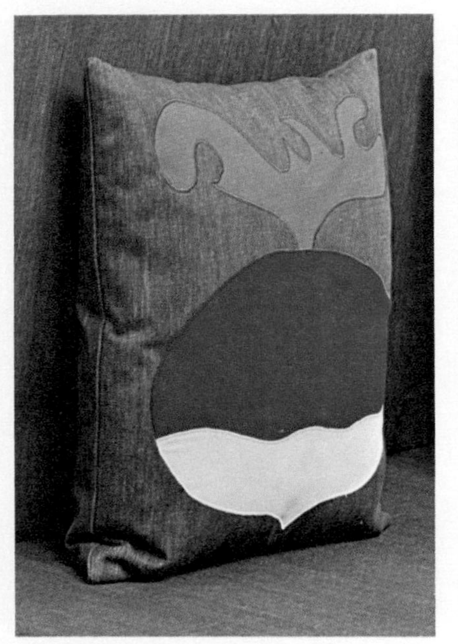

MATERIALS NEEDED

For each pillow:

½ yard of 44/45-inch fabric for cover
⅓ yard each of green, red, and white fabric for appliqué (enough for two appliqués) or assorted scraps (see Cutting for sizes)
One 14-inch pillow form *or* ½ yard of muslin and 1 bag of fiber fill batting to make a form
One 12-inch zipper
Thread in appropriate colors
Large sheet of heavy paper
Tracing wheel and carbon paper

MAKING APPLIQUÉ PATTERN

Using 1¾-inch squares, make a graph on a sheet of heavy paper and reproduce all lines of radish design. Cut out design along outer lines.

CUTTING

For each appliqué. From each of the appliqué fabrics, cut a rectangle slightly larger than the part of the design it corresponds to. For radish shown, cut a 6 x 12-inch rectangle from the green fabric; 7 x 12-inch rectangle from the red; 5 x 12-inch rectangle from the white. Using tracing wheel and carbon paper, transfer each section of the radish to the right side of the appropriate rectangle of fabric. Cut out each section, adding ¼-inch seam allowances.

For each pillow cover. Cut two 15¼-inch squares of base fabric. Center appliqué pattern on the right side of one of these squares and trace the outer lines of the design onto the fabric. This marked square is now the top piece of the pillow cover.

For each pillow form. Cut two 15¼-inch squares of muslin.

MAKING A PILLOW FORM

With right sides facing, seam muslin squares together along three edges. Turn cover right side out and stuff with batting. Turn in free seam allowances; slipstitch opening closed.

APPLIQUÉING PILLOW TOP

Lap edges of design sections and match markings. Stitch on matched lines; trim. With wrong side of the design toward right side of the pillow top, match traced lines on design to traced lines on pillow top; pin. Machine-baste design to pillow top along the outer traced lines; trim excess fabric close to stitching. Using matching thread for each section, satin-stitch over all inside and outside lines of the design, making sure the stitches cover machine-basting.

SEWING PILLOW COVER

Zipper is inserted into one of the side seams as follows: On wrong side of cover top, mark top and bottom of placket opening. With right sides together, sew cover top to cover bottom above and below placket; start at each mark and stitch to each corner's seamline. Extend the placket seam allowance of the top piece. Open zipper and place half of it face down on seam allowance, with teeth along seamline and top and bottom stops at top and bottom of opening. Stitch in place. Close zipper; spread open the cover sections and the placket seam. From right side, stitch free zipper tape to bottom of cover.

Open zipper. With right sides together, sew cover top to bottom (begin and end at placket seam); trim seams. Turn cover right side out. Insert pillow form and close zipper.

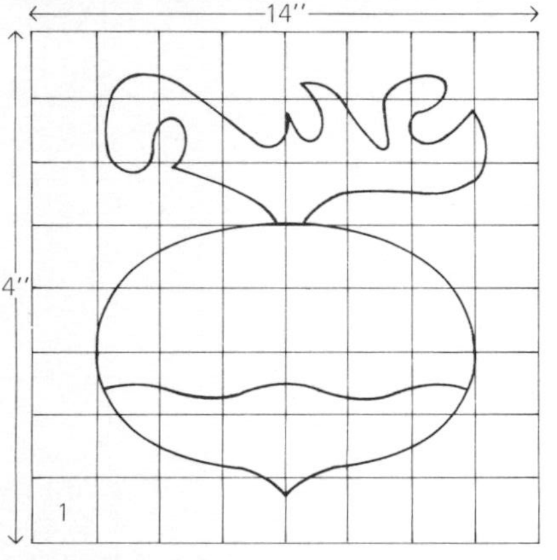

2

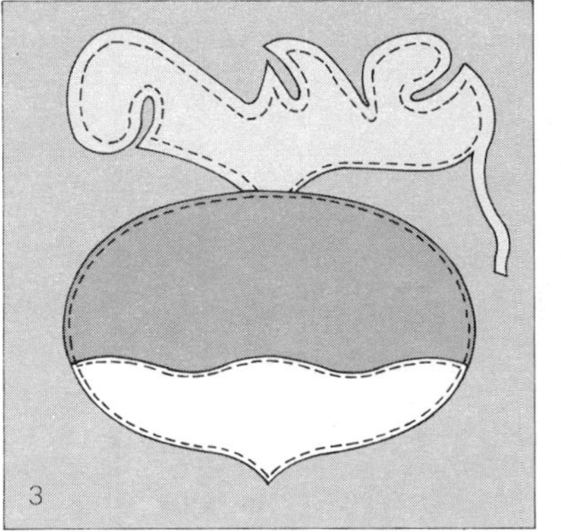

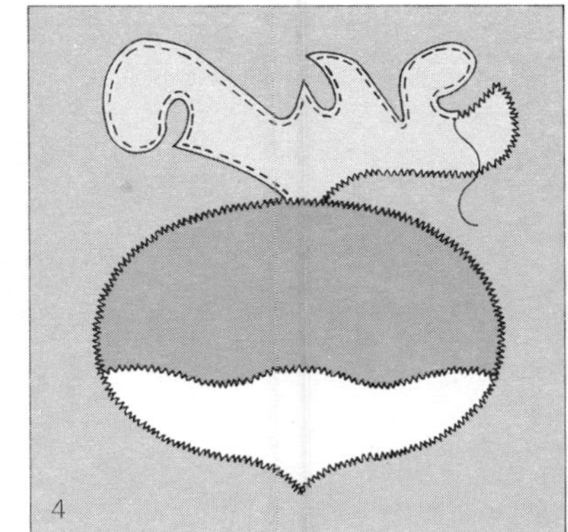

Transfer design to a graph (1). Cut out and use as a pattern for cutting out design parts. Lap and sew sections together (2). Machine-baste design onto pillow top (3). Satin-stitch over all edges of design (4).

Hassock

Centered zipper application 318
Box-edge pillow covers 420, 422

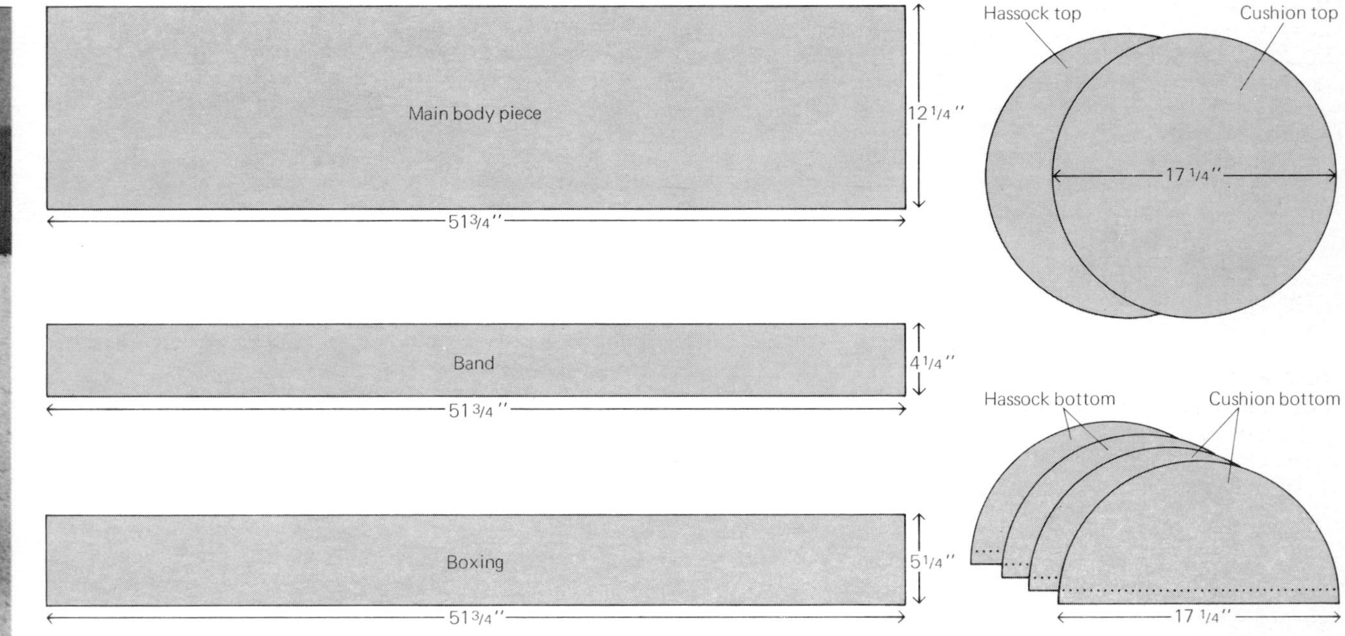

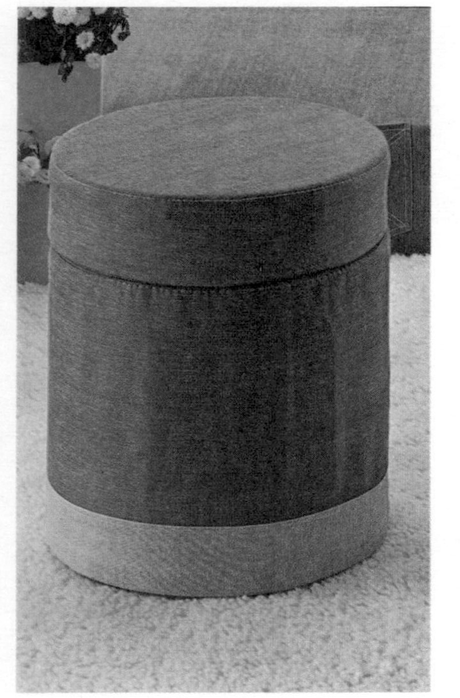

For each hassock and cushion cover, cut out all of the above pieces. Dimensions given are for a hassock and cushion of a specific size (see Cutting).

These versatile hassocks can be used in either the dining or living room as seats. Remove the cushion top and you have a side table or footstool.

MATERIALS NEEDED

For one hassock:

Hassock or cylinder 14 inches high x 16 inches in diameter
1 box-edge pillow form, 16 inches in diameter x 4 inches thick
2 yards of 44/45-inch fabric
One 12-inch zipper
Two 14-inch zippers
Appropriate thread

CUTTING

Cut a rectangle for the main body of the hassock cover measuring 51¾ x 12¼ inches; a rectangle 51¾ x 4¼ inches for the bottom band; and a 51¾ x 5¼-inch rectangle for the boxing strip of the cushion cover. Cut two circles with 17¼-inch diameters for the tops of the hassock and cushion covers. For the bottoms of these covers, cut four semicircles that are 17¼ inches in diameter but have a ⅝-inch seam allowance added on each straight edge.

If your hassock or cylinder has different dimensions than this one, cut each piece so that the body and band sections, when finished, will span the height and circumference of the cylinder, and the four circles for the top and bottom will match them in size (two of the finished circles are semicircles joined by a placket). The boxing strip should cover the height and the circumference of the pillow form. The zippers should be slightly shorter than the placket seams.

SEWING HASSOCK COVER

Match and stitch wrong side of band to right side of body along the lower edge. Staystitch and clip long edges of body. Join short ends of body and, with the top stop ¼ inch above the bottom seamline, insert a 12-inch centered zipper into this seam.

Seam two semicircles together; with top stop ¼ inch from outer seamline, insert a 14-inch zipper into seam. This circle is bottom of hassock cover. Close zippers. With right sides facing, sew bottom to body of cover. Position top stops of zippers toward each other; start and end stitching at plackets. Open zippers. With right sides facing, sew top to body of cover. Turn cover right side out. Insert hassock or cylinder into cover (if a cylinder, place open end toward bottom of cover); close zippers.

SEWING CUSHION COVER

Sew the remaining two semicircles together and apply a 14-inch centered zipper into this seam. This is the bottom of the cushion cover. Join ends of boxing strip; staystitch and clip into top and bottom edges. With right sides together, sew cover bottom to bottom seamline of boxing. Open zipper. Right sides together, sew cover top to top seamline of boxing. Turn cover right side out; insert the pillow form.

Place mats and napkins

Narrow machine-stitched hem 294

Place mats can really show off individual settings. These mats even have blue jean-style patch pockets to hold the napkins. For family dining, consider personalizing the pockets by embroidering an initial on each one, or an original abstract design.

Make the napkins from fabric that works well with its surroundings. If you rather not bother to make your own napkins, you can use ready-made napkins, cotton scarves, or big bandanna handkerchiefs.

MATERIALS NEEDED

For four place mats and napkins:

1⅓ yards of 44/45-inch fabric for the place mats
1 yard of 44/45-inch fabric for the napkins *or* four ready-made napkins or handkerchiefs
Appropriate thread

CUTTING

The place mats. Cut four rectangles, each measuring 22 inches wide x 18 inches long. For pockets, cut four rectangles, each measuring 7¼ inches wide x 8⅝ inches long. To shape the pocket bottom, mark center of bottom edge, then points on side edges 2⅝ inches up from botton. Connect bottom to side points; cut on lines.
The napkins. Cut four rectangles, each measuring 18 inches square.

SEWING

The place mats. Seam-finish all of the edges of each place mat; turn edges under 1¼ inches and press. Open the edges out. Finish each corner as follows: To form the mitering stitching lines, fold the corner diagonally to the right side, aligning the press lines; press the diagonal fold. Open out corner. Next fold the place mat down diagonally at the corner with right sides together, aligning mitering lines, press lines, and bottom edges. Stitch on the matched mitering lines. Trim seam allowances and press the seam open. Turn mitered edges to wrong side.

On the right side, stitch a double row of topstitching all around. Place the first row of stitching ½ inch from the edge; place the second row ⅜ inch from the first row.

Proceed as follows for each pocket: Seam-finish the top edge of the pocket. Turn down a 1-inch hem at the top edge; secure it with a double row of topstitching, placing one row ⅜ inch from the folded edge and the second row ¼ inch from the first. Turn in a ⅝-inch seam allowance along the remaining three sides and topstitch in place, placing the topstitching ½ inch from the edges.

Position the pocket at the top right-hand corner of the place mat so that it will be out of the way of the plate when the mat is in use. Position it 1½ inches down from the top of the mat and 1 inch in from the right-hand edge. Topstitch the pocket in place along its side and bottom edges. For reinforcement, backstitch at the top edges of the pocket.
The napkins. Form a narrow machine-stitched hem along each edge of each napkin. Hem one edge at a time as follows: Turn the edge under ¼ inch and press. Turn edge under another ¼ inch and press again. Topstitch along the edges through all layers and press. It may be necessary to trim the excess fabric at corners to turn edges properly.

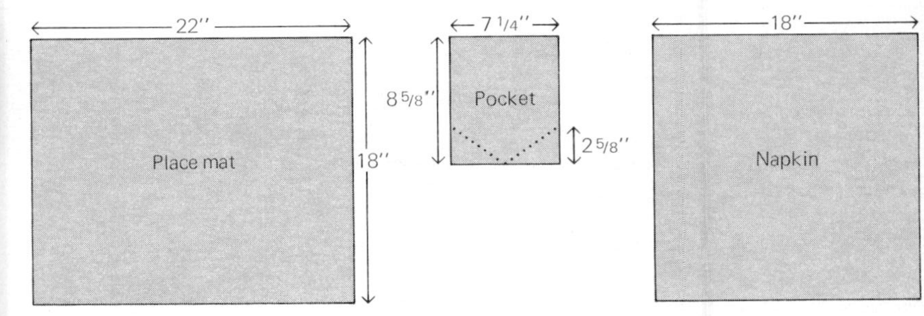

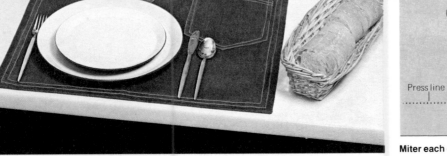

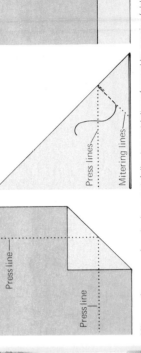

For each place mat and napkin, cut out the above pieces. Shape bottoms of pocket pieces.

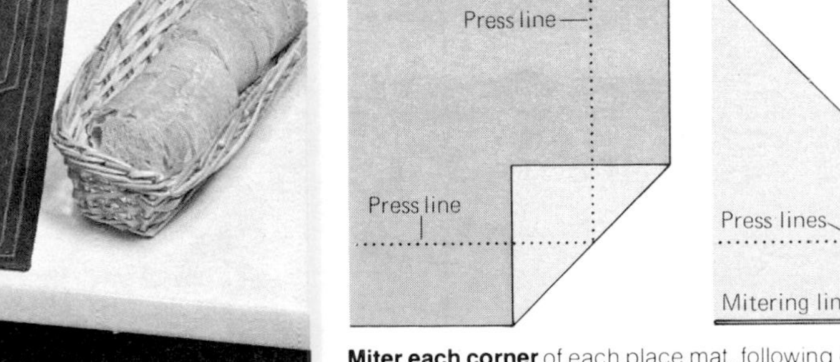

Miter each corner of each place mat, following guidelines formed by precise folding and pressing.

Classic bedroom: Spread / designer sheets / initial pillows / fake fur rug

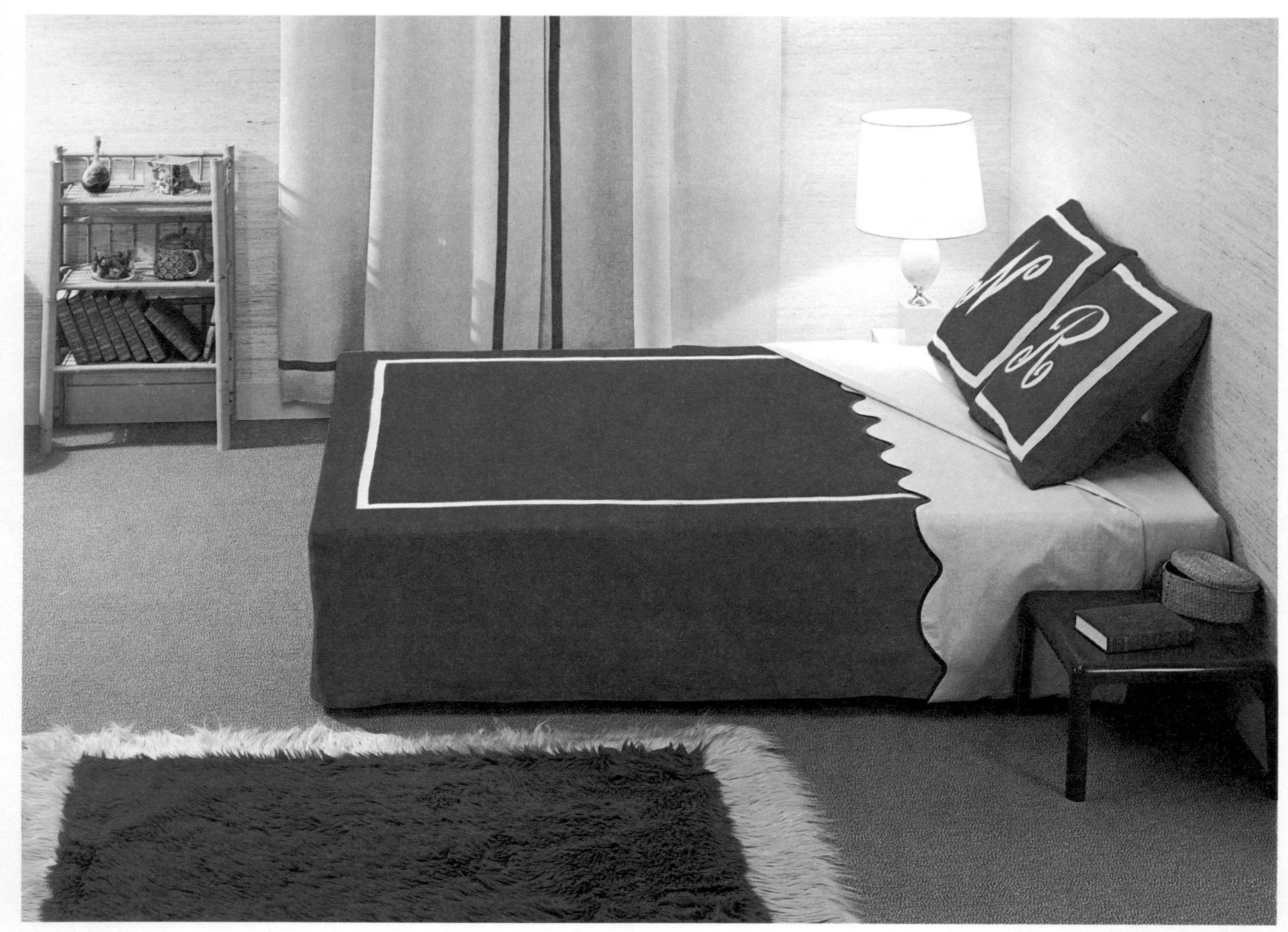

Harmony of form and color — that is the key to this serene, formal bedroom. The custom touch of coordinated linens, draperies, and rug assures its elegance; decorative bands in a contrasting color accent and emphasize the simple, classic shapes.

To reassure the practical-minded, the look of luxury is no trouble to maintain — all accessories are made of machine-wash, no-iron blends. Suggestions are a cotton-polyester for sheets and draperies; polyester-rayon for bedspread and pillow covers; modacrylic for the fake fur rug.

The **bedspread,** trimmed with white to match sheets and draperies, is neatly tailored, in keeping with the clean lines of the decor. Side drops are lined to hang smoothly; the construction method avoids the problem of hemming and encloses all seams — an advantage in laundering.

Pillow covers reflect the geometric formality of the spread; appliquéd initials add a personal touch. Choose initials from the alphabet on page 460 and enlarge them to proper size, or, if you prefer, design your own. Either way, appliqué your chosen letter with a machine satin stitch, following the instructions on page 458.

The decorative bands on pillow and spread can also be machine applied, using the same satin stitch as for the monogram. For a sleeker, more tailored look, you could straight-stitch the folded edges instead.

Sheets are the ordinary commercial kind, customized by adding a scalloped border edged in contrasting binding. An alternative idea might be to leave the hem just as it is and apply straight contrasting bands to match the spread.

Floor-length **draperies** pick up the room's colors in reverse, with white becoming the main color and red its accent. A special construction technique permits you to hem and apply the trim in a single step. For information on making unlined draperies, see pages 428-435.

Fake furs make cozy **rugs**. This one, two-toned to match the decor, is sewed either by hand or by machine to a sturdy burlap backing, its corners mitered for a trimmer fit. Add nonslip tape to help prevent skidding on bare floors. Use left-over fake fur to cover a couple of small cushions.

The linen-look chosen for spread and curtains is a crisp material that tailors well and is easy to work with. There are, of course, other possibilities, such as velveteen, sailcloth, or a polyester-linen blend, to name just a few. Suggestions for alternate color schemes are shown at the right.

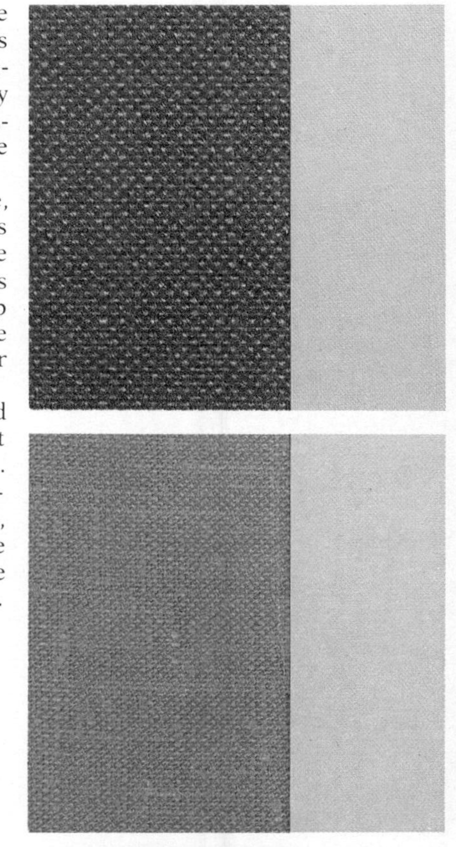

1 Spread 454
2 Designer sheets 457
3 Initial pillows 458
4 Fake fur rug 461

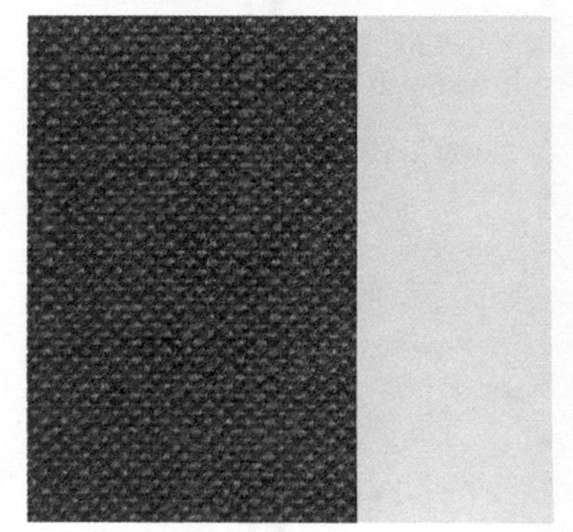

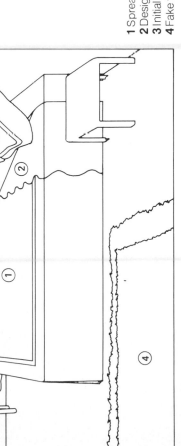

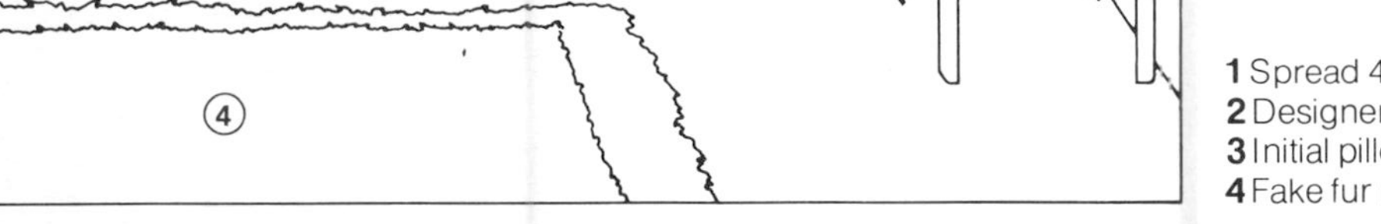

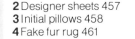

Bedspread

Measuring beds 424

Polyester-rayon makes this dramatic fitted spread practically carefree. The contrasting decorative band can be made from cut strips of linen or you can use ready-made trim.

The drops are fully lined for extra body. The lining encloses all raw edges, an asset when the spread is laundered. If your fabric is lightweight, an alternative is to self-line the bedspread drops.

The yardage and cutting dimensions given are for a 54 x 75-inch double bed that is 20 inches high. Measure your bed fully made up to determine its exact dimensions, then buy your yardage according to the width of the fabric and the width and length of the bed (see Bedspreads).

MATERIALS NEEDED

7 yards of 44/45-inch fabric
  or 6¼ yards of 60-inch fabric
  for the bedspread
3⅔ yards of 44/45-inch fabric for
  the lining drops
2⅓ yards of contrasting fabric
  for trim *or* 7 yards of 1-inch-wide
  ready-made trim
Appropriate thread

CUTTING

Cut the top part of the bedspread as follows: If the fabric is 44/45 inches wide, cut one large rectangle 89 inches long (length of bed plus 14 inches) x 44 inches wide. Cut two 89 x 6½-inch rectangles to make up the needed width for the bed. If fabric is 60 inches wide, simply cut an 89 x 55-inch rectangle.

Cut two rectangles for the side drops, each of them measuring 76 inches (bed length plus 1 inch) x 22 inches (bed height plus 2 inches). Then cut one rectangle for the foot drop that measures 55 inches (bed width plus 1 inch) x 22 inches.

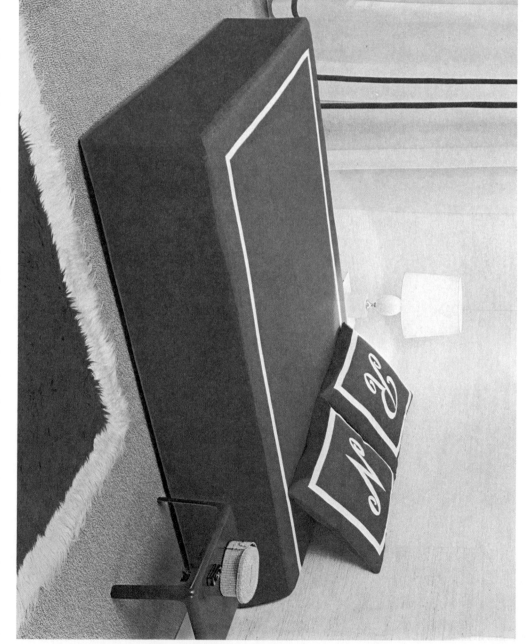

From the lining fabric, cut two side drops, each measuring 76 x 20 inches, and one foot drop measuring 55 x 20 inches. If you prefer self-lined drops, cut the drops to the given lengths, but make the width twice the bed height plus 1 inch.

To make the decorative trim, cut three strips from the contrasting fabric, each of them measuring 2 inches by the cut length of the fabric.

SEWING

If the top portion of the spread was cut in three pieces, join the narrow pieces to each side of the large piece to make up the needed width: Place the pieces together with right sides facing, and machine-stitch in a ½ inch seam. Press the seam open.

Decorative trim. If the spread top is cut as one piece, the trim will be placed 4 inches from the sides and the foot end. If the top is seamed, the trim will be placed over the seams and the same distance from the edge at the foot end.

To make decorative trim, fold long edges of strips so they meet in center. Seam strips together, mitering corners. Pin trim over seamline of bedspread.

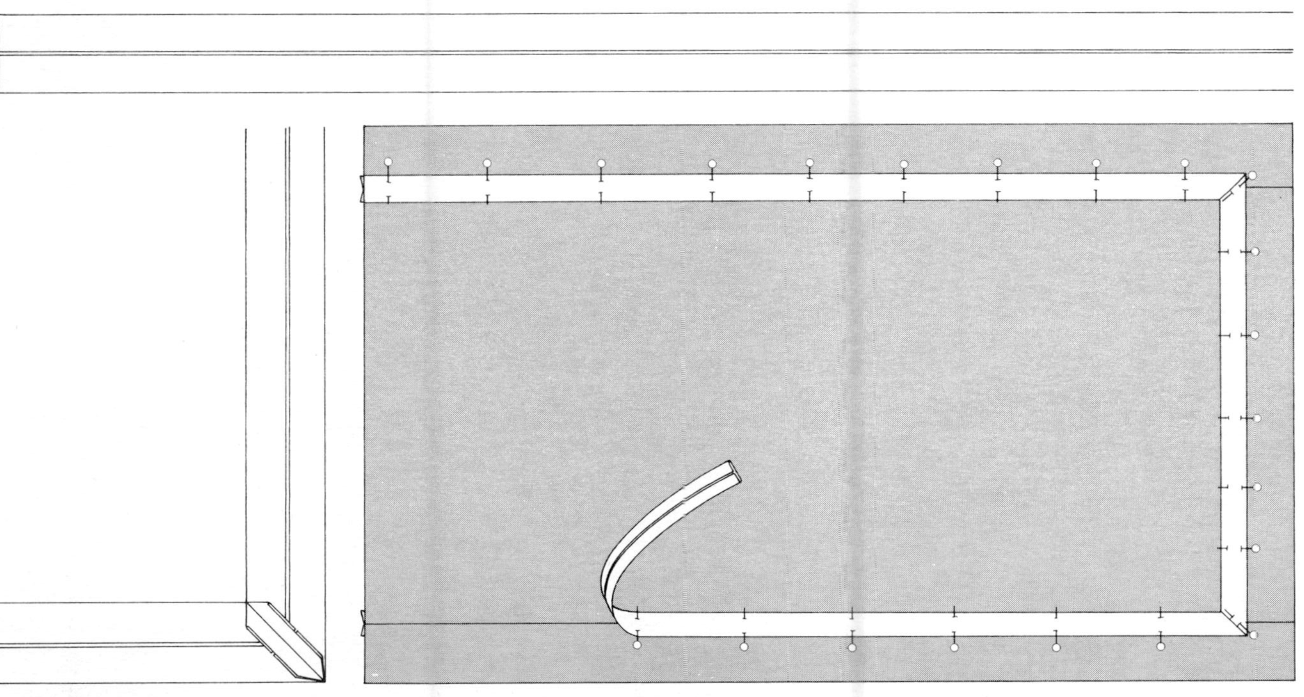

To line bedspread drops, seam side and foot drops together. Complete lining seams as well; fold top edge under. Stitch the lining to drops of bedspread.

Determine the length and width of the trim, and cut one strip to the measured width plus 1 inch for seam allowances. Cut the other two strips to the measured length plus 1 inch for seam allowances.

Lightly press each strip in half the long way to mark a center line. Press the edges of each strip in so they meet at this center foldline.

Right sides facing, place the short strip and one long strip together, raw edges even at one end. Machine-stitch diagonal seam across to make a mitered corner. Trim and taper the seam allowances, then press it open. Position and stitch the other long strip to the other end of the short strip in the same way.

Carefully position the trim onto the right side of the bedspread top. Pin in place; hand-baste as pinned. Machine-stitch near the edges on each side of the trim.

Joining the drops. With right sides facing, pin the side drops to each end of the foot drop. Machine-stitch as pinned, stopping and securing each seam ½ inch from the raw edge at the top. Join the lining pieces together. Along one long edge of the lining piece, press the seam allowance to the wrong side. (Do not press seam allowances under if you plan to line the spread top as well.)

With right sides facing, pin lining to drop along the bottom edges, aligning raw edges. Machine-stitch as pinned. Press seam open.

Fold the lining and drop so right sides are facing again, and bring the folded edge of the lining to meet at the seamline of the drop. Pin the side seams together. Machine-stitch as pinned, securing each seam at the top. Turn right side out and press; the lining should be about an inch shorter along the bottom edge.

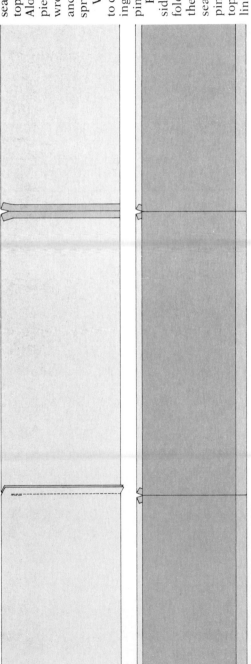

Bedspread

Curtains and draperies 428-435

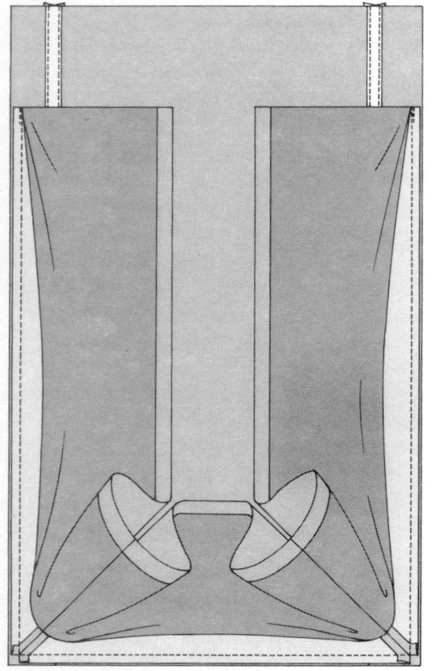

Pin and stitch the lined drops to bedspread top.

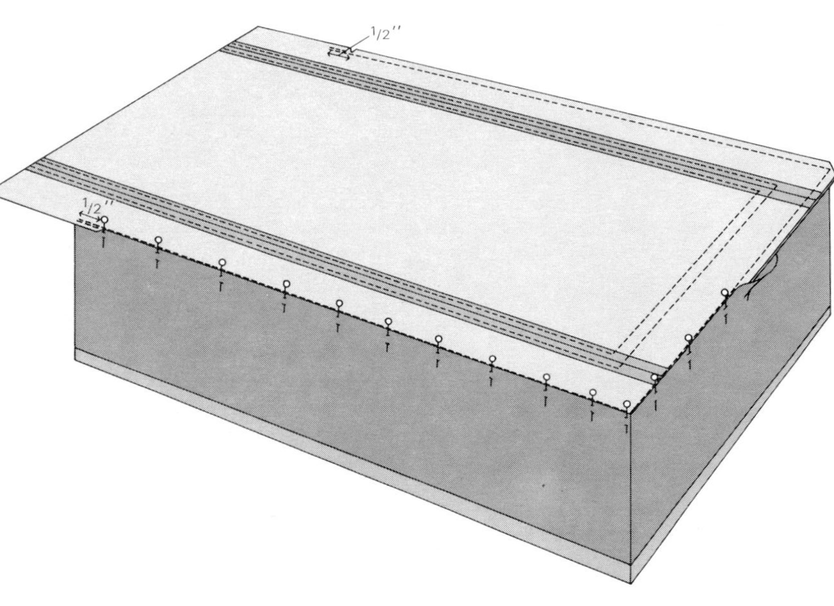

Clip seam allowances ½" from drop ends. Press seam allowances down; slipstitch lining to the seamline.

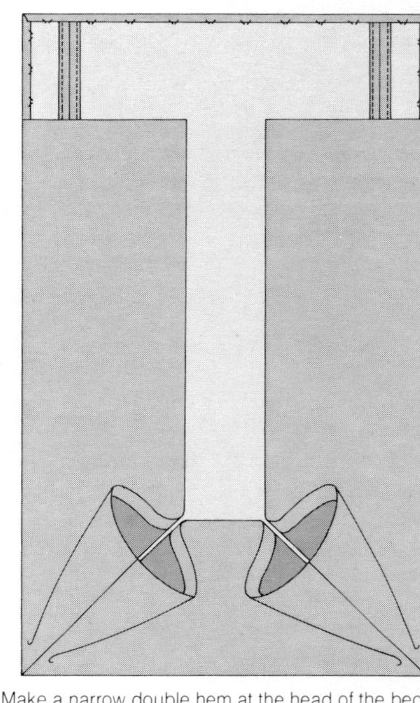

Make a narrow double hem at the head of the bed.

To join the drop to the top part of the bedspread, pin the seam allowance of the drop to the top part of the spread. Machine-stitch as pinned, pivoting for sharp corners or blunting corners if you would prefer them to curve; secure stitches at the beginning and end.

At the head of the bedspread, clip into the seam allowance of the bedspread top about ½ inch in from the end of the drop. Pull the drop down, and press the seam allowances down (trim away excess fabric at corners). Bring the folded edge of the lining to the seamline and pin in place. Slipstitch lining in place.

At the head of the bed, turn under a narrow double hem and slipstitch in place. Press well.

To make unlined draperies, see Sewing for the home, pages 428-435. Follow the instructions below for the special hemming technique used in applying the trim to these curtains. Fabric must be reversible because the hems are turned to the right side, and their edges are then covered by the decorative trim.

Allow an extra 5 inches for the width and the length of each curtain. Then cut four 2-inch wide strips, two of them measuring 4 inches less than the finished length of the curtain and the other two measuring 4 inches less than the finished width.

On each curtain, thread-trace a line 5 inches from the bottom edge and 5 inches from the side edge that will hang in the middle of the window.

At the corner of the curtain, fold the curtain diagonally (on the bias), with wrong sides together and raw edges even. Pin, then machine-stitch along the diagonal that is formed by the thread tracing. Trim the point, leaving ¼-inch seam allowance. Taper the seam allowance at the corner and press the seam open. Turn the corner to the right side.

Fold, miter, and stitch the decorative trim as described for the handling of the bedspread's trim. Pin and, if necessary, baste the trim over the raw edge of the hem, lining up the mitered corners of trim and curtain. Machine-stitch along the folded edges of the trim.

Finish the draperies as directed in section on Sewing for the home.

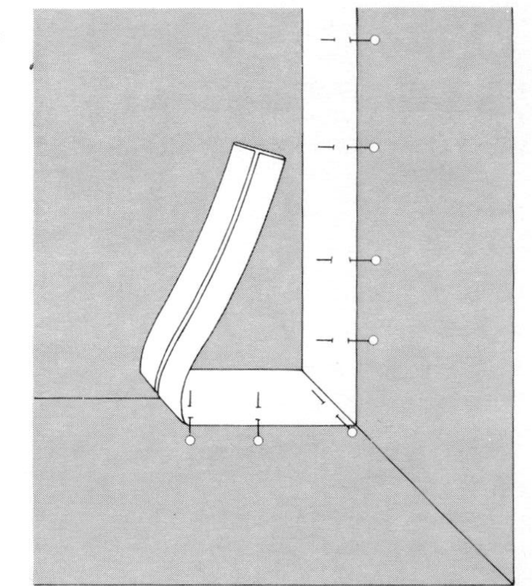

Apply trim to curtain; align both mitered corners.

Designer sheets

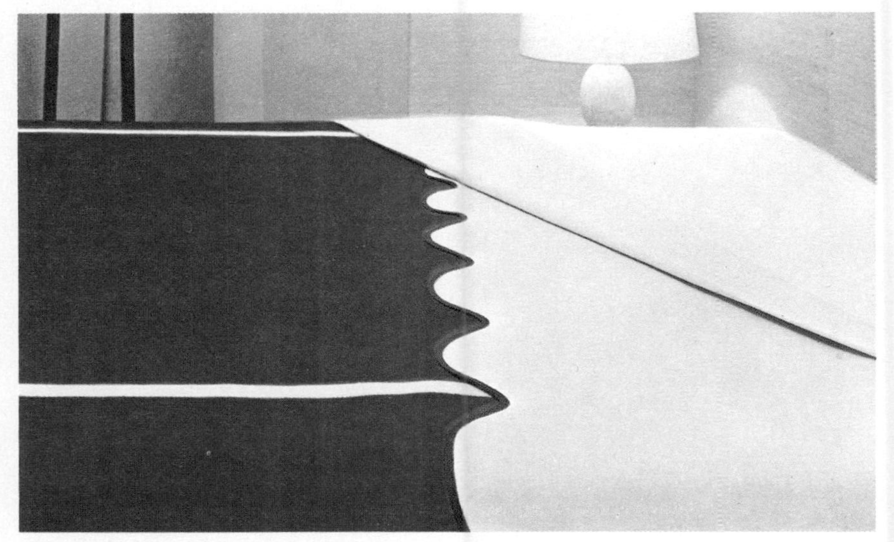

It's amazing what a simple scalloped border can do for an ordinary sheet! Accent the scallops by applying contrasting binding to their curves. Use packaged wide bias tape — it comes in many pretty colors. To apply it, follow the easy instructions below.

MATERIALS NEEDED

1 flat sheet to fit bed
Wide bias tape: 1½ times the total sheet width
18 x 5-inch piece of paper
Appropriate thread

MAKING THE PATTERN

Reproduce the scallop pattern on the piece of paper as shown; make certain the curves of each scallop are the same. Cut out scallop pattern.

CUTTING

Fold the sheet in half lengthwise and place the pattern against the foldline, with the top of the scallop touching the top edge of the sheet. Trace the scallop design, reproducing as many scallops as necessary to span the entire width of the sheet. Turn the sheet and mark the other half the same way.

Open out the sheet. Machine-stitch along the scallop design, just inside the traced lines. Then cut along the marked scallop lines.

SEWING

Fold and carefully press the width of the wide bias tape slightly off center to prepare it for binding. Starting at one end of the sheet, pin the tape along the scallop edge, encasing the raw edges; turn under a ¼ inch at the beginning and the end, and manipulate the tape to conform to the scallop curves. Hand-baste the binding in place. With the wider half of the binding below, machine-stitch as basted, using a narrow zigzag. If you do not have a zigzag machine, straight-stitch the binding in place. Press the bound edge well.

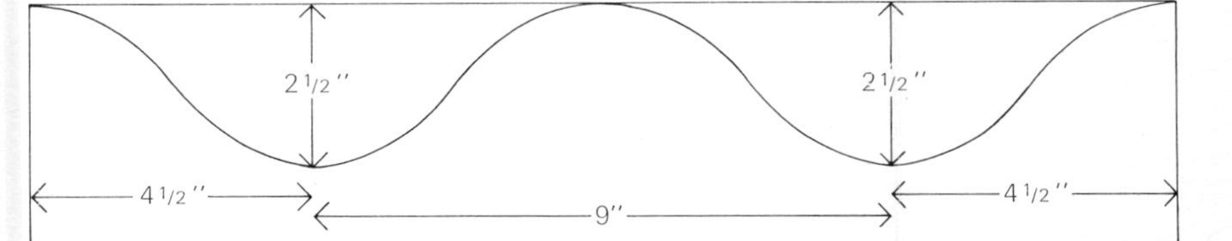

1. Follow the dimensions given above to make the scallop pattern; be sure to keep the curves even.

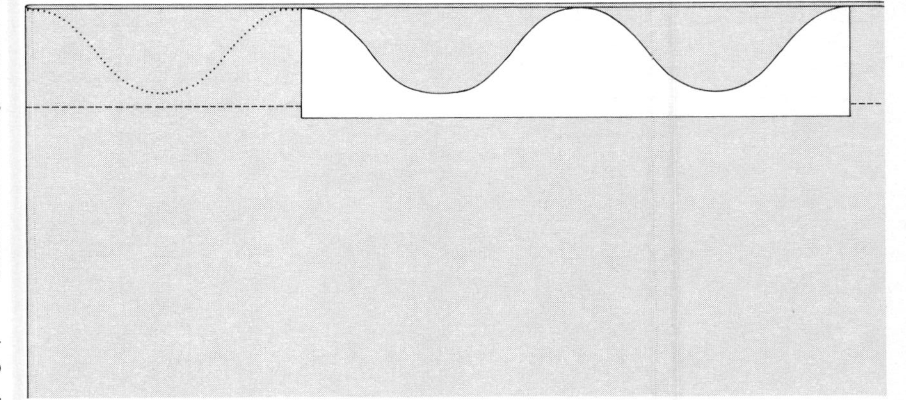

2. Fold sheet in half. Starting at fold, trace as many scallops as necessary to span the sheet width.

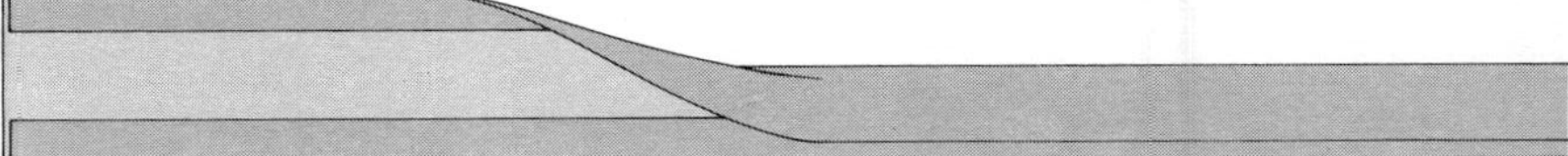

3. Press the wide bias tape slightly off center to prepare it for binding the edges of the scallops.

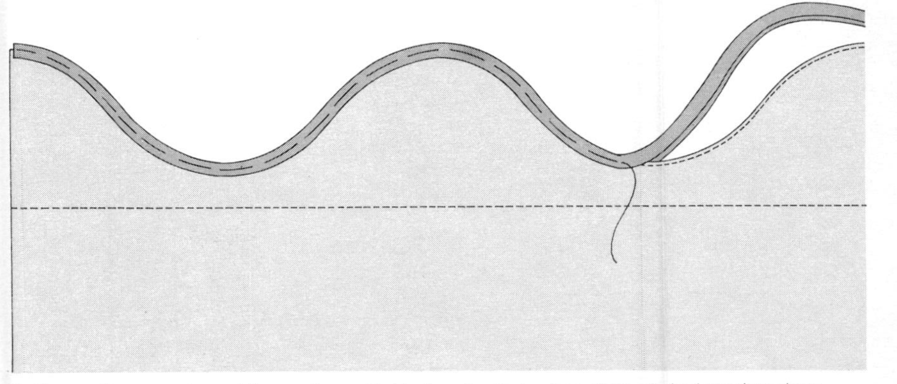

4. Encase the raw edges of the scallops with binding; baste in place, then stitch along the edges.

Initial pillows

Graceful initials are a nice personal touch, and a pleasing contrast to the straight lines of the spread. Covers are made to fit 24-inch pillow forms, but dimensions can easily be altered. Zippers are included to simplify removing the cover for laundering.

MATERIALS NEEDED
For two pillows:
2¼ yards of 44/45-inch fabric for covers
1 yard of 44/45-inch contrasting fabric for initial and trim
Two 20-inch zippers
Two 24-inch foam pillow forms
Tracing paper
Appropriate thread

CUTTING
For two pillows, cut out two 25¼-inch squares along the straight grain for the tops, and four rectangles 13¼ x 25¼ inches for the bottoms.

Also cut two 18-inch squares from the contrasting fabric, again on the straight grain; then cut eight strips from the same fabric, each 2 inches wide and about 21 inches long.

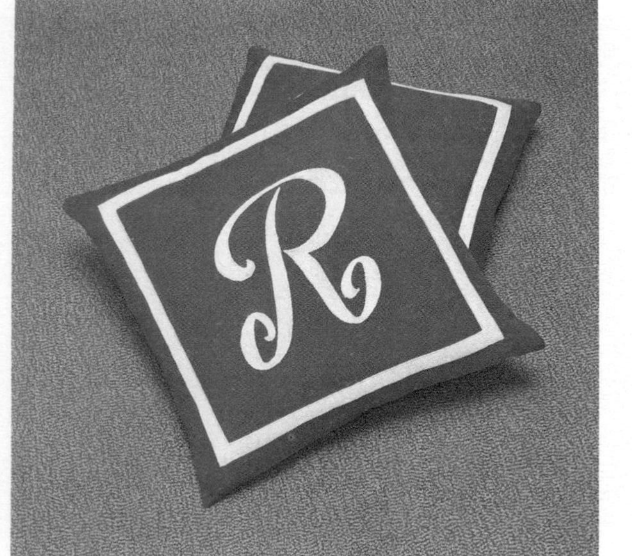

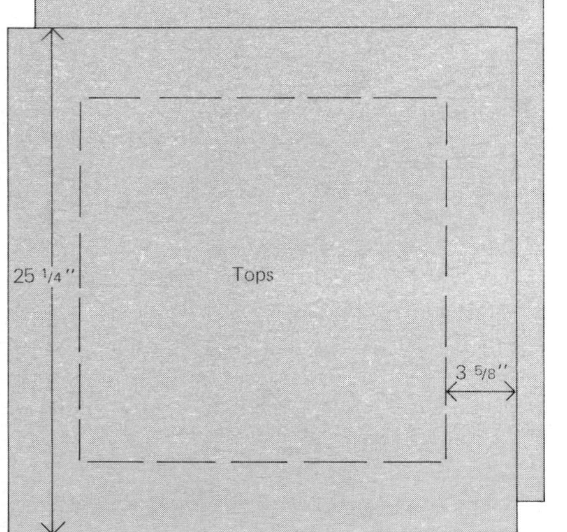

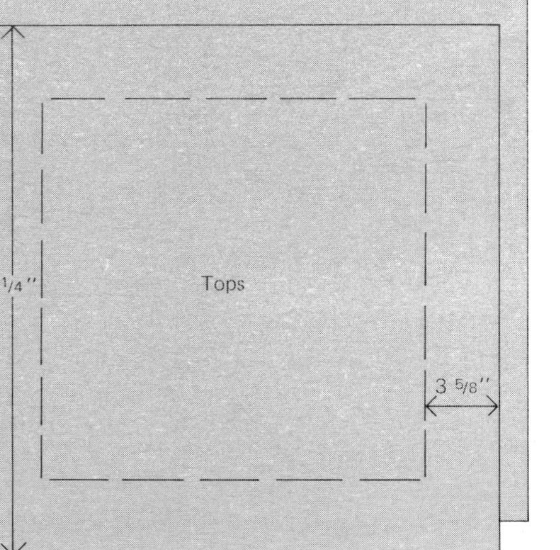

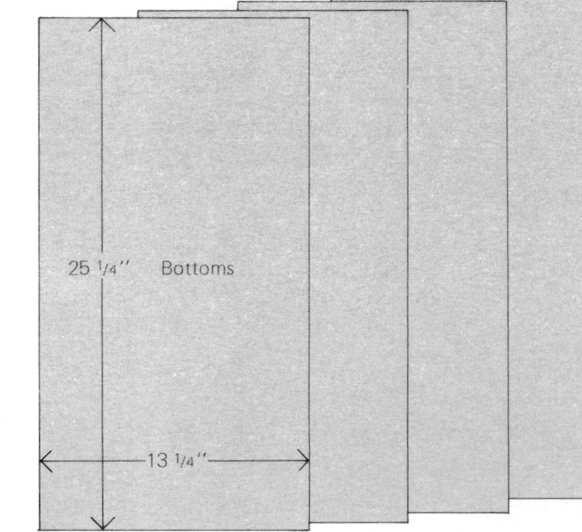

To make two 24" pillow covers, cut two large squares for the pillow tops and four rectangles for pillow bottoms as specified above.

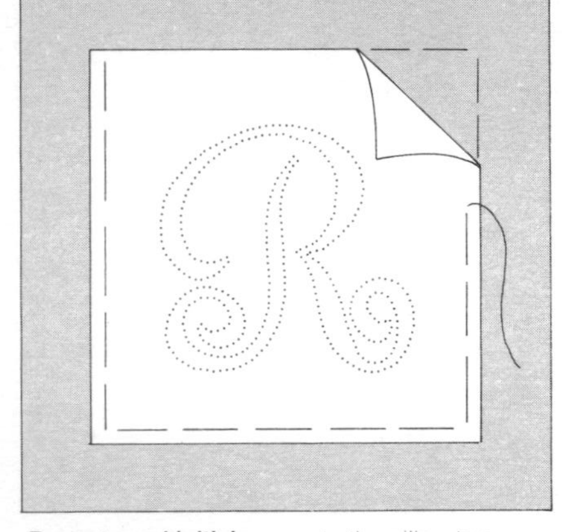

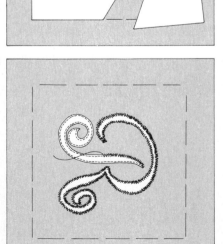

Baste traced initial square to the pillow top.

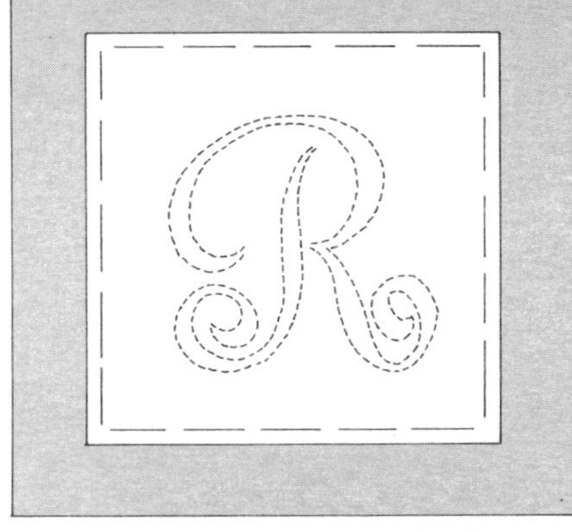

Straight-stitch along the traced initial outline.

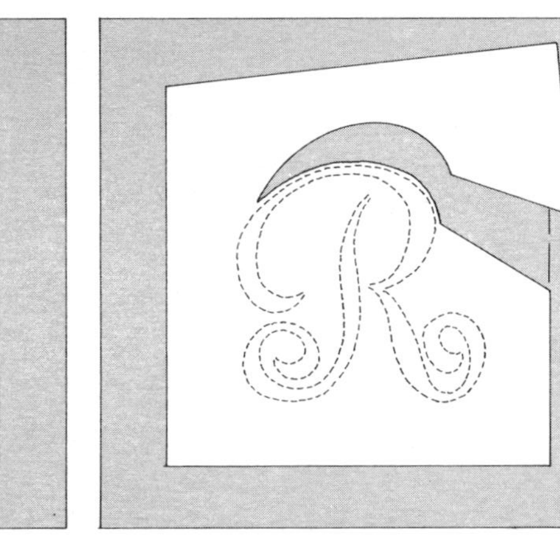

Trim away excess fabric around stitched letter.

Zigzag over the edges of the stitched letter.

Select the desired letter from the alphabet on page 460 and reproduce as directed on a sheet of paper. Center the enlarged letter on the right side of a contrasting fabric square. Slip tracing paper between and trace letter's outline onto fabric.

SEWING

Before starting, thread-trace a smaller square on each of the cover top pieces, placing the lines 3⅝ inches in from the raw edges.

The initial. Center the initialed fabric piece on a cover top piece and hand-baste around it to hold it in place. Carefully machine-stitch (straight-stitch) along the letter outline. Using embroidery scissors, trim the excess fabric as close as possible to the stitching; take care not to cut into the cover fabric. Then, using a short, medium-width satin stitch, go directly over the straight stitching and raw edges of the letter. Pull the thread ends through to the back and knot them.

Decorative trim. Lightly press each strip in half the long way to mark a center line. Press the edges in to meet at this center foldline.

Line up two strips with right sides facing and machine-stitch a diagonal seam across one end as shown to make a mitered corner. Trim and taper seam allowances; press open.

Join the other strips the same way to produce a 20-inch square "frame" on the outer edge.

Position the frame on the cover top, lining up thread-tracing with inner side of frame. Pin frame shape in place and machine-stitch on both edges of the decorative trim. Press.

The cover. With right sides facing, pin two bottom sections of each cover together. Insert a 20-inch zipper in the center of each seam.

To finish a cover, open the zipper. With right sides facing, pin the top and bottom sections together. Machine-stitch around on the seamline. Taper seam allowances at the corners. Turn cover right side out and push out corners. Insert pillow.

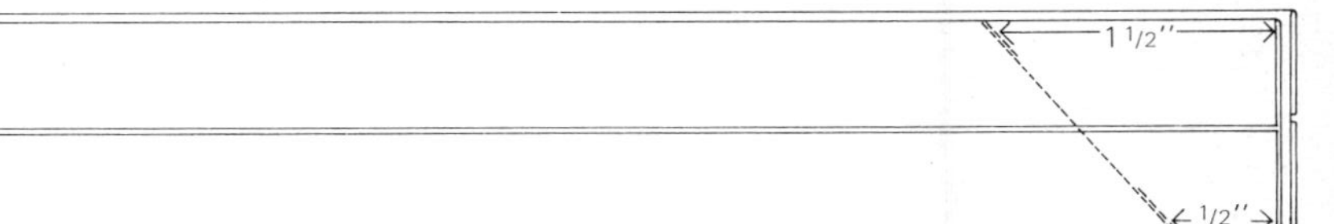

1. Prepare strips of decorative trim. Stitch the strips together in a diagonal seam to miter corners.

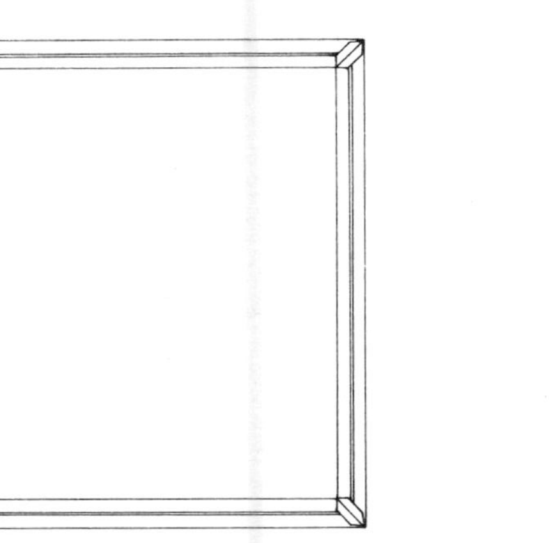

2. Trim and press the mitered seams open; a "frame" should be formed.

3. Pin trim to pillow top; align frame's inner edge to thread-traced lines.

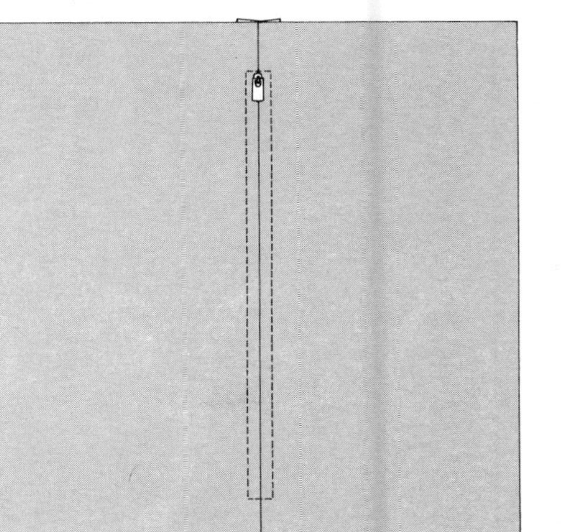

4. Join two bottom sections together inserting zipper within center of seam.

5. Open the zipper, then pin and stitch pillow top and bottom together.

Initial pillows

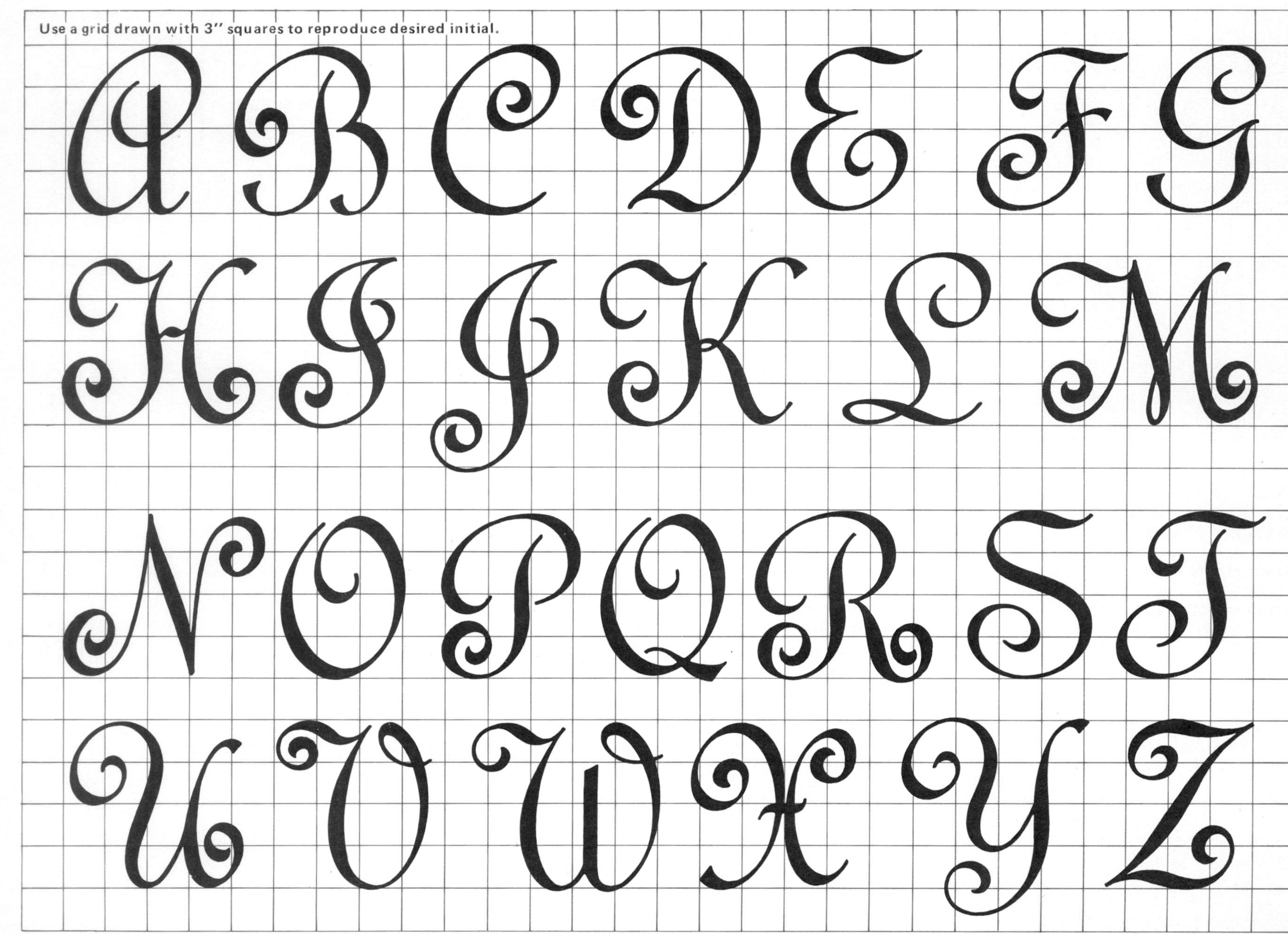

Fake fur rug

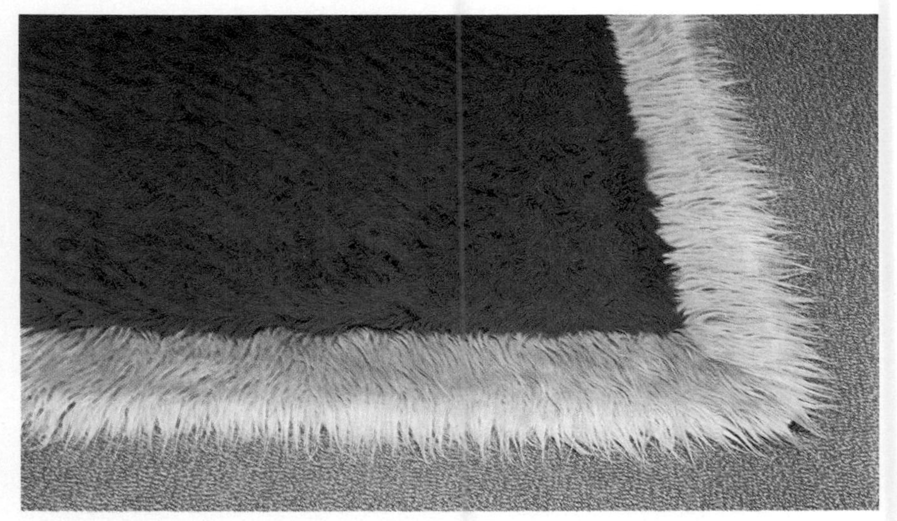

This fake fur rug is not only soft and warm for bare feet, but also sturdy, with burlap sewed to the bottom.

MATERIALS NEEDED

1⅓ yards of 54-inch fake fur for rug
1⅓ yards of 54-inch fake fur in contrasting color for the band
1⅔ yards of 60-inch burlap for backing
Appropriate thread

CUTTING

Cut a 48-inch square from the larger piece of fake fur. Cut eight band sections from the smaller piece following dimensions in the cutting diagram. For the burlap backing, cut a 58-inch square on the straight grain.

SEWING

See the section on Seams for tips on handling seams in fake fur.

With right sides facing, seam two of the trapezoids (band pieces) together along the straight ½-inch seamline to make a long band. Seam the other smaller pieces together the same way to obtain a total of four long bands. Press each seam open.

Pin the short side of each band to a side of the fur square, right sides together. Machine-stitch along the ½-inch seamline, starting and stopping ½ inch from the ends; backstitch at beginning and end.

To miter the corners, pin the diagonal ends of the bands together with right sides facing. Machine-stitch as pinned, backstitching at each seamline crossing. Press all seams open from wrong side. Trim out excess at corners so the seam allowances can lie flat. Then whipstitch the trimmed corners together.

With right sides facing, pin the rug and backing together and machine-stitch all around, leaving a 20-inch opening along one side for turning. Taper the seam allowances at the corners. Turn the rug right side out through the opening, and firmly slipstitch it closed. Press the bottom of the rug with a dry iron.

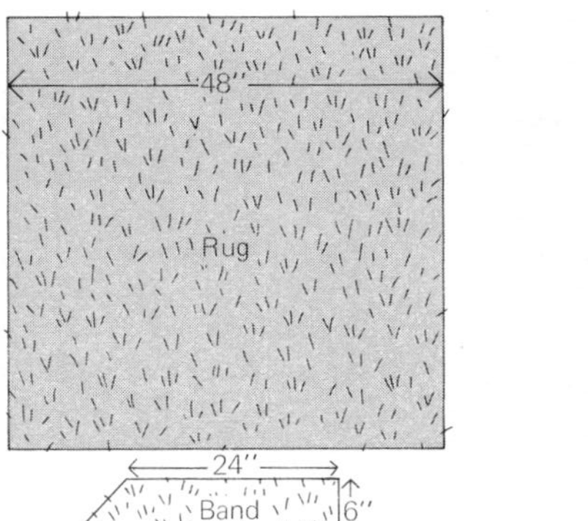

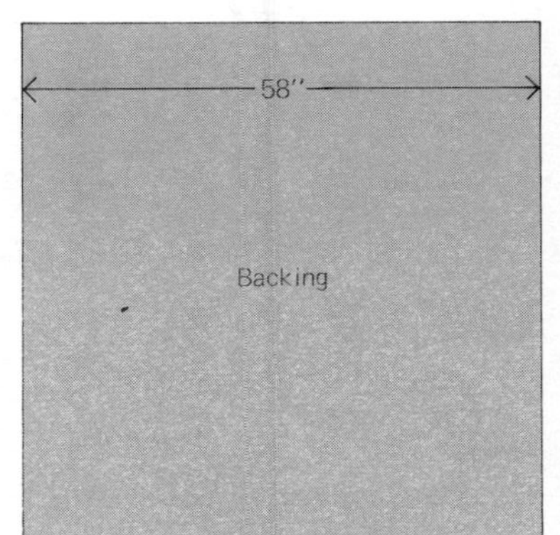

1. Cut one center square and eight band pieces from fur; cut one large burlap square for backing.

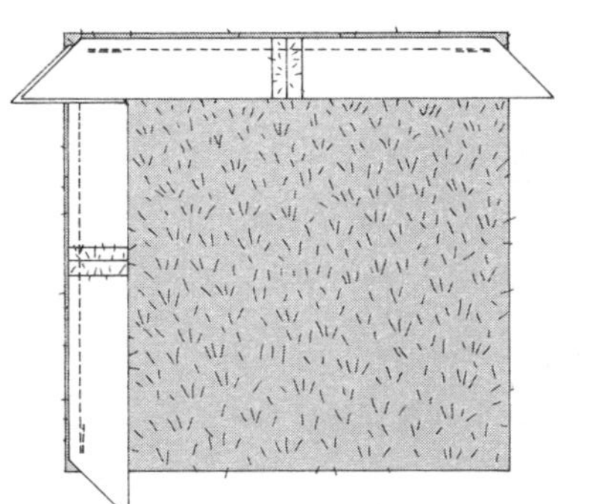

2. Sew long bands to each side of fake fur square.

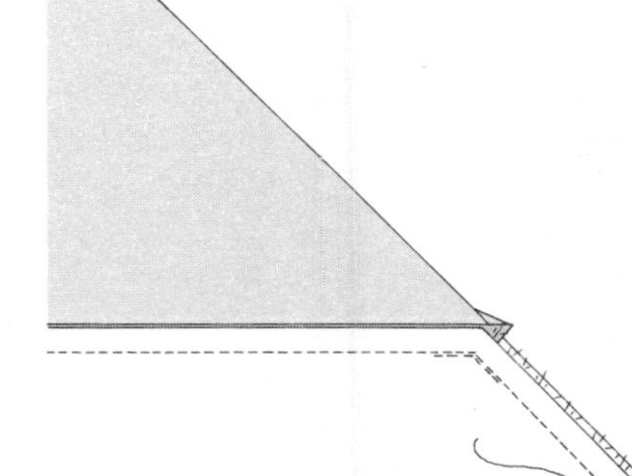

3. Join bands along the diagonal seams at corners.

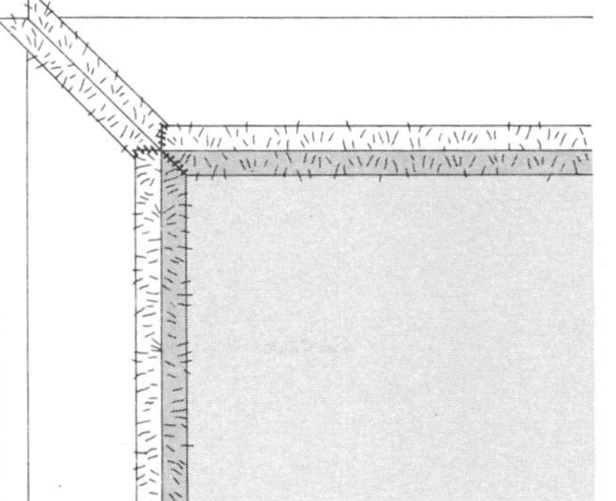

4. Trim excess; whipstitch corner edges together.

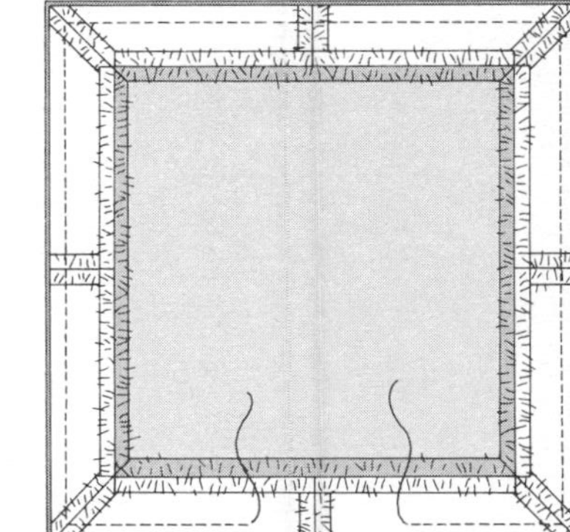

5. Pin and stitch backing to rug along outer edges.

Modern bedroom: Tone-on-tone spread / pillows / curtains / wall panel

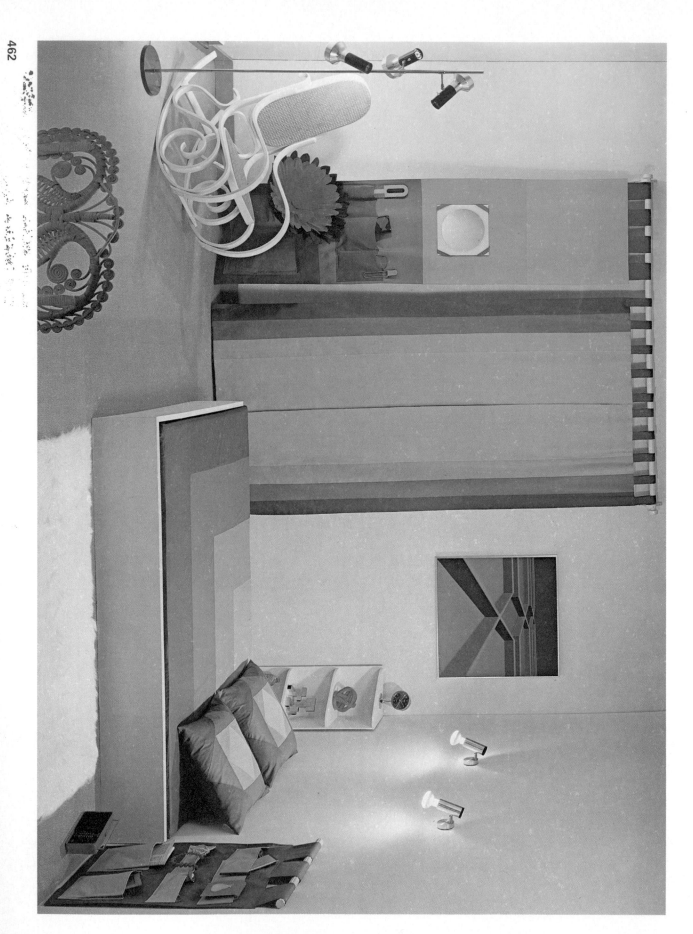

In this striking bedroom, a cool flow of blues, washing from deep navy to pale sky, shows how effective — and contemporary — a monochromatic color scheme can be.

Mitered bands of blue seamed together create the bedspread's abstract pattern. The side drops are cut separately and hang to the floor. You can, of course, shorten them if your bed requires it, as this one does. Before you start, carefully measure the dimensions of your bed, made up with sheets and blankets (see p. 424).

Pillow cases are a variation of the same scheme — progressively smaller squares satin-stitched one over the other to form a geometric design. The covers slip off easily for laundering. Dimensions given are for a 24-inch cushion but can be altered to suit. Foam pillow forms are available in a great variety of sizes. It is best to enclose foam in a muslin undercover.

For the straight, floor-length **curtains,** self-lined with sky blue fabric, bands of color are joined to produce the same gradations of tone as on the spread and pillows. Fabric loops attached at the top are sized to slide easily over a café rod.

The **pocketed wall panel** is coordinated with the curtains. It is made of rectangles of the four colors seamed together and lined. Securely attached pockets will hold magazines or paperbacks, pajamas and slippers. The mirror (optional) is held reliably in place by straps at all four corners.

The fabric here is a heavy sateen, but it could be any medium-weight fabric that offered several hues of the color of your choice. The alternate color harmonies worked out at the right will give you an idea of other monochromatic effects.

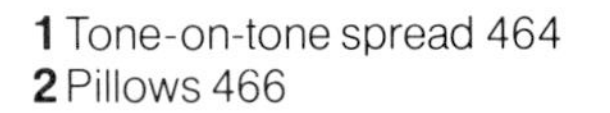

1 Tone-on-tone spread 464
2 Pillows 466
3 Curtains 467
4 Wall panel 469

Bedspread

Measuring beds 424

The top of this all-blue bedspread is made up of seven separate bands of fabric joined to form a right-angle design. The spread is also lined.

For clarity in the instructions, the colors are labeled A, B, C, and D, (from A, the lightest, to D, the darkest). When deciding on and working with your chosen color scheme, whether monochromatic or not, keep track of the colors the same way.

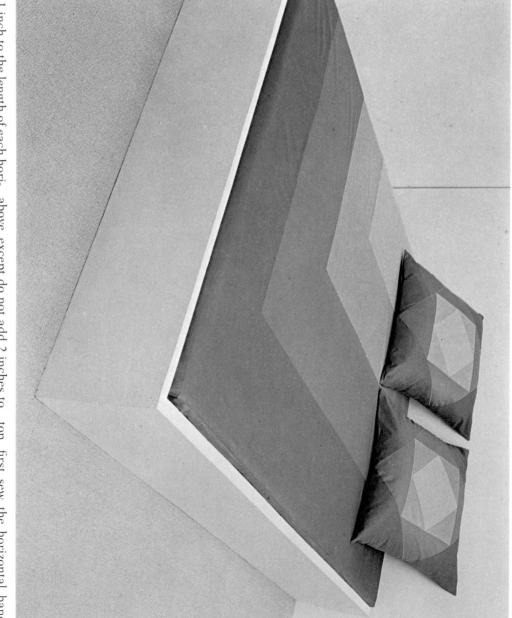

MATERIALS NEEDED

44/45-inch fabric for bedspread
- Color A, 3/5 of a bed length
- Color B, 4/5 of a bed length
- Color C, 1 bed length
- Color D, 2 bed lengths plus 1 bed width (for top design and drops)

44/45-inch fabric for lining
- 3 bed lengths plus 1 bed width (fabric A used in this spread)

1 package of seam binding
Appropriate thread

CUTTING

Before cutting the actual bands, you must determine the finished size of each. The widths of all bands will be the same (one-fourth the bed width). The lengths of both the vertical and horizontal bands will all be different, each set getting progressively shorter. Starting with the longest set (color D), the vertical band will equal the bed length and the horizontal band will equal the bed width. The vertical and horizontal bands in each successive set (C, B, A) will be cut progressively shorter, each time by the width of one band.

On the straight grain of each fabric, cut out all seven of the bands, using the given sequence of fabric colors (D, C, B, A). Add 1 inch to the width of each band (for seams); 13 inches to the length of each vertical band (for top overhang and seams); and 1 inch to the length of each horizontal band (for seams).

Cut two rectangles for the side drops, each measuring the bed length plus 1 inch by the bed height plus 2 inches. Then cut the foot drop to equal the bed width plus 1 inch by the bed height plus 2 inches.

Cut the lining for the side and foot drops, following the dimensions above, except do not add 2 inches to the height. Cut the lining for the top part of the bedspread so that it is as wide as the bed plus 1 inch and as long as the bed plus 13 inches. If necessary, piece the lining to get the proper width.

SEWING

To construct the geometric design on top, first sew the horizontal bands together, with right sides facing, in the proper sequence (B to C, C to D). Press the seams open. Join the B, C, and D vertical bands in the same way and press these seams open.

With right sides facing, pin the vertical unit to the horizontal unit, matching both the colors and the raw edges on the "stepladder" edge.

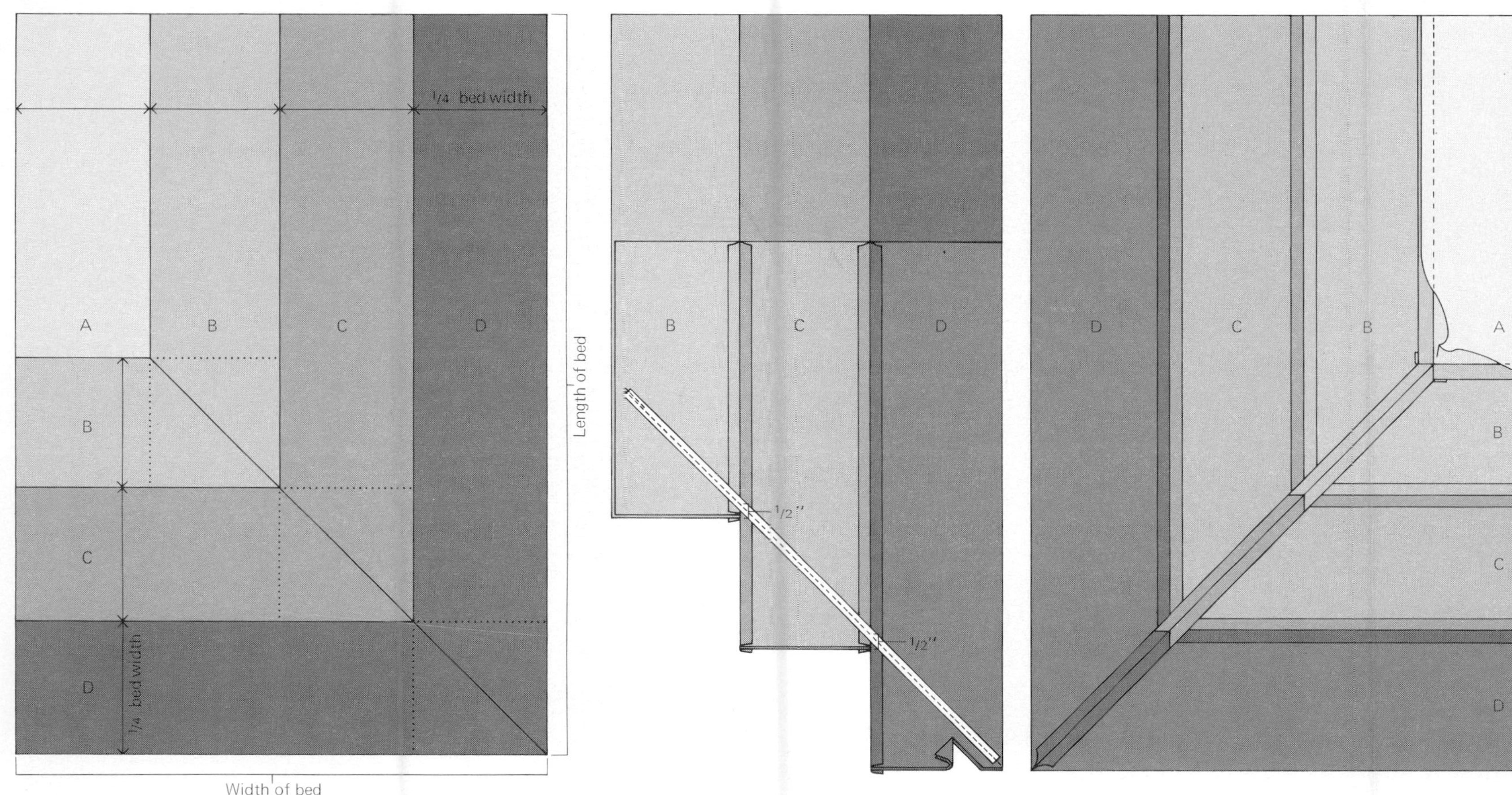

Band width equals one-fourth the bed width. D bands are full bed length and width; C, B, and A bands are progressively shorter by a band width.

Align edges of vertical and horizontal bands; stitch diagonal seam, catching in seam binding. Trim.

With right sides facing, pin and stitch the last band (A) to the edges of B bands, pivoting at the corner. Press seams toward B bands.

On one side of the pinned piece, place a mark along each stitched seamline, ½ inch up from the raw edge. Draw a diagonal line connecting the markings and the corner of the D unit. Position seam binding along the marked line and pin it in place. Stitch along the diagonal line, catching the seam binding in the stitching; stop the stitching at the seamline crossing of the B unit and secure the stitches. Trim the excess ends of the bands, leaving a seam allowance width. Press the diagonal seam open.

With right sides facing, pin the remaining band (Color A) to the edges of both B bands. Machine-stitch as pinned, pivoting at corner. Press the seams toward the B bands.

To construct the bedspread drop, pin the side drop pieces to each end of the foot drop piece, right sides together. Stitch on seamlines, stopping and securing stitches ½ inch from tops of seams. Join pieces for lining drop the same way.

To line the bedspread drop, proceed as follows: With right sides together, pin the lining drop to the bedspread drop along the bottom edges; stitch. Bring top edges of both drops together so that their raw edges are even; pin. Stitch the drops together along the two free ends. Turn the lined drop to the right side.

With right sides together, stitch the lined bedspread drop to the top of the bedspread. Proceed to line the top portion of the bedspread (see the section on Bedspreads).

Geometric pillows

Satin stitching 30, 32-35

Mitering turned-up hems 304
Centered zipper application 318

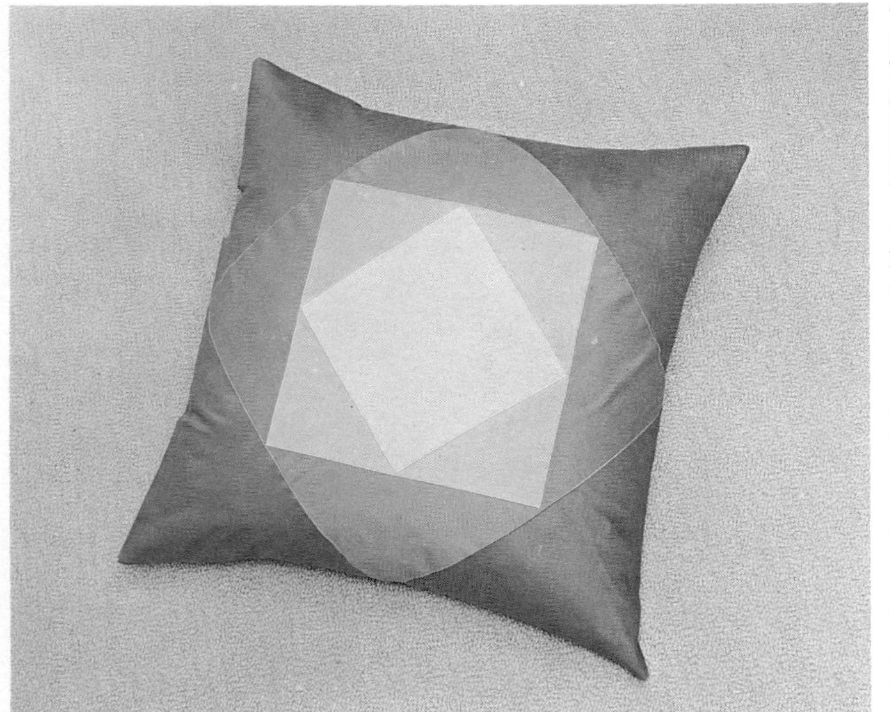

These pillow covers are a variation of the geometric spread on page 464. The colors are labeled A, B, C, and D as was done for the bedspread. Zippered for easy removal, these appliquéd covers fit a 24-inch square knife-edge pillow form.

MATERIALS NEEDED
For two pillows:
44/45-inch fabric for each color
Color A, ¼ yard
Color B, ⅜ yard
Color C, ½ yard
Color D, 2¼ yards
Two 20-inch zippers
Two 24-inch square knife-edge pillow forms (to make your own pillow forms, see page 449)
Appropriate thread

CUTTING

For each pillow cover. Cut a 25¼-inch square from color D for the top of the cover. For the cover bottom cut two 13¼ x 25¼-inch rectangles from color D. The measurements given include ⅝-inch seam allowances.

Cut squares for the appliqué as follows: From color A, a 9-inch square; from color B, a 12½-inch square; from color C, a 17½-inch square. A ¼-inch seam allowance is included in these measurements. On the right side of the fabric mark the center of each side of each square.

SEWING

To prepare squares A, B, and C for appliquéing, first press under a ¼-inch hem on all edges of each square. After the corners of each square have been mitered as shown below, hand-baste all hems in place.

With right sides up, place square A on square B, aligning corners of square A to center markings on square B; baste in place. Satin-stitch over the folded edges of square A; remove bastings. If you do not have a zigzag machine, straight-stitch close to the folded edges. Position and appliqué this stitched square on square C in the same way.

With right sides up, center the appliquéd design on the cover top (square D) and, following the same procedure as above, appliqué the design in place.

Seam the two rectangles for the bottom of the cover along two of their 25¼-inch edges, inserting a centered zipper into the seam. Position the zipper so that it is centered along the seam's length.

Open zipper. Match the raw edges of top and bottom cover sections, right sides together; pin along the ⅝-inch seamline. Stitch along the seamline, going across corners to blunt them. Trim seam allowances.

Turn cover right side out through zipper opening; push out on corners to shape cover. Insert pillow form into the cover; close zipper.

Miter each corner of each square.

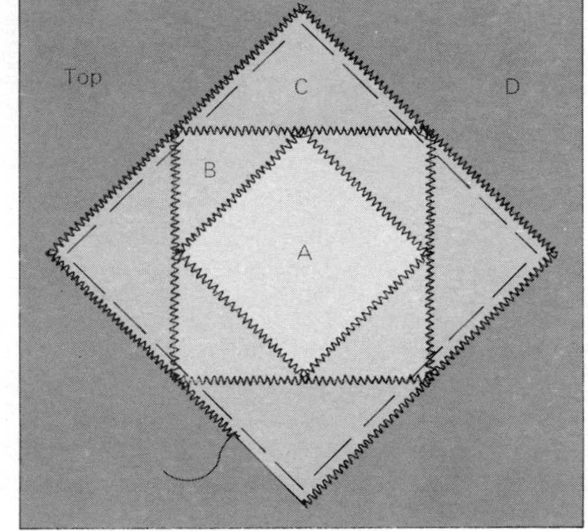

Appliqué completed design onto top of pillow cover.

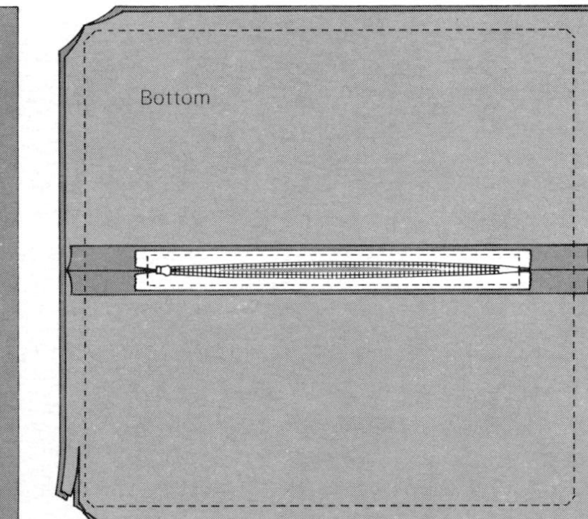

Insert zipper into bottom of cover; sew bottom to top.

Curtains

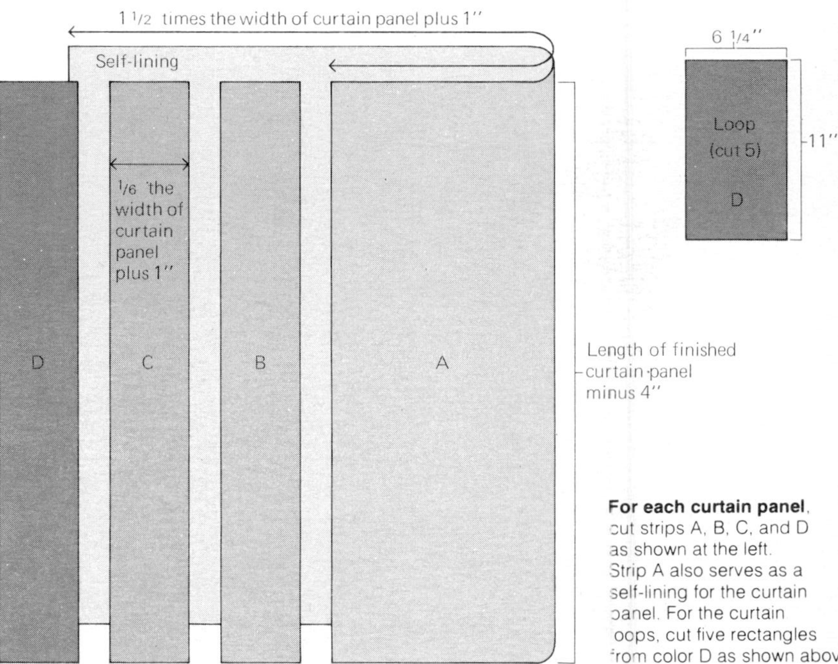

These curtains, like the other items in the bedroom, are made from separate pieces of fabric in four shades of the same color. Three bands are the same size; the fourth is wider than the others, and also acts as a self-lining. The colors, like those used elsewhere, are labeled A, B, C, and D. The extra-large loops at the top slide easily over a rod.

MATERIALS NEEDED

For two curtain panels up to 56 inches in total width:

44/45-inch fabric for each color
- Color A, 2 fabric lengths
- Colors B, C, and D, 1 fabric length each
- (a fabric length equals distance from curtain rod to floor)

Appropriate thread

CUTTING

For each curtain panel, you will need a wide band from color A, a narrow band from colors B, C, and D, and five loops from color D. Cutting length for each band should equal the desired finished length of the curtain minus 4 inches. To determine the width of the wide band, first multiply the finished width of one curtain panel by 1½, then to this number add 1 inch for seam allowances. To determine the cut width of the narrow bands, divide the width of the finished curtain panel by 6, then to this number add 1 inch for seam allowances. For the loops, cut five rectangles from color D, each of them measuring 6¼ x 11 inches. More loops may be needed if the panel is wider than 28 inches.

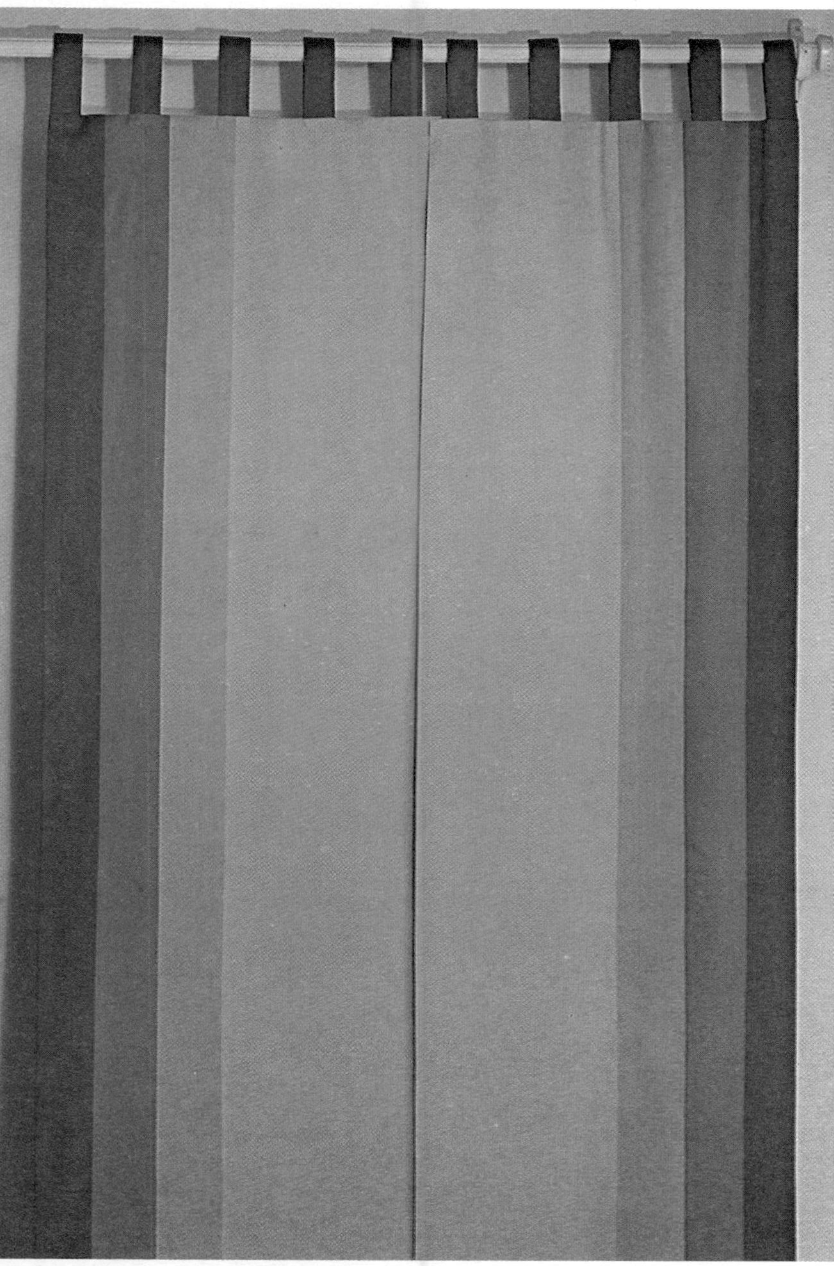

For each curtain panel, cut strips A, B, C, and D as shown at the left. Strip A also serves as a self-lining for the curtain panel. For the curtain loops, cut five rectangles from color D as shown above.

Curtains

SEWING

To make curtain loops, first press under ¼ inch along one long side of each small rectangle. Then fold each rectangle into thirds so that the raw edge of the fabric is on the inside and the folded edge on the outside. Baste, then topstitch close to edge on both long sides, through all layers. Fold each strip in half, aligning the ends; sew ends together.

For each curtain panel, join the three narrow bands in the proper color sequence — first B to C, then C to D. Then, with right sides together, sew wide band A to the free edge of band B. Press all seams open. With right sides together, fold curtain in half to bring the edge of the self-lining to the free edge of band D. Match and pin the edges together along the long side and the bottom of the curtain panel. Stitch, leaving a 12- to 14-inch opening at the center of the bottom seamline.

At the top of the panel, pin the loops between the curtain and the self-lining. Keeping the raw edges of the loops even with the raw edges of the curtain and self-lining, position the loops as follows: One loop at the seamline of band D and the self-lining; another loop 1 inch in from the fold between A and the self-lining; the remaining loops an even distance from these loops and each other. Baste, then stitch across the top seamline, through all layers.

Turn the curtain panel right side out through the opening in the bottom seam; bring the three seamlines out to the edges. Slipstitch the opening closed. Press well. Construct the other curtain panel in the same way.

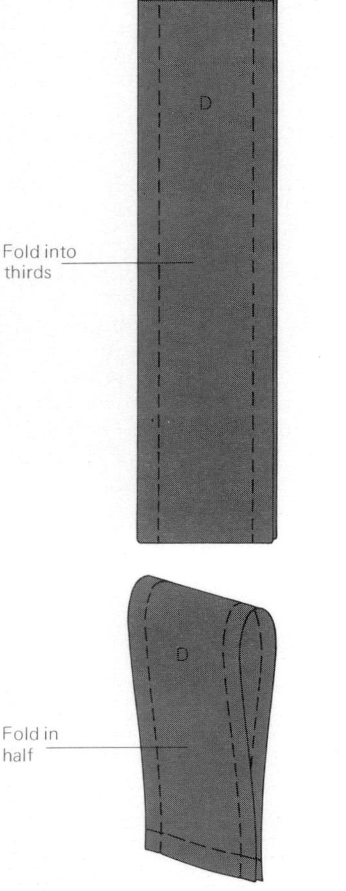

For loop, fold rectangle into thirds, then in half.

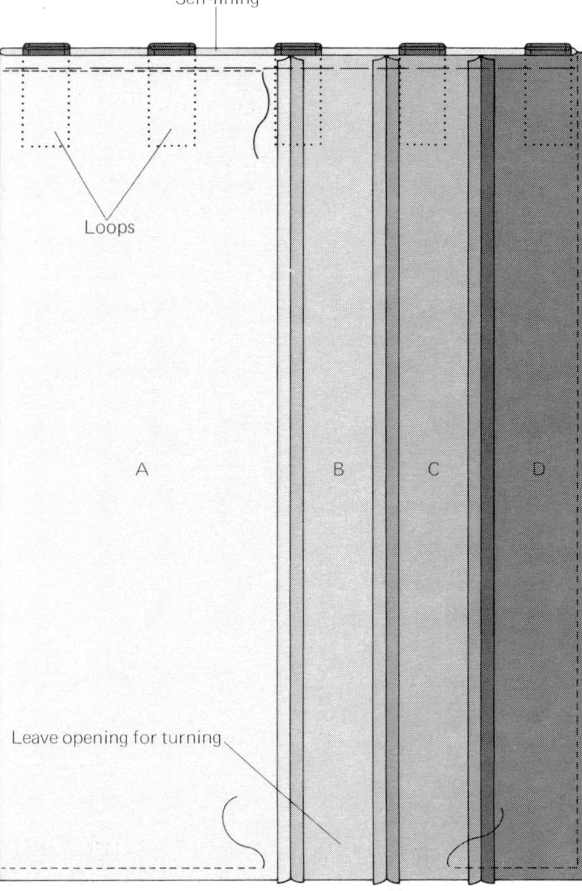

Sew panel to self-lining; at top, sew loops between panel and lining.

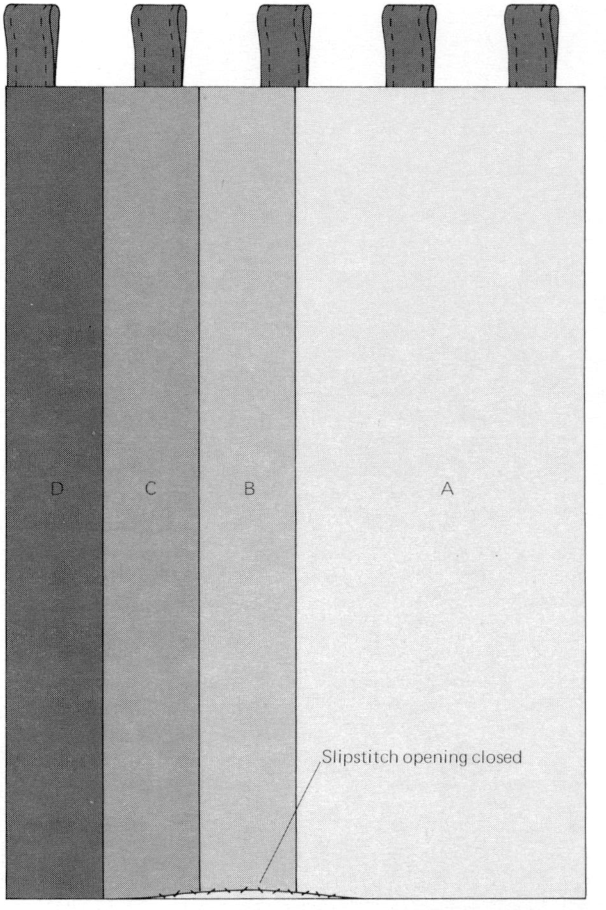

Turn panel right side out through opening; slipstitch opening closed.

Wall panel

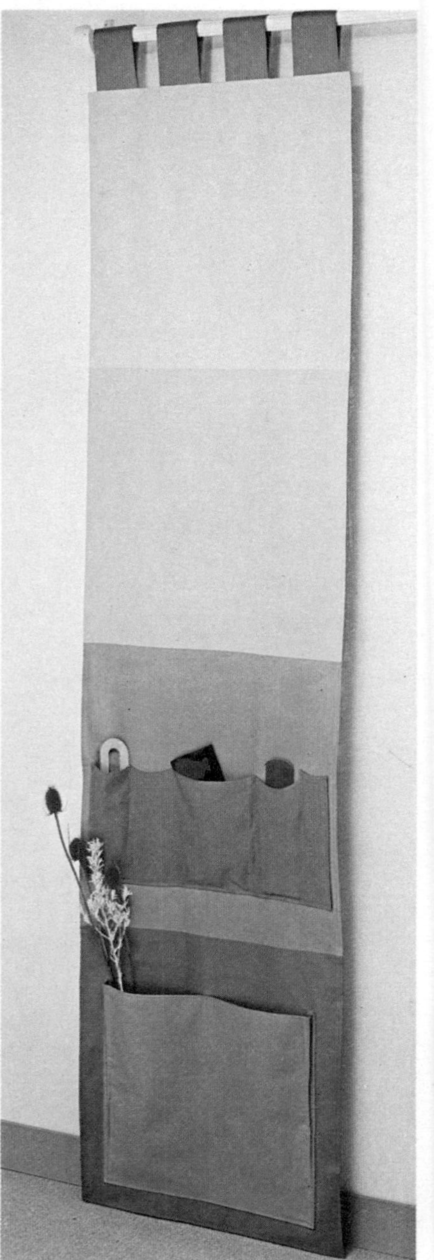

This pocketed wall panel coordinates with the rest of the blue bedroom. It can be made with or without the straps needed to hold a mirror in place; it can be hung from its own rod or the same rod as the curtains (see page 462). The wall panel is completely lined to its edges. Colors are again identified as A, B, C, and D.

MATERIALS NEEDED

44/45-inch fabric for each color
- Colors A and B, ¼-length each
- Color C, ¼-length plus 1 yard
- Color D, ¼-length plus ⅔ yard
- (a full length is equal to the distance from the curtain rod to the floor)

44/45-inch fabric for lining panel
- 1 full length

Appropriate thread

CUTTING

The measurements that follow include ½-inch seam allowances.

For the body of the wall panel, cut four identical rectangles. Each rectangle should measure 25 inches in width. To determine what length they should be, first subtract 1 inch from the finished panel length, then divide this number by four.

For the upper pocket, cut a 23 x 22-inch rectangle from color D. On it, thread-trace the vertical stitch lines that will form the pouches (see below). Cut a hexagon from color C for the lower pocket, using the dimensions below; thread-trace the stitch line that will form the pouches.

From color D, cut four rectangles, each measuring 12¼ x 11 inches. These are for the loops of the panel.

Cut the lining to measure 25 inches wide and as long as the finished panel, minus 4 inches.

SEWING

To make loops, follow instructions for curtain loops on opposite page, except press under the ¼ inch along one of the short sides rather than the long side of the rectangle.

Fold each pocket piece in half with right sides together. Stitch each on its seamlines, leaving a 4-inch opening at the bottom. Turn each pocket to the right side through opening in bottom seam; slipstitch openings closed. Topstitch ¼ inch in from the top edge of each pocket.

Center upper pocket onto the right side of body rectangle C, with the bottom of the pocket 4 inches up from the bottom edge of the rectangle; pin in place. Stitch along the side and bottom edges of the pocket. To form pouches, pin pocket to body rectangle along the thread-traced lines and stitch from top to bottom.

Center lower pocket onto the right side of body rectangle D, with the bottom edge of pocket 2½ inches up from bottom of rectangle, and the sides of the pocket parallel to the sides of the rectangle. Pin in place; stitch along side and bottom edges of pocket. To form pouches, stitch pocket to body rectangle along the center thread-traced line. Press pocket to create a pleat at each side.

Right sides together, seam body rectangles to each other in proper color sequence. Press seams open.

With right sides together, pin and stitch the lining to the panel along the sides and bottom; leave a 6-inch opening in the bottom seam.

Keeping raw edges even, pin loops between top edges of panel and lining. At each end, position a loop 1 inch from seamline; space remaining loops the same distance apart. Baste, then stitch top. Turn panel right side out through opening at bottom; slipstitch opening closed.

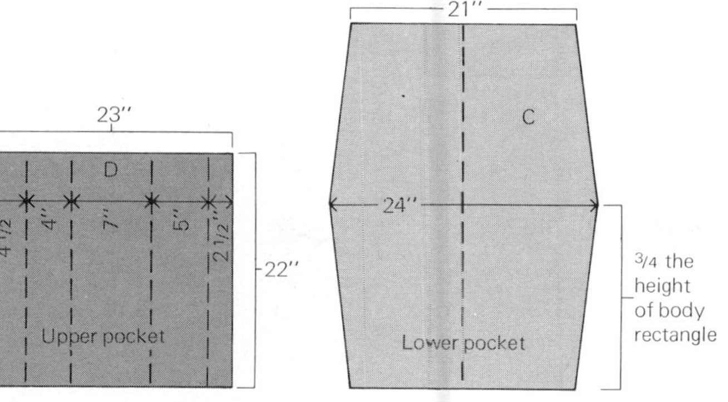

Cut and then mark both the upper and lower pockets as shown above.

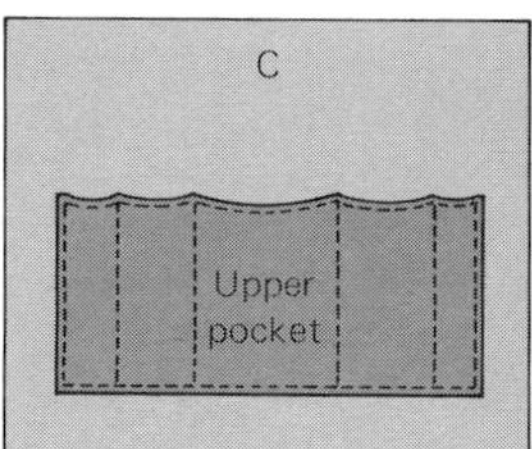

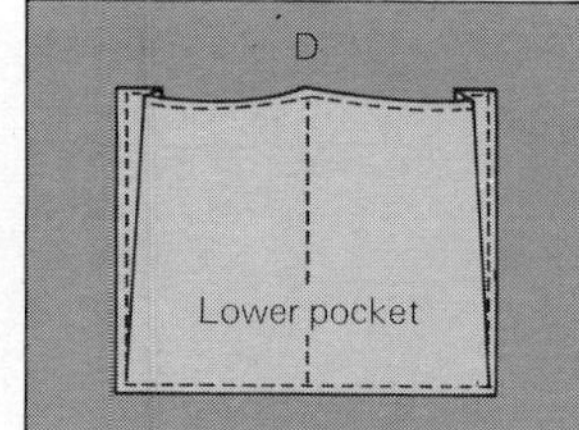

Sew upper pocket to rectangle C; sew lower pocket to rectangle D.

Girl's room: Throw spread / matching bolster / pouf floor pillow

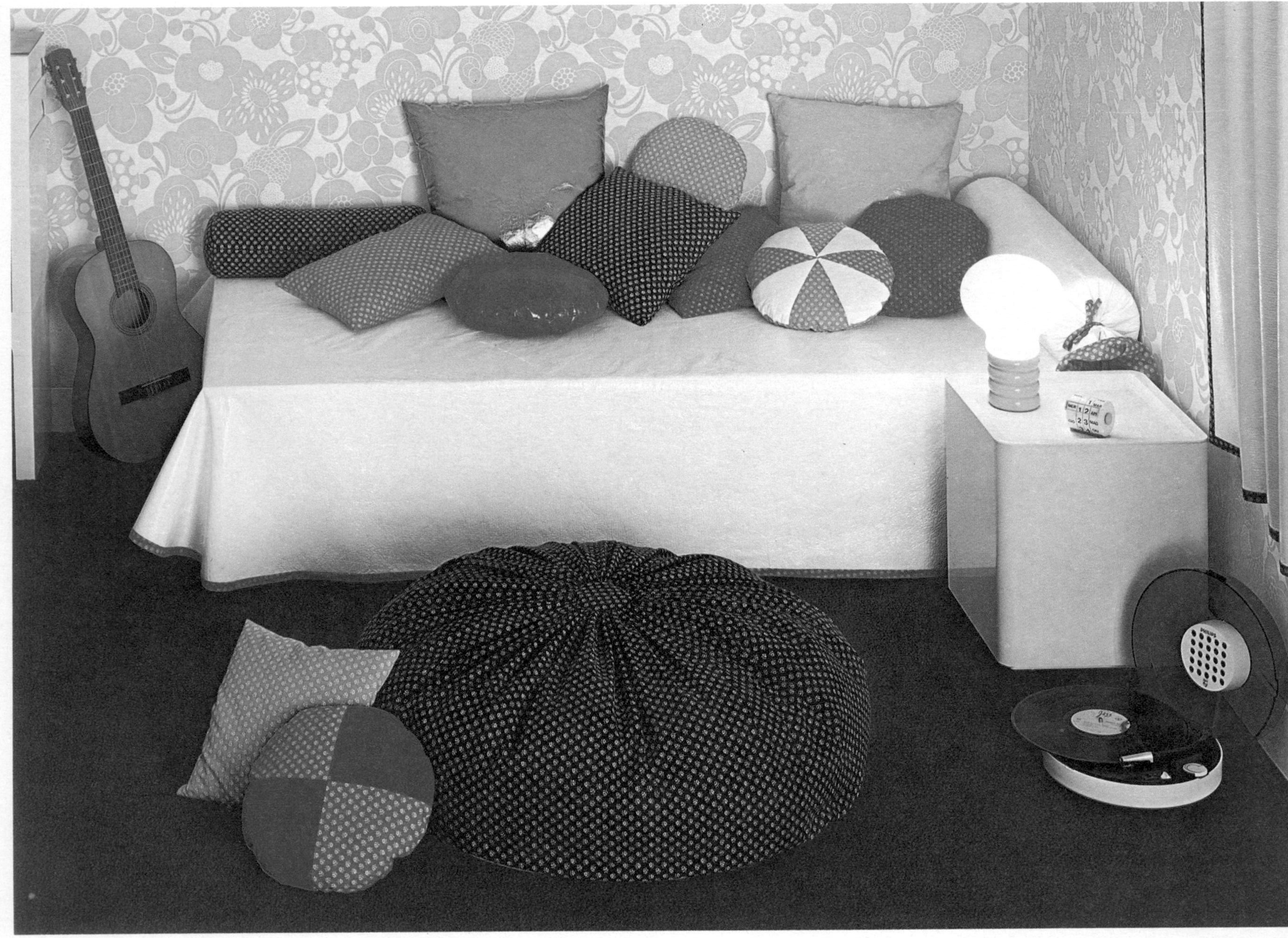

A young girl's room plays many parts. It is a place to entertain friends, finish up homework, pursue a hobby, read a book. As the setting for so many activities, such a room must have furnishings made for hard and varied wear and for easy upkeep.

A bed sometimes used for sitting should be well cushioned for comfort, and covered with a spread that takes very little fussing — when the bed is being made or at any other time. This practical **throw spread** is made of easy-to-clean vinyl, which means no worry about soft drinks or cookie crumbs — a damp sponge will wipe them away. The corners at the foot are rounded to hang gracefully, a simple effect to create, as the instructions will show. For a neat finish, bind the edges with an appropriate contrast — here a small-patterned print.

The matching **bolster** is covered "candy-wrapper" style, the ends tied to flare out and show their gaily colored linings keyed to other contrasts in the room. Use a round bolster form as long as the bed is wide.

A bouquet of throw pillows, in many shapes and colors, contrasts brilliantly with the pure white of the spread. When friends come visiting, extra seating is right at hand, in the **pouf floor pillow** form so popular with young people today. Lightweight and instantly portable, it has all the comfort of an old-fashioned armchair. You may want to make one for your own room.

The pouf pillow is simple to sew — just stitch a long rectangle of fabric firmly to a circular base, then gather it tightly around the top; a centered "button" hides gathered edges. For sturdiness, the base is made from layers of pillow fabric and interfacing; vinyl would be a practical alternative. The filling can be shredded foam or expanded polystyrene beads.

White was chosen for the spread because it coordinates so effortlessly with the many accent colors. For a change of scheme, you might consider one of the vinyl-coated fabrics that coordinate with the same fabrics minus the coating. Should you prefer a different fabric entirely, there are many of the right weight and character, among them linen, duck or comparably sturdy cotton, and corduroy.

To give you an idea of other color and pattern combinations, some suggestions are grouped at the right. You might consider, for example, a large floral pattern for the floor pillow. Small dots and stripes would combine well for throw pillows. A solid color is best for the spread in such a many-patterned scheme.

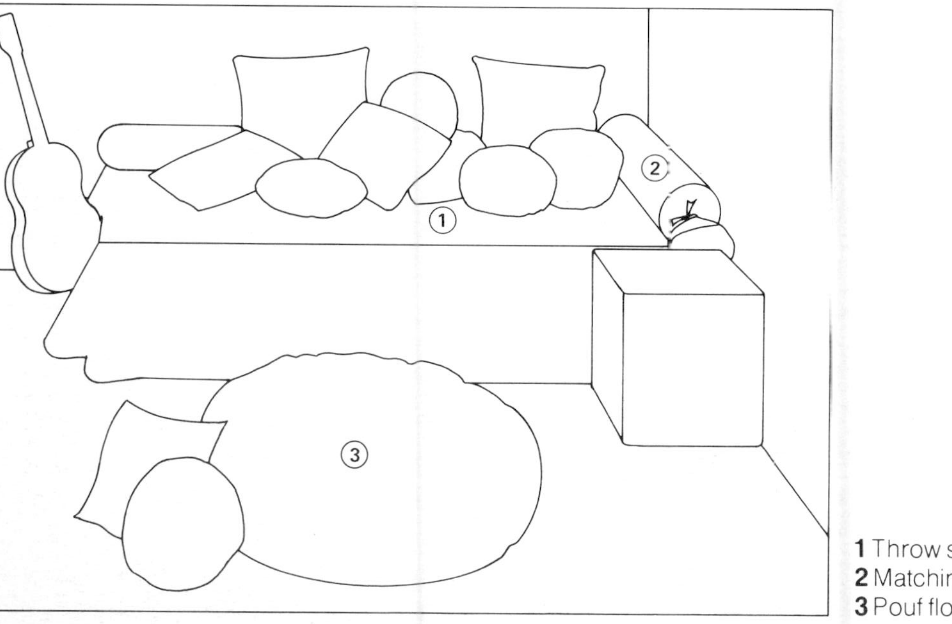

1 Throw spread 472
2 Matching bolster 472
3 Pouf floor pillow 474

Throw spread and bolster

Cutting bias strips 298-299
Mitering topstitched binding 309

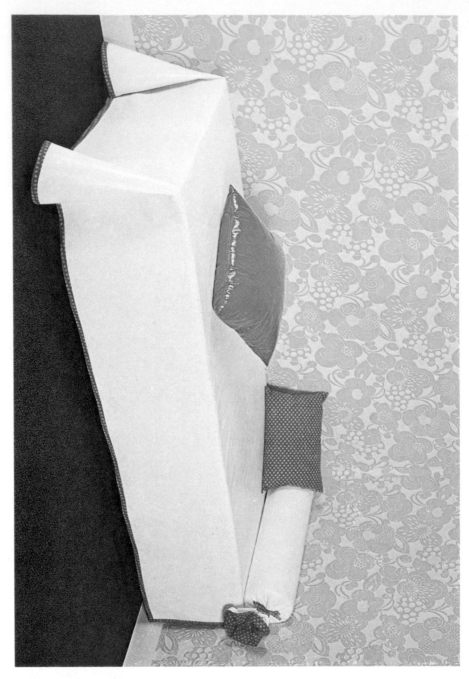

With this throw spread, it is no trouble to keep a bed looking neat all day long. The practical vinyl isn't damaged by spills as fabric can be, and you can simply wipe it clean.

The glowing white coordinates perfectly with all of the colors in the room. The contrasting trim along the bottom repeats the bolster print, but it could just as well be a solid color or another print if you prefer.

The yardage requirements given are for a twin-size bed.

MATERIALS NEEDED

For twin-size spread:

5⅓ yards of 54-inch vinyl
1½ yards of 44/45-inch fabric for bias binding
Appropriate thread

CUTTING

When you measure to determine dimensions, have the bed fully made up with sheets and blankets.

For the top (center) panel of the spread, you will need a length of fabric that equals the length of the bed plus the height of the bed, and is as wide as the bed plus a 1-inch allowance for the side seams.

To reach to the floor at the sides, you will need two side panels, each as long as the top panel and as wide as the height of the bed plus ½-inch seam allowance for joining the side panels to the top panel.

The required amount of bias binding is arrived at by adding twice the total length of the spread to twice its total width. To bind a spread for a twin bed, you will need approximately 10 yards of 4-inch-wide bias strips. To make this much binding, it is easiest to form continuous bias strips (see Hems for procedure).

SEWING

With right sides together, match and stitch a side panel to each long edge of the center panel. Finger-press the seam flat, then open. Consider using a flat-felled seam; it gives desirable sturdiness to joined panels.

To round off the two foot corners of the spread, proceed as follows: On the wrong side of the spread, mark a square at one foot corner. This square's sides should be equal to the distance from the top of the bed to the floor. Place a tape measure or yardstick at the inner corner of the square and draw a cutting line in an arc, starting and ending at opposite corners of the marked square. Cut on this curved line. Round off the other foot corner the same way.

Prepare the binding for the edge of the spread as follows: Fold the bias strip lengthwise, a little off center so that one side of the strip is approximately ⅛ inch wider than the other. Open out the pressed strip and fold the cut edges toward the pressed crease; press both edges.

With the right side of the spread up, wrap the binding around the raw edges of the bedspread, keeping the wider side of the binding underneath. Topstitch along the edge of the binding, starting and ending the binding at one of the less conspicuous seamlines; fold the end of the binding under and lap it over the beginning. Carefully miter the binding at the top corners of the bedspread (see Hems) and shape the binding to fit around curves at bottom corners.

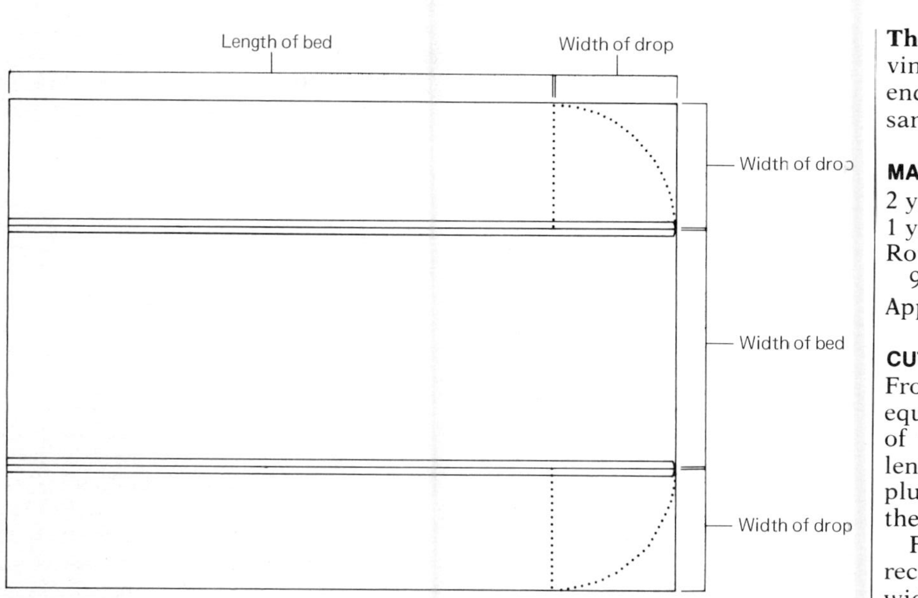

1. Join center and side panels of spread. Mark and cut curves at the foot corners.

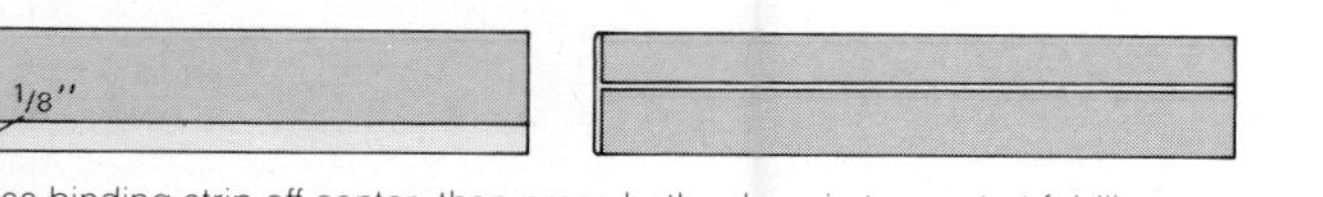

2. Press binding strip off center; then press both edges in to meet at foldline.

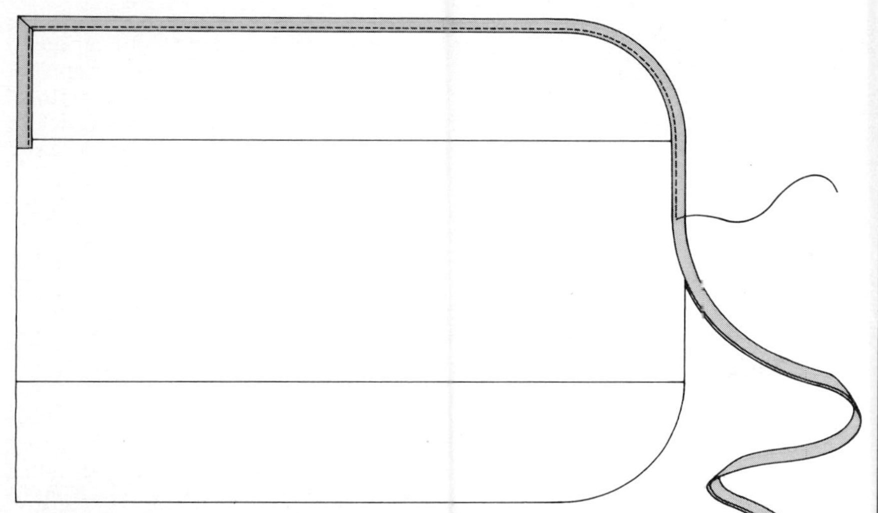

3. Wrap the binding around bottom raw edge of spread, and topstitch it in place.

The round bolster is covered in the vinyl used for the spread. The flared ends tie and untie, so it isn't necessary to install a zipper.

MATERIALS NEEDED

2 yards of 54-inch vinyl for cover
1 yard of 44/45-inch fabric for lining
Round bolster form 36 inches long x 9 inches in diameter
Appropriate thread

CUTTING

From the vinyl fabric, cut a rectangle equal in width to the circumference of the bolster plus 1 inch, and in length to the length of the bolster plus 33 inches (the extra length is for the flared ends).

From the lining fabric, cut two rectangles, each 19 inches long by the width of the large rectangle.

Also cut from the lining fabric, for the bolster ties, two strips 28 inches long and 2 inches wide.

SEWING

With right sides together, match and stitch a lining piece to each end of the bolster cover. Trim seams; press toward cover. Seam-finish raw edges at free ends of lining pieces.

Fold cover in half lengthwise with right sides facing, and stitch along the matched lengthwise edge. Trim seam; finger press open. At each end, turn lining sections down toward center of cover; tack free edges in place. Turn cover right side out.

Stitch each bolster tie as follows: First fold all edges ½ inch to wrong side and press. Then fold the tie in half lengthwise to the wrong side and press. Stitch tie through all fabric layers along all edges.

Insert bolster form into cover and center it; wrap a tie around each end of the bolster, close to the form.

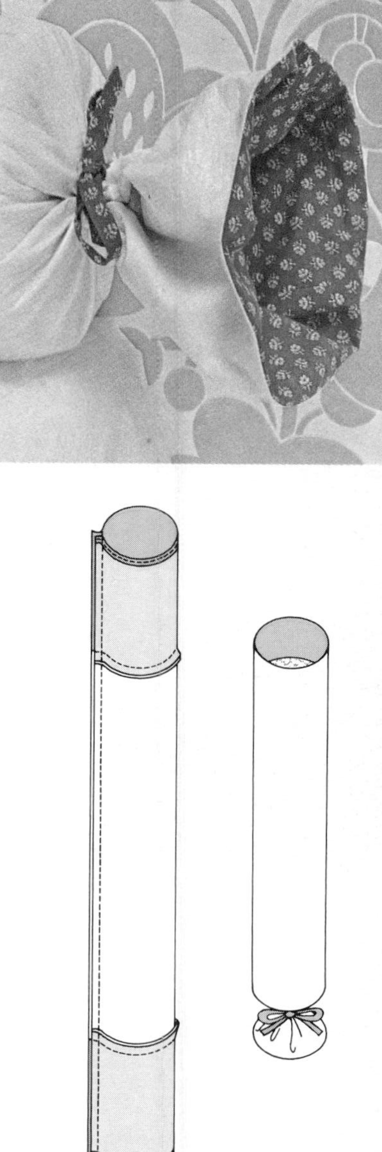

To make bolster, join lining to ends of rectangle; stitch seam. Fold lining inside; secure edges. Turn cover right side out. Insert bolster form; tie ends.

Pouf floor pillow

Lightweight, yet as comfortable as an overstuffed armchair, this floor pillow would be popular anywhere in the house. The polystyrene beads are contained in an undercover; the outer cover unzips for washing. For firmness, the base is made from several thicknesses of fabric. Fabric choice is wide; just be sure it is washable.

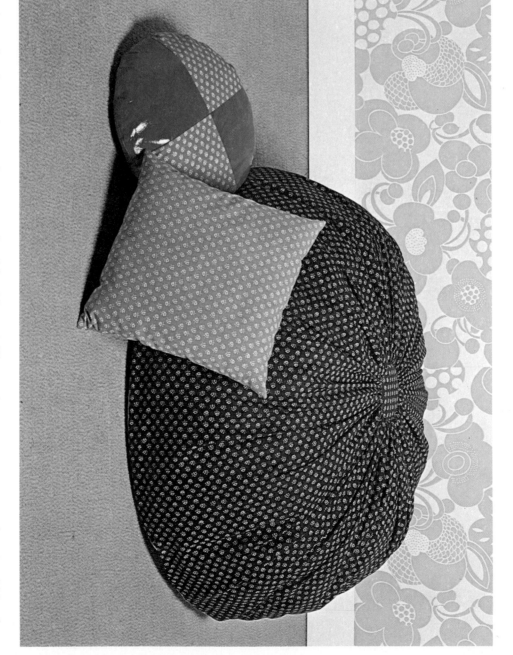

MATERIALS NEEDED

5⅓ yards of 44/45-inch fabric for outer cover
3⅔ yards of 44/45-inch fabric for undercover
2¼ yards of 26-inch fusible interfacing
One 27-inch zipper
12 inches of ½-inch twill tape
Expanded polystyrene beads or shredded foam
Appropriate thread

CUTTING

Undercover. Cut two rectangles along the lengthwise grain, each measuring 19 x 56 inches. Then cut two circles with 36½-inch diameters.

Outer cover. Cut a 25 x 114-inch rectangle along the lengthwise grain. For the base, cut four semicircles, each with a 37½-inch diameter and an added ½-inch seam allowance on the straight edges. Then cut two semicircles from fusible interfacing, each 36½ inches in diameter.

For the "button," cut two circles with 6-inch diameters from the cover fabric and two with 5½-inch diameters from fusible interfacing.

SEWING

Undercover. Staystitch the long edges of both rectangles. With right sides facing, pin and machine-stitch the ends of the two large rectangles together. Press seam open. Then pin and stitch other ends together to form a circular body; leave an 8-inch opening. Press seam open.

With right sides facing, pin one of the circles to one end of the undercover; clip the seam allowances of the undercover as necessary to go around the curves. Machine-stitch as pinned. Stitch the remaining circle to the other end of the undercover in the same way. Turn the undercover to the right side, and fill it with expanded polystyrene beads. Whipstitch the opening tightly to close.

Outer cover. Staystitch one long edge of large rectangle. With right sides facing, pin and stitch short ends together to form tube.

Fold tube in half toward seamline and mark the folds on the unstitched edge. Place two rows of gathering stitches in the unstitched seam allowance, one a thread width above seamline, the other ¼ inch higher; break stitching lines at each quarter marking (seamline serves as one marking). Leave long thread ends.

Fuse the interfacing semicircles to wrong side of two fabric semicircles. With wrong sides together, baste each of the remaining fabric semicircles to a fused semicircle.

Pin semicircles together along the

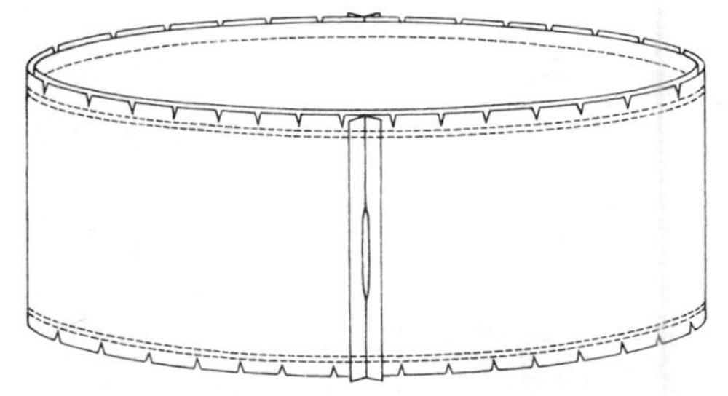

1. Make undercover as instructed, leaving an 8" opening.

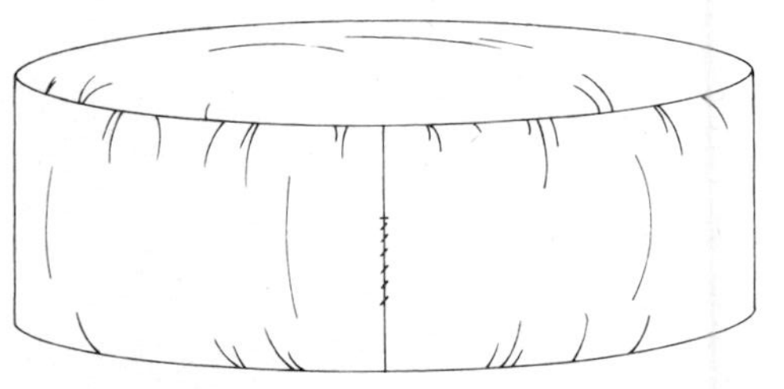

2. Stuff undercover with beads; whipstitch opening closed.

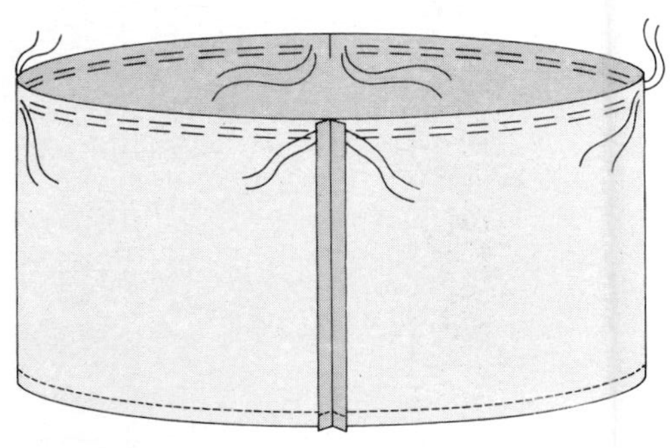

3. Join cover seam; sew gathering stitches along edge.

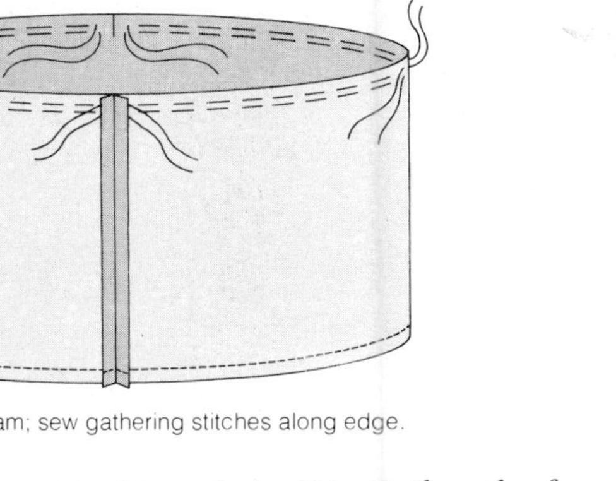

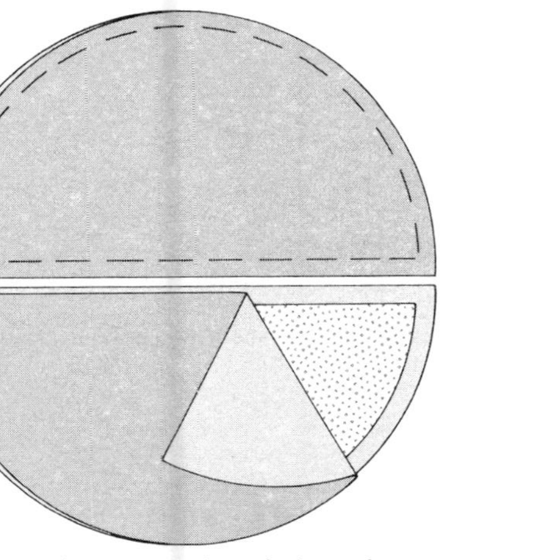

4. Fuse interfacing; layer pieces for base of cover.

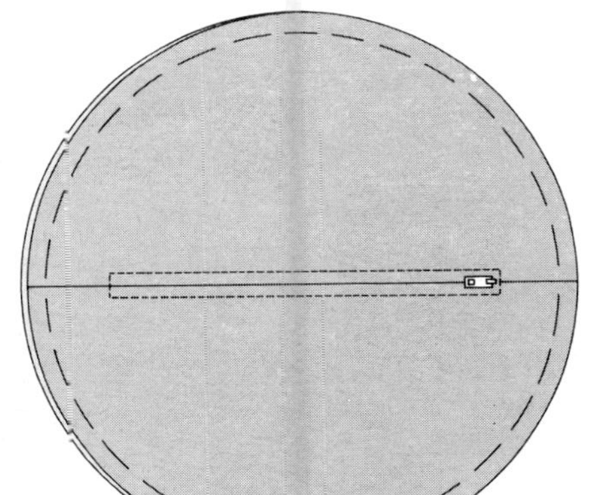

5. Insert zipper between the stitched semicircles.

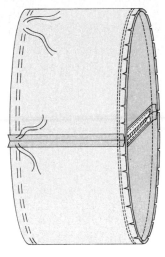

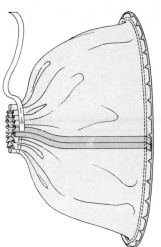

6. Sew zippered base to the staystitched edge of cover.

7. Gather up edge of cover. Pin twill tape over gathers.

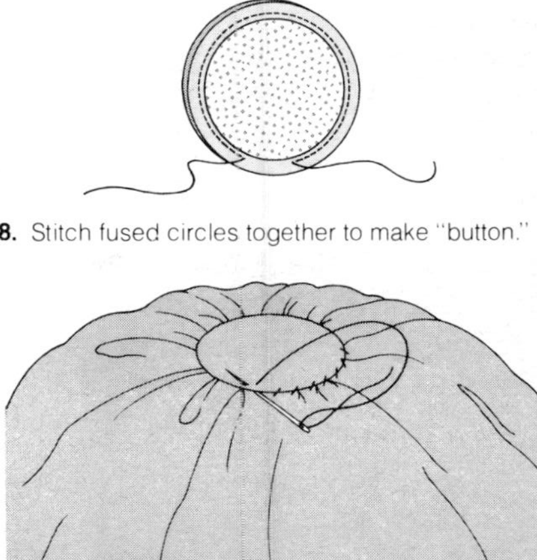

8. Stitch fused circles together to make "button."

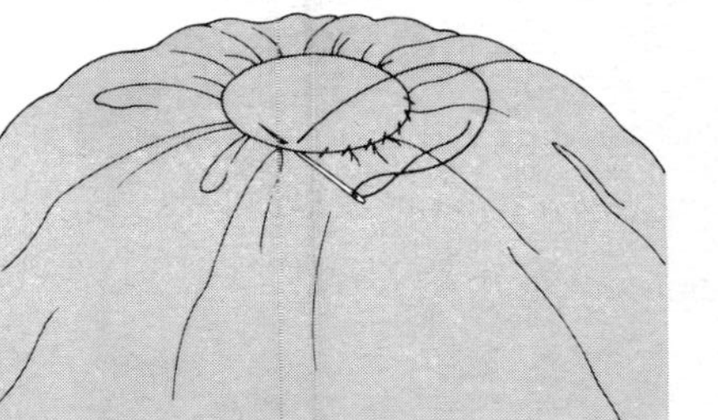

9. Whipstitch button in place over top of cover.

straight edge. Machine-stitch 5¼ inches at each end of the straight edge, leaving a 27-inch opening. Insert the zipper within the opening.

Pin and machine-stitch the staystitched edge of body to circular base, right sides together; clip the seam allowances of the body as necessary to go around the curves.

Open the zipper so you will be able to turn the cover to the right side. Gather the four sections of the top edge by gently pulling on the bobbin threads and sliding the fabric along the thread. When sections have been tightly gathered, tie thread ends.

On the wrong side, pin the twill tape over the gathers and securely hand-stitch it in place. Then turn the cover right side out.

To make the "button," first fuse a small interfacing circle to each fabric circle. Then, right sides facing, pin fused circles together. Machine-stitch along the ¼-inch seamline, leaving an opening for turning. Turn right side out; slipstitch opening closed. Center the button over the gathers, covering the gathering rows, and pin around the edges. Whipstitch button firmly in place.

Insert the bead-filled undercover through the zipper opening.

Boy's room: Spread / hassock / sailor hat cushions / fish rug / sailboat shade

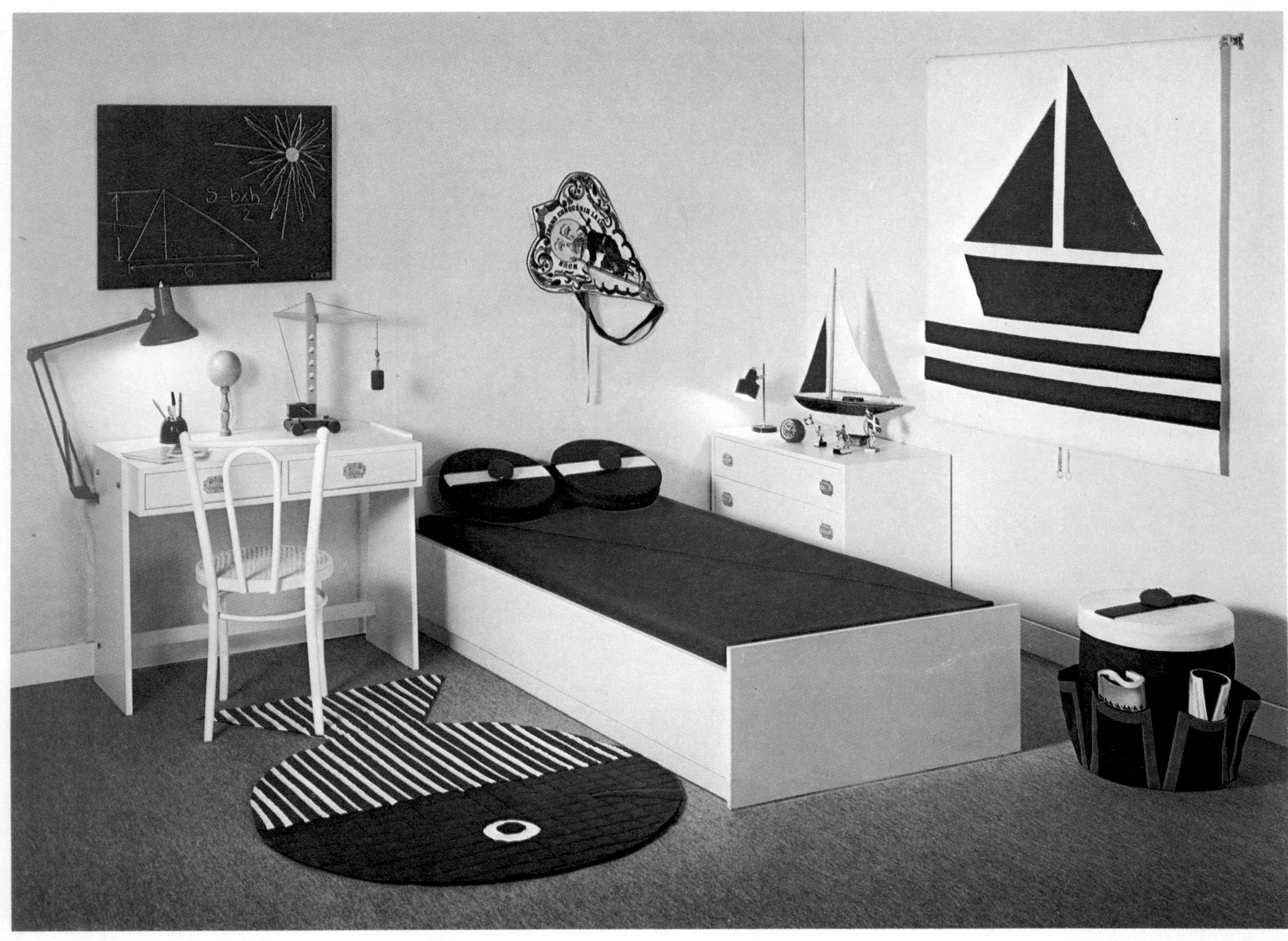

This nautical theme is just right for a young boy's room. The sailboat window shade, quilted fish rug, and French sailor hat cushions create a cheerful atmosphere with a dash of seafaring spirit. Whether only one or two objects catch your fancy, or you decide to make everything in the room, you will find these furnishings sturdy, functional, and fun to sew.

The **bedspread's** red and blue triangles, like two ship's pennants, set the color scheme. The diagonal seam is reinforced with twill tape for added strength. The side panels, cut separately from the spread top, are floor length, their corners formed by seaming. Panels may be cut shorter if needed or desired. Dimensions given are for a twin bed but can easily be altered for another size. Measure the bed fully made up with sheets and blankets (see p. 424).

Cushions, styled like a French sailor's hat, make use of fabric scraps left from the bedspread. The design is repeated for the hassock top, with the colors reversed. Foam pillow forms are readily available; a muslin undercover would be wise. The covers fit a round box-edged shape pillow and have a band appliquéd across the middle and a red wool pompon tacked in the center. To launder, unzip cushion covers; remove pompons, which are only tacked in place.

The **hassock** provides supplementary seating; its sailor hat cushion can be removed for separate use. Pouch pockets, accented with red bands, help to keep the room shipshape by providing a place for some of the objects that boys are so prone to leave lying around. Zippers are neatly concealed on both the cushion and the hassock.

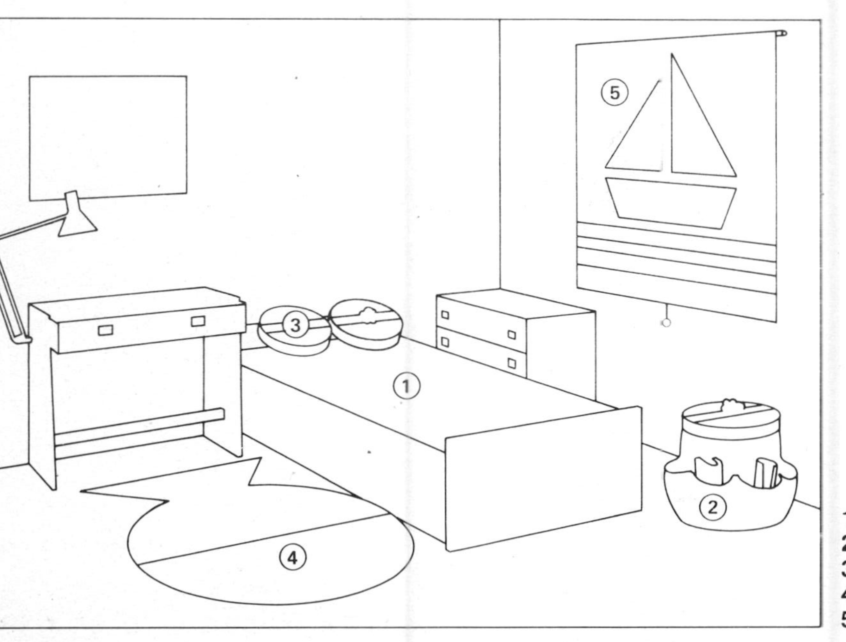

1 Spread 477
2 Hassock 479
3 Sailor hat cushions 479
4 Fish rug 482
5 Sailboat shade 484

The **fish rug** fits right in with the other marine motifs, and picks up the color scheme with its solid blue head and red and white striped body and tail. Padded for extra comfort underfoot, the quilting also brings out the fish's friendly smile. His expression can be altered if you like by simply changing the mouth pattern or its placement. You may prefer to use a print or plaid in place of the stripe, or to reverse the position of stripe and solid.

Pull down the **window shade**, and an appliqué sailboat appears. The boat design could also be used as a decorative wall hanging. To make the window shade, choose a closely woven fabric, light to medium in weight. Back it with the laminating cloth made especially for shades. Cut appliqués from colored felt and iron them in place with fusible web.

To use the sailboat motif as a wall hanging, fuse the pieces onto the background as for the window shade. Unless your fabric calls for the added body, it need not be backed for this use. (If shade is not backed, finish edges on both sides.) Follow the same instructions as for the window shade, but staple the top to a wood slat rather than to a shade roller. Or you could make a casing at the top and hang the fabric on a curtain rod.

Any durable, colorfast cotton or cotton blend is suitable for making these furnishings. Be sure the fabric is preshrunk before cutting. Red, white, and blue seems most appropriate for these designs, but you may prefer a different color scheme. Such a change would, of course, alter the room's overall personality.

For the two-color bedspread, select a medium-weight fabric, such as denim, which is sturdy and washable and comes in the necessary colors. The yardage and dimensions given below are for a twin bed.

MATERIALS NEEDED

3¾ yards of 44/45-inch fabric for each color of the bedspread
3 yards of ½-inch twill tape
Appropriate thread

CUTTING

Open out the red fabric. Straighten fabric ends and re-align if necessary. Mark off a triangle with the squared edges measuring 42 inches (wide) and 77 inches (long). From the same fabric, cut one of the side drops to measure 77 inches by the desired depth (distance from mattress to floor plus 1½ inches). Cut one of the end drops to measure 42 inches by the same desired depth. Cut blue fabric the same way.

Bedspread

SEWING
With right sides facing, pin the red end and side drops together. Stitch with a ½-inch seam allowance, starting at bottom and stopping ½ inch from the top raw edge; secure stitches. Press the seam open.

Next pin the joined drop to the squared edges of the red triangle, right sides together. Stitch together as pinned, starting the stitching from the seamline crossing at one pointed end of triangle; blunt or pivot around the square corner, and stitch to seamline crossing at other pointed end. Press the seam open.

Seam the blue end and side drops together, and stitch joined drop to the blue triangle, in the same way as described for red pieces.

Pin the two large triangles together along the diagonal seam with right sides facing. To keep the seam from stretching, pin twill tape over the seamline on one side. Stitch along the seam, catching in the twill tape as you stitch (do not catch seam allowances of drops); secure stitching at both pointed ends of the triangles. Press the seam open.

With the spread turned inside out, close the open corners: First pin the red and blue drops together with right sides facing. Stitch as pinned, and secure stitches at corner. Trim seam allowances to ½ inch and press the seams open.

At bottom edges of bedspread, turn up a double ½-inch hem and press. Machine-stitch the hem in place.

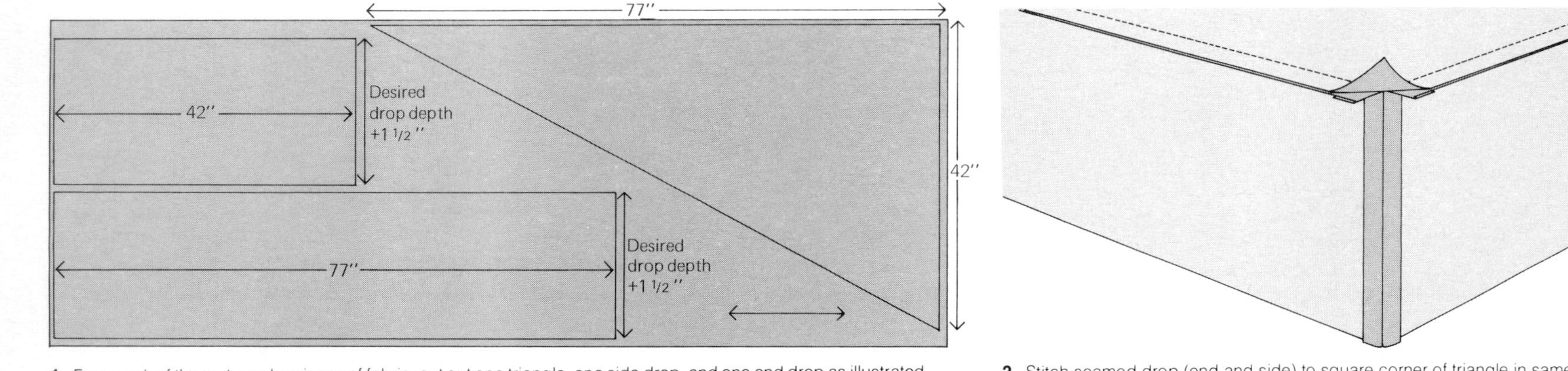

1. From each of the rectangular pieces of fabric, cut out one triangle, one side drop, and one end drop as illustrated.

2. Stitch seamed drop (end and side) to square corner of triangle in same color.

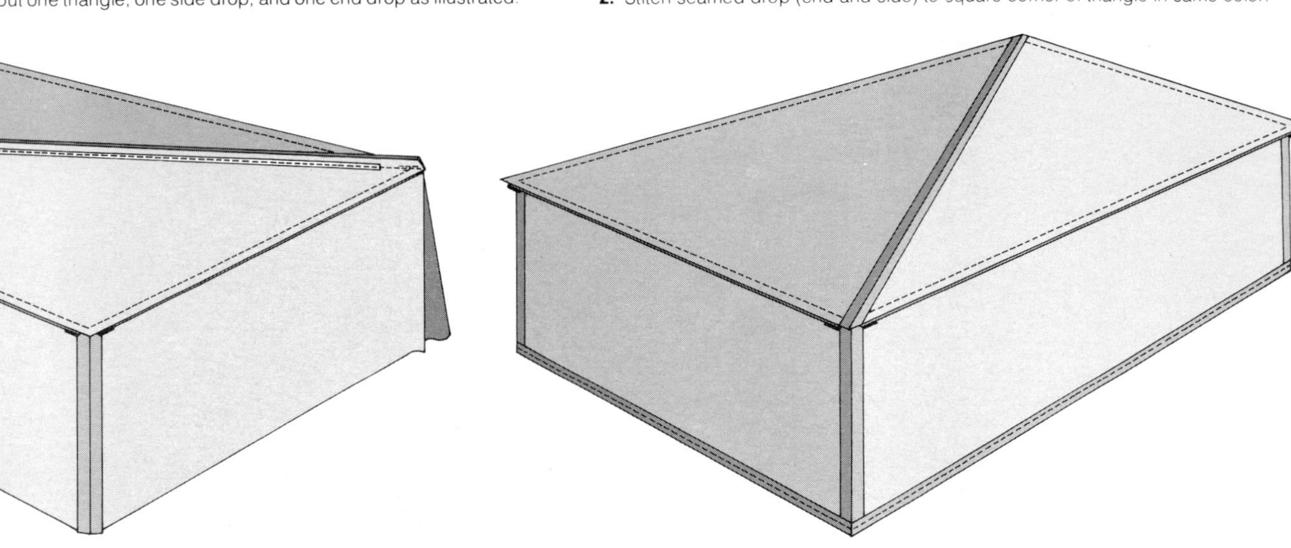

3. Pin triangular halves of spread together in a diagonal seam; stitch, catching twill tape in stitching.

4. To finish corners of spread, join free ends of drops. Press seams open. Hem bottom edge.

Hassock and cushions

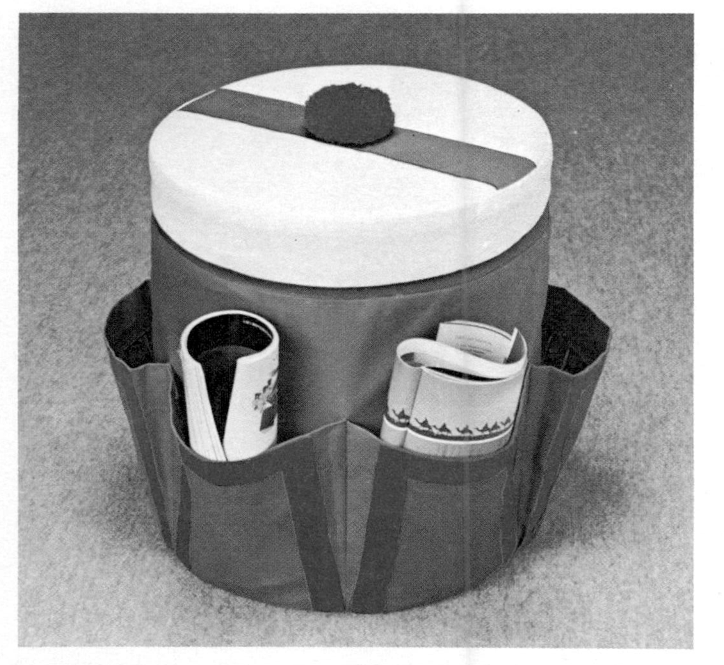

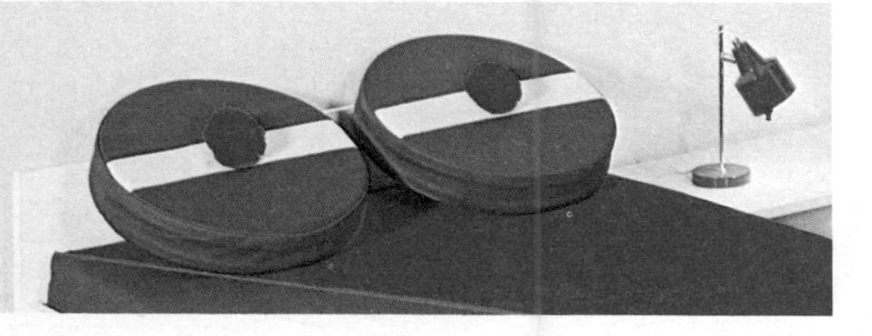

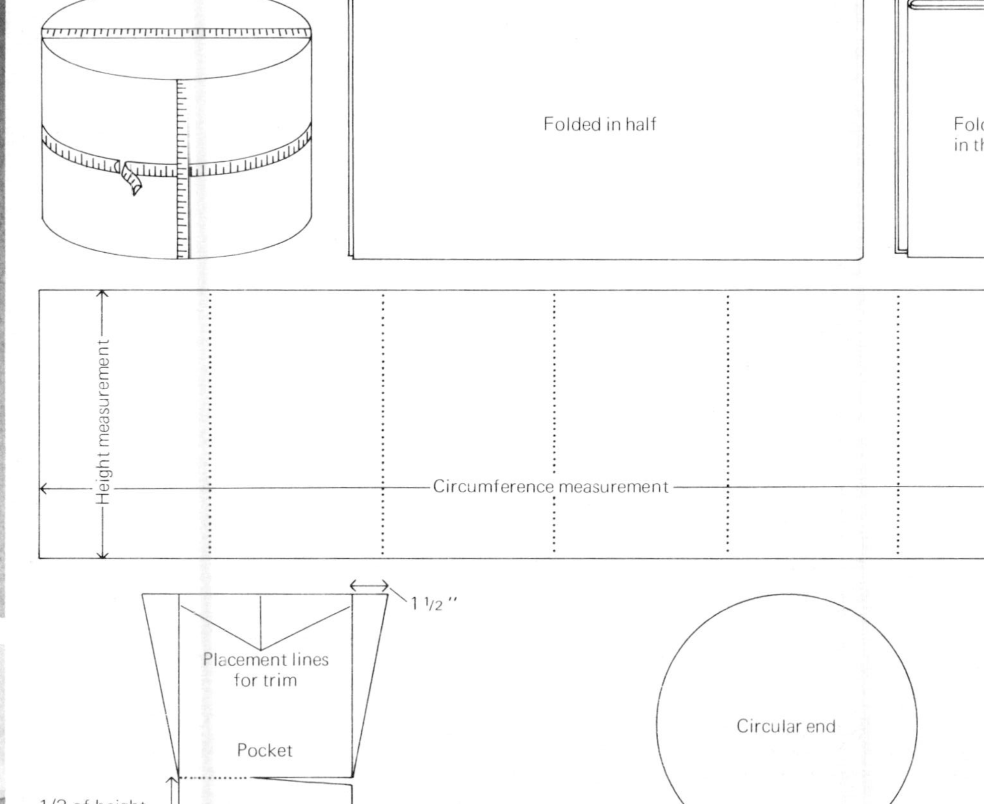

Measure cylinder. Cut pattern for body of cylinder; fold to mark pocket sections. Make pocket pattern and pattern for ends.

Hassock has pockets good for tucking away toys, comic books, many of the small objects that boys like to keep around. Zippers make it possible to remove the hassock cover for laundering. (Be sure to choose washable fabrics.) You may have an old hassock you want to re-cover, or you can purchase a fiber board cylinder. Any strong, cylindrical drum of a proper height will do; check lumberyards and hardware stores.

MATERIALS NEEDED

2 yards of 44/45-inch fabric for the hassock cover
1 zipper, slightly shorter than the cylinder diameter
1 zipper, approximately ¾ the cylinder height
Approximately 5 yards of 1-inch wide decorative trim
Hassock or sturdy cylinder
Large sheet of paper
Appropriate thread

MAKING THE PATTERN

Measure the diameter, height, and circumference of cylinder. Draw a rectangle, using the height measurement as its width and the circumference as its length. Fold the rectangle in half, then into thirds to divide it into six equal sections.

To make the pocket pattern, draw a rectangle to the dimensions of one of the sections; mark off a third from the height. Add 1½ inches to each side along the top width, and connect each side line to the base line. Use the right-angle lines within as placement lines for the trim.

For the top and bottom, draw a circle with a diameter equal to the diameter of the cylinder.

CUTTING

Cut all of the straight pieces along the straight grain of the fabric. For the body, cut out the long rectangle;

Hassock and cushions

add ⅝-inch for seam allowances. Thread-trace each section. Cut out pockets; add a ⅝-inch seam allowance all around. Mark and thread-trace the placement lines for the trim. Using the upper part of the pocket pattern, cut six pocket facings, each 1½ inches deep; add a ⅝-inch seam allowance all around.

For the top of the cover, cut a single circle with a ⅝-inch seam allowance all around. For the bottom, fold the circular pattern in half; place it on a double layer of fabric with diameter on the straight grain. Cut out two semicircles, adding a ⅝-inch seam allowance all around.

SEWING

For each pocket, pin and stitch the trim to the right side following placement lines; miter corners.

With right sides facing, pin and stitch pockets together along side seams; do not seam first and last pockets together. Press seams open.

Seam the six facing sections together in the same way. Apply a seam finish to the bottom raw edge.

With the right sides together, pin and stitch the facing unit to the pocket unit along the top edge. Trim and grade seam allowances; turn facing to the inside and press well.

Position the pocket unit onto the large rectangle; align the raw edges of the first and last pockets to the raw edges of the body, the seamline joining of each pocket to the marked division lines. Machine-stitch within the seamline groove of each pocket, backstitching at top edge. Place a row of stitching along top and bottom edges of hassock body.

With right sides facing, complete the last seam inserting one of the zippers so the top of the zipper is pointing toward the cover bottom.

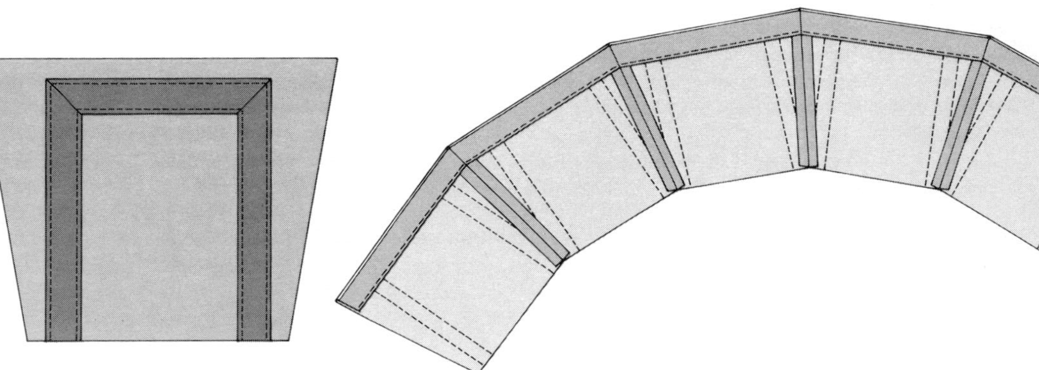

1. Apply decorative trim to the pockets.

2. Join the pockets together, then join the facing pieces together. Apply the facing to the top of the pockets.

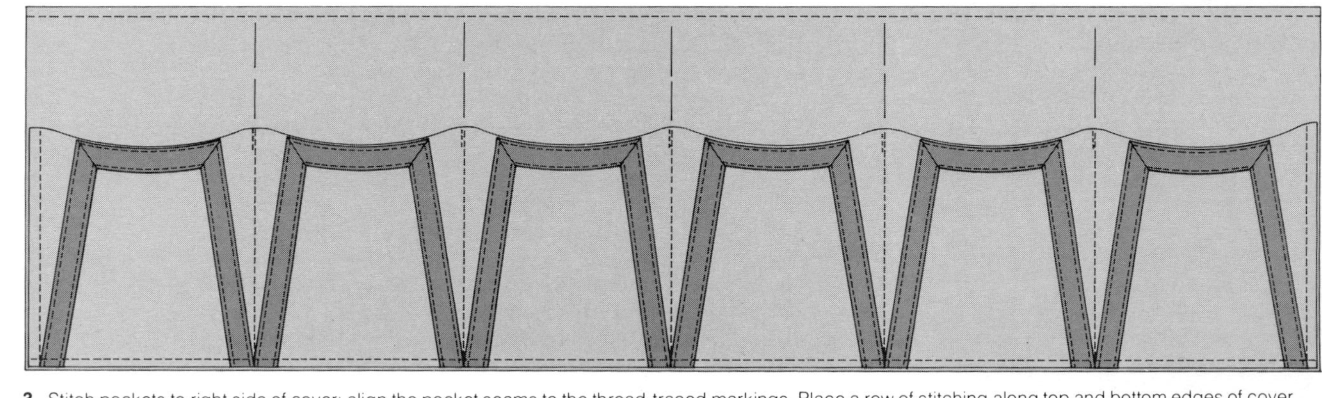

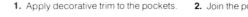

3. Stitch pockets to right side of cover; align the pocket seams to the thread-traced markings. Place a row of stitching along top and bottom edges of cover.

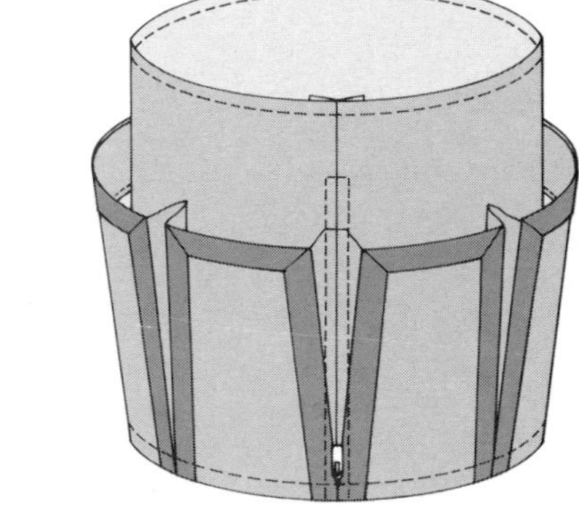

4. Insert the zipper into the side seam of cover.

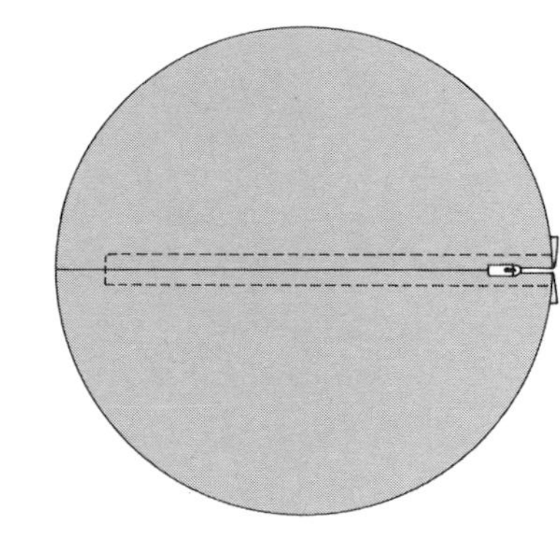

5. Insert zipper into the bottom seam of cover.

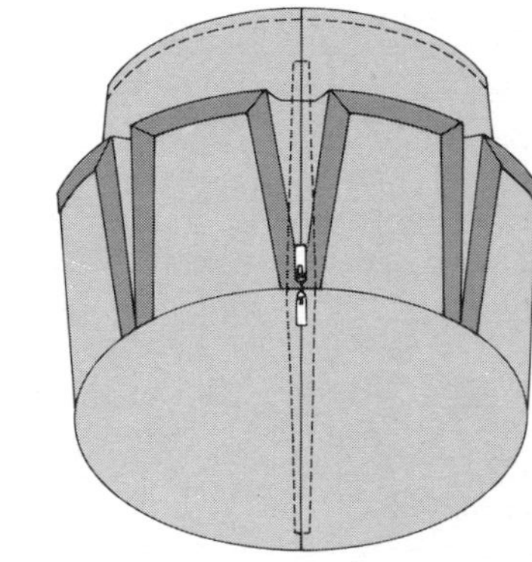

6. With zippers aligned, sew bottom end to cover.

Insert the other zipper between the two semicircles of the base.

Pin the base and main body of the cover together, right sides facing; line up the closed zippers so that the pull tabs meet; clip the seam allowance of the body unit as necessary. Machine-stitch as pinned, backstitching at either side of zippers.

Open one of the zippers. Pin and machine-stitch the top circle to the body of the cover. Turn the cover right side out and insert the cylinder.

Cushions on bed and hassock, styled to resemble a French's sailor's hat, have zippers for easy removal.

MATERIALS NEEDED
For each cushion:

½ yard of 44/45-inch fabric
Scrap of fabric in contrasting color for decorative band
One zipper, slightly shorter than the cushion diameter
¼ ounce of 4-ply yarn
3-inch piece of cardboard
Foam cushion
Appropriate thread

MAKING THE PATTERN

Measure the diameter, height, and circumference of your cushion. Draw a circle with the same diameter.

CUTTING

For the top of each cushion cover, cut a single circle by the pattern with a ⅝-inch seam allowance all around. For bottom of cover, fold the circular pattern in half; place it on a double layer of fabric with diameter on the straight grain. Cut out two semicircles, adding a ⅝-inch seam allowance around the curved as well as the cut diameter edges.

Cut one long rectangle for the boxing strip, its width equal to the cushion's height and its length to the cushion's circumference with ⅝-inch seam allowances all around.

For the decorative band, cut contrasting fabric 2½ inches wide by the diameter of top plus the seam allowances.

SEWING

With right sides facing, pin together the semicircles that make up the bottom piece, and insert the zipper into the diameter seam.

Press under ¼ inch along both long edges of the decorative band. Center the band on the right side of the top piece; pin, then machine-stitch band in place on both edges.

Place a row of staystitching along both long edges of the boxing strip. With right sides facing, pin the boxing strip ends together and stitch. Press the seam open. Pin the circular boxing strip around the top circle, right sides together; clip the boxing strip seam allowances as necessary; machine-stitch as pinned.

Open the zipper. Pin and machine-stitch the circular bottom piece to the boxing strip in the same way, lining up the seam with the zipper seam. Turn the cover right side out.

To make the 3-inch pompon, wrap the yarn over the cardboard about 50 to 60 times (more for a fuller pompon). Pull the loops off of the card, holding them together in the middle. Tie a piece of yarn around the middle of the loops, then clip the looped ends. Trim the pompon to round its edges evenly. Tack the pompon to the center of the decorative band on the top of the cover.

If you have made a muslin undercover, insert the cushion into it first, then place the cushion into the finished cover.

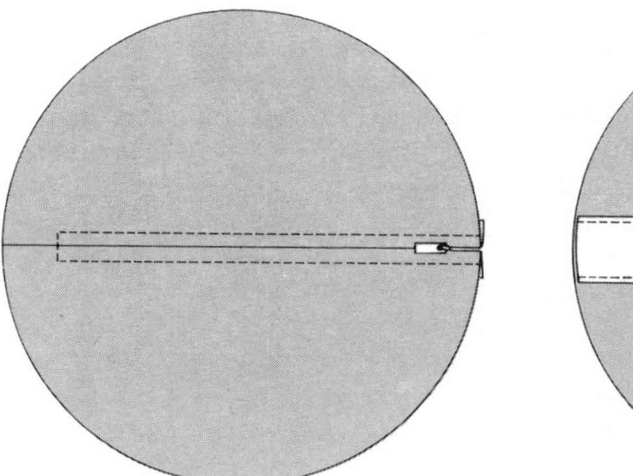

1. Insert zipper into seam in bottom of cushion.

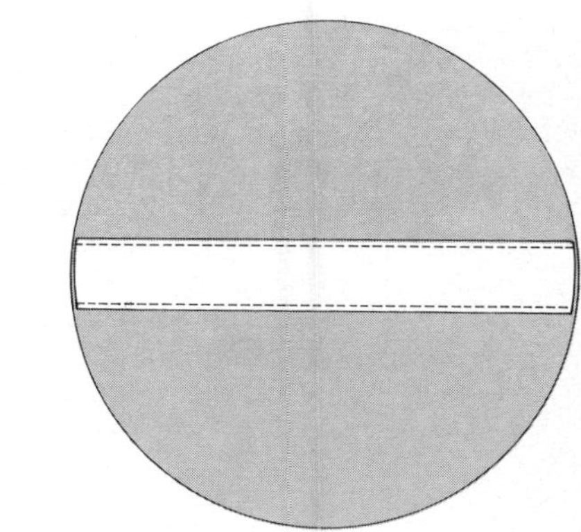

2. Apply the decorative trim to the cushion top.

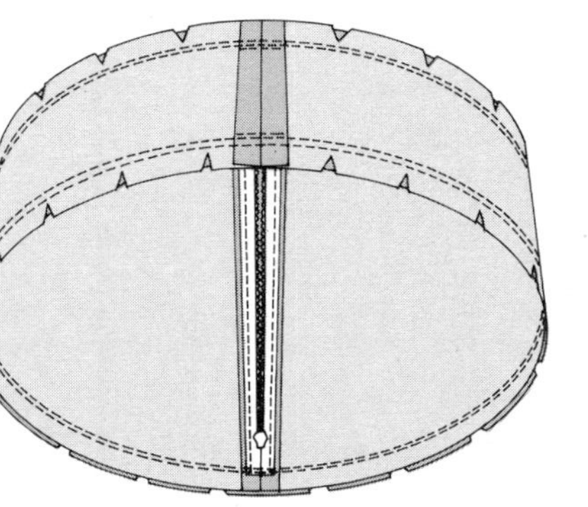

3. Seam the bottom of cushion to the boxing strip.

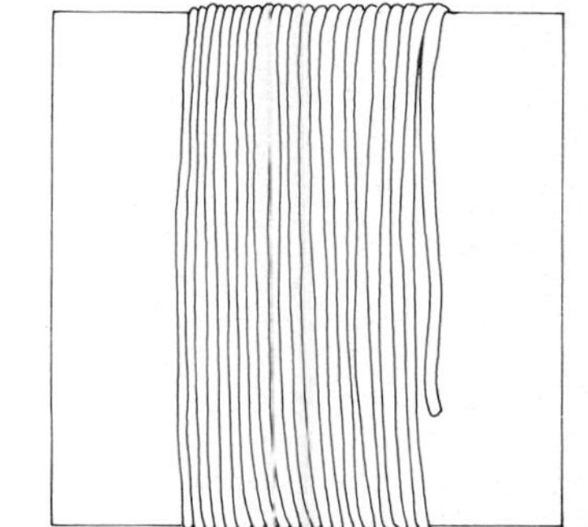

4. Wrap yarn around cardboard to make pompon.

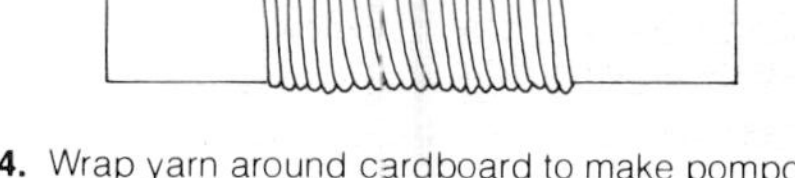

5. Trim the pompon to shape into an even ball.

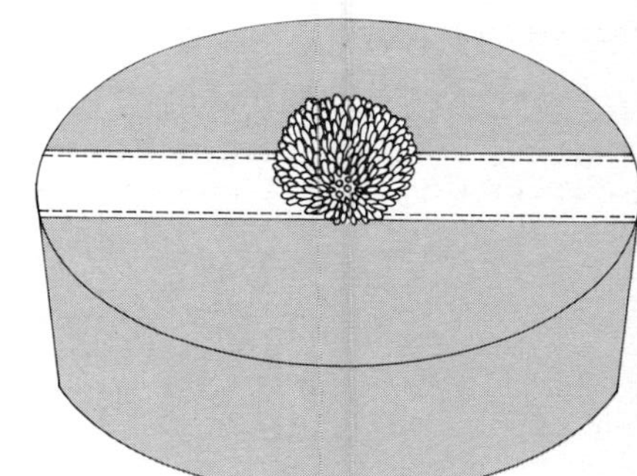

6. Tack the pompon to center of decorative trim.

Fish rug

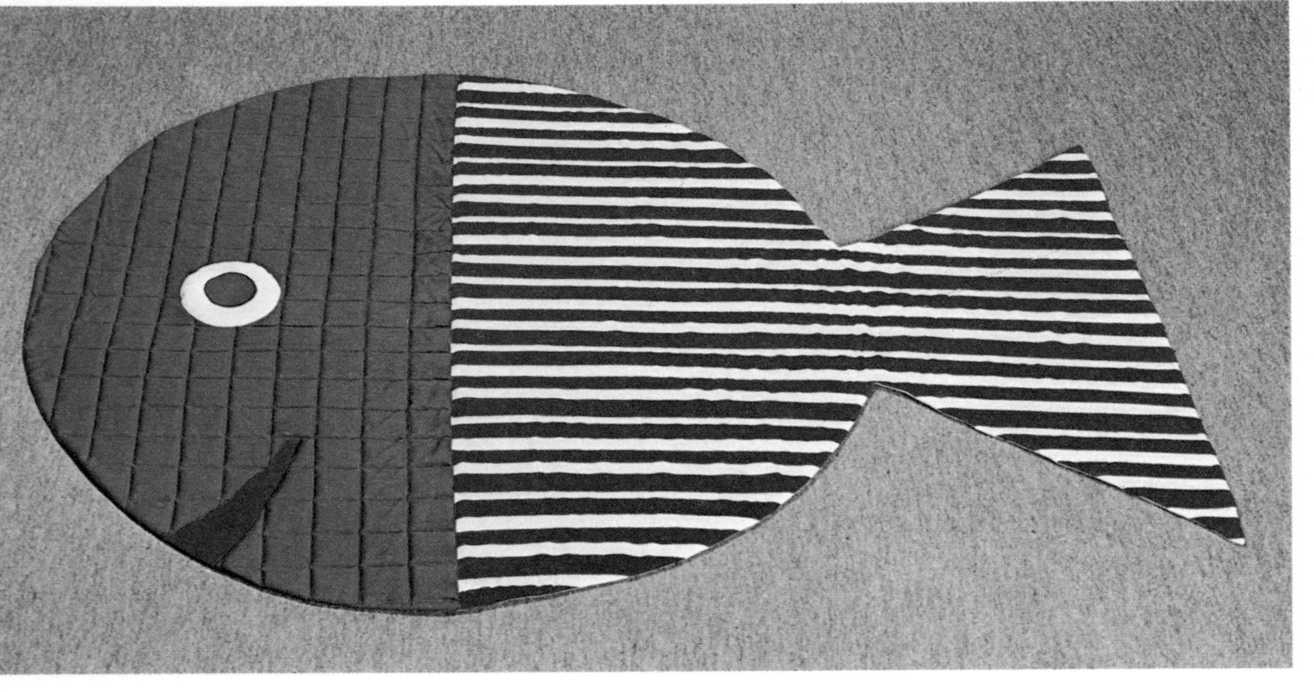

To the sharp angles of the rest of the room, the quilted fish rug adds a welcome soft touch. The stuffing is fiber fill, secured between two layers of fabric for worry-free washability. Eye and mouth are scraps of fabric, zigzagged in place.

MATERIALS NEEDED

- ¾ yard of 44/45-inch fabric for the fish's head
- 1¼ yards of 44/45-inch striped fabric for the fish's tail
- 2 yards of 44/45-inch fabric for quilt backing
- 2 yards of 44/45-inch fabric for base of rug
- Scraps of fusible web
- 45 x 62-inch sheet of fiber fill
- Heavy paper
- Appropriate thread

MAKING THE PATTERN

On heavy paper, draw a circle with a 44-inch diameter. Cut the circle in half. Along the curved edge of one semicircle, draw and center a trapezoid shape (see Drawing 1) 13 inches across the top, 33 inches along the bottom, and 17 inches high.

Following the dimensions given on the first diagram, draw the eye and mouth of the fish.

CUTTING

On a single layer of the smaller fabric piece, position and pin the semicircle so the straight edge is placed along the straight grain. Cut out the fish's head, adding ⅝ inch for seam allowances all around. Mark the placement of the fish's eye and mouth on the right side of the fabric.

Pin the tail pattern to a single layer of fabric, positioning it on the straight grain. Cut out the tail, adding an extra ⅝ inch for seam allowances all around.

Cut out the head and the tail sections from both the backing fabric and the fiber fill in the same way as described above, except do not add any allowances for seams to the cut fiber fill pieces.

For the base of the rug, lay out both pattern pieces on the straight grain so the diameters of the circles abut, and cut the base out as one piece, adding an extra ⅝ inch all around for seam allowances.

Cut out the mouth and circles for the eyes from scraps of fabric. Cut out the mouth and eye shapes from the fusible web as well.

SEWING

Fuse the blue pupil of the eye onto the white circle, and zigzag around the edges of the pupil. Then fuse the eye and mouth in place, but do not zigzag around the edges yet.

On the right side of fabric, use a chalk pencil to graph the head into 2-inch squares within the seam allowances. Do not mark over appliqués.

On wrong side of head piece, position the layer of fiber fill, then place the backing fabric over it (the fiber fill will be smaller by a seam allowance all around). Pin all layers together. Following the marked graph lines, hand-baste all the layers together along each line. From the right side, machine-stitch along each quilt line; break the stitching at the end of each appliqué and secure. When the head is completely quilted, zigzag around the eye and mouth to outline them.

Layer, baste, and quilt the tail pieces together in the same way. Use the stripes of the fabric as the quilt-lines, or mark 2-inch stripes on the tail fabric.

Line up the head and tail, right sides facing, along the center seamline. Pin them together, then machine-stitch. Press the seam open.

Right sides facing, pin base to rug. Machine-stitch around the entire fish, leaving an 18-inch opening along one side for turning. Trim the seam allowances. Clip the inner corners and taper the outer corners.

Turn the rug right side out. Push out the corners of the tail. Roll the seamline between your fingers to work it out to the edge. Press well. Press under the seam allowances of the opening and slipstitch it closed. Machine-stitch within the groove of the center seamline to hold the two layers of the rug together. Press.

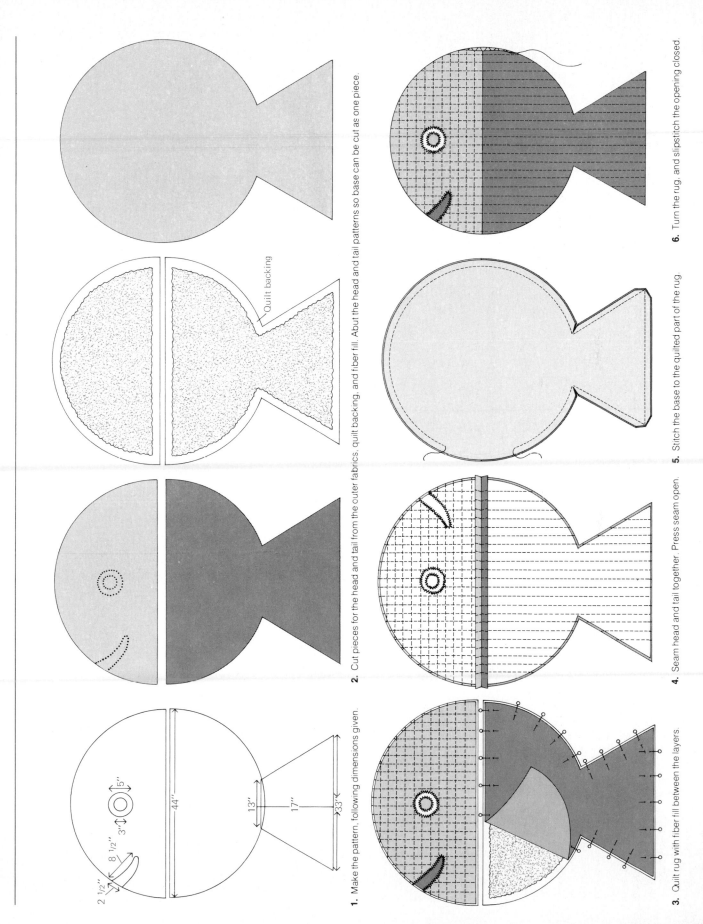

1. Make the pattern, following dimensions given.

2. Cut pieces for the head and tail from the outer fabrics, quilt backing, and fiber fill. Abut the head and tail patterns so base can be cut as one piece.

3. Quilt rug with fiber fill between the layers.

4. Seam head and tail together. Press seam open.

5. Stitch the base to the quilted part of the rug.

6. Turn the rug, and slipstitch the opening closed.

Sailboat shade

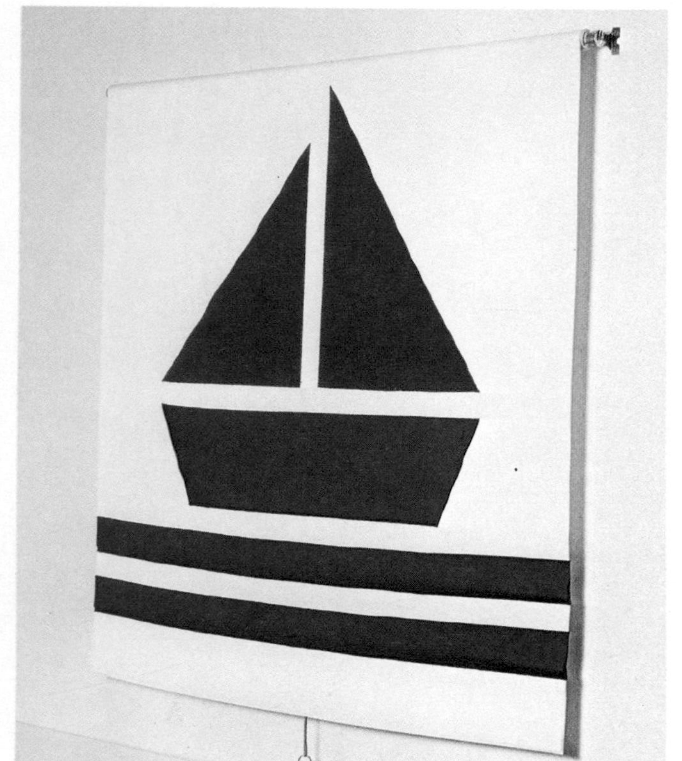

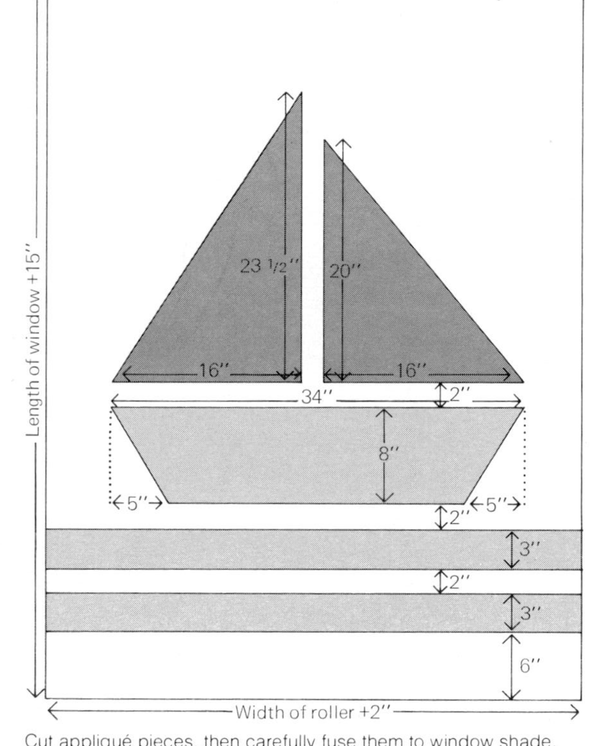

Cut appliqué pieces, then carefully fuse them to window shade.

This striking design can also be a wall hanging, if you prefer. Simply follow directions, eliminating backing unless your fabric needs body. Staple the top to a wood slat instead of a shade roller (or make a casing at the top for a curtain rod).

MATERIALS NEEDED

Special shade laminating cloth: Buy width that is at least 2 inches wider than shade roller, 15 inches longer than window
44/45-inch white fabric: Same length as laminating cloth (if shade roller is wider than 42 inches, buy two lengths and piece together)
½ yard of blue felt
¾ yard of red felt
1⅝ yards of 18-inch fusible web
1 shade roller
1 slat
1 pull cord
Tacks or staples
Appropriate thread

CUTTING

Cut all pieces along the straight grain. Cut the laminating cloth to measure 2 inches wider than the shade roller and 15 inches longer than the length of the window. From the white fabric, cut a rectangle that has the same dimensions.

From the blue felt, cut two bands 3 inches wide and as long as the width of the shade. Then cut an 8 x 34-inch rectangle. On one long edge, place a mark 5 inches in from each end. Draw a diagonal line from each point to top corner; cut on marked line.

Cut two triangles for sails from the red felt; follow the dimensions given in the diagram.

Using the felt shapes as patterns, cut similar pieces from fusible web.

SEWING

For best results, work on a surface at least as large as the total shade, such as a kitchen table or the floor. Protect the surface with several layers of old sheet or with a blanket.

Press the white fabric well to remove any wrinkles.

Position one blue band 6 inches up from the bottom edge, placing the fusible web piece underneath. Be sure the band lies straight across the shade, then fuse it in place.

Position the other band 2 inches above and parallel to the first. Fuse this band in place.

Center the body of the boat on the shade, 2 inches above and parallel to the second blue band. Fuse securely.

Position the two red sails 2 inches above and parallel to the boat. Space them 2 inches apart, so that the outer points line up with the edges of the boat. Fuse in place.

Fuse the white fabric to the laminating cloth, aligning all raw edges: Following manufacturer's directions, first partially fuse the two layers together, smoothing out any bubbles or wrinkles. Then fuse them together permanently, working from the center out. Do not move the shade until it is cool and dry.

Compare the widths of the shade and the roller. Mark trimming points on each side of the shade so shade is ¼ inch narrower than the roller at each end. Extend trimming line along each side so sides are absolutely straight and parallel. Carefully trim off the excess with a pair of sharp shears. If necessary, trim the top and bottom edges to straighten.

For the slat casing, turn up a 1½-inch hem at the bottom and secure. Insert the slat and slipstitch the opening ends closed. Hand-tack the pull cord to the bottom of the shade.

Tack or staple the shade to the roller, making sure that the fabric is on perfectly straight all the way across the roller.

Projects to sew for friends & family

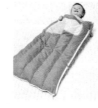

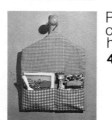

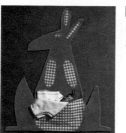

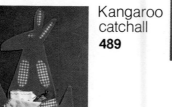

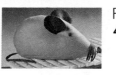

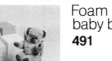

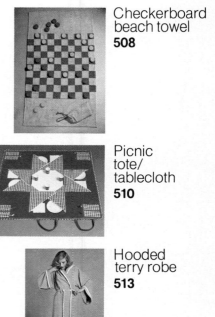

Convertible quilt

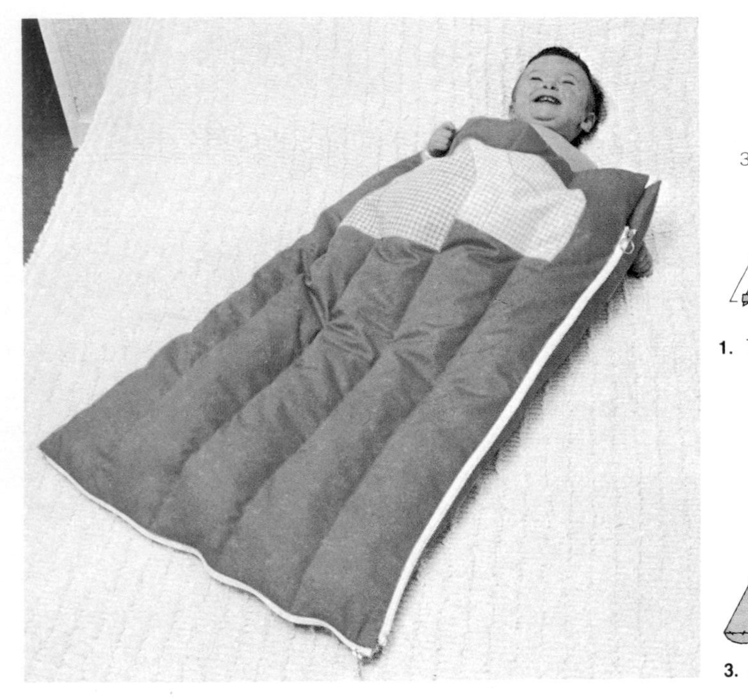

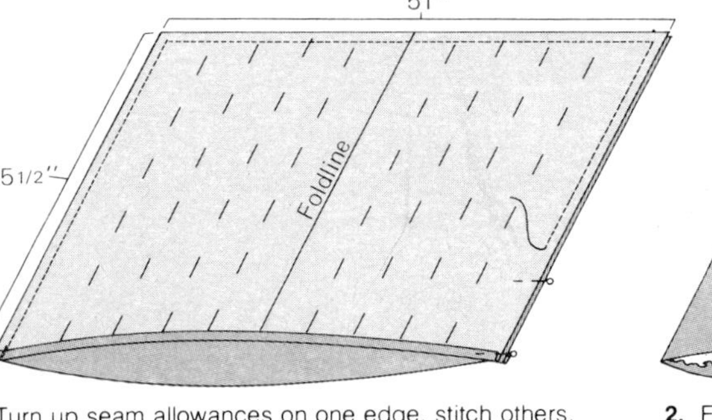
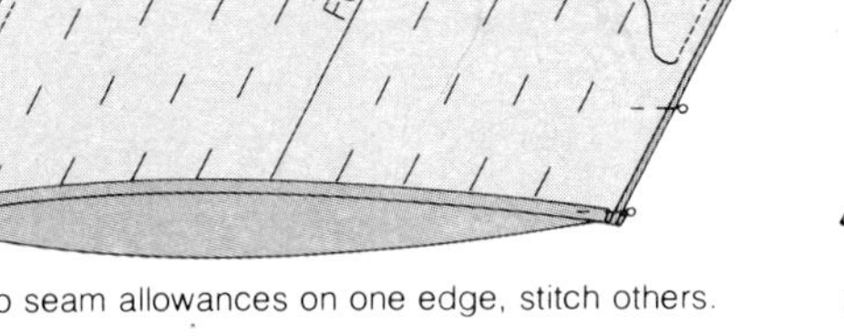

1. Turn up seam allowances on one edge, stitch others.

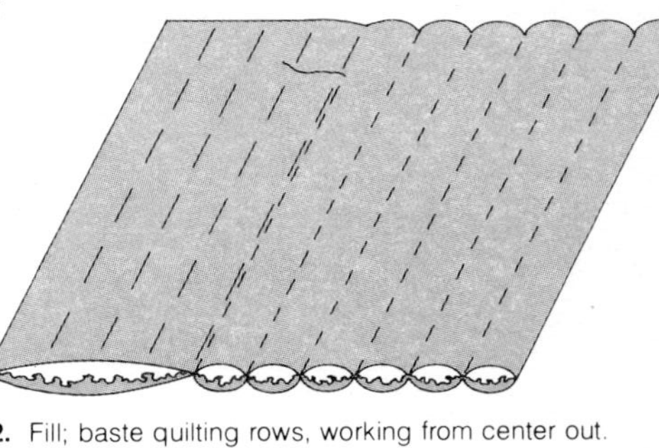

2. Fill; baste quilting rows, working from center out.

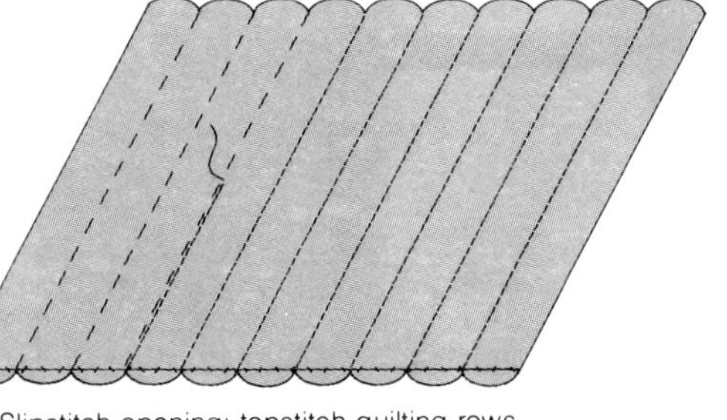
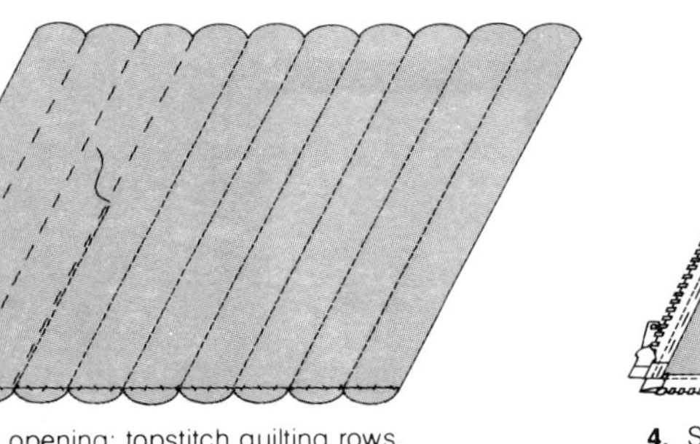

3. Slipstitch opening; topstitch quilting rows.

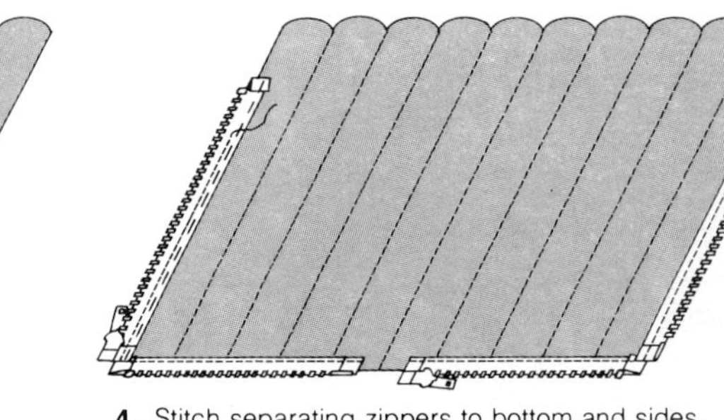

4. Stitch separating zippers to bottom and sides.

With the aid of a pair of separating zippers, this ingenious coverlet works two ways to keep a baby snug and warm. Zipped up it's a sleeping bag; unzip the bag, and it's a quilt.

Use a washable fabric such as sturdy cotton or nylon ciré for the cover, and a machine-washable fiber fill for the stuffing. A colorful bed sheet can also be used as fabric.

For a decorative touch, a free-form design, cut from gingham, can be appliquéd to the quilt before the main pieces are stitched.

MATERIALS NEEDED

2⅞ yards of 36-inch fabric
2 separating zippers (24″ and 27″)
Sheet of fiber fill, approximately 51 x 36 inches
Appropriate thread

CUTTING

From a double thickness of fabric, cut two 51 x 36-inch rectangles on the straight grain. Dimensions include half-inch seam allowances on all of the four edges.

SEWING

Fold the 51-inch width of one rectangle in half and press. (This marks the center quilting line.) Using a yardstick and pins or chalk, mark off quilting rows, working from center press line out to each side. Mark rows about 5 inches apart. Thread-trace the markings.

On each of the rectangles, turn up the seam allowance along one long edge and press. Pin the two rectangles together, right sides facing and raw edges even; machine-stitch around, leaving the turned-up seam edges open. Turn cover right side out and press. (Optional step at this point: Topstitch ⅜ inch inside the stitched edges. This will provide flat edges for easier zipper insertion.)

Through the opening in the cover, insert the fiber fill, cut slightly larger than the cover to insure a generous filling for quilting.

Baste quilting rows by hand. Baste the center row first, making sure the filling is equally divided between the two sides. Then baste the other rows, again working from the center line out. Slipstitch the open edges closed. Carefully topstitch the basted rows; remove the bastings.

The two separating zippers are attached along the sides and bottom edge of the quilt. First separate the 24-inch zipper and pin its two tapes, wrong side up, across the width, with top ends at the corners. Bottoms will almost meet at center of width. Turn under excess tape at the tops. Position the zipper on the cover so that the marked guideline of the tape is along the finished edge of the cover. Then baste zipper in place, stitching near the finished edge. It may be necessary to push filling back slightly from the edge. Machine-stitch from top to bottom, backstitching at both ends.

Follow the same procedure for the 27-inch zipper, positioning it so that its bottom end slightly overlaps the other zipper tape. Its top will fall just about 8 inches below the slipstitched edge of the rectangle. Whipstitch the overlapping ends of the zippers together.

Punching ball

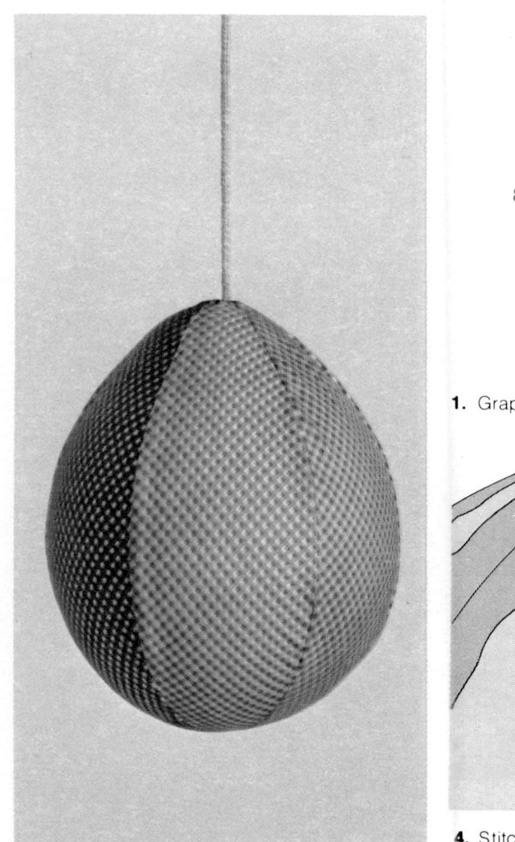

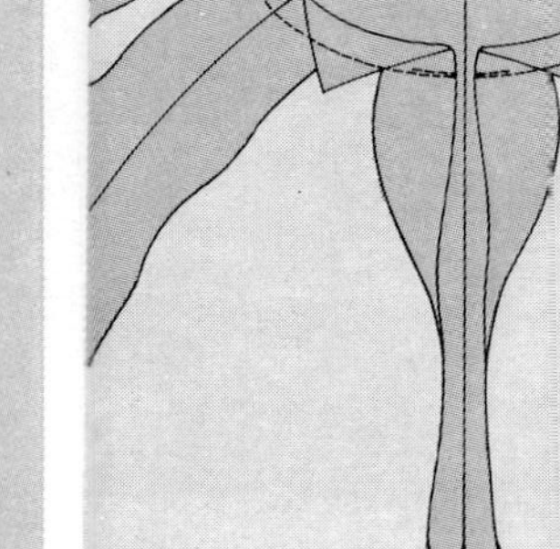

1. Graph 2″ squares on paper; draw curve.

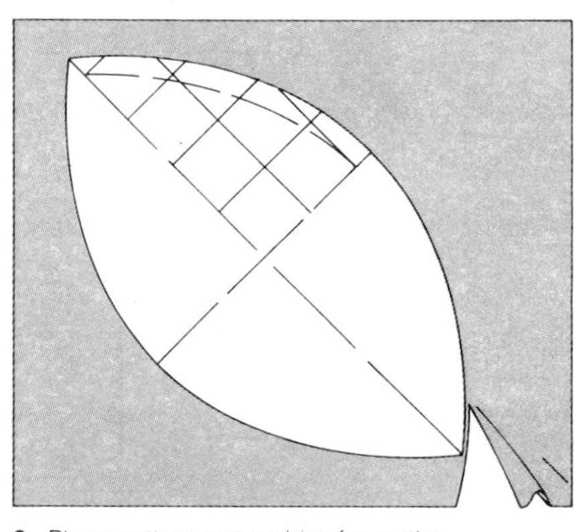

2. Place pattern on true bias for cutting.

3. Stitch sections; leave one seam open.

4. Stitch a ½″ hem/casing at the top.

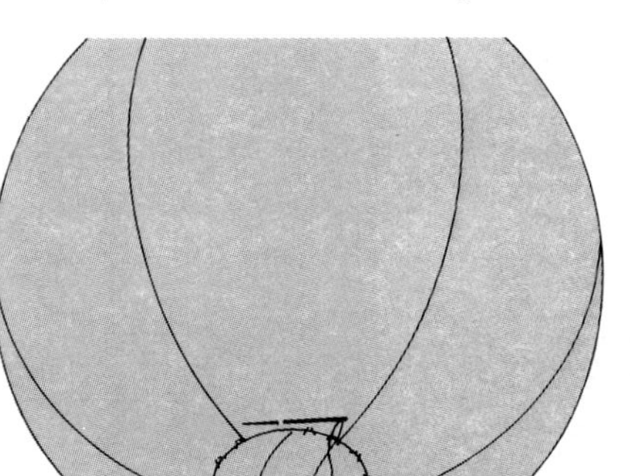

5. Slipstitch fused circles to the bottom.

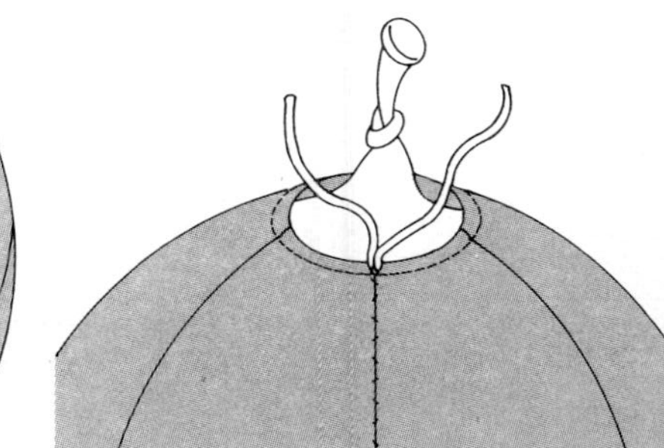

6. With balloon inserted, gather up top hem.

Balloon-filled and hung from a long string, what fun this would be in a young child's room! The ball's cover is made from six-sections, each one a different fabric. These are gingham checks, but they could be a rainbow of solids, or contrasting stripes or dots.

MATERIALS NEEDED

⅜ yard each of six different fabrics
2-inch square of fusible interfacing
Cord for gathering
Balloon
10 x 18-inch sheet of paper
Appropriate thread

MAKING THE PATTERN

Fold a 9¼ x 17¼-inch sheet of paper into quarters and graph one quarter with 2-inch squares. Work from fold-lines out; ⅝ inch will remain at each edge (for seam allowances). Transfer the pattern in Illustration 1 to your graph; cut along the solid curved line; unfold the paper. This is the pattern for one section of the cover.

CUTTING

Cut six sections, placing the length of the pattern on the true bias of each fabric. Cut out circles from the fabric and from the fusible interfacing, making each one 1¼ inches in diameter.

SEWING

With right sides facing, pin, then baste the sections together, leaving the final seam open. Machine-stitch from bottom to top, leaving ⅝ inch unstitched at the end of each seam. Carefully press seams open. At the top end of the oval, turn each little resulting flap under ½ inch and machine-stitch a scant ¼ inch from its fold. Baste, then machine-stitch the final seam, stopping 4 inches short of the folded edge. Trim seams at the bottom end. Turn the cover right side out.

Fuse interfacing and fabric circles together. Press under a small hem all around. Center the circle over the bottom of the oval, pin, then slipstitch in place. Slipstitch the opening left in the last seam closed to within ¼ inch of the folded edge.

Thread a few inches of cord through the top hem. Insert a balloon; inflate it; knot securely. Attach a cord for hanging; push knot down into cover. Pull the gathering cord tight to close up hole; knot ends and tuck inside.

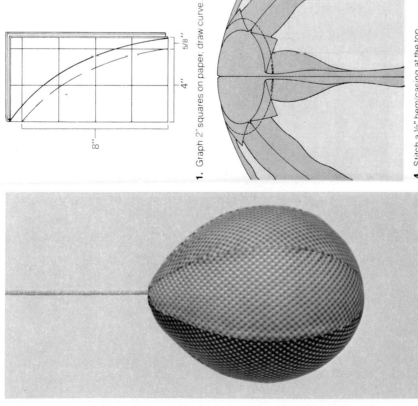

Pocketed clothes hanger

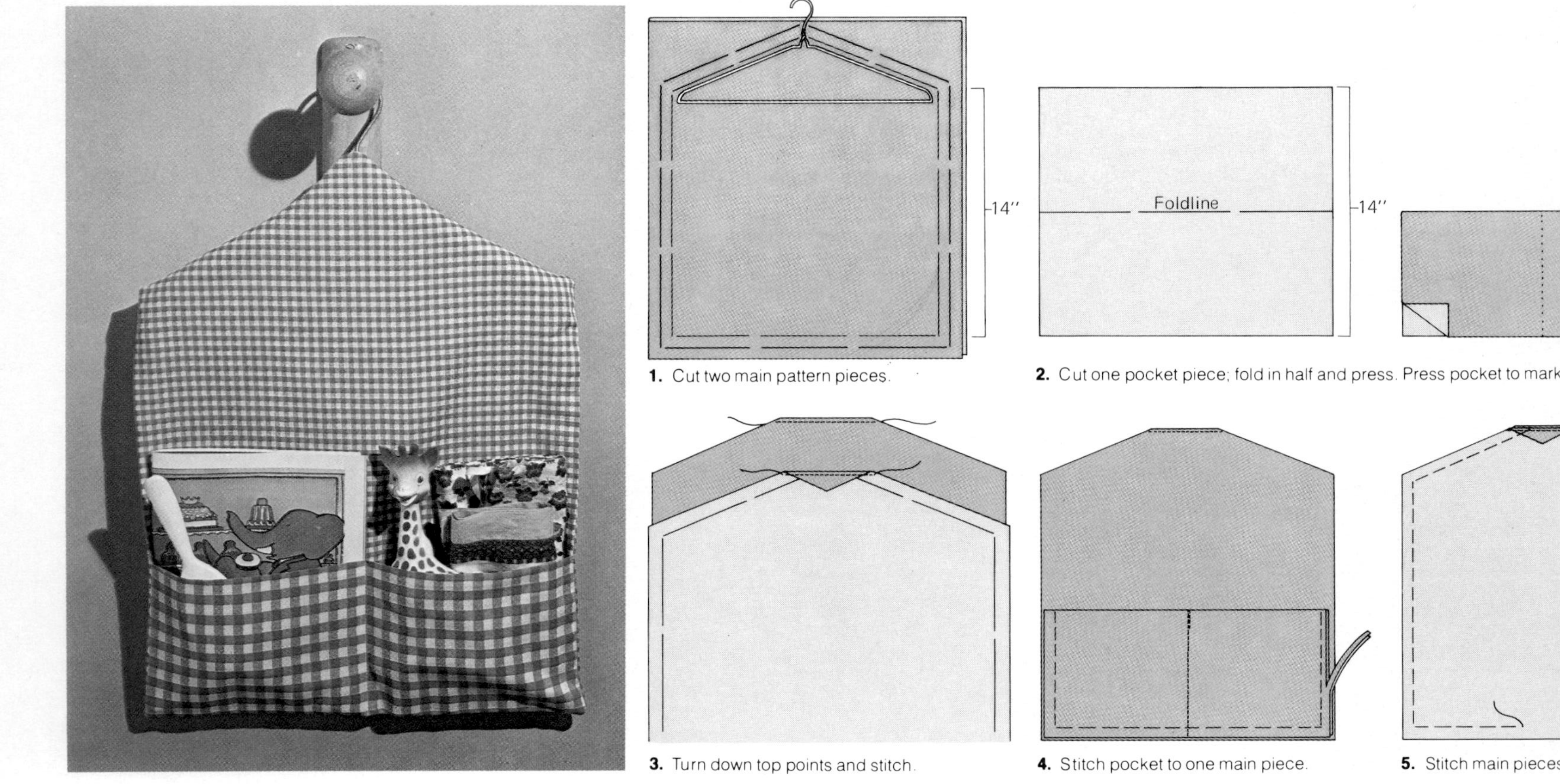

1. Cut two main pattern pieces.

2. Cut one pocket piece; fold in half and press. Press pocket to mark center.

3. Turn down top points and stitch.

4. Stitch pocket to one main piece.

5. Stitch main pieces together.

Here's a charming convenience for a little girl's closet, with pockets sized just right for her possessions. To make the pattern, simply trace the outline of a wire hanger. Appropriate materials, besides the gingham shown, would be lightweight vinyl, awning stripe canvas, or big bandanna handkerchiefs in red and blue.

MATERIALS NEEDED

⅝ yard of 36-inch fabric for cover
⅜ yard of 36-inch fabric for pocket
Wire clothes hanger
Appropriate thread

CUTTING

Fold the fabric for the main pattern piece in half lengthwise, right sides together and selvages aligned; pin to hold the layers in place. Center the clothes hanger, with its hook extending above the top edge, and carefully trace its contours. From each end of the hanger draw a 14-inch line down on the straight grain, and connect the lines at the bottom. Add a ⅝-inch seam allowance all around. Cut out, following marked cutting lines.

From the smaller piece of fabric, cut a rectangle for the pocket 14 inches by the same width as that of the main pattern piece; place and cut it on the straight grain. Fold rectangle in half lengthwise, with wrong sides together, and press the folded edge. Fold again to quarter it, and press lightly to mark the center.

SEWING

Fold each top point on the two main pieces down 1 inch to the wrong side, and stitch along the folded edge.

Position pocket on the right side of one of the main pattern pieces, aligning all raw edges at bottom and side. Pin through all three layers and baste around raw edges. Stitch in center foldline of pocket, backstitching at top edge. Grade the seam allowances of the pocket unit.

Pin and baste the two main pieces together, right sides facing. Stitch, leaving the small opening at the top and a 6-inch opening in the base for turning. Taper corners. Turn the cover right side out and press. Slip the hanger inside, extending the hook through the top opening. Turn in the raw edges at the bottom and slipstitch the opening closed.

Kangaroo catchall

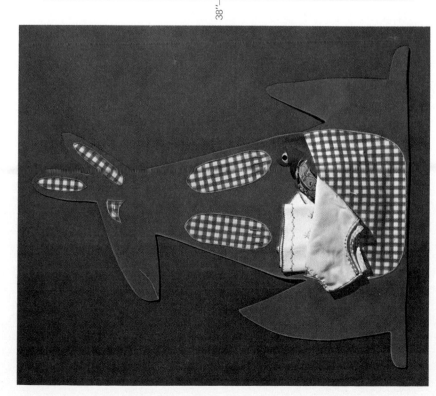

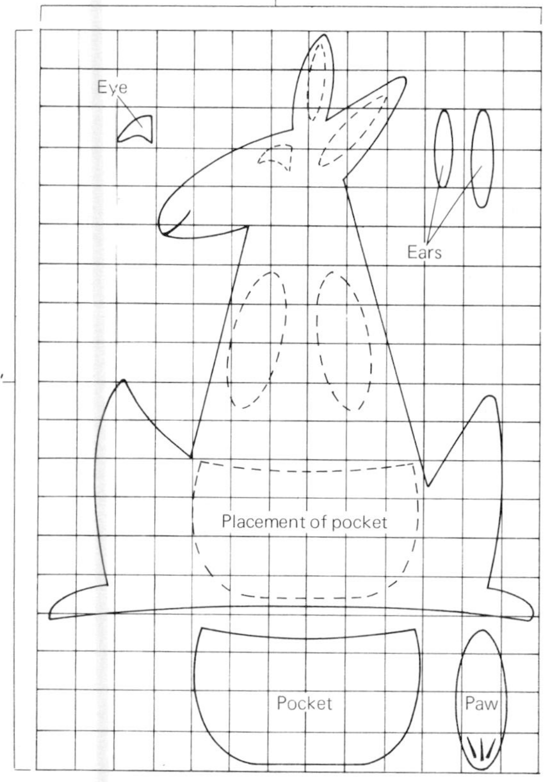

Pattern and placement of pattern pieces on kangaroo body

This friendly kangaroo, besides being very good company in a child's room, makes a handy catchall for small toys, comb and brush, perhaps even half-finished homework.

A fairly sturdy material like denim or duck is best for the body, but the appliqués can be made of any fabric you like or happen to have on hand. Fusible interfacing applied to the front body piece helps the kangaroo to keep its shape.

Satin stitching provides eye and claw details and the cheerful smile; the same stitch is used to attach the gingham appliqués. The kangaroo is equipped for hanging with loops attached to one ear and to the top of each of his haunches; to hold the loops, place stick-on picture hooks at appropriate points on the wall.

MATERIALS NEEDED

2 yards of 36-inch fabric for body
¼ yard of 36-inch fabric for the pocket and other appliqués
⅞ yard of 26-inch fusible interfacing
Scraps of fusible web
38 x 26-inch sheet of paper
Appropriate thread

MAKING THE PATTERN

Graph a 38 x 26-inch sheet of paper into 2-inch squares and reproduce on it the pieces of the pattern in the diagram above. Add a ⅝-inch seam allowance all around the body piece only; all other pieces will be satin-stitched, which both finishes and conceals the raw fabric edges. Cut the pieces out on the drawn lines.

CUTTING

To cut out the two body pieces (back and front), fold the fabric in half crosswise, with right sides together. Lay the body pieces on the doubled fabric, keeping grain lines aligned with the straight lines on the pattern piece. Pin and cut.

Remove the body pattern and place it on the interfacing. Pin and cut, making no allowance for seams.

On a single layer of fabric, lay out and cut ears, paw, eye, and pocket, cutting paw and pocket twice (the pocket is double thickness).

SEWING

Center the interfacing on the wrong side of one of the body pieces and fuse in place. For added stiffness, several layers can be used.

On the right side of the fused piece, position the ears, eye, and paws, with cut fusible web beneath them. Press in place. Satin-stitch all around.

With right sides of pocket pieces facing, pin them together. Baste, then machine-stitch ⅝ inch from the edge along the top only. Turn pocket unit right side out and press, pressing the seam out to the edge. Pin or baste pocket to the kangaroo body, then satin-stitch the raw edges.

Next, at the bottom of each of the appliquéd paws, satin-stitch three short lines to represent claws. Do the same to indicate the pupil of the eye and the smile on the muzzle.

Now, with right sides facing, pin together the front and back pieces of the kangaroo body. Baste, then machine-stitch the pieces together ⅝ inch from the edge, leaving the bottom open for turning. Clip or notch the seams at curves and sharp angles. Then turn the body right side out, manipulating the seam out to the edge; press. Turn the raw edges in along the bottom and slipstitch the opening closed. Press the body well, with special care and attention to the appliquéd areas.

Felt mouse

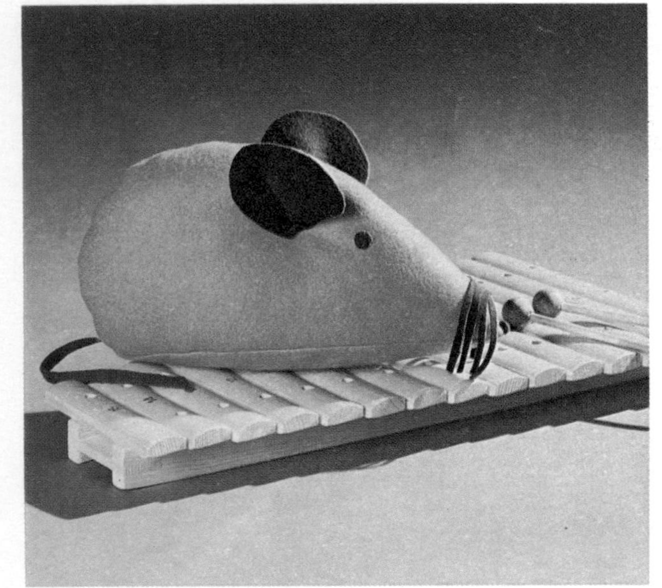

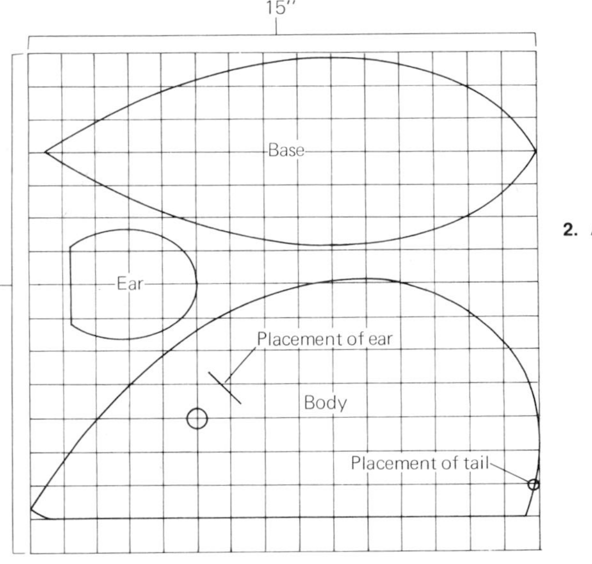

1. Draw pattern on graphed paper. Cut out all felt pieces.

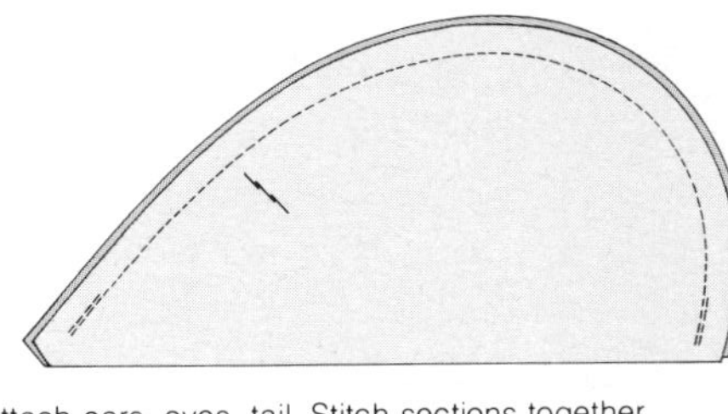
2. Attach ears, eyes, tail. Stitch sections together.

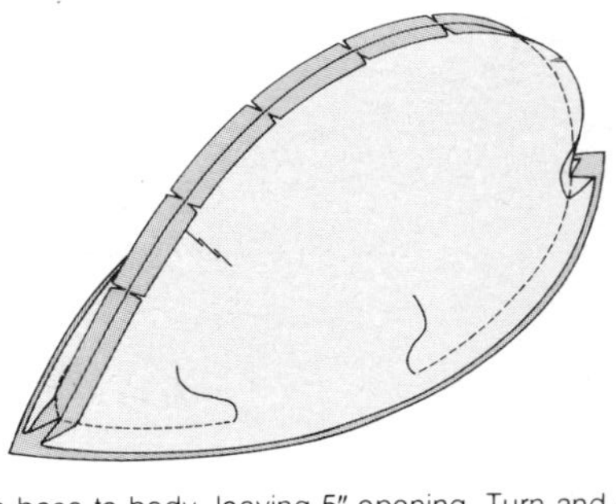
3. Stitch base to body, leaving 5" opening. Turn and stuff.

Our stuffed felt mouse is big enough to play with, but he would also make an amusing and comfortable cushion. The felt covering is well padded with fiber fill stuffing. Felt is a good fabric choice because it comes in a wide range of colors and it can often be bought in small pieces. Uncut corduroy would be a nice alternative, as would a lively printed cotton.

The pattern is a simple one to transfer, cut, and sew. The dimensions of the mouse, if desired, could easily be altered on the grid to produce a larger or smaller version.

MATERIALS NEEDED

¼ yard of 60-inch felt for body
Felt scraps for eyes, ears, and tail
Fiber fill stuffing
15 x 15-inch sheet of paper
Small (¼ inch) ball button for nose
Glue
Appropriate thread

MAKING THE PATTERN

Graph a 15 x 15-inch sheet of paper into 1-inch squares, and reproduce on it the pieces of the pattern in the first diagram above. Mark placement of eyes, ears, and tail. Add ⅝-inch seam allowance around base and side pieces. Cut pattern pieces out.

CUTTING

On a double thickness of felt, pin and cut out the two side pieces; pin and cut the base from a single layer. Mark the ⅝-inch seam allowance around the side and bottom pieces, and also mark the placement for the eyes, ears, and tail.

From the felt scraps, cut two ears, using the pattern. In addition, cut out a rectangle 7 inches long by ¾ inch wide for the whiskers, and a strip 9 inches long by ¼ inch wide for the tail. Also cut two circles, each ⅜ inch in diameter, for the eyes.

SEWING

Before attaching the ears onto the body, make a ⅜-inch pleat in the center of each ear. Pin each ear at its placement mark on the right side of the main pieces, and sew the ears in place with a half-backstitch. Glue the eyes in their proper place, using a toothpick as an applicator. Pin the tail to the right side of one of the side pieces at its placement mark; one end of the tail strip should be even with the raw edge.

With right sides facing, pin the two side pieces together along the upper curve. Machine-stitch on the ⅝-inch seamline, catching the tail in the stitching; start and stop ⅝ inch from the bottom raw edges, securing the stitching with a few backstitches at beginning and end. Press seam flat; trim to ¼ inch. Notch out the excess fullness from seam allowances and finger-press the seam open.

Then pin the base to the body, with right sides facing and the narrower end of the base toward the front of the mouse. Baste and, with body side up, machine-stitch on the ⅝-inch seamline, pivoting at the points on the front and back ends of the mouse; leave a 5-inch opening on one of the sides for turning and stuffing.

Turn the body right side out. Center and pin the rectangle for the whiskers over the center seamline, 1¼ inches from the front tip of the mouse. Securely sew whiskers in place, using half-backstitches along the seamline. Snip each side of the rectangle into ⅛-inch strips. These will represent the whiskers.

Stuff the body of the mouse with fiber fill, packing it well. Turn the raw edges in the length of the opening and slipstitch it closed. Sew the ball button onto the front tip of the mouse to represent its nose.

Foam baby blocks

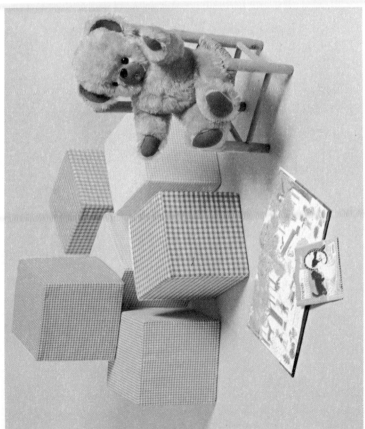

These blocks are perfect in every way for even a quite small baby. They are covered from side to side in varied patterns and gay nursery colors. The foam-rubber filling makes them soft and safe — not a sharp corner or a hard surface to be found anywhere. Foam is light, too, which makes the blocks easy for infants to handle.

Because foam is hard to find in the 8-inch thickness of the cubes, we recommend that you glue together two 4-inch layers (a far more common thickness) to make each 8-inch cube.

MATERIALS NEEDED

½ yard of 36-inch fabric
Two 8-inch squares of 4-inch thick foam rubber or polyfoam
Rubber cement
Curved needle
Appropriate thread

GLUING FOAM

Apply rubber cement to the surfaces of both of the foam sections that are to be joined. Let the glue dry until it is tacky to the touch. Then carefully line up the two foam pieces so that one is positioned right on top of the other, and press firmly together. (The bonding will be strong, so be sure positioning is correct before pressing.) Put the foam, now an 8-inch square, aside to allow the glue to dry.

CUTTING

Cut out six 8-inch squares of fabric on the straight grain. Do not add any extra for seam allowances — the cube cover will fit better if it is snug. Use a ¼-inch seam allowance when joining fabric pieces.

SEWING

To form the sides of the cover, pin and stitch four squares of fabric together, right sides facing; start and stop ¼ inch from top and bottom raw edges of each seam. Press seams open.

With right sides facing, pin and baste the fifth fabric square to the bottom edge of the cover so raw edges are even and all corners coincide (the corner seam allowances of the stitched side seams will spread). Stitch in place with the fifth square face down; shorten the stitches going around each corner. Press the seams open. Turn cube right side out.

Along three of the edges at the top of the cover and three edges of the last square, press under ¼-inch seam allowances. Pin, then stitch the raw edge of the last square to the remaining raw edge of the cube, right sides together. Press the seam down.

Insert the foam into the cover, making sure the corners of the foam fill the corners of the cover. Then, using a curved needle, whipstitch the rim of the cover invisibly to the top edges of the foam. Flap the top square down, and slipstitch its three open edges to the edges of the cube cover.

1. Seam four sides, then stitch on bottom square.

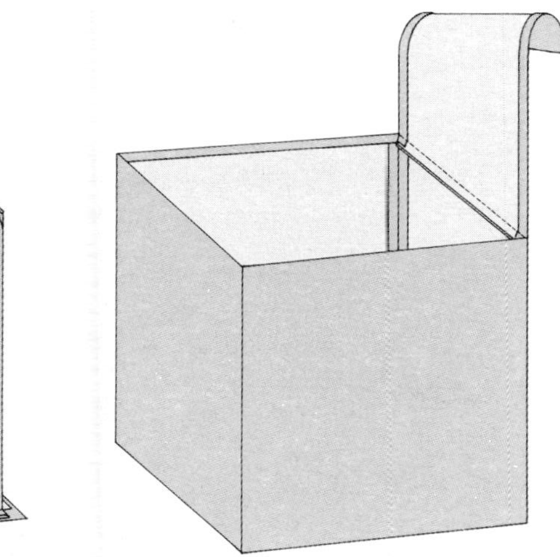

2 Turn under raw edges and stitch last square.

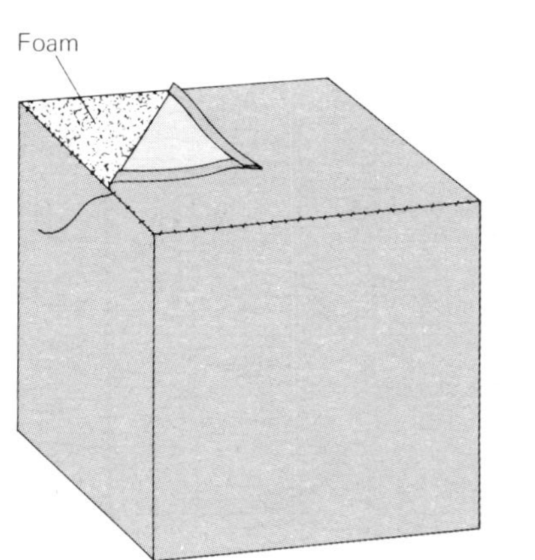

3. Insert foam; slipstitch edges of last square.

His and hers tie and scarf

Grain in fabrics 84-85
Lapped seams 153

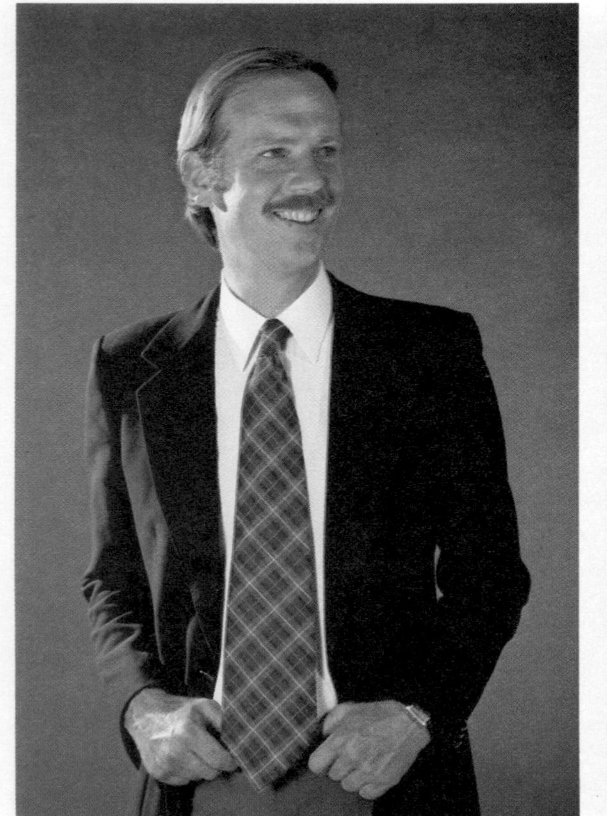

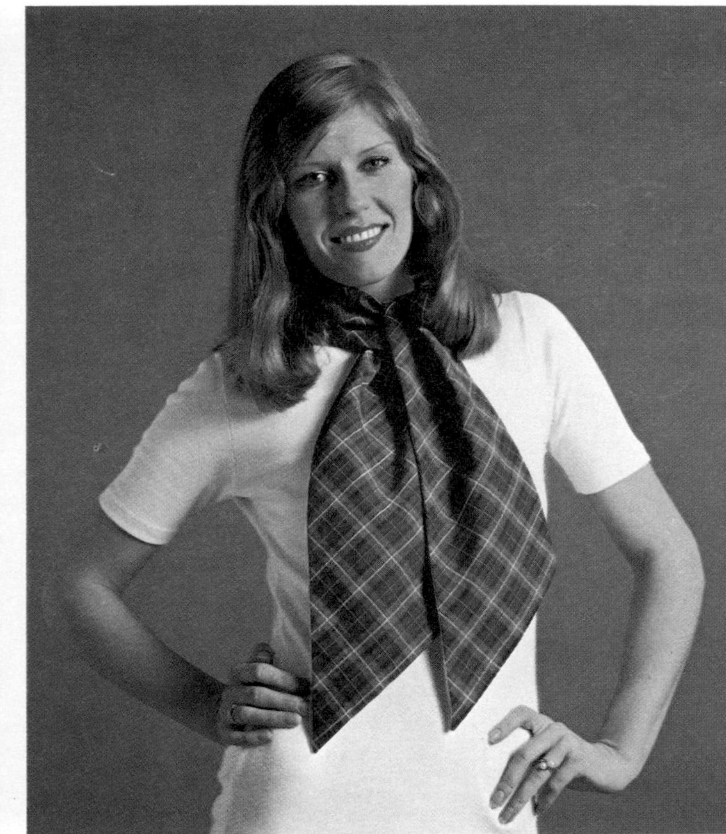

Matched sets have a "something extra" that makes them fun to wear. Both tie and scarf are cut on the bias, which calls for some special handling. Take care not to stretch or otherwise distort the fabric. Always baste before seaming and use a shorter-than-usual stitch. In choosing a fabric, remember that designs look different on the bias. A stripe, for example, becomes a diagonal. The fabric should be one that hangs softly and knots easily. Cotton, silk, wool challis are all good choices. For the tie alone, fabric can be slightly heavier.

MATERIALS NEEDED

⅝ yard of 44/45-inch fabric for tie or scarf
⅜ yard of 36-inch fabric for lining the tie
24 x 20-inch piece of interfacing made for ties
24 x 40-inch sheet of paper for tie
24 x 24-inch sheet of paper for scarf
Appropriate thread

MAKING THE PATTERNS

Graph the sheets of paper into 2-inch squares. Reproduce tie and scarf patterns from diagrams. Cut each out.

CUTTING

The scarf. On a double layer of fabric, pin the length of the pattern on the true bias of the fabric, and cut the scarf pattern twice to obtain four pieces. Mark seam allowances.

The tie. On a single layer of fabric, pin and cut the front and back tie pieces, laying their length along the true bias. Cut the lining pieces of the tie along the true bias as well. Next, pin and cut the interfacing pieces on the true bias of the interfacing fabric. Mark all pattern indications on the cut fabric pieces.

SEWING

The scarf. With right sides facing, match, pin, and machine-stitch the two scarf sections along the center seamline. Press the seam open. Stitch the remaining two sections together the same way.

Pin the two joined pieces together with right sides facing. Baste, then machine-stitch carefully around the ⅝-inch seam allowance; leave a 6-inch opening for turning at the center of one long side. Press flat. Trim the seams and taper corner points. Turn the scarf right side out. Roll seam out to edges, and press. Turn the raw edges in along the opening and slipstitch closed. Press again.

The tie. Slash into the seam allowance at the indicated marking on tie front. Press under the ⅝-inch seam allowances along front tie piece and lining; leave edges above tie slash unpressed, and neatly miter points as shown in the third drawing, bottom row, opposite page.

Center lining on front tip of tie with wrong sides together. Pin, then slipstitch in place; do not pull the stitches tight. Prepare the back tie piece and lining the same way.

With right sides facing, pin tie front to tie back and machine-stitch along straight-grain seam. Press seam open. Then join the front and back interfacing pieces in a lapped seam.

Center interfacing on wrong side of tie; slip ends in place. Work on a flat surface to keep tie from draping and stretching. Hold interfacing in place by securing it to tie's center back seam allowances with a small running stitch. Fold tie's raw edge over interfacing and press lightly; catchstitch raw edge to interfacing. Fold tie's folded edge down to overlap the raw edge; press lightly. Pin and slipstitch in place.

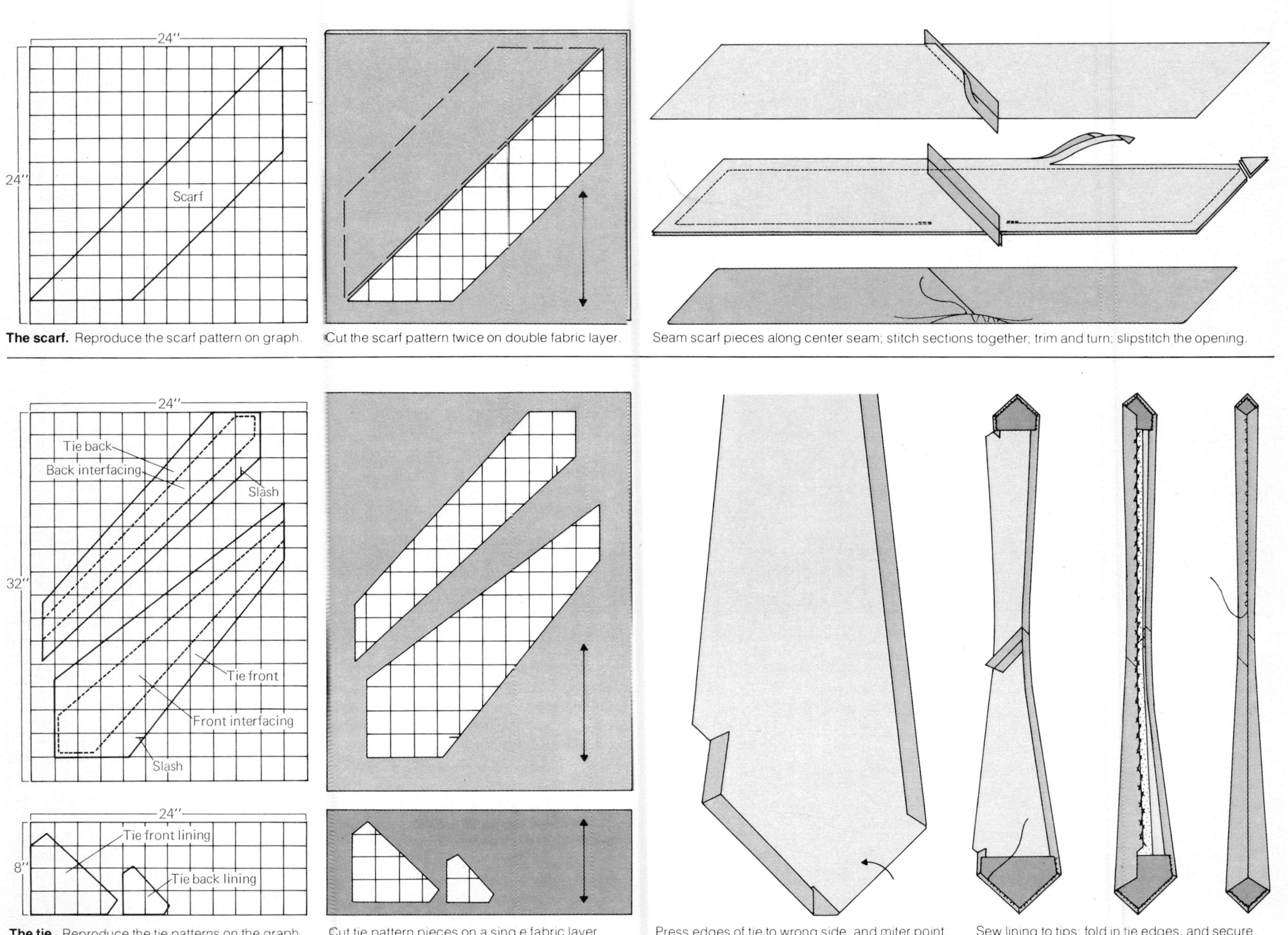

The scarf. Reproduce the scarf pattern on graph. Cut the scarf pattern twice on double fabric layer. Seam scarf pieces along center seam; stitch sections together; trim and turn; slipstitch the opening.

The tie. Reproduce the tie patterns on the graph. Cut tie pattern pieces on a sing e fabric layer. Press edges of tie to wrong side, and miter point. Sew lining to tips; fold in tie edges, and secure.

Gardening coverall

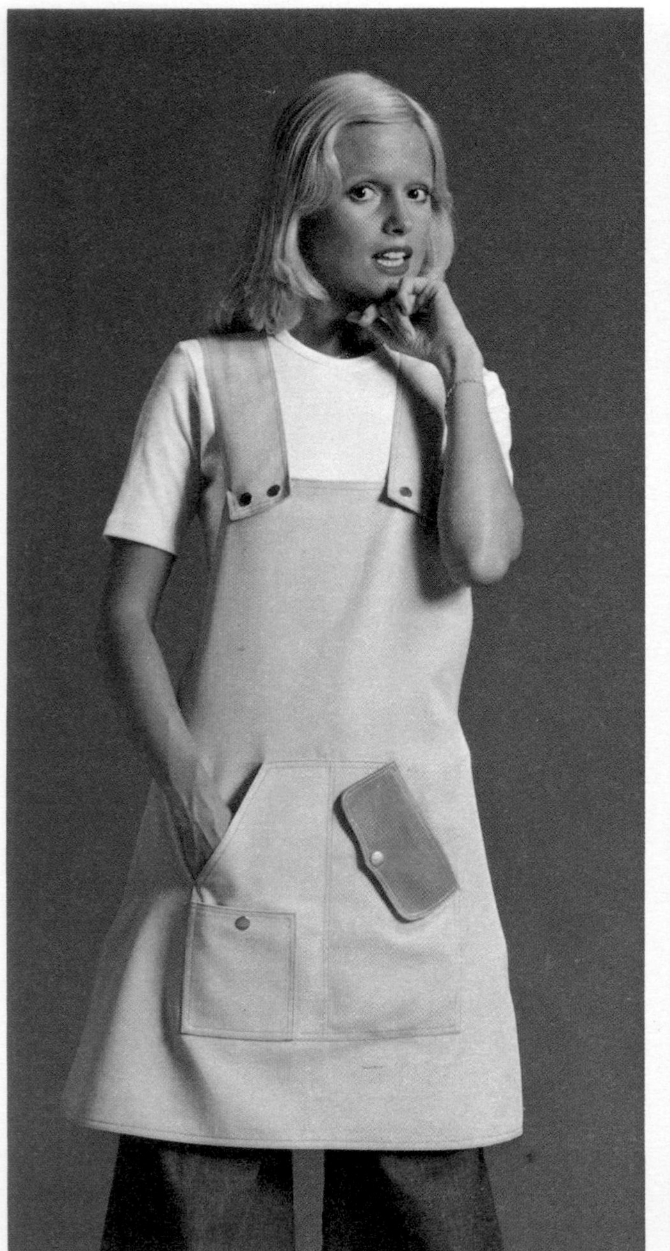

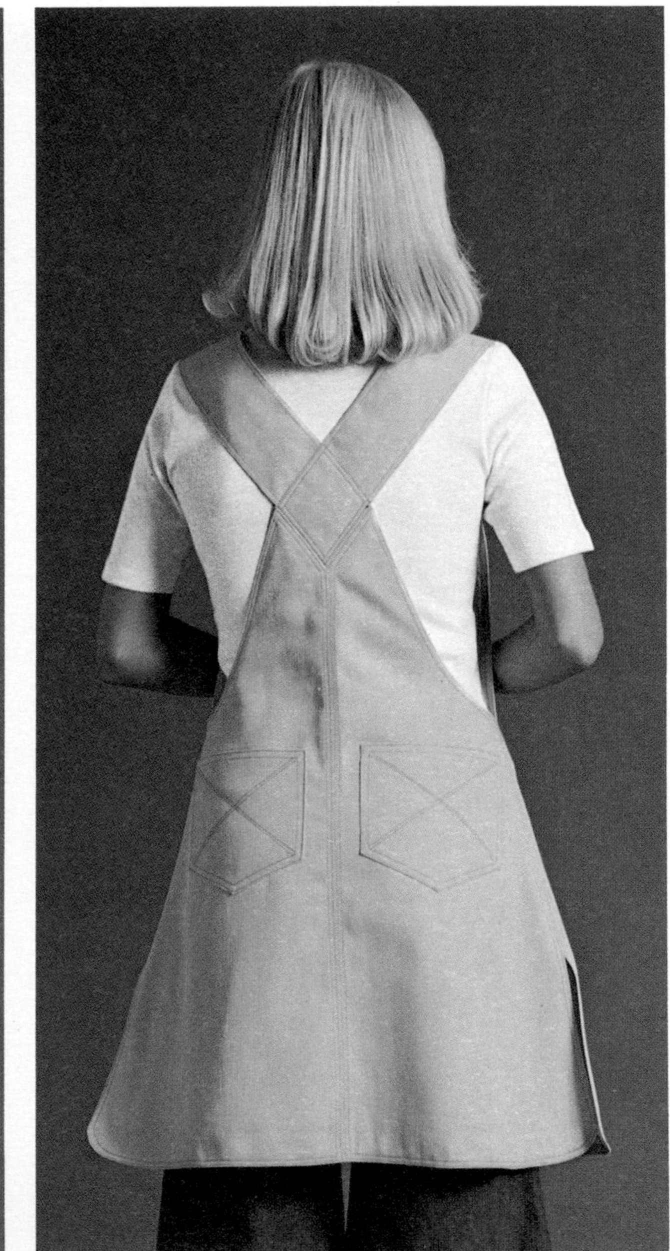

No need to change from head to toe every time you want to tend your plants. Or, for that matter, clean around the house or do a bit of barbecuing. Just slip this coverall over your clothes. It will protect them completely, and its wraparound shape fits well over skirt or pants.

Because the pattern is a one-size-fits-all type, you can make coveralls for your friends even if you have no idea of their exact sizes.

Seams are topstitched all around for looks and durability. The straps work overall-style, crisscrossing in back and snapping in front. Made in a sturdy cotton, such as duck or denim, the coverall will take long, hard wear and lots of laundering.

MATERIALS NEEDED

2 yards of 44/45-inch fabric for the coverall
16 x 5-inch piece of contrasting fabric for the flap
2 heavy decorative no-sew snaps
2 medium decorative no-sew snaps
32 x 44-inch sheet of paper
Appropriate thread

MAKING THE PATTERN

Graph the sheet of paper into 2-inch squares and reproduce the pattern pieces on it. Pieces include ⅝-inch seam allowances.

CUTTING

Fold the fabric in half lengthwise, with wrong sides together, and align the selvages. Pin the pattern pieces (except the pocket flap) along the straight grain, placing the center front and large pocket on the fold, as shown in the layout diagram. Cut out the pattern pieces.

Next fold the contrasting fabric in half, wrong sides together. Pin flap pattern to it and cut out flap.

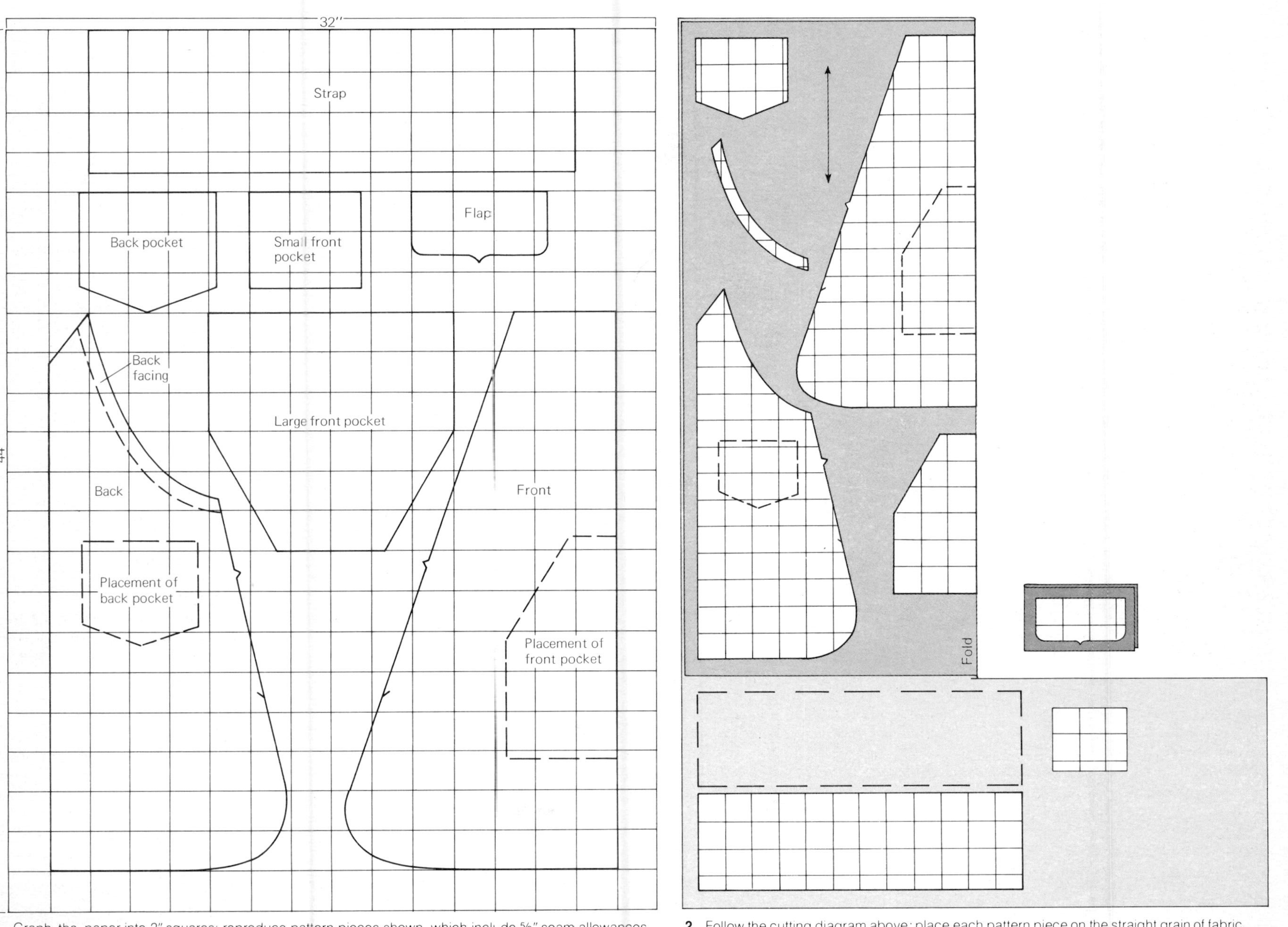

1. Graph the paper into 2″ squares; reproduce pattern pieces shown, which include ⅝″ seam allowances.

2. Follow the cutting diagram above; place each pattern piece on the straight grain of fabric.

Gardening coverall

SEWING

Staystitch the curved armhole seams of the back coverall pieces.

Pockets. With wrong side of fabric up, press under ⅜ inch across the top of the small pocket and down its left side. Place two rows of topstitching ⅛ and ¼ inch from the edge across the top, and a single row ¼ inch from the folded side edge.

With right side of fabric up, position and pin the small pocket onto the lower left-hand corner of the large pocket; align raw edges, and baste them together. Topstitch the finished side of small pocket in place, securing stitches at top.

Press under a ⅝-inch hem all the way around the large pocket, except for the upper right edge where flap is to be sewed. Topstitch around the pocket ¼ inch from the folded edge.

Pin and stitch the two flap pieces together, right sides facing; leave the top edge open. Trim the corners and turn the flap to the right side, bringing the seam out to the edge. Press. Place two rows of topstitching around the finished edges.

Pin right side of flap to wrong side of large pocket; align the raw edges. Machine-stitch along the seamline. Trim and grade the seam allowances. Fold flap over right side of pocket, and press. Place two rows of topstitching along turned edge, stitching through all thicknesses.

Position the large pocket onto the center of the apron front. Pin-baste and machine-edgestitch around the pocket, leaving the two slanted edges open; secure the stitches at each end of the opening. To divide pocket in half, place two rows of topstitching up the center of the pocket.

Press under a ⅝-inch hem around each back pocket. Topstitch all around pocket, ¼ inch from its folded edges. Place a second row of stitching along the top edge only, then crisscross two rows of topstitching through pocket center.

Position and pin pockets to each back section. Hand-baste and then edgestitch along the single-topstitched sides of each pocket.

Before constructing the straps apply the armhole facing to both back pieces: With right sides together, match and pin facings to back armhole curve. Baste and stitch; trim and clip seam allowances. Extend facing and seam allowances and understitch close to the seamline. Turn the facing to the wrong side and press.

Straps. Fold each strap in half lengthwise, right sides together. Pin, then machine-stitch along the long seamline. Press the seam open, pressing so that the seam runs down the center of each strap. Machine-stitch across one end; cut the other end off at an angle that is determined by measuring ¾ inch in from the raw edge. Turn straps to right side, and press; place two rows of topstitching along finished edges.

With right sides facing, pin and machine-stitch the back pieces together along the center back seamline; stop and secure stitches at top seamline crossing. Press seam open. Align and pin the raw edge of one strap to one of the back pointed edges, right sides together. Pin the other strap to the other back point in the same way; straps should crisscross. Machine-stitch both straps as pinned, securing stitches at beginning and end. Press seam allowances down and tack them to the armhole facing. Place two rows of topstitching around the diamond shape formed where the two straps of the coverall cross.

Assembling garment sections. Place a row of easestitching around the bottom curves of the front and back pieces. With right sides together, match and pin-baste the front to the back along the side seams. Starting from the armhole, machine-stitch down to the indicated marking; secure stitches at beginning and end. Press the seam flat, then open; continue pressing the unstitched portion of the seam allowances to the wrong side, pulling up the easestitching around the curves. Press under ⅝ inch along both the top and bottom edges of the apron.

Next place two rows of topstitching around all edges of the apron front. Then place two rows of topstitching around all edges of the apron back, including two rows down each side of the back seams.

Fasten the large snaps to the ends of the straps and to the corresponding points on the apron, the smaller snaps to the pocket flap and small pocket.

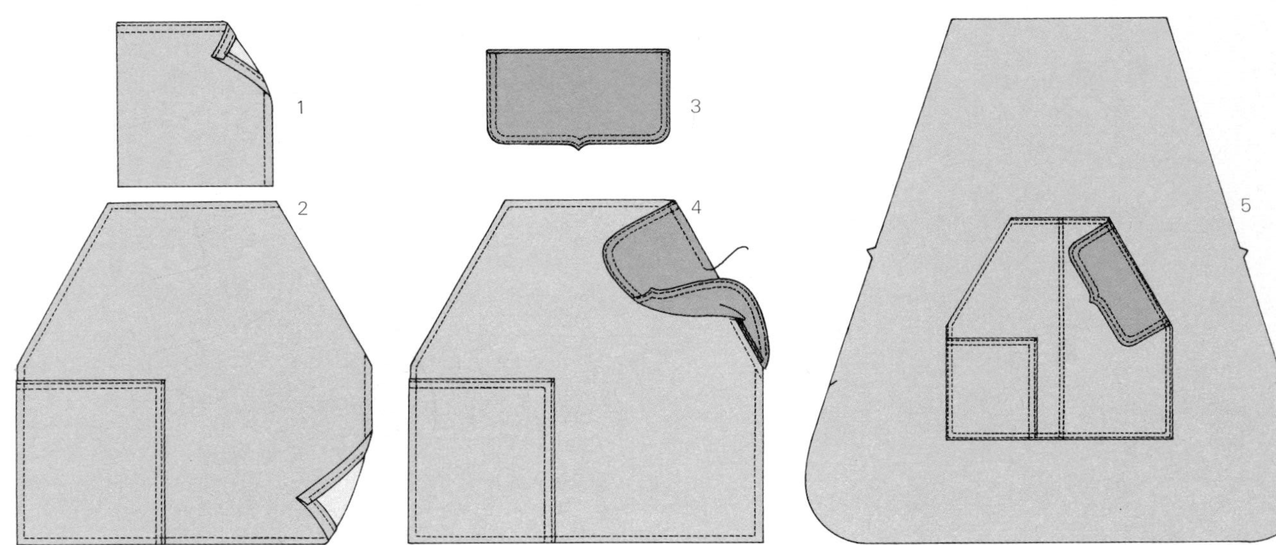

To construct front pockets, turn under edges of small pocket and stitch (1). Sew small pocket to the large pocket, and finish the edges around the large pocket (2). Complete the flap (3) and attach it to the edge of the large pocket (4). Stitch large pocket to apron front, and topstitch through center (5).

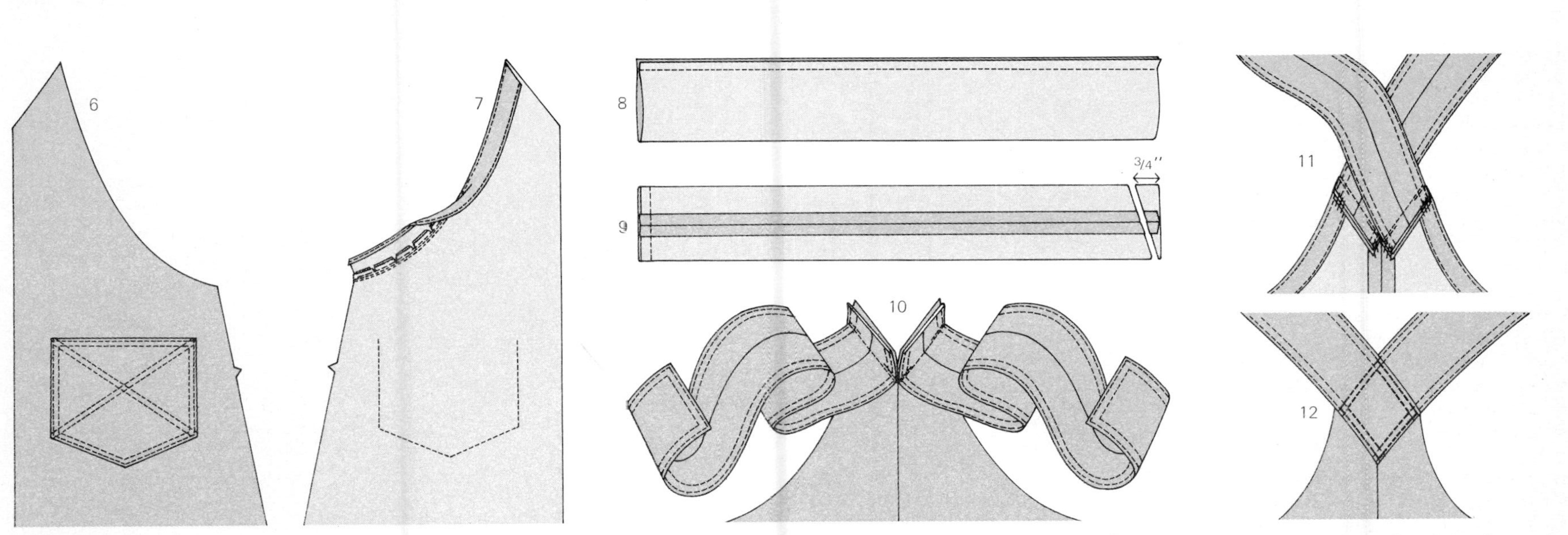

To construct back pockets, finish edges and apply topstitching; stitch pockets onto back sections (6). Apply the **armhole facings** to back pieces (7). **To construct straps,** seam each one (8) and trim off one end of each strap (9). Stitch back seams. Topstitch each strap, then apply straps to back sections (10). Press seam allowances of straps down and whipstitch in place (11). Topstitch the straps together (12).

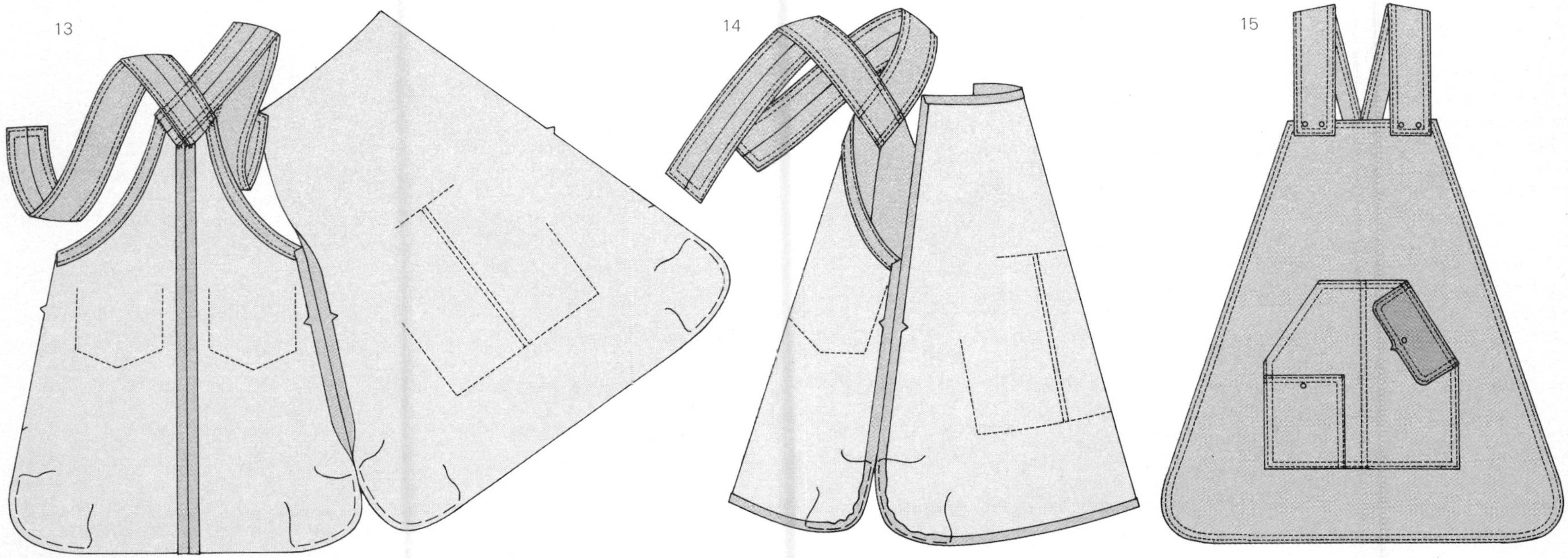

To assemble coverall, stitch back to front side seams, press seams open (13). Press all raw edges to the inside; pull easestitching threads to ease in fullness at corners (14). Complete topstitching (15).

Packable rain hat

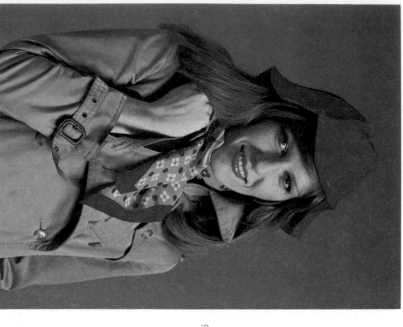

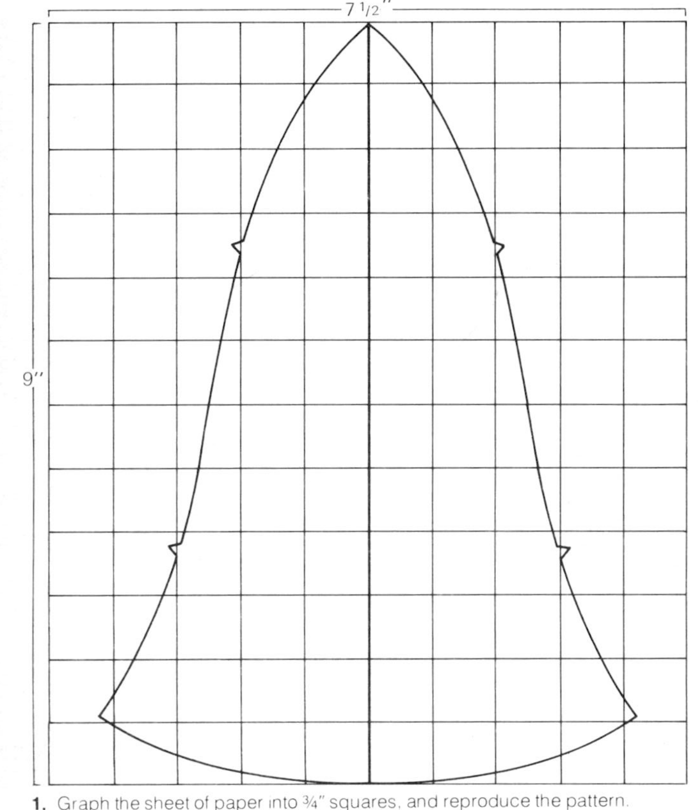

1. Graph the sheet of paper into ¾" squares, and reproduce the pattern.

2. Cut out the pattern to obtain six hat pieces.

This is surely the handiest of rain hats — designed to fold flat for easy tucking into handbag, raincoat pocket, or car. Simple to make (the waterproof nylon needs no lining), it requires only ⅓ yard of fabric. The seaming technique produces decorative ridges that also help to shape the hat. To make one for a child, adjust pattern measurements.

MATERIALS NEEDED

⅓ yard of 44/45-inch fabric
7½ x 9-inch sheet of paper
Appropriate thread

MAKING THE PATTERN

Graph the sheet of paper into ¾-inch squares; draw a line down the center. Reproduce the pattern shown in Diagram 1, taking care to match the drawn curves on both sides.

CUTTING

Fold the fabric in half along the lengthwise grain and pin selvages together. Place pattern on the straight grain. Cut the same piece three times to get six sections; to get three cuts from the width, reverse the pattern position each time.

SEWING

At the bottom edge of each hat section, turn under a double ⅛-inch hem and press. Stitch along the hem edge with a zigzag stitch, or use two rows of straight stitching.

With right sides facing, match and pin two of the sections together. Machine-stitch ¼ inch from the raw edge; stop and secure the stitches ¼ inch from the top. Join the remaining sections the same way, being particularly careful where the points meet. (If desired, at this stage narrow chin straps to hold the hat down can be inserted between two opposite seams. A ¼-inch grosgrain ribbon can be used; or you may have enough fabric left to make straps.)

Zigzag the raw edges of each seam allowance together, stopping ¼ inch from the top. If you have no zigzag stitch, place another row of straight stitching near the raw edges.

Turn hat right side out. Bring each seam out to the edge and press. Starting ¼ inch from top of hat, machine-stitch close to each seam to form decorative ridge; backstitch at bottom and tie thread ends at top.

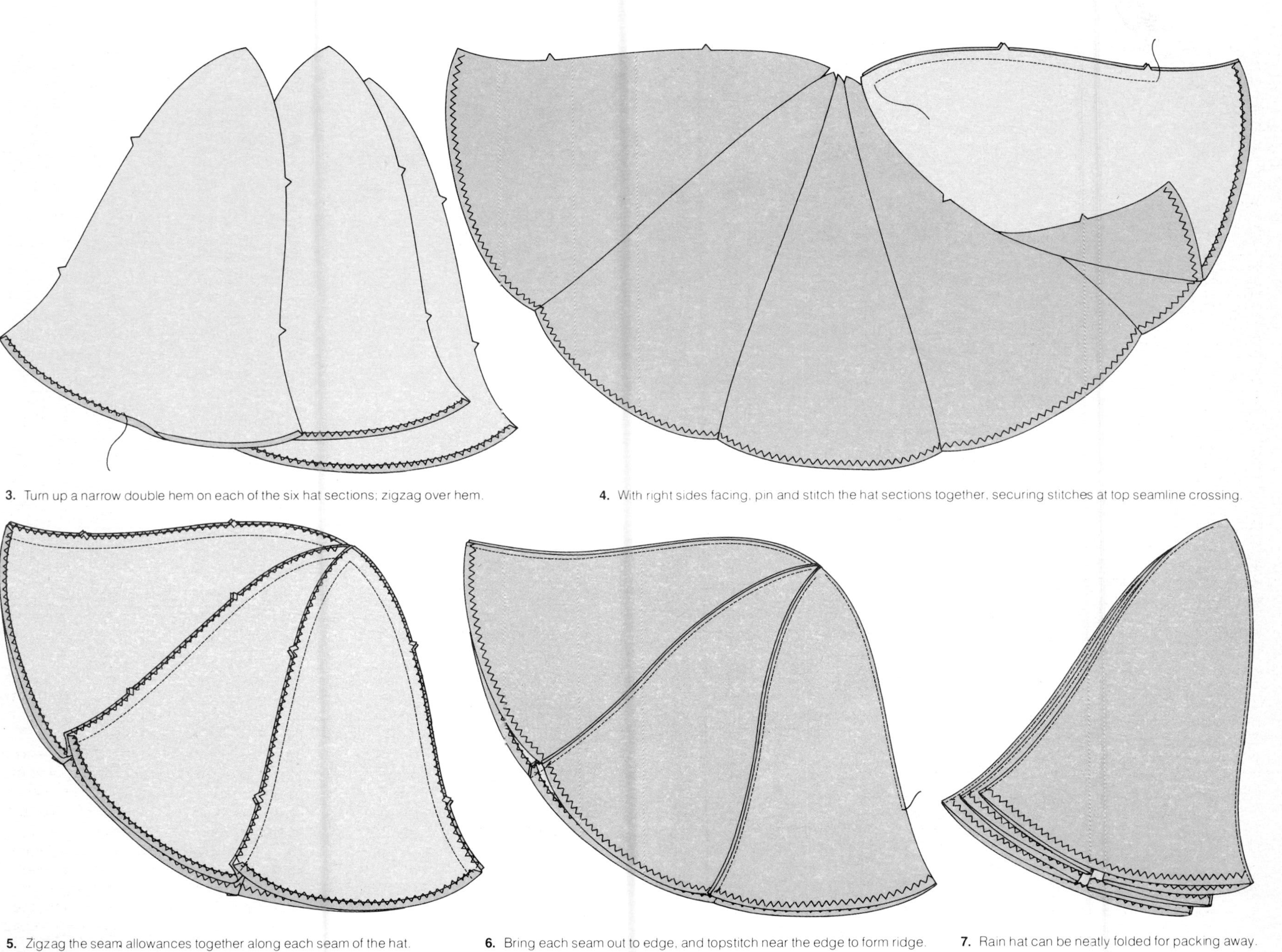

3. Turn up a narrow double hem on each of the six hat sections; zigzag over hem.

4. With right sides facing, pin and stitch the hat sections together, securing stitches at top seamline crossing.

5. Zigzag the seam allowances together along each seam of the hat.

6. Bring each seam out to edge, and topstitch near the edge to form ridge.

7. Rain hat can be neatly folded for packing away.

Barrel bag

Closing zipper tapes at top 317

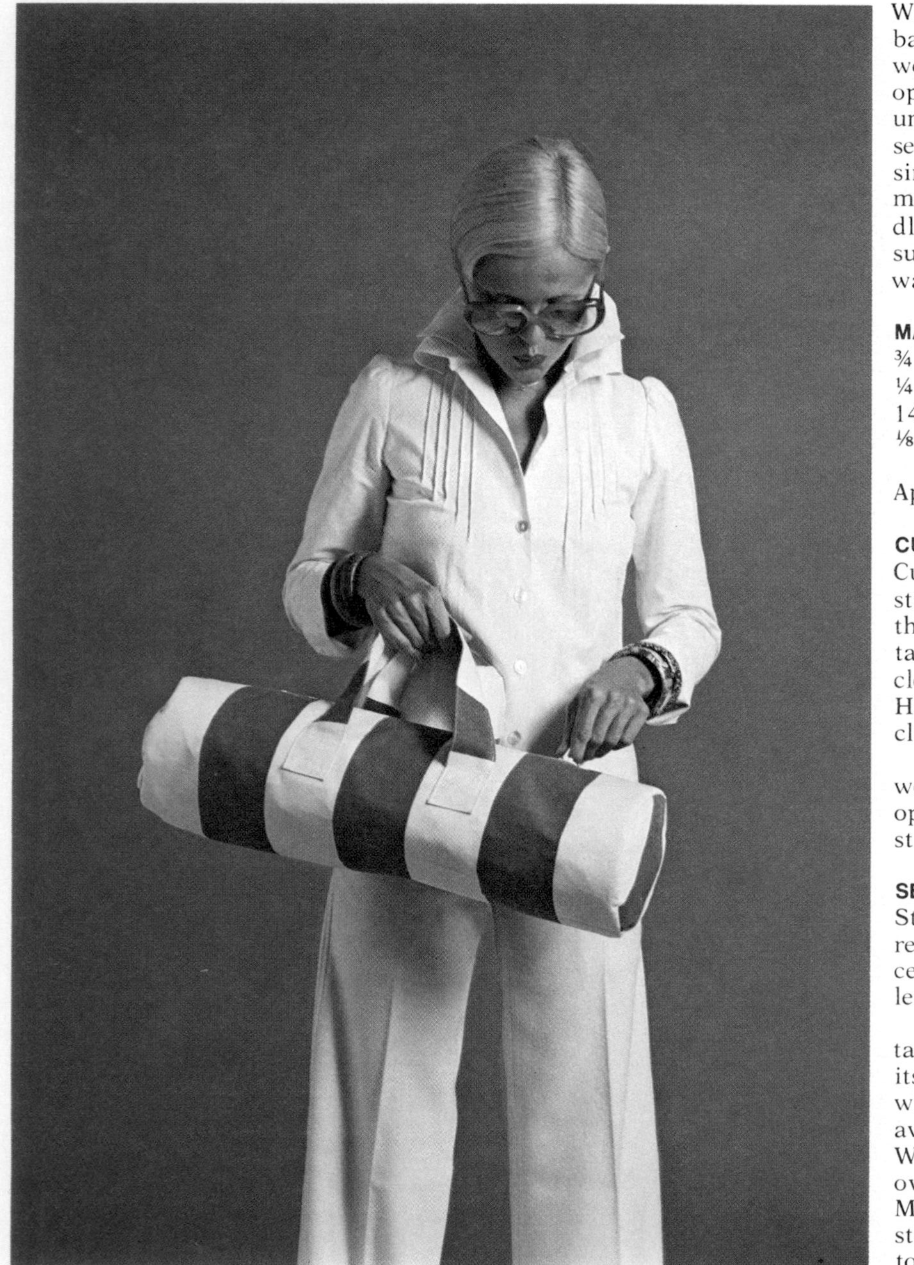

Who couldn't use a big, easy-to-carry bag like this for shopping, the beach, weekend trips? The long zippered opening makes it easy to pack and unpack. The design makes it easy to sew in a day. If you'd like it larger, simply alter the pattern measurements, and perhaps run the handles all the way around for extra support. For beach use, consider a waterproof lining.

MATERIALS NEEDED

¾ yard of 44/45-inch fabric for bag
¼ yard of 26-inch fusible interfacing
14-inch zipper
⅛ yard of lightweight fabric for zipper stay
Appropriate thread

CUTTING

Cut a 23 x 22-inch rectangle on the straight of the fabric for the body of the bag. Then cut two 20 x 5-inch rectangles for the handles, and two circles 7 inches in diameter for the ends. Half-inch seam allowances are included on all pieces.

Cut an 18 x 3-inch strip of lightweight fabric for staying the zipper opening. Also cut two 19 x 4-inch strips of fusible interfacing.

SEWING

Staystitch the two longer edges of the rectangle. Mark and thread-trace center lines between the width and length of the rectangle.

On the wrong side of the large rectangle, center the zipper and mark its position along the rectangle's width. Mark stitching lines ⅛ inch away from the centered zipper line. With right sides together, pin stay over zipper area and baste in place. Machine-stitch around on the marked stitching lines. Slash down the center to within ½ inch of both ends, then cut into corners. Turn stay to inside and press. Topstitch around the opening, placing the stitching ⅜ inch from the long edges and ½ inch from the edges at the ends. Crisscross the topstitching at each end.

Close the zipper tapes above the top stop with a bar tack. Center zipper under the opening; pin, baste, then edgestitch in place.

Handles. To make handles, center the fusible interfacing on the wrong side of each handle; press in place. Fold handle in half lengthwise, right sides together, and pin. Machine-stitch around leaving a 3-inch opening in center of long edge. Trim seam allowances and taper corners. Turn the handle right side out; pull out corners. Press the handle flat, rolling the seams out to the edges. Edgestitch around the handle. Mark handle positions so they are centered, with ends 6½ inches apart and about 4 inches from the zipper edge. Pin one of the handles to the bag; topstitch a square at each end, crisscrossing the stitching in each square. Attach the other handle to the opposite side.

Fold one circle in half, and cut a tiny notch at the foldline on each end. With right sides facing, position the circle to one end of the bag; pin bag and circle together from the top, matching the thread-traced center line with one notch. With the bag facing you, continue pinning around the entire circle, clipping the bag seam allowance as necessary to go around the curve; the bottom seam allowances of the bag should meet at the bottom notch of the circle. Baste, then stitch around circle, secure stitches at beginning and end. Finish other end of bag the same way. Open zipper; right sides together, sew bottom seam allowances. Press open; turn bag right side out.

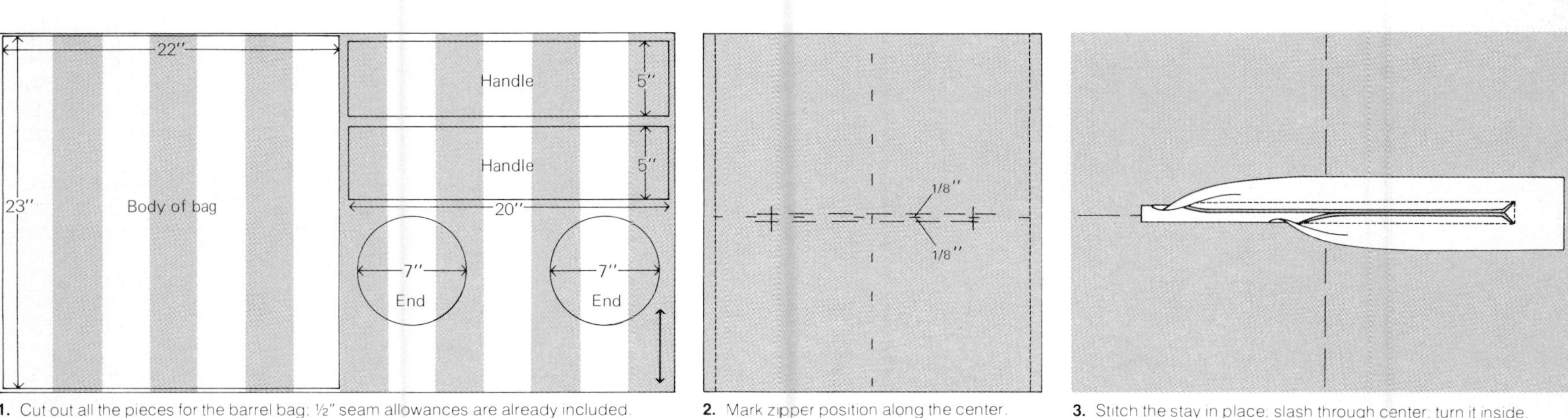

1. Cut out all the pieces for the barrel bag; ½″ seam allowances are already included.

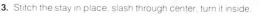

2. Mark zipper position along the center.

3. Stitch the stay in place; slash through center; turn it inside.

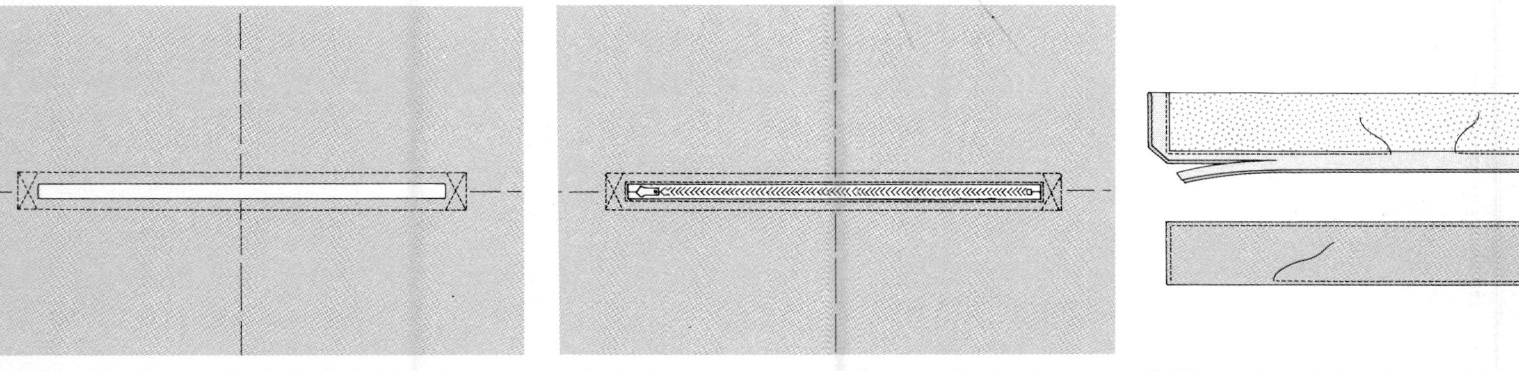

4. Topstitch around opening, crisscrossing the stitching at ends.

5. Center the zipper under opening, then edgestitch it in place.

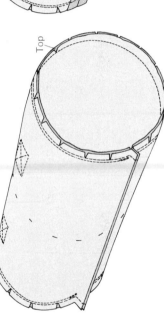

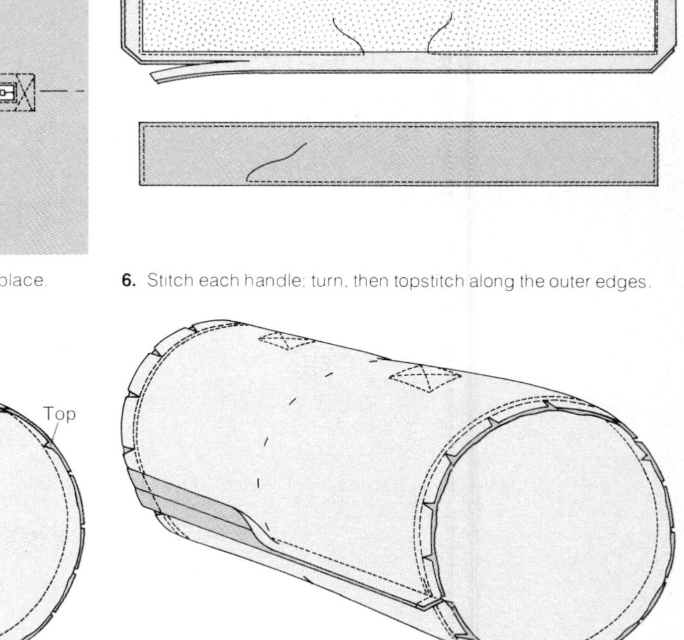

6. Stitch each handle; turn, then topstitch along the outer edges.

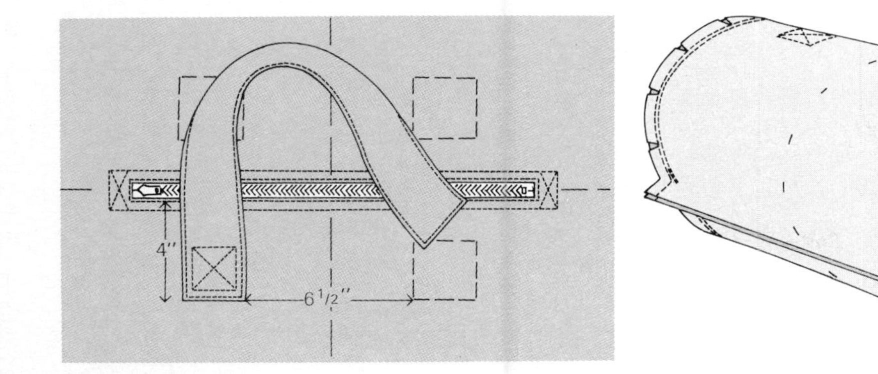

7. Pin and stitch handle in place; crisscross the stitching at ends.

8. Pin, baste, and stitch the circles to each end of the barrel bag.

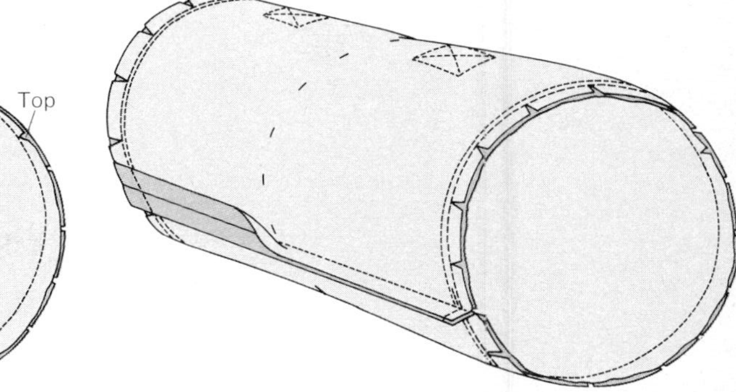

9. Complete the seam along bottom of the bag; press seam open.

Shoulder bag

Nylon tape fasteners 15
Fold-over braid 16

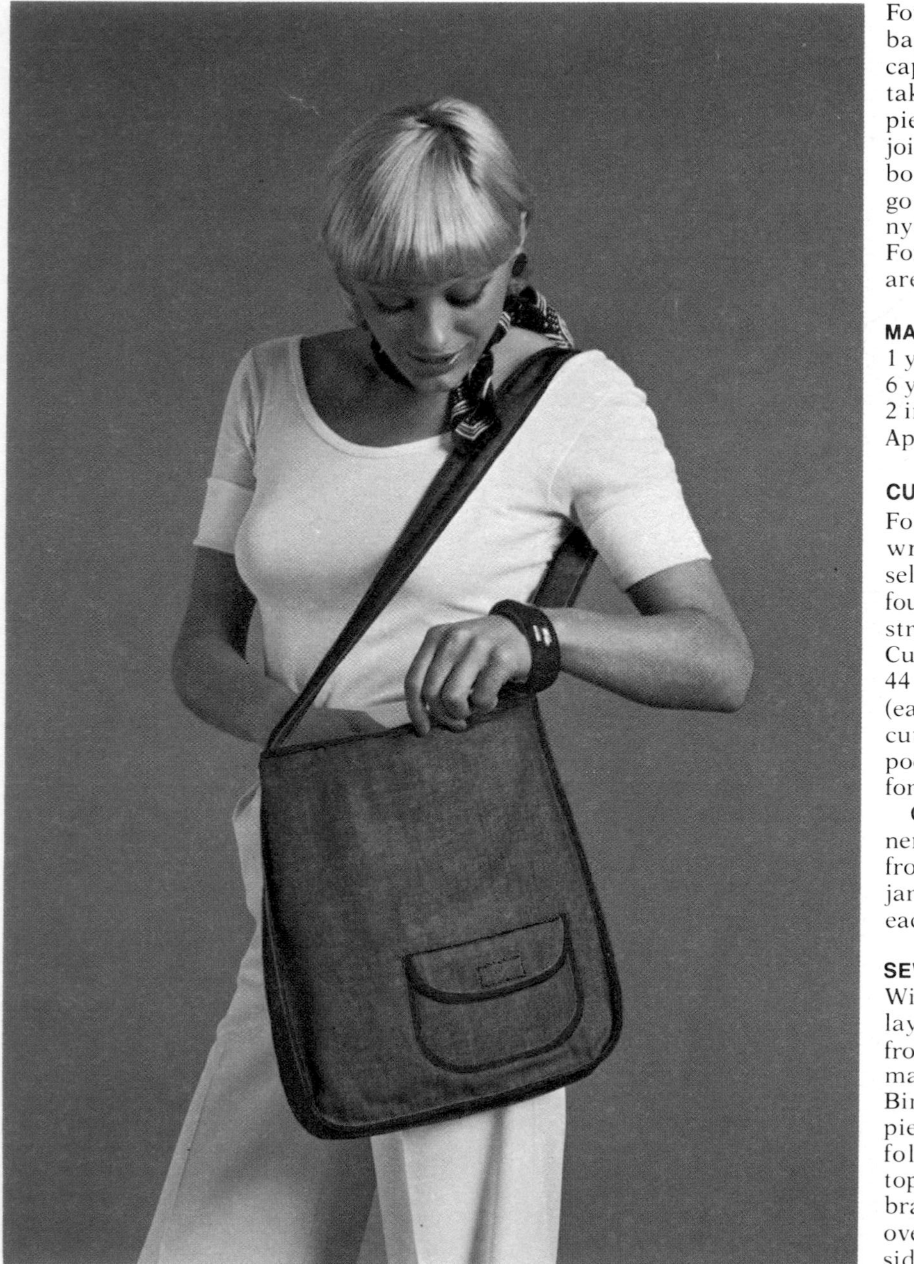

For the fashion-minded beginner, this bag should be a perfect project. Big on capacity and carrying comfort, it takes little sewing skill or time. The pieces are just a front and back, joined by circular straps that form bottom and sides. Change or keys can go in the handy outside pocket; a nylon tape closure keeps them secure. For shape and strength, fabric layers are double and edges are bound.

MATERIALS NEEDED

1 yard of 44/45-inch fabric
6 yards of fold-over braid
2 inches of nylon tape fastener
Appropriate thread

CUTTING

Fold the fabric in half lengthwise, wrong sides together, and line up the selvages. Following Diagram 1, cut four 12 x 14-inch rectangles along the straight grain for the body of the bag. Cut two long bands (each of them 2 x 44 inches) and two shorter bands (each 2 x 27 inches) for the straps. Also cut two 6 x 4-inch rectangles for the pocket and two 6 x 2-inch rectangles for the flap.

Carefully round off the bottom corners of the pocket, the flap, and the front and back pieces of the bag; use a jar lid to obtain a uniform curve on each piece.

SEWING

With wrong sides facing, pin the two layers of each piece (pocket, flap, front, and back) together and then machine-baste around the edges. Bind the tops of the front and back pieces as well as the pocket with the fold-over braid, then machine-topstitch with the wider half of the braid on the underside. Apply the fold-over braid in the same way to the sides and bottoms of the pocket, turning under ¼ inch at each end. Bind only the sides and bottoms of the flap. Pull apart the hooked and looped halves of the nylon tape fastener. Center and pin the hooked half of the tape to the underside of the flap, just above the braid. Center and pin the looped half of the tape to the top edge of the pocket, just below the braid. Machine-stitch both of the tape pieces in place.

Pin the pocket to the bottom right-hand corner of the bag front, placing the pocket 1½ inches from the bottom and 1½ inches from the side edges of the bag. Baste the pocket in place, and edgestitch around its side and bottom edges, securing the stitches at the beginning and end.

Turn and press under a ¼-inch hem at the top of the flap. Pin the flap over the pocket, aligning the surfaces of the nylon tape. Machine-stitch across the top edge of the flap with either a narrow zigzag stitch or two rows of straight stitching.

With right sides together, seam one long band to one short band to form a circular strap. Press seams open. Do the same for the remaining long and short bands. With wrong sides facing, place the two straps together, then machine-baste along both edges.

With the wrong side of the bag front against the strap, pin the two edges together; place the seams of the strap at each side of the bag. Machine-baste as pinned. Starting at the bottom of the bag, wrap and pin braid around the raw edges of the bag front and strap; before overlapping the braid ends, turn under ¼ inch on one end. Machine-topstitch the binding in place, keeping the wider half of the braid on the underside.

Using the same procedures, join the back of the bag to the strap and attach the braid.

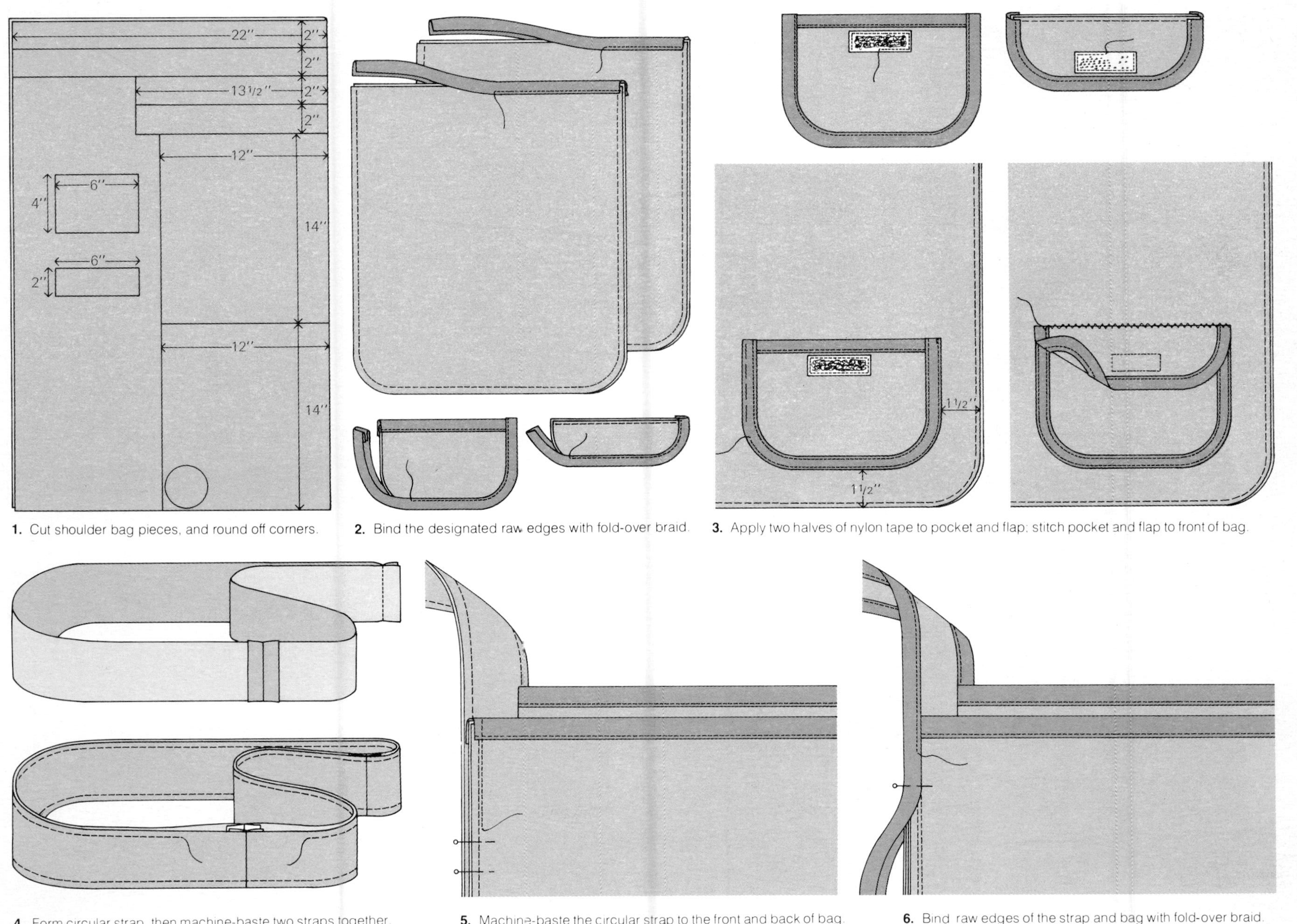

1. Cut shoulder bag pieces, and round off corners.

2. Bind the designated raw edges with fold-over braid.

3. Apply two halves of nylon tape to pocket and flap; stitch pocket and flap to front of bag.

4. Form circular strap, then machine-baste two straps together.

5. Machine-baste the circular strap to the front and back of bag.

6. Bind raw edges of the strap and bag with fold-over braid.

Skirt/cape beach coverup

Turned up hems 292-293

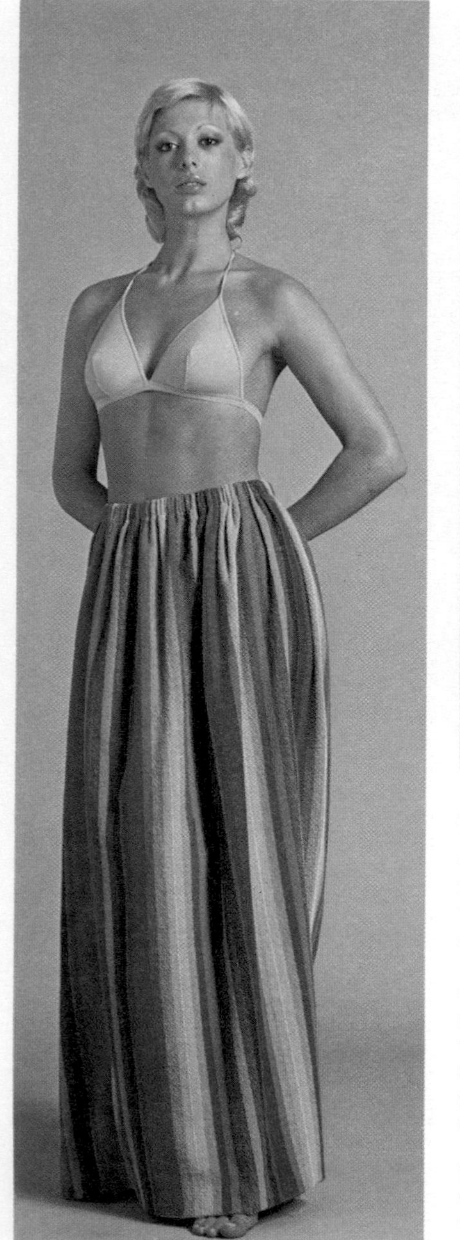

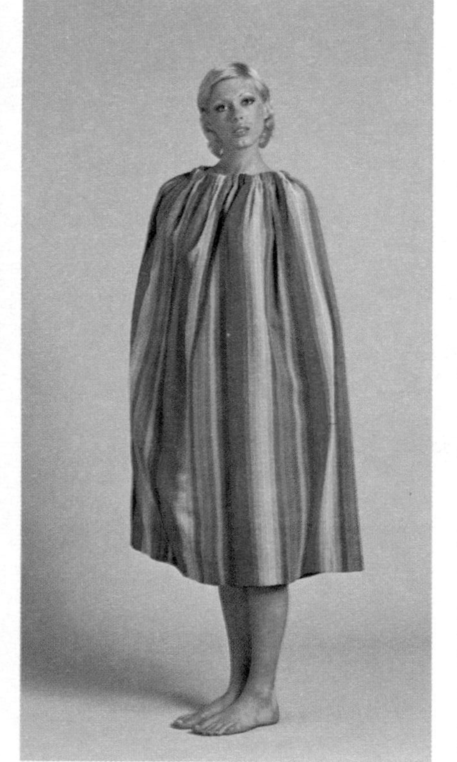

A bright idea for the young in heart, this two-way wrap also has its practical advantages. First of all, it can be run up in minutes—nothing to it but two pieces, seamed and hemmed with an elasticized casing on top.

Worn as a skirt over a swim suit, the coverup will take you in style to snack stand or parking lot. Take cover under the cape for protection against sun or breezes. In a pinch, under its generous width, you could even change from wet suit to dry clothes!

The fabric need not be terry cloth, but it is probably the best choice. Terry cloth soaks up water, isn't bothered by sand, and takes beautifully to machine washing and drying.

MATERIALS NEEDED

Two skirt lengths plus 3 inches of 44/45-inch fabric

Waist measurement plus ½ inch of 1-inch elastic

Appropriate thread

CUTTING

Cut the fabric in half along the crosswise grain to get two equal pieces. Then cut one section in half on the lengthwise grain. (Only one of the halved sections will be used.)

SEWING

Place the large piece and one of the half sections together, right sides facing; if the fabric has a nap or one-way design, make sure both pieces are lying in the same direction. Pin the pieces together, then machine-stitch the side seams.

Turn under a scant ¼ inch along the raw top edge of the skirt. Fold and press under 1½ inches for the casing; pin and machine-stitch close to the free edge, leaving a 1½-inch opening at one side seam. Machine-stitch close to the fold on the upper edge of the skirt.

Fit the elastic around your waist, add ½ inch, and cut. Attach a bodkin or safety pin to one end of the elastic and insert it into the casing. Pin the other end to the skirt to keep that end from slipping through. Work the safety pin around the casing; avoid twisting the elastic. Unpin both elastic ends, overlap them ½ inch, and pin. Stitch a square on the overlapped area, crisscrossing it for strength. Pull the joined ends of the elastic inside the casing. Stretching the elastic slightly, stitch along the casing edge to close the opening.

Finish the raw edge at the bottom of the skirt. Turn up a 1½-inch hem and secure by hand or machine.

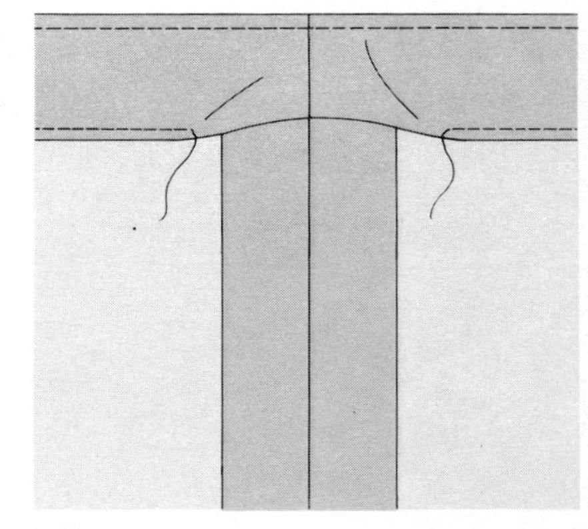

1. Turn and stitch the casing at top of the skirt.

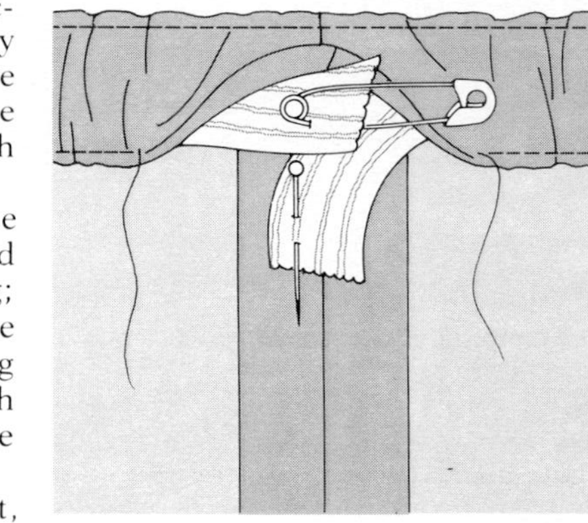

2. Insert elastic and work it through the casing.

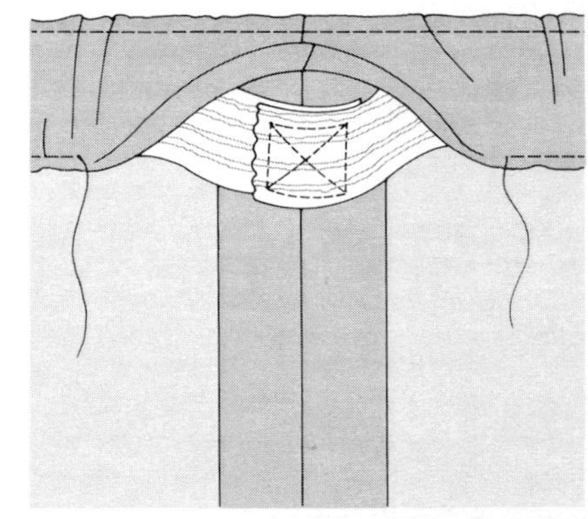

3. Stitch the ends together; pull inside the casing.

Giant pencil pillow

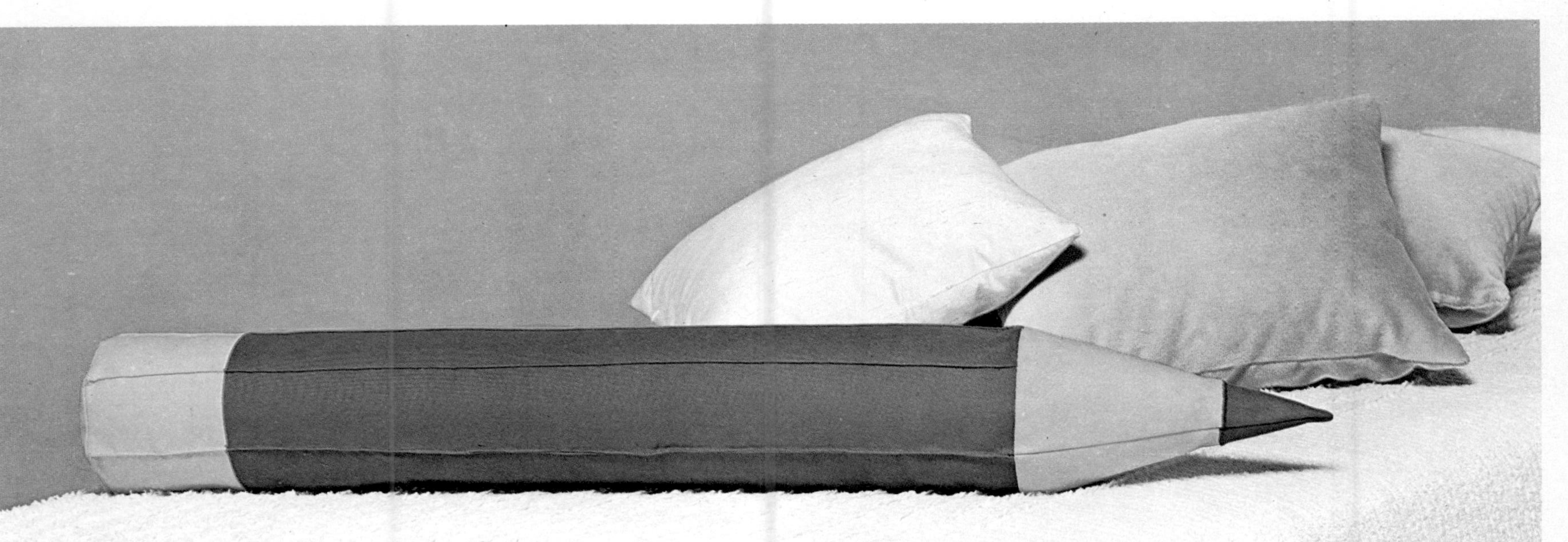

Whether you use it as a floor pillow or a bolster, this kingsize pencil will make an amusing addition to any room. The measurements given will make a pillow that is approximately 36 inches long. Choose a durable fabric, such as broadcloth, denim, or sailcloth.

MATERIALS NEEDED

½ yard of 36-inch fabric for pencil body and "lead"
½ yard of 36-inch fabric for "eraser" and pencil point
1¼ yards of 26-inch fusible interfacing
Fiber fill or foam shreds
Appropriate thread

MAKING THE PATTERN

To make the pattern piece for the pointed end and lead tip of the pencil, draw a semicircle with a 9-inch radius. Draw a small semicircle having a 3-inch radius within the larger semicircle. Use a flexible tape measure to carefully mark off 16 inches along the outer edge of the large semicircle; draw a line connecting the mark to the center point of the semicircle. Cut away the excess. The wedge that remains is the pencil top pattern; the smaller wedge drawn inside it is the lead.

CUTTING

Cut the main pieces from the fusible interfacing first; the interfacing pieces will then be used as a pattern for cutting the actual fabrics. For the body of the pencil, cut two rectangles, one 16 x 5 inches, the other 16 x 24 inches. Cut a circle 5¼ inches in diameter. Cut the pencil top from the large wedge and the pencil lead from the small wedge in the pattern.

Carefully fuse the large rectangle, on grain, to the wrong side of the fabric to be used for the pencil body. Cut the fabric out, leaving a 5/8-inch seam allowance around the interfacing. Fuse and cut the small wedge from the same fabric, leaving a 5/8-inch seam allowance all around. Fuse and cut the small rectangle, circle, and large wedge from the contrasting fabric in the same way.

SEWING

With right sides facing, pin together and machine-stitch the pencil (large rectangle) and the eraser (small rectangle). Press the seam open. Fold stitched piece in half lengthwise, and press to obtain a center foldline. On the wrong side of the pencil and eraser, draw lines that are parallel to the pressed foldline and spaced approximately 2⅝ inches apart.

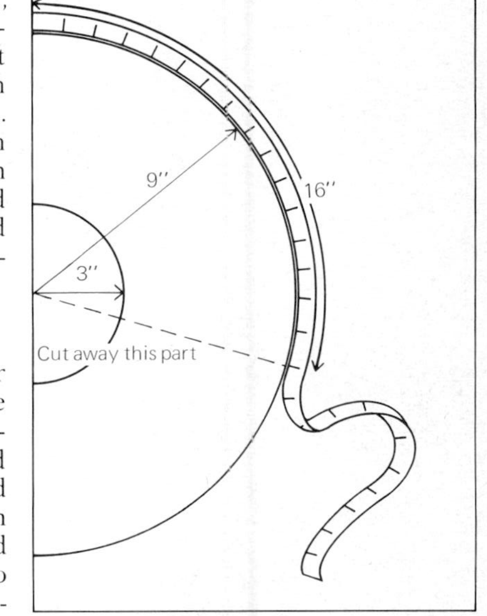

Make patterns for both the pencil point and lead

Giant pencil pillow

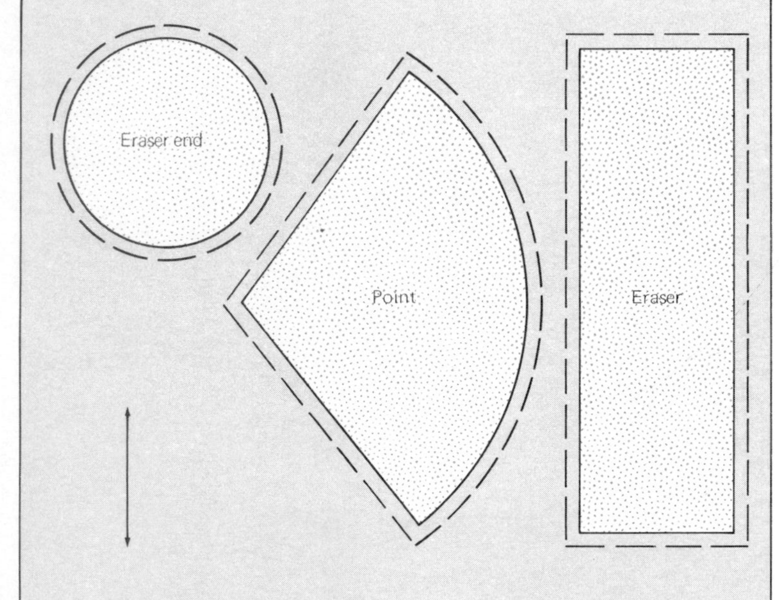

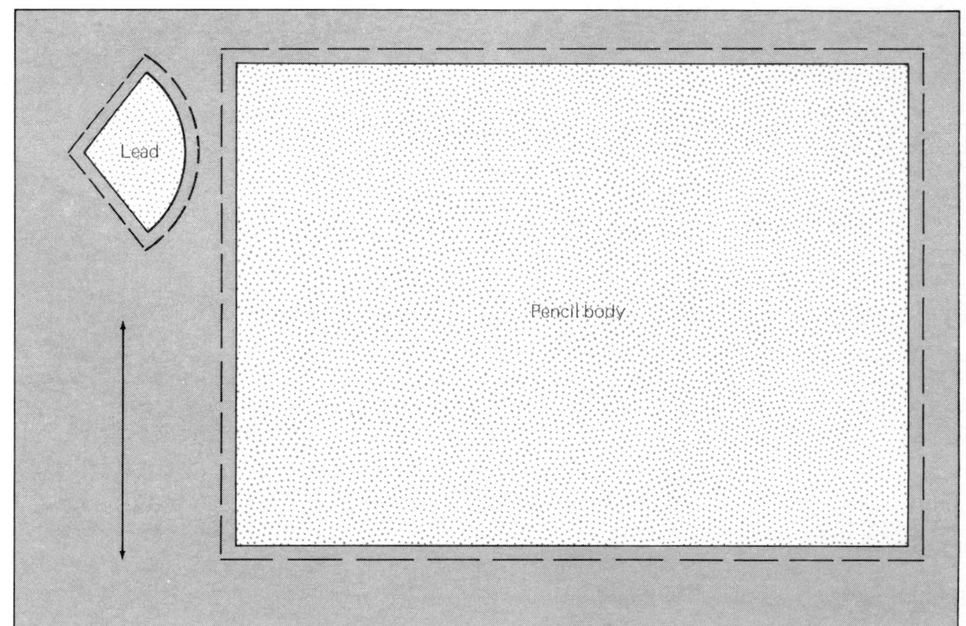

1. Cut out pencil pieces from the fusible interfacing. Fuse each piece on grain to the appropriate fabric. Mark a ⅝" seam allowance around each fused piece, then cut out the pieces along the marked lines.

Thread-trace each line. Place a row of staystitching on both ends of the pencil/eraser unit.

Press under a narrow hem along the curved edge of the pencil lead (small wedge). Pin and baste the pencil lead to tip of pencil top (large wedge), aligning the raw edges. Satin-stitch along the curved edge of the pencil lead, or use a straight stitch.

With right sides together, pin the curve of the large wedge to the pencil end of the body; clip seam allowance of pencil as needed to go around the curve. Machine-stitch as pinned. Press seam open; notch out excess.

With right sides together, pin and baste the circle to the eraser end of the body; clip the seam allowances of the eraser as necessary to go around the circle; the seamlines of the eraser should meet. Machine-stitch as basted and secure thread ends.

Pin the long seam of the entire pencil together, with right sides facing, matching cross seams. Machine-stitch, leaving an 8 to 10-inch opening in center. Turn pencil right side out.

On the right side of the pencil, fold and press each thread-traced line.

Using matching thread color for the pencil and the eraser portions, edgestitch near each fold, stopping at the base of the pencil top; secure thread ends at the begining and end of stitching lines. Edgestitch along the seamline as well, stopping at the ends of the opening.

Stuff the pencil pillow with fiber fill, packing it well and pushing the fiber fill right up into the tip. Slipstitch the opening closed.

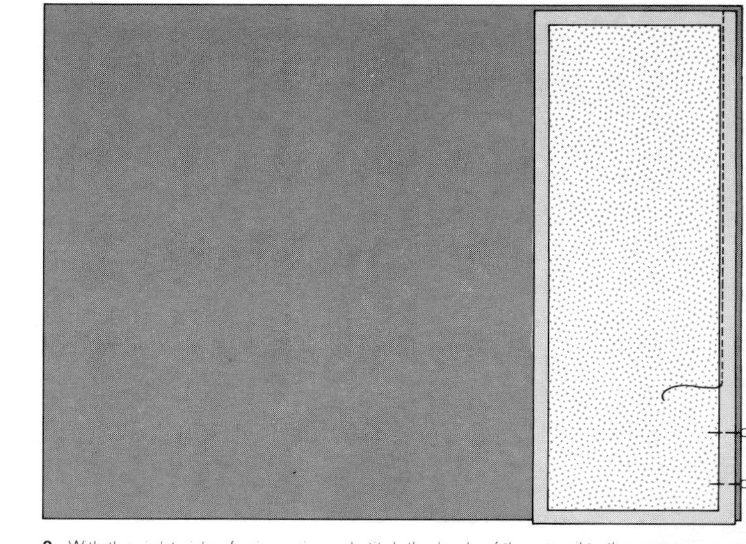

2. With the right sides facing, pin and stitch the body of the pencil to the eraser.

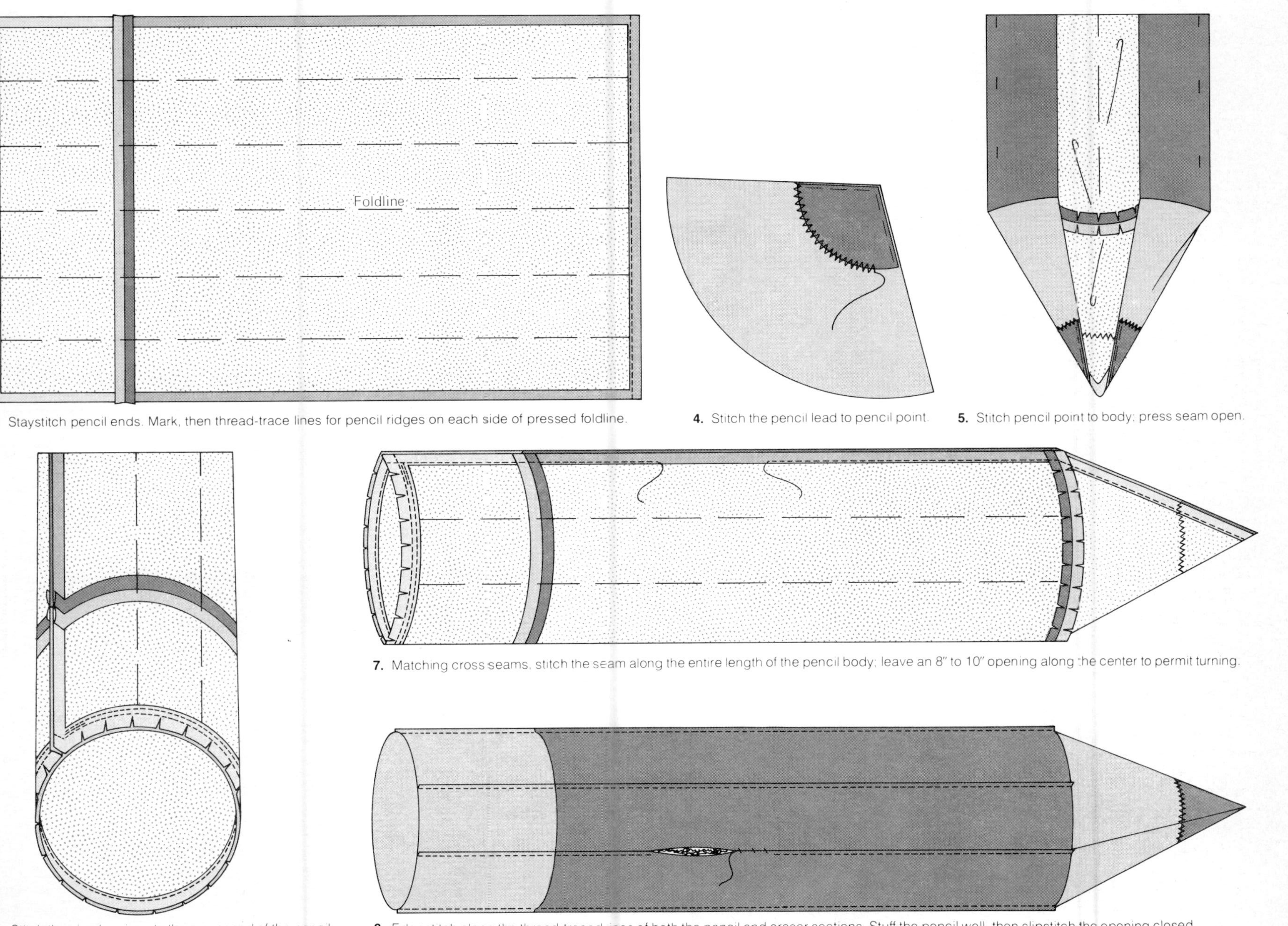

3. Staystitch pencil ends. Mark, then thread-trace lines for pencil ridges on each side of pressed foldline.

4. Stitch the pencil lead to pencil point.

5. Stitch pencil point to body; press seam open.

6. Stitch the circular piece to the eraser end of the pencil.

7. Matching cross seams, stitch the seam along the entire length of the pencil body; leave an 8" to 10" opening along the center to permit turning.

8. Edgestitch along the thread-traced lines of both the pencil and eraser sections. Stuff the pencil well, then slipstitch the opening closed.

Checkerboard beach towel

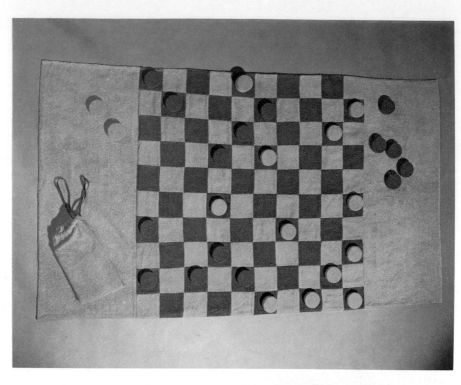

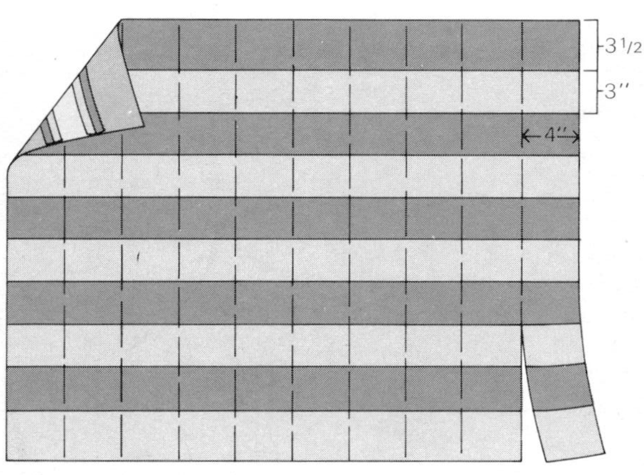

1. Sew alternate colors of strips. Mark and cut striped rectangle.

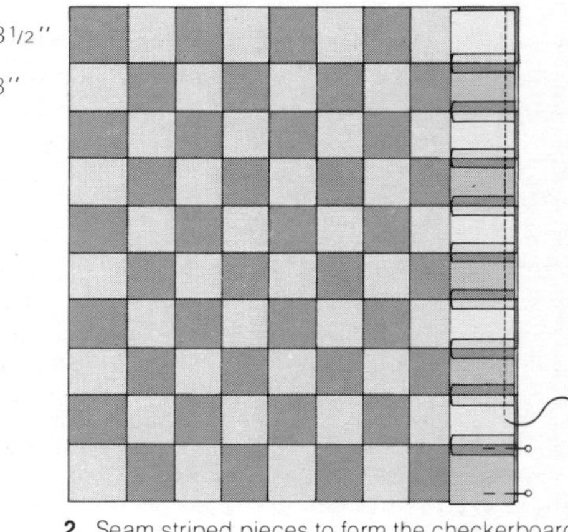

2. Seam striped pieces to form the checkerboard.

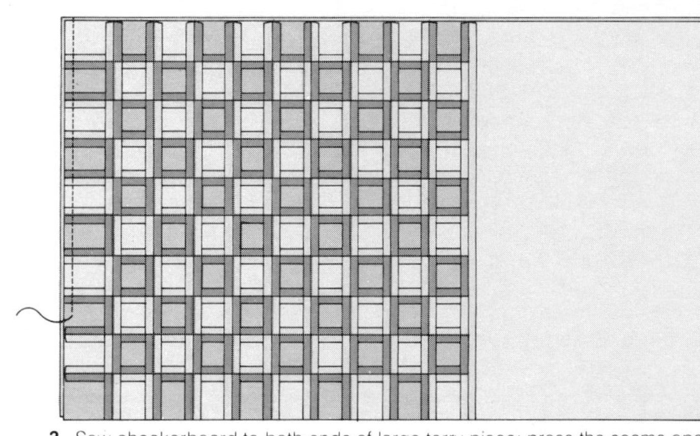

3. Sew checkerboard to both ends of large terry piece; press the seams open.

This giant checkerboard doubles as a game board and beach towel. Spread it out before you go for a swim or head for the hot-dog stand and you'll have no trouble finding your place when you come back!

The large squares and terry-covered chips (which have their own tote bag) make it easy to play checkers out of doors—the fuzzy-surfaced terry cloth tends to cling to itself.

The patchwork of orange and brown squares is seamed at each end to a length of orange terry, which also covers the back. If you prefer, appliqué the patchwork checkerboard onto a store-bought beach towel (preshrink towel and fabric).

MATERIALS NEEDED

3¼ yards of 44/45-inch terry cloth
1 yard of 44/45-inch terry cloth in a contrasting color
40 checker chips or bottle caps
1½ yards of leather thong
Appropriate thread

CUTTING

Cut two rectangles from the larger piece of terry cloth, one 31 x 83 inches (this is the towel backing) and the other 10 x 31 inches (this is for the bag). Then cut five strips from the same piece of terry cloth, each measuring 4 x 40 inches. Also from the same piece, cut twenty circles, each of them measuring approximately 5 inches in diameter.

From the smaller piece of terry cloth in the contrasting color, cut five strips and twenty circles with the same dimensions as are specified above. A ½-inch seam allowance is included for all pieces.

SEWING

The towel. With right sides facing, pin two contrasting color strips together along one of their long sides. Machine-stitch along the ½-inch seam allowance. Attach the other strips in the same way, alternating the colors each time to end up with a striped rectangle. Trim the seam allowances, and press all the seams open. The strips at each end will measure 3½ inches wide; the strips that have been seamed on both edges will measure 3 inches wide.

Divide the rectangle and mark it across into ten strips, each strip 4 inches wide and each consisting of ten squares of alternating colors. Cut each checkered strip along the lines marked on the rectangle.

With right sides facing and the raw edges aligned, pin together two of these strips, matching each colored square to a square in the contrasting color. Machine-stitch, taking a ½-inch seam. Attach the remaining strips in the same way to make the checkerboard. Press all seams open.

With right sides together, pin the raw edges of the checkerboard to the ends of the large solid-colored piece of terry cloth; machine-stitch along a ½-inch seam allowance and press the seams open; the pieces now form a large, continuous "tube."

Lay the towel out flat, with the wrong side of the checkerboard facing up; adjust the tube so there is an equal border width on each side of the checkerboard, then pin the sides of the towel together. Machine-stitch as pinned in a ½-inch seam allowance; leave a 12-inch opening along one of the edges for turning.

Turn the towel right side out. Push out the corners. Fold in the seam allowances of the opening and slipstitch it closed. Bring the seams out to the edge of the towel and baste to hold them in place; then topstitch around about ⅜ inch from the edges. Also stitch in the seam groove at both ends of the checkerboard seams to keep the tube from shifting.

The bag. Fold the 10 x 31-inch rectangle in half along its width, right sides together. Pin, then machine-stitch one side, taking a ½-inch seam. Trim the seam allowances, and zigzag them together. (If you do not have a zigzag, use a second row of straight stitching near the raw edge.) Pin the other side of the bag together and machine-stitch, stopping and backstitching about ⅝ inch from the raw edge at the top. Clip into the seam allowances about ⅜ inch below the backstitched end of the stitching. Press open the seam allowances above the clip. Trim seam allowances below the clip and zigzag (or straight-stitch) them together.

To make the casing at the top of the bag, first turn under a scant ¼ inch and press; then turn under ⅜ inch and press again. Stitch along the inner edge of the casing with a zigzag (or use straight stitching).

Tie the ends of the leather thong together; insert the double strand of thong into the casing with a bodkin or safety pin. The thong acts as a pull cord for the bag.

The chips. To cover one chip, turn under a narrow (about ⅛-inch) hem around one of the fabric circles. Using a double strand of thread, sew the hem in place with small running stitches; do not knot the thread ends. Place a chip in the center of the circle, and pull up the thread end to gather up the fabric around the chip. Pull the thread until the fabric circle is tightly wrapped around the chip, then knot the thread end securely. If the circle is too large, re-cut it smaller. Cover each of the remaining chips in the same way.

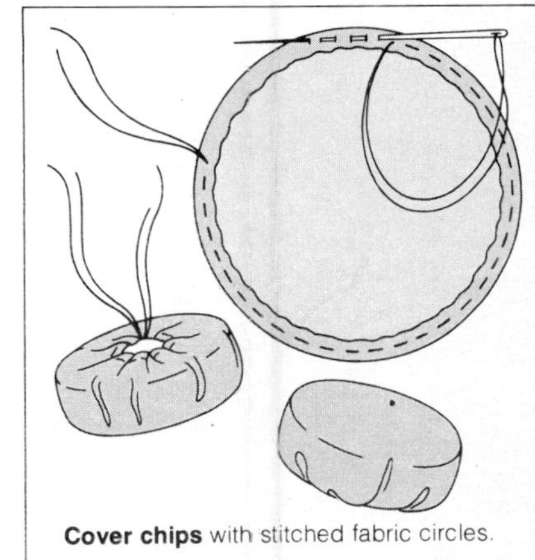

Cover chips with stitched fabric circles.

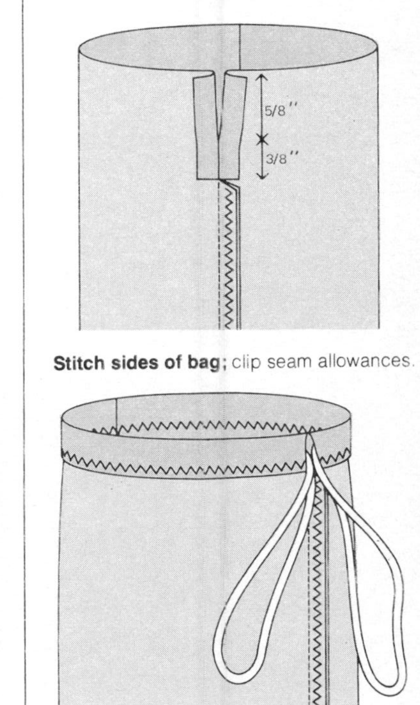

Stitch sides of bag; clip seam allowances.

Make casing at top and insert leather thong.

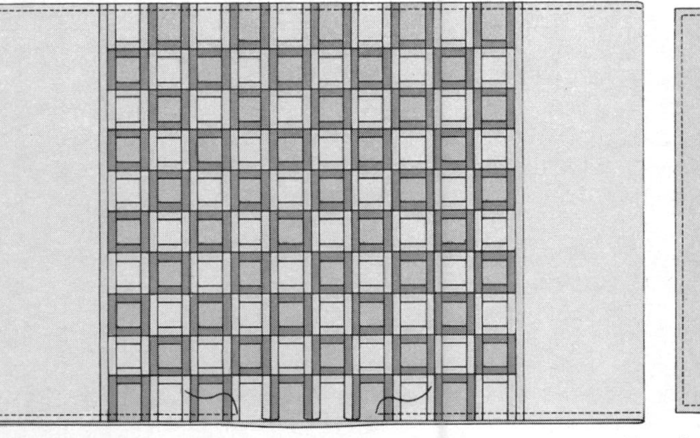

4. Stitch side edges of towel together, leaving a 12" opening along one side.

Stitching in the seam groove

5. Slipstitch opening closed. Topstitch around towel and in seam grooves.

Picnic tote/tablecloth

Cutting and making bias strips 298-299

This ingenious combination of tablecloth and picnic tote has convenient individual pockets for basic picnic necessities. The tablecloth folds up around a square of plastic laminate, which provides a firm base for setting out the picnic meal. The cheerful red denim combines attractively with gingham, but any sturdy, colorfast fabric would do just as well.

MATERIALS NEEDED

2 yards of 60-inch denim
3 yards of 44/45-inch gingham
2 packages double-fold bias binding
12 inches of ¼-inch twill tape or grosgrain ribbon
19-inch square of plastic laminate
20 x 16-inch sheet of paper
1 large hook and eye
Appropriate thread

MAKING THE PATTERN

Graph a 20 x 16-inch sheet of paper into 4-inch squares. Duplicate the pattern pieces as shown in the diagram. Cut out each pattern piece along the marked lines. A ¼-inch seam allowance is already included.

CUTTING

Cut the denim fabric into a 60-inch square. Carefully round off the corners; use a jar lid to obtain a uniform curve. From the remaining strip, cut two 2½ x 22-inch rectangles to make the handle straps.

Fold the gingham fabric along the crosswise grain. Position and cut the pattern pieces from the double layer of fabric, as shown in the diagram, to get sixteen large triangles, sixteen flatware pockets, eight small triangles, four cup holder pockets, four oil and vinegar pockets, and four salt and pepper pockets.

From the remaining gingham fabric, cut and join enough 1½-inch wide bias strips to obtain about 7 yards (see Hems). If you prefer, use ready-made bias binding.

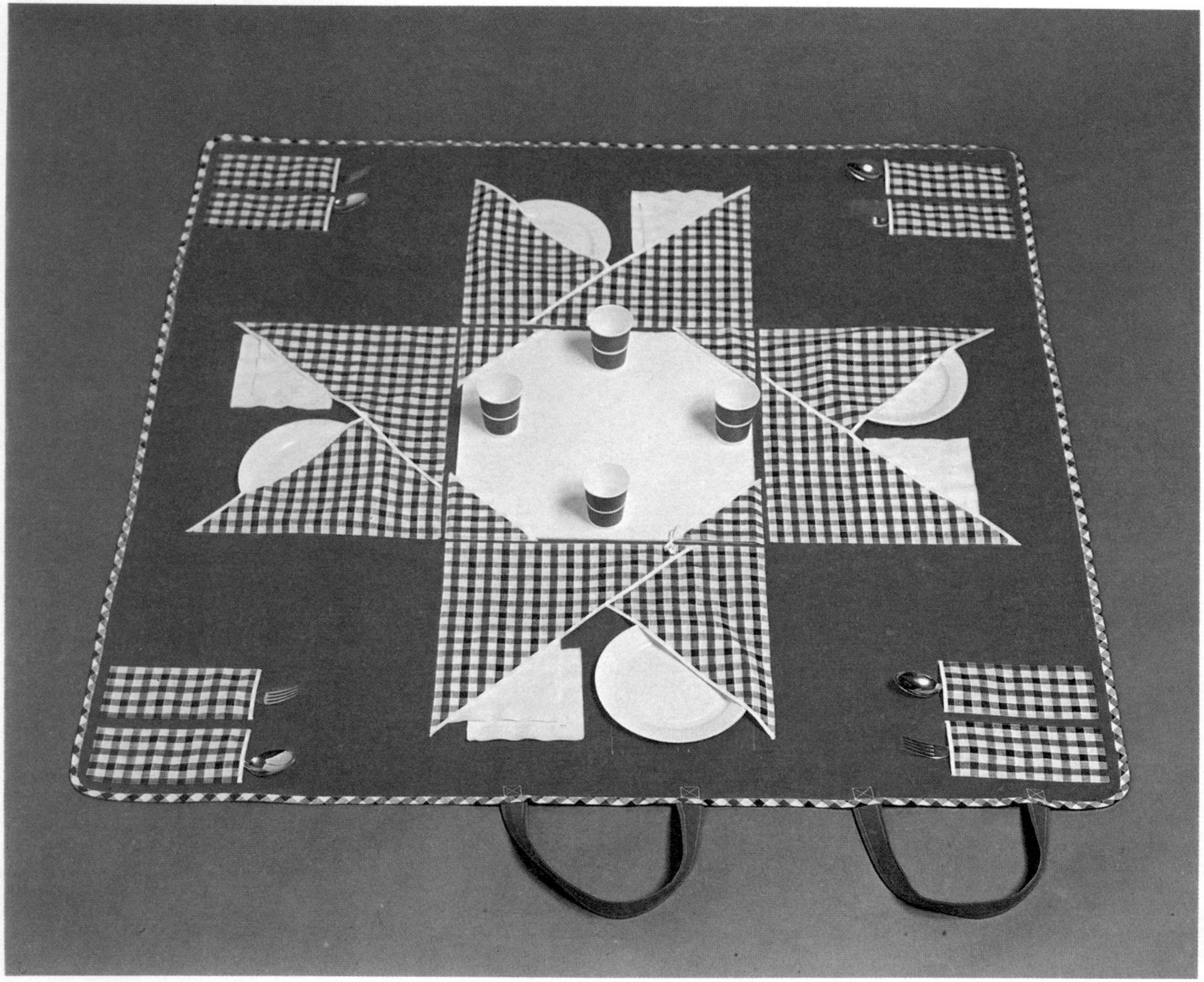

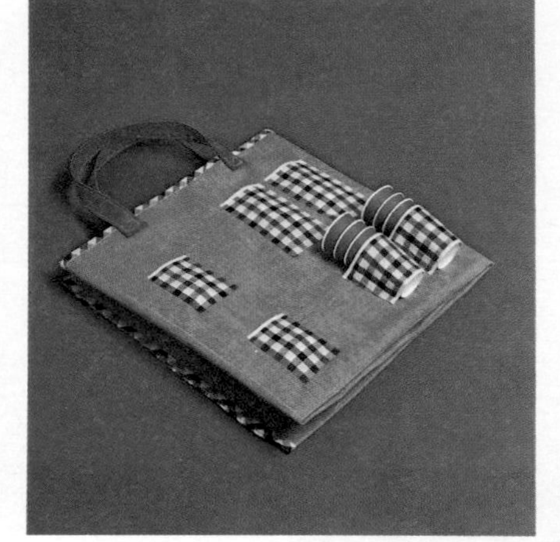

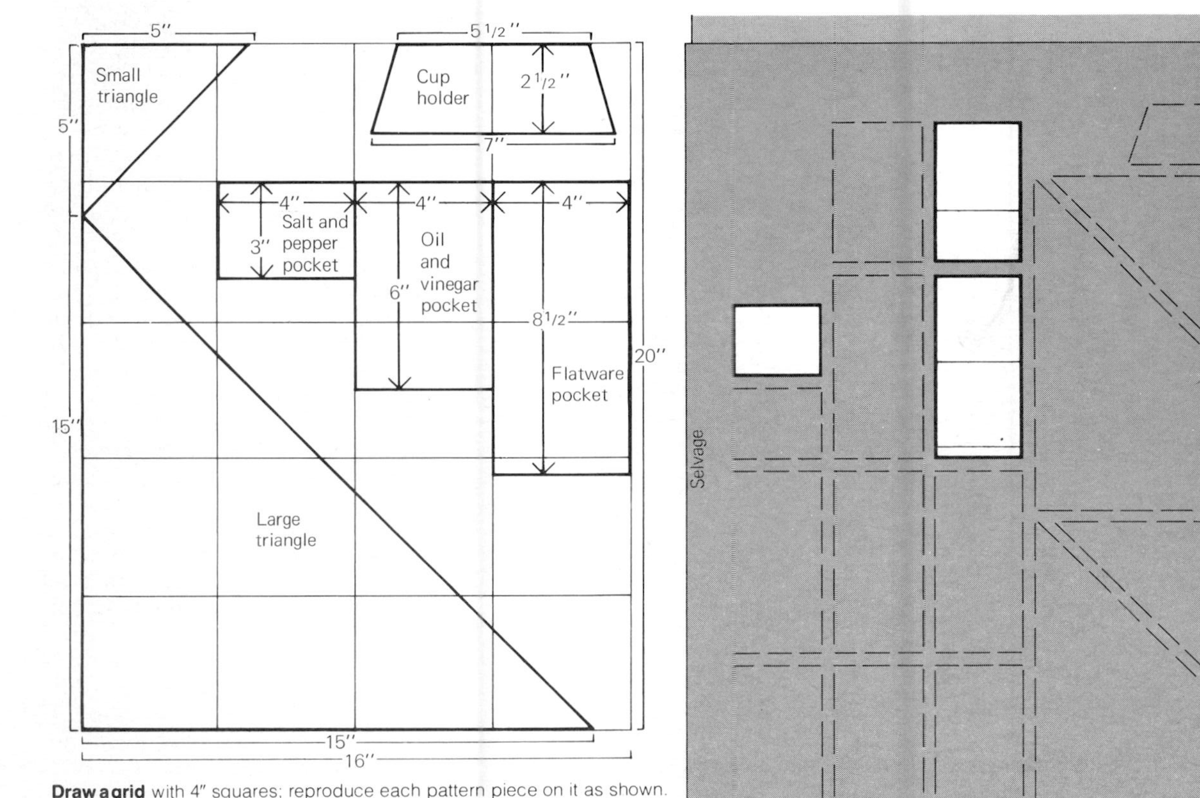

Draw a grid with 4" squares; reproduce each pattern piece on it as shown.

Fold the 44/45" fabric along its crosswise grain, and follow the cutting diagram to obtain the proper number of pieces for picnic tote.

SEWING

Pin two large triangles together with right sides facing. Machine-stitch, leaving diagonal side open. Stitch remaining large triangles, and all small triangles, the same way.

Pin two of the flatware pocket pieces together with right sides facing. Machine-stitch, leaving one end open. Stitch the remaining flatware pieces, also the vinegar and oil rectangles and the salt and pepper rectangles, the same way. Stitch the cup holders the same way, except leave both top and bottom ends open. Press all stitched pieces flat; taper corners, then turn right side out. Roll seams to edges and press.

Bind all raw edges with double-fold bias binding: Wrap binding over the raw edges, with wide half of binding beneath; machine-stitch close to the edge, folding under ¼ inch at the beginning and end.

To prepare the gingham bias strip for binding, fold the strip lengthwise, a bit off center, so that one side is ⅛ inch wider than the other; press folded strip. Then open out and fold cut edges to meet at pressed crease; press the folds again.

Bind raw edges of tablecloth, carefully manipulating binding around the rounded corners. Divide the large square into nine equal squares; then thread-trace the dividing lines.

On the outside of the tablecloth, pin the pockets for the oil, vinegar, salt, and pepper as shown in the diagram. Machine-stitch them in place along the unbound edges; secure the stitches at the opening edges. Pin the cup holder in place so that it extends out as shown in the photo. Machine-stitch its sides only.

On the inside of the tablecloth, position three of the small triangles at three corners of the middle square.

Picnic tote/tablecloth

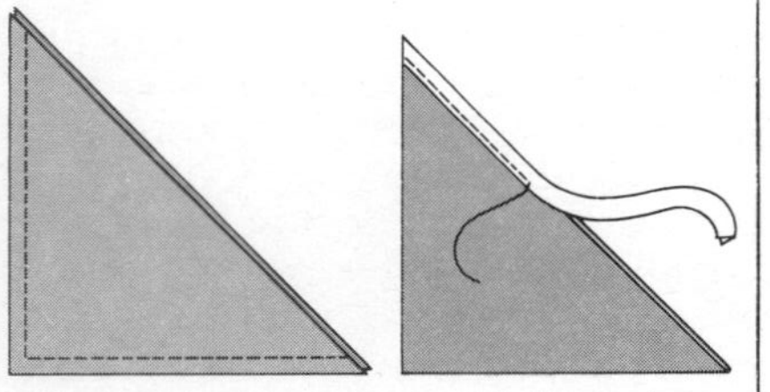

1. Stitch double layers together; bind raw edges.

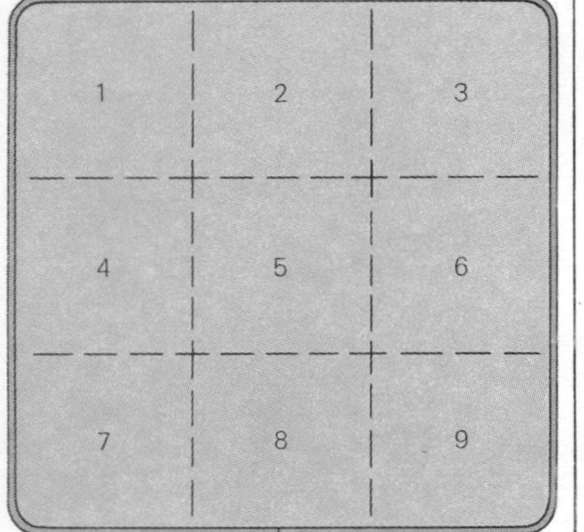

2. Bind large square, and divide into 9 sections.

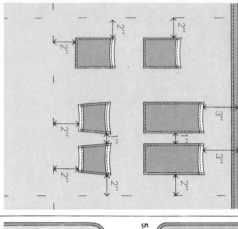

3. Attach pockets to the back of the tablecloth.

4. Sew small triangles to corners of center square.

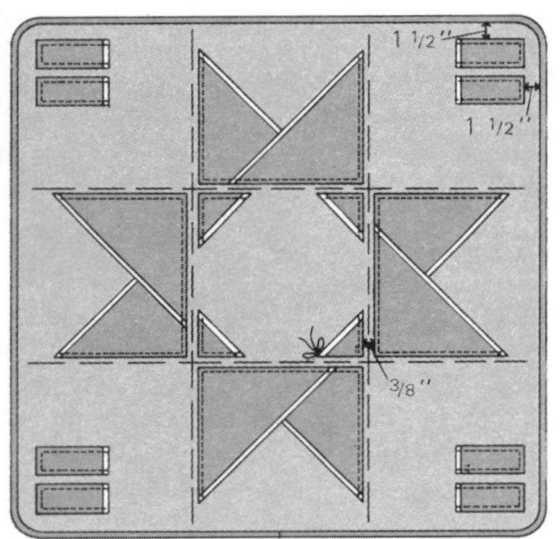

5. Sew large triangles, flatware pockets in place.

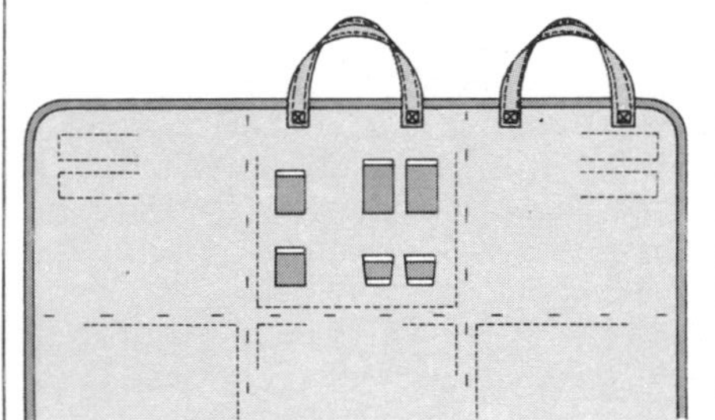

6. Attach handles to outside edge of tablecloth.

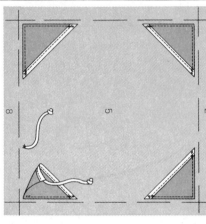

Pin and machine-stitch them in place along the two unbound edges. On the last small triangle, stitch a 6-inch length of twill tape or grosgrain ribbon at one corner. Pin this triangle in place at the remaining corner. Machine-stitch along one side only. Stitch a similar tape or ribbon tie to the tablecloth so it meets the tip of the triangle.

Pin and then baste the eight large triangles as shown, overlapping each pair to fit within a thread-traced square; keep the base of the triangles ⅜ inch away from the corner triangles. Machine-stitch along the sides and the base, securing the stitches at the beginning and end.

Position and pin a pair of flatware pockets in each corner as shown in the diagram. Place pockets with opening edges facing the center so the flatware will not fall out when the tablecloth is folded. Machine-stitch them in place, securing the stitches at the beginning and end.

To make the handle straps, fold the long rectangles in half lengthwise, with right sides together. Pin and machine-stitch along the ¼-inch seam allowance. Press the seams open, centering the seamline down the middle of the width. Stitch across one end of the strap. Turn the strap right side out; pull out the corners. Turn in the seam allowance on the open end and slipstitch it closed. Press. Topstitch around each handle.

Position and pin the handles on the wrong side of the tablecloth along one edge as shown. Machine-stitch the handles in place by topstitching a square over each end, then crisscrossing inside each square.

Fold tablecloth as shown at right. Mark fastener positions, then sew large hook and eye in place as in third step. These hold tote closed.

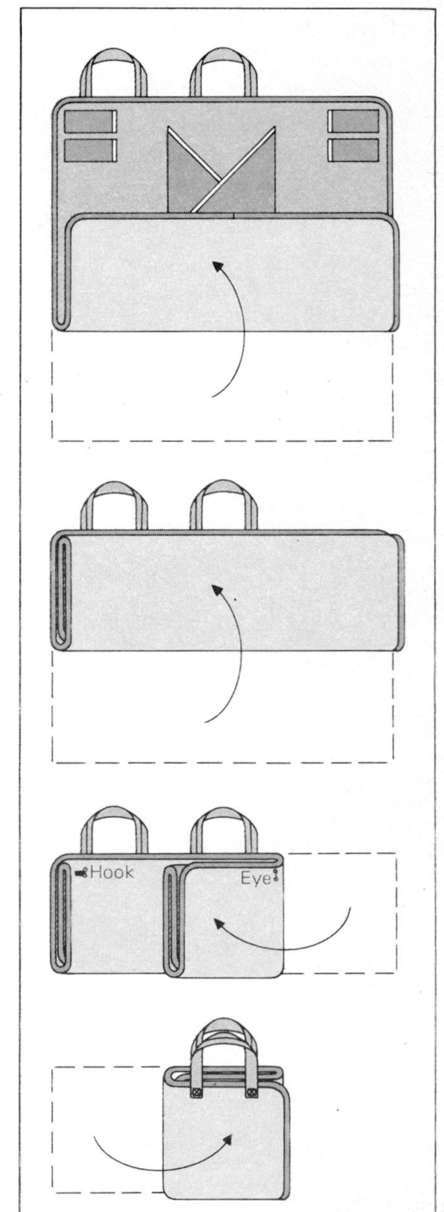

7. To fold tote, follow steps shown above.

Hooded terry robe

Mitering turned-up hems 304

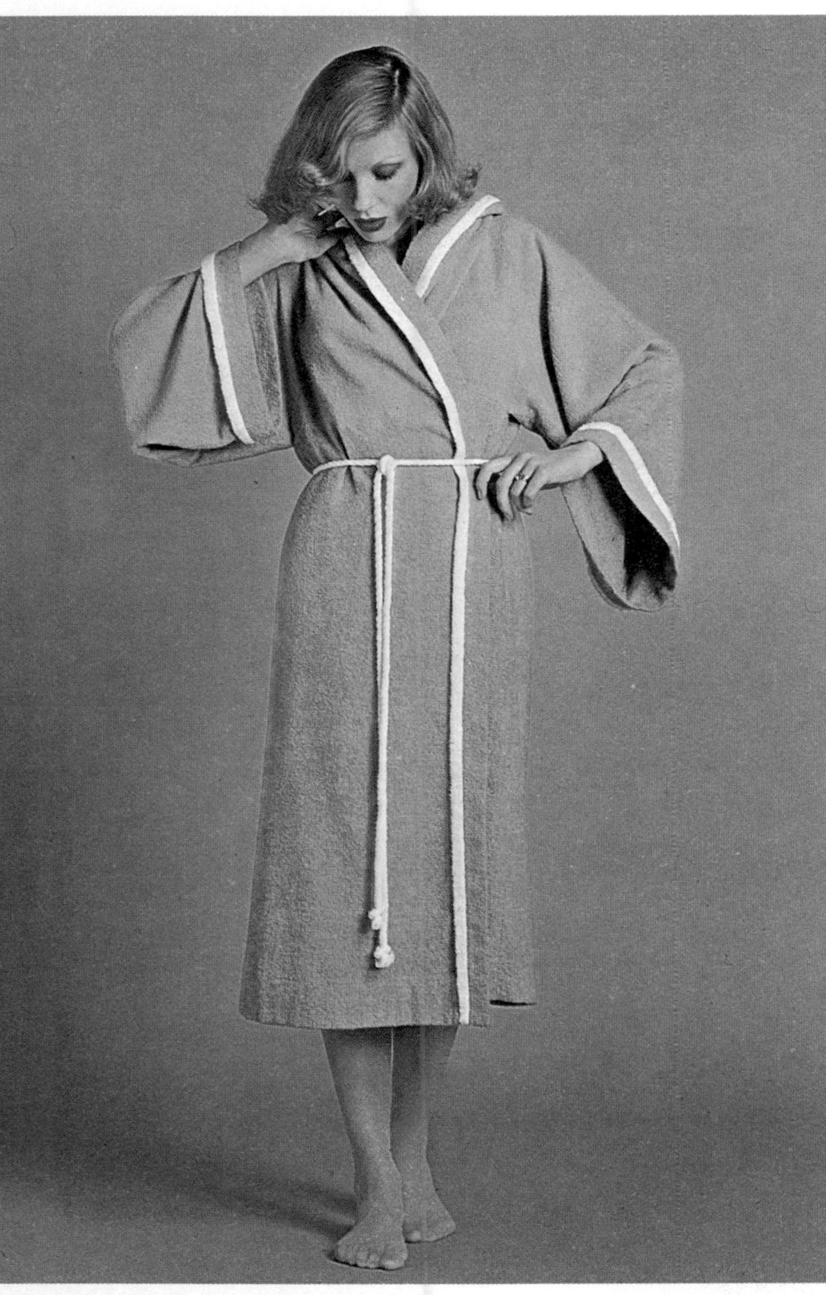

This terry robe is simply perfect for after-bath or beach wear, the hood giving protection to wet hair or just extra warmth when needed.

It is easy to make, with only four pattern pieces, which can be traced directly onto your fabric. Separate patterns are given for men and women, and for children (ages 6 to 8).

Terry cloth is, of course, an excellent choice. Sheared terry, with the sheared side out, not only has a rich velvety look, but is also snagproof. Consider also a lightweight woolen or brushed cotton for winter use.

MATERIALS NEEDED

3½ yards of 44/45-inch terry cloth for men or women
2⅔ yards of 44/45-inch terry cloth for children
½ yard of 44/45-inch terry cloth in contrasting color for banding
2¼ yards of decorative rope for belt
Appropriate thread

CUTTING

Fold the large piece of terry cloth in half lengthwise, lining up selvages. Draw the pattern pieces directly onto the fabric, following the dimensions given in the diagram on the next page. Cut out each piece, carefully notching as indicated; ⅝-inch seam allowances are included.

Cut the contrasting piece of terry cloth into strips as follows: 1½-inch strips to make about 3 yards; 3-inch strips to make about 2 yards.

SEWING

If necessary, zigzag-overcast the raw edges on each piece before beginning construction.

With right sides together, pin the sleeve extensions to the front and back sections. Machine-stitch, then press the seams open.

With right sides together, line up the front and back sections and pin the two together along the shoulder seamline. Machine-stitch, beginning 3 inches from sleeve end and stopping at the notch; secure stitches at beginning and end. Clip seam allowances at the starting point.

With right sides facing and notches matched, pin one side of the hood to one front section along the shoulder line; machine-stitch to notch and secure stitches. Pin and stitch the other side of the hood to other front section the same way. Next pin the unstitched portion of the hood to the back section, securing stitches at beginning and end of stitching line. Press all seams open.

With right sides together, pin and stitch the top of the hood. Press the seam open.

On both front and back sections, place short reinforcing stitches for 1 inch on both sides of each of the underarm corners. With right sides together, pin and stitch the front sections to the back along the underarm and side seams; start 3 inches from each sleeve end, and secure the beginning stitches. Clip into the seam allowances at the starting points and at the underarm corner. Press the stitched seams open.

Turn the robe right side out, and stitch the remaining 3 inches at the end of each sleeve seam; secure the stitches. Press seams open.

To finish the raw edges along the front, hood, and robe bottom, turn under a 2-inch hem allowance; miter the corners at the bottom (see Hems); pin, then baste along fold.

From the wrong side, machine-stitch the hem in place along the hood, the front, and the bottom edge of the robe, placing the stitching line about ⅜ inch from the raw edges.

Hooded terry robe

French tacks 134
Applying single binding 302

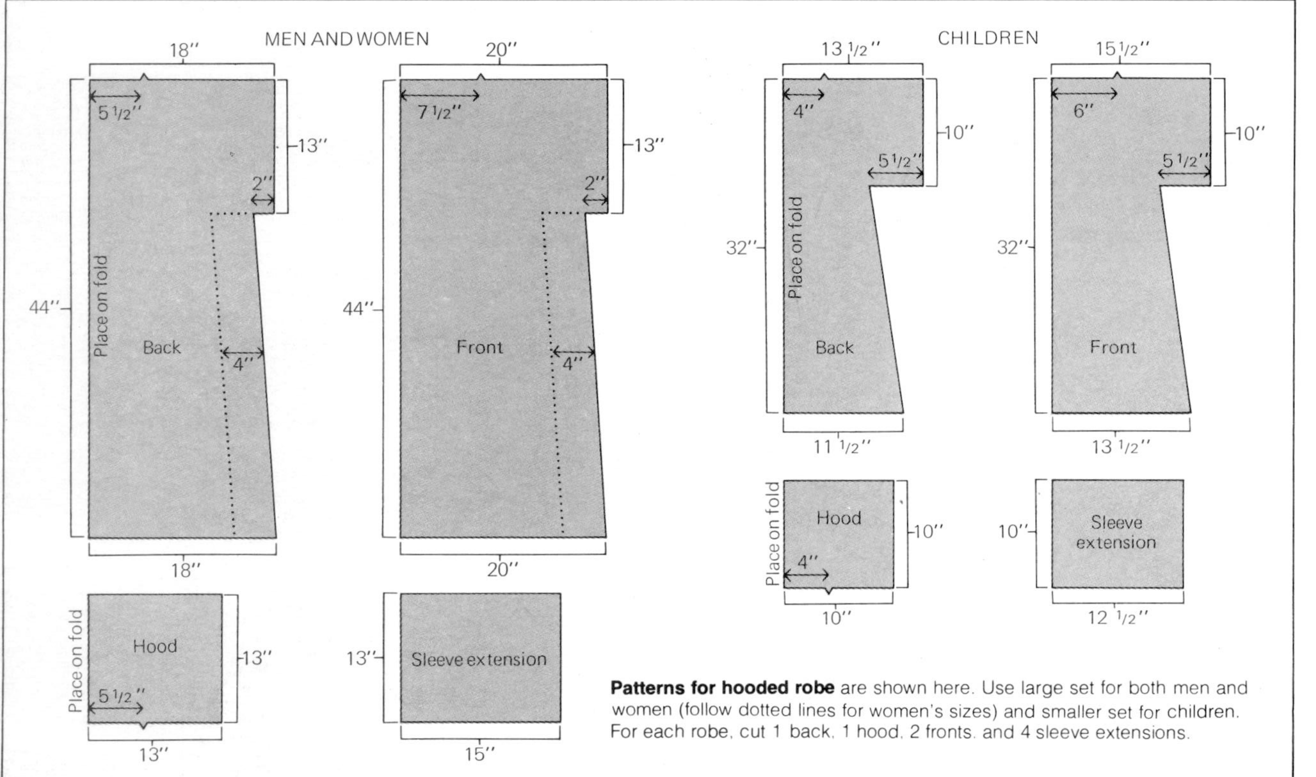

Patterns for hooded robe are shown here. Use large set for both men and women (follow dotted lines for women's sizes) and smaller set for children. For each robe, cut 1 back, 1 hood, 2 fronts, and 4 sleeve extensions.

Make the decorative bands by joining the 1½-inch fabric strips to make about 3 yards and the 3-inch fabric strips to make about 2 yards. Fold the long strips in half lengthwise and press lightly to mark center. Open them out, then press the edges in to meet at the center line.

Bind the raw edges of the sleeves with the wide strip (see Hems), keeping in mind that the sleeve will be turned back to make a cuff. Turn the sleeves back to create 2-inch cuffs. To keep the cuffs from falling, add French tacks at each seam.

To attach decorative band to front opening and hood of robe, unfold one edge of the narrow band; turn under ¼ inch at starting end; with right sides together, line up the raw edge of the band with the stitching line along the front opening. Pin the band to the robe, then machine-stitch within the foldline of the band; turn under ¼ inch at the end of the band. Turn the band to the right side and press; edgestitch along the folded edge of the band through all thicknesses; secure threads at beginning and end. Press entire robe.

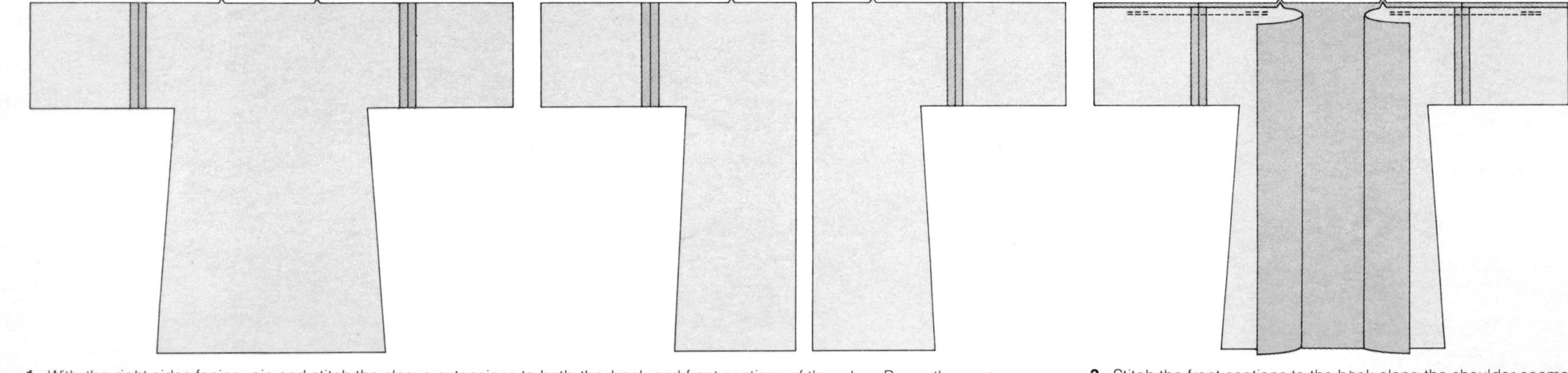

1. With the right sides facing, pin and stitch the sleeve extensions to both the back and front sections of the robe. Press the seams open. **2.** Stitch the front sections to the back along the shoulder seams.

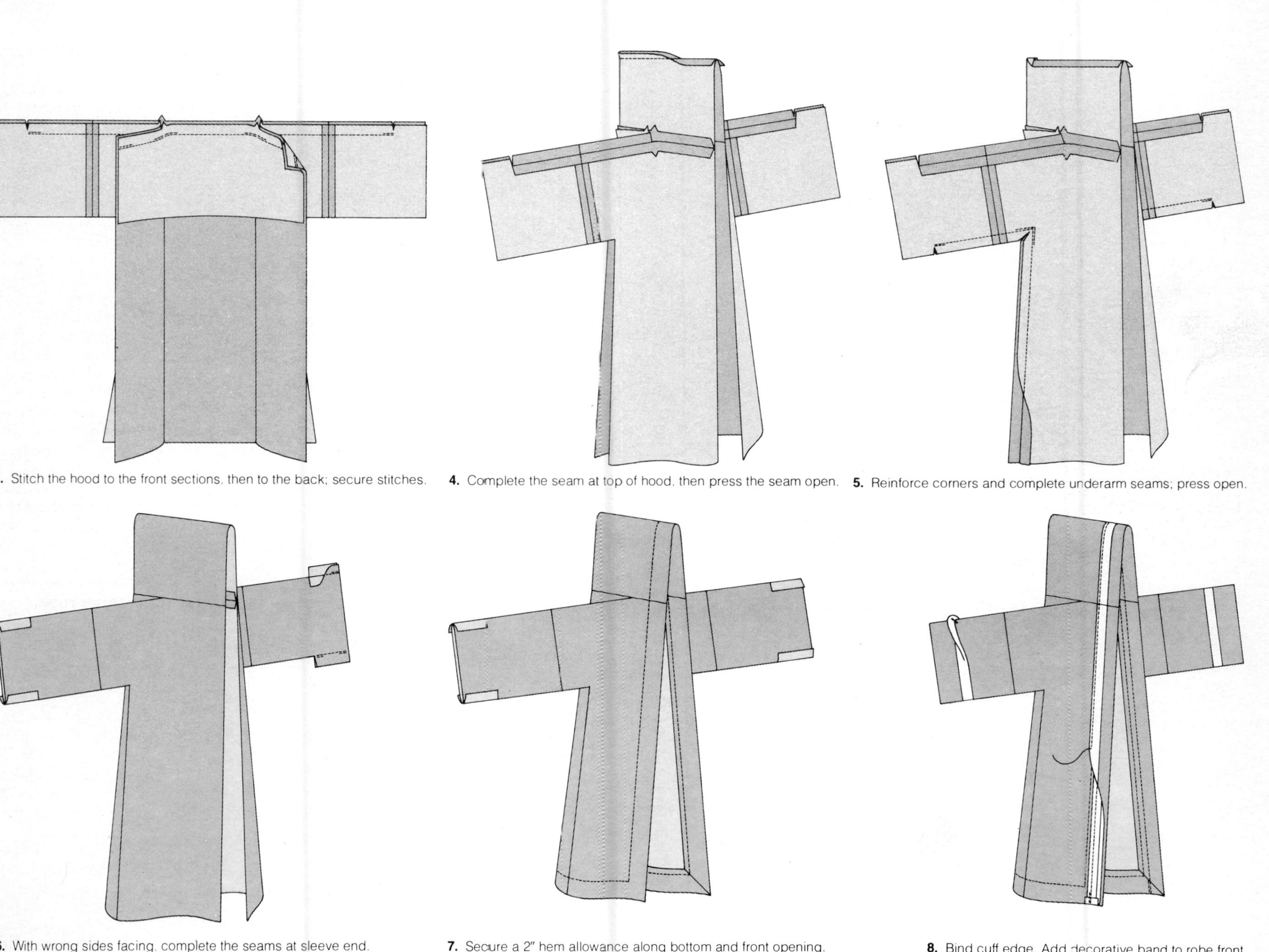

3. Stitch the hood to the front sections, then to the back; secure stitches.

4. Complete the seam at top of hood, then press the seam open.

5. Reinforce corners and complete underarm seams; press open.

6. With wrong sides facing, complete the seams at sleeve end.

7. Secure a 2" hem allowance along bottom and front opening.

8. Bind cuff edge. Add decorative band to robe front.

Duffle bag

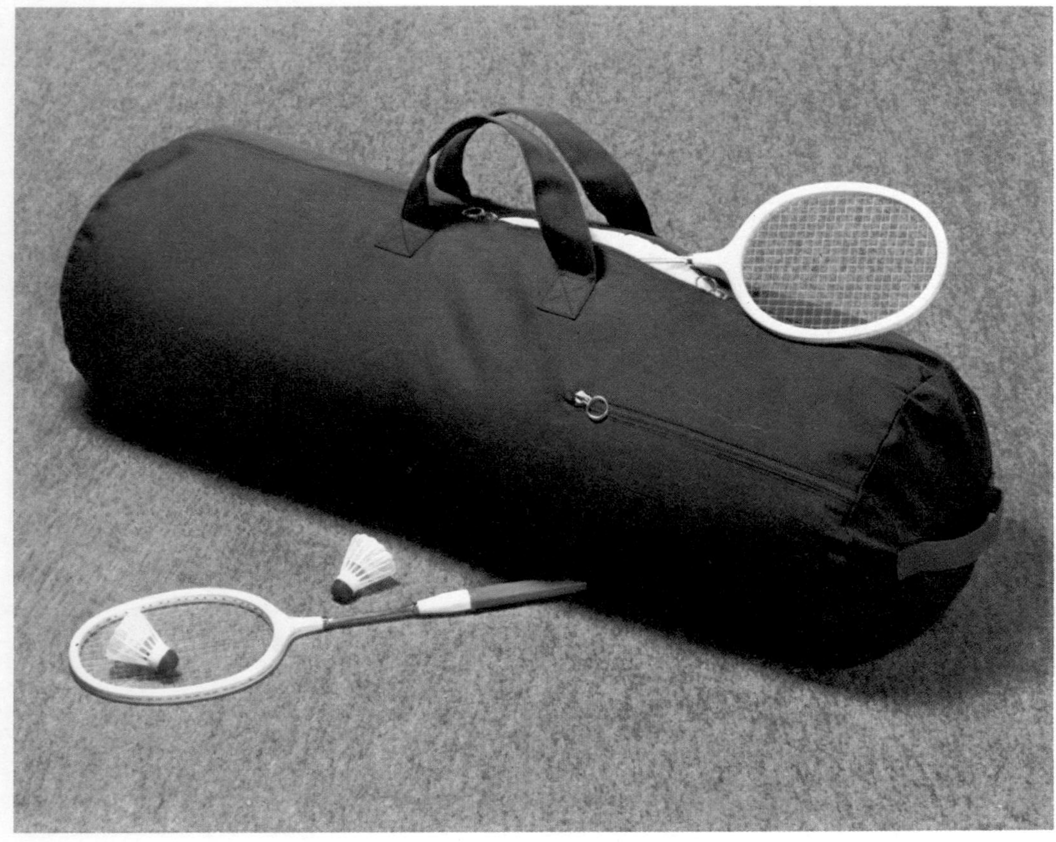

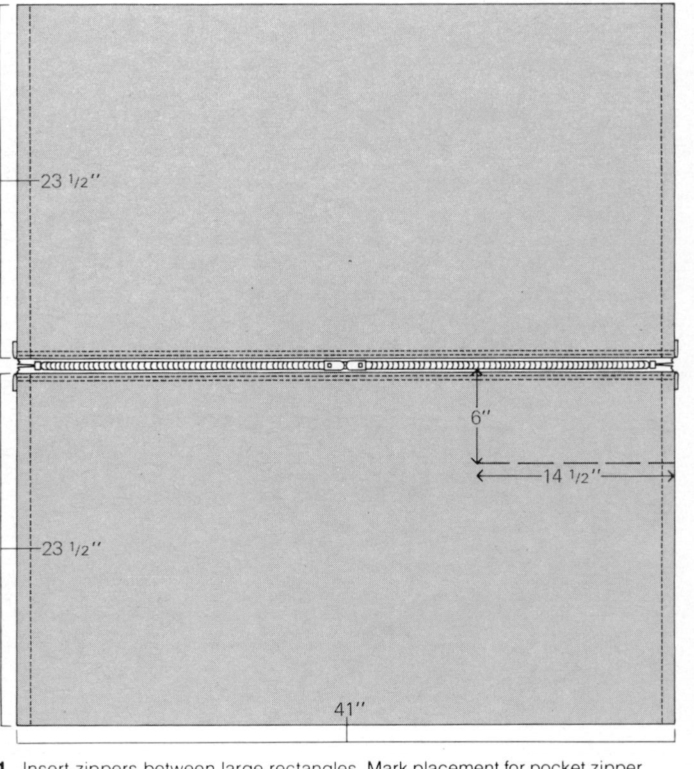

1. Insert zippers between large rectangles. Mark placement for pocket zipper.

Stout handles and plenty of room make this duffle bag great for sports and travel. It can be carried either by the top handles or by one of the handles at the end, sailor-style.

The two top zippers pull from the center of the opening, giving quick and easy access to the bag. The zippered pocket supplies an additional compartment for personal things.

Any sturdy fabric is suitable, such as denim or duck. Handles can be made of the same fabric or of strong nylon webbing. Use decorative zippers with ring-pulls and bright tapes.

MATERIALS NEEDED

2¼ yards of 44/45-inch fabric for body of bag, handles, and pockets
¼ yard of contrasting fabric for end handles
⅓ yard of 26-inch fusible interfacing
Two 20-inch and one 14-inch zippers with large plastic teeth
Appropriate thread

CUTTING

For bag, cut two 24 x 41-inch rectangles on the straight grain and two circles with 14¼-inch diameters; for pocket, cut a 15-inch square.

Then cut two 4 x 13-inch rectangles for the matching handles and, from the contrasting fabric, two 4 x 9-inch rectangles for the end handles. Also cut three 3 x 12-inch rectangles and three 3 x 8-inch rectangles from the fusible interfacing. A ½-inch seam allowance is included in the dimensions for all fabric pieces.

SEWING

Staystitch the two shorter edges of both large rectangles. Apply a seam finish to the raw edges of the fabric pieces if necessary.

Next press under the seam allowance along one long edge of each large rectangle. Position and pin the folded edge of one of the rectangles along one side of the two 20-inch zippers (have tops of the zippers meet in the center). Position and pin the other folded edge of the remaining rectangle to the other sides of the zipper tapes. Baste in place; edgestitch along both foldlines. Place another row of topstitching about ⅛ inch from first stitch line.

To construct the zippered pocket, start at right-hand edge and draw

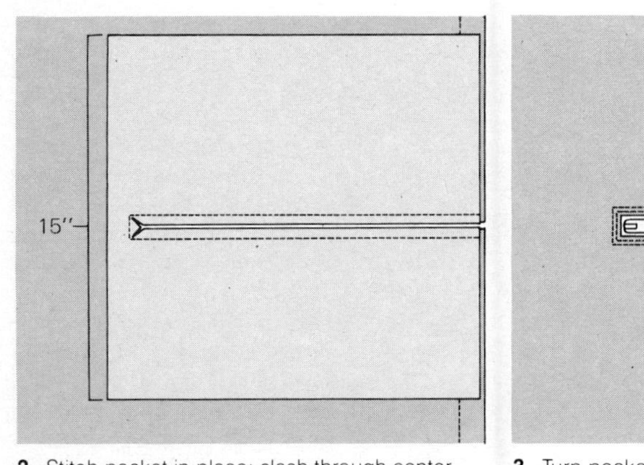

2. Stitch pocket in place; slash through center.

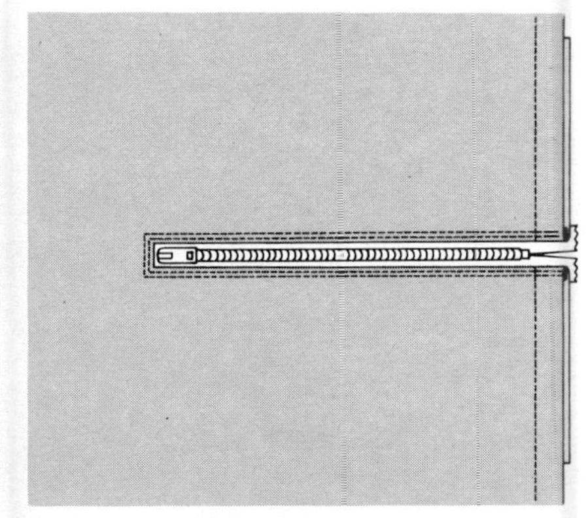

3. Turn pocket inside; stitch zipper under opening.

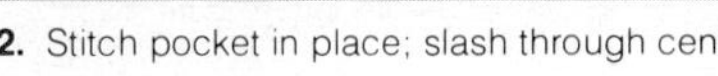

4. Stitch along pocket fold, catching zipper tape.

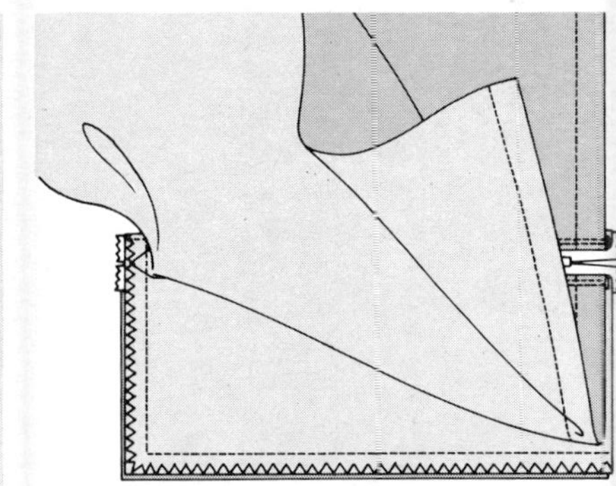

5. Stitch pocket together; zigzag around edges.

6. Mark positions, then stitch top handles in place.

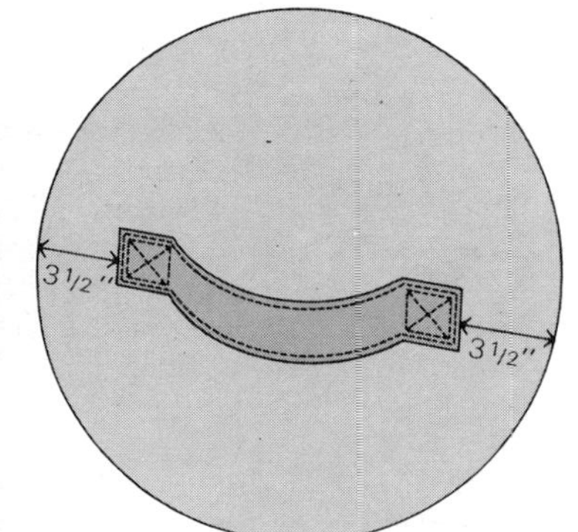

7. Stitch handles to circular end pieces of bag.

a 14½-inch line parallel to and 6 inches below the inserted zipper. Press the pocket about ¾ inch off center to mark the placement line. With right sides facing, and longer half of pocket up, pin the pocket to the bag, aligning the foldline to the marked line on the bag; the raw edges on the right-hand side should be even. Mark stitching lines ⅛ inch on each side of the folded line and ½ inch from the left edge. Machine-stitch around the marked stitching lines. Slash down the center to within ½ inch of the stitched end, then cut into the corners. Turn the pocket to the inside and press, rolling the seamline under slightly.

Close the 14-inch zipper tape above the top stop with a bar tack. Position and pin zipper under the opening so the top stop is against the finished end of the opening. Baste in place; edgestitch around. Place another row of topstitching about ⅛ inch from the first stitch line.

On the wrong side of the bag, fold top part of pocket down so the edge of the zipper tape is against the fold; the bottom raw edges of the pockets should be even (trim if they are not).

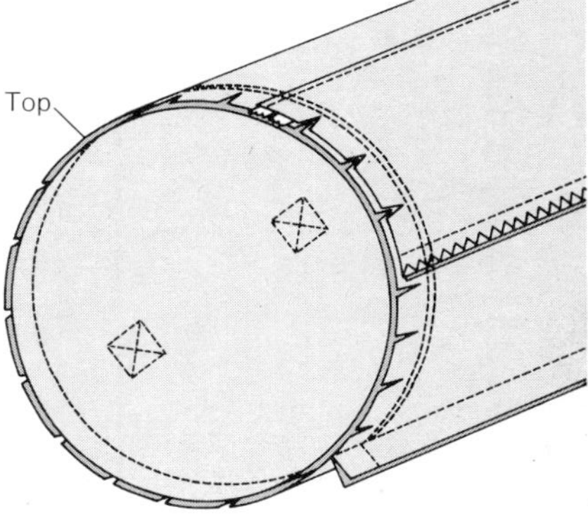

8. Stitch ends to body of bag; sew bottom seam.

Machine-stitch along the top fold of the pocket, catching zipper tape in the stitching.

Pin the bottom and inside edges of pockets together and machine-stitch. Place a second row of stitching (zigzag or straight) around the stitched pocket edges. Hold the unstitched edges of the pocket to the raw edges of the bag by pinning and stitching both edges together.

To make all handles, center and fuse three layers of interfacing to the wrong side of each handle. Proceed with handle instructions for the Barrel bag (p. 500). Mark handle positions so they are centered, with handle ends 6½ inches apart and about 4 inches from the zipper edge. Pin one of the handles to the bag; topstitch a square at each end, crisscrossing the stitching in each square. Attach the other handle to the opposite side. Attach the contrasting short handles to the center of each circle (end piece) the same way, positioning the handle ends 3½ inches from edges of circle.

Fold one circle in half and cut a tiny notch at the foldline on each end. With right sides facing, position circle to one end of the bag; pin bag and circle together from the top, matching the zippered seam with one notch. With the bag facing you, continue pinning around the circle, clipping the bag seam allowances as necessary to fit them around the curve; the bottom seam allowances of the bag should meet at the bottom notch of the circle. Baste as pinned. Machine-stitch around circle, securing stitches at beginning and end. Finish other end of bag the same way. Open the zippers; pin and stitch the bottom seam allowances together, right sides facing. Press the seam open. Turn bag right side out.

Appliqué bath towels

Mitering topstitched binding 309

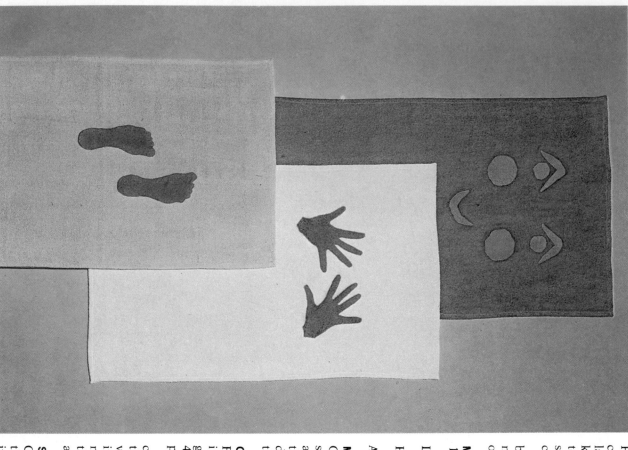

Practical and amusing, these towels can be made in any size, from extra large for the beach, to bath towels, to kitchen or guest hand towels. Patterns are provided for the appliqués shown here, but you may prefer to create your own motifs.

Terry cloth is best for large towels, but for kitchen or guest towels, you might consider an absorbent cotton or linen fabric.

MATERIALS NEEDED

1¼ yards of 44/45-inch terry cloth for each towel
Large scraps of contrasting terry cloth for appliqués
Heavy sheet of paper or lightweight cardboard
Appropriate thread

MAKING THE PATTERN

Graph the heavy paper into 2-inch squares. Then reproduce the desired appliqué design from the diagram on the next page. If desired, you can draw your own design directly onto the heavy paper. Cut out the design.

CUTTING

For each towel, cut a single 25 x 44-inch rectangle from the straight grain of the fabric. Also cut enough 4-inch strips of fabric to make approximately 4½ yards of binding.

Position the cut-out design on the contrasting terry cloth. Trace around the cut-out with a sharp pencil or with chalk. If you are using a hot-iron transfer, carefully follow the manufacturer's instructions. Cut out the design, leaving a generous inch around the traced lines.

SEWING

Carefully position the appliqué onto the large terry cloth rectangle. Pin it in place and hand-baste near the design outline. Machine-stitch, using a short stitch length, on top of the marked lines. Remove basting threads and press. Next trim away excess fabric close to stitching line. Using a short, medium-width zigzag stitch (satin stitch), carefully and slowly zigzag over the straight stitching line to cover the raw edges.

If you do not have a zigzag machine, place a row of stitching a thread's width outside the design line. Trim around appliqué, leaving a ⅛-inch hem. Then turn under the narrow hem, clipping as necessary. Baste appliqué in place, and straight-stitch around folded edges.

Join strips of fabric together to obtain about 4½ yards of binding. Prepare binding for topstitching, and apply to raw edges of towel; pay particular attention when going around the corners (see Hems).

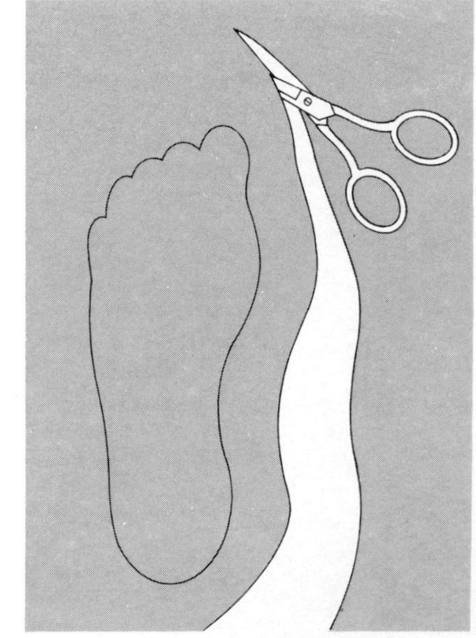

1. Cut out appliqué outside its traced markings.

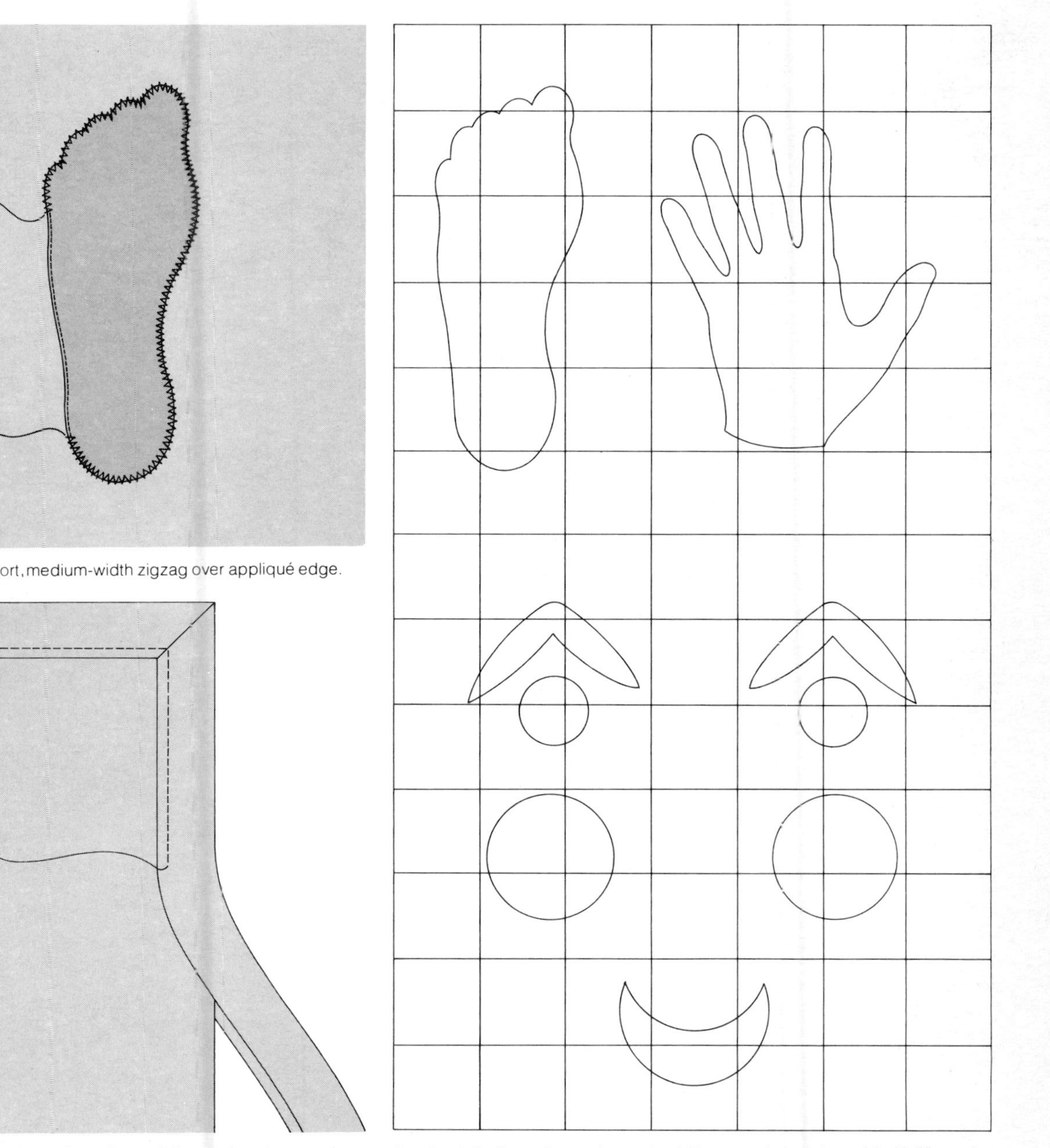

2. Stitch appliqué in place; trim excess close to stitching.

3. Use a short, medium-width zigzag over appliqué edge.

For straight-stitch machines, turn under appliqué edges.

4. Bind raw edges of towel, carefully mitering at corners.

Appliqué designs shown above should be reproduced on a grid with 2″ squares.

Index

A

B

C

D

E

F

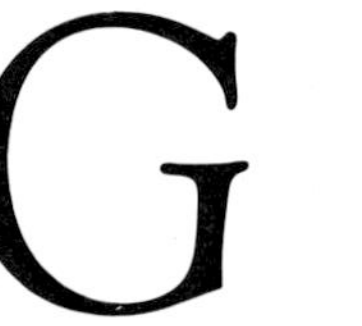

H

I

J

K

L

M

N

O

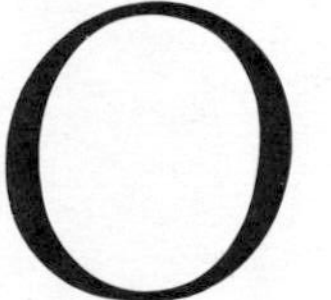

Q

R

S

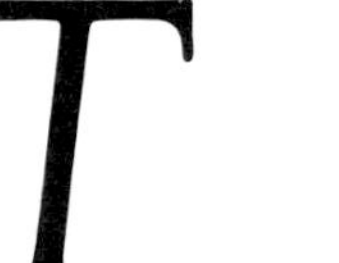

U

V

W

Y

Z